Handbook of Pesticide Toxicology
Second Edition

Handbook of Pesticide Toxicology
Second Edition

VOLUME 2
AGENTS

EDITED BY

Robert I. Krieger
University of California, Riverside

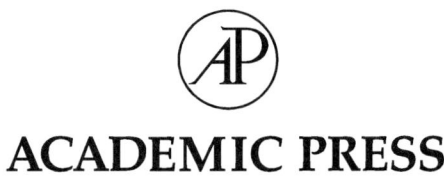

ACADEMIC PRESS

A Harcourt Science and Technology Company

San Diego San Francisco New York Boston London Sydney Tokyo

Academic Press
A Harcourt Science and Technology Company
525 B Street, Suite 1900, San Diego, California 92101-4495, USA
http://www.academicpress.com

Academic Press
Harcourt Place, 32 Jamestown Road, London NW1 7BY, UK
http://www.academicpress.com

Library of Congress Catalog Card Number: 200188747

International Standard Book Number: 0-12-426260-0 set
International Standard Book Number: 0-12-426261-9 volume 1
International Standard Book Number: 0-12-426262-7 volume 2

PRINTED IN THE UNITED STATES OF AMERICA
01 02 03 04 05 06 MM 9 8 7 6 5 4 3 2 1

In memory of
Wayland J. Hayes, Jr., M.D., Ph.D.,
who served on a grand scale to clarify the principles
of general toxicology, the epidemiology of pesticide
poisoning, and the medical management
of poisoning cases

Contents of the Handbook

Contents of Volume 2

58 Pyrethroid Chemistry and Metabolism
Hideo Kaneko and Junshi Miyamoto

59 Pyrethroid Insecticides: Mechanisms of Toxicity, Systemic Poisoning Syndromes, Paresthesia, and Therapy
David E. Ray

60 DDT and its Analogs
Andrew G. Smith

61 Inorganic and Organometal Pesticides
Thomas W. Clarkson

Contributors to the Handbook

Gail Acre (1759), Griffin LLC, Valdosta, Georgia 31603

John L. Adgate (887), University of Minnesota School of Public Health, Minneapolis, Minnesota 55455

Bruce N. Ames (799), University of California, Berkeley, California 94720

Sharada Balakrishman (747), Environmental Toxicology Graduate Program, University of California, Riverside, California 92521

Margot Barnett (603), Strategic Options Consulting, Portland, Oregon 97280

Ronald E. Baynes (515), Center for Cutaneous Toxicology and Residue Pharmacology, College of Veterinary Medicine, North Carolina State University, Raleigh, North Carolina 27606

Richard Billington (1653), Global Toxicology, Dow Agro-Sciences, LLC, Indianapolis, Indiana 46268

Jerome M. Blondell (603), Health Effects Division, Office of Pesticide Programs, U.S. Environmental Protection Agency, Washington, DC 20460

J. Scott Boone (913, 919), College of Veterinary Medicine, Mississippi State University, Mississippi State, Mississippi 39762

Ruaidhri Breathnach (1461), University College Dublin, Belfield, Dublin 4, Ireland

Charles B. Breckenridge (1157, 1511), Syngenta Crop Protection, Inc., Greensboro, North Carolina 27409

Gerald T. Brooks (1131), Center for Molecular Design, University of Portsmouth, PO1 2QF, United Kingdom

Derk H. Brouwer (457), Department of Chemical Exposure Assessment, TNO Chemistry, The Netherlands

Quang Bui (1759), Cerexagri, Inc., 100631 Beijing, China

Geoffrey M. Calvert (603), Division of Surveillance, Hazard Evaluations and Field Studies, National Institute for Occupational Safety and Health, Centers for Disease Control and Prevention, Cincinnati, Ohio 45226

Linda L. Carlock (1867), Toxicology and Regulatory Consultants, Seattle, Washington 98126

Neal Carmichael (1107), Aventis CropScience, Rhone-Poulenc, BF 153F 06903, Sophia Antipolis, France

Russell L. Carr (913, 919), College of Veterinary Medicine, Mississippi State University, Mississippi State, Mississippi 39762

Howard W. Chambers (913, 919), Department of Entomology and Plant Pathology, Mississippi State University, Mississippi State, Mississippi 39762

Janice E. Chambers (913, 919), College of Veterinary Medicine, Mississippi State University, Mississippi State, Mississippi 39762

Graham Chester (425), Syngenta Ltd., Haslemere, Surrey GU27 3JE, United Kingdom

J. Marshall Clark (203), Environmental Sciences Program, Department of Entomology, University of Massachusetts, Amherst, Massachusetts 10003

Thomas Clarkson (1357), Environmental Health Science, University of Rochester Medical School, Rochester, New York 14642

Thomas Class (671), PTRL Europe, Science Park, Ulm D-8901, Germany

Roger C. Cochran (691), California Environmental Protection Agency, Sacramento, California 95812

Franck E. Dayan (1529), USDA-ARS Natural Production Utilization Research Unit, University of Mississippi 38677

Johan S. de Cock (457), Department of Chemical Exposure Assessment, TNO Chemistry, The Netherlands

Kelly J. Dix (563), Lovelace Respiratory Research Institute, Albuquerque, New Mexico 87108

Michael Dong (479), Worker Health and Safety Branch, U.S. Environmental Protection Agency, Sacramento, California 95814

Timothy A. Dotson (1867), UCB Chemicals Corporation, Marysville, California 95901

John Doull (1), Department of Pharmacology and Toxicology, University of Kansas Medical Center, Kansas City, Kansas 66160

Jeffrey H. Driver (435), Infoscientific, Inc., Carmichael, California 95608; and risksciences.net, Arlington, Virginia 22201

Stephen O. Duke (1529), USDA-ARS Natural Production Utilization Research Unit, University of Mississippi, University, Mississippi 38677

David A. Eastmond (747), Environmental Toxicology Graduate Program, University of California, Riverside, California 92521

Donald J. Ecobichon (285, 1087), Department of Pharmacology and Toxicology, Queen's University, Kingston, Ontario K0G 1E0, Canada

Marion Ehrich (987), Department of Pharmacology and Toxicology, Virgina-Maryland Regional College of Veterinary Medicine, Virginia Polytechnic Institute and State University, Blacksburg, Virginia 24061

David L. Eisenbrandt (1881), Dow AgroSciences, LLC, Midland, Michigan 48674

J. Charles Eldridge (1511), Department of Physiology and Pharmacology, Wake Forest University School of Medicine, Winston-Salem, North Carolina 27157

Jeffrey B. Evans (435), Office of Pesticide Programs, U.S. Environmental Protection Agency, Sacramento, California 95812

Donna Farmer (1667), Monsanto Company, St. Louis, Missouri 63167

Pennelope A. Fenner-Crisp (681), U.S. Environmental Protection Agency, Washington, DC 20460

Toshio Fujita (649), EMIL Project, Fuyacho-Nishikikojiagaru, Nakagyoku, Kyoto 604-8057, Japan

Derek W. Gammon (707, 1781), Department of Pesticide Regulation, Medical Toxicology Branch, California Environmental Protection Agency, Sacramento, California 95812

V. F. Garry (1861), Lab Medicine and Pathology, University of Minnesota, Minneapolis, Minnesota 55465

Paul Glynn (953), Medical Research Council Toxicology Unit, University of Leicester, Leicester LE1 9HN, United Kingdom

B. B. Gollapudi (1849), Dow Chemical Company, Midland, Michigan, 48674

Gay Goodman (1481), Human Health Risk Resources, Inc., Seattle, Washington 98199

Elliot B. Gordon (1711), Makhteshim-Agan of North America, Inc., New York, New York 10176

Thomas R. Hanley, Jr. (1653), Global Toxicology, Dow AgroSciences, LLC, Indianapolis, Indiana 46268

Paul Harp (1639), Virginia Polytechnic Institute State University, Blacksburg, Virginia 24061

Jane E. Harris (1641), BASF Corporation, Princeton, New Jersey 08543

Wayland J. Hayes, Jr. (1), Department of Pharmacology and Toxicology, University of Kansas Medical Center, Kansas City, Kansas 66160

Leon W. Hershberger (1673), DuPont Agricultural Products, Stine-Haskell Research Center, Newark, Delaware 19714

Thomas Hertner (1701), Syngenta Crop Protection AG, Health Assessment and Environmental Safety, CH-4002 Basel, Switzerland

Frederick G. Hess (1641), BASF Corporation, Princeton, New Jersey 08543

William F. Heydens (1543), Monsanto Company, St. Louis, Missouri 63167

Ernest Hodgson (507, 531, 583), Department of Environmental and Molecular Toxicology, North Carolina State University, Raleigh, North Carolina 27695

Robert M. Hollingworth (1169), National Food Safety and Toxicology Center, Michigan State University, East Lansing, Michigan 48824

Susan Hurt (1759), Rohm and Haas Company, Philadelphia, Pennsylvania 19106

Poorni R. Iyer (375), Pesticide Regulation, California Environmental Protection Agency, Sacramento, California 95814

Richard J. Jackson (783), National Center for Environmental Health, Centers for Disease Control and Prevention, Atlanta, Georgia 30341

Martin K. Johnson (953), Medical Research Council Toxicology Unit, University of Leicester, Leicester LE1 9HN, United Kingdom

Bernard S. Jortner (987), Department of Pathobiology, Virgina-Maryland Regional College of Veterinary Medicine, Virginia Polytechnic Institute and State University, Blacksburg, Virginia 24061

Hideo Kaneko (1263), Sumitomo Chemical Co., Ltd., Kitahama, Chou-ku, Osaka 541-8550, Japan

Robert J. Kavlock (727), U.S. Environmental Protection Agency, Washington, DC 20460

Michael P. Kenna (203), Research Office, U.S. Golf Association Green Section, Stillwater, Oklahoma 74076

Elke Kennepohl (1623), Cantox Health Sciences International, Mississauga, Ontario, L5N 2X7, Canada

William C. Krieger (XXVII), Walla Walla Community College, Walla Walla, Washington 99362

Ian C. Lamb (1543), Pioneer Hi-Bred International, Inc., Des Moines, Iowa 50306

Richard L. Lampman (181), Illinois Natural History Survey, Champaign, Illinois 61820

Patricia E. Levi (531), Department of Environmental and Molecular Toxicology, North Carolina State University, Raleigh, North Carolina 27695

A. V. Lyubimov (1861), University, Minnesota, Minneapolis, Minnesota 55465

Jing Liu (1521), College of Veterinary Medicine, Oklahoma State University, Stillwater, Oklahoma 74078

Edward A. Lock (1559, 1605), Syngenta Central Toxicology Laboratory, Macclesfield, Cheshire SK10 4TJ, United Kingdom

Marcello Lotti (1043), Dipartimento di Medicina Ambientale e Sanità Pubblica, Università Degli Studi di Pasdova, 35128, Italy

Curt Lunchik (493), Aventis CropScience, Research Triangle Park, North Carolina 27709

Howard I. Maibach (905), Department of Dermatology, University of California, San Francisco, California 94143

Neela B. Manley (799), Ernest Orlando Lawrence Berkeley, National Laboratory, Berkeley, California 94720

Shajan Mannala (263), Comparative Toxicology Laboratories, Kansas State University, Manhattan, Kansas 66506

Rex E. Marsh (251), Department of Wildlife, Fish, and Conservation Biology, University of California, Davis, California 95616

Peter McCahon (1107), Aventis CropScience, Research Triangle Park, North Carolina 27709

Michael McGeehin (783), Division of Environmental Hazards and Health Effects, National Centers for Disease Control and Prevension, Atlanta, Georgia 30341

Louise N. Mehler (603), Department of Pesticide Regulation, California Environmental Protection Agency, Sacramento, California 95814

Junshi Miyamoto (1263), Sumitomo Chemical Co., Ltd., Kitahama, Chou-ku, Osaka 541-8550, Japan

Thomas B. Moore (1781), Department of Pesticide Regulation, Medical Toxicology Branch, California Environmental Protection Agency, Sacramento, California 95812

Ronald L. Mull (1673), RLM Strategies, Inc., DeLeon, Texas 76444

Ian C. Munro (1623), Cantox Health Sciences International, Mississauga, Ontario L5N 2X7, Canada

Toshio Narahashi (335), Department of Molecular Pharmacology and Biological Chemistry, Northwestern University Medical School, Chicago, Illinois 60611

Keiichiro Nishimura (649), Osaka Prefecture University, Sakai, Osaka, 599-8570, Japan

Kenneth D. Nitschke (1881), Dow Chemical Company, Midland, Michigan 48674

Robert J. Novak (181), Illinois Natural History Survey, Champaign, Illinois 61820

Michael O'Malley (299), University of California, Davis, California 95616

Frederick W. Oehme (263), Comparative Toxicology Laboratories, Kansas State University, Manhattan, Kansas 66506

Janet Ollinger (1759), Rohm and Haas Company, Philadelphia, Pennsylvania 19106

Thomas G. Osimitz (1439, 1461), S.C. Johnson Son, Inc., Racine, Wisconsin 53403

Muhilan D. Pandian (435), Infoscientific, Inc., Carmichael, California; and risksciences.net, Arlington, Virginia 22201

P. P. Parsons (1743), Syngenta Central Toxicology Laboratory

Alain F. Pelfrene (1793), Alain Pelfrene and Associated Consultants, Charbnizieres les Bain F-69260, France

Kimberly Pendino (1641), Hoffman-La Roche, Inc., Nutley, New Jersey 07110

Barbara J. Petersen (443), Novigen Sciences, Inc., Washington, DC 20036

Keith F. Pfeifer (707), Department of Pesticide Regulation, Medical Toxicology Branch, California Environmental Protection Agency, Sacramento, California 95812

Vincent J. Piccirillo (1837), NPC Incorporated, Sterling, Virginia 20164

Jack R. Plimmer (95), JRP Consultants, Tampa, Florida 33606

Kathryn Ponnock (1641), Middlesex County Community College, Edison, New Jersey 08818

Pierre-Gerard Pontal (1107), Aventis CropScience, Rhone-Poulenc, BF 153F 06903, Sophia Antipolis, France

Carey Pope (873), Department of Physiological Sciences, College of Veterinary Medicine, Oklahoma State University, Stillwater, Oklahoma 74078

David E. Ray (1289), MRC Applied Neurobiology Group, Department of Biomedical Sciences, University of Nottingham Medical School, Queens Medical Centre, Nottingham NG7 2UH, United Kingdom

Joseph P. Rieth (1107), JSC, Inc., Research Triangle Park, North Carolina 27709

Jim E. Riviere (515), Center for Cutaneous Toxicology and Residue Pharmacology, College of Veterinary Medicine, North Carolina State University, Raleigh, North Carolina 27606

Kathleen E. Rodgers (769), Keck School of Medicine, University of Southern California, Los Angeles, California 90033

Joanne G. Romagni (1529), USDA-ARS Natural Production Utilization Research Unit, University of Mississippi, University, Mississippi 38677

John H. Ross (435, 479, 493), Infoscientific, Inc., Carmichael, California 95608

Karl K. Rozman (1), Department of Pharmacology and Toxicology, University of Kansas Medical Center, Kansas City, Kansas 66160

Carol H. Rubin (783), Health Studies Branch, Division of Environmental Hazards and Health Effects, Centers for Disease Control and Prevention, Atlanta, Georgia 30333

Andrew L. Rubin (859), Medical Toxicology Branch, Department of Pesticide Regulation, California Environmental Protection Agency, Sacramento, California 95812

Michael K. Rust (243), Department of Entomology, University of California, Riverside, California 92521

Luis O. Ruzo (671), PTRL West, Inc., Hercules, California 94547

Wayne T. Sanderson (603), Division of Surveillance, Hazard Evaluations and Field Studies, National Institute for Occupational Safety and Health, Centers for Disease Control and Prevention, Cincinnati, Ohio 45226

Kai Savolainen (1013), Department of Industrial Hygiene and Toxicology, Finnish Institute of Occupational Health, Topeliukensenkatu 41B, FIN-00250 Helsinki

Gerald P. Schoenig (1439), Toxicology/Regulatory Services, Inc., Charlottesville, Virginia 22911

James N. Seiber (643), Western Regional Research Center, USDA-ARS, Albany, California 94710

Ken Sexton (887), University of Minnesota School of Public Health, Minneapolis, Minnesota 55455

Larry P. Sheets (1123), Bayer Corporation, Stilwell, Kansas 66085

James Simpkins (1511), Department of Pharmacology and Neuroscience, University of North Texas Health Sciences Center, Fort Worth, Texas 76107

Thomas H. Slone (799), University of California, Berkeley, California 94720

Paul Slovic (845), Decision Research, Inc., Eugene, Oregon 97401

Andrew G. Smith (1305), Medical Research Council Toxicology Unit, Leicester University, Leicester LE1 9HN, United Kingdom

Wayne R. Snodgrass (589), Clinical Pharmacology-Toxicology Unit, Texas Poison Center, University of Texas, Galveston, Texas 77555

Keith R. Solomon (353), Center for Toxicology, University of Guelph, Guelph, Ontario N1G 2W1, Canada

James T. Stevens (1157, 1511), Syngenta Crop Protection, Inc., Greensboro, North Carolina 27409

W. T. Stott (1849), Dow Chemical Company, Midland, Michigan 48674

Phillip L. Strong (1429), US Borax, Inc., Valencia, California 91355

Lois Swirsky Gold (799), University of California, Berkeley, California 94720

Chiyozo Takayama (649), Sumitomo Chemical Co., Ltd., Takarazuka, Hyogo, 665-8555, Japan

Charles A. Timchalk (929), Pacific Northwest National Laboratory, Richland, Washington 99352

Abraham J. Tobia (1107, 1759), Aventis CropScience, Research Triangle Park, North Carolina 27709

Matazaemon Uchida (649), Nihon Nohyaku, Co., Ltd., Kawachi-Nagano, Osaka 586-0094, Japan

István Ujváry (109), Chemical Research Center, Hungarian Academy of Sciences, H-1025 Budapest, Hungary

Joop J. van Hemmen (457), Department of Chemical Exposure Assessment, TNO Chemistry, The Netherlands

Bennard Van Ravenswaay (1759), BASF Corporation, Princeton, New Jersey 08543

Felix Waechter (1701), Syngenta Crop Protection AG, Health Assessment and Environmental Safety, CH-4002, Basel, Switzerland

Cassi L. Walls (443), Novigen Sciences, Inc., Washington, DC 20036

Edgar Weber (1701), Syngenta Crop Protection AG, Health Assessment and Environmental Safety, CH-4002, Basel, Switzerland

Ronald C. Wester (905), Department of Dermatology, University of California, San Francisco, California 94143

Gary K. Whitmyre (435, 493), risksciences, LLC, Arlington, Virginia 22201

Martin F. Wilks (1559, 1605), Syngenta Ltd., Fernhurst, Haslemere, Surrey GU27 3JE, United Kingdom

Rick Williams (1107), RTI, Inc., Research Triangle Park, North Carolina 27709

Barry W. Wilson (967), Animal Science and Environmental Toxicology, University of California, Davis, California 95616

Alan G. E. Wilson (1543), Pharmacia Corporation, Peapack, New Jersey 07977

Masanori Yoshida (649), Nihon Nohyaku, Co., Ltd., Kawachi-Nagano, Osaka 586-0094, Japan

Susan H. Youngren (443), Novigen Sciences, Inc., Washington, DC 20036

Frank G. Zalom (275), University of California, Davis, California 95616

Chemistry of Organophosphorus Insecticides

Howard W. Chambers, J. Scott Boone, Russell L. Carr, and Janice E. Chambers
Mississippi State University

44.1 INTRODUCTION

It should be emphasized at the outset that this review is not for the serious organic chemist, but for toxicologists and others desiring a basic knowledge of this important class of toxicants. Further, it is recognized that organic phosphorus chemicals have many uses other than as pesticides. Only insecticides will be considered here, with passing reference to chemical warfare agents. Finally, organophosphorus chemistry is an exceedingly complex subject and only generalizations will be made in the sections on synthesis and reactions. Other reviews (cited in the following) and numerous research articles are available that provide more detailed information.

44.2 CHEMISTRY OF ORGANOPHOSPHORUS INSECTICIDES

44.2.1 HISTORY

Organophosphorus (OP) chemistry apparently began around 1820 with the esterification of alcohols to phosphoric acid. Despite synthesis of a number of OP compounds in the early 1900s, the potential toxicity went unrecognized until the 1930s. By 1940, groups led by B. C. Saunders in England and Gerhard Schrader in Germany had produced several highly toxic compounds for possible use as chemical warfare agents. The most notable of these were sarin and soman, both phosphorofluoridates, and tabun, a phosphorocyanidate (Fig. 44.1). Schrader's group also produced the first commercial OP insecticides, including tepp in 1937, dimefox in 1940, schradan (OMPA) in 1942, and parathion in 1944.

Following World War II, with the capture of Schrader's research records, interest in OP insecticides grew rapidly. Although all of the early chemicals were effective insecticides, they were also highly toxic to mammals. In 1950, however, American Cyanamid produced malathion, one of the safest OPs ever marketed. By 1959, it was estimated that more than 50,000 OP compounds had been made. In 1970, more than 200 OP insecticides were marketed worldwide. Though development of resistance in pests and the marketing of new, safer insecticides have greatly decreased the usage of OPs and slowed the development of new products, these remain an important group of pest control agents and will probably do so for another decade or more.

44.2.2 CLASSIFICATION AND NOMENCLATURE

Because of the vast number and wide variety of organic phosphorus chemicals that can exist, any comprehensive classification system would be too complex to undertake here. Instead, a classification scheme will be presented into which all commercially important OP insecticides will fit, based on the central phosphorus atom and the four atoms immediately surrounding it. Similarly, the nomenclature of OPs will primarily address these five atoms.

The general structure of OP insecticides can be represented by

$$R_1 \underset{R_2}{\overset{}{>}} \overset{\overset{X}{\|}}{P} {-} L$$

L, the so-called leaving group, is the most reactive and most variable substituent. The term "leaving group" comes from the fact that it is the substituent that is displaced when the OP phosphorylates acetylcholinesterase, the primary target enzyme. The leaving group is also usually the most susceptible to hydrolysis. R_1 and R_2 are less reactive and are most commonly alkoxy groups, but may be alkyl, aryl, alkylthio, or alkylamino. X is either oxygen or sulfur.

OP insecticides may be considered to be derivatives of phosphoric acid (H_3PO_4) or phosphonic acid (H_3PO_3) in which all H atoms are replaced by organic moieties. Thus, phosphates are compounds in which the P atom is surrounded by

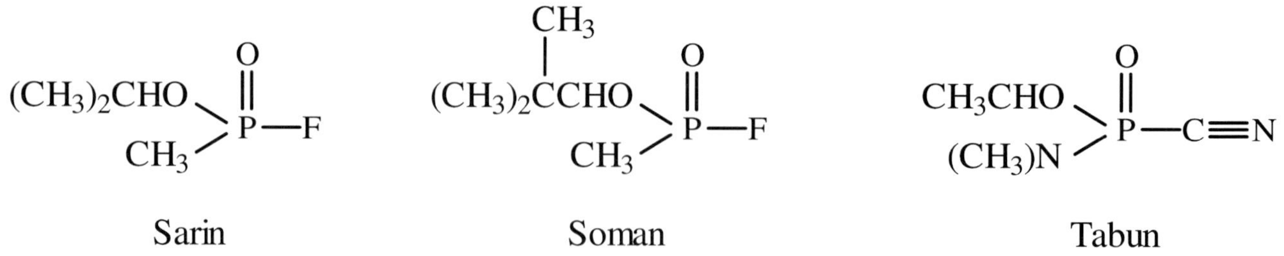

Figure 44.1 Structures of early OP nerve gases.

Table 44.1
Subclasses of OP Insecticides

Name	Atoms around P			
	O	S	N	C
Phosphate	4	0	0	0
Phosphorothioate*	3	1	0	0
Phosphorodithioate*	2	2	0	0
Phosphoramidate	3	0	1	0
Phosphorodiamidate	2	0	2	0
Phosphoramidothioate*	2	1	1	0
Phosphonate	3	0	0	1
Phosphonothioate	2	1	0	1
Phosphonodithioate	1	2	0	1

four O atoms. In phosphonates, there are three O atoms and one phosphorus–carbon bond. Phosphinates, which have two O atoms and two P—C bonds, have been investigated and show biological activity, but none have been developed commercially.

In many OPs, one or more of the oxygen atoms are replaced by sulfur and/or nitrogen. For phosphoric acid derivatives, the O, S, and N atoms can be arranged in 20 different configurations. Another 12 different configurations can exist for derivatives of phosphonic acid. Fortunately for the classification and nomenclature to be considered here, most of the 32 possible configurations have not appeared in commercial OP insecticides. Table 44.1 lists the nine subclasses of OPs for which one or more commercial insecticides are known and the numbers and types of atom attached to the phosphorus.

Subclasses with names followed by an asterisk are represented by compounds with two different configurations. For example, the S atom in a phosphorothioate may be within an ester bond (formerly called a phosphorothiolate) or may be doubly bonded to the P atom (a phosphorothionate). Similarly, a phosphorodithioate may be either a phosphorodithiolate or a phosphorothiolothionate. Recent literature has largely abandoned the thiolo and thiono terminology, however, and the positions of the atoms are designated using O- and S- prefixes before substituent names. Thus, $(Me—O)_3 P(:S)$ is named O,O,O-trimethyl phosphorothioate, whereas $(Me—O)_2 P(:O)—S—Me$ is O,O,S-trimethyl phosphorothioate. In the

first case, because the name designates a single S atom but none is within the ester linkages, the S must be doubly bonded to the P. In the second case, because the lone S atom is within an ester linkage, the doubly bonded atom must be O.

For phosphonates and phosphonothioates, the name of the substituent attached by a P—C bond is included as a single word with the root name. $(Me—O)_2 P(:O)—Me$, therefore, is dimethyl methylphosphonate and $(Me—O)_2 P(:S)—Et$ would be named O,O-dimethyl ethylphosphonothioate.

Similarly, for phosphoramides with substituents on the nitrogen atom, the names of those substituents immediately precede the phosphorus term as a single word. In this case, those names are preceded by N- to designate their attachment to the nitrogen atom. For example, $(Et—O)_2 P(:S)—N(Me)_2$ would be named O,O-diethyl N,N-dimethylphosphoramidothioate.

To further clarify the structures and nomenclature of the major subclasses of OPs, representatives of each are shown in Fig. 44.2. As will be noted, for the phosphate, phosphonate, and phosphoramidate subclasses, groups attached to oxygen atoms are not preceded by O-. In these cases, using such a prefix is unnecessary because no sulfur atoms are present in the molecules.

44.2.3 SYNTHESIS

Because of the wide variety of organophosphorus compounds known, no attempt will be made here to cover the many different pathways involved in their synthesis. Rather, the preparation of the seven most important intermediates will be presented, followed by representative examples of their use in the synthesis of specific insecticides. For additional information, the reader is referred to more comprehensive reviews by Eto (1961) and Fest and Schmidt (1982).

Initially, elemental phosphorus is converted into $P_2 S_5$ by reaction with sulfur or into PCl_3 by direct chlorination. These two materials are then converted into the following seven intermedimethyl 2,2-dichlorovinyl phosphate

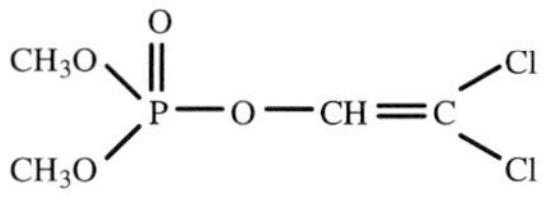

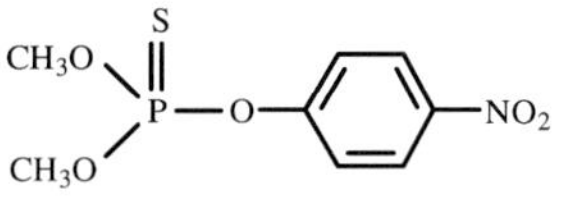

O,O-dimethyl O-(4-nitrophenyl) phosphorothioate

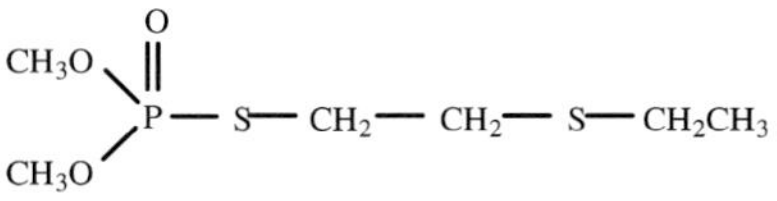

O,O-dimethyl S-(2-ethylthio)ethyl phosphorodithioate

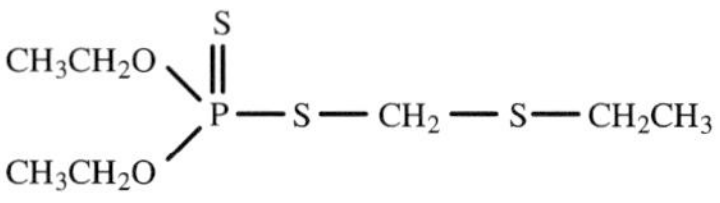

O,O-diethyl S-ethylthiomethyl phosphorodithioate

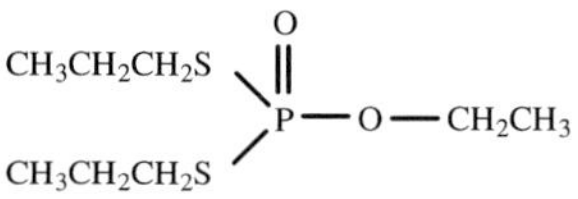

O-ethyl S,S-dipropyl phosphorodithioate

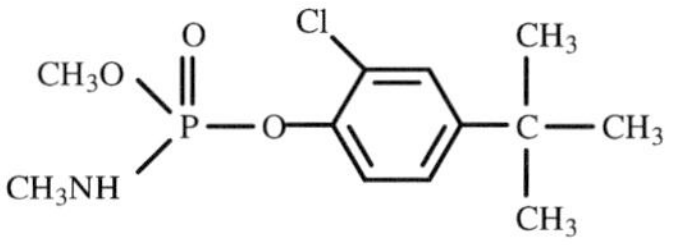

methyl 2-chloro-4-t-butylphenyl N-methylphosphoramidate

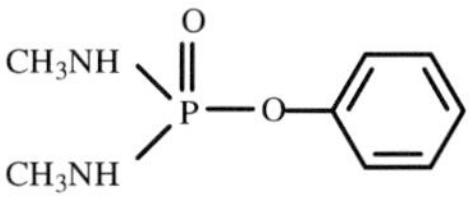

phenyl N,N-dimethylphosphorodiamidate

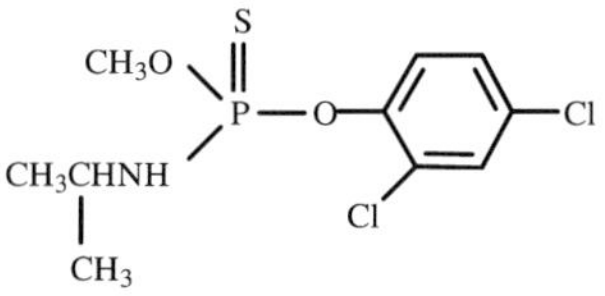

O-methyl O-(2,4-dichlorophenyl) N-isopropylphosphoramidothioate

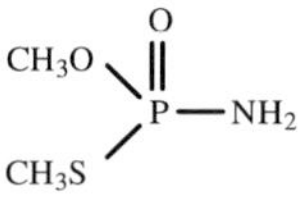

O,S-dimethyl phosphoramidothioate

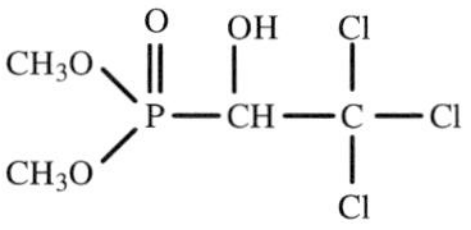

dimethyl 2,2,2-trichloro-1-hydroxyethylphosphonate

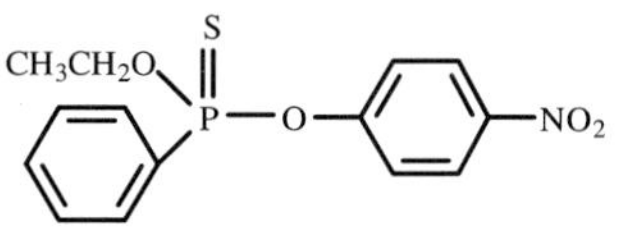

O-ethyl O-(4-nitrophenyl) phenylphosphonothioate

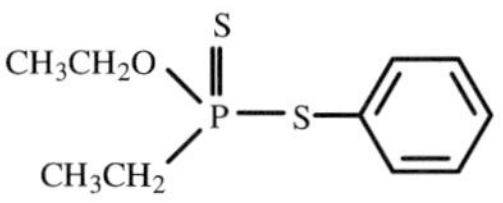

O-ethyl S-phenyl ethylphosphonodithioate

Figure 44.2   Nomenclature of major subclasses of OP insecticides.

diates from which most OP insecticides are synthesized:

$$P_2S_5 + 4\,R\!-\!OH \longrightarrow 2\,(R\!-\!O)_2\overset{\overset{\displaystyle S}{\|}}{P}\!-\!SH \qquad (1)$$

$$(R\!-\!O)_2\overset{\overset{\displaystyle S}{\|}}{P}\!-\!SH + \tfrac{1}{2}Cl_2 \longrightarrow (R\!-\!O)_2\overset{\overset{\displaystyle S}{\|}}{P}\!-\!Cl \qquad (2)$$

$$PCl_3 + \tfrac{1}{2}O_2 \longrightarrow \overset{\overset{\displaystyle O}{\|}}{PCl_3} \qquad (3)$$

$$PCl_3 + S \longrightarrow \overset{\overset{\displaystyle S}{\|}}{PCl_3} \qquad (4)$$

$$PCl_3 + 3\,R\!-\!OH \xrightarrow{\text{base}} (R\!-\!O)_3P \qquad (5)$$

$$PCl_3 + 3\,R\!-\!OH \xrightarrow{\text{no base}} (R\!-\!O)_2P\!-\!OH \qquad (6)$$

$$PCl_3 + 2\,R\!-\!OH + \tfrac{1}{2}O_2 \longrightarrow (R\!-\!O)_2\overset{\overset{\displaystyle O}{\|}}{P}\!-\!Cl \qquad (7)$$

Because there are almost as many procedures for formation of the P—C bond of phosphonates and related OPs as there are insecticides containing this bond, the synthesis of required intermediates will not be discussed. It may be noted, however, that most processes involve PCl_3, $AlCl_3$, and alkyl halides.

Trialkyl phosphites (intermediate 5) are particularly useful in the preparation of dialkyl vinyl phosphates from α-chloroaldehydes and ketones. The synthesis of DDVP serves as a good example:

$$CH_3O\!-\!\overset{\overset{\displaystyle CH_3O}{|}}{\underset{\underset{\displaystyle CH_3O}{|}}{P}} + H\overset{\overset{\displaystyle O}{\|}}{C}CCl_3 \longrightarrow \overset{\displaystyle CH_3O}{\underset{\displaystyle CH_3O}{>}}\overset{\overset{\displaystyle O}{\|}}{P}\!-\!O\!-\!CH\!=\!CCl_2$$

Interestingly, the same aldehyde reacts with dimethyl phosphite (intermediate 6) to produce the phosphonate insecticide trichlorfon:

$$\overset{\displaystyle CH_3O}{\underset{\displaystyle CH_3O}{>}}P\!-\!OH + H\overset{\overset{\displaystyle O}{\|}}{C}CCl_3 \longrightarrow \overset{\displaystyle CH_3O}{\underset{\displaystyle CH_3O}{>}}\overset{\overset{\displaystyle O}{\|}}{P}\!-\!\overset{\overset{\displaystyle OH}{|}}{C}CCl_3$$

Dialkyl phosphates may also be prepared from dialkyl phosphorochloridates (intermediate 7) by reactions analogous to the formation of carboxylic esters from acid chlorides. Paraoxon, the oxygen analog and active metabolite of parathion, is readily prepared by this reaction:

$$\overset{\displaystyle CH_3CH_2O}{\underset{\displaystyle CH_3CH_2O}{>}}\overset{\overset{\displaystyle O}{\|}}{P}\!-\!Cl + HO\!-\!\!\!\langle\bigcirc\rangle\!\!\!-\!NO_2 \xrightarrow{\text{base}} \overset{\displaystyle CH_3CH_2O}{\underset{\displaystyle CH_3CH_2O}{>}}\overset{\overset{\displaystyle O}{\|}}{P}\!-\!O\!-\!\!\!\langle\bigcirc\rangle\!\!\!-\!NO_2$$

An analogous, and more commonly used, reaction is that of dialkyl phosphorochloridothioates (intermediate 2) to produce phosphorothionates such as parathion:

$$\overset{\displaystyle CH_3CH_2O}{\underset{\displaystyle CH_3CH_2O}{>}}\overset{\overset{\displaystyle S}{\|}}{P}\!-\!Cl + HO\!-\!\!\!\langle\bigcirc\rangle\!\!\!-\!NO_2 \xrightarrow{\text{base}} \overset{\displaystyle CH_3CH_2O}{\underset{\displaystyle CH_3CH_2O}{>}}\overset{\overset{\displaystyle S}{\|}}{P}\!-\!O\!-\!\!\!\langle\bigcirc\rangle\!\!\!-\!NO_2$$

Dialkyl phosphorodithioates undergo three distinct types of reactions. The salts of these acids react with alkyl halides with

formation of the thiol ester. Disulfoton is produced in this way:

$$\overset{\displaystyle CH_3CH_2O}{\underset{\displaystyle CH_3CH_2O}{>}}\overset{\overset{\displaystyle S}{\|}}{P}\!-\!S\!-\!Na + Cl\!-\!CH_2CH_2SCH_2CH_3 \longrightarrow \overset{\displaystyle CH_3CH_2O}{\underset{\displaystyle CH_3CH_2O}{>}}\overset{\overset{\displaystyle S}{\|}}{P}\!-\!S\!-\!CH_2CH_2SCH_2CH_3$$

The free acid will add across certain carbon–carbon double bonds. Malathion is prepared from diethyl maleate by this reaction:

$$\overset{\displaystyle CH_3O}{\underset{\displaystyle CH_3O}{>}}\overset{\overset{\displaystyle S}{\|}}{P}\!-\!SH + \overset{\overset{\displaystyle O}{\|}}{\underset{\underset{\displaystyle \overset{\|}{O}}{CHC\!-\!OCH_2CH_3}}{CHC\!-\!OCH_2CH_3}} \longrightarrow \overset{\displaystyle CH_3O}{\underset{\displaystyle CH_3O}{>}}\overset{\overset{\displaystyle S}{\|}}{P}\!-\!S\!-\!\overset{\overset{\displaystyle O}{\|}}{\underset{\underset{\displaystyle \overset{\|}{O}}{CH_2C\!-\!OCH_2CH_3}}{CHC\!-\!OCH_2CH_3}}$$

Also, the free acid reacts with formaldehyde and a mercaptan to produce compounds such as phorate:

$$\overset{\displaystyle CH_3CH_2O}{\underset{\displaystyle CH_3CH_2O}{>}}\overset{\overset{\displaystyle S}{\|}}{P}\!-\!SH + CH_2O + HS\!-\!CH_2CH_3 \longrightarrow \overset{\displaystyle CH_3CH_2O}{\underset{\displaystyle CH_3CH_2O}{>}}\overset{\overset{\displaystyle S}{\|}}{P}\!-\!S\!-\!CH_2\!-\!S\!-\!CH_2CH_3$$

For OPs with three different substituents on the P atom, it is necessary to begin with P(:O) Cl_3 (from intermediate 3) or P(:S) Cl_3 (from intermediate 4). The sequence in which the groups are added varies with the specific compound. Two examples, fenamiphos and sulprofos, respectively, are as follows:

$$\overset{\overset{\displaystyle O}{\|}}{PCl_3} + (1)\ HO\!-\!\!\!\langle\bigcirc\rangle\!\!\!\overset{\displaystyle CH_3}{\underset{\displaystyle S\!-\!CH_3}{}}$$
$$+ (2)\ CH_3CH_2\!-\!OH$$
$$+ (3)\ CH_3\overset{\displaystyle}{\underset{\underset{\displaystyle CH_3}{|}}{CH}}\!-\!NH_2 \longrightarrow \overset{\displaystyle CH_3CH_2O}{\underset{\displaystyle CH_3\overset{}{\underset{\underset{\displaystyle CH_3}{|}}{CHNH}}}{>}}\overset{\overset{\displaystyle O}{\|}}{P}\!-\!O\!-\!\!\!\langle\bigcirc\rangle\!\!\!\overset{\displaystyle CH_3}{\underset{\displaystyle S\!-\!CH_3}{}}$$

$$\overset{\overset{\displaystyle S}{\|}}{PCl_3} + (1)\ CH_3CH_2\!-\!OH$$
$$+ (2)\ HO\!-\!\!\!\langle\bigcirc\rangle\!\!\!-\!S\!-\!CH_3$$
$$+ (3)\ CH_3CH_2CH_2\!-\!S\!-\!Na \longrightarrow \overset{\displaystyle CH_3CH_2O}{\underset{\displaystyle CH_3CH_2CH_2S}{>}}\overset{\overset{\displaystyle S}{\|}}{P}\!-\!O\!-\!\!\!\langle\bigcirc\rangle\!\!\!-\!S\!-\!CH_3$$

Although the preceding discussion is by no means a comprehensive treatment of OP synthesis, the reactions shown are used in the preparation of more than 90% of commercial OP insecticide compounds. One final type of reaction not previously mentioned is worthy of consideration because of its usefulness in laboratory syntheses.

Dialkyl phosphates with phenolic or heterocyclic leaving groups are easily prepared from the phenol or heterocyclic alcohol and the dialkyl phosphorochloridate. Unfortunately, the only phosphorochloridates readily available commercially are the dimethyl and the diethyl, the former being quite unstable. At least four dialkyl phosphites (dimethyl, diethyl, di-i-propyl, and di-n-butyl) are available at reasonable prices and are more stable in storage. The reaction alluded to in the previous paragraph, then, is the synthesis of dialkyl phosphates from dialkyl phosphites without independent preparation and isolation of the phosphorochloridate.

Carbon tetrachloride, in the presence of an organic base (e.g., triethylamine), will chlorinate dialkyl phosphites by the following reaction:

$$(R{-}O)_2\overset{\overset{\displaystyle O}{\|}}{P}{-}H + CCl_4 \xrightarrow{(CH_3CH_2)_3N} (R{-}O)_2\overset{\overset{\displaystyle O}{\|}}{P}{-}Cl + CHCl_3$$

This allows a one-step synthesis of many phenyl or heterocyclic dialkyl phosphates. For example, methyl paraoxon (catalog price > \$500/g) is prepared easily and inexpensively by:

$$\begin{array}{c}CH_3O\\CH_3O\end{array}\!\!>\!\!\overset{\overset{\displaystyle O}{\|}}{P}{-}H + HO{-}\!\!\left\langle\!\!\bigcirc\!\!\right\rangle\!\!{-}NO_2 \xrightarrow[\text{in } CCl_4]{(CH_3CH_2)_3N} \begin{array}{c}CH_3O\\CH_3O\end{array}\!\!>\!\!\overset{\overset{\displaystyle O}{\|}}{P}{-}O{-}\!\!\left\langle\!\!\bigcirc\!\!\right\rangle\!\!{-}NO_2$$

This synthesis has been done several times by the authors, obtaining moderate yield of product of > 98% purity. Although the process is useful on a small scale, it is rarely used in industrial syntheses because of the hazard associated with CCl_4.

44.2.4 REACTIONS

OP insecticides, when kept cool, dark, and anhydrous, are usually quite stable. Exposure to heat, light (especially ultraviolet), and/or water, however, may lead to chemical alterations. The three primary reactions involving the phosphorus atom and those immediately surrounding it are hydrolysis, oxidation, and rearrangement.

Except at very low pHs, hydrolysis of the P—O—C linkage results primarily by OH$^-$ attack on the P atom with cleavage of the P—O bond. Thus, rates of hydrolysis increase with increasing pH. Three additional generalizations may be made concerning this type of hydrolysis:

1. Compounds containing P=O hydrolyze faster than analogous compounds containing P=S.
2. Cleavage occurs between the P atom and the leaving group.
3. The hydrolysis rate decreases with increasing size of the alkyl substituents.

The most notable exception is that alkaline hydrolysis of OPs containing Me—O—P(:S)= often results in cleavage of the methyl rather than the leaving group.

Hydrolysis of the P—S—C linkage differs from that described previously in that alkaline hydrolysis results primarily in cleavage of the S—C bond. An exception to this is fonofos (*O*-ethyl *S*-phenyl ethylphosphonodithioate), which is apparently hydrolyzed at the P—S bond to yield thiophenol. Acid hydrolysis, on the other hand, consistently leads to cleavage of the P—S bond.

The P—N bond of phosphoramides is generally rather resistant to alkaline hydrolysis. Because the N atom is readily protonated, however, these compounds are quite susceptible to acid hydrolysis.

Oxidation of OPs by O_2 is enhanced by ultraviolet (UV) light. It may also be accomplished by oxidants such as HNO_3 or organic peroxyacids. These oxidations most commonly occur with P=S-type OPs, but the sulfur of the P—S—C linkage may also be oxidized. Oxidation of P=S presumably results in transient formation of the phosphooxythiirane (a three-membered ring consisting of one each of P, O, and S). This intermediate spontaneously decomposes to produce the oxon (P=O) with loss of sulfur or cleaves between the P atom and the leaving group. Oxidation of the sulfur of P—S—C produces ester-sulfoxides, which are highly reactive and usually degrade rapidly.

Upon exposure to UV or high temperatures, compounds containing C—O—P=S will undergo rearrangement in which C—S—P=O is produced. Most commonly, the C involved is in an alkyl substituent but the leaving group can also be involved. Both types of rearrangements are known for parathion as shown by

$$\begin{array}{c}CH_3CH_2O\\CH_3CH_2O\end{array}\!\!>\!\!\overset{\overset{\displaystyle S}{\|}}{P}{-}O{-}\!\!\left\langle\!\!\bigcirc\!\!\right\rangle\!\!{-}NO_2 \xrightarrow{UV}$$

$$\begin{array}{c}CH_3CH_2S\\CH_3CH_2O\end{array}\!\!>\!\!\overset{\overset{\displaystyle O}{\|}}{P}{-}O{-}\!\!\left\langle\!\!\bigcirc\!\!\right\rangle\!\!{-}NO_2$$

$$\begin{array}{c}CH_3CH_2O\\CH_3CH_2O\end{array}\!\!>\!\!\overset{\overset{\displaystyle O}{\|}}{P}{-}S{-}\!\!\left\langle\!\!\bigcirc\!\!\right\rangle\!\!{-}NO_2$$

Whether such rearrangements are intramolecular, intermolecular, or both is unclear.

Toxicologically, the chemical reactions may or may not result in loss of toxicity. Hydrolysis completely detoxifies the OP. Oxidation of P=S to P=O and both rearrangements illustrated lead to an increase in toxicity. Though other reactions of OPs may occur, those presented are the most important in the environment and in long-term storage.

REFERENCES

Eto, E. (1961). "Organophosphorus Pesticides: Organic and Biological Chemistry." CRC Press, Cleveland.

Fest, C., and Schmidt, K.-J. (1982). "The Chemistry of Organic Pesticides," 2nd ed. Springer-Verlag, Berlin/Heidelberg/New York.

CHAPTER

45

The Metabolism of Organophosphorus Insecticides

Janice E. Chambers, Russell L. Carr, J. Scott Boone,
and Howard W. Chambers
Mississippi State University

45.1 INTRODUCTION

As was illustrated in the previous chapter, the class of organophosphorus insecticides contains a diverse array of structures, all united by the presence of a pentavalent phosphorus atom with three singly bonded constituents and a coordinate covalent bond (typically drawn as a double bond) to either a sulfur or an oxygen. These insecticides or their metabolites are potent inhibitors of serine esterases through phosphorylation of the serine hydroxyl moiety within the active site of the esterase. The primary target esterase from a toxicological standpoint is acetylcholinesterase, a widely distributed enzyme within the vertebrate nervous system that mediates hydrolysis of the neurotransmitter acetylcholine throughout the central and peripheral nervous systems. The phosphorylation of acetylcholinesterase is relatively persistent, with spontaneous hydrolysis, and therefore recovery of the enzyme activity, requiring hours to days. The inhibition of acetylcholinesterase results in the accumulation of acetylcholine in cholinergic synapses and neuromuscular/glandular junctions with subsequent hypercholinergic activity. Such activity leads to a variety of signs and symptoms of intoxication, with death in mammals in lethal level poisonings resulting from respiratory failure. Other serine esterases, such as butyrylcholinesterase or carboxylesterases, can also be phosphorylated by the organophosphorus insecticides or their metabolites; however, phosphorylation of these other targets does not appear to result in toxic responses. More detailed descriptions of the neurotoxicity of organophosphorus insecticides can be found in a number of chapters and reviews, including Chambers (1992) and Ecobichon (1996). The potency of the organophosphorus insecticides or their active metabolites as inhibitors of target brain acetylcholinesterase does not correspond to the acute toxicity levels, indicating that metabolism and disposition are of great significance in determining the overall acute toxicity level of these insecticides (Chambers et al., 1990). An overview of organophosphorus insecticide chemistry, biochemistry, and toxicology can be found in Chambers and Levi (1992).

These insecticides display substantial chemical diversity, including a variety of atoms in addition to the carbon and phosphorus mandated by the compounds being "organophosphorus" compounds, such as sulfur, nitrogen, and oxygen. Therefore, the organophosphorus insecticides are subject to many metabolic pathways mediated by several of the groups of xenobiotic metabolizing enzymes. The group connected through the single bond that is the least thermodynamically stable of the three single bonds is the "leaving group" and is the group that is eliminated from the molecule as it phosphorylates its esterase targets. The leaving group may be subject to some metabolic pathways that the other substituents are not, as will be described later on. The other two substituents may be the same as one another or different and are also subject to metabolism. The organophosphorus insecticides or their metabolites are subject to oxidations, reductions, hydrolyses, and conjugations. Because of their metabolic and chemical lability, they do not readily remain intact either in the environment or in the organism. Their environmental lability was one of the factors that allowed them to replace the highly stable organochlorine insecticides as the dominant class of insecticides.

The several types of reactions that occur in the metabolic pathways of organophosphorus insecticides will be discussed later, indicating the types of enzymes involved in the reaction, some examples of these reactions with specific organophosphorus insecticides, and the toxicological outcomes of these metabolic pathways. An overview of the types of biotransformation enzymes involved in the metabolism of organophosphorus insecticides can be found in Parkinson (1996). Specific metabolic pathways for a number of specific insecticides can be found in Aizawa (1982, 1989) and Dikshith (1991).

45.2 OXIDATIONS

45.2.1 CYTOCHROMES P450

The cytochrome P450 enzymes (P450s) comprise one of the most important, if not the most important, class of xenobiotic metabolizing enzymes. The P450s are a superfamily of related enzymes characterized by the presence of a heme iron in the active site. They have a broad substrate specificity, with different enzymes (isoforms) catalyzing a variety of oxidations on phosphorus, sulfur, nitrogen, and carbon, with different substrate specificities among the isoforms. The P450s are monooxygenases and catalyze the oxidations by the addition of one atom of molecular oxygen into the substrate via an electron transport pathway with the electrons supplied by reduced nicotinamide adenine dinucleotide phosphate (NADPH) and sometimes reduced nicotinamide adenine dinucleotide (NADH). The electron transfers are catalyzed by NADPH cytochrome P450 reductase. Except for some specialized P450s, such as those involved in steroidogenesis, the P450 pathway occurs in the endoplasmic reticulum of vertebrate cells, with the highest xenobiotic metabolizing capacity in the mammalian liver and a more limited capacity observed in other mammalian tissues and in submammalian vertebrates. More detailed descriptions of P450 and associated reactions may be found in Parkinson (1996). Many of the P450-mediated reactions on organophosphorus insecticides are obvious oxidations, resulting in a more highly oxidized product with the presence of the oxygen apparent in the products. However, some of the P450-mediated reactions are not as obviously oxidations. Because of the addition of polar reactive groups by these P450-mediated reactions, some of the resultant products are more biologically reactive and therefore more toxic [such as with greater reactivity toward neural target molecules or toward deoxyribonucleic acid (DNA)] than the parent compounds were, whereas other reactions result in detoxified products; therefore, P450s mediate both bioactivations and detoxications.

One of the most important of the P450-mediated reactions involving the organophosphorus insecticides is the desulfuration reaction occurring with phosphorothionates and other compounds having the phosphorus bonded to sulfur by a coordinate covalent bond (P=S). The desulfuration reaction involves an attack of the phosphorus by oxygen, resulting in a putative phosphooxythiiran intermediate, which rearranges to a P=O group with a loss of the sulfur as illustrated in Fig. 45.1 (Neal, 1980).

The sulfur released in the desulfuration reaction is a reactive moiety and has the ability to destroy surrounding biomolecules, such as the P450s. A classic example of this desulfuration reaction is the conversion of parathion to its phosphate (oxon) metabolite, paraoxon. The P=S compounds are relatively poor anticholinesterases, whereas the oxons are potent anticholinesterases, with a three order of magnitude difference in potency with at least some of the insecticides (Forsyth and Chambers, 1989). Because so many of the most popular of the organophosphorus insecticides are

phosphorothionates or related P=S compounds, the desulfuration reaction is required for them to display appreciable anticholinesterase activity, and therefore to display classical organophosphorus insecticide neurotoxicity. Because so many of the phosphorothionate insecticides display very high acute toxicity levels (e.g., rat oral LD50s for parathion, methyl parathion, and azinphosmethyl are 2, 50, and 10 mg/kg, respectively; Meister, 1990), one can infer that the desulfuration reaction occurs *in vivo* to an appreciable extent. An example of the desulfuration of parathion is given in Fig. 45.2.

A reaction occurring parallel to the desulfuration reaction, and concurrently with it, is the dearylation reaction, occasionally termed oxidative hydrolysis, which occurs from the same putative phosphooxythiiran intermediate described previously for the desulfuration reaction. Instead of rearranging to eliminate the sulfur as occurs during the desulfuration reaction, the rearrangement in the dearylation reaction eliminates the aryl leaving group. The resultant products are the leaving group plus either the dialkyl phosphorothioate or the dialkyl phosphate; therefore, the reaction resembles a hydrolysis, but the occurrence of these reaction products is dependent on the presence of P450, oxygen, and NADPH. Additionally, classic hydrolysis reactions do not readily occur with the phosphorothionates. Therefore, the dearylation reaction appears to be an oxidation although the products do not readily suggest that an oxidation has occurred. Because the phosphate/oxon structure is required for anticholinesterase activity, the dearylation reaction is a detoxication reaction. The dearylation reaction with parathion as an example is given in Fig. 45.3.

The concurrent and competing reactions of desulfuration (activation) and dearylation (detoxication), again using parathion as an example, are illustrated in Fig. 45.4, along with the putative phosphooxythiiran intermediate. Studies conducted with purified isoforms of P450 have indicated that different isoforms have different desulfuration to dearylation ratios, indicating that substrate specificity and pathway preference among the P450 isoforms differ (Levi *et al.*, 1988). Therefore, it is expected that the activity of different isoforms of P450 would have different impacts on toxicity.

An additional P450-mediated reaction that can occur on the intact phosphorothionate or its oxon is a dealkylation reaction in which one of the carbons in an alkoxy group is oxidized to the aldehyde that is removed, leaving a hydroxyl group associated with the phosphorus (Appleton and Nakatsugawa, 1972). The oxidized product would be formaldehyde in the case of a methoxy group or acetaldehyde in the case of an ethoxy group. Using parathion as an example once again, the dealkylation reaction is illustrated in Fig. 45.5.

Oxidations of substituents in the leaving group are also possible, with a wide variety of reactions possible because of the great diversity of the leaving groups within the insecticide class. A few illustrative examples are provided in Fig. 45.6.

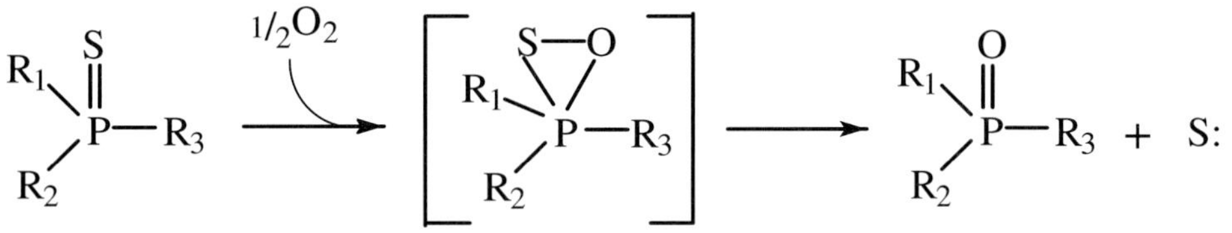

Figure 45.1 Desulfuration reaction of a phosphorothionate, illustrating the phosphooxythiiran intermediate.

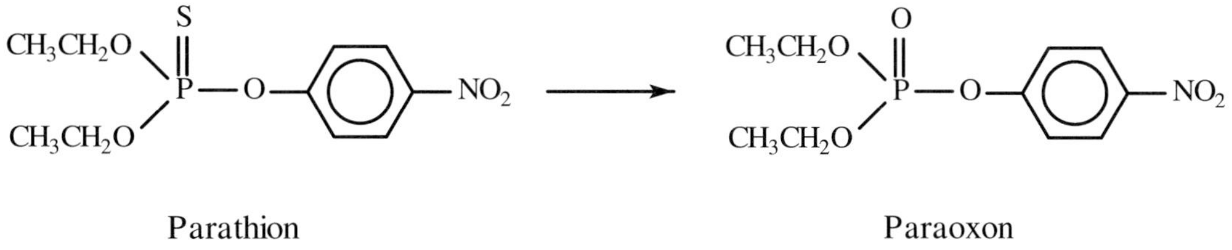

Parathion   Paraoxon

Figure 45.2 Desulfuration (activation) of parathion.

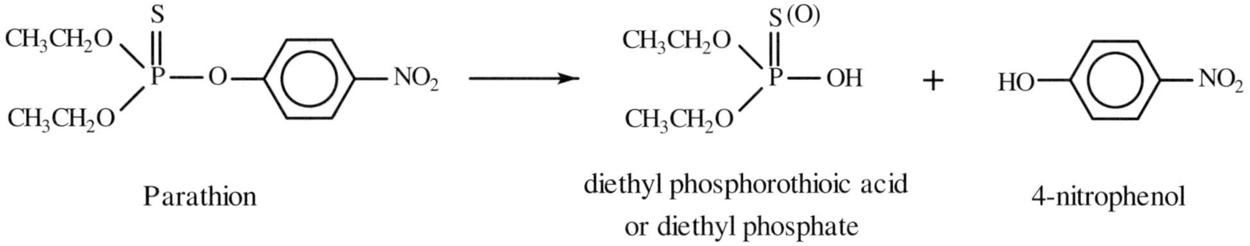

Parathion   diethyl phosphorothioic acid   4-nitrophenol
                             or diethyl phosphate

Figure 45.3 Oxidative dearylation (detoxication) of parathion.

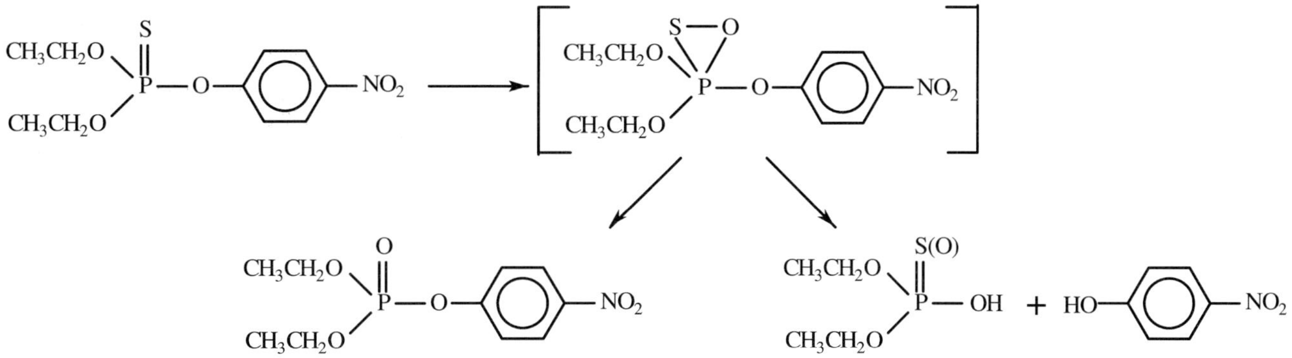

Figure 45.4 Oxidation of parathion through both the desulfuration and the dearylation pathways, arising from a common intermediate.

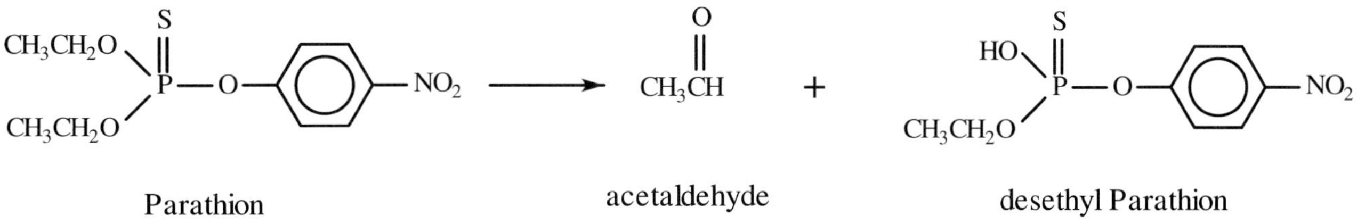

Parathion   acetaldehyde   desethyl Parathion

Figure 45.5 Oxidative deethylation of parathion.

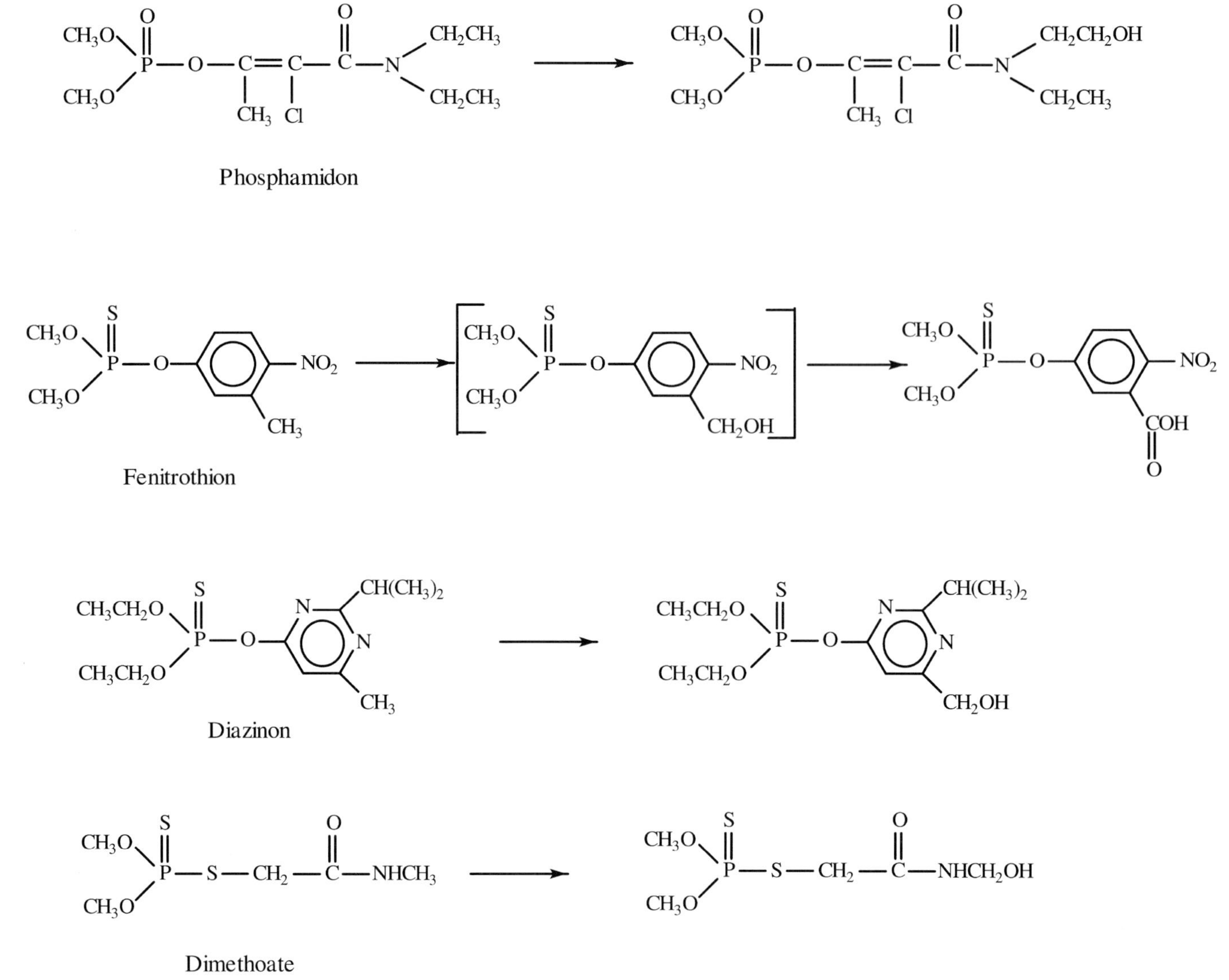

Figure 45.6 Examples of the oxidation of substituents within organophosphorus compounds.

45.2.2 FLAVIN MONOOXYGENASES

An additional class of monooxygenases capable of oxidizing N, P, or S occurring in xenobiotics are the flavin monooxygenases (FMOs), which are also microsomal, most prevalent in the mammalian liver, insert one atom of molecular oxygen into the substrate molecule, and require NADPH (Levi and Hodgson, 1992). They have a flavin group instead of a heme group to catalyze the substrate oxidations. There are fewer isoforms of the FMOs than the P450s, and they have more limited substrate specificity than the P450s. One of the more important reactions catalyzed by the FMOs is the sulfoxidation of phorate to the sulfoxide then to the sulfone (Fig. 45.7). The sulfoxidaton of the oxon of phorate to its sulfoxide, then to its sulfone, is also possible.

45.3 REDUCTIONS

Reductions are possible outcomes of P450-mediated reactions, though these would be considered rare in mammalian systems, which are oxidizing environments with few exceptions (e.g., gut contents). Nevertheless, reductive reaction products have been discovered and might be expected to occur to a limited extent. Reduction reactions are probably of greater significance environmentally because of the greater opportunity to provide reducing environments. Using, once again, parathion as an example, the nitro group on the aromatic ring of the leaving group can be reduced, yielding amino-parathion (Fig. 45.8).

45.4 HYDROLYSIS

Catalytic hydrolysis of the phosphates/oxons with elimination of the leaving group is catalyzed by the A-esterases (phos-

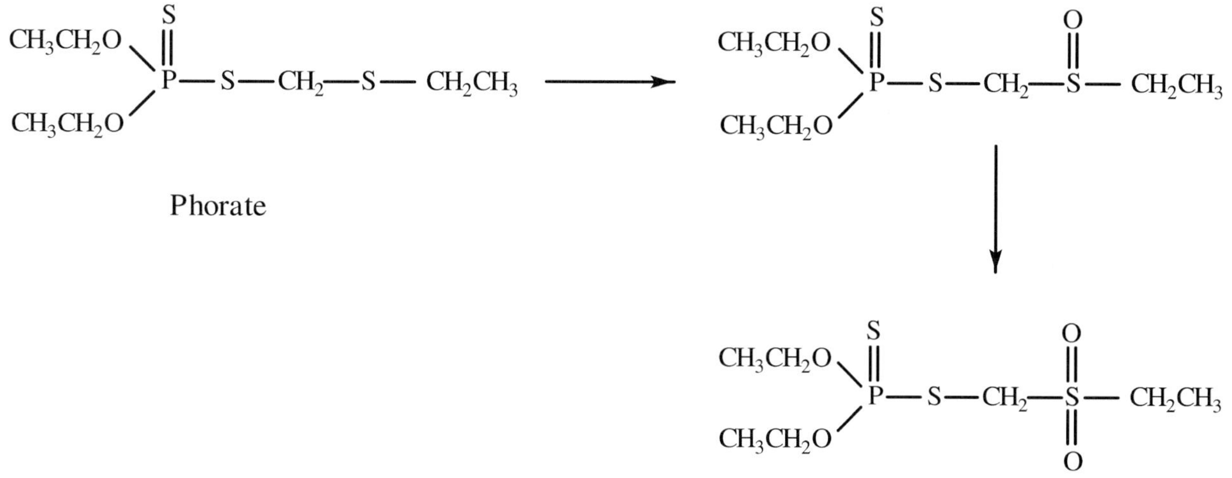

Figure 45.7 Sulfoxidation of phorate to its sulfoxide and sulfone metabolites.

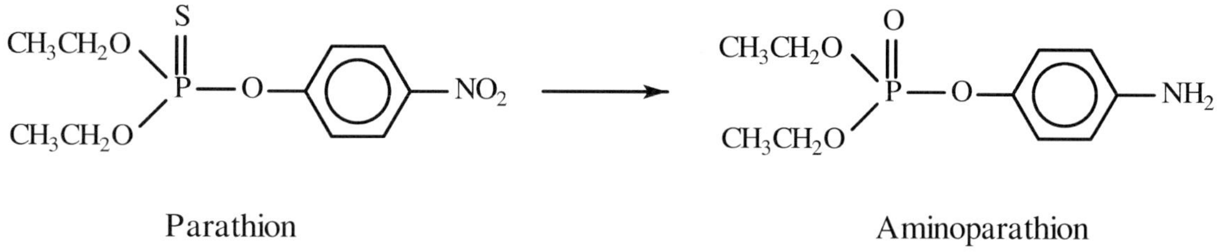

Figure 45.8 Reduction of the nitro group within parathion.

photriesterases), which are hydrolases designated as capable of hydrolyzing organophosphates and not being inhibited by them (Aldridge, 1953). In the mammalian system with the insecticidal compounds or oxons, the A-esterases are calcium dependent. Other A-esterases have greater specificity for diisopropylfluorophosphate and some of the nerve agent phosphates and have different metal cofactor requirements. The A-esterases are largely microsomal and do not appear to have the diversity of isoforms as the oxidative enzymes. Similar to the oxidation enzymes, they occur in the highest activity levels in the liver of the mammal and at lesser activity levels in extrahepatic tissues. Phosphate/oxon hydrolysis is a detoxication reaction. The A-esterases have a relatively high affinity for some phosphates/oxons, such as chlorpyrifos-oxon and diazoxon, the active metabolites of chlorpyrifos and diazinon, respectively, but only a very low affinity for many, perhaps most, of the phosphates/oxons (Chambers *et al.*, 1994; Furlong *et al.*, 1989; Pond *et al.*, 1996, 1998). Therefore, the *in vivo* importance of the A-esterases is probably great for a few insecticides, but is difficult to estimate for many of the insecticides. The A-esterases do not appear to hydrolyze P=S compounds. Even though a relatively poor substitute, for the sake of consistency throughout this chapter, the A-esterase-mediated hydrolysis of paraoxon, the active metabolite of parathion, is illustrated in Fig. 45.9.

Noncatalytic hydrolysis of the phosphates/oxons also occurs when these compounds phosphorylate serine esterases, such as carboxylesterases, butyrylcholinesterase, and even the target acetylcholinesterase; all of these esterases are classified as B-esterases, hydrolases that are inhibited by organophosphates and that cannot catalytically hydrolyze them (Aldridge, 1953). These reactions would not be considered metabolism, because the phosphorylation is persistent, leading to a stoichiometric destruction of one phosphate/oxon molecule per serine esterase molecule with enzyme incapacitation for a long period of time. Nevertheless, the phosphorylation event releases the leaving group of the molecule, which is the same product produced in dearylation and catalytic hydrolysis reactions. Therefore, serine esterase phosphorylation contributes the leaving group to the pool of metabolite formed by catalytic reactions, and this amount is sufficiently high in *in vitro* preparations to be conveniently measured (Tang and Chambers, 1999). A schematic of the phosphorylation of a serine esterase by paraoxon is given in Fig. 45.10.

The carboxylesterases also perform a very important catalytic hydrolysis of the carboxylic acid esters in malathion and contribute greatly to the low mammalian toxicity of malathion. Hydrolyses to the α- and β-monoacids and the diacid occur from the parent malathion (Fig. 45.11). In mammals, these detoxifying hydrolyses occur more readily than the P450-mediated desulfuration, allowing the malathion to be effectively detoxified prior to appreciable bioactivation and resulting in a very low acute toxicity level (rat oral LD$_{50}$ of 1200 mg/kg; Meister, 1990).

Some representative metabolic schemes for a few important organophosphorus insecticides illustrating the major oxidations and hydrolyses are given in Figs. 45.12 and 45.13.

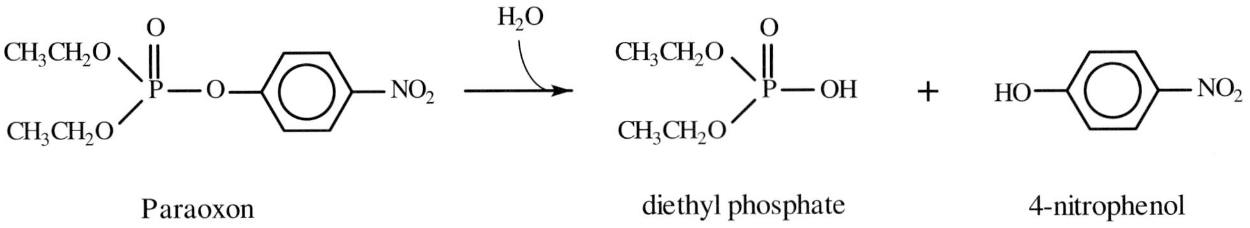

Figure 45.9 Hydrolysis of paraoxon by A-esterases.

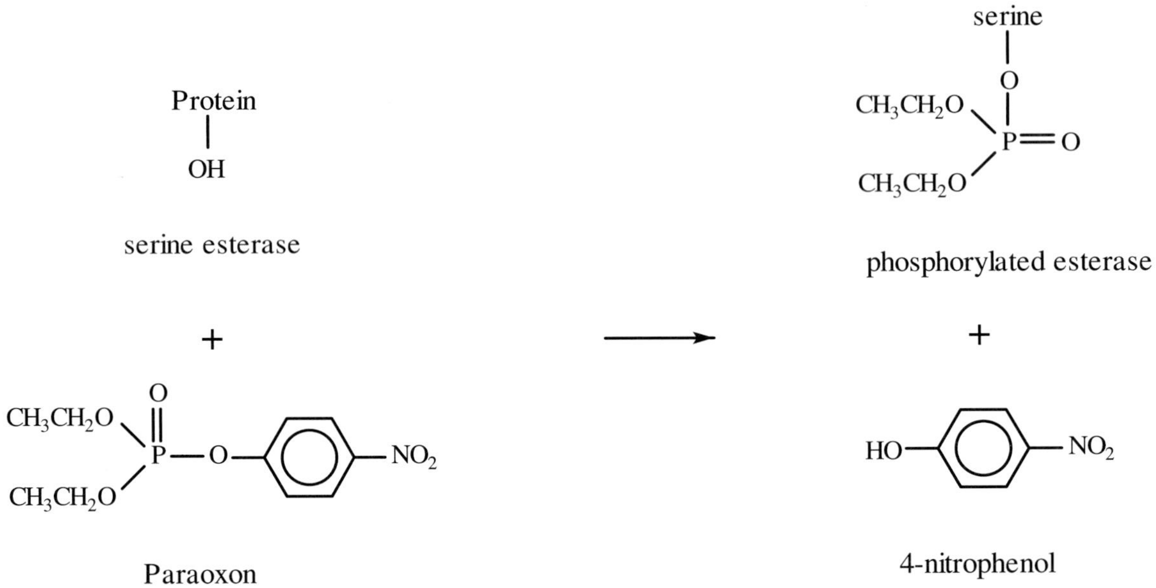

Figure 45.10 Phosphorylation of serine esterases by paraoxon.

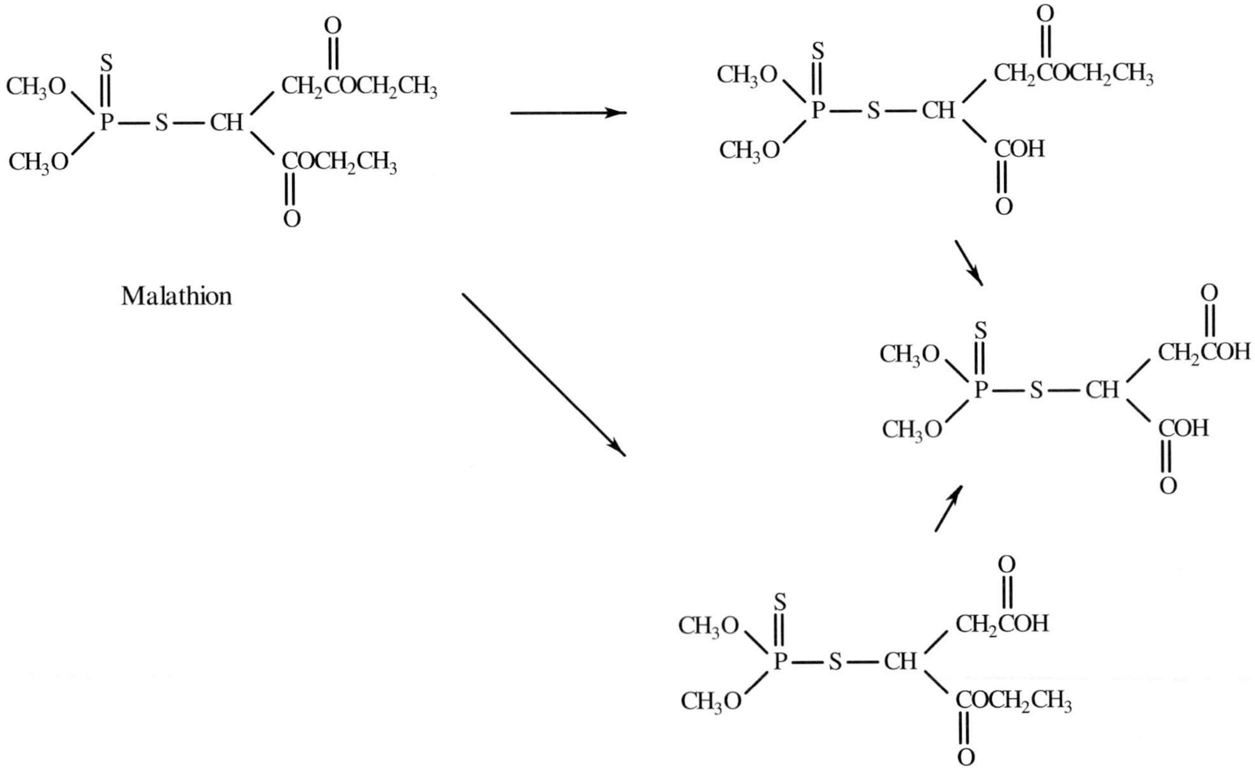

Figure 45.11 Hydrolysis of the carboxylic esters of malathion by carboxylesterases.

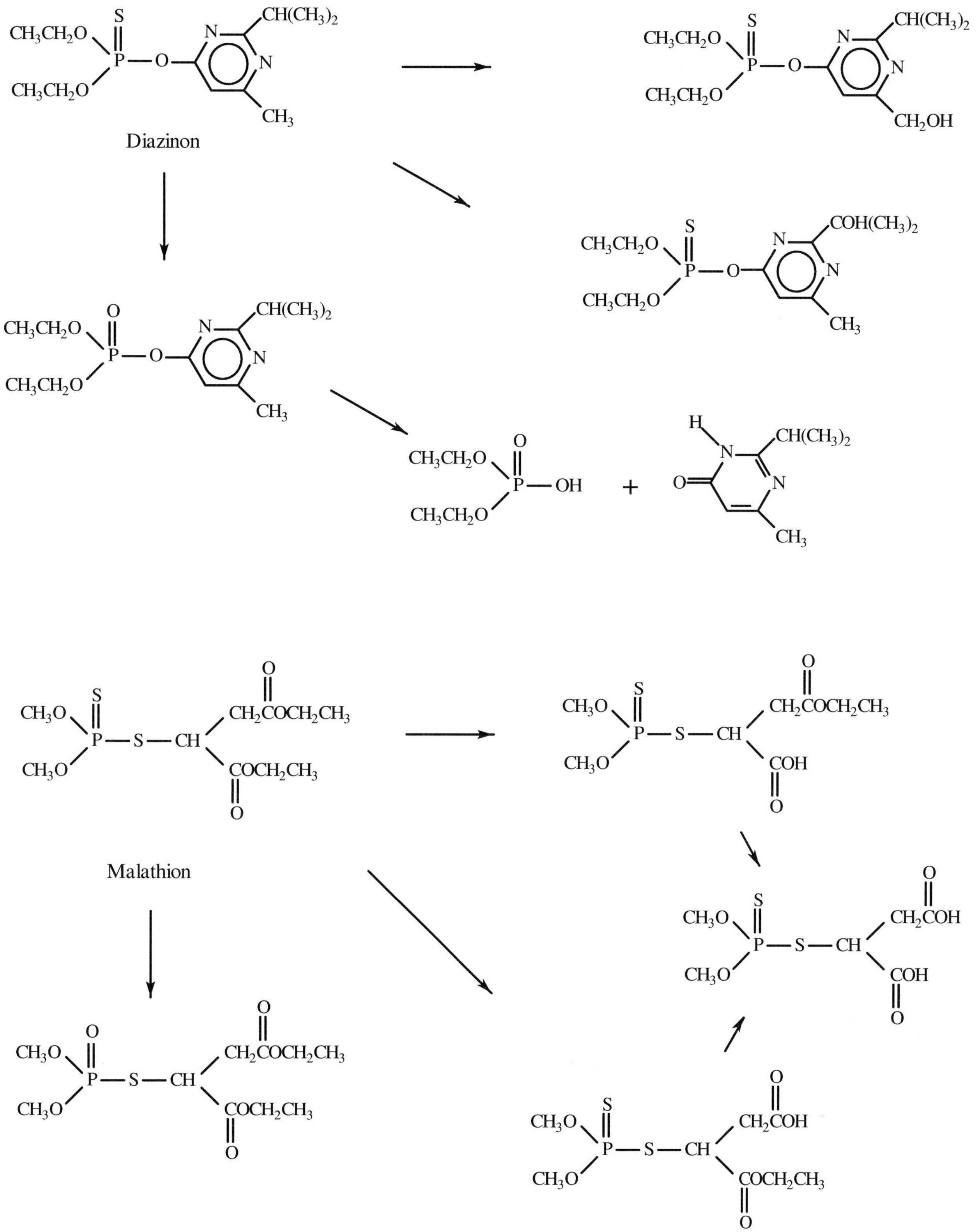

Figure 45.12   Examples of major metabolic pathways of some representative organophosphorus insecticides.

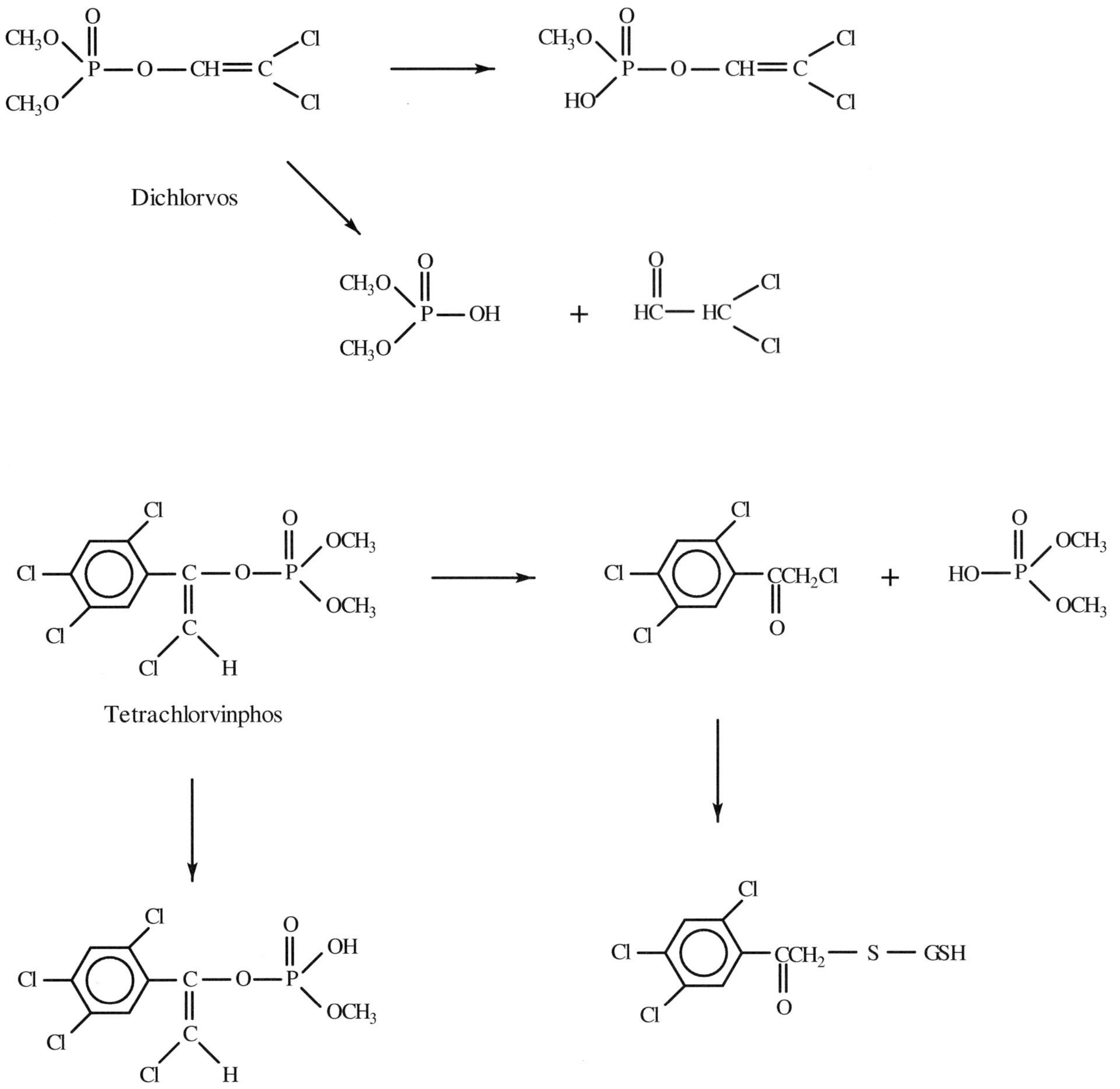

Figure 45.13 Examples of major metabolic pathways of some representative organophosphorus insecticides.

45.5 CONJUGATIONS

The Phase 2 (conjugation) reactions can render the insecticides or metabolites even more water soluble. These conjugations frequently occur with the leaving groups produced by organophosphate hydrolysis, such as some of the phenols and heterocyclic alcohols or amines. These hydrolytic metabolites would already be detoxified products, at least with respect to anticholinesterase activity, so further metabolism would not be necessary for additional detoxication. Therefore, the Phase 2 reactions have far less impact on toxicity than the Phase 1 reactions do. However, these conjugation reactions will render the metabolites more water soluble than the parent compound or the intermediate metabolites and, therefore, allow the metabolites to be readily excreted. Sulfate and glucuronide conjugates are

possible, catalyzed by sulfotransferases and glucuronosyl transferases, respectively; both types of conjugates are hydrophilic.

Glutathione conjugation is also possible. Glutathione transferases can theoretically mediate the dealkylation, primarily with methoxy compounds, of organophosphorus insecticides, such as the demethylation of methyl parathion. However, the *in vivo* significance of this reaction is controversial (Sultatos, 1992).

45.6 SUMMARY

The organophosphorus insecticides are metabolically highly labile, as illustrated by the previous discussion. This metabolic lability, along with their general lack of extreme lipophilicity, prevent their bioaccumulation. A variety of oxidation, reduction, hydrolysis, and conjugation reactions are possible within the group of organophosphorus insecticides. The mechanism of their acute toxicity is the inhibition of acetylcholinesterase. Some of the organophosphorus insecticides are active anticholinesterases, and any metabolism is therefore a detoxication. Many of the insecticides, however, are not active anticholinesterases in their parent form and require bioactivation in order to be effective anticholinesterases. The P450-mediated desulfuration reaction is responsible for the majority of these bioactivations. Most other routes of metabolism would be detoxications. The fact that many of the insecticides or the active metabolites of those insecticides requiring bioactivation are potent anticholinesterases and others are not, as well as the fact that the efficiencies of bioactivations and of detoxications vary substantially among compounds, impart to the organophosphorus insecticides a very wide range of mammalian acute toxicity levels.

REFERENCES

Aizawa, H. (1982). "Metabolic Maps of Pesticides." Academic Press, New York.

Aizawa, H. (1989). "Metabolic Maps of Pesticides," Vol. 2. Academic Press, New York.

Aldridge, W. N. (1953). Serum esterases: Two types of esterase (A and B) hydrolyzing *p*-nitrophenyl acetate, propionate and butyrate, and a method for their determination. *Biochem. J.* **53**, 110–117.

Appleton, H. T., and Nakatsugawa, T. (1972). Paraoxon deethylation in the metabolism of parathion. *Pestic. Biochem. Physiol.* **2**, 286–294.

Chambers, H. W. (1992). Organophosphorus compounds: An overview. *In* "Organophosphates: Chemistry, Fate and Effects" (J. E. Chambers and P. E. Levi, eds.), pp. 3–18. Academic Press, San Diego.

Chambers, H. W., Brown, B., and Chambers, J. E. (1990). Non-catalytic detoxication of six organophosphorus compounds by rat liver homogenates. *Pestic. Biochem. Physiol.* **36**, 308–315.

Chambers, J. E., and Levi, P. E. (eds.) (1992). "Organophosphates: Chemistry, Fate and Effects." Academic Press, San Diego.

Chambers, J. E., Ma, T., Boone, J. S., and Chambers, H. W. (1994). Role of detoxication pathways in acute toxicity levels of phosphorothionate insecticides in the rat. *Life Sci.* **54**, 1357–1364.

Dikshith, T. S. S. (ed.) (1991). "Toxicology of Pesticides in Animals." CRC Press, Boca Raton, FL.

Ecobichon, D. J. (1996). Toxic effects of pesticides. *In* "Casarett and Doull's Toxicology: The Basic Science of Poisons" (C. D. Klaassen, ed.), 5th ed., pp. 643–690. Pergamon, Elmsford, NY.

Forsyth, C. S., and Chambers, J. E. (1989). Activation and degradation of the phosphorothionate insecticides parathion and EPN by rat brain. *Biochem. Pharmacol.* **38**, 1597–1603.

Furlong, D. E., Richter, R. J., Seidel, S., and Motulsky, A. G. (1989). Spectrophotometric assays for the enzymatic hydrolysis of the active metabolites of chlorpyrifos and parathion by plasma paraoxonase/arylesterase. *Anal. Biochem.* **180**, 242–247.

Levi, P. E., and Hodgson, E. (1992). Metabolism of organophosphorus compounds by the flavin-containing monooxygenase. *In* "Organophosphates: Chemistry, Fate and Effects" (J. E. Chambers and P. E. Levi, eds.), pp. 141–154. Academic Press, San Diego.

Levi, P. E., Hollingworth, R. M., and Hodgson, E. (1988). Differences in oxidative dearylation and desulfuration of fenitrothion by cytochrome P450 isozymes and in the subsequent inhibition of monooxygenase activity. *Pestic. Biochem. Physiol.* **32**, 224–231.

Meister, R. T. (ed.) (1990). "Farm Chemicals Handbook 1990." Meister, Willoghby, OH.

Neal, R. A. (1980). Microsomal metabolism of thiono-sulfur compounds: Mechanisms and toxicological significance. *In* "Reviews in Biochemical Toxicology" (E. Hodgson, J. R. Bend, and R. M. Philpot, eds.), Vol. 2, pp. 131–172. Elsevier/North Holland, New York.

Parkinson, A. (1996). Biotransformation of xenobiotics. *In* "Casarett and Doull's Toxicology: The Basic Science of Poisons" (C. D. Klaassen, ed.), 5th ed., pp. 113–186. Pergamon, Elmsford, NY.

Pond, A. L., Chambers, H. W., Coyne, C. P., and Chambers, J. E. (1998). Purification of two rat hepatic proteins with A-esterase activity toward chlorpyrifos-oxon and paraoxon. *J. Pharmacol. Exp. Ther.* **286**, 1404–1411.

Pond, A. L., Coyne, C. P., Chambers, H. W., and Chambers, J. E. (1996). Identification and isolation of two rat serum proteins with A-esterase activity toward paraoxon and chlorpyrifos-oxon. *Biochem. Pharmacol.* **52**, 363–369.

Sultatos, L. G. (1992). Role of glutathione in the mammalian detoxication of organophosphorus insecticides. *In* "Organophosphates: Chemistry, Fate and Effects" (J. E. Chambers and P. E. Levi, eds.), pp. 155–168. Academic Press, San Diego.

Tang, J., and Chambers, J. E. (1999). Detoxication of paraoxon by rat liver homogenate and serum carboxylesterases and A-esterases. *J. Biochem. Mol. Toxicol.* **13**, 261–268.

Organophosphate Pharmacokinetics

Charles Timchalk

Pacific Northwest National Laboratory

46.1 BACKGROUND

In this chapter, an overview will be presented of the pharmacokinetic principles that are of major importance in understanding the toxicology of organophosphate (OP) insecticides in animals and humans. The approach will not entail a comprehensive review of the extensive literature, but rather a focused presentation highlighting important principles by utilizing specific examples for this class of insecticide.

Organophosphates constitute a large family of insecticides that are structurally related, pentavalent phosphorus acid esters. Their insecticidal as well as toxicological mode of action is primarily associated with their ability to target and inhibit the enzyme acetylcholinesterase (AChE) (Sultatos, 1994). In this regard, the acute toxic effects of OP insecticides are associated with the capacity of the parent chemical or an active metabolite to inhibit AChE enzyme activity within nerve tissue (Murphy, 1986; Sultatos, 1994). The three major classes of OP insecticides are the phosphorothionates, the phosphorodithioates, and the phosphoroamidothiolates (Chambers, 1992; Mileson et al., 1988). As an example, phosphorothionate insecticides such as chlorpyrifos, parathion, and diazinon are weak inhibitors of AChE, but once they undergo metabolic activation (desulfuration) to their corresponding oxygen analogs (oxon), they become extremely potent inhibitors. This enhanced toxicity is due to the oxon having a high affinity and potency for phosphorylating the serine hydroxyl group within the active site of AChE (Mileson et al., 1988; Sultatos, 1994). The toxic potency is dependent on the balance between a delivered dose to the target site and the rates of bioactivation and/or detoxification as illustrated in Fig. 46.1 (Calabrese, 1991). The pharmacokinetics and biochemical interactions between OPs and AChE and the toxicological implications of AChE inhibition are well understood. To further illustrate this point, a diagram relating OP toxicity with pharmacokinetic disposition and the formation of key OP metabolites is presented in Figs. 46.2 and 46.3. The thionophosphate pesticide diazinon [O,O-diethyl-O-(2-isopropyl-4-methyl-6-pyrimidinyl) phosphorothioate] is being utilized for illustration purposes; however, based on a common mode of action, this scheme is readily extended to other OPs.

Organophosphate insecticides, like all chemical contaminants, can gain entry into the body and, based on the detection of low levels of OP metabolites in urine within human populations, there is good evidence for widespread although low level, exposures (Aprea et al., 1999; Hill et al., 1995). These exposures can come from numerous sources. For example, ingestion of pesticide residues on foods may account for some of the low-level body burdens detected, whereas accidental or intentional ingestion of OP insecticides is associated with acute poisoning, resulting in significantly higher blood, tissue, and urine concentrations of relevant OP metabolites (Drevenkar et al., 1993). Dermal exposure represents a potential exposure route during the mixing, loading, and application of OP insecticides or from skin contact with contaminated surfaces (Knaak et al., 1993). Likewise, inhalation of airborne insecticide is feasible either during an application or as the result of exposure associated with chemical drift (Vale and Scott, 1974). Once the OP arrives at a portal of entry, it is available for absorption and, based on the bioavailability of a given OP and the exposure route, a systemic dose of the parent compound (Fig. 46.3, #1) will enter the systemic circulation. Although localized portal of entry metabolism (i.e., lung, intestines, skin) is feasible, the bulk of the metabolic activation as well as detoxification reactions occur within the liver (Sultatos, 1988; Sultatos et al., 1984). As previously mentioned, phosphorothionates like diazinon do not directly inhibit AChE, but must first be metabolized to the corresponding oxygen analog (oxon; Fig. 46.2, #2) (Iverson et al., 1975; Mücke et al., 1970; Murphy, 1986; Sultatos, 1994). Activation to the oxon metabolite (#2) is mediated by cytochrome P450 mixed-function oxidases (CYP450) primarily within the liver, although extrahepatic metabolism has been reported in other tissues, including the brain (Chambers and Chambers, 1989; Guengerich, 1977). In addition, oxidative dearylation of the parent compound, forming both 2-isopropyl-4-methyl-6-hydroxypyrimidine (IMHP, #3) and diethylthiophosphate (DETP, #4), represents a competing detoxification pathway that is likewise mediated by hepatic CYP450 (Ma and Chambers, 1994). These initial activation/detoxification reactions are believed to share a common phosphooxythiran intermediate and represent the critical biotransformation steps required for toxicity (Neal, 1980). Differences in the ratio

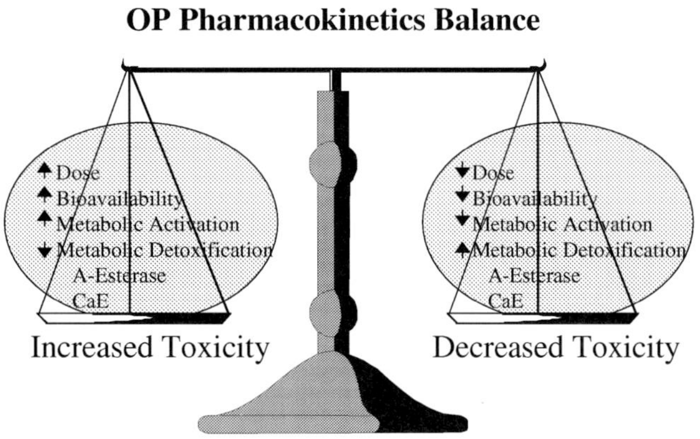

OP Pharmacokinetics Balance

Figure 46.1 Parameters impacting the organophosphate (OP) insecticide toxicity balance.

of activation to detoxification are associated with chemical-, species-, gender-, and age-dependent sensitivity to OPs (see Fig. 46.1) (Ma and Chambers, 1994). Hepatic and extrahepatic (i.e., blood and tissue) A-esterase can effectively metabolize the oxon metabolite (#2), forming IMHP (#3) and diethylphosphate (DEP, #4) metabolites. Likewise, B-esterases such as carboxylesterase (CaE) and butyrylcholinesterase (BChE) that are also well distributed across tissues can metabolize the oxon; however, these B-esterases become irreversibly bound (1:1 ratio) to the oxon and thereby become inactivated (Chanda et al., 1997; Clement, 1984). It is likewise clear from both tissue distribution and partitioning studies that phosphothionate OPs are generally well distributed in tissue throughout the body (Tomokuni et al., 1985; Wu et al., 1996). Finally, due to the extensive metabolism, little, if any, parent phosphothionate or oxon is available for excretion; however, more stable metabolites such as DEP, DETP, and IMHP are readily excreted in the urine (Iverson et al., 1975; Mücke et al., 1970).

Numerous pharmacokinetic approaches have been applied to OP insecticides, including:

1. Application of pharmacokinetics to understand the overall disposition and clearance of OPs
2. Development and application of pharmacokinetic models for quantitative biological monitoring to assess OP insecticide exposure in humans
3. Studies that facilitate extrapolation of dosimetry and biological response from animals to humans and the assessment of human health risk

To illustrate the utility of pharmacokinetics in addressing the health concerns associated with OP insecticides, several examples of these types of pharmacokinetic studies with OP insecticides will be used to illustrate both their utility and their limitations.

46.2 PHARMACOKINETIC PRINCIPLES OF IMPORTANCE TO ORGANOPHOSPHATE INSECTICIDES

Pharmacokinetics are concerned with the quantitative integration of those processes associated with the absorption, distribution, metabolism, and excretion (ADME) of drugs and xenobiotics within the body (Renwick, 1994). Studies on the pharmacokinetics of a xenobiotic provide critically useful insights into the toxicological response associated with a given agent. In this regard, pharmacokinetics provides quantitative data on the amount of toxicant delivered to a target site as well as species-, age-, and gender-specific and dose-dependent differences in biological response. An important application of pharmacokinetics within toxicology has been to provide a realistic estimate of risk by providing a means to quantitatively estimate the absorbed dose of a chemical under realistic exposure conditions (Clewell, 1995).

Toxicology studies are designed to provide a quantitative assessment of toxicity based on what the chemical agent does to the test animals. In contrast, pharmacokinetics focuses on what the animal does to the chemical. Clearly, toxicity and pharmacokinetics are integrally related because the extent of absorption, retention, metabolic activation, or detoxification is ultimately responsible for delivering a dose to a target tissue, resulting in observed effects. Pharmacokinetics represent a critically important tool that, if used correctly, can quantitatively establish a unifying model that describes both dosimetry and biological response across exposure routes, species, and chemical agents. This approach is particularly useful for OP insecticides because they share a common mode of action through their capability to inhibit AChE activity (Mileson et al., 1988). Pharmacokinetic strategies for quantitating dosimetry can be developed to measure the parent compound and its active (i.e., oxon) or inactive metabolites. It is also feasible to link dosimetry with biologically based pharmacodynamic (PD) response models based on a common mode of action (i.e., AChE inhibition). In general, pharmacokinetic modeling approaches can be characterized as empirical or physiologically based and both types of models have been applied to understand the toxicological response to OP chemicals in multiple species (Brimer et al., 1994; Gearhart et al., 1990; Pena-Egido et al., 1988; Sultatos, 1990; Tomokuni et al., 1985; Wu et al., 1996).

46.2.1 COMPARTMENTAL PHARMACOKINETIC MODELS

Compartmental models have formed the cornerstone of pharmacokinetic analysis and as such have been extensively utilized to assess bioavailability, tissue burden, and elimination kinetics in various species, including humans. All pharmacokinetics are concerned with the time course by which a chemical is absorbed into the systemic circulation, distributed throughout the body, altered through metabolic transformation, and eliminated. Compartmental models are empirical and as such

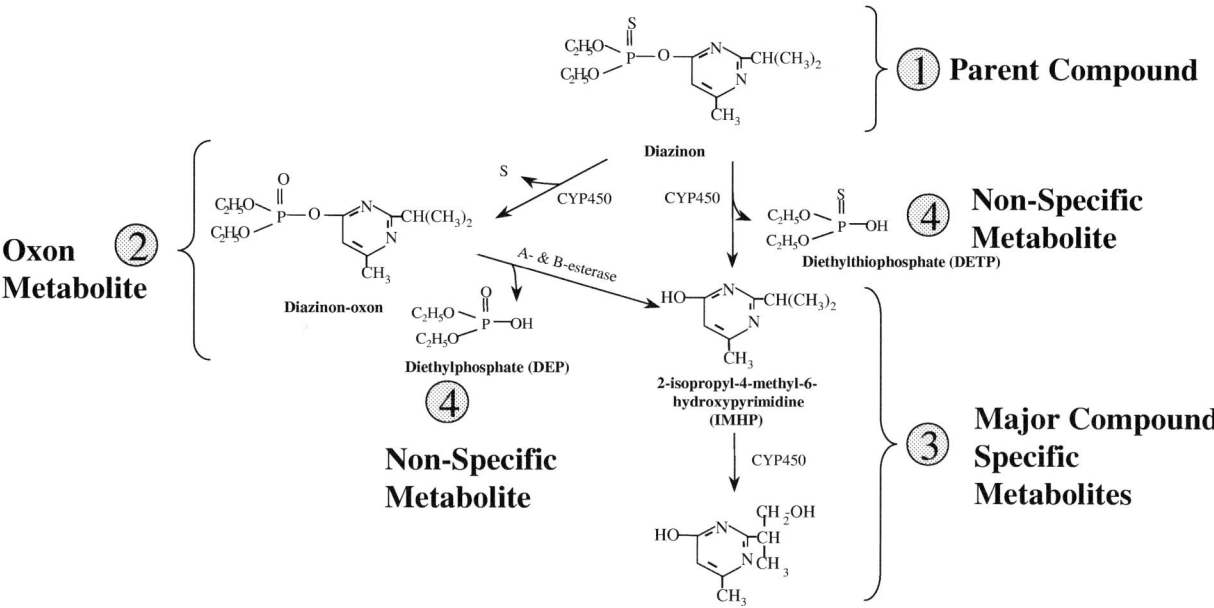

Figure 46.2 Metabolic scheme for the metabolism of the organophosphate (OP) insecticide diazinon.

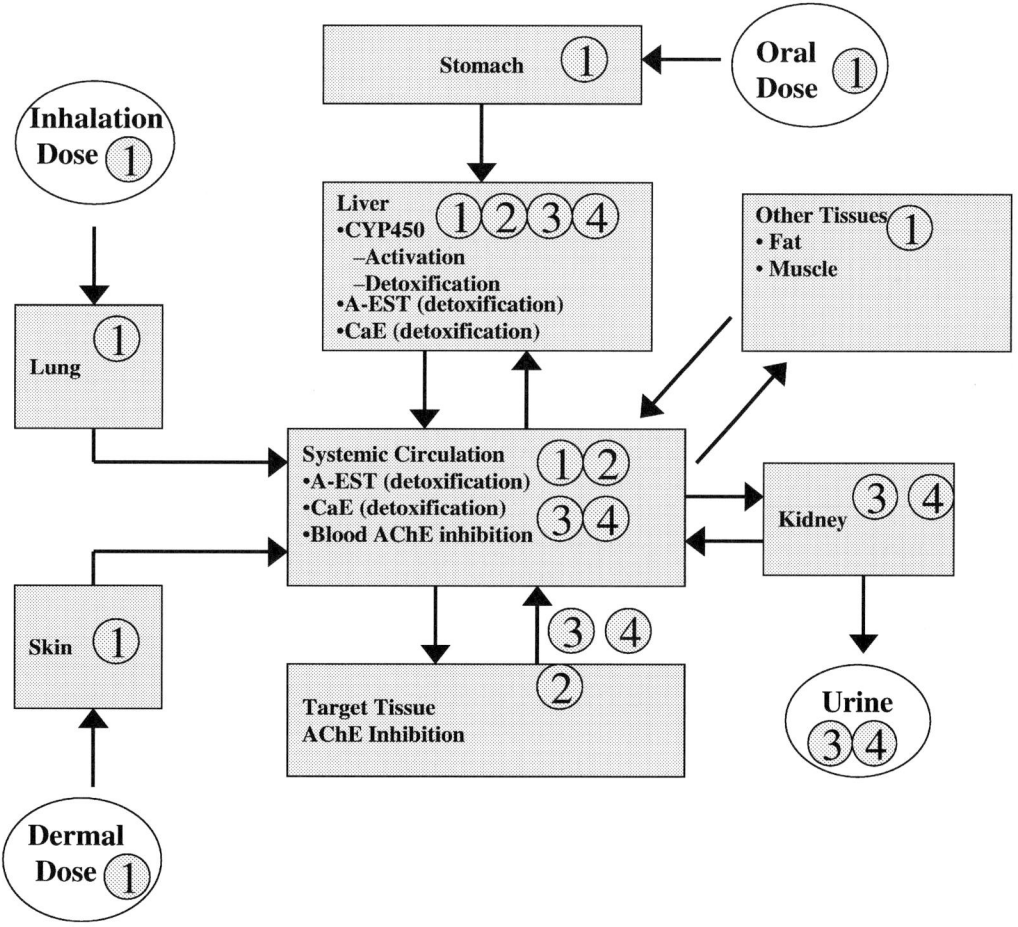

Figure 46.3 Compartmental flow diagram illustrating the critical tissue compartments associated with absorption, distribution, metabolism and excretion of organophosphate (OP) insecticides. The circled numbers (1–4) correspond to the parent compound and major metabolic products associated with metabolism of diazinon (see Fig. 46.2) that are most likely found within each compartment.

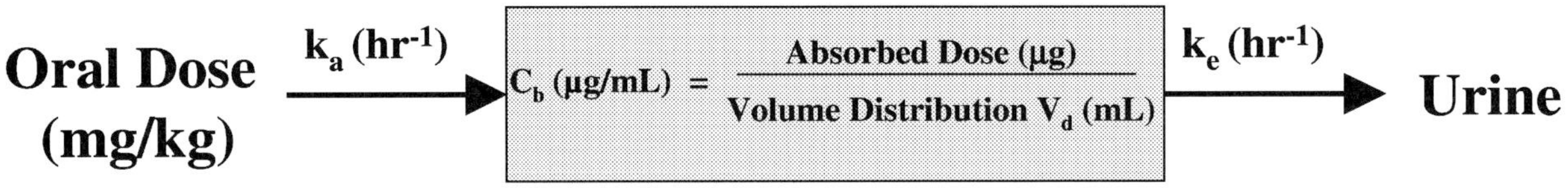

Oral Dose (mg/kg) $\xrightarrow{\mathbf{k_a}\ (\mathbf{hr^{-1}})}$ $\boxed{\mathbf{C_b}\ (\mu g/mL) = \dfrac{\text{Absorbed Dose }(\mu g)}{\text{Volume Distribution }V_d\ (mL)}}$ $\xrightarrow{\mathbf{k_e}\ (\mathbf{hr^{-1}})}$ **Urine**

$$C_{b\ (\mu g/mL)} = \frac{K_a \times \text{dose} \times F}{V_d \times (k_a - k_e)} \times \exp(k_e \times \text{time} - k_a \times \text{time}) \quad (1)$$

$$\text{Urinary Excretion Rate}_{(\mu g/hr)} = C_b \times k_e \times V_d \times \text{Body wt.} \quad (2)$$

Figure 46.4 Single compartment model used to describe the blood and urine time-course of 3,5,6-trichloropyridinol (TCP) a major metabolite of the organophosphate (OP) insecticide chlorpyrifos (CPF). Equations adapted from Nolan *et al.* (1984).

consider the organism as a single- or multicompartment homogeneous system. The number and behavior of the compartments are primarily determined by the equations chosen to describe the time-course data and not the physiological characteristics of the organism (Krishnan and Andersen, 1994). In these models, the net transfer between compartments is directly proportional to the difference in chemical concentration between compartments. However, the rate constants associated with the transfer between compartments cannot be experimentally determined (Srinivasan *et al.*, 1994).

Compartmental models range from simple well-mixed single-compartment models to more complicated multicompartment models that are used to describe the blood and/or plasma time course of a chemical or drug. These simple compartmental approaches have been broadly utilized to model the pharmacokinetics of OP insecticides and their major metabolites (Braeckman *et al.*, 1983; Drevenkar *et al.*, 1993; Nolan *et al.*, 1984; Wu *et al.*, 1996). For example, Nolan *et al.* (1984) developed a one-compartment pharmacokinetic model that accurately describes the blood and urine time course of 3,5,6-trichloropyridinol (TCP), a major metabolite of the OP insecticide chlorpyrifos, in human volunteers. A diagram of this single-compartment model is illustrated in Fig. 46.4. In this model, the blood TCP concentration and urinary excretion data were simultaneously fit to a single-compartment model using the equations shown in the figure. Absorption (k_a) and elimination (k_e) are handled as first-order processes, the blood TCP concentration is represented by C_b, and F and V_d represent the fractional absorption and the volume of distribution, respectively. To develop this model, male volunteers were orally administered a dose of 0.5 mg chlorpyrifos/kg of body weight. Then blood and urine specimens were collected at specified in-

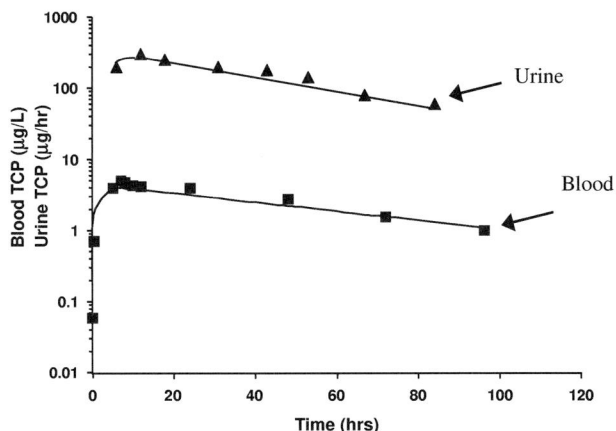

Figure 46.5 Time-course of 3,5,6-trichloropyridinol (TCP) in the blood and urine of male volunteers orally administered a 0.5 mg chlorpyrifos (CPF)/kg of body weight dose. Figure adapted from Nolan *et al.* (1984).

tervals and analyzed for TCP. The model parameters used to describe the time course of TCP and the model fit of the experimental data are presented in Table 46.1 and Fig. 46.5. The model provides an excellent fit of the experimental data and, based on the model parameters, it was determined that approximately 72% of the ingested dose was absorbed and eliminated in the urine with a half-life of 27 h. Based on this model, Nolan *et al.* (1984) suggested that the blood TCP concentration and/or urinary excretion rate could be utilized to quantify the amount of chlorpyrifos absorbed under actual use conditions.

Although compartment modeling is extremely useful for interpolation within the confines of the test species and experimental conditions (i.e., exposure routes and dose levels), these

Table 46.1
Selected Model Parameters Describing Blood Concentrations and Urinary Excretion of 3,5,6-Trichloropyridinol by Individual Volunteers Following Oral Administration of the Organophosphate Insecticide Chlorpyrifos

Parameter	Body weight (kg)	Absorption lag time (h)	Absorption rate constant k_a (h^{-1})	Absorption half-life (h)	Volume distribution V_d (ml/kg)	Elimination rate constant (h^{-1})	Elimination half-life k_e (h)	Model predicted percentage dose absorbed	Percentage dose recovered in urine
Range	72–102	0.9–1.9	0.1–2.7	0.4–6.9	160–204	0.02–0.03	21–32	52–84	49–81
Mean ± SD	83.3 ± 10.3	1.3 ± 0.4	1.5 ± 1.2	0.5	181 ± 18	0.026 ± 0.005	26.9	72 ± 11	70 ± 11

Data obtained from six male volunteers.
Data adapted from Nolan *et al.* (1984).

models are limited in their capability to extrapolate across dose levels, species, and exposure routes (Krishnan and Andersen, 1994). To enable extrapolation, physiologically based pharmacokinetic (PBPK) models have emerged as an important tool that has seen broad applications in toxicology and more specifically in human health risk assessment (Andersen, 1995; Clewell and Andersen, 1996; Krishnan and Andersen, 1994; Leung and Paustenbach, 1995; Mason and Wilson, 1999).

46.2.2 PHYSIOLOGICALLY BASED PHARMACOKINETIC MODELS

Unlike compartment modeling approaches, PBPK models utilize biologically meaningful compartments that represent individual organs such as liver and kidney or groups of organ systems (i.e., well perfused/poorly perfused) (Mason and Wilson, 1999). The general model structure is based on an understanding of comparative physiology and xenobiotic metabolism, a chemical's physical properties that define tissue partitioning, the rates of biochemical reactions determined from both *in vivo* and *in vitro* experimentation, and the physiological characteristics of the species of interest (Krishnan and Andersen, 1994). PBPK models have been developed to describe target tissue dosimetry for a broad range of environmental contaminants such as solvents, heavy metals, and pesticides, including OP insecticides (Andersen *et al.*, 1987a; Corley *et al.*, 1990; Gearhart *et al.*, 1990; O'Flaherty, 1995; Sultatos, 1990). A number of reviews have been published on the development, validation, application, and limitations of PBPK models in human health risk assessment (Andersen, 1995; Clewell, 1995; Clewell and Andersen, 1996; Frederick, 1995; Krishnan and Andersen, 1994; Leung and Paustenbach, 1995; Mason and Wilson, 1999; Slob *et al.*, 1997).

To illustrate the application of this modeling approach to OP insecticides, a PBPK model that also incorporates a pharmacodynamic (PD) component to describe AChE inhibition following diisopropylfluorophosphate exposure in rodents will be described (Gearhart *et al.*, 1990). Gearhart *et al.* (1990) developed a basic PBPK/PD model structure that described target tissue dosimetry and AChE inhibition following an acute exposure to diisopropylfluorophosphate in mice and rats. In developing this model, the authors were primarily interested in

building a structure that could readily be extended to describe the acute effects for a broad range of commercially important OP insecticides. A diagram of the PBPK/PD model for diisopropylfluorophosphate in rats is illustrated in Figs. 46.6 and 46.7. The conceptual representation of the PBPK model for diisopropylfluorophosphate is based on the anatomical and physiological characteristics of the rat and the major determinants of diisopropylfluorophosphate disposition, which include esterase binding and hydrolysis, tissue partitioning, and diisopropylfluorophosphate volatility (Gearhart *et al.*, 1990; Krishnan and Andersen, 1994). Because this OP ester does not require metabolic activation, like thionophosphate OPs, the hydrolysis of diisopropylfluorophosphate by blood and tissue A-esterase is a major factor in determining the protection against AChE inhibition.

Diisopropylfluorophosphate binds to and inhibits B-esterases, including AChE, BChE, and CaE. Although binding to AChE is associated with acute neurotoxicity, the binding to BChE and CaE is without adverse physiological effect and as such represents a detoxification pathway (Clement, 1984; Fonnum *et al.*, 1985; Pond *et al.*, 1995). The PBPK/PD model compartments included those tissues associated with toxicological response (i.e., brain, lung, and diaphragm), those containing high A-esterase activity (i.e., liver, kidney, and blood), a fat compartment having the highest tissue/blood partitioning, and the remaining tissues being collectively lumped (Gearhart *et al.*, 1990). To develop this model, tissue partitioning coefficients (PCs) were determined by the vial equilibration technique (Gargas *et al.*, 1989; Sato and Nakajima, 1979). In general, the tissue : blood PCs ranged from 0.77 to 1.63; however, the fat : blood partitioning was the highest with a coefficient of 17.6. The generalized mass balance differential equation for calculating diisopropylfluorophosphate tissue concentration and AChE tissue inhibition are also presented in Figs. 46.6 and 46.7. Within each tissue compartment, the net concentration of diisopropylfluorophosphate (mg/l) is a function of blood flow to the tissue, chemical partitioning from the blood into the tissue, and the loss of diisopropylfluorophosphate due to hydrolysis by A-esterase and inhibition of B-esterases (AChE, BChE, and CaE).

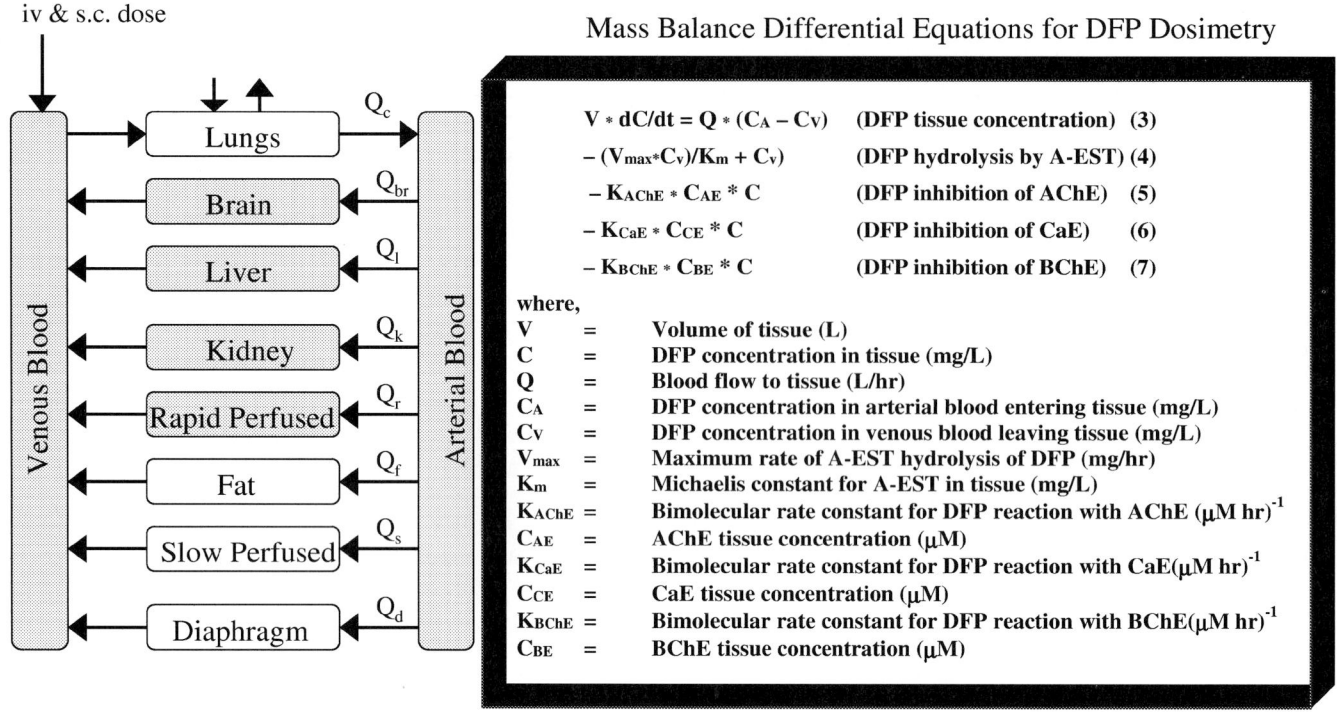

Figure 46.6 Physiologically based pharmacokinetic (PBPK) model structure and mass balance differential equations describing the distribution of diisopropylfluorophosphate (DFP) in the rat. Figure adapted from Gearhart *et al.* (1990).

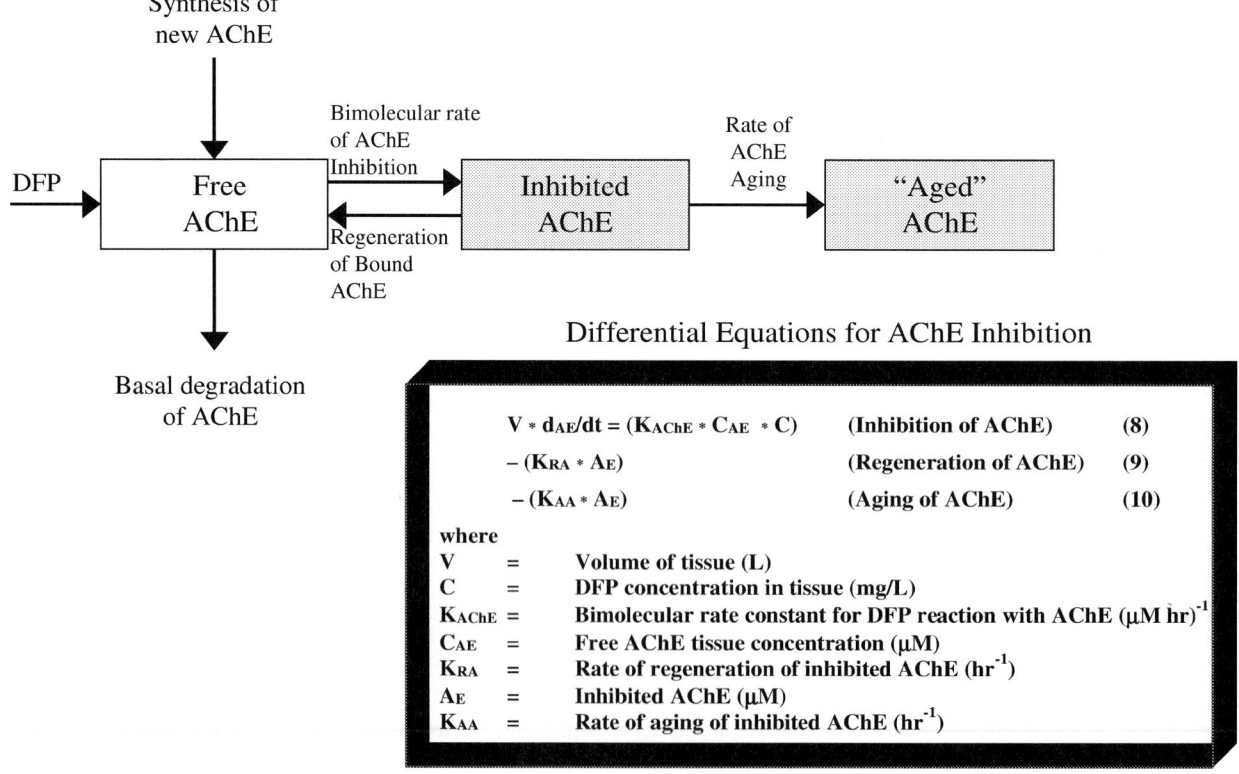

Figure 46.7 Pharmacodynamic (PD) model structure and mass balance differential equations describing the inhibition of acetylcholinesterase (AChE) by diisopropylfluorophosphate (DFP) in the rat. Figure adapted from Gearhart *et al.* (1990).

Gearhart *et al.* (1990) calculated basal AChE activity (μmol) based on a zero-order enzyme synthesis rate (μmol/h) and a first-order rate of enzyme degradation (h^{-1}). A balance between the bimolecular rate of inhibition and the rate of AChE regeneration and aging determined the amount of free AChE. Similar equations were utilized to quantify the impact of diisopropylfluorophosphate on tissue CaE and BChE activity. The capability of the diisopropylfluorophosphate model to simulate both diisopropylfluorophosphate tissue dosimetry and AChE inhibition is illustrated in Figs. 46.8 and 46.9 in mice that were administered a single intravenous (iv) dose of 1 mg diisopropylfluorophosphate/kg of body weight. The model does a reasonably good job of describing brain tissue dosimetry and AChE inhibition. In brain, the diisopropylfluorophosphate concentration rapidly falls to a fraction of its peak concentration within about 1 min, whereas AChE was rapidly inhibited to 20% of control activity. In both cases, the model simulations were consistent with the experimentally derived data.

The development and application of PBPK modeling for human health risk assessment are not without their challenges and limitations. Before a model can be used to assess risk, a determination must be made concerning the model's capability to accurately predict dosimetry and biological response (Frederick, 1995). Furthermore, PBPK/PD models are data intensive, so to adequately develop and validate a model generally requires extensive experimentation to support model parameterization and validation (Clewell, 1995). Nonetheless, a consensus opinion of an expert scientist panel concluded that biologically based risk assessments that include well-validated PBPK/PD models can provide the most accurate quantitative assessment of human health risk from exposure to environmental chemicals (Frederick, 1995).

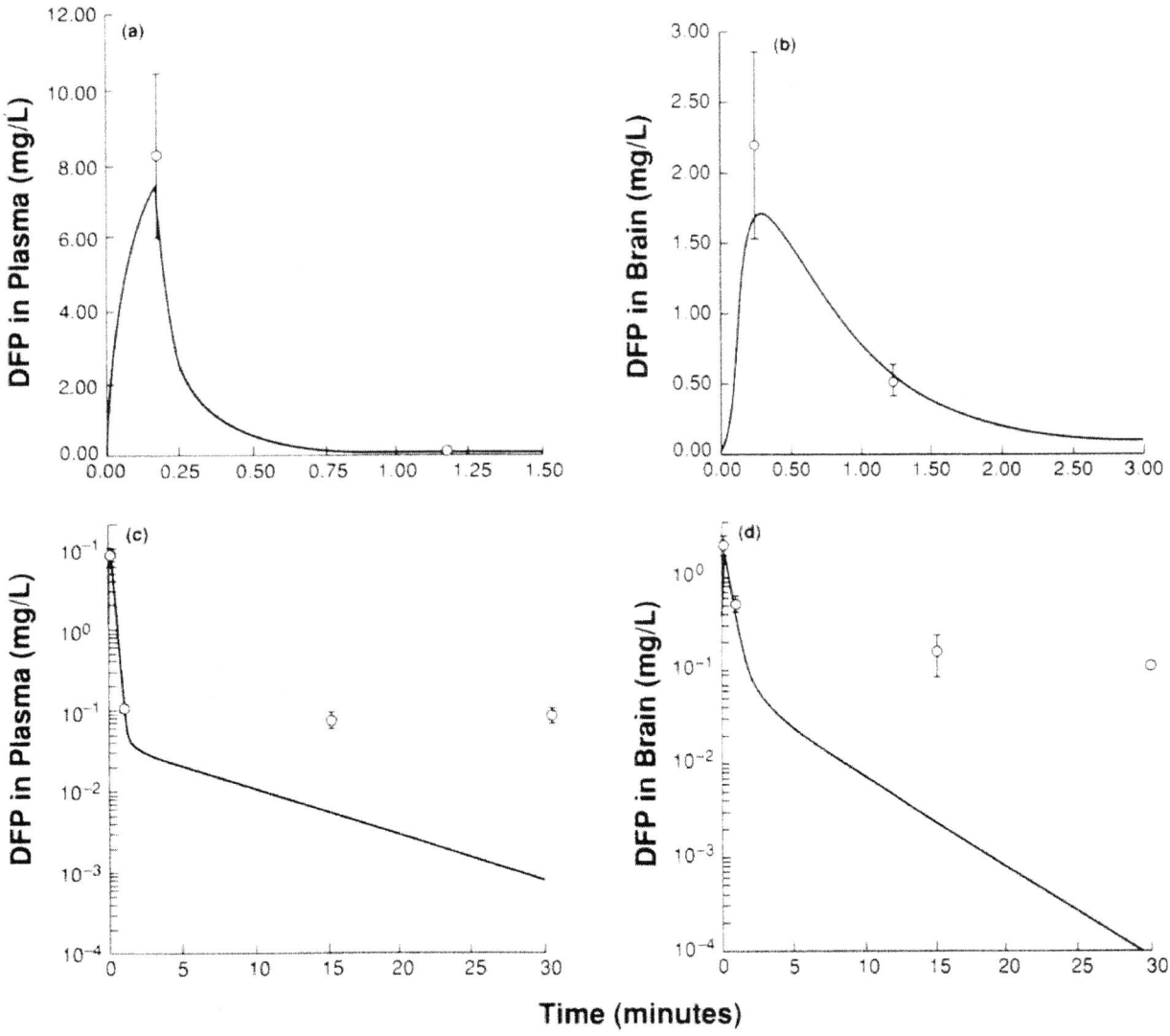

Figure 46.8   Time-course of free diisopropylfluorophosphate (DFP) concentration (mg/L) in plasma and brain in male mice after tail vein injection of 1 mg DFP/kg. Each datum represents the mean ± SD of 5 animals. Solid line depicts PBPK/PD model simulation. Figure used with permission from Gearhart *et al.* (1990).

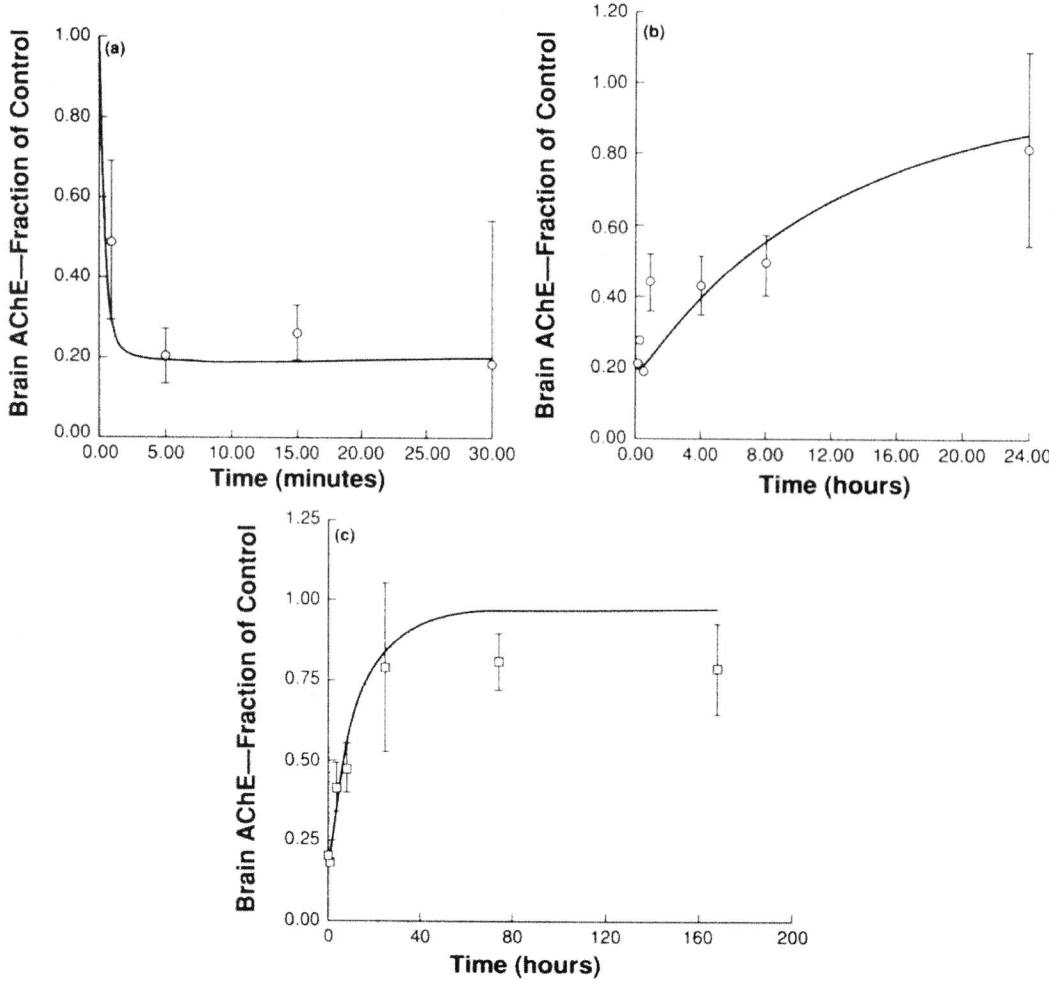

Figure 46.9 (a–c) Time-course of brain acetylcholinesterase (AChE) activity in male mice after tail vein injection of 1 mg diisopropylfluorophosphate/kg. Each datum represents the mean ± SD of 5 animals. Solid line depicts PBPK/PD model simulation. Figure used with permission from Gearhart *et al.* (1990).

46.3 PHARMACOKINETIC APPROACHES APPLIED TO ORGANOPHOSPHATE INSECTICIDES

46.3.1 APPLICATION OF PHARMACOKINETICS TO UNDERSTAND THE OVERALL DISPOSITION AND CLEARANCE OF ORGANOPHOSPHATE INSECTICIDES

Pharmacokinetic studies conducted in multiple species, at various dose levels, and across different routes of exposure can provide important insight into the *in vivo* behavior of a chemical agent and how it contributes to the observed toxicological response in a given species. To illustrate this point, a comparison is made of selected pharmacokinetic parameters obtained from a diverse group of studies conducted in animals exposed to either parathion or diazinon. As noted in Tables 46.2 and 46.3, no single study provides all the pertinent information; yet,

collectively, they provide a consistent qualitative picture of the overall pharmacokinetics of these OP insecticides.

The bioavailability of OP insecticides, defined as the amount of systemically available dose, is a function of the extent of absorption and first-pass metabolism. Braeckman *et al.* (1983) conducted a pharmacokinetic study in the dog following both oral and iv administration of parathion. Comparisons of plasma parathion areas under the curve (AUCs) indicated that 1–29% of the orally administered parathion was bioavailable. The authors suggest that the low systemic oral bioavailability of parathion is primarily associated with a rapid hepatic first-pass metabolism based on the high hepatic extraction (82–97%) that was determined after iv administration. Wu *et al.* (1996) conducted similar bioavailability studies in the rat with diazinon. The blood time course of diazinon in the rat following iv and oral doses of 10 and 80 mg/kg, respectively, is presented in Fig. 46.10. The results suggest that, following oral administration, absorption is rapid (absorption $t_{1/2} = 2.6$ h) with peak plasma concentrations of diazinon being attained within 2 h postdosing; yet a comparison of AUCs, when corrected for administered dose, indicate

Table 46.2
Selected Model Parameters Describing Blood Concentration Pharmacokinetics of Parent Compounds in Various Species Following Exposure to the Organophosphate Insecticides Parathion and Diazinon

| | | Absorption/bioavailability kinetics | | | Distribution kinetics | | Elimination kinetics | | | |
| | | | | | | | Two-compartment model | | | |
Species	Dose (route)	Bioavailability percentage	Absorption $t_{1/2}$ (h)	Hepatic extraction percentage	Volume distribution $V_{d_{ss}}$ (l/kg)	Protein binding percentage	$t_{1/2}\alpha$ (h)	$t_{1/2}\beta$ (h)	Elimination $k_e t_{1/2}$ (h)	Clearance Cl (l/h/kg)
Rabbit[a]	1.5 mg/kg (iv)	100	N/A	—	14.24 ± 6.34	—	—	5.08 ± 3.06	—	3.99 ± 1.13
Rabbit[a]	3 mg/kg (oral)	68[b]	0.021 ± 0.04	—	7.58 ± 6.45	—	0.13 ± 0.29	1.08 ± 0.27	2.54 ± 1.67	6.59 ± 3.36
Piglet[c]	0.5 mg/kg (iv)	100	N/A	—	2.6 ± 0.9	97 ± 1	—	—	3.0 ± 1.5	—
Pig[d]	1 mg/kg (iv)	100	N/A	—	9.76 ± 5.65	—	—	—	3.6 ± 1.08	4.42 ± 1.20
Pig[d]	50 mg/kg (dermal)	9.93 ± 5.28	—	—	—	—	—	—	—	—
Dog[e]	5 mg/kg (iv)	—	N/A	82–97	—	99	—	—	—	—
Dog[e]	10 mg/kg (oral)	1–29%	—	—	—	99	—	—	—	—
Rat[f]	5–10 mg/kg (iv)	100	N/A	48–55	20.01 ± 11.27	89.1	0.33 ± 0.10	4.70 ± 1.84	—	4.69 ± 0.8
Rat[f]	80 mg/kg (oral)	35.5	2.55	—	22.93 ± 4.82	89.1	—	—	2.86 ± 0.58	4.60 ± 1.05

[a] Pena-Egido et al. (1988).
[b] Estimated by comparing oral and iv AUC after adjusting for dose.
[c] Nielsen et al. (1991).
[d] Brimer et al. (1994).
[e]
[f] Wu et al. (1996).

Table 46.3
Tissue Concentration, Tissue Plasma Ratio and Partition Coefficients Following Exposure to the Organophosphate Insecticides Parathion and Diazinon

| | ^{14}C-Parathion[a] 0.5 mg/kg; iv; piglet 3 h postdosing | | Parathion[b] partition coefficient (PC) | Paraoxon[b] partition coefficient (PC) | Diazinon[c] 10 mg/kg; iv; rat 4 h postdosing | | Diazinon[d] 20 mg/kg; iv; mouse 5 h postdosing | |
Tissue	ng/g	Tissue/plasma ratio	Tissue/blood	Tissue/blood	ng/g	Tissue/plasma ratio	ng/g	Tissue/plasma ratio
Blood/plasma	262 ± 145	—	—	—	~130	—	35	—
Liver	1254 ± 638	4.78	5.21	6.62	325 ± 25	2.50	120	3.42
Kidney	1360 ± 546	5.19	5.21	6.62	790 ± 60	6.08	3000	85.7
Lung	421 ± 92	1.60	5.21[e]	6.62[e]	—	—	—	—
Muscle	484 ± 92	1.85	2.55[f]	3.62[f]	—	—	—	—
Heart	302 ± 85	1.15	—	—	—	—	—	—
Fat	—	—	101.2	10.22	—	—	—	—
Brain	215 ± 76	0.82	4.56	2.31	280 ± 10	2.15	160	4.57

[a] Nielsen et al. (1991).
[b] Gearhart et al. (1994).
[c] Wu et al. (1996).
[d] Tomokuni et al. (1985).
[e] Well-perfused tissue.
[f] Poorly perfused tissue.

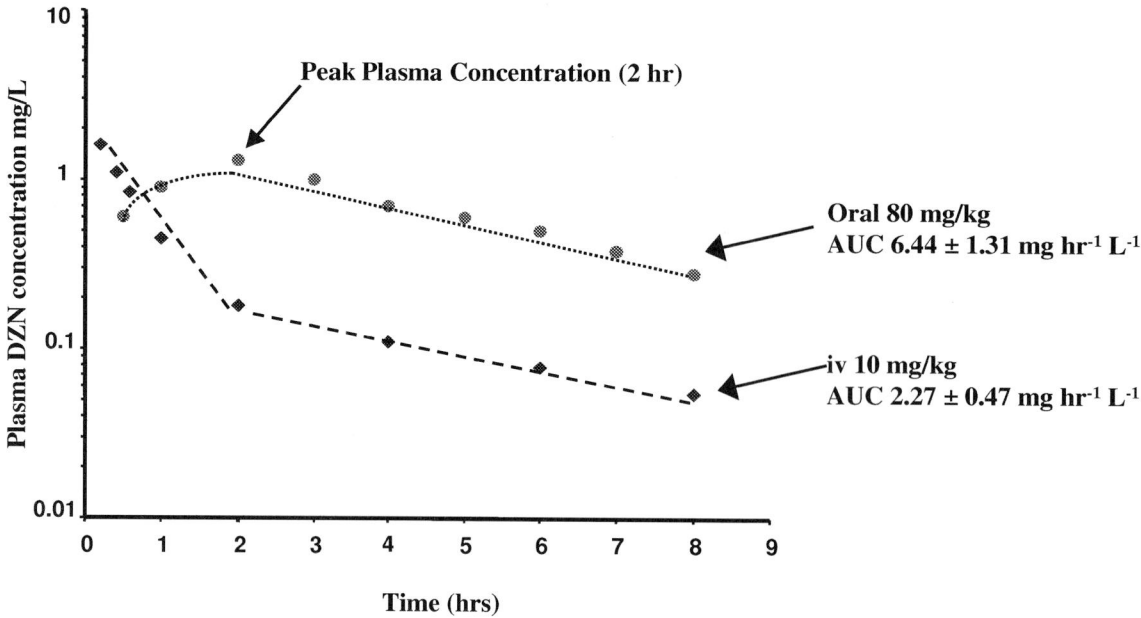

Figure 46.10 Plasma time-course of diazinon (DZN) in rats following intravenous (iv) and oral administration of 10 and 80 mg DZN/kg of body weight, respectively. Data extracted from Wu *et al.* (1996).

that only about 35% of the oral dose was systemically bioavailable. The hepatic extraction ratio for diazinon ranged from 48 to 55% and was qualitatively consistent with the findings of Braeckman *et al.* (1983) for parathion in the dog as well as chlorpyrifos in mice (hepatic extraction ratio ∼46%) (Sultatos, 1988). Rapid oral absorption ($t_{1/2} = 0.02$ h) and lower oral bioavailability (∼68%) were also demonstrated in a study in which rabbits were administered iv and oral doses of parathion (Pena-Egido *et al.*, 1988). Likewise, *in vivo* animal models also suggest that dermal absorption and systemic bioavailability of OP insecticides will be quite low (Brimer *et al.*, 1994).

Once these OP compounds have been absorbed, systemic distribution throughout the body tissues is rapid (Vale, 1998). For example, a high volume of distribution was observed ranging from 3 to 14 and from 20 to 23 l/kg in several different species administered parathion or diazinon, respectively (see Table 46.2). A cross-species comparison of the tissue distribution data following parathion or diazinon exposure is consistent with the large volume of distribution, suggesting that the OP tissue concentration follows the order of kidney > liver > lung/muscle/heart > brain (see Table 46.3). Phosphorothioates such as diazinon and parathion are more lipophilic than their respective oxon metabolites and therefore can be sequestered in the fat compartment, which may account for prolonged intoxication and observed clinical relapses (Vale, 1998). Gearhart *et al.* (1994) determined the PCs for both parathion and the toxic metabolite paraoxon (see Table 46.3). In general, the PCs for parathion and paraoxon are comparable; however, parathion has an order of magnitude (101 vs. 10.11) greater affinity than paraoxon for fat.

The systemic distribution, elimination kinetics, metabolic transformation, and target site availability of a drug or chemical

are often dependent on the extent of reversible plasma/serum protein binding (Renwick, 1994). For example, as shown in Table 46.2, parathion and diazinon are extensively bound to plasma protein (ranging from 89 to 99%) and the extent of binding is concentration independent. This response is likewise consistent with the findings of Sultatos *et al.* (1984), who reported that chlorpyrifos is approximately 97% bound to mouse plasma proteins over a broad concentration range. This high degree of protein binding in conjunction with the high volume of distribution also suggests that tissue binding may in fact be more important than plasma binding in determining the overall disposition and clearance of OPs (Braeckman *et al.*, 1983).

Although the OP insecticides parathion and diazinon are well distributed throughout the body and extensively bind to both plasma and tissue proteins, they are both rapidly cleared from the body primarily in the urine as degradation metabolites of the parent OPs [i.e., *p*-nitrophenol, 2-isopropyl-4-methyl-6-hydroxyprimidine (IMHP)] (Iverson *et al.*, 1975; Mücke *et al.*, 1970; Nielsen *et al.*, 1991; Vale, 1998). The overall systemic clearances for both parathion and diazinon are quite fast and comparable, ranging from 4 to 6.6 l/h/kg, and are consistent with the rapid blood/plasma terminal phase half-life (2.5–5 h; see Table 46.2).

As previously indicated, comparative species pharmacokinetic analysis is useful for understanding the *in vivo* behavior of OP insecticides. Although generalization to all OP agents is unwise, these types of comparative analyses do provide important insights. In summary, the oral absorption of both parathion and diazinon is rapid with peak plasma concentrations being obtained within a few hours of exposure. However, oral bioavailability is low and appears to be at least partially associated with a high rate of hepatic first-pass metabolism. Although these OP insecticides are extensively bound to plasma proteins, they are equally well distributed throughout the body's tissues and the parent phosphorothioates can sequester within the fat compartment. Nonetheless, the overall clearance is quite fast and is most likely associated with the rapid metabolism and elimination of the OP metabolites.

46.3.2 DEVELOPMENT OF PHARMACOKINETIC MODELS FOR QUANTITATIVE BIOLOGICAL MONITORING TO ASSESS ORGANOPHOSPHATE INSECTICIDE EXPOSURE IN HUMANS

In assessing human exposure to chemical agents, biological monitoring (biomonitoring) is an important quantitative measure of the amount of chemical agent that is systemically absorbed. This approach entails the quantitation of the chemical or its metabolites in biological fluids (i.e., blood, urine, exhaled breath) and offers the best means of accurately assessing exposure because it measures actual, rather than potential, exposure (Woollen, 1993). However, to accurately predict human dosimetry from occupational and/or environmental exposure to xenobiotics, human volunteer pharmacokinetic studies conducted under controlled conditions are of vital importance (Wilks and Woollen, 1994; Woollen, 1993).

Both occupational and environmental exposures to OPs are primarily associated with dermal exposure; accounting for more than 90% of the absorbed dose (Aprea *et al.*, 1994). Therefore, an understanding of the percutaneous absorption of OPs is critical for quantitatively determining a systemic dose. The extent of dermal bioavailability for a number of ^{14}C-labeled OP insecticides has been determined in humans utilizing both *in vivo* studies in volunteers and *in vitro* dermal penetration with skin obtained from cadavers (Wester *et al.*, 1983, 1992, 1993). A summary of the percentage absorption following *in vivo* and *in vitro* dermal exposure to the OP insecticides diazinon, isofenphos, and malathion is illustrated in Fig. 46.11.

The general experimental design of these studies entailed three major components. First, human volunteers were administered a topical dose of a known concentration of ^{14}C-labeled OP for a specified exposure period. The extent of absorption was determined by quantitating the amount of ^{14}C excreted in the urine and remaining on the skin surface. Second, *in vitro* percutaneous absorption was determined using a glass flow-through penetration cell in which the percentage absorption through human cadaver skin was determined by the amount of radiotracer that transferred into the receptor fluid. Finally, to calculate the *in vivo* percentage absorption, rhesus monkeys were given a ^{14}C-labeled OP as an iv dose. The percentage dose absorbed in humans was calculated from the ratio of ^{14}C excreted in the urine after topical (humans) and iv (monkey) dosing. The *in vivo* absorption for the three OP insecticides diazinon, isofenphos, and malathion in human volunteers following a topical application is very low, ranging from 2.5 to 3.9% of the applied dose. The percentage absorption as determined *in vitro*

was likewise comparable for isofenphos (3.64% ± 0.48), but slightly higher and considerably more variable for diazinon (14.1% ± 9.2). Percutaneous absorption studies conducted in humans are of particular importance because it is known that dermal absorption in animals, such as the rat, is often greater than in humans (Wester and Maibach, 1983). For example, Knaak *et al.* (1990) conducted a dermal absorption study in rats with isofenphos and reported that 47% of the applied dose was absorbed, which is 12-fold higher than the results seen in human volunteers. The major limitation associated with the experimental design of Wester *et al.* (1983, 1992, 1993) is that the quantitation of only ^{14}C provides no information on the specific form of the compound (i.e., parent or metabolite) that is systemically available. Nonetheless, these studies provide important quantitative information on the extent of dermal absorption.

To better understand the systemic pharmacokinetics of OPs and to develop pharmacokinetic models that can be utilized for biomonitoring, controlled human studies that quantitate the time course of parent chemical or metabolites in blood and urine are key. Nolan *et al.* (1984) conducted a controlled human pharmacokinetic study to follow the fate of a major metabolite, 3,5,6-trichloropyridinol (TCP), which is excreted in the urine following both oral and dermal administration of chlorpyrifos. Griffin *et al.* (1999) also conducted a controlled human study with chlorpyrifos in human volunteers, but quantitated the urinary excretion of the dialkylphosphate metabolite.

A selection of comparative pharmacokinetic parameters from the controlled human chlorpyrifos studies is presented in Table 46.4. Overall, the pharmacokinetic results obtained using TCP or dialkylphosphate in human volunteers are entirely consistent with each other. For example, following oral administration, chlorpyrifos is rapidly absorbed with maximum plasma concentration and excretion being obtained by 6 and 7 h postdosing for TCP and dialkylphosphate, respectively. The extent of absorption was quite good, based on the amount of metabolite (70–93%) recovered in the urine. In comparison, the dermal absorption was consistently slower with peak concentrations of metabolite being achieved by 17–24 h postdosing for both studies. Also, the amount recovered based on TCP and dialkylphosphate metabolites in the urine was 1.35 and 1%, respectively, suggesting limited dermal absorption of chlorpyrifos. Nolan *et al.* (1984) reported an elimination half-life of 26.9 h following oral administration, whereas Griffin *et al.* (1999) reported half-lives of 15.5 and 30 h for dialkylphosphate following oral and dermal exposure to chlorpyrifos, respectively. The increase in the urinary elimination half-life following dermal exposure is most likely associated with a delay in chlorpyrifos absorption through the skin. However, differences in the rates of TCP and dialkylphosphate kinetics are also a possible explanation (Griffin *et al.*, 1999). Nonetheless, the elimination half-life for chlorpyrifos based on either TCP or dialkylphosphate clearance is consistent.

These types of pharmacokinetic data are being used to develop models to biomonitor for OP exposure. Nolan *et al.* (1984) developed a one-compartment pharmacokinetic model having the same volume of distribution and elimination rate

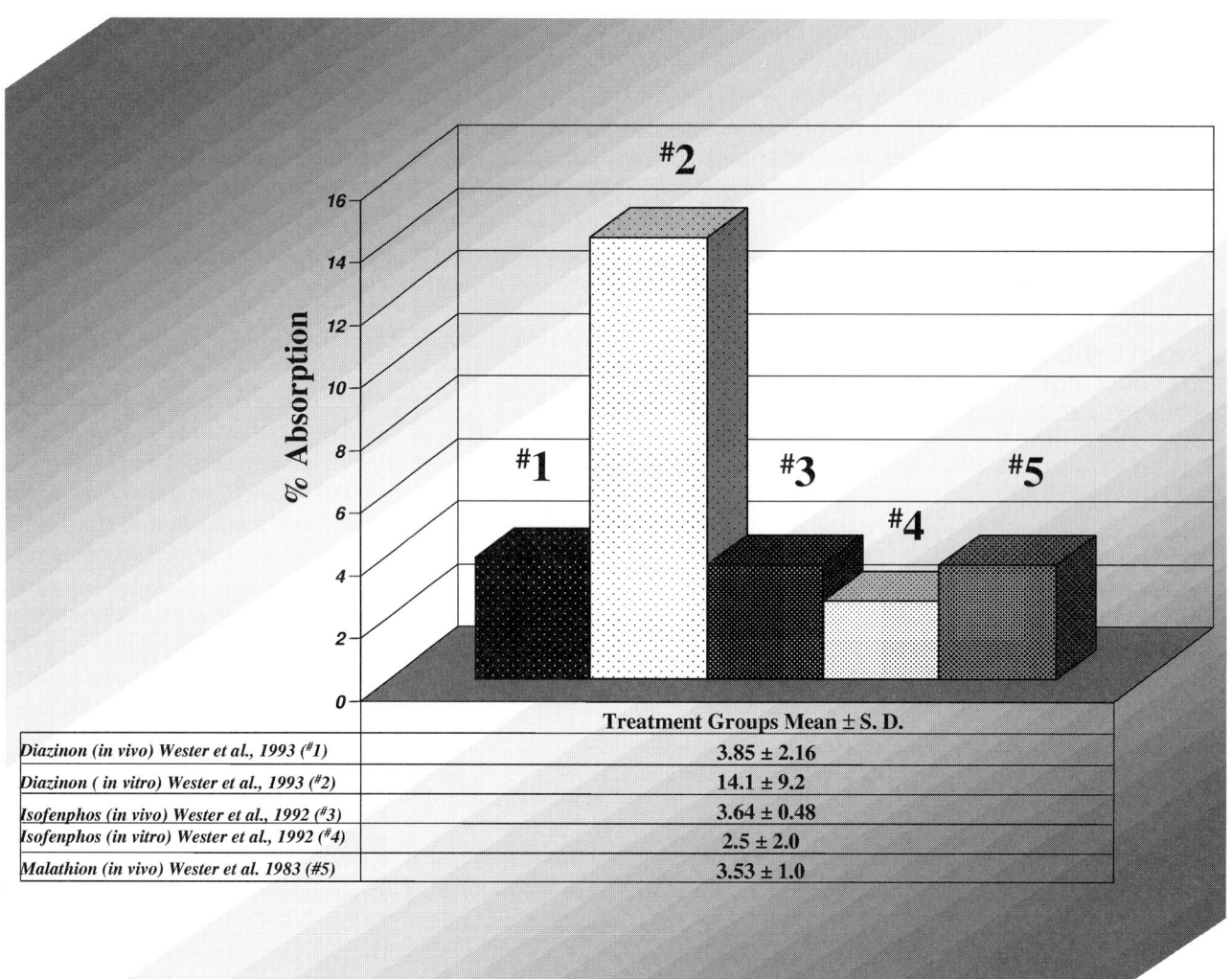

Treatment Groups Mean ± S. D.	
Diazinon (in vivo) Wester et al., 1993 (#1)	**3.85 ± 2.16**
Diazinon (in vitro) Wester et al., 1993 (#2)	**14.1 ± 9.2**
Isofenphos (in vivo) Wester et al., 1992 (#3)	**3.64 ± 0.48**
Isofenphos (in vitro) Wester et al., 1992 (#4)	**2.5 ± 2.0**
Malathion (in vivo) Wester et al. 1983 (#5)	**3.53 ± 1.0**

Figure 46.11   Summary of human dermal penetration (*in vivo/in vitro*) for the organophosphate (OP) insecticides diazinon, isofenphos and malathion.

Table 46.4

Comparison of Oral and Dermal Pharmacokinetic Parameters Describing the Blood Concentration and Urinary Excretion of 3,5,6-Trichloropyridinol (TCP) and Dialkylphosphate (DAP) by Volunteers Following Exposure to the Organophosphate Insecticide Chlorpyrifos

Exposure route/ metabolite	Dose (mg/kg)	Absorption rate (ng/cm²/h)	Absorption rate constant k_a (h⁻¹)	Absorption half-life (h)	Elimination rate constant k_e (h⁻¹)	Elimination half-life (h)	Model predicted percentage dose absorbed	Percentage dose recovered in urine
Oral								
TCP[a]	0.5	—	1.5 ± 1.2	0.5	0.0258 ± 0.0051	26.9	72 ± 11	70 ± 11
DAP[b]	0.014[c]	—	—	—	—	15.5	—	93 (range 55–115)
Dermal								
TCP[a]	5	—	0.0308 ± 0.01	22.5	—	—	1.35 ± 1.02	1.28 ± 0.83
DAP[b]	0.41	456	—	—	—	30	—	1.00

[a]Nolan *et al.* (1984).

[b]Griffin *et al.* (1999).

[c]Estimated based on average body weight (71 kg).

constant to describe blood and urinary TCP kinetics following oral and dermal exposure to chlorpyrifos (see Fig. 46.4). Similarly, the quantitative measurement of urinary dialkylphosphate is increasingly being used for biomonitoring for OP exposures (Gargas *et al.*, 1989). The development of pharmacokinetic models that are capable of describing the uptake, distribution, and elimination of OP insecticides based on the quantitation of major degradation metabolites represents an extremely useful and simple approach for exposure biomonitoring.

46.3.3 THE APPLICATION OF PHARMACOKINETICS FOR QUANTIFYING EXPOSURE TO ORGANOPHOSPHATE INSECTICIDES

The ability to more accurately quantitate human exposure to OP insecticides has been enhanced by the use of biomonitoring approaches linked to pharmacokinetic analysis. This has successfully been used to estimate agricultural worker exposures during and after the application of insecticides, to evaluate secondary exposures within cross-sectional epidemiology studies, and to assess dosimetry in persons who have been acutely poisoned either accidentally or through intentional self-administration (Drevenkar *et al.*, 1993; Lavy *et al.*, 1993; Loewenherz *et al.*, 1997).

Historically, workplace exposure to chemicals has been controlled through environmental monitoring that has primarily focused on the measurement of the chemical contaminant in the ambient air. However, because airborne concentrations may not be linearly correlated with absorption, this approach does not provide an accurate assessment of the internal dose (Franklin *et al.*, 1986). In agricultural settings, worker exposure studies have incorporated personal external monitoring to estimate the amount of chemical available from inhalation (i.e., breathing-zone sampling pumps) and dermal absorption (i.e., patch method and hand washes). Where feasible, these studies have also incorporated biomonitoring (i.e., urinary metabolites) to quantitate the amount of absorbed dose (Chester, 1993; Franklin *et al.*, 1981, 1986). Franklin *et al.* (1981, 1986) estimated exposure of workers to the OP insecticide azinphos-methyl (guthion) utilizing both external personal monitoring and urinary biomonitoring of alkylphosphate metabolite. When patch data were utilized to calculate exposure and plotted against total urinary metabolite excretion, no correlation was observed (Franklin *et al.*, 1981). However, the authors did report a much better correlation when the amount of alkylphosphate metabolite excreted in the urine was compared against the amount of active ingredient sprayed. This relationship is illustrated in Fig. 46.12, where the amount of alkylphosphate metabolite excreted in the urine increases with increasing amounts of active ingredient.

Because agricultural workers routinely apply numerous pesticides and are often sequentially exposed to OP insecticides within a relatively short time span, a number of exposure studies have been conducted to evaluate mixed OP insecticide exposures. Hayes *et al.* (1980) evaluated the occupational exposure of pest control operators in which the bulk of the pesticide applications ($\sim$ 80%) involved the combined use of the OP insecticides vaponite, diazinon, and chlorpyrifos. Worker biomonitoring was based on blood AChE determination and the quantitation of dimethyl- and diethylphosphate and dimethyl- and diethylphosphothioate metabolites in the urine. The authors reported that external air monitoring did provide information regarding the levels and types of OP exposures, but did not provide adequate information on the degree to which these OPs were absorbed. The urinary alkylphosphate levels provided sensitive quantitative information on absorption and excretion of these pesticides. However, because the alkylphosphate metabolites are not specific to any one OP, this approach is indicative only of general OP exposures to these mixtures and cannot be used to quantitatively assess individual OP dosimetry.

More recently, Lavy *et al.* (1993) conducted a comprehensive year-long biomonitoring study of tree nursery workers, who are routinely exposed to multiple pesticides. In this study, it was recognized that as many as 28 pesticides are regularly used and 17 of the most common pesticides were selected for monitoring, including a number of OPs. Evaluation of the human and animal pharmacokinetic data suggested that adequate metabolism information was available on 8 of the selected pesticides to support biomonitoring. In this year-long study, 3134 urine specimens were analyzed, but only 42 of these contained measurable pesticide metabolites (1.3%) and were composed of only three pesticides (benomyl, bifenox, and carbaryl) (Lavy *et al.*, 1993). In addition, based on a calculated margin of safety, the exposure levels were clearly below a level that would be of concern to human health.

Biomonitoring strategies have also been successfully applied to quantitatively assess secondary exposures to OP insecticides resulting from both acute and chronic exposures. Richter *et al.* (1992) quantitated diethylphosphate in the urine of individuals who were symptomatic for OP exposure and resided in a house that had been sprayed with diazinon approximately 4.5 months earlier. In this particular study, very high levels of urinary diethylphosphate were observed in family members, whereas cholinesterase activity, although slightly depressed, was well within the range of "normal." The quantitation of urinary diethylphosphate was used to establish a persistent household exposure to diazinon residues as the most likely explanation. This study clearly illustrates the utility of urinary OP metabolites for quantitative biomonitoring of exposure.

Biomonitoring based on the measurement of OP metabolites has also been used to compare pesticide exposure in children who live in proximity to high spray areas (i.e., orchards) and whose parents/guardians are pesticide applicators (Loewenherz *et al.*, 1997). Based on known pesticide use patterns, it was determined that OP insecticide exposure would be primarily associated with azinphos-methyl, chlorpyrifos, and phosmet. Therefore, the study focused on the quantitation of the alkylphosphate metabolites (dimethylthiophosphate, dimethyldithiophosphate, dimethylphosphate) in the children's urine. Loewenherz *et al.* (1997) collected and evaluated 160 spot urine specimens from 88 children and reported detectable

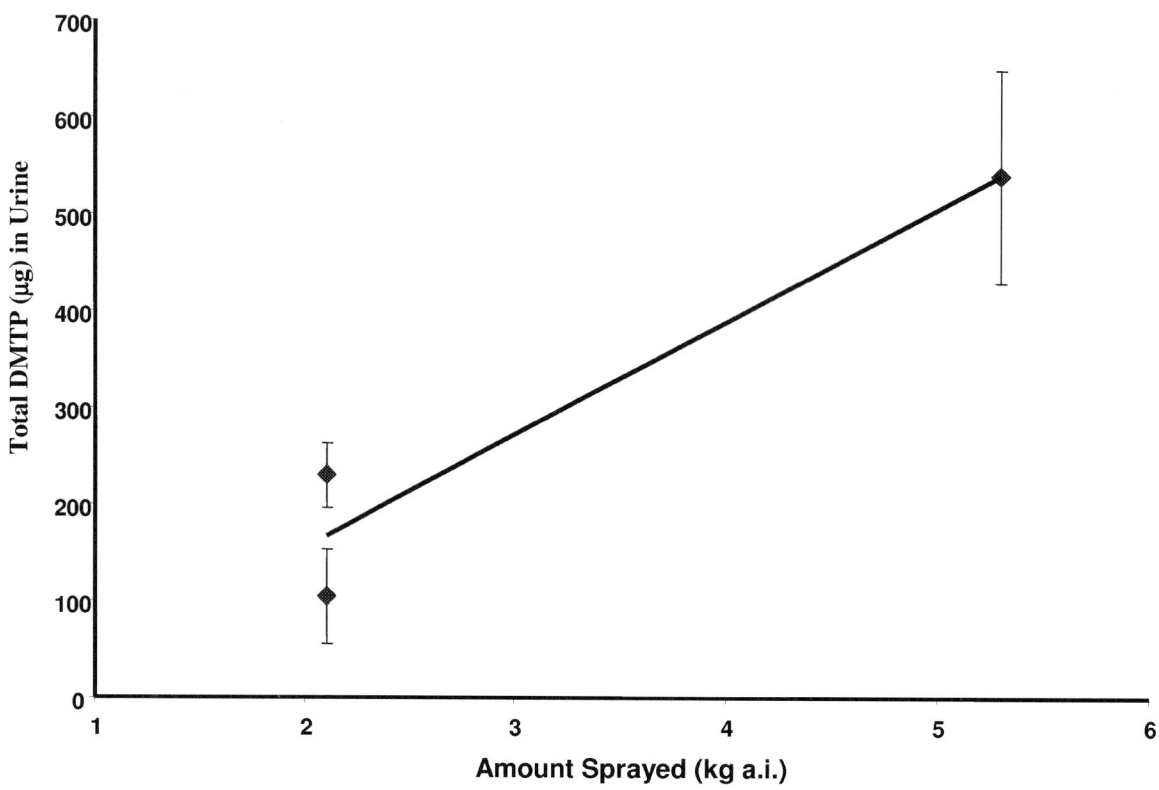

Figure 46.12 Relationship between the amount of alkyl phosphate (dimethylthiophosphate; DMTP) metabolite in urine of workers and the amount of active ingredient (a.i.) sprayed. Data obtained from Franklin *et al.* (1981).

levels of these metabolites in 27 and 47% of the reference children and applicator children, respectively. In addition, the biomonitoring data suggest that the children of applicators had a significantly higher dose than the reference children (0.021 vs. 0.005 µg/l, respectively).

Biomonitoring of parent OPs and metabolites in blood and urine has also been used to provide a quantitative assessment of dosimetry in human poisoning victims following acute high-dose exposures (Drevenkar *et al.*, 1993; Vasilic *et al.*, 1992). Although acute AChE depression (i.e., 50% of baseline) is used to substantiate OP poisoning, the analysis of intact pesticides or specific metabolites in body fluids (blood/urine) can be used to identify the specific causative chemical agent(s) (Ellenhorn and Barceloux, 1988; Lotti *et al.*, 1986). The utilization of pharmacokinetic models such as the one developed for chlorpyrifos (Nolan *et al.*, 1984) can be extremely useful for the estimation of dosimetry under these acute exposure scenarios.

To illustrate this point, a two-compartment pharmacokinetic model was used to fit pharmacokinetic data obtained from a poison victim who ingested a commercial insecticide formulation containing chlorpyrifos (Drevenkar *et al.*, 1993). These same data have been modeled utilizing a PBPK/PD model developed for the quantitation of chlorpyrifos, chlorpyrifos-oxon, and TCP in the rat and human (Timchalk and Nolan, 1998). The time course and PBPK/PD model–predicted TCP and chlorpyrifos concentration in the blood and serum of human volunteers and following oral ingestion for a single poison victim are pre-

sented in Fig. 46.13. The model adequately reflects the data from these limited human samples; more important, these examples illustrate the strength of using pharmacokinetic models for quantitating dosimetry under both controlled and noncontrolled conditions.

In summary, these examples have been presented to illustrate the practical application of pharmacokinetics to assess exposure to chemicals. Biomonitoring is clearly an integral component of the agricultural pesticide exposure assessment strategy. However, the successful application of biomonitoring for quantitative dosimetry is primarily limited by a lack of chemical-specific pharmacokinetic data in humans.

46.3.4 STUDIES THAT FACILITATE EXTRAPOLATION OF DOSIMETRY AND BIOLOGICAL RESPONSE FROM ANIMALS TO HUMANS AND THE ASSESSMENT OF HUMAN HEALTH RISK

Organophosphate insecticides constitute a large class of chemical pesticides that are widely used in the agricultural industry and in home applications. This suggests that there is significant potential for exposure and the health consequences of these exposures may be impacted by both interindividual and extrinsic variability (see Fig. 46.14). For example, extrinsic factors such as multiple exposure routes, chemical/drug interactions, and

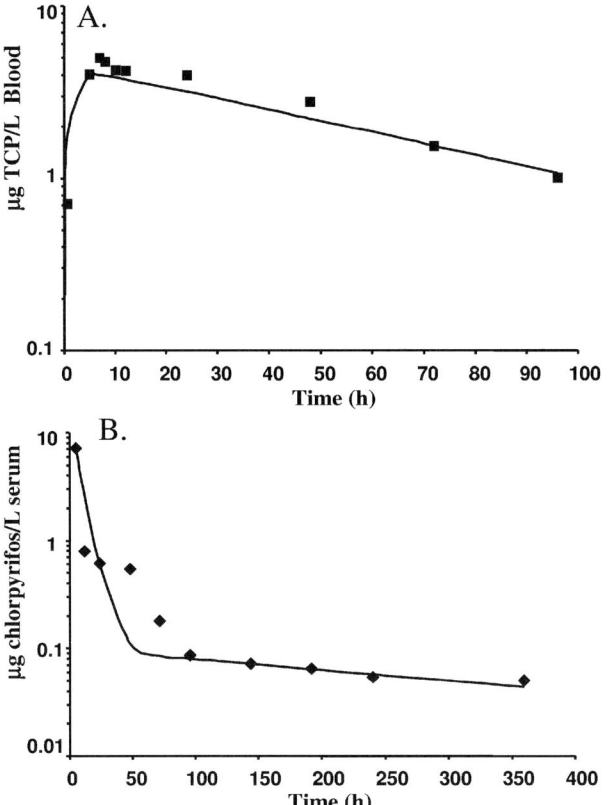

Figure 46.13   (A) Mean blood time-course of 3,5,6-trichloropyridinol (TCP) from six human volunteers administered a single oral dose of 0.5 mg chlorpyrifos (CPF)/kg of body weight. Data obtained from Nolan *et al.* (1984). (B) Time-course of CPF in the serum of a single poison victim that orally ingested a commercial insecticide product containing CPF. The symbols represent observed data while the line represents the model prediction. Data obtained from Drevenkar *et al.* (1993).

variable exposure rates may significantly modify the toxicological response to OPs. In addition, person-to-person differences in metabolism, genetic predisposition, physical environment, and age (infant, children, and elderly) are important determinants of pharmacokinetic and/or pharmacodynamic response. As previously discussed, Gearhart *et al.* (1990) developed a PBPK/PD model for quantitative OP dosimetry and AChE inhibition utilizing diisopropylfluorophosphate as a representative highly toxic OP (see Figs. 46.6 and 46.7). This PBPK/PD model was developed as a prototype that could readily be extended to the commercially important OPs. In this respect, the development and application of PBPK/PD modeling represents a logical approach for assessing risk and understanding the toxicological implications of known or suspected exposures to various OP insecticides.

To extend this initial modeling effort, Gearhart *et al.* (1994) modified their original model to incorporate the phosphorothionate insecticide parathion and its oxon, paraoxon. In addition, Timchalk and Nolan (1998) built a model to incorporate chemical-specific parameters for the OP insecticide chlorpyrifos that are based on the models of Gearhart *et al.* (1990, 1994). This model was developed to describe the time course of chlor-

pyrifos, the oxon metabolite, the elimination of TCP, and the inhibition of target esterases by the oxon. The chlorpyrifos PBPK/PD model incorporates CYP450-mediated activation of chlorpyrifos to the oxon and detoxification to TCP. In addition, hydrolysis of the oxon by B-esterases (AChE, BChE, and CaE) is modeled in the liver, blood, diaphragm, and brain. A diagram outlining the critical features of this model is presented in Fig. 46.15. Although this is a preliminary PBPK/PD model requiring further validation and refinement, it qualitatively behaves consistent with the general understanding of OP toxicity, pharmacokinetics, and pharmacodynamic responses. To illustrate this point, the model has been used to simulate the serum time course of chlorpyrifos and TCP in poisoned humans (see Fig. 46.13). In addition, a simulation of the dynamics of tissue esterase inhibition following a single acute exposure to two different doses of chlorpyrifos in the rat is qualitatively consistent with observed AChE inhibition kinetics and is illustrated in Fig. 46.16. It is anticipated that this basic model structure can be readily modified to accommodate other important phosphorothioates. Likewise, once validated, these models can be used as a foundation for understanding complex-mixture interactions, sensitive subpopulations, and the role of metabolic polymorphisms in altering dosimetry and biological response.

46.3.4.1 Organophosphate Mixtures

Both occupational and residential exposures to OP insecticides often entail simultaneous or sequential contact with OP mixtures (Hayes *et al.*, 1980; Lavy *et al.*, 1993; Loewenherz *et al.*, 1997). The potential for OP interactions has been well understood for some time. Early studies demonstrated the acute, synergistic, and toxicological interactions between the OPs malathion and EPN (ethyl-*p*-nitrophenyl phenylphosphonothionate) (Frawley *et al.*, 1957). In addition, non-OPs have been reported to influence the pharmacokinetic and toxicological response of OPs. For example, phenobarbital or alcohol pretreatment of mice protects against the acute toxicity of chlorpyrifos and parathion, respectively (O'Shaughnessy and Sultatos, 1995; Sultatos, 1988). Wu *et al.* (1996) reported that pretreatment of rats with cimetidine potentiated the acute toxicity of diazinon as a result of reducing diazinon total body clearance. Likewise, co-administration of diazinon with cocaine significantly increased the concentration of cocaine and norcocaine in the blood and tissues of mice apparently due to competition for esterase enzyme detoxification (Benuck *et al.*, 1989; Kump *et al.*, 1994). A combination of malathion and the carbamate pesticide carbaryl alters the fundamental pharmacokinetic properties of the individual compounds and it has been suggested that this may explain some of the observed toxicity seen from exposure to this chemical mixture (Waldron-Lechner and Abdel-Rahman, 1986).

OP pesticides as a class of compounds share common metabolic processes for activation and detoxification as well as a common mechanism for toxicological response through the inhibition of AChE (Murphy, 1986; Sultatos, 1994). Based on similar pharmacokinetic and mode-of-action properties,

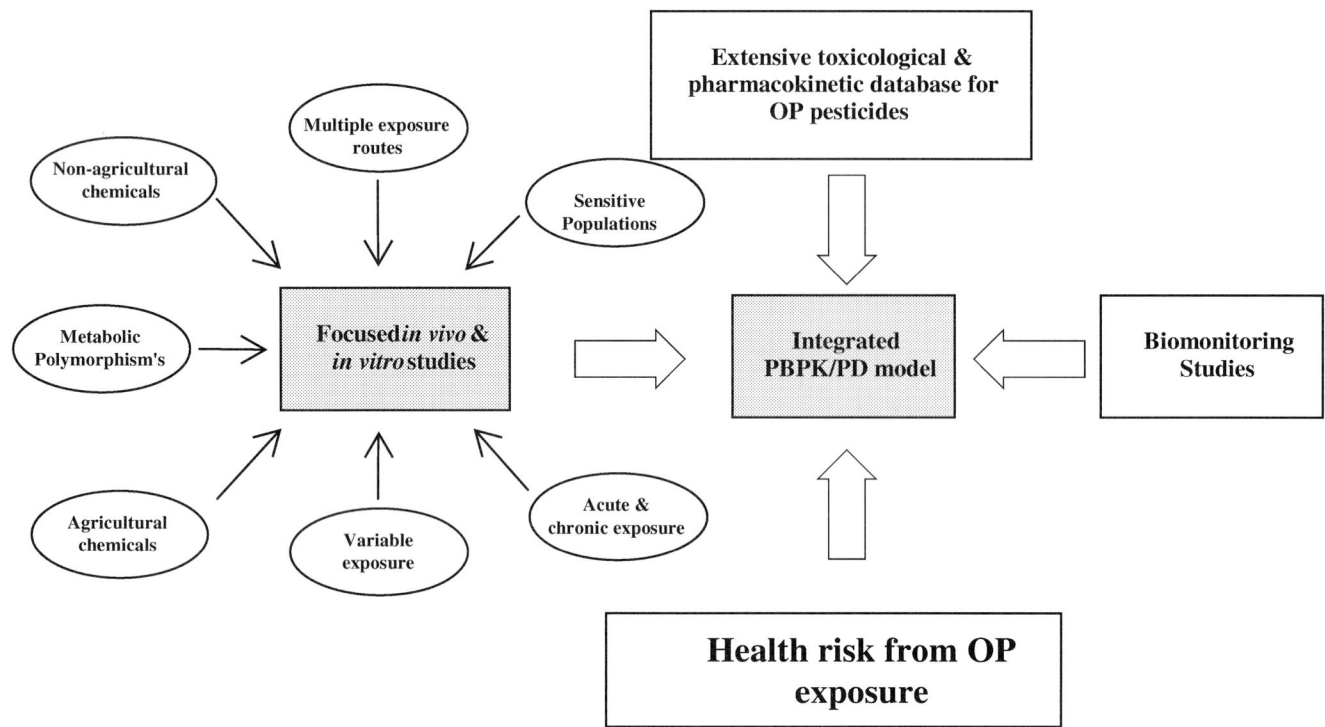

Figure 46.14 A conceptual model for evaluating the impact of intrinsic/extrinsic factors on human health risk from exposure to organophosphate (OP) insecticides.

the potential for interactions between mixtures of OPs has been hypothesized. Organophosphates can interact at a number of important metabolic steps (see Table 46.5), including (1) CYP450-mediated activation/detoxification, (2) plasma protein binding, (3) A-esterase detoxification, and (4) AChE binding/inhibition. The net effect of these interactions (additivity, synergy, or antagonism) will be dependent on the specific OP mixture, dose ranges of exposures, and sensitivity of the individual.

Several integrated approaches have been proposed to investigate the potential for toxicological interactions of chemical mixtures (El-Masri *et al.*, 1997). The proposed strategies all emphasize the utilization of PBPK modeling. Until recently, the majority of these models have focused on a single chemical exposure. However, exposure to low-dose chemical mixtures represents a more realistic exposure scenario. Although several PBPK models have been developed for binary and ternary mixtures of organic solvents, little is known about the potential metabolic and toxicological interactions of these mixtures on biological systems (Andersen *et al.*, 1987b; Pelekis and Krishnan, 1997; Purcell *et al.*, 1990; Tardif *et al.*, 1993, 1995, 1997). The evaluation of mixtures is complicated by the myriad of chemicals, doses, exposure routes, and dynamic responses observed, making it impractical to effectively test all possible permutations. In this regard, the application of PBPK models for mixtures provides a limited means to quantitatively describe the disposition of chemicals as a result of exposure to various combinations, doses, and routes of administration.

46.3.4.2 Sensitive Subpopulations (Children and Polymorphisms)

There is currently a significant focus and concern over the potential increased sensitivity of infants and children to the toxic effects of chemicals. The importance of this issue is highlighted by the National Research Council's report, *Pesticides in the Diets of Infants and Children*, and the passage of the Food Quality Protection Act. It is recognized that children are not just "small adults," but rather a unique subpopulation that may be particularly vulnerable to chemical insult. Age-dependent changes in a child's physiology (i.e., body size, blood flow, organ functions) and metabolic capacity (i.e., phase I and II metabolism) may significantly impact their response to a chemical insult, resulting in either beneficial or detrimental effects (Miller *et al.*, 1997). Clear variability in the capacity to detoxify environmental chemicals has been established in both animals and humans. However, the current risk assessment paradigms do not adequately consider the implications of these differences on the risk to infants and children. Numerous studies have demonstrated that juvenile animals are more susceptible to the acute effects of OP insecticides than adults (Benke and Murphy, 1975; Brodeur and DuBois, 1963; Gaines and Linder, 1986; Harbison, 1975; Moser and Padilla, 1998; Pope and Liu, 1997; Pope *et al.*, 1991). This greater sensitivity has primarily been attributed to the lack of complete metabolic competence during neonatal and postnatal development (Benke and Murphy, 1975).

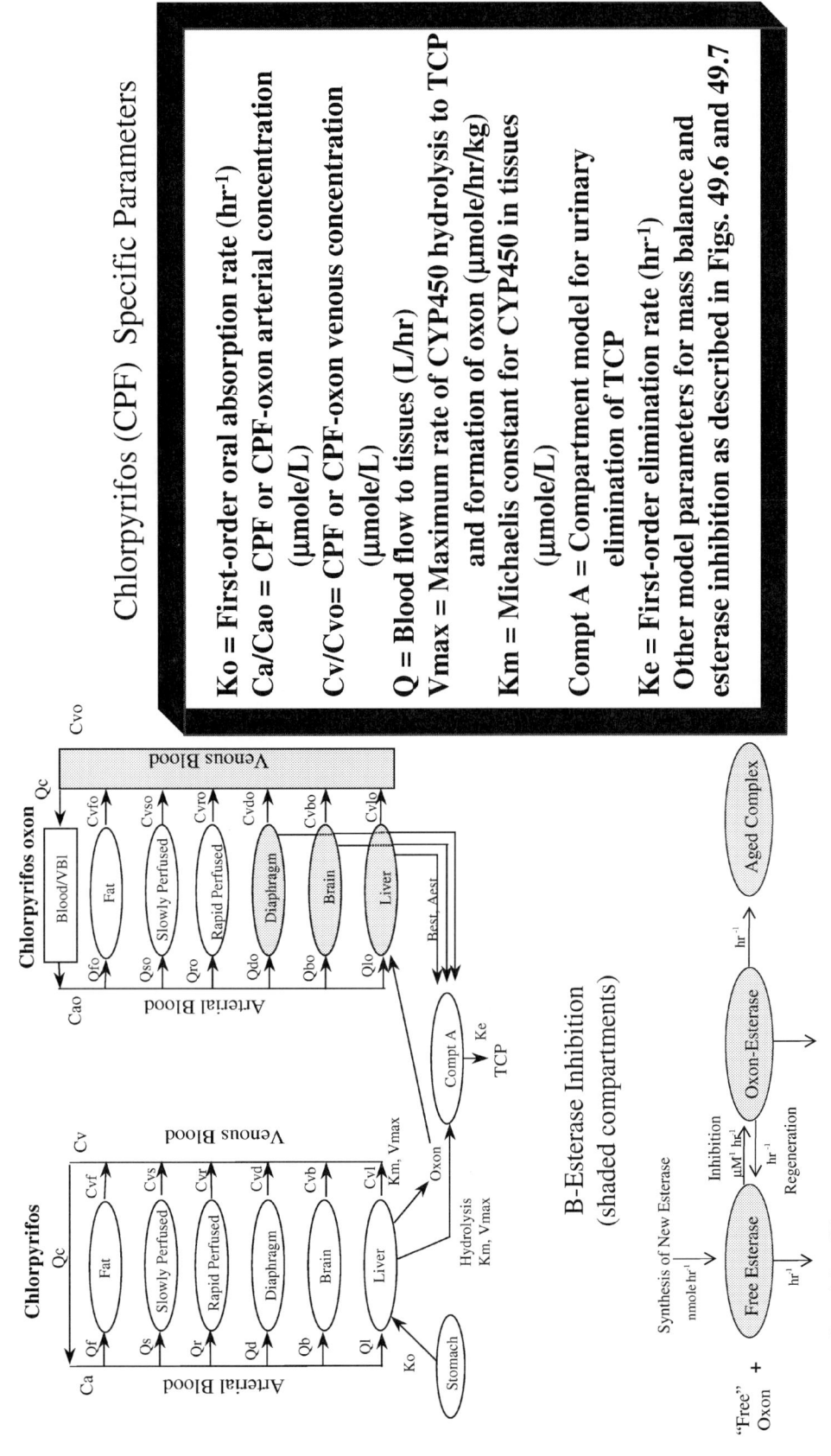

Figure 46.15 Physiologically based pharmacokinetic and pharmacodynamic (PBPK/PD) model structure describing the distribution of chlorpyrifos (CPF), CPF-oxon and 3,5,6-trichloropyridinol (TCP) in the rat.

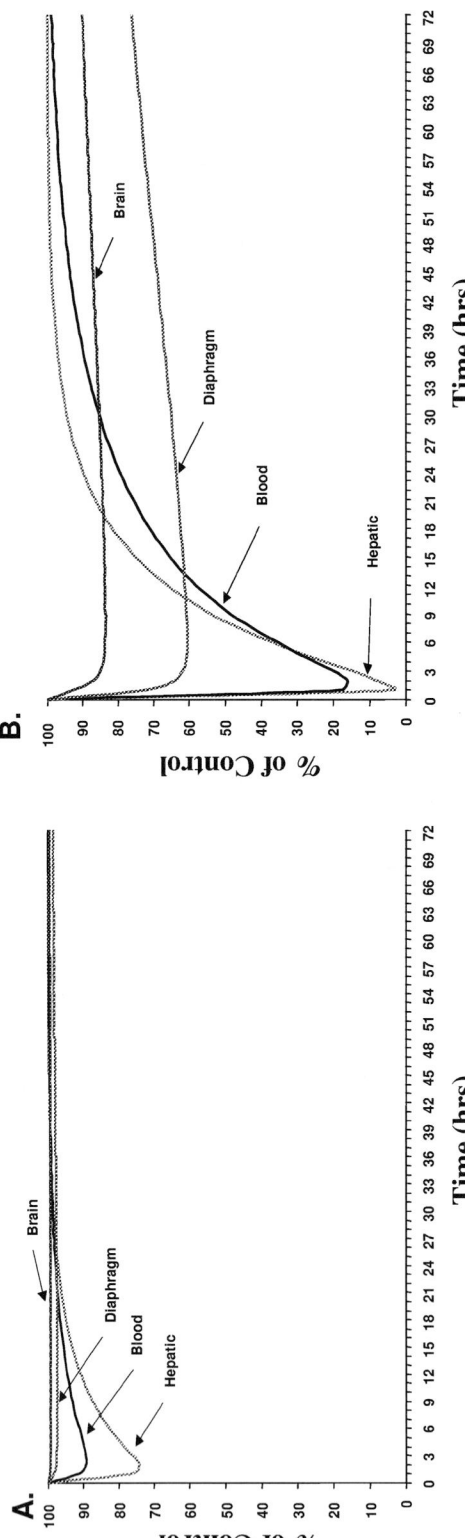

Figure 46.16 Simulated AChE inhibition in selected tissues (brain, diaphragm, blood and liver) following a single oral dose of (A) 0.5 mg and (B) 5 mg chlorpyrifos (CPF)/kg of body weight.

Table 46.5
Important Metabolic and Response Interactions for Mixtures of Organophosphate Insecticides

Parameter	Importance	Type of chemical interaction	Implication
CYP450 mixed-function oxidase metabolism	Metabolic activation/ detoxification of parent compound	Substrate (parent compound) competition for enzyme	Changes in oxon concentrations
Reversible plasma protein binding	Systemic transport of parent compound	Substrate (parent compound) competition for available protein binding sites	Increased levels of "free" parent chemical available for metabolism
A-esterase metabolism	Important metabolic step responsible for detoxification	Substrate (oxon) competition for enzyme	Changes in oxon concentrations
AChE binding/inhibition	Toxicological response	Substrates (oxon) combine to increase inhibition of AChE	Increased toxicity due to additive response

Several recent studies provide important perspective on this age-dependent sensitivity and the selected results are illustrated in Fig. 46.17. Atterberry *et al.* (1997) evaluated the developmental changes in brain AChE levels and hepatic CaE- and CYP450-mediated metabolism of chlorpyrifos in the juvenile rat. They correlated age-dependent chlorpyrifos toxicity (Fig. 46.17a) with the capacity to activate and detoxify chlorpyrifos (Fig. 46.17b and c). Their results suggest that the age-dependent sensitivity of young animals is associated with a decreased CaE-mediated hydrolysis and CYP450-mediated dearylation capacity in young animals relative to adults. In addition, it has likewise been suggested that the sensitivity of young animals is associated with a lower A-esterase activity than is found in adults (Mortensen *et al.*, 1996). The importance of A-esterase in protecting against OP toxicity has been demonstrated in several studies in which exogenous administration of A-esterase can protect against OP poisoning in rodents (Costa *et al.*, 1990; Li *et al.*, 1993, 1995; Main, 1956).

Mortensen *et al.* (1996) compared both plasma and hepatic A-esterase enzyme activity in adult and neonatal animals and reported that neonatal plasma and liver A-esterase activity were 9 and 50% of adult activity, respectively. This is consistent with the results of Li *et al.* (1997), who reported that serum A-esterase activity toward paraoxon, chlorpyrifos-oxon, and diazoxon were very low at birth, but reached adult levels of activity by about 25 days of age in rodents. This time span in rodents corresponds to *in utero* humans to approximately in 6 months old. These findings in animals are in agreement with observations in which newborns and children less than 6 months old have lower plasma A-esterase activity than adults (Augustinsson and Barr, 1963; Mueller *et al.*, 1983). In addition to age-dependent differences in A-esterase activity, a human and animal genetic polymorphism has been well established (Eckerson *et al.*, 1983; Furlong *et al.*, 1988; Geldmacher-von Mallinckrodt *et al.*, 1983). This polymorphism is known to result in the expression of a broad range of A-esterase enzyme activity within a large segment of the human population.

Although young rats appear to be more sensitive (based on LD_{50} and AChE inhibition) to the acute effects of OP insecticides relative to adults, AChE activity is reported to recover faster in young animals (Moser and Padilla, 1998; Pope *et al.*, 1991). This more rapid recovery of AChE (Lajtha and Dunlop, 1981; Moser and Padilla, 1998) is associated with a faster synthesis rate as well as higher steady-state enzyme levels. The capacity of young rats to recover AChE activity faster than adults may be of greater importance in dealing with intermittent low-dose exposure to OPs. In summary, these data suggest that the sensitivity of juvenile animals and humans to the toxic effects of OP insecticides may be a function of the maturational stage of development for a number of critical metabolic steps. These include CYP450-mediated activation/detoxification, hepatic CaE hydrolysis binding, and plasma and hepatic A-esterase detoxification.

The application of PBPK/PD modeling offers a unique opportunity to integrate age-dependent changes in OP metabolic activation and detoxification pathways into a comprehensive model that is capable of quantitating dose and response across all ages. In this context, PBPK models are being extended to the modeling of chemical exposure in developing neonatal animals. A number of these models have focused on the incorporation of xenobiotic lactational transfer to nursing pups (Byczkowski *et al.*, 1994; Fisher *et al.*, 1990; Sundberg *et al.*, 1998). Based on the potential sensitivity of children to OP insecticides, there is a need to develop quantitative models that can be used to assess the risk associated with OP exposure in infants and children. However, there are currently no published models available for OPs that are readily applicable for quantitating age-dependent changes in dose and response. For toxicants that have long residence times within the body, there is a need to develop PBPK models that appropriately incorporate growth and maturational development of physiological and metabolic function (O'Flaherty, 1991a).

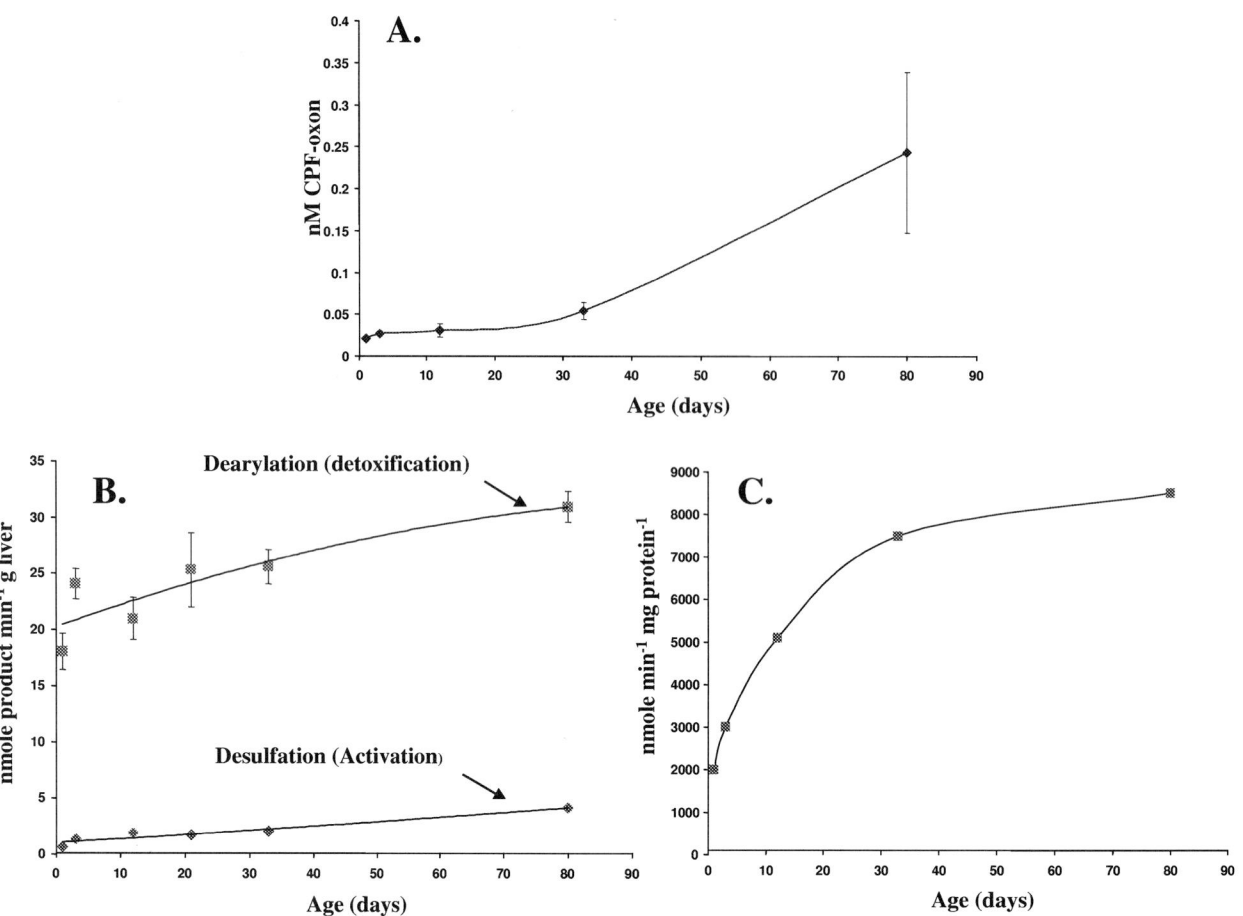

Figure 46.17 (A) Inhibitory concentration 50% (IC_{50}) of chlorpyrifos-oxon (CPF-oxon) (nM) to CaE activity in the liver of rats with increasing age, (B) CPF (50 μM) CYP450 desulfation and dearylation by rat hepatic microsomes with increasing age, (C) Developmental pattern of liver CaE activity with increasing age in the rat. All data was adapted from Atterberry *et al.* (1997).

O'Flaherty (1991a, b, 1993) has developed a series of PBPK models that begin to describe lead kinetics from birth to adulthood. Ultimately these models will enable quantitation of lead dosimetry over an entire lifetime. It is envisioned that the framework of the PBPK/PD model that has been developed for diisopropylfluorophosphate, parathion and chlorpyrifos (Gearhart *et al.*, 1990, 1994; Sultatos, 1990; Timchalk and Nolan, 1998) can readily be extended to incorporate age-dependent changes in CYP450, CaE, A-esterase and AchE activity.

In summary, pharmacokinetics and in particular the application of PBPK/PD modeling have been shown to be extremely useful approaches for dosimetry and biological response extrapolation for the assessment of human health risk from chemical exposures. The utilization of PBPK/PD modeling to address OP insecticide toxicity issues is particularly intriguing since these models can be used to assess the health consequences of both inter-individual (i.e., age, gender) and extrinsic factors (i.e., multiple exposure routes, chemical/drug interactions and variable exposure rates) that may significantly modify the toxicological response to OPs.

46.4 SUMMARY AND CONCLUSIONS

This chapter has illustrated a number of current and future applications of pharmacokinetics to assess OP dosimetry, biological response and risk in humans exposed to these insecticides. Pharmacokinetics is concerned with the quantitative integration of absorption, distribution, metabolism and excretion and can be used to provide useful insight into the toxicological responses associated with OP insecticides. Since OP insecticides share a common mode of action through their capability to inhibited AChE activity, it is feasible to develop pharmacokinetic strategies that link quantitative dosimetry with biologically based pharmacodynamic (PD) response modeling. Pharmacokinetic studies that have been conducted with OP insecticides in multiple species, at various dose levels, and across different routes of exposure have provided important insight into *in vivo* behavior of these OPs. The development and application of pharmacokinetic models capable of describing uptake, distribution, metabolism, and elimination of OP insecticides in humans represent a crucial research element needed for quantitative biomonitoring. In this regard, the successful application of biomonitoring for quantitating OP dose is primarily limited by the lack of this chemical-specific pharmacokinetic data in humans. The development and application of PBPK/PD modeling for OP insecticides represent a unique opportunity to quantitatively assess human health risk and to understand the toxicological implications of known or suspected exposures OPs. Validated PBPK/PD models for OPs can be used to consider the potential variability in human response associated with both interindividual (i.e., age, gender, polymorphism) and extrinsic variability (i.e., exposure routes and rates, single vs. multiple exposures).

In conclusion, pharmacokinetics have been successfully utilized to better understand the toxicological implications of human exposure to OP insecticides. Nonetheless, there is still a significant need to further develop and refine pharmacokinetic models that can be used to accurately assess the risk associated with OP insecticide exposures.

REFERENCES

Andersen, M. E. (1995). Physiologically based pharmacokinetic (PB-PK) models in the study of the disposition and biological effects of xenobiotics and drugs. *Toxicol. Lett.* **82/83**, 341–348.

Andersen, M. E., Clewell, H. J., III, Gargas, M. L., Smith, F. A., and Reitz, R. H. (1987a). Physiologically based pharmacokinetics and the risk assessment process for methylene chloride. *Toxicol. Appl. Pharmacol.* **87**, 185–205.

Andersen, M. E., Gargas, M. L., Clewell, H. J., III, and Severyn, K. M. (1987b). Quantitative evaluation of the metabolic interactions between trichloroethylene and 1,1-dichloroethylene *in vivo* using gas uptake methods. *Toxicol. Appl. Pharmacol.* **89**, 149–157.

Aprea, C., Betta, A., Catenacci, G., Lotti, A., Magnaghi, S., Barisano, A., Passini, V., Pavan, I., Sciarra, G., Vitalone, V., and Minoia, C. (1999). Reference values of urinary 3,5,6-trichloro-2-pyridinol in the Italian population—Validation of analytical method and preliminary results (multicentric study). *J. AOAC Int.* **82**, 305–312.

Aprea, C., Sciarra, G., Sartorelli, P., Desideri, E., Amati, R., and Sartorelli, E. (1994). Biological monitoring of exposure to organophosphate insecticides by assay of urinary alkylphosphates: Influence of protective measures during manual operations with treated plants. *Int. Arch. Occup. Environ. Health* **66**, 333–338.

Atterberry, T. T., Burnett, W. T., and Chambers, J. E. (1997). Age-related differences in parathion and chlorpyrifos toxicity in male rats: Target and nontarget esterase sensitivity and cytochrome P450-mediated metabolism. *Toxicol. Appl. Pharmacol.* **147**, 411–418.

Augustinsson, K.-B., and Barr, M. (1963). Age variation in plasma arylesterase activity in children. *Clin. Chem. Acta* **8**, 568–573.

Benke, G. M., and Murphy, S. D. (1975). The influence of age on the toxicity and metabolism of methyl parathion and parathion in male and female rats. *Toxicol. Appl. Pharmacol.* **31**, 254–269.

Benuck, M., Reith, M. E., Sershen, H., Wiener, H. L., and Lajtha, A. (1989). Oxidative metabolism of cocaine: Comparison of brain and liver. *Proc. Soc. Exp. Biol. Med.* **190**, 7–13.

Braeckman, R. A., Audenaert, F., Willems, J. L., Belpaire, F. M., and Bogaert, M. G. (1983). Toxicokinetics and methyl parathion and parathion in the dog after intravenous and oral administration. *Arch. Toxicol.* **54**, 71–82.

Brimer, L., Gyrd-Hansen, N., and Rasmussen, F. (1994). Disposition of parathion after dermal application in pigs. *J. Vet. Pharmacol. Ther.* **17**, 304–308.

Brodeur, J., and DuBois, K. P. (1963). Comparison of acute toxicity of anticholinesterase insecticides to weanling and adult male rats. *Proc. Soc. Exp. Biol. Med.* **114**, 509–511.

Byczkowski, J. Z., Kinkead, E. R., Leahy, H. F., Randall, G. M., and Fisher, J. W. (1994). Computer simulation of the lactational transfer of tetra-chloroethylene in rats using a physiologically based model. *Toxicol. Appl. Pharmacol.* **125**, 228–236.

Calabrese, E. J. (1991). Comparative metabolism: The principal cause of differential susceptibility to toxic and carcinogenic agents. *In* "Principles of Animal Extrapolation" (E. J. Calabrese, ed.), pp. 203–276. Lewis Publishers, Chelsea, MI.

Chambers, H. W. (1992). Organophosphorus compounds: An overview. *In* "Organophosphates—Chemistry, Fate and Effects" (J. E. Chambers and P. E. Levi, eds.), pp. 3–17. Academic Press, San Diego.

Chambers, J. E., and Chambers, H. W. (1989). Oxidative desulfation of chlorpyrifos, chlorpyrifos-methyl, and leptophos by rat brain and liver. *J. Biochem. Toxicol.* **4**, 201–203.

Chanda, S. M., Mortensen, S. R., Moser, V. C., and Padilla, S. (1997). Tissue-specific effects of chlorpyrifos on carboxylesterase and cholinesterase activity in adult rats: An *in vitro* and *in vivo* comparison. *Fundam. Appl. Toxicol.* **38**, 148–157.

Chandra *et al.* (1977).

Chester, G. (1993). Evaluation of agricultural worker exposure to and absorption of pesticides. *Occup. Hyg.* **37**, 509–523.

Clement, J. G. (1984). Role of aliesterase in organophosphate poisoning. *Fundam. Appl. Toxicol.* **4**, S96–S105.

Clewell, H. J., III (1995). The application of physiologically based pharmacokinetic modeling in human health risk assessment of hazardous substances. *Toxicol. Lett.* **79**, 207–217.

Clewell, H. J., III, and Andersen, M. E. (1996). Use of physiologically based pharmacokinetic modeling to investigate individual versus population risk. *Toxicology* **111**, 315–329.

Corley, R. A., Mendrala, A. L., Smith, F. A., Staats, D. A., Gargas, M. L., Conolly, R. B., Andersen, M. E., and Reitz, R. H. (1990). Development of a physiologically based pharmacokinetic model for chloroform. *Toxicol. Appl. Pharmacol.* **103**, 512–527.

Costa, L. G., McDonald, B. E., Murphy, S. D., Omenn, G. S., Richter, R. J., Motulsky, A. G., and Furlong, C. E. (1990). Serum paraoxonase and its influence on paraoxon and chlorpyrifos-oxon toxicity in rats. *Toxicol. Appl. Pharmacol.* **103**, 66–76.

Drevenkar, V., Vasilic, Z., Stengl, B., Frobe, Z., and Rumenjak, V. (1993). Chlorpyrifos metabolites in serum and urine of poisoned persons. *Chem.-Biol. Interact.* **87**, 315–322.

Eckerson, H. W., Wyte, C. M., and La Du, B. N. (1983). The human serum paraoxonase/arylesterase polymorphism. *Am. J. Hum. Genet.* **35**, 1126–1138.

Ellenhorn, M. J., and Barceloux, D. G. (1988). "Medical Toxicology—Diagnosis and Treatment of Human Poisoning," pp. 1074–1075. Elsevier, New York.

Ellman, G. L., Courtney, K. D., Andres, V., Jr., and Featherstone, R. M. (1961). A new and rapid colorimetric determination of acetylcholinesterase activity. *Biochem. Pharmacol.* **7**, 88–95.

El-Masri, H. A., Reardon, K. F., and Yang, R. S. H. (1997). Integrated approaches for the analysis of toxicologic interactions of chemical mixtures. *Crit. Rev. Toxicol.* **27**, 175–197.

Fisher, J. W., Whittaker, T. A., Taylor, D. H., Clewell, H. J., III, and Andersen, M. E. (1990). Physiologically based pharmacokinetic modeling of the lactating rat and nursing pup: A multiroute model for trichloroethylene and its metabolite, trichloroacetic acid. *Toxicol. Appl. Pharmacol.* **102**, 497–513.

Fonnum, F., Sterri, S. H., Aas, P., and Johnsen, H. (1985). Carboxyesterases, importance for detoxification of organophosphorus anticholinesterases and trichothecenes. *Fundam. Appl. Toxicol.* **5**, S29–S38.

Franklin, C. A., Fenske, R. A., Greenhalgh, R., Mathieu, L., Denley, H. V., Leffingwell, J. T., and Spear, R. C. (1981). Correlation of urinary pesticide metabolite excretion with estimated dermal contact in the course of occupational exposure to guthion. *J. Toxicol. Environ. Health* **7**, 715–731.

Franklin, C. A., Muir, N. I., and Moody, R. P. (1986). The use of biological monitoring in the estimation of exposure during the application of pesticides. *Toxicol. Lett.* **33**, 127–136.

Frawley, J. P., Fuyat, H. N., Hagen, E. C., Blake, J. R., and Fitzhugh, O. G. (1957). Marked potentiation in mammalian toxicity from simultaneous administration of two anticholinesterase compounds. *J. Pharmacol. Exp. Ther.* **121**, 96–106.

Frederick, C. B. (1995). Summary of panel discussion on the "Advantages/limitations/uncertainties in the use of physiologically based pharmacokinetic and pharmacodynamic models in hazard identification and risk assessment of toxic substances." *Toxicol. Lett.* **79**, 201–206.

Furlong, C. E., Richter, R. J., Seidel, S. L., and Motulsky, A. G. (1988). Role of genetic polymorphism of human plasma paraoxonase/arylesterase in hydrolysis of the insecticide metabolites chlorpyrifos oxon and paraoxon. *Am. J. Hum. Genet.* **43**, 230–238.

Gaines, T. B., and Linder, R. E. (1986). Acute toxicity of pesticides in adult and weanling rats. *Fundam. Appl. Toxicol.* **7**, 172–178.

Gargas, M. L., Burgess, R. J., Voisard, D. E., Cason, G. H., and Andersen, M. E. (1989). Partition coefficients of low-molecular-weight volatile chemicals in various liquids and tissues. *Toxicol. Appl. Pharmacol.* **97**, 87–99.

Gearhart, J. M., Jepson, G. W., Clewell, H. J., III, Andersen, M. E., and Conolly, R. B. (1990). Physiologically based pharmacokinetic and pharmacodynamic model for the inhibition of acetylcholinesterase by diisopropylfluorophosphate. *Toxicol. Appl. Pharmacol.* **106**, 295–310.

Gearhart, J. M., Jepson, G. W., Clewell, H. J., Andersen, M. E., and Conolly, R. (1994). Physiologically based pharmacokinetic model for the inhibition of acetylcholinesterase by organophosphate esters. *Environ. Health Perspect.* **102**, 51–59.

Geldmacher-von Mallinckrodt, M., Diepgen, T. L., Duhme, C., Hommel, G. (1983). A study of the polymorphism and ethnic distribution differences of human serum paraoxonase. *Am. J. Phys. Anthropol.* **62**, 235–241.

Griffin, P., Mason, H., Heywood, K., and Cocker, J. (1999). Oral and dermal absorption of chlorpyrifos: A human volunteer study. *Occup. Environ. Med.* **56**, 10–13.

Guengerich, F. P. (1977). Separation and purification of multiple forms of microsomal cytochrome P450. *J. Biol. Chem.* **252**, 3970–3979.

Harbison, R. D. (1975). Comparative toxicity of some selected pesticides in neonatal and adult rats. *Toxicol. Appl. Pharmacol.* **32**, 443–446.

Hayes, A. L., Wise, R. A., and Weir, F. W. (1980). Assessment of occupational exposure to organophosphates in pest control operators. *Am. Ind. Hyg. Assoc. J.* **41**, 568–575.

Hill, R. H., Jr., Head, S. L., Baker, S., Gregg, M., Shealy, D. B., Bailey, S. L., Williams, C. C., Sampson, E. J., and Needham, L. L. (1995). Pesticide residues in urine of adults living in the United States: Reference range concentrations. *Environ. Res.* **71**, 99–108.

Iverson, F., Grant, D. L., and Lacroix, J. (1975). Diazinon metabolism in the dog. *Bull. Environ. Contam. Toxicol.* **13**, 611–618.

Knaak, J. B., Al-Bayati, M. A., and Raabe, O. G. (1993). Physiologically based pharmacokinetic modeling to predict tissue dose and cholinesterase inhibition in workers exposed to organophosphorus and carbamate pesticides. *In* "Health Risk Assessment: Dermal and Inhalation Exposure and Absorption of Toxicants" (R. G. M. Wang, J. B. Knaak, and H. I. Maibach, eds.), pp. 3–29. CRC Press, Boca Raton, Fl.

Knaak, J. B., Al-Bayati, M., Raabe, O. G., and Blancato, J. N. (1990). *In vivo* percutaneous absorption studies in the rat: Pharmacokinetics and modeling of isofenphos absorption. *In* "Perdictions of Percutaneous Penetration" (R. Scott, R. Guy, and J. Hadgraft, eds.). IBC Technical Services, London.

Krishnan, K., and Andersen, M. E. (1994). Physiologically based pharmacokinetic modeling in toxicology. *In* "Principles and Methods of Toxicology" (A. Wallace Hayes, ed.), 3rd ed., pp. 149–188. Raven Press, New York.

Kump, D. F., Matulka, R. A., Edinboro, L. E., Poklis, A., and Holsapple, M. P. (1994). Disposition of cocaine and norcocaine in blood and tissues of $B_6C_3F_1$ mice. *J. Anal. Toxicol.* **18**, 342–345.

Lajtha, A., and Dunlop, D. (1981). Turnover of protein in nervous system. *Life Sci.* **28**, 755–767.

Lavy, T. L., Mattice, J. D., Massey, J. H., and Skulman, B. W. (1993). Measurements of year-long exposure to tree nursery workers using multiple pesticides. *Arch. Environ. Contam. Toxicol.* **24**, 123–144.

Leung, H. W., and Paustenbach, D. J. (1995). Physiologically based pharmacokinetic and pharmacodynamic modeling in health risk assessment and characterization of hazardous substances. *Toxicol. Lett.* **79**, 55–65.

Li, W. F., Costa, L. G., and Furlong, C. E. (1993). Serum paraoxonase status: A major factor in determining resistance to organophosphates. *J. Toxicol. Environ. Health* **40**, 337–346.

Li, W. F., Furlong, C. E., and Costa, L. G. (1995). Paraoxonase protects against chlorpyrifos toxicity in mice. *Toxicol. Lett.* **76**, 219–226.

Li, W.-F., Matthews, C., Disteche, C. M., Costa, L. G., and Furlong, C. E. (1997). Paraoxonase (PON1) gene in mice: Sequencing, chromosomal localization and developmental expression. *Pharmacogenetics* **7**, 137–144.

Loewenherz, C., Fenske, R. A., Simcox, N. J., Bellamy, B., and Kalman, D. (1997). Biological monitoring of organophosphorus pesticide exposure among children of agricultural workers in central Washington state. *Environ. Health Perspect.* **105**, 1344–1353.

Lotti, M., Moretto, A., Zoppellari, R., Dainese, R., Rizzuto, N., and Barusco, G. (1986). Inhibition of lymphocytic neropathy target esterase predicts the development of organophosphate-induced delayed neuropathy. *Arch. Toxicol.* **59**, 176–179.

Ma, T., and Chambers, J. E. (1994). Kinetic parameters of desulfuration and dearylation of parathion and chlorpyrifos by rat liver microsomes. *Food Chem. Toxicol.* **32**, 763–767.

Main, A. R. (1956). The role of A-esteraseease in the acute toxicity of paraoxon, TEPP and parathion. *Can. J. Biochem.* **34**, 197–216.

Mason, H., and Wilson, K. (1999). Biological monitoring: The role of toxicokinetics and physiologically based pharmacokinetic modeling. *Am. Ind. Hyg. Assoc. J.* **60**, 237–242.

Mileson, B. E., Chambers, J. E., Chen, W. L., Dettbarn, W., Ehrich, M., Eldefrawi, A. T., Gaylor, D. W., Kamernick, K., Hodgson, E., Karczmar, A. G., Padilla, S., Pope, C. N., Richardson, R. J., Saunders, D. R., Sheets, L. P., Sultatos, L. G., and Wallace, K. B. (1998). Common mechanism of toxicity: A case study of organophosphate pesticides. *Toxicol. Sci.* **41**, 8–20.

Miller, M. S., McCarver, D. G., Bell, D. A., Eaton, D. L., and Goldstein, J. A. (1997). Genetic polymorphisms in human drug metabolic enzymes. *Fundam. Appl. Toxicol.* **40**, 1–14.

Mortensen, S. R., Chanda, S. M., Hooper, M. J., and Padilla, S. (1996). Maturational differences in chlorpyrifos-oxonase activity may contribute to age-related sensitivity to chlorpyrifos. *J. Biochem. Toxicol.* **11**, 279–287.

Moser, V. C., and Padilla, S. (1998). Age- and gender-related differences in the time course of behavioral and biochemical effects produced by oral chlorpyrifos in rats. *Toxicol. Appl. Pharmacol.* **149**, 107–119.

Mücke, W., Alt, K. O., and Esser, H. O. (1970). Degradation of ^{14}C-labeled diazinon in the rat. *J. Agric. Food Chem.* **18**, 208–212.

Mueller, R. F., Hornung, S., Furlong, C. E., Anderson, J., Giblett, E. R., and Motulsky, A. G. (1983). Plasma paraoxonase polymorphism: A new enzyme assay, population, family, biochemical and linkage studies. *Am. J. Hum. Genet.* **35**, 393–408.

Murphy, S. D. (1986). Toxic effects of pesticides. *In* "Casarett and Doull's Toxicology: The Basic Science of Poison" (C. D. Klaassen, M. O. Amdur, and J. Doull, eds.), 3rd ed., pp. 519–581. MacMillam Co., New York.

Neal, R. A. (1980). Microsomal metabolism of thiono-sulfur compounds, mechanisms and toxicological significance. *In* "Reviews in Biochemical Toxicology" (E. Hodgson, J. R. Bend, and R. M. Philpot, eds.), Vol. 2, pp. 131–172. Elsevier–North-Holland, New York.

Nielsen, P., Friis, C., Gyrd-Hansen, N., and Kraul, I. (1991). Disposition of parathion in neonatal and young pigs. *Pharmacol. Toxicol.* **68**, 233–237.

Nolan, R. J., Rick, D. L., Freshour, N. L., and Saunders, J. H. (1984). Chlorpyrifos: Pharmacokinetics in human volunteers. *Toxicol. Appl. Pharmacol.* **73**, 8–15.

O'Flaherty, E. J. (1991a). Physiologically based models for bone-seeking elements. I. Rat skeletal and bone growth. *Toxicol. Appl. Pharmacol.* **111**, 299–312.

O'Flaherty, E. J. (1991b). Physiologically based models for bone-seeking elements. II. Kinetics of lead disposition in rats. *Toxicol. Appl. Pharmacol.* **111**, 313–331.

O'Flaherty, E. J. (1993). Physiologically based models for bone-seeking elements. II. Kinetics of lead disposition in humans. *Toxicol. Appl. Pharmacol.* **118**, 16–29.

O'Flaherty, E. J. (1995). PBK modeling for metals: Examples with lead, uranium and chromium. *Toxicol. Lett.* **82/83**, 367–372.

O'Shaughnessy, J. A., and Sultatos, L. G. (1995). Interaction of ethanol and the organophosphorus insecticide parathion. *Biochem. Pharmacol.* **50**, 1925–1932.

Pelekis, M., and Krishnan, K. (1997). Assessing the relevance of rodent data on chemical interactions for health risk assessment purposes: A case study with dichloromethane–toluene mixture. *Regul. Toxicol. Pharmacol.* **25**, 79–86.

Pena-Egido, M. J., Rivas-Gonzalo, J. C., and Marino-Hernandez, E. L. (1988). Toxicokinetics of parathion in the rabbit. *Arch. Toxicol.* **61**, 196–200.

Pond, A. L., Chambers, H. W., and Chambers, J. E. (1995). Organophosphate detoxification potential of various rat tissues via A-esterase and aliesterase activity. *Toxicol. Lett.* **78**, 245–252.

Pope, C. N., and Liu, J. (1997). Age-related differences in sensitivity to organophosphorus pesticides. *Environ. Toxicol. Pharmacol.* **4**, 309–314.

Pope, C. N., Chakraborti, T. K., Chapman, M. L., Farrar, J. D., and Arthun, D. (1991). Comparison of the *in vivo* cholinesterase inhibition in neonatal and adult rats by three organophosphorothioate insecticides. *Toxicology* **68**, 51–61.

Purcell, K. J., Cason, G. H., Gargas, M. L., Andersen, M. E., and Travis, C. C. (1990). *In vivo* metabolic interactions of benzene and toluene. *Toxicol. Lett.* **52**, 141–152.

Renwick, A. G. (1994). Toxicokinetics—Pharmacokinetics in toxicology. *In* "Principles and Methods of Toxicology" (A. Wallace Hayes, ed.), 3rd ed., pp. 101–147. Raven Press, New York.

Richter, E. D., Kowalski, M., Leventhal, A., Grauer, F., Marzouk, J., Brenner, S., Shkolnik, I., Lerman, S., Zahavi, H., Bashari, A., Peretz, A., Kaplanski, H., Gruener, N., and Ben Ishai, P. (1992). Illness and excretion of organophosphate metabolites four months after household pest extermination. *Arch. Environ. Health* **47**, 135–138.

Sato, A., and Nakajima, T. (1979). Partition coefficients of some aromatic hydrocarbons and ketones in water, blood, and oil. *Br. J. Ind. Med.* **36**, 231–234.

Slob, W., Janssen, P. H., and van den Hof, J. M. (1997). Structural identifiability of PBPK models: Practical consequences for modeling strategies and study design. *Crit. Rev. Toxicol.* **27**, 261–272.

Srinivasan, R. S., Bourne, D. W. A., and Putcha, L. (1994). Application of physiologically based pharmacokinetic models for assessing drug disposition in space. *J. Clin. Pharmacol.* **34**, 692–698.

Sultatos, L. G. (1988). Factors affecting the hepatic biotransformation of the phosphorothioate pesticide chlorpyrifos. *Toxicology* **51**, 191–200.

Sultatos, L. G. (1990). A physiologically based pharmacokinetic model of parathion based on chemical-specific parameters determined *in vitro*. *J. Am. Coll. Toxicol.* **9**, 611–619.

Sultatos, L. G. (1994). Mammalian toxicology of organophosphorus pesticides. *J. Toxicol. Environ. Health* **43**, 271–289.

Sultatos, L. G., Basker, K. M., Shao, M., and Murphy, S. D. (1984). The interaction of the phosphorothioate insecticides chlorpyrifos and parathion and their oxygen analogues with bovine serum albumin. *Mol. Pharmacol.* **26**, 99–104.

Sultatos, L. G., Shao, M., and Murphy, S. D. (1984). The role of hepatic biotransformation in mediating the acute toxicity of the phosphorothionate insecticide chlorpyrifos. *Toxicol. Appl. Pharmacol.* **73**, 60–68.

Sundberg, J., Jonsson, S., Karlsson, M. O., Palminger Hallen, I., and Oskarson, A. (1998). Kinetics of methylmercury and inorganic mercury in lactating and nonlactating mice. *Toxicol. Appl. Pharmacol.* **151**, 319–329.

Tardif, R., Charest-Tardif, G., Brodeur, J. and Krishnan, K. (1997). Physiologically based pharmacokinetic modeling of a ternary mixture of alkyl benzenes in rats and humans. *Toxicol. Appl. Pharmacol.* **144**, 120–134.

Tardif, R., Lapare, S., Charest-Tardif, G., Brodeur, J., and Krishnan, K. (1995). Physiologically-based pharmacokinetic modeling of a mixture of toluene and xylene in humans. *Risk Anal.* **15**, 335–342.

Tardif, R., Lapare, S., Krishnan, K., and Brodeur, J. (1993). Physiologically based modeling of the toxicokinetic interaction between toluene and *m*-xylene in the rat. *Toxicol. Appl. Pharmacol.* **120**, 266–273.

Timchalk, C., and Nolan, R. J. (1998). Physiologically based pharmacokinetic/pharmacodynamic (PBPK/PD) modeling of chlorpyrifos and its oxon metabolite in the rat. *Toxicol. Sci.* **42**, 693.

Tomokuni, K., Hasegawa, T., Hirai, Y., and Koga, N. (1985). The tissue distribution of diazinon and the inhibition of blood cholinesterase activities in rats and mice receiving a single intraperitoneal dose of diazinon. *Toxicology* **37**, 91–98.

Vale, J. A. (1998). Toxicokinetic and toxicodynamic aspects of organophosphate (OP) insecticide poisoning. *Toxicol. Lett.* **102–103**, 649–652.

Vale, J. A., and Scott, G. W. (1974). Organophosphate poisoning. *Guy's Hosp. Gazette* **123**, 12–25.

Vasilic, Z., Drevenkar, V., Rumenjak, V., Stengl, B., and Frobe, Z. (1992). Urinary elimination of diethylphosphorus metabolites in persons poisoned by quinalphos or chlorpyrifos. *Arch. Environ. Contam. Toxicol.* **22**, 351–357.

Waldron-Lechner, D., and Abdel-Rahman, M. S. (1986). Kinetics of carbaryl and malathion in combination in the rat. *J. Toxicol. Environ. Health* **18**, 241–256.

Wester, R. C., and Maibach, H. I. (1983). Cutaneous pharmacokinetics: 10 steps to percutaneous absorption. *Drug Metab. Rev.* **14**, 169–205.

Wester, R. C., Maibach, H. I., Bucks, D. A. W., and Guy, R. H. (1983). Malathion percutaneous absorption after repeated administration to man. *Toxicol. Appl. Pharmacol.* **68**, 116–119.

Wester, R. C., Maibach, H. I., Melendres, J., Sedik, L., Knaak, J., and Wang, R. (1992). *In vivo* and *in vitro* percutaneous absorption and skin evaporation of isofenphos in man. *Fundam. Appl. Pharmacol.* **19**, 521–526.

Wester, R. C., Sedik, L., Melendres, J., Logan, F., Maibach, H. I., and Russell, I. (1993). Percutaneous absorption of diazinon in humans. *Food Chem. Toxicol.* **31**, 569–572.

Wilks, M. F., and Woollen, B. H. (1994). Human volunteer studies with nonpharmaceutical chemicals: Metabolism and pharmacokinetic studies. *Hum. Exp. Toxicol.* **13**, 383–392.

Woollen, B. H. (1993). Biological monitoring for pesticide absorption. *Occup. Hyg.* **37**, 525–540.

Wu, H. X., Evreux-Gros, C., Descottes, J. (1996). Diazinon toxicokinetics, tissue distribution and anticholinesterase activity in the rat. *Biomed. Environ. Sci.* **9**, 359–369.

Neuropathy Target Esterase

Martin K. Johnson and Paul Glynn
Medical Research Council Toxicology, UK

47.1 INTRODUCTION

Neuropathy target esterase (NTE) is a biochemical mystery. This protein, present in neural tissue, has the capacity to catalyze rapid hydrolysis of certain (unphysiological) carboxylate ester substrates, and, similar to acetylcholinesterase (AChE), its catalytic activity is inhibited by covalent reaction with a variety of progressive inhibitors, including organophosphorus esters (OPs). However, mere loss of the catalytic activity of NTE seems not to be deleterious in adult animals. Rather, the nature of the chemical group covalently bound at the catalytic centre determines whether toxicological effects will follow. Thirty years after its discovery, there is now overwhelming evidence that initiation of OPIDN (organophosphorus ester–induced delayed neuropathy) starts with NTE: Initiation may occur within hours of ingestion of a single dose of some OPs although clinical expression is deferred for 1–4 weeks. The clinical and morphological features of OPIDN are described in Chapter 49 as are some of the biochemical and physiological changes reported to accompany (consequentially or causally) the development of the syndrome after initiation. In this chapter, we review briefly the evidence for NTE as the target and the mechanism of initiation and the possible involvement of related esterases to promotion of OPIDN. This is followed by a discussion of the application of NTE studies to human risk evaluation. Finally, we consider the nature and properties of this remarkable protein, its function in neurons, and its role in OPIDN.

47.2 BRIEF REVIEW OF THE EVIDENCE

47.2.1 ORGANOPHOSPHORUS ESTER PESTICIDES: GENERAL REACTIONS WITH SERINE ESTERASES

Acetylcholinesterase, the intended target for OP pesticides, is a member of a large family of serine esterases (Krejci *et al.*, 1991; Taylor, 1992). A particular serine residue at the active site of these enzymes is rendered reactive by the presence of a histidine and a glutamate or aspartate, the components of the catalytic triad. Serine esterases catalyze hydrolysis of carboxylate esters by the mechanism shown, in highly simplified form, in Fig. 47.1a, which involves formation of a covalent acyl enzyme intermediate. This mechanism is essentially the same in serine proteases such as chymotrypsin, which cleave peptide bonds with intermediate formation of a covalent acyl enzyme (Aldridge and Reiner, 1972).

OP pesticides have been made from a variety of organophosphates, -phosphonates, -phosphinates, or -phosphoramidates. As a class, these compounds are hydrolyzable esters and act as pseudo-substrates for a variety of serine esterases and proteases. As an example, the reaction of an organophosphate with a serine esterase is shown in simplified form in Fig. 47.1b. The rate of hydrolysis of the phosphorylated enzyme is greatly (6–10 orders of magnitude) reduced compared to that of the acyl enzyme. Thus, the enzyme becomes virtually permanently inhibited, although certain nucleophilic agents such as oximes or fluoride anion can catalyze a speedier dephosphorylation—hence the therapeutic use of oximes in the treatment of acetylcholinesterase poisoning. However, the phosphorylated enzyme can subsequently undergo a second reaction, known as aging, which, in the case shown of an organophosphate, results in the liberation of one of the bound R groups into solution (Fig. 47.1b). This leaves the active-site serine covalently attached to a negatively charged monoorganophosphoryl moiety, which is significantly more resistant to removal by therapeutic nucleophiles. Organophosphinates, in which both R groups are directly attached to the phosphorus atom, also covalently react with the active-site serine but cannot undergo the aging reaction (Fig. 47.1c).

47.2.2 NEUROPATHY TARGET ESTERASE AS THE TARGET FOR INITIATION OF ORGANOPHOSPHORUS ESTER-INDUCED DELAYED NEUROPATHY

Elucidation of the events that initiate OPIDN involved a sequence of observations *in vitro* and *ex vivo* on the interaction of radiolabeled diisopropyl phosphorofluoridate (DFP) and other

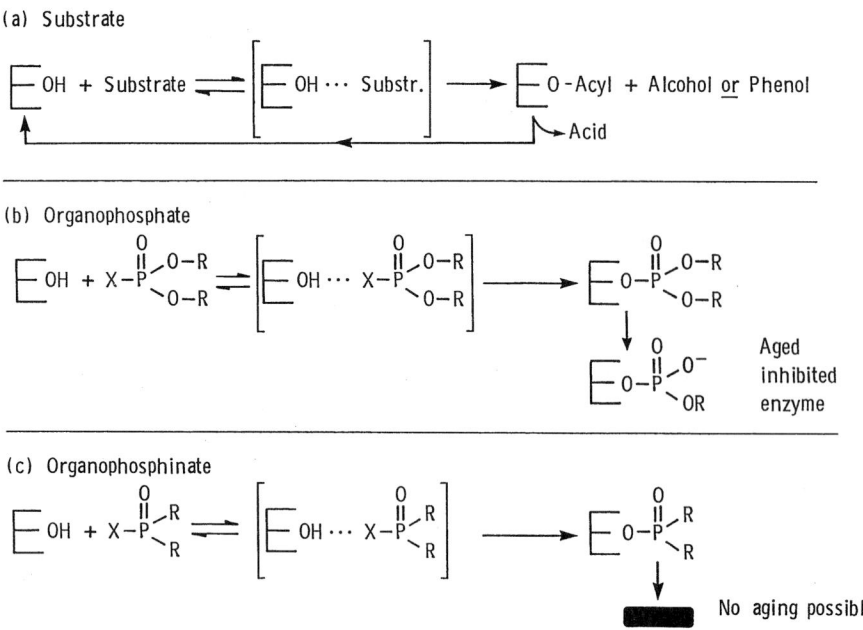

Figure 47.1 Reaction of a serine esterase with a carboxylate ester substrate and with organophosphate and organophosphinate inhibitors. The reactive serine residue at the enzyme active site is represented by —OH. (a) Following reversible formation of an enzyme–substrate Michaelis complex (in square brackets), the serine residue makes a nucleophilic attack on the acyl carbon of the ester and forms a tetrahedral hemiacetal intermediate (not shown). The alcohol moiety is rapidly expelled from this intermediate to produce a covalent acyl enzyme. Rapid aqueous hydrolysis of the acyl enzyme liberates the carboxylic acid and regenerates free enzyme. (b) Part of the efficacy of OP esters as serine esterase inhibitors results from their structural resemblance to the tetrahedral hemiacetal intermediate formed between the enzyme and the carboxylate ester substrate. The rate of hydrolysis of the organophosphorylated or organophosphinylated enzyme is much slower than that of the acyl enzyme, resulting in essentially irreversible inhibition. In addition, organophosphates, but not organophosphinates, are able to undergo a second reaction termed aging. This entails loss of one of the R groups from the organophosphorylated enzyme leaving a negatively charged species attached to the active site.

(unlabeled) esterase inhibitors (OPs, carbamates, and sulfonyl fluorides) with homogenized whole brain of adult chickens: The evidence, doubts, and arguments are detailed by Johnson (1990). In brief, because preliminary study showed that DFP bound only to proteins, criteria were adopted for a putative target site which would be a protein able to undergo the same set of general reactions shown in Fig. 47.1. It was found that about 5% of total DFP-labeling sites in hen brain were not covalently blocked by a variety of OPs known not to cause OPIDN but were inhibited at toxicologically relevant doses by neuropathic compounds. Extensive screening then showed that only two out of more than 60 hydrolyzable esters, lipids, and or peptides competed with labeling of that subset, suggesting that only these two had significant affinity for the relevant DFP-reactive sites. Finally, only one of several esterases that could hydrolyze these competitors (phenyl esters of phenylacetic acid and valeric acid) shared the same inhibitor responses as the apparently homogeneous target site (Johnson, 1969a, b, 1970). This esterase was dubbed NTE for neurotoxic esterase and, later, neuropathy target esterase; its ability to hydrolyze phenyl valerate (PV) in a reaction sensitive to neuropathic OPs forms the basis for a widely used *in vitro* screening test for such OPs. A threshold level of about 70–90% inhibition of NTE in the brain and spinal cord of test adult chickens has been found to be the

norm for precipitation of clinically visible OPIDN, and this criterion has been incorporated into current regulatory guidelines (see Section 47.3).

Progressive inhibitors of NTE were found to fall into two classes: Some were neuropathic but others, which were unable because of their chemical structure to undergo an aging reaction analogous to that shown in Fig. 47.1b, were not only not neuropathic, but they were actually specifically prophylactic against OPIDN (not against acute anticholinesterase effects) if given to chickens prior to a neuropathic OP. These prophylactic compounds included carbamates (Johnson and Lauwerys, 1969), sulfonyl fluorides (Johnson, 1970), and phosphinates (as in Fig. 47.1c; Johnson, 1974). The most striking evidence for the validity of NTE as the true target has been the correlation in time of the degree of inhibition of NTE (and of the radiolabeled target) by the nonaging compounds with their prophylactic effect: both short-term (hours) and long-term (up to 5 days) prophylaxis is possible according to the structure of the agent and the "window" correlates with the persistence of inhibition until about 70–80% of NTE is again available to neuropathic challenge by virtue of reactivation or turnover of the inhibited enzyme [summarized by Johnson (1990)].

OPIDN prophylaxis by nonaging NTE inhibitors led to the proposal that generation of a negative charge at the active site of NTE was critical for initiation of OPIDN (Johnson, 1974). A neat confirmation of the importance of the aging reaction in initiation is the demonstration that, in the case of chiral phosphonates such as the oxon of EPN (*O*-ethyl *O*-4-nitrophenyl phenylphosphonothioate), both enantiomers can inhibit NTE at tolerable doses *in vivo*, but the one that engages in the subsequent aging reaction causes OPIDN whereas the other is prophylactic (Johnson and Read, 1987). This raises special questions about the interpretation of regulatory tests for chiral compounds (see Section 47.3.3.3).

47.2.3 POSSIBLE INVOLVEMENT OF OTHER ESTERASES IN ORGANOPHOSPHORUS ESTER-INDUCED DELAYED NEUROPATHY

Accumulated evidence has supported the early identification of NTE as the site for initiation of OPIDN. However, although all detectable binding sites for [^{32}P]-labeled DFP in brain were dissected, it has been proposed that further sites were actually present at such low concentration that they were undetectable but might have equal claim to be the initiating site. No convincing evidence for this idea has emerged over many years, but the role of the recently identified "soluble NTE" is worthy of further consideration (Vilanova *et al.*, 1999). NTE is only one of at least six distinct phenyl valerate hydrolases easily demonstrated to be present in hen brain (Johnson, 1982a) and, until recently, no association of any of these with normal or abnormal processes had been demonstrated. However, Vilanova and colleagues have made extensive studies of NTE and related enzymes in sciatic nerve of the hen because that tissue undergoes more obvious degenerative changes in OPIDN than does brain [reviewed by Vilanova *et al.* (1999)]. They have identified and studied what appears to be a freely soluble enzyme behaving rather like NTE according to inhibition characteristics. Apart from having a lower apparent molecular size than the NTE subunit from brain particles (Escudero and Vilanova, 1997), the most striking characteristic of this and related soluble sciatic nerve PV hydrolases is the sensitivity of one or more of these esterases to paraoxon with which they react rapidly and progressively to form covalently inhibited enzymes, which then spontaneously reactivate within a few hours at body temperature. Thus, in the standard *in vitro* laboratory assay for NTE, such enzymes are excluded by the paraoxon preincubation but, *in vivo*, they would, for practical purposes, appear to be insensitive to that OP and could therefore be added to the list of putative targets for the site of initiation of OPIDN (Barril *et al.*, 1999). The uncovering of these enzymes is a tribute to more careful kinetic analysis of the OP/enzyme interaction than has been possible in some general screening operations. Furthermore, these researchers have shown that paraoxon competes strongly with substrate in the assay of soluble NTE so that the activity in sciatic nerve has routinely been underestimated by 20-fold or more (Barril and Vilanova, 1997). Fortunately, neither of these confusing factors seems to exist with regard to

particulate NTE. The possible relevance of any of these soluble enzymes to either initiation of OPIDN or to its promotion (a phenomenon discussed in Chapter 49) requires evaluation by structure–activity studies using autopsy tissue from hens dosed with a battery of neuropathic and nonneuropathic OPs. Thus far, studies *in vitro* with the soluble enzymes (Vilanova *et al.*, 1999) discourage an association because sensitivity to mipafox *in vitro* is so considerable (I$_{50}$ less than 0.1 μM compared with 7 μM for NTE) that one might expect that such activities would be fully inhibited *in vivo* at doses that would barely affect NTE and would be well below the neuropathic or promoting dose.

Lotti and colleagues have produced some correlative structure–activity evidence to suggest that the target for promotion of OPIDN by certain OPs is not one of the two paraoxon-sensitive hydrolases first identified by Poulsen and Aldridge (1964) but may be a component of the particulate PV hydrolases, which they have dubbed "M-200" on the basis of its comparatively low sensitivity to mipafox. M-200 is a portion of the *C* activity (see Section 47.4.2), which can be segregated in assays where mipafox concentration is raised (from the 50 μM used in standard assays) to detect an enzyme with an I$_{50}$ of 200 μM (Lotti and Moretto, 1999; Milatovic *et al.*, 1997). Further evaluation of these encouraging observations is in progress (M. Lotti, private communication). Also, Vilanova and colleagues have identified a component of soluble PV hydrolases that fits the characteristics of the target for promoters rather than initiators of OPIDN (Céspedes *et al.*, 1997; Vilanova *et al.*, 1999).

47.3 TOXOLOGICAL APPLICATIONS

47.3.1 HEN TEST

As noted in Chapter 49, OP pesticides are screened for their relative abilities to inhibit acetylcholinesterase and to cause OPIDN; consequently, humans and susceptible animals are unlikely to develop OPIDN without acute cholinergic toxicity following OP pesticide exposure. The hen test has developed in sophistication from its origins in studies in the early 1930s, which showed that mature adult chickens were the most satisfactory animals to detect the OPIDN potential of various OPs found in the toxic "Ginger Jake" drink that paralyzed thousands of people in the southern United States (Smith *et al.*, 1930). OPIDN in the adult chicken is, at present, the best available model for the human syndrome. Historically, it was found that hens responded positively and uniformly in tests of compounds suspected of causing OPIDN in humans. The best known examples were tri-cresyl phosphates (not insecticides) and mipafox and leptophos which were pesticides responsible for OPIDN incidents in the United Kingdom and the United States. The spinal tracts, which are known to suffer selective damage in human OPIDN, are well-developed in hens and damage to these regions is easily detected by standard techniques (see Chapter 49). Furthermore, slight abnormalities of gait are easily detected in these bipeds. Biochemically, the sensitivity of hen and human NTE to inhibition by OP inhibitors is similar (Lotti and Johnson, 1978).

Since the 1950s, the UK Ministry of Agriculture Fisheries and Food has required information about the OPIDN potential of OP pesticides submitted for registration. Briefly, batches of hens are required to be dosed with about the maximum tolerable dose accompanied by therapeutic measures to carry them through the inevitable cholinergic crisis. After observation over a period of 21 days for signs of ataxia, positively affected birds are autopsied and histopathological signs are sought: Unaffected birds are redosed and the observation is continued for an additional 21 days with sample birds being autopsied at the conclusion regardless of the presence or absence of clinical signs. Since the 1970s, the U.S. Environmental Protection Agency (U.S. EPA) has required clinical and histopathological tests after long-term (often 90 days) feeding of tolerable low levels of OPs. However, in spite of such testing procedures becoming mandatory, reports continue to appear of occasional cases of full-blown OPIDN resulting from occupational exposure or suicide attempts with pesticides, including methamidophos, leptophos, dichlorvos, trichlorphon, chlorpyrifos, and EPN (Lotti, 1992). The possibility of less severe clinical cases being overlooked has caused concern, and improvements in the discriminatory power of regulatory tests for OPIDN are clearly desirable.

Assay of NTE activity in appropriate autopsy samples taken soon after dosing became first an optional extra, then recommended, and finally a required component of OPIDN toxicity tests over a period of about 20 years following the first reports of the enzyme in 1969, although some manufacturers adopted the procedure voluntarily very early (U.S. EPA, 1991; OECD, 1995). The biochemical test does not replace clinical and histopathological observation but, rather, complements them (ECETOC, 1998; Johnson, 1984). It has the advantage that, unlike those subjective and qualitative tests, it is quantitative so that the degree of risk of OPIDN arising from a defined dose can be assessed: hitherto the conclusion from tests could only be 'Yes/No" or occasionally "Marginal." Furthermore, sufficient data on the relationship of chemical structure to neuropathic response have been accumulated in experimental studies *in vivo* (Johnson, 1975a) and *in vitro* (the latter using both human and animal tissues; Johnson, 1975b, 1988; Lotti and Johnson, 1978) that fairly confident predictions of the OPIDN potential of an untested compound can be made: Monitoring of NTE activity in accessible tissue samples taken from a few patients who have deliberately ingested known OPs confirms the relationship (Moretto and Lotti, 1998).

Although the early work studied brain tissue only, it is accepted that clinical signs of OPIDN reflect the fact that neuropathic lesions are scarce in brain and more marked in spinal cord and peripheral nerve (see Chapter 49). In some early experiments with dichlorvos (Johnson, 1978), the dose (although many times the LD_{50}) appeared not to have reached the spinal cord sufficiently to inhibit NTE and no clinical signs developed in pair-dosed birds although brain NTE was in-

hibited. A further dose was necessary to increase inhibition in spinal cord and to precipitate clinical neuropathy. For this reason, it is now customary for *ex vivo* assays from dosed birds to study both tissues and it is not uncommon to find slightly less inhibition in cord than in brain: The threshold figure of inhibition is accordingly set a little lower for spinal cord.

47.3.2 STRUCTURE–ACTIVITY RELATIONSHIPS AND PREDICTION OF ORGANOPHOSPHORUS ESTER-INDUCED DELAYED NEUROPATHY POTENTIAL IN HENS

The ability to analyze both positive and negative clinical responses in terms of the degree of effect on NTE during OPIDN tests made it possible to review a large amount of test data and to define guidelines for predicting neuropathic potential of both the plasticizer and the pesticide types of OP esters (Johnson, 1975a, 1982a). Guidelines (to be taken in concert) concerning the likelihood that a pesticide-type OP ester with general structure $R^1R^2P(O \text{ or } S)X$ will cause neuropathy at less than lethal doses are as follows:

1. Factors that *increase* OPIDN potential more than acute toxicity include:

   a. Choice of phosphonates or phosphoramidates rather than analogous phosphates
   b. Increase in chain length or hydrophobicity of R^1 and R^2
   c. A leaving group X that does not sterically hinder approach to the active site of NTE

2. Factors that *decrease* the comparative potential include:

   a. The converse of factors 1a–c
   b. Choice of R or X groups that are very bulky (naphthyloxy) or nonplanar
   c. Choice of a nitrophenyl group at X
   d. Choice of comparatively more hydrophilic X groups (oximes or heterocyclics)
   e. Choice of thioether linkages at X

Although inclusion of NTE assays in toxicological tests is now mandatory for all OP pesticides submitted for registration or re-registration, most data do not reach the open literature. Table 47.1 lists the results for compounds reported for 1975–1981 (Johnson, 1982a). Considering the structure–activity factors, it is clear why malathion, parathion, fenitrothion, and diazinon among the compounds listed are all far below the hazard line for OPIDN and why EPN, a phosphonothioate with a hydrophobic phenyl group at R, is neuropathic even with a 4-nitrophenyl leaving group. Also, it is not surprising that other phenylphosphonothioates such as desbromo-leptophos or cyanofenphos are also neuropathic (Johnson, 1975a; Soliman *et al.*, 1986) and

Table 47.1
NTE and Clinical OPIDN Responses of Pesticides Reported 1975–1981[a]

Pesticide	Dose (mg/kg)^3	Brain enzyme inhibition (%)		Clinical response (+ or −)
		AChE	NTE	
Diazinon	20	55	0	−
(EtO)$_2$ · P(S)·O-[6-Me-2-(1-methylethyl)]-4-pyrimidinyl	50**			−
Malathion	1000*	97	15	−
(MeO)$_2$ · P(S)·S · CH · CO · OEt				
CH$_2$ · CO · OEt				
Chlorpyrifos	100*		51	−
(EtO)$_2$ · P(S) · O-(3,5,6-Cl$_3$)-2-pyrimidinyl				
Methamidophos	50***		50	−
MeO · P · (O) · (NH$_2$) · SMe				
Methyl parathion	100**	85	12	−
(MeO)$_2$ · P(S) · O-(4-NO$_2$ · Ph)				
Fenitrothion	500*	78	8	−
(MeO)$_2$ · P(S) · O-(3-Me-4-NO$_2$ · Ph)				
Cyanophos	20*	75	0	−
(MeO)$_2$ · P(S) · O-(4-CN · Ph)				
Salithion	100*	76	72	−
(MeO) · P(S) · O-C$_6$H$_4$-2-CH$_2$O				
Cyanofenphos	100	74	75	−
EtO · (Ph) · P(S) · O-(4-CN · Ph)	303		83–90	+
EPN (racemic)	50*		60	−
EtO · (Ph) · P(S) · O-(4-NO$_2$ · Ph)	53–69*			±
EPN (+)	50**		45	−
	69–89***			−
	10–20 × 5			±
EPN (−)	50*		75	±
	69*			+
Omethoate	75*	>90	0	−
(MeO)$_2$ · P(O) · S · CH$_2$ · C(O) · NH · CH$_3$	150–300***	>90	0	−
Carbophenothion (Trithion)	90 × 50***		0	−
(EtO)$_2$ · P(S) · S-(4-Cl · Ph)				
Parathion	Range +		Low	−
(EtO)$_2$ · P(S) · O-(4-NO$_2$ · Ph)	55 × 6***			

[a]From Johnson (1982a). All doses were administered orally in corn oil (or glycerol formal). NTE reponse was measured 1–2 days after dosing; for several compounds, inhibition peaked at day 2. Where clinical response was negative, the dose is marked according to whether it was about LD$_{50}$, *; 1–2 × LD$_{50}$, **; or more than twice the LD$_{50}$, ***.

that, in its homologous series, only dichlorvos is not neuropathic at the LD$_{50}$ dose (Table 47.2). Apart from the obvious correlation with clinical effects at both ends of the range of inhibition, there was a valuable warning of risk with chlorpyriphos dosed to hens at about LD$_{50}$: At that time, this pesticide was regarded as nonneuropathic on the basis of approved tests involving only clinical and histopathological measures. The risk indication was vindicated by positive OPIDN seen in both hens given higher doses and in a failed human suicide attempt (Capodicasa *et al.*, 1991; Moretto and Lotti, 1998).

47.3.3 APPLICATION OF NEUROPATHY TARGET ESTERASE STUDIES TO HUMAN RISK ASSESSMENT

47.3.3.1 *In Vitro* Comparison of Enzyme Targets

When OP esters that exert biological effects *in vivo* are administered to animals, they are subjected to a variety of processes (absorption, metabolic activation and/or deactivation, distribution and/or excretion, etc.) before a certain amount of a proximal toxin is delivered to the ultimate targets—acetylcholinesterase

Table 47.2
Relative Effects of Some OP Esters against Two Toxicity Targets of the Hen Assessed *in vitro* and *in vivo*[a]

Compound	*In vitro* AChe I_{50}/NTE I_{50}	*In vivo* LD_{50}/NTD
Dimethyl 2,2-dichlorovinyl phosphate	0.02	0.05
Diethyl 2,2-dichlorovinyl phosphate	0.16	0.17
Di-*n*-propyl 2,2-dichlorovinyl phosphate	2.6	5
Di-*n*-pentyl 2,2-dichlorovinyl phosphate	32	13
Leptophos oxon	0.2	nd*
Leptophos	*b*	0.8
Trichloronate oxon[c]	0.1	nd*
Trichloronate	*b*	0.15
Mipafox	5.9	>1
DFP	0.9	1

[a] From Johnson (1982a) who compiled *in vivo* data from several sources. NTD is that dose that caused severe ataxia in the majority of hens tested.
[b] Thionates free of oxons have negligible antiesterase activity *in vitro*.
[c] Trichloronate oxon is ethyl 2,4,5-trichlorophenyl ethylphosphonate.
*nd: not determined.

in the case of acute toxicity and NTE for delayed neuropathy. However, because the targets for both acute and delayed toxicity are associated with nervous tissue, it seems reasonable to propose that whatever percentage of a dose ultimately reached the nervous system in appropriately reactive form, then that amount would prefer to react with AChE or NTE according to the relative potencies demonstrable with these enzymes *in vitro*. Table 47.2 demonstrates a fair correlation between the *relative potencies in vitro* and *in vivo* of a variety of compounds not restricted to one homologous series. Use of the *in vitro* ratios, which can be determined easily and very early in a development program, may serve to guide synthetic chemists away from structures carrying neuropathic hazard.

Although such *in vitro/in vivo* correlations have been obtained, the following assumptions built into the system need to be recognized:

1. For compounds that require metabolic activation *in vivo,* the actual inhibitor species must be identified and tested *in vitro*.
2. The inhibitor has equal access to both enzymes in the brain.
3. The rates of synthesis of fresh NTE and AChE are sufficiently slow not to affect the prognosis after an intoxication that causes massive inhibition of enzymes.
4. The rate of aging of NTE is rapid compared with the rates of synthesis of new enzymes.
5. The extent of spontaneous reactivation of inhibited enzymes *in vivo* is small.
6. The hen is an adequate model for humans.

Assumption 1 is often possible for OP pesticides. There is good evidence to support assumptions 2–4. Assumption 5 appears true for NTE in our experience; inhibited NTE ages with a half-life of less than 1 h to a nonreactivatable form in most cases tested and there is little spontaneous reactivation of NTE. However, assumption 5 is not true in all cases of AChE inhibition. For example, after poisoning with haloxon, the di-2-chloroethylphosphorylated acetylcholinesterase has a half-life of approximately 22 min. Consequently, the acute toxicity of haloxon is less than might have been predicted and although the ratio of I_{50}s for this compound is 0.01, it is, in fact, neuropathic at less than the LD_{50} dose (Johnson, 1982a). For a similar reason, methamidophos has caused OPIDN in humans, although in hens neuropathy is not caused by doses less than 6–8 times the unprotected LD_{50} given with massive treatment to prevent cholinergic death (Johnson, 1981; Lotti, 1992; Senanayake and Johnson, 1982a). Assumption 6 is considered in more detail later in the chapter.

The previous considerations led to the suggestion that any compound for which the ratio is more than 0.05 should be viewed with strong suspicion and that neuropathy may be caused in atropinized birds with single doses of compounds where the ratio is as low as 0.01.

In spite of such a large difference in species type, it has been shown that the target enzymes in humans and hens are similar in their response to OP inhibitors; the I_{50}s for both AChE and NTE differed between species by no more than a factor of 4 and often by less (Lotti and Johnson, 1978). However, these variations were not identical for each enzyme so that ratios of I_{50}s diverged up to eightfold in some cases. For cases where the ratio is lower for humans, one might predict it would be comparatively more difficult to produce neuropathy in humans than in hens. However, in the case of trichlorphon (dichlorvos being the active inhibitory species), the *in vitro* ratio is 3 times higher for humans than for hens. There is increasing evidence that trichlorphon in single massive doses can produce neuropathy in humans (Johnson, 1981), whereas it requires more than one dose in hens. This may reflect the greater relative sensitivity of the human target or it may indicate that a lower proportion of NTE in the human nervous system is required to be phosphorylated and aged to reach the initiation threshold.

47.3.3.2 Neuropathy Target Esterase and the Evaluation of Organophosphorus Ester–Induced Delayed Neuropathy in Humans

Lotti (1992) listed 10 different pesticides that have been reported to cause OPIDN in humans, and isofenphos has been added to the list subsequently (Moretto and Lotti, 1998). According to the structure–activity relationships (SARs) listed previously, nine of these have molecular structures indicative of significant neuropathic potential, which has also been confirmed in laboratory studies involving assay of NTE in hen autopsy samples: Lotti noted that a case report naming omethoate (*not* significantly anti-NTE) as a causative agent had no sound evidence to identify the poison. A case of OPIDN believed to be due to a suicide attempt with a massive dose of parathion (De Jager *et al.*, 1981) was highly unusual in that it appeared to be a solitary event although acute poisoning with this pesticide is probably the most common of all reported OP intoxications. Parathion and paraoxon have very low anti-NTE potential, but the oxon derived from the impurity ethyl bis-(4-nitrophenyl) phosphorothioate is a potent inhibitor (Johnson, 1982b) and this could well have been the actual causative agent.

The threshold of NTE inhibition that precipitates OPIDN in humans might be established if the following steps were taken more often following severe poisonings due to OPs:

1. The actual agent involved should be identified by chemical analysis.
2. The sample should be analyzed for major and minor OP constituents.
3. Lymphocyte NTE as well as erythrocyte AChE should be assayed in (serial) blood samples during treatment.
4. In the event of fatal poisoning, immediate autopsy samples should be obtained from brain and spinal cord and deep-frozen until AChE and NTE assays can be performed.

A few such investigations have been performed with patients who did and others who did not suffer a neuropathic consequence of severe OP poisoning (Lotti *et al.*, 1981; Moretto and Lotti, 1998). The authors concluded that only substantial peak inhibition of NTE was associated with expression of frank clinical OPIDN. On the basis of the preceding limited information, the application of the *in vitro* ratios of enzyme sensitivity appears to be an acceptable procedure in predictive toxicology and in clinical prognosis.

47.3.3.3 Neuropathy Target Esterase and the Assessment of Chiral Compounds

One currently unresolved toxicological issue is the problem of chiral compounds (Johnson, 1987). The relative sensitivities of AChE and NTE in humans and hens to most tested OPs are not greatly different, so that the measured relative susceptibility of hens to cholinergic or OPIDN effects can be transposed to humans. The actual dose effective in these species may differ because, in general, mammals have greater capacity for both bioactivation and detoxification of chemicals, but this does not alter the relative anti-esterase activities of these products. However, chiral OPs are a 50/50 mixture of two distinct chemicals that may be metabolized differently and to different extents in hens Johnson *et al.* (1991) and differently yet again in humans. Furthermore, the relative anti-AChE/anti-NTE potencies of the various metabolic products are unlikely to be all the same. Thus, in a worst case scenario, the predominant form of the anti-esterase compound(s) circulating in a dosed hen may dominantly affect AChE, whereas a different (anti-NTE) compound(s) might predominate in humans. Although the problems of doing full toxicological evaluations of resolved isomers would be immense, the following comparatively easy investigations could be useful:

1. Perform assays of AChE and NTE in autopsy samples from a few mammals (rats) dosed with racemic compound and run in parallel with the full OPIDN evaluation in hens: Neither clinical nor histopathological examination is needed because the object is to decide whether the mammal produces markedly different *relative effects* on the enzyme targets than does the hen.
2. Run assays *in vitro* for the potency against AChE and NTE of resolved isomers of whatever anti-esterase compounds have been identified during routine metabolism studies of the unresolved compound: These assays are straightforward and require only a very few milligrams of material, whereas whole-animal studies might require many grams.

Taken together, these two limited studies should indicate whether or not the hen study with racemic compound is indicative of the human situation.

47.3.3.4 Neuropathy Target Esterase and the Assessment of Effects of Long-Term, Low-Level Exposure

A significant concern is whether short-term, high-dose experiments in hens are appropriate to assess the possible neuropathic hazard of long-term human exposure to relatively lower levels of OP pesticides, with the possibility of cumulative effects. The quantitative data on inhibition of NTE that emerge after short-term tests, even when no other effects are seen, go some way in providing a useful assessment. Thus, whereas a single dose of 50 mg/kg of mono-*o*-cresyl diphenyl phosphate (MOCP) caused OPIDN in hens, a total of 175 mg/kg dosed daily over 10 weeks did not; monitoring brain and spinal cord NTE activity over this period showed that inhibition reached a stable equilibrium after 1–2 weeks at a value (45–60%) below the threshold (70–90%) required to initiate OPIDN (Lotti and Johnson, 1980a). Current Organization for Economic Cooperation and Development (OECD) Guideline 419 restricts multidose tests to 28 days unless special exposure conditions pertain and suggests that negative results on the biochemical, histopathological, and behavioral endpoints indicate that further testing of the compound is not required (OECD, 1995).

47.4 NATURE AND PROPERTIES OF NEUROPATHY TARGET ESTERASE

47.4.1 BIOCHEMICAL STUDIES

Until quite recently, all studies on NTE relied on detection of its esterase activity or labeling by [³H]DFP. Using these methods, it was shown that, in the adult chicken, the highest specific activities of NTE were found in brain whereas spinal cord and sciatic nerve contained substantially less (Johnson, 1982a). In dissected areas of human brain, NTE varied by a factor of 2 with cerebral cortex the highest and cerebellum the least (Lotti and Johnson, 1980b). Relatively high levels of NTE were present in several nonneural chicken tissues, including intestine, spleen, and thymus (Johnson, 1982a), and extremely high levels have been found in bovine adrenal medulla (Sogorb et al., 1994). Cultured bovine chromaffin cells and human neuroblastoma cell lines have been shown to have substantial NTE activity and have been suggested as in vitro systems for assessment of neuropathic OPs (Sogorb et al., 1997; Veronesi et al., 1997).

Biochemical fractionation of chicken brain homogenates showed that NTE is enriched in microsomal membrane fractions (Richardson et al., 1979). [³H]DFP-labeling indicated that NTE comprised less than 0.1% of total microsomal protein (Williams and Johnson, 1981). NTE is an integral membrane protein as indicated by its requirement for detergent for solubilization. The type and concentration of detergent were shown to be important for the maintenance of NTE activity (Davis and Richardson, 1987); fractionation of the solubilized material generally led to substantial loss in NTE activity, which could be partially ameliorated by the addition of phospholipids (Pope and Padilla, 1989a). On sodium dodecyl sulfate–polyacrylamide gel electrophoresis (SDS–PAGE), [³H]DFP-labeled NTE runs as a 155-kDa polypeptide (Williams and Johnson, 1981) whereas, on gel filtration, detergent-solubilized NTE migrates as a complex with an apparent molecular weight greater than 850 kDa (Pope and Padilla, 1989b; Thomas et al., 1990).

47.4.2 ENZYMOLOGY OF NEUROPATHY TARGET ESTERASE

Enzymically, NTE behaves as a typical B-esterase (i.e., it is sensitive to OP). No physiological substrate has been identified, but it rapidly hydrolyzes certain hydrophobic artificial substrates of which phenyl valerate (PV) has the best combination of sensitivity and specificity under appropriate assay conditions. Even with PV, a differential assay is necessary to distinguish NTE from other esterases that can hydrolyze the same substrate but do not have the appropriate inhibition characteristics to qualify as a target for OPIDN. Thus, when total hydrolytic activity in the absence of inhibitors is dubbed A, the paraoxon-resistant activity is dubbed B, and the residual activity resistant to both paraoxon and mipafox (either together or in sequence) is C, then the activity of NTE is determined as $B - C$ and specificity as the ratio $(B - C)/B$. In an assay of hen brain PV hydrolases, after preincubation of the tissue with paraoxon, the substrate specificity is about 65%, which allows quite accurate determination of NTE by the $B - C$ calculation even when overall activity is low as in some autopsy samples from birds dosed with neuropathic compounds.

Extensive structure–activity studies for both substrates and inhibitors in vitro were reported by Johnson (1975b, 1988), Thomas et al. (1990), Wu and Casida (1992), and Borhan et al. (1995); these identified substrates more sensitive than PV (catalytic center activity up to two- to threefold greater) but all were less than 50% specific. For routine investigations, PV is accepted as widely tested and approved but some of these alternatives may be useful for specific studies, such as for a partly purified enzyme free of interfering esterases or when tissue activity is very low or for kinetic investigations that require substrate to have sufficiently low K_m to ensure complete quench of any progessive inhibition at the instant of the addition of substrate. It is a fact that the K_m of PV for NTE is high (about 10 mM compared with about 0.1 mM for phenyl phenylacetate, which was used in early studies but which lacked both sensitivity and specificity; Johnson, 1982a).

The aging reaction (cf. Fig. 47.1b) of DFP-inhibited NTE is very rapid with a half-life of a few minutes and the aged isopropyl group is quantitatively transferred to a covalent acceptor site, dubbed site Z, within NTE itself; this contrasts with a much slower rate of aging for DFP-inhibited cholinesterases in which the aged isopropyl group is liberated into free solution (Clothier and Johnson, 1979). Yoshida et al. (1995) have investigated the reaction of chicken brain NTE with tritiated octyl cyclic saligenin phosphonate; these authors report that only about 15% of the aged saligenin group is transferred to site Z. The identity of site Z in NTE is unknown but clearly it is a residue that is in close proximity to the active site in the native folded protein; there is evidence from proteolysis of SDS-solubilized preparations of [³H]DFP-labeled chicken brain microsomes that site Z lies within 150 residues of the active site serine residue (Glynn et al., 1993).

Although the rapidity of aging of covalently bound OP and the intramolecular transfer of alkyl groups appears to be a unique feature of NTE, it has been concluded that the generation of a negatively charged species at the active site, rather than the modification of site Z, is the critical event in initiation of OPIDN (Johnson, 1990). In the case of phosphoramidates such as mipafox, it has been proposed that aging involves loss of a proton, rather than an alkyl/aryl group, to leave an electronegative species attached to the active-site serine (Richardson, 1995).

47.4.3 ISOLATION AND IMMUNOHISTOCHEMICAL LOCALIZATION

The low abundance and apparent requirement for membrane lipid to maintain NTE activity impeded its isolation for several years. A fraction substantially enriched in [^{3}H]DFP-labeled NTE, but far from homogeneous, was isolated from chicken brain (Rueffer-Turner et al., 1992). An apparently homogeneous NTE preparation from phospholipase A2-solubilized embryonic chicken brain had a specific activity about half that in the initial crude solubilized extract (Mackay et al., 1996). A breakthrough was finally achieved by the synthesis of a novel reagent, S9B [1-(saligenin cyclic phosphoro)-9-biotinyldiaminononane], for affinity purification of NTE (Glynn et al., 1994). S9B reacted rapidly and specifically with NTE in brain microsomes and resulted in the covalent attachment, via a long alkyl spacer, of a biotin molecule to the active-site serine residue. Microsomal proteins, quantitatively solubilized by boiling in dilute SDS, were then subjected to affinity chromatography with avidin–Sepharose, which binds biotinylated polypeptides. S9B-labeled NTE was eluted from the avidin by boiling in SDS. Two polypeptides (carboxylases) with endogenous covalent biotin prosthetic groups that co-eluted from avidin–Sepharose with NTE were removed by subsequent preparative electrophoresis (Glynn et al., 1994).

Isolated chicken NTE was digested with endoproteinase Glu-C and the resulting peptide fragments resolved by SDS–PAGE. The N-terminal amino acid sequence of one of these fragments provided sufficient information to synthesize an 11-residue peptide, which was used to raise a rabbit antiserum to NTE (Glynn et al., 1998). An immunohistochemical survey of the chicken nervous system using this antiserum showed that NTE was present in essentially all neurons but was absent from glia. NTE immunostaining could not be detected in normal sciatic nerve but accumulated at the constriction site 8 h after nerve ligation, indicating that NTE undergoes fast axonal transport. NTE immunostaining filled neuronal cell bodies (except the nucleus) and sometimes extended into the proximal axon; this pattern, taken together with the biochemical data on NTE in microsomal fractions, indicated that NTE is probably associated with the endoplasmic reticulum. These immunostaining characteristics were not detectably altered in chickens 1 or 3 days after treatment with a neuropathic OP, suggesting that OP-modified NTE was neither grossly redistributed nor degraded faster than native NTE (Glynn et al., 1998).

47.4.4 MOLECULAR CLONING OF HUMAN NEUROPATHY TARGET ESTERASE: IMPLICATIONS FOR STRUCTURE AND FUNCTION

The N-terminal sequence of an endoproteinase Glu-C fragment of S9B-labeled pig brain NTE was found to be very similar to a human-expressed sequence tag cDNA; the latter was used to

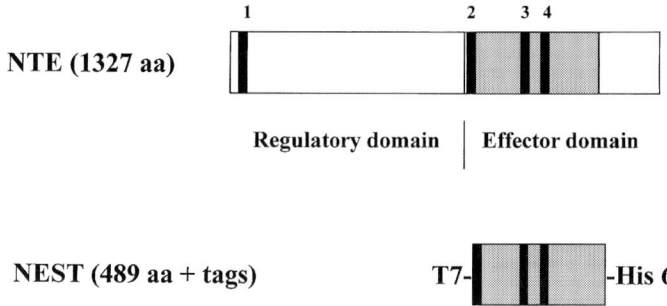

Figure 47.2 Predicted secondary structure of NTE and NEST. NTE is shown as a linear polypeptide of 1327 amino acids with two major functional domains: an N-terminal regulatory domain, which contains regions with some similarity to cyclic AMP-binding proteins, and a C-terminal effector domain (shown in gray), which contains the esterase activity. Four transmembrane segments predicted by TM-pred analysis are shown as thick vertical bars. The active-site serine (Ser 966) lies at the center of putative transmembrane segment 4. NTE residues 727–1216 have been cloned into a pET vector and expressed in E. coli with a short N-terminal (T7) tag sequence and a C-terminal His-6 tag; this construct, dubbed NEST, has all the OP-sensitive phenyl valerate hydrolase activity of full-length NTE (Atkins and Glynn, 2000).

initiate screening of human brain cDNA libraries from which a full-length NTE cDNA clone was finally isolated (Lush et al., 1998). The NTE cDNA clone D16 encoded a polypeptide of 1327 amino acids, and analysis of this sequence with the transmembrane prediction (TM-pred) program indicated the presence of four potential transmembrane segments (see Fig. 47.2). Biochemical experiments indicated that the active-site serine residue labeled by S9B lay between residues 955 and 1033, and attention was drawn to Ser 966, which lay in the motif Gly-Xxx-Ser-Xxx-Gly, common to all serine hydrolases (Lush et al., 1998). Ser 966 has subsequently been confirmed as the active-site residue by [^{3}H]DFP-labeling and protease digestion of a recombinant form of NTE (Atkins and Glynn, 2000). Interestingly, Ser 966 is at the center of the fourth predicted transmembrane segment in NTE (Lush et al., 1998). Whether the segment of NTE containing the active-site serine is actually located within a membrane lipid bilayer is currently under investigation in this laboratory. If this proves to be the case, then, in order to achieve hydrolysis of the acyl enzyme intermediate (Fig. 47.1a), the active-site serine of NTE would have to line an aqueous transmembrane pore. In turn, this structure would suggest NTE's physiological function may not be due simply to its esterase activity. Alternatively, this secondary structure prediction may simply indicate that the active-site serine lies in a hydrophobic helical segment, akin to the arrangement in some lipases (Derewenda and Sharp, 1993). Whichever possibility is correct, it is clear that placing a negatively charged group in this location—the result of OP-mediated aging—would be expected to have a drastic effect on the structure of NTE.

Human NTE is highly homologous (41% identical) to a Drosophila neuronal protein called swiss cheese (SWS; Lush et al., 1998). The sws mutation results in glial hyperwrapping of neurons, which, in turn, leads to apoptotic death of both cell types; the name "swiss cheese" derives from the vacuolated appearance of the mutant brains (Kret-

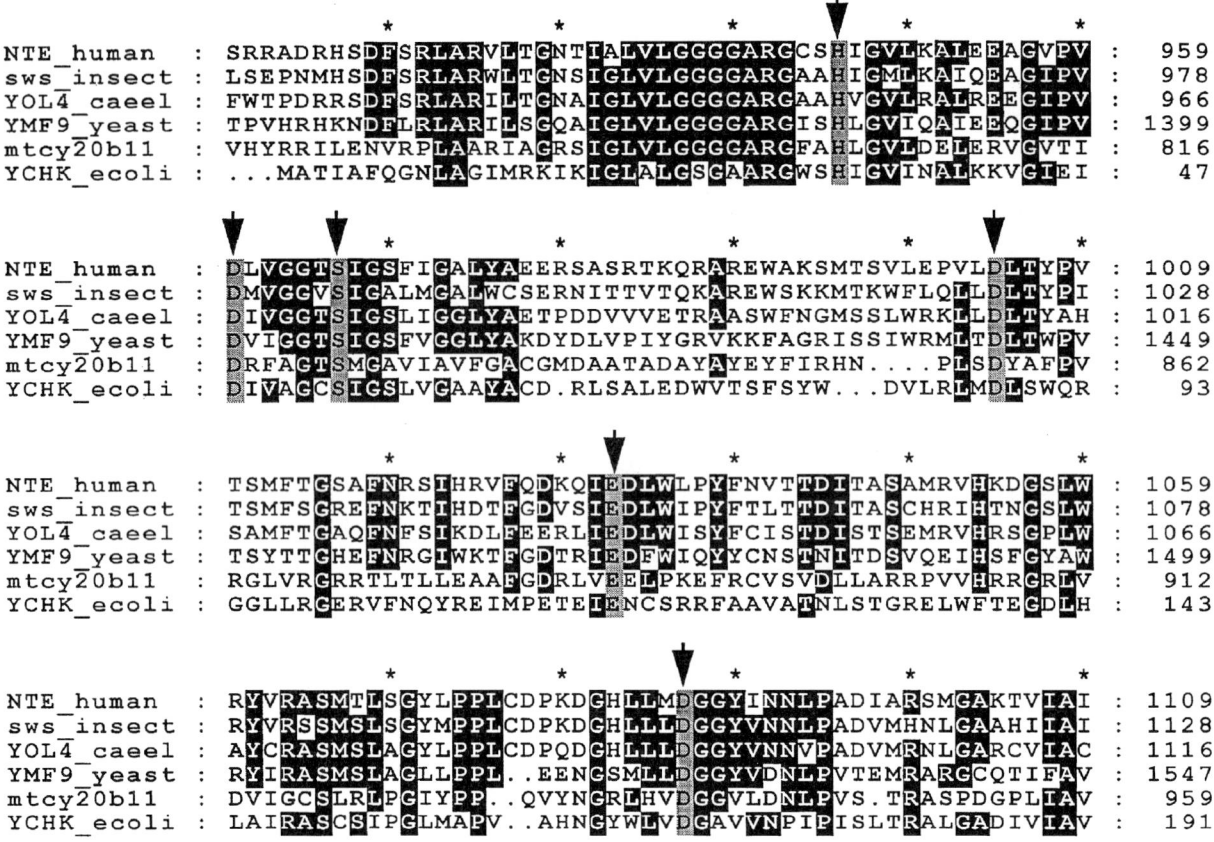

Figure 47.3 Alignment of amino acid sequences in the highly conserved C-terminal region of NTE with homologous proteins from various species. Amino acids (aa) 910–1109 of NTE (complete sequence = 1327 aa) are aligned with homologous regions from SWS (*Drosophila*; 1425 aa), YOL4 (*Caenorhabditis elegans*; 1351 aa), YMF9 (*Saccharomyces cerevisiae*; 1679 aa), MTCY20B11.14c (*Mycobacterium tuberculosis*; 1048 aa), and YCHK (*E. coli*; 314 aa). Residues identical in at least four of the proteins are shown white on black. The positions of the active-site serine (Ser 966) and of conserved His, Asp, and Glu residues are shown black on grey and are indicated by an arrow.

zschmar *et al.*, 1997). It has been suggested that the SWS protein is involved in a cell-signaling pathway, and attention has been drawn to the similarity between an N-terminal domain of SWS (also present in NTE) that resembles the cyclic AMP-binding regulatory subunit of protein kinase A (Kretzschmar *et al.*, 1997). In addition to sharing sequence homology, biochemical assays have shown that NTE-like phenyl valerate hydrolase activity is present in wild-type *Drosophila* but absent from *sws* mutants (Moser *et al.*, 2000). is the *Drosophila* homolog of NTE and, by analogy, NTE may mediate cell signaling in the developing vertebrate brain. *In situ* hybridization experiments on mouse embryos show that NTE mRNA is expressed in neurons from their earliest appearance in the developing nervous system (Moser *et al.*, 2000).

Sequence database searches revealed that NTE is not related to any known serine esterases or proteases but, in addition to its close similarity with *Drosophila* SWS, it shares homology with a number of polypeptides predicted from the sequencing of genomes of bacteria, yeast, and nematodes (Lush *et al.*, 1998). In particular, a 200-amino-acid domain, cor-

responding to NTE residues 910–1109, is highly conserved (29% identity between human NTE and the *Escherichia coli* homolog YCHK) and, notably, all the homologous proteins contain a serine residue in the same position as Ser 966 of NTE. In addition, a completely conserved His and several acidic (Asp and Glu) residues are found within this domain, which, together with the serine, could comprise a catalytic triad as found in conventional serine hydrolases (Fig. 47.3; Lush *et al.*, 1998). Thus, NTE is a member of a novel protein family that appears to comprise potential serine hydrolases. However, although recombinant fragments of both NTE (residues 727–1216) and SWS (residues 746–1235) show substantial PV hydrolase activity when expressed in the pET vector/*E. coli* system, we have been unable to detect PV hydrolase activity for analogous portions of the bacterial or yeast homologues expressed in the same system (Fig. 47.3; J. Atkins, Y. Li, and P. Glynn, unpublished). Whether this result simply reflects the differing substrate specificity of these potential esterases or, alternatively, indicates that this domain has been conserved for a nonesteratic function is currently under investigation.

Table 47.3
Species Susceptibility to Single-Dose OPIDN and Brain NTE Levels

Species	Susceptibility	Brain NTE (nmol/min/g)
Human	+	2400
Chicken	+	2400
Cat	+	2200
Pig	+	2000
Sheep	+	1850
Marmoset	−	2000
Quail	−	2000
Guinea pig	−	1000
Rat	−	950
Mouse	−	700
Rabbit	−	600
Gerbil	−	400

Data from Johnson (1982a) and Read and Glynn (unpublished).

47.4.5 ROLE OF NEUROPATHY TARGET ESTERASE IN ORGANOPHOSPHORUS ESTER-INDUCED DELAYED NEUROPATHY: A TOXIC GAIN OF FUNCTION?

The close similarity between NTE and *Drosophila* SWS suggests that NTE may have an important function during brain development through involvement in a cell-signaling pathway; a number of experimental approaches are currently investigating this possibility. The role of NTE in OPIDN is a rather different issue. It has long been clear that prolonged inhibition of NTE's esterase activity has no obvious adverse effects in the adult chicken (Johnson, 1990). Thus, it may be that NTE no longer has a vital role in adult animals but rather it acquires a novel toxic function on modification by a neuropathic OP.

Data on species variation in susceptibility to OPIDN and in brain levels of NTE are shown in Table 47.3. Susceptible species are generally larger and hence have longer axons than resistant species. This is particularly apparent, for instance, when adult chickens are compared with quails—both have relatively high levels of brain NTE activity and yet the latter birds are resistant. However, an additional consistent observation is that animals with relatively low levels of NTE (<1000 nmol/min/g) are relatively resistant to OPIDN. Furthermore, we have found that in mice (a particularly resistant species) NTE appears to turn over faster ($t_{1/2} = 2$ days; D. J. Read and P. Glynn, unpublished) than in chickens ($t_{1/2} = 4$–5 days; Johnson, 1974; Meredith and Johnson, 1988). This would be consistent with a mechanism whereby a certain threshold level of OP-modified NTE must be achieved and then maintained for a finite period in order to initiate OPIDN. Experiments are now underway attempting to generate transgenic mice expressing very high levels of NTE to determine whether these animals show a heightened susceptibility to OPIDN.

47.5 SUMMARY

Neuropathy target esterase is a high-molecular-weight integral membrane protein present in neurons. It was defined originally by its uniquely selective reactivity with those organophosphorus esters that induce delayed onset neuropathy in humans and various test animals, of which the adult chicken is the most convenient and reproducible in showing the effect. Initiation of OPIDN by a pesticide requires that the compound be in its oxon (P=O) form, which can react covalently with NTE to modify the protein in two steps: (1) organophosphorylation of the serine residue at the catalytic centre of the enzyme (which inhibits the esterase activity) and (2) a rapid intramolecular rearrangement of the bound OP to generate a negatively charged group attached to the serine. Certain classes of NTE inhibitors (carbamates, sulfonyl fluorides, and phosphinates) can inhibit catalytic activity by progressive covalent reaction at the serine but are structurally incapable of undergoing step 2. Doses of these compounds do not cause neuropathy but act as prophylactic compounds against OPIDN by virtue of their ability to block the target site in an apparently innocuous fashion. It appears that the ability of NTE to catalyze hydrolysis of esters is redundant in the adult and it is possible that the initiation of OPIDN involves a toxic gain of function initiated by generation of the negative charge on the NTE molecule very soon after ingestion of the pesticide.

Assay of the degree of inhibition of NTE in autopsy samples of brain and spinal cord from dosed animals provides quantifiable biochemical data as a valuable adjunct to clinical and morphological assessment of the effects in tests of the neuropathic potential of OPs. The NTEs of hen and human brain are similar in sensitivity to many OPs. Studies *in vitro* have provided structure–activity relationships, and comparison of the sensitivities of NTE and acetylcholinesterase enable predictions of the relative acute/neuropathic potential of candidate pesticides, including chiral compounds, which present peculiar problems to regulatory toxicologists. Assays of NTE in accessible lymphocytes from a few poisoned patients suggest that there is predictive value in the procedure and that OPIDN in humans, as in hens, requires a high level of inhibition to precipitate frank clinical neuropathy. Assessment of long-term, low-level exposure to OPs indicates that inhibition of NTE is not totally cumulative and may reach an equilibrium level below that needed to initiate OPIDN.

As an enzyme, NTE behaves as a typical B-esterase that rapidly hydrolyzes phenyl valerate and related esters, but no physiological substrate has been identified; related enzymes may be involved in the mechanism of promotion of OPIDN by some inhibitors that are unable to initiate the process. Although attempts to isolate catalytically active enzyme failed, an affinity-labeled form has been purified and antibodies raised: Immunohistochemical study shows NTE confined largely to the endoplasmic reticulum of neuronal cell bodies and to be transported rapidly down axons.

The primary sequence of NTE has been determined from its cDNA and shown to be unrelated to any known serine esterases or proteases. NTE is the vertebrate homolog of the swiss cheese protein (SWS) of *Drosophila*: SWS resides in neurons and appears to be involved in signaling between these cells and glia in the developing fly brain. In embryonic mice, NTE is expressed in neurons from their earliest appearance in the nervous system where it could function in analogous fashion to SWS. Conceivably, the esterase function of NTE is required during neural development but not in later life. The active-site serine of NTE is located in a C-terminal domain that is conserved in proteins expressed by organisms from bacteria to humans; however, unlike NTE and SWS, homologs from unicellular organisms appear to lack phenyl valerate hydrolase activity. The active-site serine of NTE lies at the center of a hydrophobic segment of the polypeptide chain; generation of a negative charge by a bound neuropathic OP in this location would probably have drastic effects on the structure and function of NTE.

REFERENCES

Aldridge, W. N., and Reiner, E. (1972). "Enzyme Inhibitors as Substrates." Elsevier/North-Holland, Amsterdam.

Atkins, J., and Glynn, P. (2000). Membrane association and critical residues in the catalytic domain of human neuropathy target esterase. *J. Biol. Chem.* **275**, 24477–24483.

Barril, J., and Vilanova, E. (1997). Reversible inhibition can profoundly mislead studies on progressive inhibition of enzymes: The interaction of paraoxon with soluble neuropathy target esterase. *Chem.-Biol. Interact.* **108**, 19–25.

Barril, J., Estevez, J., Escudero, M. A., Cespedes, M. V., Niguez, N., Sorgob, A., Monroy, A., and Vilanova, E. (1999). Peripheral nerve soluble esterases are spontaneously reactivated after inhibition by paraoxon: Implications for a new definition of NTE. *Chem.-Biol. Interact.* **119–120**, 541–550.

Borhan, B., Ko, Y., Wilson, B. W., Kurth, M. J., and Hammock, B. D. (1995). Development of surrogate substrates for neuropathy target esterase. *Biochim. Biophys. Acta* **1250**, 171–182.

Capodicasa, E., Scapellato, M. L., Moretto, A., Caroldi, S., and Lotti, M. (1991). Chlorpyrifos-induced delayed polyneuropathy. *Arch. Toxicol.* **65**, 150–155.

Céspedes, M. V., Escudero, M. A., Barril, J., Sogorb, M. A., Vicedo, J. L., and Vilanova, E. (1997). Discrimination of carboxylesterases of chicken neural tissue by inhibition with neuropathic and non-neuropathic organophosphorus compounds and a neuropathy promoter. *Chem.-Biol. Interact.* **106**, 191–200.

Clothier, B., and Johnson, M. K. (1979). Rapid aging of neurotoxic esterase after inhibition by di-isopropyl phosphorofluoridate. *Biochem. J.* **177**, 549–558.

Davis, C. S., and Richardson, R. J. (1987). Neurotoxic esterase: Characterisation of the solubilised enzyme and the conditions for its solubilisation from chicken brain microsomal membranes with ionic, zwitterionic or non-ionic detergents. *Biochem. Pharmacol.* **36**, 1393–1399.

De Jager, A. E. J., Van Weerden, T. W., Houthhoff, H. J., and de Monchy, J. G. R. (1981). Polyneuropathy after massive exposure to parathion. *Neurology* **31**, 603–605.

Derewenda, Z. S., and Sharp, A. M. (1993). News from the interface: The molecular structures of triacylglceride lipases. *Trends Biochem. Sci.* **18**, 20–25.

Escudero, M. A., and Vilanova, E. (1997). Purification and characterisation of naturally soluble neuropathy target esterase from chicken sciatic nerve by HPLC and Western blot. *J. Neurochem.* **69**, 1975–1982.

European Centre for Ecotoxicology and Toxicology of Chemicals (ECETOC) (1998). "Organophosphorus Pesticides and Long-Term Effects on the Nervous System." Technical Report 75, European Centre for Ecotoxicology and Toxicology of Chemicals, Brussels.

Glynn, P., Holton, J. L., Nolan, C. C., Read, D. J., Brown, L., Hubbard, A., and Cavanagh, J. B. (1998). Neuropathy target esterase: Immunolocalisation to neuronal cell bodies and axons. *Neuroscience* **83**, 295–302.

Glynn, P., Read, D. J., Guo, R., Wylie, S., and Johnson, M. K. (1994). Synthesis and characterisation of a biotinylated organophosphorus ester for detection and affinity purification of a brain serine esterase: Neuropathy target esterase. *Biochem. J.* **301**, 551–556.

Glynn, P., Rueffer-Turner, M., Read, D. J., Wylie, S., and Johnson, M. K. (1993). Molecular characterisation of neuropathy target esterase: Proteolysis of the [^{3}H]DFP-labelled polypeptide. *Chem. Biol. Interact.* **87**, 361–367.

Johnson, M. K. (1969a). A phosphorylation site in brain and the delayed neurotoxic effect of some organophosphorus compounds. *Biochem. J.* **111**, 487–495.

Johnson, M. K. (1969b). The delayed neurotoxic effect of some organophosphorus compounds: Identification of the phosphorylation site as an esterase. *Biochem. J.* **114**, 711–714.

Johnson, M. K. (1970). Organophosphorus and other inhibitors of "neurotoxic esterase" and the development of delayed neurotoxicity in hens. *Biochem. J.* **120**, 523–531.

Johnson, M. K. (1974). The primary biochemical lesion leading to the delayed neurotoxic effects of some organophosphorus esters. *J. Neurochem.* **23**, 785–789.

Johnson, M. K. (1975a). Organophosphorus esters causing delayed neurotoxic effects: Mechanism of action and structure/activity relationships. *Arch. Toxicol.* **34**, 259–288.

Johnson, M. K. (1975b). Structure–activity relationships for substrates and inhibitors of hen brain neurotoxic esterase. *Biochem. Pharmacol.* **24**, 797–805.

Johnson, M. K. (1978). The anomalous behaviour of some dimethyl-phosphates in the biochemical test for delayed neurotoxicity potential. *Arch. Toxicol.* **41**, 107–110.

Johnson, M. K. (1981). Delayed neurotoxicity—do trichlorphon and/or dichlorvos cause delayed neuropathy in man or in test animals? *Acta Pharmacol. Toxicol.* **49**, 87–98.

Johnson, M. K. (1982a). The target for initiation of delayed neurotoxicity by organophosphorus esters: Biochemical studies and toxicological applications. *In* "Reviews in Biochemical Toxicology" (E. Hodgson, J. R. Bend, and R. M. Philpot, eds.), Vol. 4, pp. 141–212. Elsevier, New York.

Johnson, M. K. (1982b). Check your paraoxon and parathion for neurotoxic impurities. *Veterin. and Hum. Toxicol.* **24**, 220a.

Johnson, M. K. (1984). Delayed neurotoxicity tests of organophosphorus esters: A proposed protocol integrating neuropathy target esterase (NTE) assays with behaviour and histopathology tests to obtain more information more quickly from fewer animals. *In* "Proceedings of the International Conference on Environmental Hazards of Agrochemicals in Developing Countries, Alexandria, Egypt, November 8–12, 1983" (A. H. El-Sebae, ed.), pp. 474–493. Univ. of Alexandria, Alexandria, Egypt.

Johnson, M. K. (1987). The importance of chirality in influencing both acute and delayed neuropathic toxicity of organophosphorus esters. *Toxicol. Environ. Chem.* **14**, 321–335.

Johnson, M. K. (1988). Sensitivity and selectivity of compounds interacting with neuropathy target esterase: Further structure/activity studies. *Biochem. Pharmacol.* **37**, 4095–4104.

Johnson, M. K. (1990). Organophosphates and delayed neuropathy—Is NTE alive and well? *Toxicol. Appl. Pharmacol.* **102**, 385–399.

Johnson, M. K., and Lauwerys, R. R. (1969). Protection by some carbamates against the delayed neurotoxic effect of di-isopropyl phosphorofluoridate. *Nature* (London) **222**, 1066–1067.

Johnson, M. K., and Read, D. J. (1987). The influence of chirality on the delayed neuropathic potential of some organophosphorus esters: Neuropathic and prophylactic effects of stereoisomers of ethyl phenylphosphonic acid (EPN oxon and EPN) correlate with quantities of aged and unaged neuropathy target esterase *in vivo*. *Toxicol. Appl. Pharmacol.* **90**, 103–115.

Johnson, M. K., Vilanova, E., and Read, D. J. (1991). Anomalous biochemical responses in tests of the delayed neuropathic potential of methamidophos (*O,S*-dimethyl phosphorothioamidate), its resolved isomers and of some higher 0-alkyl homologues. *Arch. Toxicol.* **65**, 618–624.

Krejci, E., Duval, N., Chatonnet, A., Vincens, P., and Massoulie, J. (1991). Cholinesterase-like domains in enzymes and structural proteins: Functional and evolutionary relationships and identification of a catalytically essential aspartic acid. *Proc. Natl. Acad. Sci. U.S.A.* **88**, 6647–6651.

Kretzschmar, D., Hasan, G., Sharma, S., Heisenberg, M., and Benzer, S. (1997). The swiss cheese mutant causes glial hyperwrapping of and brain degeneration in *Drosophila. J. Neuroscience* **17**, 7425–7432.

Lotti, M. (1992). The pathogenesis of organophosphate polyneuropathy. *Crit. Rev. Toxicol.* **21**, 465–487.

Lotti, M., and Johnson, M. K. (1978). Neurotoxicity of organophosphorus pesticides: Predictions can be based on *in vitro* studies with hen and human enzymes. *Arch. Toxicol.* **41**, 215–221.

Lotti, M., and Johnson, M. K. (1980a). Repeated small doses of a neurotoxic organophosphate: Monitoring of neurotoxic esterase in brain and spinal cord. *Arch. Toxicol.* **45**, 263–271.

Lotti, M., and Johnson, M. K. (1980b). Neurotoxic esterase in human nervous tissue. *J. Neurochem.* **34**, 747–749.

Lotti, M., and Moretto, A. (1999). Promotion of organophosphate induced polyneuropathy by certain esterase inhibitors. *Chem.-Biol. Interact.* To appear.

Lotti, M., Ferrara, S. D., Caroldi, S., and Sinigaglia, F. (1981). Enzyme studies with human and hen autopsy tissue suggest omethoate does not cause delayed neuropathy in man. *Arch. Toxicol.* **48**, 265–270.

Lush, M. J., Li, Y., Read, D. J., Willis, A. C., and Glynn, P. (1998). Neuropathy target esterase and a homologous *Drosophila* neurodegeneration mutant protein contain a domain conserved from bacteria to man. *Biochem. J.* **332**, 1–4.

Mackay, C. E., Hammock, B. D., and Wilson, B. W. (1996). Identification and isolation of a 155kDa protein with neuropathy target esterase activity. *Fundam. Appl. Toxicol.* **30**, 23–30.

Meredith, C., and Johnson, M. K. (1988). Neuropathy target esterase: Rates of turnover *in vivo* following covalent inhibition with phenyl di-*n*-pentylphosphinate. *J. Neurochem.* **51**, 1097–1101.

Milatovic, D., Moretto, A., Osman, K. A., and Lotti, M. (1997). Phenyl valerate esterases other than neuropathy target esterase and the promotion of organophosphate polyneuropathy. *Chem. Res. Toxicol.* **10**, 1045–1048.

Moretto, A., and Lotti, M. (1998). Poisoning by organophosphorus insecticides and sensory neuropathy. *J. Neurol. Neurosurg. Psychiat.* **64**, 463–468.

Moser, M., Stempl, T., Li, Y., Glynn, P., Buttner, R., and Kretzschmar, D. (2000). Molecular cloning of the mouse NTE/SWS gene. *Mech. Dev.* **90**, 279–282.

Organization for Economic Co-operation and Development (OECD) (1995). "Delayed Neurotoxicity of Organophosphorus Substances Following Acute Exposure" and "Delayed Neurotoxicity of Organophosphorus Substances: 28-Day Repeated Dose Study." Guidelines for Testing of Chemicals 418 and 419, Environmental Health and Safety Division, Organization for Economic Co-operation and Development, Paris.

Pope, C. N., and Padilla, S. S. (1989a). Modulation of neurotoxic esterase activity *in vitro* by phospholipids. *Toxicol. Appl. Pharmacol.* **97**, 272–278.

Pope, C. N., and Padilla, S. S. (1989b). Chromatographic characterisation of neurotoxic esterase. *Biochem. Pharmacol.* **38**, 181–188.

Poulsen, E., and Aldridge, W. N. (1964). Studies on esterases in the chicken nervous system. *Biochem. J.* **90**, 182–189.

Richardson, R. J. (1995). Assessment of the neurotoxic potential of chlorpyrifos relative to other organophosphorus compounds: A critical review of the literature. *J. Toxicol. Environ. Health* **44**, 135–165.

Richardson, R. J., Davis, C. S., and Johnson, M. K. (1979). Subcellular distribution of marker enzymes and of neurotoxic esterase in adult hen brain. *J. Neurochem.* **32**, 607–615.

Rueffer-Turner, M. E., Read, D. J., and Johnson, M. K. (1992). Purification of neuropathy target esterase from avian brain after prelabelling with [3H]diisopropyl phosphorofluoridate. *J. Neurochem.* **58**, 135–141.

Senanayake, N., and Johnson, M. K. (1982). Acute polyneuropathy after poisoning by a new organophosphorus insecticide. *N. Engl. J. Med.* **306**, 155–156.

Smith, M. I., Elvove, E., and Frazier, W. H. (1930). The pharmacological action of certain phenol esters with special reference to the etiology of the so-called ginger paralysis. *Public Health Rep.* **45**, 2509–2524.

Sogorb, M. A., Bas, S., Gutierrez, L. M., Vilanova, E., and Viniegra, S. (1997). Bovine chromaffin cells as an *in vitro* model for the study of non-cholinergic toxic effects of organophosphorus compounds. *Arch. Toxicol. Suppl.* **19**, 347–355.

Sogorb, M. A., Viniegra, S., Reig, J. A., and Vilanova, E. (1994). Partial characterisation of neuropathy target esterase and related phenyl valerate esterases from bovine adrenal medulla. *J. Biochem. Toxicol.* **9**, 145–152.

Soliman, S. A., Curley, A., Farmer, J., and Novak, R. (1986). *In vivo* inhibition of chicken brain acetylcholinesterase and neurotoxic esterase in relation to the delayed neurotoxicity of leptophos and cyanophenphos. *J. Environ. Pathol. Toxicol. Oncol.* **7**, 211–224.

Taylor, P. (1992). Impact of recombinant DNA technology and protein structure determination on past and future studies on acetylcholinesterase. *In* "Multidisciplinary Approaches to Cholinesterase Functions" (A. Shafferman and B. Velan, eds.), pp. 1–15. Plenum, New York.

Thomas, T. C., Szekacs, A., Rojas, S., Hammock, B. D., Wilson, B. W., and MacNamee, M. G. (1990). Characterisation of neuropathy target esterase using trifluoromethyl ketones. *Biochem. Pharmacol.* **40**, 2587–2596.

U.S. Environmental Protection Agency (EPA) (1991). "Pesticide Assessment Guidelines, Subdivision F; Hazard Evaluation: Human and Domestic Animals: Addendum 10, Neurotoxicity," Series 81, 82, and 83, pp. 3–12. EPA 540/09-91-123, PB 91-154617, Health Effects Division, Office of Pesticide Programs, U.S. Environmental Protection Agency, Washington, DC.

Veronesi, B., Ehrich, M., Blusztajn, J. K., Oortgiesen, M., and Durham, H. (1997). Cell culture models of interspecies selectivity to organophosphorus insecticides. *Neurotoxicology* **18**, 283–297.

Vilanova, E., Escudero, M. A., and Barril, J. (1999). NTE soluble isoforms: New perspectives for targets of neuropathy inducers and promoters. *Chem.-Biol. Interact.* **119–120**, 525–540.

Williams, D. G., and Johnson, M. K. (1981). Gel electrophoretic identification of hen brain neurotoxic esterase labelled with tritiated di-isopropyl phosphorofluoridate. *Biochem. J.* **199**, 323–333.

Wu, S.-Y., and Casida, J. E. (1992). Neuropathy target esterase inhibitors: 2-Alkyl-, 2-alkoxy-, and 2-(aryloxy)-4*H*-1,3,2-benzodioxaphosphorin 2-oxides. *Chem. Res. Toxicol.* **5**, 680–684.

Yoshida, M., Tomizawa, M., Wu, S.-Y., Quistad, G. B., and Casida, J. E. (1995). Neuropathy target esterase of hen brain: Active site reactions with 2-[octyl-^{3}H]octyl-4*H*-1,3,2-benzodioxaphosphorin 2-oxide and 2-octyl-4*H*-1,3,2-[aryl-^{3}H]benzodioxaphosphorin 2-oxide. *J. Neurochem.* **64**, 1680–1687.

CHAPTER

48

Cholinesterases

Barry W. Wilson
University of California, Davis

48.1 INTRODUCTION

Cholinesterases (ChEs) are specialized carboxylic ester hydrolases that break down esters of choline. Two of special concern to the toxicology of pesticides are acetylcholinesterase (AChE, acetylcholine hydrolase, EC 3.1.1.7) and butyrylcholinesterase (BuChE, acylcholine acylhydrolase, EC 3.1.1.8). BuChE is also known as nonspecific cholinesterase or pseudocholinesterase. The preferred substrate for AChE enzymes is acetylcholine (ACh); nonspecific cholinesterase BuChE enzymes prefer butyrylcholine and/or propionylcholine, depending on the species (Silver, 1974). This chapter discusses these enzymes, their importance in understanding the toxicity of organophosphate esters (OPs) and carbamate pesticides (CBs), and their application to risk assessment of anticholinesterase pesticides and other agents (Taylor, 1999).

ChEs are classed among the B-esterases, enzymes inhibited by OPs, and possessing a serine catalytic site (Aldridge and Reiner, 1972; Ballantyne and Marrs, 1992; Chambers and Levi, 1992; Ecobichon, 1996; Gallo and Lawryk, 1991). Other B-esterases include the broad class of carboxylesterases (CarbE, EC 3.1.1.1.), one of which is neuropathy target esterase (NTE), the enzyme associated with organophosphate-induced delayed neuropathy (OPIDN) discussed in other chapters. A different group of enzymes known as A-esterases (e.g., arylesterases, paraoxonases, and DFPases) actively hydrolyze OPs. They represent an important means of detoxification (Furlong et al., 2000; La Du et al., 1999; Haley et al., 1999).

There has been an immense amount of research on ChEs since 1914 when Sir Henry Dale (Dale, 1914) suggested there was an esterase capable of hydrolyzing acetylcholine in blood, and Abderhalden and Paffrath (1925) and Loewi and Navratil (1926) demonstrated tissue extracts that broke down the chemical. [There are over 14,000 research reports on ChEs listed in an ACS on-line database (Sci Finder Scholar, 1999) from 1992 through late 2000.] In the past decade, the tertiary structure and amino acid and DNA sequences of several ChEs have been elucidated. (For reviews, see Doctor et al., 1998; Reiner et al., 1999; Taylor, 1994, 1996.) Today, techniques such as site-directed mutagenesis and knock-out mutants enable investigators to dissect the form and function of these proteins lit-

erally one amino acid at a time (e.g., Faerman et al., 1996; Gnatt et al., 1994). Tomorrow, this knowledge will help design chemicals specifically targeted for the tertiary structure of these proteins. Specific reviews (e.g., Massoulie et al., 1999; Taylor, 1996), conferences (e.g., Doctor et al., 1998; Reiner et al., 1999), and even full-color molecular structures displayed on the Internet, help bring the reader the latest information in this rapidly moving research area. [For brevity, only selected references to a topic may be cited here. The reader is referred to these references and to the article of Gallo and Lawryk (1991), in a previous edition of this book, for citations to earlier work.]

OPs with high toxicity were synthesized as chemical warfare agents in the late 1930s and early 1940s (Ecobichon, 1996; Holmstedt, 1963; Koelle, 1963). Their offspring have been adapted to agricultural use as pesticides. Synthetic CBs modeled on the natural carbamate physostigmine and specifically designed to inhibit ChEs have been in commercial use as pesticides since the 1950s (Ecobichon, 1996). Because of their potential as weapons, much research has focused on antidotes (e.g., oximes) and prophylactics to OP chemical warfare agents (e.g., National Academy of Sciences Report, 1999).

48.2 DISTRIBUTION

ChEs are widely distributed across animal species (Ecobichon, 1996). Their presence in insects and other invertebrate pests have made anti-ChE agents popular and effective pesticides. Molecular forms of ChE similar to those in vertebrates have been studied in animals as varied as nematodes (e.g., Caenorhabditis; Culetto et al., 1999), squid (e.g., Talesa et al., 1999), and Amphioxus, a protochordate (Pezzementi et al., 1998). Vertebrate-like AChE forms have been reported from Paramecium, a ciliated protozoan (Delmonte Corrado et al., 1999).

AChEs in the nervous system regulate excitation by destroying the neurotransmitter ACh. They are found at synapses, neuromuscular and myotendinous junctions, cerebrospinal fluid, central nervous system (CNS) neuron cell bodies, and axons, skeletal and smooth muscles (Silver, 1974). AChEs also are present on the surface of erythrocytes (RBCs) of mammals, megakaryocytes, lymphocytes, and platelets (Husain, 1994; Paulus *et al.*, 1981; Zajicek, 1957). Some research has been done on ChE in saliva (Ryhanen *et al.*, 1983; Yamalik *et al.*, 1990).

Blood ChE forms are often used as surrogates for CNS enzymes in studies of toxicants. The AChE activity of human blood is restricted to its formed elements; most of the activity is vested in the RBCs (Wills, 1972). Plasma ChEs of other vertebrates (e.g., birds) often hydrolyze ACh too (Augustinsson, 1948, 1959a, b), and specific AChE enzyme activity is present in the plasma of some mammals. For example, the plasma ChE activity of rodents such as the laboratory rat is high in both AChE and BuChE (Traina and Serpietri, 1984). Neglecting plasma AChE activity may lead to misinterpretations of the extent of ChE inhibition in animals used for pesticide research and in the setting of regulations for food safety and human exposure (Wilson *et al.*, 1996). AChE activity also has been found in the serum of embryo mammals and birds, decreasing to adult levels after birth. AChE activity in fetal calf serum is high enough to be used as a source for purifying the enzyme (De la Hoz *et al.*, 1986). In contrast, adult bovine blood has relatively high RBC AChE and very low plasma ChE levels (Zajicek, 1957). Other species have a mixture establishable by studies of substrate and inhibitor specificity and, recently, by DNA analyses (Bartels *et al.*, 2000).

Table 48.1 compares adult levels of RBC AChE for several species. The human has the highest activity. The rat has one of the lowest RBC AChE levels even though it is often used in biomedical research on anti-ChE agents.

BuChEs are also found at synapses, motor endplates, and muscle fibers together with AChE (Silver, 1974). BuChE activity in blood is restricted to serum. The physiological functions of RBC and serum ChEs are unclear. The primary structure of ChEs is homologous to proteases and lipases (Taylor, 1996). One possibility is that blood ChEs evolved to protect the body from natural anti-ChE agents. A number of plant toxins have anti-ChE activity; these include the solanaceous glycoalkaloids, naturally occurring steroids in potatoes and related plants (Krasowski *et al.*, 1997; McGehee *et al.*, 2000),

and the fungal territrems (Chen and Ling, 1996). The Calabar bean, *Physostigma venenosum*, was once used by West Africans in a "trial by ordeal" (O'Brien, 1967). Study of the action of its active anticholinergic ingredient, the CB physostigmine (eserine), helped to establish the roles of ACh and AChE in the nervous system (Engelhart and Loewi, 1930). Other examples of naturally occurring anti-ChE agents are: fasciculin from Elapsid snake venom (Marchot *et al.*, 1998), chaconine and solancine from tubers and nightshades (Nigg *et al.*, 1996), and huperzine from moss (Patocka, 1998). The association of cholinergic transmission with Alzheimer's disease is serving as a stimulus to modern studies of natural anti-ChE agents (e.g., Francis *et al.*, 1999; Nordberg and Svensson, 1998) as part of the search for treatments of this common disorder.

Tissue ChEs may have specific but still unknown roles in addition to their regulation of neural transmission. For example, evidence has been amassing (e.g., Anderson and Key, 1999; Chiappa and Brimijoin, 1998; Layer *et al.*, 1998; Robitzki *et al.*, 1997; Sharma and Bigbee, 1998) for a developmental function for ChEs based on studies of neurite outgrowth in retinal and dorsal root ganglion cultures and embryos using immunological, sense and anti-sense oligonucleotides and inhibitors (reviewed by Layer *et al.*, 1998). Nevertheless, the successful development and survival of a knock-out mouse mutant lacking AChE indicates that other enzymes such as BuChE can function in its stead (Li *et al.*, 2000; Xie *et al.*, 2000).

There have been persistent reports concerning pesticide induced ocular damage (recognized clinically as Saku disease in Japan). These studies, reviewed by Dementi (1994), have stimulated studies by the U.S. EPA (Atkinson *et al.*, 1994; Boyes *et al.*, 1994), although without striking results. However, there are reports of visual changes and damage during growth and development (Geller *et al.*, 1998; Wyttenbach and Thompson, 1985). Hamm *et al.* (1998) found that diazinon, a widely used pesticide, damaged the development of the neural retina in Medaka, a fish.

Table 48.1
Relative RBC AChE Levels of Adults of Selected Species

Species	Sex	AChE levels (%)
Human	M/F	100 ± 8.7
Cow	F	87.6 ± 1.9
Guinea pig	M/F	32.7 ± 3.5
Horse	M/F	28.8 ± 9.0
Rabbit	M/F	21.7 ± 5.3
Rat	M	12.6 ± 3.0
Cat	M/F	30^a

Source: Adapted from Zajicek (1957).
Notes: Manometric assay at $N = 3$. Mean human AChE was 2180 µl CO_2/30 min/mg nitrogen. ACh substrate.
$^a N = 2.$

Table 48.2
Plasma Hydrolysis of Choline Esters of Selected Species of Mammals

Species	ACh	PrCh	BuCh	MeCh	BzCh
Man	135	310	360	2	60
Cow	3	4	2	0	0
Guinea pig	50	130	170	5	20
Horse	130	225	365	2	40
Rabbit	16	16	10	4	2
Rat	20	30	15	15	10
Dog	70	115	180	6	30
Cat	50	75	150	5	12

Source: Augustinsson (1959a).
Notes: Manometric assay. µl CO_2/0.1 ml plasma/30 min. $N = 3$ or more animals. ACh: acetylcholine; PrCh: propionylcholine; BuCh: butyrylcholine; MeCh: methylcholine; BzCh: benzoylcholine.

Table 48.3
Plasma Hydrolysis of Choline Esters of Selected Species of Birds, Reptiles, Amphibians, and Fish

Species	ACh	PrCh	BuCh	MeCh	BzCh
Chicken	37	71	36	19	2
Duck	43	74	67	7	8
Turtle	14	103	27	7	1
Rana	40	90	87	2	10
Xenopus	2	5	9	—	—
Pike	12	2	1	1	1

Source: Augustinsson (1959b).
Notes: Manometric assay. $\mu l CO_2/0.1$ ml plasma/30 min. $N = 3$ or more animals. ACh: acetylcholine; PrCh: propionylcholine; BuCh: butyrylcholine; MeCh: methylcholine; BzCh: benzoylcholine.

48.3 SUBSTRATE PREFERENCES AND SELECTIVE INHIBITORS

AChEs prefer ACh as a substrate. Substrate preferences and activities of BuChEs vary with the species. For example, rat plasma BuChE activity has been reported to favor propionyl rather than butyryl substrates, and cows have hardly any plasma ChE activity at all (Tables 48.2 and 48.3). An important distinction between the AChEs and BuChEs is their response to substrate concentration. AChEs are inhibited by substrate in excess of a few mM; BuChEs are less sensitive (Hoffmann *et al.*, 1989; Wilson, 1999). In general, mammalian and avian AChEs rapidly hydrolyze ACh and its thiocholine analog acetylthiocholine (ACTh). Mammalian, but not avian, AChEs preferentially hydrolyze acetyl-β-methylcholine. AChEs are selectively inhibited by several agents. One is the CB BW284c51 (1,5-bis(4-allyldimethylammoniumphenyl)pentan-3-one dibromide) (Austin and Berry, 1953; Holmstedt, 1957; Silver, 1974); another is ARA 1327 (Augustinsson *et al.*, 1978). BuChEs are preferentially inhibited by iso-OMPA (tetraisopropylpyrophosphoramide; Austin and Berry, 1953), ethopropazine (Mikalsen *et al.*, 1986), and quinidine (Wright and Sabine, 1948). Effective concentrations for these selective inhibitors may vary by species. Useful starting points for testing are 0.1 to 0.01 mM.

48.4 MULTIPLE MOLECULAR FORMS AND LIFE HISTORY

ChEs are polymorphic proteins; they occur in multiple molecular forms. AChEs consist of asymmetric and globular forms (Figs. 48.1, 48.2). The asymmetric forms tend to be localized at synapses and motor endplates. They have glycosylated heads joined by sulfhydryl groups and collagen tails. The heads contain the active sites; the collagen tails attach the enzymes to cell surfaces. The globular forms are made up of the catalytic subunits (Taylor, 1996). Although these forms have similar kinetic properties, they differ in their ionic and hydrophobic interactions.

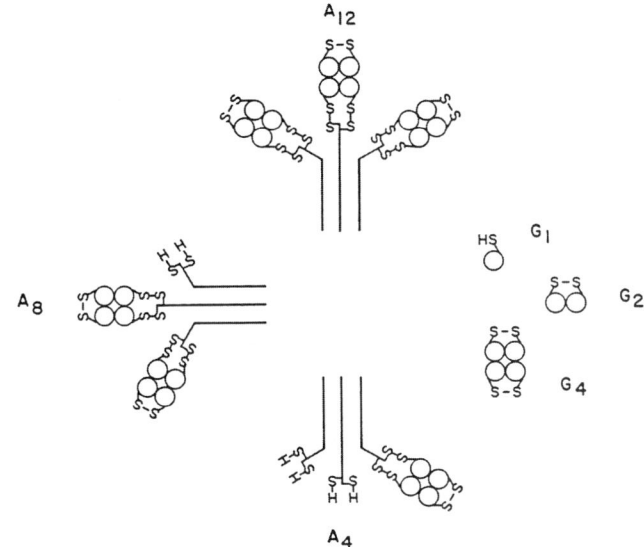

Figure 48.1 Organization of subunits in the molecular forms of ChEs. Each circle represents a catalytic subunit. Globular forms are represented by "G." Asymmetric forms are designated by "A." Linear elements represent collagen-like tails. Disulfide bridge locations from studies of eel electroplax AChE, assumed to reflect ChEs from many sources. (After Brimijoin, 1992.)

ChE forms (Massoulie *et al.*, 1993, 1999) are synthesized as catalytic globular monomers (G1) that oligomerize via disulfide bonds into multiple G2 and G4 forms (Fig. 48.1). The G1 subunits are synthesized within cells (e.g., nerve, muscle, and liver), glycosylated, and then secreted. Collagen tails are

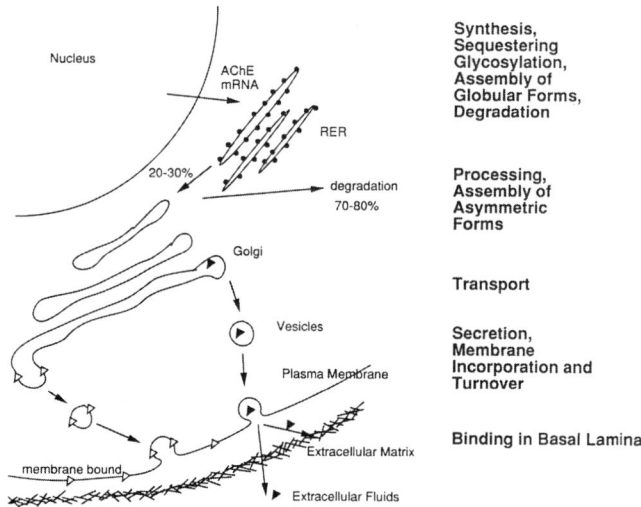

Figure 48.2 Life history of ChEs. Enzyme is synthesized as a monomeric globular form (G1). Up to 80% of the enzyme is degraded by intracellular proteases after ribosomal translation and before transit of the Golgi. In the Golgi, secretory forms (black triangles) are sequestered from membrane bound forms (open triangles), collagen-like tails are added to asymmetric forms, the peptide backbone is glycosytated, and the ChE becomes enzymatically active. Globular secretory forms may escape the synaptic cleft to enter extracellular fluids, blood, or external secretions. Asymmetric forms are probably bound quantitatively by adsorption or entrapment in the polyanion-rich, fibrous matrix of the extracellular synaptic basal lamina. (After Brimijoin, 1992.)

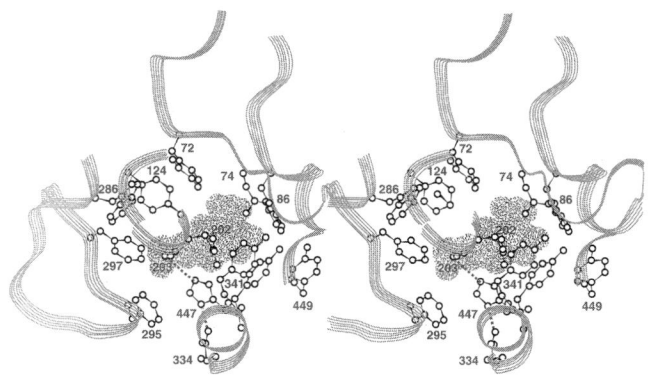

Figure 48.3 Three-dimensional view of the active center of AChE. Modeled from Torpedo AChE with the addition of amino acid side chains of the mammalian enzyme. Amide backbone shown by the ribbons. The catalytic triad of the enzyme is Glu_{334}, His_{447}, Ser_{203} with hydrogen bonds indicated by dotted lines. The acyl pocket is Phe_{295} and Phe_{297}; the choline subsite is Trp_{86}, Glu_{202}, and Tyr_{337}; the peripheral site is Trp_{286}, Tyr_{72}, Tyr_{124}, and Asp_{74}. Tyrosines 341 and 449 may help to stabilize some ligands. The catalytic triad, choline subsite, and acyl pocket are at the base of the 18-20 A gorge; the peripheral site is at its lip. (One way to see the diagram in three dimensions is to use 3-D glasses; another is to move the page toward your eyes until the images superimpose, keeping your head level. If there appear to be three images, concentrate on the middle one.) (After Taylor, 1996.)

attached to one, two, or three catalytic tetramers to yield A4, A8, and A12 asymmetric forms. Collagen-tailed forms become attached to the cell surface at specific binding sites. Globular forms are released into body fluids or bind to cell surfaces through hydrophobic amino acid sequences or glycophospholipids (Taylor, 1996). Antibodies have been prepared to several purified AChEs and BuChEs; specific protein and nucleic acid sequences have been determined and altered by site-directed mutagenesis (Doctor *et al.*, 1998).

AChE and BuChE forms are each coded by single genes. The gene coding sequence for the collagen-tailed forms contains a C-terminal extension of 40 amino acids, the T-peptide, that interacts by a short proline rich attachment domain (PRAD) with the collagen. A single collagen gene (ColQ) is associated with both the AChE and BuChE collagen-tailed forms. The globular forms are synthesized by an alternative splice variant, the H-exon, that is expressed instead of the T-exon [see Krejci (1998) for a model and Massoulie *et al.* (1999) for further information].

The three-dimensional structures (Fig. 48.3) of ChEs are subjects of intense investigation (Doctor *et al.*, 1998; Massoulie *et al.*, 1999). In the past, the active site of AChE was loosely described by models based on work of Nachmansohn and Wilson (1951), in which there was a negatively charged "anionic" site and an "esteratic" site of catalytic residues. The positively charged choline moiety of ACh was hypothesized to bind to the negatively charged anionic site. A nucleophilic group, assumed to be a serine residue at the esteratic (acylation) site, was proposed to catalyze the hydrolysis [see Silman and Sussman (1998) for a more detailed historical perspective].

Recently, the crystallization of ChE proteins such as the dimeric AChE form of *Torpedo californica* has led to a more detailed understanding of the form/function relationships of the enzyme (Doctor *et al.*, 1998). An important feature is the embedding of the active site of AChE in a "gorge" lined with 14 aromatic residues, about 20 A from the surface of the protein (Fig. 48.3). The quaternary nitrogen of choline binds through interactions with π electrons of tryptophan residues (Sussman *et al.*, 1991) at the "peripheral site" at the mouth of the gorge, a region conceptually corresponding to the historical concept of an "anionic site." One current view of the molecular mechanism has the ester substrate led down the gorge by molecular interactions to become hydrolyzed at the bottom by a catalytic triad of glutamate 334, histidine 447, and serine 203 residues (Doctor *et al.*, 1998; Taylor, 1996). Matters of current research include whether the products are ejected via a "side" door to make room for the next substrate molecule or are rapidly moved to the entrance of the gorge.

The amino acid sequences around the entrance to the gorge that comprise the "peripheral site" may be important in determining the differences in substrate specificity and inhibition by excess substrate between AChE and BuChE forms (Doctor *et al.*, 1998; Reiner *et al.*, 1999). Figure 48.3 provides a three-dimensional diagram of an AChE molecule. (Other depictions may be found on the Internet by searching for "acetylcholinesterase.")

48.5 MECHANISM OF HYDROLYSIS

$$E + AX \underset{k_{-1}}{\overset{k_{+1}}{\rightleftharpoons}} EAX \overset{k_2}{\to} EA + X \overset{k_3}{\to} E + A$$

E: Enzyme; AX is substrate (ACh, acetylcholine) or inhibitor; EAX is reversible enzyme complex; X is Ch (choline); ks are reaction rate constants (see Rosenberry *et al.*, 1998; Taylor, 1996).

The kinetics of ACh hydrolysis is a complicated multistep process [Fig. 48.4 from Taylor (1996) is one depiction]. It is discussed here in abbreviated form. The first step is a nucleophilic attack of the carbonyl carbon resulting in the formation of a reversible enzyme–substrate complex (EAX), acylation of the catalytic site (EA), and liberation of choline. This is followed by a rapid hydrolysis of the acylated enzyme, producing acetic acid and regenerating the enzyme (E + A). A similar reaction scheme applies to BuChEs (Taylor, 1996). The real-time kinetics of the enzyme reactions has been described by one biochemist (Quinn, personal communication) as "approaching catalytic perfection." The rate of ACh turnover (described by k_{cat}/K_m) is extremely rapid, where $k_{cat} = k_2k_3/k_2 + k_3$ (the geometric mean of the two rate constants). AChE is capable of hydrolyzing 6×10^5 molecules of ACh per molecule of enzyme per minute, a turnover time of 150 microseconds (Taylor, 1996). The upshot of this rapid rate of hydrolysis is that k_1 becomes the rate-limiting step for hydrolysis of ACh and its analog acetylthiocholine (AcTC). Perhaps this represents the diffusion of substrate to the active center. The deacylation step

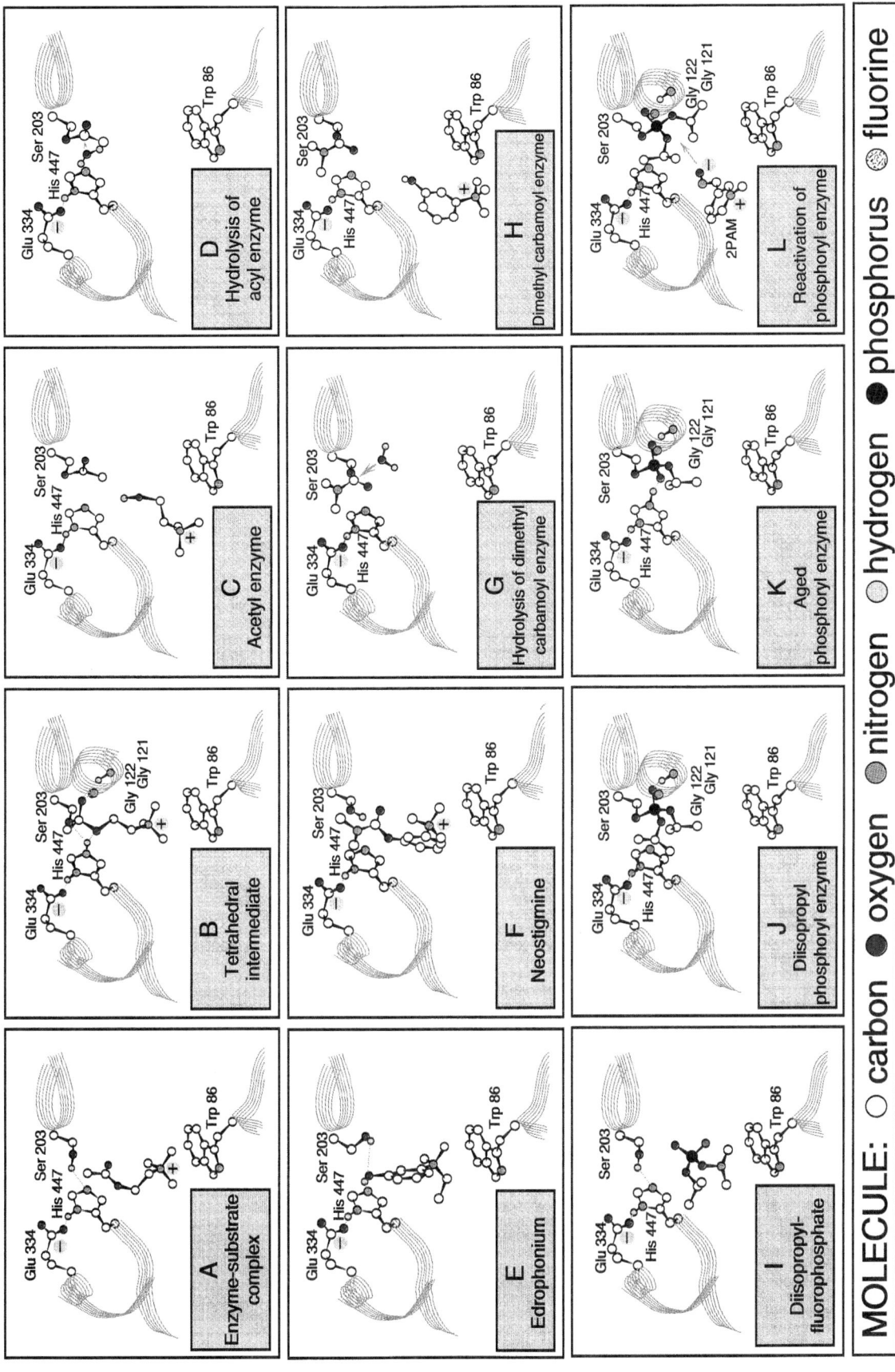

Figure 48.4 Hydrolysis of ACh by AChE and inhibition and reactivation of the enzyme. (A) Binding of ACh. (B) Attack by the serine hydroxyl, formation of a transient tetrahedral intermediate. (C) Loss of choline and formation of the acylated enzyme. (D) Deacylation of the enzyme by H_2O attack. (E) Binding of the reversible inhibitor edrophonium. (F) Binding of neostigmine. (G) Formation of the carbamoylated enzyme. (H) Hydrolysis of the carbamoylated enzyme. (I) Binding of diisopropyl fluorophosphate. (J) Formation of the phosphoryl enzyme. (K) Formation of the aged form of the phosphoryl enzyme. (L) Attack by pralidoxime (2-PAM) to regenerate active enzyme. (After Taylor, 1996.)

MOLECULE: ○ carbon ● oxygen ● nitrogen ○ hydrogen ● phosphorus ◉ fluorine

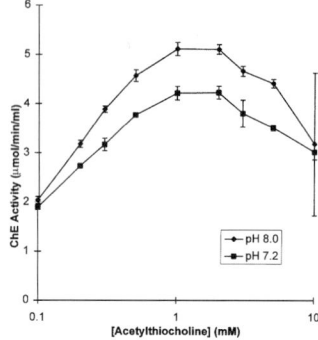

Figure 48.5 Effect of substrate concentration on activity of human blood AChE at pH 8.0 and pH 7.2. Ellman assay, pooled blood. (After Wilson *et al.*, 1997.)

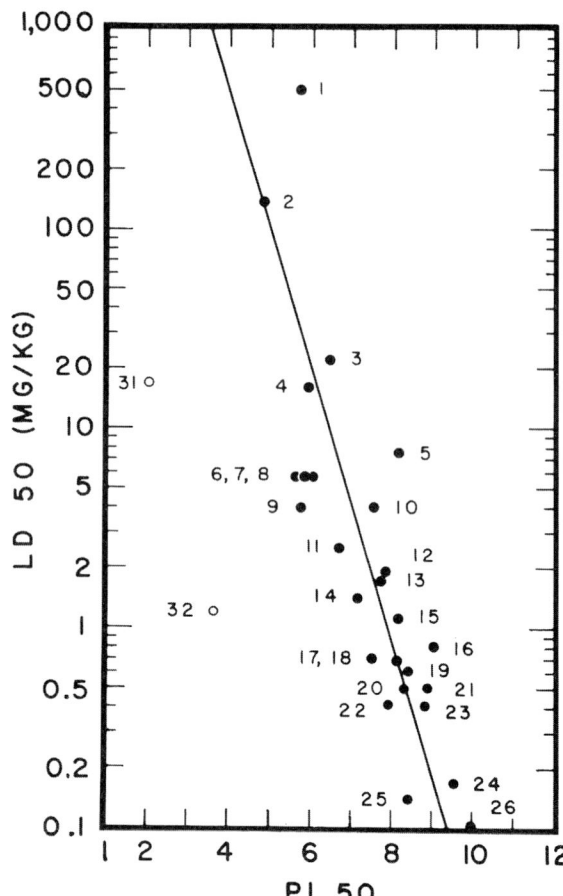

Figure 48.6 Toxicity *in vivo* of directly acting OPs versus their inhibition of AChE *in vitro*. (1) Dipterex. (2) O,O-diethyl-4-chlorophenylphosphate. (3) O,O-diethyl-bis-dimethyl pyrophosphorodiamide (sym). (4) TIPP. (5) O,O-diethylphosphostigmine. (6) Isodemeton sulfoxide. (7) Isodemeton. (8) Isodemeton sulfone. (9) DFP. (10) Diethylamidoethoxy-phosphoryl cyanide. (11) O,O-dimethyl-O,O-diisopropyl pyrophosphate (asy). (12) Diethyl; amido-methoxy-phosphoryl cyanide. (13) Tetramethyl pyrophospnate. (14) O,O-diethyl phosphorocyanidate. (15) O,O-dimethyl-O,O-diethyl pyrophosphate (asym). (16) Soman. (17) TEPP. (18) O-isopropyl-ethylphosphone-fluoridate. (19) Tabun. (20) Amiton. (21) Diethylamido-isopropoxy-phosphoryl cyanide. (22) O,O-diethyl-S-(2-diethylaminoethyl))phosphorothioate. (23) Sarin. (24) O,O-diethyl-S-(2-triethylammoniumethyl)thiophosphate iodide. (25) Echothiophate. (26) Methylfluorophosphorylcholine iodide. (27) Methylfluorophosphoryl-beta-methylcholine iodide. (28) O-ethyl-methylphosphorylthiocholine iodide. (29) Methylfluorophosphoryl-homo-choline iodide. (27), (28), and (29) with LD50 values from 0.03–0.07 mg/kg are not shown. (31) Schradan and (32) dimefox shown on the graph were not used to calculate the regression. (After Hayes as shown in Gallo and Lawryk, 1991.)

(k_3) is considered rate limiting to carbamoylating and phosphorylating agents.

A major distinction between AChEs and BuChEs is the inhibition of AChE activity with increasing substrate concentration [S]. A plot of activity versus [S] for ACh, AcTC, and, in mammals, acetyl-β-methylcholine, yields a curve with a maximum at 1–3 mM, whereas BuChE activity increases with [S] to at least 10 mM. These effects are illustrated in Fig. 48.5 from data of Wilson *et al.* (1997) for the human. The late Dr. A. R. Main (Hoffmann *et al.*, 1989) pointed out: "Because of this inhibition, methods for determining AChE activities should employ substrate concentrations at or below [S]$_{opt}$." Unfortunately, his advice has not always been followed.

The phenomenon of inhibition with excess substrate may be due to interactions at the peripheral site. Rosenberry *et al.* (1998) present evidence that excess substrate inhibition and the action of peripheral site inhibitors such as propidium are brought about by the imposition of a steric blockade in the catalytic pathway. Figuratively, a chemical cork blocks the gorge.

48.6 TOXICITIES OF ANTICHOLINESTERASES

The knowledge of the three-dimensional structure of the ChEs has led to a better understanding of the mechanisms of action of drugs and chemical agents that inhibit the hydrolysis of choline esters. In general, there are three major domains for inhibitors to bind. They are the acyl and choline pockets of the active center and the peripheral anionic site. Taylor (1996) uses edrophonium and tacrine as examples of reversible inhibitors that bind to the choline subsite near tryptophan 86 and glutamate 202; other reversible inhibitors such as fasciculin and propidium bind to the peripheral anionic site on AChE at the lip of the gorge encompassed by tryptophan 286 and tyrosines 72 and 124.

CBs and OP pesticides inhibit enzyme activity by acting as alternate substrates to ACh. Carbamates give rise to a carbamoylated enzyme that is more stable than the acylated enzyme, taking minutes instead of milliseconds to rehydrolyze. Organophosphate esters are true hemisubstrates; they covalently bind with the serine at the active center, forming a tetrahedral configuration that resembles the transition state formed during hydrolysis of ACh. If the alkyl groups on the OP are methyl or ethyl, spontaneous regeneration may require hours, and may be even longer if tertiary alkyl groups are involved. Loss of one of the alkyl groups, a phenomenon known as aging, further stabilizes the phosphorylated enzyme, to all intents and purposes permanently inhibiting its catalytic ability. It is not appropriate to use the terms "reversible" and "irreversible"

Table 48.4
Tissue IC50 Values for 4-Day and Adult Mice after Chlorpyrifos-Oxon

Tissue	Neonate	Adult
Brain	9.6 ± 0.1	10 ± 0.2
Liver	96 ± 3	530 ± 50
Plasma	18 ± 1.5	330 ± 28
Purified	3 nM for all tissues	

Source: Mortinsen *et al.* (1998).
Note: Values are nM, means $\pm$ SE.

Table 48.5
Necrosis of Rat Muscle after DFP and Botulinum Toxin (Btx)

Treatment	EDL	SOL
Saline	0	0
DFP	85.5	28.0
Btx	0	0
DFP + Btx	0	1.59

Source: Sket *et al.* (1991).
Notes: Necroses/1000 fibers; DFP injected 48 hours after Btx, sampled 24 hours later 1.5 mg/kg sc. EDL: extensor digitorum longus; SOL: soleus musce.

to refer to the inhibitions brought about by CBs and OPs, respectively. Both classes of chemicals react covalently with the active center of the enzyme, and at some stage of the sequence of reactions, both enzyme-inhibitor complexes are rehydrolyzable.

The toxicities of OPs and CBs often are correlated with the extent of their inhibitions of brain AChE. Figure 48.6 depicts the relationship between the toxicity *in vivo* of 30 directly acting OPs and their inhibition of AChE *in vitro*. However, such relationships do not necessarily signify that there are simple relationships between inhibition of AChE activity in an organ or tissue and in the test tube. For example, Mortinsen *et al.* (1998) measured IC50 values for chlorpyrifos-oxon with tissues from 4-day-old and adult rats (Table 48.4). The IC50s from young and adult brains were similar; the IC50s from the other tissues were not, differing by 5.5 (liver) and 20 (plasma) fold even though the IC50s of immunoprecipitated purified AChEs were the same, regardless of tissue or age. Possible interference of BuChE activities were excluded by using the specific BuChE inhibitor iso-OMPA. Factors such as A-esterase destruction, carboxyesterase binding, and sequestration of the lipophilic OP were considered possible factors to account for the differences between the *in vitro* and *in vivo* findings.

One example of a carboxyesterase is serum paraoxonase (PON1), an A-esterase associated with high-density plasma lipoproteins; PON1 destroys OPs such as the oxon analogs of parathion and chlorpyrifos. Direct evidence for its role in detoxifying OPs was provided by showing that mice exposed to chlorpyrifos were protected against cholinesterase inhibition and toxicity by administration of purified PON1 (Li *et al.*, 1995). Shih *et al.* (1998) demonstrated that knock-out PON1-deficient mice were more sensitive to chlorpyrifos and chlorpyrifos-oxon than genetically unaltered mice. Blood ChEs also have been shown to protect animals from OP toxicity. Studies on chemical warfare agents, led by the initial report of Wolfe *et al.* (1987), have shown that injection with purified AChE can protect mice and other animals from exposure to OPs (see Doctor *et al.*, 1991).

Many physiological actions of anti-ChEs are those expected from an excess of ACh caused by the inhibition of its catalysis. Specific symptoms depend on the chemicals and the receptors concerned (discussed elsewhere in this volume). Early signs of cholinergic poisoning likely involve stimulation of muscarinic neuroeffectors of the parasympathetic system. Symptoms include slowing of the heart (bradycardia), constriction of the pupil of the eye (miosis), diarrhea, urination, lacrimation, and salivation (Spencer *et al.*, 2000; Taylor, 1996). Overstimulation at skeletal nicotinic neuromuscular junctions (motor endplates) causes muscle fasciculation (disorganized twitching) and, at higher doses, muscle paralysis. Increased ACh at cholinergic junctions of the sympathetic and parasympathetic autonomic ganglia affect the eye, bladder, heart, and salivary glands. Finally, anti-ChEs affect junctions of the central nervous system (CNS), producing hypothermia, tremors, headache, anxiety, convulsions, coma, and death. Whether or not there are consistent behavioral effects at low dose levels of OPs and CBs, such as deficits in learning and memory, is a matter of current research.

In addition to affecting the nervous system, the excess ACh brought about by anticholinergic agents can cause a transient myopathy (Dettbarn, 1984). *In vivo* studies of Meshul (1989) and *in vitro* studies of the late Miriam Salpeter and colleagues using ACh receptor antagonists (Leonard and Salpeter, 1979) show this is due to an influx of Ca^{+2} and other cations into the postsynaptic cell. For example, necrosis due to diisopropyl fluorophosphate (DFP) was prevented *in vivo* by treatment with alpha-bungarotoxin, a snake venom agent that binds irreversibly to the nicotonic ACh receptor (Kasprzak and Salpeter, 1985). Further evidence that the necrosis is ACh mediated was provided by Sket *et al.* (1991). They demonstrated that botulinum toxin (a presynaptic inhibitor of ACh release) prevented muscle necrosis induced by diisopropyl fluorophosphate (DFP) in the rat (Table 48.5).

ACh-induced myopathy may cause necrosis in 10 to 30 percent of the muscle fibers around the motor endplates (Dettbarn, 1984). Prolonged muscle weakness and muscle damage lasting several weeks or longer may occur. A similar transient muscle damage in humans has been termed Intermediate Syndrome (Senanayake and Karalliedde, 1987).

Although it is generally accepted that most of the effects of OPs and CBs are due to inhibition of AChE, there is evidence for other modes of action of these agents. Anti-ChE pesticides have been shown to directly affect pre- and postsynaptic events (Pope, 1999). Electrophysiological studies suggest that choline itself may act as a regulator of nicotinic receptors in the CNS (Albuquerque *et al.*, 1998; Alkondon *et al.*, 1997). Malathion and other OPs have been shown to affect the immune responses of mammals and fish (Beaman *et al.*, 1999; Rodgers and Ellefson, 1990; Rodgers and Xiong, 1997). A few OPs, including some pesticides (e.g., isofenphos, chlorpyrifos) and at least one chemical warfare agent (sarin), have been shown to cause OPIDN (organophosphate induced delayed neuropathy), a distal axonopathy. (This topic is discussed elsewhere in this volume.)

Inhibition of ChEs plays a role in drug interactions. For example, cocaine is both detoxified by and is itself a reversible inhibitor of BuChEs. Studies on experimental animals indicate that depressing ChEs with anti-ChE treatments intensifies the toxic effect of cocaine (Hoffman *et al.*, 1992).

Genetic variation between individuals can play an important role in the toxicity of anti-ChEs. One example is humans with inherited low levels of plasma BuChEs. Although usually symptomless, patients with genetically low BuChE given succinylcholine (or a similar drug) during surgery to induce relaxation of muscles are unable to speedily destroy the drug, intensifying and prolonging its activity, sometimes with serious consequences. People with such a genetic makeup can be detected by assays using dibucaine and fluoride (Silk *et al.*, 1979). At least two genetic polymorphisms, that of low BuChE and PON1, are considered risk factors for OP and CB pesticide exposures (Shih *et al.*, 1998).

48.7 ASSAY TECHNIQUES

The history of ChE assays has been reviewed previously (e.g., Hoffmann *et al.*, 1989; Silver, 1974; Wills, 1972; Wilson, 1999; Witter, 1963). Some are "end-point" assays; others record the time course of the hydrolyses. One early assay to determine the hydrolysis of acetylcholine used a Warburg manometer to measure the CO^2 released from a bicarbonate containing buffer (Ammon, 1933). Although accurate, it is little used today. The particulars of this method are outlined by Wills (1972).

Following World War II, there was a widespread development of OPs for pest control. A veritable OP race ensued. By 1950, scientists were seeking rapid, accurate, and convenient clinical assays for blood ChE levels. Metcalf (1951) expressed the rationale for monitoring: "Since the cholinesterases of human blood are very sensitive to the presence of cholinesterase inhibitors, it appears that periodic estimation of blood cholinesterase levels may provide an indication of dangerous levels of overexposure to these toxicants." Several of the methods developed are still in use today. Hestrin (1949) determined the ACh remaining after incubation by reacting it with hydroxylamine under alkaline conditions to form a reddish-purple complex read at 515 nm. Metcalf (1951) adapted the method for drops of blood obtained with a spring-loaded lancet. Okabe *et al.* (1977) oxidized the choline released during ACh hydrolysis; the hydrogen peroxide produced was determined with an indicator reaction at 500 nm (see Abernathy *et al.*, 1988).

Three kinds of ChE assays are commonly used today; one utilizes electrometric (pH), another uses radiometric, and a third

Table 48.6
Common ChE Assays

Test	Basis	Conditions	Analysis
Johnson and Russell (1975)	Radiometric 3H-ACh	End point	Micro, fast, costly disposal
Michel (1949)	pH	Rate, ACh	Simple, slow, cheap
Ellman *et al.* (1961)	Colorimetric	Rate, ATCh	Micro, rapid

Adapted from Wilson and Henderson (1992).

uses colorimetric methodologies. Specific examples are listed in Table 48.6.

48.7.1 RADIOMETRIC

An example of a radiometric technique is that of Johnson and Russell (1975). It is based on the differential solubility of ACh and its hydrolysis products in organic and aqueous media. Sample and tritiated ACh are reacted together; an organic solvent is added when the assay is completed. The radioactive acetate remains in the aqueous phase, quenching its scintillation; the radioactive ACh that remains in the organic phase is counted. The values are compared to a totally hydrolyzed ACh sample, usually accomplished by incubation with an excess of eel AChE. This and similar assays have high sensitivity, problems with dilution of samples encountered with "reversible" carbamate chemicals are minimized, many tubes may be measured at once, the sample size is small, and readouts may be computerized. However, radioactive assays involve a high initial investment and costly disposal of radioactive waste. Being an end-point assay, many duplicate samples are needed to run a kinetic analysis. Potter *et al.* (1993) applied a radioactive assay similar to that of Thomsen *et al.* (1988, 1989) in a field study of applicators of OPs and fumigants. In this radiometric end-point method, ^{14}C-labeled ACh hydrolysis was stopped by ethanol/glacial acetic acid, the labeled acetic acid was evaporated, and the unhydrolyzed ACh counted.

48.7.2 pH

The modified Michel method (Michel, 1949) directly determines the change in pH due to ACh hydrolysis with a pH meter or by titrating the acetic acid produced with NaOH, while keeping the pH constant (Groff *et al.*, 1976; Nabb and Whitfield, 1967). Potentiometric methods are reliable, they use simple reagents, and they are relatively inexpensive. However, they are limited by their relative insensitivity; they often have larger sample requirements and lower outputs than radiometric methods. Several micro pH methods have been described (see Gage, 1967); one using 10 μl of capillary blood was described by Mosca *et al.* (1995).

pH assays can have relatively low variability. An early pH assay study of Rider *et al.* (1957) of 12 males and 12 females

Table 48.7
Plasma and RBC ACh Hydrolysis Levels for 40-Year-Old Blood Donors

	Men	Women
RBC ChE	0.766 ± 0.081	0.750 ± 0.082
Plasma ChE	0.953 ± 0.157	$0.817 + 0.187$

Source: Rider *et al.* (1957).
Notes: ΔpH/hour/0.02 ml red cells or plasma, 25°C, Mean $\pm$ S.D.

aged 40 years, taken from a study of 800 donors at a San Francisco blood bank, is shown in Table 48.7. Whether or not there is a difference between male and female subjects (as suggested in Table 48.7) is not clear. Many studies have noted a higher variability of plasma than RBC ChE activities. Gage (1967) points out that "... population averages obtained by different investigators ... depend to some extent upon the method of assay used." Even so, Gage concluded on the basis of the studies available to him, that "an individual in good health with a plasma ChE 33 percent below the population average, or a red cell cholinesterase more than 20 percent below, has an abnormally low value and has probably been exposed to a ChE inhibitor." Such "red-alert level" estimates have changed little in more than 30 years.

48.7.3 THIOL SUBSTRATES AND THE ELLMAN ASSAY

Thiocholine substrate assays based on the work of Ellman *et al.* (1961) may be the most popular of ChE assays, replacing the pH methods. Many variations of the original Ellman assay have been published. The conditions of three popular commercial assays are shown in Table 48.8. Several automated versions (e.g., those of Technicon and COBIAS) are no longer marketed. The basis for the thiocholine assays is the hydrolysis of acetylthiocholine (ACTh) or related substrates by the enzyme, producing a thiol group that reacts with a sulfhydryl-sensitive chromogen such as dithiobisnitrobenzoate (DTNB). In this case, peak absorption of the thionitrobenzoate produced is at 410–412 nm. The original Ellman assay used cuvettes; some

Table 48.8
Common Thiocholine-Based Assays

Parameter	Ellman	B/M Manual	B/M Auto	Sigma
Wavelength (nm)	412	405	480	405
Substrate (mM)	ATCh	ATCh	ATCh	PrTh
	0.5–1.0	5.4	5.4	5.0
pH	8.0	7.2	7.2	7.2
DTNB (mM)	0.32	0.24	0.24	0.25

Source: Wilson (1999).
Notes: ATCh: acetylthiocholine; PrTh: propionylthiocholine; B/M: Boehringer–Mannheim (Roche); DTNB: dithionitrobenzoate.

laboratories have modified the assay for a 96-well microplate reader in a manner similar to that described by Doctor *et al.* (1987). The Boehringer–Mannheim (Roche Diagnostics) kits (1981), Nos. 124117 and 450035, use ACTh as a substrate; the Sigma Diagnostic Cholinesterase (PTC) kit Procedure No. 422 uses propionylthiocholine (Sigma Diagnostics, 1989) for both AChE and BuChE. The Boehringer–Mannheim version used with a Hitachi automated spectrophotometer reads the reaction at 480 nm. This avoids possible interference of the Soret band of hemoglobin (Hb), but at the expense of reducing the sensitivity of the assay (Wilson and Henderson, 1992). The manual instrument kits recommend 405 nm. Instructions for both Boerhinger–Mannheim (Roche Diagnostics) and Sigma kits are for human blood. The reader is cautioned that the kits may not be suited to the needs of clinical veterinary laboratories or researchers without modification. In the case of the human, Wilson *et al.* (1997) showed that the high substrate concentration and low pH of the Boerhinger–Mannheim (Roche Diagnostics) kit introduce a difference of 40 percent in the manual assay compared to the Ellman assay run under optimum conditions (Fig. 48.5) . This is because the optimum concentration of substrate for human AChE is 1–2 mM and the optimum pH for the assay is pH 8.0, whereas the kit uses a substrate concentration of 5.4 mM and a pH of 7.2. Absorbances would have been even more reduced if the measurements for the Boerhinger–Mannheim (Roche Diagnostics) substrate and pH conditions were read at 480 nm (Wilson and Henderson, 1992).

There have been recommendations that the Ellman assay be modified to use dithionitrobenzoic acid (DTNA), a chromogen that absorbs in the near-ultraviolet at 340 nm, to avoid the interference of Hb at 410 nm, thus divorcing the wavelength of the assay from the Soret band of Hb (Christenson *et al.*, 1994; Loof, 1992; Willig *et al.*, 1996). However, instruments reading in the near-ultraviolet are often more costly than those that register in the visual range. The stability of modern instruments should be sufficient to overcome the increased noise level of the assay at 410 nm, providing activity levels are sufficiently high. The substrate and pH of the Sigma Diagnostics Kit are optimal for neither RBC nor plasma BuChE. Augustinsson *et al.* (1978) proposed using propionylthiocholine, the Sigma kit substrate, as a compromise substrate for both enzymes. Under the conditions of their assay, it was no better a substrate for one than it was for the other. They recommended measuring the reaction in the ultraviolet, avoiding Hb interference that might well play a role, given the reduced sensitivity of the assay. The Sigma kit is no doubt excellent as a screen for patients with reduced BuChE activities before they undergo surgery and treatment with muscle relaxants like succinylcholine and mivacurium, but its use may be more difficult to justify, given the excellence of today's instrumentation, for the determination of RBC AChE activities to detect exposures to pesticides, since the conditions are not optimum for the enzyme. What to do? With blood enzyme assays, no one size seems to fit all. One approach is to focus on ACTh hydrolysis, and specific inhibitors such as iso-OMPA or quinidine to inhibit BuChE, establishing an estimate of BuChE

Table 48.9
Relative Substrate Specificity of Plasma ChEs

Species	Propionyl	Butyryl	Benzoyl
Butyryl Favoring			
Dog	150	253	60
Horse	161	231	28
Cat	111	211	27
Man	155	192	36
Duck	139	153	25
Squirrel	122	144	14
Ferret	122	139	28
Propionyl Favoring			
Hamster	153	128	24
Rat	211	119	17
Chicken	147	83	6
Mouse	139	75	11

Source: Adapted from Hoffmann *et al.* (1989, Table 11.4) and Myers (1953).
Note: Normalized to plasma ChE hydrolysis of ACh = 100%.

by difference, accepting, for convenience, the use of an inappropriate substrate and substrate concentration.

The problems of using commercial kits with conditions designed for the human may be exacerbated when applied to other species. Many studies (some of which are summarized in Tables 48.9 and 48.10) indicate that, with other species, the relative activities of AChE and BuChEs, and even the properties of BuChEs, may differ from those of human enzymes. Lack of consideration for this may result in possible discrepancies and misinformation. For example, Harlin and Ross (1990) used adult bovine blood to establish conditions for the determination of cholinesterase activities in the only approved AOAC assay with ACTh as substrate and bovine blood. This excellent round-robin study did not discuss the report of Augustinsson (1959a, Table 51.2) that bovines had hardly any plasma cholinesterase activity. Further study is needed to establish whether the assay was determining only RBC AChE, and is useful for assaying it when serum cholinesterase is low or absent. Another problem arises when studies are undertaken with species that lack RBC AChE; the literature examined by the author suggests that only mammals have RBC AChE and that the properties of serum ChEs may vary with the species (Table 48.9).

Table 48.10
Relative Acetyl Ester Hydrolysis Levels of Several Species

Species	RBC	N	Plasma	N
Human	135 ± 29	60	37 ± 9.3	56
Dog	17.9 ± 3.5	18	25.4 ± 5.5	18
Male rat	9.0 ± 1.3	24	4.3 ± 1.0	45

Source: Adapted from Humiston and Wright (1967, Table 4).
Notes: ACTh 0.8 mM (RBC); 7 mM (plasma) Autotechnicon analyzer, Mean± SD, N = Trials.

Table 48.11
AChE/BuChE Activity of Rat Plasma

Total ChE	BuChE	AChE
452 ± 17	175 ± 12	210 ± 8

Source: Traina and Serpietri (1984).
Notes: Mean±S.E. mU/ml; 18 rats, Ellman assay. Total with acetylthiocholine; BuChE with butyrylthiocholine; AChE with acetylthiocholine + 0.1 mM iso-OMPA.

A further problem arises when, as is common in studies of laboratory animals that play a role in pesticide registration, the investigators assume AChE activity is restricted to the RBCs. Table 48.10 illustrates the wide differences between AChE activity in blood for humans and for two species often used in registration-geared research, the dog and the rat. Of the three, only the human has a relatively low ACTh hydrolysis rate in the plasma. Indeed, the AChE activity of rat plasma (Table 48.11) may exceed the activity of plasma BuChE.

Another source of plasma AChE is the platelets (Table 48.12). Although the AChE activity per platelet is high, its relative contribution to blood ChE is low, since the platelet content of blood is several orders of magnitude less than its content of RBCs. Studies of the particular AChE forms in the plasma of many species are lacking.

An important and often unrecognized problem with thiocholine-based assays is the presence of a transient nonlinear "thiol oxidase" reaction with the color reagent DTNB in RBCs of some species. It is necessary that assays with species such as the rat that have such high "tissue blanks" be designed to either circumvent or correct for them since they can lead to indeterminate errors greater than 70 percent (Table 48.13). One way is to include the appropriate blank in the assay. Another is to preincubate the samples for a few minutes before adding substrate until the nonlinear first 5–10 minutes of the assay are over (e.g., Chaney *et al.*, 2000). Lack of consideration of such problems in clinical assays of experimental animals submitted for regulatory purposes may have played a role in the difficulties encountered when the EPA tried to compare data from different laboratories on the rat (EPA, 1992). Errors may be compounded. For

Table 48.12
Comparison of RBC and Platelet Activities of Several Species

Species	Sex	Red blood cell	Platelet
Man	M/F	2180 ± 189	0
Cow	F	1910 ± 42	53 ± 21
Guinea pig	M/F	713 ± 76	493 ± 119
Horse	M/F	627 ± 200	1500 ± 252
Rabbit	M/F	473 ± 116	3930 ± 208
Rat	M	274 ± 64	4240 ± 1070
Cat	M/F[a]	30	5450

Source: Adapted from Zajicek (1957).
Notes: Manometric, $\mu l CO_2$/30 min/mgN; N = 3.
[a] N = 2.

Table 48.13
RBC DTNB Background Reaction in Various Species

Species	Percent total activity
Man	<10
Monkey	18–27
Dog	30–60
Rabbit	50–70
Rat	60–75
Mouse	<4
Brain (all species)	N/A

Source: Loof (1992).
Notes: Transient activity, first 5–10 minutes, Ellman method.

Table 48.14
Average Values of Cholinesterase Activity in Fasting Healthy Humans

Subjects	Men	Women
N	40	38
BuChE	8920 ± 2500	7490 ± 1950
AChE	1210 ± 200	1220 ± 123
AChE (Hb)	37.6 ± 4.91	39.3 ± 4.49

Source: Sidell and Kamiskis (1975).
Notes: BuChE in U/L, butyrylthiocholine, Boeringher/Mannheim (Roche) Kit; AChE in nU/RBC and U/g Hb (Hb), acetylthiocholine according to Ellman. Mean ± standard deviation.

example, a large and indeterminate error will occur when the Boehringer–Mannheim (Roche Diagnostics) kit assays are applied to rats without preincubating the samples. Such an error could be exacerbated by the low RBC activities and the misinterpreted plasma "BuChE" activities that are actually due to a mixture of the AChE and BuChE activities. The lesson is that, whatever the assay, it is critical that its conditions be validated for each species, tissue, and chemical under study.

CBs represent a special problem because of the ease of rehydrolysis of carbamate–ChE complexes. The sensitivity of the assay requires dilution of the enzyme samples, but the act of dilution itself promotes rehydrolysis of the enzyme. Several investigators have suggested ways to minimize the problem, including Thomsen et al. (1988) for the radiometric assays and Nostrandt et al. (1993) for Ellman-type thiocholine-based assays.

Regardless of the assay used, samples should be kept iced from the time of their collection to their assay. It is unfortunate that some are under the impression that OP exposures lead to "irreversible" inhibitions, and that icing a blood sample is unnecessary so long as an anticlotting agent such as EDTA or heparin has been used. To the contrary, as discussed elsewhere in this volume, ChE inhibitions by methyl-OPs such as azinphosmethyl (Guthion) have relatively rapid rates of spontaneous reactivation at room temperature; in this case, the half-life of recovery of activity for azinphos-methyl is approximately 2.5 hours (Wilson et al., 1992b). The lack of a requirement to keep samples on ice as a part of assay protocols makes it difficult to interpret the results of otherwise excellently designed and executed studies such as that of Yeary et al. (1993). Although the instructions that accompany the commercial ChE monitoring kits discussed in this chapter recommend storing samples under refrigeration [4°C, Boerhinger–Mannheim (Roche Diagnostics), 2–6°C or −20°C (Sigma Diagnostics)], several clinical laboratories we contacted said they did not specify that samples be delivered to them on ice.

48.7.4 VARIABILITY

When it comes to studies using the Ellman assay, a paraphrase from George Orwell's classic "Animal Farm" (1945)

might be that "All Ellman thiocholine assays are created equal, but some are more equal than others." The variety of conditions used in field studies and laboratory experiments with thiocholine substrates, and the lack of an accepted standard assay and enzyme, make it difficult to compare the activities obtained from one experiment to another (Carakostas and Landis, 1991; Wilson et al., 1992a). Perhaps this is what has led to the idea that thiocholine-based ChE studies are "too variable" to be relied upon for population exposure research and regulatory decisions, even though a number of carefully performed studies such as Sanz et al. (1991) indicate that ChE assays of populations can be performed with satisfactory results. For example, Sidell and Kamiskis (1975) measured RBC and plasma ChEs of a group of 22 subjects biweekly for a year, using the Technicon autoanalyzer. They found that RBC AChE levels varied less than hematocrit, Hb, or RBC counts. The annual average range of AChE values was 8% for men, 12% for women. The corresponding plasma ChE values were 25% for men, 24% for women. In general, as was true for the pH methods discussed earlier, plasma ChE values appear more variable than RBC AChE activities, whether the data are expressed on a per cell or a per Hb basis (Table 48.14).

Bellino et al. (1978) used fingersticks and saponin-hemolyzed human blood to carefully determine the optimum conditions for the Ellman assay for human red blood cells and

Table 48.15
ChE Activities of Healthy Human Subjects

Enzyme	Mean ± SE	n
AChE		
Male	4.99 + 0.14	72
Female	5.18 + 0.18	71
Pooled	5.08 + 0.11	143
BuChE		
Male	2.26 + 0.04	101
Female	2.46 + 0.09	71
Pooled	2.34 + 0.05	172

Source: Modified from Bellino et al. (1978).
Note: IU/ml whole blood; Ellman assay.

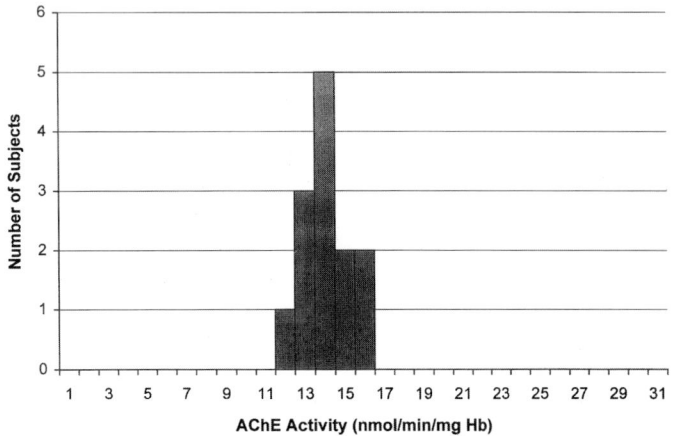

Figure 48.7 Fingerstick AChE activities of UC Davis volunteers. Whole blood hemolyzed with Triton X 100 and assayed according to Ellman modified for a multiple plate reader. Activity is 14.6 ± 1.2 nmoles/min/mg hemoglobin. $N = 13$. (After Wilson *et al.*, © 1998, Plenum.)

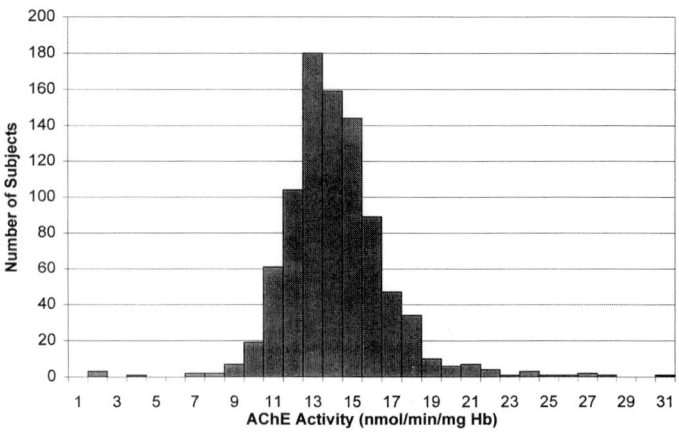

Figure 48.8 Fingerstick AChE activities of migrant family center residents. Blood filled capillaries kept on ice before returning to the laboratory. Whole blood assayed as in Fig. 48.7. Activity is 14.6 ± 2.6 nmoles/min/mg hemoglobin. $N = 894$. (After Wilson *et al.*, © 1998, Plenum.)

plasma, demonstrating inhibition of AcTh hydrolysis with excess substrate, and an S-shaped substrate–concentration curve with butyrylthiocholine. They established that 0.01 mM eserine inhibited AChE and 0.3 mM eserine inhibited BuChE. Similarly, they found that 7.0 mM totally inhibited both AChE and BuChE activity, and 2.8 mM of sodium dodecylsulphate inhibited AChE but not BuChE. Their study of healthy men and women showed relatively low variability. See Table 48.15.

Large sample numbers were obtained in a study of farm worker families from migrant housing centers in California by Wilson *et al.* (1998), in which almost 900 volunteers contributed fingersticks of blood. Ten microliters of blood were hemolyzed at the site, transported on ice to the laboratory, stored at −70°C, analyzed under optimum assay conditions for RBC AChE using quinidine to inhibit plasma BuCh, and expressed on a Hb basis. Mean activity of the migrant housing center families ($n = 894$) was 14.6 ± 2.6 nmol/min/mg Hb, virtually the same as those from fingersticks and venous blood draws of approximately a dozen UC Davis volunteers. See Figs. 48.7 and 48.8.

One problem to circumvent is the possible contamination of the sample with pesticide on the skin (Yuknavage *et al.*, 1997).

48.8 STANDARDS

Several companies provide AChE standards for laboratory use using human and other species ChE preparations. Wilson *et al.* (2000) have been testing an AChE standard prepared by hemolyzing washed bovine RBCs. These RBC ghosts showed low variability when stored either at refrigeration (+4°C) or low-temp (−75°C) freezer temperatures for more than 250 days, suggesting that such preparations are suitable for laboratory standards. Similar results have been obtained in shorter-term studies for a lyophilized AChE from Sigma Inc.

48.9 FIELD KITS

Well-designed, reliable field kits for cholinesterase determinations would be valuable for monitoring the health of those who apply pesticides and those who work in agricultural workplaces subject to pesticide spraying. Enzyme-impregnated filter paper, potentiometric sensors, and colorimetric comparisons have been used in the past (e.g., Collombel and Perrot, 1970; Dahlgren, 1983; Gamson *et al.*, 1973; Rogers *et al.*, 1991). A farely new device is the EQM Test-Mate kit (Magnotti *et al.*, 1988; Magnotti and Eberly, 1996). It uses a solid-state device and the Ellman method to measure ChE activity in a drop of whole blood obtained by a fingerstick. Several models have been marketed. The Test-Mate has the advantages of portability, relative low cost, conveniently prepared reagents, and small sample volumes. Field and laboratory studies have been conducted with it (Keifer *et al.*, 1996; Prall *et al.*, 1998). Nevertheless, the current model (Model ChE) is not recommended by the manufacturer for field use; the instructions advise it be operated in the laboratory by a trained technician. One difficulty with using whole blood is sensitivity; blood samples are not diluted as much as they would be using a larger, more sensitive device. Under these conditions, readings may be affected by the relatively high absorption of the Soret band of Hb at 412 nm, the optimum absorbance of DTNB, the Ellman colorimetric reagent. The Test-Mate models have attempted to circumvent this by using higher wavelengths, sacrificing sensitivity of the chromogen for a lower noise level (Wilson and Henderson, 1992). A second problem with the device is that the Test-Mate does not display the raw absorbance values of the reaction. Instead, it displays values normalized to those expected at 25°C, employing a temperature sensor and a built-in algorithm that has been criticized for accuracy temperature (Amaya *et al.*, 1996; London *et al.*, 1995; Wilson *et al.*, 1998).

48.10 REGULATORY MATTERS: ARE ChE INHIBITIONS ADVERSE EFFECTS?

Shortly after the introduction of OP pesticides, the experiences of University of California scientists led to a recommendation that "... individuals showing a 20 percent or more depletion from normal pre-exposure plasma ChE levels should discontinue participation in the work ... until cholinesterase levels have returned to normal" (Metcalf, 1951). Almost 50 years and many studies and task forces later, similar guidelines are still used. The rationale for choosing one specific decrease in ChE level over another as constituting a health hazard is not clear. One theory is that since most clinical laboratories should be able to detect a 20 percent decrease in ChE activity, and since dose/response curves for many anti-ChEs tend to be steep, this level provides a realistic statistically significant difference between test groups suitable for regulatory purposes.

48.11 BLOOD ChEs AND DETECTION OF EXPOSURE

Whether or not a decrease in ChE activity in the blood constitutes an "adverse effect" raises questions concerning the short- and long-term health of individuals, populations, and their progeny that have yet to be answered to the satisfaction of most investigators. Detecting a statistically significant decrease in blood ChE levels between a putative exposed group and an unexposed group, or compared to an accepted "normal" range, is usually accepted as indicating that a potentially hazardous exposure to an anti-ChE chemical has occurred. Anti-ChE chemicals are not usually long-lasting within the body, and blood ChE activity can be expected to recover relatively rapidly from inhibition by an OP or CB. In the human, RBCs (and their AChE activities) are replaced at approximately 0.9 percent per day (a 120-day life span). Plasma BuChE is replaced even more rapidly (Boyer *et al.*, 1977).

48.12 REACTIVATION OF INHIBITED AChE

The discovery of Wilson and Ginsburg (1955) that oximes could displace OPs from the active site of ChEs, restoring enzyme activity, provided an important treatment for OP poisonings. It also opened the door to using reactivation of inhibited enzymes to establish that exposure had occurred when reliable unexposed control data or normal ranges of activity were lacking (Hansen and Wilson, 1999) reviewed by Wilson *et al.*, 1992b. Useful as it may be, the application of reactivation techniques is not currently performed on a routine basis by clinical laboratories known to the author. Benschop and colleagues treated OP-inhibited serum ChE with potassium fluoride at pH 4 to chemically detect the presence of the inhibited OP-ChE. The fluoride ions reactivated the inhibited enzyme, converting the OP moiety into the corresponding phosphofluoridate and permitting its subsequent identification. Benschop's

group applied the technique to obtain direct evidence of exposure to sarin in several victims of the release of the nerve gas in a Tokyo subway in 1986, and from an earlier incident in Matsumoto Japan (Polhuijs *et al.*, 1997, 1999).

48.13 SIGNIFICANCE OF BLOOD ChEs

Even if ChEs were not the targets of a multibillion-dollar, worldwide pesticide industry, they would still be of great interest to physiologists, cell biologists, and biochemists. ChEs have important roles in regulating neural transmission, and they are targets for pharmacological interventions in disorders such as glaucoma, myasthenia gravis, and Alzheimer's (Taylor, 1996). The widespread use of OP and CB pesticides and the dangers attendant upon their applications have resulted in ChE enzymes being used as biomarkers of both exposure and effect in assessing the risks to workers in agriculture and to consumers. ChEs enter into the picture in several ways. One is in the use of experimental animals, most often rats, but also dogs, rabbits, and other species, to determine no-effect levels that can be extrapolated to the human. Another is in the recommendation of safe residue levels in food. A third role is to help provide a safe agricultural workplace by monitoring those who could be exposed to dangerous levels of anti-ChE chemicals (i.e., mixer loaders, applicators). A fourth role is to decide whether poisoning episodes have involved ChE-inhibiting agents. One factor in favor of using ChEs for such clinical and regulatory ends is the ease with which they may be rapidly and inexpensively assayed compared to analyzing for the cholinergic chemicals themselves. Generations of toxicologists and public officials have worked to establish ChE assays as a simple way to help provide answers to complicated questions of health effects, exposures, and risk. Today, agencies require submission of blood and brain ChE levels from experimental animals after short- and long-term experiments as part of the registration process for pesticides. Most agree with the position that statistically significant decreases in brain ChE activities, when accompanied by knowledge of the doses involved, are useful for establishing quantitative toxicity indices. Even so, issues such as the significance of ChE levels in specific parts of the brain and the applicability of one animal model over another are unresolved.

There is continuing discussion of the significance of monitoring blood ChEs of humans and other animals. One issue is the role of no observable adverse effect levels (NOAELs, the highest dose levels at which no important effect of a drug is observed) in assigning safe levels for toxic chemicals. One way to establish NOAELs is by batteries of behavioral tests under controlled laboratory conditions. Another is to measure residues on skin and clothing, urinary metabolites of agricultural workers, and fecal metabolites of laboratory and wild animals. Blood ChE levels represent standardized, relatively inexpensive measurements of a biochemical effect due to an exposure to a toxic chemical, in addition to providing evidence of the exposure itself (Nigg and Knaak, 2000). But some do not agree. For example, an industry "Acute Cholinesterase Risk Assessment

Work Group" has published a review of RBC AChE, plasma ChE, and brain AChE activities focusing on their use in risk assessment (Carlock *et al.*, 1999). The review drew upon the literature and a compilation of toxicity data from previously unpublished industry sources in which the chemicals were listed by code and category. The work group concluded in part that: (*a*) plasma ChE should not be used in risk assessments since it is not an adverse effect; (*b*) RBC inhibition is not *per se* an adverse effect; (*c*) when available, cholinergic effects or brain AChE levels should be used ahead of RBC AChE values in setting NOELs, and that human data should take precedence over animal-derived results. In their discussion of NOELs, the group did not take into account that much of the data were derived from studies of rats and dogs and were not corrected for blood AChE levels or thiol oxidase activities of the RBCs, as discussed earlier in this chapter.

A moderate position might be to use blood ChE values as biomarkers of exposure to anti-ChE inhibitors, rather than to insist they be considered quantitative indicators of physiological effects, thus supporting their use as early warning signs and as important weight-of-evidence factors.

48.14 DIRECT EFFECTS

Although much of the attention of neurotoxicologists has been directed toward understanding the nature of the inhibition of ChEs and their toxicological consequences, a number of neuroscientists have been studying direct effects of anti-ChE agents on the presynaptic release of ACh (e.g., Rocha *et al.*, 1996) and on the postsynaptic target receptors of ACh. For example, van den Beukel *et al.* (1998) found that micromolar levels of physostigmine, parathion, paraoxon, and phenyl saligenin cyclic phosphate blocked ACh-induced transient nicotinic inward currents in mouse N1E-115 and human neuroblastoma and locust thoracic ganglion cells. The Eldefrawis' and colleagues (Katz *et al.*, 1997) demonstrated that chlorpyrifos, parathion, and their oxons bind to and desensitize the nicotinic receptor (nAChR) of Torpedo, the electric ray. Narahashi's group (Nagata *et al.*, 1997) used rat clonal phaeochromocytoma (PC12) cells to demonstrate that neostigmine and carbaryl blocked nAChR channels. In contrast, Albuquerque's group (Camara *et al.*, 1997) found that methamidophos did not affect neurotransmitter release or act directly on rat nAChR but that choline itself affected the response of the receptors (Albuquerque *et al.*, 1998). The low levels at which these electrophysiological effects occur strongly suggest they should be taken into consideration when considering the effects of ChE-inhibiting OPs and carbamates, such as the report of Burruel *et al.* (2000) of effects of methamidophos on sperm in mice.

48.15 ANTIDOTES

ChE inhibitions by OPs and CBs are one of the few examples of enzyme inhibitions for which there are specific antidotes. Two drugs in use are atropine and pralidoxime (2-PAM). Doses depend on the extent of exposure and species. Atropine binds to the muscarinic ACh receptor (mAChR), reducing the effectiveness of the excess ACh generated by the inhibition of AChE. It is given intravenously as required to relieve the symptoms of excess ACh in cases of pesticide poisoning. Oximes directly reactivate OP-inhibited AChEs (Wilson and Ginsburg, 1955; reviewed in Wilson *et al.*, 1992b). 2-PAM Cl (Protopam) is the oxime registered for use in the United States; its methanesulfonate salt (P2S) is used in Europe. Reactivation of the enzyme involves transfer of the substituted phosphate or phosphonate residue from the catalytic site of the enzyme to the oxime.

There has been much research on treatment of exposure to ChE inhibitors focusing on chemical warfare agents (e.g., Hille *et al.*, 1995; Raveh *et al.*, 1996). One of the U.S. Department of Defense kits is "Convulsion Antidote for Nerve Agents (CANA)." It has 2 ml of the anticonvulsant diazepam, and "Nerve Agent Antidote Kit (NAAK)" containing autoinjectors with 2 mg of atropine and 600 mg of pralidoxime. Another kit, "Nerve Agent Pre-treatment Tablets (NAPS)" contains 30-mg tablets of pyridostigmine bromide to be taken orally three times a day. A Swedish auto-injector contains HI-6 (500 mg), an oxime not available in the United States, and atropine (2 mg). The logic behind the use of pyridostigmine bromide is that this CB AChE inhibitor will reduce the extent to which AChE becomes irreversibly inhibited by rapidly aging chemical warfare agents such as soman, by virtue of its ability to temporarily occupy the catalytic site of AChE, interfering with its more permanent phosphorylation by soman and other OPs (Tuovinen *et al.*, 1999). Three 30-mg doses of pyridostigmine bromide per day were given to the Allied Forces during the Gulf War under an experimental-drug FDA license. This led to speculations that the interaction of this CB with other neuroactive chemicals present in the sector was a factor in the cluster of symptoms termed the Gulf War Syndrome (Abou-Donia *et al.*, 1996a, b; Kurt, 1998). An alternative approach to OP poisoning is to destroy the agent within the body. Two of the most successful treatments are to inject purified ChEs to bind the agents and phosphotriesterases to destroy them (e.g., Tuovinen *et al.*, 1999; Wolfe *et al.*, 1987).

Experimental evidence of nerve damage (in this case to chickens) was reported by Abou-Donia and co-workers after combined treatments of pyridostigmine bromide, DEET (an insect repellent), chlorpyrifos (Abou-Donia *et al.*, 1996a), or permethrin (Abou-Donia *et al.*, 1996b).

48.16 RISK ASSESSMENT AND ChEs

ChE activity has been used for many years as a biomarker of exposure and effect for setting regulations for anti-ChE pesticide use and for safe levels of such pesticides in foods and in the environment. Almost three-quarters of a century of research has provided tools to qualitatively establish whether exposure has occurred to man and other animals in the laboratory, the clinic, and the environment. Nevertheless, problems arise when data are used quantitatively, such as in setting NOAELs of a pesticide in food, or in estimating lifetime exposure levels of a chemical warfare agent. The lack of universally acceptable standards for ChE assays and the difficulty in deciding whether ChE levels are, in and of themselves, an adverse effect are two of the difficulties encountered when using ChE activities for regulatory purposes. Even so, cholinergic mechanisms became a criterion for creating a category of aggregate pesticide use in the new Food Quality and Protection Act (Mileson *et al.*, 1998).

The U.S. Food Quality and Protection Act was passed unanimously by Congress on August 3, 1996. It created a single health-based safety standard for pesticide residues in food and removed the regulation that specified zero tolerance from pesticides that may be concentrated in processed commodities. It required a "reasonable certainty" that no harm will result from aggregate exposures, that is, exposures from chemicals with a common mode of action. The Act was health based; that is, exposures from diet, including drinking water, and nonfood exposures (e.g., residential, lawn, garden, indoor, institutional, industrial uses) were all to be considered. Children received special treatment; up to 10 additional uncertainty factors could be added for them. The Act specifies the use of sound science in making the determinations and requires a focus on health-based approaches to food safety and the promotion of safer, effective pest control methods.

Applying the policies delineated by the FQPA may occupy the attention of the agricultural community, government regulators, and toxicologists specializing in agricultural chemicals for the next decade. It is safe to predict that there will continue to be sticky issues at each step of the risk assessment process, in the assessments of hazard, dose–response and exposure, and the characterization of risk.

A special problem will involve determining aggregate exposures, deciding which chemicals should be included as part of a common "Risk Cup." ChE-inhibiting chemicals played a leading role in this venture when a panel of distinguished toxicologists asserted that inhibition of AChE was a "common mechanism of toxicity" for OPs. They concluded "that OP pesticides act by a common mechanism of toxicity if they inhibit phosphorylation and elicit any spectrum of cholinergic effects" (Mileson *et al.*, 1998). It may be too soon to say whether such a pharmacologically simplistic, but regulatorily valuable, view will win the day. Pope (1999), one of the authors of the "common mechanism" review, concluded in a separate article that "additional macromolecular targets for some OP pesticides . . . may alter the cascade of events following AChE phosphorylation and thereby modify that common mechanism. . . ." His review analyzed the comparative toxicity of 38 OP AChE inhibitors currently in use in pesticides. Demonstrated direct effects of anticholinesterases on receptors and transmitter release discussed earlier in this chapter, and the evidence of groups like Albuquerque's that choline itself may have an effect on ACh receptors (Albuquerque *et al.*, 1998; Alkondon *et al.*, 1997), suggest that there may be holes in the "Risk Cup." Whether the leaks are large enough to lead to a modification of the "common mechanism" policy is a matter for the future.

48.17 CHOLINESTERASES TOMORROW

The specific course of research on ChEs parallels, indeed has been at the cutting edges of some of the advances of the 20th century in biochemistry, pharmacology, physiology, cell biology, and toxicology. Many of today's disciplines had not yet been christened when ChEs were first recognized as special proteins intimately associated with the regulation of the nervous system. Although it is likely that some anticholinergic agricultural chemicals will be replaced by newer agents with different modes of action, ChEs are not likely to languish. (Registrations of several OPs already have been cancelled or restricted in use in the last ten years in the United States.) Nevertheless, use of OPs and CBs elsewhere on the planet will certainly continue for the foreseeable future, if only because some countries may not be able to afford the new generations of chemicals. The rapid development of cDNA microarrays suggests that studies of the impact of anticholinergic chemicals will soon be routinely conducted on the level of responsive genes (Gupta *et al.*, 1999). The advent of probabilistic methods of assessing risk of pesticides to human health and wildlife will create opportunities to apply sophisticated methods of determining risk from anticholinergic agents based on the population distributions of exposures and effects (Boyce, 1998). Research into the molecular bases of pharmaceuticals, enzyme action, development of the nervous system, and many other basic features of living systems will benefit from studies of ChEs for many years to come. And, dismayingly, the simplicity of synthesizing and deploying anti-ChEs as weapons of war and terror is likely to be as tempting to governments and terrorists of the 21st century as they have been to some in the 20th. Today's scientists leave a legacy of knowledge for those who come after, but the gift of wisdom is not theirs to bestow, much as they might wish to do so.

REFERENCES

Abderhalden, E., and Paffrath, H. (1925). Beitrag der Frage der Inkret(Hormon)-Wirkung aud die motorischen Funktionen des Verdauungskanales V. Uber die synthese von cholinestern aus Cholin und Fettsauren mittels Fermenten des Dunndarm. *Fermentforsch* **8**, 299.

Abernathy, M. H., Fitzgerald, H. P., and Ahern, K. M. (1988). An enzymatic method for erythrocyte acetylcholinesterase. *Clinical Chemistry* **34**, 1055–1057.

Abou-Donia, M. B., Wilmarth, K. R., Abdel-Rahman, A. A., Jensen, K. F., Oehme, F. W., and Kurt, T. L. (1996a). Increased neurotoxicity following concurrent exposure to pyridostigmine bromide, DEET, and chlorpyrifos. *Fund. Appl. Toxicology,* **34**, 201–222.

Abou-Donia, M. B., Wilmarth, K. R., Jensen, K. F., Oehme, F. W., and Kurt, T. L. (1996b). Neurotoxicity resulting from coexposure to pyridostigmine bromide, deet, and permethrin, implications of Gulf War chemical exposures. *J. Toxicology Environ. Health,* **48**, 35–56.

Albuquerque, E. X., Pereira, E. F., Braga, M. F., and Alkondon, M. (1998). Contribution of nicotinic receptors to the function of synapses in the central nervous system, the action of choline as a selective agonist of alpha 7 receptors. *J. de Physiologie* **92**, 309–316.

Aldridge, W. N., and Reiner, E. (1972) "Enzyme Inhibitors as Substrates." North-Holland/American Elsevier, Amsterdam.

Alkondon, M., Pereira, E. F., Cortes, W. S., Maelicke, A., and Albuquerque, E. X. (1997). Choline is a selective agonist of alpha7 nicotinic acetylcholine receptors in the rat brain neurons. *Eur. J. Neurosci.* **12**, 2734–2742.

Amaya, A., Keifer, M., and McConnell, R. (1996). Comment on EQM Testmate OP cholinesterase kit. *Occupat. Environ. Medicine* **53**, 358.

Ammon, R. (1933). Die fermentative spaltung des acetylcholins. *Arch. ges. Physiol. Menschen Tiere* **233**, 486–491.

Anderson, R. B., and Key, B. (1999). Role of acetylcholinesterase in the development of axon tracts within the embryonic vertebrate brain. *Int. J. Devel. Neurosci.* **17**, 787–793.

Atkinson, J. E., Bolte, H. F., Rubin, L. F., and Sonawane, M. (1994). Assessment of ocular toxicity in dogs during 6 months' exposure to a potent organophosphate. *J. Appl. Toxicol.* **14**, 145–152.

Augustinsson, K.-B. (1948). Cholinesterases, a study in comparative enzymology. *Acta Physiol. Scand.* **15**(Suppl 52), 1–182.

Augustinsson, K.-B. (1959a). Electrophoresis studies on blood plasma esterases. I. Mammalian plasmata. *Acta Chem. Scand.* **13**, 571–592.

Augustinsson, K.-B. (1959b). Electrophoresis studies on blood plasma esterases. II. Avian, reptilian, amphibian and pisacine plasmata. *Acta Chem. Scand.* **13**, 1081–1096.

Augustinsson, K.-B., Eriksson, H., and Faijersson, Y. (1978). A new approach to determining cholinesterase activities in samples of whole blood. *Clin. Chim. Acta* **89**, 239–252.

Austin, L., and Berry, W. K. (1953). Two selective inhibitors of cholinesterase. *Biochem. J.* **54**, 695–700.

Ballantyne, B., and Marrs, T. C. (1992). "Clinical and Experimental Toxicology of Organophosphates and Carbamates." Butterworth-Heinemann Ltd., Oxford.

Bartels, C. F., Xie, W., Miller-Lindholm, A. K., Schopfer, L. M., and Lockridge, O. (2000). Determination of the DNA sequences of acetylcholinesterase and butyrylcholinesterase from cat and demonstration of the existence of both in cat plasma. *Biochem. Pharmacol.* **60**(4), 479–487.

Beaman, J. R., Finch, R., Gardner, H., Hoffmann, F., Rosencrance, A., and Zelikoff, J. T. (1999). Mammalian immunoassays for predicting the toxicity of malathion in a laboratory fish model. *J. Toxicol. Environ. Health* **56**, 523–542.

Bellino, M., Ficarra, M., Frontali, N., Ghezzo, F., Guarcini, A. M., Orecchio, F., Serpietri, L. A., and Traina, M. E. (1978). A quick and simple method for the routine determination of acetyl- and butyrylcholinesterase in blood. *Brit. J. Ind. Med.* **35**, 161–167.

Boehringer Mannheim Diagnostics. (1981). Reagenset cholinesterase 124117. Boehringer Mannheim Diagnostics Division, Indianapolis, IN.

Boyce, C. P. (1998). Comparison of approaches for developing distributions for carcinogenic slope factors. *Hum. Ecol. Risk Assess.* **4**(2), 527–577.

Boyer, A. C., Brown, L. J., Slomka, M. B., and Hine, C. H. (1977). Inhibition of human plasma cholinesterase by ingested dichlorvos, effect of formulation vehicle. *Toxicol. Appl. Pharmacol.* **41**, 389–394.

Boyes, W. K., Tandon, P., Barone, Jr., S., and Padilla, S. (1994). Effects of organophosphates on the visual system of rats. *J. Appl. Toxicol.* **14**, 135–143.

Brimijoin, S. (1992). Enzymology and biology of cholinesterases. *In* "Proceedings of the U.S. EPA Workshop on Cholinesterase Methodologies," p. 30. U.S. Environmental Protection Agency, Washington, DC.

Burruel, V. R., Raabe, O. G., Overstreet, J. W., Wilson, B. W., and Wiley, L. M. (2000). Paternal effects from methamidophos administration in mice. *Toxicol. Appl. Pharmacol.* **165**, 148–157.

Camara, A. L., Braga, M. F., Rocha, E. S., Santos, M. D., Cortes, W. S., Cintra, W. M., Aracava, Y., Maelicke, A., and Albuquerque, E. X. (1997). Methamidophos, an anticholinesterase without significant effects on postsynaptic receptors or transmitter release. *Neurotoxicology* **18**, 589–602.

Carakostas, M. C., and Landis, M. A. (1991). Modification of an automated method for determining plasma and erythrocyte cholinesterase activity in laboratory animals. *Vet. Hum. Toxicol.* **33**, 450–456.

Carlock, L. L., Chen, W. L., Gordon, E. B., Killeen, J. C., Manley, A., Meyer, L. S., Mullin, L. S., Pendino, K. J., Percy, A., Sargent, D. E., Seaman, L. R., Svanborg, N. K., Stanton, R. H., Tellone, C. I., and Van Goethem, D. L. (1999). Regulating and assessing risks of cholinesterase-inhibiting pesticides, divergent approaches and interpretations. *J. Toxicol. Environ. Health Part B* **2**, 105–160.

Chambers, J. E., and Levi, P. E. Eds. (1992). "Organophosphates: Chemistry, Fate, Effects." Academic Press, New York.

Chaney, L. A., Wineman, R. W., Rockhold, R. W., and Hume, R. S. (2000). Acute effects of an insect repellant, N,N-Diethyl-m-toluamide, on cholinesterase inhibition induced by pyridostigmine bromide in rats. *Toxicol. Appl. Pharm.* **165**, 107–114.

Chen, J.-W., and Ling, K.-H. (1996). Territrems, naturally occurring specific irreversible inhibitors of acetylcholinesterase. *J. Biomed. Sci.* **3**, 54–58.

Chiappa, S., and Brimijoin, S. (1998). Pharmacologic tests of a role for acetylcholinesterase in promoting neurite outgrowth by dorsal root ganglia. *In* "Structure and Function of Cholinesterases and Related Proteins" (B. P. Doctor *et al.*, eds.), pp. 585–592. Plenum Press, New York.

Christenson, W. R., Van Goethem, D. L., Schroeder, R. S., Wahle, B. S., Dass, P. D., Sangha, G. K., and Thyssen, J. H. (1994). Interlaboratory comparison determinations and the effect on the results of statistical evaluation of cholinesterase inhibition. *Toxicol. Lett.* **71**, 139–150.

Collombel, C., and Perrot, L. (1970). Determination of the cholinesterase activity of whole blood removed by pricking the skin and deposited on filter paper. Application to the detection of organophosphorus insecticide poisonings. *J. Eur. Toxicol.* **3**, 368–372.

Culetto, E., Combes, D., Fedon, Y., Roig, A., Toutant, J. P., and Arpagaus, M. (1999). Structure and promoter activity of the 5′ flanking region of ace-1, the gene encoding acetylcholinesterase of class A in Caenorhabditis elegans. *J. Molec. Biol.* **290**, 951–966.

Dahlgren, E. (1983). "Recent Research in Sweden on Chemical Detection." Nat. Def. Res. Inst., Umea, Sweden. FOA Rep. C 40171-C2, C3, Proc. Int. Symp. Prot. Against Chem. Warf. Agents, pp. 77–82.

Dale, H. H. (1914). The action of certain esters and ethers of choline and their relation to muscarine. *J. Pharmacol. Exp. Ther.* **6**, 147–190.

De la Hoz, D., Doctor, B. P., Ralston, J. S., Rush, R. S., and Wolfe, A. D. (1986). A simplified procedure for the purification of large quantities of fetal bovine serum acetylcholinesterase. *Life Sci.* **39**, 195–199.

Delmonte Corrado, M. U., Politi, H., Trielli, F., Angelini, C., and Falugi, C. (1999). Evidence for the presence of a mammalian-like cholinesterase in Paramecium primaurelia (Protista, Ciliophora) developmental cycle. *J. Exper. Zool.* **283**(1), 102–105.

Dementi, B. (1994). Ocular effects of organophosphates, a historical perspective of Saku disease. *J. Appl. Toxicol.* **14**, 119–129.

Dettbarn, W. D. (1984). Pesticide induced muscle necrosis: Mechanisms and prevention. *Fund. Appl. Toxicol.* **4**(2 Pt 2), S18–26.

Doctor, B. P., Taylor, P., Quinn, D. M., Rotundo, R. L., and Gentry, M. K. (1998). "Structure and Function of Cholinesterases and Related Proteins." Plenum Press, New York.

Doctor, B. P., Raveh, L., Wolfe, A. D., Maxwell, D. M., and Ashani, Y. (1991). Enzymes as pretreatment drugs for organophosphate toxicity. *Neurosci. and Biobehavioral Rev.* **15**, 123–128.

Doctor, B. P., Toker, L., Roth, E., and Silman, I. (1987). Microtiter assay for acetylcholinesterase. *Analyt. Biochem.* **166**, 399–403.

Ecobichon, D. J. (1996). Toxic effects of pesticides. *In* "Cassarett and Doull's Toxicology," 5th ed., (C. D. Klassen, ed.), pp. 655-666. McGraw-Hill, New York.

Ellman, G. L., Courtney, K. D., Andres, Jr., V., and Featherstone, R. M. (1961). A new rapid colorimetric determination of acetylcholinesterase activity. *Biochem. Pharm.* **7**, 88–95.

Engelhart, E., and Loewi, O. (1930). Fermentative azetylcholinspaltung im blut und ihre hemmung. *Naunyn-Schiedeberg's Arch. Exptl. Pathol. Pharmakol.* **150**, 1–13.

Faerman, C., Ripoll, D., Bon, S., Le Feuvre, Y., Morel, N., Massoulie, J., Sussman, J. L., and Silman, I. (1996). Site-directed mutants designed to test back-door hypotheses of acetylcholinesterase function. *FEBS Lett.* **386**, 65–71.

Francis, P. T., Palmer, A. M., Snape, M., and Wilcock, G. K. (1999). The cholinergic hypothesis of Alzheimer's disease, a review of progress. *J. Neurology, Neurosurgery Psychiatry* **66**, 137–147.

Furlong, C. E., Li, W.-F., Richter, R. J., Shih, D. M., Lusis, A. J., Alleva, E., and Costa, L. G. (2000). Genetic and temporal determinants of pesticide sensitivity, role of paraoxonase (PON1). *Neurotoxicology* **21**(1 & 2), 91–100.

Gage, J. C. (1967). The significance of blood cholinesterase activity measurements. *Residue Rev.* **18**, 159–173.

Gallo, M. A., and Lawryk, N. J. (1991). Organic phosphorus pesticides. In "Handbook of Pesticide Toxicology" (W. J. Hayes, Jr. and E. R. Laws, Jr., eds.), pp. 917–1123. Academic Press, New York.

Gamson, R. M., Robinson, D. W., and Goodman, A. (1973). Test for anticholinesterase materials in water. *Environ. Sci. Technol.* **7**, 1137–1140.

Geller, A. M., Abdel-Rahman, A. A., Peiffer, R. L., Abou-Donia, M. B., and Boyes, W. K. (1998). The organophosphate pesticide chlorpyrifos affects form deprivation myopia. *Investigative Ophthalmol. Visual Sci.* **39**, 1290–1294.

Gnatt, A., Lowenstein, Y., Yaron, A., Schwarz, M., and Soreq, H. (1994). Site-directed mutagenesis of active site residues reveals plasticity of human butyrylcholinesterase in substrate and inhibitor interactions. *J. Neurochem.* **62**, 749–755.

Groff, W. A., Kaminskis, A., and Ellin, R. I. (1976). Interconversion of cholinesterase enzyme activity units by the manual $^{\wedge}$pH method and recommended automated method. *Clin. Toxicol.* **9**, 353–358.

Gupta, P. K., Roy, J. K., and Prasad, M. (1999). DNA chips, microarrays and genomics. *Curr. Sci.* **77**, 875–884.

Haley, R. W., Billecke, S., and LaDu, B. N. (1999). Association of low PON1 Type Q (Type A) arylesterase activity with neurologic symptom complexes in Gulf War veterans. *Toxicol. Appl. Pharmacol.* **157**, 227–233.

Hamm, J. T., Wilson, B. W., and Hinton, D. E. (1998). Organophosphate-induced acetylcholinesterase inhibition and embryonic retinal cell necrosis in vivo in the teleost (Oryzias latipes). *Neurotoxicology* **19**, 853–869.

Hansen, M. E., and Wilson, B. W. (1999). Oxime reactivation of RBC acetylcholinesterases for biomonitoring. *Arch. Environ. Contamination Toxicol.* **37**, 283–289.

Harlin, K. S., and Ross, P. F. (1990). Enzymatic-spectrophotometric method for determination of cholinesterase activity in whole blood, collaborative study. *J. Assoc. Off. Anal. Chem.* **73**, 616–619.

Hestrin, S. (1949). The reaction of acetylcholine and other carboxylic acid derivatives with hydroxylamine, and its analytical application. *J. Biol. Chem.* **180**, 249–261.

Hille, T., Mueller, W., Asmussen, B., Levy, A., and Meshulam, Y. (1995). Pharmaceutical formulation for prophylaxis or preliminary treatment against poisoning by organophosphorus cholinesterase inhibitors. *Ger. Offen.* 6 pp.

Hoffman, R. S., Henry, G. C., Wax, P. M., Weisman, R. S., Howland, M. A., and Goldfrank, L. R. (1992). Decreased plasma cholinesterase activity enhances cocaine toxicity in mice. *J. Pharmacol. Exper. Therapeutics* **263**, 698–702.

Hoffmann, W. E., Kramer, J., Main, A. R., and Torres, J. L. (1989). "Clinical Enzymology in The Clinical Chemistry of Laboratory Animals" (W. F. Loeb and F. W. Quimby, eds.), pp. 217–278. Pergamon Press, New York.

Holmstedt, B. (1957). A modification of the thiocholine method for the determination of cholinesterase. I. Biochemical evaluation of selective inhibitors. *Acta Physiol. Scand.* **40**, 322–330.

Holmstedt, B. (1963). Structure-activity relationships of the organophosphorus anticholinesterase agents. In "Cholinesterases and Anticholinesterase Agents," Handbuch der Experimentellen Pharmakologie (G. B. Koelle, ed.), Vol. XV, pp. 428–485. Springer-Verlag, Berlin.

Humiston, C. G., and Wright, G. W. (1967). An automated method for the determintion of cholinesterase activity. *Toxicol. Appl. Pharmacol.* **10**, 467–480.

Husain, K. (1994). Phenylvalerate and choline ester hydrolases in the platelets of human, hen, rat and mouse. *Hum. Exp. Toxicol.* **13**, 157–159.

Johnson, C. D., and Russell, R. L. (1975). Rapid simple radiometric assay for cholinesterase, suitable for multiple determinations. *Anal. Biochem.* **64**(1), 229–238.

Kasprzak, H., and Salpeter, M. M. (1985). Recovery of acetylcholinesterase at intact neuromuscular junctions after in vivo inactivation with diisopropylfluorophosphate. *J. Neurosci.* **5**, 951–955.

Katz, E. J., Cortes, V. I., Eldefrawi, M. E., and Eldefrawi, A. T. (1997). Chlorpyrifos, parathion, and their oxons bind to and desensitize a nicotinic acetylcholine receptor, relevance to their toxicities. *Toxicol. Appl. Pharmacol.* **146**, 227–236.

Keifer, M., Rivas, F., Moon, J. D., and Checkoway, H. (1996). Symptoms and cholinesterase activity among rural residents living near cotton fields in Nicaragua. *Occupat. Environ. Med.* **53**, 726–729.

Koelle, G. B. (1963). "Cholinesterases and Anticholinesterase Agents," Handbuch der Experimentellen Pharmakologie, Vol. XV. Springer-Verlag, Berlin.

Krasowski, M. D., McGehee, D. S., and Moss, J. (1997). Natural inhibitors of cholinesterases, implications for adverse drug reactions. *Can. J. Anaesthesia* **44**(5 Pt 1), 525–534.

Krejci, E. (1998). The building of acetylcholinesterase collagen-tailed forms. In "Structure and Function of Cholinesterases and Related Proteins" (B. P. Doctor *et al.*, eds.), pp. 57–63. Plenum Press, New York.

Kurt, T. L. (1998). Epidemiological association in US veterans between Gulf War illness and exposures to anticholinesterases. *Toxicol. Lett.* **102-103**, 523–526.

La Du, B. N., Aviram, M., Billecke, S., Navab, M., Primo-Parmo, S., Sorenson, R. C., and Standiford, T. J. (1999). On the physiological role(s) of the paraoxonases. *Chemical-Biological Interactions* **119-120**, 379–388.

Layer, P. G., Keller, M., Mack, A., Willbold, E., and Robitzki, A. (1998). Nonenzymatic roles of cholinesterases in avian neurogenesis. In "Structure and Function of Cholinesterases and Related Proteins" (B. P. Doctor *et al.*, eds.), pp. 569–576. Plenum Press, New York.

Leonard, J. P., and Salpeter, M. M. (1979). Agonist-induced myopathy at the neuromuscular junction is mediated by calcium. *J. Cell Biol.* **82**, 811–819.

Li, B., Stribley, J. A., Ticu, A., Xie, W., Schopfer, L. M., Hammond, P., Brimijoin, S., Hinrichs, S. H., and Lockridge, O. (2000). Abundant tissue butyrylcholinesterase and its possible function in the acetylcholinesterase knockout mouse. *J. Neurochem.* **75**(3), 1320–1331.

Li, W. F., Furlong, C. E., and Costa, L. G. (1995). Paraoxonase protects against chlorpyrifos toxicity in mice. *Toxicol. Lett.* **76**, 219–226.

Loewi, O., and Navratil, E. (1926). Uber humorale Ubertragbarkeit der Herzenwirkung X. Uber das Schicksal des Vagusstoffes. *Arch. Ges. Physiol.* **214**, 678.

London, L., Thompson, M. L., Sacks, S., Fuller, B., Bachman, O. M., and Myers, J. E. (1995). Repeatability and validity of a field kit for estimation of cholinesterase in whole blood. *Occ. Env. Med.* **52**, 57–64.

Loof, I. (1992). Experience with the Ellman method, proposal for a modification and an alternative method (PAP). In "U.S. Environmental Protection Agency (EPA) Workshop on Cholinesterase Methodologies," pp. 119–139. Office of Pesticide Programs, U.S. Environmental Protection Agency, Washington, DC.

Magnotti, Jr., R. A., Dowling, K., Eberly, J. P., and McConnell, R. S. (1988). Field measurement of plasma and erythrocyte cholinesterases. *Clin. Chim. Acta* **176**(3), 315–332.

Magnotti, R. A., and Eberly, J. P. (1996). Test-mate ChE, new simplified cholinesterase assay system. *Med. Def. Biosci. Rev. Proc.* **3**.

Marchot, P., Bourne, Y., Prowse, C. N., Bougis, P. E., and Taylor, P. (1998). Inhibition of mouse acetylcholinesterase by fasciculin, crystal structure of the complex and mutagenesis of fasciculin. *Toxicon* **36**, 1613–1622.

Massoulie, J., Pezzementi, L., Bon, S., Krejci, E., and Vallette, F. M. (1993). Molecular and cellular biology of cholinesterases. *Progr. Neurobiol.* **41**, 31–91.

Massoulie, J., Anselmet, A., Bon, S., Krejci, E., Legay, C., Morel, N., and Simon, S. (1999). The polymorphism of acetylcholinesterase post-translational processing, quaternary associations and localization. *Chemical-Biological Interactions* **119-120**, 29–42.

McGehee, D. S., Krasowski, M. D., Fung, D. L., Wilson, B., Gronert, G. A., and Moss, J. (2000). Cholinesterase inhibition by potato glycoalkaloids slows mivacurium metabolism. *Anesthesiology* **93**, 510–519.

Meshul, C. K. (1989). Calcium channel blocker reverses anticholinesterase-induced myopathy. *Brain Res.* **497**, 142–148.

Metcalf, R. L. (1951). The colorimetric microestimation of human blood cholinesterases and its application to poisoning by organic phosphate insecticides. *J. Econ. Entomol.* **44**, 883–890.

Michel, H. O. (1949). An electrometric method for the determination of red blood cell and plasma cholinesterase activity. *J. Lab. Clin. Med.* **34**, 1564–1568.

Mikalsen, A., Andersen, R. A., and Alexander, J. (1986). Use of ethopropazine and BW 284C51 as selective inhibitors for cholinesterases from various species. *Compar. Biochem. Physiol. C Compar. Pharmacol.* **83**, 447–449.

Mileson, B. E., Chambers, J. E., Chen, W. L., Dettbarn, W., Ehrich, M., Eldefrawi, A. T., Gaylor, D. W., Hamernik, K., Hodgson, E., Karczmar, A. G., Padilla, S., Pope, C. N., Richardson, R. J., Saunders, D. R., Sheets, L. P., Sultatos, L. G., and Wallace, K. B. (1998). Common mechanism of toxicity, a case study of organophosphorus pesticides. *Toxicol. Sci.* **41**, 8–20.

Mortinsen, S. R., Brimijoin, S., Hooper, M. J., and Padilla, S. (1998). Comparison of the in vitro sensitivity of rat acetylcholinesterase to chlorpyrifos-oxon. What do tissue IC50 values represent? *Toxicol. Appl. Pharmacol.* **148**, 46–49.

Mosca, A., Onelli, E., Rosti, E., Paleari, R., Luzzana, M., and Imbimbo, B. P. (1995). A patient-side technique for real-time measurement of acetylcholinesterase activity during monitoring of eptastigmine treatment. *Therapeut. Drug Monitor.* **17**, 230–238.

Myers, D. K. (1953). Studies on cholinesterase. Species variation in the specificity patterns of the pseudo-cholinesterase. *Biochem. J.* **55**, 67–69.

Nabb, D. P., and Whitfield, F. (1967). Determination of cholinesterases by an automated pH stat method. *Arch. Envir. Health* **15**, 147–154.

Nachmansohn, D., and Wilson, I. B. (1951). The enzymic hydrolysis and synthesis of acetylcholine. *Adv. Enzymol.* **12**, 259–339.

Nagata, K., Huang, C. S., Song, J. H., and Narahashi, T. (1997). Direct actions of anticholinesterases on the neuronal nicotinic acetylcholine receptor channels. *Brain Res.* **769**, 211–218.

National Academy of Sciences (1999). "Review of the US Army's Health Risk Assessments for Oral Exposure to Six-Chemical Warfare Agents" (R. Snyder, ed.). National Academy Press, Washington, DC.

Nigg, H. N., and Knaak, J. B. (2000). Blood cholinesterase as human biomarkers of organophosphorus pesticide exposure. *Rev. Environ. Contamin. Toxicol.* **163**, 29–111.

Nigg, H. N., Ramos, L. E., Graham E. M., Sterling, J., Brown, S., and Cornell, J. A. (1996). Inhibition of human plasma and serum butyrylcholinesterase (EC 3.1.1.8) by alpha-chaconine and alpha solanine. *Fund. Appl. Pharmacol.* **33**, 272–281.

Nordberg, A., and Svensson, A. L. (1998). Cholinesterase inhibitors in the treatment of Alzheimer's disease, a comparison of tolerability and pharmacology. *Drug Safety* **19**, 465–480.

Nostrandt, A. C., Duncan, J. A., and Padilla, S. (1993). A modified spectrophotometric method appropriate for measuring cholinesterase activity in tissue from carbaryl-treated animals. *Fund. Appl. Toxicol.* **21**, 196–203.

O'Brien, R. D. (1967). "Insecticides, Actions and Metabolism," p. 83. Academic Press, New York.

Okabe, H., Sagesaka, K., Nakajima, N., and Noma, A. (1977). New enzymatic assay of cholinesterase activity. *Clin. Chim. Acta* **80**, 87–94.

Orwell, G. (1945). "Animal Farm; A Fairy Story." Secker & Warburg, London.

Patocka, J. (1998). Huperzine A—An interesting anticholinesterase compound from the Chinese herbal medicine. *Acta Medica (Hradec Kralove)* **41**(4), 155–157.

Paulus, J.-M., Maigne, J., and Keyhani, E. (1981). Mouse megakaryocytes secrete acetylcholinesterase. *Blood* **58**, 1100–1106.

Pezzementi, L., Sutherland, D., Sanders, M., Soong, W., Milner, D., McClellan, J. S., Sapp, M., Coblentz, W. B., Rulewicz, G., and Merritt, S. (1998). Structure and function of cholinesterases from agnathans and cephalochordates: Implications for the evolution of cholinesterases. *In* "Structure and function of cholinesterases and related proteins" (B. P. Doctor *et al.*, eds.), pp. 105–110. Plenum Press, New York.

Polhuijs, M., Langenberg, J. P., and Benschop, H. P. (1997). New method for retrospective detection of exposure to organophosphorus anticholinesterases, application to alleged sarin victims of Japanese terrorists. *Toxicol. Appl. Pharmacol.* **146**, 156–161.

Polhuijs, M., Langenberg, J. P., Noort, D., Hulst, A. G., Benschop, H. P., and De Jong, L. P. A. (1999). Retrospective detection of exposure to organophosphates: Analyses in blood of human beings and rhesus monkeys. *NATO Sci.* *Ser., 1, 25 (NBC Risks: Current Capabilities and Future Perspectives for Protection)*, pp. 513–521.

Pope, C. N. (1999). Organophosphorus pesticides: Do they all have the same mechanism of toxicity? *J. Toxicol. Environ. Health. Part B, Critical Rev.* **2**, 161–181.

Potter, W. T., Garry, V. F., Kelly, J. T., Tarone, R., Griffith, J., and Nelson, R. L. (1993). Radiometric assay of red cell and plasma cholinesterase in pesticide appliers from Minnesota. *Toxicol. Appl. Pharmacol.* **119**, 150–155.

Prall, Y. G., Gambhir, K. K., and Ampy, F. R. (1998). Acetylcholinesterase, an enzymatic marker of human red blood cell aging. *Life Sci.* **63**, 177–184.

Raveh, L., Cohen, G., Grauer, E., Alkali, D., Chapman, S., Kapon, Y., Sahar, R., Kadar, T., and Shapira, S. (1996). Efficacy of prophylactic treatments against sarin poisoning in rats. *Med. Def. Biosci. Rev. Proc.* **1**, 539–547.

Reiner, E., Rudolf, V. S., Doctor, B. P., Furlong, C. E., Johnson, M. K., Lotti, M., Silman, I., and Taylor, P. (1999). Esterases reacting with organophosphorus compounds. *Chemico-Biological Interactions* **119-120**, 1–619.

Rider, J. A., Hodges, J. L., Swader, J., and Wiggins, A. D. (1957). Plasma and red cell cholinesterase in 800 "healthy" blood donors. *J. Lab. Clin. Med.* **50**, 376–383.

Robitzki, A., Mack, A., Hoppe, U., Chatonnet, A., and Layer, P. G. (1997). Regulation of cholinesterase gene expression affects neuronal differentiation as revealed by transfection studies on reaggregating embryonic chicken retinal cells. *Eur. J. Neurosci.* **9**, 2394–2405.

Rocha, E. S., Swanson, K. L., Aracava, Y., Goolsby, J. E., Maelicke, A., and Albuquerque, E. X. (1996). Paraoxon, cholinesterase-independent stimulation of transmitter release and selective block of ligand-gated ion channels in cultured hippocampal neurons. *J. Pharmacol. Exper. Therapeut.* **278**, 1175–1187.

Rodgers, K. E., and Ellefson, D. D. (1990). Modulation of respiratory burst activity and mitogenic response of human peripheral blood mononuclear cells and murine splenocytes and peritoneal cells by malathion. *Fund. Appl. Toxicol.* **14**, 309–317.

Rodgers, K., and Xiong, S. (1997). Effect of administration of malathion for 14 days on macrophage function and mast cell degranulation. *Fund. Appl. Toxicol.* **37**, 95–99.

Rogers, K. R., Cao, C. J., Valdes, J. J., Eldefrawi, A. T., and Eldefrawi, M. E. (1991). Acetylcholinesterase fiber-optic biosensor for detection of anticholinesterases. *Fund. Appl. Toxicol.* **16**, 810–820.

Rosenberry, T. L., Mallender, W. D., Thomas, P. J., and Szegletes, T. (1998). Substrate binding to the peripheral site occurs on the catalytic pathway of acetylcholinesterase and leads to substrate inhibition. *In* "Structure and Function of Cholinesterases and Related Proteins" (B. P. Doctor *et al.*, eds.), pp. 189–196. Plenum Press, New York.

Ryhanen, R., Narhi, M., Puhakainen, E., Hanninen, O., and Kontturi-Narhi, V. (1983). Pseudocholinesterase activity and its origin in human oral fluid. *J. Dental Res.* **62**, 20–23.

Sanz, P., Rodriguez-Vicente, M. C., Diaz, D., Repetto, J., and Repetto, M. (1991). Red blood cell and total acetylcholinesterase and plasma pseudocholinesterase in humans, observed variances. *Clin. Toxicol.* **29**, 81–90.

Sci Finder Scholar, American Chemical Society, Copyright 1999.

Senanayake, N., and Karalliedde, L. (1987). Neurotoxic effects of organophosphorus insecticides. An intermediate syndrome. *New England J. Med.* **316**, 761–763.

Sharma, K. V., and Bigbee, J. W. (1998). Acetylcholinesterase antibody treatment results in neurite detachment and reduced outgrowth from cultured neurons, further evidence for a cell adhesive role for neuronal acetylcholinesterase. *J. Neurosci. Res.* **53**, 454–464.

Shih, D. M., Gu, L., Xia, Y.-R., Navab, M., Li, W.-F., Hama, S., Castellani, L. W., Furlong, C. E., Costa, L. G., Fogelman, A. M., and Lusis, A. J. (1998). Mice lacking serum paraoxonase are susceptible to organophosphate toxicity and atherosclerosis. *Nature (London)* **394**, 284–287.

Sidell, F. R., and Kamiskis, A. (1975). Temporal intrapersonal physiological variability of cholinesterase activity in human plasma and erythrocytes. *Clin. Chem.* **21**, 1961–1963.

Sigma Diagnostics (1989). Cholinesterase (PTC) Procedure no. 422, *Sigma Diagnostics*, PO Box 14508, St Louis, MO 63178.

Silk, E., King, J., and Whittaker, M. (1979). Assay of cholinesterase in clinical chemistry. *Ann. Clin. Biochem.* **16**, 57–75.

Silman, I., and Sussman, J. L. (1998). Structural and functional studies on acetylcholinesterase: A perspective. *In* "Structure and Function of Cholinesterases and Related Proteins" (B. P. Doctor *et al.*, eds.), pp. 25–33. Plenum Press, New York.

Silver, A. (1974). "The Biology of Cholinesterases." Frontiers of Biology, Vol. 36. North-Holland, Amsterdam.

Sket, D., Dettbarn, W.-D., Clinton, M. E., Misulis, K. E., Sketelj, J., Cucke, D., and Brizin, M. (1991). Prevention of diisopropylphosphorofluoridate-induced myopthy by botulinum toxin type A blockage of quantal release of acetylcholine. *Acta Neuropathologia* **82**, 134–142.

Spencer, P. S., Schaumburg, H. H., and Ludolph, A. C. (2000). "Experimental and Clinical Neurotoxicology," 2nd ed. Oxford University Press, New York.

Sussman, J. L., Harel, M., Frolow, F., Oefner, C., Goldman, A., Toker, L., and Silman, I. (1991). Atomic structure of acetylcholinesterase from Torpedo californica: A prototypic acetylcholine-binding protein. *Science* **253**, 872–879.

Talesa, V., Grauso, M., Arpagaus, M., Giovannini, E., Romani, R., and Rosi, G. (1999). Molecular cloning and expression of a full-length cDNA encoding acetylcholinesterase in optic lobes of the squid Loligo opalescens, a new member of the cholinesterase family resistant to diisopropyl fluorophosphate. *J. Neurochem.* **72**(3), 1250–1258.

Taylor, P. (1999). Esterases reacting with organophosphorus compounds. *Chemical-Biological Interactions* **119-120**, 1–620.

Taylor, P. (1996). Cholinesterase agents. *In* "Goodman and Gilman's The Pharmacological Basis of Therapeutics," 9th ed. (J. G. Hardman *et al.*, eds.), pp. 161–176. McGraw-Hill, New York.

Taylor, P. (1994). The cholinesterases: From genes to proteins. *Ann. Rev. Pharmacol. Toxicol.* **34**, 281–320.

Thomsen, T., Kewitz, H., and Pleul, O. (1989). A suitable method to monitor inhibition of cholinesterase activities in tissues as induced by reversible enzyme inhibitors. *Enzyme*, **42**, 219–224.

Thomsen, T., Kewitz, H., and Pleul, O. (1988). Estimation of cholinesterase activity (EC 3.1.17; 3.1.1.8) in undiluted plasma and erythrocytes as a tool for measuring in vivo effects of reversible inhibitors. *J. Clin. Chem. Clin. Biochem.* **26**, 469–475.

Traina, M. E., and Serpietri, L. A. (1984). Changes in the levels and forms of rat plasma cholinesterases during chronic diisopropylphosphofluoridate intoxication. *Biochem. Pharmacol.* **33**, 645–653.

Tuovinen, K., Kaliste-Korhonen, E., Raushel, F. M., and Hanninen, O. (1999). Success of pyridostigmine, physostigmine, eptastigmine and phosphotriesterase treatments in acute sarin intoxication. *Toxicology* **134**, 169–178.

U.S. Environmental Protection Agency (EPA) (1992). "Workshop on Cholinesterase Methodologies." Office of Pesticide Programs, U.S. Environmental Protection Agency, Washington, DC.

van den Beukel, I., van Kleef, R. G., and Oortgissen, M. (1998). Differential effects of physostigmine and organophosphates on nicotinic receptors in neuronal cells of different species. *Neurotoxicology* **19**, 777–787.

Willig, S., Hunter, D. L., Dass, P. D., and Padilla, S. (1996). Validation of the use of 6,6′-dithiodinicotinic acid as a chromogen in the Ellman method for cholinesterase determinations. *Veterinary Human Toxicol.* **38**, 249–253.

Wills, J. H. (1972). The measurement and significance of changes in the cholinesterase activities of erythrocytes and plasma in man and animals. *CRC Crit. Rev. Toxicol.* **1**, 153–199.

Wilson, B. W. (1999). Cholinesterases. *In* "Clinical Chemistry of Laboratory Animals," 2nd ed. (E. Quimby and W. Loeb, eds.), pp. 430–440. Taylor and Francis Inc., Philadelphia.

Wilson, B. W., and Henderson, J. D. (1992). Blood esterase determinations as markers of exposure. *Rev. Environ. Contam. Toxicol.* **128**, 55–69.

Wilson, B. W., Henderson, J. D., Bosworth, D. H., and Oliveira, G. H. (2000). Standardization of cholinesterase measurements for monitoring human exposures. Book of Abstracts, 219th ACS National Meeting, San Francisco, CA, March 26–30.

Wilson, B. W., Hooper, M. J., Hansen, M. E., and Nieberg, P. S. (1992b). Reactivation of organophosphate inhibited AChE with oximes. *In* "Organophosphates, Chemistry, Fate and Effects" (J. E. Chambers and P. E. Levi, eds.), pp. 107–137. Academic Press, New York.

Wilson, B. W., Jaeger, B., and Baetcke, K., Eds. (1992a). "Proc. U.S. EPA Workshop on Cholinesterase Methodologies," Arlington, VA, Dec. 4–5, 1991. Office of Pesticide Programs, U.S. Environmental Protection Agency, Washington, DC.

Wilson, B. W., McCurdy, S. A., Henderson, J. D., McCarthy, S. A., and Billitti, J. E. (1998). Cholinesterases and agriculture, humans, laboratory animals and wildlife. *In* "Structure and Function of Cholinesterases and Related Proteins" (B. P. Doctor *et al.*, eds.), pp. 539–546. Plenum Press, New York.

Wilson, B. W., Padilla, S., and Henderson, J. D. (1996). Factors in standardizing automated cholinesterase assays. *J. Toxicol. Environ. Health* **48**, 187–195.

Wilson, B. W., Sanborn, J. R., O'Malley, M. A., Henderson, J. D., and Billitti, J. R. (1997). Monitoring the pesticide-exposed worker. *Occupat. Med.* **12**, 347–363.

Wilson, I. B., and Ginsburg, S. (1955). A powerful reactivator of alkyl phosphate-inhibited acetylcholinesterase. *Biochim. Biophys. Acta* **18**, 168–170.

Witter, R. F. (1963). Measurement of blood cholinesterase. *Arch. Environ. Health* **6**, 537–563.

Wolfe, A. D., Rush, R. S., Doctor, B. P., Koplovitz, I., and Jones, D. (1987). Acetylcholinesterase prophylaxis against organophosphate toxicity. *Fund. Appl. Toxicol.* **9**, 266–270.

Wright, C. I., and Sabine, J. C. (1948). Cholinesterases of human erythrocyte and plasma and their inhibition by antimalarial drugs. *J. Pharmacol.* **93**, 230–239.

Wyttenbach, C. R., and Thompson, S. C. (1985). The effects of the organophosphate insecticide malathion on very young chick embryos, malformations detected by histological examination. *Am. J. Anatomy* **174**, 187–202.

Xie, W., Stribley, J. A., Chatonnet, A., Wilder, P. J., Rizzino, A., McComb, R. D., Taylor, P., Hinrichs, S. H., and Lockridge, O. (2000). Postnatal developmental delay and supersensitivity to organophosphate in gene-targeted mice lacking acetylcholinesterase. *J. Pharmacol. Exper. Therapeut.* **293**(3), 896–902.

Yamalik, N., Ozer, N., Caglayan, F., and Caglayan, G. (1990). Determination of pseudocholinesterase activity in the gingival crevicular fluid, saliva, and serum from patients with juvenile periodontitis and rapidly progressive periodontitis. *J. Dental Res.* **69**, 87–89.

Yeary, R. A., Eaton, J., Gilmore, E., North, B., and Singell, J. (1993). A multiyear study of blood cholinesterase activity in urban pesticide applicators. *J. Toxicol. Environ. Health* **39**, 11–25.

Yuknavage, K. L., Fenske, R. A., Kalman, D. A., Keifer, M. C., and Furlong, C. E. (1997). Simulated dermal contamination with capillary samples and field cholinesterase biomonitoring. *J. Toxicol. Environ. Health* **51**, 35–55.

Zajicek, J. (1957). Studies on the histogenesis of blood platelets and megakaryocytes. *Acta Physiol. Scand.* **40**(Suppl. 138), 1–32.

Organophosphorus-Induced Delayed Neuropathy

Marion Ehrich and Bernard S. Jortner
Virginia-Maryland Regional College of Veterinary Medicine, Virginia Tech

49.1 HISTORY

Neuropathy due to exposure to organophosphorus (OP) compounds was first reported in 1899, many years before this class of chemical agents was recognized for its insecticidal capabilities (Abou-Donia, 1981, 1995; Cherniack, 1986, 1988; Davis and Richardson, 1980; Ecobichon, 1994; Gallo and Lawryk, 1991; Goldstein *et al.*, 1988; Johnson, 1982; Lotti, 1992; Metcalf, 1984). Until the 1930s, however, organophosphorus-induced delayed neuropathy (OPIDN) appeared as isolated incidents and attracted little attention from the biomedical community. In the 1930s, between 4000 and 20,000 residents of the United States, which was under Prohibition at the time, were affected when a tricresyl phosphate–containing preparation was used as an alcohol substitute (Kidd and Langworthy, 1933). This product, called Ginger Jake, caused limb weakness and ataxia in exposed individuals from which they did not fully recover.

Since the 1930s, other situations in which exposure to OP compounds has caused delayed neuropathy in humans have been identified; for relatively recent reviews, see Abou-Donia and Lapadula (1990) and Ecobichon (1994). Some of these have been isolated incidents, involving intentional or accidental exposures of individuals (Abou-Donia, 1981; Cherniack, 1988; Goldstein *et al.*, 1988; Lotti, 1992; Lotti *et al.*, 1986, 1995; Osterloh *et al.*, 1983). Others have resulted in the exposure of numerous people, such as those who consumed tricresyl phosphate–contaminated cooking oil in Europe, Africa, and Asia (Abou-Donia and Lapadula, 1990), those who used an adulterated abortifacient (Abou-Donia and Lapadula, 1990), and shoe-manufacturing workers in Italy exposed to an OP agent used as a plasticizer (Cavalleri and Cosi, 1980). These incidents put over 10,000 people at risk for OPIDN (Hierons and Johnson, 1978). Animals, too, can be susceptible to OPIDN following accidental exposures, and reports of OPIDN in water buffalo, cattle, horses, and sheep appear in the literature (Beck *et al.*, 1977; El-Sebae *et al.*, 1977; Perdrizet *et al.*, 1985; Sanders *et al.*, 1985).

Most of the recent victims of OPIDN have been people and animals exposed to OP agents that are used as lubricants and plasticizers, rather than insecticides. Current federal testing of OP compounds under the U.S. Federal Insecticide, Fungicide, and Rodenticide Act (FIFRA) requires that those proposed for use as insecticides be examined for their capability to cause OPIDN in relation to their capability to inhibit acetylcholinesterase, which is their insecticidal mechanism of action (EPA, 1991). Consequently, unless exposure is at concentrations that are above those necessary to cause signs of acute toxicity due to acetylcholinesterase inhibition, humans and susceptible animals are unlikely to develop OPIDN following insecticide exposure.

Recent reports have suggested that OPIDN could contribute to symptoms seen in veterans of the Gulf War, based on self-reports provided by veterans (Haley *et al.*, 1997). Soldiers on active duty were exposed to a variety of chemicals, including OP insecticides, pyrethrin insecticides, insect repellents, petroleum products, and sand dust. They were also at risk for exposure to OP compounds used as chemical warfare agents (potent acetylcholinesterase inhibitors), and, to prevent toxicity associated with such, the carbamate acetylcholinesterase inhibitor pyridostigmine was used to protect them preexposure. Soldiers were vaccinated against infectious diseases, anthrax, and botulinum toxin (NIH, 1994; President's Advisory, 1996). Investigations have determined that OP chemical warfare agents were released during this conflict; exposure levels were not determined but levels were too low to cause immediate physical symptoms. Although OPIDN appears weeks to months after exposure to some OP compounds, the OP insecticides used in the Persian Gulf and the OP chemical warfare agents are unlikely to cause this syndrome, especially in the absence of clinical signs of acute acetylcholinesterase inhibition (President's Advisory, 1996). Neurological examination of Gulf War veterans and animal studies do not appear to support the assertion that OPIDN is a clinical entity associated with soldiers that participated in the Gulf War (Abou-Donia *et al.*, 1996; Haley and Kurt, 1997).

49.2 CHEMISTRY OF ORGANOPHOSPHORUS COMPOUNDS

Not all organophosphorus (OP) compounds are capable of causing organophosphorus-induced delayed neuropathy (OPIDN). Lists of neuropathy-inducing OP compounds are contained in the 1991 edition of the *Handbook of Pesticide Toxicology* (Gallo and Lawryk, 1991) and other reviews of OPIDN (Abou-Donia, 1981; Abou-Donia and Lapadula, 1990; Cherniack, 1988; Hollingshaus, 1983; Johnson, 1975b, 1982). Among the OP compounds responsible for reported incidents of OPIDN in man and animals or OP compounds used for laboratory studies of OPIDN are the protoxicants leptophos (*O*-4-bromo-2,5-dichlorophenyl *O*-methyl phenylphosphorothioate) and tri-*ortho*-cresyl phosphate (TOCP, also known as tri-*ortho*-tolyl phosphate, TOTP), which is metabolized to a cyclic saligenin phosphate responsible for inducing the OPIDN. Active OPIDN-inducing agents used for many experimental studies include mipafox (*N*, *N'*-diisopropylphosphorodiamidic fluoride), diisopropyl phosphorofluoridate (DFP), and di-*n*-dibutyl-2,2-dichlorovinyl phosphate (DBDCVP) (Fig. 49.1). None of these are currently used as insecticides. Several reports and reviews, including those listed previously and others (Abou-Donia, 1995; Davis and Richardson, 1980; Ecobichon, 1994; Johnson *et al.*, 1991; Lotti, 1992; Richardson *et al.*, 1993; Wu and Casida, 1994; Yoshida *et al.*, 1994), have examined structure–activity relationships among compounds that cause OPIDN, with the following points noted:

1. For OPIDN, sometimes referred to as Type I OPIDN (Abou-Donia and Lapadula, 1990), phosphorus must be in the pentavalent state.

2. The atom with the coordinate covalent bond attached to the phosphorus must be an oxygen; protoxicants with sulfur attached by a coordinate covalent bond can be oxidized to active neurotoxicants.

3. The neuropathy-inducing OP compounds all have at least one oxygen or amine bridge linking an R group to phosphorus. Therefore, the major subgroups producing OPIDN are either phosphates (derivatives of phosphoric acid, which has four oxygens on the phosphorus), phosphonates (derivatives of phosphonic acid, which has three oxygens on the phosphorus), phosphoramidates (derivatives of phosphoramidic or phosphorodiamidic acids, with one or two nitrogens and two or three oxygens on the phosphorus), or phosphorofluoridates (three oxygens and a fluoride on the phosphorus) (Fig. 49.2).

4. Alkyl substitution on an *ortho* site of phenyl phosphates increases the likelihood that the compound can be metabolized to a neurotoxicant. *Ortho* methyl substitution rather than longer chain substitution on the phenyl ring(s) of triphenyl phosphates increases the capability to cause OPIDN. However, not all *ortho*-methyl-substituted phenyl phosphates induce neuropathy. Substitution at other sites on the *ortho*-substituted ring decreases the neurotoxicity.

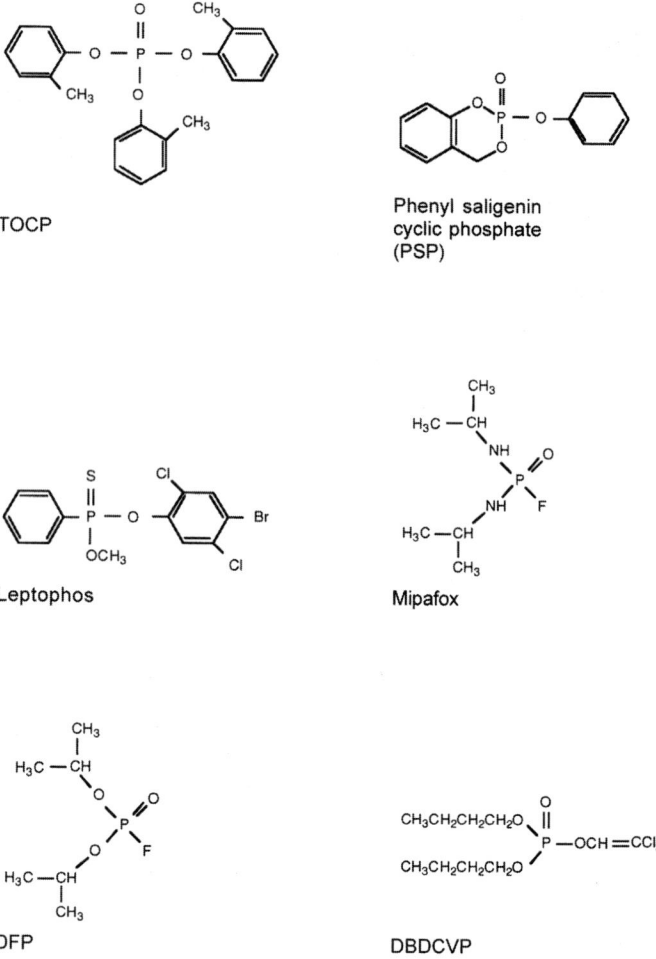

Figure 49.1 Chemical structures of organophosphorus compounds commonly used in laboratory studies. Included are tri-*ortho*-cresyl phosphate (TOCP, also known as tri-*ortho*-tolyl phosphate, TOTP), PSP, a cyclic saligenin phosphate metabolite congener of TOCP, leptophos, mipafox, diisopropyl phosphorofluoridate (DFP), and di-*n*-dibutyl-2,2-dichlorovinyl phosphate (DBDCVP).

5. Increasing the size of the alkyl substituents (up to four or five) on phosphoro- and phosphonofluoridates, phosphorodiamidofluoridates, and dichlorovinyl phosphates increases the hydrophobicity and increases the capability to cause OPIDN.

6. Chirality can contribute to neurotoxicity. Racemic mixtures tend to be less potent as inducers of OPIDN; for compounds tested to date, one enantiomer generally appears to be a more potent neuropathy-inducing agent than the other (Hollingshaus, 1983; Johnson and Read, 1987; Johnson *et al.*, 1991; Lotti *et al.*, 1995).

Neuropathy-inducing OP compounds have a leaving group attached to a labile oxygen or nitrogen bond (Johnson, 1982). Dealkylation at this site results in a negatively charged phosphoryl group, and formation of this chemical species is needed if a phosphate or phosphonate is to induce classical delayed

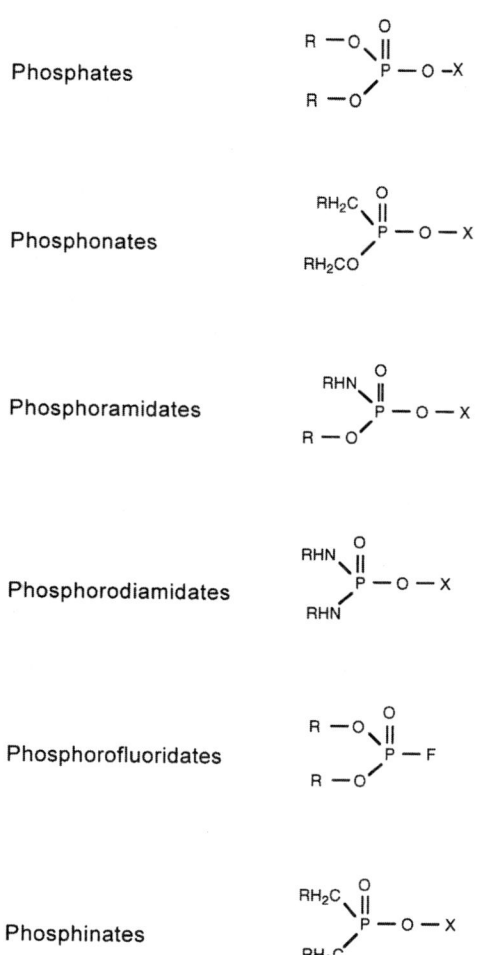

Figure 49.2 Basic structures of organophosphorus compounds. Phosphates, phosphonates, phosphoramidates, phosphorodiamidates, and phosphorofluoridates cause classical OPIDN (Type I OPIDN); phosphinates do not.

neuropathy [sometimes designated Type I OPIDN (Abou-Donia and Lapadula, 1990)]. Deprotonation rather than dealkylation is thought to provide the necessary negative charge for neuropathy-inducing phosphoramidates (Richardson, 1995). This dealkylation occurs after the OP inhibits an esterase, specifically, neuropathy target esterase (NTE, also known as neurotoxic esterase). It has been suggested that another site on this enzyme, one other than the serine active site of NTE, is altered after this dealkylation occurs (Johnson, 1982). The NTE inhibition and the dealkylation reaction render the structure capable of essentially irreversibly binding to NTE, which is a necessary prerequisite to OPIDN (see Section 49.7).

Another type of neuropathy induced by OP compounds, referred to as Type II OPIDN (Abou-Donia and Lapadula, 1990), has been reported for four trivalent phosphites [triphenyl phosphite and the tricresyl phosphites (*o*, *m*, or *p*)]. The chemistry of their interaction(s) with esterases such as NTE has not been delineated in the detail provided for OP compounds that induce Type I OPIDN (Abou-Donia, 1995).

49.3 CLINICAL MANIFESTATIONS (HUMAN)

Descriptions of the clinical manifestations of OPIDN in humans can be found in several reviews (Abou-Donia, 1995; Cherniack, 1986; Ecobichon, 1994; Gallo and Lawryk, 1991). These descriptions follow a similar scenario. Some days (usually 6–14) after exposure, humans note tingling of the hands and feet, followed by sensory loss in the hands and feet. Electromyograms and nerve conduction studies indicate decreased firing of motor units and slowed motor conduction. It is, however, the appearance days to weeks after exposure of bilateral and symmetrical weakness progressing to flaccidity of the distal skeletal muscles of the lower and upper extremities that is characteristic of this disorder. Ataxia can be noted. Even though this may resolve with time, victims of OPIDN may still have abnormal reflexes and spasticity.

49.4 CLINICAL MANIFESTATIONS (ANIMAL)

The adult hen is the recognized animal model for OPIDN (Abou-Donia, 1981; EPA, 1991). This is because clinical signs, which occur after a delay period similar to that which occurs in humans, are easy to observe as they progress, and the associated histopathologic changes are easily identified. In addition, the hen provides readily reproducible results in a relatively small, relatively accessible animal model.

In the hen, a lag period of several days is needed before any clinical alterations appear. Early signs of OPIDN in this species are abnormal foot placement and leg weakness, which may affect balance. As OPIDN progresses, hens become reluctant to walk, show incoordination when they do, and may have wing droop and/or use wings for balance. More severe signs include loss of upright posture when walking, followed by loss of ability to walk. Eventually, the wings also become involved. These clinical deficits can be differentiated, using designations that range from mild effects to paralysis on a scoring system that ranges from 1 to 5 or from 1 to 8 (Sprague *et al.*, 1980) (Fig. 49.3).

It is, however, only the adult chicken that shows these clinical signs upon exposure to neuropathy-inducing organophosphorus compounds. This manifestation of OPIDN does not seem to appear in chickens under 55–60 days of age (Funk *et al.*, 1994a; Moretto *et al.*, 1991).

Clinical manifestations of OPIDN are seen in a variety of other species (Abou-Donia, 1981; Johnson, 1982), including other avians such as the pheasant and turkey (Johnson, 1982; Larsen *et al.*, 1986). Humans (see the previous section) and mammals such as sheep, pigs, cattle, water buffalo, horses, cats, dogs, and ferrets are susceptible to clinical manifestations of OPIDN, as indicated by progressive ataxia (Abou-Donia, 1995; Johnson, 1982; Jortner *et al.*, 1983; Stumpf *et al.*, 1989; Tanaka *et al.*, 1994). Clinical manifestations specifically associated with OPIDN are not, however, generally seen in laboratory

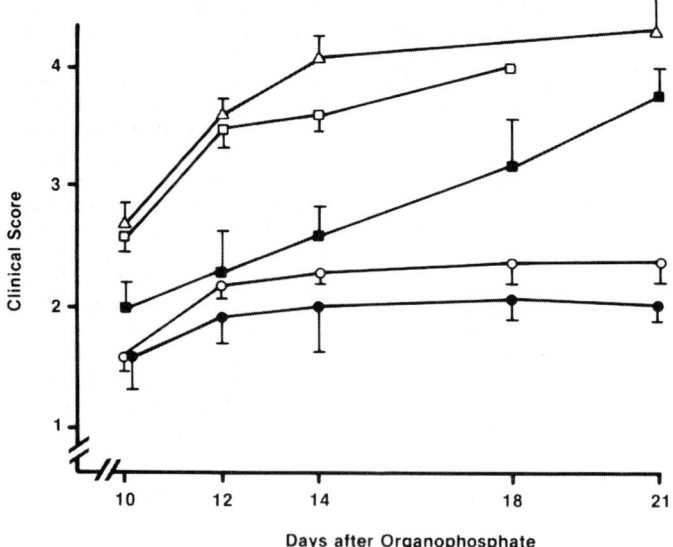

Figure 49.3 Development of clinical signs in chickens after administration of phenyl saligenin phosphate (PSP) and tri-*ortho*-tolyl phosphate (TOTP). Results are presented as the mean ± SD, n = 3–9, on a scale of 1–5. PSP im 2 mg/kg (○—○), 3 mg/kg (□—□), 10 mg/kg (△—△); TOTP 360 mg/kg po (●—●), 500 mg po (■—■). Increasing clinical scores reflect progression of deficits. Reproduced with permission from Jortner, B. S., and Ehrich, M. (1987). Neuropathological effects of phenyl saligenin phosphate in chickens. *NeuroToxicology* **8**, 303–314. Copyright © 1987 by Intox Press, Little Rock, AR.

rodents (Ehrich *et al.*, 1993b, 1995; Lehning *et al.*, 1996; Padilla and Veronesi, 1985; Somkuti *et al.*, 1988; Veronesi *et al.*, 1991), although they have been reported to appear in rats over 6 months old or mice dosed for over 200 days (Lapadula *et al.*, 1985; Moretto *et al.*, 1992b).

There have been suggestions that there are actually two types of OPIDN—OPIDN induced by pentavalent phosphorus compounds (phosphates, phosphonates, and phosphoramidates; Type I OPIDN) and OPIDN that can induced by phosphites (trivalent phosphorus compounds, with most studies done with triphenyl phosphite; Type II OPIDN) (Abou-Donia and Lapadula, 1990). Triphenyl phosphite has been reported to cause ataxia in species both susceptible to (hens, ferrets) and relatively resistant to (rats, Japanese quail) Type I OPIDN. The latent period is, however, shorter than that of Type I OPIDN, as seen in hen studies (Carrington *et al.*, 1988). In contrast to the minimal clinical neuropathy induced by pentavalent phosphorus compounds in rats, triphenyl phosphite elicited prominent clinical manifestations, such as hyperexcitability, spasticity, tail-kinking, side-to-side movements, circling, ataxia, and flaccid paralysis in these rodents (Lehning *et al.*, 1996; Veronesi and Dvergsten, 1987). Pathological manifestations of phosphite neurotoxicity, too, differ from those characteristic of OPIDN (see Section 49.5) (Abou-Donia and Lapadula, 1990; Lehning *et al.*, 1996). We have used the terms Type I and Type II OPIDN in this review. Some investigators feel that based on differences in species susceptibility, magnitude of NTE inhibition, onset and nature of clinical signs, and extent and nature of

brain and spinal cord lesions, these are not two types of OPIDN, but represent separate categories of organophosphorus-induced neurotoxicity (Lehning *et al.*, 1996).

49.5 NEUROPATHOLOGY

Neuropathologic studies of experimental OPIDN induced by pentavalent phosphorus compounds (Type 1 OPIDN) have revealed a consistent pattern of lesions, which is felt to represent the morphologic substrate of the entity. The test compounds most often used to elicit these lesions were tri-*ortho*-cresyl (or tolyl) phosphate (TOCP), its neurotoxic cyclic congener phenyl saligenin phosphate (PSP), diisopropyl phosphorofluoridate (DFP), or mipafox, with the chicken and cat being the major experimental animal subjects (Bischoff, 1967, 1970; Cavanagh, 1954, 1964; Cavanagh and Patangia, 1965; Illis *et al.*, 1966; Itoh *et al.*, 1984; Jortner and Ehrich, 1987; Krinke *et al.*, 1979; Prineas, 1969; Tanaka and Bursian, 1989). This body of work reveals that the primary lesion is a bilateral degenerative change in distal levels of axons and their terminals, primarily affecting larger/longer myelinated central and peripheral nerve fibers, leading to breakdown of affected neuritic segments and secondarily of their myelin sheaths. These lesions generally begin to develop at or near the end of the postdosing symptom-free period. In experimental studies of chickens, this distal pattern of injury is manifest by clinical neuropathy associated with bilateral central nervous system long-tract involvement, such as in cervical spinal cord, medullary, and cerebellar levels of the ascending spinocerebellar tracts and fasciculus gracilis, and lumbar levels of the descending medial pontine spinal tracts (Abou-Donia and Preissig, 1976a, 1976b; Cavanagh, 1954; Classen *et al.*, 1996; Itoh *et al.*, 1984; Jortner and Ehrich, 1987; Tanaka and Bursian, 1989; Tanaka *et al.*, 1990a) (Fig. 49.4). The most sensitive histological indicator of OPIDN was felt to be degenerating cerebellar fibers, especially in folia IV and V (Classen *et al.*, 1996).

Use of Fink–Heimer silver impregnation histological techniques in hens dosed with TOCP or DFP revealed more extensive distribution of central nervous system axonal and terminal degeneration, particularly extension of alterations of the lumbar medial pontine spinal tract into ventral gray matter laminae VI and VII and those of the rostral spinocerebellar system, which were seen in the deep cerebellar nuclei and mossy fiber projections to the anterior lobe of the cerebellar cortex (Tanaka and Bursian, 1989; Tanaka *et al.*, 1990a). Terminal and preterminal degeneration was also noted in a number of medullary structures such as the spinal lemniscus and lateral vestibular, inferior olivary, gracile, external cuneate, and lateral cervical nuclei. Degenerating presynaptic boutons and small axons (Bischoff, 1970; Dyer *et al.*, 1996) are the likely ultrastructural substrate of these silver-impregnated altered gray matter neurites in hens.

In addition to these central nervous system lesions of OPIDN, distal regions of long peripheral nerve myelinated fibers in chickens, particularly in the legs, are similarly affected

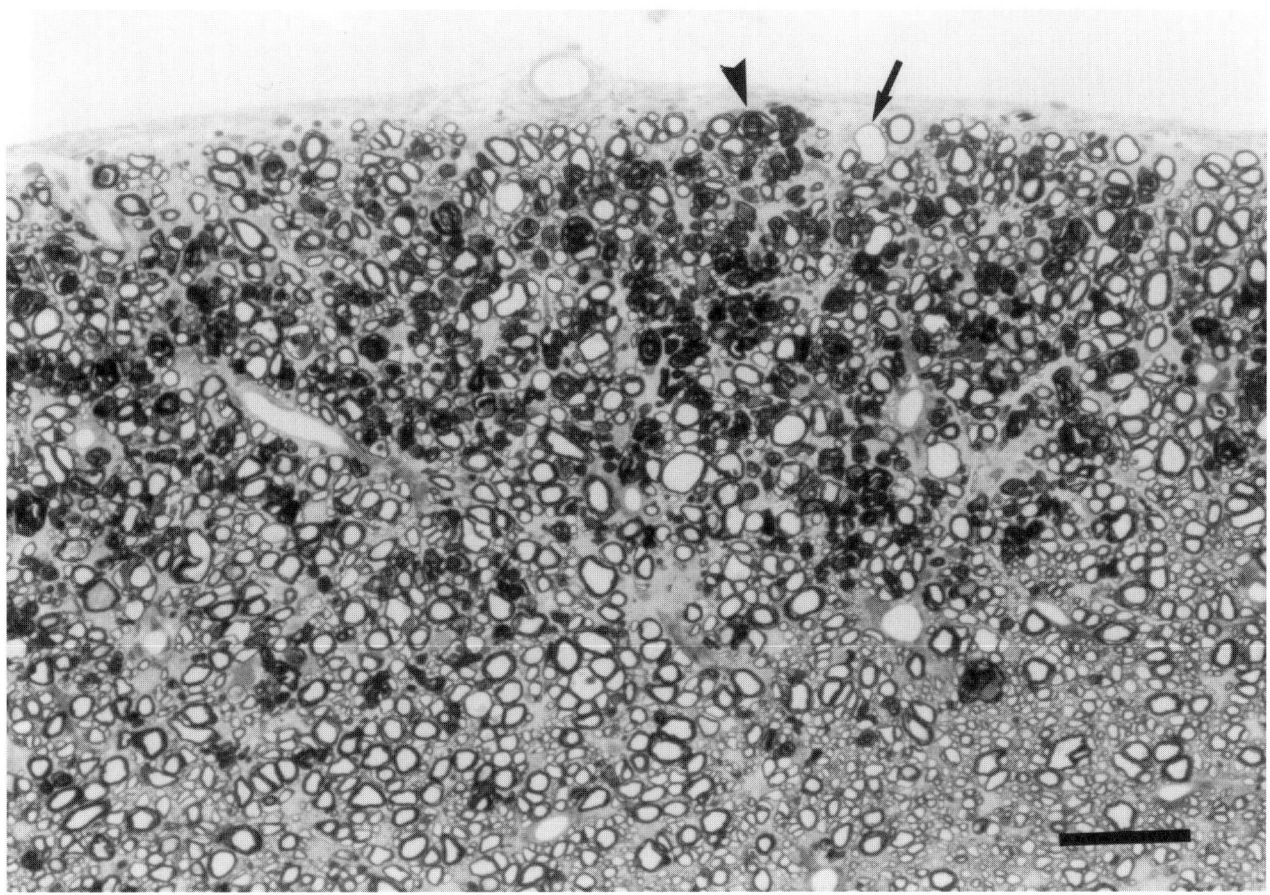

Figure 49.4 Cross section of a spinocerebellar tract in the cervical level of spinal cord from a hen 21 days after exposure to a neurotoxic dose of mipafox (30 mg/kg ip). The section shows extensive myelinated fiber degeneration, manifest by pale-staining swollen axons (arrow) or dark-staining fibers with collapsed axons and disordered myelin sheaths (arrowhead). Toluidine blue–safranin stain; bar = 25 μm.

(Cavanagh, 1954; Dyer *et al.*, 1991, 1992; El-Fawal *et al.*, 1988, 1990b, 1990c; Jortner, 1984; Jortner and Ehrich, 1987; Prineas, 1969). Attention has been directed to the sensitivity of the nerve supplying the biventer cervicis muscle and the large-diameter myelinated fibers of the tibial nerve branch to the lateral head of the gastrocnemius muscle in this species (El-Fawal *et al.*, 1988, 1990c; Krinke *et al.*, 1979).

A similar neuropathologic pattern has been noted in cats exposed to neurotoxic doses of DFP or TOCP. This is manifest by distal degeneration mainly affecting large, long myelinated fibers, involving rostral (cervical, medullary, and, for some, cerebellar) levels of ascending tracts (fasciculus gracilis, spinocerebellar tracts, spino-olivary tract) and thoracolumbar spinal cord levels of descending tracts (corticospinal, reticulospinal, rubrospinal) (Abou-Donia *et al.*, 1986; Cavanagh and Patangia, 1965). Degenerating nerve fiber terminals were seen in gray matter afferent nuclei (Cavanagh and Patangia, 1965; Illis *et al.*, 1966; Prineas, 1969). Distal levels of long peripheral nerve myelinated fibers and their terminals, such as in the hind legs and in recurrent laryngeal nerves, were similarly affected (Bouldin and Cavanagh, 1979a, 1979b; Ca-

vanagh, 1964; Drakontides *et al.*, 1982; Glazer *et al.*, 1978; Prineas, 1969).

By light microscopy, the qualitative changes were best demonstrated in sections from epoxy resin–embedded preparations of spinal cord and medullary white matter, and peripheral nerve. These included axonal swelling with attenuated myelin sheaths (Figs. 49.5–49.7). The swollen axons were pale staining or debris laden and dark staining (Figs. 49.5–49.8). Another feature, common in central nervous system myelinated tracts, was the presence of contracted dark-staining axons with disordered myelin sheaths (Figs. 49.4 and 49.5). These lesions increased in affected regions as the clinical neuropathy advanced. Later lesions included fragmentation of affected fiber segments as the process of Wallerian-like degeneration ensued (Figs. 49.8 and 49.9). This was associated with formation of myelin-rich ovoids and phagocytosis of the degraded element by macrophages or Schwann cells (the latter in peripheral nerve) (Figs. 49.8 and 49.9).

Ultrastructurally, changes in axonal membrane systems were early morphologic events in OPIDN. This includes proliferation of intra-axonal tubules and cisterns, resembling smooth endo-

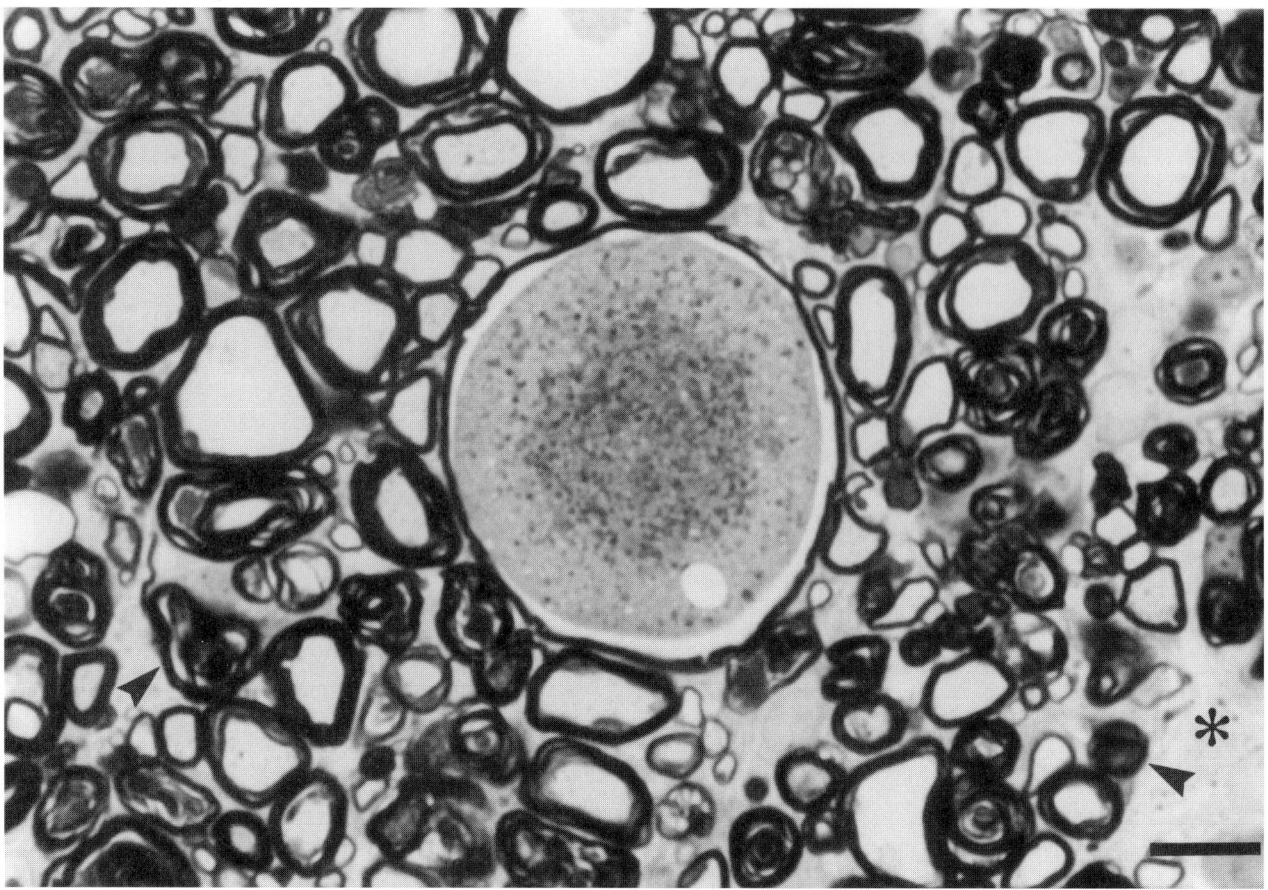

Figure 49.5   High-power view of spinal cord long-tract degeneration in cross section from a chicken given mipafox (30 mg/kg ip) 21 days earlier shows a large central swollen axon with moderately dense staining axoplasm containing particulate material and a vacuole. The myelin sheath is thin. Many of the adjacent degenerating fibers have contracted, dark-staining axons with disordered dark-staining myelin sheaths (arrowhead). Pale-staining regions of myelinated fiber loss with associated gliosis are present (asterisk). Toluidine blue–safranin stain; bar = 10 μm.

plasmic reticulum, and vesicles in hens and cats receiving toxic doses of TOCP or DFP (Bischoff, 1967, 1970; Bouldin and Cavanagh, 1979a, 1979b; LeVay *et al.*, 1971; Prineas, 1969) (Fig. 49.10).

Other early changes, seen in cats dosed with DFP, were peripheral myelinated fiber distal, nonterminal varicosities due to the presence of abnormal membrane-lined vacuoles in axons, inner myelin sheaths, or both, which preceded fiber degeneration (Bouldin and Cavanagh, 1979a, 1979b). These workers suggest such vacuolar alterations represent a "chemical transection" of the fiber, leading to its subsequent breakdown.

Following these early ultrastructural events, a variety of subsequent degradative axonal changes are seen, progressing to fiber degeneration. One sequence involves axonal swelling with secondary attenuation of the myelin sheath. Electron microscopic study revealed that numbers of these swollen axons contained disorganized masses of normal and altered mitochondria, cytoskeletal components (neurofilaments), lysosome-like dense bodies, and membranous multilamellar bodies (Bischoff,

1967, 1970; Bouldin and Cavanagh, 1979b; Jortner and Ehrich, 1987; Prineas, 1969) (Fig. 49.11). A second appearance of the swollen axons, which may be derived from the preceding, is one in which there has been granular degeneration of its contents due to lysis of the cytoskeleton and other axonal contents, leading to swollen electron-lucent axons (Jortner and Ehrich, 1987) (Fig. 49.12). This is thought to be an advanced manifestation of the neuropathy (Prineas, 1969) and may be related to increased activity of calcium-activated proteinases, associated with toxicant-induced intra-axonal elevations of calcium ions (El-Fawal *et al.*, 1990a). Yet a third ultrastructural appearance of degenerating fibers, particularly prominent in the central nervous system, is distal axonal collapse with ill-defined electron-dense axoplasm and disordered myelin sheaths (Fig. 49.11). These axonal changes are associated with aggregation of membranous masses, altered mitochondria, and dense bodies in degenerating axon terminals (Drakontides *et al.*, 1982; Glazer *et al.*, 1978; Prineas, 1969). Some workers suggest that axon terminals are the initial site of degeneration, with sub-

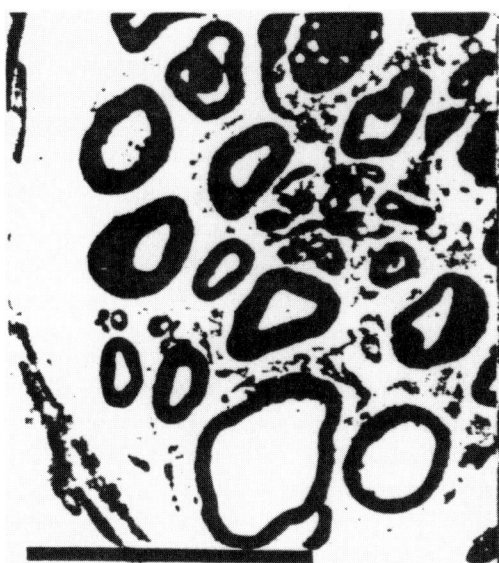

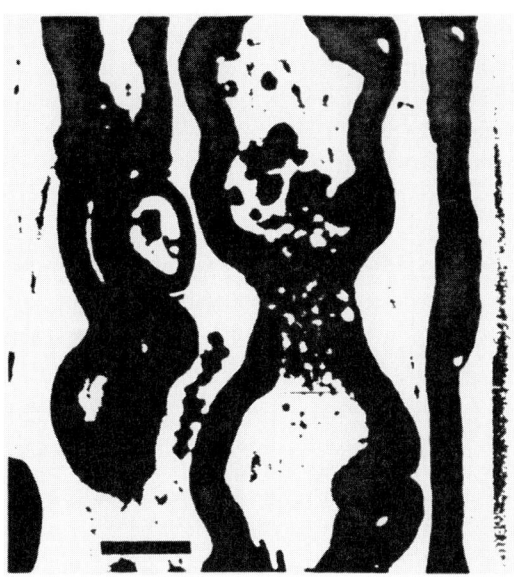

Figure 49.6 Cross-sectioned distal (dorsal metatarsal nerve) peripheral nerve from a chicken given 2 mg/kg of phenyl saligenin phosphate 14 days earlier. Fiber degeneration is manifest by swollen, pale-staining axons and thin myelin sheaths. Toluidine blue–safranin stain; bar = 100 μm. Reproduced with permission from Jortner, B. S., and Ehrich, M. (1987). Neuropathological effects of phenyl saligenin phosphate in chickens. *NeuroToxicology* **8**, 303–314. Copyright © 1987 by Intox Press, Little Rock, AR.

Figure 49.7 Longitudinal section of a dorsal metatarsal nerve from a chicken 21 days after exposure to a toxic dose (10 mg/kg) of phenyl saligenin phosphate, showing dark-staining axonal debris in the paranodal region of a large myelinated fiber. Toluidine blue–safranin stain; bar = 10 μm. Reproduced with permission from Jortner, B. S., and Ehrich, M. (1987). Neuropathological effects of phenyl saligenin phosphate in chickens. *NeuroToxicology* **8**, 303–314. Copyright © 1987 by Intox Press, Little Rock, AR.

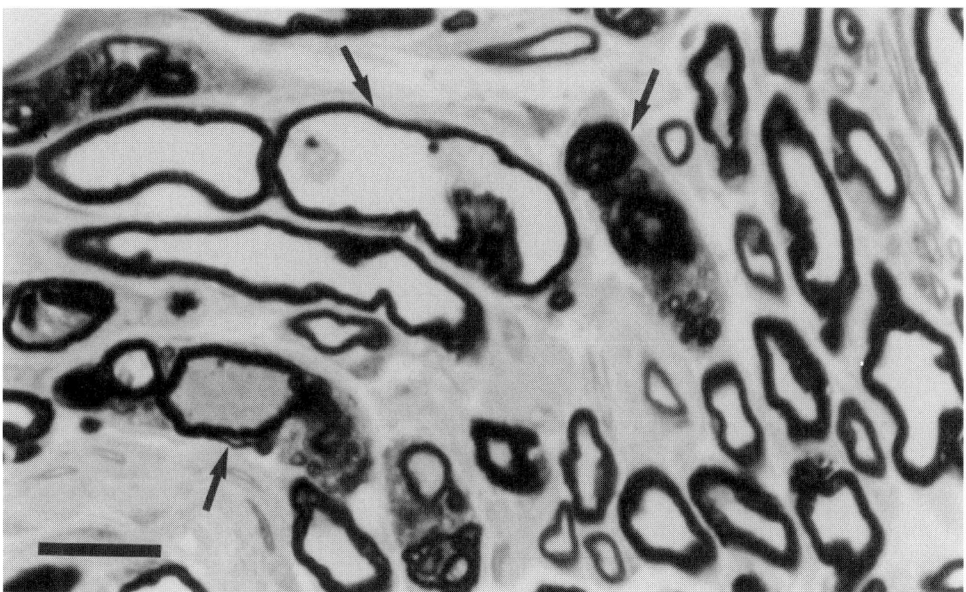

Figure 49.8 This tangentially sectioned tibial nerve branch to the lateral head of the gastrocnemius muscle from a chicken 15 days after dosing with 2.5 mg/kg of phenyl saligenin phosphate shows several stages of myelinated nerve fiber degeneration (arrows). These include swollen axons with pale or moderate staining of their contents and formation of myelin-rich segments (ovoids) of Wallerian-like degeneration. Toluidine blue–safranin stain; bar = 25 μm.

sequent involvement of terminal portions of the axon, creating a true "dying-back" neuropathy (Tanaka and Bursian, 1989). This contrasts with another view, that the terminal lesions are secondary to injury in the distal, nonterminal portions of the axon (Bouldin and Cavanagh, 1979a, 1979b; Prineas, 1969).

Eventually, the degrading segments of affected myelinated fibers are phagocytized, an event occurring more rapidly in peripheral than central regions of the nervous system (Fig. 49.13). In the former, most fiber debris was phagocytized and degraded by 4 weeks following a single toxic dose in hens, but these damaged neurites may persist much longer in the central nervous system (Jortner *et al.*, 1989). In peripheral nerve, the damaged fiber swells, fragments, and is phagocytized by macrophages or Schwann cells within the column formed by the original Schwann cell basal lamina. This resembles events in Wallerian

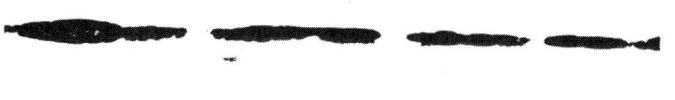

Figure 49.9 Teased peripheral nerve myelinated fiber from the tibial nerve branch to the lateral head of the gastrocnemius muscle from a chicken dosed with 10 mg/kg phenyl saligenin phosphate 14 days earlier. The nerve is fragmented into myelin ovoids typical of the Wallerian-like degeneration of OPIDN. Osmium tetroxide stain; bar = 100 μm. Reproduced with permission from Jortner, B. S., and Ehrich, M. (1987). Neuropathological effects of phenyl saligenin phosphate in chickens. *NeuroToxicology* **8**, 303–314. Copyright © 1987 by Intox Press, Little Rock, AR.

(hence the term Wallerian-like) degeneration. With advanced breakdown of the fiber in OPIDN, proliferation of Schwann cells in their basal lamina forms the band of Büngner. The latter is a site of subsequent nerve fiber regeneration, which is robust in OPIDN following a single dose of the toxicant (Jortner *et al.*, 1989). The bands of Büngner (columns of proliferating Schwann cells) provide an appropriate structural and growth-enhancing environment to permit re-innervation to occur. This regeneration included replacement of degenerated peripheral axon terminals as well (Glazer *et al.*, 1978; Illis *et al.*, 1966).

Consistent with other forms of nerve fiber degeneration, there is a failure of such axonal regeneration in the central nervous system in OPIDN (Jortner *et al.*, 1989). The prominence of spinal cord lesions relative to those in sciatic nerve of hens sacrificed 1 month or more following dosing with OPIDN-inducing insecticides was attributed to peripheral nerve regeneration (Abou-Donia and Graham, 1978; Abou-Donia and Preissig, 1976a, 1976b; Abou-Donia *et al.*, 1979). In the central nervous system, macrophages provide the phagocytic element acting on degraded myelinated fibers, and there is prominent

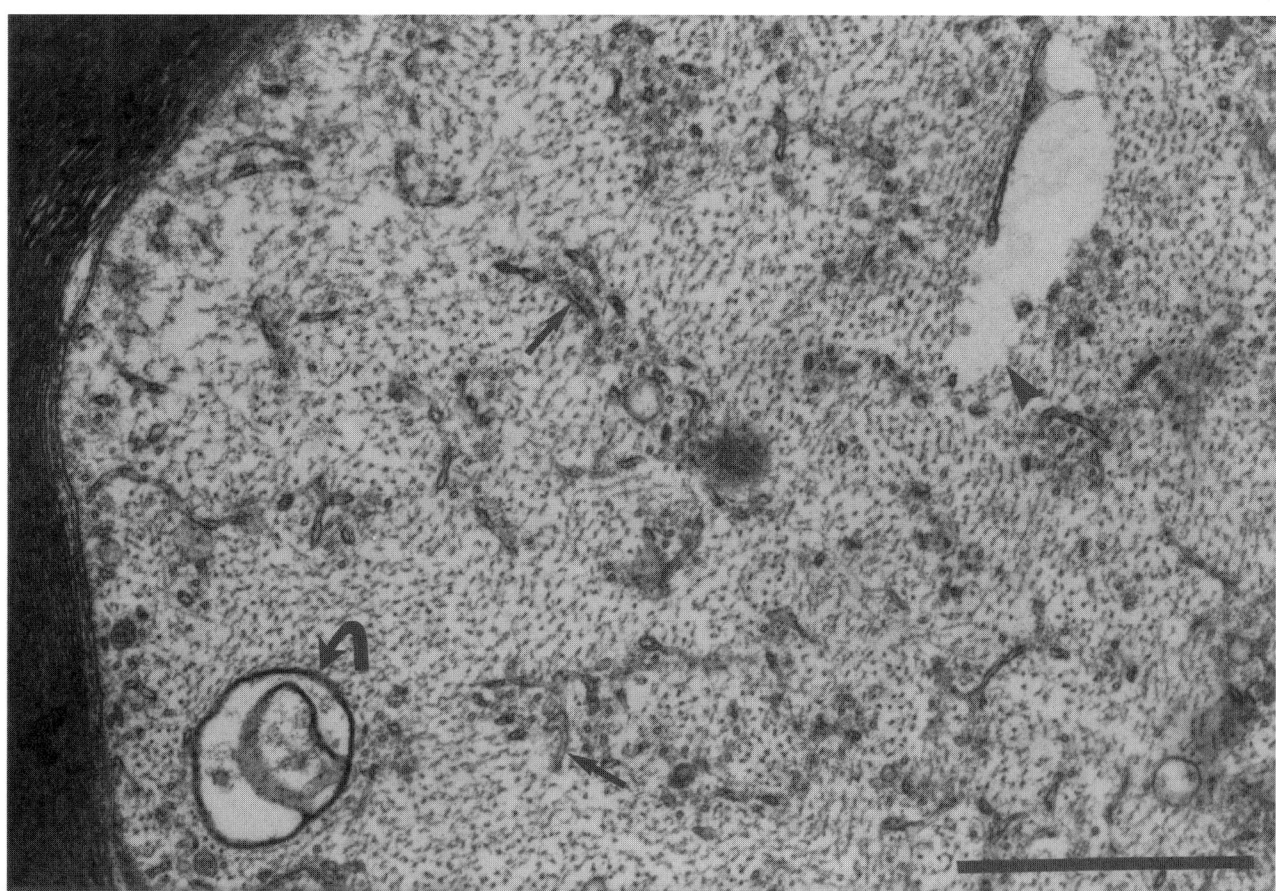

Figure 49.10 Electron micrograph showing early ultrastructural axonal changes of OPIDN (hen given PSP 2.5 mg/kg im). An increase in membrane-lined tubules and cisterns suggestive of proliferation of agranular endoplasmic reticulum is noted (straight arrow). In addition, there is a focus of granular degeneration of the cytoskeleton (arrowhead) and a small lamellar body (curved arrow). Bar = 1 μm.

astrocytic proliferation in the damaged levels of spinal cord and brainstem (Jortner *et al.*, 1989) (Figs. 49.5 and 49.13).

In contrast to the lesions induced by pentavalent organophosphorus compounds (the Type I OPIDN described previously), another morphologic pattern of the neuropathy is induced by exposure to trivalent organophosphates. This has been designated Type II OPIDN (Abou-Donia, 1995; Abou-Donia and Lapadula, 1990) and is produced by aryl phosphites, mainly triphenyl phosphite, in monkeys, cats, rats, and chickens. The histological lesions have best been described in the latter two species. Those in the rat consist of delayed-onset, dose-related bilateral alteration of myelinated fibers and neuronal cell bodies. The fiber lesions have qualitative similarity to those of Type I OPIDN, in that intra-axonal aggregates of agranular reticulum and masses of tubulovesicular elements are seen, and the lesions progress over time to fiber degeneration (Veronesi and Dvergsten, 1987). The extent and distribution of these lesions differ from those of Type I OPIDN in rats (see the following discussion). In the brainstem, in addition to involving the spinocerebellar tracts, lesions were seen in the medial and lateral reticular formation, medial longitudinal fasciculus, and medial vestibular nucleus. Spinal cord white matter fiber degeneration involved the ventral and ventrolateral funiculi housing the spinocerebellar, spinothalamic, tectospinal, and reticulospinal tracts, at all levels. They were also noted in several gray matter laminae. In contrast, the prominent involvement of the rostral (cervicomedullary) levels of the fasciculus gracilis seen in Type I OPIDN was absent.

Neuronal cell body lesions of chromatolysis and necrosis were a prominent feature of Type II OPIDN, being seen in the medial vestibular and lateral reticular nuclei and, on occasion, in the lumbosacral gray matter, associated with nerve fiber degeneration (Veronesi and Dvergsten, 1987). Such neuronal lesions are not a feature of the Type I form of the neuropathy in rats.

Type II OPIDN has also been induced in chickens by a single 1000-mg/kg dose of triphenyl phosphite (Carrington *et al.*, 1988). This avian model is characterized by neuronal cell body chromatolysis and necrosis in the anterior horns of the spinal cord gray matter and dorsal root ganglia. In addition, myelinated fiber degeneration involving the cerebellar peduncle, reticular formation, ventral and lateral spinal cord white

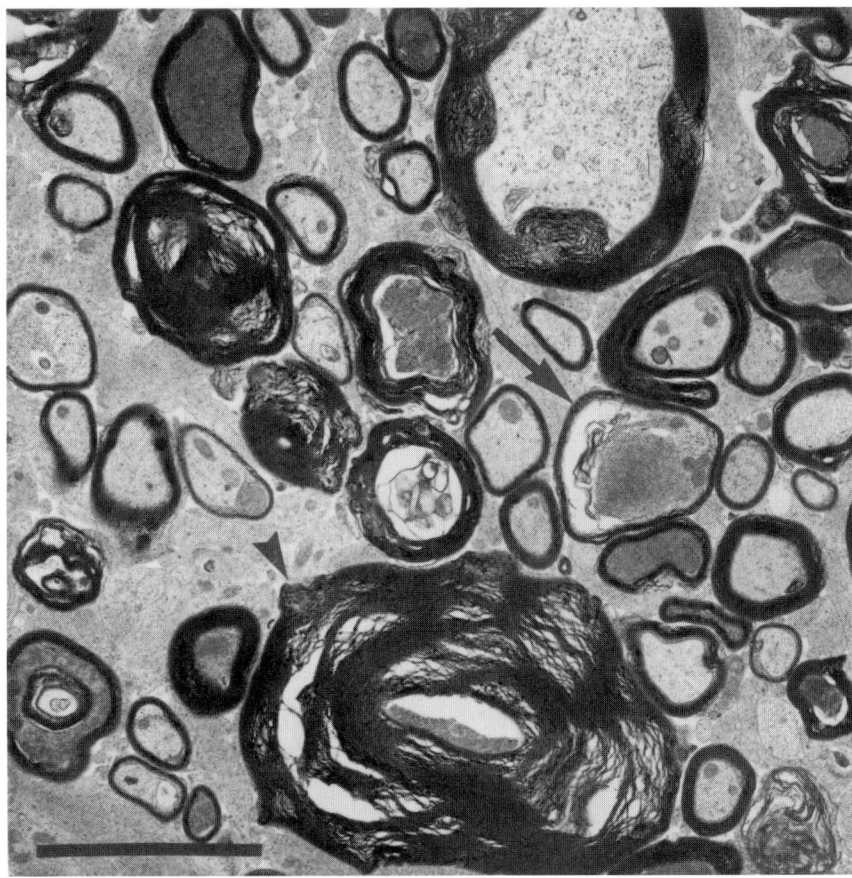

Figure 49.11 Electron micrograph demonstrating extensive myelinated fiber degeneration in a cross section of the medullary (distal) level of the fasciculus gracilis from a chicken administered a toxic dose (500 mg/kg po) of tri-*ortho*-tolyl-phosphate 21 days earlier. The morphologic presentations of fiber degeneration include swollen axons with multilamellar membranous aggregates (arrow) and contracted electron-dense axons with disordered myelin sheaths (arrowhead). Bar = 5 μm.

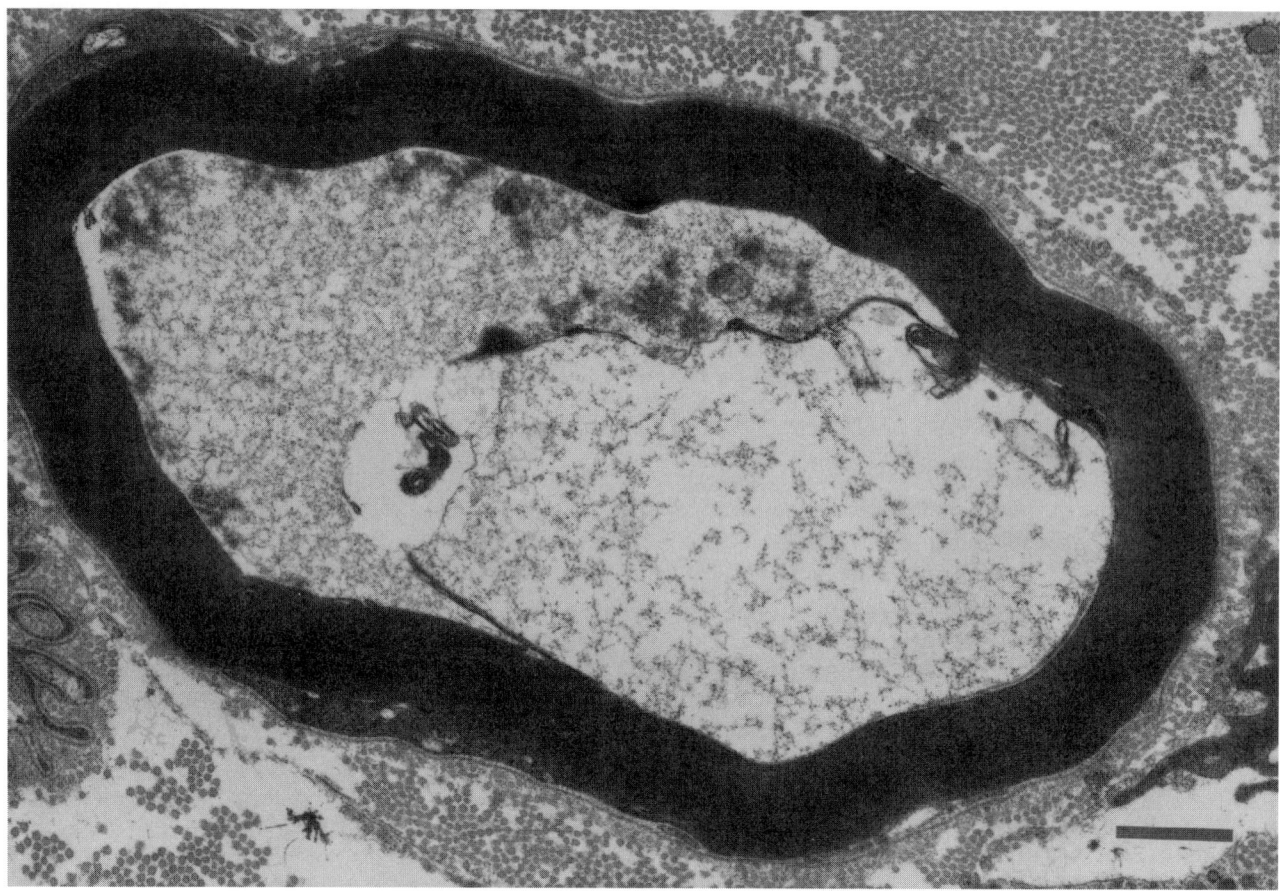

Figure 49.12 Electron micrograph demonstrating one pattern of advanced axonal alteration. This is manifest by extensive granular degeneration of the axoplasm and axonal organelles in this cross-sectioned myelinated fiber from the dorsal metatarsal nerve of a chicken dosed with 10 mg/kg of phenyl saligenin phosphate 14 days earlier. Bar = 1 μm.

matter funiculi, spinal cord gray matter, and peripheral nerve is seen (Abou-Donia and Lapadula, 1990; Carrington *et al.*, 1988). This spectrum of lesions is somewhat different from that induced in chickens by pentavalent organophosphorus compounds, as described previously.

The Fink–Heimer silver impregnation method was also employed to study the lesions of Type II (triphenyl phosphite induced) OPIDN in chickens (Tanaka *et al.*, 1992). This procedure revealed extensive evolving terminal and axonal degeneration, prominent in the spinal cord gray and white matter, selected medullary nuclei and fiber tracts, cerebellar granular layer in folia I–VI, and several midbrain and forebrain regions. Major systems affected included descending brainstem–spinal pathways originating in the lateral vestibular nuclei, mossy fiber afferents to the anterior lobe of the cerebellum, afferents to the lateral mesencephalic nuclei, and tracts associated with the basal ganglia and its optic tectal pathways. This represented more widespread injury than seen in Type I OPIDN, in that higher order centers responsible for processing and integrating sensorimotor, visual, and auditory information were involved (Tanaka *et al.*, 1992).

Neuropathological studies of triphenyl phosphite–induced delayed neuropathy in the rat, Japanese quail, and ferret have utilized the Fink–Heimer technique (Lehning *et al.*, 1996; Stumpf *et al.*, 1989; Tanaka *et al.*, 1990b, 1991; Varghese *et al.*, 1995). Although there were some species variations in affected tracts and nuclei, lesions of axonal and terminal degeneration were noted at multiple levels of the central nervous system and included thalamic and cerebral cortical (in mammals) regions in these studies. As with chickens (discussed previously), these included higher order centers.

49.6 NEUROPATHOLOGY OF MAMMALIAN ANIMAL MODELS

The most reliable experimental animal model of OPIDN is obtained by single or multiple dosing in the domestic adult chicken (hen), and the spectrum of nervous system alterations in that species has been documented previously in some detail. A good deal of earlier work has employed the domestic cat, which, along with other susceptible mammalian species (sheep,

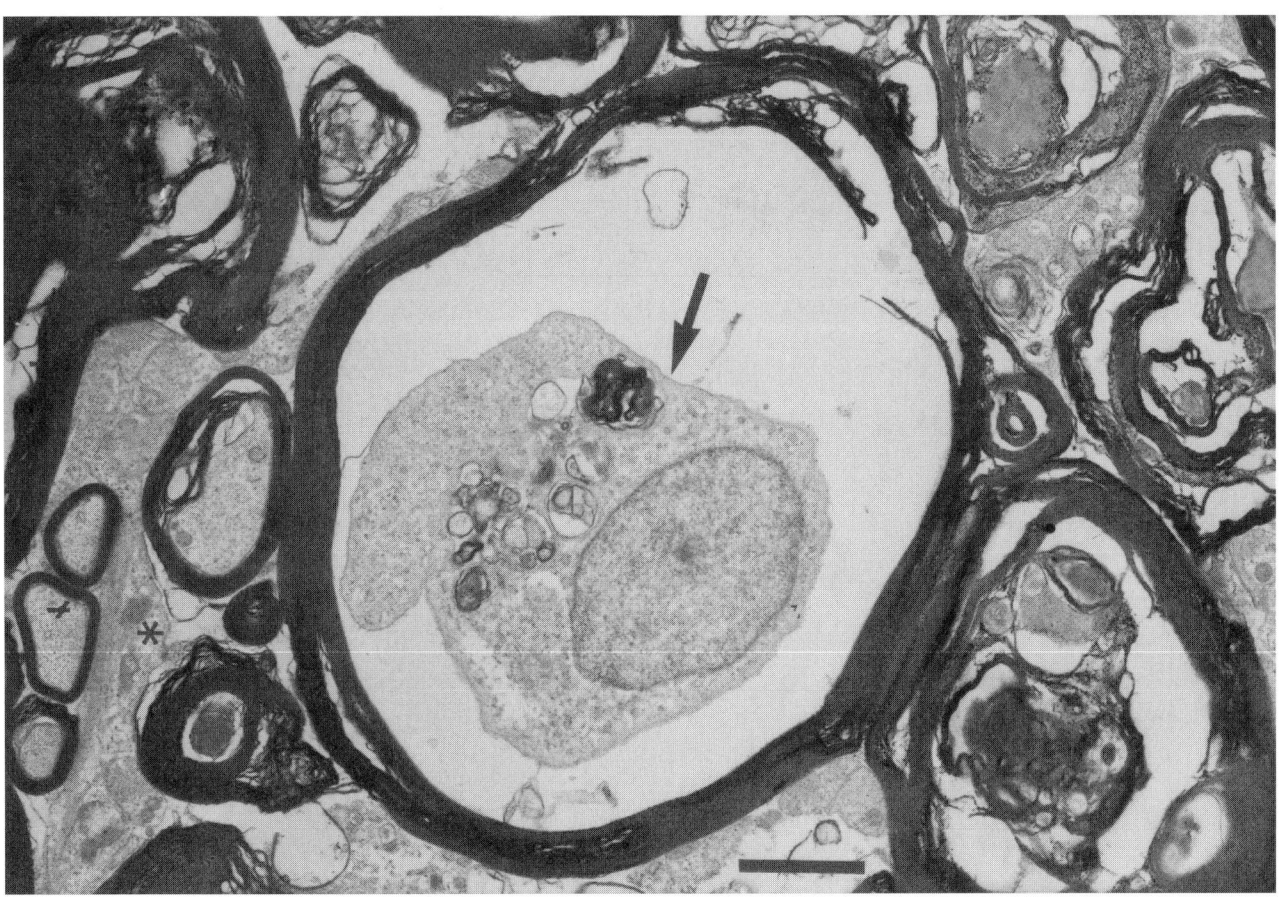

Figure 49.13   This electron micrograph shows a cross-sectioned myelinated fiber in the medullary level of the fasciculus gracilis from a chicken 21 days after a neurotoxic dose of tri-*ortho*-tolyl-phosphate (500 mg/kg po). The degenerated axonal contents have been phagocytized by a macrophage (arrow) within the myelin tube. Processes of reactive astrocytes are seen in adjacent tissue (asterisk). Bar = 2 μm.

cattle, nonhuman primates, etc.), has a qualitative and distributive pattern of lesions that follows that of the hen (Abou-Donia, 1981; Cavanagh and Patangia, 1965; Jortner, 1984; Jortner *et al.*, 1983; Prineas, 1969). Thus, the basic nature of changes in these mammalian species has already been considered. Due to concern about regulatory reliance on an avian experimental model, there has been considerable interest in the evaluation of laboratory rodents as potential model systems for OPIDN. Most of this attention has focused on the laboratory rat (Jortner, 1988).

In a series of studies in the Long–Evans strain of rat, using several dosing paradigms of TOCP, bilateral distal myelinated fiber alterations were demonstrated (Padilla and Veronesi, 1985; Veronesi, 1984). These involved distal levels of long spinal cord myelinated tracts, including ascending and descending spinal cord tracts (demonstrated in cervical levels of fasciculus gracilis and dorso- and ventrolateral white matter columns and in lumbar dorsolateral, ventrolateral, and ventral columns, respectively). This largely recapitulated the distribution of lesions seen in hens (Cavanagh, 1954; Jortner and Ehrich, 1987). The fiber lesions developed after a postdosing

latent period and were associated with a transient postdosing inhibition of whole brain neuropathy target esterase (NTE). No definitive clinical deficits were observed in affected rats. The lesions were seen in larger myelinated nerve fibers and consisted of giant axonal swellings containing accumulations of tubulovesicular profiles of smooth endoplasmic reticulum and/or vacuoles, progressing to massive accumulations of mitochondria, vesicular profiles, and amorphous bodies in granular axoplasm (Veronesi, 1984). The swellings were associated with attenuation of their myelin sheaths.

Other pathological studies of rats with OPIDN, using a variety of strains (Wistar, Long–Evans, Sprague–Dawley) and TOCP or mipafox as toxicants, did not demonstrate this extensive distribution of myelinated nerve fiber lesions (Carboni *et al.*, 1992; Dyer *et al.*, 1992; Ehrich *et al.*, 1993a, 1993b, 1995; Inui *et al.*, 1993; Itoh *et al.*, 1985; Lehning *et al.*, 1996). The lesions were, in fact, primarily found in the medullary and cervical (distal) levels of the fasciculus gracilis and its afferent target nucleus, and axonal vacuolization and swelling were prominent features (Carboni *et al.*, 1992; Dyer *et al.*, 1992) (Fig. 49.14). Studies by Veronesi and colleagues using mipafox

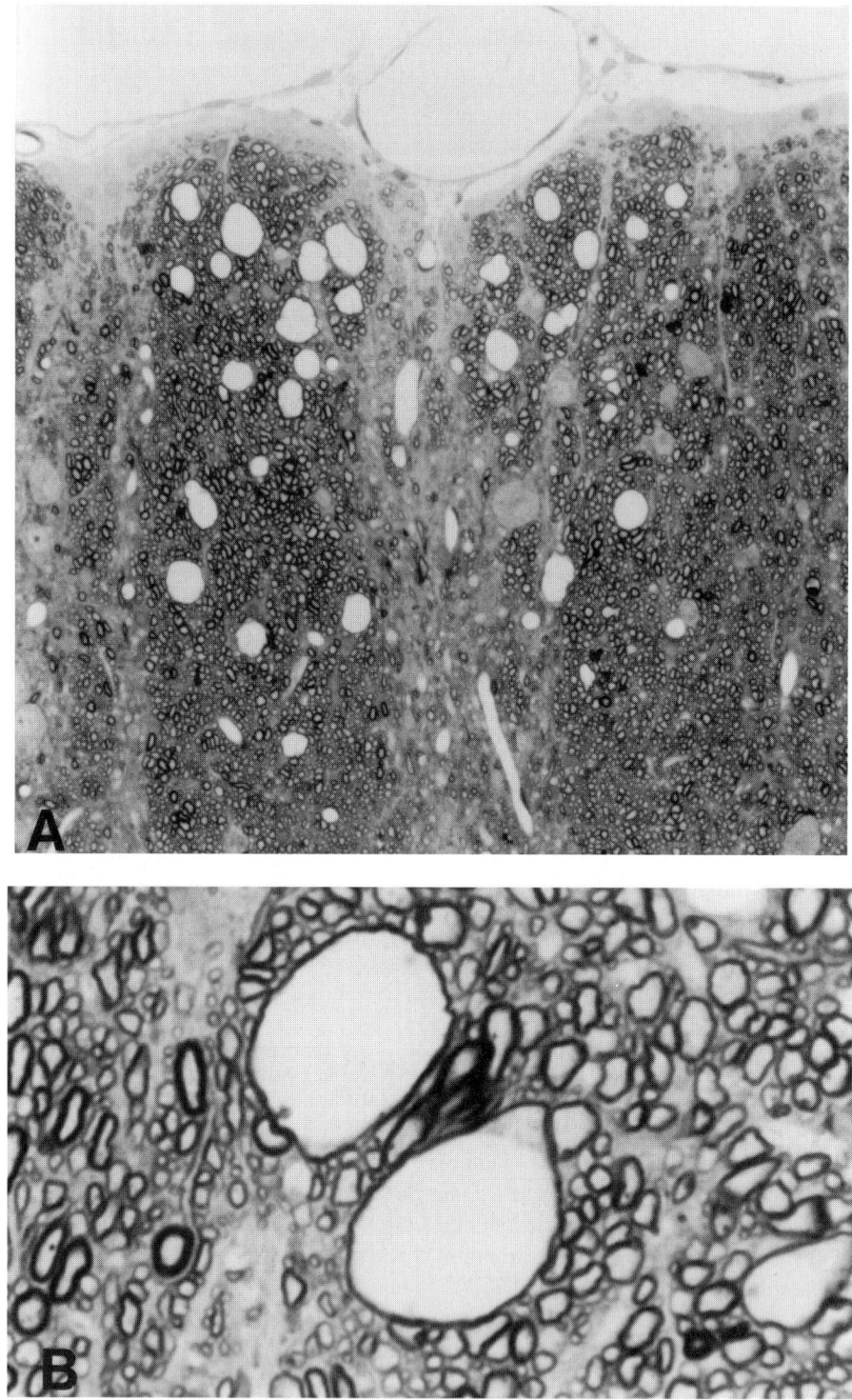

Figure 49.14 Medullary (terminal) level of the fasciculus gracilis from a Long–Evans rat that had been given a toxic dose (30 mg/kg ip) of mipafox 21 days earlier. There are numerous pale-staining swollen axons seen bilaterally (A). Higher power of the lesion (B) shows associated thin myelin sheaths. Toluidine blue–safranin stain.

in rats demonstrated a similar distribution of lesions (Veronesi et al., 1986). The fate of affected fibers in this rodent model is still in question, in that one study suggests they are reversible, whereas another indicates progression to degeneration and loss of affected segments (Carboni et al., 1992; Itoh et al., 1984). One of the problems in evaluating neuropathic changes of this nature in the rostral fasciculus gracilis is the presence of some swollen, vacuolated axons in this region in normal rats (Carboni *et al.*, 1992; Eisenbrandt *et al.*, 1990; Veronesi *et al.*, 1986). In addition, rats generally required higher dosages of toxicant to elicit pathological changes than did chickens (Ehrich *et al.*, 1993a, 1995). These findings, clinical insensitivity and restricted lesions, limit the utility of the laboratory rat as a model for OPIDN.

Neuropathologic studies of a putative OPIDN model in laboratory mice have been done in animals dosed with 580–3480 mg/kg TOCP (Veronesi *et al.*, 1991). Lesion distribution was not consistent with that seen in other models of the neuropathy, although myelinated fibers had qualitatively the same axonal pathology. The latter included intra-axonal vacuoles, neurofilament masses, and floccular degeneration, which were noted in cervical spinal cord white matter, medullary inferior olivary nucleus, and the fasciculus gracilis. The lesions were not associated with a specific pattern of toxicant-induced inhibition of neuropathy target esterase (NTE). The mouse, therefore, is not considered to be an acceptable model of OPIDN.

Several studies of OPIDN in the ferret have brought to light another animal model of this neuropathy (Stumpf *et al.*, 1989; Tanaka *et al.*, 1991). These utilized tri-*ortho*-tolyl phosphate administered either orally or dermally (250, 500, or 1000 mg/kg) or DFP (2 or 4 mg/kg) given subcutaneously. The former compound was more toxic via the dermal route and, indeed, had little effect orally. Tri-*ortho*-tolyl phosphate–dosed animals in the 1000-mg/kg dermal group had 46% inhibition of brain neurotoxic esterase and associated clinical signs of rear leg ataxia and weakness progressing over the 11- to 49-day postdosing period. These were seen in a dose- and lesion-related fashion. Spinal cord lesions of bilateral, degenerating axons in the cervical level of the fasciculus gracilis and lumbar regions of the dorsal spinocerebellar tract, and, on occasion, in the lumbar ventral gray matter were noted. Because these lesions were delineated using the Fink–Heimer silver impregnation method, no qualitative histological details of the lesions were detectable.

The DFP-induced neuropathy in ferrets was associated with a dose-related wider spectrum of lesions, along with associated clinical deficits and inhibition of medullary/cerebellar neurotoxic esterase (Tanaka *et al.*, 1991). A single dose of 4 mg/kg inhibited this esterase by 86% at 4 h, with recovery of activity by 4 days. There was more prolonged acetylcholinesterase inhibition as well. These animals had rear leg ataxia, which progressed to paralysis in the 14- to 28-day postdosing period (the study was terminated at that point). Lesions detected by the Fink–Heimer method included dense axonal and terminal degeneration seen in the animals sacrificed at 21 and 28 days. In the spinal cord, these were seen in laminae VI–VII of the gray matter, in the ventral motor nucleus at the cervical level, and (as axonal degeneration) in the lateral corticospinal tract at the lumbar levels, and fasciculus gracilis and dorsal spinocerebellar tract in the cervical region. The medulla has both axonal and terminal alterations in the gracile, inferior vestibular, lateral reticular, and inferior olivary nuclei, as did the cerebellar folia of the anterior lobe. These studies indicate that the ferret has the spectrum of lesions, along with detectable clinical signs and ap-

propriate inhibition of brain esterases, to make it an appropriate model of OPIDN, although it has other limitations (availability, husbandry concerns) regarding its use as a standard test animal for safety assessment.

49.7 PATHOGENESIS

Factors important in the development of organophosphorus-induced delayed neuropathy (OPIDN) have been discussed in a number of previous reviews (Abou-Donia, 1981, 1995; Abou-Donia and Lapadula, 1990; Carrington, 1989; Cherniack, 1986; Cranmer and Hixson, 1984; Davis and Richardson, 1980; Ecobichon, 1994; Ehrich, 1996; Gallo and Lawryk, 1991; Hollingshaus, 1983; Johnson, 1975a, 1982, 1992, 1993; Jortner, 1984, 1988; Lotti, 1992, 1995, 1997; Lotti *et al.*, 1993; Richardson, 1995; see Chapter 50). A number of events that occur during the development of the neuropathy have been identified, yet the precise mechanism(s) remains elusive.

One factor known to be important in the initiation of OPIDN is inhibition of neuropathy target esterase (NTE, also known as neurotoxic esterase). This enzyme has been suggested to be the molecular target of neuropathy-inducing OP compounds with a pentavalent phosphorus atom, yet recent evidence has suggested that NTE may be a biomarker rather than the single, specific target that initiates OPIDN (Ehrich, 1996; Johnson, 1982; Lotti, 1992; Lotti and Moretto, 1993; Lotti *et al.*, 1993). What is certain, however, is that NTE must be phosphorylated and extensively inhibited by the OP compound before notable OPIDN develops. In addition to inhibiting NTE, the OP compounds inducing delayed neuropathy must bind sufficiently strongly to the NTE that it is difficult to impossible to remove them (Clothier and Johnson, 1979; Johnson, 1980, 1982; Milatovic and Johnson, 1993; Nostrandt and Ehrich, 1993; Richardson, 1995). For this type of binding to occur, the pentavalent OP compound (phosphate, phosphonate, phosphoramidate) must have a leaving group whose removal or rearrangement results in a negatively charged moiety on the enzyme (Johnson, 1982, 1992, 1993). This process has been called "aging." Whether typical "aging" occurs with phosphoramidates has been debated (Johnson, 1993; Johnson and Safi, 1993; Milatovic and Johnson, 1993; Richardson, 1995), but, in any case, a strong attachment of OP compound to NTE must be part of the process between exposure and development of OPIDN.

Although a 70% threshold for NTE inhibition was once thought necessary before ataxia and nervous system degeneration could occur, OPIDN induced by OP compounds with pentavalent phosphorus atoms actually follows a dose–response curve (Ehrich *et al.*, 1993a, 1995). The correlation between early NTE inhibition and OPIDN is sufficiently strong that registration of OP insecticides under the U.S. Federal Insecticide, Fungicide, and Rodenticide Act (FIFRA) requires that data on NTE inhibition and on doses required for its inhibition relative to acetylcholinesterase inhibition be obtained as a biochemical determinant of potential to cause OPIDN (Ehrich, 1996; EPA, 1991).

Neuropathy-inducing phosphites also inhibit NTE (Abou-Donia, 1995; Abou-Donia and Lapadula, 1990), yet they do not have a leaving group as do the OP compounds with a pentavalent phosphorus atom. This distinction, as well as differences in clinical and pathological presentation (see Section 49.5), place the phosphite-induced disorder (Type II OPIDN) in a different category than classical OPIDN (Lehning et al., 1996; Varghese et al., 1995; Veronesi and Dvergsten, 1987).

To say that NTE is or is not the precise target for initiation of neuropathy induced by OP compounds is difficult. The physiological functions of NTE are unknown. It is a carboxylesterase, a class of enzymes responsible for the hydrolysis of a wide variety of compounds, including OP compounds, carboxylesters, thioesters, and aromatic amides. Its molecular weight is in the range of 150,000 Da. This enzyme is found in brain, spinal cord, peripheral nerves, and in nonnervous tissue, such as the adrenal gland, lymphocytes, and platelets (Bertoncin et al., 1985; Dudek and Richardson, 1982; Ehrich, 1996; Maroni and Bleecker, 1986; Schwab and Richardson, 1986). Suggestions have been made that activity in the peripheral nerve has a differential sensitivity than tissue from the central nervous system and that this tissue may be more predictive of potential for OPIDN (Barril et al., 1988; Caroldi and Lotti, 1982; Carrera et al., 1992; Lotti et al., 1987; Moretto et al., 1989). The nerve used for assay, however, is the sciatic nerve, which does not show exceptional pathogenic effects, except in its distal branches, following administration of neuropathy-inducing OP compounds (Dyer et al., 1991). Furthermore, the sciatic nerve is relatively small and more difficult to use for assay than brain without providing generally recognized additional benefit (Barril et al., 1988; Correll and Ehrich, 1991; Ehrich, 1996; Johnson, 1982).

Purification of NTE has been a long and difficult process, and no studies examining the effects of a purified enzyme on cellular functions have yet been reported. NTE is a membrane-associated enzyme, and early attempts to purify the protein resulted in loss of activity when attempts were made to separate the enzyme protein from the membrane phospholipid (Clothier and Johnson, 1979; Davis and Richardson, 1987; Davis et al., 1980; Ishakawa et al., 1983; Pope and Padilla, 1989a, 1989b; Ruffer-Tumer et al., 1992; Schwab et al., 1985; Thomas et al., 1989, 1990; Williams and Johnson, 1981). Early studies with brain tissue suggested NTE could exist in multiple forms (Chemnitius et al., 1983; Zech and Chemnitius, 1987), but later studies determined that such was not the case (Carrington and Abou-Donia, 1986; Richardson, 1992), except, perhaps, in peripheral nerve, where recent studies suggest that soluble and membrane-associated enzymes exist in that tissue (Carrera et al., 1994; Escudero et al., 1997; Tormo et al., 1993; Vilanova et al., 1990, 1993).

Only recently have reports appeared that suggest an active enzyme could be purified (Glynn et al., 1993, 1994; Johnson and Glynn, 1995; Mackay et al., 1996; Seifert and Wilson, 1994; Thomas et al., 1993), cloned (Glynn et al., 1999; Lush et al., 1998), and localized in neuronal cell bodies (Glynn et al., 1998). Purification, characterization, and physiological effects of OP phosphorylation and aging of NTE may be aided by use of new, very potent probes and sensitive substrates (Borhan et al., 1995; Wu and Casida, 1994, 1995; Yoshida et al., 1994, 1995). NTE, its biochemistry, enzymology, and isolation are discussed in more detail in Chapter 50.

Although early and significant inhibition of NTE is an excellent predictor of potential for developing OPIDN, the relationship between NTE inhibition and OPIDN itself is less clear. These items have been summarized in recent reviews (Ehrich, 1996; Lotti, 1992; Lotti et al., 1991, 1993; Richardson, 1992; see Chapter 50). For example, although NTE is inhibited shortly after OP administration, it may no longer be inhibited some days to weeks later when clinical and pathological manifestations of OPIDN are evident. If NTE were a target, its inhibition would need to initiate some series of events that no longer required its inhibition. Furthermore, NTE inhibition predictive for OPIDN is usually measured in brain and spinal cord, tissues that have a relatively low proportion of their nerve fiber population affected. The most concentrated nerve fiber lesions of OPIDN are found in distal levels of peripheral nerves, such as branches of the tibial or in the biventer cervicis in the hen, and these tissues are too small for measurement of NTE activity (El-Fawal et al., 1988, 1990c; Jortner and Ehrich, 1987).

Another consideration with the designation of NTE as the specific target for initiation of OPIDN is that this enzyme in brain, spinal cord, and/or peripheral nerve can be inhibited in species and age groups of animals that do not show notable clinical signs or pathological manifestations of OPIDN (e.g., chicks, rats, mice, and, possibly, quail [Ehrich, 1996; Funk et al., 1994a; Padilla and Veronesi, 1985, 1988; Peraica et al., 1993; Varghese et al., 1995; Veronesi et al., 1991]). It appears, for instance, that chickens need to be 55–60 days of age before clinical signs indicative of OPIDN appear. Some pathological evidence of OPIDN, however, can be seen in the spinal cord of chicks that were only 2 weeks old when exposed to diisopropyl phosphorofluoridate (DFP), suggesting that age susceptibility in this animal model of OPIDN needs reevaluation (Funk et al., 1994a).

Further discordance between NTE inhibition and OPIDN can be noted in other situations. For example, clinical and pathological manifestations of OPIDN that follow administration of a single OP compound can increase in a dose-related manner when NTE is already maximally inhibited in both hens and rats (Ehrich et al., 1993a, 1995).

Although the relationship to OPIDN has not yet been proven to be direct, there are events that do occur between NTE inhibition and the development of neuropathic lesions that define the ensuing syndrome as OPIDN. These include depression of nerve muscle conduction, inhibition of retrograde transport, and perturbations of calcium-mediated intracellular biochemical processes.

A number of studies, although not all (Chemnitius et al., 1988; Shell et al., 1988), have indicated that administration of neuropathy-inducing OP compounds altered nerve and/or muscle electrophysiological responses in humans (Roberts, 1977; Vasilescu et al., 1984), hens (Anderson et al., 1988; Durham and Ecobichon, 1984; El-Fawal *et al.*, 1988, 1989, 1990b, 1990c; Lidsky *et al.*, 1990; Robertson *et al.*, 1987, 1988), dogs (Schaeppi *et al.*, 1984), and cats (Abou-Donia *et al.*, 1986; Baker *et al.*, 1980; Drakontides and Baker, 1983; Lapadula *et al.*, 1982). For example, an increase in threshold excitability was noted in peripheral nerves (sciatic, tibial), biventer cervicis) of the hen, which is the accepted animal model for OPIDN early (1–4 days) after administration of the OP neurotoxicants phenyl saligenin phosphate (PSP) and di-*n*-butyryl dichlorovinyl phosphate (DBDCVP) (El-Fawal *et al.*, 1988, 1989, 1990b, 1990c; Robertson *et al.*, 1987, 1988). Morphological damage was seen in the biventer cervicis nerve as early as 4 days after administration of PSP, even though clinical manifestations of OPIDN were not evident before day 10 (El-Fawal *et al.*, 1990c).

Alteration of axonal transport following administration of neuropathy-inducing OP compounds has also been investigated. NTE itself was reported to be carried by anterograde axonal transport (Carrington and Abou-Donia, 1985a). Studies in the cat sciatic nerve indicated that anterograde axonal transport was accelerated 7 days after administration of diisopropyl phosphorofluoridate (DFP), an effect the investigators suggested was secondary to the pathologic effect, as the effect was relatively small (Carrington *et al.*, 1989). More recent studies from this laboratory, however, suggest that sciatic nerve transport of neurofilament protein in the hen is first increased (at 3 days) and then decreased (>7 days) after exposure to DFP (Gupta *et al.*, 1997). Another laboratory examined retrograde transport in hens given di-*n*-dibutyl-2,2-dichlorovinyl phosphate (DBDCVP). Retrograde transport decreased in the ventral spinal cord 3 days after treatment. Maximal effects were noted 7 days after dosing, with effects both in the ventral spinal cord and in the dorsal root ganglia (Moretto *et al.*, 1987). Clinical deficits were not reported before day 10 after dosing.

Effects of neuropathy-inducing OP compounds have also been examined on lipid constituents of axonal membranes, including cholesterol, gangliosides, and other lipids (Bush *et al.*, 1995; Morazina and Rosenberg, 1970; Williams *et al.*, 1966). Although membrane changes are evident in OPIDN, only the relatively recent work on ganglioside profiles suggests that these particular membrane lipids may be specifically involved as OPIDN develops.

Much of the work on perturbations of calcium-mediated intracellular biochemical processes has been done in the laboratory of M. B. Abou-Donia, who has summarized the work in several reviews (Abou-Donia, 1993, 1995; Abou-Donia and Lapadula, 1990). The investigators in this laboratory first noted that radiolabeled neuropathy-inducing OP compounds could bind to proteins other than NTE (Carrington and Abou-Donia, 1985b). Spinal cords collected from hens exposed to 750 mg/kg tri-*o*-cresyl phosphate (TOCP) only 1 day previously had some increase in capability to incorporate ^{32}P, an effect that was enhanced in the presence of calcium and that increased as ataxia developed. Increased protein phosphorylation was not noted 3 weeks after treatment with a nonneuropathy-inducing OP compound (Patton *et al.*, 1983, 1985, 1986).

The investigators proceeded to attempt to identify the protein(s) phosphorylated following exposure to a neuropathy-inducing OP, TOCP. Gel electrophoresis indicated that exposure of hens to TOCP 1, 6, or 21 days previously enhanced *in vitro* phosphorylation of tubulin, microtubule-associated protein-2 (MAP-2), and neurofilament proteins of 70, 160, and 210 kDa. These are cytoskeletal proteins important in the maintenance of axonal integrity. Because only Ca^{2+}-calmodulin (CaM) kinase II activity catalyzes the phosphorylation of these cytoskeletal proteins, effects of neuropathy-inducing OP compounds on this enzyme were examined (Lapadula *et al.*, 1991, 1992; Suwita *et al.*, 1986a, 1986b). Further experimentation indicated that there was an increase in calmodulin binding following administration of diisopropyl phosphorofluoridate (DFP), suggesting that DFP caused conformational changes that could enhance *in vitro* phosphorylation of cytoskeletal proteins in tissues removed from OP-treated hens. For example, phosphorylation of tubulin and all three neurofilament subunits was enhanced *in vitro* by treatment with CaM kinase II purified from hens that had OPIDN from DFP treatment 18–21 days previously (Abou-Donia *et al.*, 1993; Gupta and Abou-Donia, 1993, 1994, 1995b; Gupta *et al.*, 1992). The investigators suggested that the hyperphosphorylation of cytoskeletal proteins decreases their ability to be transported down the axon, causing accumulation (Abou-Donia, 1993; Gupta *et al.*, 1997).

The preceding studies measured phosphorylation of cytoskeletal proteins *in vitro* in tissues from animals exposed to neuropathy-inducing OP compounds. To verify if excess phosphorylation of neurofilaments actually occurred in nervous tissue, immunohistochemical techniques were used to determine the status of phosphorylated neurofilaments in affected myelinated nerve fibers of hens exposed to neuropathy-inducing OP compounds (Jensen *et al.*, 1992). This study demonstrated an excess accumulation of phosphorylated neurofilaments in swollen axons at 21 (distal sciatic nerve) or 7 (spinal cord dorsal columns) days after administration of 750 mg/kg TOCP. This accumulation, presumably antecedent to fiber degeneration, was thought to be related to toxicant-induced conformational change of CaM kinase II, leading to excessive phosphorylation of neurofilaments (Jensen *et al.*, 1992). Immunohistochemical studies in another laboratory did not demonstrate prominent excessive phosphorylated neurofilament aggregates prior to fiber degeneration in susceptible axonal populations of hens given a neuropathic dosage of PSP (Jortner *et al.*, 1999; Perkins *et al.*, 1995).

49.8 FACTORS INFLUENCING THE DEVELOPMENT OF ORGANOPHOSPHORUS-INDUCED DELAYED NEUROPATHY

Although a number of events that occur between OP exposure and development of OPIDN have been identified, questions remain about susceptibilities. It is evident that certain species (e.g., the accepted animal model, the hen, as well as humans, cats, ferrets, sheep, dogs, turkeys) are more susceptible than others (e.g., rats, mice) to clinical manifestations of the toxicity (Johnson, 1982). Certain strains of hens, the animal model of OPIDN, also appear to be differentially affected (Bursian *et al.*, 1989; Dunnington *et al.*, 1989; Ehrich *et al.*, 1986a), Furthermore, young animals appear to be relatively resistant to clinical manifestations of toxicity (Davis and Richardson, 1980; Funk *et al.*, 1994a; Johnson, 1982; Moretto *et al.*, 1991; Peraica *et al.*, 1993). NTE inhibition, however, can be significant in most susceptible and nonsusceptible species and age groups. In addition, although different and less extensive than that seen in the hen, neuropathological manifestations can be noted in populations once thought not susceptible to OPIDN (e.g., rats, young chicks) (Ehrich *et al.*, 1993a, 1993b, 1995; Funk *et al.*, 1994a; Padilla and Veronesi, 1985, 1988).

Comparative studies on the effects of neuropathy-inducing OPs in hens and rats have been done, including studies of the progression and regression of lesions (Carboni *et al.*, 1992; Dyer *et al.*, 1991, 1992; Ehrich *et al.*, 1993a, 1995; El-Fawal *et al.*, 1990c; Jortner *et al.*, 1989). These studies were done with hens 18 months old and rats more than 60 days old. Indications were that lesions could repair in both species over time, with repair occurring considerably earlier in the rat than in the hen. The reason for that is that, in hens, repair is manifest only in peripheral nerve, where myelinated nerve fiber regeneration is seen over a period of weeks following fully developed OPIDN (Jortner *et al.*, 1989). The repair of rat lesions is thought to be related to return of swollen, vacuolated fasciculus gracilis axons to the normal state, a more rapid process (Carboni *et al.*, 1992). It has been suggested that such capability for repair could at least partially explain species and age differences to induction of OPIDN, including the low susceptibility of chicks and increased susceptibility of older rats (>6 months) as measured by clinical evidence of neurological damage following treatment with neuropathy-inducing OP compounds (Funk *et al.*, 1994a; Lotti, 1992; Moretto *et al.*, 1992b; Peraica *et al.*, 1993).

Although repair may play a role in age and species susceptibilities to clinical and pathological manifestations of OPIDN, this process may be less significant in the treatment of OPIDN. Amelioration of OPIDN has been examined in animal models of this disorder (hen, cat) using agents suggested to provide therapeutic advantage in people or experimental animals with natural or experimentally induced neurological disorders (Capildeo, 1989; Drug Facts and Comparisons, 2001; Schlimmer and Parker, 1996; USP DI, 2001).

Glucocorticoids are used in the treatment of patients with acute traumatic injuries of the nervous system (Capildeo, 1989; Drug Facts and Comparisons, 2001; Schlimmer and Parker, 1996). The first studies examining the potential of glucocorticoids to ameliorate OPIDN were done in cats (Baker and Stanec, 1985; Baker *et al.*, 1982; Drakontides *et al.*, 1982). Glucocorticoids were administered shortly after diisopropyl phosphorofluoridate (DFP) and treatments continued over the next 19–20 days. The depression of repetitive neural discharges and muscle contractile response usually seen in cats with OPIDN

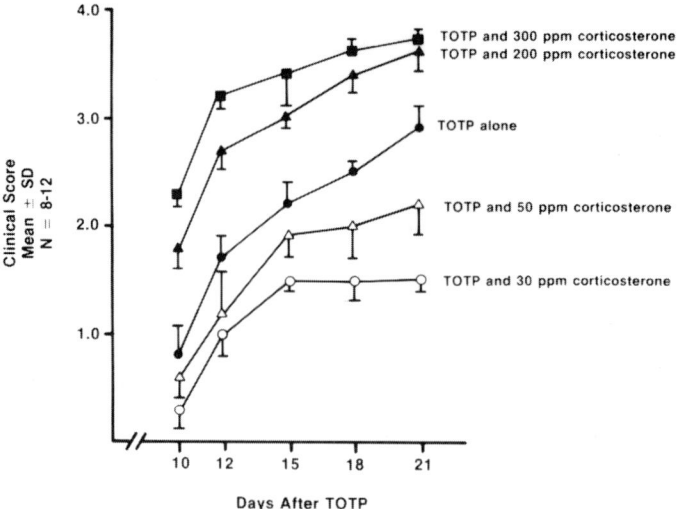

Figure 49.15 Effect of 30–300 ppm corticosterone on clinical signs of delayed neuropathy induced by po administration of TOTP (360 mg/kg) to chickens. Results are presented as mean±SD, $n = 8$–12. A score of 0 = no clinical signs, 1 = mild ataxia, 2 = moderate ataxia, 3 = severe ataxia, 4 = paralysis. Chickens given corn oil or corticosterone without TOTP had scores of 0. Reproduced with permission from Ehrich, M., Jortner, B. S., and Gross, W. B. (1986). Dose-related beneficial and adverse effects of dietary corticosterone on organophosphorus-induced delayed neuropathy in chickens. *Toxicol. Appl. Pharmacol.* **83**, 250–260. Copyright © 1986 by Academic Press, San Diego.

did not appear and morphological damage to motor nerve terminals was much attenuated. Glucocorticoids could also ameliorate OPIDN in hens, an effect that was dependent on dose of both corticoid and OP compound. Doses of OP compound that were not overwhelming but still sufficient to induce neuropathy and relatively low concentrations of glucocorticoids were protective, as indicated by clinical, electrophysiological, and morphological endpoints (Ehrich and Gross, 1982; Ehrich *et al.*, 1986b, 1988; Lidsky *et al.*, 1990). When doses were higher, glucocorticoids (and extreme stress) could exacerbate OPIDN (Ehrich and Gross, 1983, 1986; Ehrich *et al.*, 1985, 1986a, 1986b, 1988) (Fig. 49.15). The myopathy caused by large doses of glucocorticoids could have been exaggerating the neuropathic effects of the OP compounds in this situation (Schlimmer and Parker, 1996). The mechanism for glucocorticoid-induced alteration of OPIDN was not related to its effect on esterase activities, as NTE was equivalently inhibited whether or not the hens received corticoids. Measurements of esterase and microsomal enzyme activities also suggested that the glucocorticoids did not affect the metabolism of the neuropathy-inducing OP compound. However, even though the mechanism(s) for the interaction of neuropathy-inducing OP compounds and glucocorticoids remains undefined, the possibility remains that stress and/or corticoids could be a contributing factor in OPIDN.

Calcium channel blockers are also used to treat neurological disorders, especially those related to ischemia (Brailowsky, 1988; Drug Facts and Comparisons, 2001; USP DI, 2001). The rationale for studies on amelioration of OPIDN is based on the general role of calcium in neuronal degradation (Schlaepfer, 1971, 1987; Schlaepfer and Hasler, 1979; Schlaepfer and Zimmerman, 1984). Axonal degeneration, which is a feature of OPIDN (see Section 49.5), has been suggested to result from an increase in calcium-dependent proteinase (CANP or calpain) activity (Schlaepfer, 1987). Calpain activity increased in brain, sciatic nerve, and muscle of hens treated with TOTP or PSP, with activity significantly increased in sciatic nerve as early as 2 days after treatment with PSP (El-Fawal *et al.*, 1990a). Total nerve calcium was also increased, with this effect noted 4 days after PSP treatment. Increases in calpain activity were blocked by administration of 4 daily doses of the calcium channel blocker nifedipine, when initiated 1 day before PSP treatment. Calcium channel blockers were demonstrated to ameliorate PSP- and TOTP-induced OPIDN, as indicated by clinical, electrophysiological, and morphological endpoints (El-Fawal and Ehrich, 1993; El-Fawal *et al.*, 1989, 1990a, 1990b). Clinical signs developed later in hens treated with the calcium channel blockers verapamil and nifedipine. In addition, excitability thresholds of nerve–muscle preparations from hens given PSP and calcium channel blockers approached levels in preparations from control animals, and the pathological effects of PSP on myelinated fibers of the biventer cervicis nerve were markedly attenuated (Figs. 52.16 and 49.17). Calcium channel blockers have also been demonstrated to decrease lethal effects of DFP, another neuropathy-inducing OP compound (Dretchen *et al.*, 1986). In another laboratory, however, using a different approach, a slight decrease in calpain activity was reported along with a decrease in certain cytoskeletal proteins (e.g., a neurofilament subunit, NF-H, vimentin, GFAP), with the suggestion made that the proteinase was being degraded, and that axonal degeneration was related to decreased cytoskeletal proteins (Gupta and Abou-Donia, 1995a).

The amelioration of OPIDN by calcium channel blockers may, be related to their effects on calpain (El-Fawal and Ehrich, 1993; El-Fawal *et al.*, 1990a) or to their action against differential vascular effects induced by neuropathic and nonneuropathic OP compounds (McCain *et al.*, 1995, 1996). Calcium channel blockers did not affect NTE. Neuropathy-inducing PSP increased peripheral vascular resistance, response to vasoactive agents, and circulating levels of norepinephrine and epinephrine. The calcium channel blocker verapamil attenuated all of these responses. The effects of PSP on the cardiovascular system did not occur in hens exposed to paraoxon, an OP compound that does not cause OPIDN, suggesting that OP effects on the cardiovascular system may contribute to development of OPIDN.

As noted previously both inhibition and "aging" of NTE are expected before OPIDN will occur. OP compounds that do not age do not cause OPIDN (Johnson, 1982). In fact, nonaging inhibitors of NTE, given prior to neuropathy-inducing OPs, will prevent OPIDN. These NTE inhibitors include carbamates, phosphinates, and sulfonyl fluorides. These compounds appear to protect the NTE from the OP compound; that these compounds protect this enzyme has been a primary reason for designating NTE as the primary target for initiation of OPIDN (Johnson, 1980, 1982, 1993; Johnson and Read, 1993; Richardson, 1992).

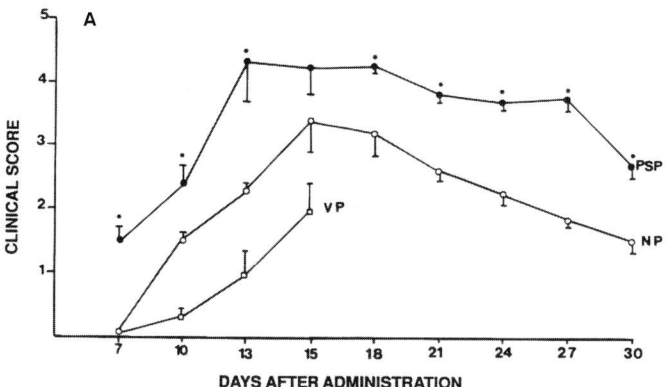

Figure 49.16A Development of clinical deficits and partial recovery after administration of phenyl saligenin phosphate (PSP = ●—●), nifedipine plus PSP (NP = ○—○), or verapamil plus PSP (VP = □—□). Verapamil, 7 mg/kg/day im, was given for 4 days beginning one day before PSP, 2.5 mg/kg im. Nefedipine, 10 mg/kg/day, was given for 5 days beginning one day before PSP. Results are presented as mean±SE, n = 5–10. Differences between the group of hens given only PSP and hens given nifedipine or verapamil plus PSP are denoted by asterisks (ANOVA with Newman–Keuls test for multiple comparisons, $p < 0.05$). 1 = altered gait, 2 = difficulty in walking and standing; 3 = severe ataxia, 4 = leg paralysis, 5 = paralysis with both leg and wing involvement. Hens not given PSP had scores of 0. Reproduced with permission from El-Fawal, H. A., Jortner, B. S., and Ehrich, M. (1990). Modification of phenyl saligenin phosphate–induced delayed effects by calcium channel blockers: *in vivo* and *in vitro* electrophysiological assessment. *NeuroToxicology* **11**, 573–592. Copyright © 1990 by Intox Press, Little Rock, AR.

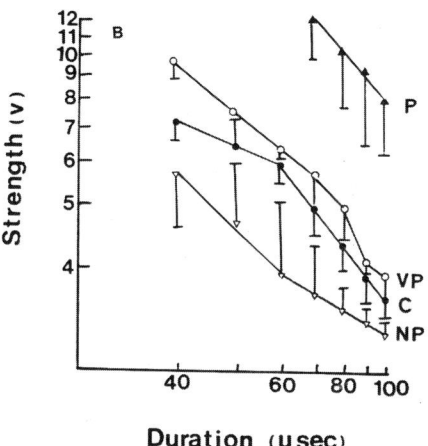

Figure 49.16B Log–log plot for inflection region (40–500 μs) of strength–duration curves from biventer cervices nerve muscle preparation days 15–16 after treatment of hens with PSP (2.5 mg/kg im). The dosing regimen is given in the legend to Fig. 49.16A. Control (C) ●—●, PSP (P) = ▲—▲, nifedipine plus PSP (NP) = ▽—▽, verapamil plus PSP (VP) = ○—○. Reproduced with permission from El-Fawal, H. A., Jortner, B. S., and Ehrich, M. (1990). Modification of phenyl saligenin phosphate–induced delayed effects by calcium channel blockers: *in vivo* and *in vitro* electrophysiological assessment. *NeuroToxicology* **11**, 573–592. Copyright © 1990 by Intox Press, Little Rock, AR.

Recently, it was discovered that administration of certain NTE inhibitors after neuropathy-inducing OP compounds will initiate or exacerbate clinical manifestations of OPIDN (Lotti *et al.*, 1991; Pope and Padilla, 1990). This phenomenon, called

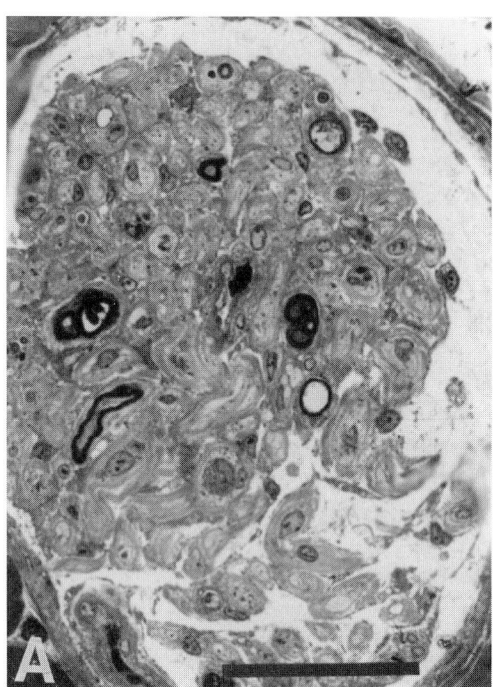
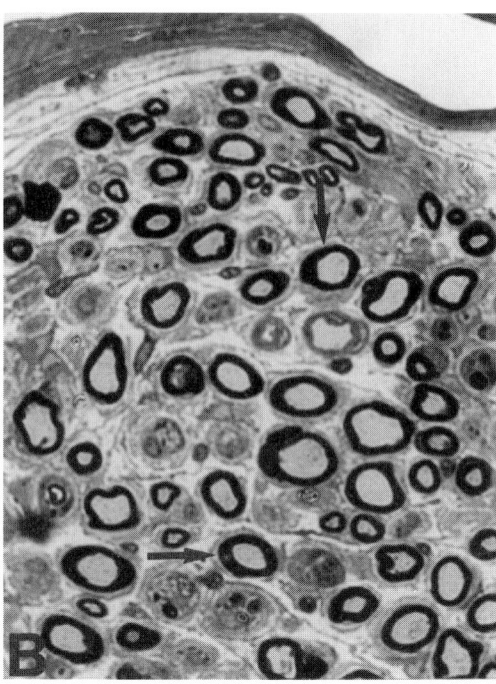

Figure 49.17 Cross sections of distal levels of the biventer cervicis nerve from chickens dosed with 2.5 mg/kg im of phenyl saligenin phosphate 15 days earlier. The nerve in A is from a hen that only received the toxicant and shows extensive loss of myelinated fibers. The nerve in B was from a hen that had received the toxicant, plus the calcium channel blocker verapamil at 7 mg/kg/day for 4 days, beginning one day prior to the phenyl saligenin phosphate administration. Examination of this nerve (B) shows that the verapamil dosing was protective to the myelinated nerve fibers, many of which have a normal morphological appearance (arrow). Toluidine blue–safranin stain; bar = 100 μm.

promotion or potentiation, has subsequently been reproduced in other laboratories, with clinical manifestations and nervous system lesions included among the endpoints (Johnson and Read, 1993; Massicotte *et al.*, 1999; Pope *et al.*, 1992; Randall *et al.*, 1997; Richardson, 1995). With administration of NTE inhibitors after dosing with a neuropathy-inducing OP compound, OPIDN in hens has been exaggerated beyond what would be expected if the neuropathy-inducing OP compound were given alone. The exacerbation of OPIDN appears to be due to a quantitative rather than qualitative difference, as observed in hens given several different OP compounds (e.g., DFP, DBD-CVP, PSP) and several different NTE inhibitors, with phenyl methanesulfonyl fluoride (PMSF) being used most often (Massicotte *et al.*, 1999; Moretto *et al.*, 1992a; Osman *et al.*, 1996; Peraica *et al.*, 1995; Randall *et al.*, 1997). To date, all promotors of OPIDN are NTE inhibitors, yet most are those that do not lose a side group after attachment to the enzyme (in other words, the promotor–enzyme complex does not have to "age"). There have been reports recently of promotion occurring with a dose of an NTE inhibitor below that necessary for inhibition of the enzyme (Moretto *et al.*, 1994; Osman *et al.*, 1996). During promotion, OPIDN can appear at subclinical doses of a neuropathy-inducing OP compound or in test subjects normally not susceptible to this condition (e.g., chicks, rats) (Harp *et al.*, 1997; Lotti *et al.*, 1993, 1995; Moretto *et al.*, 1992a,

1992b; Pope *et al.*, 1992, 1993, 1995). A recent report indicated that the only enzyme consistently inhibited by promoters was NTE, suggesting that some fraction or isoform of NTE may be the molecular target for promotion of OPIDN (Milatovic *et al.*, 1997). However, because NTE can be maximally inhibited without subsequent OPIDN by the OP compound first given, with administration of a second NTE inhibitor being followed by OPIDN, others have suggested that NTE is unlikely to be the target of OPIDN for promotion (Gardiman *et al.*, 1999; Johnson, 1993; Lotti, 1992, 1995, 1997; Lotti and Moretto, 1999; Lotti *et al.*, 1993; Moretto *et al.*, 1994; Osman *et al.*, 1996; Pope *et al.*, 1993). Factors other than NTE inhibition may be involved in OPIDN and promotion of OPIDN, because a recent study indicated that a soluble factor released in the spinal cord after exposure to a neuropathic OP compound had dramatic effects on cell growth (Pope *et al.*, 1995).

49.9 TESTING FOR ORGANOPHOSPHORUS-INDUCED DELAYED NEUROPATHY

Registration of OP compounds for pesticide use under FIFRA recommends that they be tested in hens 8–14 months old without designation of breed or strain. Since 1991, this testing has

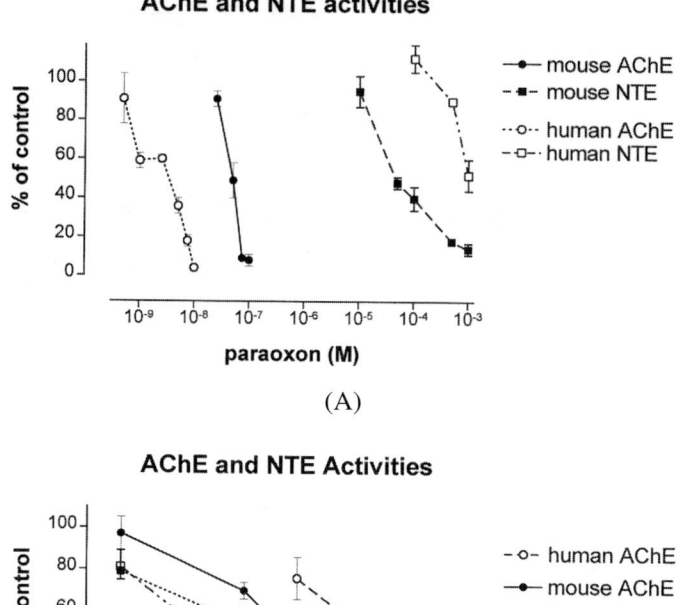

AChE and NTE activities

(A)

AChE and NTE Activities

(B)

Figure 49.18 Concentration response curves for inhibition of acetyl-cholinesterase (AChE) and neuropathy target esterase (NTE) in neuroblastoma cells of human and murine origin by organophosphorus compounds. Cells were incubated with OP compounds for 1 h before assay. Paraoxon causes acute cholinergic crisis (AChE inhibition) rather than organophosphorus-induced delayed neuropathy (OPIDN); PSP causes OPIDN. Point-to-point composite curves are provided to aid visualization (Prism; GraphPad, San Diego). Each curve represents at least three different assays that included at least three concentrations of OP compounds that provided values between 10 and 90% of values in vehicle-treated cells. Reproduced with permission from Ehrich, M., Correll, L., and Veronesi, B. (1997). Acetylcholinesterase and neuropathy target esterase inhibitions in neuroblastoma cells to distinguish organophosphorus compounds causing acute and delayed neurotoxicity. *Fundam. Appl. Toxicol.* **38**, 55–63. Copyright © 1997 by Academic Press, San Diego.

included NTE and acetylcholinesterase determinations, clinical observations, and neuropathology following single- and multiple-dosing procedures (EPA, 1991). In the initial testing procedure, brain and spinal cord samples are collected from a subset of the dosed hens within 48 h of administration of a single dose of the test OP insecticide and NTE and acetylcholinesterase activities determined. The remaining hens are observed over the next 3 weeks, with *in situ* perfusion-fixation and removal of brain, spinal cord, and peripheral nerves for histopathological examination at that time. Multiple-dose testing (28 days) may also be necessary. With these tests, the relative sensitivity of NTE to inhibition compared to acetylcholinesterase inhibition identifies those OP compounds

capable of causing OPIDN even before clinical signs and morphological changes appear.

Suggestions have been made that NTE measurements in cultured cells could be used to predict potential for OPIDN without the need to run this test in animals (Barber *et al.*, 1999a, 1999b; Ehrich and Veronesi, 1995, 1999; Ehrich *et al.*, 1994, 1997; Funk *et al.*, 1994b, 1994c; Knoth-Anderson and Abou-Donia, 1993; Knoth-Anderson *et al.*, 1992; Nostrandt and Enrich, 1992, 1993; Sogorb *et al.*, 1996, 1997; Veronesi, 1992; Veronesi and Ehrich, 1993; Veronesi *et al.*, 1997). Investigations indicated that NTE activity could be found in both primary cultures of avian and bovine origin and continuous cell lines of human and rodent origin (e.g., SH-SY5Y, PC-12, NB41A3). A recent, thorough concentration–response study with 11 active esterase inhibitors, including 7 that cause OPIDN and 4 that do not, indicated that either a human cell line or a murine cell line was capable of identifying the neuropathy-inducing OP compounds based on the relative sensitivity of NTE to inhibition compared to acetylcholinesterase (Ehrich *et al.*, 1997) (Fig. 49.18). Concentrations of OP compounds needed to inhibit NTE and acetylcholinesterase were far below those cytotoxic to the cultures. A similar result was noted in another study in which new, very sensitive NTE inhibitors were examined in cell lines of rodent origin (Li and Casida, 1997). Although it appeared that cell cultures did not have sufficient oxidative capability to convert protoxicant phosphorothioates to active enzyme inhibitors (Ehrich, 1995; Ehrich and Veronesi, 1995; Ehrich *et al.*, 1994, 1997), recent studies have indicated that this can be overcome by preincubation of OP protoxicants with a bromine solution or a microsomal preparation (Barber *et al.*, 1999a, 1999b). The results of recent studies enhance the possibility that OP compounds may one day be screened for potential to induce OPIDN by using an *in vitro* system.

49.10 SUMMARY

Organophosphorus-induced delayed neuropathy (OPIDN) is a generally progressive, irreversible disorder that causes clinical manifestations appearing days to weeks after humans and certain species of animals are exposed to OP compounds that can essentially irreversibly inhibit most of the available neuropathy target esterase (NTE, neurotoxic esterase). The severity of OPIDN, as indicated by clinical and anatomical manifestations, depends on species and age of test animals and extent of NTE inhibition. Chickens have proven the most sensitive test species. OPIDN is manifest clinically by ataxia and weakness progressing to paralysis, associated with bilateral degeneration of distal and terminal regions of long myelinated nerve fibers. The neuropathy can be prevented by pretreatment with NTE inhibitors; yet these same compounds promote OPIDN when given after a neuropathy-inducing OP compound. Although the precise mechanism of OPIDN has not been determined, there appears to be a role for calcium, as calcium blockers ameliorated the effect, and changes on CaM kinase II activity and cytoskeletal protein phosphorylation appear after administration of neuropathy-inducing OP compounds. Recent studies indicate that NTE purification is imminent, and that neuropathy-inducing OP compounds and their effects on NTE can be studied in cultured cells.

REFERENCES

Abou-Donia, M. B. (1981). Organophosphorus ester–induced delayed neurotoxicity. *Annu. Rev. Pharmacol. Toxicol.* **21**, 511–548.

Abou-Donia, M. B. (1993). The cytoskeleton as a target for organophosphorus ester–induced delayed neurotoxicity (OPIDN). *Chem.–Biol. Interact.* **87** 383–393.

Abou-Donia, M. B. (1995). Organophosphorus pesticides. *In* "Handbook of Toxicology" (L. W. Chang and R. S. Dyer, eds.), pp. 419–473. Dekker, New York.

Abou-Donia, M. B., and Graham, D. G. (1978). Delayed neurotoxicity from long-term low-level topical administration of leptophos to the comb of hens. *Toxicol. Appl. Pharmacol.* **46**, 199–213.

Abou-Donia, M. B., and Lapadula, D. M. (1990). Mechanisms of organophosphorus ester–induced delayed neurotoxicity: Type I and type II. *Annu. Rev. Pharmacol. Toxicol.* **30**, 405–440.

Abou-Donia, M. B., and Preissig, S. H. (1976a). Delayed neurotoxicity of leptophos: Toxic effects on the nervous system of hens. *Toxicol. Appl. Pharmacol.* **35**, 269–282.

Abou-Donia, M. B., and Preissig, S. H. (1976b). Delayed neurotoxicity from continuous low-dose oral administration of leptophos to hens. *Toxicol. Appl. Pharmacol.* **38**, 595–608.

Abou-Donia, M. B., Graham, D. G., and Komeil, A. A. (1979). Delayed neurotoxicity of *O*-ethyl *O*-2,4-dichlorophenyl phenylphosphonothioate: Effects of a single oral dose on hens. *Toxicol. Appl. Pharmacol.* **49**, 293–303.

Abou-Donia, M. B., Trofatter, L. P., Graham, D. G., and Lapadula, D. M. (1986). Electromyographic, neuropathologic, and functional correlates in the cat as the result of tri-*o*-cresyl phosphate delayed neurotoxicity. *Toxicol. Appl. Pharmacol.* **83**, 126–141.

Abou-Donia, M. B., Viana, M. E., Gupta, R. P., and Anderson, J. K. (1993). Enhanced calmodulin binding concurrent with increased kinase-dependent phosphorylation of cytoskeletal proteins following a single subcutaneous injection of diisopropyl phosphorofluoridate in hens. *Neurochem. Int.* **22**, 165–173.

Abou-Donia, M. B., Wilmarth, K. R., Abdel-Rahman, A. A., Jensen, K. F., Oehme, F. W., and Kurt, T. L. (1996). Increased neurotoxicity following concurrent exposure to pyridostigmine bromide, DEET, and chlorpyrifos. *Fundam. Appl. Toxicol.* **34**, 201–222.

Anderson, R. J., Robertson, D. G., Henderson, J. D., and Wilson, B. W. (1988). DFP-induced elevation of strength–duration threshold in hen peripheral nerve. *NeuroToxicology* **9**, 47–52.

Baker, T., and Stanec, A. (1985). Methylprednisolone treatment of an organophosphorus-induced delayed neuropathy. *Toxicol. Appl. Pharmacol.* **79**, 348–352.

Baker, T., Drakontides, A. B., and Riker, W. F. (1982). Prevention of the organophosphorus neuropathy by glucocorticoids. *Exp. Neurol.* **78**, 397–408.

Baker, T., Lowndes, H. E., Johnson, M. K., and Sandborg, I. C. (1980). The effects of phenylmethanesulfonyl fluoride on delayed organophosphorus neuropathy. *Arch. Toxicol.* **46**, 305–311.

Barber, D., Correll, L, and Ehrich, M. (1999a). Comparison of two *in vitro* activation systems for protoxicant organophosphorous esterase inhibitors. *Toxicol. Sci.* **47**, 16–22.

Barber, D., Correll, L, and Ehrich, M. (1999b). Comparative effectiveness of organophosphorous protoxicant activating systems in neuroblastoma cells and brain homogenates. *J. Toxicol. Environ. Health* **56**, 101–112.

Barril, J. B., Vilanova, E., and Pellin, M. (1988). Sciatic nerve neuropathy target esterase: Methods of assay, proximo-distal distribution and regeneration. *Toxicology* **49**, 107–114.

Beck, B. E., Wood, C. D., and Whanham, G. R. (1977), Triaryl phosphate poisoning in cattle. *Vet. Pathol.* **14**, 128–137.

Bertoncin, D., Russolo, A., Caroldi, S., and Lotti, M. (1985). Neuropathy target esterase in human lymphocytes. *Arch. Environ. Health* **40**, 139–144.

Bischoff, A. (1967). The ultrastructure of tri-*ortho*-cresyl phosphate poisoning. I. Studies on myelin and axonal alterations in the sciatic nerve. *Acta Neuropathol.* **9**, 158–174.

Bischoff, A. (1970). Ultrastructure of tri-*ortho*-cresyl phosphate poisoning in the chicken. II. Studies on spinal cord alterations. *Acta Neuropathol.* **15**, 142–155.

Borhan, B., Ko, Y., Mackay, C., Wilson, B. W., Kurth, M. J., and Hammock, B. D. (1995). Development of surrogate substrates for neuropathy target esterase. *Biochim. Biophys. Acta* **1250**, 171–182.

Bouldin, T. W., and Cavanagh, J. B. (1979a). Organophosphorus neuropathy. I. A teased-fiber study of the spatio-temporal spread of axonal degeneration. *Am. J. Pathol.* **94**, 241–252.

Bouldin, T. W., and Cavanagh, J. B. (1979b). Organophosphorus neuropathy. II. A fine-structural study of the early stages of axonal degeneration. *Am. J. Pathol.* **94**, 253–270.

Brailowsky, S. (1988). Therapeutic approaches in subjects with brain lesions. *In* "Pharmacological Approaches to the Treatment of Brain and Spinal Cord Injury" (D. G. Stein and B. A. Sabel, eds.), pp. 1–21. Plenum, New York.

Bursian, S. J., Lehning. E. J., Correll, L., and Ehrich, M. (1989). Effect of beta-naphthoflavone on *o*-tolyl saligenin phosphate–induced delayed neuropathy in two lines of chickens. *J. Toxicol. Environ. Health* **28**, 461–471.

Bush, D. M., Lehning, E. J., and Bursian, S. J. (1995). The effects of diisopropylphosphorofluoridate (DFP) on the ganglioside profile in the chicken (*Gallus domesticus*) hindbrain. *NeuroToxicology* **16**, 55–61.

Capildeo, R. (1989). "Steroids in Diseases of the Central Nervous System." Wiley, New York.

Carboni, D., Ehrich, M., Dyer, K., and Jortner, B. S. (1992). Comparative evolution of mipafox-induced delayed neuropathy in rats and hens. *NeuroToxicology* **13**, 723–733.

Caroldi, S., and Lotti, M. (1982). Neurotoxic esterase in peripheral nerve: Assay, inhibition, and rate of resynthesis. *Toxicol. Appl. Pharmacol.* **62**, 498–501.

Carrera, V., Barril, J., Mauricio, M., Pellin, M., and Vilanova, E. (1992). Local application of neuropathic organophosphorus compounds to hen sciatic nerve: Inhibition of neuropathy target esterase and peripheral neurological impairments. *Toxicol. Appl. Pharmacol.* **117**, 218–225.

Carrera, V., Diaz-Alejo, N., Sogorb, M. A, Vicedo, J. L., and Vilanova, E. (1994). *In vivo* inhibition by mipafox of soluble and particulate forms of organophosphorus neuropathy target esterase (NTE) in hen sciatic nerve. *Toxicol. Lett.* **71**, 47–51.

Carrington, C. D. (1989). Prophylaxis and the mechanism for the initiation of organophosphorus compound–induced delayed neurotoxicity. *Arch. Toxicol.* **63**, 165–172.

Carrington, C. D., and Abou-Donia, M. B. (1985a). Axoplasmic transport and turnaround of neurotoxic esterase in hen sciatic nerve. *J. Neurochem.* **44**, 616–621.

Carrington, C. D., and Abou-Donia, M. B. (1985b). Characterization of [^{3}H]diisopropyl phosphorofluoridate–binding proteins in hen brain: Rates of phosphorylation and sensitivity to neurotoxic and non-neurotoxic organophosphorus compounds. *Biochem. J.* **228**, 537–544.

Carrington, C. D., and Abou-Donia, M. B. (1986). Kinetics of substrate hydrolysis and inhibition by mipafox of paraoxon-preinhibited hen brain esterase activity. *Biochem. J.* **236**, 503–507.

Carrington, C. D., Brown, H. R., and Abou-Donia, M. B. (1988). Histopathological assessment of triphenyl phosphite neurotoxicity in the hen. *NeuroToxicology* **9**, 223–233.

Carrington, C. D., Lapadula, D. M., and Abou-Donia, M. B. (1989). Acceleration of anterograde axonal transport in cat sciatic nerve by diisopropyl phosphorofluoridate. *Brain Res.* **476**, 179–182.

Cavalleri, A., and Cosi, V. (1980). Polyneuropathy in shoe factory workers. *In* "Advances in Neurotoxicology" (L. Manzo, ed.), pp. 193–200. Pergamon, New York.

Cavanagh, J. B. (1954). The toxic effects of tri-*ortho*-cresyl phosphate on the nervous system: An experimental study in hens. *J. Neurol. Neurosurg. Psych.* **17**, 163–172.

Cavanagh, J. B. (1964). Peripheral nerve changes in *ortho*-cresyl phosphate poisoning in the cat. *J. Pathol. Bacteriol.* **87**, 365–383.

Cavanagh, J. B., and Patangia, G. N. (1965). Changes in the central nervous system in the cat as the result of tri-*o*-cresyl phosphate poisoning. *Brain* **88**, 165–180.

Chemnitius, J. M., Haselmeyer, K. H., and Zech, R. (1983). Neurotoxic esterase, identification of two isoenzymes in hen brain. *Arch. Toxicol.* **53**, 235–244.

Chemnitius, J. M., Holling, M., Meyer, J. H., Schmidt, P. F., Schomburg, E. D., Steffens, H., and Zech, R. (1988), Influence of the organophosphorus compound DFP on inhibitory motor systems and esterase activity in the spinal cord of cats. *Neurosci. Res.* **6**, 257–263.

Cherniack, M. G. (1986). Organophosphorus esters and polyneuropathy. *Ann. Int. Med.* **104**, 264–266.

Cherniack, M. G. (1988). Toxicological screening for organophosphorus-induced delayed neurotoxicity: Complications in toxicity testing. *Neuro-Toxicology* **9**, 249–272.

Classen, W., Gretener, P., Rauch, M., Weber, E., and Krinke, G. J. (1996). Susceptibility of various areas of the nervous system of hens to TOCP-induced delayed neuropathy. *NeuroToxicology* **17**, 597–604.

Clothier, B., and Johnson, M. K. (1979). Rapid aging of neurotoxic esterase after inhibition by di-isopropyl phosphorofluoridate. *Biochem. J.* **177**, 549–558.

Correll, L., and Ehrich, M. (1991). A microassay method for neurotoxic esterase determinations. *Fundam. Appl. Toxicol.* **16**, 110–116.

Cranmer, J. M., and Hixson, E. J. (1984). "Delayed Neurotoxicity." Intox Press, Little Rock, AR.

Davis, C. S., and Richardson, R. J. (1980). Organophosphorus compounds. *In* "Experimental and Clinical Neurotoxicology" (P. S. Spencer and H. H. Schaumburg, eds.), pp. 527–544. Williams and Wilkins, Baltimore.

Davis, C. S., and Richardson, R. J. (1987). Neurotoxic esterase: Characterization of the solubilized enzyme and the conditions for its solubilization from chicken brain microsomal membranes with ionic, zwitterionic, or nonionic detergents. *Biochem. Phamacol.* **36**, 1393–1399.

Davis, C. S., Barth, M. L., Dudek, B. R., and Richardson, R. J. (1980). Inhibitor characteristics of native, solubilized, and lipid-reconstituted neurotoxic esterase. *Dev. Toxicol. Environ. Sci.* **8**, 63–66.

Drakontides, A B., and Baker, T. (1983). An electrophysiologic and ultrastructural study of the phenylmethanesulfonyl fluoride protection against a delayed organophosphorus neuropathy. *Toxicol. Appl. Pharmacol.* **70**, 411–422.

Drakontides, A B., Baker, W., and Riker, W. F. (1982). A morphological study of the effect of glucocorticoid treatment on delayed organophosphorus neuropathy. *NeuroToxicology* **3**, 165–178.

Dretchen, K. L., Bowles, A. M., and Raines, A. (1986). Protection by phenytoin and calcium channel blocking agents against the toxicity of diisopropylfluorophosphate. *Toxicol. Appl. Pharmacol.* **83**, 584–589.

"Drug Facts and Comparisons" (2001). Facts and Comparisons, St. Louis.

Dudek, B. R., and Richardson, R. J. (1982). Evidence for the existence of neurotoxic esterase in neural and lymphatic tissue of the adult hen. *Biochem. Pharmacol.* **31**, 1117–1121.

Dunnington, E. A., Siegel, P. B., and Ehrich, M. (1989). Differences in response of chickens from two genetic lines to diisopropyl phosphorofluoridate. *NeuroToxicology* **10**, 71–78.

Durham, H. D., and Ecobichon, D. J. (1984). The function of motor nerves innervating slow tonic skeletal muscle in hens with delayed neuropathy induced by tri-*o*-tolyl phosphate. *Can. J. Physiol. Pharmacol.* **62**, 1268–1273.

Dyer, K., Ehrich, M., and Jortner, B. S. (1996). Neuropathology of organophosphorus ester induced delayed neuropathy (OPIDN) in hens, lesions of spinal cord gray matter revisited. *Fundam. Appl. Toxicol.* **30S**, 300.

Dyer, K. R., El-Fawal, H. A., and Ehrich, M. F. (1991). Comparison of organophosphate-induced delayed neuropathy between branches of the tibial nerve and the biventer cervicis nerve in chickens. *NeuroToxicology* **12**, 687–695.

Dyer, K. R., Jortner, B. S., Shell, L. G., and Ehrich, M. (1992). Comparative dose–response studies of organophosphorus ester–induced delayed neuropathy in rats and hens administered mipafox. *NeuroToxicology* **13**, 745–755.

Ecobichon, D. J. (1994). Organophosphorus insecticides. *In* "Pesticides and Neurological Diseases" (D. J. Ecobichon and R. M. Joy, eds.), pp. 171–249. CRC Press, Boca Raton, FL.

Ehrich, M. (1995). Using neuroblastoma cell lines to address differential specificity to organophosphates. *Clin. Exp. Pharmacol. Physiol.* **22**, 291–292.

Ehrich, M. (1996). Neurotoxic esterase inhibition: Predictor of potential for organophosphorus-induced delayed neuropathy. *In* "Biomarkers for Agrochemicals and Toxic Substances" (J. N. Blancato, R. N. Brown, C. C. Dary, and M. A. Saleh, eds.), pp. 79–93. Am. Chem. Soc., Washington, DC.

Ehrich, M., and Gross, W. B. (1982). Effect of corticosterone on toxicity of malathion and TOTP in hens. *Neurobehav. Toxicol. Teratol.* **4**, 789–792.

Ehrich, M., and Gross, W. B. (1983). Modification of tri-*ortho*-tolyl phosphate toxicity in chickens by stress. *Toxicol. Appl. Pharmacol.* **70**, 249–254.

Ehrich, M., and Gross, W. B. (1986). Effect of supplemental corticosterone and social stress on organophosphorus-induced delayed neuropathy in chickens. *Toxicol. Lett.* **31**, 9–13.

Ehrich, M., and Veronesi, B. (1995). Esterase comparison in neuroblastoma cells of human and rodent origin. *Clin. Exp. Pharmacol. Physiol.* **22**, 385–386.

Ehrich, M., and Veronesi, B. (1999). *In vitro* neurotoxicology. *In* "Neurotoxicology" (H. A. Tilson and G. J. Harry, eds.), 2nd ed., pp. 37–51. Taylor & Francis, Philadelphia.

Ehrich, M., Brites, R. W., Briles, W. E., Dunnington, E. A., Martin, A., Siegel, P. B., and Gross, W. B. (1986a). Neurotoxicity of tri-*ortho*-tolyl phosphate in chickens of different genotypes in the presence and absence of deoxycorticosterone. *Poult. Sci.* **65**, 375–379.

Ehrich, M., Correll, L., and Veronesi, B. (1994). Neuropathy target esterase inhibition by organophosphorus esters in human neuroblastoma cells. *NeuroToxicology* **15**, 309–313.

Ehrich, M., Correll, L., and Veronesi, B. (1997). Acetylcholinesterase and neuropathy target esterase inhibitions in neuroblastoma cells to distinguish organophosphorus compounds causing acute and delayed neurotoxicity. *Fundam. Appl. Toxicol.* **38**, 55–63.

Ehrich, M., Jortner, B. S., and Gross, W. B. (1985). Absence of a protective effect of corticosterone on *O-O*-diisopropyl phosphorofluoridate (DFP) induced delayed neurotoxicity in chickens. *NeuroToxicology* **6**, 87–92.

Ehrich, M., Jortner, B. S., and Gross, W. B. (1986b). Dose-related beneficial and adverse effects of dietary corticosterone on organophosphorus-induced delayed neuropathy in chickens. *Toxicol. Appl. Pharmacol.* **83**, 250–260.

Ehrich, M., Jortner, B. S., and Gross, W. B. (1988). Types of adrenocorticoids and their effect on organophosphorus-induced delayed neuropathy in chickens. *Toxicol. Appl. Pharmacol.* **92**, 214–223.

Ehrich, M., Jortner, B. S., and Padilla, S. (1993a). Relationship of neuropathy target esterase inhibition to neuropathology and ataxia in hens given organophosphorus esters. *Chem.-Biol. Interact.* **87**, 431–437.

Ehrich, M., Jortner, B. S., and Padilla, S. (1995). Comparison of the relative inhibition of acetylcholinesterase and neuropathy target esterase in rats and hens given cholinesterase inhibitors. *Fundam. Appl. Toxicol.* **24**, 94–101.

Ehrich, M., Shell, L., Rozum, M., and Jortner, B. S. (1993b). Short-term clinical and neuropathologic effects of cholinesterase inhibitors in rats. *J. Am. Coll. Toxicol.* **12**, 55–68.

Eisenbrandt, D. L., Mattsson, J. L., Albee, R. R., Spencer, P. J., and Johnson, K. A. (1990). Spontaneous lesions in subchronic neurotoxicity testing of rats. *Toxicol. Pathol.* **18**, 154–164.

El-Fawal, H. A., and Ehrich, M. F. (1993). Calpain activity in organophosphorus-induced delayed neuropathy (OPIDN): Effects of a phenylalkylamine calcium channel blocker. *Annu. N. Y. Acad. Sci.* **679**, 325–329.

El-Fawal, H. A., Correll, L., Gay, L., and Ehrich, M. (1990a). Protease activity in brain, nerve, and muscle of hens given neuropathy-inducing organophosphates and a calcium channel blocker. *Toxicol. Appl. Pharmacol.* **103**, 133–142.

El-Fawal, H. A., Jortner, B. S., and Ehrich, M. (1989). Effect of verapamil on organophosphorus-induced delayed neuropathy in hens. *Toxicol. Appl. Pharmacol.* **97**, 500–511.

El-Fawal, H. A., Jortner, B. S., and Ehrich, M. (1990b). Modification of phenyl saligenin phosphate–induced delayed effects by calcium channel blockers: *in vivo* and *in vitro* electrophysiological assessment. *NeuroToxicology* **11**, 573–592.

El-Fawal, H. A., Jortner, B. S., and Ehrich, M. (1990c). Use of the biventer cervicis nerve–muscle preparation to detect early changes following exposure to organophosphates inducing delayed neuropathy. *Fundam. Appl. Toxicol.* **15**, 108–120.

El-Fawal, H. A., Jortner, B. S., Eyre, P., and Ehrich, M. (1988). The biventer cervicis nerve–muscle preparation of adult hens: Effects of phenyl saligenin phosphate administration. *NeuroToxicology* **9**, 625–636.

El-Sebae, A. H., Soliman, S. A., Abo El-Amayen, M., and Ahmed, N. S. (1977). Neurotoxicity of organophosphorus insecticides leptophos and EPN. *J. Environ. Sci. Healt, B* **12**, 269–288.

Environmental Protection Agency (EPA) (1991). "Pesticide Assessment Guidelines, Subdivision E. Hazard Evaluation: Human and Domestic Animals. Addendum 10: Neurotoxicity, Series 81, 82, and 83." National Technical Information Service, Springfield, VA.

Escudero, M. A., Cespedes, M. V., and Vilanova, E. (1997). Chromatographic discrimination of soluble neuropathy target esterase isoenzymes and related phenyl valerate esterases from chicken brain, spinal cord, and sciatic nerve. *J. Neurochem.* **68**, 2170–2176.

Funk, K. A., Henderson, J. D., Liu, C. H., Higgins, R. J., and Wilson, B. W. (1994a). Neuropathology of organophosphate-induced delayed neuropathy (OPIDN) in young chicks. *Arch. Toxicol.* **68**, 308–316.

Funk, K. A., Liu, C. H., Higgins, R. J., and Wilson, B. W. (1994b). Avian embryonic brain reaggregate culture system. II. NTE activity discriminates between effects of a single neuropathic or nonneuropathic organophosphorus compound exposure. *Toxicol. Appl. Pharmacol.* **124**, 159–163.

Funk, K. A., Liu, C. H., Wilson, B. W., and Higgins, R. J. (1994c). Avian embryonic brain reaggregate culture system. I. Characterization for organophosphorus compound toxicity studies. *Toxicol. Appl. Pharmacol.* **124**, 149–158.

Gallo, M. A., and Lawryk, N. J. (1991). Organic phosphorus pesticides. *In* "Handbook of Pesticide Toxicology" (W. J. Hayes and E. R. J. Laws, eds.), Vol. 2, pp. 917–1123. Academic Press, San Diego.

Gardiman, G., Moretto, A., and Lotti, M. (1999). Influence of dithiocarbamates on the development of organophosphate induced delayed polyneuropathy (OPIDP). *Toxicol. Sci.* **48S**, 100.

Glazer, E. J., Baker, T., and Riker, W. F., Jr. (1978). The neuropathology of DFP at cat soleus neuromuscular junction. *J. Neurocytol.* **7**, 741–758.

Glynn, P., Hotton, J. L., Nolan, C. C., Read, D. J., Brown, L., Hubbard, A., and Cavanagh, J. B. (1998). Neuropathy target esterase: Immunolocalization to neuronal cell bodies and axons. *Neuroscience* **83**, 295–302.

Glynn, P., Read, D. J., Quo, R., Wylie, S., and Johnson, M. K. (1994). Synthesis and characterization of a biotinylated organophosphorus ester for detection and affinity purification of a brain serine esterase: Neuropathy target esterase. *Biochem. J.* **301**, 551–556.

Glynn, P., Read, D. J., Lush, M. J., Li, Y., and Atkins, J. (1999). Molecular cloning of neuropathy target esterase (NTE). *Chem.-Biol. Interac.* **119–120**, 513–518.

Glynn, P., Ruffer-Tumer, M., Read, D., Wylie, S., and Johnson, M. K. (1993). Molecular characterisation of neuropathy target esterase: Proteolysis of the [^{3}H]DFP-labelled polypeptide. *Chem.-Biol. Interact.* **87**, 361–367.

Goldstein, D. A., McGuigan, M. A., and Ripley, B. D. (1988). Acute tricresylphosphate intoxication in childhood. *Hum. Toxicol.* **7**, 179–182.

Gupta, R. P., and Abou-Donia, M. B. (1993). Comparison of Ca^{2+}/calmodulin-dependent protein kinase II purified from control and diisopropyl phosphorofluoridate (DFP)-treated hens. *Neurochem. Res.* **18**, 259–269.

Gupta, R. P., and Abou-Donia, M. B. (1994). *In vivo* and *in vitro* effects of diisopropyl phosphorofluoridate (DFP) on the rate of hen brain tubulin polymerization. *Neurochem. Res.* **19**, 435–444.

Gupta, R. P., and Abou-Donia, M. B. (1995a). Diisopropyl phosphorofluoridate (DFP) treatment alters calcium-activated proteinase activity and cytoskeletal proteins of the hen sciatic nerve. *Brain Res.* **677**, 162–166.

Gupta, R. P., and Abou-Donia, M. B. (1995b). Neurofilament phosphorylation and [^{125}I]calmodulin binding by Ca^{2+}/calmodulin-dependent protein kinase in the brain subcellular fractions of diisopropyl phosphorofluoridate (DFP)-treated hen. *Neurochem. Res.* **20**, 1095–1105.

Gupta, R. P., Abdel-Rahman, A., Wilmarth, K. W., and Abou-Donia, M. B. (1997). Alteration in neurofilament axonal transport in the sciatic nerve of the diisopropyl phosphorofluoridate (DFP)-treated hen. *Biochem. Pharmacol.* **53**, 1799–1806.

Gupta, R. P., Lapadula, D. M., and Abou-Donia, M. B. (1992). Ca^{2+}/calmodulin-dependent protein kinase II from hen brain: Purification and characterization. *Biochem. Pharmacol.* **43**, 1975–1988.

Haley, R. W., and Kurt, T. L. (1997). Self-reported exposure to neurotoxic chemical combinations in the Gulf War. *J. Am. Med. Assoc.* **277**, 231–237.

Haley, R. W., Horn, J., Roland, P. S., Bryan, W. W., Van Ness, P. C., Bonte, F. J., Devous, M. D., Mathews, D., Fleckenstein, J. L., Wians, F. H., Wolfe, G. I., and Kurt, T. L. (1997). Evaluation of neurologic function in Gulf War veterans. *J. Am. Med. Assoc.* **277**, 223–230.

Harp, P., Tanaka, D., Jr., and Pope, C. N. (1997). Potentiation of organophosphorus-induced delayed neurotoxicity following phenyl saligenin phosphate exposures in 2-, 5-, and 8-week-old chickens. *Fundam. Appl. Toxicol.* **37**, 64–70.

Hierons, R., and Johnson, M. K. (1978). Clinical and toxicological investigations of a case of delayed neuropathy in man after acute poisoning by an organophosphorus pesticide. *Arch. Toxicol.* **40**, 279–284.

Hollingshaus, J. G. (1983). Chemistry and metabolism of delayed neurotoxic organophosphorus esters. *In* "14th Conference on Environmental Toxicology," pp. 76–105. National Technical Information Service, Springfield, VA.

Illis, L., Pantangia, G. N., and Cavanagh, J. B. (1966). Boutons terminaux and tri-*ortho*-cresyl phosphate neurotoxicity. *Exp. Neural.* **14**, 160–174.

Inui, K., Mitsumori, K., Harada, T., and Maita, K. (1993). Quantitative analysis of a neuronal damage induced by tri-*ortho*-cresyl phosphate in Wistar rats. *Fundam. Appl. Toxicol.* **20**, 111–119.

Ishakawa, Y., Chow, E., McNamee, M. G., McChesney, M., and Wilson, B. W. (1983). Separation of paraoxon and mipafox sensitive esterases by sucrose density gradient sedimentation. *Toxicol. Lett.* **17**, 315–320.

Itoh, H., Kishida, H., Tadokoro, M., and Oikawa, K. (1984). Studies on the delayed neurotoxicity of organophosphorus compounds. II. *J. Toxicol. Sci.* **9**, 37–50.

Itoh, H., Kishida, H., Takeuchi, E., Tadokoro, M., Uchikoshi, T., and Oikawa, K. (1985). Studies on the delayed neurotoxicity of organophosphorus compounds. III. *J. Toxicol. Sci.* **10**, 67–82.

Jensen, K. F., Lapadula, D. M., Anderson, J. K., Haykal-Coates, N., and Abou-Donia, M. B. (1992). Anomalous phosphorylated neurofilament aggregations in central and peripheral axons of hens treated with tri-*ortho*-cresyl phosphate (TOCP). *J. Neurosci. Res.* **33**, 455–460.

Johnson, M. K. (1975a). The delayed neuropathy caused by some organophosphorus esters: Mechanism and challenge. *Crit. Rev. Toxicol.* **3**, 289–316.

Johnson, M. K. (1975b). Structure–activity relationships for substrates and inhibitors of hen brain neurotoxic esterase. *Biochem. Pharmacol.* **24**, 797–805.

Johnson, M. K. (1980). Irreversible phosphorylation of brain neurotoxic esterase: The primary event leading to the delayed neuropathy caused by some organophosphorus esters. *Mon. Neural Sci.* **7**, 99–105.

Johnson, M. K. (1982). The target for initiation of delayed neurotoxicity by organophosphorus esters: Biochemical studies and toxicological application. *In* "Reviews in Biochemical Toxicology" (E. Hodgson, J. R. Bond, and R. M. Philpot, eds.), Vol. 4, pp. 141–212. Elsevier Biomedical, New York.

Johnson, M. K. (1992). Molecular events in delayed neuropathy: Experimental aspects of neuropathy target esterase. *In* "Clinical and Experimental Toxicology of Organophosphates and Carbamates" (B. Ballantyne and T. C. Marrs, eds.), pp. 90–113. Butterworth–Heinemann, Oxford.

Johnson, M. K. (1993). Symposium introduction: Retrospect and prospects for neuropathy target esterase (NTE) and the delayed polyneuropathy (OPIDP) induced by some organophosphorus esters. *Chem.-Biol. Interact.* **87**, 339–346.

Johnson, M. K., and Glynn, P. (1995). Neuropathy target esterase (NTE) and organophosphorus-induced delayed polyneuropathy (OPIDP): Recent advances. *Toxicol. Lett.* **82–83**, 459–463.

Johnson, M. K., and Read, D. J. (1987). The influence of chirality on the delayed neuropathic potential of some organophosphorus esters: Neuropathic and prophylactic effects of stereoisomeric esters of ethyl phenylphosphonic acid (EPN oxon and EPN) correlate with quantities of aged and unaged neuropathy target esterase *in vivo*. *Toxicol. Appl. Pharmacol.* **90**, 103–115.

Johnson, M. K., and Read, D. J. (1993). Prophylaxis against and promotion of organophosphate-induced delayed neuropathy by phenyl di-*n*-pentylphosphinate. *Chem.-Biol. Interact.* **87**, 449–455.

Johnson, M. K., and Safi, J. M. (1993). The R-(+)isomer of *O-n*-hexyl *S*-methyl phosphorothioamidate causes delayed neuropathy in hens after generation of a form of inhibited neuropathy target esterase (NTE) which can be reactivated *ex vivo*. *Chem.-Biol. Interact.* **87**, 443–448.

Johnson, M. K., Vilanova, E., and Read, D. J. (1991). Anomalous biochemical responses in tests of the delayed neuropathic potential of methamidophos (*O,S*-dimethyl phosphorothioamidate), its resolved isomers and of some higher *O*-alkyl homologues. *Arch. Toxicol.* **65**, 618–624.

Jortner, B. S. (1984). Pathology of organophosphorus-induced delayed neurotoxicity. *In* "14th Conference on Environmental Toxicology," pp. 106–117. National Technical Information Service, Springfield, VA.

Jortner, B. S. (1988). Organophosphorus ester–induced delayed neuropathy, rat. *In* "Monographs on Pathology of Laboratory Animals—Nervous System" (T. C. Jones, U. Mohr, and R. D. Hunt, eds.), pp. 41–47. Springer-Verlag, New York.

Jortner, B. S., and Ehrich, M. (1987). Neuropathological effects of phenyl saligenin phosphate in chickens. *NeuroToxicology* **8**, 303–314.

Jortner, B. S., Perkins, S. K., and Ehrich, M. (1999). Immunohistochemical study of phosphorylated neurofilaments during the evolution of organophosphorus ester-induced delayed neuropathy (OPIDN). *NeuroToxicology* **20**, 971–976.

Jortner, B. S., Pope, A. M., and Heavner, J. E. (1983). Haloxon-induced delayed neurotoxicity: Effect of plasma A (aryl) esterase activity on severity of lesions in sheep. *NeuroToxicology* **4**, 241–246.

Jortner, B. S., Shell, L., El-Fawal, H., and Ehrich, M. (1989). Myelinated nerve fiber regeneration following organophosphorus ester–induced delayed neuropathy. *NeuroToxicology* **10**, 717–726.

Kidd, J. G., and Langworthy, O. R. (1933). Jake paralysis: Paralysis following the ingestion of Jamaica ginger extract adulterated with tri-*ortho*-cresyl phosphate. *Bull. Johns Hopkins Hosp.* **52**, 39–65.

Knoth-Anderson, J., and Abou-Donia, M. B. (1993). Differential effects of triphenylphosphite and diisopropyl phosphorofluoridate on catecholamine secretion from bovine adrenomedullary chromaffin cells. *J. Toxicol. Environ. Health* **38**, 103–114.

Knoth-Anderson, J., Veronesi, B., Jones, K., Lapadula, D. M., and Abou-Donia, M. B. (1992). Triphenyl phosphite–induced ultrastructural changes in bovine adrenomedullary chromaffin cells. *Toxicol. Appl. Pharmacol.* **112**, 110–119.

Krinke, G., Ullmann, L., Sachsee, K., and Hess, R. (1979). Differential susceptibility of peripheral nerves of the hen to tri-*ortho*-cresyl phosphate and to trauma. *Agents Actions* **9**, 227–231.

Lapadula, D. M., Kinnes, C. G., Somjen, G. G., and Abou-Donia, M. B. (1982). Monosynaptic reflex depression in cats with organophosphorus neuropathy: Effects of tri-*O*-cresyl phosphate. *NeuroToxicology* **3**, 51–61.

Lapadula, D. M., Patton, S. E., Campbell, G. A., and Abou-Donia, M. B. (1985). Characterization of delayed neurotoxicity in the mouse following chronic oral administration of tri-*o*-cresyl phosphate. *Toxicol. Appl. Pharmacol.* **79**, 83–90.

Lapadula, E. S., Lapadula, D. M., and Abou-Donia, M. B. (1991). Persistent alterations of calmodulin kinase II activity in chickens after an oral dose of tri-*o*-cresyl phosphate. *Biochem. Pharmacol.* **42**, 171–180.

Lapadula, E. S., Lapadula, D. M., and Abou-Donia, M. B. (1992). Biochemical changes in sciatic nerve of hens treated with tri-*o*-cresyl phosphate: Increased phosphorylation of cytoskeletal proteins. *Neurochem. Int.* **20**, 247–255.

Larsen, C., Jortner, B. S., and Ehrich, M. (1986). Effect of neurotoxic organophosphorus compounds in turkeys. *J. Toxicol. Environ. Health* **17**, 365–374.

Lehning, E. J., Tanaka, D., Jr., and Bursian, S. J. (1996). Triphenyl phosphite and diisopropylphosphorofluoridate produce separate and distinct axonal degeneration patterns in the central nervous system of the rat. *Fundam. Appl. Toxicol.* **29**, 110–118.

LeVay, S., Meier, C., and Glees, P. (1971). Effects of tri-*ortho*-cresyl-phosphate on spinal ganglia and nerves of chickens. *Acta Neuropathol.* **17**, 103–113.

Li, W., and Casida, J. E. (1997). Actions of two highly potent organophosphorus neuropathy target esterase inhibitors in mammalian cell lines. *Toxicol. Lett.* **92**, 123–130.

Lidsky, T. I., Manetto, C., and Ehrich, M. (1990). Nerve conduction studies in chickens given phenyl saligenin phosphate and corticosterone. *J. Toxicol. Environ. Health* **29**, 65–75.

Lotti, M. (1992). The pathogenesis of organophosphate polyneuropathy. *Crit. Rev. Toxicol.* **21**, 465–488.

Lotti, M. (1995). A key step forward in understanding the pathogenesis of organophosphate polyneuropathy. *Hum. Exp. Toxicol.* **14**, 69–70.

Lotti, M. (1997). The concept and target of promotion of axonopathies. *Arch. Toxicol. Suppl.* **19**, 331–336.

Lotti, M., and Moretto, A. (1993). The search for the physiological functions of NTE: Is NTE a receptor? *Chem.-Biol. Interact.* **87**, 407–416.

Lotti, M., and Moretto, A. (1999). Promotion of organophosphate induced polyneuropathy by certain esterase inhibitors. *Chem.-Biol. Interact.* **119–120**, 513–518.

Lotti, M., Caroldi, S., Capodicasa, E., and Moretto, A. (1991). Promotion of organophosphate-induced delayed polyneuropathy by phenylmethanesulfonyl fluoride. *Toxicol. Appl. Pharmacol.* **108**, 234–241.

Lotti, M., Caroldi, S., Moretto, A., Johnson, M. K., Fish, C. J., Gopinath, C., and Roberts, N. L. (1987). Central–peripheral delayed neuropathy caused by diisopropyl phosphorofluoridate (DFP): Segregation of peripheral nerve and spinal cord effects using biochemical, clinical, and morphological criteria. *Toxicol. Appl. Pharmacol.* **88**, 87–96.

Lotti, M., Moretto, A., Bertolazzi, M., Peraica, M., and Fioroni, F. (1995). Organophosphate polyneuropathy and neuropathy target esterase: Studies with methamidophos and its resolved optical isomers. *Arch. Toxicol.* **69**, 330–336.

Lotti, M., Moretto, A, Capodicasa, E., Bertolazzi, M., Peraica, M., and Scapellato, M. L. (1993). Interactions between neuropathy target esterase and its inhibitors and the development of polyneuropathy. *Toxicol. Appl. Pharmacol.* **122**, 165–171.

Lotti, M., Moretto, A., Zoppellari, R., Dainese, R., Rizzuto, N., and Barusco, G. (1986). Inhibition of lymphocytic neuropathy target esterase predicts the development of organophosphate-induced delayed polyneuropathy. *Arch. Toxicol.* **59**, 176–179.

Lush, M. J., Li, Y., Read, D. J., Willis, A. C., and Glynn, P. (1998). Neuropathy target esterase and a homologous *Drosophila* neurodegeneration-associated mutant protein contain a novel domain conserved from bacteria to man. *Biochem. J.* **332**, 1–4.

Mackay, C. E., Hammock, B. D., and Wilson, B. W. (1996). Identification and isolation of a 155-kDa protein with neuropathy target esterase activity. *Fundam. Appl. Toxicol.* **30**, 23–30.

Maroni, M., and Bleecker, M. L. (1986). Neuropathy target esterase in human lymphocytes and platelets. *J. Appl. Toxicol.* **6**, 1–7.

Massicotte, C., Dyer Inzana, K., Ehrich, M., and Jortner, B. S. (1999). Neuropathologic effects of phenylmethylsulfonyl fluoride (PMSF)–induced promotion and protection in organophosphorus ester–induced delayed neuropathy (OPIDN) in hens. *NeuroToxicology*, **20**, 749–760.

McCain, W. C., Flaherty, D. M., Correll, L., Jortner, B., and Ehrich, M. (1996). Catecholamine concentrations and contractile responses of isolated vessels from hens treated with cyclic phenyl saligenin phosphate or paraoxon in the presence or absence of verapamil. *J. Toxicol. Environ. Health* **48**, 397–411.

McCain, W. C., Wilcke, J., Lee, J. C., and Ehrich, M. (1995). Effect of cyclic phenyl saligenin phosphate and paraoxon treatment on vascular response to adrenergic and cholinergic agents in hens. *J. Toxicol. Environ. Health* **44**, 167–187.

Metcalf, R. L. (1984). Historical perspective of organophosphorus ester–induced delayed neurotoxicity. *In* "Delayed Neurotoxicity" (J. M. Cranmer and E. J. Hixson, eds.), pp. 7–22. Intox Press, Little Rock, AR.

Milatovic, D., and Johnson, M. K. (1993). Reactivation of phosphorodiami-dated acetylcholinesterase and neuropathy target esterase by treatment of inhibited enzyme with potassium fluoride. *Chem.-Biol. Interact.* **87**, 425–430.

Milatovic, D., Moretto, A., Osman, K. A., and Lotti, M. (1997). Phenyl valer-ate esterases other than neuropathy target esterase and the promotion of organophosphate polyneuropathy. *Chem. Res. Toxicol.* **10**, 1045–1048.

Morazina, R., and Rosenberg, P. (1970). Lipid changes in tri-*o*-cresyl phosphate–induced neuropathy. *Toxicol. Appl. Pharmacol.* **16**, 461–471.

Moretto, A., Bertolazzi, M., Capodicasa, E., Peraica, M., Richardson, R. J., Scapellato, M. L., and Lotti, M. (1992a). Phenylmethanesulfonyl fluoride elicits and intensifies the clinical expression of neuropathic insults. *Arch. Toxicol.* **66**, 67–72.

Moretto, A., Bertolazzi, M., and Lotti, M. (1994). The phosphorothioic acid *O*-(2-chloro-2,3,3-trifluorocyclobutyl) *O*-ethyl *S*-propyl ester exacerbates organophosphate polyneuropathy without inhibition of neuropathy target esterase. *Toxicol. Appl. Pharmacol.* **129**, 133–137.

Moretto, A., Capodicasa, E., and Lotti, M. (1992b). Clinical expression of organophosphate-induced delayed polyneuropathy in rats. *Toxicol. Lett.* **63**, 97–102; Erratum (1992). *Toxicol. Lett.* **63**, 355.

Moretto, A., Capodicasa, E., Peraica, M., and Lotti, M. (1991). Age sensitiv-ity to organophosphate-induced delayed polyneuropathy: Biochemical and toxicological studies in developing chicks. *Biochem. Pharmacol.* **41**, 1497–1504.

Moretto, A., Lotti, M., Sabri, M. I., and Spencer, P. S. (1987). Progressive deficit of retrograde axonal transport is associated with the pathogenesis of di-*n*-butyl dichlorvos axonopathy. *J. Neurochem.* **49**, 1515–1522.

Moretto, A., Lotti, M., and Spencer, P. S. (1989). *In vivo* and *in vitro* regional differential sensitivity of neuropathy target esterase to di-*n*-butyl-2,2-dichlorovinyl phosphate. *Arch. Toxicol.* **63**, 469–473.

National Institutes of Health (NIH) (1994). "The Persian Gulf Experience and Health." National Institutes of Health, Bethesda, MD.

Nostrandt, A. C., and Ehrich, M. (1992). Development of a model cell culture system in which to study early effects of neuropathy-inducing organophos-phorus esters. *Toxicol. Lett.* **60**, 107–114.

Nostrandt, A. C., and Ehrich, M. (1993). Modification of mipafox-induced inhi-bition of neuropathy target esterase in neuroblastoma cells of human origin. *Toxicol. Appl. Pharmacol.* **121**, 36–42.

Osman, K. A., Moretto, A., and Lotti, M. (1996). Sulfonyl fluorides and the pro-motion of diisopropyl fluorophosphate neuropathy. *Fundam. Appl. Toxicol.* **33**, 294–297.

Osterloh, J., Lotti, M., and Pond, S. M. (1983). Toxicologic studies in a fatal overdose of 2,4-D, MCPP, and chlorpyrifos. *J. Anal. Toxicol.* **7**, 125–129.

Padilla, S., and Veronesi, B. (1985). The relationship between neurological damage and neurotoxic esterase inhibition in rats acutely exposed to tri-*ortho*-tolyl phosphate. *Toxicol. Appl. Pharmacol.* **78**, 78–87.

Padilla, S., and Veronesi, B. (1988). Biochemical and morphological valida-tion of a rodent model of organophosphorus-induced delayed neuropathy. *Toxicol. Ind. Health* **4**, 331–337.

Patton, S. E., Lapadula, D. M., and Abou-Donia, M. B. (1986). Relationship of tri-*o*-cresyl phosphate–induced delayed neurotoxicity to enhancement of *in vitro* phosphorylation of hen brain and spinal cord proteins. *J. Pharmacol. Exp. Ther.* **239**, 597–605.

Patton, S. E., Lapadula, D. M., O'Callaghan, J. P., Miller, D. B., and Abou-Donia, M. B. (1985). Changes in *in vitro* brain and spinal cord protein phosphorylation after a single oral administration of tri-*o*-cresyl phosphate to hens. *J. Neurochem.* **45**, 1567–1577.

Patton, S. E., O'Callaghan, J. P., Miller, D. B., and Abou-Donia, M. B. (1983). Effect of oral administration of tri-*o*-cresyl phosphate on *in vitro* phosphorylation of membrane and cytosolic proteins from chicken brain. *J. Neurochem.* **41**, 897–901.

Peraica, M., Capodicasa, E., Moretto, A., and Lotti, M. (1993). Organophos-phate polyneuropathy in chicks. *Biochem. Pharmacol.* **45**, 131–135.

Peraica, M., Moretto, A., and Lotti, M. (1995). Selective promotion by phenylmethanesulfonyl fluoride of peripheral and spinal cord neuropathies initiated by diisopropyl phosphorofluoridate in the hen. *Toxicol. Lett.* **80**, 115–121.

Perdrizet, J. A., Cummings, J. E., and Lahunta, A. (1985). Presumptive organophosphate-induced delayed neurotoxicity in a paralyzed bull. *Cor-nell Veterinarian* **75**, 401–410.

Perkins, S. K., Ehrich, M., and Jortner, B. S. (1995). Morphological and im-munocytochemical study of phosphorylated neurofilaments during the evo-lution of organophosphorus ester–induced delayed neuropathy (OPIDN). *Toxicologist* **15**, 209.

Pope, C., diLorenzo, K., and Ehrich, M. (1995). Possible involvement of a neurotrophic factor during the early stages of organophosphate-induced de-layed neurotoxicity. *Toxicol. Lett.* **75**, 111–117.

Pope, C. N., and Padilla, S. (1989a). Modulation of neurotoxic esterase activity *in vitro* by phospholipids. *Toxicol. Appl. Pharmacol.* **97**, 272–278.

Pope, C. N., and Padilla, S. S. (1989b). Chromatographic characterization of neurotoxic esterase. *Biochem. Pharmacol.* **38**, 181–188.

Pope, C. N., and Padilla, S. (1990). Potentiation of organophosphorus-induced delayed neurotoxicity by phenylmethylsulfonyl fluoride. *J. Toxicot. Envi-ron. Health* **31**, 261–273.

Pope, C. N., Chapman, M. L., Tanaka, D., and Padilla, S. (1992). Phenylmethyl-sulfonyl fluoride alters sensitivity to organophosphorus-induced delayed neurotoxicity in developing animals. *NeuroToxicology* **13**, 355–364.

Pope, C. N., Tanaka, D., and Padilla, S. (1993). The role of neurotoxic esterase (NTE) in the prevention and potentiation of organophosphorus-induced de-layed neurotoxicity (OPIDN). *Chem.-Biol. Interact.* **87**, 395–406.

President's Advisory Council on Gulf War Veterans (1996). "Final Report." U.S. Gov. Printing Office, Washington, DC.

Prineas, J. (1969). The pathogenesis of dying-back polyneuropathies. I. An ul-trastructural study of experimental tri-*ortho*-cresyl phosphate intoxication in the cat. *J. Neuropathol. Exp. Neurol.* **28**, 571–597.

Randall, J. C., Yano, B. L., and Richardson, R. J. (1997). Potentiation of organophosphorus compound–induced delayed neurotoxicity (OPIDN) in the central and peripheral nervous system of the adult hen: Distribution of axonal lesions. *J. Toxicot. Environ. Health* **51**, 571–590.

Richardson, R. J. (1992). Interactions of organophosphorus compounds with neurotoxic esterase. *In* "Organophosphates: Chemistry, Fate, and Effects" (J. E. Chambers and P. E. Levi, eds.), pp. 299–323. Academic Press, San Diego.

Richardson, R. J. (1995). Assessment of the neurotoxic potential of chlorpyri-fos relative to other organophosphorus compounds: A critical review of the literature. *J. Toxicol. Environ. Health* **44**, 135–165.

Richardson, R. J., Moore, T. B., Kayyali, U. S., and Randall, J. C. (1993). Chlorpyrifos: Assessment of potential for delayed neurotoxicity by repeated dosing in adult hens with monitoring of brain acetylcholinesterase, brain and lymphocyte neurotoxic esterase, and plasma butyrylcholinesterase ac-tivities. *Fundam. Appl. Toxicol.* **21**, 89–96.

Roberts, D. V. (1977). A longitudinal electromyographical study of six men occupationally exposed to organophosphorus compounds. *Int. Arch. Occup. Environ. Health* **38**, 221–229.

Robertson, D. G., Mattson, A. M., Bestervelt, L. L., Richardson, R. J., and An-derson, R. J. (1988). Time course of electrophysiologic effects induced by di-*n*-butyl-2,2-dichlorovinyl phosphate (DBCVP) in the adult hen. *J. Toxi-col. Environ. Health* **23**, 283–294.

Robertson, D. G., Schwab, B. W., Sills, R. D., Richardson, R. J., and An-derson, R. J. (1987). Electrophysiologic changes following treatment with organophosphorus-induced delayed neuropathy-producing agents in the adult hen. *Toxicol. Appl. Pharmacol.* **87**, 420–429.

Ruffer-Tumer, M. E., Read, D. J., and Johnson, M. K. (1992). Purification of neuropathy target esterase from avian brain after prelabelling with [^{3}H]diisopropyl phosphorofluoridate. *J. Neurochem.* **58**, 135–141.

Sanders, D. E., Lahunta, D. E., Cummings, J. F., and Sanders, J. A. (1985). Pro-gressive paresis in sheep due to delayed neurotoxicity of triaryl phosphates. *Cornell Veterinarian* **75**, 493–504.

Schaeppi, U., Krinke, G., and Kobel, W. (1984). Prolonged exposure to tri-ethylphosphate induces sensory motor neuropathy in the dog. *Neurobehav. Toxicol. Teratol.* **6**, 39–50.

Schlaepfer, W. W. (1971). Experimental alterations of neurofilaments and neu-rotubules by calcium and other ions. *Exp. Cell Res.* **67**, 73–80.

Schlaepfer, W. W. (1987). Neurofilaments: Structure, metabolism and implications in disease. *J. Neuropathol. Exp. Neurol.* **46**, 117–129.

Schlaepfer, W. W., and Hasler, M. B. (1979). Characterization of the calcium-induced disruption of neurofilaments in rat peripheral nerve. *Brain Res.* **168**, 299–309.

Schlaepfer, W. W., and Zimmerman, U. P. (1984) Calcium activated protease and the regulation of the axonal cytoskeleton. *In* "Axonal Transport in Neuronal Growth and Regeneration" (J. S. Elam and P. Cancalon, eds.), pp. 261–273. Plenum, New York.

Schlimmer, B. P., and Parker, K. I. (1996). Adrenocorticotropic hormone; adrenocortical steroids and their synthetic analogs; inhibitors of the synthesis and actions of adrenocortical hormones. *In* "Goodman & Gilman's The Pharmacological Basis of Therapeutics" (J. G. Hardman, L. E. Limbird, P. B. Molinoff, R. W. Ruddon, and A. G. Gilman, eds.), 9th ed., pp. 1459–1485. McGraw–Hill, New York.

Schwab, B. W., and Richardson, R. J. (1986). Lymphocyte and brain neurotoxic esterase: Dose and time dependence of inhibition in the hen examined with three organophosphorus esters. *Toxicol. Appl. Pharmacol.* **83**, 1–9.

Schwab, B. W., Davis, C. S., Miller, P. H., and Richardson, R. J. (1985). Solubilization of hen brain neurotoxic esterase in dimethylsulfoxide. *Biochem. Biophys. Res. Commun.* **132**, 81–87.

Seifert, J., and Wilson, B. W. (1994). Solubilization of neuropathy target esterase and other phenyl valerate carboxylesterases from chicken embryonic brain by phospholipase A2. *Comp. Biochem. Physiol.* **108**, 337–341.

Shell, L., Jortner, B. S., and Ehrich, M. (1988). Assessment of organophosphorus-induced delayed neuropathy in chickens using needle electromyography. *J. Toxicol. Environ. Health* **25**, 21–33.

Sogorb, M. A., Bas, S., Gutierrez, L. M., Vilanova, E., and Viniegra, S. (1997). Bovine chromaffin cells as an *in vitro* model for the study of non-cholinergic toxic effects of organophosphorus compounds. *Arch. Toxicol. Suppl.* **19**, 347–355.

Sogorb, M. A., Vilanova, E., Quintanar, J. L., and Viniegra, S. (1996). Bovine chromaffin cells in culture show carboxylesterase activities sensitive to organophosphorus compounds. *Int. J. Biochem. Cell Biol.* **28**, 983–989.

Somkuti, S. G., Tilson, H. A., Brown, H. R., Campbell, G. A., Lapadula, D. M., and Abou-Donia, M. B. (1988). Lack of delayed neurotoxic effect after tri-o-cresyl phosphate treatment in male Fischer 344 rats: Biochemical, neurobehavioral, and neuropathological studies. *Fundam. Appl. Toxicol.* **10**, 199–205.

Sprague, G. L., Sandvik, L. L., Bickford, A. A., and Castles, T. R. (1980). Evaluation of a sensitive grading system for assessing acute and subchronic delayed neurotoxicity in hens. *Life Sci.* **27**, 2523–2528.

Stumpf, A. M., Tanaka, D. J., Aulerich, R. J., and Bursian, S. J. (1989). Delayed neurotoxic effects of tri-o-tolyl phosphate in the European ferret. *J. Toxicol. Environ. Health* **26**, 61–73.

Suwita, E., Lapadula, D. M., and Abou-Donia, M. B. (1986a). Calcium and calmodulin stimulated *in vitro* phosphorylation of rooster brain tubulin and MAP-2 following a single oral dose of tri-o-cresyl phosphate. *Brain Res.* 374, 199–203.

Suwita, E., Lapadula, D. M., and Abou-Donia, M. B. (1986b). Calcium and calmodulin-enhanced *in vitro* phosphorylation of hen brain cold-stable microtubules and spinal cord neurofilament triplet proteins after a single oral dose of tri-o-cresyl phosphate. *Proc. Natl. Acad. Sci. U.S.A.* **83**, 6174–6178.

Tanaka, D., Jr., Bursian, S. J., and Aulerich, R. J. (1994). Age-related effects of triphenyl phosphite–induced delayed neuropathy on central visual pathways in the European ferret (*Mustela putorius furo*). *Fundam. Appl. Toxicol.* **22**, 577–587.

Tanaka, D., Bursian, S. J., and Lehning, E. J. (1992). Neuropathological effects of triphenyl phosphite on the central nervous system of the hen. *Fundam. Appl. Toxicol.* **18**, 72–78.

Tanaka, D., Bursian, S. J., and Lehning, E. (1990a). Selective and terminal degeneration in the chicken brainstem and cerebellum following exposure to bi(1-methylethyl)phosphorofluoridate (DFP). *Brain Res.* **519**, 200–208.

Tanaka, D., Bursian, S. J., Lehning, E. J., and Aulerich, R. J. (1990b). Exposure to triphenyl phosphite results in widespread degeneration in the mammalian central nervous system. *Brain Res.* **531**, 294–298.

Tanaka, D. J., and Bursian, S. J. (1989). Degeneration patterns in the chicken central nervous system induced by ingestion of the organophosphorus delayed neurotoxin tri-*ortho*-tolyl phosphate: A silver impregnation study. *Brain Res.* **484**, 240–256.

Tanaka, D. J., Bursian, S. J., Lehning, E. J., and Auterich, R. J. (1991). Delayed neurotoxic effects of bis(1-methylethyl) phosphorofluoridate (DFP) in the European ferret: A possible mammalian model for organophosphorus-induced delayed neurotoxicity. *NeuroToxicology* **12**, 209–224.

Thomas, T. C., Ishakawa, Y., McNamee, M. G., and Wilson, B. W. (1989). Correlation of neuropathy target esterase activity with specific tritiated di-isopropyl phosphorofluoridate–labelled proteins. *Biochem. J.* **257**, 109–116.

Thomas, T. C., Szekacs, A., Hammock, B. D., Wilson, B. W., and McNamee, M. G. (1993). Affinity chromatography of neuropathy target esterase. *Chem.-Biol. Interact.* **87**, 347–360.

Thomas, T. C., Szekacs, A., Rojas, S., Hammock, B. D., Wilson, B. W., and McNamee, M. G. (1990). Characterization of neuropathy target esterase using trifluoromethyl ketones. *Biochem. Pharmacol.* **40**, 2587–2596.

Tormo, N., Gimeno, J. R., Sogorb, M. A., Diaz-Alejo, N., and Vilanova, E. (1993). Soluble and particulate organophosphorus neuropathy target esterase in brain and sciatic nerve of the hen, cat, rat, and chick. *J. Neurochem.* **61**, 2164–2168.

"USP DI" (2001). United States Pharmacopia, Micromedix, Englewood, CO.

Varghese, R. G., Bursian, S. J., Tobias, C., and Tanaka, D., Jr. (1995). Organophosphorus-induced delayed neurotoxicity: A comparative study of the effects of tri-*ortho*-tolyl phosphate and triphenyl phosphite on the central nervous system of the Japanese quail. *NeuroToxicology* **16**, 45–54.

Vasilescu, C., Alexianu, M., and Dan, A. (1984). Delayed neuropathy after organophosphorus insecticide (Diperterex) poisoning: A clinical, electrophysiological and nerve biopsy study. *J. Neurol. Neurosurg. Neuropsych.* **47**, 543–548.

Veronesi, B. (1984). Effect of metabolic inhibition with piperonyl butoxide on rodent sensitivity to tri-*ortho*-cresyl phosphate. *Exp. Neurol.* **85**, 651–660.

Veronesi, B. (1992). The use of cell culture for evaluating neurotoxicity. *In* "Neurotoxicology" (H. A Tilson and C. L. Mitchell, eds.), pp. 21–49. Raven Press, New York.

Veronesi, B., and Dvergsten, C. (1987). Triphenyl phosphite neuropathy differs from organophosphorus-induced delayed neuropathy in rats. *Neuropathol. Appl. Neurobiol.* **13**, 193–208.

Veronesi, B., and Ehrich, M. (1993). Using neuroblastoma cell lines to examine organophosphate neurotoxicity. *In Vitro Toxicol.*, **6**, 57–65.

Veronesi, B., Enrich, M., Blusztajn, J. K., Oortgiesen, M., and Durham, H. (1997). Cell culture models of interspecies selectivity to organophosphorous insecticides. *NeuroToxicology* **18**, 283–297.

Veronesi, B., Padilla, S., Blackmon, K., and Pope, C. (1991). Murine susceptibility to organophosphorus-induced delayed neuropathy (OPIDN). *Toxicol. Appl. Pharmacol.* **107**, 311–324.

Veronesi, B., Padilla, S., and Lyerly, D. (1986). The correlation between neurotoxic esterase inhibition and mipafox-induced damage in rats. *NeuroToxicology* **7**, 207–216.

Vilanova, E., Barril, J., and Carrera, V. (1993). Biochemical properties and possible toxicological significance of various forms of NTE. *Chem.-Biol. Interact.* **87**, 369–381.

Vilanova, E., Barril, J., Carrera, V., and Pellin, M. C. (1990). Soluble and particulate forms of the organophosphorus neuropathy target esterase in hen sciatic nerve. *J. Neurochem.* **55**, 1258–1265.

Williams, C. H., Johnson, H. J., and Casterline, J. L. (1966). Cholesterol content of spinal cord and sciatic nerve of hens after organophosphate and carbamate administration. *J. Neurochem.* **13**, 471–474.

Williams, D. G., and Johnson, M. K. (1981). Gel-electrophoretic identification of hen brain neurotoxic esterase, labelled with tritiated di-isopropyl phosphorofluoridate. *Biochem. J.* **199**, 323–333.

Wu, S. Y., and Casida, J. E. (1994). Neuropathy target esterase inhibitors: Enantiomeric separation and stereospecificity of 2-substituted-4H-1,3,2-benzodioxaphosphorin 2 oxides. *Chem. Res. Toxicol.* **7**, 77–81.

Wu, S. Y., and Casida, J. E. (1995). Ethyl octylphosphonofluoridate and analogs: Optimized inhibitors of neuropathy target esterase. *Chem. Res. Toxicol.* **8**, 1070–1075.

Yoshida, M., Tomizawa, M., Wu, S. Y., Quinstad, G. B., and Casida, J. E. (1995). Neuropathy target esterase of hen brain: Active site reactions with 2-[octyl-^{3}H]octyl-4H-,3,2-benzodioxaphosphorin 2 oxide and 2-octyl-4H-,3,2-[aryl-^{3}H]benzodioxaphosphorin 2 oxide. *J. Neurochem.* **64**, 1680–1687.

Yoshida, M., Wu, S. Y., and Casida, J. E. (1994). Reactivity and stereospecificity of neuropathy target esterase and α-chymotrypsin with 2-substituted-4H-1,3,2-benzodioxaphosphorin 2 oxides. *Toxicol. Lett.* **74**, 164–176.

Zech, R., and Chemnitius, J. M. (1987). Neurotoxicant sensitive esterase: Enzymology and pathophysiology of organophosphorus ester–induced delayed neuropathy. *Prog. Neurobiol.* **29**, 191–218.

CHAPTER

50

Understanding the Toxic Actions of Organophosphates

Kai Savolainen
Finnish Institute of Occupational Health

50.1 INTRODUCTION

Organophosphates (OP) are widely used as insecticides and thus exposure to these compounds still represents a genuine health risk. The overall mechanisms of action of organophosphate-induced neurotoxic effects are well known, but the underlying molecular mechanisms of toxic actions are surprisingly poorly known. However, the introduction of a number of OP pesticides and highly toxic OP nerve agents has emphasized the importance of understanding the mechanisms of toxicity of these OP compounds in detail. It is fundamental to appreciate that their toxicity stems largely from excess acetylcholine (ACh) due to the inhibition of acetylcholinesterase (AChE) and subsequent accumulation of ACh in the target tissues, especially those cells in the vicinity of cholinergic receptors that are responsible for mediating the effects of ACh. The dramatic effects seen in OP intoxication include brain activation, epileptiformic convulsions, muscular tremors, which lead ultimately to flaccid paralysis, increased sweating and salivation, profound bronchial secretion, bronchoconstriction, increased activity of the intestine and diarrhea, miosis, hypertension, lowered body temperature, and hyperglycemia. When the effects of OP compounds are compared, marked differences are evident between them. This is most likely due to the marked differences in their ability to bind with their prime target, AChE, and the differences in the rapidity of ACh accumulation in and close to the targets of ACh. The consequences of excess ACh are primarily mediated via cholinergic muscarinic and nicotinic receptor activation. Muscarinic receptors are found in the central nervous system (CNS), blood vessel walls, and endocrine and exocrine glands. Nicotinic receptors are located in autonomic nervous ganglia, in the CNS, in the adrenals, and in the neuromuscular junction, the area specialized for transmission of neuronal impulses to striated muscles. Muscarinic receptors are G-protein-coupled, slow reacting transmembrane proteins. After activation, their effects are mediated into the cells via formation of calcium-mobilizing phosphoinositide-derived second

messengers or inhibition of adenylate cyclase, leading to increased formation of cyclic adenosine monophosphate (cAMP).

Nicotinic receptors are ion channels. Their activation leads to increased influx of sodium into the cell. There are several subtypes of both receptors, and the mode of action of different muscarinic receptors and different nicotinic receptors may markedly differ from each other. In the CNS, there are more muscarinic than nicotine receptors, and muscarinic receptor activation in the brain, as in peripheral tissue, has profound effects on neuronal signalling, and can alter the numbers of many different receptors, as well as modify gene expression and the expression of proteins encoded by these genes.

Cholinergic muscarinic activation also dramatically facilitates brain metabolism and induces major electrophysiological effects, often associated with overt convulsions. The CNS effects of OPs can be modified by drugs, typically cholinergic antagonists such as atropine, but also with γ-aminobutyric acidergic (GABAergic) agonists such as benzodiazepines and antagonists of glutamatergic receptors. In fact, anticholinergics, like atropine, and diazepam, which belong to the benzodiazepine group of drugs, are the most effective antidotes against OP poisoning. In addition, interaction of cholinergic stimulation with lithium markedly amplifies cholinergic-induced neuronal signalling and convulsions, most likely due to an interaction at the G-protein level.

Nicotinic receptors have their most dramatic effects in autonomic ganglia and the neuromuscular endplates. These alterations are characterized by a decrease in membrane potential, membrane resistance, and a decrease in afterhyperpolarization. Many of these effects can, surprisingly, be inhibited by atropine, most likely due to an interaction of muscarinic and nicotinic receptors in autonomic ganglia. The most effective blockers of nicotinic receptors are d-tubocurarine and its more modern analogs. At the neuromuscular endplate, OPs induce (1) repetitive activity in response to single nerve stimulus and (2) decremental responses to repetitive nerve stimulation. OPs typically also induce accelerated spontaneous release of ACh, leading to increases in the miniature endplate potentials

(MEPP) frequency, but at high OP concentrations, the end result is depolarization of the neuromuscular endplate and endplate regions. The effects of OPs on neuromuscular endplates can be prevented with AChE reactivators such as pyradine-2-aldoxime methiodide (2-PAM) that can restore, in part, neuromuscular transmission. The cardiovascular and respiratory systems are particularly sensitive to the effects of OPs because both are under strict cholinergic control. A more detailed understanding of the effects of these toxic agents seems to be warranted because of their dramatic effects on the CNS. In particular, muscarinic receptor-mediated effects have been overlooked in the past. Recent observations also suggest that cholinergic stimulation of cholinergic muscarinic receptors might, in fact, be a trigger that activates many other neurotransmitter systems. For example, it is now becoming clear that cholinergic brain stimulation is the trigger that sets off the propagation of convulsive waves.

50.2 HISTORY AND BACKGROUND

Organophosphorous compounds were first synthetized in 1854, but their remarkable toxicity was not recognized until the 1930s (see Minton and Murray, 1988). The first synthesized OP pesticide, tetraethyl pyrophosphate (TEPP), was developed in Germany before World War II to replace the highly toxic and lipid-soluble botanical insecticide, nicotine. At the same time, the highly toxic nerve gas agents, tabun and sarin, also were developed, but they were not used during the war (Minton and Murray, 1988).

Anticholinesterase OP compounds have been widely used as insecticides because it was quickly appreciated that insects are highly susceptible to these agents, even though their toxicity to mammals also proved to be high (Minton and Murray, 1988). OPs represent a large group, many members of which cause toxicity by inhibiting the key enzyme, acetylcholinesterase. This enzyme promotes the hydrolysis of acetylcholine, the principal physiological cholinergic agonist of nicotinic and muscarinic receptors in the body. Thus, the toxicity of OP compounds in many respects can be considered to be ACh toxicity.

Due to the ubiquitous distribution of both nicotinic and muscarinic cholinergic receptors throughout the body, exposure to OP compounds has widespread toxic consequences in several target organs. The actions of OPs include neuronal excitation in the brain and subsequent epileptic convulsions, muscular tremors, increased sweating and salivation, increased bronchial secretion, bronchoconstriction, increased activity of the intestine and diarrhea, miosis of the eyes, blurred vision, tachycardia and hypertension, hyperglycemia, and lowered body temperature. For example, when adult baboons were exposed to soman, a highly toxic anticholinesterase OP nerve agent (for soman, see Churchill *et al.*, 1985), via an intravenous infusion, the animals had a very rapid onset of OP-type cholinergic signs of intoxication, including overt muscular fasciculations resembling epileptic convulsions, stridorous breathing, copious secretions, and atrioventricular arrhythmias (Anzueto *et al.*, 1986).

Table 50.1

Major Actions of Organophosphate Anticholinesterases at Various Sites in the Body

Receptor	Target organ	Symptoms and signs
Central	Central nervous system	Giddiness, anxiety, restlessness, headache, tremor, confusion, failure to concentrate, convulsions, respiratory depression
Muscarinic	Glands	
	Nasal mucosa	Rhinorrhea
	Bronchial mucosa	Bronchorrhea
	Sweat	Sweating
	Lachrymal	Lachrymation
	Salivary	Salivation
	Smooth muscle	
	Iris	Miosis
	Ciliary muscle	Failure of accommodation
	Gut	Abdominal cramps, diarrhea
	Bladder	Frequency, involuntary micturition
	Heart	Bradycardia
Nicotinic	Autonomic ganglia	Sympathetic effects: pallor, tachycardia, hypertension
	Skeletal muscle	Weakness, fasciculation

Source: Modified from Fuortes *et al.* (1993), and Marrs (1996).

OP-induced effects are mediated through the activation of nicotinic or muscarinic receptors. The distribution of these receptors varies in different parts of the body. Table 50.1 summarizes the most important toxic actions of OP compounds and classifies them according to the receptor type that is behind each toxic action. A number of recent reviews have summarized the key toxic actions of different OP compounds (Choi *et al.*, 1995; De Bleecker *et al.*, 1992; Ecobichon, 1996; Fuortes *et al.*, 1993; Gunderson *et al.*, 1992; Gutmann and Besser, 1990; Marrs, 1996; McDonough and Shih, 1997; Minton and Murray, 1988).

Intoxication with OPs can take place a number of ways. Previously, when less was known about their toxicity, careless use of OPs often lead to accidental acute poisonings, and even some deaths of workers using these agents. It was estimated in 1990 that the number of annual pesticide poisonings was about 3 million cases in the world and that the incidence was thus about 57 cases per potentially exposed 100,000 individuals. There were about 20,000 cases of pesticide-induced fatalities in the world, most due to excessive exposure to OP compounds. In industrialized countries, occupational exposure to OP compounds is, for the most part, well controlled and the number of poisonings is relatively small. However, in developing countries, in which the use of OP compounds is particularly widespread because of the hot climatic conditions, the number of deaths may be high. For example, pesticide poisonings are relatively common in countries such as Sri Lanka, Venezuela, Indonesia, South Africa, and Brazil (see Choi *et al.*, 1995).

Whereas OP compounds are usually highly lipid-soluble, they readily penetrate the skin, and exposure in the occupational environment takes place mainly through the skin. This is illustrated in Fig. 50.1 by the excellent correlation between alterations of the levels of mevinphos, a highly toxic OP insecticide, on the foliage in greenhouses, and the dermal contamination rate, as well as the decline in the acetylcholinesterase activity in red blood cells in the exposed workers as a function of time (Kangas *et al.*, 1993). In some cases, exposure via the lungs also may play a role, but it is usually of minor importance (Savolainen and Kangas, 1995). In some cases, inhalation can be relatively important as the route of the compound into the body. These situations are, however, unlikely to be associated with an exposure to OP that would have remarkable health consequences. A rare example could be the use of OP nerve agents when OP concentrations in the air are likely to be high. However, in occupational environments and in situations in which OP-induced effects are likely to take place, dermal exposure predominates (Kangas *et al.*, 1993; Savolainen and Kangas, 1995; Storm *et al.*, 2000). Exposure to OPs via food, in household use, and thorough oral routes is nonsignificant when suicidal cases are excluded.

Lethalities associated with OPs in the past contained a large number of suicides; for example, in the 1950s, parathion-containing formulations became popular for this purpose in several countries (Choi *et al.*, 1995; Hayes *et al.*, 1978; Jovanovic *et al.*, 1990), including Finland, until their availability was strictly restricted (Alha, 1967; Minton and Murray, 1988; Marrs, 1996). However, the most toxic OP compounds are the anticholinesterase OP nerve agents, which were created by defence industries of many countries. These include sarin (isopropyl methylphosphonofluoridate), soman (pinacolyl methylphosphonofluoridate), tabun (ethyl N−dimethylphosphoramidocyanidate), and VX (O-ethyl-S-[2(diisopropyl-amine)-ethyl)methyl-phosphonothionate) (see Abdallah *et al.*, 1992). Even though these compounds have been used rarely (e.g., the Iraqis against the Iranians and the Kurds, as well as in the well known attack by a terrorist group in a Tokyo underground station), their very existence carries a potential continuous threat (Gunderson *et al.*, 1992; Ecobichon, 1996). The extreme toxicity of many OP compounds highlights the need for a more complete understanding of their mechanisms of toxic actions. Even though the overall toxicity and the general mechanisms of toxic actions of OP compounds have been rather well clarified over the years and seem to be quite similar within the group, a more thorough understanding of the cascades of cellular and subcellular toxic events of these compounds in the nervous systems is needed for effective prevention and treatment of OP-induced poisonings. For this purpose, studies on mechanisms of OP nerve agents are important, because state-of-the-art studies on mechanisms of occupationally used OPs are, for the most part, lacking.

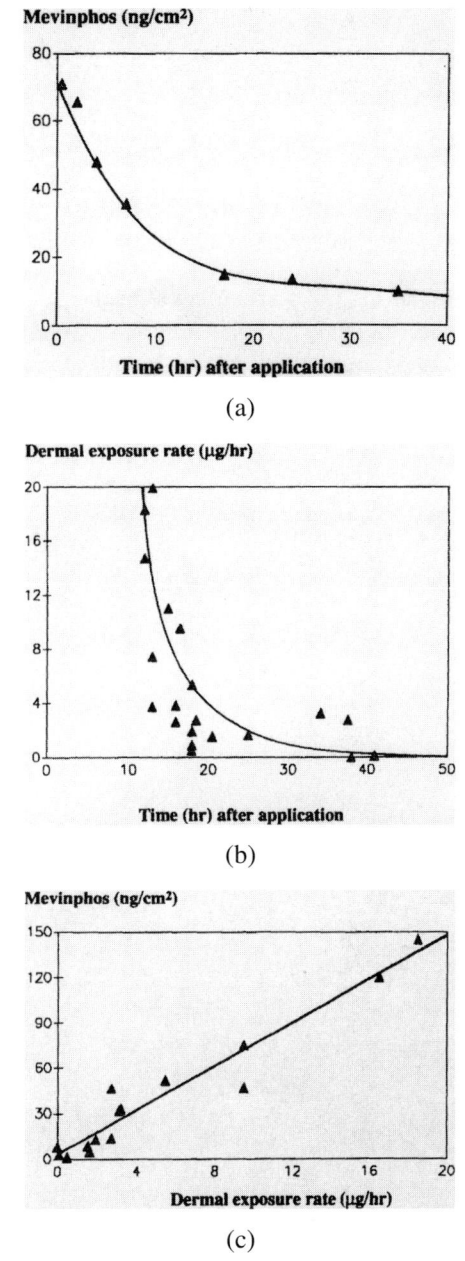

Figure 50.1 Dermal absorption is important in the absorption of organophosphates. Absorption of mevinphos into the body after exposure in greenhouses is used as an example in an occupational setting. (a) The decrease in the amount of mevinphos in foliar samples from flowers grown in greenhouses as a function of time. The equation of the curve is $y = -0.026 + 1.789$; $r = 0.96$. (b) The dermal exposure rate of workers exposed to mevinphos after the application of the compound to flowers grown in greenhouses. The equation of the curve is $y = 3352.7^{-2.4}$; $r = -0.67$. (c) The correlation ($y = 7.2 + 3.5$; $r = 0.97$) between the decrease of the amount of mevinphos on the foliage and the dermal exposure rate to mevinphos via the hands. These data provide evidence that in this situation the skin is the most important exposure route to mevinphos. Reprinted with permission from J. Kangas *et al.*, *Am. J. Ind. Hyg.* **54**(4), 150–157 (1993).

50.3 CHEMISTRY OF ORGANOPHOSPHORUS COMPOUNDS

Anticholinesterase OPs are derivatives of phosphonic or phosphoric acid or their sulfur-containing analogs, notably phosphorothioic, phosphonothionic, phosphorodithioic, or phosphonodithioic acids (see Fig. 50.2). Phosphonic acid or its derivatives does not generally inhibit AChE activity. OPs with AChE activity usually have two alkyl groups and a third group, the leaving group, that is often an aryl group or a heterocyclic group. However, in most of the OP warfare nerve agents, the leaving group contains fluorine (see Fig. 50.3; Holmstedt, 1963; Marrs, 1996; Minton and Murray, 1988; World Health Organization, 1986). The leaving group is more susceptible to hydrolysis than the alkyl groups. Typically, OPs with the P=S

configuration have little or no inhibitory action on AChE unless they have been activated through enzymatic or nonenzymatic oxidative desulfuration to the corresponding oxon that contains the P=O configuration. Such compounds are termed indirect inhibitors of AChE, and include many important insecticides such as malathion and parathion (Aldridge, 1996; Ecobichon, 1996; Hirvonen et al., 1993; Savolainen et al., 1991).

Holmstedt (1963) classified the OPs into four categories based on the structure of the leaving group. In category I, the leaving group contains a quaternary nitrogen. An example of the compounds in this group is the drug ecothiopate. Category II includes the warfare nerve agents soman and sarin, as well as diisopropyl phosphofluoridate (DFP) (see Churchill et al., 1987; Savolainen et al., 1988a, b), where the leaving group is fluorine. In category III, the leaving group is cyanide, cyanate, thio-

Type of OP	Structure	Example
Phosphates	RO—P(=O)—OR, OR	Monocrotophos, Chlorfenvinphos, Chlorpyrifos-methyl, Dichlorvos, Tri-o-cresyl phosphate
Phosphonates	RO—P(=O)—R, OR	Trichlorfon
Phosphinates	R—P(=O)—R, OR	Glufosinate[a]
Phosphorothioates (S=)	RO—P(=S)—OR, OR	Pirimiphos-methyl, Bromophos, Diazinon, Triazophos
Phosphonothioates (S=)	RO—P(=S)—R, OR	EPN, Leptophos
Phosphorothioates (S-substituted)	RS—P(=O)—OR, OR	Demeton-S-methyl, Ecothiopate
Phosphonothioates (S-substituted)	RS—P(=O)—R, OR	VX

(continued)

Figure 50.2 Organic derivatives of phosphoric acid.

cyanate, or a halogen other than fluorine. For example, the nerve agent tabun belongs to category III (see Holmstedt, 1963). The fourth group, category IV, is the most heterogeneous in terms of the structure of the leaving group, and contains a large number of pesticides. Derivatives of pyrophosphoric acid include compounds such as TEPP, sulfotep, monothiotep, schradan, and tetraisopropyl pyrophosphoramide (iso-OMPA) that is extensively used in laboratories as a specific inhibitor of butyrylcholinesterase (see Koelle, 1963; Savolainen *et al.*, 1984). These compounds do not, in fact, conveniently fit into the classification created by Holmstedt (1963). What they have in common is an ability to inhibit AChE activity (Marrs, 1996). Some of the other OPs that express some AChE activity do not have a clearly defined leaving group. For example, *S,S,S*-tributyl phosphorotrithioite (DEF) and phosphorotrithioite (merphos), where all three substituents are *S*-butyl moieties, and perhaps ethephon, an accelerator of fruit ripening and a mono(chloroalkyl)

derivative of phosphonic acid, all belong to this poorly defined group of OPs (Marrs, 1996).

In terms of OP chemistry and nonenzymatic degradation, it is important to keep in mind that most OPs are poorly water-soluble, have a high oil–water partition coefficient, and a low vapor pressure. Most of the OPs, with the exception of dichlorvos, are not particularly volatile, and all are degraded by hydrolysis, especially in alkalic conditions, yielding water-soluble products that are generally considered to be nontoxic. Knowledge of these general chemical properties of OPs has practical implications in decontamination of skin exposed to OP compounds because scrubbing the skin with (an alkali) soap causes rapid hydrolysis of the compound. Extensive reviews on the treatment and management of acute OP compound poisoning are available (see De Bleecker *et al.*, 1992; Ecobichon, 1996; Marrs, 1996; McDonough and Shih, 1997; Minton and Murray, 1988; World Health Organization, 1986).

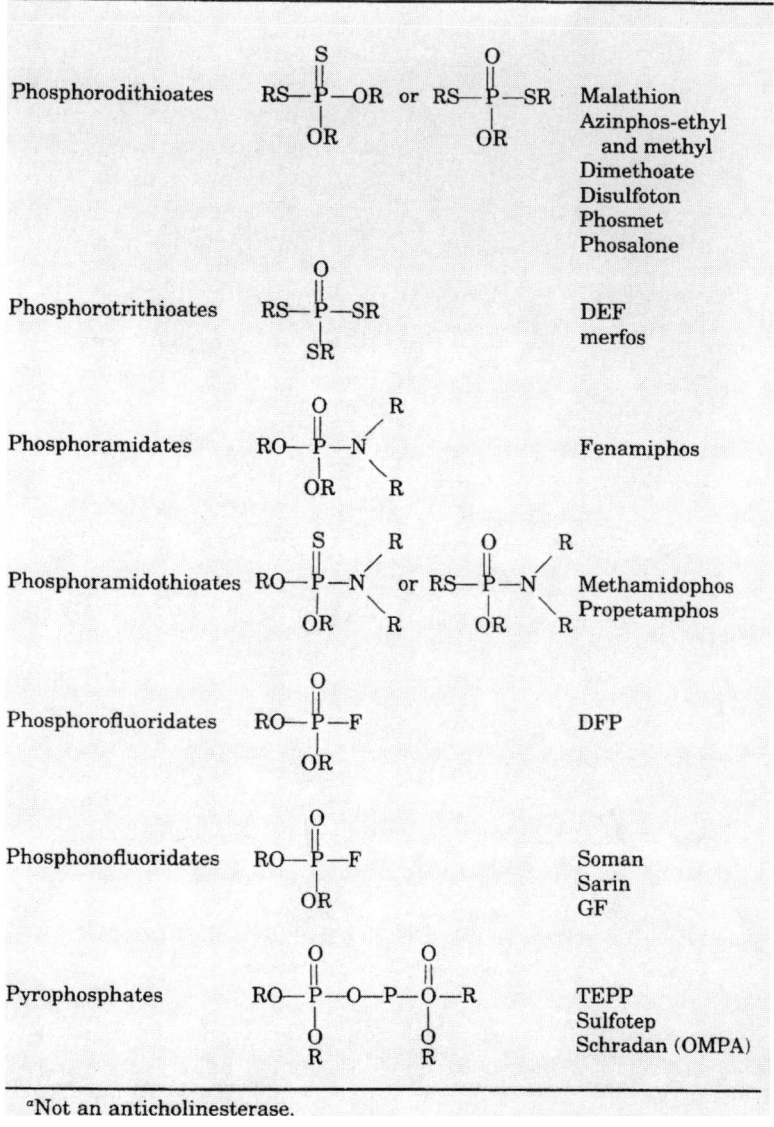

*Not an anticholinesterase.

Figure 50.2   (Continued).

Examples of the Four Main Categories of Organic Phosphorus Compounds

Group	X constituents	Example
I	substituted quaternary nitrogen	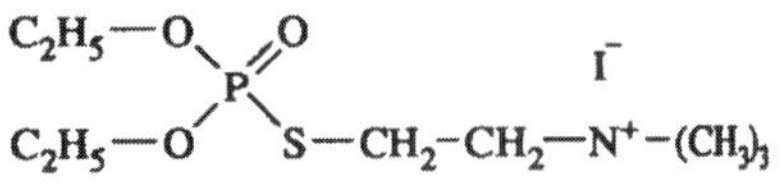 C_2H_5—O P O C_2H_5—O S—CH_2–CH_2—N^+–$(CH_3)_3$ I^- **Ecothiopate isodide**
II	F	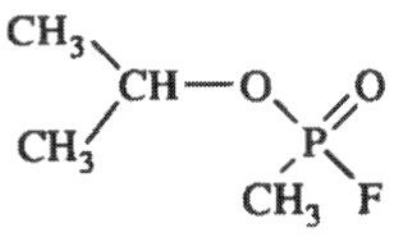 CH_3 CH—O P O CH_3 CH_3 F **Sarin** $(iC_3H_7O)_2 P(O)$—F **DFP**
III	CN, OCN, SCN, or halogen other than F	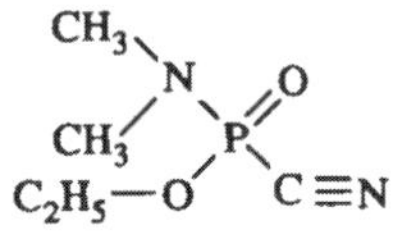 CH_3 N P O CH_3 C_2H_5—O C ≡ N **Tabun** C_2H_5—O S P C_2H_5—O O —NO_2 **Parathion**
IV	alkyl; alkoxy or alkylthio; aryl or heterocyclic; aryloxy, arylthio, or one of their heterocyclic analogs; nitrogen; or disubstituted phosphoryl groups	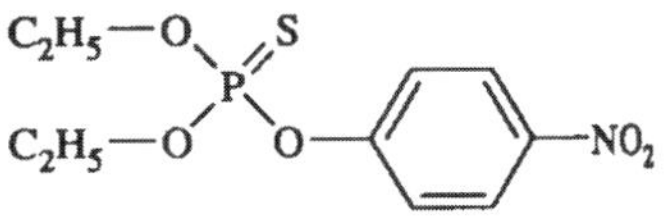 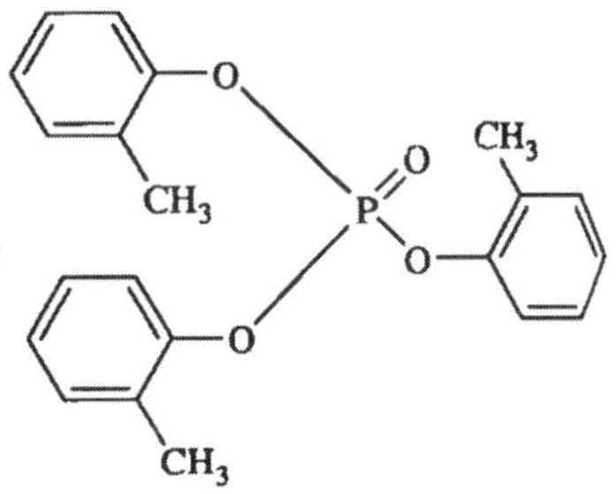 CH_3 O O CH_3 P O O CH_3 **Triorthocresyl phosphate**

Figure 50.3 Examples of the four main categories of organic phosphorous compounds according to Holmstedt (1963). Reprinted with permission from *Handbook of Pesticide Toxicology*, Vol. 2, p. 918, Academic Press, San Diego (1991).

50.4 ACETYLCHOLINE AND ACETYLCHOLINESTERASE, THE TARGET OF ANTICHOLINESTERASE ORGANOPHOSPHOROUS COMPOUNDS

ACh is one of the most important neurotransmitters in the human body. It can be considered an excitotoxic transmitter because when it is present in excess, it readily causes toxicity (Jope *et al.*, 1989; Lallement *et al.*, 1994a; McDonough and Shih, 1997; Meldrum and Garthwaite, 1990; Naarala *et al.*, 1997; Olney *et al.*, 1986; Savolainen *et al.*, 1991, 1998; Solberg and Belkin, 1997). The term excitotoxicity implies that a receptor agonist, usually a physiological neurotransmitter or

its analog, causes overt excitation of neuronal cells through receptor activation. This overt neuronal excitation then usually leads to elevated levels of intracellular calcium, activation of proteases and endonucleases, and ultimately cell death through apoptosis (programmed cell data) or necrosis (Meldrum and Garthwaite, 1990; Olney *et al.*, 1986; Savolainen *et al.*, 1998; Solberg and Belkin, 1997).

The toxicity induced by OP compounds is, in fact, the toxicity of excess free ACh in the target tissues because hydrolysis by ACh is by far the most important route for inactivation ACh accumulates (Ecobichon, 1996; McDonough and Shih, 1997; Savolainen *et al.*, 1995). In man, the neurotransmitter ACh is present in cholinergic nerves in the CNS, at the terminal nerve endings on all postganglionic parasympathetic nerves (where it activates muscarinic receptors), innervating salivary, lacrimal, and sweat glands, at neuromuscular junctions (activating nicotinic receptors), and in the autonomic nervous system, that is, sympathetic and parasympathetic ganglia (activating nicotinic receptors). The loss of activity of AChE due to the accumulation of ACh results in excessive nervous system stimulation that may rapidly lead to respiratory failure and death (Ecobichon, 1996; Marrs, 1996; Minton and Murray, 1988). The signs of OP-induced toxicity include those that result from stimulation of muscarinic receptors in the parasympathetic nervous system (increased secretions, bronchoconstriction, miosis, gastrointestinal cramps, diarrhea, urination, bradycardia) and those that result from the stimulation and subsequent blockade of nicotinic receptors. Nicotinic receptor stimulation excites receptors in the ganglia of the sympathetic and parasympathetic divisions of the autonomic nervous system, as well as the junctions between nerves and muscles (tachycardia, hypertension, muscle fasciculations, tremors, weakness, and/or flaccid paralysis). Furthermore, stimulation of cholinergic receptors in the CNS results in restlessness, emotional lability, ataxia, lethargy, mental confusion, loss of memory, generalized weakness, convulsions, cyanosis, and coma (see also Ecobichon, 1996).

50.4.1 ACETYLCHOLINE SYNTHESIS IS CATALYZED BY CHOLINE ACETYLTRANSFERASE

ACh synthesis is catalyzed by the enzyme, choline acetyltransferase (CAT). Synthesis is regulated by the availability of choline and acetyl coenzyme A (CoA) (Jope, 1979). Choline for ACh synthesis is supplied by active choline uptake into the cell, membrane phospholipid breakdown, and blood-derived lysophosphatidylcholine (see Pepeu, 1983). Choline is taken up by cholinergic neurons from the extracellular space by active high and low affinity uptake systems (Antonelli *et al.*, 1981). The supply of choline, which is directly proportional to the effectiveness of choline uptake into the cell, is rate limiting for *de novo* ACh synthesis. There is also evidence that some of the choline for acetylcholine synthesis can come from removal at the head group of the membrane phospholipid, phosphalidylcholine (Caulfield, 1993; Gutmann and Besser, 1990).

Normally, the concentration of choline in the plasma is about 10 μmol/l. Choline does not cross-diffuse through the blood–brain barrier and, therefore, it requires an active transport system to help it cross biological membranes. Cholinergic neurons have a membrane-bound, energy- and Na$^+$-dependent, active choline transport system. The K_m of the choline pump is 1–5 μmol/l (i.e., less than the concentration of choline in the extracellular space), and thus the availability of choline is not likely to be a limiting factor in the synthesis of ACh, even though it is possible that the rate of ACh, synthesis in the neurons is regulated by altering the transport capacity (V_{max}) of the choline pump.

50.4.2 CHOLINE UPTAKE IS A TARGET FOR THE EFFECTS OF ORGANOPHOSPHOROUS COMPOUNDS

Choline uptake by neuronal cells may also be a target for the effects of OP compounds. In synaptosomes obtained from rats injected with 120 μg/kg of sarin or soman subcutaneously (s.c.) and studied *ex vivo*, sodium-dependent, high-affinity choline uptake was transiently but markedly decreased in the cortex and the hippocampus, and increased in the striatum. Similar effects on high-affinity choline uptake by soman or sarin could not be demonstrated in rat synaptosomes *in vitro*. The authors concluded that the OP effect was not due to a direct action of these compounds on the uptake process nor did it depend on AChE inhibition (Whalley and Shih, 1989). Earlier, Harris *et al.* (1982) showed that inhibition of ACh synthesis with hemicholinium, a competitive inhibitor of carrier-mediated uptake of choline across the nerve endings, effectively inhibited soman-induced elevations in cerebral ACh levels and also protected against soman toxicity. These authors concluded that excess ACh is the primary cause of OP intoxication and that the CNS is very sensitive to excess ACh. The possibility that these effects are compensatory and are aimed at protecting the organism against excessive accumulation of ACh in target tissues cannot be excluded. Liu and Pope (1998) exposed adult male rats to high doses of OP anticholinesterase compounds, chlorpyrifos (280 mg/kg) or parathion (6.6 mg/kg). They found that when AChE was maximally (82–96%) inhibited, both compounds markedly inhibited high-affinity choline uptake in striatal synaptosomes *ex vivo*, although chlorpyrifos was less effective than parathion. Both OPs prevented ACh release in the presence of physostigmine and the muscarinic agonist atropine; thus both chlorpyrifos and parathion most likely affected muscarinic presynaptic autoreceptor activity.

ACh released from postsynaptic nerve endings binds to postsynaptic muscarinic and nicotinic receptors. Receptor activation is followed by inhibition of the hydrolysis of ACh by AChE due to ACh accumulation (Massoulié and Bon, 1982). With a continuous accumulation of free ACh at the nerve ending of all cholinergic nerves, there is a continuous activation of the postsynaptic neurons or activation of other types of postsynaptic cells, notably ganglion cells, muscle cells, or endocrine or exocrine gland cells (Ecobichon, 1996). There are several excellent reviews on the role and characteristics of ACh and AChE (Ecobichon, 1996; Erulkar, 1989) and reference will be made to these sources.

50.4.3 REACTION OF ANTICHOLINESTERASE ORGANOPHOSPHOROUS COMPOUNDS WITH ACETYLCHOLINESTERASE

The reaction between an OP compound and the active site in the AChE protein, a serine hydroxyl group, leads to the formation of a transient intermediate complex that partially hydrolyzes the leaving group. The resulting stable, phosphorylated, and largely unreactive inhibited enzyme can be reactivated, under normal circumstances, only at a very slow rate. In many cases, reaction with a number of anticholinesterase OP compounds will lead to irreversible inhibition of the enzyme (Fig. 50.4), and the signs and symptoms will be prolonged and persistent, requiring vigorous medical attention and active treatment with specific antidotes of cholinergic receptor stimulation and enzyme reactivation (Choi *et al.*, 1995; Gutmann and Besser, 1990). Also, once an irreversibly inhibited OP compound–enzyme complex is formed, synthesis of new AChE enzyme molecules is required to restore the normal rapid hydrolysis of ACh. Before that, several events, including cholinergic receptor desensitization (see Gutmann and Besser, 1990) and downregulation (Churchill *et al.*, 1984a), will take place (see later) to attenuate the effects of ACh-induced excitation of postsynaptic cholinergic receptors and subsequent excitotoxicity (Savolainen *et al.*, 1995), and other toxic events (McDonough and Shih, 1997).

Even though much is known about the effects of OPs on AChE in animals and in *in vitro* systems, there is very limited information available on the effects of OP compounds on AChE in the human CNS. Postmortem examination of the distribution of AChE inhibition in the brains of two victims of parathion intoxication and of two control brains, matched for age and sex, indicated that paraoxon-induced AChE inhibition was regionally selective. The largest decrease (60–85%) occurred in the cerebellum, in some thalamic nuclei, and the cortex. Only a moderate decrease (10–30%) was detected in the substantia nigra and basal ganglia, and no effects were seen in the white matter. The authors (Finkelstein *et al.*, 1988) concluded that a detailed knowledge of the brain regions affected by OP poisoning may explain some of the clinical manifestations of poisonings by these compounds. These results were in partial agreement with findings obtained in experimental animal studies (Churchill *et al.*, 1985, 1987).

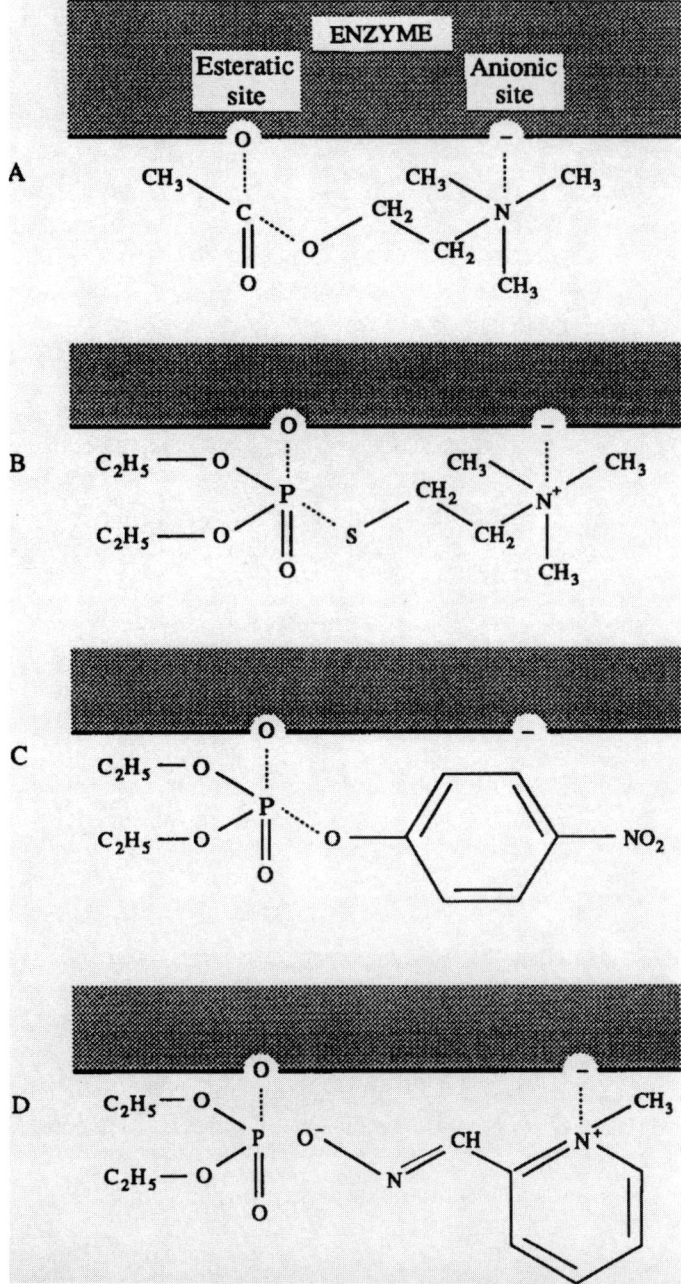

Figure 50.4 Reaction of acetylcholine (A), ecthiopate (B), and paraoxon (C) with acetylcholinesterase and positioning of 2-PAM (see Section 50.8.2) for reactivation of the enzyme inhibited by diethoxyphosphate (D) derived from either of the two inhibitors. Reprinted with permission from *Handbook of Pesticide Toxicology*, Vol. 2, p. 922, Academic Press, San Diego (1991).

50.4.4 ORGANOPHOSPHOROUS COMPOUND DIFFERENTIALLY INHIBIT ACETYLCHOLINESTERASE

There are marked differences between different OP compounds in their ability to inhibit AChE. In fact, some of the dramatic differences between OP compounds that cause some of their serious toxic effects such as convulsions are related to their affinities for AChE (see Churchill *et al.*, 1987; Savolainen *et al.*,

1988a, b). This is because the rate of AChE inhibition and subsequent ACh accumulation may be critical for these effects (Olney *et al.*, 1986). In a number of studies, DFP failed to produce convulsions, whereas both paraoxon and soman readily induced tonic–clonic convulsions in a subpopulation of rats; these differences may be explained by the rate of AChE inhibition by various OPs (see Savolainen *et al.*, 1991; 1988a, b). The rate of AChE inhibition with paraoxon is at least 45 times greater than which can be achieved with DFP over a wide range $(10^{-6}-10^{-10}$ M) of paraoxon concentrations *in vitro* (Chemnitius *et al.*, 1983; Liu and Tsou, 1986). Soman inhibits AChE even more effectively than paraoxon (Aldridge and Reiner, 1972; Hoskins *et al.*, 1986; Koelle, 1963; Sterri *et al.*, 1985). In addition, soman increases brain ACh concentrations much more rapidly than DFP (Fonnum and Guttormsen, 1969; Shih, 1982). Hence, the OP-induced inhibition rate for AChE may be important for OP-induced toxic effects such as convulsions and may explain some of the differences in the seizurogenic potentials of DFP, paraoxon, soman, and other OP compounds. It is also important to keep in mind that several OP-induced effects may, in fact, have an association, or even a causal relationship, with OP-induced alterations in brain metabolic events and neuronal signalling, in addition to convulsions and other behavioral effects.

50.5 DISTRIBUTION OF CHOLINERGIC SYSTEMS IN THE CENTRAL NERVOUS SYSTEM

Because the emphasis of this review will be on the mechanisms of toxic actions of OP compounds in the CNS, central cholinergic pathways will be discussed in more detail. Central cholinergic pathways were initially identified by CAT immunochemistry in cat (Kimura *et al.*, 1981), guinea pig, and rat (Kimura *et al.*, 1980) brains. CAT reactive cells are found throughout the medial septal nucleus, diagonal band area, neostriatum (caudoputamen), nucleus accumbens, olfactory tubercle region, and fields of the medial forebrain bundle. CAT reactive neurons are not found in other areas, such as neo- and piriform cortex (Kimura *et al.*, 1980). These immunohistochemical techniques have identified several important cholinergic pathways in the brain, such as the septohippocampal pathway, and intrinsic cholinergic neurons in the caudate–putamen complex (Pepeu, 1983).

In addition to immunohistochemical identification of CAT reactive neurons, information on the distribution of cholinergic receptors in the central nervous also provides insight into the cholinergic connections in the CNS and helps provide an understanding of the unique effects of OP- and other cholinergic-mediated toxic actions in the CNS. It is noteworthy that the density of muscarinic receptors in the CNS as determined by $[^3H]ACh$ binding is about 100 times greater than that of the nicotinic receptors (Schwarz and Kellar, 1982).

Autoradiographic techniques show the highest densities of brain muscarinic receptors in the corpus striatum (nucleus caudatus–putamen), the cerebral cortex, and the hippocampal formation (Churchill *et al.*, 1984a, b; Kuhar and Yamamura, 1975). More specifically, stratum oriens, radiatum, and molecular layer in the hippocampus, and cingulate cortex and piriform cortex in the cerebral cortex contain particularly high densities of muscarinic receptors (Kuhar and Yamamura, 1975). The density of muscarinic receptors is low in the thalamus, and very low or nonexistent in the midbrain and the cerebellum (Churchill *et al.*, 1984a, b; Kuhar and Yamamura, 1975). Thus, the distribution of muscarinic receptors resembles the distribution of the histochemical and immunohistochemical markers of cholinergic neurons (Jacobowitz and Palkovits, 1974; Kimura *et al.*, 1980; Palkovits and Jacobowitz, 1974; Pepeu, 1983). Particularly in the hippocampus, the muscarinic receptor distribution corresponds to that of cholinergic nerve terminals (Kuhar and Yamamura, 1976). M_1 (specific pharmacological agonist pirenzepine; Caulfield, 1993) and M_2 (specific pharmacological agonists are experimental drugs AF-DX 116 and methoctramine) receptors are distributed heterogeneously (for characteristics of the various muscarinic receptors, see the next chapter) (Mash and Potter, 1986). High densities of M_1 muscarinic receptors exist in olfactory tubercle, caudate putamen, nucleus accumbens, hippocampus, amygdala, and cerebral cortex. M_2 receptors are distributed throughout the brain with high densities in regions that contain large numbers of cholinergic nerve bodies (Hammer *et al.*, 1980; Mash and Potter, 1986).

The density of receptors with a stereospecific binding site for nicotine (Romano and Goldstein, 1980) in the mammalian brain is only 1% of that of muscarinic receptors (Pepeu, 1983). In the brain, the highest concentrations of nicotinic receptors are found in the thalamus, cortex, superior colliculus, and striatum, whereas the lowest concentrations occur in the piriform cortex and hippocampus (Schwarz and Kellar, 1982). Thus, the distribution of nicotinic receptors in the CNS clearly differs from that of muscarinic receptors. It is also quite evident that most of the cholinergic effects of OPs in the CNS are mediated via muscarinic rather than nicotinic receptors. This is important because the most dramatic toxic actions of OPs are mediated via their effects on cholinergic receptors in the CNS and subsequent stimulation of other neurotransmitter systems in the brain, as well as via cholinergic receptor stimulation in other target organs, subsequent to the initial effects of OPs on AChE and the cholinergic systems (see Savolainen *et al.*, 1995).

50.6 RECEPTORS AS TARGETS OF ACETYLCHOLINE-MEDIATED ORGANOPHOSPHORUS COMPOUND EFFECTS

Based on the great diversity of pharmacological and toxicological actions of ACh, it was not difficult to conclude that several types of receptors that mediate the effects of ACh must exist in different organs of the body. Muscarinic receptors predominate in the target tissues innervated by the parasympathetic nervous system, endocrine and exocrine glands, and vessel walls. Furthermore, muscarinic receptors also predominate in the CNS. The effects of ACh on muscarinic receptors can in most cases be blocked by atropine. Nicotinic receptors predominate in autonomic nervous ganglia, in the adrenals, and within the neuromuscular junction, in the muscular endplate. The effects of ACh on nicotinic receptors cannot be blocked by atropine (Caulfield, 1993).

50.6.1 MUSCARINIC RECEPTORS

Muscarinic receptors (mAChRs) are the main cholinergic receptors in the CNS and are expressed at high concentrations (Fisher *et al.*, 1983). The nicotinic receptor differs and is much like the other ligand-gated ion channels, such as the GABA acid receptor, causing rapid signal transduction in response to ligand binding. The muscarinic receptor is a member of the family of (7-transmembrane (7-TM)) surface proteins (Perelta *et al.*, 1988). Muscarinic receptors transduce their signals across the membrane by interacting with guanosine 5′-triphosphate (GTP) binding proteins (G proteins) (see Gilman, 1987). There is a cascade that involves a number of macromolecular interactions in muscarinic receptor activation, which means that the responses of muscarinic receptors are slow compared with those mediated through the nicotinic receptors. The mAChRs are also termed calcium-mobilizing receptors, because they are usually coupled with phosphoinositide (PI) signalling and may either excite or inhibit neurons (Putney, 1987). At somatic neuromuscular junctions, mAChRs also mediate a diverse range of physiological actions, including the regulation of cardiac and smooth muscle contraction, and exocrine gland secretion (Leiber *et al.*, 1990).

The stimulation of mAChR leads to activation of membrane integral PI-specific phospholipase C (PLC), which in turn promotes facilitated bifurcating PI metabolism and increased formation of two second messengers, inositol-1,4,5-trisphosphate ($InsP_3$), and diacylglycerol (DAG). This latter compound activates a key cellular enzyme, protein kinase C (PKC), which is involved in cell activation, regulation of differentiation, and even apoptosis (Dypbukt *et al.*, 1994; Orrenius, 1997). Furthermore, the activation of mAChRs leads to the inhibition of guanylate cyclase (Felder *et al.*, 1989; Gilman, 1987; Hanley and Iversen, 1978), the activation of cAMP-specific phosphodiesterase (Meeker and Harden, 1982), and the synthesis of prostanoids (Busija *et al.*, 1988). The relationships between these responses are not well understood and, in fact, multiple mAChRs may be responsible. Also, the mAChRs seem to be involved in the regulation of Ca^{2+}-dependent K^+ channels (Baraban *et al.*, 1985) and voltage-dependent Ca^{2+} channels (Hesheler *et al.*, 1987).

Due to their structural characteristics, muscarinic receptors are also termed seven transmembrane-domain receptors, indicating that the receptor has seven hydrophobic transmembrane segments that penetrate the cell membrane (Fig. 50.5; Caulfield, 1993). Guanine nucleotides inhibit muscarinic agonists from

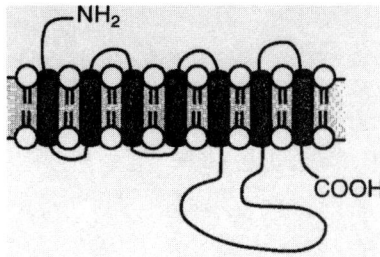

Figure 50.5 G-protein-coupled seven transmembrane domain receptors are composed of a single subunit with seven presumptive transmembrane domains. Muscarinic receptors belong to this category of receptors that are coupled through G proteins to an effector enzyme, phospholipase C. Its activation leads to increased formation of calcium-mobilizing second messengers, hence also the name calcium-mobilizing receptor (for functional details, see Fig. 50.7).

Table 50.2

Muscarinic Acetylcholine Receptor Subtypes, Localization, and Effects on Second Messenger Systems

Receptor subtype	M_1	M_2	M_3	?	?
Gene	m_1	m_2	m_3	m_4	m_5[b]
Gene localization[c]					
Brain	+	−	+	+	−
Heart	−	+	−	−	−
Salivary glands	+	−	+	−	−
Intestines	+−	+	+	−	
Trachea		−	+	+	−
Urinary bladder	−	+	+	−	
Cell line (NG108-15)	−	−	−	+	
Effects on second messengers[d]					
PI	*	*	*	*	
cAMP	*	−	*	−	

[a]For references, see the text.

[b]The gene m_5 has been cloned from a rat brain cDNA library (Liao *et al.*, 1989).

[c]+, detectable; +−, barely detectable; −, not detectable.

[d]*, stimulation.

binding to cell membrane receptors, but they do not prevent the binding of muscarinic antagonists to these receptors (Hesheler *et al.*, 1987). Muscarinic receptor signalling is discussed in more detail in Section 50.7.1, which deals mainly with PI metabolism and events associated with PI signalling. This is because PI signalling-related events are more relevant to OP-induced neuronal excitation than inhibition of adenylate cyclase (Cockcroft, 1986; Mei *et al.*, 1989).

Initially, mAChRs were classified into two groups according to their pharmacological properties: one in the brain with a high affinity for pirenzepine (M_1) and the other in the peripheral organs with a low affinity for pirenzepine (M_2; Cross *et al.*, 1984). Activation of M_1 receptors most likely stimulates PI metabolism and formation of the two second messengers, InsP$_3$ and DAG (Berridge, 1989), whereas M_2 receptors inhibit cAMP formation. However, today three types of mAChRs can be defined based on their affinities toward selective agonists. In addition, five genes that code for the muscarinic receptors have been identified (Liu *et al.*, 1986; Mei *et al.*, 1989). The different types of mAChRs are coupled with different and specific second messenger systems (see Table 50.2). It is evident that the M_1 and M_2 receptors are encoded by m_1 and m_2 genes, respectively (Perelta *et al.*, 1987). Later, the protein encoded by the m_3 gene was identified as the M_3 mAChR (Buckley *et al.*, 1989; Pinkas-Kramarski *et al.*, 1988). The specific pharmacological antagonist of the M_3 receptor is hexahydrociladephinole (Caulfield, 1993). The pharmacology of the mAChRs encoded by the m_4 and m_5 genes is not clear. When expressed in cells, the m_4 gene-encoded receptor shows a relatively high affinity for pirenzepine and thus resembles the M_1 receptor, which is coupled with PI hydrolysis and formation of InsP$_3$ and DAG. These two receptors are, however, two distinct receptor subtypes because the m_4 encoded receptor seems to couple to adenylate cyclase instead of PLC (Ashkenazi *et al.*, 1989). The possibility that different muscarinic receptor subtypes differ in their ability to couple with different G proteins cannot be exclude. The mAChR subtypes also exhibit a distinct regional distribution in the brain. The main consideration with ACh-induced stimulation of mAChRs is the subsequent activation of the target cells, which may lead to overt excitation and toxicity, especially in the CNS.

Direct effects of OP compounds on muscarinic receptors were studied by using rat brain membranes or cultures of human neuroblastoma N1E-115 cells (Bakry *et al.*, 1988). Sarin, soman, or tabun had no effect on the receptors, but VX and echothiopate inhibited, in a competitive manner, the binding of 1-quinuclidinyl(phenyl-4[^{3}H])-benzilate ([^{3}H]QNB) and of [^{3}H]pirenzepine ([^{3}H]PZ) to muscarinic receptors, with VX being the most potent in this respect. The authors (Bakry *et al.*, 1988) suggested that OP compounds may directly act on muscarinic receptors if their concentration in the circulation is at or above micromolar levels. However, the mechanism of this receptor–OP compound interaction remains to be elucidated. Ward *et al.* (1993) explored the interaction of eight OP compounds with muscarinic receptors with regard to their ability to inhibit AChE activity *in vitro* in tissue homogenates from rat hippocampus and frontal cortex. Of the compounds tested, only ecotbiopate competed for [^{3}H]QNB binding and only at concentrations exceeding 100 μM. The OP anticholinesterases did compete, however, with a muscarinic receptor agonist, [^{3}H]CD ([^{3}H]*cis*-methyldioxolane) that binds with a high affinity to 10 and 3% of muscarinic receptors in the frontal cortex and hippocampus, respectively. Ecothiopate and DFP were potent inhibitors of [^{3}H]CD binding as were the active oxon forms of parathion, malathion, and disulfoton. A similar pattern of potency was observed for the inhibition of brain AChE activity, indicating that there was a strong correlation between the abilities of OP compounds to inhibit [^{3}H]CD binding and to inhibit AChE activity.

50.6.2 NICOTINIC RECEPTORS

The nicotinic ACh receptor is the best characterized neurotransmitter receptor, and understanding its function is essential for understanding the mechanisms of action of OP compounds. Electric organs of the *Torpedo* species have served as a rich source of nicotinic receptors. The electrical discharge of *Torpedo* depends solely on a postsynaptic excitatory potential that results from depolarization of the postsynaptic membrane due to an interaction between the receptor and a nicotinic receptor agonist. Depolarization arises directly from the opening of receptor channels. In skeletal muscle and in the fresh water electric eel, *Electrophorus electricus*, depolarization at the endplate activates a voltage-sensitive Na^+ channel that causes the depolarization to spread across the surface of the muscle or electric organ. The density of receptors in *Torpedo* electrical organs is about 100 pmol/mg protein, as compared with 0.1 pmol/mg protein in skeletal muscle (see Taylor and Brown, 1989). Several snake α toxins, including α-bungarotoxin, irreversibly inactivate receptor function in intact skeletal muscle, and this property of the toxin has been utilized to identify and isolate the nicotinic ACh receptor from *Torpedo* (Changeux *et al.*, 1984). Labeled α toxins have been utilized as markers of the nicotinic receptor during its solubilization and purification.

The nicotinic ACh receptor belongs to the group of ligand-gated ion channels and consists of five subunits arranged around a pseudoaxis of symmetry. In the nicotinic receptors of skeletal muscles and the electric organ of *Torpedo*, one of the subunits, designated α, is expressed in two copies; the other three subunits, β, ε/γ, and δ, are present as single copies (see Fig. 50.6; Taylor and Brown, 1989). The receptor is thus a pentamer of molecular mass near 280 kDa. However, the neuronal nicotinic receptors contain only α and β subunits in different combinations with two α subunits and three β subunits. Structural studies have shown that the subunits are arranged around a central cavity, with the largest portion of the protein exposed toward the extracellular surface. The central cavity is most likely the ion channel that, in its resting state, is impermeable to ions. However, once activated, it opens to form a 6.5 Å diameter pore. The open channel is selective for cations, and permeation of the channel by a particular cation seems to be controlled by the diameter of the open channel. Both of the α subunits have a site for binding ACh (plus other nicotinic agonists). ACh must occupy both sites to permit receptor activation and subsequent channel opening (Maelicke, 1986). This then leads to a brief surge of Na^+ ions into the cell. The influx of Na^+ ions causes a change in membrane potential, and this induces a localized depolarization of one part of the cell membrane. This depolarization of the neuromuscular endplate is termed the endplate potential (epp). If this local depolarization is sufficiently large, it can trigger an action potential that spreads throughout the cell. In a muscle cell, the generation of an action potential leads to muscular contraction. Compounds that are competitive antagonists of ACh, such as d-tubocurarine, compete for the ACh binding site in the α subunit of the nicotinic receptor. They are

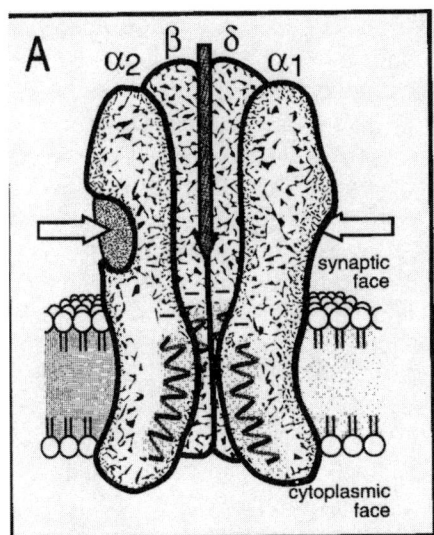

Figure 50.6 Molecular structure of the nicotinic cholinergic receptor. The structure of the receptor is described in the text. The figure shows a longitudinal view with the γ subunit removed. The remaining subunits, two copies of α, one of β, and one of γ, surround an internal channel with an outer vestibule and a narrowing located deep in the membrane bilayer region. Acetylcholine binding sites, indicated by arrows, are found at the $\alpha\gamma$ and $\alpha\delta$ (not visible) interfaces. Reprinted with permission from N. Unwin, *J. Mol. Biol.* **229**, 1101–1124 (1993).

termed competitive inhibitors because they can be displaced from the binding site by increasing the concentration of ACh in the vicinity of the receptor (see Taylor and Brown, 1989).

It is noteworthy that α and β subunits of neuronal nicotinic receptors differ from those in skeletal muscle nicotinic receptors, but are structurally and chemically identical in their amino acid content, and they are evolutionary homologs (Unwin *et al.*, 1988). Neuronal nicotinic receptors differ in structure and pharmacological characteristics from skeletal muscle nicotinic receptors. Ca^{2+} ions permeate more easily through neuronal nicotinic receptors than they pass through skeletal muscle nicotinic receptors; changes in the levels of free intracellular Ca^{2+} concentrations may markedly modify those responses mediated through neuronal nicotinic receptors.

The problem with nicotinic receptors is, in fact, more complex than described above. To date, genes that encode 16 different subunits of vertebrate nicotinic receptors have been cloned. These subunits are identified as $\alpha1$–$\alpha9$, $\beta1$–$\beta4$, γ, δ, and ε. However, because neither the subunit stochiometry nor the arrangement of most of the receptors is known with certainty, this issue will not be tackled in more depth in this context (Lukas *et al.*, 1999; McGehee and Role, 1995; Sargent, 1993). Instead, a simplified approach will be utilized.

OP anticholinesterases may have direct actions on nicotinic receptors. There are data to suggest that OP anticholinesterases bind to allosteric sites of the cholinergic nicotinic receptors as identified by inhibition of [³H]phencyclidine binding, but some can also bind to the receptor's recognition site because they inhibit [¹²⁵I]α-bungarotoxin binding (Bakry *et al.*, 1988). Soman and ecothiopate at micromolar concentrations acted like partial agonists of the nicotinic receptors and induced receptor desensitization. On the other hand, VX acted like an open channel blocker of the activated receptor (i.e., a compound that can only gain access to the ion channel when it is in the open configuration) and also enhanced receptor desensitization. The authors (Bakry et al., 1988) suggested that the toxicity of OP compounds may include some direct actions on the nicotinic receptor if their concentration in the circulation exceeds the micromolar level. The mechanism of this nicotinic receptor–OP compound interaction remains to be elucidated. Chi and Sun (1995) found that soman, sarin, tabun, and phencyclidine did not modify the binding of $[^{25}I]\alpha$-cobratoxin to the nicotinic receptor.

Katz et al. (1997) also reported that incubation of Torpedo membrane-bound nicotinic receptors with the muscarinic agonist carbacholine stimulated the binding of $[^3H]$thienyl-cyclohexylpiperidine ($[^3H]$TCP), which binds to the receptor's noncompetitive agonist binding site in its ionic channel. This agonist stimulated binding of $[^3H]$TCP was inhibited in a dose-dependent manner by OPs such as chlorpyrifos oxon, chlorpyrifos, parathion, and paraoxon. The OPs did not have any effect on equilibrium binding of $[\alpha^{125}I]$bungarotoxin to the receptor's ACh binding site, but preincubation of the membranes with OPs increased the site's affinity for carbachol. In the absence of an agonist, the OPs increased the binding of $[^3H]$TCP markedly. These data suggest that, in addition to AChE inhibition, OPs bind directly to a site on the nicotinic receptor that is distinct from the ACh or TCP binding sites and that this binding induces nicotinic receptor desensitization. In summary, these results indicate that OP compounds may exert direct actions on nicotinic receptors.

50.7 CENTRAL NERVOUS SYSTEM CHOLINERGIC EFFECTS OF ORGANOPHOSHOROUS COMPOUNDS AND OTHER CHOLINERGIC AGONISTS

Stimulation of neuronal cholinergic, predominantly muscarinic receptors (Pepeu, 1983) in the CNS with high doses of direct or indirect cholinergic agonists such as ACh, OP compounds, pilocarpine, carbachol, and oxotremorine has profound effects on neuronal aerobic glucose, phospholipid, sphingolipid, and RNA metabolism, neuronal signalling, and osmoregulation (Churchill et al., 1984a, b; Hoskins et al., 1986; Jope and Morrisett, 1986; Jope et al., 1986; Pazdernik et al., 1985; Savolainen et al., 1988a, b; Wade et al., 1987), as well as a having a profound impact on neuronal electrophysiological effects (see, e.g., Gutmann and Besser, 1990). These events are associated with dramatic behavioral effects such as generation of epileptic foci, and clonic and tonic–clonic convulsions. If these effects are not interrupted, they inevitably lead to the demise of experimental animals and humans (Churchill et al., 1984a, b; McDonough and Shih, 1997; Pazdernik et al., 1985, 1986;

Savolainen et al., 1988a, b; Wade et al., 1987). Long-lasting convulsions are often associated with serious cell losses and brain damage, in addition to dramatic downregulation of cholinergic muscarinic receptors (Churchill et al., 1985; Pazdernik et al., 1985). In the following section, some of the most important effects of cholinergic brain stimulation will be described, with a special emphasis on OP compounds.

50.7.1 EFFECTS ON CEREBRAL CHOLINERGIC SIGNALLING

It can be said that OP-induced brain stimulation is predominantly a consequence of the activation of cerebral mAChRs and, hence, activation of receptor-coupled G protein (Fain et al., 1988; Gilman, 1987) and subsequent activation of PLC-mediated PI signalling (Berridge and Irvine, 1989). Thus, events associated with facilitated PI hydrolysis play an crucial role in OP-induced brain effects. The following paragraphs give a brief description of the signalling cascade.

PIs play a key role in muscarinic cell signalling as precursors of second messengers that are responsible for transducing the signal from the cell surface muscarinic receptors into the cell (Berridge, 1989). PIs are different from all other membrane phospholipids because kinases are able to further phosphorylate their inositol head groups. Although PIs account for about 10% of the total phospholipid composition of the cell membrane in most cells, phosphatidylinositol-4,5-bisphosphate (PIP_2) is a minor membrane component that makes up between 1 and 10% of the total PI pool. Its concentration is higher in the brain than in any other tissue, which suggests that it plays an important role in the specialized functions of the nervous system. Stimulation of calcium-mobilizing receptors, to which muscarinic receptor subtypes belong, initiates a bifurcating hydrolysis pathway of PIP_2, an acidic membrane-bound phospholipid. Hydrolysis of this membrane phospholipid results in the formation of two second messengers, $InsP_3$ and DAG (Downes and Michell, 1981). DAG stimulates PKC, an enzyme vital for several important cellular functions, including receptor-mediated activation (Nishizuka, 1988), whereas $InsP_3$ diffuses into the cytosol to release calcium from nonmitochondrial internal stores and, perhaps indirectly, to stimulate the entry of extracellular calcium into the cell (Berridge, 1987). Ultimately, the PI pathway leads to the reformation of PIP_2, and the cycle is again primed. Lithium inhibits the metabolism of inositol phosphates in the final dephosphorylation step (see Fig. 50.7). Thus, lithium is likely to reduce the supply of free inositol required to maintain the formation of lipid precursors used for cell signalling. These pathways regulate several cellular processes, including metabolism, contraction, neural activity, and cell proliferation (Berridge, 1989; Berridge and Irvine, 1989).

OP compounds induce their effects by inhibiting AChE, leading to accumulation of ACh and excessive activation of mAChRs. Thus, OP-induced brain effects and neurotoxicity are, in fact, the toxicity of excess ACh (Savolainen et al., 1998). Katz and Marquis (1992) exposed human SK–N–SH

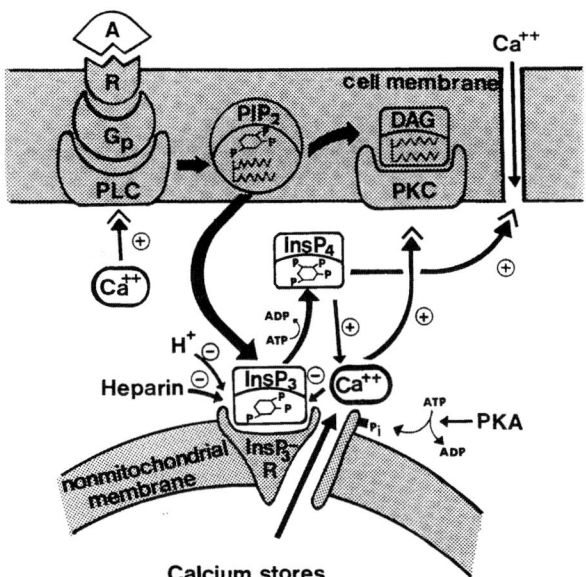

Calcium stores

Figure 50.7 Receptor-mediated phosphoinositide turnover: An agonist (A) such as ACh binds to receptor (R), causing the activation of a G protein (G_p) that, in turn, stimulates PLC. The PLC hydrolyses PIP_2, generating $InsP_3$ and DAG. $InsP_3$ binds to a specific receptor on the membrane of a nonmitochondial cell organelle that contains Ca^{2+}, causing the release of calcium from the intracellular stores. The binding of $InsP_3$ to its receptors is inhibited by heparin and increased intracellular H^+ and Ca^{2+}. $InsP_3$ can further be phosphorylated to $InsP_4$, which may facilitate the entry of calcium into the cell through the plasma membrane or may trigger the movement of calcium within the cell. DAG activates PKC, which phosphorylates a large number of substrates. Activation of cAMP-dependent protein kinase A (PKA) leads to phosphorylation of $InsP_3$ receptor protein.

neuroblastoma cells to low concentrations of paraoxon or carbachol, a direct muscarinic agonist. Paraoxon inhibited the N-[^{3}H]methylscopolamine ([^{3}H]NMS) muscarinic receptor binding. Paraoxon, also at low concentrations (0.1 nM), caused a time-dependent increase in the PI turnover, whereas high concentrations of carbachol were required for the same effect. Both pertussis toxin, a G-protein inhibitor, and neomycin, a PLC inhibitor, inhibited cholinergic-induced facilitation of PI hydrolysis. It seems that paraoxon may modulate signal transduction in neuronal cells by indirect activation of muscarinic receptors, that is, by elevating levels of ACh, as well as by acting at a site distal to the receptor (Katz and Marquis, 1992). Bodjarian *et al.* (1992) demonstrated that soman also facilitates PI hydrolysis in hippocampal slices from rats. The effect was mediated through muscarinic receptor subtypes M_1 and M_3 subsequent to AChE inhibition and ACh accumulation. Even though the M_2 muscarinic receptor subtype is preferentially coupled with inhibition of adenylate cyclase, leading to reduction of levels of cAMP, it was also shown to be associated with PLC-mediated hydrolysis of PIs (Mei *et al.*, 1989). Thus, findings from *in vitro* studies are consistent with the assumption that OP compounds affect neuronal PI signalling and that this is mediated via cholinergic muscarinic receptor activation.

Savolainen and co-workers have shown in a series of *in vivo* studies that exposure of experimental animals to several OP

compounds, such as DFP, malaoxon, paraoxon, and soman, dramatically increases PI signalling, as measured by the accumulation of inositol-1-monophosphate, that is closely associated with cholinergic-induced clonic or tonic–clonic convulsions (Hirvonen *et al.*, 1989, 1990, 1993; Savolainen *et al.*, 1988a, b, 1991; Savolainen and Hirvonen, 1992). In these studies, rats were usually pretreated with lithium (3–5 mequiv/kg), because lithium amplifies the cholinergic-induced PI turnover and its associated convulsions (Hirvonen *et al.*, 1990; Honchar *et al.*, 1983; Savolainen *et al.*, 1988a, b). When rats were given soman with or without lithium pretreatment, tonic–clonic convulsions and increased PI turnover could be prevented by pretreating the animals with atropine or benzodiazepine, indicating that the events are associated with stimulation of mAChR and are modifiable by increasing the GABAergic tone in the CNS (Savolainen *et al.*, 1988a, b). In another study (Hirvonen *et al.*, 1990), malaoxon-induced convulsions were associated with marked increases in PI signalling and early neuronal injury, especially in the hippocampus (Hirvonen *et al.*, 1990). During an investigation of the differences between male and female rats, Savolainen and Hirvonen (1992) observed that malaoxon stimulates PI signalling in the brain of the rats' offspring and that females seem to be more sensitive than males toward the OP-induced cholinergic brain stimulation and alterations in PI signalling. Lithium seemed to increase the sensitivity of experimental animals toward OP-induced convulsions. Furthermore, increased PI turnover in the hippocampus may indicate a lithium-induced lowering of the seizure threshold for OP in limbic regions (Savolainen *et al.*, 1991).

Hirvonen *et al.* (1993) gave a single convulsive dose of pilocarpine and then overt convulsions were abruptly terminated with diazepam after 15 min. This did not prevent the occurrence of serious brain damage and facilitated PI signalling was still seen 5 days after the cessation of the convulsions and exposure to pilocarpine. At this stage, the entire dose of pilocarpine had been excreted via urine and all convulsions had been over for 5 days. The authors concluded that pilocarpine served as a trigger for seizures and convulsions, and, subsequently, other neurotransmitter systems, most likely systems coupled to PI turnover, became activated and were responsible for the residual stimulation of PI turnover as well as the associated brain damage.

The candidate receptors most likely to become activated after initial cholinergic neuronal stimulation are the glutamatergic receptors (see Savolainen *et al.*, 1998). The hypothesized pathway is as follows: AChE inhibition by OP compounds leads to ACh accumulation and subsequent excessive cholinergic muscarinic stimulation. There are convulsions that lead to release of glutamate, activation of glutamate receptors, influx of calcium into the neurons, and neuronal apoptosis or necrosis. Similar effects can also be induced by stimulating neuronal cells with direct cholinergic muscarinic agonists such as pilocarpine or carbachol (Felipo *et al.*, 1998; Hirvonen *et al.*, 1993; Savolainen *et al.*, 1995, 1998; Solberg and Belkin, 1997). Bodjarian *et al.* (1995) provided evidence that, in addition to cholinergic receptors, histamine H_1 subtypes and glutamate metabotropic receptors also are involved in the facilitated PI signalling that is associated with soman-induced convulsions. In contrast, 5-HT$_2$ or α_1 adrenoreceptors—receptors also coupled to PI signalling—were not associated with these soman-induced signalling events.

Cholinergic brain stimulation by OP compounds also affects the levels of cyclic nucleotides—AMP and cyclic GMP—in different brain regions due to inhibition of the cyclase enzymes (Liu *et al.*, 1986). In another study, Liu *et al.* (1988) observed that decreases in the levels of AMP or cyclic GMP in the striatum, cerebellum, and spinal cord were not related to soman-induced convulsions in rats. This is consistent with the assumption that the facilitation of PI signalling, rather than the activity of adenylate cyclase, is essential for cholinergic-induced convulsions, associated second messenger formation, and neuropathology (Hirvonen *et al.*, 1990, 1993).

50.7.2 EFFECTS ON RECEPTORS

The density of various receptors and their subtypes in different brain regions markedly affects brain cholinergic signalling and subsequent metabolic events, and the pathological consequences. Yagle and Costa (1996) exposed Sprague Dawley (SD) rats to doses of 2 mg/kg per day of disulfoton (*S*-(2-(ethylthio)ethyl)phosphorothionate) for 14 consecutive days, and measured messenger ribonucleic acid (mRNA) levels of muscarinic receptor m$_1$, m$_2$, and m$_3$ subtypes, immediately after the cessation of the exposure, as well as after a 28-day recovery period. There was a marked reduction in the levels of muscarinic receptor subtypes in several brain regions immediately after the exposure, but after the recovery period, only the m$_2$ subtype mRNA levels remained decreased, indicating that this receptor subtype may be more sensitive than the others toward OP-induced alterations. Also, marked reductions in [^{3}H]QNB binding were seen immediately after the cessation of the exposure, indicating a marked reduction in muscarinic receptor numbers. The findings of Yagle and Costa (1996) are consistent with earlier observations by Doebler *et al.* (1983a), who showed that repetitive s.c. injections of soman at a 0.5 LD$_{50}$ dose level caused a marked and progressive RNA depletion in caudate and cortex. Soman-induced reductions of overall brain RNA levels were mediated via muscarinic receptor stimulation because they could be completely blocked by pretreatment with atropine when given together with pralidoxime (Doebler *et al.*, 1983b). Feeding mice with parathion (0.4–500 mg/kg/day) in their diet for 14 days inhibited mouse brain AChE activity and transiently reduced the maximal binding of [^{3}H]QNB, [^{3}H]NMS, and [^{3}H]4-DAMP ([^{3}H]-4-diphenylacetoxy-*N*-methylpiperidine methiodide) binding without affecting receptor affinities for these ligands (Jett *et al.*, 1993). Inhibition of whole brain AChE varied between 10 and 80% in a dose-dependent fashion. These results suggest that dietary doses of parathion induced a transient downregulation of different muscarinic receptor subtypes in the mouse brain.

Churchill *et al.* (1984a, b) found that [^{3}H]QNB binding to muscarinic receptors in the rat forebrain decreased after con-

vulsions induced by a single dose of soman, as well as after a single dose of conic acid, an analog of an excitotoxic neurotransmitter, glutamate (Churchill *et al.*, 1990). The reason for the decreased binding of [^{3}H]QNB was a decrease in the number of muscarinic receptors rather than the affinity for the ligand. Blockade of the convulsions by diazepam also inhibited alterations in the [^{3}H]QNB binding. Consistent with the findings of Churchill *et al.* (1990), Chaudhuri *et al.* (1993) found that high doses of parathion or chlorpyriphos, both anticholinesterase OP compounds, markedly inhibited [^{3}H]QNB binding in cortex and striatum.

Abdallah *et al.* (1992) found that 100 μM paraoxon markedly reduced the B_{max} of [^{3}H]4-DAMP binding, an M$_3$ muscarinic receptor subtype-specific antagonist, without any significant alterations in its affinity toward the receptor in rat submaxillary gland (SMG) cells, indicative of a noncompetitive inhibition of the binding by paraoxon in these cells. The authors suggested that paraoxon may bind to two different sites in these SMG cells. One might be an allosteric site on the M$_3$ muscarinic receptor that modulates receptor function. The other site could be in the G$_i$ protein–adenylate cyclase complex (Gilman, 1987). These findings complicate our understanding of OP toxicity, because they also mean that OPs can have direct effects on muscarinic receptors. Viana *et al.* (1988) demonstrated that when PC12 pheochromocytoma cells were treated with nerve growth factor (NGF), the number of [^{3}H]NMS binding sites increased twofold, but NGF did not change the K_d for this ligand. Exposure of these cells to 50 μM soman decreased the number of binding sites in both cells with and without NGF treatment. Other OP compounds, including sarin, tabun, and VX, also reduced [^{3}H]NMS binding. These reductions in muscarinic binding were not reversed by atropine. Interestingly, similar changes induced by carbacholine were reversed by atropine. It thus seems that the decreases in muscarinic receptor binding in PC12 cells induced by OP compounds occur via a mechanism that does not necessarily involve agonist-induced receptor desensitization. Blanchet *et al.* (1986) previously reported results that concurred with those of Viana *et al.* (1988) that exposure of mouse NS-20 and N1E-115 neuroblastoma cells to soman markedly reduced the number of [^{3}H]NMS binding sites and inhibited carbacholine-induced cyclic GMP formation. Thus, exposure of neuronal cells to an OP was able to induce muscarinic receptor downregulation and subsequent desensitization of muscarinic receptor-mediated responses. Low levels of paraoxon also have been found to block M$_2$ and M$_3$ muscarinic receptors in homogenates of calf caudate nuclei as indicated by modulation of paraoxon-induced inhibition of [^{3}H]QNB binding by specific antagonists of M$_2$ (AF-DX116) and M$_3$ (4-DAMP) receptors (Katz and Marquis, 1989).

To explore whether a critical period exists for OP-induced alterations in the density of mAChRs and spontaneous behavior, neonatal mice were exposed to a single dose of 1.5 mg/kg of DFP on neonatal days 3, 10, or 19, and followed for changes in receptor density and behavioral alterations at the age of 4 months (Ahlbom *et al.*, 1995). Mice exposed on days 3 or 10 showed a decrease in mAChR density and spontaneous motor behavior, but those exposed on day 19 no longer showed any effects. The lack of effects in mice exposed on neonatal day 19 was not due to differences in AChE activity; thus, we cannot exclude the possibility that a critical period exists for OP-induced cholinergic effects during neonatal life. Jett *et al.* (1994) found that high doses of parathion, resulting in 84–90% inhibition of AChE, to adult male rats for 21 days did not affect the affinities of different mAChR subtypes toward ligands. However, there was a significant downregulation of the m_4 receptor subtype gene product, and m_1 mRNA and m_3 mRNA in the frontal cortex as well as the m_4 mRNA in the striatum. However, no changes in mAChR subtype gene products or mRNAs were found in the hippocampus. These findings indicate that paraoxon-induced ACh accumulation causes a marked depletion in the numbers of receptors of several muscarinic receptor subtypes. Whereas the degree of AChE inhibition in all brain areas was of the same magnitude, differences in parathion concentrations do not explain the lack of effect in the hippocampus, a key brain region in the regulation of seizure and convulsive activity. One possibility, though, is that in the hippocampus, OP-induced effects were less severe because of quicker renewal of the muscarinic receptors in this brain region.

Churchill *et al.* (1985) used muscarinic receptor autoradiography after soman administration sufficient to cause a pronounced weight loss in a subgroup of rats to reveal a consistent pattern of cell loss with extensive neuronal necrosis. Receptor autoradiography indicated that these changes were associated with a dramatic decrease in the numbers of muscarinic receptors in the piriform cortex and the thalamus. These authors concluded that quantitative receptor autoradiography provides, in addition to kinetic information and topographical distribution, radiohistochemical evidence of neuronal damage that most likely took place subsequent to early effects of soman, such as alterations in total or muscarinic receptor-specific mRNA levels. Aas *et al.* (1987) demonstrated, however, that exposure to a low concentration of soman in the inhalaled air did not induce any marked reduction in muscarinic receptor binding characteristics in the hippocampus and the neostriatum of rats. This finding emphasized a fundamental aspect of toxicology—the significance of dose—even when we are dealing with highly toxic agents such as soman.

Rocha *et al.* (1996) investigated the presynaptic effects of paraoxon in rat cultured hippocampal neurons, and found that paraoxon (30 μmol–1 mM) blocked the ion channels of glycine, γ-aminobutyric acid$_A$ (GABA$_A$), N-methyl-D-aspartic acid (NMDA; glutamate receptor subtype), and nicotinic ACh receptors, but not the ion channels of kainate- and α-amino-3-hydroxy-5-methyl-4-isoxazolepropionic acid -(AMPA) -like glutamate receptors. The authors suggested that the combined effects of paraoxon on the functions of several ligand-gated receptors may constitute actions relevant to the neurotoxicity of paraoxon. Even if these findings that reflect the direct effects of paraoxon on a number of ligand-gated ion channels are difficult to interpret, they are consistent with a number of recent observations that implicate the involvement of glutamate receptors in the effects of cholinergic neuronal stimulation (Jope *et al.*,

1986; Loikkanen *et al.*, 1998; Naarala *et al.*, 1997; Savolainen *et al.*, 1998; Solberg and Belkin, 1997). It is also of interest that the nerve agent, VX, but not soman or sarin, markedly inhibited [^{3}H]NMS binding to muscarinic receptors and also reduced [^{3}H]s-piperone binding to dopamine D_2 receptors in the rat striatum (Naseem, 1990). This OP seemed to differ somewhat from other OPs because they did not mirror its effects.

It seems that OP compounds have both direct and indirect effects, mediated mainly via ACh accumulation subsequent to AChE inhibition. Even if OPs have some direct effects on a wide variety of receptors and their subtypes, it seems that they only slightly modify the overall effects of these agents. The vast majority of their actions are attributable to ACh accumulation on cholinergic receptors and subsequent glutamatergic activation.

50.7.3 EFFECTS OF BRAIN METABOLISM

Chemical-induced seizures, and pure cholinergic agonist-induced brain activation, also in the absence of seizures, increase functional brain activity when assessed by local cerebral glucose utilization (LCGU; Churchill *et al.*, 1984a, b). Churchill *et al.* (1987) gave s.c. injections of soman or DFP to SD rats. Soman rapidly induced tonic–clonic convulsions, whereas DFP only occasionally induced transient seizurelike activity. Soman induced LCGU in most of the cortex, striato–pallido–nigral pathway, limbic system and thalamic nuclei, whereas DFP increased LCGU in a very limited fashion, primarily in the dorsal striato–pallido–nigral pathway. Both soman- and DFP-induced facilitation of LCGU could be blocked or markedly inhibited by a mixture of muscarinic agonists, trimedoxime, atropine, and benactyzine, indicating that cholinergic stimulation was responsible for the activation of the striato–pallido–nigral pathway, which is known to be important in muscarinic receptor-mediated convulsions. These authors suggested that even though soman and DFP activate this cholinergic pathway, only soman causes the spread of activity throughout the pathway, leading to overt motor convulsions. Possible explanations for this difference in response to these OPs are differential responses in cholinergic actions within specific brain regions or some noncholinergic action of soman. Also, delayed effects of soman on LCGU were studied by giving rats [^{14}C]2-deoxyglucose (2-DG) prior to a single s.c. dose of 120 μg/kg ($0.9 \times$ LD$_{50}$) sarin and by following the rats for up to 72 h. At later time points, there was a marked reduction in the LGGU, and this was associated with neuropathology in many brain regions, with the most marked damage occurring in the piriform cortex and the amygdala (Pazdernik *et al.*, 1985; Samson *et al.*, 1985). These data suggest (Samson *et al.*, 1985) that shortly after OP administration, there is an initial and marked increase of LCGU that reflects cerebral activation. Later there is a secondary reduction in cerebral LCGU. This is most likely due to convulsion-associated neuropathology and subsequent cell loss in the most severely affected brain regions.

Khan and Hasan (1988) investigated the effects of methyl parathion at doses of 1.0, 1.5, or 2.0 mg/kg on the levels of gangliosides and glycogen in the cerebral hemisphere, cerebellum, brain stem, and spinal cord following seven daily i.p. injections. The authors observed a marked and dose-dependent decrease in the levels of gangliosides in all brain regions. An identical decrement in the levels of glycogen was found in different brain regions. The authors concluded that the OP-induced, dose-dependent, cholinergic brain stimulation was responsible for the changes in the levels of gangliosides and glycogen in different brain regions. The applied dose induced overt toxicity in the rats, including hyperexcitability, muscular fasciculations, tremors, and convulsions. After 6–7 days, all experimental rats became lethargic. Control rats exhibited no abnormality.

50.7.4 EFFECTS ON GENE EXPRESSION

Convulsions may be associated with rapid and major increases in gene expression. This may be a direct consequence of convulsions, or at least be causally associated with them (Ceccatelli *et al.*, 1989; Zimmer *et al.*, 1997a, b). A high dose of soman [77.7 μg/kg body weight (bw)] caused tonic–clonic convulsions in the exposed rats and induced a robust progressive expression of an immediate early gene, *c-fos*, a reliable indicator of neuronal activation (Greenberg *et al.*, 1986; Murphy *et al.*, 1994), in the piriform cortex and the noradrenergic locus coereleus. Later, *c-fos* expression also occurred in the entorhinal cortex, the endopiriform nucleus, the olfactory tubercle, the anterior olfactory nucleus, and the main olfactory bulb. At 2 h the *c-fos* expression achieved its maximum and was then present also in the cerebral cortex, thalamus, caudate–putamen, and the hippocampus, brain regions, typically metabolically activated subsequent to soman exposure (Pazdernik *et al.*, 1985). At 8 h and beyond, *c-fos* expression returned to the control level (Zimmer *et al.*, 1997a, b). In general, *c-fos* promotes the transcription of additional genes, including those that encode proteins that are required for metabolic and physiologic activities of the cell. Thus, *c-fos* expression indicates that the cell is adapting to external stimuli by producing the proteins necessary for continued cellular function. Under extreme stress, *c-fos* also promotes the transcription of genes that encode proteins that are critical to cell survival (Sheng and Greenberg, 1990). Several other investigators (Arenander *et al.*, 1989; Greenberg *et al.*, 1986; Seuwen *et al.*, 1990) also have shown that muscarinic receptor-mediated activation of PKC induces the immediate early genes *c-fos* and *c-jun*. These are genes that encode nuclear proteins (Maki *et al.*, 1987) and act in tandem as a dimeric complex that binds to a specific DNA consensus sequence in target genes to stimulate their transcription.

Muscarinic receptor activation has induced *c-fos* expression in PC12 pheochromocytoma cells (Arenander *et al.*, 1989; Greenberg *et al.*, 1986), and both *c-fos* and *c-jun* expression in fibroblasts that express M_1 muscarinic receptors (Seuwen *et al.*, 1990) and glial cell lines (Ashkenazi *et al.*, 1989). The changes induced by OPs may produce permanent changes in the gene levels in these cells. It is clear that cholinergic-induced convulsions are associated with increased expression of immediate early genes. The exact role of these genes, whether they are consequences of neuronal excitation or causally linked with it, remains to be elucidated.

50.7.5 EFFECTS ON NEUROTRANSMITTER LEVELS IN THE BRAIN

Exposure to OP compounds also has been shown to markedly affect the release and metabolism of a number cerebral neurotransmitters. Convulsive doses of soman (31.2 μg/kg) inhibited guinea pig brain AChE by 90%, and elevated ACh levels in most brain areas, with levels of ACh remaining high for long periods of time. In all brain regions, soman reduced noradrenaline (NA) levels and the levels of dopamine (DA) were unchanged, but the levels of dopamine metabolites increased. The levels of 5-HT were unchanged, but those of its metabolites showed a modest increase. Changes in the levels of amino acid neurotransmitters correlate well with alterations in ACh levels: aspartate levels fell whereas those of GABA rose. It was concluded that these changes in the levels of several cerebral neurotransmitters are secondary to the initial increase in ACh content, and include an increased DA and 5-HT turnover, and release of NA and excitatory and inhibitory amino acid neurotransmitters (Fosbraey *et al.*, 1990). In contrast, a reversible AChE inhibitor, physostigmine, decreased levels of GABA in the hypothalamus, striatum, cerebellum, and the rest of the brain, whereas OP compounds paraoxon and soman had no effect on brain GABA levels. The lack of any effect of OPs on brain GABA levels may have been due to short-term exposure to paraoxon and soman (Coudray-Lucas *et al.*, 1984).

Fosbraey *et al.* (1990) and El-Etri *et al.* (1992) both reported that a dose of soman that induced tonic–clonic convulsions in most of the exposed animals also decreased cerebral noradrenaline levels in several brain regions in convulsing rats, but no change in NA was seen in nonconvulsing rats. Also consistent with the observations of Fosbraey *et al.* (1990), levels of DA and 5-HT were unaltered, but the levels of corresponding metabolites were elevated (El-Etri *et al.*, 1992). Thus, it is possible that rapid and sustained NA release plays a role in the induction and/or maintenance of OP-induced convulsions, whereas the changes in the levels of the other neurotransmitters, notably 5-HT and DA are likely to be secondary to the convulsions. Consistent with the observations of El-Etri *et al.* (1992), Shih and McDonough (1997) found that ACh levels increased rapidly after soman administration and that NA levels already started to decline 5 min after seizure onset and this process continued. However, levels of DA and its metabolites 3,4-dihydroxyphenylacetic acid and homovanillic acid also were elevated 5 min after seizure onset and thereafter. The brain aspartate levels were decreased within 20 min after the onset of seizures, and those of glutamate were decreased within 80 min after seizure initiation. Levels of GABA were markedly increased in the cortex, but concentrations of glutamine, glycine, and taurine were unchanged. The results are consistent with the notion that inhibition of AChE and elevation of ACh initiate the seizure process, resulting in secondary changes in DA turnover and release of NE, and later changes in excitatory (aspartate, glutamate) and inhibitory (GABA) amino acid neurotransmitters.

Thomsen and Wilson (1986) found earlier that repeated sublethal doses (300 µg/kg bw) of paraoxon decreased transmitter release as measured via MEPPs. The authors suggested that this effect was attributable to a decrease in the transmitter store and mobilization ability that could account for the behavioral tolerance observed during long-term OP intoxication. Liu *et al.* (1994) studied catecholamine secretion and calcium influx in bovine adrenal chromaffin cells after their exposure to OP compounds, and found that catecholamine secretion and $^{45}Ca^{2+}$ uptake evoked by a nicotinic receptor agonist DMPP (1,1-dimethyl-4-phenylpiperazinium) were inhibited by both methyl parathion and malathion. The authors suggested that in addition to AChE, voltage-gated Ca^{2+} channels and nicotinic receptors also may be sites of OPs action in the mammalian nervous system.

50.7.6 EFFECTS ON ELECTROPHYSIOLOGY AND ASSOCIATED EVENTS

A supralethal dose of soman (180 µg/kg bw), 1 min prior to a 2 mg/kg dose of atropine and 30 min after a dose of the oxime HI-6 (125 mg/kg) caused epileptiform tonic–clonic seizures in rats. The convulsions were associated with extensive neuronal damage 1, 3, 10, or 30 days later. The severity of neuronal damage was associated with significantly, but transiently, increased δ (0–3.5 Hz) frequency in the electroencephalographs (EEGs) recorded 24 h after the exposure. Particularly sustained damage occurred in cortical areas, with piriform and perirhinal cortices exhibiting the most serious morphological alterations (McDonough *et al.*, 1998). Even though there was a clear correlation between the occurrence of δ frequency and the severity of damage, EEG alterations could not be used to predict the morphological alterations. The EEG normalized within 10 days. When two doses of chlorphenvinfos, an OP insecticide [(2-chloro-1-(dichlorophenyl)vinyl ethyl phosphate) (CVP)], were given at a 3 month intervals, EEG and behavioral alterations were induced in rabbits. The effects were less pronounced after the second dose. In rats, a symptomatic dose of 3 mg/kg of CVP given s.c. on 10 consecutive days induced subtle changes in complex behavior—neophobia in the open field test—and increased the EEG arousal response to an external painful stimulus (Gralewicz and Socko, 1997).

Generalized convulsive status epilepticus is the most common and potentially most damaging form of status epilepticus. It exhibits a typical electrophysiological pattern: phases 1–5 are seen in the EEGs. Koplovitz and Skvorak (1998) found that soman induced all stages in 12 out of 15 rats, but phases 2–5 occurred in all rats. The findings suggest that the sequence of EEG changes is independent of the initiating cause, reflect a common electrical response to generalized convulsive status epilepticus and point to a common underlying neurochemical

mechanism. These conclusions do not conflict with the hypotheses that acetylcholine and the convulsive excitatory amino acids may be the common final pathway in generalized convulsions even if the agent that initiates the cascade of events differs (Savolainen *et al.*, 1998; Solberg and Belkin, 1997).

OP compounds also induce more subtle electrophysiological changes, which can be reflected in potential problems with learning and memory. Subchronic *ex vivo* and *in vitro* exposure to parathion resulted in an increase of the field excitatory postsynaptic potentiation (EPSP) after a subthreshold tetanic stimulation. Furthermore, the occurrence of a late effect reduced long-term potentiation (LTP; Schmuck *et al.*, 1998). LTP is a long-lasting increase in the efficacy of synaptic transmission that is considered to underlie the plastic changes associated with learning and memory (Doyere and Laroche, 1992). In the CA1 region of the hippocampus, tetanus-induced LTP is dependent on activation of the NMDA receptors and on the rise in intracellular calcium concentration (Collingridge *et al.*, 1992; Lynch *et al.*, 1983). Schmuck *et al.* (1998), suggested that the effects of parathion on EPSP and LTP may be due to elevated synaptic ACh and stimulation of cholinergic muscarinic receptors, even if no persistent neurobehavioral changes that correlate with these electrophysiological effects have been demonstrated (Ivens *et al.*, 1998).

50.7.7 SEIZUROGENIC AND BEHAVIORAL EFFECTS

Dissociation between the motor and electrical aspects of convulsive status epilepticus induced by OP compounds is problematic in many cases. Sparenborg *et al.* (1993) used the nerve agent soman (200 µg/kg bw) to induce cholinergic convulsions and electrical brain discharges in guinea pigs, and administered cholinergic or GABAergic antagonists to investigate the association between behavior and electrical brain events. All animals that received soman without other treatments developed severe status epilepticus associated with continuous electrographic seizure activity. Despite the presence of continual motor convulsions in all animals challenged with soman and pretreated with diazepam, increased electrographic seizure activity did not take place in most of these animals. Likewise, scopolamine also inhibited soman-induced increased electrographic activity, even though it did not terminate the motor convulsions. Neuronal necrosis was found in the hippocampus, thalamus, amygdala, and cerebral and piriform cortices in animals that exhibited both increased electrographic activity and motor convulsions, but not in those that exhibited motor convulsions alone. Thus, it is important to note that overt convulsions may take place, at least in experimental animals, with no electrographic alterations present in the brain that lead to actual necrosis. Soman given as an infusion at a dose of 13.1 µg/kg bw to adult baboons induced the onset of intoxication within 2–3 min, manifested as hyperactivity and severe grand mal convulsions (Anzueto *et al.*, 1986).

Stamper *et al.* (1988) exposed preweanling rat pups to daily doses of 1.3 or 1.0 mg/kg of parathion during postnatal days

5–20, a time period critical for development of behavior and biochemical maturation of the cholinergic systems in the brain. Even though the doses of parathion were quite high, they were not lethal to these experimental animals. Had the exposure been to paraoxon, the situation would have been different. The exposure resulted in a dose-dependent reduction in AChE activity and muscarinic receptor binding in the brain, and was later associated with multiple deficits in spatial memory. Thus, impairment of memory functions due to alterations in brain cholinergic systems were seen even though the doses of OP did not provoke severe signs of toxicity.

Repeated sublethal doses of DFP or soman were given to rats for 4 weeks to explore behavioral tolerance toward anticholinesterase OP compounds (Van Dongen and Wolthuis, 1989). Even though there was progressive AChE inhibition, the rats' behavior, as measured with shuttle-box performance, remained virtually normal 24 h after the DFP injections throughout the study. However, behavioral tolerance did not develop toward soman. The results indicate that the differences between DFP- and soman-induced behavioral tolerance could not be explained by (1) inhibition of AChE *de novo* synthesis, (2) muscarinic receptor downregulation, (3) differences in the number of nicotinic receptors, or (4) the activity of phosphorylphosphatase (DFPase or somanase) in different organs. The authors concluded that the behavioral tolerance induced by DFP is probably due to presynaptic alterations or increased synthesis of *de novo* synthesis of OP-binding proteins (see also Meldrum and Garthwaite, 1990).

50.8 MODULATION OF EFFECTS OF ORGANOPHOSPHOROUS COMPOUNDS

Whereas OP anticholinesterase compounds are indirect cholinergic agonists that induce their effects through stimulation of cholinergic muscarinic and nicotinic receptors, it is conceivable that modulation of the responses of these receptors could be used to modulate the effects of these agents. The cholinergic muscarinic receptors also communicate with other receptor systems, especially glutamatergic (Felipo *et al.*, 1998; Savolainen *et al.*, 1998; Solberg and Belkin, 1997) and GABAergic receptors (Hirvonen *et al.*, 1993; McDonough and Shih, 1997; Savolainen *et al.*, 1988a, b), and thus their responses can be modulated not only by antagonists of muscarinic receptors, but also with agonists or antagonists of other receptors. Furthermore, because muscarinic receptors are G-protein-coupled (Gilman, 1987) Ca^{2+} mobilizing receptors (Berridge, 1989), they permit modulatory interactions with compounds that affect this protein (Jope *et al.*, 1989). It is not likely that nicotinic receptors can be modulated other than via their antagonists such as d-tubocurarine and its analogs (Taylor and Brown, 1989). However, nicotinic receptor functions may be modulated directly by OP compounds and indirectly by cholinergic muscarinic agonists (see Katz *et al.*, 1997).

50.8.1 ATTENUATION OF CHOLINERGIC EFFECTS BY MUSCARINIC RECEPTOR INHIBITION

Several studies indicate that atropine, the nonsubtype-selective antagonist of all muscarinic receptors, is effective in blocking muscarinic receptor-mediated effects of OP compounds (Johnson and Lowndes, 1974; Lundy *et al.*, 1978; Savolainen *et al.*, 1988b; Shih, 1990, 1991; Shih *et al.*, 1991a, b). High doses of atropine (32 mg/kg) given prior to soman (100 mg/kg) effectively blocked soman-induced convulsions in rats and attenuated the increased cerebral PI hydrolysis (Savolainen *et al.*, 1988a, b). In another rat study (Shih, 1990), atropine (12 mg/kg) given prior to soman (100 µg/kg) did not block soman-induced convulsions and did not affect AChE activity or degree of OP-induced inhibition. The difference in the effectiveness of atropine to prevent soman-induced convulsions in these two studies (Savolainen *et al.*, 1988a, b; Shih, 1990) may have been due to the different doses of atropine used. Long-term exposure to sublethal doses of soman results in behavioral supersensitivity to atropine, possibly due to downregulation in the number of muscarinic receptors in the brain (Modrow and McDonough, 1986).

Pazdernik *et al.* (1983) reported that administration of large doses of soman ($2 \times LD_{50}$) to rats protected with TAB [a mixture of trimedoxime (TMB-4), atropine, and benactyzine] resulted in approximately twofold reductions of LCGU in most brain regions. This was in contrast to the marked increase in LCGU that occurred in conjunction with the convulsions after a LD_{50} dose of soman. The results indicated that TAB is effective in protecting against soman-induced convulsions, but only at the expense of a severe decrease in LCGU after soman exposure. These findings are consistent with those of Shih *et al.* (1991a, b) (see subsequent text), who demonstrated a marked protection against soman-induced toxicity by atropine or benactyzine. When rats were given a convulsive dose of soman subsequent to pretreatment by diazepam, atropine, or benactyzine, both diazepam and benactyzine prevented convulsive activity, but atropine had no effect. All pretreatments attenuated LCGU with a unique pattern. In the pathology phase, 72 h postsoman, the marked reduction in LCGU and the conspicious brain damage associated with soman-induced convulsions was minimized with all three pretreatments (Pazdernik *et al.*, 1986).

Shih *et al.* (1991a, b) studied the efficacy of several drugs, especially antagonists of cholinergic muscarinic receptors, to prevent soman-induced toxicity, OP-induced convulsions, and death. In the absence of atropine sulfate, only tertiary anticholinergic drugs (scopolamine, trihexyphenidyl, biperidene, benactyzine, bentzatropine, azaprophen and aprophen), ceramiphen, carbetapentane, and the NMDA–receptor antagonist MK-801 were effective anticonvulsants. In the presence of atropine sulfate, the benzodiazepines (diazepam, midazolam, clonazepam, loprazolam, and alprazolam), mecamylamine, flunazirine, phenytoin, clonidine, CGS 19755 and Organon 6370 protected against soman-induced convulsions. The authors concluded that central muscarinic cholinergic mechanisms are primarily involved in eliciting the convulsions following exposure to soman and that subsequent recruitment of other excitatory neurotransmitter systems and loss of inhibitory control may be responsible for sustaining the convulsions and for producing the subsequent brain damage. These overall conclusions are consistent with a number of research articles (see Hirvonen *et al.*, 1993; Olney *et al.*, 1986; Savolainen *et al.*, 1988a, b, 1995, 1998; Solberg and Belkin, 1997).

50.8.2 ATTENUATION OF CHOLINERGIC EFFECTS BY ACETYLCHOLINESTERASE REACTIVATION

Because OP-induced cholinergic intoxication is due to inhibition of the enzyme that hydrolyzes ACh (i.e., AChE), it is natural that attempts have been made to develop drugs that alleviate OP-induced AChE inhibition (Shih *et al.*, 1991a, b). Emergency treatment is always necessary when dealing with OP poisoning. Even if cholinergic muscarinic agonists such as atropine and scopolamine are the first line of treatment in these cases, a supplementary treatment goal is AChE reactivation, which is necessary in many cases (see Shih *et al.*, 1991a, b; Ecobichon, 1996). Oximes (pralidoxime chloride or 2-PAM, pralidoxime methanesulfonate or P2S) are give intravenously to reactivate the nervous tissue AChE, and to alleviate nicotinic and muscarinic symptoms. The use of oximes is not necessary in mild intoxications, but may greatly amplify the effect of direct cholinergic antagonists to attenuate the cholinergic symptoms.

The therapeutic action of oximes is due to its ability to reactivate AChE without having marked toxic actions of their own. The basic requirements for a reactivating molecule of AChE consist of a rigid structure with a quaternary ammonium group and an acidic nucleophile. This nucleophile must be complementary to the phosphorylated (i.e., deactivated) enzyme in such a way that the nucleophilic oxygen is positioned close to the electrophilic phosphorus atom. These requirements lead to the development of 2-PAM. The reactivation is an equilibrium reaction, where the oxime reacts with the phosphorylated enzyme or with the free unbound OP ester. Development of new oximes has produced P2S, obidoxime [bis(4-formyl-*N*-methyl-pyridinium oxime)ether dichloride], TMB-4 [*N*,*N*-trimethylene bis(pyridine-4-aldoxime)bromide], and, more recently, the H-series compounds (Ecobichon, 1996; Shih *et al.*, 1991a, b; see subsequent text).

Ligtenstein and Moes (1991) utilized two OPs as AChE inhibitors. One is *S*-diethylaminoethyl-*O*-cyclohexyl-methyl-phosphonothionate, a tertiary amine that readily penetrates the CNS and, therefore, exhibits both central and peripheral AChE inhibiting properties. The other compound is the methiodide derivative of this agent, which has a strong and pH-independent ionic character that does not allow it to penetrate though the blood–brain barrier (BBB); thus, it does not gain access to the brain. Atropine sulfate inhibited convulsions and

toxicity induced by the former compound, but not lethality induced by the latter. The oxime (HI-6) used as the reactivator of AChE was more effective than atropine in both cases. Atropine and HI-6 together had a synergistic effect in the case of brain-penetrating compounds, but not in the case of an ionized OP agent. The authors concluded that a combination of atropine and an oxime is an effective combination when an OP has both central and peripheral actions. Several other investigators have confirmed the synergistic protective effect of the combination of atropine and various oximes against OP-induced poisoning in both humans and experimental animals (De Neef and Porsius, 1982; Endres *et al.*, 1989; Lallement *et al.*, 1997; Shih *et al.*, 1991a, b; Singh *et al.*, 1998). When diazepam was combined with atropine and an oxime, it further amplified the protection offered by the atropine–oxime combination (Lallement *et al.*, 1994a, b, 1997). In humans, administration of the oxime pralidoxime produced neurophysiological amelioriation in 11 out of 15 cases. The authors (Singh *et al.*, 1998) also emphasized that although the administration of three compounds—pralidoxime, magnesium sulfate, and pancuronium—resulted in the reversal of the neuroelectrophysiological defects, only pralidoxime was of true therapeutic value, but because of its short duration of action, frequent administration is required.

50.8.3 ATTENUATION OF CHOLINERGIC EFFECTS BY INCREASING GABAERGIC TONE IN THE CNS

Diazepam (5 mg/kg) effectively prevented soman-induced (100 μg/kg) overt convulsions, consistent with earlier observations (Lundy *et al.*, 1978), and markedly attenuated the soman-induced facilitation of PI signalling in rat brains (Savolainen *et al.*, 1988a, b). Doebler *et al.* (1985), in turn, observed that diazepam almost completely prevented soman-induced depletion of RNA in two brain regions, but did not affect the mean time of soman-induced death or 24-h survival. These data suggest that excessive neuronal activity *per se* may underlie the genesis of soman-induced central metabolic impairments. We could also conclude from these results that it is possible to dissociate epileptiform activity from the lethal action of soman. These data also provide evidence that cerebral GABAergic tone is involved in controlling brain metabolic events and the initiation of convulsions. These conclusions are in agreement with the findings of Gant *et al.* (1987), who suggested that there may be an interaction between GABA receptors and OP compounds in a manner that modifies OP toxicity.

50.8.4 THE ROLE OF EXCITATORY AMINO ACIDS

Excitatory amino acid (EAA) neurotransmitters have been implicated in the initiation and propagation of seizures, and the involvement of the NMDA class of glutamatergic EAA receptors has been demonstrated in several models of seizures (Dingledine *et al.*, 1990). Glutamate, acting through a number of EAA receptor subtypes including NMDA receptors, is known to evoke neuronal cell death (Meldrum and Garthwaite, 1990). Glutamate also has been implicated in cholinergic agonist-induced seizures (Hirvonen *et al.*, 1990, 1993; McDonough and Shih, 1997; Savolainen *et al.*, 1988a, b, 1998; Solberg and Belkin, 1997).

Dizocilpine (MK-801), a noncompetitive inhibitor of NMDA receptors, was given to guinea pigs either before or after a convulsive dose of soman. Pretreatment of the animals with MK-801 did not prevent or delay the onset of electrical seizure activity, but did diminish its intensity and led to its rapid termination. A large dose of MK-801 (5 mg/kg) was even able to prevent the appearance of seizures. Posttreatment of the animals with MK-801 prevented, arrested, or reduced seizure activity, convulsions, and neuronal death in a dose-dependent manner, pointing to a possible role for the NMDA receptor in the spread and maintenance of cholinergically induced seizures, although NMDA receptors themselves are not involved in seizure initiation. Shih (1990) made similar observations on the effects of MK-801 on soman-induced convulsions in a rat model. He found that MK-801 was an especially effective antidote against soman-induced convulsions when administered in conjunction with diazepam. Deshpande *et al.* (1995) observed that soman did not induce cytotoxicity in cultured hippocampal neurons, whereas exposure of these cells to glutamate did not induce death in 80% of the exposed cells. Memantine, a glutamate receptor antagonist, significantly protected the neurons against glutamate toxicity. When rats were pretreated with memantine 1 h prior to soman ($0.9 \times \mathrm{LD}_{50}$), the severity of convulsions as well as brain damage were significantly reduced, indicative of a role for glutamatergic receptors in soman-induced neurotoxicity. The role of glutamatergic receptors in soman-induced chlolinergic neurotoxicity was emphasized by the finding that a noncompetitive antagonist of NMDA receptors (thienylcyclohexylpiperidine) offered useful protection against soman-induced (62.5 µg/kg) seizures and lethality in guinea pigs (Carpentier *et al.*, 1994; Lallement *et al.*, 1994a, b).

Lallement *et al.* (1994a, b) found that administration of NBQX (2,3-dihydroxy-6-nitro-7-sulfamoylbenzoquinoxaline), a selective inhibitor of AMPA glutamatergic receptors, prevented the onset of soman-induced convulsions in rats. When NBQX was given after the soman injection, it also reduced the intensity of convulsions. These results clearly indicate that glutamatergic receptors are involved in OP-induced convulsions. This conclusion can be extended from NMDA glutamatergic receptors (see Carpentier *et al.*, 1994; Loikkanen *et al.*, 1998; Naarala *et al.*, 1997) to include non-NMDA glutamatergic receptors (Lallement *et al.*, 1994a, b) also. These studies (Carpentier *et al.*, 1994; Lallement *et al.*, 1994a, b) also indicate that atropine amplifies the attenuation of soman-induced convulsions obtained with both glutamatergic NMDA (TCP) and non-NMDA-receptors (NBQX) antagonists, highlighting the interaction between glutamatergic and cholinergic receptors in the initiation and propagation of convulsions (see Felipo *et al.*, 1998; Fig. 50.8).

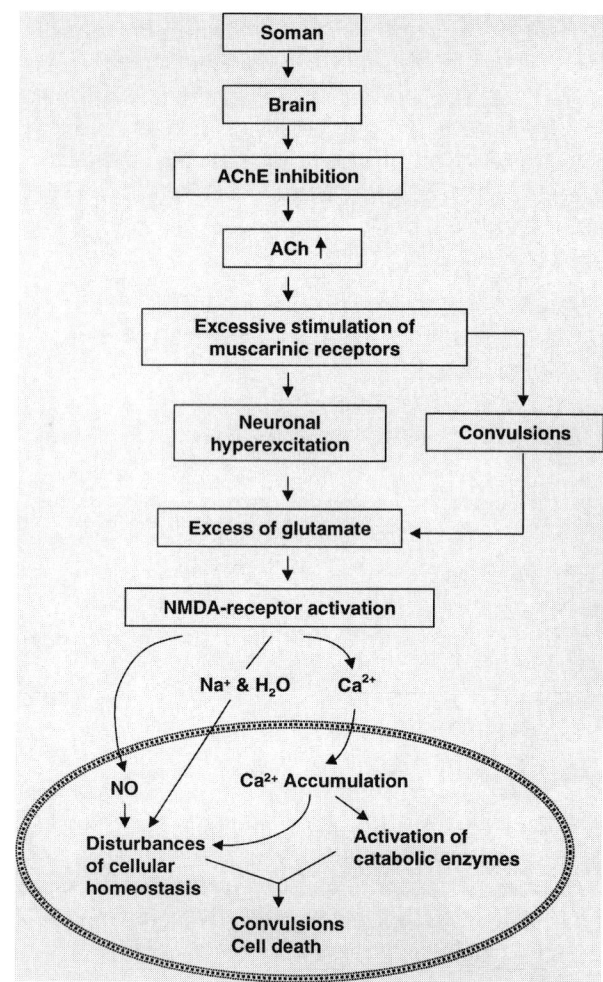

Figure 50.8 Pictorial representation of the role of glutamate in neuronal damage caused by intoxication with an organophosphate nerve agent, soman, subsequent inhibition of acetylcholinesterase, and acetylcholine accumulation in the central nervous system. Typically, excessive activation of muscarinic receptors leads to neuronal stimulation, subsequent convulsions, release of excessive amounts of glutamate, and NMDA receptor activation, which is followed by an influx of calcium to the neurons and subsequent programmed (apoptotic) or necrotic neuronal death. These terminal events are preceded by increased production of cellular messengers, such as nitric oxide and phosphoinositides, accumulation of free calcium in the cell, oxidative stress, alterations in gene expression, and serious dysfunction in the maintenance of cellular homeostasis.

50.8.5 DOWNREGULATION OF MUSCARINIC RECEPTORS

Lim *et al.* (1991) observed that simultaneous and continuous administration of physostigmine and trihexyphenidyl had protective effects against soman-induced toxicity in guinea pigs. Combination of these two compounds provided greater protection against soman-induced toxicity than either of the compounds alone. The antimuscarinic properties of trihexyphenidyl and protection of AChE activity by physostigmine against irreversible enzyme inhibition by soman may be responsible for the protective effect of this drug combination. When physostigmine was given alone, it also provided protection against soman toxicity; this protection was amplified when scopolamine was given simultaneously with physostigmine. Physostigmine-induced protection was due to the well-known tolerance toward its AChE-inhibiting properties, whereas scopolamine-induced protection was due to its antimuscarinic effects. Jointly these protective effects seem to provide marked protection against soman-induced convulsions and lethality (Philippens *et al.*, 1998). Shih *et al.* (1993) reported that the antiparkinsonian drugs biperidene and trihexyphenidyl provide protection against soman-induced toxicity; this is likely due to their antimuscarinic effects rather than their secondary effects of cerebral dopamine turnover. Aronstam *et al.* (1987) even found that clonidine, a centrally acting α-2 adrenergic agonist (Buccafusco and Aronstam, 1986), given prior to soman administration prevented the decrease in receptor number and decreased the extent of AChE inhibition caused by soman. The authors concluded that clonidine may protect AChE from irreversible inhibition by soman, thereby decreasing the extent of cholinergic overstimulation with its attendant downregulation of muscarinic receptors. Buccafusco and Aronstam (1986) found that clonidine provided protection against soman-induced toxicity including tremors, convulsions, and Straub tail, as well as excessive salivation that results from activation of peripheral muscarinic receptors. Atropine further amplified the clonidine-induced protection against soman intoxication. Clonidine noncompetitively inhibited AChE *in vitro* and *in vivo*, and also inhibited ligand binding to cortical muscarinic receptors *in vitro*. The authors concluded that the protective effects of clonidine are likely to involve multiple effects, including blockade of acetylcholine release and postsynaptic muscarinic receptors, and transient inhibition of AChE.

50.8.6 AMPLIFICATION OF CHOLINERGIC-INDUCED CONVULSIONS

Inhibition or attenuation of receptor-mediated responses is usually easier than amplification. In the case of cholinergic receptors, a number of antagonists exist for both cholinergic muscarinic and nicotinic receptors (McDonough and Shih, 1997; Minton and Murray, 1988). Even if amplification of cholinergic receptor-mediated responses does not have any therapeutic or practical value, understanding the mechanisms involved in amplification of cholinergic-induced responses may provide valuable insight into the receptor mechanisms. Amplification of muscarinic receptor-mediated cellular and molecular events, and subsequent behavioral changes such as convulsions have been intensively investigated. Honchar *et al.* (1983) initially showed that pretreatment of rats with lithium chloride greatly amplified cholinergic-induced convulsions and further facilitated the associated cerebral PI signalling. Savolainen *et al.* (1988a, b, 1991) and Hirvonen *et al.* (1989, 1990, 1993) showed in a number of studies that lithium pretreatment greatly amplified convulsions induced in rats by OPs such as soman, DFP, paraoxon, and malaoxon, as well as convulsions produced by

a direct cholinergic agonist, pilocarpine. In the case of several OPs, pretreatment of rats with lithium increased their sensitivity to cholinergic-induced convulsions by about two- to threefold (Savolainen *et al.*, 1991). Several investigators (Honchar *et al.*, 1983; Berridge, 1989) hypothesized that lithium's ability to decrease the threshold for cholinergic-induced convulsions or amplify these convulsions is due to the noncompetitive inhibition of PI metabolism. This blockade of myo-inositol-1-phosphatase leads to a dramatic accumulation of myo-inositol-1-phosphate in the brain. Later studies provided evidence that most likely this is not the case. Instead, the interaction between lithium and cholinergic stimulation seems to take place at the G-protein level, that is, lithium may affect the coupling mechanisms of cholinergic muscarinic receptors (Jope, 1988; Jope *et al.*, 1986; Savolainen *et al.*, 1995).

50.9 EFFECTS ON AUTONOMIC GANGLIA

Heppner and Fiekers (1992) explored the prevention and the reversal of the effects of soman on the electrical properties of sympathetic ganglion neurons *in vitro* from the adult bullfrog *Rana catesbeiana*. Atropine pretreatment (10 μM) blocked the soman-induced decrease in the membrane potential, membrane resistance, and duration of the afterhyperpolarization. Atropine posttreatment restored the soman-induced decrease in the membrane potential, but was ineffective in reversing either the change in membrane resistance or the duration of the afterhyperpolarization. These authors concluded that the effects of soman on the electrical properties of these neurons are mediated by the activation of muscarinic receptors, and that following receptor activation, different cellular mechanisms may be involved in the regulation of the electrical properties of the neuron. The results also indicated that pre-OP rather than post-OP treatment with atropine was more effective in blocking these direct effects of soman.

50.10 EFFECTS ON THE NEUROMUSCULAR ENDPLATE AND MUSCLE CELLS

Acetylcholinesterase inhibition can lead to severe neuromuscular dysfunction. For example, the OP anticholinesterase, paraoxon, produces a dose-dependent necrosis in the rat skeletal muscle fibers even after a single administration. The pathology, initially concentrated around the neuromuscular endplate region, already is evident 30 min after paraoxon administration. By 24 h, a generalized breakdown of muscle fiber architecture is apparent with an accompanying infiltration of phagocytes. Electrophysiological studies indicate that paraoxon increases neurotransmitter release and causes spontaneous and impulse-related antidromic nerve activity, both of which can be reduced markedly by reactivation of inhibited AChE with the oxime 2-PAM. Furthermore, the severity of the pathology is positively correlated to the degree and duration of AChE inhibition: the critical loss of AChE activity is 85% provided the inhibition lasts at least for 2 h (see Wecker *et al.*, 1978).

50.10.1 ELECTROPHYSIOLOGICAL EFFECTS

Electromyographic (EMG) features of OP poisoning include (1) repetitive activity (RA) in response to single nerve stimuli and (2) two types of decremental responses to repetitive nerve stimulation (RNS). The smallest amplitude can either occur in the second response, with a subsequent gradual recovery (decrement–increment phenomenon), or the amplitude can progressively decline toward further responses (decrement phenomenon; Besser *et al.*, 1989). Paraoxon and fenthion both induced RA and decrements in RNS in rats as the main EMG findings in both types of OP intoxications. Various types of impairment of neuromuscular transmission seem to coexist, most likely due to variations present at distinct stages of anticholinesterase poisoning (De Bleecker *et al.*, 1994). Paraoxon (10^{-9}–10^{-3} M) produced repetitive nerve terminal activity as well as accelerated MEPP frequency at the neuromuscular junction in an isolated muscle. At high concentrations, paraoxon also depolarized the muscle membrane, especially in the endplate regions. The depolarizing effects of paraoxon, due to ACh accumulation, are mediated through nicotinic ACh receptors because they can be attenuated by d-tubocurarine. They occur when muscle membrane AChE is inhibited to about 32% of the control levels. The fact that pretreatment with 2-PAM prevented paraoxon-induced depolarization indicates that AChE on the outer membrane was essential for the effect because 2-PAM, which is a quaternary ammonium compound, does not cross the cellular membrane. These findings support the proposal that both the pre- and the postsynaptic actions of paraoxon are consequences of AChE inhibition and are not caused by any direct effects of paraoxon (Laskowski and Dettbarn, 1979).

50.10.2 NEUROMUSCULAR TRANSMISSION

Van Dongen *et al.* (1988) explored the role of *de novo* synthesis of AChE in the spontaneous recovery of neuromuscular transmission in isolated diaphragms from soman-intoxicated rats. Within 10 min after soman administration, neuromuscular transmission was completely blocked, but AChE activity in endplate and endplate-free regions recovered linearly during the next 3 h, and neuromuscular transmission also improved. This recovery could not be attributed to synthesis of AChE because *de novo* synthesis of AChE had been blocked by cycloheximide and reinhibition of AChE was ensured with an additional dose of soman. Thus, this recovery in muscular activity seemed to be independent of AChE activity. Smith and Wolthuis (1983) exposed rhesus monkeys to soman and then treated the animals with the oxime HI6. Soman exposure induced neuromuscular blockade in intercostal and diaphragm muscle strips that could be partially relieved by their exposure to the AChE activating oxime.

50.10.3 EFFECTS OF ACETYLCHOLINESTERASE REACTIVATORS

Rats poisoned with sarin, soman, or VX and then administered two bispyridium oximes, BDB-27 and HGG-12, were tested for their ability to restore neuromuscular function in isolated phrenic nerve–diaphragm preparations. These results were compared with the traditional oximes HI-6 and TMB-4. BDB-27 was equal or superior to HI-6 in sarin, soman, and VX poisoning and better than TMB-4 in tabun poisoned animals. However, recovery of function after HGG-12 was equal to HI-6 only in soman poisoning, but much less pronounced against neuromuscular blockade induced by the three other OPs (Jovanovic, 1983). Several investigators (Bhattacharyya *et al.*, 1990; Ozkutlu *et al.*, 1995) also showed that hemicholinium-3 and its analogs provide protection against OP-induced toxicity. These drugs, which block choline uptake, were able to provide significant antagonism against OPs and also to produced a profound nicotinic receptor desensitization as reflected in reductions to indirect or directly evoked EPC (endplate current). Whereas these effects were voltage-dependent, they may be due to reduction of endplate permeability, rather than to blockage of ACh synthesis, because it has been claimed that hemicholinium can also block nicotinic receptor associated ion channels in their open form (Bhattacharyya *et al.*, 1990).

50.10.4 MUSCARINIC RECEPTOR DOWNREGULATION

Single and short-term inhalation of soman in rats reduced subsequent sensitivity of smooth muscle to contraction induced by cholinergic stimulation. A single exposure to 8.51 mg/m^3 of soman for 45 min inhibited bronchial smooth muscle AChE by 85% and reduced the contraction induced by carbachol and/or ACh by 70–80%. This exposure did not induce alterations in [^{3}H]QNB binding. However, consecutive exposures to low doses of soman (0.45–0.63 mg/m^3) markedly reduced [^{3}H]QNB binding in bronchial smooth muscle, in addition to evoking AChE inhibition and inhibiting the ACh- and carbachol-induced concentration of smooth muscle (Aas *et al.*, 1987). These results indicate that short-term inhalation of relatively low concentrations of soman reduces the number of cholinergic muscarinic receptors in the peripheral cholinergic system.

50.11 EFFECTS ON CARDIOVASCULAR AND RESPIRATORY SYSTEMS AND TEMPERATURE CONTROL

Anticholinesterase OP compounds have widespread effects on both the cardiovascular and respiratory systems because both are under the control of the parasympathetic and sympathetic divisions of the autonomic nervous system. In autonomic ganglia, ACh serves as the primary neurotransmitter. Furthermore, ACh also serves as a transmitter at the neuromuscular endplate in both skeletal and smooth muscles. Administration of 32, 80, or 160 µg/kg of soman to guinea pigs resulted in respiratory arrest followed by circulatory failure and death. Atropine treatment restored the circulatory parameters and improved respiration. However, atropine was ineffective after very high doses of soman ($10 \times LD_{50}$). These results indicate that soman-induced respiratory depression is mainly due to CNS affects and that a significant neuromuscular block develops only at very high doses of soman. The circulatory disturbances are mainly caused by bradycardia that results from peripheral muscarinic stimulation in the heart (Worek and Szinicz, 1993). ACh reduced atrial contraction by 82.5, 50.8, and 41.5% in rats, guinea pigs, and rabbits, respectively. The EC_{50} values for the negative inotropic effect of ACh were 3.3×10^{-7} M in rat and guinea pig atria, and 4.1×10^{-6} M in rabbit atria. However, there was no correlation between the species differences in the negative inotropic effect of ACh in the atria and the density or affinity of AChE or the characteristics of muscarinic receptors. Inhibition of atrial AChE with soman reduced the EC_{50} of ACh by threefold in all species, but did not change the maximal inotropic effect of ACh. The authors hypothesized that species differences in the negative inotropic effect of ACh may be due to differences in the coupling between myocardial muscarinic receptors and the ion channels that mediate negative inotropy (Maxwell *et al.*, 1991).

Worek *et al.* (1994) observed that atropine treatment was very effective in improving the respiratory function after a dose of 60 µg/kg of tabun, but ineffective when tabun was given at a dose of 300 µg/kg. However, the circulatory parameters were restored almost completely in all atropine treated groups. However, when atropine was combined with an oxime, such as obidoxime, Hlö 7, or HI 6, the antidotal efficacy of the combination was markedly improved over atropine alone. Atropine was especially effective in restoring circulation, but respiration could be improved only in cases of intoxication with low doses of tabun. The results of this study demonstrated the remarkable synergistic protective effect of atropine and an AChE reactivator against tabun-induced circulatory and respiratory failure, both of which seem to be strictly mediated via the cholinergic system.

Chiou and Li (1994) studied the effects of cholinolytic agents (i.e., ganglion blocking drugs) on cardiovascular effects of DFP intoxication in rats. The lethal action of DFP (8 mg/kg) was partially or completely prevented by pretreatment with hexamethonium (10 mg/kg), trimethaphan (80 mg/kg), and mecamylamine (30 mg/kg). The combined effects of these drugs with an AChE reactivator 2-PAM (100 mg/kg) greatly improved the prophylaxis of presynaptic cholinolytic drugs against DFP intoxication. Even though the exact mechanism of action of these drugs remains to be elucidated, DFP induced cardiovascular suppression before neuromuscular blockade, indicating that the cardiovascular system is more sensitive to the effects of OPs than the neuromuscular junction. Kubinec *et al.* (1987) found that when rats were treated with paraoxon, signif-

icant decreases in heart cholinergic muscarinic receptor densities occurred both in the atria and ventricles after several daily injections; these changes were associated with decreased levels of cardiac AChE activity. Thus, we cannot exclude the possibility that downregulation of cholinergic muscarinic receptors may be involved in the effects of OPs on the cardiovascular system.

Bartholomew *et al.* (1985) explored the mechanism of OP-induced depression of the respiratory center in the brain stem, bronchoconstriction, increased secretions in the airways, and paralysis of the respiratory musculature in rats. After 14 daily doses of malathion (400 mg/kg), the activities of AChE were 26–28% in the striatum (ST), hippocampus (HI), and cortex (CX), but 41% in the brain stem of the corresponding control values. Furthermore, there was a marked reduction in the numbers of mAChRs in ST, HI, and CX, but not in the brain stem. The authors concluded that the mechanisms by which the respiratory center in the brain stem adapts to the effects of OP exposure differ from responses to OPs in the rest of the CNS.

Clement (1991, 1993a, b) studied the effects of OP anticholinesterase agents on temperature control in experimental animals. Several studies have shown that subchronic administration of a cholinergic agonist or an AChE inhibitor frequently results in tolerance to its behavioral effects. Tolerance to the OP compound DFP was characterized by a decrease in the symptoms of poisoning, such as salivation, lacrimation, and hypothermia (Gupta and Dettbarn, 1986; Lomax *et al.*, 1986; Overstreet *et al.*, 1973), and a decrease in the number but no change in the affinity of muscarinic receptors in various regions in the brain (Churchill *et al.*, 1984a, b; Yamada *et al.*, 1983). Likewise, following acute (Aronstam *et al.*, 1987) or subchronic (Churchill *et al.*, 1984a, b) administration of soman, there was a decrease in the number of muscarinic receptors in the brain (i.e., receptor downregulation). Repeated administration of soman and DFP induced tolerance toward OP-induced hypothermia after a few doses, and this effect showed cross-tolerance with a direct cholinergic agonist, oxotremorine (Clement, 1991). In later studies, Clement (1993a) suggested that soman-induced hypothermia may be due to the recovery of AChE, perhaps from the assembly of previously synthesized precursors. Soman hypothermia appears to be due to muscarinic receptor activation and can be partially, but not completely, antagonized by atropine. Thus, soman-induced hypothermia is primarily a muscarinic receptor-related event (Clement, 1993b).

50.12 SUMMARY AND CONCLUSIONS

Insecticidal OPs and nerve gases cause their effects by inhibiting AChE, thereby leading to ACh accumulation. The rapidity of this accumulation depends on the inhibition rate of the AChE by the OP; thus, different OPs can have different effects. The signs and symptoms of OP intoxication are due to activation of cholinergic muscarinic and nicotinic receptors. Muscarinic receptor-mediated effects include convulsions, smooth muscle activation, and increased secretions, whereas nicotinic receptor-induced effects are due to activation of autonomic ganglia and neuromuscular endplates, leading to muscular dysfunctions and cardiovascular effects such as bradycardia. Muscarinic receptors are membrane integral proteins, so-called transmembrane G-protein-coupled receptors, most of which mediate their effects through generation of calcium-mobilizing second messengers, inositol phosphates. Some of the muscarinic receptors, however, mediate their effects by inhibiting adenylate cyclase, thereby decreasing cellular cAMP levels. Nicotinic receptors are ion channels that open to permit preferential influx of sodium into the cell. Muscarinic receptor activation can be blocked by muscarinic antagonists such as atropine, but atropine is not effective in inhibiting nicotinic receptor activation. d-Tubocurarine and its analogs can be used to block nicotinic receptors. Both receptor systems contribute to OP-induced lethalities. The muscarinic receptors are involved in convulsions and their associated neuronal damage—depression of the respiratory center, and increased bronchoconstriction and bronchial secretions. Nicotinic receptors cause muscle fasciculations, flaccid paralysis, and hypertension. Cholinergic muscarinic receptors have widespread effects on cellular function in the CNS and periphery by altering cell signalling, gene expression, cellular metabolism, levels of brain neurotransmitters, and brain electrophysiology. Muscarinic receptor activation can be modulated by a number of antagonists, including muscarinic antagonists, which may be especially effective when combined with oximes, so-called AChE reactivators. Whereas brain cholinergic systems seem to be at least under partial GABAergic control, benzodiazepines can also be used as antidotes for OP-induced convulsions. Recent observations indicate that cholinergic muscarinic stimulation may be the trigger that evokes convulsions, but that subsequent glutamate release may be necessary for their maintenance and propagation. Antagonists of both NMDA and non-NMDA glutamate receptor antagonists have been proven to be effective antagonists of muscarinic receptor-mediated intoxication, including OP-induced intoxication. Glutamate also may be important in cholinergic-induced toxicity because this amino acid transmitter is involved in neuronal programmed cell death, or apoptosis (see Nicotera *et al.*, 1999). This OP-induced neurotoxicity can be prevented at least partially by using glutamatergic antagonists. This information provides new insights into cholinergic toxicity and also opens new vistas for research to explore mechanisms of OP toxicity. The essential elements of apoptosis, such as DNA fragmentation, mitochondrial failure, activation of caspases, and cytochrome *c* release, need to be clarified in this context. The role of nicotinic receptors, which are also important in OP-induced intoxication, has been better clarified, but it also requires further research. Nicotinic receptor activation in autonomic ganglia and neuromuscular endplates can be blocked by nicotinic antagonists, although this is more difficult to achieve than blockade of muscarinic receptors. Because many OP compounds, especially the insecticides and nerve agents, are often extremely toxic, a thorough understanding of their basic mechanisms of action is

necessary if effective therapeutic agents and measures are to be developed.

REFERENCES

Aas, P., Veiteberg, T. A., and Fonnum, F. (1987). Acute and sub-acute inhalation of an organophosphate induced alteration of cholinergic muscarinic receptors. *Biochem. Pharmacol.* **36**(8), 1261–1266.

Abdallah, E. A. M., Jett, D. A., Eldefrawi, M. E., and Eldefrawi, A. T. (1992). Differential effects of paraoxon on the M_3 muscarinic receptor and its effector system in rat submaxillary gland cells. *J. Biochem. Toxicol.* **7**(2), 125–132.

Ahlbom, J., Fredriksson, A., and Eriksson, P. (1995). Exposure to an organophosphate (DFP) during a defined period in neonatal life induces permanent changes in brain muscarinic receptors and behaviour in adult mice. *Brain Res.* **677**, 13–19.

Aldridge, W. N., ed. (1996). "Mechanisms and Concepts in Toxicology." Taylor & Francis, London.

Aldridge, W. N., and Reiner, E. (1972). "Enzyme Inhibitors as Substrates. Interaction of Esterases of Organophosphorus and Carbamic Esters." North-Holland, Amsterdam.

Alha, A. (1967). Forensic-chemically detected poisonings in Finland in 1966. *Acta Neurol. Scand.* **43**(Suppl. 31), 133.

Antonelli, T., Beani, L., Bianchi, L., Pedata, F., and Pepeu, G. (1981). Changes in synaptosomal high affinity choline uptake following electrical stimulation of guinea-pig cortical slices: Effect of atropine and physostigmine. *Br. J. Pharmacol.* **74**, 525–531.

Anzueto, A., Berdine, G. G., Moore, G. T., Gleiser, C., Johnson, D., White, C. D., and Johanson, W. G., Jr. (1986). Pathophysiology of soman intoxication in primates. *Toxicol. Appl. Pharmacol.* **86**, 56–68.

Arenander, A. T., de Vellis, J., and Hershiman, H. R. (1989). Induction of *c-fos* and TIS genes in cultured rat astrocytes by neurotransmitters. *J. Neurosci. Res.* **24**, 107–114.

Aronstam, R. S., Smith, M. D., and Buccafusco, J. L. (1987). Clonidine prevents the short-term down regulation of muscarinic receptors in the mouse brain induced by the acetylcholinesterase inhibitor soman. *Neurosci. Lett.* **78**, 107–112.

Ashkenazi, A., Ramachandron, J., and Capon, D. J. (1989). Acetylcholine analogue estimates DNA synthesis in brain-derived cells via specific muscarinic receptor subtypes. *Nature* **340**, 146–150.

Bakry, N. M. S., El-Rashidy, A. H., Eldefrawi, A. T., and Eldefrawi, M. E. (1988). Direct actions of organophosphate anticholinesterases on nicotinic and muscarinic acetylcholine receptors. *J. Biochem. Toxicol.* **3**, 235–259.

Baraban, J. M., Snyder, S. H., and Alger, B. E. (1985). Protein kinase C regulates ionic conductance in hippocampal pyramidal neurons: Electrophysiological effects of phorbol esters. *Proc. Natl. Acad. Sci. U.S.A.* **82**, 2538–2542.

Bartholomew, P. M., Gianutsos, G., and Cohen, S. D. (1985). Differential cholinesterase inhibition and muscarinic receptor changes in CD-1 mice made tolerant to malathion. *Toxicol. Appl. Pharmacol.* **81**, 147–155.

Berridge, M. J. (1987). Inositol triphosphate and diacylglycerol: Two interacting second messengers. *Ann. Rev. Biochem.* **56**, 159–193.

Berridge, M. J. (1989). Inositol trisphosphate, calcium, lithium, and cell signalling. *JAMA* **262**, 1834–1841.

Berridge, M. J., and Irvine, R. F. (1989). Inositol phosphates and cell signalling. *Nature* **341**, 97–205.

Besser, R., Gutmann, L., Dillmann, U., Weilemann, L. S., and Hopf, H. C. (1989). End-plate dysfunction in acute organophosphate intoxication. *Neurology* **39**, 561–567.

Bhattacharyya, B., Sokoll, M. D., Flynn, S. J. R., Nyanda, A. M., Lee, T., Cannon, J. G., and Long, J. P. (1990). Mechanism for antagonism of paraoxon by hemicholinium-3 analogues. *Arch. Int. Pharmacodyn.* **308**, 149–167.

Blanchet, G., Baubichon, D., Mavet, S., Morelis, P., and Lemercier, G. (1986). Modulation of the number of muscarinic receptors in mouse neuroblastoma cells by soman. *Biochem. Pharmacol.* **35**(22), 4077–4081.

Bodjarian, N., Lallement, G., Carpentier, P., Baubichon, D., and Blanchet, G. (1992). Soman-induced phosphoinositide hydrolysis in rat hippocampal slices: Biochemical characterization. *NeuroToxicology* **13**, 715–722.

Bodjarian, N., Carpentier, P., Baubichon, D., Blanchet, G., and Lallement, G. (1995). Involvement of non-muscarinic receptors in phosphoinositide signalling during soman-induced seizures. *Eur. J. Pharmacol.* **289**, 291–297.

Buccafusco, J. J., and Aronstam, R. S. (1986). Clonidine protection from the toxicity of soman, an organophosphate acetylcholinesterase inhibitor, in the mouse. *J. Pharmacol. Exp. Ther.* **239**(1), 43–47.

Buckley, N. J., Bonner, T. I., Buckley, C. M., and Brann, M. R. (1989). Antagonist binding properties of five cloned muscarinic receptors expressed in CHO-K1 cell. *Mol. Pharmacol.* **35**, 469–476.

Busija, D. W., Wagerle, L. C., Pourcyrous, M., and Leffler, C. W. (1988). Acetylcholine dramatically increases prostanoid synthesis in piglet parietal cortex. *Brain Res.* **439**, 122–126.

Carpentier, P., Foquin-Tarricone, A., Bodjarian, N., Rondouin, G., Lerner-Natoli, M., Kamenka, J.-M., Blanchet, G., Denoyer, M., and Lallement, G. (1994). Anticonvulsant and antilethal effects of the phencyclidine derivative TCP in soman poisoning. *NeuroToxicology* **15**(4), 837–852.

Caulfield, M. P. (1993). Muscarinic receptors–characterization, coupling and function. *Pharmacol. Ther.* **58**(3), 319–379.

Ceccatelli, S., Villar, M. J., Goldstein, M., and Hökfelt, T. (1989). Expression of c-Fos immunoreactivity in transmitter-characterized neurons after stress. *Proc. Natl. Acad. Sci. U.S.A.* **86**, 9569–9573.

Changeux, J.-P., Devilers-Thierry, A., and Chemuivilli, P. (1984). Acetylcholine receptor: An allosteric protein. *Science* **25**, 1335–1345.

Chaudhuri, J., Chakraborti, T. K., Chanda, S., and Pope, C. N. (1993). Differential modulation of organophosphate-sensitive muscarinic receptors in rat brain by parathion and chlorpyrifos. *J. Biochem. Toxicol.* **8**(4), 207–216.

Chemnitius, J.-M., Haselmeyer, K.-H., and Zech, R. (1983). Brain cholinesterases: Differentiation of target enzymes for toxic organophosphorus compounds. *Biochem. Pharmacol.* **32**, 1693–1699.

Chi, M., and Sun, M. (1995). Action of organophosphate anticholinesterases on the three conformational states of nicotinic receptor. *Adv. Exp. Med. Biol.* **363**, 65–73.

Chiou, G. C. Y., and Li, B. H. (1994). Prevention of organophosphate intoxication with presynaptic cholinergic blockers. *Life Sci.* **55**(1), 69–75.

Choi, P. T.-L., Quinonez, L. G., and Cook, D. J. (1995). Acute organophosphate insecticide poisoning. *Clin. Intensive Care* **6**, 228–235.

Churchill, L., Pazdernik, T. L., Jackson, J. L., Nelson, S. R., Samson, F. E., and McDonough, J. H., Jr. (1984a). Topographical distribution of decrements and recovery in muscarinic receptors from rat brains repeatedly exposed to sublethal doses of soman. *J. Neurosci.* **4**, 2069–2079.

Churchill, L., Pazdernik, T. L., Samson, F., and Nelson, S. R. (1984b). Topographical distribution of down-regulated muscarinic receptors in rat brains after repeated exposure to diisopropyl phosphorofluoridate. *J. Neurosci.* **11**, 463–472.

Churchill, L., Pazdernik, T. L., Jackson, J. L., Nelson, S. R., Samson, F. E., McDonough, J. H., Jr., and McLeod, C. G., Jr. (1985). Soman-induced brain lesions demonstrated by muscarinic receptor autoradiography. *NeuroToxicology* **6**(3), 81–90.

Churchill, L., Pazdernik, T. L., Cross, R. S., Giesler, M. P., Nelson, S. R., and Samson, F. E. (1987). Cholinergic systems influence local cerebral glucose use in specific anatomical areas: Diisopropyl phosphorofluoridate versus soman. *Neuroscience* **20**(1), 329–339.

Churchill, L., Pazdernik, T. L., Cross, R. S., Nelson, S. R., and Samson, F. E. (1990). Soman- or kainic acid-induced convulsions decrease muscarinic receptors but not benzodiazepine receptors. *NeuroToxicology* **11**, 57–72.

Clement, J. G. (1991). Hypothermia: Limited tolerance to repeated soman administration and cross-tolerance to oxotremorine. *Pharmacol., Biochem. Behav.* **39**, 305–312.

Clement, J. G. (1993a). Recovery from soman-induced hypothermia is due to an increase in acetylcholinesterase activity but not new protein synthesis. *NeuroToxicity* **14**(4), 411–416.

Clement, J. G. (1993b). Pharmacological nature of soman-induced hypothermia in mice. *Pharmacol., Biochem. Behav.* **44**, 689–702.

Cockcroft, S. (1986) The dependence on CA^{2+} of the guanine-nucleotide-activated polyphosphoinositide phosphodiesterase in neutrophil plasma membranes. *Biochem. J.* **249**, 503–507.

Collingridge, G. L., Harvey, J., Frenguelli, B. G., Bortolotto, Z. A., Bashir, Z. I., and Davies, C. A. (1992). Amino acid receptors and long term potentiation: Targets for the development of cognitive enhancers. *Int. Acad. Biomed. Drug Res.* **2**, 41–49.

Coudray-Lucas, C., Prioux-Guyonneau, M., Sentenac, H., Cohen, Y., and Wepierre, J. (1984). Effects of physostigmine, paraoxon and soman on brain GABA level and metabolism. *Acta Pharmacol. Toxicol.* **55**, 153–157.

Cross, A. J., Johnson, J. A., Frith, C., and Taylor, G. R. (1984). Muscarinic cholinergic receptors in a rat phaeochromocytoma cell line. *Biochem. Biophys. Res. Commun.* **119**(1), 163–167.

De Bleecker, J. L., De Reuck, J. L., and Willems, J. L. (1992). Neurological aspects of organophosphate poisoning. *Clin. Neurol. Neurosurg.* **94**, 93–103.

De Bleecker, J. L., Van Den Abeele, K., and De Reuck, J. (1994). Electromyography in relation to end-plate acetylcholinesterase in rats poisoned by different organophosphates. *NeuroToxicology* **15**(2), 331–340.

De Neef, J. H., and Porsius, A. J. (1982). The influence of obidoxime, diacetylmonoxime, pralidoxime, and two less hydrophilic derivatives of pralidoxime upon the cholinesterase inhibition and the pressor effect by paraoxon in the rat. *Toxicol. Appl. Pharmacol.* **66**, 244–251.

Deshpande, S. S., Smith, C. D., and Filbert, M. G. (1995). Assessment of primary neuronal culture as a model for soman-induced neurotoxicity and effectiveness of memantine as a neuroprotective drug. *Arch. Toxicol.* **69**, 384–390.

Dingledine, R., McBrain, C. J., and McNamara, J. O. (1990). Excitatory amino acid receptors in epilepsy. *Trends Pharmacol. Sci.* **11**, 334–338.

Doebler, J. A., Moore, R. A., Wall, T. J., and Anthony, A. (1983a). Brain neuronal RNA metabolism during sustained low-level soman toxication. *Life Sci.* **34**, 659–667.

Doebler, J. A., Bocan, T. M. A., Moore, R. A., Shih, T.-M., and Anthony, A. (1983b). Brain neuronal RNA metabolism during acute soman toxication: Effects of antidotal pretreatments. *Neurochem. Res.* **8**(8), 997–1011.

Doebler, J. A., Wall, T. J., Martin, L. J., Shih, T.-M. A., and Anthony, A. (1985). Effects of diazepam on soman-induced brain neuronal RNA depletion and lethality in rats. *Life Sci.* **36**, 1107–1115.

Downes, C. P., and Michell, R. H. (1981). The polyphosphoinositide phosphodiesterase of erythrocyte membranes. *Biochem. J.* **203**, 169–177.

Doyere, V., and Laroche, S. (1992). Linear relationship between maintenance of hippocampal long-term potentiation and retention of an associative memory. *Hippocampus* **2**, 39–48.

Dypbukt, J. M., Ankarcrona, M., Burkitt, M., Sjöholm, Å., Ström, K., Orrenius, S., and Nicotera, P. (1994). Different prooxidant levels stimulate growth, trigger apoptosis, or produce necrosis of insulin-secreting RINm5F cells. *J. Biol. Chem.* **269**, 30553–30560.

Ecobichon, D. J. (1996). Toxic effects of pesticides. In "Casarett & Doull's Toxicology: The Basic Science of Poisons" (C. D. Klaassen, ed.), pp. 643–689. McGraw-Hill, New York.

El-Etri, M. M., Nickell, W. T., Ennis, M., Skau, K. A., and Shipley, M. T. (1992). Brain norepinephrine reductions in soman-intoxicated rats: Association with convulsions and AChE inhibition, time course, and relation to other monoamines. *Exp. Neurol.* **118**, 153–163.

Endres, W., Spuler, A., and ten Bruggencate, G. (1989). Acetylcholinesterase reactivators antagonize epileptiform bursting induced by paraoxon in guinea pig hippocampal slices. *J. Pharmacol. Exp. Ther.* **251**(3), 1181–1186.

Erulkar, S. D. (1989). Chemically mediated synaptic transmission: An overview. In "Basic Neurochemistry" (G. Sieger, B. Agranoff, R. W. Albers, and P. Molinoff, eds.), 4th ed., pp. 151–182. Raven Press, New York.

Fain, J. N., Wallace, M. A., and Wojcikiewicz, R. J. H. (1988). Evidence for involvement of guanine nucleotide-binding regulatory proteins in the activation of phospholipases by hormones. *FASEB J.* **2**, 2569–2574.

Felder, C. C., Kanterman, R. Y., Ma, A. L., and Axelrod, J. (1989). A transfected M1 muscarinic acetylcholine receptor stimulates adenylate cyclase via phosphatidylinositol hydrolysis. *J. Biol. Chem.* **264**, 20,365–20,362.

Felipo, V., Hermenegildo, C., Montoliu, C., Llansola, M., and Minana, M.-D. (1998). Neurotoxicity of ammonia and glutamate: molecular mechanisms and prevention. *NeuroToxicology* **19**(4-5), 675–682.

Finkelstein, Y., Wolff, M., and Biegon, A. (1988). Brain acetylcholinesterase after acute parathion poisoning: A comparative quantitative histochemical analysis post mortem. *Ann. Neurol.* **24**(2), 252–257.

Fisher, S. K., Klinger, P. D., and Agranoff, B. W. (1983). Muscarinic agonist binding and phospholipid turnover in brain. *J. Biol. Chem.* **258**, 7358–7363.

Fonnum, F., and Guttormsen, D. M. (1969). Changes in acetylcholine content of rat brain by toxic doses of di-isopropyl phosphorofluoridate. *Experientia* **25**, 505–506.

Fosbraey, P., Wetherell, J. R., and French, M. C. (1990). Neurotransmitter changes in guinea-pig brain regions following soman intoxication. *J. Neurochem.* **54**(1), 72–79.

Fuortes, L. J., Ayebo, A. D., and Kross, B. C. (1993). Cholinesterase-inhibiting insecticide toxicity. *Am. Fam. Physician* **47**(7), 1613–1620.

Gant, D. B., Eldefrawi, M. E., and Eldefrawi, A. T. (1987). Action of organophosphates on $GABA_A$ receptor and voltage-dependent chloride channels. *Fundam. Appl. Toxicol.* **9**, 698–704.

Gilman, A. G. (1987). G proteins: Transducers of receptor-generated signals. *Annu. Rev. Biochem.* **56**, 615–649.

Gralewicz, S., and Socko, R. (1997). Persisting behavioural and electroencephalographic effects of exposure to chlorphenvinphos, an organophosphorous pesticide, in laboratory animals. *Int. J. Occup. Med. Environ. Health* **10**(4), 375–394.

Greenberg, M. E., Ziff, E. B., and Greene, L. A. (1986). Stimulation of neuronal acetylcholine receptors induces rapid gene transcription. *Science* **3**, 80–83.

Gunderson, C. H., Lehmann, C. R., Sidell, F. R., and Jabbari, B. (1992). Nerve agents: A review. *Neurology* **42**, 946–950.

Gupta, R. C., and Dettbarn, W.-D. (1986). Role of uptake of [^{14}C]valine into protein in the development of tolerance to diisopropylphosphorofluoridate (DFP) toxicity. *Toxicol. Appl. Pharmacol.* **84**, 551–560.

Gutmann, L., and Besser, R. (1990). Organophosphate intoxication: Pharmacologic, neurophysiologic, clinical, and therapeutic considerations. *Semin. Neurol.* **10**(1), 46–51.

Hammer, R., Berrie, C. P., Birdsal, N. J. M., Burgen, A. S. V., and Hulme, E. C. (1980). Pirenzepine distinguishes between different subclasses of muscarinic receptors. *Nature (London)* **283**, 90–92.

Hanley, M. R., and Iversen, L. L. (1978). Muscarinic cholinergic receptors in rat corpus striatum and regulation of guanosine cyclic 3,5-monophosphate. *Mol. Pharmacol.* **14**, 246–255.

Harris, L. W., Stitcher, D. L., and Heyl, W. C. (1982). Effects of inhibitors of acetylcholine synthesis on brain acetylcholine and survival in soman-intoxicated animals. *Life Sci.* **30**, 1867–1873.

Hayes, M. M. M., Van der Westhuizen, N. G., and Gelfand, M. (1978). Organophosphate poisoning in Rhodesia. A study of the clinical features and management of 105 patients. *S. Afr. Med. J.* **54**, 230–234.

Heppner, T. J., and Fiekers, J. F. (1992). Comparison of atropine pre- and post-treatment in ganglion neurons exposed to soman. *Brain Res. Bull.* **28**, 849–852.

Hesheler, J., Rosenthal, W., Trautwein, W., and Schultz, G. (1987). The GTP-binding protein, G_o, regulates neuronal calcium channels. *Nature* **325**, 445–447.

Hirvonen, M.-R., Komulainen, H., Paljärvi, L., and Savolainen, K. (1989). Time-course of malaoxon-induced alterations in brain regional inositol-1-phosphate levels in convulsing and nonconvulsing rats. *Neurochem. Res.* **14**(2), 143–147.

Hirvonen, M.-R., Paljärvi, L., Naukkarinen, A., Komulainen, H., and Savolainen, K. (1990). Potentiation of malaoxon-induced convulsions by lithium: Early neuronal injury, phosphoinositide signalling, and calcium. *Toxicol. Appl. Pharmacol.* **104**, 276–289.

Hirvonen, M.-R., Paljärvi, L., and Savolainen, K. M. (1993). Malaoxon-induced neurotoxicity in old rats: Alterations in cerebral inositol lipid signalling, brain tissue calcium levels and early neuronal injury. *Toxicology* **79**, 157–167.

Holmstedt, B. (1963). Structure activity relationship of the organophosphorus anticholinesterase agents. *In* "Handbuch der Experimentellen Pharmakologie" (O. Eichler and A. Farah, eds.), pp. 428–485. Springer-Verlag, Berlin.

Honchar, M. P., Olney, J. W., and Sherman, W. R. (1983). Systemic cholinergic agents induce seizures and brain damage in lithium-treated rats. *Science* **220**, 323–325.

Hoskins, B., Fernando, J. C. R., Dulaney, M. D., Lim, D. K., Liu, D. D., Watanabe, H. K., and Ho, I. K. (1986). Relationship between the neurotoxicities of soman, sarin and tabun, and acetylcholinesterase inhibition. *Toxicol. Lett.* **30**, 121–129.

Ivens, I., Schmuck, G., and Machemer, L. (1998). Learning and memory of rats after long term administration of low doses of parathion. *Toxicol. Sci.* **46**(1), 101–111.

Jacobowitz, D. M., and Palkovits, M. (1974). Topographic atlas of catecholamine and acetylcholinesterase-containing neurons in the rat brain. I. Forebrain (telencephalon, diencephalon). *J. Comp. Neurol.* **157**(1), 13–28.

Jett, D. A., Hill, E. F., Fernando, J. C., Eldefrawi, M. E., and Eldefrawi, A. T. (1993). Down-regulation of muscarinic receptors and the M3 subtype in white-footed mice by dietary exposure to parathion. *J. Toxicol. Environ. Health* **39**, 395–415.

Jett, D. A., Eldefrawi, M. E., and Eldefrawi, A. T. (1994). Differential regulation of muscarinic receptor subtypes in rat brain regions by repeated injections of parathion. *Toxicol. Lett.* **73**, 33–41.

Johnson, D. D., and Lowndes, H. E. (1974). Reduction by diazepam of repetitive electrical activity and toxicity resulting from soman. *Eur. J. Pharmacol.* **28**, 245–250.

Jope, R. S. (1979). Effects of lithium treatment *in vitro* and *in vivo* on acetylcholine metabolism in rat brain. *J. Neurochem.* **33**, 487–495.

Jope, R. S. (1988). Modulation of phosphoinositide hydrolysis by NaF and aluminum in rat cortical slices. *J. Neurochem.* **51**, 1731–1736.

Jope, R. S., and Morrisett, R. A. (1986). Neurochemical consequences of status epilepticus induced in rats by coadministration of lithium and pilocarpine. *Exp. Neurol.* **93**, 404–414.

Jope, R. S., Morrisett, R. A., and Snead, O. C. (1986). Characterization of lithium potentiation of pilocarpine induced status epilepticus in rats. *Exp. Neurol.* **91**, 471–480.

Jope, R. S., Miller, J. M., Ferraro, T. N., and Hare, T. A. (1989). Chronic lithium treatment and status epilepticus induced by lithium and pilocarpine cause selective changes of amino acid concentrations in rat brain regions. *Neurochem. Res.* **14**(9), 829–834.

Jovanovic, D. (1983). The effect of bis-pyridinium oximes on neuromuscular blockade induced by highly toxic organophosphates in rat. *Arch. Int. Pharmacodyn.* **262**, 231–241.

Jovanovic, D., Randjelovic, S., and Joksovic, D. (1990). A case of unusual suicidal poisoning by the organophosphorus insecticide dimethoate. *Hum. Exp. Toxicol.* **9**, 49–51.

Kangas, J., Laitinen, S., Jauhiainen, A., and Savolainen, K. (1993). Exposure to sprayers and plant handlers to mevinphos in Finnish greenhouses. *Am. J. Ind. Hyg.* **54**, 150–157.

Katz, L. S., and Marquis, J. K. (1989). Modulation of central muscarinic receptor binding *in vitro* by ultralow levels of the organophosphate paraoxon. *Toxicol. Appl. Pharmacol.* **101**, 114–123.

Katz, L. S., and Marquis, J. K. (1992). Organophosphate-induced alterations in muscarinic receptor binding and phosphoinositide hydrolysis in the human SK-N-SH cell line. *NeuroToxicology* **13**, 365–378.

Katz, E. J., Cortes, V. I., Eldefrawi, M. E., and Eldefrawi, A. T. (1997). Chlorpyrifos, parathion, and their oxons bind to and desensitize a nicotinic acetylcholine receptor: relevance to their toxicities. *Toxicol. Appl. Pharmacol.* **146**, 227–236.

Khan, N. A., and Hasan, M. (1988). Dose-related neurochemical changes in the levels of gangliosides and glycogen in various regions of the rat brain and spinal cord following methyl parathion administration. *Exp. Pathol.* **35**, 61–65.

Kimura, H., McGeer, P. L., Peng, F., and McGeer, E. G. (1980). Choline acetyltransferase-containing neurons in rodent brain demonstrated by immunohistochemistry. *Science* **208**, 1057–1059.

Kimura, H., McGeer, P. L., Peng, J. H., and McGeer, E. G. (1981). The central cholinergic system studied by choline acetyltransferase immunohistochemistry in the cat. *J. Comp. Neurol.* **200**, 151–201.

Koelle, G. B., ed. (1963). Cholinesterases and anticholinesterase agents. *In* "Handbuch der Experimentellen Pharmakologie." Springer-Verlag, Berlin.

Koplovitz, I., and Skvorak, J. P. (1998). Electrocorticographic changes during generalized convulsive status epilepticus in soman intoxicated rats. *Epilepsy Res.* **30**, 159–164.

Kubinec, J., Vrana, K. E., and Roskoski, R., Jr. (1987). Paraoxon-induced decrease in the muscarinic acetylcholine receptor content in rat heart. *Eur. J. Pharmacol.* **136**, 295–301.

Kuhar, M. I., and Yamamura, H. I. (1975). Light autoradiographic localization of cholinergic muscarinic receptors in rat brain by specific binding of a potent antagonist. *Nature (London)* **253**, 560–561.

Kuhar, M. J., and Yamamura, H. I. (1976). Localization of cholinergic muscarinic receptors in rat brain by light microscopic radioautography. *Brain Res.* **110**, 229–243.

Lallement, G., Pernot-Marino, I., Foquin-Tarricone, A., Baubichon, D., Piras, A., Blanchet, G., and Carpentier, P. (1994a). Antiepileptic effects of NBQX against soman-induced seizures. *Neuroreport* **5**, 425–428.

Lallement, G., Pernot-Marino, I., Foquin-Tarricone, A., Baubichon, D., Piras, A., Blanchet, G., and Carpentier, P. (1994b). Coadministration of atropine, NBQX and TCP against soman-induced seiqures. *Neuroreport* **5**, 1113–1117.

Lallement, G., Clarencon, D., Brochier, G., Baubichon, D., Galonnier, M., Blanchet, G., and Mestries, J.-C. (1997). Efficacy of atropine/pralidoxime/diazepam or atropine/HI-6/prodiazepam in primates intoxicated by soman. *Pharmacol. Biochem. Behav.* **56**(2), 325–332.

Laskowski, M. B., and Dettbarn, W.-D. (1979). An electrophysiological analysis of the effects of paraoxon at the neuromuscular junction. *J. Pharmacol. Exp. Ther.* **210**(2), 269–274.

Leiber, D., Marc, S., and Harbon, S. (1990). Pharmacological evidence for distinct muscarinic receptor subtypes coupled to the inhibition of adenylate cyclase and to increased generation of inositol phosphates in the guinea pig myometrium. *J. Pharmacol. Exp. Ther.* **252**, 800–809.

Liao, C. F., Themmen, A. P. N., Joho, R., Barberis, C., Birnbaumer, M., and Birnbaumer, L. (1989). Molecular cloning and expression of a fifth muscarinic acetylcholine receptor. *J. Biol. Chem.* **264**, 7328–7337.

Ligtenstein, D. A., and Moes, G. W. H. (1991). The synergism of atropine and the cholinesterase reactivator HI-6 in counteracting lethality by organophosphate intoxication in the rat. *Toxicol. Appl. Pharmacol.* **107**, 47–53.

Lim, D. K., Hoskins, B., and Ho, I. K. (1991). Trihexyphenidyl enhances physostigmine prophylaxis against soman poisoning in guinea pigs. *Fundam. Appl. Toxicol.* **16**, 482–489.

Liu, D. D., Watanabe, H. K., Ho, I. K., and Hoskins, B. (1986). Acute effects of soman, sarin and tabun on cyclic nucleotide metabolism in rat striatum. *J. Toxicol. Environ. Health* **19**, 23–32.

Liu, D. D., Ueno, E., Ko, I. K., and Hoskins, B. (1988). Evidence that changes in levels of cyclic nucleotides in the CNS are not related to soman-induced convulsions. *NeuroToxicology* **9**(1), 23–38.

Liu, J., and Pope, C. N. (1998). Comparative presynaptic neurochemical changes in rat striatum following exposure to chlorpyrifos or parathion. *J. Toxicol. Environ. Health A* **53**, 531–544.

Liu, P.-S., Kao, L.-S., and Lin, M.-K. (1994). Organophosphates inhibit catecholamine secretion and calcium influx in bovine adrenal chromaffin cells. *Toxicology* **90**, 81–91.

Liu, W., and Tsou, C. (1986). Determination of rate constants for the irreversible inhibition of acetylcholine esterase by continuously monitoring the substrate reaction in the presence of the inhibitor. *Biochim. Biophys. Acta* **870**, 185–190.

Loikkanen, J., Naarala, J., and Savolainen, K. M. (1998). Modification of glutamate-induced oxidative stress by lead: The role of extracellular calcium. *Free Rad. Biol. Med.* **24**, 377–384.

Lomax, P., Kokka, N., and Lee, R. J. (1986). Acetylcholinesterase inhibitors and thermoregulation. *In* "Homeostasis and Thermal Stress. Experimental and Therapeutic Advances" (K. Cooper, P. Lomax, E. Schonbaum, and W. Veale, eds.), pp. 108–112. Karger, Basel.

Lukas, R. J., Changeaux, J.-P., Le Novere, N., Albuquerque, E. X., Balfour, D. J. K., Berg, D. K., Bertrand, D., Chiappinelli, V. A., Clarke, P. B. S., Collins, A. C., Dani, J. A., Grady, S. R., Kellar, K. J., Lindstrom, J. M., Marks, M. J., Quick, M., Taylor, P. W., and Wonnacott, S. (1999). International Union of Pharmacology. XX. Current Status of the Nomenclature for Nicotinic Acetylcholine Receptors and their Subunits. *Pharmacol. Rev.* **51**, 397–401.

Lundy, P. M., Magor, G., and Shaw, R. K. (1978). Gamma aminobutyric metabolism in different areas of rat brain at the onset of soman-induced convulsions. *Arch. Int. Pharmacodyn.* **234**, 64–73.

Lynch, G., Larson, J., Kelso, S., Barrionuevo, G., and Schottler, F. (1983). Intracellular injections of EGTA block induction of hippocampal long-term potentiation. *Nature* **305**, 719–721.

Maelicke, A., ed. (1986). "Nicotinic Acetylcholine Receptor Structure and Function," NATO ASI Series, Vol. H-3. Springer-Verlag, Berlin.

Maki, Y., Bos, T. J., Davis, C., Statbuck, M., and Vogt, P. K. (1987). Avian sarcoma virus 17 carries the *jun* oncogene. *Proc. Natl. Acad. Sci. U.S.A.* **84**, 2848–2852.

Marrs, T. C. (1996). Organophosphate anticholinesterase poisoning. *Toxic Substance Mechanisms* **15**, 357–388.

Mash, D. C., and Potter, L. T. (1986). Autoradiographic localization of M1 and M2 muscarine receptors in the rat brain. *Neuroscience* **19**, 551–564.

Massoulié, J., and Bon, S. (1982). The molecular forms of cholinesterase and acetylcholinesterase in vertebrates. *Ann. Rev. Neurosci.* **5**, 57–100.

Maxwell, D. M., Thomsen, R. T., and Baskin, S. I. (1991). Species differences in the negative inotropic effect of acetylcholine and soman in rat, guinea pig, and rabbit hearts. *Comp. Biochem. Physiol.* **100C**(3), 591–595.

McDonough, J. H., Jr., and Shih, T.-M. (1997). Neuropharmacological mechanisms of nerve agent-induced seizure and neuropathology. *Neurosci. Biobehav. Rev.* **21**(5), 559–579.

McDonough, J. H., Jr., Clark, T. R., Slone, T. W., Jr., Zoeffel, D., Brown, K., Kim, S., and Smith, C. D. (1998). Neural lesions in the rat and their relationship to EEG delta activity following seizures induced by the nerve agent soman. *NeuroToxicology* **19**(3), 381–392.

McGehee, D. S., and Role, L. W. (1995). Physiological diversity of nicotinic acetylcholine receptors expressed by vertebrate neurons. *Annu. Rev. Physiol.* **57**, 521–546.

Meeker, R. B., and Harden, T. K. (1982). Muscarinic cholinergic receptor-mediated activation of phosphodiesterase. *Mol. Pharmacol.* **22**, 310–319.

Mei, L., Roeske, W. R., and Yamamura, H. I. (1989). Molecular pharmacology of muscarinic receptor heterogeneity. *Life Sci.* **45**, 1831–1851.

Melchers, B. P. C., and van Helden, H. P. M. (1990). On the development of behavioral tolerance to organophosphates II: Neurophysiological aspects. *Pharmacol. Biochem. Behav.* **35**, 321–325.

Meldrum, B., and Garthwaite, J. (1990). Excitatory amino acid neurotoxicity and neurodegenerative disease. *Trends Pharmacol. Sci.* **11**, 379–387.

Minton, N. A., and Murray, V. S. G. (1988). A review of organophosphate poisoning. *Med. Toxicol.* **3**, 350–375.

Modrow, H. E., and McDonough, J. H. (1986). Change in atropine dose effect curve after subacute soman administration. *Pharmacol. Biochem. Behav.* **24**, 845–848.

Murphy, A. Z., Ennis, M., Shipley, M. T., and Behbehani, M. M. (1994). Directionally specific changes in arterial pressure induce differential patterns of *fos* expression in discrete areas of the rat brainstem: A double-labeling study for *fos* and catecholamines. *J. Comp. Neurol.* **349**, 36–50.

Naarala, J., Tervo, P., Loikkanen, J., and Savolainen, K. (1997). Cholinergic-induced oxidative burst in human neuroblastoma cells. *Life Sci.* **60**, 1905–1914.

Naseem, S. M. (1990). Effect of organophosphates on dopamine and muscarinic receptor binding in rat brain. *Biochem. Int.* **20**(4), 799–806.

Nicotera, P., Leist, M., and Manzo L. (1999). Neuronal cell death: A demise with different shapes. *Trends Pharmacol. Sci.* **20**, 46–51.

Nishizuka, Y. (1988). The molecular heterogeneity of protein kinase C and its implications for cellular regulation. *Nature* **334**, 661–665.

Olney, J. W., Collins, R. C., and Sloviter, R. S. (1986). Excitotoxic mechanisms of epileptic brain damage. *Adv. Neurol.* **44**, 857–878.

Orrenius, S. (1997). The living and dying cell. *Acta Anaesthesiol. Scand. Suppl.* **110**, 84.

Overstreet, D. H., Kozar, M. D., and Lynch, G. S. (1973). Reduced hypothermic effects of cholinomimetic agents following chronic anticholinesterase treatment. *Neuropharmacology* **12**, 1017–1032.

Ozkutlu, U., Long, J. P., Cannon, J. G., Sahin, M. F., and Liang, C. (1995). Prevention of organophosphate-induced toxicity in mice. *Arch. Int. Pharmacodyn.* **329**, 331–342.

Palkovits, M., and Jacobowitz, D. M. (1974). Topographic atlas of catecholamine and acetylcholinesterase-containing neurons in the rat brain. II. Hindbrain (mesencephalon, rhombencephalon). *J. Comp. Neurol.* **157**(1), 29–42.

Paxinos, G., and Watson, C. (1982). "The Rat Brain in Stereotaxic Coordinates." Academic Press, New York.

Pazdernik, T. L., Cross, R., Nelson, S., Samson, F., and McDonough, J., Jr. (1983). Soman-induced depression of brain activity in TAB-pretreated rats: 2-Deoxyglucose study. *NeuroToxicology* **4**(4), 27–34.

Pazdernik, T. L., Cross, R., Giesler, M., Nelson, S., Samson, F., and McDonough, J., Jr. (1985). Delayed effects of soman: Brain glucose use and pathology. *NeuroToxicology* **6**(3), 61–70.

Pazdernik, T. L., Nelson, S. R., Cross, R., Churchill, L., Giesler, M., and Samson, F. E. (1986). Effects of antidotes on soman-induced brain changes. *Arch. Toxicol. (Suppl.)* **9**, 333–336.

Pellegrino, L. J., Pellegrino, A. S., and Cushman, A. J. (1979). "A Stereotaxic Atlas of the Rat Brain," 2nd ed. Plenum, New York.

Pepeu, G. (1983). Brain acetylcholine: An inventory of our knowledge on the 50th anniversary of its discovery. *Trends Pharmacol. Sci.* **5**, 416–418.

Perelta, E. G., Winslow, J. W., Peterson, G. L., Smith, D. H., Ashkenazi, A., Ramachandran, J., Schmerlik, M. I., and Capon, D. J. (1987). Primary structure and biochemical properties of an M_2 muscarinic receptor. *Science* **236**, 600–605.

Perelta, E., Winslow, J., Ashkenazi, A., Smith, D., Ramachandran, J., and Capon, D. (1988). Structural basis of muscarinic acetylcholine receptor subtype diversity. *Trends Pharmacol. Sci. Suppl* III, 6–11.

Philippens, I. H. C. H. M., Busker, R. W., Wolthuis, O. L., Olivier, B., Bruijnzeel, P. L. B., and Melchers, B. P. C. (1998). Subchronic physostigmine pretreatment in guinea pigs: Effective against soman and without side effects. *Pharmacol. Biochem. Behav.* **59**(4), 1061–1067.

Pinkas-Kramarski, R., Stein, R., Zimmer, Y., and Sokolowsky, M. (1988). Cloned rat M3 muscarinic receptors mediate phosphoinositide hydrolysis but not adenylate cyclase inhibition. *FEBS* **239**, 174–178.

Putney, J. W., Jr. (1987). Formation and actions of calcium-mobilizing messenger, inositol 1,4,5-triphosphate. *Am. J. Physiol.* **252**, G149–G157 (*Gastrointest. Liver Physiol.* **15**).

Rocha, E. S., Swanson, K. L., Aracava, Y., Goolsby, J. E., Maelicke, A., and Albuquerque, E. X. (1996). Paraoxon: Cholinesterase-independent stimulation of transmitter release and selective block of ligand-gated ion channels in cultured hippocampal neurons. *J. Pharmacol. Exp. Ther.* **278**(3), 1175–1187.

Romano, C., and Goldstein, A. (1980). Stereospecific nicotine receptors in rat brain membranes. *Science* **220**, 647–650.

Samson, F., Pazdernik, T. L., Cross, R. S., Churchill, L., Giesler, M. P., and Nelson, S. R. (1985). Brain regional activity and damage associated with organophosphate induced seizures: Effects of atropine and benactyzine. *Proc. West. Pharmacol. Soc.* **28**, 183–185.

Sargent, P. (1993). The diversity of neuronal nicotinic acetylcholine receptors. *Annu. Rev. Neurosci.* **16**, 403–443.

Savolainen, K. M., and Hirvonen, M.-R. (1992). Effects of malaoxon on phosphatidylinositol signalling in convulsing and non-convulsing non-pregnant and pregnant female rats and their offspring. *NeuroToxicology* **13**, 295–300.

Savolainen, K., and Kangas, J. (1995). Strategies for biological monitoring of workers exposed to pesticides. *In* "Bioindicators of Environmental Health" (M. Munawar, O. Hänninen, S. Roy, N. Munawar, L. Kärenlampi, and D. Brown, eds.), Ecovision World Monograph Series, pp. 165–178. SPB Academic Publishing, Amsterdam.

Savolainen, K., Hervonen, H., Lehto, V.-P., and Mattila, M. J. (1984). Neurotoxic effects of disulfiram on autonomic nervous system in rat. *Acta Pharmacol. Toxicol.* **55**, 339–344.

Savolainen, K. M., Nelson, S. R., Samson, F. E., and Pazdernik, T. L. (1988a). Soman-induced convulsions affect the inositol lipid signalling system: Potentiation by lithium; attenuation by atropine and diazepam. *Toxicol. Appl. Pharmacol.* **96**, 305–314.

Savolainen, K. M., Terry, J. B., Nelson, S. R., Samson, F. E., and Pazdernik, T. L. (1988b). Convulsions and cerebral inositol-1-phosphate levels in rats treated with diisopropyl fluorophosphate. *Pharmacol. Toxicol.* **63**, 137–138.

Savolainen, K. M., Muona, O., Nelson, S. R., Samson, F. E., and Pazdernik, T. L. (1991). Lithium modifies convulsions and brain phosphoinositide turnover induced by organophosphates. *Pharmacol. Toxicol.* **69**, 346–354.

Savolainen, K. M., Loikkanen, J., and Naarala, J. (1995). Amplification of glutamate-induced oxidative stress in neuronal cells. *Toxicol. Lett.* **82/83**, 399–405.

Savolainen, K. M., Loikkanen, J., Eerikäinen, S., and Naarala, J. (1998). Interactions of excitatory neurotransmitters and xenobiotics in excitotoxicity and oxidative stress: Glutamate and lead. *Toxicol. Lett.* **102-103**, 363–367.

Schmuck, G., Schürmann, A., Ivens, I., and Machemer, L. (1998). *In vitro* investigations on long-term potentiation and neuronal cell cultures of the rat hippocampus after treatment with parathion *in vivo* and *in vitro*. *In vitro Mol. Toxicol.* **11**(2), 139–152.

Schwarz, R. D., and Kellar, K. J. (1982). Nicotinic cholinergic receptor binding sites in the brain: Regulation *in vivo*. *Science* **220**, 214–216.

Seuwen, K., Kahan, C., Hartman, T., and Poryssegur, J. (1990). Strong and persistent activation of inositol breakdown induces early mitogenic events but not Go to S phase progression in hamster fibroblasts. *J. Biol. Chem.* **265**, 22,292–22,299.

Sheng, M., and Greenberg, M. E. (1990). The regulation and function of c-fos and other immediate early genes in the nervous system. *Neuron* **4**, 477–485.

Shih, T.-M. (1982). Time course effects of soman on acetylcholine and choline levels in six discrete areas of the rat brain. *Psychopharmacology* **78**, 170–175.

Shih, T.-M. (1990). Anticonvulsant effects of diazepam and MK-801 in soman poisoning. *Epilepsy Res.* **7**, 105–116.

Shih, T.-M. (1991). Cholinergic actions of diazepam and atropine sulfate in soman poisoning. *Brain Res. Bull.* **26**, 565–573.

Shih, T.-M., and McDonough, J. H. (1997). Neurochemical mechanisms in soman-induced seizures. *J. Appl. Toxicol.* **17**(4), 255–264.

Shih, T.-M., Koviak, T. A., and Capacio, B. R. (1991a). Anticonvulsants for poisoning by the organophosphorus compound soman: Pharmacological mechanisms. *Neurosci. Biobehav. Rev.* **15**, 349–362.

Shih, T.-M., Whalley, C. E., and Valdes, J. J. (1991b). A comparison of cholinergic effects of HI-6 and pralidoxime-2-chloride (2-PAM) in soman poisoning. *Toxicol. Lett.* **55**, 131–147.

Shih, T.-M., Capacio, B. R., and Cook, L. A. (1993). Effects of anticholinergic-antiparkinsonian drugs on striatal neurotransmitter levels of rats intoxicated with soman. *Pharmacol. Biochem. Behav.* **44**, 615–622.

Singh, G., Avasthi, G., Khurana, D., Whig, J., and Mahajan, R. (1998). Neurophysiological monitoring of pharmacological manipulation in acute organophosphate (OP) poisoning. The effects of pralidoxime, magnesium sulphate and pancuronium. *Electroencephalogr. Clin. Neurophysiol.* **107**, 140–148.

Smith, A. P., and Wolthuis, O. L. (1983). H16 as an antidote to soman poisoning in rhesus monkey respiratory muscles in-vitro. *J. Pharm. Pharmacol.* **35**, 157–160.

Solberg, Y., and Belkin, M. (1997). The role of excitotoxicity in organophosphorous nerve agents central poisoning. *Trends Pharmacol. Sci.* **18**(6), 183–185.

Sparenborg, S., Brennecke, L. H., and Beers, E. T. (1993). Pharmacological dissociation of the motor and electrical aspects of convulsive status epilepticus induced by the cholinesterase inhibitor soman. *Epilepsy Res.* **14**, 95–103.

Stamper, C. R., Balduini, W., Murphy, S. D., and Costa, L. G. (1988). Behavioral and biochemical effects of postnatal parathion exposure in the rat. *Neurotoxicol. Teratol.* **10**, 261–266.

Sterri, S. H., Berge, G., and Fonnum, F. (1985). Esterase activities and soman toxicity in developing rat. *Acta Pharmacol. Toxicol.* **57**, 136–140.

Storm, J. E., Rozman, K. K., and Doull, J. (2000). Occupational exposure limits for 30 organophosphate pesticides based on inhibition of red blood cell acetylcholinesterase. *Toxicology* **150**, 1–29.

Taylor, P., and Brown, J. H. (1989). Acetylcholine. *In* "Basic Neurochemistry" (G. Sieger, B. Agranoff, R. W. Albers, and P. Molinoff, eds.), 4th ed., pp. 203–232. Raven Press, New York.

Thomsen, R. H., and Wilson, D. F. (1986). Chronic effects of paraoxon on transmitter release and the synaptic contribution to tolerance. *J. Pharmacol. Exp. Ther.* **237**(3), 689–694.

Unwin, N., Toyoshima, C., and Kubalek, E. (1988). Arrangement of the acetylcholine receptor subunits in the resting and desensitized states, determined by cryoelectron microscopy of crystallized Torpedo postsynaptic membranes. *J. Cell Biol.* **107**(3), 1123–1138.

Van Dongen, C. J., Valkenburg, P. W., and van Helden, H. P. M. (1988). Contribution of de novo synthesis of acetylcholinesterase to spontaneous recovery of neuromuscular transmission following soman intoxication. *Eur. J. Pharmacol.* **149**, 381–384.

Van Dongen, C. J., and Wolthuis, O. L. (1989). On the development of behavioral tolerance to organophosphates I: Behavioral and biochemical aspects. *Pharmacol. Biochem. Behav.* **34**, 473–481.

Viana, G. B., Davis, L. H., and Kauffman, F. C. (1988). Effects of organophosphates and nerve growth factor on muscarinic receptor binding number in rat pheochromocytoma PC12 cells. *Toxicol. Appl. Pharmacol.* **93**, 257–266.

Wade, J. V., Samson, F. E., Nelson, S. R., and Pazdernik, T. L. (1987). Changes in extracellular amino acids during soman- and kainic acid-induced seizures. *Journal of Neurochemistry* **49**(2), 645–650.

Ward, T. R., Ferris, D. J., Tilson, H. A., and Mundy, W. R. (1993). Correlation of the anticholinesterase activity of a series of organophosphates with their ability to compete with agonist binding to muscarinic receptors. *Toxicol. Appl. Pharmacol.* **122**, 300–307.

Wecker, L., Laskowski, M. B., and Dettbarn, W.-D. (1978). Neuromuscular dysfunction induced by acetylcholinesterase inhibition. *Federat. Proc.* **37**(14), 2818–2822.

Whalley, C. E., and Shih, T.-M. (1989). Effects of soman and sarin on high affinity choline uptake by rat brain synaptosomes. *Brain Res. Bull.* **22**, 853–858.

Worek, F., and Szinicz, L. (1993). Analysis of cardiovascular and respiratory effects of various doses of soman in guinea-pigs: Efficacy of atropine treatment. *Arch. Int. Pharmacodyn.* **325**, 96–112.

Worek, F., Kirchner, T., and Szinicz, L. (1994). Treatment of tabun poisoned guinea-pigs with atropine, HLö 7 or HI 6: Effect on respiratory and circulatory function. *Arch. Toxicol.* **68**, 231–239.

World Health Organization (1986). "Organophosphorus insecticides: A general introduction." Environmental Health Criteria 63, World Health Organization, Geneva.

Yagle, K., and Costa, L. G. (1996). Effects of organophosphate exposure on muscarinic acetylcholine receptor subtype mRNA levels in the adult rat. *NeuroToxicology* **17**(2), 523–530.

Yamada, S., Isogai, M., Okudaira, H., and Hayashi, E. (1983). Correlation between cholinesterase inhibition and reduction in muscarinic receptors and choline uptake by repeated diisopropylfluorophosphate administration: Antagonism by physostigmine and atropine. *J. Pharmacol. Exp. Ther.* **226**, 519–525.

Zimmer, L. A., Ennis, M., El-Etri, M., and Shipley, M. T. (1997a). Anatomical localization and time course of *fos* expression following soman-induced seizures. *J. Comp. Neurol.* **378**, 468–481.

Zimmer, L. A., Ennis, M., and Shipley, M. T. (1997b). Soman-induced seizures rapidly activate astrocytes and microglia in discrete brain regions. *J. Comp. Neurol.* **378**, 482–492.

Clinical Toxicology of Anticholinesterase Agents in Humans

Marcello Lotti

Università degli Studi di Padova

Several chemicals display anticholinesterase activity among which organophosphorus esters (OPs) represent the vast majority because they are widely used and easily available. Since their introduction after World War II as insecticides (Khurana and Prabhakar, 2000), countless publications have described their clinical toxicology in humans. Initially, most case reports dealt with accidental and occupational poisoning, whereas later the majority of poisonings were the result of suicide attempts. Most recently, attention has been directed to possible subtle effects caused by low-level long-term exposures such as those encountered in the workplace. Concurrently, an even larger amount of experimental studies have contributed to our understanding of anticholinesterase toxicology.

Therefore, anticholinesterase agents, and OPs in particular, undoubtedly represent the most extensively studied class of chemicals in toxicology and it is not surprising that a very large number of reviews, textbooks, book chapters, and other general publications, in addition to research papers, have appeared over the years on their clinical toxicology (the most recent reviews include: Bardin *et al.*, 1994; Brown and Brix, 1998; De Bleecker *et al.*, 1992a; ECETOC, 1998; Eyer, 1995; Gunderson *et al.*, 1992; Jamal, 1997; Karalliede, 1999; Karalliedde and Senanayake, 1999; Marrs, 1993; Millard and Broomfield, 1995; Ray, 1998a, b; Steenland, 1996). Nevertheless, some controversies still exist on some aspects of both the clinical toxicology and the treatment of OP poisoning. In particular, conflicting results have been published on long-term sequelae of acute exposure and on possible effects of long-term exposures that do not cause overt cholinergic toxicity, and different opinions exist on the uses of antidotes in the treatment of acute poisonings.

This chapter deals with the clinical aspects of OP toxicology in humans, mentioning, where appropriate, those of other anticholinesterase agents and supporting experimental evidence in animals as well. Moreover, this chapter does not replace the specific chapters of the previous editions of this book (Hayes,

1982; Hayes and Laws, 1991), where additional details on OP toxicology, as derived from the older literature, can be found.

51.1 THE CHOLINERGIC SYNDROME

The cholinergic syndrome is characterized by overstimulation of cholinergic receptors throughout the body. It may be the consequence of single or repeated exposures to a variety of chemicals such as OPs and carbamates, which inhibit acetylcholinesterase (AChE) at the synaptic level. As a consequence, the level of acetylcholine increases, although the amount and time course of neurotransmitter accumulation may vary widely among various districts of the cholinergic system (Stavinoha *et al.*, 1976). Thus, the clinical picture that results from this excess of neurotransmitter may be quite variable in presentation of signs and symptoms, at the onset, in time course, and in outcome. This clinical polymorphism largely depends on the chemical involved and on the dose.

51.1.1 ETIOLOGY

51.1.1.1 Anticholinesterases as Pesticides and Warfare Agents

Although the use of anticholinesterase OP insecticides has declined during the last two decades, particularly in agriculture, they still represent an important class of pesticides, which account for about 10% of all active ingredients currently used as pesticides. However, several OPs that caused poisoning in humans in the past are believed to be no longer manufactured or marketed (Tomlin, 1997).

The long inventory of acute intoxications in humans involves a variety of OPs. Table 51.1 lists examples of OPs, ranked according to their chemical structure, that caused acute toxicity in humans. Most compounds that belong to group A are chemical warfare agents and are highly toxic. Most pesticides belong

Table 51.1
Classification of Organophosphorus Esters;[a] General Formula:

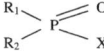

A. Compounds where X = halogen or CN, CNS, etc.

  1. R_1 = alkoxy, R_2 = alkyl

    Example: sarin (isopropyl methylphosphonofluoridate), nerve gas (Okumura *et al.*, 1996)

  2. R_1 and R_2 = alkoxy

    Example: DFP (diisopropyl phosphorofluoridate), laboratory chemical and discontinued drug (Moore, 1956)

  3. R_1 = alkylamide, R_2 = alkoxy

    Example: tabun (ethyl *N*-dimethylphosphoroamido cyanidate), nerve gas (Compton, 1987)

  4. R_1 and R_2 = mono- or dialkylamido

    Example: mipafox (*N N'*-diisopropyl phosphorodiamido fluoridate), laboratory chemical (Bidstrup *et al.*, 1953).

B. Compounds where X = alkyl, alkoxy, or aryloxy

  1. Alkoxydialkyl or dialkoxyalkyl compounds

    Example: trichlorfon (dimethyl (2,2,2-trichloro-1-hydroxyethyl) phosphonate), insecticide and drug (Vasilescu and Florescu, 1980)

  2. Trialkyl compounds and dialkoxy, aryloxy compounds

    Example: dichlorvos (dimethyl 2,2 dichlorovinyl phosphate), insecticide (Wadia *et al.*, 1987)

C. Thiol- and thiono-phosphorus compounds

  1. Thiol compounds

    Example: demeton-*S*-methyl (*S*-[2-(ethylthio)ethyl] dimethyl phosphorothioate), insecticide (Weir *et al.*, 1992)

  2. Thiono compounds

    Example: parathion (diethyl *O*-(4-nitrophenyl)phosphorothioate), insecticide (Namba *et al.*, 1971)

  3. Thiol – thiono compounds

    Example: malathion (dimethyl *S*-(1,2-dicarboxylethyl) phosphorodithioate), insecticide (Baker *et al.*, 1978)

D. Derivatives of pyrophosphorous acid

    Example: sulfotepp (tetraethyl dithionopyrophosphate), insecticide (Namba *et al.*, 1971)

E. Compounds containing a quaternary nitrogen

    Example: ecothiophate (diethyl-*S*-2-trimethyl ammonium-ethyl phosphorothioate iodide), drug (Gesztes, 1966).

---

[a]Nerve gases belong to group A, whereas most common pesticides belong to groups B and C. Examples of OPs which caused poisoning in humans are given.
Source: Holmstedt (1963).

---

to groups B and C, among which dimethoxy OPs are the most common. In contrast to other OPs, dimethoxy OPs are less toxic because of certain biochemical characteristics (i.e., relative high speed of reactivation of dimethoxyphosphorylated AChE; see Section 51.1.2.2). In Table 51.2, the World Health Organization (WHO) recommended classification of OP pesticides by hazard is reported. The classification is based on acute oral and dermal toxicity in rats and the physical state of product or formulation. Confirmation of the hazard severity of these chemicals has often been obtained from clinical observations.

OPs have also been used as warfare agents and large amounts are thought to be stockpiled in arsenals worldwide. They were developed during the 1950s and were used as recently as the early 1990s in a terrorist attack in a Tokyo subway (Suzuki *et al.*, 1995). Moreover, during the Persian Gulf War, soldiers were thought to have been exposed to low levels of nerve gases (NIH, 1994).

51.1.1.2 Anticholinesterases as Drugs

Anticholinesterase drugs have a variety of indications in clinical medicine, and toxicity may arise from their therapeutic uses. However, although used in the past, nowadays drugs do not include OPs, but use reversible inhibitors of AChE such as physostigmine, pyridostigmine, neostigmine, and edrophonium. Their acceptability has been established in four areas: atony of the smooth muscle of the intestinal tract and urinary bladder, myasthenia gravis, glaucoma, and termination of effects of competitive neuromuscular blocking drugs (Taylor, 1996a). Moreover, reversible anticholinesterases are also used for treatment of overdoses of atropine and other anticholinergic drugs (such as phenothiazines and tricyclic antidepressant; Nilsson, 1982). Pyridostigmine was administered on a large scale during the Persian Gulf War to soldiers as a prophylaxis for nerve gas attacks to obtain reversible carbamylation of AChE, thereby preventing irreversible phosphorylation (Keeler *et al.*, 1991).

Several AChE inhibitors have been used or are on clinical trial for the treatment of Alzheimer's disease. The rationale is to ameliorate cognitive performance in these patients by increasing synaptic levels of acetylcholine (Summers *et al.*, 1986). Tacrine (tetrahydroaminoacridine) is the most extensively studied drug; however, controversies arose from initial

Table 51.2
Organophosphorus Pesticides and Risk of Cholinergic Syndrome[a]

Classification	Common name
Extremely hazardous	Chlorethoxyfos, chlormephos, coumaphos, disulfoton, EPN, ethoprophos, fenamiphos, fonofos, mevinphos, parathion, parathion-methyl, phorate, phosphamidon, sulfotepp, tebupirimfos, terbufos
Highly hazardous	Azinphos-ethyl, azinphos-methyl, cadusafos, chlorfenvinphos, demeton-S-methyl, dichlorvos, dicrotophos, edifenphos, famphur, heptenophos, isazofos, isofenphos, isoxathion, mecarbam, methamidophos, methidation, monocrotophos, omethoate, oxydemeton-methyl, pirimiphos-ethyl, propaphos, propetamphos, thiometon, triazophos, vamidothion
Moderately hazardous	Anilofos, bilanafos, butamifos, chlorpyrifos, cyanophos, diazinon, dimethoate, ethion, etrimfos, fenitrothion, fenthion, formothion, methacrifos, naled, phenthoate, phosalone, phosmet, phoxim, piperophos, profenofos, prothiofos, pyraclofos, pyrazophos, quinalphos, sulprofos
Slightly hazardous	Acephate, azamethiphos, iprobenfos, malathion, pirimiphos-methyl, pyridaphenthion, trichlorfon

[a]WHO recommended classification by hazard (WHO, 1998). Based on acute oral and dermal toxicity in rats and the physical state of product or formulation, pesticides are ranked as follows:

   Extremely hazardous: 5 mg/kg or less if solid; 20 mg/kg or less if liquid
   Highly hazardous: 5–50 mg/kg if solid; 20–200 mg/kg if liquid
   Moderately hazardous: 50–500 mg/kg is solid; 200–2000 mg/kg if liquid
   Slightly hazardous: over 500 mg/kg if solid; over 2000 mg/kg if liquid
Only compounds in use or being developed are reported (Tomlin, 1997).

reports (Relman, 1991) and clinical results have so far not been convincing (Davis *et al.*, 1992; Maltby *et al.*, 1994).

Finally, pyridostigmine salicylate was shown to rapidly reverse clinical signs of central and peripheral anticholinergic toxicity caused by a variety of drugs, such as antidepressants, antiparkinsonians, antihistamines, and antispasmodics, and toxic plants, such as mushrooms, potato sprouts, and bittersweet (Granacher and Baldessarini, 1975).

51.1.2 PATHOGENESIS

OPs exert their toxic action by interfering with cholinergic transmission. The molecular mechanism of cholinergic toxicity involves the interaction of OPs with AChE, which almost completely explains all the signs and symptoms of acute OP poisoning. Symptoms and signs are related to excess acetylcholine and the consequent overstimulation in all districts of the central and peripheral nervous systems (CNS and PNS) where acetylcholine acts as a neurotransmitter.

51.1.2.1 Acetylcholinesterase and Cholinergic Functions

AChE is an elongated molecular structure formed by heterologous subunits that is localized mainly in the outer basal lamina of the synapse. The enzyme is highly concentrated at the neuromuscular junction, and it is synthesized in both nerve and muscle. A single gene encodes the catalytic subunits of AChE (Taylor, 1996a). The atomic structure, determined by x-ray analysis, reveals that the active site catalytic triad (serine, histidine, and glutamate) lies near the bottom of a deep and narrow gorge that reaches halfway into the protein. Substrates and inhibitors are drawn to the active site of the enzyme by an aromatic guidance mechanism that is formed by 14 aromatic residues that line about 40% of the gorge, providing an array of low-affinity binding sites (Sussman *et al.*, 1991).

The synaptic function of AChE is to remove the neurotransmitter acetylcholine. The hydrolysis of acetylcholine involves acetylation of the serine residue followed by restoration of the active center of AChE. The time required for hydrolysis of acetylcholine at the neuromuscular junction is less than a millisecond (Taylor, 1996a). However, because the cholinergic transmission is involved in a variety of functions that require specific features at different sites, AChE distribution and hydrolysis time may vary, depending on the type of response needed in a given district. Moreover, differences in the cholinergic transmission also depend on several other factors, including synthesis storage and release of acetylcholine, distribution of different receptors, and types of signal transduction (Brown and Taylor, 1996; Taylor, 1996a, b).

Cholinergic transmission is involved in the stimulation of skeletal muscle and autonomic ganglia (nicotinic), autonomic effector cells in the white muscles, cardiac conduction system, and secretory glands (muscarinic), and CNS neurons.

51.1.2.2 Chemistry and Biochemistry of Anticholinesterases

OPs that display anticholinesterase activity are triesters of phosphoric acid with the general structure shown in Table 51.1 and in Figs. 51.1 and 51.2. R_1 and R_2 vary (e.g., alcohols, amides) as does the X moiety (e.g., fluorine, phenoxy). The nomenclature of OPs and other anticholinesterases, and their classification may follow various schemes (Chambers, 1992; Edmundson, 1988; Holmstedt, 1963). Figure 51.3 and Table 51.3 illustrate the biochemical interactions between OPs and AChE, and Table 51.3 offers some examples of them.

OPs react covalently with AChE by phosphorylating the serine residue at the catalytic center. This occurs essentially in the same manner that acetylcholine acetylates AChE (Aldridge and Reiner, 1972; reactions 1 and 2 in Fig. 51.3). Affinity constants vary, depending on the OP involved. However, in contrast to the acetylated enzyme, which rapidly yields acetic acid and restores the catalytic center, the phosphorylated enzyme is stable and catalytic activity recovers very slowly (reaction 3 in Fig. 51.3). The rate of spontaneous reactivation depends on the chemistry of the attached phosphoryl residue. In the case of dimethoxy-phosphorylated AChE, rates are much higher compared with those of phosphoryl residues with longer carbon chains (diethoxy, dipropoxy, etc.), where reactivation might not occur at all. Rates of spontaneous reactivation are even higher for carbamylated AChE, which restores its catalytic activity more rapidly than the phosphorylated enzyme, although still much more slowly than acetylated AChE. For this reason, carbamates are defined as reversible AChE inhibitors. Rates of spontaneous reactivation should be considered in conjunction with those of a further nonenzymatic reaction that occurs on phosphorylated AChE. This reaction, called aging, involves the loss of one alkyl group and leads to stabilization of the phosphorylated

enzyme (reaction 4 in Fig. 51.3). The degree of AChE inhibition and its duration *in vivo* largely depend on these rates: when the rate of spontaneous reactivation is higher than that of the aging reaction, almost complete recovery of activity is expected. On the contrary, if the rate of aging is higher than that of spontaneous reactivation, then irreversible inhibition takes place (Table 51.3). Rates of spontaneous reactivation and aging may have clinical relevance in the case of poisoning by dimethoxy OPs (and by carbamates, where carbamylated AChE does not undergo aging) because diagnostic and therapeutic attitudes may differ from those in cases of poisoning by other OPs (see Section 51.1.3.8).

51.1.3 CLINICAL MANIFESTATIONS

51.1.3.1 General Features

The clinical pictures of acute OP poisoning reflect the degree of accumulation of neurotransmitter that causes cholinergic overstimulation in various organs. Early effects are characterized by stimulation or facilitation at various sites, which are followed, at higher concentrations of anticholinesterases, by inhibition or paralysis (Taylor, 1996a). The relationship between OP toxicity and nervous tissue AChE inhibition is influenced by many factors. In general, 50–80% of AChE must be inactivated before symptoms are noted. Brain AChE activity around 10–15% of normal is associated with severe toxicity, and below 10% with coma, seizures, respiratory failure, and death. Lethal exposures in the absence of treatment have been estimated to correspond to approximately 30–50 times the minimal symptomatic exposure for most OPs (Holmstedt, 1959). A pharmacological description of acute poisoning is reported in Table 51.4, where signs and symptoms are ranked as muscarinic, nicotinic, and CNS.

Signs and symptoms of acute poisoning usually appear within minutes or a few hours of exposure, depending on the chemical involved, route of exposure, and dose. Unusual cases of suicide attempts by intravenous injections of OPs have been reported, where symptoms and signs appeared quite early even if doses were (probably) small (Güven *et al.*, 1997; Lyon *et al.*, 1987).

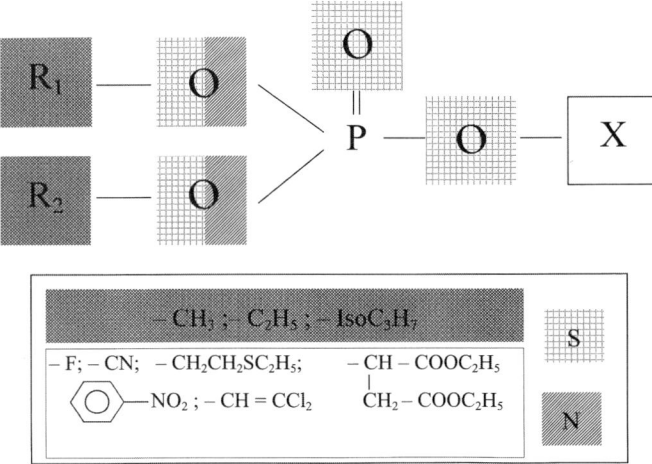

Figure 51.1 Chemical structure of organophosphorus esters. Oxygen can be replaced with sulfur at all sites. Oxygen atoms bound to R_1 and R_2 can also be replaced with nitrogen or may be absent on one (phosphonates) or both groups (phosphinates). R groups can be the same or different. Examples of the chemistry of R groups and of leaving groups (X) are also given (also see Table 51.1).

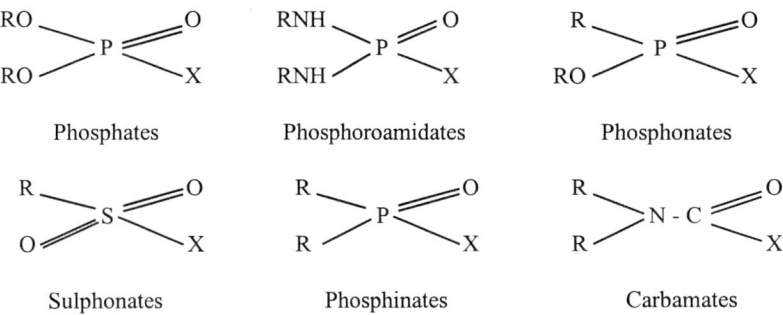

Figure 51.2 Chemical structure of anticholinesterase agents. Some are pesticides (phosphates, phosphoroamidates, phosphonates and carbamates); others are not (phosphinates and sulfonates). Carbamates are reversible inhibitors of AChE.

Cases have been reported of delayed onset of symptoms and signs often associated with prolonged toxicity and relapses. Five patients displayed mild cholinergic toxicity within a few hours of ingestion of dichlofenthion, but severe toxicity did not appear until 40–48 h afterward (Davies *et al.*, 1975). Two patients died and cholinergic symptomatology persisted up to 48 days in the survivors. In one patient, blood dichlofenthion was detected for 75 days after poisoning, whereas in another patient, inhibition of both plasma and red blood cell (RBC) cholinesterases was detected for 66 days.

In another case of combined dermal and inhalation exposure to fenitrothion, mild symptoms appeared after 2 days and more severe symptoms appeared over the next 3 days. Relapses of cholinergic signs occurred on days 11 and 17 (Ecobichon *et al.*, 1977). In a case of ingestion of fenitrothion, delayed onset of poisoning was confirmed (Sakamoto *et al.*, 1984).

A case of suicide attempt was described where the patient started to complain of symptoms 5 days after ingestion of fenthion and relapse of cholinergic toxicity occurred on day 24 (Merrill and Mihm, 1982). In another suicide attempt with fenthion, the patient had initial symptoms a few minutes after ingestion that became severe 31 h later and lasted for 18 days (Mahieu *et al.*, 1982). In a further case of poisoning by fenthion, blood levels of the chemical measured 11 days after intoxication were 1000 times higher than those measured upon admission to the hospital (Martinez-Chuecos *et al.*, 1992). In a case of suicide attempt with isofenphos, severe symptoms occurred 24 h after intramuscular injection and lasted for 10 days (Zoppellari *et al.*, 1997).

All these cases involved OPs with slow disposal and long persistence in the fat; both these pharmacokinetic characteristics are justified by the high partition coefficient of these

Table 51.3
Examples of Interactions of Some OPs with Human AChE[a]

Organophosphates		Inhibition	Phosphorylated AChE	Spontaneous reactivation	Aging
		(AChE I_{50} 10^{-6} M)		($t_{1/2}$ hours)	($t_{1/2}$ hours)
CH_3O, CH_3O > P–O–CH=CCl$_2$ (=O)	Dichlorvos	0.95	E–O–P(=O)(OCH$_3$)(OCH$_3$)	0.85	3.9
C_2H_5O, C_2H_5O > P–O– (=O) pyridinyl Cl,Cl,Cl	Clorpyrifos-oxon	0.007	E–O–P(=O)(OC$_2$H$_5$)(OC$_2$H$_5$)	58	41
i-C_3H_7O, i-C_3H_7O > P–F (=O)	DFP	0.83	E–O–P(=O)(OC$_3$H$_7$-i)(OC$_3$H$_7$-i)	No reactivation at 6	4.6

[a]Data from Lotti and Johnson (1978), Capodicasa *et al.* (1991), and EPA (1992).

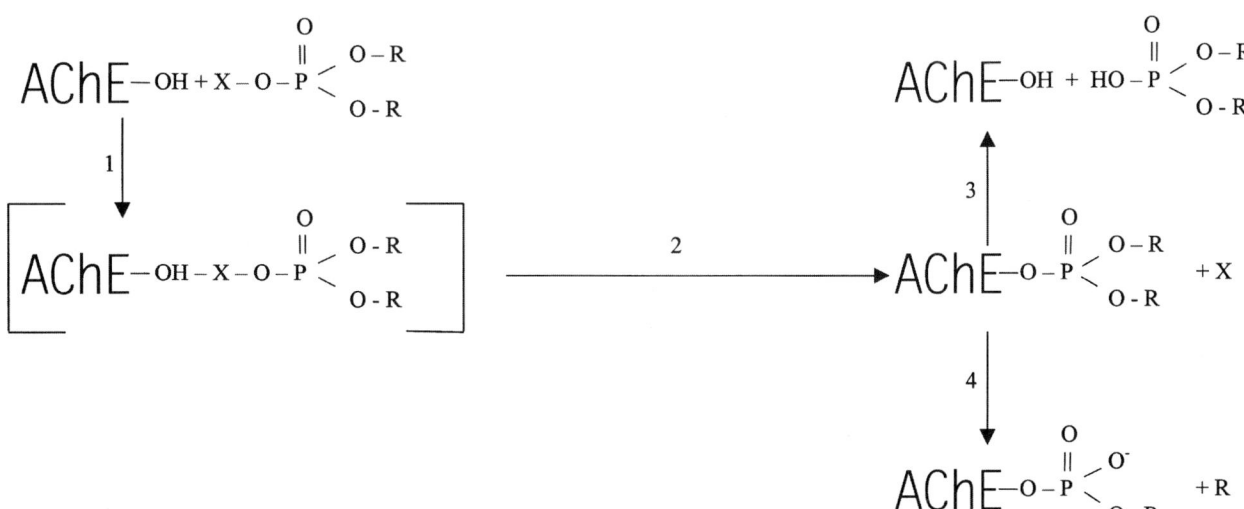

Figure 51.3 General representation of biochemical interactions between OPs and AChE. Reaction 1 leads to the formation of Michaelis complex and reaction 2 leads to phosphorylated AChE. Rates of these reactions indicate the affinity of enzyme for a given OP. Reaction 3 is spontaneous reactivation of AChE, which is usually very slow, although in the case of dimethoxy phosphorylated AChE the speed of reactivation is higher. Reaction 4 leads to a stable, negatively charged phosphorylated AChE (aging of phosphorylated AChE).

Table 51.4
Signs and Symptoms of Organophosphate Poisoning

Manifestations	Signs and symptoms
Muscarinic	
Respiratory system	Wheezing, dyspnea, cyanosis, bronchorrhea, bronchospasm, pulmonary edema
Gastrointestinal system	Anorexia, nausea, vomiting, diarrhea, abdominal pain, fecal incontinence
Cardiovascular system	Bradycardia, hypertension
Urinary system	Urinary incontinence
Glands	Hypersalivation, hyperlacrimation, increased sweating
Pupils	Miosis, unreactive to light
Nicotinic	
Red muscles (including respiratory muscles)	Weakness, fasciculations, twitching, tachycardia, hypertension
Central nervous system	Headache, drowsiness, dizziness, confusion, blurred vision, slurred speech, ataxia, coma, convulsions, depression and block of respiratory center

compounds (Tomlin, 1997). These chemical and toxicological characteristics of certain OPs should be kept in mind either when patients are first observed or when antidotal treatment is discontinued.

The first signs to appear are usually muscarinic, which may or may not be in combination with nicotinic signs. The incidence of signs and symptoms is variable, depending on the dose, the chemical involved, and the time after exposure when detected. Respiratory failure is the hallmark of the clinical picture of severe OP poisoning, whereas mild poisoning and/or early stages of an otherwise severe poisoning may display no clear-cut signs and symptoms. Therefore, diagnosis is made through symptom recognition, followed by grading of poisoning severity, although the latter is only a guide for immediate treatment and has no prognostic value (Bardin *et al.*, 1987; Bardin and van Eeden, 1990; Lotti, 1991; Minton and Murray, 1988). Miosis is observable in more than 80% of patients and in the case of mild poisoning, may represent the only sign (Rengstorff, 1985, 1994). Anorexia, nausea, and vomiting are reported in 40–80% of patients and may also be the only and earliest signs of poisoning (Bardin *et al.*, 1987; Grob and Harvey, 1958; Hayes *et al.*, 1978; Namba *et al.*, 1971; Ohbu *et al.*, 1997; Okumura *et al.*, 1996; Saadeh *et al.*, 1996; Tafuri and Roberts, 1987; Tsao *et al.*, 1990). Diarrhea and abdominal pain are also reported in 20–60% of patients. Hypersalivation is reported in more than 60% and excessive sweating in more than 30% of patients. Hyperlacrymation is less frequent (10–30%). Bronchial hypersecretion and respiratory distress usually follow other muscarinic signs, but not always. Urinary and fecal incontinence can be observed in the most severe cases.

Weakness is the only nicotinic symptom that appears at early stages of poisoning. Muscle fasciculations appear later when the clinical picture becomes more severe. CNS signs such as coma and convulsions appear after muscarinic and nico-

tinic symptoms, although early CNS symptoms may include headache, dizziness, and blurred vision.

Based on the recording and evaluation of this constellation of signs and symptoms, and on the circumstantial evidence of exposure, diagnosis is relatively easy. The course of the illness depends on the toxicological characteristics of the OP, on the severity of the clinical picture, and on the promptness and efficacy of treatment.

51.1.3.2 Respiratory Failure

As result of combined nicotinic, muscarinic, and CNS cholinergic overstimulation, severe OP poisoning results in respiratory failure. Thus, bronchoconstriction, bronchorrhea, pulmonary edema, fasciculations and paralysis of respiratory muscles (the diaphragm in particular), and depression of the brain respiratory center all contribute to respiratory insufficiency. This clinical condition usually develops within 24 h of exposure and within a shorter period from the onset of signs and symptoms. It should be distinguished from a somewhat delayed respiratory failure (one to several days after poisoning) that characterizes the intermediate syndrome, which has a different pathophysiology (see Sections 51.2.2 and 51.2.3.1). The severity of respiratory failure in 52 patients with acute OP poisoning was graded according to the presence/absence of acidosis, which in turn predicted the survival rate, which is much higher in patients with hypoxemia only (Goswamy *et al.*, 1994). In the same study some markers at the time of physical examination were identified as indicative of the need for artificial ventilation. These markers include miosis, hypotension, fasciculations, unconsciousness, and low plasma cholinesterases. As a single sign, fasciculation was the most significant prognostic marker for ventilator requirement and final outcome. This observation indirectly suggests that respiratory muscle failure is more important than any other factor in causing respiratory insufficiency. However, some authors indicated the failure of central respiratory drive as the important factor (Grob, 1956; Tsao *et al.*, 1990; see Section 51.1.3). The use of plasma cholinesterase (ChE) levels to assess poisoning severity and to predict the development of respiratory failure, as also suggested by others (Tsao *et al.*, 1990), should be discouraged because low plasma ChE do not necessarily correlate with the severity of cholinergic overstimulation (see Section 51.1.3.5 and 51.4.3.2).

51.1.3.3 Cardiac Manifestations

Given the cholinergic innervation of the heart (Lefkowitz *et al.*, 1996), several types of cardiac alterations are included in the clinical picture of acute poisoning. In a review of 168 cases of acute poisoning that involved a variety of OPs (including dimethoate, methylparathion, trichlorphon, sevin, mevinphos, dichlorvos, and malathion), 134 patients showed electrocardiographic abnormalities, including prolonged QT interval and ST and T abnormalities. Fifty-six patients had arrhythmias 3–15 days after poisoning: ventricular extrasystoles and ventricular tachycardia with "torsade de pointes" characteristics have been observed. Bradyarrhythmias were less frequent, although two cases of AV block occurred (Kiss and Fazekas, 1979). QT prolongation and/or polymorphous ventricular arrhythmias also were observed in 14 patients of another series of 15 cases of OP poisoning that involved phosdrin, parathion, and phosphamidon (Ludomirsky *et al.*, 1982).

A case in which sinus bradycardia, AV dissociation, idioventricular rhythm, multiform ventricular extrasystoles, and prolongation of the PR, QRS, and QT intervals was observed. Polymorphic ventricular tachycardia, characterized by extreme variability of QRS morphology and changes in the RR interval, was also present (Brill *et al.*, 1984). QT prolongation was recorded in 97 patients in a series of 223 OP poisonings, when electrocardiograms (ECGs) were examined in retrospect (Chuang *et al.*, 1996). Mevinphos, parathion, methamidophos, ethyl 4-nitrophenyl phenylphosphonothioate (EPN), and other unspecified OPs were involved. The authors concluded that patients who presented with such ECG changes have higher mortality and a higher incidence of respiratory failure compared with those without QT prolongation. These patients were also among those who had the highest plasma cholinesterase inhibition. However, whereas patient ranking was based on plasma cholinesterase levels, and QT changes and respiratory failure also were detected in patients graded as having very mild to moderate poisoning, it is not possible to appreciate the prognostic value, if any, of these ECG changes.

In another review of 46 cases of OP and carbamate poisoning, 31 patients developed QT prolongation with or without ST and T changes, among which, 4 had ventricular tachycardia and 2 had ventricular fibrillation. Sinus tachycardia and bradycardia were equally represented (Saadeh *et al.*, 1997).

In 50 fatal cases of OP intoxication, focal myocardial damage was observed at autopsy, including pericapillar hemorrhage, micronecrosis, and patchy fibrosis (Kiss and Fazekas, 1982).

Post mortem ultrastructural examination of the heart was also performed on 10 patients who died of acute poisoning by azinphos-ethyl (9) or dimethoate (Pimentel and Carrington da Costa, 1992). Patients died 3–17 days after poisoning, all having shown ECG changes during the illness. Lysis of myofibrils, swollen and fragmented mitocondria, disorganization of nuclear chromatin, and Z band abnormalities were observed. Whether these changes are primarily related to cholinergic overstimulation of the heart and subsequent arrhythmias or are secondary to the general condition of the patients cannot be ascertained.

In conclusion, several types of arrhythmias may develop during acute OP poisoning. Therefore, patients must be carefully monitored and promptly treated.

51.1.3.4 Central Nervous System Manifestations

Various manifestations of CNS involvement that grossly reflect the severity of poisoning have been described. Thus symptoms and signs range from headache, anxiety, confusion, sleep disturbances, and blurred vision to tremor and convulsions to coma, hypothermia, and central respiratory depression.

Some authors believe the failure of the central respiratory drive is an important factor in causing respiratory failure (Grob, 1956; Tsao *et al.*, 1990), although clinical discrimination of the selective effects of anticholinesterases on the CNS is difficult, particularly in assessing their relative importance in causing death (Lotti, 1992a), because toxicity to the CNS, in general (Norton, 1986), and of anticholinesterases, in particular (Glow and Rose, 1965), always holds a strong peripheral component (see also Section 51.1.3.2).

Early CNS signs and symptoms may last for several days, in which only moderate additional cholinergic symptomatology may be detectable (Grob and Harvey, 1958). Electroencephalogram (EEG) abnormalities can be detected at the onset of symptoms and are characterized by irregularities in rhythm, variation and increase in potential, and intermittent bursts of abnormally slow waves of elevated voltage similar to those seen in epilepsy; these symptoms usually persist for about a week or longer (Grob *et al.*, 1947).

Coma is usually due to direct CNS depression by OPs, although hypoxia that derives from respiratory failure may contribute. In this condition, EEGs show profound depression of cortical activity (Lotti and Becker, 1982a). OPs vary in their potency to induce seizures (Hoskins *et al.*, 1986) and perhaps this manifestation is not entirely due to AChE inhibition (Van Meter *et al.*, 1978), considering that it is blocked by benzodiazepines, which is known to act via γ-aminobutyric acidergic (GABAergic) mechanisms (Lipp, 1973; see also Section 51.1.3.8).

Occasionally, during the acute phase of OP intoxication, patients displayed opsoclonus (De Bleecker, 1992; Hata *et al.*, 1986; Pullicino and Aquilina, 1989). Opsoclonus is an abnormal, rapid, involuntary, repetitive, chaotic, and conjugated ocular movement. Different OPs were involved in reported cases; the onset was from 3 to 48 h and there no was correlation with the typical symptomatology, although all patients were severely poisoned. Opsoclonus is most likely another sign of cholinergic overstimulation, which lasts for several hours to a few days and recovers spontaneously.

One case of poisoning with chlorpyrifos and two others with unknown OPs presented with choreo-athetosis (Joubert *et al.*, 1984; Joubert and Joubert, 1988). Extrapyramidal signs lasted a few days during recovery from acute intoxication. Similar signs also have been reported several days after the onset of cholinergic toxicity (see Section 51.1.3.6).

51.1.3.5 Laboratory Findings

Red Blood Cell and Plasma Cholinesterases In addition to synapses, AChE is also present in the outer membrane of red blood cells and, to a lesser extent, in plasma. Its physiological functions in blood are unknown. Plasma butyrylcholinesterase (BuChE), also known as pseudocholinesterase, has a different substrate specificity because it hydrolyzes butyrylcholine. Its physiological functions also are not known in plasma or elsewhere. BuChE inhibition by OPs is, therefore, not necessarily indicative of exposures high enough to cause poisoning. Moreover, certain diseases and genetic conditions are characterized

Table 51.5
Correlation between Severity of Poisoning, Inhibition of RBC AChE, and Symptoms and Signs of OP Poisoning[a]

Severity of poisoning (approximate activity of RBC AChE)	Symptoms and signs		
	Muscarinic	Nicotinic	Central nervous system
Mild (RBC AChE > 40%)	Nausea, vomiting, diarrhea, salivation/lachrymation, miosis bronchoconstriction, increased bronchial secretions, bradycardia	Usually none	Headache, dizziness
Moderate (20% < RBC AChE < 40%)	Same as above plus pupils unreactive to light, urinary/fecal incontinence	Muscle fasciculation (fine muscles)	Same as above plus dysarthria, ataxia
Severe (RBC AChE < 20%)	Same as above	Same as above plus muscle fasciculation (diaphragm and respiratory muscles)	Same as above plus coma, convulsions

[a]Modified from Lotti (1991).

by low levels of plasma BuChE (see Section 51.4.3.2). Several methods are available to measure these blood enzymes (among the many are Doctor *et al.*, 1987; Ellman *et al.*, 1961; Garcia-Lopez and Monteoliva, 1988; Lewis *et al.*, 1981; London *et al.*, 1995; St. Omer and Rottinghaus, 1992; Wilson *et al.*, 1996). However, because hospital laboratories rarely measure RBC AChE activity, in most circumstances one should rely on measurements of plasma BuChE, for which kits are easily available.

RBC AChE inhibition confirms the diagnosis of acute OP poisoning. Whole blood AChE also may be measured, considering that only about 10% of the activity is due to the plasma enzyme (Worek *et al.*, 1999b). Usually there is a good correlation between the severity of signs and symptoms of poisoning and the degree of inhibition of RBC AChE (Table 51.5). Nevertheless, because acute poisoning usually requires prompt treatment, treatment should not be delayed while laboratory confirmation is sought. Therefore, measurement of RBC AChE has limited value in an emergency because diagnosis is exclusively clinical and severe poisoning is inevitably associated with high RBC AChE inhibition.

It is more difficult to interpret the relatively low levels of RBC and plasma cholinesterases such as those observed in cases of poisoning that present with equivocal symptoms. This may be the case in mild poisoning or in the initial phase of poisoning caused by OPs that are slowly disposed. Reasons for these difficulties are manyfold and include the following:

- Large inter- and intraindividual variability of both RBC AChE and plasma BuChE, making the distinction between physiologically low and inhibited activities impossible. Methods to address these difficulties have recently been developed but they have not been applied yet in clinical settings (Polhuijs *et al.*, 1997; see Section 51.4.3.2).
- Different sensitivity of AChE and BuChE to the same inhibitor. In many cases, the identity of the chemical involved and knowledge of its biochemical characteristics are unknown, thus hampering the interpretation of a significant inhibition of plasma BuChE associated with little

or no inhibition of RBC AChE. This may be the case in both a mild poisoning or the early phase of a more severe poisoning when poisonings are caused by OPs that preferentially inhibit BuChE (see Section 51.4.3.2).

- The ratio between the inhibition of RBC AChE and that in the synapses may vary according to the compound. Inhibition of the RBC enzyme may be detected without clinical signs of toxicity in cases of exposures to OPs that do not easily cross the blood–brain barrier (see Section 51.4.3.2).
- If reactivators (oximes) are administered, the pharmacological effect depends on the ratio between inhibited and aged enzyme. This ratio may be different in blood and in the nervous tissue, and the pharmacological reactivation of inhibited blood enzymes will be more effective than that of enzymes in the nervous system. Under these circumstances relatively small inhibition in blood enzymes would not correlate with symptomatology (see Section 51.4.3.2).
- The method of cholinesterase measurement involves dilutions, which in the case of inhibitors such as carbamates and dimethyl phosphates, may favor the spontanous reactivation of inhibited enzymes (see Section 51.1.2.2). These assay related problems would understimate the actual *in vivo* inhibition.

In conclusion, measurements of blood cholinesterases may confirm the diagnosis, but are not essential: clinical observation remains the cornerstone for diagnosis. For the same reasons, repeated measurements of blood cholinesterase during poisoning have no prognostic value (Nouira *et al.*, 1994) and they cannot be used to assess the efficacy of treatment. When AChE is irreversibly inhibited by OPs, the reappearance of RBC activity depends on new erythrocytes entering the blood stream. Whereas the average lifespan of RBCs is 120 days, in most cases, observed reappearance of RBC AChE occurs at a rate of about 1% per day. The corresponding rate for plasma BuChE, which derives from liver synthesis, is about 5% per day (see Section 51.4.3.2).

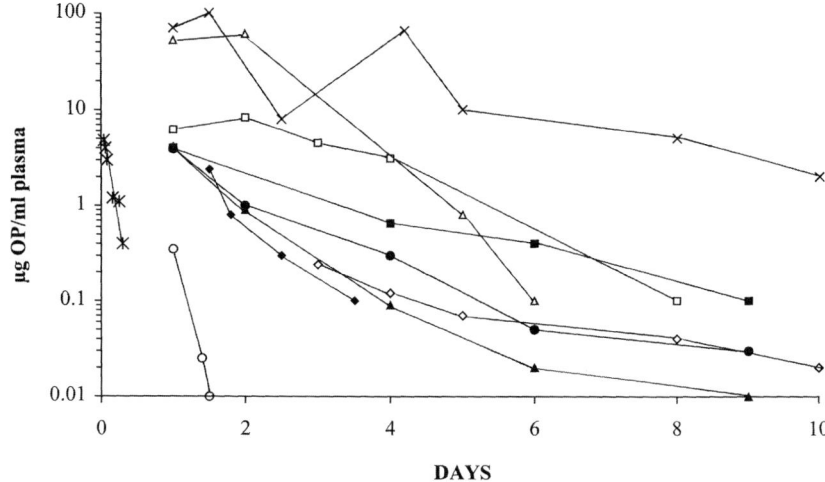

Figure 51.4 Time course of blood concentration of several OPs in acutely poisoned patients. Data for (◆) methamidophos, (■) fenitrothion, (▲) methylparathion, and (●) parathion from (Lotti, 2000); (◇) chlorpyrifos from (Lotti *et al.*, 1986); (□) methidation, (△) dimethoate, and (×) mecarbam from (Tsatsakis *et al.*, 1996); (○) malathion from (Lyon *et al.*, 1987); (∗) trichlorfon from (Nordgren *et al.*, 1980).

Measurements of OPs and Metabolites in the Blood and Urine Several analytical methods based on chromatographic techniques are available for quantitative and qualitative measurements of OPs and their metabolites in body fluids (Tomlin, 1997). These measurements have confirmatory uses in clinical toxicology although they are rarely performed because they are not easily available. Nevertheless, serial measurements of the parent compound in blood (Fig. 51.4) identifies the compound(s) and provides information about its pharmacokinetics in humans.

Metabolites of OPs can be measured in the urine. They are products of hydrolytic reactions, and include the alkylphosphate and the alcoholic moieties. Because the kinetics of urinary excretion of metabolites differ, quantitative extrapolations are almost impossible unless complete urine collection is performed over several days and both metabolites are measured. Moreover, if only one of these metabolites is measured, the results may be less specific because different OPs can share identical acidic or alcoholic moieties. Thus, two parent OP compounds that display quite different acute toxicity may produce the same amount of the same metabolite, thereby further hampering quantitative extrapolations (see Section 51.4.3.1). In conclusion, measurements of OPs and their metabolites have a limited value for diagnosis of acute OP poisoning. They may be useful for confirmatory purposes and research.

Routine Hematological and Biochemical Tests Abnormalities of almost all common laboratory tests have been reported during the course of acute OP poisoning. None of them is specific and they may reflect either somewhat typical short-term complications (pancreatitis and myopathy; see Section 51.1.3.6) or the general clinical conditions of the patient (degree of respiratory failure, changes in organ perfusion, concurrent infections, iatrogenic consequences, etc.). Isolated reports indicate that activation of blood coagulation was ob-

served in cases of parathion and dimethoate poisoning, and in one case the patient was treated with eparine (Jastrzebski *et al.*, 1994; Kaulla and Holmes, 1961). However, when studies were performed on a series of 31 patients moderately poisoned with either parathion or sarin, both hyper- and hypocoagulability were observed (Kaulla and Holmes, 1961). The clinical and toxicological relevance of these isolated observations remains unclear. In conclusion, changes in common laboratory tests are not specific for the diagnosis of OP poisoning.

Electrophysiology The electrophysiological consequences of AChE inhibition at the neuromuscular junction have been reviewed (Singh *et al.*, 1998b), and are characterized by single electrical stimulus-induced repetitive compound muscle action potentials (CMAPs) and, in response to repetitive nerve stimulation, by a decrement of the CMAP (Besser *et al.*, 1989a, b; Maselli *et al.*, 1986). These events reflect the excess of acetylcholine at synaptic levels and subsequent alteration of nicotinic receptor responses. The repetitive muscle response to a single nerve stimulus is thought to result from reexcitation of the muscle by the prolonged endplate potentials brought about by the excess of acetylcholine. At relatively low AChE inhibition, repetitive stimulation causes a decrement followed by complete recuperation of CMAP amplitudes. However, at higher AChE inhibition, repetitive stimulation results in an unimodal pattern of progressive decrements of CMAP amplitudes. Experimental studies demonstrated that in the former case, impaired neuromuscular transmission is caused by transient depolarization of the endplate region, whereas in the latter, direct blockade is due to desensitization of postsynaptic nicotinic receptors (Maselli and Leung, 1993; Maselli and Soliven, 1991).

Decremental response to repetitive nerve stimulation dramatically worsened after injection of edrophonium (Maselli *et al.*, 1986), indicating the effects of a further excess of acetylcholine, whereas the administration of pancuronium improved neuromuscular transmission, indicating a blockade of nicotinic receptors (Besser *et al.*, 1990, 1991). Distinction between these findings and those detected during the intermediate syndrome may be difficult (see Section 51.2.3.2).

Other Tests   On a small series of patients poisoned with OPs, cerebral perfusion was investigated by brain single photon emission computerized tomography (Yilmazalar and Özyurt, 1997). The authors concluded that in severe cases of poisoning, patients showed perfusion defects, especially in the parietal lobe. This study is difficult to assess because some patients who had normal plasma cholinesterase and some mild symptoms probably were not poisoned. Moreover, the patients who had major perfusion deficits were the oldest and almost no improvement was detected 3 months after poisoning.

Pathology   Gross pathology and histological examination performed at autopsy after fatal poisoning were either unremarkable or nonspecific (Maresch, 1957). In particular, given the mechanism by which OPs cause death, neuropathology is not observed unless severe hypoxia or convulsions occurred (McLeod, 1985). A common nonspecific feature of CNS histopathology is vascular damage associated with increased permeability of the vessel walls, suggesting major changes in the blood–brain barrier that might occur during OP poisoning (see Section 51.1.3.8).

51.1.3.6 Short-Term Complications

Neurological   Fatal encephalopathy was reported in two cases of acute OP poisoning (de Reuck *et al.*, 1979). These patients, after an initial recovery from cholinergic toxicity, developed a severe encephalopathy within 3–4 days and died 9–20 days after admission. Necroscopy showed severe hemorrhagic necrosis of the ventricles, resembling lesions observed in Wernicke's encephalopathy. There is no explanation for such findings, although it was reported that one patient had a history of alcoholism and the other of recurrent depression.

Neuroleptic malignant-like syndromes following organophosphate poisoning have been reported in the Japanese literature (Ochi *et al.*, 1995). In one case, a 60-year-old schizophrenic patient who had undergone a frontal lobotomy at the age of 20, but was free of medications since then, attempted suicide by ingesting a large amount of methidathion. About a week after full recovery from symptoms and signs of OP poisoning, the patient developed a high fever, extrapyramidal rigidity, and coma. Serum CPK and LDH were increased, and high urinary myoglobin was detected, whereas plasma cholinesterase was back to normal. The patient was treated successfully with dandrolene. A correlation with OP poisoning is difficult to ascertain because this clinical picture is also consistent with lethal catatonia, a rare and potentially lethal syndrome that occurs in schizophrenic patients (Castillo *et al.*, 1989).

Extrapyramidal manifestations that complicate OP poisoning were described in six patients poisoned with fenthion (Senanayake and Sanmuganathan, 1995). Patients had moderate to severe cholinergic signs and all developed intermediate syndrome subsequently. Dystonia was observed in all patients, and the most common signs were tremor, choreo-athetosis, and cog-wheel rigidity. Onset of these extrapyramidal signs was variable (4–40 days) and spontaneous recovery was observed within 4 weeks. Although the development of extrapyramidal signs is rarely described in OP poisoned patients (and in these cases, it may be compound specific), a possible relationship with inadequate oxime therapy has been inferred.

Transient bilateral vocal cord paralysis has been reported after OP poisoning, although the reports are inconsistent and describe different clinical characteristics. A 3-year-old boy severely poisoned with chlorpyrifos was intubated and artificially ventilated (Aiuto *et al.*, 1993). On day 3, immediately after extubation, the boy developed stridor and was reintubated. He was reextubated on day 6 and specific treatment for OP poisoning was halted. Occasional stridor was treated conservatively until day 11, when he needed intubation again. Tracheostomy was performed on day 19 and maintained for more than 50 days. Generalized areflexia was observed on day 18 that rapidly recovered within a week. Follow-up was not reported. Although the authors suggested that organophosphate-induced delayed polyneuropathy (OPIDP) developed, the distribution of weakness and the time course of events is not characteristic (see Section 51.3.3.1).

Three cases of delayed recurrent laryngeal nerve paralysis (25–35 days from the onset poisoning) were observed in subjects severely poisoned with three different OPs (chlorpyrifos, methamidophos, and parathion) who required intubation and artificial ventilation (de Silva *et al.*, 1994). At the onset of stridor, no other nerve was involved and the patients had been extubated 14–26 days earlier. One patient required tracheostomy, whereas the others were treated conservatively. Recovery occurred within 4–15 weeks. Although OPIDP was suggested as the cause of laryngeal nerve paralysis, the isolated involvement of this nerve speaks against it. Moreover, parathion is not known to cause OPIDP (see Section 51.3.1). Another case of isolated bilateral vocal cord paralysis was associated with OP exposure (Thompson and Stocks, 1997). However, exposure was anecdotal and there was no evidence of OP poisoning.

In further case of poisoning with unspecified OPs, bilateral vocal fold palsy was reported (Indudharan *et al.*, 1998). Palsy was observed at extubation, about 10 days after poisoning, and required tracheostomy that was maintained for 2 months. The authors suggested intermediate syndrome, but it was unknown when, after poisoning, this palsy occurred (because the patient was intubated) and if other signs of proximal weakness were detected (see Section 51.2.3.1).

Cortical visual loss was observed in two patients poisoned with OPs (Wang *et al.*, 1999). One patient had cortical visual loss as shown with positron emission tomography (PET) scan 1 year after poisoning with EPN. During this period, blurred vision was the main symptom and was not clear how long she was hypoxic. Another patient had similar effects that were detected 2 months after acute poisoning with mevinphos. She was reported to have had apnea, but the duration was unspecified. Therefore, it is likely that these two cases represent consequences of secondary hypoxia, although selectivity for this cortical area is unusual.

A case of moderate poisoning with a mixture of dimethoate, diazinon, and methoxychlor was reported where the patient was markedly hypothermic 1 h after ingestion in addition to having miosis and diffuse fasciculations. She had a rectal temperature of 33°C, which normalized within 1 h after passive rewarming (Hantson *et al.*, 1996).

In conclusion, there is no strong evidence for any neurological short-term complication directly linked to OP toxicity, except, perhaps, hypothermia, which has been consistently reported in animal studies as a compound-specific effect of certain OPs (Coudray-Lucas *et al.*, 1983).

Pancreatitis   Although it is uncommon, pancreatitis has been consistently associated with acute OP poisoning. Nevertheless, because the diagnosis of pancreatitis is usually established by detection of an increased level of serum amylase, quite often the roles of salivary gland overstimulation and/or of acidosis, both present in OP poisoning, have been overlooked as a cause of increased serum amylase. Additionally, in most reports there is no information on possible alternative causes of pancreatitis, including anoxia, hypoperfusion, infections, and concurrent treatment. The latter is important for a differential diagnosis of toxic pancreatitis, because about 5% of causes of acute pancreatitis are related to commonly used drugs (Greenberger *et al.*, 1998). Transient hyperglycemia and glycosuria, which are often found in severe OP poisoning (Namba *et al.*, 1971; Zadik *et al.*, 1983), are also common in acute pancreatitis. Hypotheses have been formulated that link the pathophysiology of the triad of pancreatitis, hyperamylasemia, and hyperglycemia in acute and severe OP poisoning (Haubenstock *et al.*, 1983).

The first case was reported on a patient who was anoxic for an unspecified period, was misdiagnosed as acute kerosene inhalation, and was later found to be intoxicated with OPs. High serum amylase levels were almost immediately detected and after 9 days, a pancreatic pseudocyst was drained (Dressel *et al.*, 1979). A case of OP poisoning by coumaphos was reported where the patient with severe respiratory failure had elevated serum amylase on admission that returned to normal 20 h later (Moore and James, 1981). Another case of pancreatitis was less convincingly attributed to cutaneous exposure to an organophosphate insecticide. Symptomatology was mild though consistent with OP poisoning but there was no evidence of poisoning and medical history suggested a very mild exposure, if any. Symptoms of pancreatitis persisted for 6 months (Marsh *et al.*, 1988).

Acute painless pancreatitis developed in a patient soon after severe intoxication with mevinphos (Hsiao *et al.*, 1996). RBC AChE was inhibited, serum amylase and lipase were elevated, and a computed axial tomography (CT) scan indicated pancreatitis. Persistent hyperglycemia developed. Two cases of acute severe pancreatitis, complicated by pancreatic necrosis and retroperitoneal sepsis were described in patients with severe poisoning by unspecified OPs (Panieri *et al.*, 1997). In both cases, diagnosis of pancreatitis was made several weeks after admission (2 and 5, respectively) and confirmed at surgery.

On a series of 75 patients admitted to the hospital for malathion poisoning, serum amylase was serially measured (Dagli and Shaikh, 1983): 47 patients had a mildly raised amylase that reversed within 2 days. Mild symptoms compatible with OP poisoning were reported in most patients, but it is not clear if they were the same patients with elevated amylase. Apparently none had severe poisoning and no toxicological evidence of OP poisoning was provided.

In another series of nine patients poisoned with parathion, painless acute hemorrhagic pancreatitis was manifested by ileus in two cases (Lankisch *et al.*, 1990). Patients were severely ill, requiring artificial ventilation, and had depressed plasma cholinesterase levels. One subject developed persistent ileus 1 week after admission and hemorrhagic pancreatitis was observed at surgery. The other patient presented with severe shock and paralytic ileus. Blood lipase and amylase were elevated and the CT scan indicated pancreatitis.

A series of 17 children poisoned with OPs was compared with a matched control group with similar abdominal symptoms (Weizman and Sofer, 1992). Compounds were identified in nine cases and included parathion, malathion, and diazinon. Five poisoned children were diagnosed with acute pancreatitis based on elevated serum amylase trypsin and glucose. Ultrasonography was not performed. None of the controls developed pancreatitis. It is not clear when pancreatitis developed after exposure, if adominal pain in these patients was, due to either pancreatitis or cholinergic overstimulation, how severe the poisoning was and what disease was diagnosed in controls.

In a retrospective study on 32 cases of OP poisoning (unspecified chemicals), 16 patients developed respiratory failure (Matsumiya *et al.*, 1996). The average levels of plasma amylase of these patients on admission was higher than that of patients who did not developed respiratory failure. The authors concluded that high amylase was predictive of subsequent respiratory failure. However, several patients with respiratory failure had normal plasma amylase and several patients without respiratory failure had elevated plasma amylase.

In a retrospective study on 159 patients admitted to the hospital for OP poisoning, Lee *et al.* (1998) found hyperamylasemia in 44 patients (out of 121 for which data were available) and hyperlypasemia in 9 (out of 28). Nine patients were diagnosed as having pancreatitis and two of them died. The incidence of hyperamylasemia was related to the clinical severity of poisoning.

It is difficult to conclude from the described clinical data whether OPs are directly toxic to the pancreas. Different OPs have been involved in these cases, the onset of pancreatitis seems to be quite variable after the beginning of cholinergic symptomatology, and important details are missing in many reports. Moreover, there are indications that in most circumstances, shock and subsequent hypoperfusion preceded the development of pancreatitis. In conclusion, although pancreatitis is consistently reported, there is no strong evidence that it is a characteristic feature of acute OP toxicity.

Myopathy On several occasions, junctional myopathy, that is, muscle damage that originates in the endplate region, has been observed in poisoned patients. The first description of muscle fiber necrosis was obtained from a case of severe parathion poisoning (de Reuck and Willems, 1975). The patient was admitted with severe respiratory failure and was artificially ventilated. Myoclonic jerks and fasciculations were present and blood cholinesterases were profoundly depressed. Episodes of irregular tachycardia developed on day 4 and the patient died of cardiac arrest on day 9. Post mortem examination revealed patchy and focal areas of necrosis of muscle fibers in the diaphragm. Nerve endings in the segmental necrotic zones of the muscle fibers were degenerated, whereas normal motor endplates were observed in the nonnecrotic muscle fibers.

Similar lesions involving muscles other than the diaphragm were reported after acute poisoning with trichlornate (de Reuck et al., 1979). The patient had moderate signs of acute OP poisoning including muscle fasciculations. After an initial improvement, the patient became comatose and required artificial ventilation on day 6, and eventually died 20 days after admission because of Gram-negative sepsis. Post mortem examination revealed waxy degeneration and lysis of individual fibers in the quadriceps femori muscle and, to a lesser degree, in the deltoid, diaphragm, and intercostal muscles. Nerve fibers were normal. In another study, samples of intercostal muscles were obtained at autopsy from a subject who died after an unquantified exposure to malathion and diazinon. Toxicological evidence of exposure and information on the severity of cholinergic overstimulation were scanty. Moreover, the patient died of brain hemorrhage. Histopathology of muscles showed basophilic inclusions and scattered necrotic fibers. It is difficult to attribute these changes to OP exposures and even more difficult to attributed them to prolonged AChE inhibition. In fact, muscular AChE was inhibited to about 50% and plasma cholinesterases were inhibited perhaps a little more (Wecker et al., 1985).

Another case report associated myopathy with OP exposure, although it was much less convincing (Ahlgren et al., 1979). The patient, who was working as an exterminator, had never had acute poisoning. Sometimes he exhibited symptoms compatible with cholinergic overstimulation, but they rapidly subsided. He presented with a 2-year history of muscle weakness, involving mainly the trunk, the shoulders and the pelvic girdle. Several muscle biopsies performed during the course of the disease revealed necrotic fibers, inflammatory reactions, and fibrotic changes in the deltoid muscle and quadriceps femoris muscles. Five years after the onset of symptoms, this patient died of progressive respiratory failure. At autopsy generalized atrophy and fibrosis of striated muscles was observed; and in particular, the diaphragm was almost entirely fibrotic. It is difficult to judge whether chronic exposure to OP caused the progressive myopathy. Clinical expression of any toxic disease is usually complete after cessation of exposure, and this patient reduced and eventually halted the exposure because of the clinical condition. No other reports indicate the progression of acute myopathy beyond the initial period of cholinergic overstimulation. There is

no quantitative evidence of exposure, which was presumably low and comprised several pesticides, although the patient reported that he most frequently sprayed diazinon.

In conclusion, there is limited evidence that acute OP poisoning causes myopathy in humans and it may be the consequence, in the cases described, of either fasciculations or sepsis. Muscle necrosis, the human equivalent of a well known effect observed in experimental animals (Dettbarn, 1992), was thought to be a possible cause of intermediate syndrome (Karalliedde and Henry, 1993; Senanayake and Karalliedde, 1987; see Section 51.2.2). However, although clinical signs suggestive of red muscle damage (such as elevated CPK) have been observed in some patients who displayed signs of intermediate syndrome (He et al., 1998), muscle biopsies suggest that the lesions were too sparse to justify clinically detectable muscle weakness (De Bleecker, 1993; De Bleecker et al., 1993).

Others Severe intoxications carry obvious risks of several secondary manifestations. Examples include a case of diazinon poisoning characterized by loss of fluids complicated with acute renal failure (Abend et al., 1994), a case of acute dimethoate poisoning complicated with Gram-negative pneumonia, acute respiratory distress syndrome, and acute renal failure (Betrosian et al., 1995), and two fatal cases of poisoning with diazinon presenting with severe hyperglycemia, metabolic acidosis, and hypoalkalemia (Hui, 1983). Preexisting diseases may also be worsened by OP poisoning as described in cases of cardiovascular disorders, which have precipitated cerebral infarction and gangrene (Buckley et al., 1994). All these and other complications should be expected in any severe case of poisoning treated in an intensive care unit.

The low levels of plasma cholinesterase caused by OP exposure change the pharmacokinetics of drugs that are substrates for these enzymes. Thus, neuromuscular blocking agents, which are widely used in anesthesia, will be slowly metabolized, thereby prolonging their pharmacological action (Østergaard et al., 1992). The first case was described in a patient severely poisoned with parathion who had undetectable plasma cholinesterase activity. In an effort to control the patient's convulsions, small doses of succinylcholine were administered (Quinby et al., 1963). The patient became suddenly apneic and completely flaccid, and the marked neuromuscular block lasted for about 2 h. A patient suspected of having a partial obstruction of the small intestine underwent emergency laparotomy and the anesthesia was induced with thiopentone and suxamethonium (Gesztes, 1966). At inspection, no obstruction was observed and the patient had a prolonged apnea when treatment was discontinued. It was later recognized that the patient had been treated with eye drops that contained ecothiopate iodide—an anticholinesterase drug—that was systemically absorbed. This clinical case is fully justified by the toxicity of ecothiopate. Thus, the pseudo-obstruction associated with the diarrhea was likely a sign of cholinergic overstimulation by ecothiopate and the prolonged apnea was the consequence of plasma cholinesterase inhibition, eventually leading to reduced metabolism of the suxamethonium.

A similar case was reported in a girl severely poisoned with chlorpyrifos following administration of succinylcholine for airway management (Selden and Curry, 1987). A patient exposed to malathion underwent surgery for acute appendicitis. Because he had no signs of cholinergic overstimulation, suxamethonium was given to facilitate tracheal intubation (Guillermo et al., 1988). He suffered prolonged apnea due to low plasma cholinesterase activity, which most likely was due to relatively low exposure to malathion because he had a normal plasma cholinesterase phenotype.

Another case of a boy who suffered relatively mild exposure to chlorpyrifos and propetamphos, and exhibited no symptoms of cholinergic overstimulation, showed prolonged apnea following suxamethonium treatment (Weeks and Ford, 1989).

These cases represent one of several possible conditions in which low plasma cholinesterase activity prolongs the pharmacological effects of neuromuscular blocking agents (Davies and Landy, 1998; Hart et al., 1995; Kopman et al., 1978; see Sections 51.4.3.2 and 51.4.3.3).

OP intoxication seems to have no effect on pregnancy if patients are properly treated. Pregnant women, between 9 and 36 weeks of gestation, intoxicated with OPs (sarin, methamidophos and fenthion) who received appropriate management completely recovered from the poisoning, allowing the pregnancies to continue to term unaffected and the delivery of healthy babies (Karalliedde et al., 1988; Ohbu et al., 1997).

51.1.3.7 Differential Diagnosis

Needless to say, it is vital to distinguish OP poisoning from other diseases, particularly when the differential diagnosis may be hampered by unusual scenarios. Thus, when observing a severely ill patient, an exposure to OPs may not be suspected at first glance (Björnsdóttir and Smith, 1999). Conversely, patients known to have been exposed to OPs may present with illnesses that are unrelated to exposure.

Although diagnosis of acute OP poisoning is straightforward, difficulties have been reported. In 20 children transferred from other hospitals, correct diagnosis of OP poisoning was made in only 4, whereas the others had diagnoses of pneumonia, various infectious diseases, encephalopathy and head trauma (Zwiener and Ginsburg, 1988). Conversely, in another series of 78 patients admitted to the hospital with diagnoses of pesticide poisoning (among which 34 were thought to be caused by OPs), only 36 (among which 18 were due to OPs) were confirmed as clinical poisoning (Lamminpää and Riihimäki, 1992). Reasons for misdiagnosis included other illnesses, no evidence of exposure, or proven limited absorption. Although the signs of cholinergic overstimulation are characteristic, they must be actively sought when OP poisoning is suspected, particularly in mild cases, because they are rarely isolated. Detection of concurrent signs would help, for instance, to ascertain the toxic nature of respiratory failure, which should be distinguished from other respiratory and circulatory causes and, similarly, for differential diagnosis of the most serious CNS manifestation such as seizures and coma (Greenaway and Orr, 1996; Hollis, 1999).

51.1.3.8 Treatment

Prompt treatment of OP poisoning is lifesaving. Several procedures are available, the sequence of which depends solely on the severity of poisoning. Special attention should be exercised by medical personnel caring for these patients, because passive contamination may occur (Ohbu et al., 1997).

Minimizing Further Exposure Procedures aimed at decontamination and/or at minimizing absorption depend on the route of exposure. Thus, in the case of dermal exposure, contaminated clothing should be removed and the skin should be washed with alkaline soap. When the skin appears to be clear, the patient should be bathed or swabbed, because most OPs are more soluble in alcohol than in water (Durham and Hayes, 1962). In the case of eye contamination, extensive irrigation with water or saline should be performed for several minutes.

In case of ingestion, various procedures have been recommended to reduce absorption from the gastrointestinal tract, although there is limited evidence of their efficacy (Johnson and Vale, 1992; Lotti, 1991). In conscious patients, vomiting is usually induced with syrup of ipecacuanha (10–30 ml followed by 2–300 ml of water). This treatment is contraindicated if the patient is semiconscious, has difficulty swallowing, or if the pesticide is dissolved in hydrocarbon solvents or is corrosive, given the high incidence of pneumonitis/atelectasias due to insecticides that contain petroleum distillate (Zwiener and Ginsburg, 1988). In these circumstances, the increased probability of aspiration pneumonia largely exceeds that of potential benefits. Gastric lavage with instillation of activated charcoal should be performed after the patient's airway has been protected with an endotracheal tube. It has been suggested that this procedure be repeated every few hours, as long as the chemical is detectable in the lavage fluid, because it may persist for several days (Futagami et al., 1995; Willems, 1981). Although the value of this continuous lavage is not proven, empirical evidence and the slow absorption characteristic of some OPs (see Section 51.1.3.1) suggest this option be considered. Moreover, complications due to administration of activated charcoal, in addition to aspiration, may also include intestinal ulceration and massive bleeding due to constipation (Mizutani et al., 1991). In fact, when these patients are treated with atropine concurrently, they display decreased bowel peristalsis. Thus, although the use of vigorous cathartic treatment has been suggested as an adjunct to charcoal to hasten the elimination of the charcoal–poison complex, studies in humans have failed to demonstrate any substantial benefit from this combination (Neuvonen and Olkkola, 1988). Other procedures aimed at removing the absorbed OP, for example, hemoperfusion or hemodialysis, have been suggested (Luzhnikov et al., 1977; Verpooten and De Broe, 1984; Yokoyama et al., 1995), but it is doubtful that these methods achieve higher clearance of OPs from the blood than that which occurs spontaneously (Nagler et al., 1981). Moreover, because of the high reactivity and large volume of distribution of OPs, even a high blood clearance will not significantly reduce the total amount of the compound. In a retrospective study on the effects of hemoperfusion, it was shown that this procedure did not remove significant amounts of various insecticides (fenitrothion, methylparathion, fenthion, chlorpyrifos, trichlorphon, diazinon, omethoate and fenamiphos) from the body of 10 patients (Martinez-Chuecos *et al.*, 1992). High plasma concentration of OPs reappeared after the last hemoperfusion, symptoms and signs did not ameliorate, and prolonged clinical course and complications were not avoided. Similar results were reported in a fatal case of fenitrothion poisoning treated with combined hemoperfusion and hemodialysis (Yoshida *et al.*, 1987).

Atropine   Atropine represents the cornerstone of the treatment for poisoning by anticholinesterase. Other available drugs, such as reactivators of inhibited AChE, which are very effective, should be considered, in principle, as valid adjuncts to atropine administration.

Atropine is a muscarinic receptor antagonist that prevents the effects of acetylcholine by blocking its binding to muscarinic cholinergic receptors (Brown and Taylor, 1996). It is a racemic mixture of active l-hysocyamine and inactive d-hysocyamine that should be stored at 15–30°C and protected from light. Freezing should be avoided. The shelf life is 24 months from the date of manufacture if it is kept under the recommended conditions (Heath and Meredith, 1992).

Pharmacokinetic data about atropine are limited. The kinetics of distribution of atropine seem to be dose dependent: about 20% of the drug is bound in plasma and two phases, with apparent half-lives of 1 and 140 min, respectively, have been identified after intravenous injection (Hinderling *et al.*, 1985). However, for practical purposes, the reported plasma half-lives after both intravenous and intramuscular injections, varying between 1.3 and 4.3 h, should be considered. Differences are due to assay methods and to a considerable intra- and interindividual variability (Adams *et al.*, 1982; Kanto and Klotz, 1988; Kentala *et al.*, 1990). In children and in the elderly, the plasma half-life may be longer. The reported apparent volume of distribution is quite large (2–3.5 liter kg^{-1}), implying significant intra- and extracellular binding and partitioning of the drug. In children, higher volumes of distribution than in adults have been reported. About 50% of atropine is eliminated unchanged in the urine. There is no correlation between plasma levels and maximal pharmacological effects after intravenous injections (Adams *et al.*, 1982); therefore, the dose of atropine cannot be titrated by means of plasma concentration. For practical purposes, however, one should consider that the effects of intravenous atropine begin within 3–4 min and are maximal about 12–16 min after injection.

Atropine is less effective in blocking certain muscarinic effects (for example, effects on the gastrointestinal and urinary tracts) than others effects (for example, effects on the heart and the salivary glands). Atropine has no effect on nicotinic symptoms, and central muscarinic effects may be undetectable, perhaps reflecting the difficulty of penetration of atropine into the CNS, which can be achieved only by large doses (Taylor, 1996a).

Caution should be exercised in the use of atropine in hypoxic patients because it may cause ventricular fibrillation due to the increased myocardial oxygen demand brought about by the increased heart rate produced by atropine (Massumi *et al.*, 1972). Therefore, in severe cases of OP poisoning, anoxia should be corrected before atropine is administered (Durham and Hayes, 1962). However, when arterial oxygen has been normalized, there is no reason to avoid the use of atropine because of the suggested risk of ventricular fibrillation (Kecik *et al.*, 1993).

Atropine is preferably given intravenously, although the intramuscular route is also effective. Satisfactory absorption also can be achieved by inhalation, and the pharmacokinetic characteristics are similar to those that occur after intramuscular injection (Harrison *et al.*, 1986). However, atropine administration by inhalation has not been tested in cases of OP poisoning. Although several dosage regimens have been proposed and some caution was suggested in the dosage of atropine (de Kort *et al.*, 1988), the best clinical approach is to administer doses of atropine large enough to achieve clinical evidence of atropinization, that is, flushing, dry mouth, changes in pupil size, bronchodilation and increased heart rate. If such signs are undetected, the dose of atropine is assumed to be insufficient and it must be increased (Barr, 1966). A mild degree of atropinization should be maintained for at least 48 h and withdrawal of atropine should be very carefully monitored because relapse can occur, particularly when OPs are stored in fat (see Section 51.1.3.1). In case of relapse, atropinization should be immediately reestablished. In patients with mild cholinergic signs, it is appropriate to start with a test dose of atropine (1 mg in the adult and 0.01 mg kg^{-1} in children, intravenously). If signs of atropinization occur rapidly, severe poisoning is unlikely, although observation of the patient for at least 24 h is mandatory. In moderately to severely poisoned adult patients, 2–5 mg of atropine should be given intravenously and repeated every 10–20 min (0.02–0.05 mg kg^{-1} in children at the same intervals). Continuous intravenous infusion may be required in severe cases. Because patients poisoned with OPs are tolerant to the effects of atropine, quite large doses of the drug have been used in cases of severe and prolonged poisoning (Golsousidis and Kokkas, 1985; Lotti *et al.*, 1986). In a case of dimethoate poisoning, 30 g of atropine were given over 35 days with maximum daily dosage of 3.5 g (Le Blanc *et al.*, 1986). Indicated dosages of atropine in accord with the severity of the clinical picture are summarized in Table 51.6. Overdosage with

Table 51.6

Indicative Dosage of Atropine in OP Poisoning According to Severity[a]

Poisoning	Adults (mg)	Children (mg kg^{-1} i.v.)
Mild	1.0	0.01
Moderate	2.0–5.0	0.02–0.05
Severe	20 h^{-1} (infusion)	0.2 h^{-1} (infusion)

[a] See Table 51.5 for grading of poisoning severity.

atropine is rarely serious in OP poisoned patients. On the contrary, patients frequently die because of insufficient atropine. When massive tachycardia is produced by atropine, it may be corrected by propanolol (Valero and Golan, 1967), thus avoiding the need to reduce the amount of atropine. It has also been suggested that using a combination of atropine and glycopyrrolate might offer an advantage over atropine alone, inasmuch as tachycardia could be avoided and adequate antimuscarinic effects still could be provided (Tracey and Gallagher, 1990), and that glucopyrrolate may better alleviate some signs of cholinergic overstimulation (Choi *et al.*, 1998).

Oximes Oximes are nucleophilic chemicals that remove the phosphoryl group from the inhibited enzyme, thus restoring the catalytic site of AChE and its function (Bismuth *et al.*, 1992). However, this chemical reaction occurs only when the phosphorylated AChE has not undergone the intramolecular rearrangement known as aging (Fig. 51.3 and Table 51.3; Aldridge and Reiner, 1972; Holmstedt, 1959; Taylor, 1996a). Whereas this reaction is fast (usually within a few minutes), oximes should be available at the synaptic cleft as long as there is newly inhibited AChE. Therefore, oximes should be administered over the first several hours after poisoning, although treatment may be prolonged in cases of massive poisoning and in poisonings by OPs with slow pharmacokinetics.

Several oximes have been synthesized and are available (Bismuth *et al.*, 1992; Dawson, 1994): pralidoxime (2-pyridine aldoxime or 2-PAM) is the most commonly used. Oximes currently in use are pralidoxime chloride (Protopam) in the United States, pralidoxime methylsulfate (Contrathion) in France and Italy, obidoxime chloride (Toxogonin) in Germany and Sweden, and pralidoxime methanesulfonate (P2S) in the United Kingdom. The availability of these oximes, including others such pralidoxime iodide, varies according to national pharmacopeas. Other oximes have been designed for the treatment of nerve gases, but they are not available for civilian uses (Kušić *et al.*, 1985).

The pharmacokinetics of oximes has been studied mostly in normal volunteers and a few studies have compared these results with those observed in poisoned patients. In studies that involved 15 volunteers given pralidoxime (single intravenous doses 2.5, 5.0, 7.5, and 10.0 mg), the plasma half-life was about 1.3 h and the apparent volume of distribution was 0.8 liter kg^{-1} (Sidell and Groff, 1971; Sidell *et al.*, 1972). Pharmacokinetic parameters have been derived after intravenous injection of obidoxime in five healthy volunteers. The half-life (mean ± SD) was 1.2 ± 0.16 h and the volume of distribution (steady state) was 0.17 liter kg^{-1} (Sidell *et al.*, 1972). Pharmacokinetic data are also available for P2S (Holland and Parkes, 1976; Sundwall, 1960, 1961).

A short infusion regimen of pralidoxime chloride was compared with administration of a loading dose followed by continuous infusion in healthy volunteers (Medicis *et al.*, 1996). Plasma levels above 4 mg liter^{-1} were maintained with the latter regime for twice as long as with the former (257 vs. 118 min). The pharmacokinetics of pralidoxime chloride was

compared in nine healthy volunteers and six severely poisoned patients (Jovanović, 1989). Compounds involved in the poisonings were malathion, quinalfos, and dimethoate, and pharmacokinetic data were obtained after a single intramuscular dose of 1 g 2-PAM. The pharmacokinetic parameters (means ± SD) in volunteers were different from those previously reported in the literature: plasma half-lives were 148 ± 65 min, volume of distribution was 2.7 liter kg^{-1}, and total body clearance was 9±4 ml min^{-1} kg^{-1}. Nevertheless, when these parameters were compared with those in poisoned patients, significant differences were found. Thus, mean plasma concentrations of 2-PAM were one and a half times higher in patients than in volunteers at each time point and remained above 4 mg liter^{-1} for 239 and 137 min, respectively. Elimination of oxime was greatly reduced in poisoned patients as compared with controls.

Different pharmacokinetics of pralidoxime chloride also were reported in a series of children poisoned to a different degrees of severity with parathion, dichlorvos, diazinon, chlorfenvinfos, dicrotofos, and other OPs (Schexnayder *et al.*, 1998). Continuous intravenous infusion of 10–20 mg kg^{-1} h^{-1} pralidoxime following a loading dose of 15–50 mg kg^{-1} gave the following results: mean (±SD) steady state plasma concentration of pralidoxime was 22.2 mg liter^{-1} ± 12.3 (range 6.9–47.4 mg liter^{-1}), mean (±SD) plasma half-life was 3.6 ± 0.8 h (range 2.4–5.3 h), mean clearance (±SD) was 0.88 ± 0.55 liter kg^{-1} h^{-1} (range 0.28–2.2 liter kg^{-1} h^{-1}), and mean volume of distribution (±SD) was 5.5±4 liter kg^{-1} (range 1.7–13.8 liter kg^{-1}). The large clearance and the high variability of volume of distribution found in these children should be noted. These differences of 2-PAM pharmacokinetics as compared with that in normal subjects are likely to be due to changes in hemodynamics during OP poisoning.

A study that involved nine patients poisoned with various OPs (dimethoate, ethyl parathion, methyl parathion, and bromophos) indicated that pharmacokinetic data after intravenous pralidoxime methylsulfate were similar to those of pralidoxime chloride (Willems *et al.*, 1992). Thus, after a loading dose of 4.42 mg kg^{-1} pralidoxime methylsulfate, followed by a maintenance dose of 2.14 mg kg^{-1} h^{-1}, plasma levels in these patients ranged from 2.12 to 9 mg liter^{-1}. Calculated pharmacokinetic data (means ± SD) were total body clearance of 0.57 ± 0.27 liter kg^{-1} h^{-1}, elimination half-life of 3.44 ± 0.9 h, and volume of distribution of 2.77 ± 1.45 liter kg^{-1}.

Pharmacokinetic differences between healthy volunteers (see previous discussion) and poisoned patients also have been reported for obidoxime. Pharmacokinetic parameters were calculated under a steady state condition in the case of a patient severely poisoned with methamidophos and complicated by renal failure. This patient was given 4 mg kg^{-1} obidoxime intravenously over 30 min every 6 h (Bentur *et al.*, 1993). The obidoxime half-life was 6.9 h, the volume of distribution was 0.845 liter kg^{-1}, and the total body clearance 85.4 ml min^{-1}. Obidoxime plasma concentrations ranged from a preinfusion value of 5.6 μg ml^{-1} to 20.8 μg ml^{-1} during the infusion. These values are comparable to the reported values in healthy volunteers. On the contrary, the plasma half-life was longer, the clearance was lower, and the volume of distribution was larger. The most likely explanation for such differences is the renal insufficiency that affected this patient. In conclusion, pharmacokinetic parameters should be assessed cautiously because of changes in hemodynamics, particularly because of the reduction of renal blood flow produced by severe OP intoxication (Green *et al.*, 1985; Jovanović, 1989).

Each oxime has different reactivation power on a given phosphorylated AChE and different phosphoryl residues attached to AChE are not equally susceptible to the same oxime (Aldridge and Reiner, 1972; Durham and Hayes, 1962; Kassa and Cabal, 1999; Worek *et al.*, 1996, 1998a, b, 1999a). Several authors reported limited or no efficacy of oximes in the treatment of OP poisoning (Besser *et al.*, 1995; Bismuth *et al.*, 1992; de Silva *et al.*, 1992; Erdmann *et al.*, 1966; Singh *et al.*, 1995; Tafuri and Roberts, 1987; Willems *et al.*, 1993). Poisonings thought to be resistant to reactivation therapy involved chrotoxyphos, demeton, dimethoate, dimefox, methyl-phenkapton, shradan, prothoate, and triamiphos (summarized in Bismuth *et al.*, 1992). Whereas these compounds form phosphoryl–AChE complexes that are identical to those formed by other OPs for which oximes have been found effective (Worek *et al.*, 1999a), it seems to be inappropriate to consider resistance as the cause of lack of effects; other reasons should be sought, including the dose of oxime and duration of treatment, which are often insufficient (Johnson *et al.*, 1992; Willems *et al.*, 1993), the pharmacokinetics of the oxime, which may be quite variable depending on the clinical conditions of the patient, and the rates of oxime-induced reactivation of AChE (Worek *et al.*, 1996). In this respect, the plasma concentration of the OP is relevant. In cases of ethyl and methyl parathion poisonings, oximes were shown to be ineffective as long as OP concentrations remained above 30 μg liter^{-1} (Willems *et al.*, 1993; also see subsequent text).

In one study, 21 severe to moderately poisoned patients treated with atropine alone were compared with 24 patients treated with atropine plus pralidoxime (de Silva *et al.*, 1992). Patients were poisoned by a variety of OPs, including malathion, methamidophos, fenthion, dimethoate, phoxim, phentoate, and trichlorfon. Because the clinical outcomes were similar in the two groups, the authors cast doubt on the necessity of cholinesterase reactivators for the treatment of acute OP poisoning. This report was criticized because of the high mortality in both groups and because low doses of pralidoxime were used (Johnson *et al.*, 1992). Moreover, given the specific characteristics of the phosphoryl residue attached to the enzyme in the rates of aging and of reactivatibility of AChE, the lack of measurement of plasma concentrations of OPs, and the different dosages of atropine, the study and the control groups are not comparable. Finally, there is no precise endpoint to assess the efficacy for a given oxime treatment when key variables that influence the clinical outcome are involved, such as mechanical ventilation.

In conclusion, data on the inefficacy of oximes are not convincing and this potentially lifesaving therapy cannot be dismissed. On the contrary, such a course is highly recommended

in any case of severe OP poisoning and treatment should continue as long as there is circulating OP. However, because OP plasma concentrations cannot be obtained easily, some empirical approaches have been suggested to assess the need for oxime treatment. For instance, measurements of RBC AChE before and after a bolus of oximes, or *in vitro* reactivatibility of AChE from RBC sampled from the patient may indicate whether newly inhibited AChE can be reactivated (Lotti, 1995). Other methods have been described based on *in vitro* inhibition of cholinesterases by the plasma of the patient (Dawson *et al.*, 1997; Mahieu *et al.*, 1982). Nevertheless, because reactivation of blood enzymes may not strictly reflect that in the synapses and because even minimal reactivation in the nervous system is likely to be beneficial, these approaches and their results should be regarded as a guide and not as a rule.

Dosing regimes for various oximes that depend on the severity of poisoning have been suggested. The following regimes are recommended by the manufacturers.

- *Pralidoxime chloride*: Start with 1 g intravenously, followed by another 1 g after 15–30 min if no improvement. If still no improvement, start an infusion of 0.5 g h^{-1}. Slow intravenous administration is preferable, but intramuscular injection also is an option. In healthy volunteers, the pharmacokinetics of pralidoxime chloride was similar with either route of administration (Sidell and Groff, 1971).
- *Pralidoxime methylsulfate*: Start with 400 mg, followed by 200 mg after 0.5, 4, 6, and 12 h. In severe cases, start with 500 mg, repeat the same dose after 30 min, and then give 200 mg in repeated doses up to 2 g in 24 h. Continuous infusions also may be used (Willems *et al.*, 1993), up to 500 mg/h in cases of slowly disposed OPs (Tush and Amstead, 1997).
- *Obidoxime chloride*: Start with 250 mg and repeat the same dose within 2 h, or 3–6 mg kg^{-1} once or twice after poisoning.
- In children, a loading dose of 25–50 mg kg^{-1} pralidoxime chloride is recommended followed by a continuous infusion of 10–20 mg kg^{-1} h^{-1}.

All these recommended dosage schedules are aimed at achieving a plasma oxime concentration of 4 mg liter^{-1}, which was shown to be effective when using pralidoxime methanesulfonate (Sundwall, 1961). This concentration subsequently has been used a target reference value for all oximes. Nevertheless, this reference plasma level cannot be generalized because the molar concentrations of 2-PAM, obidoxime, and other oximes are different. Moreover, when the effects of various salts are compared, their different water solubilities should be taken into account because the amount of free base may vary considerably in the administered dose (Durham and Hayes, 1962). In some patients with ethyl and methyl parathion poisoning, enzyme reactivation could be obtained with pralidoxime methyl sulfate concentrations as low as 2.88 mg liter^{-1}, whereas in other patients, oxime concentrations as high as 14.6 mg liter^{-1} had no effect. In such cases, the therapeutic effect of the oxime depends on the plasma concentration of ethyl and methyl parathion (Willems *et al.*, 1993).

Insufficient oxime therapy also has been considered as a possible cause of the intermediate syndrome (Benson *et al.*, 1992). However, such a hypothesis does not explain why the intermediate syndrome is not influenced by atropine or why this condition selectivity affects certain neuromuscular junctions (see Section 51.2.3.1).

Treatment with oximes is not reccommended in carbamate poisoning and in moderate poisoning by dimethylphosphate OPs because the rates of spontanous reactivation of dimethoxyphosphorylated and carbamylated AChE are fast. Moreover, with certain carbamates, more toxic complexes with oximes may be formed (Sterri *et al.*, 1979). Pralidoxime is thought to be effective only on peripherally inhibited AChE because the quaternary nitrogen atom does not allow the drug to cross the blood–brain barrier. However, clinical observation in humans and some experimental data on animals point to the contrary (Lotti and Becker, 1982a; Namba *et al.*, 1971). A possible explanation is an alteration of the blood–brain barrier brought about by OP poisoning.

The toxicity of oximes was studied in human volunteers and iatrogenic effects were reported after treatment in some cases of OP poisoned patients (Marrs, 1991). In a study on volunteers, the acute and chronic toxicities of 2-PAM, P2S and 1,1′-trimethylenebis(4-formylpyridinium chloride) (TMB4Cl2) were compared. TMB4Cl2 and, to a lesser extent, P2S (doses higher than 2.5 g a day) were found to cause marked gastrointestinal disturbances. Minor reversible cardiovascular effects also were noted (Calesnick *et al.*, 1967).

In a patient severely poisoned with coumaphos, sudden cardiac arrest was observed 2 min after beginning an infusion of pralidoxime methyliodide, initiated about 4 h after poisoning. Trifluperazine and chloropromazine were also found in the blood of the patient. After restoring cardiac activity oxime infusion was started again but asystole recurred (Scott, 1986). The presence of phenothiazines might have potentiated the OP toxicity. However, this effect was shown in humans only in a single case report (Arterberry *et al.*, 1962) and results from research on experimental animals are conflicting (Fernández *et al.*, 1975; Michaleck and Stavinoha, 1978). Cardiac arrest was probably coincidental.

Another case of worsening symptomatology coincident with the beginning of 2-PAM treatment was reported, although there were some notable differences (Good *et al.*, 1993). A 51-year-old man presented at the hospital with limited signs consistent with moderate acute OP toxicity after several weeks of exposure to phosmet. RBC AChE was normal. Within several minutes of 2-PAM infusion, the patient had systemic and ventilatory weakness that required intubation. Electrophysiology revealed a subacute postsynaptic neuromuscular syndrome associated with some CNS dysfunctions that lasted for several weeks. One suggestive explanation offered by authors is that desensitization cholinergic receptors was produced by prolonged excess cholinergic stimulation and calcium influxes damaged the neuromuscular junction. The recommendation

was made not to use oximes in the presence of postsynaptic dysfunction because of the possible direct effects of oximes on the receptor itself (Alkondon and Albuquerque, 1989). It remains to be explained why this patient had normal RBC AChE at the onset and during the entire course of the illness.

There is some indication that further inhibition of AChE might occur during reactivation with 2-PAM (de Jong and Ceulen, 1978). Two phosphoryl oximes that formed during reactivation of the ethoxy methylphosphonyl–AChE conjugate by two oximes (LüH6 and TMB4) have been detected; they have not been detected during the reactivation of diethylphosphoryl–AChE conjugates. These phosphoryl oximes were found to be potent inhibitors of AChE, although usually they are likely to be hydrolyzed by paraoxonase (Luo *et al.*, 1999). The worsening of symptomatology after treatment of massive poisonings with certain oximes may be due to accumulation of phosphoryloximes that occurs fast enough to saturate paraoxonase activity. It has been suggested that these events might also explain the pathogenesis of intermediate syndrome (Luo *et al.*, 1999), although intermediate syndrome has been observed in many patients poisoned with diethyl OPs (see Section 51.2.3).

Mild biochemical signs of liver toxicity have been related to the use of oximes. The symptoms disappeared when treatment was discontinued and seemed more frequent with obidoxime (Balali-Mood and Shariat, 1998; de Kort *et al.*, 1988).

Diazepam Diazepam must be included in the treatment of acute OP poisoning in all but the mildest cases (WHO, 1986). Diazepam relieves anxiety in mild cases, and reduces muscle fasciculations and antagonizes convulsions in the more severe cases (Johnson and Vale, 1992; Namba *et al.*, 1971; Willems and Belpaire, 1992), although OP-induced convulsions are usually reduced by large doses of atropine (Vale and Scott, 1974). Moreover, animal data indicate that benzodiazepines improve morbidity and mortality in OP poisoning (Bošković *et al.*, 1984).

Doses of diazepam (10–20 mg) given subcutaneously or intravenously are recommended and may be repeated as needed (Minton and Murray, 1988). Rarely, other anticonvulsants such as phenytoin have been used successfully in OP poisoning cases (Sellström, 1992).

Supportive Treatment The cornerstone of supportive treatment for severe poisoning is artificial ventilation, which must be started at the first signs of respiratory insufficiency. In such cases, admission to intensive care facilities is mandatory. Supplemental oxygen may be required to correct hypoxemia, and adjustments of fluid intake and electrolyte balance should be made as necessary. In severely ill patients, it may be necessary to maintain cardiac and urinary output pharmacologically. Prophylaxis of infections and *ad hoc* treatment of cardiac arrhythmias are also necessary.

Sequence of Treatment The sequence of first aid maneuvers depends on the circumstances and on the severity of poisoning. In cases of poisoning in the field, where antidotes are rarely

Table 51.7
Suggested Sequence of Therapeutic Approaches to Acute OP Poisoning According to Severity[a]

	What to do				
Clinical conditions	First	Second	Third	Fourth	Fifth
Mild	Decontamination	Atropine[b] (bolus)	Diazepam[c]	Observation	
Moderate	Atropine[b]	Decontamination	Diazepam[c]	Pralidoxime[d]	Observation
Severe	Artificial ventilation	Diazepam[c]	Atropine[b] (infusion)	Pralidoxime[d]	Decontamination

[a] Modified from Lotti (1991). See Table 51.5 for grading severity.
[b] See Table 51.6 for dose.
[c] 10 mg s.c.
[d] See dose in the text.

available, the patient should be rushed to the hospital: very cautious decontamination may be tried in the case of dermal exposure, but in the case of ingestion, vomiting should not be induced. After the patient is evaluated in the hospital, the sequence of treatment is dictated by the severity of the clinical picture. Suggestions are given in Table 51.7.

51.1.3.9 Late Complications

Neurological   Although it is known that the recovery time for some effects exceeds, to a limited extent, the time to replace AChE (Bowers *et al.*, 1964; Namba *et al.*, 1971; Whorton and Obrinsky, 1983), these cholinergic signs and symptoms that last up to several weeks after peak effects will not be considered. Moreover, OPIDP, a well established toxicity of some OPs, will be discussed separately (see Section 51.3). Several neurologic, psychiatic, and neurobehavioral abnormalities have been observed in patients who suffered previous acute poisoned with OPs, although prospective studies are not available. These symptoms and signs recently were conceptualized as a syndrome called chronic OP-induced neuropsychiatric disorders (COPIND; Jamal, 1997), together with similar symptoms also observed after long-term low-level exposures. COPIND after acute poisoning has been labeled phenomenon 1, whereas that after long-term exposure has been labeled phenomenon 2. Similarities between the two phenomena are few and superficial, many findings are contradictory and inconsistent, and given the different types of exposures, there is no reason to believe that they belong to the same entity. Moreover, possible neurological, psychiatric, and behavioral effects either after acute or after low-level long-term exposures would be better appreciated if a distinction is maintained (see Section 51.4.1).

Like any condition associated with prolonged hypoxia, severe OP poisoning obviously could lead to various persistent neurological disorders of the CNS. Therefore, in cases of late CNS disturbances, assessments of the severity of the poisoning and of time elapsed between onset of symptoms and the beginning of treatment are required to distinguish between primary and secondary effects of OPs. For instance, a patient severely poisoned with sarin during the terrorist attack in Tokyo presented 6 months later with retrograde amnesia (Hatta *et al.*, 1996). Because the patient was hypoxic for several minutes, it is impossible to ascertain whether the cause of amnesia was a direct biochemical effect of sarin.

An unusual syndrome was reported in a patient 10 weeks after discharge from the hospital following acute poisoning with dimethoate (Sahin *et al.*, 1994). The patient presented with erythema edema and hyperesthesia in the hands associated with pain and limited movements. Upper arm electrophysiological studies revealed bilateral neuropathy and a bone scan detected increased osteoblastic activity of the hand bones. A diagnosis was made of reflex sympathetic dystrophy, which was associated with the previous poisoning. This was probably a coincidental association because the report was isolated, dimethoate does not cause OPIDP, and when OPIDP does occurs it does not exclusively affect the upper limbs or the bones (see Section 51.3).

After ingestion of bromophos, a patient presented with no signs of cholinergic overstimulation and the only evidence of exposure was a reduction of plasma cholinesterases to about 10% of normal values. Oxime was given, but no atropine (Michotte *et al.*, 1989). The patient was under treatment with maprotiline for a recurrent unipolar depressive disorder. Five weeks later the patient developed a cerebellar ataxia that subsided after 5 weeks. This case was likely a casual association, perhaps due to uncontrolled dosing with maprotiline.

EEG changes in industrial workers with past repeated accidental exposures to the warfare agent sarin have been reported (Duffy *et al.*, 1979). These exposures were not quantified, occurred at least 1 year prior to examination, and caused symptoms as well as significant RBC AChE inhibition. However, it is not clear whether cases of frank poisoning occurred. Some individuals had up to six such episodes. A number of differences, derived from complex analysis of EEG spectra, were observed between 77 exposed workers and 38 controls from the same factory but not exposed to sarin. These changes include increased β activity, increased δ and θ slowing, decreased α activity, and increased amounts of rapid eye movement sleep. Most of these changes were detected in the temporal and occipital lobes. Some controversies exist concerning the value of computerized analysis of brain wave topography (American Electroencephalographic Society, 1987; Duffy et al., 1986; Oken and Chiappa, 1986). In a commentary on these and similar results observed in animals (Burchfiel et al., 1976) the toxicological significance of these findings was questioned (Duffy and Burchfiel, 1980).

The EEGs of 100 individuals with previous acute OP poisoning (one or more episodes occurring from 3 months up to 25 years before the survey) were compared with those of matched controls (Savage et al., 1988). Several OPs were involved in the poisonings, including methylparathion, parathion, malathion, disulfoton, mevinphos, dicrotophos, TEPP, dioxathion, DEF, and phorate. Poisoned cases had slightly more abnormal EEGs, but results were not significantly different between the matched cases and the control cohort. Although the authors stated that poisoning documentation was screened for completeness, some information was missing, such as the clinical severity of poisoning, the toxicological evidence of poisoning, and the nature of intercurrent diseases. For instance, one exclusion criterion was head trauma with period of unconsciousness totaling more than 15 min, but the clinical conditions of cases with unconsciousness less than that were unreported.

A retrospective study examined the vibrotactile thresholds in three groups of subjects: (1) previously poisoned with a variety of OPs (15 subjects), (2) poisoned with methamidophos (21 subjects), and (3) a matched control (35 subjects; McConnell et al., 1994). The results indicated that over one-fourth of the subjects previously poisoned with methamidophos, known to cause OPIDP (Senanayake and Johnson, 1982), had higher vibrotactile thresholds, but similar though less pronounced effects were seen in subjects poisoned with other OPs not known to cause OPIDP. The authors concluded that classical OPIDP is only the worst disease caused by methamidophos in a spectrum of peripheral nervous system impairments that represent the sequelae of poisoning. However, toxicological and clinical assessment of the poisoning episodes were not reported, and the elevated vibrotactile threshold was not symmetrical and also detected in the fingers. In mild toxic axonopathies, lesions are confined to the lower limbs and are characteristically symmetrical; hence, the described findings are not consistent with a toxic neuropathy. Moreover, subjects were examined 1–3 years after the acute poisoning and a toxic peripheral neuropathy is likely to recover over this period of time if exposure ceases.

In a retrospective study (Steenland et al., 1994), 83 subjects exposed to a variety of OPs (among which only chlorpyrifos, which accounted for 10 cases, is known to cause OPIDP), who had one or more symptoms compatible with poisoning and documented inhibition of either RBC AChE or plasma BuChE (more than 20% of baseline or below normal range), showed significant alterations of vibrotactile sensitivity of fingers and toes compared with a control group (90 subjects). It is not clear when testing was performed, although it appears that it was done several years later. Because actual electrophysiological and vibration sensitivity data were not reported, and the clinical and toxicological data are not comprehensive, it is difficult to assess the biological significance of such changes. Moreover, as

stated before, involvement of the arms is not expected in OPIDP unless it is extremely severe and a toxic peripheral neuropathy is expected to have recovered years after cessation of exposure.

A similar retrospective study was reported by the same group of investigators (Ames et al., 1995). In 45 asymptomatic subjects who had a history of cholinesterase inhibition short of frank poisoning (RBC $\leq$ 70% of baseline or plasma cholinesterase $\leq$60% of baseline), some electrophysiological parameters were measured and no differences were found between cases and 90 controls. The OPs involved were not identified. The difference between cases in this study and those of the preceding study seems to be due to the presence of at least one symptom of cholinergic overstimulation in the subjects of the former study group, whereas the latter group had none. Cholinesterase inhibitions were overlapping in the two studies. The authors concluded that preventing acute organophosphate poisoning also prevents neurological sequelae.

Knowing the limitations of measurements of cholinesterase inhibition, of reporting symptoms common to both OP toxicity and to a variety of other conditions, and of electrophysiological studies on the upper limbs, and in the absence of detailed clinical data in one of the studies, it is difficult to compare the two studies or to agree with the authors' conclusions about the existence of chronic sequelae of acute OP poisoning, which would not occur unless substantial AChE inhibition had occurred.

In a study carried out in 1983–1984 and published in 1996, volunteers exposed to sarin concentrations that caused 30–40% RBC AChE inhibition showed mild electrophysiological changes up to 15 months after a single exposure. The small number of subjects, the high variability of changes, and the fact that only three out of eight subjects displayed persistent changes make this study difficult to interpret (Baker and Sedgwick, 1996).

In a cross-sectional study on 164 pesticide workers, a correlation was found between past OP poisoning and increased incidence of symptoms such as dizziness, sleepiness, and headache (London et al., 1998; see also Section 51.4.1.2). No evidence of correlation with past poisoning was found when vibration sense and tremor were evaluated and found to be unaltered. Moreover, clinical details of OP acute poisoning were not given.

Psychiatric Follow up studies based on interview, physical examination, and blood chemistry on long-term sequelae of acute OP poisoning revealed no significant serious neuropsychiatric effect in a group of 114 individuals, 6 of whom had severe poisoning and the others mild to moderate poisoning (Tabershaw and Cooper, 1966). An array of different symptoms reported by subjects was not considered to be associated with the poisoning. However, the authors conceded that their study would not reveal minor after effects or those of low incidence.

Preexisting psychiatric symptomatology has been reported to have worsened over 2 years after OP poisoning and whenever small further exposures to OPs occurred (Rosenthal and Cameron, 1991). Details of the poisoning of this patient were not given.

Neurobehavioral In the study described previously, combined clinical and neuropsychological evaluations were used to detect changes in the cognitive functions in a group of 100 subjects with previous acute OP poisonings compared with a matched control group (Savage *et al.*, 1988). In this study, however, the limitations already outlined raise the question whether these changes represent a consequence of brain hypoxia or of other intercurrent factors, given the very large variability in the time elapsed from poisoning to assessment. Most differences between the two groups, detected on a number of tests, were within normal variability. Certainly other factors such as educational differences might account for differences in comprehension, arithmetic, vocabulary, etc. Moreover, toxicological analysis showed that blood levels of organochlorine pesticides in the study group were about twice those of the controls. Whereas statistical analysis failed to show any association between such blood levels and the results of neuropsychological tests, the authors ruled out organochlorine as the causative agent of such impairments. However, from a toxicological viewpoint, organochlorine exposure might have been more relevant, given the pharmacokinetic differences between these pesticides and OPs, especially because organochlorine is more easily stored in the body.

In a retrospective cohort study (Rosenstock *et al.*, 1991), a group of 36 subjects previously poisoned with OPs were tested on average about 2 years after the episode of poisoning and compared with a matched control group. The poisoned group did much worse than the control group on several neuropsychological tests (visual and verbal attention, visual memory, visuomotor activities, and dexterity). The type of OPs involved and the severity of poisoning were not reported, and the design and statistical significance of the study were criticized (Schuman and Wagner, 1991). Moreover, subjects in the control group (a close friend or sibling in the same community who had never been treated for pesticide poisoning) were also occupationally exposed to OPs. Given the endpoints used (for instance, visuomotor performance) and the lack of follow-up studies, it is possible that the neuropsychological deficits were a cause rather than a consequence of OP poisoning.

A neuropsychological test battery was administered to 21 migrant farm workers who had been acutely exposed to phosdrin and other pesticides (lannate and maneb) and to matched controls (Reidy *et al.*, 1992). Two acute exposures occurred 3 years apart and subjects were examined 2 years after the second exposure on the occasion of a worker's litigation. The exposed group was significantly more impaired than controls on tests of psychomotor speed, dexterity, and visuospatial memory. Although symptomatic, RBC AChE and plasma BuChE were normal on both occasions. Therefore, if related these changes were to pesticide exposures, they cannot be a consequence of OP poisoning, but perhaps of the other involved pesticides.

In the previously quoted study (Steenland *et al.*, 1994), several behavioral parameters were tested, but only sustained activity was found to be worse in the case group than in the controls. In another previously mentioned study (Ames *et al.*, 1995), a number of neurobehavioral tests were performed on subjects who had a history of cholinesterase inhibition "short of frank poisoning." Only one test (serial digit performance) was statistically significant, but it was opposite to the hypothesized direction.

In conclusion, there is little evidence to support the notion that acute OP poisoning may result in late permanent toxic effects other than OPIDP if hypoxia and/or severe uncontrolled convulsions did not occur or did not last for sufficient time. Similar conclusions have been reached by others (Ray, 1998a, b). Moreover, ranking all these effects under one syndrome (COPIND phenomenon 1) is inappropriate and may be misleading.

51.2 THE INTERMEDIATE SYNDROME

The intermediate syndrome is characterized by weakness of respiratory, neck, and proximal limb muscles. It is not a direct effect of AChE inhibition and appears several hours after the beginning of signs and symptoms of severe cholinergic overstimulation. It is caused by a variety of OPs and seems to be related to postsynaptic effects.

This form of OP toxicity was first conceptualized by Senanayake and Karalliedde (1987), although the first accurate description of the syndrome was given by (Wadia *et al.*, 1974), who categorized the neurological manifestations of acute OP poisoning into two groups. Type 1 signs are the classical signs of cholinergic overstimulation, whereas type 2 signs, which appear later and while undergoing atropine treatment, are characterized by proximal weakness and cranial nerve palsies. New case reports and prospective studies or cases derived from retrospective analysis of medical records have been reported.

51.2.1 ETIOLOGY

Intermediate syndrome seems to occur in 20–50% of acute OP poisoning cases (Sedgwick and Senanayake, 1997). It has been observed after exposures to several OPs, including fenthion (De Wilde *et al.*, 1991; Karademir *et al.*, 1990; Senanayake and Karalliedde, 1987), omethoate (He *et al.*, 1998), dimethoate (De Bleecker *et al.*, 1993; He *et al.*, 1998; Senanayake and Karalliedde, 1987), methamidophos, monocrotophos (Senanayake and Karalliedde, 1987), diazinon (Wadia *et al.*, 1974), demeton *S*-methylsulfone (Besser *et al.*, 1989a), trichlorfon (Karademir *et al.*, 1990), parathion (De Bleecker *et al.*, 1993; He *et al.*, 1998), methylparathion (De Bleecker *et al.*, 1993) dichlorvos (He *et al.*, 1998), phosmet (Good *et al.*, 1993), and malathion (Gadoth and Fisher, 1978), and to various mixtures of OPs (De Bleecker *et al.*, 1993; He *et al.*, 1998).

51.2.2 PATHOGENESIS

The mechanism by which the intermediate syndrome develops is unknown. The first characterization of the syndrome suggested a postsynaptic effect based on electromyographic evidence of fade on tetanic stimulation, absence of fade on low-frequency stimulation, and absence of posttetanic facilitation (Senanayake and Karalliedde, 1987). This concept was further supported by morphological and electrophysiological studies, both in humans (De Bleecker *et al.*, 1992b, 1993; Sedgwick and Senanayake, 1997; Singh *et al.*, 1998a, b) and animals (Engel *et al.*, 1973), suggesting that muscle weakness may result from cholinergic receptor desensitization due to prolonged cholinergic stimulation. Therefore, the hypothesis was put forward that the pathophysiology of intermediate syndrome is the result of a time-confined phenomenon that includes both changes in the postsynaptic structures by desensitization and restoring the ratio of acetylcholine to AChE (De Wilde *et al.*, 1991). This process may explain the observation of an unusual case of respiratory failure precipitated by 2-PAM in a patient thought to have had prolonged cholinergic overstimulation by phosmet (Good *et al.*, 1993). Neuromuscular block may have been increased because of a sudden reduction of acetylcholine levels that had caused the postsynaptic dysfunction. Similarly, a patient poisoned with oxydemeton-*S*-methyl was comatose shortly after poisoning, but responded to noxious stimuli. However, such response decreased suddenly 42 h after intoxication and the electrophysiological investigation performed 66 h after poisoning detected severe neuromuscular dysfunction characterized by the decrement phenomenon after repetitive nerve stimulation. At this point in time, obidoxime was given and the neuromuscular block worsened (Besser *et al.*, 1995). With this interpretation, the hypothesis that the intermediate syndrome may result from excessive and persistent acetylcholine levels due to insufficient oxime therapy during the early acute phase of cholinergic toxicity might have some validity (Gadoth and Fisher, 1978; Benson *et al.*, 1992).

Another hypothesis relates the development of intermediate syndrome to the formation of oxime–phosphoryl complexes, which greatly inhibit AChE and not efficiently cleaved by paraoxonase (Luo *et al.*, 1999; see Section 51.1.3.8). Muscle necrosis, the human equivalent of a well known effect observed in experimental animals (Dettbarn, 1992), was also thought to be a possible cause of intermediate syndrome. Myopathy was described by de de Reuck and Willems (1975), Ahlgren *et al.* (1979), de Reuck *et al.* (1979), and Wecker *et al.* (1985; see Section 51.1.3.6). However, the clinical evidence of muscle necrosis was not consistent in a 21 case series because only about one-half of the patients had elevated CPK and LDH (He *et al.*, 1998). Moreover, the histopathological lesions were too limited (De Bleecker *et al.*, 1993) to support the notion that intermediate syndrome is due to muscle necrosis.

In conclusion, in support of the explanation that intermediate syndrome is a consequence of desensitization of nicotinic receptors is the observation that several OPs, quite different chemically and toxicologically, did produce intermediate syndrome and that all patients had a prolonged AChE inhibition and consequent high levels of acetylcholine. However, the reasons for the selectivity for some nicotinic receptors only, as shown by the clinical features of intermediate syndrome, remain unexplained.

51.2.3 CLINICAL MANIFESTATIONS

51.2.3.1 Clinical Signs and Course

The intermediate syndrome develops during recovery from cholinergic manifestations, one to several days after the poisoning. Distinction should be made between this syndrome and the recurrence of cholinergic toxicity, which may occur with OPs that display prolonged disposal (Davies *et al.*, 1975; Ecobichon *et al.*, 1977; Gadoth and Fisher, 1978; Molphy and Rathus, 1964; Perron and Johnson, 1969; see Section 51.1.3.1). In some cases, the sudden onset of intermediate syndrome occurs in patients when they are completely recovered from the initial cholinergic crisis (Senanayake and Karalliedde, 1987; Wadia *et al.*, 1974), whereas in others, it is concurrent with muscarinic signs of toxicity or with superimposed muscarinic relapses (De Bleecker *et al.*, 1993). Concurrent and recurrent cholinergic signs are controlled by atropine, whereas those of the intermediate syndrome are not.

A constant feature in all patients is a marked weakness of neck flexion and of proximal limb muscles. These patients are unable to raise their head off the pillow, to abduct their shoulders' or to flex their hips. A sudden respiratory failure due to weakness of respiratory muscles also characteristically occurs in 70–100% of the cases, often drawing attention to the onset of the syndrome. Upper and lower limb reflexes are often reduced or absent, and in several patients there was evidence of weakness of muscles innervated by cranial nerves. One or more nerves may be involved, including the III, IV, VII, IX, X, and XI. There is no distinct pattern in the development of these signs.

Mortality due to respiratory paralysis and complications ranges from 15 to 40%. The clinical course in surviving patients lasts up to 30–40 days. Regression of cranial nerve palsies appears first, followed by improvement of respiratory insufficiency and recovery of strength in the proximal limb muscles. Neck flexion is the last function to recover.

51.2.3.2 Electrophysiology

Electrophysiological studies have been performed on a few patients with intermediate syndrome (De Bleecker *et al.*, 1993; Sedgwick and Senanayake, 1997; Senanayake and Karalliedde, 1987; Singh *et al.*, 2000; Wadia *et al.*, 1987). Nerve conduction velocity was normal and distal latencies were either normal or slightly reduced. No signs of spontaneous activity, such as fibrillation potentials or positive sharp waves, were observed. Repetitive stimulation showed decrements of CMAP at low and/or intermediate frequencies in most patients (10–50 Hz), lasting for several days, but always disappearing before clinical normalization, indicating that the neuromuscular junctional dysfunction in the intermediate syndrome is likely postsynaptic.

Electrophysiological changes that occur after repetitive stimulation have been detected both in poisoned patients with clinical evidence of intermediate syndrome and in patients with acute poisoning without subsequent development of intermediate syndrome (De Bleecker *et al.*, 1993). In the latter group, these changes followed recovery from initial depolarization block due to acetylcholine excess (see Section 51.1.3.5). It is, therefore, not clear whether this postsynaptic block is always present in all cases of acute OP poisoning, beginning a few days from the initial cholinergic syndrome. In such a case, the reasons for the switch from subclinical to a clinically evident intermediate syndrome are unknown.

51.2.3.3 Pathology

Muscle histopathology was performed in very few patients (De Bleecker *et al.*, 1992a, b, 1993). Few and scattered necrotic muscle fibers were observed. Histochemical endplate AChE staining was variable in intensity. Ultrastructural examination showed neuromuscular junctions that contained numerous synaptic vesicles, swollen mitochondria, and synaptic clefts with well established basal lamina. Some endplates showed vesiculations and phagocytic lysosomal activity suggestive of degeneration. Some of the synaptic clefts were widened and filled with debris, junctional folds were simplified, and postsynaptic areas were denuded and degenerated.

51.2.3.4 Treatment

Treatment is exclusively supportive because there is no specific treatment for the intermediate syndrome and atropine is not effective. Endotracheal intubation and mechanical ventilation are lifesaving.

51.3 DELAYED POLYNEUROPATHY

Organophosphate-induced delayed polyneuropathy is a rare toxic effect in humans, although some epidemics have occurred in the past such as the famous Ginger–Jake paralysis when thousands of patients were intoxicated with triorthocresyl phosphate (TOCP; Morgan, 1982; Inoue *et al.*, 1988). Neuropathy is characterized by a symmetric, distal sensory–motor, central–peripheral axonopathy that affects the legs and, in the most severe cases, also the arms. OPIDP is mechanistically unrelated to cholinergic and intermediate syndromes, and, therefore, it is not necessarily associated with the anticholinesterase activity of OPs. In fact, several OPs (such as triarylphosphates) are devoid of this activity, but may cause OPIDP. A large body of experimental data indicate that this axonopathy is likely to be correlated with effects on a neural esterase known as neuropathy target esterase (NTE; Johnson, 1990; Lotti, 1992b). Clinical onset is delayed for up to 10–20 days after a single exposure and for an unspecified period after continuous exposures.

51.3.1 ETIOLOGY

Not all OPs are capable of causing OPIDP and in the case of OP insecticides currently in use, polyneuropathy develops exclusively after a severe episode of cholinergic toxicity. Because OPIDP is not a consequence of acute cholinergic toxicity,

Table 51.8
Comparative Sensitivities of Human AChE and NTE for Various Inhibitors[a]

Compound[b]	AChE I$_{50}$ (μM)	NTE I$_{50}$ (μM)	$\dfrac{\text{AChE I}_{50}}{\text{NTE I}_{50}}$
Dichlorvos	0.95	16	0.06
Methamidophos (L isomer)	100	400	0.2
Chlorpyrifos-oxon	0.01	0.2	0.05
Mipafox	>100	12	>1
Phenylsaligenin phosphate	0.12	0.003	39

[a]Data from Lotti and Johnson (1978), Bertolazzi *et al.* (1991), and Capodicasa *et al.* (1991).
[b]Direct acting OPs or metabolites (chlorpyrifos oxon from chlorpyrifos and phenylsaligenin phosphate from TOCP).

but just another toxic effect of OPs, in the case of insecticides it will develop at a much higher dose than that which causes cholinergic overstimulation. This is indirectly shown in Table 51.8, where sensitivity to various inhibitors of AChE (target of cholinergic toxicity) and of NTE (target of OPIDP) derived from human tissues are compared. OP insecticides that caused OPIDP in humans (Table 51.9) produced OPIDP only after cholinergic toxicity. Mipafox was never developed as an insecticide and caused OPIDP after mild cholinergic toxicity. Phenylsaligenin phosphate is the active metabolite of TOCP (not an insecticide), which caused several cases of OPIDP without cholinergic toxicity. Similar differences were seen with hen enzymes, which in turn correlate with the capability of a given OP to cause OPIDP, relative to that of causing death (Lotti and Johnson, 1978). Therefore, compounds with AChE I$_{50}$/NTE I$_{50}$ ratios > 1 may cause OPIDP without cholinergic toxicity, whereas those with a ratio < 1 will cause OPIDP only after cholinergic toxicity and appropriate antidotal treatment.

OPIDP displays a characteristic age-related sensitivity in both experimental animals and humans. Children are resistant to OPIDP (Goldstein *et al.*, 1988) and when they are affected, they recover much quicker than adults, usually within a few months (Senanayake, 1981).

In addition to the case reports listed in Table 51.9, other reports can be found where development of OPIDP was associated with single or short-term exposures to certain OPs, although clinical and toxicological evidence was not convincing. EPN and leptophos cause OPIDP in hens and are NTE inhibitors, but only at doses that cause severe cholinergic toxicity (Johnson, 1975; Ohkawa *et al.*, 1980). However, a report of OPIDP that involved several workers who had long-term exposure to EPN indicated little or no evidence of cholinergic overstimulation and most clinical details were missing. Moreover, during the release of EPN, these workers were also exposed to other chemicals derived from an explosion and fire in a manufacturing facility (Xintaras and Burg, 1980).

An outbreak of neurological disorders occurred in a plant that manufactured leptophos (Xintaras *et al.*, 1978), which is

Table 51.9
OP Insecticides that Cause Delayed Polyneuropathy in Humans[a]

Compound	Number of cases	Circumstances	References
Chlorpyrifos	2	Suicide	Lotti *et al.*, 1986; Martinez-Chuecos *et al.*, 1992
Dichlorvos	3	Suicide	Vasilescu and Florescu, 1980; Wadia *et al.*, 1985
Isofenphos[b]	3	Suicide	Catz *et al.*, 1988; Tracey and Gallagher, 1990; Moretto and Lotti, 1998
Methamidophos	Several	Suicide/occupational	Senanayake and Johnson, 1982; Moretto and Lotti, 1998; McConnell *et al.*, 1999
Mipafox	2	Occupational	Bidstrup *et al.*, 1953
Trichlorfon	Several	Suicide	Hierons and Johnson, 1978; Johnson, 1981; Shiraishi *et al.*, 1983; Niedziella *et al.*, 1985; Csik *et al.*, 1986
Trichlornate	2	Suicide	Jedrzejowska *et al.*, 1980; Willems, 1981

[a]Modified from Lotti (2000). All cases displayed preceding cholinergic toxicity.
[b]One of these cases was a combined exposure with phoxim.

known to cause OPIDP in experimental animals (Hollingshaus *et al.*, 1981). Three subjects had signs compatible with OPIDP at medical examination and six had symptoms in a retrospective study. Several subjects, however, had neurological signs unrelated to OPIDP and all were exposed to a variety of neurotoxic chemicals, including *n*-hexane.

Another group of case reports suggested OPIDP development after exposures to omethoate, parathion, mecarbam, fenthion, and mevinphos. However, these pesticides are not NTE inhibitors and negative results have always been reported in the hen test (FAO/WHO, 1987, 1996, 1997; Johnson, 1975; Lotti, 1992b).

A polyneuropathy compatible with OPIDP developed after a suicide attempt with omethoate (Curtes *et al.*, 1981), but in a subsequent report of a man who died shortly after an acute omethoate poisoning, no NTE inhibition was detected in post mortem nerve tissues (Lotti *et al.*, 1981). Parathion was associated with OPIDP after massive poisoning together with methanol (de Jager *et al.*, 1981). Toxicological evidence of parathion in body fluids was missing and the clinical description does not support evidence of RBC AChE inhibition or methanol poisoning (Lotti and Becker, 1982b). Moreover, several cases of severe parathion poisoning resulted in no OPIDP (Namba *et al.*, 1971). Mecarbam was reported to cause neuropathy, but nerve biopsy revealed segmental demyelination without axonal degeneration (Stamboulis *et al.*, 1991), a morphological lesion not expected in OPIDP (see Section 51.3.3.3).

A case of delayed neuropathy apparently developed 1 month after acute poisoning by fenthion, which was followed by intermediate syndrome (Karademir *et al.*, 1990). It is not clear whether diagnosis was made on clinical grounds or exclusively on electromyography (EMG). Because the results of EMG studies were not reported, interpretation of this case is difficult. One further case of delayed polyneuropathy by fenthion was reported (Martinez-Chuecos *et al.*, 1992), but no clinical details were given. Moreover, another patient poisoned with fenthion, and belonging to the same series, did not develop neuropathy.

A female patient who attempted suicide with methylparathion, fell into a deep coma that lasted 4 weeks (Nisse *et al.*,

1998). Electromyography was normal 3 weeks after poisoning, whereas 1 week later it showed signs of mild distal sensory motor polyneuropathy. Diffuse myogenic alterations were also detected, but electrophysiological data were not reported. Because the neuropathy disappeared within 4 weeks, this was unlikely a case of OPIDP and was probably a consequence of prolonged coma.

A case of severe poisoning by mevinphos was reported to have been complicated by polyneuropathy (Hsiao *et al.*, 1996). No clinical or electrophysiological data were given. It is said that nerve conduction studies confirmed the neuropathy. In such a case, OPIDP would be unlikely, because conduction is usually, at the most, slightly affected in axonopathy. No followup was reported.

An isolated case of Guillan–Barré-like syndrome was described in a patient after exposure to merphos, a defoliant with little anticholinesterase activity (Fisher, 1977). Exposure was dermal and likely very low. Four days later the patient started complaining of upper and lower limb weakness; 14 days after exposure, he developed facial diplegia. EMG and clinical features were suggestive of Guillan–Barré syndrome. This is the only case in the literature of Guillan–Barré-like signs after acute exposure to OP, but the clinical and electrophysiological characteristics of OPIDP are quite different.

In conclusion, combined clinical and experimental evidence allows firm conclusions on OPIDP only for a few chemicals (Table 51.9). Nevertheless, it should be pointed out that neuropathic impurities may be present in commercial formulations, which perhaps accounts for some of these cases (Johnson, 1984).

51.3.2 PATHOGENESIS

The initial event in OPIDP is the inhibition of NTE, followed by aging of the phosphoryl NTE complex. These molecular changes occur within a few hours of exposure, but almost nothing is known about what happens between these events and the clinical, morphological, and electrophysiological onset of

OPIDP 2–3 weeks later (Johnson, 1990; Lotti, 1992b). Limited evidence suggests that development of OPIDP in humans also involves inhibition of NTE. In two fatal cases of OP poisoning, NTE activity was measured post mortem in the peripheral nerve. As expected from animal studies, NTE was found to be inhibited in a case of chlorpyrifos poisoning (Osterloh *et al.*, 1983), whereas it was not in a case of omethoate poisoning (Lotti *et al.*, 1981). Lymphocytic NTE (see Section 51.3.3.2) was found to be inhibited soon after exposure in one case of poisoning with chlorpyrifos (Lotti *et al.*, 1986) and in two cases with methamidophos that all developed OPIDP weeks later (Moretto and Lotti, 1998; McConnell *et al.*, 1999). Lymphocytic NTE inhibition was also found in a patient poisoned with isofenphos who died on day 32; OPIDP might have developed after this time. In severe poisoning by compounds not known to cause OPIDP, lymphocytic NTE inhibition was not detected (Moretto and Lotti, 1998). After occupational exposures to DEF, substantial NTE inhibition in lymphocytes was measured, but found not to be associated with the development of OPIDP or with electrophysiological changes. In this case, lymphocytic NTE did not represent a good mirror of peripheral nerve NTE, probably because of the particular pharmacokinetics of this compound (Lotti *et al.*, 1983).

51.3.3 CLINICAL MANIFESTATIONS

51.3.3.1 General Features

Symptoms of OPIDP begin 2–3 weeks after single doses when, as in the case of insecticides, cholinergic symptoms have subsided (Lotti *et al.*, 1984). The lag time between single or short-term exposure and the clinical onset of OPIDP depends on both the chemical involved and the dose (Bidstrup *et al.*, 1953; Lotti *et al.*, 1986; Senanayake and Johnson, 1982). OPs with slow pharmacokinetics may cause OPIDP after a prolonged period following exposure (up to 4 weeks), whereas higher doses of OPs that are powerful in causing OPIDP may shorten this period to about 10 days. Clinical features of OPIDP are usually fully expressed within a few days of the onset of symptoms and signs, and no progression has been observed in the absence of further exposure. After repeated exposures, such as those to nonanticholinesterase OPs, the onset of symptoms and their full development is more variable and less definible (Vasilescu, 1982).

The usual initial complaint is cramping muscle pain in the legs (Susser and Stein, 1957), followed by distal numbness and paresthesia (Senanayake and Jeyaratnam, 1981; Vasilescu *et al.*, 1984). Progressive leg weakness occurs, together with depression of tendon reflexes. Symptoms and signs may also appear in the arms and forearms following those in the legs, but always after severe exposures (Bidstrup *et al.*, 1953; Moretto and Lotti, 1998; Senanayake and Jeyaratnam, 1981; Vasilescu, 1982; Vasilescu *et al.*, 1984).

Physical examination reveals distal symmetrical predominantly motor polyneuropathy, with wasting and flaccid weakness of distal limbs muscles, especially in the legs. Signs

include a characteristic high-stepping gait associated with bilateral foot drop (Senanayake and Jeyaratnam, 1981). Severe OPIDP may result in quadriplegia with foot and wrist drop as well as mild pyramidal signs. In time, there is complete functional recovery if spinal cord axons have been spared by smaller doses (Senanayake, 1981); otherwise, pyramidal and other signs of central neurological involvement may become more evident. The degree of pyramidal involvement determines the prognosis for functional recovery, and spastic ataxia may represent a permanent outcome of severe OPIDP (Morgan and Penovich, 1978; Tosi *et al.*, 1994; Vasilescu, 1982). Objective evidence of sensory loss is usually slight or absent. In one group of patients poisoned with methamidophos, some sensory symptoms, but no objective signs, were recorded (Senanayake and Johnson, 1982). In two patients who developed OPIDP after exposure to chlorpyrifos and isofenphos, slight sensory alterations were detected during both physical and electrophysiological examination (Moretto and Lotti, 1998). However, in a series of patients, cases were reported where purely sensory peripheral neuropathy was displayed after repeated low exposures to chlorpyrifos that caused some symptomatology, and no signs or mild signs of cholinergic overstimulation (Kaplan *et al.*, 1993). This contrasts with the known toxicological characteristics of chlorpyrifos, which is a better inhibitor of AChE than NTE (Capodicasa *et al.*, 1991; Richardson, 1995), and the clinical features observed in two cases of OPIDP induced by chlorpyrifos, where OPIDP was always preceded by severe cholinergic overstimulation (Lotti *et al.*, 1986; Martinez-Chuecos *et al.*, 1992). Whereas the exposure assessment in the Kaplan series was limited and based almost exclusively on medical history, interpretation of these discrepancies is difficult.

51.3.3.2 Laboratory Findings

They are no specific changes in common laboratory tests, including chemical and morphological analysis of spinal fluid. Increased serum levels of immunoglobulin G autoantibodies to glial fibrillary acidic protein and to neurofilament 200 have been detected in a case of methamidophos poisoning after the development of OPIDP (McConnell *et al.*, 1999), probably reflecting peripheral nerve damage.

Lymphocytic NTE NTE activity was found in lymphatic tissues in humans (Moretto and Lotti, 1988) and its characteristics in circulating lymphocytes led to the conclusion that the level of this blood enzyme is similar to that in the nervous system (Bertoncin *et al.*, 1985). On this basis, suggestions were made to measure and use lymphocytic NTE like RBC AChE activity is used in the clinical setting and in the biomonitoring of occupational exposures (Lotti, 1987). NTE activity has also been detected in humans platelets (Maroni and Bleecker, 1986). Only on one occasion has the ratio between NTE inhibition in lymphocytes and peripheral nerves been measured, and it was found to be about 1 (Osterloh *et al.*, 1983), although it is anticipated that it will not be always so, given the different pharmacokinetics of OPs. Inhibition of lymphocytic NTE soon after poisoning was predictive of OPIDP development when measured several days before the onset of OPIDP in two cases (McConnell *et al.*, 1999; Moretto and Lotti, 1998).

Given the relatively high turnover of blood lymphocytes and the usually rapid disappearance of OPs from the blood, measurement of lymphocytic NTE should be made in the early days after poisoning because the activity may be back to almost normal at the onset of OPIDP. However, because no treatment for OPIDP is available, the detection of lymphocytic NTE soon after poisoning has limited clinical value. Similarly, measurements of lymphocytic NTE to monitor occupational exposures to OP insecticides have no practical value because such exposures preferentially inhibit blood cholinesterases and, therefore, lymphocytic NTE rarely would be affected (see Section 51.3.1).

Electrophysiology Electrophysiological changes are usually detected concurrently with the onset of clinical symptoms and signs of OPIDP. When performed during the symptom-free period between the disappearance of cholinergic toxicity and the clinical onset of OPIDP, the electrophysiological examination is normal (Lotti *et al.*, 1986). The electrophysiological picture accords well with the histopathological findings of distal axonopathy (Jedrzejowska *et al.*, 1980; Lotti *et al.*, 1986; Moretto and Lotti, 1998; Vasilescu and Florescu, 1980; Vasilescu *et al.*, 1984; see Section 51.3.3.3). The evaluation reveals partial denervation of affected muscles, with increased insertional activity, abnormal spontaneous activity (fibrillation potentials and positive sharp waves), and a reduced interference pattern; large polyphasic motor unit potentials also may be found after a few weeks. The compound muscle action potentials to supramaximal stimulation of motor nerves are reduced in amplitude, and terminal motor latencies are delayed; maximal conduction velocity is usually normal or slightly reduced. Minimal electrophysiological abnormalities of sensory function are occasionally detected.

About 1 year after poisoning, normalization of electrophysiological parameters parallels that of clinical signs unless the pyramidal tract is involved. In such a case, findings may resemble those of amyotrophic lateral sclerosis (Vasilescu, 1982).

51.3.3.3 Pathology

The histopathology of OPIDP has rarely been described in humans (Aring, 1942; Jedrzejowska *et al.*, 1980; Lotti *et al.*, 1986; Vasilescu *et al.*, 1984), although there are no major differences from what has been extensively observed in experimental animals (Abou-Donia and Lapadula, 1990; Cavanagh, 1973; Tanaka and Bursian, 1989). The central peripheral distribution of lesions is similar to that of toxic neuropathies of other origins. The vulnerability of nerve fibers is directly related to axonal length and diameter; large-diameter and long fibers are more susceptible than small and short ones. Spinal cord changes involve mainly the anterior horn cells and the pyramidal tracts. Lesions in the tract of Goll were less constant and no lesions were seen in the tract of Burdach (Aring, 1942).

Sural nerve biopsies indicated axonal-type lesions with an even degree of involvement of myelinated fibers of differ-

ent sizes and a lesser degree of involvement of unmyelinated fibers. Dark and swollen axoplasm due to the accumulation of axoplasmic organelles can be observed association with aspects of axonal degeneration. On teased fiber preparations, some ovoids arranged in linear rows were identified. Electron microscopy found myelin debris in the Schwannian profiles. Depending on the time of biopsy after poisoning, various stages of regeneration and remyelination can be observed. Segmental demyelination is not observed (Jedrzejowska *et al.*, 1980; Lotti *et al.*, 1986). These changes indicate a process that is a primary distal axonopathy with moderate, secondary, and distal loss of myelin.

51.3.3.4 Differential Diagnosis

The unequivocal suggestion for diagnosis of OPIDP caused by insecticides is the presence of an episode of acute cholinergic toxicity in the recent past medical history. More difficult is differential diagnosis when substantial exposures to nonanticholinesterase OPs that cause OPIDP is overlooked. Symmetrical leg involvement with additional involvement of upper limbs only in severe cases, lack of involvement of cranial nerves and the autonomic system, and electromyographic changes consistent with distal axonal neuropathy are all indicative of OPIDP. Medical history aimed at identification of possible sources of OP exposure remains, in these cases, the only way to etiologically attribute neuropathy.

51.3.3.5 Treatment

There is no specific treatment for OPIDP. Intensive programs of physical therapy are indicated to ameliorate muscle trophism during the recovery from peripheral nerve lesions. In later stages, if spasticity develops, GABA antagonists may be used.

51.4 LONG-TERM EXPOSURES

Long-term exposures to OPs may cause cholinergic syndrome if both the size of repeated doses and the intervals between them overcome AChE resynthesis in the nervous tissues. In such a case, a buildup of AChE inhibition may occur and when threshold is reached, symptoms that are indistinguishable from those observed after single or short-term exposures are produced. Therefore, only signs and symptoms unrelated to overt cholinergic toxicity will be considered in this section.

Many reports on the effects of long-term exposures to OPs lack follow up studies, particularly after cessation of exposures. Therefore, most of the described effects may not be chronic (i.e., longstanding or irreversible) and probably reflect the effects of current exposures. Therefore, it is advisable not to talk about chronic effects, but rather of effects of low-level exposures, either during exposure or shortly afterward, and keep them distinct from effects detectable several months or years after cessation of exposure. Moreover, the major problem of these studies is often the insufficient assessment of exposures, that obviously hampers the interpretation of results.

51.4.1 NEUROLOGICAL, PSYCHIATRIC, AND BEHAVIORAL EFFECTS

The large amount of literature that describes neurological, psychiatric, and behavioral effects has been reviewed in several articles (Brown and Brix, 1998; ECETOC, 1998; Eyer, 1995; Steenland, 1996; Ray, 1998a, b). In one review, these effects were all ranked under the heading of chronic OP-induced neuropsychiatric disorders (COPIND, phenomenon 2; Jamal, 1997). As previously discussed (see Section 51.1.3.9), the various effects will be discussed separately for better comprehension and because there is no evidence that they collectively represent a single nosological entity.

51.4.1.1 Neurological Effects on Central Nervous System

Clinical reports   A case of parkinsonism was described in a subject with reported past and prolonged exposure to OPs. Apparently he also had several episodes of acute poisoning with parathion and malathion said to have required treatment with oral doses of atropine to control symptoms and signs (Davis *et al.*, 1978). The past history was not fully reported and it is doubtful that oral atropine would have been effective because it is known to be poorly and unreliably absorbed. Consequently, this case remains an isolated and anecdotal report.

A visual syndrome, known as Saku disease, which is characterized by reduced visual field, myopia, astigmatism, lesions of the optic nerve, and abnormal retinal functions, was associated with the extensive use of OPs during the 1960s in one area of Japan (Saku). These effects, exclusively reported by Japanese investigators, have been summarized by Pleština and Piuković-Pleština (1978) and Dementi (1994). However, the symptoms were not consistant among various OPs to which patients were allegedly exposed and often, but not always, associated with AChE inhibition. This inconsistency raises the question whether the effects are compound-specific and related to RBC AChE inhibition. These results have been criticized and the etiological link between OPs and Saku disease remains, for the time being, speculative (Erikson-Lamy and Grant, 1992).

Veterans who took part in the Persian Gulf War reported higher rates of many symptoms, including neurological ones, and had a decreased perception of well-being (Ismail *et al.*, 1999; NIH, 1994). Although a single consistent pattern of symptoms and signs is far from being defined (Gray *et al.*, 1996), this mysterious ailment is now known as the Gulf War syndrome or illness, and several hypotheses have been made concerning causes (Lotti, 1999). One theory states that wartime exposure to a combination of OPs and other cholinesterase inhibiting chemicals synergistically produced the syndrome and the neurological signs in particular, (Haley and Kurt, 1997). Among these chemicals, pyridostigmine bromide was the only defined risk factor (Shen, 1998) because it was given to soldiers who served in the Gulf, apparently for several weeks, as prophylaxis for possible nerve gas attacks. The dosing regime was a 30 mg tablet every 8 hours and it aimed to cause reversible inhibition of AChE at nerve endings, thereby preventing irreversible inhibition of the enzyme by OP weapons. None of the soldiers ever experienced acute cholinergic symptoms and signs compatible with OP or pyridostigmine poisoning.

In a study based on a questionnaire submitted by 249 Gulf War veterans from a single battalion of 606 soldiers, factor analysis of symptoms yielded several syndrome factors (possibly variants of a single syndrome) that suggested various neurological dysfunctions (Haley *et al.*, 1997a). Subjects with the highest factor scores on syndrome 1 (impaired cognition), syndrome 2 (confusion–ataxia), and syndrome 3 (arthro-myo-neuropathy), for a total of 23 cases, were evaluated for neurological functions and compared with 20 controls from the same battalion, 10 of whom had been deployed in the war region but had no complaints and 10 of whom had not been deployed (Haley *et al.*, 1997b). Brain dysfunction was evidenced by changes in auditory evoked potentials, interocular asymmetry of nystagmic velocity, asymmetry of saccadic velocity, and somatosensory evoked potentials. However, no clinical differences between cases and controls were detected on neurological examination. Exposures to anticholinesterase chemicals of either cases or controls were not reported. Therefore, whether the Gulf War syndrome exists, whether it affects the nervous system, and whether the clinical findings are due to anticholinesterases cannot be ascertained from these studies.

Occupational Exposure Studies   Minimal EEG disturbances were reported in a study on 50 workers engaged in the manufacture of a range of unspecified OPs (Metcalf and Holmes, 1969). These changes were not seen in 22 controls and mirrored, to a lesser degree, the more severe disturbances usually seen after acute exposures. Work history and exposure data were insufficient, although it was claimed that the workers were also exposed to chlorinated hydrocarbons. Certain neuropsychological changes were also reported, but it is not clear whether they were associated with such persistent EEG changes.

In another study, 32 workers exposed to both OPs and organochlorine (dieldrin) pesticides were subdivided into two equal groups, low and high exposure, based on occupational history. Plasma cholinesterase levels were the same in both groups. EEG and neuropsychological changes were found in the high exposure group (Korsak and Sato, 1977). Quantitative exposure data were not given and EEG changes were different from those reported in the above-mentioned study. A selective effect on the left frontal hemisphere, as derived from EEG and neuropsychological results, was detected. This seems inconsistent with a toxic effect.

In a seven country biomonitoring and cross-sectional epidemiological survey of low-dose occupational exposure to OPs, changes in EEG were reported only from some countries. Data from one country showed postseason slow wave activity, whereas data from another country reported different changes (Richter, 1993). These results are difficult to assess given the lack of information on exposure and other confounding factors at the time of testing.

51.4.1.2 Neurological Effects on Peripheral Nervous System

Clinical Reports In a study on volunteers, mevinphos (25 μg kg^{-1}) was administered daily for 28 days to eight subjects, whereas placebo was given to eight controls (Verberk and Sallé, 1977). RBC AChE was depressed by 19%, but no correlation was found with the detected changes. At the end of exposure, a 7% decrease in slow fiber motor nerve conduction velocity and a 38% increase in Achilles tendon reflex force were found (as percentages of preexposure values). No effects on neuromuscular transmission were detected. The authors concluded that the significance of such effects with regard to health is unclear.

Sensory neuropathies on a series of patients with low-level exposures to chlorpyrifos have been consistently associated with mild or no cholinergic symptoms (Kaplan *et al.*, 1993) although there is little evidence, if any, for a causal relationship between sensory neuropathy and low-level exposures to chlorpyrifos (see Section 51.3.3.1).

In a pilot study, 14 Gulf War veterans were examined for peripheral nerve dysfunction and compared with a control group. Although differences were detected in some parameters (cold threshold, sural nerve latencies, and median nerve sensory action potential), the authors' conclusion was that there may be dysfunction in veterans, but more studies are required (Jamal *et al.*, 1996). Moreover, the hypothesis that anticholinesterases, other than pyridostigmine, represented a risk factor for veterans of the Gulf War remains to be demonstrated.

A clinical study was performed on 72 selected subjects with long-term exposure to sheep dip OPs identified in pilot field studies (Pilkington *et al.*, 1999). According to defined criteria and neuropathy scores, 23 workers were ranked as having probable/definite neuropathy, 34 workers had possible neuropathy, and 15 workers had no neuropathy. Clinical evaluation, quantitative sensation testing, nerve conduction studies, and electromyography were performed. Results showed neurological signs in 10% of subjects and some small fiber abnormalities in 65% of electrophysiological tests. None of subjects with symptoms was in the no neuropathy subgroup. This neuropathy was thought to be different from classical OPIDP (see Section 51.2), because sensory fiber almost exclusively and small fiber more than large fiber populations were affected. Clinical and electrophysiological assessments were apparently performed at variable times after cessation of peak exposures (up to 1.5 years). Unlike other toxic neuropathies, this apparently new entity also affected upper limbs at early stages, but unlike OPIDP caused by commercial OP pesticides, there was no preceding cholinergic toxicity. Results from this study are difficult to evaluate because they are not presented analytically. Electrophysiological changes were overwhelmingly more frequent than neurological ones, but it is impossible to derive what electrophysiological abnormalities were found in patients with clinically detectable neuropathy. Moreover, the relevance of electrophysiological alterations that are not associated with signs and symptoms is unclear. According to the criteria of

sample selection, a causal relationship with exposure cannot be inferred; there is also a lack of relationship with the estimated cumulative dose. Finally, we should ask why, after such a long period since cessation of exposure, a very mild neuropathy did not recover. It seems that perhaps the study better represents a validation of a screening system to detect minor electrophysiological signs to be used in the field than a demonstration of a causal relationship between low-level exposure to OPs during sheep dipping and the development of a new form of toxic peripheral sensory neuropathy.

Occupational Exposure Studies Neuromuscular function was assessed with surface electrodes on the upper limbs of workers exposed to OPs and organochlorine pesticides (Jager *et al.*, 1970). A higher incidence of electromyographic changes (repetitive activity and reduced amplitude) was detected in workers exposed to both chemical classes ($n = 36$) as compared to those exposed to organochlorine only ($n = 24$) and controls ($n = 28$). The biological significance of these small changes is unclear, in part because of the use of surface electrodes. There was insufficient information, only statements, concerning exposures. Changes were thought to be related to synaptic dysfunction because they were similar to changes found in myastenic patients who were overtreated with anticholinesterase drugs. However, when observed in such patients, these changes are associated with substantial inhibition of AChE, whereas changes in workers were not associated with whole blood AChE inhibition.

Fifty-three workers exposed to both OPs and organochlorine were examined shortly after the start and toward the end of a spraying season (Drenth *et al.*, 1972). Surface electrode electromyography records of 12 subjects changed from normal to abnormal, whereas those of 13 subjects changed from abnormal to normal. No differences in blood AChE were detected. No evidence of exposure was given. Therefore, the conclusion of the authors that electromyography abnormalities represent only an indication of the need for more protection of workers and no evidence of immediate health problems is not substantiated.

Minimal electromyographic changes were detected by surface electrodes in 102 workers exposed to OPs when compared to an unmatched control group of 75 subjects (Roberts, 1976). Fifty-six workers were examined before and after a holiday period. Subjects who displayed these changes somewhat improved after the holidays, whereas some unspecified variability was observed in exposed subjects with normal electromyography. No exposure data were available.

In a longitudinal study on six workers exposed to OPs over a 7–9 month period, surface electrode electromyography indicated that voltages varied in a manner that reflected a vague assessment of the pattern of exposure (Roberts, 1977). It is difficult to evaluate these results given the lack of exposure data and the methods used.

Neuromuscular function was assessed with surface electrodes in a group of 11 spraymen exposed to OPs (including bromophos, diazinon, chlorpyrifos, and malathion) on a recurrent basis (Stålberg *et al.*, 1978). Plasma cholinesterases were significantly reduced after work, whereas RBC AChE was not. A slight reduction in sensory conduction velocity and increased fiber density was detected in some workers, but was unrelated to lowered plasma cholinesterase activity. Although exposure was not assessed in this study, plasma enzyme inhibition indirectly suggests a lack of correlation between degree of exposure and detected electrophysiological changes.

Another study was conducted on four groups of subjects in which approximate exposure was assessed: 42 highly exposed to OP pesticides, 14 seasonal workers exposed to OPs and reexamined after exposure, 129 agricultural workers with low exposure to OPs, and 26 agricultural workers not exposed (Jušić *et al.*, 1980). The authors concluded that synapse testing with needle electromyography and clinical examination did not detect latent OP intoxication.

A study was conducted on workers exposed to the defoliant DEF, where needle electromyography and biochemical studies (lymphocytic NTE and blood cholinesterases) were performed before and after the spraying season (Lotti *et al.*, 1983). Air and dermal exposure were measured on a typical working day. No electrophysiological changes were detected, although lymphocytic NTE was about 60% inhibited. NTE inhibition after exposure without correlation with electrophysiological changes was explained by the pharmacokinetics of DEF, which requires metabolic activation to be an esterase inhibitor and occurs mainly in the liver; the active metabolite formed is extremely reactive and unless large amounts are formed, it will not reach the nervous system, but will reach the blood, where it inhibits lymphocytic NTE.

Twenty-four workers exposed to fenthion were examined with surface electromyography before and after exposure and compared with 19 unexposed controls (Misra *et al.*, 1988). Serum AChE was also measured. Electrophysiological findings after exposure were no different from controls. However, mean values of some electrophysiological parameters were altered in the exposed group when results obtained during exposure were compared with follow-up data collected 3 weeks after withdrawal from exposure. Also, mean cholinesterase values increased after the end of exposure, but remained within the normal range. Although each exposed individual was his or her own control, results are difficult to interpret because the intraindividual variability of measured parameters of controls was not reported.

Two-hundred twenty-nine workers at a pesticide plant were examined clinically (for neurological impairment) and biochemically (lymphocytic NTE and plasma cholinesterase), and tested for tactile sensitivity and motor performance (Otto *et al.*, 1990). These workers were engaged in the production of a variety of OPs including diazinon, dimethoate, malathion, phentoate, EPN, leptophos, methamidophos, and trichorfon. Results were compared with those obtained from 180 workers from a fertilizer plant and 167 workers from a textile plant. Mean serum cholinesterases and lymphocytic NTE were lower in pesticide workers, although they were within normal ranges.

The proportion of workers with abnormal neurological findings (involuntary tremors and vibration sense) varied between plants. Tactile thresholds in the finger of the nondominant hand were higher in workers in the pesticide plant and the authors stated that this symptom was the most sensitive index of pesticide neurotoxicity. Toes were not tested. No changes were detected in the neurobehavioral tests. Assessment of exposure was missing (although some OPs that potentially cause OPIDP were manufactured), the incidence of various diseases, including neurological ones, was particularly high (in both cases and controls), and the fact that upper limb neuropathy is not expected in mild OPIDP creates problems in interpretating results.

An epidemiological study on 90 pesticide applicators (Stokes *et al.*, 1995) led to the conclusion that prolonged OP exposure is associated with loss of peripheral nerve function. Exposure was assessed by means of urinary excretion of dimethylthiophosphate, one metabolite of azinphos-methyl. However, workers had been exposed to several other OPs and pesticides. The authors' conclusion was based on a significant increase in mean vibration threshold sensitivity for applicators' hands as compared to a matched control group. Feet were not affected. Long-term exposure was determined by questionnaire, but it is unclear whether poisonings had occurred in the past. Subjective symptoms were collected off and on season: headache, weight loss, and nightmares were reported more frequently among pesticide workers, but only headache was statistically increased during the season. Because toxic polyneuropathy does not exclusively affect upper limbs and because workers were exposed to many chemicals, there is no evidence that long-term low-level exposures to OPs cause loss of peripheral nerve functions.

A cross-sectional study compared 168 spray operators with long-term exposures to OPs with 84 controls (London *et al.*, 1997). No evidence was found between exposure and loss of vibration sense. However, small differences were found on neurobehavioral test batteries based on information-processing parameters. The authors concluded that there was a small overall evidence of chronic effects of OP exposures, but indicated that exposure misclassification may have contributed to these findings.

In another study, the same authors (London *et al.*, 1998) investigated neurological symptoms, vibration sense, and tremors in much the same population during the peak spraying season. Eighty-three nonspraying workers were used as the control group. Exposure, as in the previous study, was derived from a job-exposure matrix for pesticides in agriculture. Applicators significantly reported more dizziness, sleepiness, and headache, and had a higher overall neurological symptom score. Vibration sense and tremor outcome were not associated with past long-term OP exposure. A correlation was found between symptoms and either current exposure or episodes of past OP poisoning (see also Section 51.1.3.9).

The effects of low-level exposure to foliar OP residues (primarily to azinphos methyl and possibly to phosmet and methylparathion) during one season were assessed in a cross-sectional study on 67 workers and 68 matched controls (Engel *et al.*, 1998). Sensory and motor nerve conduction velocities, neuromuscular junction testing, and RBC AChE were measured. No differences were found between exposed and controls.

51.4.1.3 Psychiatric Effects

Clinical Reports Schizophrenic and depressive reactions, with severe impairment of memory and difficulty in concentration were reported in 16 workers after variable exposures to OPs (Gershon and Shaw, 1961). This report was criticized because of serious flaws, including the lack of evidence for exposure, the detailed clinical description of only a few cases, and the inconsistency with larger studies (Barnes, 1961; Bidstrup, 1961).

An anecdotal report suggested a causal relationship between psychiatric disturbances and exposure to a variety of pesticides including OPs in two pilots (Dille and Smith, 1964).

Another anecdotal report linked the onset of psychosis in a farmer with previous spraying of demeton-*S*-methyl, but no casual relationship was established (Bradwell, 1994).

Geographical Studies A geographical study was carried out to determine whether areas of high OP usage in Australia had a higher proportion of admissions for psychiatric disorders than low-usage areas (Stoller *et al.*, 1965). No evidence was found that schizophrenia, depressive states, psychoneuroses, or personality disorders were more common in high-usage areas than elsewhere.

Increased risk of suicide was associated to pesticide exposure (mainly OPs) in an agricultural area (Parrón *et al.*, 1996a). The rate of suicides was compared with rates where exposure to pesticides was low. Most suicide cases involved pesticides, but other factors that influenced suicide attitudes were not analyzed.

Occupational Exposure Studies Workers who had unspecified exposures to OPs were compared with a control group on personality tests, structured interview, and cholinesterase levels (Levin *et al.*, 1976). Commercial sprayers, but not farmers, showed higher levels of anxiety and lower plasma cholinesterase than controls. The authors concluded that these findings were tentative until confirmed by additional studies.

The effect of exposure stress in the absence of exposure was reported during a manufacturing accident with malathion (Markowitz *et al.*, 1986). The reactions of allegedly exposed workers were compared with a matched group. The exposed group showed high demoralization scores, particularly among those who admitted to little knowledge about toxic chemicals.

Twenty-five greenhouse workers were compared to controls and showed a higher incidence of symptoms of depression and tremors (Parrón *et al.*, 1996b). Exposure was not measured and blood cholinesterases were normal.

Two groups, one of pesticide formulators (208 individuals) and another of applicators (172 individuals), were compared with matched controls (72 and 151 individuals, respectively; Amr *et al.*, 1997). Exposures to a variety of pesticides, including OPs, carbamates, organochlorine, and pyrethroids, were not quantified. Both exposed groups had a higher incidence of total psychiatric disorders, whereas formulators had a higher incidence of depressive neurosis that was related to the duration of employment. It is difficult to assess the role, if any, of the OPs, given the variety of pesticides to which these workers were exposed.

A case control study investigated the link between exposure to pesticides and suicide in Canadian farmers (Pickett *et al.*, 1998). Results excluded exposure to pesticides as an important risk factor for suicide among farmers. However, the chemicals used were not identified and were only divided between herbicides and insecticides. The latter certainly included OPs. Therefore, it cannot be ascertained from this study whether exposures to OPs were involved.

51.4.1.4 Neurobehavioral Effects

The neurobehavioral effects of long-term exposures to low levels of OPs have been extensively reviewed over the last few years (D'Mello, 1993; ECETOC, 1998; Eyer, 1995; Jamal, 1995; Mearns *et al.*, 1994; Ray, 1998a, b; Steenland, 1996). Although much information has been published, results are contradictory and whether such exposures are linked with an increased risk of behavioral effects in humans is controversial.

A study compared two groups of 53 and 68 asymptomatic workers with varying degrees of unquantified and unspecified exposure to OPs to controls (25 and 22 subjects, respectively) on a complex reaction time test. Results showed there was no indication that exposure at levels insufficient to produce clinical illness had any important effect on mental alertness (Durham *et al.*, 1965).

Another study selected 23 workers who regularly used OPs and had used them within 2 weeks of the testing date (Rodnitzky *et al.*, 1975). Recent exposure was confirmed by lower plasma cholinesterase, but RBC AChE was normal. Types of pesticides were not reported. The results of tests for memory, signal processing, vigilance, language, and proprioceptive performance were no different from those of a matched control group.

Neurobehavioral tests were performed before and after work shifts on 99 pest control workers with low-level, short-term exposure to diazinon (Maizlish *et al.*, 1987). Exposure was measured by means of the urinary metabolite diethylthiophosphate before and after the end of shifts. No changes in neurobehavioral functions were detected on a battery of seven tests. Similarly, no changes were seen when workers were subdivided according to the degree of exposure.

Neuropsychological performance was assessed by test battery in a group of 49 pesticide applicators prior to and 1 month after the end of a 6-month pesticide spraying season. Results were compared with 40 controls (Daniell *et al.*, 1992). The nature and extent of pesticide exposure were assessed and reported in another paper (Karr *et al.*, 1992). The comparison of seasonal RBC AChE changes according to exposure levels showed lower cholinesterase among higher exposure groups compared with lesser exposure group. No evidence of significant decrements in neuropsychological performance was reported.

The neurobehavioral status was assessed in workers and kibbutz residents differently exposed to OPs and other pesticides (Richter *et al.*, 1992). Subjects were examined during the spraying season and afterward. Most neurobehavioral scores were poorer during the season. Exposure data were not reported and the authors drew attention to other risk factors such as work load and heat stress.

In a cross-sectional study, neuropsychological performance in 146 sheep farmers was compared to 143 quarry workers (Stephens *et al.*, 1995a, b). The selection and the testing procedures for workers who belonged to the experimental group were different from those of controls. Long-term exposure data were assessed by means of a retrospective exposure questionnaire that used the number of sheep, dips, and years of employment as a surrogate. Farmers performed significantly worse than controls in tests to assess sustained attention and speed of information processing (simple reaction time, symbol digit substitution, and syntactic reasoning). A dose–response relationship was found only for one test (syntactic reasoning). Moreover, in another article, no association was found between the experience of acute symptoms and performance on neuropsychological tests (assessed on a subset of workers), and it was concluded that neuropsychological data reflect chronic effects that occur independently of acute effects (Stephens *et al.*, 1996). Given the large differences between OP and quarry workers, it is doubtful that the small changes detected in the former should be attributed to low-level long-term exposures to OPs.

Fifty-seven licensed applicators were compared on several neuropsychological tests to a control group of 34 farmers who had no exposure to pesticides (Fiedler *et al.*, 1997). Exposure to OPs was assessed with a questionnaire on work history, but details were not given. None of the applicators had episodes of acute poisoning, and RBC AChE values were normal. Except for slower reaction time, no other difference in neuropsychological performances was detected between exposed and nonexposed subjects.

Subclinical morbidity patterns, including symptoms, aiming at digit symbol tests, and measurement of RBC AChE, were investigated in 226 established farm workers and were compared with an equal number of controls and with 92 new farm workers (Gomes *et al.*, 1998). Results indicated a higher incidence of symptoms (irritated conjunctiva, watery eyes, blurred vision, dizziness, headache, and muscular pain and weakness), reduced performance on the aiming and digit symbol tests, and reduced AChE activity in the group of established farmworkers. Although RBC AChE inhibition implies OP exposure, no actual exposure data were reported. Moreover, reduction of AChE was still within the coefficient of variation of the test. Nevertheless, because the above-reported symptoms are consistent with cholinergic overstimulation, it is likely that differences between groups reflect the effects of current exposures to OPs.

51.4.2 OTHER EFFECTS

Several toxic effects have been associated with long-term exposures to OPs. However, most of them are either isolated reports or are based on circumstantial evidence of exposure and probably are simply coincidental. A case report, for instance, suggested congestive cardiomyopathy caused by long-term exposure to OPs without signs of severe acute poisoning. Evidence of exposure was limited and the patient had a previous myocardial infarction, therefore, cardiomyopathy was likely a consequence of myocardial infarction rather than OP exposure (Fazekas and Kiss, 1980). Several cases of influenza-like symptoms associated with OP use in farmers during the sheep dipping season apparently were unrelated to RBC AChE inhibition (Murray *et al.*, 1992).

Contact dermatitis and asthma have been linked to exposures to OP pesticides (Bryant, 1985; Deschamps *et al.*, 1994; Xue, 1992). Whether the effects are due to sensitization or irritation, or if they are linked to other ingredients always present in commercial formulations of pesticides is unclear.

Immunotoxicity of OPs has been suggested, although human data are mostly based on *in vitro* studies (Newcombe and Esa, 1992; Rodgers *et al.*, 1992; Sharma and Tomar, 1992). Hypotheses propose that exposures to OPs are linked to cancer development (Newcombe, 1992). One study was performed on workers engaged in the production of several OPs (trichlorfon, chlorfenvinphos, malathion, dichlorvos, fenitrothion, and formothion; Hermanowicz and Kossman, 1984). Exposure involved other chemicals and its assessment was rather approximate. RBC AChE and plasma ChE were reported on a group basis and correlated with the assessment of exposure. A marked impairment in neutrophil chemotaxis was found in workers who were likely to be exposed to OPs. The frequency of upper respiratory tract infections was higher in the exposed group compared with controls. No other types of infections showed increased frequency. The authors themselves concluded that a distinction cannot be made between OPs and other chemicals as possible factors for the described effects. Certainly more information is needed to ascertain whether immunotoxicity is an effect of OPs and what pathophysiological significance should be attributed to it. There is no evidence so far that any form of immunomediated clinical effect is linked to OP exposures.

51.4.3 BIOMONITORING OCCUPATIONAL EXPOSURES

Long-term occupational exposures to OPs are commonly monitored by measuring either urinary excretion of alkylphosphates or blood cholinesterases. The goal is to prevent adverse effects from OPs.

51.4.3.1 Assessment of Urinary Alkylphosphates

Although OPs may be excreted unchanged, they are usually hydrolyzed, and the acidic and alcoholic moieties can be found in the urine of exposed subjects. Measurement of metabolites is common practice in workers exposed to OPs, and several alkylphosphates have been identified, including dimethylphosphates, dimethylthiophosphates, dimethyldithiophosphates, and dimethylphosphorothioates derived from dimethylated OPs and the corresponding metabolites derived from diethylated OPs (Coye *et al.*, 1986). Several gas-chromatographic methods to measure urinary dialkylphosphates have been developed (Aprea *et al.*, 1996; Nutley and Cocker, 1993).

Measurement of excretion of the alcoholic moiety in exposed workers has been used less frequently. Examples include the measurement of 3,5,6-trichloropyridinol after exposure to chlorpyrifos and chlorpyrifos-methyl (Nolan *et al.*, 1984), *p*-nitrophenol after exposure to parathion and parathion-methyl (Morgan *et al.*, 1977), and mono- and dicarboxylic acid after exposure to malathion (Bradway and Shafik, 1977).

Despite the numerous field studies where exposures have been assessed by means of urinary metabolites, not many data are suitable for a toxicological interpretation. The reasons are many. The first problem is related to usual agricultural practices, which lead to concurrent exposures to several OPs. As stated earlier, different OPs, each with its own toxicity, may be metabolized, yielding the same product. It is, therefore, difficult to assess the toxicological risk associated with such exposures. For instance, certain exposures to either parathion-methyl or chlorpyrifos-methyl caused comparable excretion of dimethylphosphates and dimethylthiophosphates. However, the risk derived from each OP is quite different, because they display a 3 orders of magnitude difference in acute toxicity (Moretto *et al.*, 1995).

Depending on the OP, route of exposure, metabolism, and distribution, peak metabolite excretion might be reached at different times after the end of exposure. For instance, certain compounds such as chlorpyrifos show peak urinary excretion of ethylphosphates several hours after the end of exposure (Fenske and Elkner, 1990; Moretto *et al.*, 1995). On the contrary, peak excretion of ethylphosphates derived from exposures to parathion occurs within a much shorter time (Morgan *et al.*, 1977). Moreover, alkylphosphates may have a different time course of excretion. For instance, diethylphosphate peaks earlier than diethylphosphorothioate after exposure to diazinon (Sewell *et al.*, 1999). Therefore, the timing of urine sampling is crucial to assess the significance of a given concentration; for many OPs, the relevant timing information is missing.

Finally, very little is known about the correlation between urinary metabolite excretion and the inhibition of AChE and/or plasma BuChE. In many cases, enzyme inhibition was not found (Griffin *et al.*, 1999; Kraus *et al.*, 1977, 1981; Krieger and Thongsinthusak, 1993; Popendorf *et al.*, 1979); in a few cases, minimal inhibition was found (Jauhiainen *et al.*, 1992; Spear *et al.*, 1977). Only at a time when occupational exposures were probably much more severe than nowadays, was a good correlation found between *p*-nitrophenol and RBC AChE inhibition in parathion exposed workers (Arterberry *et al.*, 1961). In conclusion, for the time being, it is difficult to give these data a toxicological significance beyond that of being a qualitative exposure index.

51.4.3.2 Monitoring Blood Cholinesterase

Blood cholinesterase activities have been used extensively to monitor the effects of occupational exposures to OPs. Guidelines have been developed on methods, interpretation of results, and actions to be taken (EPA, 1992; Pleština, 1984; WHO, 1986). However, these suggestion should be taken as general indications, particularly when interpreting single data, because the following issues must be considered (Lotti, 1995).

Relationship between Inhibition of Blood Enzymes and Cholinergic Toxicity The postulate for using blood cholinesterases to biomonitor occupational exposures to OPs is that inhibition of these enzymes reflects either or both the degree of exposure or the corresponding enzyme inhibition in the nervous tissues. Because no physiological functions have been attributed to BuChE (confirmed by the fact that homozygote carriers of defective BuChE are healthy subjects; see succeeding text), the inhibition of this enzyme in any tissue most likely has no significance in terms of health. However, its inhibition in plasma means that exposure has occurred. This statement may not be true in the case of diseases (unlikely in occupational exposures) that cause depression of plasma BuChE, such as parenchimal liver diseases, acute infections, some anemias, and malnutrition. In this respect, an interesting observation is that patients with liver diseases not only have low plasma cholinesterases, but also may show a further reduction as a result of a level of exposure to OPs that causes no change of enzyme activity in normal persons or in persons affected by other diseases (Hayes, 1982). A possible explanation is the reduced ability of patients affected by liver diseases to detoxify certain OPs.

Obviously, if BuChE inhibition is associated with inhibition of RBC AChE, then different conclusions should be drawn. How accurately inhibition of RBC AChE reflects that in the synapses is unknown and extrapolation is difficult, given the different access various OPs have to the blood and the nervous system. Animal data suggest that sometimes inhibition is similar, more often, inhibition of blood enzyme is higher (Su *et al.*, 1971) due to the particular protection of the nervous system that is offered by the blood–brain barrier.

After recovery from exposure, extrapolation is even more difficult, given the different rates of recovery of AChE in the RBCs and nervous tissues, respectively. Nevertheless, based on clinical and toxicological data, a rough estimate of the levels of RBC AChE inhibition that require action are reported in the Table 51.10. It is also clear that because the access of xenobiotics to blood is always easier than to brain and because no evidence exists that OPs accumulate in the nervous system, the inhibition of RBC AChE usually overestimates the level in the brain.

Spontaneous Reactivation and Reappearance of Blood Enzymes When measuring blood cholinesterase for biomonitoring purposes, the rates of reappearance of activities after inhibition should be taken into account. Such rates depend on spontaneous reactivation (in the case of carbamates and

Table 51.10

Relationship between RBC AChE Inhibition and Preventive Actions When Monitoring Occupational Exposures to OPs[a]

RBC AChE (% inhibition from preexposure values)	Significance	Preventive action
20–29	Evidence of exposure	Improve hygenic conditions
30–50	Hazard	As above plus removal of subject from exposure
>50	Poisoning	Admit subject to the hospital

[a]Data from WHO (1986) and Lotti (1995).

Table 51.11

Sensitivity of Plasma BuChE and RBC AChE in Humans to Various Insecticides[a]

RBC AChE most inhibited	Plasma cholinesterase most inhibited
Dimefox (Edson, 1964)	Chlorfenvinphos (FAO/WHO, 1995)
Mevinphos (Rider et al., 1972, 1975)	Chlopyrifos (Eliason et al., 1969)
Methyl-parathion (Rider et al., 1970)	Demeton (Moeller and Rider, 1965)
Parathion (Hayes, 1982)	Diazinon (FAO/WHO, 1967)
	Dichlorvos (Rasmussen et al., 1963)
	Fenitrothion (Vandekar, 1965)
	Malathion (Elliot and Barnes, 1963)
	Monocrotophos (FAO/WHO, 1996)
	Trichlorfon (Abdel-Al et al., 1970)

[a]Circumstances of exposure vary.

dimethylphosphates) and resynthesis of new enzymes. As previously discussed (Section 51.1.2), the rate constants of spontaneous reactivation and of aging vary according to the phosphorylating agent. Because rate constants also depend on the enzyme that is phosphorylated, they will be different when measured in RBC AChE or plasma BuChE (Aldridge and Reiner, 1972). However, the few studies in humans do not necessarily confirm these theoretical considerations. Data from school children treated orally with trichlorfon against schistosomiasis showed that plasma BuChE as well as RBC AChE recovered much slower than was predicted from *in vitro* spontanous reactivation studies (Reiner and Pleština, 1979).

The synthesis of AChE occurs in the bone marrow, and its presence in the blood depends on the normal turnover of RBCs (i.e., 120 days). The synthesis of BuChE occurs in the liver and its turnover in plasma corresponds to about 20 days. Resynthesis of both enzymes after irreversible inhibition by OPs in the nervous systems of animals seems to occur at similar rates, corresponding to a half-life of 5–7 days. However, resynthesis is reflected in the blood quite differently because the localizations of AChE and BuChE differ. Thus, the reappearance of RBC AChE has been shown to occur at a rate of about 1% per day, whereas the rate of plasma BuChE is about 5% per day (Hayes, 1982).

Sensitivity of Blood Enzymes to Inhibitors   As stated previously, RBC AChE and plasma BuChE are different enzymes, and, therefore, they display different substrate specificity. Whereas interactions of OPs with esterases are analogous to interactions of substrates with esterases, it is clear that blood cholinesterases are differently inhibited by a given OP. As shown in Table 51.11, plasma BuChE is generally more sensitive to inhibition than RBC AChE by most OPs used as insecticides.

In cases of mild exposures, plasma BuChE may be the only inhibited enzyme. This observation should be interpreted as a sign of exposure, but not of poisoning. In cases of severe exposures, profound inhibition of plasma BuChE is always associated with similar inhibition of RBC AChE as it occurs in poisoned patients. The situation may be more complex when substantial repeated exposures are involved. In such a case, even if the plasma enzyme is more sensitive, a buildup of RBC

AChE inhibition can occur, thus equalizing the inhibition of both enzymes at a certain time because of the different rates of reappearance of the two enzymes. Therefore, equal inhibition of the enzymes may represent the consequence of either a single substantial exposure or less severe but repeated exposures.

Finally, RBC AChE may be more inhibited, even if the plasma enzyme is more sensitive when subjects are recovering from substantial exposures, given the prolonged life of the RBCs that carry inhibited AChE.

Inter- and Intraindividual Variability of Blood Enzymes   Intraindividual variability of both plasma BuChE and RBC AChE is high. Samples taken at intervals ranging from a few days to several years indicate that the coefficients of variation of both enzymes in unexposed subjects vary from 7 to 11%. In some cases, an intraindividual variability of plasma enzyme up to 100% was detected in the course of several months (Hayes, 1982). Interindividual variability of these enzymes is even greater. The coefficients of variation of RBC AChE in unexposed subjects vary from 10 to 40%, whereas the corresponding values for plasma enzyme vary from 12 to 46%. Minor differences exist according to gender, age, and race (Hayes, 1982).

A few people who have normal levels of RBC AChE are genetically deprived of plasma BuChE (Østergaard et al., 1992). It was observed that some of these people who were treated with succinylcholine during surgery exhibited an abnormal prolonged period of muscular paralysis after usual dosages of the drug. These patients were found to have a plasma BuChE much lower than normal (Bourne et al., 1952). Moreover, the enzyme is also qualitatively different from the norm, as for instance, in sensitivity to inhibitors. Because of this, a test was developed based upon lesser inhibition of the enzyme by dibucaine (Kalow and Staron, 1957). The dibucaine number (degree of plasma cholinesterase inhibition by dibucaine) discriminates three phenotypes: normal, intermediate, and atypical. The approximate frequency of these phenotypes has been estimated at 96, 3.9, and 0.05%, respectively (Harris and Whittaker, 1962). Other tests are available to discriminate abnormal BuChE, based upon fluoride number (Harris and Whittaker, 1961), chloride number (Whittaker, 1968), scoline number (King and Griffin, 1973), and urea number (Hanel and Viby-Mogensen, 1977; see Section 1.3.6.4).

51.4.3.3 Detection of Hypersusceptible Subjects

Whereas OPs are inhibitors of plasma BuChE and are largely hydrolyzed by A-esterases, such as paraoxonase (PON1) and other carboxylesterases (aliesterases), inherited or acquired deficits of scavenger (plasma BuChE) or detoxifying (esterases) abilities have been suggested as potential factors for increased susceptibility to OPs (Loewenstein-Lichtenstein *et al.*, 1996; Saxena *et al.*, 1997). Although there is some evidence in experimental animals for hypersusceptibility based upon reduced ability to detoxify OPs, only one example is known in humans. An unexpected outbreak of malathion poisoning arose in workers occupationally exposed to commercial brands of malathion that contained high amounts of impurities. Among these, iso-malathion was the most relevant because it inhibited the carboxylesterases that inactivivate malathion by hydrolyzing its carboxyl–ester linkages (Baker *et al.*, 1978). Recurrent suggestions have been made that genetically determined low levels of plasma BuChE increased the susceptibility to OP toxicity because of a reduced scavenger capability. However, a relationship between abnormal plasma BuChE and hypersusceptibility to OP poisoning has never been reported. Hypersusceptibility to succinylcholine would never have been discovered if some unusual people had not undergone succinylcholine treatment, an event that is probably no more common than heavy exposure to OPs. Moreover, when the biochemical characteristics of the normal and of the genetically determined defective enzymes were compared stoichiometrically with the plasma concentrations of inhibitors, no scavenger functions to plasma BuChE could be detected (Lotti and Moretto, 1995).

Based on the polymorphism of PON1 in human populations and the known role of this enzyme in the detoxification of some OPs (Davies *et al.*, 1996; Mueller *et al.*, 1983), it has been inferred that the expression of this enzyme is involved in determining hypersusceptibility to OPs (Mackness *et al.*, 1998). However, so far, proof for this has been obtained only in animals (Costa *et al.*, 1999).

REFERENCES

Abdel-Al, A. M. A., El-Hawary, M. F. S., Kamel, H., Abdel-Khalek, M. K., and El-Diwany, K. M. (1970). Blood cholinesterases, hepatic, renal and haemopoietic functions in children receiving repeated doses of "Dipterex." *J. Egypt. Med. Assoc.* **53**, 265–271.

Abend, Y., Goland, S., Evron, E., Sthoeger, Z. M., and Geltner, D. (1994). Acute renal failure complicating organophosphate intoxication. *Renal. Fail.* **16**, 415–417.

Abou-Donia, M. B., and Lapadula, D. M. (1990). Mechanisms of organophosphorus ester-induced delayed neurotoxicity: Type I and type II. *Ann. Rev. Pharmacol. Toxicol.* **30**, 405–440.

Adams, R. G., Verma, P., Jackson, A. J., and Miller, R. L. (1982). Plasma pharmacokinetics of intravenously administered atropine in normal human subjects. *J. Clin. Pharmacol.* **22**, 477–481.

Ahlgren, J. D., Manz, H. J., and Harvey, J. C. (1979). Myopathy of chronic organophosphate poisoning: A clinical entity? *S. Afr. Med. J.* **72**, 555–563.

Aiuto, L. A., Pavlakis, S. G., and Boxer, R. A. (1993). Life-threatening organophosphate-induced delayed polyneuropathy in a child after accidental chlorpyrifos ingestion. *J. Pediatr.* **122**, 658–660.

Aldridge, W. N., and Reiner, E. (1972). "Enzyme Inhibitors as Substrates." North-Holland, Amsterdam.

Alkondon, M., and Albuquerque, E. X. (1989). The nonoxime bispyridinium compound SAD-128 alters the kinetic properties of the nicotinic acetylcholine receptor ion channel: A possible mechanism for antidotal effects. *J. Pharmacol. Exp. Ther.* **250**, 842–852.

American Electroencephalographic Society (1987). Statement on the clinical use of quantitative EEG. *J. Clin. Neurophysiol.* **4**, 75.

Ames, R. G., Steenland, K., Jenkins, B., Chrislip, D., and Russo, J. (1995). Chronic neurologic sequelae to cholinesterase inhibition among agricultural pesticide applicators. *Arch. Environ. Health* **50**, 440–443.

Amr, M. M., Halim, Z. S., and Moussa, S. S. (1997). Psychiatric disorders among Egyptian pesticide applicators and formulators. *Environ. Res.* **73**, 193–199.

Aprea, C., Sciarra, G., and Lunghini, L. (1996). Analytical method for the determination of urinary alkylphosphates in subjects occupationally exposed to organophosphorus insecticides and in the general population. *J. Anal. Toxicol.* **20**, 559–563.

Aring, C. D. (1942). The systemic nervous affinity of triorthocresyl phosphate (Jamaica Ginger Palsy). *Brain* **65**, 34–47.

Arterberry, J. D., Durham, W. F., Elliot, J. W., and Wolfe, H. R. (1961). Exposure to parathion: Measurement by blood cholinesterase level and urinary *p*-nitrophenol excretion. *Arch. Environ. Health* **3**, 112–121.

Arterberry, J. D., Bonifaci, R. W., Nash, E. W., and Quinby, G. E. (1962). Potentiation of phosphorus insecticides by phenothiazine derivatives. Possible hazard, with report of a fatal case. *JAMA* **182**, 848–850.

Baker, D. J., and Sedgwick, E. M. (1996). Single fibre electromyographic changes in man after organophosphate exposure. *Human Exp. Toxicol.* **15**, 369–375.

Baker, E. L., Zack, M., Miles, J. W., Alderman, L., Warren, M., Dobbin, R. D., Miller, S., and Teeters, W. R. (1978). Epidemic malathion poisoning in Pakistan malaria workers. *Lancet* **i**, 31–34.

Balali-Mood, M., and Shariat, M. (1998). Treatment of organophosphate poisoning. Experience of nerve agents and acute pesticide poisoning on the effects of oximes. *J. Physiol. Paris* **92**, 375–378.

Bardin, P. G., and van Eeden, S. F. (1990). Organophosphate poisoning: Grading the severity and comparing treatment between atropine and glycopyrrolate. *Crit. Care Med.* **18**, 956–960.

Bardin, P. G., van Eeden, S. F., and Joubert, J. R. (1987). Intensive care management of acute organophosphate poisoning. A 7-year experience in the western Cape. *S. Afr. Med. J.* **72**, 593–597.

Bardin, P. G., van Eden, S. F., Moolman, J. A., Foden, A. P., and Joubert, J. R. (1994). Organophosphate and carbamate poisoning. *Arch. Intern. Med.* **154**, 1433–1441.

Barnes, J. M. (1961). Psychiatric sequelae of chronic exposure to organophosphorus insecticides. *Lancet* **ii**, 102–103.

Barr, A. M. (1966). Further experience in the treatment of severe organic phosphate poisoning. *Med. J. Aust.* **1**, 490–492.

Benson, B. J., Tolo, D., and McIntire, M. (1992). Is the intermediate syndrome in organophosphate poisoning the result of insufficient oxime therapy? *Clin. Toxicol.* **30**, 347–349.

Bentur, Y., Nutenko, I., Tsipiniuk A., Raikhlin-Eisenkraft, B., and Taitelman, U. (1993). Pharmacokinetics of obidoxime in organophosphate poisoning associated with renal failure. *Clin. Toxicol.* **31**, 315–322.

Bertolazzi, M., Caroldi, S., Moretto, A., and Lotti, M. (1991). Interaction of methamidophos with hen and human acetylcholinesterase and neuropathy target esterase. *Arch. Toxicol.* **65**, 580–585.

Bertoncin, D., Russolo, A., Caroldi, S., and Lotti, M. (1985). Neuropathy target esterase in human lymphocytes. *Arch. Environ. Health* **40**, 139–144.

Besser, R., Gutmann, L., and Weilemann, L. S. (1989a). Inactivation of end-plate acetylcholinesterase during the course of organophosphate intoxications. *Arch. Toxicol.* **63**, 412–415.

Besser, R., Gutmann, L., Dillmann, U., Weilemann, L. S., and Hopf, H. C. (1989b). End-plate dysfunction in acute organophosphate intoxication. *Neurology* **39**, 561–567.

Besser, R., Vogt, T., and Gutmann, L. (1990). Pancuronium improves the neuromuscular transmission defect of human organophosphate intoxication. *Neurology* **40**, 1275–1277.

Besser, R., Vogt, T., Gutmann, L., and Wessler, I. (1991). High pancuronium sensitivity of axonal nicotinic-acetylcholine receptors in humans during organophosphate intoxication. *Muscle Nerve* **14**, 1197–1201.

Besser, R., Weilemann, L. S., and Gutmann, L. (1995). Efficacy of obidoxime in human organophosphorus poisoning: Determination by neuromuscular transmission studies. *Muscle Nerve* **18**, 15–22.

Betrosian, A., Balla, M., Kafiri, G., Kofinas, G., Makri, R., and Kakouri, A. (1995). Multiple systems organ failure from organophosphate poisoning. *Clin. Toxicol.* **33**, 257–260.

Bidstrup, P. L. (1961). Psychiatric sequelae of chronic exposure to organophosphorus insecticides. *Lancet* **ii**, 103.

Bidstrup, P. L., Bonnell, J. A., and Beckett, A. G. (1953). Paralysis following poisoning by a new organic phosphorus insecticide (mipafox). Report on two cases. *Brit. Med. J.* **1**, 1068–1072.

Bismuth, C., Inns, R. H., and Marrs, T. C. (1992). Efficacy, toxicity and clinical use of oximes in anticholinesterase poisoning. In "Clinical & Experimental Toxicology of Organophosphates and Carbamates" (B. Ballantyne and T. C. Marrs, eds.), pp. 555–577. Butterworth–Heinemann, Oxford.

Björnsdóttir, U. S., and Smith, D. (1999). South African religious leader with hyperventilation, hypophosphataemia, and respiratory arrest. *Lancet* **354**, 2130.

Bošković, B., Kovačević, V., and Jovanović, D. (1984). PAM-2 Cl, HI-6, and HGG-12 in soman and tabun poisoning. *Fundam. Appl. Toxicol.* **4**, S106–S115.

Bourne, J. E., Collier, H. O. J., and Somers, G. F. (1952). Succinylcholine (succinoylcholine). Muscle relaxant of short action. *Lancet* **i**, 1225–1229.

Bowers, M. B., Jr., Goodman, E., and Sim, V. M. (1964). Some behavioral changes in man following anticholinesterase administration. *J. Nerv. Mental. Dis.* **138**, 383–389.

Bradway, D. E., and Shafik, T. M. (1977). Malathion exposure studies. Determination of mono- and dicarboxylic acids and alkyl phosphates in urine. *Agr. Food Chem.* **25**, 1342–1344.

Bradwell, R. H. (1994). Psychiatric sequelae of organophosphorus poisoning: A case study and review of the literature. *Behav. Neurol.* **7**, 117–122.

Brill, D. M., Maisel, A. S., and Prabhu, R. (1984). Polymorphic ventricular tachycardia and other complex arrhythmias in organophosphate insecticide poisoning. *J. Electrocardiol.* **17**, 97–102.

Brown, J. H., and Taylor, P. (1996). Muscarinic receptor agonists and antagonists. In "Goodman and Gilman's the Pharmacological Basis of Therapeutics" (J. G. Hardman and L. E. Limbird, eds.), 9th ed., pp. 141–160. McGraw–Hill, New York.

Brown, M. A., and Brix, K. A. (1998). Review of health consequences from high-, intermediate- and low-level exposure to organophosphorus nerve agent. *J. Appl. Toxicol.* **18**, 393–408.

Bryant, D. H. (1985). Asthma due to insecticide sensitivity. *Aust. N. Z. J. Med.* **15**, 66–68.

Buckley, N. A., Dawson, A. H., and Whyte, I. M. (1994). Organophosphate poisoning: Peripheral vascular resistance—a measure of adequate atropinization. *Clin. Toxicol.* **32**, 61–68.

Burchfiel, J. L., Duffy, F. H., and Sim, V. M. (1976). Persistent effects of sarin and dieldrin upon the primate electroencephalogram. *Toxicol. Appl. Pharmacol.* **35**, 365–379.

Calesnick, B., Christensen, J. A., and Richter, M. (1967). Human toxicity of various oximes. 2-Pyridine aldoxime methyl chloride, its methane sulfonate salt, and 1,1′-trimethylenebis-(4-formylpyridinium chloride). *Arch. Environ. Health* **15**, 599–608.

Capodicasa, E., Scapellato, M. L., Moretto, A., Caroldi. S., and Lotti, M. (1991). Chlorpyrifos-induced delayed polyneuropathy. *Arch. Toxicol.* **65**, 150–155.

Castillo, E., Rubin, R. T., and Holsboer-Trachsler, E. (1989). Clinical differentiation between lethal catatonia and neuroleptic malignant syndrome. *Am. J. Psychiatry* **146**, 324–328.

Catz, A., Chen, B., Jutrin, I., and Mendelson, L. (1988). Late onset of isofenphos neurotoxicity. *J. Neurol. Neurosurg. Psychiatry* **51**, 1338–1340.

Cavanagh, J. B. (1973). Peripheral neuropathy caused by toxic agents. *Crit. Rev. Toxicol.* **2**, 365–417.

Chambers, H. W. (1992). Organophosphorus compounds: An overview. In "Organophosphates. Chemistry, Fate, and Effects" (J. E. Chambers and P. E. Levi, eds.), pp. 3–17. Academic Press, San Diego.

Choi, P. T.-L., Quinonez, L. G., Cook, D. J., Baxter, F., and Whitehead, L. (1998). The use of glycopyrrolate in a case of intermediate syndrome following acute organophosphate poisoning. *Can. J. Anaesth.* **45**, 337–340.

Chuang, F. R., Jang, S. W., Lin, J. L., Chern, M. S., Chen, J. B., and Hsu, K. T. (1996). QT$_c$ prolongation indicates a poor prognosis in patients with organophosphate poisoning. *Am. J. Emerg. Med.* **14**, 451–453.

Compton, J. A. F. (1987). "Military Chemical and Biological Agents." Telford Press, Caldwell, NJ.

Costa, L. G., Li, W. F., Richter, R. J., Shih, D. M., Lusis, A., and Furlong, C. E. (1999). The role of paraoxonase (PON1) in the detoxication of organophosphates and its human polymorphism. *Chem.-Biol. Interact.* **119-120**, 429–438.

Coudray-Lucas, C., Prioux-Guyonneau, M., Sentenac, H., Cohen, Y., and Wepierre, J. (1983). Brain catecholamine metabolism changes and hypothermia in intoxication by anticholinesterase agents. *Acta Pharmacol. Toxicol.* **52**, 224–229.

Coye, M. J., Lowe, J. A, and Maddy, K. J. (1986). Biological monitoring of agricultural workers exposed to pesticides: II. Monitoring of intact pesticides and their metabolites. *J. Occup. Med.* **28**, 628–636.

Csik, V., Motika, D., and Marosi, G. Y. (1986). Delayed neuropathy after trichlorfon intoxication. *J. Neurol. Neurosurg. Psychiatry* **49**, 222.

Curtes, J. P., Develay, P., and Hubert, J. P. (1981). Late peripheral neuropathy due to an acute voluntary intoxication by organophosphorus compounds. *Clin. Toxicol.* **18**, 1453–1462.

Dagli, A. J., and Shaikh, W. A. (1983). Pancreatic involvement in malathion–anticholinesterase insecticide intoxication: A study of 75 cases. *Br. J. Clin. Pract.* **37**, 270–272.

Daniell, W., Barnhart, S., Demers, P., Costa, L. G., Eaton, D. L., Miller, M., and Rosenstock, L. (1992). Neuropsychological performance among agricultural pesticide applicators. *Environ. Res.* **59**, 217–228.

Davies, H. G., Richter, R. J., Keifer, M., Broomfield, C. A., Sowalla, J., and Furlong, C. E. (1996). The effect of human serum paraoxonase polymorphism is reversed with diazoxon, soman and sarin. *Nat. Genet.* **14**, 334–336.

Davies, J. E., Barquet, A., Freed, V. H., Haque, R., Morgade, C., Sonneborn, R. E., and Vaclavek, C. (1975). Human pesticide poisonings by a fat-soluble organophosphate insecticide. *Arch. Environ. Health* **30**, 608–613.

Davies, P., and Landy, M. (1998). Suxamethonium and mivacurium sensitivity from pregnancy-induced plasma cholinesterase deficiency. *Anaesthesia* **53**, 1109–1116.

Davis, K. L., Yesavage, J. A., and Berger, P. A. (1978). Possible organophosphate-induced parkinsonism. *J. Nerv. Ment. Dis.* **166**, 222–225.

Davis, K. L., Thal, L. J., Gamzu, E. R., Davis, C. S., Woolson, R. F., Gracon, S. I., Drachman, D. A., Schneider, L. S., Whitehouse, P. J., Hoover, T. M., Morris, J. C., Kawas, C. H., Knopman, D. S., Earl, N. L., Kumar, V., Doody, R. S., and the Tacrine Collaborative Study Group. (1992). A double blind, placebo-controlled multicenter study of tacrine for Alzheimer's disease. *N. Engl. J. Med.* **327**, 1253–1259.

Dawson, A., Buckley, N., and Whyte, I. (1997). What target pralidoxime concentration? *Clin. Toxicol.* **35**, 227–228.

Dawson, R. M. (1994). Review of oximes available for treatment of nerve agent poisoning. *J. Appl. Toxicol.* **14**, 317–331.

De Bleecker, J. L. (1992). Transient opsoclonus in organophosphate poisoning. *Acta Neurol. Scand.* **86**, 529–531.

De Bleecker, J. L. (1993). Intermediate syndrome: Prolonged cholinesterase inhibition. *Clin. Toxicol.* **31**, 197–199.

De Bleecker, J. L., De Reuck, J. L., and Willems, J. L. (1992a). Neurological aspects of organophosphate poisoning. *Clin. Neurol. Neurosurg.* **94**, 93–103.

De Bleecker, J., Vogelaers, D., Ceuterick, C., Van Den Neucker, K., Willems, J. L., and De Reuck, J. L. (1992b). Intermediate syndrome due to prolonged parathion poisoning. *Acta Neurol. Scand.* **86**, 421–424.

De Bleecker, J., Van Den Neucker, K., and Colardyn, F. (1993). Intermediate syndrome in organophosphorus poisoning: A prospective study. *Crit. Care Med.* **21**, 1706–1711.

de Jager, A. E. J., van Weerden, T. W., Houthoff, H. J., and de Monchy, J. G. R. (1981). Polyneuropathy after massive exposure to parathion. *Neurology* **31**, 603–605.

de Jong, L. P. A., and Ceulen, D. I. (1978). Anticholinesterase activity and rate of decomposition of some phosphylated oximes. *Biochem. Pharmacol.* **27**, 857–863.

de Kort, W. L. A. M., Kiestra, S. H., and Sangster, B. (1988). The use of atropine and oximes in organophosphate intoxications: A modified approach. *Clin. Toxicol.* **26**, 199–208.

Dementi, B. (1994). Ocular effects of organophosphates: A historical perspective of Saku disease. *J. Appl. Toxicol.* **14**, 119–129.

de Reuck, J., and Willems, J. (1975). Acute parathion poisoning: Myopathic changes in the diaphragm. *J. Neurol.* **208**, 309–314.

de Reuck, J., Colardyn, F., and Willems, J. (1979). Fatal encephalopathy in acute poisoning with organophosphorus insecticides. A clinico-pathologic study of two cases. *Clin. Neurol. Neurosurg.* **81**, 247–254.

Deschamps, D., Questel, F., Baud, F. J., Gervais, P., and Dally, S. (1994). Persistent asthma after acute inhalation of organophosphate insecticide. *Lancet* **344**, 1712.

de Silva, H. J., Wijewickrema, R., and Senanayake, N. (1992). Does pralidoxime affect outcome of management in acute organophosphorus poisoning? *Lancet* **339**, 1136–1138.

de Silva, H. J., Sanmuganathan, P. S., and Senanayake, N. (1994). Isolated bilateral recurrent laryngeal nerve paralysis: A delayed complication of organophosphorus poisoning. *Hum. Exp. Toxicol.* **13**, 171–173.

Dettbarn, W. D. (1992). Anticholinesterase induced myonecrosis. *In* "Clinical & Experimental Toxicology of Organophosphates and Carbamates" (B. Ballantyne and T. C. Marrs, eds.), pp. 167–179. Butterworth–Heinemann, Oxford.

De Wilde, V., Vogelaers, D., Colardyn, F., Vanderstraeten, G., Van Den Neurcker, K., De Bleecker, J., De Reuck, J., and Van den Heede, M. (1991). Postsynaptic neuromuscular dysfunction in organophosphate induced intermediate syndrome. *Klin. Wochenschr.* **69**, 177–183.

Dille, J. R., and Smith, P. W. (1964). Central nervous system effects of chronic exposure to organophosphates insecticides. *Aerospace Med.* **35**, 475–478.

D'Mello, G. D. (1993). Behavioural toxicity of anticholinesterases in humans and animals—A review. *Hum. Exp. Toxicol.* **12**, 3–7.

Doctor, B. P., Toker, L., Roth, E., and Silman, I., (1987). Microtiter assay for acetylcholinesterase. *Anal. Biochem.* **166**, 399–403.

Drenth, H. J., Ensberg I. F. G., Roberts, D. V., and Wilson, A. (1972). Neuromuscular function in agricultural workers using pesticides. *Arch. Environ. Health* **25**, 395–398.

Dressel, T. D., Goodale, R. L., Jr., Arneson, M. A., and Borner, J. W. (1979). Pancreatitis as a complication in anticholinesterase insecticide intoxication. *Ann. Surg.* **189**, 199–204.

Duffy, F. H., and Burchfiel, J. L. (1980). Long term effects of the organophosphate sarin on EEGs in monkeys and humans. *Neurotoxicology* **1**, 667–689.

Duffy, F. H., Burchfiel, J. L., Bartels, P. H., Gaon, M., and Sim, V. M. (1979). Long-term effects of an organophosphate upon the human electroencephalogram. *Toxicol. Appl. Pharmacol.* **47**, 161–176.

Duffy, F. H., Bartels, P. H., and Neff, R. (1986). A response to Oken and Chiappa. *Ann. Neurol.* **19**, 494–496.

Durham, W. F., and Hayes, W. J., Jr. (1962). Organic phosphorus poisoning and its therapy. *Arch. Environ. Health* **5**, 21–47.

Durham, W. F., Wolfe, H. R., and Quinby, G. E. (1965). Organophosphorus insecticides and mental alertness. Studies in exposed workers and in poisoning cases. *Arch. Environ. Health* **10**, 55–66.

ECETOC (1998). "Organophosphorus Pesticides and Long-Term Effects on the Nervous System." Tech. Rep. 75, European Center for Ecotoxicology and Toxicology of Chemicals, Brussels.

Ecobichon, D. J., Ozere, R. L., Reid, E., and Crocker, J. F. S. (1977). Acute fenitrothion poisoning. *Can. Med. Assoc. J.* **116**, 377–379.

Edmundson, R. S. (1988). "Dictionary of Organophosphorus Compounds." Chapman and Hall, London.

Edson, E. F. (1964). No-effect levels of three organophosphates in the rat, pig, and man. *Food Cosmet. Toxicol.* **2**, 311–316.

Eliason, D. A., Cranmer, M. F., von Windeguth, D. L., Kilpatrick, J. W., Suggs, J. E., and Schoof, H. F. (1969). Dursban premises application and their effect on the cholinesterase levels in spraymen. *Mosq. News* **29**, 591–595.

Elliot, R., and Barnes, J. M. (1963). Organophosphorus insecticides for the control of mosquitos in Nigeria. *Bull. W.H.O.* **28**, 35–54.

Ellman, G. L., Courtney, K. D., Andres, V., Jr., and Featherstone, R. M. (1961). A new and rapid colorimetric determination of acetylcholinesterase activity. *Biochem. Pharmacol.* **7**, 88–95.

Engel, A. G., Lambert E. H., and Santa, T. (1973). Study of long-term anticholinesterase therapy. Effects on neuromuscular transmission and on motor end-plate fine structure. *Neurology* **23**, 1273–1281.

Engel, L. S., Keifer, M. C., Checkoway, H., Robinson, L. R., and Vaughan, T. L. (1998). Neurophysiological function in farm workers exposed to organophosphate pesticides. *Arch. Environ. Health* **53**, 7–14.

EPA (1992). *In* "Proceedings of the EPA Workshop on Cholinesterase Methodologies," Office of Pesticide Programs, United States Environmental Protection Agency, Washington, DC.

Erdmann, W. D., Zech, R., Franke, P., and Bosse, I. (1966). Zur Frage der therapeutischen Wirksamkeit von Esterase-Reaktivatoren bei der Vergiftung mit Dimethoat. *Arzneimittelforschung* **16**, 492–494 (in German).

Erikson-Lamy, K., and Grant, W. M. (1992). Ophthalmic toxicology of anticholinesterases. *In* "Clinical & Experimental Toxicology of Organophosphates and Carbamates" (B. Ballantyne and T. C. Marrs, eds.), pp. 180–194. Butterworth–Heinemann, Oxford.

Eyer, P. (1995). Neuropsychopathological changes by organophosphorus compounds—A review. *Hum. Exp. Toxicol.* **14**, 857–864.

FAO/WHO (1967). Evaluations of some pesticide residues in food. 1966. *In* "Joint Meeting of the Food and Agriculture Organization Working Party and the World Health Organization Expert Committee on Pesticide Residues," World Health Organization, Geneva, WHO/FoodAdd./667.32.

FAO/WHO (1987). Pesticide residues in food, 1986. *In* "Evaluations of the Joint Meeting of the Food and Agriculture Organization Panel of Experts on Pesticide Residues in Food and Environment and the Food and Agriculture Organization Expert Group on Pesticide Residues. Part II—Toxicology," Food and Agriculture Organization, Rome, Plant Production and Protection Paper 78/2, pp. 90–91.

FAO/WHO (1995). Pesticide residues in food, 1994. Report. *In* "Joint Meeting of the Food and Agriculture Organization Panel of Experts on Pesticide Residues in Food and Environment and the Food and Agriculture Organization Expert Group on Pesticide Residues," Food and Agriculture Organization, Rome, FAO Plant Production and Protection Paper 127.

FAO/WHO (1996). "Pesticide residues in food, 1995. *In* "Evaluations of the Joint Meeting of the Food and Agriculture Organization Panel of Experts on Pesticide Residues in Food and Environment and the Food and Agriculture Organization Expert Group on Pesticide Residues. Part II—Toxicological and Environmental," World Health Organization, Geneva, WHO/PCS/96.48, pp. 141–142.

FAO/WHO (1997). Pesticide residues in food, 1996. *In* "Evaluations of the Joint Meeting of the Food and Agriculture Organization Panel of Experts on Pesticide Residues in Food and Environment and the Food and Agriculture Organization Expert Group on Pesticide Residues. Part II—Toxicological and Environmental," World Health Organization, Geneva, WHO/PCS/97.1, pp. 187–188.

Fazekas, T., and Kiss, Z. (1980). Organophosphate cardiomyopathy. Congestive cardiomyopathy caused by long-term organic phosphoric acid ester exposure. *Z. Kardiol.* **69**, 584–586 (in German).

Fenske, R. A., and Elkner, K. P. (1990). Multi-route exposure assessment and biological monitoring of urban pesticide applicators during structural control treatments with chlorpyrifos. *Toxicol. Ind. Health* **6**, 349–371.

Fernández, G., Díaz Gómez, M. I., and Castro J. A. (1975). Cholinesterase inhibition by phenothiazine and nonphenothiazine antihistaminics: Analysis of its postulated role in synergizing organophosphate toxicity. *Toxicol. Appl. Pharmacol.* **31**, 179–190.

Fiedler, N., Kipen, H., Kelly-McNeil, K., and Fenske, R. (1997). Long-term use of organophosphates and neuropsychological performance. *Am. J. Ind. Med.* **32**, 487–496.

Fisher, J. R. (1977). Guillain–Barré syndrome following organophosphate poisoning. *JAMA* **238**, 1950–1951.

Futagami, K., Otsubo, K., Nakao, Y., Aoyama, T., Iimori, E., Urakami, S., Ide, M., and Oishi, R. (1995). Acute organophosphate poisoning after disulfoton ingestion. *Clin. Toxicol.* **33**, 151–155.

Gadoth, N., and Fisher, A. (1978). Late onset of neuromuscular block in organophosphorus poisoning. *Ann. Intern. Med.* **88**, 654–655.

Garcia-Lopez, J. A., and Monteoliva, M. (1988). Physiolagial changes in human erythrocyte cholinesterase as measured with the "pH-stat." *Clin. Chem.* **34**, 2133–2135.

Gershon, S., and Shaw, F. H. (1961). Psychiatric sequelae of chronic exposure to organophosphorus insecticides. *Lancet* **i**, 1371–1374.

Gesztes, T. (1966). Prolonged apnoea after suxamethonium injection associated with eye drops containing an anticholinesterase agent. *Br. J. Anaesth.* **38**, 408–409.

Glow, P. H., and Rose, S. (1965). Effects of reduced acetylcholinesterase levels on extinction of a conditioned response. *Nature* **206**, 475–477.

Goldstein, D. A., McGuigan, M. A., and Ripley, B. D. (1988). Acute tricresylphosphate intoxication in childhood. *Human Toxicol.* **7**, 179–182.

Golsousidis, H., and Kokkas, V. (1985). Use of 19 590 mg of atropine during 24 days of treatment, after a case of unusually severe parathion poisoning. *Human Toxicol.* **4**, 339–340.

Gomes, J., Lloyd, O., Revitt, M. D., and Basha, M. (1998). Morbidity among farm workers in a desert country in relation to long-term exposure to pesticides. *Scand. J. Environ. Health* **24**, 213–219.

Good, J. L., Khurana, R. K., Mayer, R. F., Cintra, W. M., and Albuquerque, E. X. (1993). Pathophysiological studies of neuromuscular function in subacute organophosphate poisoning induced by phosmet. *J. Neurol. Neurosurg. Psychiatry* **56**, 290–294.

Goswamy, R., Chaudhuri, A., and Mahashur, A. A. (1994). Study of respiratory failure in organophosphate and carbamate poisoning. *Heart Lung* **23**, 466–472.

Granacher, R. P., and Baldessarini, R. J. (1975). Physostigmine. Its use in acute anticholinergic syndrome with antidepressant and antiparkinson drugs. *Arch. Gen. Psychiatry* **32**, 375–380.

Gray, G. C., Coate, B. D., Anderson, C. M., Kang, H. K., Berg, S. W., Wignall, F. S., Knoke, J. D., and Barrett-Connor, E. (1996). The postwar hospitalization experience of U.S. veterans of the Persian Gulf War. *N. Engl. J. Med.* **335**, 1505–1513.

Green, M. D., Jones, D. E., and Hilmas, D. E. (1985). Sarin intoxication elevates plasma pralidoxime. *Toxicol. Lett.* **28**, 17–21.

Greenaway, C., and Orr, P. (1996). A foodborne outbreak causing a cholinergic syndrome. *J. Emerg. Med.* **14**, 339–344.

Greenberger, N. J., Toskes, P. P., and Isselbacher, K. J. (1998). Acute and chronic pancreatitis. *In* "Harrison's Principles of Internal Medicine" (A. S. Fauci, E. Braunwald, K. J. Isselbacher, J. D. Wilson, J. B. Martin, D. L. Kasper, S. L. Hauser, and D. L. Longo, eds.), 14th ed., pp. 1741–1752. McGraw–Hill, New York.

Griffin, P., Mason, H., Heywood, K., and Cocker, J. (1999). Oral and dermal absorption of chlorpyrifos: A human volunteer study. *Occup. Environ. Med.* **56**, 10–13.

Grob, D. (1956). The manifestations and treatment of poisoning due to nerve gas and other organic phosphate anticholinesterase compounds. *Arch. Intern. Med.* **98**, 221–239.

Grob, D., and Harvey, J. C. (1958). Effects in man of the anticholinesterase compound sarin (isopropyl methyl phosphonofluoridate). *J. Clin. Invest.* **37**, 350–368.

Grob, D., Harvey, A. M., Langworthy, O. R., and Lilienthal, J. L., Jr. (1947). The administration of di-isopropyl fluorophosphate (DFP) to man. III. Effect on the central nervous system with special reference to electrical activity of the brain. *Bull. Johns Hopkins Hosp.* **81**, 257–266.

Guillermo, F. P., Pretel, C. M. M., Royo, F. T., Macias, M. J. P., Ossorio, R. A., Gomez, J. A. A., and Vidal, J. C. (1988). Prolonged suxamethonium-induced neuromuscular blockade associated with organophosphate poisoning. *Br. J. Anaesth.* **61**, 233–236.

Gunderson, C. H., Lehmann, C. R., Sidell, F. R., and Jabbari, B. (1992). Nerve agents: A review. *Neurology* **42**, 946–950.

Güven, M., Ünlühizarci, K., Göktaş, Z., and Kurtoðlu, S. (1997). Intravenous organophosphate injection: An unusual way of intoxication. *Human Exp. Toxicol.* **16**, 279–280.

Haley, R. W. and Kurt, T. L. (1997). Self-reported exposure to neurotoxic chemical combinations in the Gulf War. A cross sectional epidemiologic study. *JAMA* **277**, 231–237.

Haley, R. W., Kurt, T. L., and Hom, J. (1997a). Is there a Gulf War Syndrome? Searching for syndromes by factor analysis of symptoms. *JAMA* **277**, 215–222.

Haley, R. W. Hom, J., Roland, P. S., Bryan, W. W., VanNess, P. C., Bonte, F. J., Devous, M. D., Mathews, D., Fleckenstein, J. L., Wians, F. H., Wolfe, G. I., and Kurt, T. L. (1997b). Evaluation of neurologic function in Gulf War Veterans. A blinded case-control study. *JAMA* **277**, 223–230.

Hanel, H. K., and Viby-Mogensen, J. (1977). The inhibition of serum cholinesterase by urea. Mechanism of action and application in the typing of abnormal genes. *Br. J. Anaesth.* **49**, 1251–1257.

Hantson, P., Hainaut, P., Vander Stappen, M., and Mahieu, P. (1996). Regulation of body temperature after acute organophosphate poisoning. *Can. J. Anaesth.* **43**, 755.

Harris, H., and Whittaker, M. (1961). Differential inhibition of human serum cholinesterase with fluoride. Recognition of two new phenotypes. *Nature* **191**, 469–498.

Harris, H., and Whittaker, M. (1962). The serum cholinesterase variants. Study of twenty-two families selected via the "intermediate" phenotype. *Ann. Human Genet.* **26**, 59–72.

Harrison, L. I., Smallridge, R. C., Lasseter, K. C., Goldlust, M. B., Shamblen, E. C., Gam, V. W., Chang, S. F., and Kvam, D. C. (1986). Comparative absorption of inhaled and intramuscularly administered atropine. *Am. Rev. Respir. Dis.* **134**, 254–257.

Hart, P. S., McCarthy, G. J., Brown, R., Lau, M., and Fisher, D. M. (1995). The effect of plasma cholinesterase activity on mivacurium infusion rates. *Anesth. Analg.* **80**, 760–763.

Hata, S., Bernstein, E., and Davis, L. E. (1986). Atypical ocular bobbing in acute organophosphate poisoning. *Arch. Neurol.* **43**, 185–186.

Hatta, K., Miura, Y., Asukai, N., and Hamabe, Y. (1996). Amnesia from sarin poisoning. *Lancet* **347**, 1343.

Haubenstock, A., Hruby, K., and Jager, U. (1983). More on the triad of pancreatitis, hyperamylasemia, and hyperglycemia. *JAMA* **249**, 1563.

Hayes, M. M. M., Van der Westhuizen, N. G., and Gelfand, M. (1978). Organophosphate poisoning in Rhodesia. A study of the clinical features and management of 105 patients. *S. Afr. Med. J.* **54**, 230–234.

Hayes, W. J., Jr. (1982). "Pesticides Studies in Man." William and Wilkins, Baltimore.

Hayes, W. J., Jr., and Laws, E. R. (1991). "Handbook of Pesticide Toxicology." Academic Press, San Diego.

He, F., Xu, H., Qin, F., Xu, L., Huang, J., and He, X. (1998). Intermediate myasthenia syndrome following acute organophosphates poisoning—An analysis of 21 cases. *Human Exp. Toxicol.* **17**, 40–45.

Heath, A. J. W., and Meredith, T. (1992). Atropine in the management of anticholinesterase poisoning. *In* "Clinical & Experimental Toxicology of Organophosphates and Carbamates" (B. Ballantyne and T. C. Marrs, eds.), pp. 543–554. Butterworth–Heinemann, Oxford.

Hermanowicz, A., and Kossman, S. (1984). Neutrophil function and infectious disease in workers occupationally exposed to phosphoorganic pesticides:

Role of mononuclear-derived chemotactic factor for neutrophils. *Clin. Immunol. Immunopathol.* **33**, 13–22.

Hierons, R., and Johnson, M. K. (1978). Clinical and toxicological investigations of a case of delayed neuropathy in man after acute poisoning by an organophosphorus pesticide. *Arch. Toxicol.* **40**, 279–284.

Hinderling, P. H., Gundert-Remy, U., and Schmidlin, O. (1985). Integrated pharmacokinetics and pharmacodynamics of atropine in healthy humans I: Pharmacokinetics. *J. Pharm. Sci.* **74**, 703–710.

Holland, P., and Parkes, D. C. (1976). Plasma concentrations of the oxime pralidoxime mesylate (P2S) after repeated oral and intramuscular administration. *Br. J. Ind. Med.* **33**, 43–46.

Hollingshaus, J. G., Nishioka, T., March, R. B., and Fukuto, T. R. (1981). Effect of impurities on the delayed neurotoxicity of *O*-(4-bromo-2,5-dichlorophenyl) *O*-ethyl phenylphosphonothioate administered orally to hens. *J. Agric. Food Chem.* **29**, 593–600.

Hollis, G. J. (1999). Organophosphate poisoning versus brainstem stroke. *Med. J. Aust.* **170**, 596–597.

Holmstedt, B. (1959). Pharmacology of organophosphorus cholinesterase inhibitors. *Pharmacol. Rev.* **11**, 567–688.

Holmstedt, B. (1963). Structure–activity relationships of the organophosphorus anticholinesterase agents. *In* "Handbuch der Experimentellen Pharmakologie. Cholinesterases and Anticholinesterase Agents" (O. Eichler, A. Farah, and G. B. Koelle, eds.), pp. 428–485. Springer-Verlag, Berlin.

Hoskins, B., Fernando, J. C. R., Dulaney, M. D., Lim, D. K., Liu, D. D., Watanabe, H. K., and Ho, I. K. (1986). Relationship between the neurotoxicities of soman, sarin and tabun, and acetylcholinesterase inhibition. *Toxicol. Lett.* **30**, 121–129.

Hsiao, C.-T., Yang, C.-C., Deng, J. F., Bullard, M. J., and Liaw, S.-J. (1996). Acute pancreatitis following organophosphate intoxication. *Clin. Toxicol.* **34**, 343–347.

Hui, K. S. (1983). Metabolic disturbances in organophosphate insecticide poisoning. *Arch. Pathol. Lab. Med.* **107**, 154.

Indudharan, R., Win, M. N., and Noor, A. R. (1998). Laryngeal paralysis in organophosphorus poisoning. *J. Laryngol. Otol.* **112**, 81–82.

Inoue, N., Fujishiro, K., Mori, K., and Matsuoka, M. (1988). Triorthocresyl phosphate poisoning. A review of human cases. *J. UOEH* **10**, 433–442.

Ismail, K., Everitt, B., Blatchley, N., Hull, L., Unwin, C., David, A., and Wessley, S. (1999). Is there a Gulf War Syndrome? *Lancet* **353**, 179–182.

Jager, K. W., Roberts, D. V., and Wilson, A. (1970). Neuromuscular function in pesticide workers. *Br. J. Industr. Med.* **27**, 273–278.

Jamal, G. A. (1995). Long term neurotoxic effects of organophosphate compounds. *Adverse Drug React. Toxicol. Rev.* **14**, 85–99.

Jamal, G. A. (1997). Neurological syndromes of organophosphorus compounds. *Adverse Drug React. Toxicol. Rev.* **16**, 133–170.

Jamal, G. A., Hansen, S., Apartopoulos, F., and Peden, A. (1996). The "Gulf War Syndrome." Is there evidence of dysfunction in the nervous system? *J. Neurol. Neurosurg. Psychiatry* **60**, 449–451.

Jastrzebski, J., Zlotorowicz, M., and Szczepański, M. (1994). Activation of blood coagulation induced by organophosphate pesticide. *Mater. Med. Pol.* **26**, 33–34.

Jauhiainen, A., Kangas, J., Laitinen, S., and Savolainen, K. (1992). Biological monitoring of workers exposed to mevinphos in greenhouses. *Bull. Environ. Contam. Toxicol.* **49**, 37–43.

Jedrzejowska, H., Rowińska-Marcińska, K., and Hoppe, B. (1980). Neuropathy due to phytosol (agritox). Report of a case. *Acta Neuropathol. (Berlin)* **49**, 163–168.

Johnson, M. K. (1975). Organophosphorus esters causing delayed neurotoxic effects. Mechanism of action and structure/activity studies. *Arch. Toxicol.* **34**, 259–288.

Johnson, M. K. (1981). Delayed neurotoxicity—Do trichlorphon and/or dichlorvos cause delayed neuropathy in man or in test animals? *Acta Pharmacol. Toxicol.* **49**(Suppl V), 87–98.

Johnson, M. K. (1984). Check your paraoxon and parathion for neurotoxic impurities. *In* "Delayed Neurotoxicity Workshop. Proceedings of the Delayed Neurotoxicity Workshop" (J. M. Crammer and J. E. Hixson, eds.). IUTOX Press, Little Rock, AK.

Johnson, M. K. (1990). Organophosphates and delayed neuropathy—Is NTE alive and well? *Toxicol. Appl. Pharmacol.* **102**, 385–399.

Johnson, M. K., and Vale, J. A. (1992). Clinical management of acute organophosphate poisoning: An overview. *In* "Clinical & Experimental Toxicology of Organophosphates and Carbamates" (B. Ballantyne and T. C. Marrs, eds.), pp. 528–535. Butterworth–Heinemann, Oxford.

Johnson, M. K., Vale, J. A., Marrs, T. C., and Meredith, T. J. (1992). Pralidoxime for organophosphorus poisoning. *Lancet* **340**, 64.

Joubert, J., and Joubert, P. H. (1988). Chorea and psychiatric changes in organophosphate poisoning. A report of 2 further cases. *S. Afr. Med. J.* **74**, 32–34.

Joubert, J., Joubert, P. H., van der Spuy, M., and van Graan, E. (1984). Acute organophosphate poisoning presenting with choero-athetosis. *Clin. Toxicol.* **22**, 187–191.

Jovanović, D. (1989). Pharmokinetics of pralidoxime chloride. A comparative study in healthy volunteers and in organophosphorus poisoning. *Arch. Toxicol.* **63**, 416–418.

Jušić, A., Jurenić, D., and Milić, S. (1980). Electromyographical neuromuscular synapse testing and neurological findings in workers exposed to organophosphorus pesticides. *Arch. Environ. Health* **35**, 168–175.

Kalow, W., and Staron, N. (1957). On the distribution and inheritance of atypical forms of human serum cholinesterase as indicated by dibucaine numbers. *Can. J. Biochem. Physiol.* **35**, 1305–1320.

Kanto, J., and Klotz, U. (1988). Pharmacokinetic implications for the clinical use of atropine, scopolamine and glycopyrrolate. *Acta Anaesthesiol. Scand.* **32**, 69–78.

Kaplan, J. G., Kessler, J., Rosenberg, N., Pack, D., and Schaumburg H. H. (1993). Sensory neuropathy associated with Dursban (chlorpyrifos) exposure. *Neurology* **43**, 2193–2196.

Karademir, M., Ertük, F., and Koçak, R. (1990). Two cases of organophosphate poisoning with development of intermediate syndrome. *Human Exp. Toxicol.* **9**, 187–189.

Karalliede, L. (1999). Organophosphorus poisoning and anaesthesia. *Anaesthesia* **54**, 1073–1088.

Karalliede, L., and Henry, J. A. (1993). Effects of organophosphates on skeletal muscle. *Human Exp. Toxicol.* **12**, 289–296.

Karalliede, L., and Senanayake, N. (1999). Organophosphorus insecticide poisoning. *JIFCC* **11**, 4–9.

Karalliede, L., Senanayake, N., and Ariaratnam, A. (1988). Acute organophosphorus insecticide poisoning during pregnancy. *Human Toxicol.* **7**, 363–364.

Karr, C., Demers, P., Costa, L. G., Daniell, W. E., Barnhart, S., Miller, M., Gallagher, G., Horstman, S. W., Eaton, D., and Rosenstock, L. (1992). Organophosphate pesticide exposure in a group of Washington State orchard applicators. *Environ. Res.* **59**, 229–237.

Kassa, J., and Cabal, J. (1999). A comparison of the efficacy of acetylcholinesterase reactivators against cyclohexyl methylphosphonofluoridate (GF agent) by *in vitro* and *in vivo* methods. *Pharmacol. Toxicol.* **84**, 41–45.

Kaulla, K., and Holmes, J. H. (1961). Changes following anticholinesterase exposures. *Arch. Environ. Health.* **2**, 168–177.

Kecik, Y., Yorukoglu, D., Saygin, B., and Sekerci, S. (1993). A case of acute poisoning due to organophosphate insecticide. *Anaesthesia* **48**, 141–143.

Keeler, J. R., Hurst, C. G., and Dunn, M. A. (1991). Pyridostigmine used as a nerve agent pretreatment under wartime conditions. *JAMA* **266**, 693–695.

Kentala, E., Kaila, T., Iisalo, E., and Kanto, J. (1990). Intramuscular atropine in healthy volunteers: A pharmacokinetic and pharmacodynamic study. *Int. J. Clin. Pharmacol. Ther. Toxicol.* **28**, 399–404.

Khurana, D., and Prabhakar, S. (2000). Organophosphorus intoxication. *Arch. Neurol.* **57**, 600–602.

King, J., and Griffin, D. (1973). Differentiation of serum cholinesterase variants by succinylcholine inhibition. *Br. J. Anaesth.* **49**, 450–454.

Kiss, Z., and Fazekas, T. (1979). Arrhythmias in organophosphate poisonings. *Acta Cardiol.* **34**, 323–330.

Kiss, Z., and Fazekas, T. (1982). Organophosphate poisoning and complete heart block. *J. R. Soc. Med.* **73**, 138–139.

Kopman, A. F., Strachovsky, G., and Lichtenstein, L. (1978). Prolonged response to succinylcholine following physostigmine. *Anesthesiology* **49**, 142–143.

Korsak, R. J., and Sato, M. M. (1977). Effects of chronic organophosphate pesticide exposure on the central nervous system. *Clin. Toxicol.* **11**, 83–95.

Kraus, J. F., Richards, D. M., Borhani, N. O. Mull, R., Kilgore, W. W., and Winterlin, W. (1977). Physiological response to organophosphate residues in field workers. *Arch. Environ. Contam. Toxicol.* **5**, 471–485.

Kraus, J. F., Mull, R., Kurts, P., Winterlin, W., Franti, C. E., Borhani, N., and Kilgore, W. (1981). Epidemiologic study of physiological effects in usual and volunteer citrus workers from organophosphate pesticide residues at reentry. *J. Toxicol. Environ. Health* **8**, 169–184.

Krieger, R. I., and Thongsinthusak, T. (1993). Metabolism and excretion of dimethoate following ingestion of overtolerance peas and a bolus dose. *Food Chem. Toxicol.* **31**, 177–182.

Kušić, R., Bošković, B., Vojvodić, V., and Jovanović, D. (1985). HI-6 in man: Blood levels, urinary excretion, and tolerance after intramuscular administration of the oxime to healthy volunteers. *Fund. Appl. Toxicol.* **5**, S89–S97.

Lamminpää, A., and Riihimäki, V. (1992). Pesticide-related incidents treated in Finnish hospitals—A review of cases registered over a 5-year period. *Human Exp. Toxicol.* **11**, 473–479.

Lankisch, P. G., Müller C.-H., Niederstadt, H., and Brand, A. (1990). Painless acute pancreatitis subsequent to anticholinesterase insecticide (parathion) intoxication. *Am. J. Gastroenterol.* **85**, 872–875.

Le Blanc, F. N., Benson, B. E., and Gilg, A. D. (1986). A severe organophosphate poisoning requiring the use of an atropine drip. *J. Toxicol. Clin. Toxicol.* **24**, 69–76.

Lee, W.-C., Yang, C.-C., Deng, J.-F., Wu, M.-L., Ger, J., Lin, H.-C., Chang, F.-Y., and Lee, S.-D. (1998). The clinical significance of hyperamylasemia in organophosphate poisoning. *Clin. Toxicol.* **36**, 673–681.

Lefkowitz, R. J., Hoffman, B. B., and Taylor, P. (1996). Neurotransmission. The autonomic and somatic motor nervous systems. *In* "Goodman and Gilman's the Pharmacological Basis of Therapeutics" (J. G. Hardman and L. E. Limbird, eds.), 9th ed., pp. 105–139. McGraw-Hill, New York.

Levin, H. S., Rodnitzky, R. L., and Mick, D. L. (1976). Anxiety associated with exposure to organophosphate compounds. *Arch. Gen. Psychiatry* **33**, 225–228.

Lewis, P. J., Lowing, R. K., and Gompertz, D. (1981). Automated discrete kinetic method for erythrocyte acetylcholinesterase and plasma cholinesterase. *Clin. Chem.* **27**, 929–929.

Lipp, J. A. (1973). Effect of benzodiazepine derivatives on soman-induced seizure activity and convulsions in the monkey. *Arch. Int. Pharmacodyn.* **202**, 244–251.

Loewenstein-Lichtenstein, Y., Glick, D., Gluzman, N., Sternfeld, M., Zakut, H., and Soreq, H. (1996). Overlapping drug interaction sites of human butyrylcholinesterase dissected by site-directed mutagenesis. *Mol. Pharmacol.* **50**, 1423–1431.

London, L., Thompson, M. L., Sacks, S., Fuller, B., Bachmann, O. M., and Myers, J. E. (1995). Repeatability and validity of a field kit for estimation of cholinesterase in whole blood. *Occup. Environ Med.* **52**, 57–64.

London, L., Meyers, J. E., Nell, V., Taylor, T., and Thompson, M. L. (1997). An investigation into neurologic and neurobehavioral effects of long-term agrichemical use among deciduous fruit farm workers in the Western Cape, South Africa. *Environ. Res.* **73**, 132–145.

London, L., Nell, V., Thompson, M. L., and Meyers, J. E. (1998). Effects of long-term organophosphate exposures on neurological symptoms, vibration sense and tremor among South African farm workers. *Scan. J. Work Environ. Health* **24**, 18–29.

Lotti, M. (1987). Organophosphate-induced delayed polyneuropathy in humans: Perspectives for biomonitoring. *Trends Pharmacol. Sci.* **8**, 175–176.

Lotti, M. (1991). Treatment of acute organophosphate poisoning. *Med. J. Aust.* **154**, 51–55.

Lotti, M. (1992a). Central neurotoxicity and behavioural effects of anticholinesterases. *In* "Clinical & Experimental Toxicology of Organophosphates and Carbamates" (B. Ballantyne and T. C. Marrs, eds.), pp. 75–83. Butterworth–Heinemann, Oxford.

Lotti, M. (1992b). The pathogenesis of organophosphate delayed polyneuropathy. *Crit. Rev. Toxicol.* **21**, 465–487.

Lotti, M. (1995). Cholinesterase inhibition: Complexities in interpretation. *Clin. Chem.* **41**, 1814–1818.

Lotti, M. (1999). Causes of the Gulf War Syndrome: testing hypotheses. *Muscle Nerve* **22**, 663–665.

Lotti, M. (2000). Organophosphorus compounds. *In* "Experimental and Clinical Neurotoxicology" (P. S. Spencer, H. S. Schaumburg, and A. C. Ludolph, eds.), 2nd ed., pp. 898–925. Oxford University Press, New York.

Lotti, M., and Becker, C. E. (1982a). Treatment of acute organophosphate poisoning: Evidence of a direct effect on central nervous system by 2-PAM (pyridine-2-aldoxime methyl chloride). *J. Toxicol.-Clin. Toxicol.* **19**, 121–127.

Lotti, M., and Becker, C. E. (1982b). Polyneuropathy and exposure to parathion. *Neurology* **32**, 217.

Lotti, M., and Johnson, M. K. (1978). Neurotoxicity of organophosphorus pesticides: Predictions can be based on *in vitro* studies with hen and human enzymes. *Arch. Toxicol.* **41**, 215–221.

Lotti, M., and Moretto, A. (1995). Cholinergic Symptom and Gulf War Syndrome. *Nature Med.* **1**, 1225–1226.

Lotti, M., Ferrara, S. D., Caroldi, S., and Singaglia, F. (1981). Enzyme studies with human and hen autopsy tissue suggest omethoate does not cause delayed neuropathy in man. *Arch. Toxicol.* **48**, 265–270.

Lotti, M., Becker, C. E., Aminoff, M. J., Woodrow, J. E., Seiber, J. N., Talcott, R. E., and Richardson, R. J. (1983). Occupational exposure to the cotton defoliants DEF and merphos. A rational approach to monitoring organophosphorus-induced delayed neurotoxicity. *J. Occup. Med.* **25**, 517–522.

Lotti, M., Becker, C. E., and Aminoff, M. J. (1984). Organophosphate polyneuropathy: Pathogenesis and prevention. *Neurology* **34**, 658–662.

Lotti, M., Moretto, A., Zoppellari, R., Dainese, R., Rizzuto, N., and Barusco, G. (1986). Inhibition of lymphocytic neuropathy target esterase predicts the development of organophosphate-induced delayed polyneuropathy. *Arch. Toxicol.* **59**, 176–179.

Ludomirsky, A., Klein, H. O., Sarelli, P., Becker, B., Hoffman, S., Taitelman, U., Barzilai, J., Lang, R., David, D., Disegni, E., and Kaplinsky, E. (1982). Q-T prolongation and polymorphous ("Torsade de Pointes") ventricular arrhythmias associated with organophosphorus insecticide poisoning. *Am. J. Cardiol.* **49**, 1654–1658.

Luo, C., Saxena, A., Smith, M., Garcia, G., Radiæ, Z., Taylor, P., and Doctor, B. P. (1999). Phosphoryl oxime inhibition of acetylcholinesterase during oxime reactivation is prevented by edrophonium. *Biochemistry* **38**, 9937–9947.

Luzhnikov, E. A., Yaroslavsky, A. A., Molodenkov, M. N., Shurkalin, B. K., Evseev, N. G., and Barsukov, U. F. (1977). Plasma perfusion through charcoal in methylparathion poisoning. *Lancet* **i**, 38–39.

Lyon, J., Taylor, H., and Ackerman, B. (1987). A case report of intravenous malathion injection with determination of serum half-life. *Clin. Toxicol.* **25**, 243–249.

Mackness, B., Durrington, P. N., and Mackness, M. I. (1998). Human serum paraoxonase. *Gen. Pharmacol.* **31**, 329–336.

Mahieu, P., Hassoun, A., Van Binst, R., Lauwerys, R., and Deheneffe, Y. (1982). Severe and prolonged poisoning by fenthion. Significance of the determination of the anticholinesterase capacity of plasma. *J. Toxicol. Clin. Toxicol.* **19**, 425–432.

Maizlish, N., Schenker, M., Weisskopf, C., Seiber, J., and Samuels, S. (1987). A behavioral evaluation of pest control workers with short-term, low-level exposure to the organophosphate diazinon. *Am. J. Ind. Med.* **12**, 153–172.

Maltby, N., Broe, G. A., Creasey, H., Jorm, A. F., Christensen, H., and Brooks, W. S. (1994). Efficacy of tacrine and lecithin in mild to moderate Alzheimer's disease: Double blind trial. *Br. Med. J.* **308**, 879–883.

Maresch, W. (1957). Die Vergiftung durch Phosphorsäureester (E 605, Parathion, Thiophos). *Archiv für Toxikologie* **16**, 285–319 (in German).

Markowitz, J. S., Gutterman, E. M., and Link, B. G. (1986). Self-reported physical and psychological effects following a malathion pesticide incident. *J. Occup. Med.* **28**, 377–383.

Maroni, M., and Bleecker, M. L. (1986). Neuropathy target esterase in human lymphocytes and platelets. *J. Appl. Toxicol.* **6**, 1–7.

Marrs, T. C. (1991). Toxicology of oximes used in treatment of organophosphate poisoning. *Adverse Drug React. Toxicol. Rev.* **10**, 61–72.

Marrs, T. C. (1993). Organophosphate poisoning. *Pharmac. Ther.* **58**, 51–66.

Marsh, W. H., Vukov, G. A., and Conradi, E. C. (1988). Acute pancreatitis after cutaneous exposure to an organophosphate insecticide. *Am. J. Gastroenterol.* **83**, 1158–1160.

Martinez-Chuecos, J., Jurado, M. C., Gimenez, M. P., Martinez, D., and Menendez, M. (1992). Experience with hemoperfusion for organophosphate poisoning. *Crit. Care Med.* **20**, 1538–1543.

Maselli, R. A., and Leung, C. (1993). Analysis of anticholinesterase-induced neuromuscular transmission failure. *Muscle Nerve* **16**, 548–553.

Maselli, R. A., and Soliven, B. C. (1991). Analysis of the organophosphate-induced electromyographic response to repetitive nerve stimulation: Paradoxical response to edrophonium and d-tubocurarine. *Muscle Nerve* **14**, 1182–1188.

Maselli, R. A., Jacobsen, J. H., and Spire, J.-P. (1986). Edrophonium: An aid in the diagnosis of acute organophosphate poisoning. *Ann. Neurol.* **19**, 508–510.

Massumi, R. A., Mason, D. T., Amsterdam, E. A., DeMaria A., Miller, R. R., Scheinman, M. M., and Zelis, R. (1972). Ventricular fibrillation and tachycardia after intravenous atropine for treatment of bradycardias. *N. Engl. J. Med.* **287**, 336–338.

Matsumiya, N., Tanaka, M., Iwai, M., Kondo, T., Takahashi, S., and Sato, S. (1996). Elevated amylase is related to the development of respiratory failure in organophosphate poisoning. *Human Exp. Toxicol.* **15**, 250–253.

McConnell, R., Keifer, M., and Rosenstock, L. (1994). Elevated quantitative vibrotactile threshold among workers previously poisoned with methamidophos and other organophosphate pesticides. *Am. J. Ind. Med.* **25**, 325–334.

McConnell, R., Delgado-Téllez, E., Cuadra, R., Tórres, E., Keifer, M., Almendárez, J., Miranda, J., El-Fawal, H. A. N., Wolff, M., Simpson, D., and Lundberg, I. (1999). Organophosphate neuropathy due to methamidophos: Biochemical and neurophysiological markers. *Arch. Toxicol.* **73**, 296–300.

McLeod, C. G., Jr. (1985). Pathology of nerve agents: Perspectives on medical management. *Fund. Appl. Toxicol.* **5**, S10–S16.

Mearns, J., Dunn, J., and Lees-Haley, P. R. (1994). Psychological effects of organophosphate pesticides: A review and call for research by psychologists. *J. Clin. Psychol.* **50**, 286–294.

Medicis, J. J., Stork, C. M., Howland, M. A., Hoffman, R. S., and Goldfrank, L. R. (1996). Pharmacokinetics following a loading plus a continuous infusion of pralidoxime compared with the traditional short infusion regimen in human volunteers. *Clin. Toxicol.* **34**, 289–295.

Merrill, D. G., and Mihm, F. G. (1982). Prolonged toxicity of organophosphate poisoning. *Crit. Care Med.* **10**, 550–551.

Metcalf, D. R., and Holmes, J. H. (1969). EEG, psychological, and neurological alterations in humans with organophosphorus exposure. *Ann. N.Y. Acad. Sci.* **160**, 357–365.

Michaleck, H., and Stavinoha, W. B. (1978). Effect of chlorpromazine pre-treatment on the inhibition of total cholinesterases and butyrylcholinesterase in brain of rats poisoned by physostigme or dichlorvos. *Toxicology* **9**, 205–218.

Michotte, A., Van Dijck, I., Maes, V., and D'Haenen, H. (1989). Ataxia as the only delayed neurotoxic manifestation of organophosphate insecticde poisoning. *Eur. Neurol.* **29**, 23–26.

Millard, C. B., and Broomfield, C. A. (1995). Anticholinesterases: Medical applications of neurochemical principles. *J. Neurochem.* **64**, 1909–1918.

Minton, N. A., and Murray, V. S. G. (1988). A review of organophosphate poisoning. *Med. Toxicol.* **3**, 350–375.

Misra, U. K., Nag, D., Khan, W. A., and Ray, P. K. (1988). A study of nerve conduction velocity, late responses and neuromuscular synapse functions in organophosphate workers in India. *Arch. Toxicol.* **61**, 496–500.

Mizutani, T., Naito, H., and Oohashi, N. (1991). Rectal ulcer with massive haemorrhage due to activated charcoal treatment in oral organophosphate poisoning. *Human Exp. Toxicol.* **10**, 385–386.

Moeller, H. C., and Rider, J. A. (1965). Further studies on the anticholinesterase effect of systox and methyl parathion in humans. *Fed. Proc., Fed. Am. Soc. Exp. Biol.* **24**, 641.

Molphy, R., and Rathus, E. M. (1964). Organic phosphorus poisonings and therapy. *Med. J. Aust.* **2**, 337–340.

Moore, W. K. S. (1956). Two cases of poisoning with di-isopropylfluorophosphonate (D.F.P.). *Br. J. Industr. Med.* **13**, 214–216.

Moore, P. G., and James, O. F. (1981). Acute pancreatitis induced by acute organophosphate poisoning. *Postgrad. Med. J.* **57**, 660–662.

Moretto, A., and Lotti, M. (1988). Organ distribution of neuropathy target esterase in man. *Biochem. Pharmacol.* **37**, 3041–3043.

Moretto, A., and Lotti, M. (1998). Poisoning by organophosphorus insecticides and sensory neuropathy. *J. Neurol. Neurosurg. Psychiatry* **64**, 463–468.

Moretto, A., Capodicasa, E., Bertolazzi, M., De Paris, P., Saia, B. O., and Lotti, M. (1995). Biological monitoring of occupational exposures to organophosphorus insecticides. In "Agriculture Health and Safety: Workplace, Environment, Sustainability" (H. H. McDuffie, J. A. Dosman, K. M. Semchuk, S. A. Olenchock, and A. Senthilselvan, eds.), pp. 217–221. CRC Press, Boca Raton, FL.

Morgan, J. P. (1982). The Jamaica ginger paralysis. *JAMA* **248**, 1864–1867.

Morgan, J. P., and Penovich, P. (1978). Jamaica ginger paralysis. Forty-seven-year follow-up. *Arch. Neurol.* **35**, 530–532.

Morgan, D. P., Hetzler, H. L., Slach, E. F., and Lin, L. I. (1977). Urinary excretion of paranitrophenol and alkyl phosphates following ingestion of methyl or ethyl parathion by human subjects. *Arch. Environ. Contam. Toxicol.* **6**, 159–173.

Mueller, R. F., Hornung, S., Furlong, C. E., Anderson, J., Giblett, E. R., and Motulsky, A. G. (1983). Plasma paraoxonase polmorphism: A new enzyme assay, population, family, biochemical, and linkage studies. *Am. J. Hum. Genet.* **35**, 393–408.

Murray, V. S. G., Wiseman, H. M., Dawling, S., Morgan, I., and House, I. M. (1992). Health effects of organophosphate sheep dips. *Br. Med. J.* **305**, 1090.

Nagler, J., Braeckman, R. A., Willems, J. L., Verpooten, G. A., and De Broe, M. E. (1981). Combined hemoperfusion–hemodialysis in organophosphate poisoning. *J. Appl. Toxicol.* **1**, 199–201.

Namba, T., Nolte, C. T., Jackrel, J., and Grob, D. (1971). Poisoning due to organophosphate insecticides. Acute and chronic manifestations. *Am. J. Med.* **50**, 475–492.

Neuvonen, P. J., and Olkkola, K. T. (1988). Oral activated charcoal in the treatment of intoxications. Role of single and repeated doses. *Med. Toxicol.* **3**, 33–58.

Newcombe, D. S. (1992). Immune surveillance, organophosphorus exposure, and lymphomagenesis. *Lancet* **339**, 539–541.

Newcombe, D. S., and Esa, A. H. (1992). Immunotoxicity of organophosphorus compounds. In "Clinical Immunotoxicology" (D. S. Newcombe, N. R. Rose, and J. C. Bloom, eds.), pp. 349–364. Raven Press, New York.

Niedziella, S. W., Göpel, W., and Banzhaf, E. (1985). Akute Alkylphosphat-intoxikation (Trichlorphon) mit intervallärem Polyneuropathie-Syndrom. *Z. Ges. Inn. Med. Jahrg.* **40**, 237–239 (in German).

NIH Technology Assessment Workshop Panel (1994). The Persian Gulf experience and health. *JAMA* **272**, 391–395.

Nilsson, E. (1982). Physostigmine treatment in various drug-induced intoxications. *Ann. Clin. Res.* **14**, 165–172.

Nisse, P., Forceville, X., Cezard, C., Ameri, A., and Mathieu-Nolf, M. (1998). Intermediate syndrome with delayed distal polyneuropathy from ethyl parathion poisoning. *Vet. Human Toxicol.* **40**, 349–352.

Nolan, R. J., Rich, D. L., Freshour, N. L., and Saunders, J. H. (1984). Chlorpyrifos: Pharmacokinetics in human volunteers. *Toxicol. Appl. Pharmacol.* **73**, 8–15.

Nordgren, I., Holmstedt, B., Bengtsson, E., and Finkel, Y. (1980). Plasma levels of metrifonate and dichlorvos during treatment of schistosomiasis with bilarcil®. *Am. J. Trop. Med. Hyg.* **29**, 426–430.

Norton, S. (1986). Toxic responses of the central nervous system. In "Casarett and Doull's Toxicology" (C. D. Klaassen, M. O. Amdur, and J. Doull, eds.), 3rd ed., pp. 359–386. Macmillan, New York.

Nouira, S., Abroug, F., Elatrous, S., Boujdaria, R., and Bouchoucha, S. (1994). Prognostic value of serum cholinesterase in organophosphate poisoning. *Chest* **106**, 1811–1814.

Nutley, B., and Cocker, J. (1993). Biological monitoring of workers occupationally exposed to organophosphorus pesticides. *Pest. Sci.* **38**, 315–322.

Ochi, G., Watanabe, K., Tokuoka, H., Hatakenaka, S., and Arai, T. (1995). Neuroleptic malignant-like syndrome: A complication of acute organophosphate poisoning. *Can. J. Anaesth.* **42**, 1027–1030.

Ohbu, S., Yamashina, A., Takasu, N., Yamaguchi, T., Murai, T., Nakano, K., Matsui, Y., Mikami, R., Sakurai, K., and Hinohara, S. (1997). Sarin poisoning on Tokyo subway. *S. Afr. Med. J.* **90**, 587–593.

Ohkawa, H., Oshita, H., and Miyamoto, J. (1980). Comparison of inhibitory activity of various organophosphorus compounds against acetylcholinesterase and neurotoxic esterase of hens with respect to delayed neurotoxicity. *Biochem. Pharmacol.* **29**, 2721–2727.

Oken, B. S., and Chiappa, K. H. (1986). Statistical issues concerning computerized analysis of brainwave topography. *Ann. Neurol.* **19**, 493–497.

Okumura, T., Takasu, N., Ishimatsu, S., Miyanoki, S., Mitsuhashi, A., Kumada, K., Tanaka, K., and Hinohara, S. (1996). Report on 640 victims of the Tokyo subway sarin attack. *Ann. Emerg. Med.* **28**, 129–135.

Østergaard, D., Jensen, F. S., Jenson, E., Skovgaard, L. T., and Viby-Mogensen, J. (1992). Influence of plasma cholinesterase activity on recovery from mivacurium-induced neuromuscular blockade in phenotypically normal patients. *Acta Anaesthesiol. Scand.* **36**, 702–706.

Osterloh, J., Lotti, M., and Pond, S. M. (1983). Toxicologic studies in a fatal overdose of 2,4-D, MCPP, and chlorpyrifos. *J. Analyt. Toxicol.* **7**, 125–129.

Otto, D. A., Soliman, S., Svendsgaard, D., Soffar, A., and Ahmed, N. (1990). Neurobehavioral assessment of workers exposed to organophosphorus pesticides. *In* "Advances in Neurobehavioural Toxicology: Applications in Environmental and Occupational Health" (B. L. Johnson, ed.), pp. 305–322 Lewis Publishers, Chelsea, MI.

Panieri, E., Krige, J. E., Bornman, P. C., and Linton, D. M. (1997). Severe necrotizing pancreatitis caused by organophosphate poisoning. *J. Clin. Gastroenterol.* **25**, 463–465.

Parrón, T., Hernández, A. F., and Villanueva, E. (1996a). Increased risk of suicide with exposure to pesticides in an intensive agricultural area. A 12-year retrospective study. *Foren. Sci. Int.* **79**, 53–63.

Parrón, T., Hernández, A. F., Pla, A., and Villanueva, E. (1996b). Clinical and biochemical changes in greenhouse sprayers chronically exposed to pesticides. *Human Exp. Toxicol.* **15**, 957–963.

Perron, R., and Johnson, B. B. (1969). Insecticide poisoning. *N. Engl. J. Med.* **281**, 274–275.

Pickett, W., King, W. D., Lees, R. E. M., Bienefeld, M., Morrison, H. I., and Brison, R. J. (1998). Suicide mortality and pesticide use among Canadian farmers. *Am. J. Ind. Med.* **34**, 364–372.

Pilkington, A., Jamal, G. A., Gilham, R., Hansen, S., Buchanan, D., Kidd, M., Azis, M. A., Julu, P. O., Al-Rawas, S., Ballantyne, J. P., Hurley, J. F., and Soutar, C. A. (1999). "Epidemiological Study of the Relationshps between Exposure to Organophosphate Pesticides and Indices of Chronic Peripheral Neuropathy, and Neurophysiological Abnormalities in Sheep Farmers and Dippers. Phase 3. Clinical Neurological, Neurophysiological and Neuropsychological Study." Technical Memorandum Series TM/99/02c, Institute of Occupational Medicine, Edinburgh.

Pimentel, J. M., and Carrington da Costa, R. B. (1992). Effects of organophosphates on the heart. *In* "Clinical & Experimental Toxicology of Organophosphates and Carbamates" (B. Ballantyne and T. C. Marrs, eds.), pp. 145–148. Butterworth–Heinemann, Oxford.

Pleština, R. (1984). "Prevention, Diagnosis and Treatment of Insecticide Poisoning." Report WHO/VBC/84.889, World Health Organization, Geneva.

Pleština, R., and Piuković-Pleština, M. (1978). Effect of anticholinesterase pesticides on the eye and on vision. *Crit. Rev. Toxicol.* **6**, 1–23.

Polhuijs, M., Langenberg, J. P., and Benschop, H. P. (1997). New method for retrospective detection of exposure to organophosphorus anticholinesterases: Application to alleged sarin victims of Japanese terrorists. *Toxicol. Appl. Pharmacol.* **146**, 156–161.

Popendorf, W. J., Spear, R. C., Leffingwell, J. T., Yager, J., and Kahn, E. (1979). Harvester exposure to Zolone® (phosalone) residues in peach orchards. *J. Occup. Med.* **21**, 189–194.

Pullicino, P., and Aquilina, J. (1989). Opsoclonus in organophosphate poisoning. *Arch. Neurol.* **46**, 704–705.

Quinby, G. E., Loomis, T. A., and Brown, H. W. (1963). Oral occupational parathion poisoning treated with 2-PAM iodide (2-pyridine aldoxime methiodide). *N. Engl. J. Med.* **268**, 639–643.

Rasmussen, W. A., Jensen, J. A., Stein, W. J., and Hayes, W. J., Jr. (1963). Toxicological studies of DDVP for disinsection of aircraft. *Aerosp. Med.* **34**, 594–600.

Ray, D. E. (1998a). "Organophosphorus Esters: An Evaluation of Chronic Neurotoxic Effects." MRC Institute for Environment and Health, Leicester, UK.

Ray, D. E. (1998b). Chronic effects of low level exposure to anticholinesterases—A mechanistic view. *Toxicol. Lett.* **102-103**, 527–533.

Reidy, T. J., Bowler, R. M., Rauch, S. S., and Pedroza, G. I. (1992). Pesticide exposure and neuropsychological impairment in migrant farm workers. *Arch. Clin. Neuropsychol.* **7**, 85–95.

Reiner, E., and Pleština, R. (1979). Regeneration of cholinesterase activities in humans and rats after inhibition by *O,O*-dimethyl-2,2-dichlorovinyl phosphate. *Toxicol. Appl. Pharmacol.* **49**, 451–454.

Relman, A. S. (1991). Tacrine as a treatment for Alzheimer's dementia. *N. Engl. J. Med.* **324**, 349.

Rengstorff, R. H. (1985). Accidental exposure to sarin: vision effects. *Arch. Toxicol.* **56**, 201–203.

Rengstorff, R. H. (1994). Vision and ocular changes following accidental exposure to organophosphates. *J. Appl. Toxicol.* **14**, 115–118.

Richardson, R. J. (1995). Assessment of the neurotoxic potential of chlorpyrifos relative to other organophosphorus compounds: A critical review of the literature. *J. Toxicol. Environ. Health* **44**, 135–165.

Richter, E. (1993). "Organophosphorus Pesticides: A Multinational Epidemiologic Study." World Health Organization, Copenhagen, Denmark.

Richter, E. D., Chuwers, P., Levy, Y., Gordon M., Grauer, F., Marzouk, J., Levy, S., Barron, S., and Gruener, N. (1992). Health effects from exposure to organophosphate pesticides in workers and residents in Israel. *Isr. J. Med. Sci.* **28**, 584–597.

Rider, J. A., Swader, J. I., and Puletti, E. J. (1970). Methyl parathion and guthion anticholinesterase effects in human subjects. *Fed. Prod. Fed. Am. Soc. Exp. Biol.* **29**, 349.

Rider, J. A., Swader, J. I., and Puletti, E. J. (1972). Anticholinesterase toxicity studies with guthion, phosdrin, di-syston, and trithion in human subjects. *Fed. Prod. Fed. Am. Soc. Exp. Biol.* **31**, 520.

Rider, J. A., Puletti, E. J., and Swader, J. I. (1975). The minimal oral toxicity level for mevinphos in man. *Toxicol. Appl. Pharmacol.* **32**, 92–100.

Roberts, D. V. (1976). E. M. G. voltage and motor nerve conduction velocity in organophosphorus pesticide factory workers. *Int. Arch. Occup. Environ. Health* **36**, 267–274.

Roberts, D. V. (1977). A longitudinal electromyographic study of six men occupationally exposed to organophosphorus compounds. *Int. Arch. Occup. Environ. Health* **38**, 221–229.

Rodgers, K. E., Devens, B. H., and Imamura, T. (1992). Immunotoxic effects of anticholinesterases. *In* "Clinical & Experimental Toxicology of Organophosphates and Carbamates" (B. Ballantyne and T. C. Marrs, eds.), pp. 211–222. Butterworth–Heinemann, Oxford.

Rodnitzky, R. L., Levin, H. S., and Mick, D. L. (1975). Occupational exposure to organophosphate pesticides. A neurobehavioral study. *Arch. Environ. Health* **30**, 98–103.

Rosenstock, L., Keifer, M., Daniell, W. E., McConnell, R., Claypoole, K., and the Pesticide Health Effects Study Group (1991). Chronic central nervous system effects of acute organophosphate pesticide intoxication. *Lancet* **338**, 223–227.

Rosenthal, N. E., and Cameron, C. L. (1991). Exaggerated sensitivity to an organophosphate pesticide. *Am. J. Psychiatry* **148**, 270.

Saadeh, A. M., Al-Ali, M. K., Farsakh, N. A., and Ghani, M. A. (1996). Clinical and sociodemographic features of acute carbamate and organophosphate poisoning: A study of 70 adult patients in North Jordan. *Clin. Toxicol.* **34**, 45–51.

Saadeh, A. M., Farsakh, N. A., and Al-Ali, M. K. (1997). Cardiac manifestations of acute carbamate and organophosphate poisoning. *Heart* **77**, 461–464.

Sahin, M., Bernay, I., Cantürk, F., and Demircali, A. E. (1994). Reflex sympathetic dystrophy syndrome secondary to organophosphate intoxication induced neuropathy. *Ann. Nucl. Med.* **8**, 299–300.

Sakamoto, T., Sawada, Y., Nishide, K., Sadamitsu, D., Yoshioka, T., Sugimoto, T., Nishii, S., and Kishi, H. (1984). Delayed neurotoxicity produced by an organophosphorus compound (Sumithion). A case report. *Arch. Toxicol.* **56**, 136–138.

Savage, E. P., Keefe, T. J., Mounce, L. M., Heaton, R. K., Lewis, J. A., and Burcar, P. J. (1988). Chronic neurological sequelae of acute organophosphate pesticide poisoning. *Arch. Environ. Health* **43**, 38–45.

Saxena, A., Maxwell, D. M. Quinn, D. M., Radić, Z., Taylor, P., and Doctor, B. P. (1997). Mutant acetylcholinesterase as potential detoxification agents for organophosphate poisoning. *Biochem. Pharmacol.* **54**, 269–274.

Schexnayder, S., James, L. P., Kearns, G. L., and Farrar, H. C. (1998). The pharmacokinetics of continuous infusion pralidoxime in children with organophosphate poisoning. *Clin. Toxicol.* **36**, 549–555.

Schuman S. H., and Wagner, S. L. (1991). Pesticide intoxication and chronic CNS effects. *Lancet* **338**, 948.

Scott, R. J. (1986). Repeated asystole following PAM in organophosphate self-poisoning. *Anaesth. Int. Care* **14**, 458–460.

Sedgwick, E. M., and Senanayake, N. (1997). Pathophysiology of the intermediate syndrome of organophosphorus poisoning. *J. Neurol. Neurosurg. Psychiatry* **62**, 201–202.

Selden, B. S., and Curry, S. C. (1987). Prolonged succinylcholine-induced paralysis in organophosphate insecticide poisoning. *Ann. Emerg. Med.* **16**, 215–217.

Sellström, Å. (1992). Anticonvulsants in anticholinesterase poisoning. *In* "Clinical & Experimental Toxicology of Organophosphates and Carbamates" (B. Ballantyne and T. C. Marrs, eds.), pp. 578–586. Butterworth–Heinemann, Oxford.

Senanayake, N. (1981). Tri-cresyl phosphate neuropathy in Sri Lanka: A clinical and neurophysiological study with a three year follow up. *J. Neurol. Neurosurg. Psychiatry* **44**, 775–780.

Senanayake, N., and Jeyaratnam, J. (1981). Toxic polyneuropathy due to gingili oil contaminated with tri-cresyl phosphate affecting adolescent girls in Sri Lanka. *Lancet* **i**, 88–89.

Senanayake, N., and Johnson, M. K. (1982). Acute polyneuropathy after poisoning by a new organophosphate insecticide. *N. Engl. J. Med.* **306**, 155–157.

Senanayake, N., and Karalliedde, L. (1987). Neurotoxic effects of organophosphorus insecticides. An intermediate syndrome. *N. Engl. J. Med.* **316**, 761–763.

Senanayake, N., and Sanmuganathan, P. S. (1995). Extrapyramidal manifestations complicating organophosphorus insecticide poisoning. *Human Exp. Toxicol.* **14**, 600–604.

Sewell, C., Pilkington, A., Buchanan, D., Tannahill, S. N., Kidd, M., Cherrie, B., and Robertson, A., (1999). "Epidemiological Study of the Relationships between Exposure to Organophosphate Pesticides and Indices of Chronic Peripheral Neuropathy, and Neuropsychological Abnormalities in Sheep Farmers and Dippers. Phase 1. Development and Validation of an Organophosphate Uptake Model for Sheep Dippers." Technical Memorandum Series, Institute of Occupational Medicine, Edinburgh.

Sharma, R. P., and Tomar, R. S. (1992). Immunotoxicity of anticholinesterase agents. *In* "Clinical & Experimental Toxicology of Organophosphates and Carbamates" (B. Ballantyne and T. C. Marrs, eds.), pp. 203–210. Butterworth–Heinemann, Oxford.

Shen, Z.-X. (1998). Pyridostigmine bromide and Gulf War syndrome. *Med. Hypothesis* **51**, 235–237.

Shiraishi, S., Inoue, N., Murai, Y., Onishi. A., and Noda, S. (1983). Dipterex (trichlorfon) poisoning. Clinical and pathological studies in human and monkeys. *J. UOEH* **5**(Suppl.), 125–132.

Sidell, F. R., and Groff, W. A. (1971). Intramuscular and intravenous administration of small doses of 2-pyridinium aldoxime methochloride to man. *J. Pharm. Sci.* **60**, 1224–1228.

Sidell, F. R., Groff, W. A., and Kaminskis, A. (1972). Toxogonin and pralidoxime: Kinetic comparison after intravenous administration to man. *J. Pharmacol. Sci.* **61**, 1765–1769.

Singh, G., Avasthi, G., Khurana, D., Whig, J., and Mahajan, R. (1998a). Neurophysiological monitoring of pharmacological manipulation in acute organophosphate (OP) poisoning. The effects of pralidoxime, magnesium sulphate and pancuronium. *Electroenceph. Clin. Neurophysiol.* **107**, 140–148.

Singh, G., Mahajan, R., and Whig, J. (1998b). The importance of electrodiagnostic studies in acute organophosphate poisoning. *J. Neurol. Sci.* **157**, 191–200.

Singh, G., Sidhu, U. P. S., Mahajan, R., Avasthi, G., and Whig, J. (2000). Phrenic nerve conduction studies in acute organophosphate poisoning. *Muscle Nerve* **23**, 627–632.

Singh, S., Batra, Y. K., Singh, S. M., Wig, N., and Sharma, B. K. (1995). Is atropine alone sufficient in acute severe organophosphorus poisoning?: Experience of a North West Indian Hospital. *Int. J. Clin. Pharmacol. Ther.* **33**, 628–630.

Spear, R. C., Popendorf, W. J., Leffingwell, J. T., Milby, T. H., Davies, J. E., and Spencer, W. F. (1977). Fieldworker's response to weathered residues of parathion. *J. Occup. Med.* **19**, 406–410.

Stålberg, E., Hilton-Brown, P., Kolmodin-Hedman, B., Holmstedt, B., and Augustinsson, K. B. (1978). Effect of occupational exposure to organophosphorus insecticides on neuromuscular function. *Scand. J. Work. Environ. Health* **4**, 255–261.

Stamboulis, E., Psimaras, A., Vassilopoulos, D., Davaki, P., Manta, P., and Kapaki, E. (1991). Neuropathy following acute intoxication with mecarbam (OP ester). *Acta Neurol. Scand.* **83**, 198–200.

Stavinoha, W. B., Modak, A. T., and Weintraub, S. T. (1976). Rate of accumulation of acetylcholine in discrete regions of the rat brain after dichlorvos treatment. *J. Neurochem.* **27**, 1375–1378.

Steenland, K. (1996). Chronic neurological effects of organophosphate pesticide. *Br. Med. J.* **312**, 1312–1313.

Steenland, K., Jenkins, B., Ames, R. G., O'Malley, M., Chrislip, D., and Russo, J. (1994). Chronic neurological sequelae to organophosphate pesticide poisoning. *Am. J. Public Health* **84**, 731–736.

Stephens, R., Spurgeon, A., Beach, J., Calvert, I., Berry, H., Levy, L., and Harrington, J. M. (1995a). "An Investigation into the Possible Chronic Neuropsychological and Neurological Effects of Occupational Exposure to Organophosphates in Sheep Farmers." Contract Research Report 74/1995, Health & Safety Executive, Sheffield, UK.

Stephens, R., Spurgeon, A., Calvert, I. A., Beach, J., Levy, L. S., Berry, H., and Harrington, J. M. (1995b). Neuropsychological effects of long term exposure to organophosphates in sheep dip. *Lancet* **345**, 1135–1139.

Stephens, R., Spurgeon, A., and Berry, H. (1996). Organophosphates: The relationship between chronic and acute exposure effects. *Neurotoxicol. Teratol.* **18**, 449–453.

Sterri, S. H., Rognerud, B., Fiskum, S. E., and Lyngaas, S. (1979). Effects of toxogonin and P2S on the toxicity of carbamates and organophosphorus compounds. *Acta Pharmacol. Toxicol.* **45**, 9–15.

Stokes, L., Stark, A., Marshall, E., and Narang, A. (1995). Neurotoxicity among pesticide applicators exposed to organophosphates. *Occup. Environ. Med.* **52**, 648–653.

Stoller, A., Krupinski, J., Christophers, A. J., and Blanks, G. K. (1965). Organophosphorus insecticides and major mental illness. An epidemiological investigation. *Lancet* **i**, 1387–1388.

St. Omer, V. E. V., and Rottinghaus, G. E. (1992). Biochemical determination of cholinesterase activity in biological fluids and tissues. *In* "Clinical & Experimental Toxicology of Organophosphates and Carbamates" (B. Ballantyne and T. C. Marrs, eds.), pp. 15–27. Butterworth–Heinemann, Oxford.

Su, M.-Q., Kinoshita, F. K., Frawley, J. P., and DuBois, K. P. (1971). Comparative inhibition of aliesterases and cholinesterase in rats fed eighteen organophosphorus insecticides. *Toxicol. Appl. Pharmacol.* **20**, 241–249.

Summers, W. K., Majovski, L. V., Marsh, G. M., Tachiki, K., and Kling, A. (1986). Oral tetrahydroaminoacridine in long-term treatment of senile dementia, Alzheimer type. *N. Engl. J. Med.* **315**, 1241–1245.

Sundwall, A. (1960). Plasma concentration curves of P2S after intramuscular, intravenous and oral administration in man. *Biochem. Pharmacol.* **8**, 413–417.

Sundwall, A. (1961). Minimum concentrations of *N*-methylpyridinium-2-aldoxime methane sulphonate (P2S) which reverse neuromuscular block. *Biochem. Pharmacol.* **8**, 413–417.

Susser, M., and Stein, Z. (1957). An outbreak of tri-ortho-cresyl phosphate (T. O. C. P.) poisoning in Durban. *Br. J. Indust. Med.* **14**, 111–120.

Sussman, J. L., Harel, M., Frolow, F., Oefner, C., Goldman, A., Toker, L., and Silman, I. (1991). Atomic structure of acetylcholinesterase from *Torpedo californica*: A prototypic acetylcholine-binding protein. *Science* **253**, 872–879.

Suzuki, T., Morita, H., and Ono, K. (1995). Sarin poisoning in Tokyo subway. *Lancet* **345**, 980.

Tabershaw, I. R., and Cooper, W. C. (1966). Sequelae of acute organic phosphate poisoning. *J. Occup. Med.* **8**, 5–20.

Tafuri, J., and Roberts, J. (1987). Organophosphate poisoning. *Ann. Emerg. Med.* **16**, 193–202.

Tanaka, D., Jr., and Bursian, S. J. (1989). Degeneration patterns in the chicken central nervous system induced by ingestion of the organophosphorus delayed neurotoxin tri-*ortho*-tolyl phosphate. A silver impregnation study. *Brain Res.* **484**, 240–256.

Taylor, P. (1996a). Anticholinesterase agents. *In* "Goodman and Gilman's the Pharmacological Basis of Therapeutics" (J. G. Hardman and L. E. Limbird, eds.), 9th ed., pp. 161–176. McGraw–Hill, New York.

Taylor, P. (1996b). Agents acting at the neuromuscular junction and autonomic ganglia. *In* "Goodman and Gilman's the Pharmacological Basis of Therapeutics" (J. G. Hardman and L. E. Limbird, eds.), 9th ed., pp. 177–197. McGraw–Hill, New York.

Thompson, J. W., and Stocks, R. M. (1997). Brief bilateral vocal cord paralysis after insecticide poisoning. A new variant of toxcity syndrome. *Arch. Otolaryngol. Head Neck Surg.* **123**, 93–96.

Tomlin, C. D. S. (1997). "The Pesticide Manual," 11th ed. British Crop Protection Council, Surrey, UK.

Tosi, L., Righetti, C., Adami, L., and Zanette, G. (1994). October 1942: A strange epidemic paralysis in Saval, Verona, Italy. Revision and diagnosis 50 years later of tri-ortho-cresyl phosphate poisoning. *J. Neurol. Neurosurg. Psychiatry* **57**, 810–813.

Tracey, J. A., and Gallagher, H. (1990). Use of glycopyrrolate and atropine in acute organophosphorus poisoning. *Human Exp. Toxicol.* **9**, 99–100.

Tsao, T. C.-Y., Juang, Y.-C., Lan, R.-S., Shieh, W.-B., and Lee, C.-H. (1990). Respiratory failure of acute organophosphate carbamate poisoning. *Chest* **98**, 631–636.

Tsatsakis, A. M., Aguridakis, P., Michalodimitrakis, M. N., Tsakalov, A. K., Alegakis, A. K., Koumantakis, E., and Troulakis, G. (1996). Experiences with acute organophosphate poisonings in Crete. *Vet. Human Toxiciol.* **38**, 101–107.

Tush, G. M., and Amstead, M. I. (1997). Pralidoxime continuous infusion in the treatment of organophosphate poisoning. *Ann. Pharmacother.* **31**, 441–444.

Vale, J. A., and Scott, G. W. (1974). Organophosphorus poisoning. *Guy's Hosp. Rep.* **123**, 13–25.

Valero, A., and Golan, D. (1967). Accidental organic phosphorus poisoning: The use of propranolol to counteract vagolytic cardiac effects of atropine. *Isr. J. Med. Sci.* **3**, 582–584.

Vandekar, M. (1965). "Observations of the Toxicity of Two Organophosphorus and One Carbamate Insecticide in a Village Trial Performed by WHO Insecticide Testing Unit in Lagos During 1964", WHO Work. Doc. 65/Tox/2.64, U.S. Govt. Printing Office, Washington, DC.

Van Meter, W. G., Karczmar, A. G., and Fiscus, R. R. (1978). CNS effects of anticholinesterases in the presence of inhibited cholinesterases. *Arch. Int. Pharmacodyn.* **231**, 249–260.

Vasilescu, C. (1982). Neuropathy after organophosphorus compounds poisoning. *J. Neurol. Neurosurg. Psychiatry* **45**, 942.

Vasilescu, C., and Florescu, A. (1980). Clinical and electrophysiological study of neuropathy after organophosphorus compounds poisoning. *Arch. Toxicol.* **43**, 305–315.

Vasilescu, C., Alexianu, M., and Dan, A. (1984). Delayed neuropathy after organophosphorus insecticide (dipterex) poisoning: A clinical, electrophysiological and nerve biopsy study. *J. Neurol. Neurosurg. Psychiatry* **47**, 543–548.

Verberk, M. M., and Sallé, H. J. A. (1977). Effects of nervous function in volunteers ingesting mevinphos for one month. *Toxicol. Appl. Pharmacol.* **42**, 351–358.

Verpooten, G. A., and De Broe, M. E. (1984). Combined hemoperfusion–hemodialysis in severe poisoning: Kinetics of drug extraction. *Resuscitation* **11**, 275–289.

Wadia, R. S., Sadagopan, C., Amin, R. B., and Sardesai, H. V. (1974). Neurological manifestations of organophosphorus insecticide poisoning. *J. Neurol. Neurosurg. Psychiatry* **37**, 841–847.

Wadia, R. S., Shinde, S. N., and Vaidya, S. (1985). Delayed neurotoxicity after an episode of poisoning with dichlorvos. *Neurol. India* **33**, 247–253.

Wadia, R. S., Chitra, S., Amin, R. B., Kiwalkar, R. S., and Sardesai, H. V. (1987). Electrophysiological studies in acute organophosphate poisoning. *J. Neurol. Neurosurg. Psychiatry* **50**, 1442–1448.

Wang, A.-G., Liu, R.-S., Liu, J.-H., Teng, M. M.-H., and Yen, M. Y. (1999). Positron emission tomography scan in cortical visual loss in patients with organophosphate intoxication. *Ophthalmology* **106**, 1287–1291.

Wecker, L., Mrak, R. E., and Dettbarn, W. D. (1985). Evidence of necrosis in human intercostal muscle following inhalation of an organophosphate insecticide. *J. Environ. Pathol. Toxicol. Oncol.* **6**, 171–175.

Weeks, D. B., and Ford, D. (1989). Prolonged suxamethonium-induced neuromuscular block associated with organophophate poisoning. *Br. J. Anaesth.* **62**, 327.

Weir, S., Minton, N., and Murray, V. (1992). Organophosphate poisoning in the U.K.: The National Poisons Information Service experience during 1984–1987. *In* "Clinical & Experimental Toxicology of Organophosphates and Carbamates" (B. Ballantyne and T. C. Marrs, eds.), pp. 463–470. Butterworth–Heinemann, Oxford.

Weizman, Z., and Sofer, S. (1992). Acute pancreatitis in children with anticholinesterase insecticide intoxication. *Pediatrics* **90**, 204–206.

Whittaker, M. (1968). The pseudocholinesterase variants. Differentiation by means of sodium chloride. *Acta Genet.* **18**, 566–562.

WHO (1986). "Organophosphorus Insecticides: A General Introduction." Environmental Health Criteria 63, World Health Organization, Geneva.

WHO (1998). "The WHO Recommended Classification of Pesticides by Hazard and Guidelines to Classification 1998–1999." WHO/PCS/98.21, World Health Organization, Geneva.

Whorton, M. D., and Obrinsky, D. L. (1983). Persistence of symptoms after mild to moderate acute organophosphate poisoning among 19 farm field workers. *J. Toxicol. Environ. Health* **11**, 347–354.

Willems, J. L. (1981). Poisoning by organophosphate insecticide: Analysis of 53 human cases with regard to management and drug treatment. *Acta Med. Milit. (Belg)* **134**, 7–14.

Willems, J. L., and Belpaire, F. M. (1992). Anticholinesterase poisoning: An overview of pharmacotherapy. *In* "Clinical & Experimental Toxicology of Organophosphates and Carbamates" (B. Ballantyne and T. C. Marrs, eds.), pp. 536–544. Butterworth–Heinemann, Oxford.

Willems, J. L., Langenberg, J. P., Verstraete, A. G., De Loose, M., Vanhaesebroeck, B., Goethals, G., Belpaire, F. M., Buylaert, W. A., Vogelaers, D., and Colardyn, F. (1992). Plasma concentrations of pralidoxime methylsulphate in organophosphorus poisoned patients. *Arch. Toxicol.* **66**, 260–266.

Willems, J. L., De Bisschop, H. C., Verstraete, A. G., Declerck, C., Christiaens, Y., Vanscheeuwyck, P., Buylaert, W. A., Vogelaers, D., and Colardyn, F. (1993). Cholinesterase reactivation in organophosphorus poisoned patients depends on the plasma concentrations of the oxime pralidoxime methylsulphate and of the organophosphate. *Arch. Toxicol.* **67**, 79–84.

Wilson, B. W., Padilla, S., Henderson, J. D., Brimijoin, S., Dass, P. D., Elliot, G., Jaeger, B., Lanz, D., Pearson, R., and Spies, R. (1996). Factors in standardizing automated cholinesterase assays. *J. Toxicol. Environ. Health* **48**, 187–195.

Worek, F., Kirchner, T., Bäcker, M., and Szinicz, L. (1996). Reactivation by various oximes of human erythrocyte acetylcholinesterase inhibited by different organophosphorus compounds. *Arch. Toxicol.* **70**, 497–503.

Worek, F., Eyer, P., and Szinicz, L. (1998a). Inhibition, reactivation and aging kinetics of cyclohexylmethylphosphonofluoridate-inhibited human cholinesterases. *Arch. Toxicol.* **72**, 580–587.

Worek, F., Widmann, R., Knopff, O., and Szinicz, L. (1998b). Reactivating potency of obidoxime, pralidoxime, HI 6 and HLö 7 in human erythrocyte acetylcholinesterase inhibited by highly toxic organophosphorus compounds. *Arch. Toxicol.* **72**, 237–243.

Worek, F., Diepold, C., and Eyer, P. (1999a). Dimethylphosphoryl-inhibited cholinesterases: Inhibition, reactivation, and aging kinetics. *Arch. Toxicol.* **73**, 7–14.

Worek, F., Mast, U., Kiderlen, D., Diepold, C., and Eyer, P. (1999b). Improved determination of acetylcholinesterase activity in human whole blood. *Clin. Chim. Acta* **288**, 73–90.

Xintaras, C., and Burg, J. R. (1980). Screening and prevention of human neurotoxic outbreaks: Issues and problems. *In* "Experimental and Clinical Neurotoxicology" (P. S. Spencer and H. H. Schaumburg, eds.), pp. 663–674. Williams & Wilkins, Baltimore.

Xintaras, C., Burg, J. R., Tanaka, S., Lee, S. T., Johnson, B. L., Cottrill, C. A., and Bender, J. (1978). "NIOSH Health Survey of Velsicol Pesticide Workers, Occupational Exposure to Leptophos and Other Chemicals. " DHEW (NIOSH) Publication 78–136, U.S. Govt. Printing Office, Washington, DC.

Xue, S. Z. (1992). Acute anticholinesterase poisoning in China. *In* "Clinical & Experimental Toxicology of Organophosphates and Carbamates" (B. Ballantyne and T. C. Marrs, eds.), pp. 502–510. Butterworth–Heinemann, Oxford.

Yilmazalar, A., and Özyurt, G. (1997). Brain involvement in organophosphate poisoning. *Environ. Res.* **74**, 104–109.

Yokoyama, K., Ogura, Y., Kishimoto, M., Hinoshita, F., Hara, S., Yamada, A., Mimura, N., Seki, A., and Sakai, O. (1995). Blood purification for severe sarin poisoning after the Tokyo subway attack. *JAMA* **274**, 379.

Yoshida, M., Shimada, E., Yamanaka, S., Aoyama, H., Yamamura, Y., and Owada, S. (1987). A case of acute poisoning with fenitrothion (sumithion). *Human Toxicol.* **6**, 403–406.

Zadik, Z., Blachar, Y., Barak, Y., and Levin, S. (1983). Organophosphate poisoning presenting as diabetic ketoacidosis. *J. Toxicol.-Clin. Toxicol.* **20**, 381–385.

Zoppellari, R., Borron, S. W., Chieregato, A., Targa, L., Scaroni, I., and Zatelli, R. (1997). Isofenphos poisoning: Prolonged intoxication after intramuscular injection. *Clin. Toxicol.* **35**, 401–404.

Zwiener, R. J., and Ginsburg, C. M. (1988). Organophosphate and carbamate poisoning in infants and children. *Pediatrics* **81**, 121–126.

Carbamate Insecticides

Donald J. Ecobichon
Queen's University

52.1 INTRODUCTION

Early testing of the natural carbamate, physostigmine (eserine) from the calabar bean (*Physostigma venenosum*) and the synthetic derivative, neostigmine, revealed that these highly polar compounds possessed no insecticidal activity. Aliphatic esters of carbamic acid were synthesized in the early 1930s and, while showing herbicidal and fungicidal activities, were not insecticidal. These agents will be discussed in other chapters (Chapter 66 for herbicides and Chapter 77 for fungicides). Interest in the carbamates was not renewed until the mid-1950s when there was a search for insecticides having anticholinesterase activity, more selectivity, and less mammalian toxicity than some of the organophosphorus esters then in use. This led to the synthesis of several potent aryl esters of methyl carbamic acid, these agents becoming the insecticides of the 1960s and 1970s. While a large number of carbamates have been synthesized, relatively few were developed further, the pesticide market being limited to less than 20 agents. The early history of carbamate insecticide development has been discussed by Kuhr and Dorough (1976) and Cremlyn (1978).

52.2 NOMENCLATURE

As is shown in Fig. 52.1, the structure of all carbamate insecticides is based on carbamic acid (the monoamide of carbon dioxide), a highly unstable compound decomposing into carbon dioxide and ammonia. Carbamic acid may be stabilized by forming salts such as ammonium carbamate or by synthesizing alkyl or aryl esters. Replacement of one hydrogen associated with the nitrogen by a methyl group results in the formation of N-monomethylcarbamic acid which, when combined with an aryl ester substituent, results in significant alterations in various physicochemical properties and introduces insecticidal activity (e.g., bendiocarb, carbaryl, propoxur). An additional group of carbamate insecticides are derivatives of aliphatic oximes rather than esters, resembling aldehydes or ketones, known collectively as methylcarbamoyloximes, and possessing a high degree of toxicity (e.g., aldicarb and methomyl).

The majority of the carbamate insecticides in use are N-monomethyl carbamates, frequently referred to as N-methylcarbamates or just methylcarbamates. In this chapter, the insecticides will be referred to by the name commonly used in the literature, thereby simplifying discussion. Table 52.1 lists the methylcarbamates currently used in pest control with their chemical names and chemical structures (Baron, 1991).

52.3 CHEMISTRY

The nature of the substituent groups alters both the physicochemical properties of the insecticide and the biological activity. Most of these insecticides dissolve readily in organic solvents but are only slightly soluble in water, thereby conferring varying degrees of lipid solubility. The exceptions are the methylcarbamoyloximes, the "oxime" carbamates aldicarb and methomyl, which are highly water soluble. A wide range of melting points (50 to 150°C) is found for these agents, determined largely by the size of the substituent group. Vapor pressures range from less than 5×10^{-6} to 5×10^{-2} mmHg (Melnikov, 1971). While high melting points and low vapor pressures enhance the environmental stability of the compound, decomposition can be markedly enhanced by increased temperatures, a 10°C increase raising the hydrolysis rate two- to three-fold (Aly and El-Dib, 1971; Fukuto *et al.*, 1967). The environmental stability of carbamates is severely affected by photodegradation at short ultraviolet wavelengths (254 nm) and by oxidation upon exposure to air. These aspects of decomposition are discussed succinctly by Kuhr and Dorough (1976).

Alkyl esters tend to be relatively unstable in the environment, in contrast to aryl esters. Stability can be enhanced by attaching additional substituents either to the aryl structure or to the carbamoylated nitrogen. While carbamates decompose slowly in water at an acidic pH, alkalinity enhances degradation since the substituent groups tend to draw electrons from around the ester linkage, thereby weakening it and accelerating the hydrolysis by hydroxide ions. Considering some of the structurally different agents shown in Table 52.1, incubation in an alkaline solution (0.01 M sodium barbital buffer, pH 9.3)

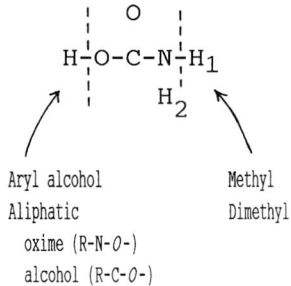

Figure 52.1 The basic structure of carbamic acid, the monoamide of carbon dioxide, shoving the positions of substituant methyl, aryl, or aliphatic groups to produce methylcarbamate insecticides.

resulted in the determination of biological half-lives for methiocarb, carbaryl, mexacarbate, and propoxur of 0.4, 0.5, 2.3, and 3.1 hours, respectively (Abdel-Wahab *et al.*, 1966). Mono- or dimethylation of the carbamoyl nitrogen results in stabilization of the ester bond. N-monomethylcarbamates degrade slowly in the environment; for example, carbaryl at pH 7.0 has a half-life of 10 days. Dimethylcarbamates are exceedingly stable, the half-life of dimetilan (1-dimethyl-carbamoyl-5-methylpyrazol-3-yl dimethylcarbamate) being approximately 100 days at pH ranging from 6 to 10 (Kuhr and Dorough, 1976).

In addition to the direct-acting, anticholinesterase methylcarbamates, certain derivative agents such as benfuracarb, carbosulfan, mecarbam, and thiodicarb, known as procarbamates, have insecticidal activity but low mammalian toxicity until they are biotransformed to release biologically active agents or to yield nontoxic, readily excreted products. Fukuto (1983) showed that substitution of the remaining hydrogen on the carbamyl nitrogen of methylcarbamates reduced the mammalian toxicity due to slower conversion of the derivative to the original toxic insecticide. For example, carbosulfan and thiocarb are sulfide derivatives of carbofuran and methomyl, respectively.

Most of the carbamate ester insecticides have low vapor pressures, which results in poor volatility at usual temperatures (Fig. 52.2). However, as is shown for aldicarb, oxamyl, and pirimicarb, increasing the temperature can markedly alter the vapor pressure, a factor that must be considered when using these agents in tropical countries. If other carbamate esters behave in the same manner, many would become highly volatile in climates having high temperatures. The propoxur toxicity incident in southern Nigeria, discussed by Vandekar (1965), is an example in point. Propoxur has a vapor pressure of 6.5×10^{-6} mmHg at 20°C; spraying huts and roofs at ambient temperatures of 70°C (140°F) caused acute toxicity among spraymen who wore some protective equipment. The effects were considered to be due to revolatilized propoxur from surfaces rather than from the suspended spray aerosol.

Most of the carbamates in commercial use have relatively low water solubility (Table 52.2), a high level of solubility in polar solvents (ethanol, isopropanol, methanol, acetone), and limited-to-moderate solubility in nonpolar solvents (benzene, toluene, xylenes). This lipophilicity enhances the insec-

ticidal potency, the agents readily penetrating insect cuticles and tissues, but it also presents problems of oral and/or dermal absorption in other animal species, and enhanced storage in tissues. There are, however, exceptions, the high water solubility of some carbamates playing important roles in absorption, distribution (both *in vivo* and environmental), storage, and elimination, as well as governing the regulation of use. Example: note the degree of water solubility of the "oxime" carbamates, aldicarb, methomyl, oxamyl (Table 52.2). These agents are restricted for use on crops with a low water content. There has been illegal use of aldicarb resulting in consumer poisonings from melons and hydroponically grown cucumbers and widespread contamination of groundwater and community drinking water (Fiore *et al.*, 1986; Goes *et al.*, 1980; Goldman *et al.*, 1990a, 1990b; Zaki *et al.*, 1982).

52.4 TOXICOKINETICS

52.4.1 ABSORPTION

The most likely route of exposure to carbamates is via the skin in an occupational setting. The lipophilicity of this class of agents and the fact that most formulations contain organic solvents and emulsifiers insure a rapid dermal penetration and absorption into the systemic circulation. Temperature and humidity play important roles; high temperature and relative humidity enhance absorption, environmental conditions being reflected in less clothing being worn, greater areas of skin being exposed, and greater subdermal vasodilatation and perspiration, all resulting in a more complete absorption.

Carbamates are readily absorbed in the gastrointestinal tract, the efficiency of absorption being somewhat guided by the vehicle(s) in which they are administered or are formulated. Exposure to low levels of carbamate residues in fresh fruits and vegetables may occur where regulatory tolerances have been established for food crop use. Residues in edible foods may be less efficiently absorbed, being trapped or bound in the food bolus.

Under certain circumstances, inhalation may be an important route of exposure. The vapor pressures of some carbamates (Fig. 52.2) make them vulnerable to rapid revolatilization when applied under climatic conditions of high temperature in excess of 60–70°C. The previously mentioned accidental poisonings by propoxur in southern Nigeria are a case in point (Vandekar, 1965). The spraymen, applying a 5.0% suspension of propoxur on hut walls and roofs, had to terminate the operation within 2 to 3 hours when severe symptoms of toxicity were observed due to revolatilized agent rather than to the spray aerosol. Similar conditions would be encountered in greenhouses and mushroom barns, areas of high temperature and high humidity. These conditions alter the behavior of aerosols, the change being primarily to keep them suspended in air for long periods of time.

Table 52.1
Structure, Common Names, and Chemical Names of Carbamate Insecticides

Agent	CAS number	Structure	IUPAC chemical name
Aldicarb TEMIK™	CAS 116-06-3	MeS.C.CH:N.O.CO.NHMe (with Me groups)	2-methyl-2-(methylthio)pro-pionaldehyde O-methyl-carbamoyloxime
Bendiocarb FICAM™ ROTATE™	CAS 22781-23-3		2,2-dimethyl-1,3-benzodioxol-4-yl methylcarbamate
Carbaryl SEVIN™	CAS 63-25-2	O.CO.NHMe	1-naphthyl methylcarbamate
Carbofuran FURADAN™	CAS 1563-66-2	MeNHCO.O	2,3-dihydro-2,2-dimethyl-7-benzofuranyl methylcarbamate
Carbosulfan ADVANTAGE™ MARSHAL™	CAS 55285-14-8	$(CH_3-CH_2-CH_2-CH_2-)_2-N$	2,3-dihydro-2,3-dimethyl-7-benzofuranyl((dibutyl-amino)thio) methylcarbamate
Formetanate HCl CARZOL™ DICARZOL™	CAS 23422-53-9 HCl	$N:CH.NMe_2$ O.CO.NHMe	3-dimethylaminomethylene-aminophenyl methylcarbamate hydrochloride
Methiocarb MESUROL™	CAS 2032-65-7	MeS, OCNHMe	4-methylthio-3,5-xylyl methylcarbamate
Methomyl LANNATE™	CAS 16752-77-5	MeS C=N-OCNHMe	S-methyl N-(methylcarbamoyl-oxy) thioacetimidate
Mexacarbate ZECTRAN	CAS 315-18-4	Me_2N OCNHMe	3,5-dimethyl-4-(dimethyl-amino)phenyl methylcarbamate
Oxamyl VYDATE™	CAS 23135-22-0	$Me_2N.C.C=N.O.C.NHMe$ SMe	N,N-dimethyl-2-methylcar-bamoyloxyimino-2-(methyl-thio)acetamide
Pirimicarb ABOL™ APHOX™	CAS 23103-98-2	$O.C.NMe_2$ NMe_2	2-dimethylamino-5,6-dimethyl-pyrimidin-4-yl dimethyl-carbamate

(*continues*)

Table 52.1

(*continued*)

Agent	CAS number	Structure	IUPAC chemical name
Propoxur BAYGON™	CAS 114-26-1		2-isopropoxyphenyl methyl- carbamate
Thiodicarb LARVIN™	CAS 59669-26-0		Dimethyl N,N-(thiobis(methyl- imino)carbonyloxy)-bis- (ethanimidothioate)

52.4.2 BIOTRANSFORMATION

A number of excellent reviews consider the biotransformation of carbamate insecticides, including those of Knaak (1971), Ryan (1971), Fukuto (1972), Kuhr and Dorough (1976), Wilkinson (1976), Kulkarni and Hodgson (1980), and the IPCS (1986). The initial response of any species exposed to a carbamate ester is to convert the chemical into more polar forms for ready excretion via the urine. To achieve this, the organism calls upon Phase I and Phase II detoxification mechanisms in tissues to create water-soluble, easily excreted, and less toxic by-products. While these insecticidal esters are suscep-

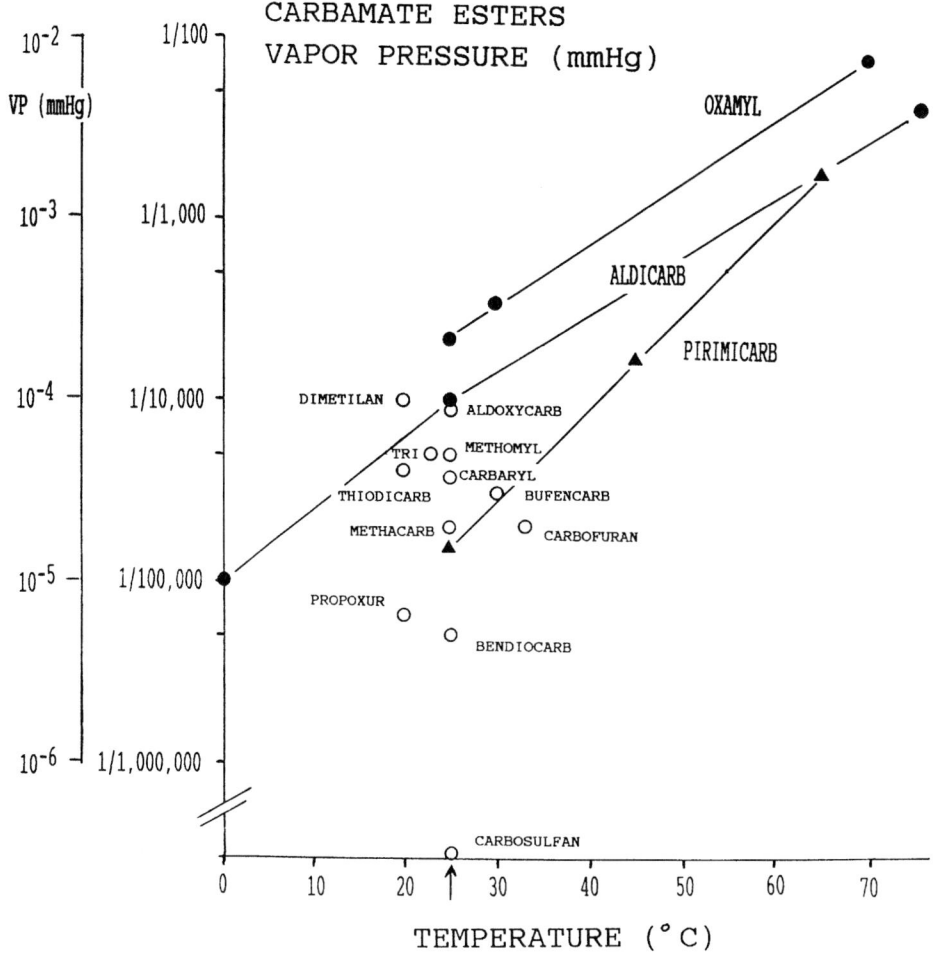

Figure 52.2   The vapor pressures of carbamate insecticides determined at 20°C, 25°C, or 30°, with examples of altered vapor pressures at elevated temperatures as might be encountered in tropical countries.

Table 52.2
Relative Water Solubility of Carbamate Ester Insecticides[a,b]

Agent	Solubility (g/L)
Aldicarb	6.0
Bendiocarb	0.04
Carbaryl	0.7
Carbofuran	0.7
Carbosulfan	0.0003
Formetanate HCl	>500
Methiocarb	0.01
Methomyl	58
Mexacarbate	0.1
Oxamyl	280
Pirimicarb	2.75
Propoxur	2.0
Thiodicarb	0.035

[a] Data from Baron (1991) and the Merck Index, 12th edition (1996).
[b] Measured at 20–25°C.

tible to a variety of enzyme-catalyzed detoxification reactions, the principal biotransformation pathways involve oxidation and hydrolysis, with conjugation of some of the cleaved products (Ecobichon, 1994a). The nature and position of the substituent groups on the ether oxygen or the nitrogen exert an important role over the rate and pathway of biotransformation.

Being esters, carbamate insecticides are susceptible to hydrolysis by nonspecific carboxylesterases ubiquitously distributed throughout the tissues of species from insects to humans. The products formed are identical to many of those produced by chemical (alkali, water) hydrolysis in that an aryl alcohol plus methyl- or dimethyl-carbamic acid will be formed. The unstable methylated carbamic acids will rapidly decompose into carbon dioxide and mono- or dimethylamine. Rates of hydrolysis in vivo are governed by the molecular structure of the agent, the specificity or selectivity of the carboxylesterases for particular agents, and interspecies differences. Carbamate esters are actually poor substrates for many tissue esterases. The hydrolysis of the various carbamate esters is highly individualistic, only a certain percent hydrolysis occurring with different agents (Schlagbauer and Schlagbauer, 1972). A generalization that carbamates can be hydrolyzed by tissue enzymes requires rigorous testing with several carbamates as substrates.

The ubiquitous distribution of the reactive hemoprotein, cytochrome P-450, and the various isoenzymatic forms in tissues of all life forms, point to a commitment to the oxidative detoxification of a broad spectrum of both endogenous and exogenous chemicals as a protective measure. These hemoprotein isoenzymes, in conjunction with molecular oxygen, flavoproteins, cytochrome-b$_5$ and reduced nicotinamide adenine dinucleotide phosphate (NADPH), can initiate a variety of enzymatic oxidative/reductive reactions depending upon the nature of the substituent groups on the carbamate ester. Oxidative reactions can be simplified into two groups: (1) oxidation of appropriate side chains, for example, hydroxylation of N-methyl groups

and/or hydroxylation of methyl substituents on aryl moieties to form hydroxymethyl groups, N-demethylation of secondary amines attached to the aryl moiety; and (2) ring hydroxylation through the formation of an epoxide intermediate. In addition, thiocarbamates may undergo S-oxidation by these same oxidative mechanisms; for example, aldicarb can be converted into a sulfoxide and/or a sulfone, depending upon the species being studied.

In conjugative or Phase II detoxification reactions, a functional group on the molecule, introduced as a consequence of hydrolytic or oxidative biotransformation, is enzymatically reacted with an endogenous substance in the tissues of the life form to produce water-soluble, biologically inactive, and readily excreted products. Depending upon the species of plant or animal being studied, a variety of products may be formed but, in general, the products may be classified as sulfates, glucuronides, glucosides, amino acid conjugates, acetylated amines, or glutathione conjugates, the last being excreted as mercapturic acid derivatives. In mammalian species, the cleaved aryl substituent(s) are conjugated to produce sulfates, glucuronides, and mercapturates.

Biotransformation/degradation in aquatic systems, plants, and by microorganisms has been reviewed (IPCS, 1986). Hydrolysis of the carbamate ester bond is the major degradation pathway in soils. In plants, oxidative processes result in ring hydroxylation followed by conjugation with either amino acids (cysteine), phosphates, or sugars to form glycosides. Hydrolysis can occur in some plant species.

52.4.3 ELIMINATION

There is little evidence of extensive carbamate bioaccumulation since biotransformation is relatively rapid. There is at least one report of persistent toxicity in a human intoxication, the signs and symptoms disappearing slowly when the afflicted individual was removed from the source (Branch and Jacqz, 1986a). However, this effect might have been related to slow recovery from agent-induced neuropathy, or altered metabolism, rather than the clearance of any body burden.

Excretion of the water-soluble by-products of detoxification occurs relatively rapidly via the urine and/or feces in most vertebrate species. Glucuronide and sulfate derivatives of the aryl substituents are the major products found in the urine. Small amounts of the parent carbamate may be excreted in the urine. Mercapturates are usually found in mammalian feces if they are not broken down in the intestinal tract, reabsorbed systemically, and recycled to form other products to be excreted in the urine.

52.5 MECHANISM

Like the organophosphorus ester insecticides, the carbamates elicit toxicity by inhibiting nervous tissue acetylcholinesterase (AChE). However, it is a transient, reversible inhibition, since there is a relatively rapid reactivation of the enzyme in the

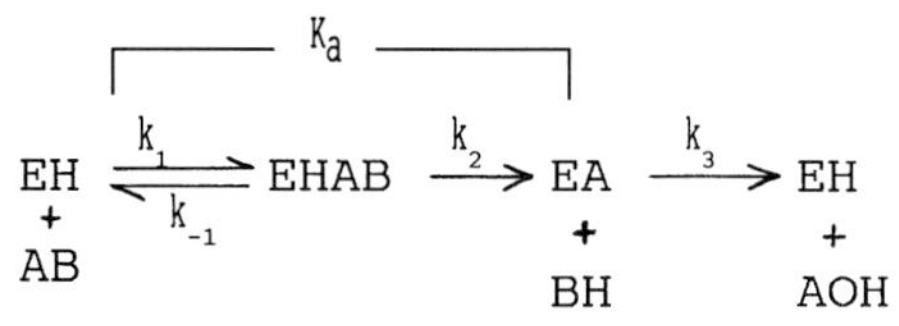

$$EH + AB \xrightleftharpoons[k_{-1}]{k_1} EHAB \xrightarrow{k_2} EA + BH \xrightarrow{k_3} EH + AOH$$

with K_a spanning from EH to EA.

Figure 52.3 A schematic diagram showing the mechanism of interaction between a methylcarbamate insecticide (AB) and acetylcholinesterase (EH), depicting the unstable intermediate complex (EHAB), the carbambylated enzyme (EA), the leaving group (BH), and the spontaneously decarbamoylated enzyme (EH) and the released methylcarbamic acid (AOH).

Table 52.3

Kinetic Rates of Inhibition of Cholinesteerases By Carbamate and Organophosphorus Esters

Parameter	Kinetic constants[a]	Organophosphorus	Carbamate
		Reaction rates	
Complex Formation	k_{-1}/k_1	Rapid (high affinity)	Rapid (high affinity)
Inhibition Rate	k_2	Rapid to moderately rapid	Variable
Reactivation Rate	k_3	Slow to extremely slow	Relatively rapid

[a] See Fig. 52.3.

presence of "tissue" water. The biological effects of the accumulating acetylcholine (ACh) tend to be of short duration, in terms of hours rather than in days to weeks as is seen with organophosphorus esters.

As is shown in Fig. 52.3, a reversible carbamate-AChE complex (EHAB) is formed, followed by the hydrolysis of the ester bond and the loss of the aryl or alkyl substituent (BH), the result being a carbamylated enzyme (EA) which is unstable and hydrolyzes in the presence of water to release free and active enzyme (EH) (Ecobichon, 1996). The differences between organophosphorus and carbamate ester inhibitors lie in the rate constants for the various steps in the reaction(s) (Table 52.3). Both classes of insecticides have high affinity constants ($K_a = k_{-1}/k_1$) for the active center of the enzyme, the interaction with the enzyme (EHAB) being almost instantaneous (Hastings *et al.*, 1970; Reiner, 1971). The rate of carbamylation of the enzyme depends largely on molecular complementarity and reactivity, the latter depending on the nature of the leaving group, for example, phenolic and oxime substituents being somewhat better than benzyl alcohols. While carbamylation appears to be reversible from the point of view of the enzyme, it is not reversible from the point of view of the carbamate which is cleaved and loses anticholinesterase potency in the process (Baron, 1991). Thus, the carbamylation constant, K_2, will vary considerably between carbamate esters. Acetylcholinesterase inhibition varies in degree with the rate of the EHAB-to-EA complex formation and the relative K_a of each compound. The decarbamylation constant, K_3, would be the same for all N-methylcarbamates, the moiety (A) adhering to the enzyme being identical in all cases, with aqueous hydrolysis at the same rate resulting in the formation of free, uninhibited enzyme (EH). By contrast, the phosphorylation of AChE is regulated by (1) the electron-withdrawing power of the "leaving" substituent, which is highly variable between chemicals; and (2) the nature of the alkyl (methyl, ethyl, isopropyl, methylamido, ethylamido, etc.) substituents on the ester. The rate of reactivation of AChE is governed by the rate constants, K_2 and K_3, frequently quite different from those for carbamate esters (Table 52.2). The phosphorylated enzyme can be quite stable, aqueous hydrolysis being very slow in many cases.

The degree of inhibition of nervous tissue AChE and/or plasma pseudocholinesterase (PChE) by carbamates is variable, being dependent upon the specificity of the agent for the active site of the enzyme, the rate constants for complex formation,

spontaneous reversal of the complex, the carbamylation of the enzymes, and the decarbamylation stage. Carbamate variability is reflected in the relative rate(s) of recovery of AChE and PChE and the level of exposure. In mild-to-moderate cases of intoxication, carbamates may have little effect on PChE while severely inhibiting the AChE (both erythrocytic and nervous tissue). In severe intoxications, both PChE and AChE will be markedly inhibited. As an example, in a case of a suicidal attempt with a propoxur formulation, the blood sample taken within an hour of visiting the emergency room revealed no activity of either erythrocytic AChE or PChE, but the sample taken 6 hr later showed 60% inhibition of erythrocytic AChE and no residual inhibition of PChE (Ecobichon, unpublished).

The transient nature of carbamate-induced inhibition of AChE poses several problems in the attempt to measure the level of inhibition. Care must be taken to keep blood and tissue samples cold or frozen during transportation to the laboratory prior to analysis. For example, blood samples should be kept on ice, centrifuged under refrigerated conditions to recover both the plasma and the erythrocyte fractions, and frozen at $-20°C$ immediately until assayed. Spontaneous reversal of the inhibition is rapid and can be accelerated by (1) the time interval between sampling and analysis; (2) the dilution of the sample; (3) the addition of substrate, usually acetylcholine at high concentration, which competes successfully for the enzymatic active site in either of the EHAB and EA complexes; and (4) the duration of the assay time. Laboratory assays of cholinesterase inhibition must be very rapid (less than 3 minutes), and must employ minimal dilution and minimal amounts of substrate. Modifications can be made to the colorimetric assay of Ellman *et al.* (1961) to meet the restrictive criteria mentioned above.

It is fallacious to measure cholinesterase activities in biological fluids and tissues collected in subchronic and chronic exposure studies 24 hours after the last exposure. Such assays should be done immediately following the last treatment since, as was seen in the case of acute aminocarb (4-dimethylamino-m-tolyl methylcarbamate) toxicity in rats, recovery of the vital cholinesterases was complete by 6 hours post-treatment (Vassilieff and Ecobichon, 1983). Little or no inhibition would be observed if the activities were measured 24 hours following the last exposure.

Table 52.4
Signs and Symptoms of Anticholinesterase Insecticide Poisoning

Nervous tissue and receptors affected	Site affected	Manifestations
Parasympathetic autonomic (muscarinic receptors) postganglionic nerve fibers	Exocrine glands	Increased salivation, lacrimation, perspiration
	Eyes	Miosis (pinpoint and nonreactive), ptosis, blurring of vision, conjunctival injection, "bloody tears"
	Gastrointestinal tract	Nausea, vomiting, abdominal tightness, swelling and cramps, diarrhea, tenesmus, fecal incontinence
	Respiratory tract	Excessive bronchial secretions, rhinorrhea, wheezing, edema, tightness in chest, bronchospasms, bronchoconstriction, cough, bradypnea, dyspnea
	Cardiovascular system	Bradycardia, decrease in blood pressure
	Bladder	Urinary frequency and incontinence
Parasympathetic and sympathetic autonomic fibers (nicotinic receptors)	Cardiovascular system	Tachycardia, pallor, increase in blood pressure
Somatic motor nerve fibers (nicotinic receptors)	Skeletal muscles	Muscle fasciculations (eyelids, fine facial muscles), cramps, diminished tendon reflexes, generalized muscle weakness in peripheral and respiratory muscles, paralysis, flaccid or rigid tone
		Restlessness, generalized motor activity, reaction to acoustic stimuli, tremulousness, emotional lability, ataxia
Brain (acetylcholine receptors)	Central nervous system	Drowsiness, lethargy, fatigue, mental confusion, inability to concentrate, headache, pressure in head, generalized weakness
		Coma with absence of reflexes, tremors, Cheyne–Stokes respiration, dyspnea, convulsions, depression of respiratory centers, cyanosis

Source: From Ecobichon and Joy (1982).

The toxicity of carbamates in mammals can be predicted *in vitro* by the degree to which they inhibit AChE activity, and *in vivo* by the severity of the clinical manifestations (Feldman, 1999).

52.6 TOXICOLOGY

52.6.1 MODE OF ACTION

The insecticidal carbamates, like organophosphorus esters, exert their effects by inhibiting nervous tissue AChE found in the synaptic spaces and on the postsynaptic membranes of all neurons, using acetylcholine as a chemical neurotransmitter. The role of this enzyme is to terminate, by hydrolysis, the biological actions of the neurotransmitter, thereby restoring the acetylcholine receptors to a state where they can receive the next chemical stimulus. With the loss of this regulating mechanism, the accumulating, nondetoxified acetylcholine (ACh) continues to stimulate specific receptor types, eliciting a spectrum of characteristic clinical signs and symptoms of intoxication (Cranmer, 1986; Ecobichon, 1994b, 1996). Due to the transient nature of carbamate-inhibited nervous tissue AChE, acute intoxication by carbamates is generally resolved within a few hours. Depending upon the level of exposure, the clinical signs and symptoms may appear quite rapidly, be of mild-to-severe intensity, but last for a relatively short duration, disappearing within six hours.

Acetylcholine is an important neurotransmitter at parasympathomimetic, postganglionic nerve endings that are not under voluntary control (autonomic pathways) and which include the exocrine glands, the eyes, the gastrointestinal tract, the respiratory tract secretions, the cardiovascular system, and the bladder (Ecobichon, 1994b). Such neuronal junctions are stimulated specifically by the chemical muscarine and are blocked by atropine, an agent used in treating intoxications to alleviate what are called muscarinic effects, which frequently appear early in any carbamate intoxication.

Acetylcholine is also a neurotransmitter at the interneuron ganglia of both the parasympathomimetic and the sympathomimetic divisions of the autonomic nervous system, the major effects seen being a stimulation of the ganglia of sympathetic, adrenergic neurons and the adrenal medulla (releasing epinephrine), with observed clinical signs in the cardiovascular system (tachycardia, vasoconstriction) resulting in increased heart rate and blood pressure and pallor. These neuronal junctions are also stimulated by nicotine, giving rise to the term nicotinic receptors.

Acetylcholine stimulates skeletal neuromuscular junctions under voluntary control (the somatic nervous system), these neuromuscular receptors characteristically being stimulated by nicotine and blocked by the agents d-tubocurarine and succinyldicholine. These receptors are known as nicotinic receptors. Overstimulation of such receptors by acetylcholine causes generalized increased motor activity with muscle fasciculations. An excess of neurotransmitter may lead to receptor blockade, the evident clinical signs being skeletal muscle paralysis and/or generalized muscle weakness, as well as respiratory distress due to paralysis of the diaphragmatic and intercostal muscles (Ecobichon, 1996).

Acetylcholine has important roles in the central nervous system, cholinergic brain receptors being both muscarinic and nicotinic in nature. The respiratory center is cholinergic in nature, controls the respiratory rate (overstimulation causes blockade, respiration is impaired or stops), and responds to atropine treatment. Convulsions are elicited through centrally located neurons, and a host of other effects (disorientation, anxiety, memory loss, drowsiness, lethargy, fatigue, general malaise) appear to have central origins.

The acronym "MUDDLES" (i.e., **m**iosis, **u**rination, **d**iarrhea, **d**iaphoresis, **l**acrimation, **e**xcitation of the CNS, **s**alivation) is an accurate description of the principal effects of AChE inhibition (O'Malley, 1997). A detailed listing of clinical signs and symptoms observed in animals and humans is presented in Table 52.4 (Ecobichon, 1996). The appearance of none, some, or all of the symptomatology is largely dependent upon the compound and the level of exposure (Cranmer, 1986; Vandekar, 1965; Vassilieff and Ecobichon, 1983). The rate(s) of recovery will be dependent upon the rate(s) of biotransformation and excretion of the particular chemical, most intoxications being brief but with some signs, particularly in humans, persisting for weeks after exposure. The persistent peripheral- and central-mediated symptoms will be addressed in a later section.

The acute toxicity of different carbamate insecticides correlates well with their anticholinesterase activity, particularly with the inhibition of erythrocytic AChE (Vandekar et al., 1971; Vassilieff and Ecobichon, 1983). Intoxications showing obvious cholinergic signs of toxicity may be accompanied by little or no inhibition of cholinesterase activity, this phenomenon being due to a number of assay problems: (1) the selection of the proper enzyme for assay, the plasma PChE being less sensitive to carbamates than the erythrocytic AChE; (2) the selection of an inappropriate substrate for the enzyme being assayed; (3) the ease with which the carbamoylated cholinesterase spontaneously reactivates following dilution, lysis in the case of erythrocytes, or addition of substrate, all factors related to the assay method being used; and (4) the interval between exposure and blood sampling, during which time the carbamate may be degraded or the inhibition may be reversed in vivo (Berry, 1971; Ecobichon and Comeau, 1973; Iverson, 1975; Reiner, 1971; Wilhelm and Reiner, 1973). Particular attention should be paid to the analytical method, which should incorporate minimum exposure-to-collection intervals, minimum dilution of sample, minimum assay time, minimum substrate concentration, and the appropriate pH.

52.6.2 ACUTE TOXICITY—ANIMAL

One index of acute toxicity is reflected by an LD_{50} value determined in suitable animal species, the agent being administered

Table 52.5
Acute Oral Toxicity of Carbamate Insecticides (Technical)[a]

Chemical	Species	Sex	LD_{50} (mg/kg)[b]
Aldicarb	rat	both	0.46–1.23
	mouse	both	0.38–1.50
	rabbit	?	1.3
	guinea pig	?	1.0
Bendiocarb	rat	both	34–156
		M	138
		both	350–657
	mouse	both	28–45
		M	175
		both	173–380
	rabbit	both	35–40
	guinea pig	F	35
	dog	both	ca. 300
Carbaryl	rat	both	233–850
	mouse	both	108–650
	rabbit	?	710
	guinea pig	?	280
	dog	?	250–795
	cat	?	125–250
	swine	?	1500–2000
	monkey		>1000
Carbofuran	rat	M	5.3–13.2
	mouse	?	2.0
	dog	?	19
Carbosulfan	rat	both	90–250
	mouse	both	33–124
	rabbit	both	37–53
Formetanate HCl	rat	both	15–26
	mouse	both	13–25
	dog	both	19
Methiocarb	rat	both	13–135
	guinea pig	both	14–100
	dog	both	10–25
Methomyl	rat	both	12–48
Mexacarbate	rat	both	8.5–12.0
Oxamyl	rat	both	2.5–16.0
	mouse	both	2.3–3.3
	guinea pig	M	7.1
Pirimicarb	rat	F	68–221
	mouse	F	107
	dog	both	100–200
Propoxur	rat	both	80–191
	mouse	both	37–109
	guinea pig	?	40
Thiodicarb	rat	both	39–136
	mouse	both	226
	guinea pig	M	160
	rabbit	both	556
	monkey	both	467.2

[a] Data modified from Baron (1991).
[b] Values determined using different vehicles.

Table 52.6
Acute Dermal Toxicity of Carbamate Insecticides (Technical)[a]

Chemical	Species	Sex	LD$_{50}$ (mg/kg)[b]
Aldicarb	rat	both	3.2–>10
	rabbit	M	5.0–20
Bendiocarb	rat	both	566
Carbaryl	rat	both	>5000
Carbofuran	rat	both	>1000
	rabbit	both	>2000
Carbosulfan	rabbit	both	>2000
Formetanate HCl	rabbit	both	>10200
Methiocarb	rat	both	>300–>5000
	rabbit	both	>2000
Methomyl	rat	M	>1000–>2400
	rabbit	both	556–>1500
Mexacarbate	rabbit	both	>2000
Oxamyl	rat	M	>1200
	rabbit	M	740
Pirimicarb	rat	F	>500
	rabbit	?	>500
Propoxur	rat	both	1000–>2400
	rabbit	M	>500
Thiodicarb	rat	M	2540
	rabbit	both	>6310

[a] Data modified from Baron (1991).
[b] Values determined using different vehicles.

via the route(s) by which humans are most likely to acquire the chemical (Ecobichon, 1996). To this end, for comparative purposes, Tables 52.5, 52.6, and 52.7 list the oral, dermal, and inhalation LD$_{50}$s of the carbamate ester insecticides of commercial interest, these tables being reproduced from the 1991 edition of Hayes' and Laws' *Handbook of Pesticide Toxicology* (Baron, 1991). The specific references for any particular LD$_{50}$ may be found in that text.

Table 52.7
Acute Inhalation Toxicity of Carbamate Insecticides (Technical)[a]

Chemical	Species	Sex	LD$_{50}$ (mg/L)[b]
Carbaryl	rat	?	0.005–0.023
Carbosulfan	rat	both	0.61–1.53
Formetanate HCl	rat	both	0.29–2.8
Methiocarb	rat	both	>0.322
Methomyl	rat	M	0.45
Oxamyl	rat	both	0.12–0.17
		M	0.064
Pirimicarb	rat	?	ca. 0.3
Propoxur	rat	M	>1.44
Thiodicarb	rat	both	0.116–0.22
		?	>0.20

[a] Data modified from Baron (1991).
[b] Values determined over different time intervals (1–6 hr).

The signs and symptoms of carbamate-induced, acute toxicity observed in various animal species should be comparable for the different insecticides, given that adequate, toxic doses have been administered. Considering carbaryl as a prototype carbamate ester of moderate toxicity, the following signs will be seen in mammals in approximate order of appearance, beginning some 15 to 30 minutes after oral administration: salivation, lacrimation, increased respiration with rales due to bronchial secretions, urination, defecation, and muscle fasciculations and tremors progressing to mild-to-moderate convulsions within 90 minutes of treatment. More severe intoxications may be characterized by pupillary constriction, profuse salivation, chromodacryorrhea, respiratory difficulty, loss of bladder and bowel control, muscular spasms and weakness, prostration, and incoordination. While most of the symptoms will disappear within 6 hours of exposure, a few, such as diarrhea, chromodacryorrhea, and muscle weakness, may persist beyond 24 hours posttreatment. Death is due to respiratory collapse if intoxication is severe.

A number of studies have examined the behavioral effects of anticholinesterase-type insecticides immediately following treatment. Carbaryl produces CNS depressant effects, making it obvious that ACh plays a significant role in memory, cognitive, and motor functions; many of the adverse effects are ameliorated by such cholinolytic agents as atropine or scopolamine (Kurtz, 1977; Takahashi *et al.*, 1991).

The acute administration of carbaryl (1.0, 3.0, 5.0, and 10 mg/kg) to rats resulted in a dose-related decrease in variable interval response rates in a learned procedure of pushing a lever to receive a food pellet (Anger and Wilson, 1980). The rate decreases were 55 to 77, 81 to 94, and 88 to 100 percent at 3.0, 5.0, and 10 mg/kg, depending upon the route (ip or im) of administration. In other acute experiments, both propoxur and carbaryl caused post-treatment reductions in motor activity (open field and figure eight mazes) in a dose-dependent manner (Ruppert *et al.*, 1983). However, maze activity recovered within 30 and 60 minutes, while the brain AChE activities remained depressed for 120 to 240 minutes for propoxur and carbaryl, respectively. These results suggest several possibilities, including no association between behavior and AChE or some threshold effect of ACh counteracted by the spontaneous recovery of sufficient AChE activity.

A more recent intoxication in both sheep and humans involved aldicarb contamination of a buckwheat field into which the sheep had been moved (Grendon *et al.*, 1994). Of the 318 sheep, 288 died rapidly from acute poisoning, exhibiting respiratory distress, hypersalivation, miosis, diarrhea, and seizures. Reduced erythrocytic AChE activity was measured in five animals tested, and levels of aldicarb ranging from 0.19 to 344 ppm were detected in the rumen contents of 13 of the exposed animals. The remaining live sheep, given atropine, showed some clinical improvement but continued to have poor appetites, showed body weight loss, and, within 3 weeks, either had died or were euthanized. The shepherd was affected with difficulty in breathing and a burning sensation in his throat. Those arriving to assist the owner experienced classical acute signs and symptoms. Chronic symptoms, evident in some of the humans, will be considered in a later section.

From acute animal studies, reports in the literature suggest that carbamates possess another mechanism of action in addition to that of inhibition of nervous tissue AChE. In some experiments, animals died within a few minutes of receiving the agent, seemingly from a marked anesthetic-like or "narcotic" effect accompanied by severe respiratory difficulty (dyspnea) and eventual respiratory failure (Vandekar et al., 1971). These effects have been observed with intravenous and intraperitoneal administration but not with oral administration. The "narcotic" effect was produced only by carbamates of low toxicity (high LD$_{50}$ values) (Ecobichon, 1994a). Hypotheses have suggested that such agents cause a complete blockade of nerve conduction by direct action at the level of sodium ion transport across axonal membranes and/or at motor end plate, postsynaptic, ACh receptors, both effects indicating a possible interaction of the agent with membranes to cause perturbation. A similar effect was noted following the intravenous injection of some organophosphorus ester insecticides of low toxicity (Heath, 1961).

52.6.3 ACUTE TOXICITY—HUMAN

Despite statements to the effect that "most" carbamate ester insecticides are relatively safe and produce only transient, short-term toxicity in animals following acute administration, carbamate toxicity does occur in humans, particularly in cases of ingestion by accident or with suicidal intent (Ecobichon, 1994a; Hayes, 1982). Invariably, acute toxicity in humans is associated with one of the more acutely toxic carbamates such as aldicarb, methomyl, or propoxur.

Because of long and extensive use, several reported carbaryl intoxications have been summarized in the literature (Cranmer, 1986; Dickoff et al., 1987; Farago, 1969; Hayes, 1982). Fatalities have occurred, one particular case being well documented (Farago, 1969). In this situation, a 39-year-old male purposefully drank approximately 500 mL of Sevin-80™ (80% concentration of carbaryl), with death occurring some 6 hours after ingestion, even with prompt hospitalization, gastric lavage, and antidote administration. Quantitative analysis of tissues and fluids revealed carbaryl concentrations (ppm): stomach lavage fluid (2,446), stomach contents (148), intestinal contents (176), blood (14), liver (29), kidney (25), and urine (31). No measurements of cholinesterases were reported (Farago, 1969).

Overexposure to mexacarbate as a consequence of leakage from a high-pressure pump line in a cockpit resulted in acute intoxication of a copilot (Richardson and Batteese, 1973). Approximately 110 minutes post-exposure, the copilot experienced the characteristic cholinergic symptoms. On landing, the affected individual was unable to stand, shook uncontrollably, and developed paresthesia and paralysis of the hands and arms and slurred speech while in transit to the hospital. After atropine treatment was initiated at the hospital, the symptoms disappeared rapidly and the patient was discharged three hours

after admission, the only residual effects being headache and weakness for the remainder of the day.

Carbofuran-induced occupational intoxication has occurred, two plant employees being affected while preparing a 10% granular formulation (Tobin, 1970). Taken to their respective physicians within 3 hours after the onset of symptoms, one patient received atropine, while the second was not treated since the symptoms appeared to be regressing. The atropine-treated patient recovered fully within 30 minutes, while the untreated patient recovered over the course of 2 to 3 hours.

Hayes (1982) reported several interesting poisoning and voluntary consumption cases never published in the literature, giving insight to the amount(s) required to elicit toxicity. In one case, a physician, testing the efficacy of carbaryl as an anthelmintic, ingested 250 mg of carbaryl (2.8 mg/kg) and experienced sudden, violent epigastric pain and profuse sweating within 20 to 30 minutes, followed by a gradually developing lassitude and vomiting (twice). By 3 hours after self-administration, and after having taken 3.0 mg of atropine, improvement of the symptoms occurred and, by 4 hours, the individual had recovered completely. In a second case described by Hayes (1982), arising from a personal communication from a professional colleague who was also testing the anthelmintic efficacy of carbaryl, an oral dose of 420 mg of carbaryl (5.45 mg/kg) was ingested on an empty stomach. The signs and symptoms appeared in the order shown in Table 52.8. The severity of the symptoms reached a maximum by 120 minutes after ingestion of the carbaryl. By the third hour after ingestion, the symptoms were dissipating, and the patient felt "practically normal" by the fourth hour. In a limited volunteer study reported by Wills et al. (1968), volunteers receiving acute oral doses of carbaryl (0.5, 1.0, and 2.0 mg/kg) showed

Table 52.8

Time Sequence of Appearance of Symptoms in a Carbaryl Intoxication[a]

Time interval (min)	Symptoms observed
5	Blurred vision persisting for 10 to 15 min
10[b]	Nausea
	Lightheaded
17[b]	Nausea, lightheaded, continuing sweating
	Hyperperistalsis
120	Persistent nausea without vomiting or diarrhea
	Weakness
	Pulse rate—normal 64/min
	Respiratory rate—18/min
	No pinpoint pupil
	No lacrimation, salivation or rales
	Answered questions readily and correctly
180	Improvement of symptoms
	Some increase in strength
240	Practically normal, walking about

[a] Data from Hayes, Jr. (1982).
[b] Atropine administered, 20 mg at 10 min 2.8 mg at 17 min.

no subjective or objective effects. In a further study in which carbaryl doses of 0.06, 0.12, and 0.13 mg/kg/day were administered for six consecutive days to volunteers, few conclusive abnormalities attributable to carbaryl were observed. The suicidal poisoning described by Dickoff *et al.* (1987) details the case of a 23-year-old male who swallowed 100 mL of Ortho-Liquid Sevin™ containing 27% carbaryl, showed the classical signs and symptoms reported earlier but, following recovery from the acute cholinergic toxicity, developed an acute weakness in the arms and legs associated with a peripheral, axonal neuropathy. The apparent delayed neurotoxicity will be addressed in a later section.

One unpublished incident reported by Hayes (1982) involved the aerial application of carbofuran in place of carbaryl on corn, with the rapid onset of mild-to-moderate symptoms and the rapid recovery from the intoxication. Within 12 hours of application, 142 teenaged boys and girls entered the sprayed field to remove tassels from the plants. Within 6 hours, 74 complained of dizziness, nausea and/or blurred vision; some 45 received medical aid, with 29 being hospitalized and all but one individual being released within a few hours.

Propoxur has frequently been associated with occupational intoxications, volunteer trials, accidents and suicidal attempts (Hayes, 1982; Vandekar *et al.*, 1968, 1971). Voluntary ingestion of propoxur at concentrations of 1.5 mg/kg resulted in a depression of erythrocytic AChE to 27% of normal at 15 minutes, with a return to normal activity by 120 minutes post-ingestion. Symptoms such as discomfort, head pressure, blurred vision, pallor, nausea, sweating, increased pulse rate (from 76 to 140/minute), increased blood pressure (from 130/90 to 175/95 mmHg) were observed by 60 minutes after ingestion and, by 30 minutes, pronounced nausea, repeated vomiting, and profuse sweating were observed, these symptoms persisting through 45 minutes after ingestion. By 60 minutes, the individual was feeling better, the signs and symptoms disappearing and, by 120 minutes, was feeling well enough to eat (Vandekar *et al.*, 1971). Ingestion of propoxur at a level of 0.36 mg/kg caused a rapid decrease in erythrocytic AChE to 57% of normal activity within 10 minutes and recovery within 180 minutes, and produced initial abdominal discomfort, blurred vision, moderate facial redness, and sweating lasting about 5 minutes, with recovery by 3 hours after ingestion (Vandekar *et al.*, 1971). A more recent, suicidal attempt, using a tick-and-flea preparation of propoxur, has been described, giving a detailed list of classic signs and symptoms of severe toxicity over an 8-hour period, including: unconsciousness, labored breathing, bilateral pinpoint pupils, salivation, reduced respiratory movements, regular heart rhythm but with frequent premature ventricular contractions, incontinence with watery stool, cyanosis in the extremities, sweating, no response to painful stimuli, no gag or deep-tendon reflexes, downward deflection of toes during the plantar reflex, myotonic jerks of all extremities, and grand-mal seizure (Remaley *et al.*, 1988). The patient spontaneously awakened approximately 8 hours after hospital admission and was discharged 4 days after the episode.

The most toxic of the carbamate esters is the systemic insecticide aldicarb, registered for use on citrus fruits, cotton, potatoes, peanuts and soybeans. It is not registered for use on any fruits or vegetables having a high water content. Surprisingly, this highly water-soluble chemical has been the source of periodic outbreaks of poisoning, usually associated with the inappropriate, even illegal, use in hydroponically grown cucumbers (CDC, 1979; Goes *et al.*, 1980), various melons (CDC, 1986; Goldman *et al.*, 1990a, b), or the contamination of drinking water in New York and Wisconsin (Fiore *et al.*, 1986; Sterman and Varma, 1983; Zaki *et al.*, 1982). Levels of aldicarb in cucumbers ranged from 6.6 to 10.7 ppm (Goes *et al.*, 1980). In the melons, the active ingredient was not the parent insecticide but the equally water-soluble, biologically active metabolite, aldicarb sulfoxide (Goldman *et al.*, 1990a). Estimates of the amounts of aldicarb sulfoxide ingested and responsible for intoxications ranged from 0.0011 to 0.06 mg/kg body weight (Goldman *et al.*, 1990a). In drinking water derived from groundwater sources, levels of aldicarb ranged between 8 and 75 µg/L in Suffolk County, NY, while in Wisconsin, the levels ranged between 1.0 and 61 µg/L (Fiore *et al.*, 1986; Zaki *et al.*, 1982). In all of the cucumber and melon intoxications, classic cholinergic symptoms (diarrhea, nausea, vomiting, sweating, blurred vision, abdominal pain, dyspnea, muscle fasciculations, headache, and, in some cases, loss of function of arms and legs) were observed, persisting some 4 to 12 hours followed by complete recovery (Risher *et al.*, 1987). The exposures to aldicarb in drinking water were less conclusively related to specific signs and symptoms of intoxication (Sterman and Varma, 1983; Zaki *et al.*, 1982). In an experimental study with human subjects, aldicarb was administered in single oral doses of 0.025, 0.05, 0.1 mg/kg body weight, with consequent manifestations of a variety of cholinergic symptoms at the highest level, all of which disappeared by 6 hours after administration (Union Carbide report quoted by Risher *et al.*, 1987). While abnormal reductions in erythrocytic AChE activity (25% of pre-exposure activity) were measured at the highest dose, the inhibition was rapidly reversible and preceded the disappearance of the symptoms.

Methomyl appears periodically as an insecticidal toxicant in humans, either from occupational exposure or through accidental or suicidal ingestion (Simpson and Bermingham, 1977). One recorded acute poisoning in Jamaica involved unleavened bread prepared with methomyl mistakenly used in place of common table salt, a level of some 1000 ppm being detected (Liddle *et al.*, 1979). Consumption of the bread was rapidly fatal to three individuals; another was asymptomatic, while the fifth showed generalized muscle fasciculations and respiratory distress. It was estimated that, in those who died, the amounts ingested were equivalent to 12 to 15 mg/kg body weight. In Japan, a 31-year-old woman committed suicide by incorporating methomyl in food, this being eaten by her three children as well (Araki *et al.*, 1982). A 9-year-old child survived. Autopsies revealed congestion of the stomach lining and lungs, edema, and hemorrhaging due to acute circulatory failure. The amounts ingested were estimated at 55 mg/kg for the mother and 13 mg/kg for a 6-year-old child.

Concerning the more toxic carbamate ester insecticides, aldicarb and methomyl, it has been demonstrated that central effects of these toxicants are more severe in children than in adults; symptoms in adults were miosis, muscle fasciculations, slowing of the heart, and broncorrhea, whereas in children, stupor/coma, hypotonia, and diarrhea were significant effects. Feldman (1999) suggested that the observed differences might be reflected in differences in the permeability of the blood–brain barrier of children and adults.

52.6.4 CHRONIC TOXICITY—ANIMAL

Subchronic and chronic studies have been conducted in various animal species, including mice, rats, dogs, swine, and monkeys, although many have never been published since they were confidential documents submitted to regulatory agencies in support of product registrations. Summaries of the general chronic effects of carbamate insecticides on various target sites have been published (Cranmer, 1986; Ecobichon, 1994a; IPCS, 1986). Much of the toxicity is associated with the nervous systems, neuromuscular dysfunction, and neurobehavioral changes. The chronic toxicity of carbaryl has been the most extensively reviewed (Cranmer, 1986).

Baron (1991) has published a relatively complete inventory of the effects resulting from the subchronic and chronic treatment of mice, rats, and dogs with several carbamate insecticides; much of this data was gleaned from unpublished reports from chemical manufacturers submitted at the time of product registration. Consistently, depression of erythrocytic and plasma cholinesterases were seen associated with cholinergic effects, particularly at higher dosages. Only with some agents were changes seen in food consumption, growth and development, organ weights, hematological and clinical chemistry measurements, urinalysis, and gross and histopathological parameters. The data from chronic dietary exposure studies are summarized in Table 52.9.

52.6.4.1 Neurophysiological Effects

There is evidence from animal studies that long-term exposure to carbamates such as sodium diethylthiocarbamate (a copper-chelating agent) and tetraethylthiuram (a rubber vulcanizer and a therapeutic agent in chronic alcoholism) can elicit neurological effects, possibly due to metabolism to carbon disulfide, a neuropathic agent (Barry, 1953; Gardner-Thorpe and Benjamin, 1971; Moddel et al., 1978; Waibel et al., 1957; Watson et al., 1980). Detailed descriptions of anatomic lesions including degeneration and vacuolization in the peripheral and central nervous systems of rabbits and chickens have been published, suggesting that the lesion pattern was similar to the "dying back" process described for some organophosphorus esters (Cavanagh, 1969, 1973; Edington and Howell, 1966, 1969; Howell and Edington, 1968). The elicited neurotoxicity has been attributed to the biotransformation of the dithiocarbamates to yield carbon disulfide, a known neuropathic agent (Brugnone et al., 1993; Johnson et al., 1998).

Miller et al. (1969) demonstrated that a single dose of carbaryl (20 mg/kg) given to miniature swine caused a 44% and 75% inhibition of cerebral cortex and brain stem AChE, respectively, and caused a hindlimb paralysis even though no obvious effects were seen upon histopathological examination. Severe carbaryl-induced neuromuscular effects were observed in another study in swine (Smalley et al., 1969). High dosages (150 mg/kg/day over 73 to 83 days or 150 mg/kg daily for 28 days followed by 300 mg/kg/day over the next 18 or 57 days) caused severe neuromuscular effects. Reluctance to stand was observed first, followed by a peculiar stance, the rear legs being carried well forward under the body, the animals appearing to be "walking" on their dew claws. There was greatly exaggerated flexion of the rear legs, the animals having difficulty in backing up or sitting down. Forcing the animals to move caused marked incoordination, ataxia, muscle tremors, and clonic contractions. Muscular lesions consisted of a myodegeneration of traumatic or ischemic nature, an acute hyaline and vacuolar degeneration, and an acute degenerative process associated with dystrophic calcification (Smalley et al., 1969).

Carbamate esters have caused severe neuropathy in adult chickens following repeated oral administration, although this neuropathy is different from organophosphorus-induced delayed neuropathy (OPIDN) (Fisher and Metcalf, 1983; Hollingshaus and Fukuto, 1982). In young (3-week-old) chicks, both carbaryl and aldicarb affected locomotor activity for 6 weeks after cessation of the subacute (7 days) exposure (Farage-Elawar, 1989a, 1989b). The treated chicks walked with an abnormal gait, taking shorter steps but with a wider stance suggestive of ataxia. Some paralysis was seen for up to 40 days post-treatment. Once again, this neuropathy was unlike that seen in OPIDN.

While the short-term exposure of rats and dogs to repeated oral doses of carbaryl, carbofuran, and propoxur resulted in the inhibition of plasma, erythrocytic, and brain cholinesterases accompanied by typical acute signs of toxicity, there was little evidence of persistent effects on the central and/or peripheral nervous systems (Cranmer, 1986; IPCS, 1986; Krechniak and Foss, 1982). While rats dying in an acute carbaryl study showed congestion of the brain and meninges, such morphological changes have not been reported in animals treated with less than near-lethal concentrations (Boyd and Boulanger, 1968). Cranmer (1986) cited studies in which morphological changes in the brain ganglia in rabbits and increased brain protein in rats were reported, but suggested that such effects occurred only at doses that reduced cholinesterase activities. Rats and dogs receiving oral aldicarb for up to two years showed no adverse effects (Risher et al., 1987).

Two studies have suggested that long-term exposure to carbamate esters can cause neurotoxicity. In a two-year rat study of carbaryl at levels causing no inhibition of blood cholinesterases or clinical signs, the animals showed electroencephalographic (EEG) changes and had a decreased maze performance (Desi et al., 1974). In monkeys, the EEG patterns were not adversely affected at carbaryl levels of 1.0 mg/kg/day (Santolucito and Morrison, 1971). Tolerance to carbamates has been reported

Table 52.9
Chronic Toxicity of Carbamate Insecticides[a]

Chemical	Species	Max. dosage (mg/kg)	Food consump.	Organ			Hema-tology	Clin. chem.	Urina-ysis	Path-ology
				Growth	Wt.	Death				
Aldicarb	Rat	0.5	+	−	−	+	−	−	−	−
	Rat	0.3	−	−	−	−	−	−	−	−
	Dog	0.25	−	−	−	−	−	−	−	−
Bendiocarb	Rat	200 ppm	+	+	+	−	+	+	+	−
	Dog	500 ppm	−	−	−	−	−	+	+	−
Carbaryl	Rat	400 ppm	−	+	+	−	−			−
	Dog	1250 ppm		+	−		+	−		−
Carbofuran	Mouse	500 ppm	−	+	−	−	−	−	−	−
	Rat	100 ppm	−	+	−	−	−	+	−	−
	Dog	500 ppm	+	+	+	−	+	+		+
Carbosulfan	Rat	500 ppm	+	+						−
		2500 ppm	+	+	+		+	+		−
	Dog	1000 ppm	+	+	+					+
	Mouse	2500 ppm	+	+	+	−		+		+
Methiocarb	Rat	600 ppm	−	+	+	−	−	−	−	−
	Dog	60 ppm	−	−	−	−	−	−	−	−
Methomyl	Mouse	800 ppm	−	−	−	+	−	−	−	−
	Rat	20–26	+	−	−	−	−	−	−	−
	Dog	1000 ppm				+	+	+		+
Mexacarbate	Mouse	300 ppm	+	+	−	−	−	−	−	−
	Rat	250 ppm	+	+	−	−	−	−	−	−
	Dog	325 ppm	+	+	+	+		+		+
Oxamyl	Rat	150 ppm	+	+	+	−	−	−	+	−
	Dog	150 ppm	−	−	−	−		+		−
Pirimicarb	Rat	250–750 ppm	−	−	+	−	−	−		−
	Dog	4.0 ppm	−	−	−	−	−	−		−
Propoxur	Rat	2000 ppm	+							+
	Rat	750 ppm			+					+
	Dog	2000 ppm		+	−	−	−	−		−

[a]Data derived from Baron (1991). Positive effects on a parameter are indicated by "+," while no effects are represented by "−." Maximum dosage is in milligram per kilogram of body weight (mg/kg) unless presented as parts per million (ppm) in food.

(Costa et al., 1982). For example, male rats receiving carbaryl (200 mg/kg/day) orally for 3 days/week for 90 days showed no overt toxicity (Dikshith et al., 1976).

In the above-mentioned carbaryl swine study, Smalley et al. (1969) described a clinical syndrome of chronic intoxication characterized by progressive myasthenia, incoordination, ataxia, intention tremor, and clonic muscular contractions terminating in paraplegia and prostration. Moderate-to-severe edema was found in myelinated tracts of the cerebellum, brain stem, and upper spinal cord, as well as fragmentation of myelin sheaths, moderate swelling and rupture of axons, necrosis of cellular components in spinocerebellar tracts, and vascular congestion, hypertrophic endothelium, and vascular degeneration and hemorrhage in the gray columns. The authors attributed the pathological effects to vascular changes induced by carbaryl (Smalley et al., 1969).

52.6.4.2 Neurobehavioral Effects

Behavioral changes have been associated with carbamate exposure in many animal studies, although such adverse effects were usually detected immediately following acute administration of sufficient chemical to inhibit cholinesterases, suggesting that the effects were the result of cholinergic-mediated stress. Most studies have involved carbaryl (Cranmer, 1986).

Single intraperitoneal doses of carbaryl (8.0 mg/kg) reduced shock avoidance by 50% in treated rats for 30 minutes, while a dose of 7.3 mg/kg caused a 50% reduction in a positive reward response test (food presentation) (Goldberg et al., 1965). In a food reward test in cats, inhaled carbaryl (40 mg/m^3) caused a deficit only immediately after exposure (Yakim, 1967). Spontaneous locomotor activity was reduced in rats in a 60-minute period after acute oral carbaryl (0.56 and 2.24 mg/kg), whereas the daily administration of a higher dose for 14 consecutive days had no effect on "wheel-turning" (Singh, 1973). In contrast, acute intoxication of rats with carbaryl (10 mg/kg) resulted in increased locomotor activity in a familiar environment but reduction in exploratory activity in a new environment (Singh, 1973). A decrease in rats' working memory was carbaryl dose-dependent shortly after treatment (Heise and Hudson, 1985). In a feeding study of carbaryl and arprocarb (2-isopropoxyphenyl-N-methylcarbamate) in rats, the amounts given in the diet to achieve body dosages of 10 and 20 mg/kg over 50 days resulted in the animals showing increased difficulty in performing tasks, forgetting already learned skills (Desi *et al.*, 1974). Over 4-month periods, rats inhaling carbaryl (12 to 23 mg/m^3 for 4 hours daily) showed decreased performance in a maze task for food reward, but if the treatment was extended every two weeks for four months, performance was normal (Viter, 1978). A possible association could be suggested between behavioral alterations and cholinesterase inhibition/acute toxicity, the adverse effects being ACh-related.

Learning in monkeys appeared to be affected by small, chronic doses of carbaryl. This led to the use of the technique called "chain acquisition" task in which monkeys learned one set of equivalent response sequences each day; they were trained to make four out of the 12 possible response sequences in a certain order, with the correct responses being changed

every day (Anger and Setzer, 1979). Carbaryl was administered orally (up to 50 mg/kg) or intramuscularly (1.0, 3.0, 5.0, and 10 mg/kg) to trained macaque monkeys. Oral carbaryl caused no consistent effects on performance, whereas the injected carbaryl elicited significant decreases in total session time and increased errors in performance at and above dosages of 3.0 mg/kg.

52.6.4.3 Mutagenicity

As a class, methylcarbamates are not mutagenic, negative results being obtained in an overwhelming majority of *in vitro* gene mutation assays using microbial systems, cultured mammalian cells, and such *in vivo* systems as Drosophila and dominant lethal mutation tests (Baron, 1991; IPCS, 1986). Table 52.10 lists the methylcarbamate insecticides that showed mutagenicity in *in vitro* and *in vivo* test systems. While weak mutagenicity has been identified as a property of several carbamates, high, almost toxic dosages were used and, frequently, the results either could not be replicated or were derived from nonstandardized protocols that could not be compared with results from acceptable techniques.

Table 52.10
Mutagenic Potential of Carbamate Insecticides

Chemical	Test systems	Effects[a]	References
Aldicarb	S. typhimurium	DNA damage	Rashid and Mumma (1986)
	Mouse bone marrow cells	CA	Debuyst and Van Larebeke (1983)
	Cultured human lymphocytes	SCE	Gonzales and Matos (1984)
Carbaryl	Saccharomyces cerevisiae	M	Guerzoni *et al.* (1976)
	S. typhimurium	M	Egert and Greim (1976)
	Cultured rodent cells	M	Ahmed *et al.* (1977)
	Cultured rodent cells	CA	Ishidate and Odashima (1977)
	Cultured rodent cells	spindle poison	Onfelt (1983)
	Human fibroblasts	DNA damage	Ahmed *et al.* (1977)
	D. melanogaster	CA	Hoque (1972)
	Rats	mitotic abnormalities	Baron (1991)
Carbofuran	S. typhimurium	M	Moriya *et al.* (1983)
	Cultured rodent cells	M	Wojciechowski *et al.* (1982)
	Cultured rodent cells	CA	Debuyst and Van Larebeke (1983)
Formetanate HCl	Cultured human lymphocytes	M	Baron (1991)
Methomyl	Saccharomyces cerevisiae	M	Guerzoni *et al.* (1976)
	Human lymphocytes	SCE	Debuyst and Van Larebeke (1983)
Mexacarbate	Cultured mammalian cells	CA	Baron (1991)
Propoxur	Saccharomyces cerevisiae	M	Guerzoni *et al.* (1976)
	Mouse dominant lethal	CA	Baron (1991)
Pirimicarb	Cultured mammalian cells	CA	Pilinskaya (1981, 1982)
	Human lymphocytes	CA	Pilinskaya (1981)
Thiodicarb	Saccharomyces cerevisiae	DNA damage	Baron (1991)

[a] Abbreviations: M, mutagenic; CA, chromosomal aberrations; SCE, sister-chromatid exchanges.

52.6.4.4 Reproductive Effects

There is little evidence that methylcarbamate insecticides cause reproductive anomalies in mammals. The common, positive findings have been embryotoxicity and/or fetotoxicity associated with the administration of high dosages and concomitant maternal and possibly nutritional toxicity (IPCS, 1986). There is little evidence of these carbamates causing teratogenicity other than through nutrition-related problems (IPCS, 1986).

52.6.4.5 Carcinogenicity

There has been no evidence of the potential of methylcarbamate insecticides to cause carcinogenicity (IPCS, 1986). However, in studies where positive effects have been found, caution must be observed in interpreting the data because of design inadequacies (limited dosage range, duration of study, numbers of animals, etc.) and the extremely high doses administered. Most of these studies are summarized in the IPCS document (IPCS, 1986); more recent reports have not been seen.

52.6.5 CHRONIC TOXICITY—HUMAN

As has been observed with organophosphorus ester intoxications, persistent effects may result following either acute, single, high-level or repeated, even long-duration, low-level exposure to carbamate esters (Ecobichon, 1994a, b). Involvement of both the peripheral and central nervous systems has given rise to distinctive neurophysiological and/or behavioral anomalies.

In 1982, a bizarre case of a 55-year-old male was described following a thorough soaking of skin and clothing by a water-wettable preparation of carbaryl (Ecobichon, 1982). Within 3 to 4 weeks of initial antibiotic treatment for "bacterial meningitis," the patient was reporting headaches, blurred vision, photophobia, peripheral numbness, tingling sensations in the hands and legs, muscle weakness, vertigo, incoordination, lethargy, tiredness, forgetfulness, and loss of recent memory. More alarmingly, behavioral changes persisting for several months manifested themselves as frustrated rage, inability to control temper, severe headaches, and short periods of blackouts. Even at 18 months post-exposure, the patient was unable to drive a car, still experienced photophobia, had persistent short-term memory loss and mild peripheral paresthesia, and suffered from lassitude, lethargy, and muscle weakness. The behavioral aspects persisted, being partially controlled by anticonvulsant and antipsychotic drugs. At the time of this case, no other reports had been published concerning slow developing and/or persistent symptoms arising from exposure to carbamate ester insecticides. Subsequently, a number of such cases have appeared in the literature, all reporting persistent adverse effects (Ecobichon, 1994a; Feldman, 1999).

52.6.5.1 Neurophysiological Effects

Indicative of delayed neurotoxicity following acute exposure to high levels of carbamate insecticides, Dickoff et al. (1987) reported a case involving the ingestion of a liquid preparation of carbaryl (500 mg/kg), showing a weakness in the arms and legs as well as sensory loss following the acute cholinergic crisis, with electrophysiological alterations consistent with a peripheral axonal neuropathy. Recovery began one week after exposure and progressed for 9 months. However, while recovery appeared to be complete, bilateral severe ankle and toe weakness persisted, accompanied by reduced propioception in the toes and tactile preception below mid-calf. In a second, suicidal case, the ingestion of a metolcarb (m-tolyl-methylcarbamate) formulation (estimated dosage of 1.0–1.2 mg/kg) resulted in neurological damage (Umehara et al., 1991). Fibrillation potentials and sharp positive waves were observed at rest, with reduced recruitment patterns during muscle contractions. A sural nerve biopsy, performed 38 days after the poisoning, revealed reduced densities of large and small myelinated fibers, degenerated axons, and denervated Schwann cell clusters. At 3 months post-exposure, motor symptoms had improved, with a reduction in numbness, although deep tendon reflexes in the extremities were absent. By 6 months, upper motor neuronal signs were no longer observed. In a more recent case of acute exposure to aldicarb, men handling poisoned sheep showed persistent symptoms similar to those mentioned above, five of the six individuals still experiencing persistent neurotoxicity some three years after exposure (Grendon et al., 1994).

Feldman (1999) described two cases of chronic symptoms following an aerial overspray of carbaryl in a forest spraying program. Both individuals had symptoms persisting for more than six years after the exposure, one (a 35-year-old male) showing hoarseness, bronchorrhea, dizziness, and a peripheral neuropathy. The second individual (a 53-year-old male) suffered recurrent bouts of abdominal cramps and diarrhea, anxiety attacks with associated flashback memories, fatigue, numbness in the feet which gradually affected the hands, a clumsy gait, reduced sensation to mid-calf developing within three months of exposure, and some effects (slowed nerve conduction, reduced muscle action potential amplitude and motor activity in the lower extremities) for some five years post-exposure. Electromyographical and nerve conduction studies indicated a peripheral neuropathy with chronic denervation and reinnervation in distal muscles.

In contrast to the acute-exposure situation, reports linking incidents of-low-to-moderate, subchronic or chronic exposure to chronic toxicity are almost nonexistent. In one study in which volunteers took daily oral doses of carbaryl (0.06 or 0.13 mg/kg) for six weeks, with concomitant monitoring of plasma and whole blood cholinesterase activities, other blood and urinary biochemical parameters, and electroencephalograms, no deleterious changes were attributable to the agent (Wills et al., 1968). However, the level of exposure could be considered to be low. One case report of a low-level exposure to carbaryl stands out as being contrary to everything known and expected of carbamate-related toxicity. The propositus patient, a 75-year-old male, and his family (wife and son) were exposed over a period of 8 to 10 months to carbaryl (a 10% dust formulation) applied some six times to the basement area of a home to control fleas (Branch and Jacqz, 1986a). The insecticide was dispersed throughout the home by the central air conditioning located in the basement. While the entire family experienced a range of acute influenza-like symptoms (headache, malaise, epigastric discomfort, abdominal colic, diarrhea, nausea, muscle spasms, cough) within 3 days of the initial application, the wife and son appeared to recover. However, the father's signs and symptoms became progressively more severe (headache with intense pressure, tinnitus, vertigo, mild ataxia, rhinorrhea, excessive lacrimation, weakness in major skeletal muscle groups, fasciculations, somnolence, agitation, mental confusion). Both the plasma and erythrocytic cholinesterase activities were below normal values and consistent with an anticholinesterase intoxication. During intervals of living away from the home, the patient's symptoms dissipated, but they returned when he reentered the house for any extended period. Leaving the house permanently, the patient's well-being improved, but it was two months before the plasma PChE was within normal range. Symptoms that failed to abate included alterations in sleep patterns (episodic awakening with headache and tinnitus) and mental confusion that persisted for a further two years. A computerized tomographic scan revealed cerebral atrophy which had not been observed on a pre-exposure scan. A persistent, neurological deficit became more severe, being defined as a stocking-and-glove peripheral neuropathy.

There has been considerable criticism of this last case report, including that of drawing a valid inference of carbaryl intoxication based on one case in the absence of any occupational exposure literature of similar agent-related toxicity. No indoor measurements of aerial or surface concentrations of carbaryl were ever made, thereby preventing an estimation of exposure. The advanced age of the patient could have played a role in the rate of carbaryl detoxification. The concomitant treatment of the patient with cimetidine, an H_2-receptor antagonist used in treating gastric acidity and peptic ulcers, might have had an effect. In animal studies, cimetidine has been shown to inhibit carbaryl biotransformation, thereby increasing the systemic bioavailability of the agent (Branch and Jacqz, 1986b). However, taken in context with other case reports, the claim of a carbaryl-induced intoxication appears valid.

Regular occupational exposure to methomyl, particularly in the packaging area of the manufacturing plant, resulted in a high incidence of anticholinesterase symptoms (constricted pupils, nausea, vomiting, blurred vision, increased salivation, muscle weakness, fatigue) and a high number of hospitalizations (Morse et al., 1979). A decreased vibratory sensation was noted in 19.8% of the workforce, with hospitalized workers having significantly more vibratory sensory loss than nonhospitalized workers. However, no depression of either plasma or erythrocytic cholinesterase activities was noted.

It is of interest to note that some acute carbamate intoxications have resulted in the later development of persistent respiratory problems that were exacerbated by exposure to other chemicals such as solvents, household pesticides, hairsprays, and perfumes (Feldman, 1999; Grendon et al., 1994). The descriptions are reminiscent of multiple chemical sensitivity, an olfactory sensitizing and triggering phenomenon described by

Ashford and Miller (1998). One of the earliest reports of odor aversion as a consequence of pesticide exposure was that of Tabershaw and Cooper (1966), who reported that several of their cases could no longer tolerate smelling or contact with pesticides, reacting with nausea and vomiting after even a whiff of the agents and being forced to give up work involving contact with agrochemicals. The genesis of this idiosyncratic reaction has not yet been ascertained but appears to have both neurological and psychogenic components.

52.6.5.2 Neurobehavioral Effects

Sufficient numbers of cases of both acute and chronic intoxications by organophosphorus ester, anticholinesterase insecticides have revealed a recognizable pattern of delayed and/or persistent neurobehavioral anomalies that can be detected and assessed by appropriate neuropsychological evaluation (Ecobichon, 1994b, 1999; Feldman, 1999). Not surprisingly, close examination of acute and chronic carbamate insecticide intoxications reveals a similar pattern of persistent behavioral effects even though neuropsychological testing of affected individuals has not been reported.

The long-term follow-up of acutely or chronically carbamate-exposed individuals has been poor but, in several of the incidents discussed in the previous section, observed symptoms have included vertigo, incoordination, disturbed sleep patterns, anxiety attacks, mood changes, chronic lethargy and fatigue, agitation, mental confusion, and difficulty in performing simple tasks or making decisions (Branch and Jacqz, 1986a; Ecobichon, 1982; Grendon et al., 1994). Feldman (1999) describes the detailed neuropsychological assessment of two individuals some five or six years following an overspraying by carbaryl applied aerially, using the Wechsler Adult Intelligence Scale (WAIS) test battery. As has been observed with organophosphorus ester insecticide intoxications, many of the component tests were within normal values, but impairment, deficiency, or slowing of performance were detected in: a confrontational naming task (Boston Naming Test), memory tests requiring a delayed recall of information; psychomotor (Digit Symbol Test) evaluation, and tasks of visual spatial organization, cognitive tracking, and reasoning. The Profile of Mood States (POMS) and the Minnesota Multiphasic Personality Inventory (MMPI) revealed persistent fatigue, depression and/or anxiety states. Discrepancies were revealed between verbal and performance intelligence quotients. It is obvious that greater use could be made of refined neurological and behavioral test batteries to evaluate short- and long-term neurological effects of carbamate exposure.

52.6.5.3 Reproductive Effects

Few specifics are known about the potential of short- and long-term influence of carbamate insecticide exposure on any aspects of reproduction in either male or female agricultural workers. One paper has reported an increase in sperm abnormalities (abnormally shaped heads) in production workers who had been exposed to carbaryl at the time of sampling (Wyrobek et al., 1981). Neither the sperm count nor the presence of double fluorescent bodies was changed. Formerly exposed workers, removed from carbaryl-related occupational activities for an average of 6.3 years, showed only a marginally significant elevation in sperm abnormalities, results suggesting that the carbaryl-induced morphological effects may not be reversible or may be only slowly so. A dose-dependent change in sperm morphology could not be established. More research needs to be conducted in this area of toxicology.

52.7 TREATMENT

The symptoms (Table 52.8) associated with carbamate insecticide intoxication are associated with the accumulating, unmetabolized neurotransmitter ACh at the nerve endings of the parasympathetic and sympathetic autonomic ganglia, the post-ganglionic parasympathetic nerve endings, and the neuromuscular junctions of the somatic, motor neurons, as a consequence of the inhibition of the nervous tissue AChE. The reversible nature of the AChE inhibition would suggest that the symptoms would be transient although, depending upon the level of exposure, possibly moderate to severe in nature.

Atropine is the antidote of choice, antagonizing the action of ACh by blocking the receptor site for the transmitter at parasympathetic nerve fibers innervating exocrine glands, gastrointestinal tract, respiratory tract, eyes, heart, and bladder, as well as exerting a direct, central effect on the respiratory center (Ecobichon et al., 1977; Feldman, 1999; Namba et al., 1971). Alleviation of these muscarinic signs will be best achieved by administering frequent small doses (0.5 to 1.0 mg) subcutaneously until there is dilatation (mydriasis) of the pupils and the face becomes flushed and/or sweating disappears. The patient should be carefully titered using these signs as physiological endpoints since excess atropine can cause severe toxicity. This is of particular importance in carbamate ester poisoning where the enzyme–insecticide complex is unstable; the enzyme may be decarbamoylated by the excess ACh and the carbamate ester may be metabolized in a short period of time. Atropine is ineffective in counteracting the nicotinic, neuromuscular effects of the accumulated ACh.

Acetylcholinesterase reactivators such as the pyridinium oximes, 2-PAM, P2S, and toxogonin, have been used in carbamate-induced intoxications but with mixed results, their use remaining controversial. Signal animal (rats, dogs) experiments involving carbaryl intoxications revealed that the protective effect of atropine was markedly reduced by the concomitant administration of 2-PAM (Carpenter et al., 1961; Natoff and Reiff, 1973; Sanderson, 1961). This observation was confirmed in one human carbaryl-related poisoning where it was noted that the patient's condition deteriorated rapidly following the administration of 2-PAM (Farago,1969). This led to a generalized condemnation of oxime use as an antidote in carbamate insecticide intoxication (Harris et al., 1989; Lifshitz et al., 1994; Natoff and Reiff, 1973; Sterri et al., 1979). However, beneficial effects of oxime treatment were seen in treating aldicarb,

Table 52.11
Exposure Limits For Carbamate Insecticides[a]

Chemical	OSHA (PEL)	NIOSH REL	NIOSH IDLH	ACGIH (TLV)
Carbaryl	5.0	5.0	100	5.0
Carbofuran	0.1[b]	0.1	ND	0.1
Methomyl	2.5[b]	2.5	ND	2.5
Propoxur	0.5[b]	0.5	ND	0.5

[a] Values represent concentrations (mg/m^3) in air. REL values represent a time-weighted average for a 10-hr exposure, while TLV values represent a time-weighted average for an 8-hr exposure.
[b] Values "vacated" by OSHA in 1993.

mecarbam (S-(N-ethoxycarbonyl-N-methyl-carbamoylmethyl) O,O-diethyl phosphorodithioate) and methomyl intoxications (Natoff and Reiff, 1973; Sterri et al., 1979). In cases involving carbofuran, methiocarb, mexacarbate, thiodicarb, and trimethacarb, 2-PAM was ineffective but did not exacerbate the clinical symptoms or interfere with the antidotal effectiveness of atropine (Baron, 1991; FAO/WHO, 1982). Similar results were seen for P2S with pirimicarb and for toxogonin with methomyl (FAO/WHO, 1982; Sanderson, 1961). Overall, the studies to date suggest the efficacious use of oximes with aliphatic oxime carbamate (aldicarb, methomyl, and possibly mecarbam) intoxications but not their use in carbaryl- or other carbamate-related intoxications (Feldman, 1999). The myorelaxant agent, diazepam, should be considered in treatment regimens of all but the mildest cases of carbamate intoxications to relieve anxiety, to counteract some central nervous system-related symptoms not affected by atropine.

52.8 EXPOSURE LIMITS

Given the importance of methyl carbamate insecticides in the agricultural industry, it is surprising that so few exposure limit values have been established for these agents by the Occupational Safety and Health Administration (OSHA), the National Institute for Occupational Safety and Health (NIOSH), and the American Conference of Governmental Industrial Hygienists (ACGIH). As is shown in Table 52.11, the promulgated values for a few carbamates include permissible exposure levels (PELs), recommended exposure limits (RELs), immediately dangerous to life and health (IDLH) levels, and threshold limit values (TLVs) or time-weighted average (TWA) exposure levels for 8 to 10 hours. In addition, the U.S. Environmental Protection Agency (EPA) has introduced maximum drinking water contamination levels (MCLs) only for aldicarb (0.007 mg/L) and carbofuran (0.04 mg/L), chemicals that have been associated with problems of surface and groundwater contamination.

REFERENCES

Abdel-Wahab, A. M., Kuhr, R. J., and Casida, J. E. (1966). Fate of ^{14}C-carbonyl-labeled aryl methylcarbamate insecticide chemicals in and on bean plants. *J. Agric. Food Chem.* **14**, 290–298.

Ahmed, F. E., Lewis, N. J., and Hart, R. W. (1977). Pesticide-induced ouabain resistant mutants in Chinese hamster V79 cells. *Chem. Biol. Interact.* **19**, 369–374.

Aly, O. M., and El-Dib, M. A. (1971). Studies on the persistence of some carbamate insecticides in the aquatic environment. I. Hydrolysis of Sevin[TM], Baygon[TM], Pyrolan[TM] and Dimetilan[TM] in waters. *Water Res.* **5**, 1191–1200.

Anger, W. K., and Setzer, J. V. (1979). Effect of oral and intramuscular carbaryl administration on repeated acquisition in monkeys. *J. Toxicol. Environ. Health* **5**, 793–808.

Anger, W. K., and Wilson, S. M. (1980). Effect of carbaryl on variable interval response rates in rats. *Neurobehav. Toxicol.* **2**, 21–24.

Araki, M., Yonemitsu, K., Kambe, T., Idaka, D., Tsunenari, S., Kanda, M., and Kambara, T. (1982). Forensic toxicological investigations on fatal cases of carbamate pesticide methomyl (Lannate®) poisoning. *Jpn. J. Legal Med.* **36**, 584–588.

Ashford, N., and Miller, C. (1998). "Chemical Exposures. Low Levels and High Stakes," 2nd ed. Van Nostrand Reinhold, New York.

Baron, R. L. (1991). Carbamate insecticides. *In* "Handbook of Pesticide Toxicology" (W. J. Hayes, Jr. and E. R. Laws, Jr., eds.), Vol. 3, Ch. 17, pp. 1125–1189. Academic Press, New York.

Barry, W. K. (1953). Peripheral neuritis following tetraethylthiuram-disulfide treatment. *Brit. Med. J.* **2**, 937.

Berry, W. K. (1971). Acceleration by free carbamate of the spontaneous reactivation of carbamylated acetylcholinesterase. *Biochem. Pharmacol.* **20**, 3236–3238.

Boyd, E. M., and Boulanger, M. A. (1968). Insecticide toxicology. Augmented susceptibility to carbaryl toxicity in albino rats fed purified casein diets. *J. Agric. Food Chem.* **16**, 834–838.

Branch, R. A., and Jacqz, E. (1986a). Subacute neurotoxicity following long-term exposure to carbaryl. *Am. J. Med.* **80**, 741–745.

Branch, R. A., and Jacqz, E. (1986b). Is carbaryl as safe as its reputation? Does it have a potential for causing chronic neurotoxicity in humans? *Am. J. Med.* **80**, 659–664.

Brugnone, F., Maranelli, G., Guglielmi, G., Ayyad, K., Soleo, L., and Elia, G. (1993). Blood concentrations of carbon disulfide in dithiocarbamate exposure and in the general population. *Int. Arch. Occup. Environ. Health* **64**, 503–507.

Carpenter, C. P., Weil, C. S., Palm, P. E., Woodside, M. W., Nair, III, J. H., and Smyth, Jr., H. F. (1961). Mammalian toxicity of 1-naphthyl-N-methylcarbamate (Sevin insecticide). *J. Agric. Food Chem.* **9**, 30–38.

Cavanagh, J. B. (1969). Toxic substances and the nervous system. *Brit. Med. Bull.* **25**, 268–273.

Cavanagh, J. B. (1973). Peripheral neuropathy caused by chemical agents. *CRC Crit. Rev. Toxicol.* **2**, 365–417.

Centers for Disease Control (CDC) (1979). Suspected carbamate intoxications—Nebraska. *Morbidity and Mortality Weekly Report* **28**, 133–134.

Centers for Disease Control (CDC) (1986). Aldicarb food poisoning from contaminated melons—California. *Morbidity and Mortality Weekly Report* **35**, 254–255.

Costa, L. G., Schwab, B. W., and Murphy, S. D. (1982). Tolerance to anticholinesterase compounds in mammals. *Toxicology* **25**, 79–97.

Cranmer, M. F. (1986). Carbaryl: A toxicological review and risk analysis. *Neurotoxicology* **7**, 247–328.

Cremlyn, R. (1978). "Pesticides. Preparation and Mode of Action." John Wiley and Sons, New York.

Debuyst, B., and Van Larebeke, N. (1983). Induction of sister-chromatid exchanges in human lymphocytes by aldicarb, thiofonax and methomyl. *Mutat. Res.* **113**, 242–243.

Desi, I., Gonczi, L., Simon, G., Farkas, I., and Kneffel, Z. (1974). Neurotoxicologic studies of two carbamate pesticides in subacute animal experiments. *Toxicol. Appl. Pharmacol.* **27**, 465–476.

Dickoff, D. J., Gerber, O., and Turovsky, Z. (1987). Delayed neurotoxicity after ingestion of carbamate pesticide. *Neurology* **37**, 1229–1231.

Dikshith, T. S. S., Gupta, P. K., Gaur, J. S., Datta, K. K., and Mathur, A. K. (1976). Ninety day toxicity of carbaryl in male rats. *Environ. Res.* **12**, 161–170.

Ecobichon, D. J. (1982). Carbamic Acid Ester Pesticides. *In* "Pesticides and Neurological Diseases" (D. J. Ecobichon and R. M. Joy, eds.), Ch. 6, pp. 220–221. CRC Press, Boca Raton, FL.

Ecobichon, D. J. (1994a). Carbamic acid ester insecticides. *In* "Pesticides and Neurological Diseases" (D. J. Ecobichon and R. M. Joy, eds.), 2nd ed., Ch. 5, pp. 258–262. CRC Press, Boca Raton, FL.

Ecobichon, D. J. (1994b). Organophosphorus ester insecticides. *In* "Pesticides and Neurological Diseases" (D. J. Ecobichon and R. M. Joy, eds.), 2nd ed., Ch. 4, pp. 211–220. CRC Press, Boca Raton, FL.

Ecobichon, D. J. (1996). Toxic effects of pesticides. *In* "Casarett and Doull's Toxicology. The Basic Science of Poisons" (C. D. Klaassen, ed.), 5th ed., Ch. 22, pp. 655–662. McGraw-Hill, New York.

Ecobichon, D. J. (1999). Biological monitoring: Neurophysiological and behavioral assessments. *In* "Occupational Hazards of Pesticide Exposures: Sampling, Monitoring, Measuring" (D. J. Ecobichon, ed.), Ch. 8, pp. 209–230. Taylor and Francis, Philadelphia.

Ecobichon, D. J., and Comeau, A. M. (1973). Pseudocholinesterases of mammalian plasma: Physicochemical properties and organophosphate inhibition in eleven species. *Toxicol. Appl. Pharmacol.* **24**, 92–100.

Ecobichon, D. J., and Joy, R. M. (1982). Carbamic acid ester pesticides. *In* "Pesticides and Neurological Diseases." CRC Press, Boca Raton, FL.

Ecobichon, D. J., Ozere, R. L., Reid, E., and Crocker, J. F. S. (1977). Acute fenitrothion poisoning. *Can. Med. Assoc. J.* **116**, 377–379.

Edington, N., and Howell, J. M. (1966). Changes in the nervous system of rabbits following the administration of sodium-diethylthiocarbamate. *Nature* **210**, 1060–1062.

Edington, N., and Howell, J. M. (1969). The neurotoxicity of sodium diethylthiocarbamate in the hen. *Acta Neuropathol.* **12**, 339–347.

Egert, G., and Greim, H. (1976). Formation of mutagenic nitroso-compounds from ephedrine and the pesticides carbaryl, dodin and prometryn in the presence of nitrite at pH 1. *Naunyn-Schmiedberg's Arch. Pharmacol.* **293**, Supp. R66.

Ellman, G. L., Courtney, K. D., Andres, Jr., V., and Featherstone, R. M. (1961). A new and rapid colorimetric determination of acetylcholinesterase activity. *Biochem. Pharmacol.* **7**, 88–95.

Farage-Elawar, M. (1989a). Enzyme and behavioral changes in young chicks as a result of carbaryl treatment. *J. Toxicol. Environ. Health* **26**, 119–131.

Farage-Elawar, M. (1989b). Toxicity of aldicarb in young chicks. *Neurotox. Teratol.* **10**, 549–554.

Farago, A. (1969). Suicidal, fatal Sevin® (1-naphthyl-N-methyl carbamate) poisoning. *Arch. Toxicol.* **24**, 309–315.

Feldman, R. G. (1999). Carbamates. *In* "Occupational and Environmental Neurotoxicology" (R. G. Feldman, ed.), Ch. 23, pp. 442–465. Lippincott-Raven Publishers, Philadelphia.

Fiore, M. C., Anderson, H. A., Hong, Z., Golubjatnikov, R., Seiser, J. E., Nordstrom, D., Hanrahan, L., and Belluck, D. (1986). Chronic exposure to aldicarb-contaminated groundwater and human immune function. *Environ. Res.* **41**, 633–645.

Fisher, S. W., and Metcalf, R. L. (1983). Production of delayed ataxia by carbamic acid esters. *Pestic. Biochem. Physiol.* **19**, 243–253.

Food and Agricultural Organization/World Health Organization (FAO/WHO) (1982). "Pesticide Residues in Food: 1981 Evaluations: The Monographs." FAO Plant Product Protection Paper No. 42. Food Agric. Organ. U.N., Rome.

Fukuto, T. R. (1972). Metabolism of carbamate insecticides. *Drug Metab. Rev.* **1**, 117–150.

Fukuto, T. R. (1983). Structure-activity relationships in derivative of anticholinesterase insecticides. *In* "Pesticide Chemistry: Human Welfare and the Environment" (J. Miyamoto and P. C. Kearney, eds.), Vol. 1, pp. 203–213. Pergamon Press, New York.

Fukuto, T. R., Fahmy, M. A. H., and Metcalf, R. L. (1967). Alkaline hydrolysis, anticholinesterase and insecticidal properties of some nitro-substituted phenyl carbamates. *J. Agric. Food Chem.* **15**, 273–277.

Gardner-Thorpe, C., and Benjamin, S. (1971). Peripheral neuropathy after disulfiram adminstration. *J. Neurol. Neurosurg. Psychiat.* **34**, 253–259.

Goes, A. E., Savage, E. P., Gibbons, G., Arronson, M., Ford, S. A., and Wheeler, H. W. (1980). Suspected foodborne carbamate pesticide intoxications with the ingestion of hydroponic cucumbers. *Am. J. Epidem.* **111**, 254–259.

Goldberg, M. E., Johnson, H. E., and Knaak, J. B. (1965). Inhibition of discrete avoidance behavior by three anticholinesterase agents. *Psychopharmacologia* **7**, 72–76.

Goldman, L. R., Beller, M., and Jackson, R. J. (1990a). Aldicarb food poisonings in California, 1985–1988: Toxicity estimates for humans. *Arch. Environ. Health* **45**, 141–147.

Goldman, L. R., Smith, D. F., Neutra, R. R., Saunders, L. D., Pond, E. M., Stratton, J., Walker, K., Jackson, R. J., and Kizer, K. W. (1990b). Pesticide food poisoning from contaminated watermelons in California. *Arch. Environ. Health* **45**, 229–236.

Gonzales, C. M., and Matos, E. (1984). Induction of sister-chromatid exchanges in cultured human lymphocytes by aldicarb, a carbamate pesticide. *Mutat. Res.* **138**, 175–179.

Grendon, J., Frost, F., and Baum, L. (1994). Chronic health effects among sheep and humans surviving an aldicarb poisoning incident. *Vet. Human Toxicol.* **36**, 218–223.

Guerzoni, M. E., DelCupolo, L., and Ponti, I. (1976). Mutagenic activity of pesticides. *Riv. Sci. Tecnol. Alimenti. Nutr.* **6**, 161–165.

Harris, L. W., Talbot, B. G., Lennox, W. J., and Anderson, D. R. (1989). The relationship between oxime-induced reactivation of carbamylated acetylcholinesterase and antidotal efficacy against carbamate intoxication. *Toxicol. Appl. Pharmacol.* **98**, 128–133.

Hastings, F. L., Main, A. R., and Iverson, F. (1970). Carbamylation and affinity constants of some carbamate inhibitors of acetylcholinesterase and their relation to analogous substrate constants. *J. Agric. Food Chem.* **18**, 497–502.

Hayes, Jr., W. J. (1982). Carbamate pesticides. *In* "Pesticides Studied in Man" (W. J. Hayes, Jr., ed.), Ch. 8, pp. 436–462. Williams and Wilkins, Baltimore.

Heath, D. F. (1961). Abnormal effects. *In* "Organophosphorus Poisons. Anticholinesterases and Related Compounds," Ch. XVI, pp. 338–339. Pergamon Press, New York.

Heise, G. A., and Hudson, J. D. (1985). Effects of pesticides and drugs on working memory in rats: Continuous delayed response. *Pharmacol. Biochem. Behav.* **23**, 591–598.

Hollingshaus, J. G., and Fukuto, T. R. (1982). The effect of exposure to pesticides on delayed neurotoxicity. *In* "Effects of Chronic Exposures to Pesticides on Animal Systems" (J. Chambers and J. D. Yarborough, eds.), pp. 85–120. Raven Press, New York.

Hoque, M. Z. (1972). Carbaryl, a new chemical mutagen. *Curr. Sci.* **41**, 855–856.

Howell, J. M., and Edington, N. (1968). The neurotoxicity of sodium diethyldithiocarbamate in the hen. *J. Neuropathol. Exp. Neurol.* **27**, 464–472.

International Program on Chemical Safety (IPCS) (1986). "Carbamate Pesticides: A General Introduction." Environmental Health Criteria 64. World Health Organization, Geneva.

Ishidate, Jr., M., and Odashima, S. (1977). Chromosome tests with 134 compounds on Chinese hamster cells *in vitro*. A screening for chemical carcinogens. *Mutat. Res.* **48**, 337–354.

Iverson, F. (1975). Affinity and carbamylation rate constants of propoxur in reaction with erythrocyte and serum cholinesterase. *Biochem. Pharmacol.* **24**, 1537–1538.

Johnson, D. J., Graham, D. G., Amarnath, V., Amarnath, K., and Valentine, W. M. (1998). Release of carbon disulfide is a contributing mechanism in the axonopathy produced by N,N-diethyldithiocarbamate. *Toxicol. Appl. Pharmacol.* **148**, 288–296.

Knaak, J. B. (1971). Biological and nonbiological modifications of carbamates. *Bull. W.H.O.* **44**, 121–131.

Krechniak, J., and Foss, W. (1982). Cholinesterase activity in rats treated with propoxur. *Bull. Environ. Contam. Toxicol.* **29**, 599–604.

Kuhr, R. J., and Dorough, H. W. (1976). "Carbamate Insecticides: Chemistry, Biochemistry and Toxicology." CRC Press, Boca Raton, FL.

Kulkarni, A. P., and Hodgson, E. (1980). Metabolism of insecticides by mixed function oxidase systems. *Pharmacol. Ther.* **8**, 379–475.

Kurtz, P. J. (1977). Behavioral and biochemical effects of the carbamate insecticide, Mobam. *Pharmacol. Biochem. Behav.* **6**, 303–310.

Liddle, J. A., Kimbrough, R. D., Needham, L. L., Cline, R. E., Smrek, A. L., Yert, L. W., and Bayse, D. D. (1979). A fatal episode of accidental methomyl poisoning. *Clin. Toxicol.* **15**, 159–167.

Lifshitz, M., Rotenberg, M., Sofer, S., Tamiri, T., Shahak, E., and Almog, S. (1994). Carbamate poisoning and oxime treatment in early children: A clinical and laboratory study. *Pediatrics* **93**, 652–655.

Lifshitz, M., Shahak, E., Bolotin, A., and Sofer, S. (1997). Carbamate poisoning in early childhood and in adults. *Clin. Toxicol.* **35**, 25–27.

Lima, J. S., Alberto, C., and Reis, G. (1995). Poisoning due to illegal use of carbamates as a rodenticide in Rio de Janeiro. *Clin. Toxicol.* **33**, 687–690.

Melnikov, N. N. (1971). Chemistry of pesticides. *Residue Rev.* **36**, 1–480.

Merck Index, 12th ed. (1996). Merck Research Laboratories, Division of Merck and Co., Inc., Whitehouse Station, NJ.

Miller, E., Reinwall, J., Brouwer, J., Ear, F. L., and Loon, E. J. (1969). Effects of acute administration of carbaryl on cholinesterase levels in the CNS of swine. *Toxicol. Appl. Pharmacol.* **14**, 622–623.

Moddel, G., Bilbao, J. M., Payne, D., and Ashby, P. (1978). Disulfiram neuropathy. *Arch. Neurol.* **35**, 658–660.

Moriya, M., Ohta, T., Watanabe, K., Miyazawa, T., Kato, K., and Shirasu, Y. (1983). Further mutagenicity studies on pesticides in bacterial reversion assay systems. *Mutat. Res.* **116**, 185–216.

Morse, D. L., Baker, E. L., Kimbrough, R. D., and Wisseman, C. L. (1979). Propanil-chloracne and methomyl toxicity in workers of a pesticide manufacturing plant. *Clin. Toxicol.* **15**, 13–21.

Namba, T., Nolte, C. T., Jackrel, J., and Grob, D. (1971). Poisoning due to organophosphate insecticides. *Am. J. Med.* **50**, 475–492.

Natoff, I. L., and Reiff, B. (1973). Effect of oximes on the acute toxicity of anticholinesterase carbamates. *Toxicol. Appl. Pharmacol.* **25**, 569–573.

O'Malley, M. (1997). Clinical evaluation of pesticide exposure and poisonings. *Lancet* **349**, 1161–1166.

Onfelt, A. (1983). Spindle disturbances in mammalian cells. I. Changes in the quantity of free sulfhydryl groups in relation to survival and C-mitosis in V79 Chinese hamster cells after treatment with colcemid, diamide, carbaryl and methyl mercury. *Chem. Biol. Interact.* **46**, 201–217.

Pilinskaya, M. A. (1981). Study of the cytogenetic effect of a number of pesticides in human peripheral blood lymphocyte culture at various initial levels of chromosomal aberrations. *Cytol. Genet.* **15**, 74–76.

Pilinskaya, M. A. (1982). The cytogenetic effect of pesticide pirimor in a human peripheral blood lymphocyte culture *in vivo* and *in vitro*. *Cytol. Genet.* **16**, 45–49.

Rashid, K. A., and Mumma, R. O. (1986). Screening pesticides for their ability to damage bacterial DNA. *J. Environ. Sci. Health Part B* **21**, 319–334.

Reiner, E. (1971). Spontaneous reactivation of the phosphorylated and carbamylated cholinesterases. *Bull. W.H.O.* **44**, 109–112.

Remaley, A. T., Hicks, D. G., Kane, M. D., and Shaw, L. M. (1988). Laboratory assessment of poisoning with a carbamate insecticide. *Clin. Chem.* **34**, 1933–1936.

Richardson, E. M., and Batteese, R. I. (1973). An incident of Zectran poisoning. *J. Maine Med. Assoc.* **64**, 158–159.

Risher, J. F., Mink, F. L., and Stara, J. F. (1987). The toxicologic effects of the carbamate insecticide aldicarb in mammals: A review. *Environ. Health Res.* **72**, 267–281.

Ruppert, P. H., Cook, L. L., Dean, K. F., and Reiter, L. W. (1983). Acute behavioral toxicity of carbaryl and propoxur in adult rats. *Pharmacol. Biochem. Behav.* **18**, 569–584.

Ryan, A. J. (1971). The metabolism of pesticidal carbamates. *CRC Crit. Rev. Toxicol.* **1**, 33–54.

Sanderson, D. M. (1961). Treatment of poisoning by anticholinesterase insecticides in the rat. *J. Pharm. Pharmacol.* **13**, 435–442.

Santolucito, J. A., and Morrison, G. (1971). EEG of Rhesus monkeys following prolonged low-level feeding of pesticides. *Toxicol. Appl. Pharmacol.* **19**, 147–154.

Schlagbauer, B. G. L., and Schlagbauer, A. W. J. (1972). The metabolism of carbamate pesticides—A literature analysis. Part I and Part II. *Residue Rev.* **42**, 1–84; **42**, 85–90.

Simpson, G. R., and Bermingham, S. (1977). Poisoning by carbamate pesticides. *Med. J. Austr.* **2**, 148–149.

Singh, J. M. (1973). Decreased performance behavior with carbaryl—An indication of clinical toxicity. *Clin. Toxicol.* **6**, 97–108.

Smalley, H. E., O'Hara, P. J., Bridges, C. H., and Radeleff, R. D. (1969). The effect of chronic carbaryl administration on the neuromuscular system of swine. *Toxicol. Appl. Pharmacol.* **14**, 409–419.

Sterman, A. B., and Varma, A. (1983). Evaluating human neurotoxicity of the pesticide aldicarb: When man becomes the experimental animal. *Neurobehav. Toxicol. Teratol.* **5**, 493–495.

Sterri, S. H., Rognerud, B., Fiskum, S. E., and Lyngaas, S. (1979). Effect of toxogonin and P2S in the toxicity of carbamates and organophosphorus compounds. *Acta Pharmacol. Toxicol.* **45**, 9–15.

Tabershaw, I. R., and Cooper, W. C. (1966). Sequelae of acute organic phosphate poisoning. *J. Occup. Med.* **8**, 5–20.

Takahashi, R. N., Poli, A., Morato, G. S., Lima, T. C. M., and Zanin, M. (1991). Effect of age on behavioral and physiological responses to carbaryl in rats. *Neurotox. Teratol.* **13**, 21–26.

Tobin, J. S. (1970). Carbofuran a new carbamate insecticide. *J. Occup. Med.* **12**, 16–19.

Umehara, F., Izumo, S., Arimura, K., and Osame, M. (1991). Polyneuropathy induced by m-tolyl methyl carbamate intoxication. *J. Neurol.* **238**, 47–48.

Vandekar, M. (1965). Observations on the toxicity of carbaryl, folithion and 3-isopropoxyphenyl-N-methylcarbamate in a village-scale trial in Southern Nigeria. *Bull. W.H.O.* **33**, 107–115.

Vandekar, M., Heyadat, S., Plestina, R., and Ahmady, G. (1968). A study of the safety of O-isopropoxyphenyl-methylcarbamate in an operational field trial in Iran. *Bull. W.H.O.* **38**, 609–623.

Vandekar, M., Plestina, R., and Wilhelm, K. (1971). Toxicity of carbamates for mammals. *Bull. W.H.O.* **44**, 241–249.

Vassilieff, I., and Ecobichon, D. J. (1983). Acute toxicity of aminocarb in male rats and inhibition of their esterases. *Bull. Environ. Contam. Toxicol.* **31**, 326–330.

Viter, V. F. (1978). Continuous and intermittent effect of carbaryl on certain behavior reactions of experimental animals. *Gig. Sanit.* **43**, 33–34.

Waibel, P. E., Johnson, E. L., Pomeroy, B. S., and Howard, L. B. (1957). Toxicity of tetraethylthiuram disulfide in chicks, poults and goslings. *Poultry Sci.* **36**, 697–701.

Watson, C. P., Ashby, P., and Bilbao, J. M. (1980). Disulfiram neuropathy. *Can. Med. Assoc. J.* **123**, 123–126.

Wilhelm, K., and Reiner, E. (1973). Effect of sample storage on human blood cholinesterase activity after inhibition by carbamates. *Bull. W.H.O.* **48**, 235–238.

Wilkinson, C. F., ed. (1976). "Insecticide Biochemistry and Physiology." Plenum Press, New York.

Wills, J. H., Jameson, E., and Coulston, F. (1968). Effects of oral doses of carbaryl on man. *Clin. Toxicol.* **1**, 265–271.

Wojciechowski, J. P., Kaur, P., and Sabharwal, P. S. (1982). Induction of ouabain resistance in V79 cells by four carbamate pesticides. *Environ. Res.* **29**, 48–53.

Wyrobek, A. J., Watchmaker, G., Gordon, L., Wong, K., Moore, II, D., and Whorton, D. (1981). Sperm shape abnormalities in carbaryl-exposed employees. *Environ. Health Perspec.* **40**, 255–265.

Yakim, V. S. (1967). The maximum permissible concentration of Sevin in the air of the work zone. *Hyg. Sanit.* **32**, 32–37.

Zaki, M. H., Moran, D., and Harris, D. (1982). Pesticides in ground-water: The aldicarb story in Suffolk County, New York. *Am. J. Public Health* **72**, 1391–1395.

CHAPTER

53

Aldicarb: Current Science-Based Approaches in Risk Assessment

Abraham J. Tobia, Pierre-Gerard Pontal, Peter McCahon and Neil G. Carmichael
Aventis CropScience

Joseph P. Rieth
JSC, Inc.

Rick Williams
RTI, Inc.

53.1 INTRODUCTION

Toxicology-based human health risk assessment is evolving continuously. As new data are developed allowing greater understanding of chemical effects, dose relationships, and modes of action, improvements in the reliability of the subsequent risk assessments follow. This is particularly true in the case of pesticides, because this class of chemicals has undergone a virtually continuous process of registration and reregistration since the advent of the Environmental Protection Agency in the United States (U.S. EPA) as well as increased regulatory activity in Europe and Japan since the early 1970s. As a result, each currently registered pesticide has a very robust toxicological database from which one can assess potential health risks, and the wealth of information continues to grow as new study types are developed and conducted.

With the advent of the Food Quality Protection Act of 1996 (FQPA) in the United States further emphasis has been placed on the quality of the risk assessment. Whereas previous risk assessment practices did indeed ensure the protection of infants and children, with FQPA emphasis is now placed on increasing the certainty of the assessment. A variety of new science-based techniques have been and are being developed to increase the certainty of the risk assessment process.

This chapter describes new approaches, which reduce the uncertainty in the risk assessment of aldicarb. It begins with a description of aldicarb chemistry, uses, and biological mode of action. This is followed by a brief overview of risk assessment practices in the crop protection industry. The next section describes the available toxicology and exposure studies used to evaluate the potential risk of the product. Finally, two elements of aldicarb risk assessment are presented. The first demonstrates the use of the pharmacokinetics of reversibility of cholinesterase inhibition following aldicarb exposure to adjust the exposure component of the risk assessment. The second describes special dermal toxicity studies used to evaluate the potential toxicity to occupational users of the aldicarb-formulated product Temik

53.2 ALDICARB: DESCRIPTION, USE AND BIOLOGICAL MODE OF ACTION

Technical aldicarb belongs to the *N*-methyl carbamate chemical family. The pure (technical) material is a white crystalline solid with a water solubility of approximately 6000 ppm at 25°C and is stable at room temperature. The empirical formula of aldicarb is $C_7H_{14}N_2O_2S$, with a molecular weight of 190.3. The structural formula is shown in Fig. 53.1, and the (IUPAC) and Chemical Abstract Service (CAS) names are as follows:

IUPAC—2-methyl-2-(methylthio)propionaldehyde *O*-(methylcarbamoyl) oxime

CAS—2-methyl-2-(methylthio)propanal *O*-[(methylamino) carbonyl]

CAS number—116-06-30

Aldicarb is a carbamate insecticide used in agriculture for the control of insects, mites, and nematodes. The product is mar-

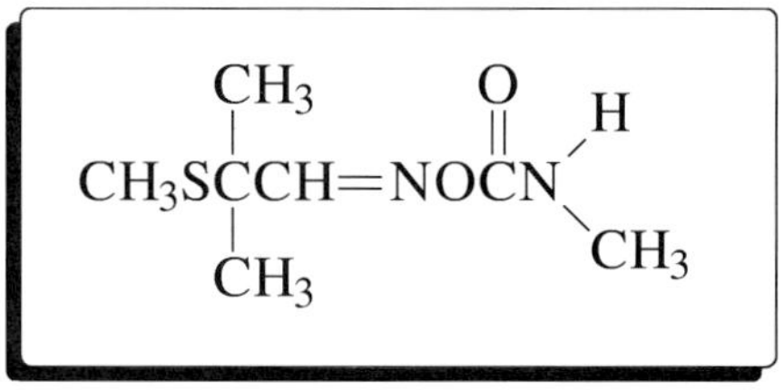

$$CH_3SCCH=NOCN$$

Figure 53.1 Structural formula of aldicarb.

keted under the trade name Temik as a 15% (active ingredient) granule in the United States, and as a 5, 10, or 15% granule worldwide. Aldicarb has a number of unique characteristics which make it an invaluable tool for crop protection. First, aldicarb controls pests from three divergent animal groups: insects, mites, and nematodes. This range of activity for a single product is rare for this class of crop protection chemicals, and because of it, a single application of aldicarb can replace two or more applications of alternative pesticides. Second, aldicarb has systemic activity whereby the product can be applied beneath the soil, and uptake through the roots allows distribution throughout the plant, with subsequent control of chewing and sucking pests. Aldicarb is formulated solely as a dust-free granule and is not produced as a liquid formulation. This type of formulation significantly reduces potential dermal and inhalation exposures, which makes the product much safer from an occupational perspective. Granular Temik is also much safer for the environment than liquid-formulated insecticides. It affords longer control, reducing the number of applications. Also, it is applied beneath the surface of the soil to a depth of up to several inches. Both of these factors significantly reduce the negative impact on beneficial insects, fish, birds, and other wildlife because the product is not available for exposure.

Aldicarb was discovered by Union Carbide Corporation in 1962. The first U.S. registration of Temik was received in 1970 for use on cotton. The four major crops on which Temik is currently used are citrus, cotton, peanuts, and potatoes, and it is also registered for use on nine other crops in the United States. Temik is typically applied via tractor-mounted equipment used to place the granules at a depth of 2–6 inches beneath the surface of the soil. Developments in positive displacement metering devices allow the application of precise amounts of the material into the application area. It is often applied in conjunction with other cultural practices such as planting, cultivating, or fertilizing. Most often, application is once per use season.

Technical aldicarb is produced as an integrated 35% solution and then formulated into a granular product. Two types of granules are produced, one made of corncob grit and the other with gypsum clay. Both granules have binding agents and the production method produces a virtually dust-free product.

Carbamate insecticides are reversible cholinesterase inhibitors for which recovery is primarily a function of the rate at which the active chemical is hydrolytically decarbamylated by the cholinesterase enzyme (Alvarez, 1992; O'Brien, 1967; Rotenberg and Almog, 1995). This process, commonly called spontaneous reactivation, is often measured in minutes. This is in contrast to the organophosphates, which are generally irreversible inhibitors of cholinesterase; the inhibition is due to significantly stronger binding between the chemical and enzyme by the process of phosphorylation. Recovery following exposure to organophoshates is primarily through prolonged reactivation of the inactivated enzyme and synthesis of new enzyme, and is typically measured in days or weeks. It is primarily because of the difference in recovery times that carbamates are considered to pose significantly less risk to exposed humans, relative to organophosphate repeated exposure.

53.3 CURRENT PRACTICES IN PESTICIDE RISK ASSESSMENT

The general process of human health risk assessment based on toxicological data is similar for all chemicals, that is, for pharmaceuticals, crop protection chemicals and industrial and naturally occurring chemicals.

At a minimum, two types of information are required for a reliable risk assessment, knowledge of the "hazard" the chemical may cause, and data on possible levels of exposure to humans (Cohrssen and Covello, 1989). Hazard refers to the potential toxic effect or effects the material may cause; this information is typically gleaned either from descriptive toxicity tests in animals or from controlled studies in humans such as clinical trials or epidemiological studies (or a combination of both). Exposure data may be known exactly, as in the case of the prescribed dose of a pharmaceutical, or can be measured on those individuals coming into contact with the chemical, using a variety of techniques (U.S. EPA, 1987).

In essence, human health risk assessment involves the determination of a level of exposure to a chemical which is expected to be safe for humans. This process is based on the well-established principles that for every toxic effect there must be a dose sufficiently large to cause that effect. Comparison of hazard and exposure data will not provide a safe exposure level, but can indicate if an exposure level is safe.

Hazard information for registered pesticides is based on a very extensive toxicological database. Table 53.1 provides a listing of the types of toxicological studies conducted on aldicarb, which have been cited, reviewed and accepted by multiple international regulatory authorities [Baron, 1994; California EPA, 1998; Food and Agriculture Organization–World Health Organization (FAO/WHO), 1992; International Agency for Research on Cancer (IARC), 1991; International Programme on Chemical Safety (IPCS), 1991]. Studies are performed to examine the full spectrum of possible toxicological effects. These include acute, short-term, and long-term studies; tests for carcinogenicity and mutagenicity; reproductive and developmental effects; and neurotoxicity tests. The studies are conducted by various routes of exposure, for example, oral, dermal, and inhalation, and the studies are typically designed to approximate the route and duration of a potential human exposure.

Table 53.1
Toxicological Studies Conducted on Aldicarb

Acute
   Oral LD_{50}
   Dermal LD_{50}
   Inhalation LC_{50}
   Potential for eye irritation
   Potential for skin irritation
   Potential for sensitization
Subchronic
   7-day dietary study in rats
   90-day dietary study in rats
   7-day dietary study in mice
   14-day dietary study in dogs
   90-day dietary study in dogs
Chronic
   2-year dietary study in rats (two studies)
   2-year dietary study in rats with a mixture of aldicarb, aldicarb sulfoxide, and aldicarb sulfone
Neurotoxicity
   Acute neurotoxicity study
   90-day neurotoxicity study
   Developmental neurotoxicity study
Human volunteer studies
   Controlled clinical studies (two studies)
   Worker exposure monitoring
Studies on product formulations
   21-day dermal study
   Oral LD_{50}
   Dermal LD_{50}
   Inhalation LC_{50}
   Potential for eye irritation
   Potential for skin irritation

Table 53.2
Human Health Risk Assessments for Aldicarb

Acute dietary exposure
Chronic dietary exposure

Short-term dermal occupational exposure
Intermediate-term dermal occupational exposure
Long-term dermal occupational exposure

Short-term inhalation occupational exposure
Intermediate-term inhalation occupational exposure
Long-term inhalation occupational exposure

The risk assessment is performed by first determining the human exposure scenario of interest and then selecting the toxicological study of most relevance to the human situation as well as the relevant end point in this study (usually the most sensitive). Thus, human health risk assessment involves a number of different risk assessments, which reflect each particular human exposure scenario. A listing of the types of risk assessments required for aldicarb can be found in Table 53.2. The potential routes of exposure for aldicarb include oral exposure, from low-level residues in food, and dermal and inhalation exposure of workers handling the product.

Once the end point and study of interest for the appropriate risk assessment have been determined, the next step in the process is the determination of the no-observed-adverse-effect level (NOAEL). The NOAEL for the study is the dose level at which no hazard has been detected. Because these studies are generally conducted in animals, the NOAEL for a given study represents a safe dose for the species tested. The prediction of a safe dose for humans is derived by dividing the NOAEL from the animal study by an appropriate safety factor (also called

uncertainty factor); thus the safe human dose is lower than the NOAEL from the animal study. The safe dose for human intake is described in a number of ways, for example, a dose "without appreciable health risk" (WHO, 1987) and reference dose (RfD; U.S. EPA, 1993), which was previously known as allowable or acceptable daily intake (ADI).

The safety factor historically considered appropriate to provide a safe dose for human exposure for pesticides is 100 when it is derived from an appropriate animal study; typically the RfD is set as the NOAEL from an appropriate animal study divided by 100. For excellent reviews of the origin and justification for the use of a 100-fold safety factor in human health risk assessment see Swartout et al. (1998), Dourson et al. (1992), and Renwick and Lazarus (1998). The 100-fold safety factor takes into consideration two sources of uncertainty in the risk assessment: (*i*) the toxicology study was conducted in animals but the objective is the protection of humans (interspecies extrapolation); (*ii*) there is variability in the human population and sensitive individuals need to be protected (intraspecies extrapolation). A 10-fold margin of safety is generally considered to provide adequate protection for each of these sources of uncertainty, hence the margin of safety of 100, which accounts for both sources simultaneously in the risk assessment. For the protection of infants and children, an additional safety factor with a default value of $10\times$ has been mandated by FQPA (1996). When implemented, this will create a safety margin of 1000.

Once the RfD has been established, it can be compared to the expected exposure. If anticipated human exposures are less than the RfD, then such exposures are considered safe. A related approach is to divide the NOAEL by the exposure value and calculate the margin of safety value directly. With this method, also called the margins of exposure (MOE) approach, values greater than 100 (or other numbers if considered appropriate) are considered adequate to protect human health.

In cases where the initial risk assessment indicates that the exposure is higher than the RfD, additional measures must be taken to ensure human safety. The risk assessment can be improved by reducing the uncertainty contained within it. This can be accomplished by developing new information, which allows a better understanding of the biological processes resulting in the hazard, and also by improving the knowledge of the exposures actually taking place. Direct measurement of the true exposure levels through the conduct of a worker exposure study may demonstrate that the real exposure values are less than the estimated values. In addition exposure levels can be closely estimated from knowledge of related products for which exposure studies have been conducted.

There are also ways in which improved toxicology information can be used to increase the accuracy of risk assessments by reducing the uncertainty. For example, if the mechanism of toxicity in the animal model can be demonstrated with certainty, and if it can be shown that this mechanism does not exist in humans, then a higher NOAEL based on another toxicity end point may be appropriate. This would have the effect of increasing the safety relative to the exposure value. Another way to reduce the uncertainty is to study the effects of the chemical in humans if human exposure will occur as a result of the product use. If the information used in the risk assessment has been determined in a well-conducted study in humans and demonstrates that there is concordance between the animal and human databases, then the safety factor used for the interspecies extrapolation is not necessary, and a safety factor of 10 (for the intraspecies extrapolation only) is considered adequate. Therefore, it is normal and appropriate practice to utilize the human study to augment the derivation a NOAEL and the RfD.

In the past, risk assessments were conducted primarily for long-term or lifetime exposure to pesticides. However, more recently, regulatory agencies (such as U.S. EPA) have also begun to conduct risk assessments for acute (1 day), short-term (1–7 days), and intermediate (7 days to 3 months) time periods for oral (dietary), dermal, and inhalation routes of exposure. The process is generally the same as described previously, except that the RfD approach is used to assess chronic risk whereas the MOE approach is used for the short-term and intermediate assessments. There are other methodologies used to calculate the short-term assessments, but this chapter will focus mainly on the methodology utilized by the U.S. EPA.

It should be noted that there are other risk assessment methods which do not rely on the NOAEL, such as the benchmark dose (BMD) approach, which describe the dose–response data mathematically; then a point-of-departure (POD) approach is used in which a predefined effect level, such as dose predicted to give a 10% effect (ED_{10}), is used rather than the NOAEL. The safety factor is then applied to the dose–response curve with the POD as the starting point for the hazard component of the risk assessment. These types of models have advantages in certain situations, for example, where no NOAEL has been established in a study. These models have not been widely used in a regulatory context because there is currently no scientific consensus to drive policy decisions.

53.4 ALDICARB TOXICOLOGY PROFILE

53.4.1 SUMMARY OF ALDICARB TOXICITY

Aldicarb has a very robust toxicity database including developmental, reproductive, and neurotoxicity studies, as well as a developmental neurotoxicity study. Aldicarb has high acute toxicity. Toxicity is that commonly associated with acetylcholinesterase inhibition (ChEI) caused by a carbamate pesticide, that is, cholinergic symptoms. These symptoms are dose-dependent, are rapidly reversible, and do not occur at expected human exposure levels. Aldicarb is neither genotoxic nor carcinogenic. It does not cause developmental or reproductive effects in the absence of maternal toxicity.

The degradation pathway for aldicarb involves a combination of oxidation to aldicarb sulfoxide and then aldicarb sulfone and hydrolysis of parent, sulfoxide, and sulfone, to low toxicity compounds.

53.4.2 ALDICARB ACUTE TOXICITY

Tables 53.3 and 53.4 provide acute toxicity data for aldicarb technical and for the formulated product Temik 15G. Aldicarb technical is highly toxic by the oral, dermal, and inhalation routes. Aldicarb is not a sensitizer. Aldicarb sulfoxide has similar potency with regard to acetylcholinesterase inhibition as aldicarb itself. Aldicarb sulfone is approximately 25 times less toxic than either aldicarb or aldicarb sulfoxide.

53.4.3 ALDICARB SUBCHRONIC TOXICITY

In assessing the subchronic toxicity of aldicarb, the most sensitive indicator of exposure is cholinesterase inhibition. A number of subchronic and subacute (e.g., 14-day) oral studies have been conducted on aldicarb, aldicarb sulfoxide, and aldicarb sulfone. Results from study to study are consistent; for the sake of simplicity, only the longer term oral studies and a 21-day dermal study are discussed. Table 53.5 provides a summary of these studies.

In an oral study, rats were fed aldicarb in their diet for 93 days at dose levels of 0, 0.02, 0.1, and 0.5 mg/kg/day. The no-

Table 53.3

Acute Toxicity Data for Aldicarb Technical[a]

Study	Species	Findings	Toxicity category
Acute oral toxicity	Rat	$LD_{50} = 1.2$ mg/kg	1
Acute dermal toxicity	Rabbit	$LD_{50} = 544$ mg/kg	II
Acute inhalation toxicity	Rat	$LC_{50} = 0.0039$ mg/l	I
Primary eye irritation	Rabbit	Moderately irritating	III
Primary dermal irritation	Rabbit	Slightly irritating	IV
Dermal sensitization	Guinea pig	Not a sensitizer	Not applicable

[a] Aldicarb technical is approximately 35% aldicarb in dichloromethane.

Table 53.4
Acute Toxicity Data For Temik 15 G

Study	Species	Findings[a]	Toxicity category
Acute oral toxicity	Rat	$LD_{50} = 2.14$ (m)/2.46 (f) mg/kg	I
Acute dermal toxicity	Rabbit	$LD_{50} > 2000$ mg/kg	III
Acute inhalation toxicity	Rat	Not applicable— granular product	
Primary eye irritation	Rabbit	Moderately irritating	III
Primary dermal irritation	Rabbit	Not irritating (21-day dermal study)	IV
Dermal sensitization	Guinea pig	No data—technical is not a sensitizer	Not applicable

[a] m = male; f = female.

observed-adverse-effect level was 0.5 mg/kg/day based on the lack of effects on red blood cell ChE. In addition, body weight and food consumption were decreased at the highest dose level.

An oral dog study was conducted to investigate the ChEI dose–response curve of aldicarb. During the 5-week study, the dogs were fed diets mixed with aldicarb technical at levels of 0, 0.35, 0.7, and 2 ppm (0.013, 0.023, and 0.069 mg/kg/day in males, and 0.012, 0.025, and 0.067 mg/kg/day in females). There was neither mortality nor any changes in body weight, food consumption, or clinical observation data indicative of a compound effect. A NOAEL based on erythrocyte cholinesterase was established at 0.07 mg/kg/day.

There have been a number of subchronic and subacute studies using aldicarb sulfoxide and aldicarb sulfone. As stated in the acute toxicity section, the sulfoxide metabolite is comparable in toxicity to aldicarb; the sulfone metabolite is less toxic. In each case, ChEI is the most sensitive indicator of exposure.

Table 53.6
Acute Neurotoxicity Study in Rats: Cholinesterase Inhibition in Females—Percentage Relative to Control, 0.75 h

Dose (mg/kg)	% Inhibition		
	Plasma	RBC	Brain
0.05	46.6	8.6	5.1
0.1	73.3	30.6	15.6
0.5	94.1	54.2	50.4

53.4.4 ALDICARB NEUROTOXICITY STUDIES

There is a complete neurotoxicity database on aldicarb consisting of acute, subchronic, and developmental neurotoxicity studies. In addition, there is a "time to peak behavioral effects" study of a single oral administration of aldicarb technical. Also, there are acute neurotoxicity studies on both aldicarb sulfoxide and aldicarb sulfone. As discussed earlier, effects on ChEI are always the most sensitive indicators of both exposure and toxicity in the case of aldicarb.

The aldicarb dose–effect relationship for ChEI is consistent across studies. A dose of 0.05 mg/kg/day gives the first indications of erythrocyte cholinesterase inhibition with no concomitant brain cholinesterase inhibition or behavioral changes. At 0.2 mg/kg/day, marked erythrocyte ChEI is observed accompanied by measurable inhibition in the brain and moderate clinical signs. Higher dose levels result in marked erythrocyte and brain ChEI and clinical signs, the magnitude of which increases with dose.

A summary of the ChEI effects from three aldicarb neurotoxicity studies is provided in Tables 53.6–53.8. In these tables, data on ChEI are shown for females only, to simplify the presentation, but the effects for males show the same magnitude of effects.

Table 53.5
Subchronic Toxicity Data for Aldicarb

Study	Species	Dose Level (mg/kg/day)	NOAEL[a] (mg/kg/day)	LOEL[a] (mg/kg/day)	Toxicological endpoints
Oral toxicity, 93-day	Rat	0, 0.02, 0.1, 0.5	0.1	0.5	Plasma ChEI at the highest dose tested. In addition, food consumption and body weight were decreased at this dose level. RBC ChEI was not affected at all dose levels.
Oral toxicity, 5-week	Dog	0, 0.35, 0.7, and 2 ppm; 0, 0.013, 0.023, and 0.069 mg/kg/day (m); 0, 0.012, 0.025, and 0.067 mg/kg/day (f)	0.023 (m), 0.025 (f)	0.069 (m), 0.067 (f)	Plasma ChEI was over 20% compared to controls at the highest dose tested. RBC ChEI was not affected at all dose levels.
Dermal toxicity, 21-day, Temik 15G	Rat	0, 100, 250, 500	100	250	Plasma ChEI at 250 mg/kg/day dose level. RBC NOAEL was 250 mg/kg/day; brain ChEI NOAEL was at least 500 mg/kg/day.

[a] m = male; f = female.

Table 53.7
Time to Peak Behavioral Effects Study in Rats, Females—Percentage Relative to Predose Value, 1 h

DOSE (mg/kg)	% Inhibition plasma	% Inhibition RBC
0.1	79.7	39.5
0.4	93.1	62.2
0.6	93.9	78.4

In an oral feeding developmental neurotoxicity study in rats, the dose levels were 0, 0.05, 0.1, and 0.3 mg/kg/day. This study provides strong evidence that aldicarb does not cause permanent effects on the nervous system, and that the young are not more sensitive to the effects of aldicarb than mature animals. The maternal NOAEL was 0.05 mg/kg/day based on miosis at 0.1 mg/kg/day. The developmental NOAEL was 0.05 mg/kg/day based on postweaning body weight decrement, reduced hindlimb grip strength, and foot splay in F_1 females on postpartum day 35.

Cholinesterase (ChE) activity was measured in the maternal animals on gestation day 7, and lactation days 7 and 11. Cholinesterase inhibition was not detected at 0.05 mg/kg/day, probably because the blood was collected two hours postdose and the enzyme had spontaneously reactivated by this time. In a subchronic toxicity study, this same dose level resulted in 24% erythrocyte ChEI. Thus, the systemic toxicity NOAEL was 0.05 mg/kg/day and the maternal NOAEL for red blood cell (RBC) ChEI was similar.

These results demonstrate the lack of increased sensitivity to developing animals relative to adults because there were no developmental effects even in the presence of slight maternal ChEI.

In an acute gavage study, rats were treated with aldicarb sulfoxide at doses of 0, 0.05, 0.1, and 0.5 mg/kg/day. Cholinesterase activity was not measured in this study. There were no deaths in the study and no significant effects on body weights or body weight gain. Food intake values were reduced for males in the 0.5 mg/kg/day dose. Significant functional observation battery (FOB) effects were seen at the 0.5-mg/kg/day dose level at the time of peak effect. Significant decreases in motor activity were also seen at this same dose. There were no neuropathology effects. The NOAEL for FOB and motor activity was 0.1 mg/kg/day; the NOAEL for histopathology was 0.5 mg/kg/day.

Table 53.8
13-Week Neurotoxicity Study in Rats: Cholinesterase Inhibition Females at 4 Weeks Relative to Control, 0.75 h

Dose (mg/kg/day)	% Inhibition		
	Plasma	RBC	Brain
0.05	64.9	24.0	2.1
0.2	92.7	71.1	33.1
0.3	94.9	70.3	56.7

In an acute neurotoxicity gavage study in rats, the dose levels for aldicarb sulfone were 0, 1, 10, and 20 mg/kg/day. Cholinesterase activity was not measured in this study. No deaths occurred in the study. At the 20-mg/kg/day dose level, males and females showed significant decreases in food consumption, and males exhibited a significant reduction in body weight gain. At the time of peak effect, significant FOB effects were seen at the 10- and 20-mg/kg/day dose levels. Neuropathological evaluations revealed no effects at any dose. The NOAEL for FOB and motor activity was 1 mg/kg/day; the NOAEL for histopathology was 20 mg/kg/day.

53.4.5 ALDICARB DEVELOPMENTAL AND REPRODUCTIVE TOXICITY STUDIES

There is a complete developmental and reproductive toxicity database including a developmental neurotoxicity study (discussed in the previous section). Aldicarb does not cause developmental or reproductive effects in studies in the absence of maternal (or parental) toxicity. The following section discusses the study results, and these are summarized in Table 53.9.

In an oral gavage developmental study, rats were given doses of 0, 0.125, 0.25, and 0.5 mg/kg/day. Maternal toxicity was indicated by maternal death and clinical signs were observed at the upper dose levels. Gestational parameters were not affected. No increased incidence of malformations was observed in the absence of clear maternal toxicity. The NOAEL for fetal toxicity was 0.25 mg/kg/day; fetal effects at the highest dose included dilated ventricles.

In an oral gavage rabbit developmental study with doses of 0, 0.1, 0.25, and 0.5 mg/kg/day, there were no fetal effects. Maternal toxicity was clearly established in the upper two dose levels with an increase in severity being observed at the highest dose level tested. The maternal NOAEL was 0.1 mg/kg/day based on decreased body weight and clinical signs.

In a two-generation reproductive toxicity study, rats were fed a diet with 0, 2, 5, 10, or 20 ppm (ca. 0, 0.1, 0.25, 0.5, or 1.0 mg/kg/day). Cholinesterase inhibition and body weight changes in parents were observed at the upper dose levels. The maternal NOAEL was 0.25 mg/kg/day. The reproductive NOAEL was 0.5 mg/kg/day based on decreased pup weight and reduced viability. There were no reproductive effects in the absence of parental toxicity.

53.4.6 ALDICARB MUTAGENICITY STUDIES

Studies covering gene mutations, chromosomal aberrations, unscheduled DNA synthesis, and dominant lethal effects were all negative for aldicarb. There is no concern for mutagenicity for aldicarb. A limited battery of genotoxicity studies on aldicarb sulfoxide and sulfone are also negative.

Table 53.9
Developmental and Reproductive Toxicity Data for Aldicarb

Study	Species	Dose level	NOAEL (mg/kg/day)	LOEL (mg/kg/day)	Toxicological endpoints
Developmental toxicity	Rat	0, 0.125, 0.25, 0.5 mg/kg/day	Maternal toxicity, 0.125; fetal toxicity, 0.25	Maternal, 0.25; fetal, 0.5	Maternal toxicity was indicated by death, reduced body weight gain and food consumption, and clinical signs of cholinesterase inhibition at 0.5 mg/kg/day, and reduced food consumption and body weights at 0.25 mg/kg/day. Fetal toxicity was indicated by increased dilated ventricles and reduced ossification of the 6th sternebrae.
Developmental toxicity	Rabbit	0, 0.1, 0.25, 0.5 mg/kg/day	Maternal toxicity, 0.1; fetal toxicity: 0.5	Maternal, 0.25; fetal, >0.5	Signs of maternal toxicity included pale kidneys, hydroceles on oviducts, and decreased body weight. There was no fetal toxicity.
Two-generation reproductive toxicity	Rat	0, 2, 5, 10, 20 ppm; ca. 0, 0.1, 0.25, 0.5, 1.0 mg/kg/day	Parental, 0.25; reproductive, 0.5	Parental: 0.5; reproductive, 1.0	Maternal toxicity included plasma and RBC Cheri and body weight changes at the upper dose levels. The reproductive LOEL is based on decreased pup weights and reduced viability.

53.4.7 ALDICARB CHRONIC TOXICITY AND ONCOGENICITY STUDIES

Aldicarb has been shown to have no oncogenic potential when administered to rats and mice in lifetime experiments. Cholinesterase inhibition is the most sensitive indicator of exposure in chronic studies in rats and dogs. A discussion of chronic toxicity and oncogenicity data follows and Table 53.10 summarizes the study results.

In a 2-year study, rats were fed aldicarb at levels of 0, 1, 10, and 30 ppm in the diet (equivalent to ca. 0, 0.05, 0.5, and 1.5 mg/kg/day). There were no compound-related effects on sur-

Table 53.10
Chronic Toxicity and Oncogenicity Data for Aldicarb

Study	Species	Dose levels	NOAEL[a] (mg/kg/day)	LOEL[a] (mg/kg/day)	Toxicological endpoints
Chronic toxicity or oncogenicity	Rat	0, 1, 10, 30 ppm; ca. 0, 0.05, 0.5, 1.5 mg/kg/day	0.05 (m), 0.59 (f)	0.5 (m), 1.5 (f)	Highest dose tested equivalent to greater than an LD_{50} dosage when administered by gavage. Only clinical effect was limited use of the tail at the highest dose tested. Body weights and body weight gains reduced at this dose level. Atrophy of the iris at the high dose.
Oncogenicity	Rat	0, 2, 6 ppm; ca. 0, 0.1, 0.3	Not evaluated	Not evaluated	None.
Chronic toxicity or oncogenicity	Rat	0, 0.3 mg/kg/day for aldicarb; other doses for other materials (e.g., aldicarb sulfoxide)	Not evaluated	Not evaluated	There were slight increases in mortality and slight depressions in growth at certain stages for some of the test materials.
Oncogenicity	Mouse	0, 0.1, 0.3, 0.7 mg/kg/day	Not evaluated	Not evaluated	Mortality and an increase in hematomas and lymphoid neoplasia were observed at the highest dose tested.
Oncogenicity	Mouse	0, 2, 6 ppm; ca. 0, 0.29, and 0.86 mg/kg/day	Not evaluated	Not evaluated	None.
Chronic toxicity	Dog	0, 1, 2, 5, 10 ppm; ca. 0, 0.027, 0.055, 0.13 mg/kg/day	0.027	0.055	Plasma ChEI occurred at 0.055 mg/kg/day. Brain ChEI occurred at 0.13 mg/kg/day.

[a]m = male; f = female.

vival. It should be noted that the high dose of 1.5 mg/kg/day was greater than the LD_{50} and was tolerated every day over the course of the study. This was possible because the aldicarb was administered via the diet, and the total dose was ingested in fractionated amounts throughout the day, allowing for ChEI reversibility between consumption periods. The principal clinical effect observed was limited use of the tail in high-dose males and females. Body weights and body weight gains were reduced in high-dose males and females. Also, atrophy of the iris occurred in this dose group. There was no evidence of direct organ toxicity, and no evidence of oncogenic effects. The NOAELs were 0.05 mg/kg/day in males and 0.59 mg/kg/day in females based on erythrocyte ChEI. It is noteworthy that the rats could tolerate such a dosing regimen over their entire lifespan, demonstrating that recovery is complete, accumulation of aldicarb does not occur, and there are no persistent effects following such exposure.

In a National Cancer Institute (NCI) study, rats were fed aldicarb in the diet at concentrations of 0, 2, and 6 ppm (equivalent to ca. 0, 0.1, and 0.3 mg/kg/day). There was no mortality attributed to aldicarb and no effect on body weight was noted. It was concluded that aldicarb was not oncogenic; the NOAEL was the highest dose tested.

In a third rat study, rats were fed aldicarb at dose levels of 0 and 0.3 mg/kg/day. In addition, other groups were fed aldicarb sulfoxide at dose levels of 0, 0.3, and 0.6 mg/kg/day, aldicarb sulfone at dose levels of 0, 0.6, and 0.24 mg/kg/day, or a mixture of aldicarb sulfoxide and aldicarb sulfone at doses of 0, 0.5, and 1.2 mg/kg/day. Neither aldicarb nor either of its major metabolites was found to be oncogenic. There were slight increases in mortality and slight depressions in growth at certain stages for some of the test materials. Cholinesterase activity was measured at 6, 12, and 24 months during the study. Plasma, erythrocyte, and brain ChE activity were examined 24 hours after animals were removed from test diets. No ChEI was noted other than a possible slight inhibition with respect to plasma ChE.

There have been three mouse oncogenicity studies conducted on aldicarb. The first is a National Cancer Institute study in which mice were fed 0, 2, or 6 ppm of aldicarb in the diet (equivalent to ca. 0, 0.29, and 0.86 mg/kg/day). It was concluded that aldicarb was not oncogenic. No effects on mortality or body weights were noted.

In a second study, mice were fed aldicarb at doses of 0, 0.1, 0.2, 0.4, and 0.7 mg/kg/day. Mortality was evident in males at the two highest dose levels, and in females at the three highest dose levels during the first few months of the study. Following this period, aldicarb was mixed in the diet in a different manner which eliminated the acute toxicity. Based on the mortality observed in the study, these data are not considered appropriate for the evaluation of an oncogenic response.

In a third study, mice were fed aldicarb at dose levels of 0, 0.1, 0.3, and 0.7 mg/kg/day. There was no effect on mortality or growth. Inclusion of aldicarb in the diet did not result in an increased incidence of oncogenic response.

In a one-year study in dogs, groups of beagles were fed dietary concentrations of 0, 1, 2, 5, and 10 ppm daily for 52 weeks (equivalent to ca. 0, 0.027, 0.055, 0.13, and 0.24 mg/kg/day). The study was designed to produce maximum ChEI by limiting feeding time to 2 hours per day to mimic a bolus administration of aldicarb. Cholinesterase activity was measured from blood samples approximately 2 hours after the feeding period. There were no observable effects other than ChEI. The NOAEL for erythrocyte ChEI was 0.027 mg/kg/day. The lowest observed effect levels (LOELs) for erythrocyte and brain ChEI were 0.055 and 0.24 mg/kg/day, respectively.

In another one-year dog feeding study, aldicarb sulfone was administered at dietary concentrations of 0, 5, 25, and 100 ppm (ca. 0, 0.125, 0.625, and 2.5 mg/kg/day). Cholinesterase determinations were taken approximately 2 hours after feeding to measure maximum ChEI. No mortality or treatment related clinical signs were seen. At the high dose, slight changes in spleen and thyroid–parathyroid weights and slight effects in the mandibular lymph nodes and adrenal cortex were observed. The NOAEL based on erythrocyte ChEI was 0.625 mg/kg/day.

53.4.8 HUMAN VOLUNTEER STUDIES

In a series of studies reported in 1973, groups of four adult male volunteers were administered aldicarb orally in aqueous solution at dose levels of 0.025, 0.05, and 0.1 milligram per kilogram of body weight (mg/kg bw). Clinical signs were recorded and whole blood cholinesterase activity was measured up to 6 hours after administration of the sample. Total urine voided was collected and aldicarb-excretion patterns for the initial 8 hours after dosing were evaluated. In addition, spot samples were taken at 12 and 24 hours. In other studies, two additional subjects were administered aldicarb in water solution at dose levels of 0.05 and 0.26 mg/kg bw. Dose levels of 0.1 and 0.26 mg/kg bw are considered to be high doses. Acute signs, typical of anticholinesterase agents, were observed at the high-dose levels (0.1 and 0.26 mg/kg bw) within 1 hour of aldicarb administration. Cholinesterase depression at these very high dose levels was observed in all volunteers within 1–2 hours after treatment. Within the first 6 hours of treatment, cholinesterase depression and clinical signs of poisoning were within normal levels. There were no signs of treatment observed at the 0.05-mg/kg bw dose level. Urine analysis showed that approximately 10% of the administered dose was excreted as carbamates within the first 8-hour interval. Cholinesterase analyses confirmed the same rapid inhibition and recovery pattern with man as had been observed in experimental animals.

In 1992 Aventis CropScience conducted a human volunteer study, which was conducted and performed under globally accepted ethical guidelines established for such work. This was a double blind, placebo controlled study, in which aldicarb was administered as a single oral dose to healthy male and female subjects. The doses administered were: placebo (22 subjects—16 males and 6 females); 0.01 mg/kg bw (8 males); 0.025 mg/kg bw (8 males and 4 females); 0.05 mg/kg bw (8 males and 4 females); and 0.075 mg/kg bw (4 males). Volunteers were screened before entry for general medical history by examination and laboratory tests including hematology, clinical chemistry, and urinalysis. Clinical measurements were made at intervals before and after dosing. These included vital signs (systolic and diastolic blood pressure, pulse rate), pulmonary function tests, pupil size, electrocardiographs (ECGs), salivation, and clinical signs of nausea, vomiting, diarrhea, sweating, abdominal cramps, involuntary movement, or slurred speech. Samples were taken for urinalysis, clinical chemistry (including red blood cell and plasma cholinesterase activity), and hematology before and after dosing. There were no clinically significant changes in vital signs, pupil size, pulmonary function, ECGs, salivation, clinical signs, clinical chemistry (apart from cholinesterase), hematology, or urinalysis in the study. Cholinesterase activity was the only parameter affected during the study. Red blood cell and plasma cholinesterase was maximally depressed at 1 hour after dosing and had recovered by 8 hours in all subjects. The fall in cholinesterase activity and recovery was dose-related. No biologically significant depression of erythrocyte cholinesterase activity ($>20\%$) was seen in subjects treated with 0.01 or 0.025 mg/kg bw or in plasma cholinesterase at 0.01 mg/kg bw. Depression in cholinesterase activity $>20\%$ was seen in erythrocytes at 0.05, and 0.075 mg/kg bw and in plasma at 0.025, 0.05, and 0.075 mg/kg bw. A single volunteer (0.075-mg/kg bw group, actual dose 0.06 mg/kg bw) reported some sweating, which is not considered to be related to aldicarb. Nevertheless, the NOAEL for clinical signs was reported as 0.05 mg/kg bw and the NOAEL based on erythrocyte cholinesterase inhibition was 0.025 mg/kg bw.

53.5 USE OF PHARMACOKINETICS IN ALDICARB RISK ASSESSMENTS

Although it has been known since the initial discovery of the carbamates that this class of compounds present reduced risk compared to organophosphates due to the rapid reversibility of cholinesterase inhibition, a quantitative analysis of ChE reversibility is desirable because it allows the conduct of more precise risk assessments taking into account the exposure patterns (route of exposure, duration, and repetition).

The kinetics of reversibility of cholinesterase inhibition for aldicarb has been studied through the development of a mathematical model, which describes the reversal of inhibition using data generated during the 1992 study in human volunteers. As previously described, healthy male and female volunteers were administered aldicarb in a study to evaluate its effects on plasma (PChE) and red blood cell (RChE) cholinesterase activity. Cholinesterase activity was measured at three pretreatment time points (-16 and -3 hr, and immediately predose) and 1, 2, 4, 6, 8, and 21 hr post dose. Measurement of PChE and RChE activity at these time points allowed the determination of the maximum inhibitory effect for each dose level as well as the time required for spontaneous reactivation of the enzyme activity through hydrolysis of the carbamate. In addition, samples were taken for urinalysis, clinical chemistry, and hematology evaluations.

The data presented in this chapter will focus on the male RChE data because these are more robust (a larger number of male than female subjects were observed), and because RChE data are generally considered to have more biological relevance than PChE in regard to potential peripheral and central nervous system effects (Carlock *et al.*, 1999; U.S. EPA, 2000). A graphical representation of the male RChE data in the volunteer study is shown in Fig. 53.2. The data show a very stable baseline activity level and rapid decrease in RChE activity following exposure to the bolus dose. The RChE inhibition is then subsequently reversed during a time period ranging from minutes to approximately 2 hours depending on the magnitude of the initial inhibition event (i.e., the smaller the inhibition, the faster the recovery time).

The mathematical model was developed to quantitatively describe the data from the study. With such a model, one can predict the degree of cholinesterase inhibition which would be expected to occur following exposure to a dose that had not been tested experimentally. Additionally, one can calculate the time needed to completely reverse the effects of cholinesterase inhibition following exposure to a given dose. The approach presented here is based on the knowledge that the clinical determination of the reversal of cholinesterase inhibition following exposure to a carbamate is in effect the measurement of the removal of the carbamate from the body. This is so because the reactivation of the cholinesterase enzyme occurs via hydrolysis of the carbamate; hydrolysis results in the production of inactive metabolites and the full restoration of the functional capability of the enzyme. If the enzyme is not inhibited, then there is no longer free aldicarb in the blood compartment available for binding to the enzyme. Thus a mathematical description of the reactivation of cholinesterase activity following cholinesterase inhibition due to carbamate exposure can be regarded as the inverse of the model for removal of the carbamate. The latter model can be used in risk assessments for human health issues surrounding carbamate exposure because, when the initial exposure level is known, the amount remaining after a given point in time can be calculated. In general terms, the model is

$$f(t_1\phi_1, \phi_2, \phi_3) = \phi_1\{1 - \phi_2 \exp[-\phi_3(t - 1)]\}$$

where t is time in hours after exposure ($t \geq 1$), ϕ_1 is the horizontal asymptote that is approached over time ($t \to \infty$), $\phi_1(1 - \phi_2)$ is the minimum value at 1 hour, and ϕ_3 is a scale parameter related to the rate of recovery. The value $100\phi_2$ is the percentage reduction from the asymptotic maximum value to the minimum value at time 1 hour. In biological terms, ϕ_1 is the baseline cholinesterase activity level, ϕ_2 is a parameter describing the degree of inhibition as a function of dose, and ϕ_3 describes the rate of recovery of enzymatic activity (Williams *et al.*, 2000).

The model belongs to the general class of nonlinear mixed effects growth curve models containing both fixed and random effects. The fixed effects permit estimation of the average curves describing the cholinesterase activity levels following exposure to a given dose; the random effects account for individual variability observed in a repeated measures study of

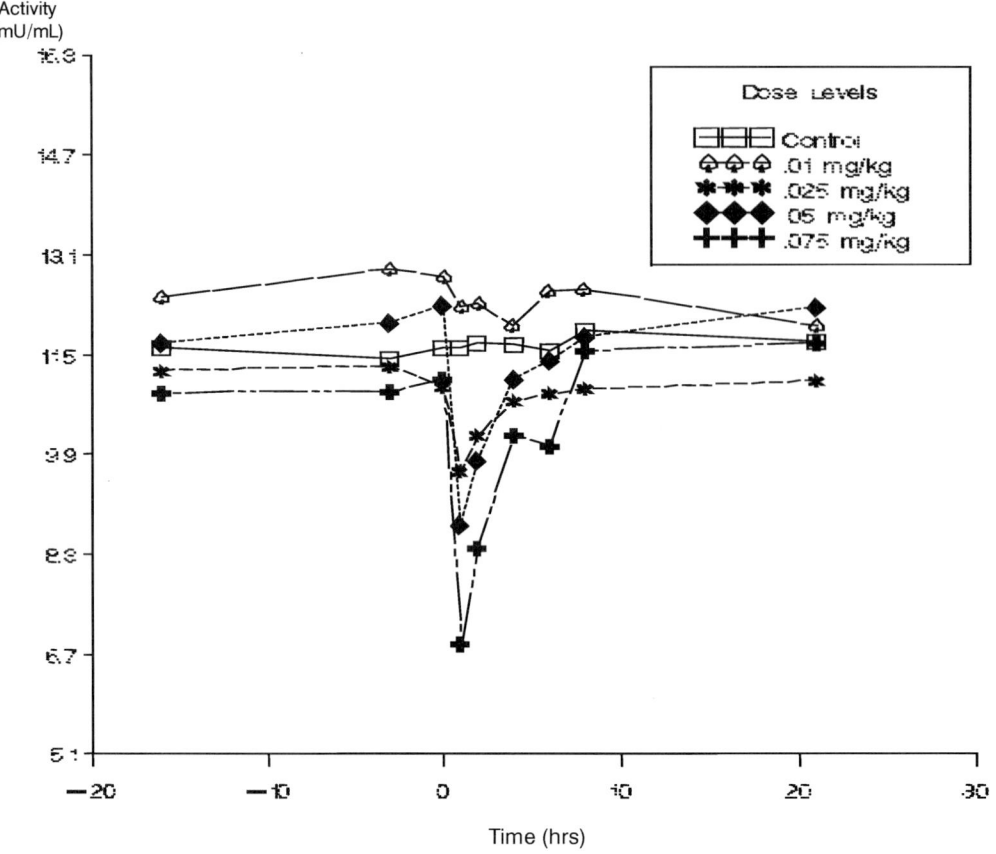

Figure 53.2 Male red blood cell cholinesterase activity from the human volunteer study on aldicarb.

this type. Although the model was developed and validated empirically, it can be thought of as a mechanistic model in the sense that assumptions regarding what was known about the biological system were used in its development. For example, the degree of cholinesterase inhibition was assumed to be a function of the exposure dose, and it was also assumed that cholinesterase returned to predose activity levels over time. Both of these assumptions were tested by the model and validated.

The rate of change (as cholinesterase activity returned to baseline levels following inhibition) predicted from the model was calculated as follows. The rate of change, or the first derivative, of the predicted activity for a particular person is a function of the person's normal cholinesterase activity. The basic model used for activity level is

$$y_{it} = \phi_{1i}\{1 - \phi_{2i}\exp[-\phi_{3i}(t-1)]\}$$

The models for the ϕs are as follows. For baseline activity level,

$$\phi_{1I} = \beta_1 m_i + u_{1I}$$

where m_i is the typical, nonexposed, cholinesterase activity for person i, β_1 is the proportion of the preexposure activity, and u_{1I} is a random effect specific to session I, which a person should reach for the recovery to be considered complete. To test time to recovery, one must specify what percentage of the

preexposure activity is considered the normal state, if β_1 is estimated in the model to be 1, and then recovery has completely returned to predose levels. Finally, u_{1I} accounts for random effects associated with person i. For the magnitude of the inhibition,

$$\phi_{2I} = \exp[\beta_2 + u_{2I}]d_i$$

where β_2 is a fixed value for a typical subject, u_{2I} is a random effect specific to session I, and d_i is the dosage person i ingests. Thus the degree of inhibition is a simple multiple of the dose to which the person is exposed. Finally, for the rate of recovery,

$$\phi_{3I} = \exp[\beta_3 + \beta_4 d_4 + u_{3I}]$$

where β_3 and β_4 are fixed values for each subject. β_4 was included in the model to test if there was an effect of dosage on the rate of recovery; the model was found to be very close to 1, indicating that the rate of recovery was independent of dose-estimated β_4; u_{3I} is a random effect specific to session I.

Thus, taking the derivative of the full model gives

$$\frac{dy_{it}}{dt} = m_i d_i \beta_1 \exp(\beta_2 + \beta_3)\exp[-\beta_3(t-1)].$$

This shows that the rate of change in activity after exposure is a function of the normal cholinesterase activity particular to person i (m_i), and that the derivative changes with time (t). The

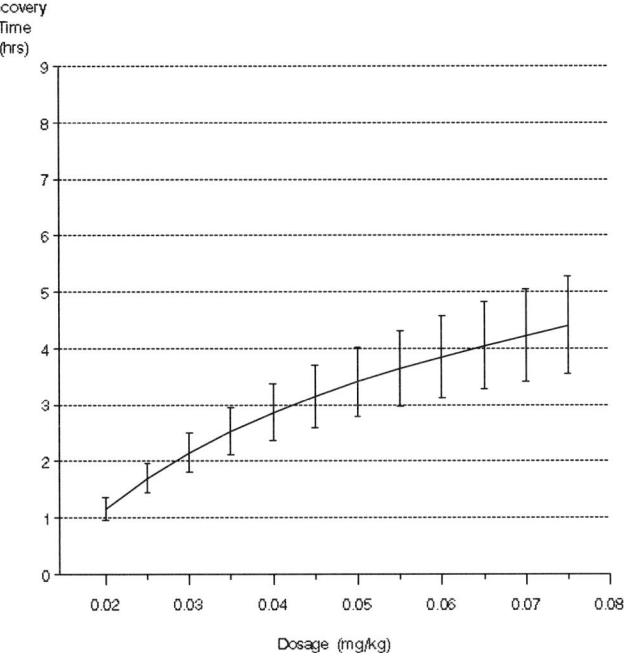

Figure 53.3   Model predicted recovery curves based on the male red blood cell cholinesterase activity from the human volunteer study on aldicarb.

model was validated using two methods for variance estimation, by comparing observed versus expected values directly and through residuals, and was shown to have a good fit to the experimental values. Model-predicted recovery curves are shown in Fig. 53.3.

The model demonstrated that there was full recovery following exposure to aldicarb. This was evaluated by examination of the parameter β_1 in the model. β_1 as predicted by the model was virtually identical to 1, and β_1 is a multiplier of the baseline value; any deviation from return to baseline would have been indicated by a model-predicted β_1 being different from 1. This was predicted by simple examination of the ChE activity graphs following aldicarb exposure, and has now been validated both mathematically and statistically.

The model also demonstrated that recovery rate was not affected by administered dose; the rate of recovery for all doses was the same. This again was predicted because first-order kinetics would be presumed for the hydrolysis reaction between the cholinesterase enzyme and the aldicarb substrate. Because the rate of recovery is not affected by dose, the time to recovery is dependent solely on the initial magnitude of inhibition (i.e., the smaller the dose, the lower degree of inhibition, and thus the faster the recovery time).

53.5.1 REPEATED EXPOSURE MODELING

The time to recovery for the critical toxicological effect is important in the evaluation of the effects of multiple exposures to a chemical because if the effect has completely reversed prior to a subsequent exposure, then the two exposures can be

considered separate events. If, however, the effect has not completely reversed because a certain amount of the dose remains in the system, then the second dose may be additive with however much of the first dose remains. The steps in establishing whether or not two separate exposures can be considered separate events are as follows:

- Determination of the critical toxicological effect
- Development of a method to measure the critical toxicological effect
- Establishing that the critical toxicological effect does in fact reverse completely
- Demonstrating the time to reversal

In the case of aldicarb, the existing toxicological database provides clear answers to the first three of these questions, and the model provides the time to reversal.

53.5.2 CRITICAL EFFECTS

The critical toxicological effect is inhibition (i.e., ChEI), which is not in fact a toxic effect, but a marker of exposure. The toxicological studies described in this review covering carcinogenic, reproductive, neurotoxic, genotoxic, and chronic effects generated no effects other than those which are typically associated with acetylcholinesterase inhibition, as a marker of exposure. The most sensitive indicator of acetylcholinesterase inhibition is measurement of RBC cholinesterase activity. The detailed neurotoxicity studies conducted on aldicarb show that the first indicator following exposure is a decrease in RBC ChE activity. At higher doses, effects on the central and peripheral nervous systems become evident. The studies also demonstrate that the degree of central nervous system (CNS) ChEI for a given dose is less than that measured in RBCs. Thus measurement of RBC ChE activity provides the most sensitive indication of exposure to aldicarb. In addition, RBC ChE activity is readily measurable with a variety of analytical techniques.

53.5.3 REVERSIBILITY

The fact that the reversal of RBC ChE inhibition is complete was demonstrated empirically with a mathematical model. The toxicological database clearly demonstrates no persistence of aldicarb. For example, it would not have been possible to dose every day at such high levels in the 2-year rat study were there any cumulative effects of aldicarb. Also, these animals received multiple doses within each day because they were administered aldicarb ad libitium via the diet and rats eat sporadically during the night. Similarly, the two-generation reproduction, the developmental neurotoxicity, and the subchronic neurotoxicity studies all used repeated daily dosing and gave no evidence of any cumulative effects. Thus it has been adequately demonstrated that the effects of aldicarb exposure are the same either following repeated within-day dosing or following administra-

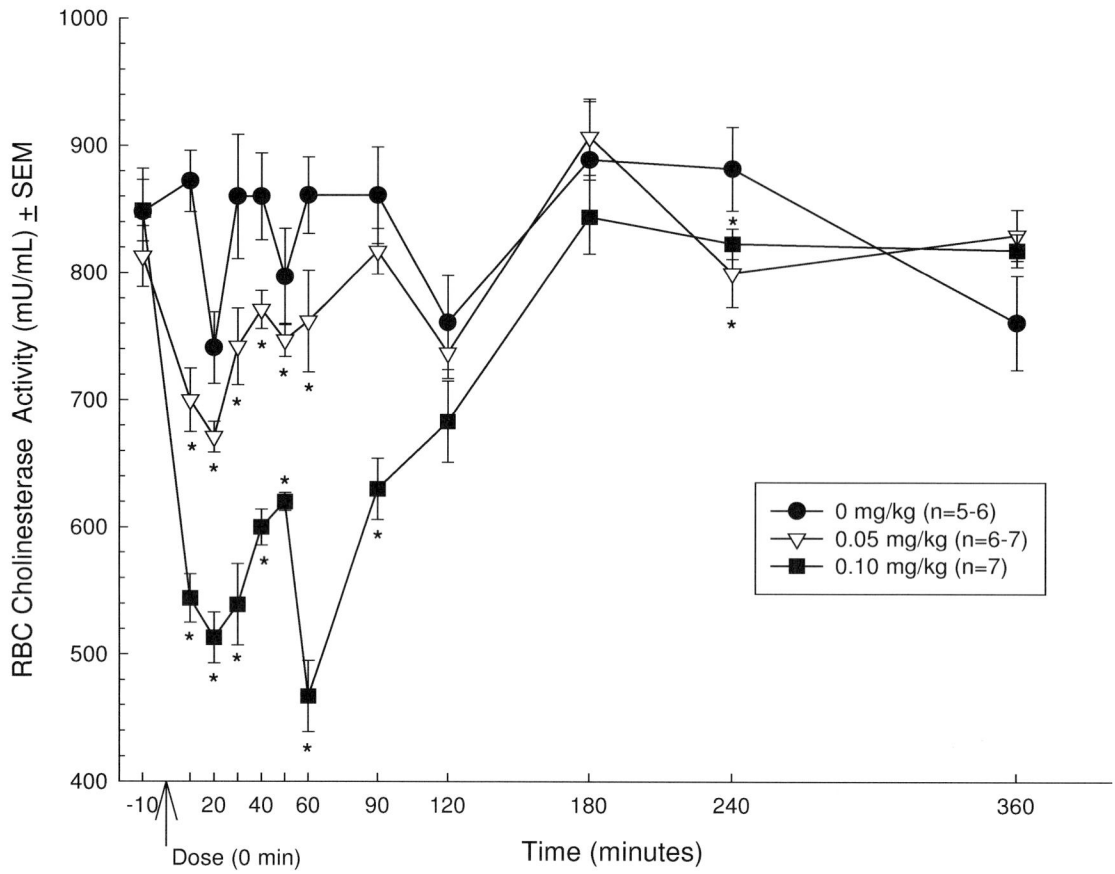

Figure 53.4   Phase I—mean RBC cholinesterase activity in cannulated adult male CD rats following a single oral administration of aldicarb: (∗) significantly different from control within time point ($p < 0.05$).

tion over multiple days up to and including the lifespan of the animals.

More recently, a pharmacokinetic reversibility study was completed using single and multiple dosing of aldicarb in rats to further validate the reversibility. The purpose of this study was to determine the time course of inhibition and recovery of cholinesterase activity after a single or repeated administration of aldicarb for both plasma and RBC. Aldicarb was orally administered once in Phase I and twice in Phase II to cannulated adult male CD® rats at three dose levels (0, 0.05, and 0.10 mg/kg). Red blood cell cholinesterase was inhibited 10 minutes after oral administration of aldicarb in both dose groups and had returned to baseline levels within 180 minutes (see Fig. 53.4).

In Phase II, two consecutive administrations at 4-hour intervals, RBC cholinesterase activity was inhibited after the first dose in a manner similar to the single administration study. Cholinesterase returned to baseline levels of activity by 120 minutes for the low-dose group and 240 minutes for the high-dose group (see Fig. 53.5). Following the second dose, approximately 4.5 hours after the first, inhibition occurred through 40 and 120 minutes for the low- and high-dose groups, respectively. When comparing the cholinesterase inhibition curves following the first and second dose administration for each dose group, no significant differences were detected. Thus, the

pattern of RBC cholinesterase inhibition following a second administration of aldicarb was not different from the single administration. As was shown in the chronic study, no accumulation was observed in this acute pharmacokinetic reversibility study.

To assess the recovery time following aldicarb exposure, it was of interest to know the time to recovery of ChEI at dose levels that a human might possibly be exposed to. The model was used to answer the question: What is the time to recovery for an individual exposed to the U.S. EPA reference dose (0.001 mg/kg/day)? Recovery is defined as the return to 99% of the individual's baseline RBC ChE level. The RfD was chosen because this dose would be expected to give the longest recovery time within the range of regulatory relevant dose levels. Return to 99% of baseline was chosen because this is a conservative cutoff criteria insofar as normal RBC ChE levels can vary as much as or more than 10% or in nonexposed individuals.

The model predicted that recovery time for someone exposed to the full reference dose is instantaneous. This is because no deviation from baseline ChE activity is predicted at the RfD. This is, of course, what one would expect given that the RfD was set at a level 10-fold lower than the human NOAEL for the effect. The conclusion to be drawn is that, for acute dietary exposure to aldicarb where all exposures are less than the ref-

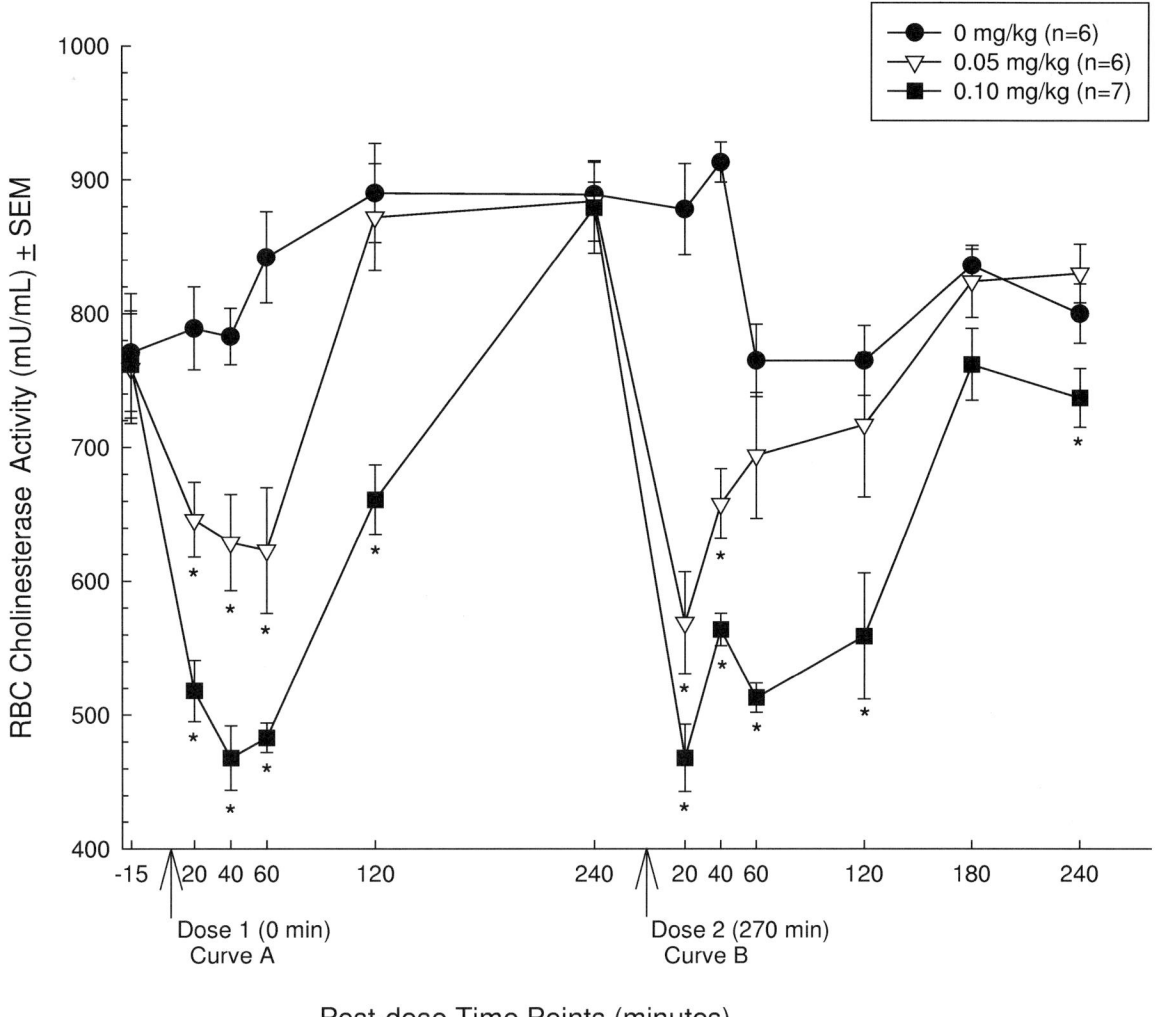

Figure 53.5   Phase II—mean RBC cholinesterase activity in cannulated adult male CD rats following repeated oral administration of aldicarb: (∗) significantly different from control within time point ($p < 0.05$).

erence dose, each meal should be considered a separate eating event for the dietary risk assessment. Any aldicarb exposure encountered in a given meal will be removed from the body prior to any subsequent exposure. Thus acute risk assessments for aldicarb should be based on the amount received in any individual meal and the exposures from meal to meal should not be added together over the course of a 24-hour day.

53.6 ALDICARB DERMAL EXPOSURE RISK ASSESSMENT

Aldicarb is formulated solely as a granular product thus greatly reducing the possibility of occupational exposure. A hazard assessment for potential dermal exposure of agricultural workers has typically been conducted one of two ways. These assessments are based on subchronic toxicity studies conducted by either the oral or the dermal route of exposure; in both cases the studies are normally conducted with the technical material.

When an oral study is used for a dermal risk assessment, the oral NOAEL can be converted to dermal equivalents through the use of a dermal absorption factor. This is typically determined experimentally by using radiolabeled test material applied to the skin and measuring the levels of radioactivity, which has been absorbed through the skin, at varying time intervals. The percentage absorbed can then be used to modify the dose from the oral study. This first approach, however, is not appropriate for aldicarb because the compound is rapidly hydrolyzed in the body and, soon after exposure, the radiolabel is no longer attached to active aldicarb and, thus, cannot be used as a reliable indicator of the amount of active aldicarb in the body.

The second approach involves repeated dermal dosing with the technical material and determination of the NOAEL by this route of exposure. The risk assessment is then conducted by applying the safety factor directly to the dermal NOAEL. This method has the advantage of not relying on a dermal equivalent dose. However, it is also not appropriate for aldicarb, because the granular product is specifically designed to minimize exposure by adhering the technical material to the granule with a binding agent and removing any excess dust after the product is manufactured. Thus a study with the technical material would be expected to greatly overestimate the amount of material absorbed in an agricultural application situation.

Because of the problems with the traditional study designs used for the hazard assessment component of the occupational risk assessments, a 21-day dermal study with the granular product was conducted and used this study as the basis for the risk assessment. The effect of Temik grit (containing 14.75% aldicarb), administered by semioccluded topical application on peripheral (erythrocyte and plasma) and brain cholinesterase activities, was evaluated in CD (Sprague-Dawley) rats. The granular Temik grit was applied to the shaved dorsum, and the site moistened with saline to ensure good contact with the skin.

Eight rats per sex per dose were exposed topically 6 hours/day, 5 days/week (Monday through Friday) for three consecutive weeks at 0, 100, 250, and 500 mg/kg/day. Body weights and clinical observations were recorded daily, and feed consumption was recorded twice weekly (Mondays and Fridays). Blood samples (0.25 ml) were taken from the lateral tail vein of each rat 1 hour postdosing on day 1 (Monday) and day 5 (Friday) on each of the three weeks of exposure. On the last day of exposure, after the blood sampling, the animals were sacrificed and the brains were weighed and analyzed for cholinesterase activity.

For the males, there were no effects on daily body weights or daily weight changes. Absolute and relative brain weights were equivalent across all groups. Feed consumption was equivalent across groups for all intervals. There were no dose-related clinical signs of toxicity. Plasma cholinesterase levels were significantly reduced at 250 mg/kg/day on days 1, 5, 8, 12, and 19 (but not on day 15 when the level was reduced, but not statistically significantly, to 81.4% of controls). Erythrocyte cholinesterase levels were not statistically different across all groups at all time points evaluated, but the mean activity at 500 mg/kg/day was clearly reduced relative to the control group values on all days evaluated. Brain cholinesterase activity on day 19 at termination of the study was not affected at any treatment level.

For the females, there were no effects of treatment on body weights, weight changes, absolute or relative brain weights, or on feed consumption for any group at any time point during the study. There were also no dose-related clinical signs of toxicity. Plasma cholinesterase levels were reduced at 250 and 500 mg/kg/day on all days evaluated (days 1, 5, 8, 12, 15, and 19). Erythrocyte cholinesterase levels were reduced at 500 mg/kg/day. Brain cholinesterase activity on day 19 was not affected at any treatment level.

In conclusion, the study evaluating Temik 15G grit, administered by occluded topical application, demonstrated that effects on peripheral and brain cholinesterase activity were rapidly reversible, and that there were no cumulative effects on these parameters over time. A NOAEL was established for erythrocyte cholinesterase activity at 250 mg/kg/day, and for brain cholinesterase activity of at least 500 mg/kg/day, for both male and female rats.

The NOAEL for RBC cholinesterase activity of 100 mg/kg/day Temik grit corresponds to a NOAEL for aldicarb of 15 mg/kg/day because the granule is 15% aldicarb. The NOAEL for aldicarb when administered orally is 0.025 mg/kg/day based on RBC cholinesterase inhibition in the study with human volunteers. Thus the dermal study with the formulated product gives $15/0.025 = 600$ extra margin of safety relative to oral dosing. In other words the risk assessment for occupational exposure for the granular product using an appropriate toxicity study provides a more realistic margin of safety. This is based on the fact that the release of aldicarb from the granule is very slow and thus the amount absorbed is extremely low. Therefore, any inhibition which occurs is rapidly reversed within seconds.

One could argue that because the dermal study was conducted in the rat, an extra 10-fold margin of safety should be applied to the risk assessment to account for the interspecies extrapolation. This is clearly not necessary for aldicarb as the entire toxicology database demonstrates that animals and humans respond very similarly to the effects of exposure. In fact, in this case, the only expected interspecies difference is a lower dermal absorption through human skin compared to rat skin. However, even if an extra 10-fold interspecies safety factor is applied to the risk assessment, the granular product and dermal exposure provide at least 150 extra margins of safety relative to an assessment, which assumes oral dosing with the technical material. Furthermore, the modeling work supports and strengthens the results of this dermal toxicity study based on a hypothesis for total dermal absorption of the material and the hypothesis that this absorption would be constant over the maximum 8-hour workday.

53.7 CONCLUSION

Aldicarb is an economically important and scientifically interesting pest control chemical. Were this material not available, in many cases a suitable alternative is not available. The alternative control strategies would require treatment with a number of different chemicals, resulting in a concomitant increase in potential exposure as well as cost. Aldicarb has high acute toxicity, so it must be carefully managed and used according to label instructions to ensure its safe use for crop protection. The following are the major conclusions of this chapter:

1. The biomarker effect observed in all animal and human testing demonstrated that ChEI is the only effect observed.

2. To assess the recovery time following aldicarb exposure, it is important to know the time to recovery of ChEI following exposure. A model was used to clearly answer the question: What is the time to recovery for an individual exposed to the U.S. EPA reference dose (0.001 mg/kg/day)? The model predicted that recovery time for someone exposed to the full reference dose is instantaneous. This is because no deviation from baseline ChE activity is predicted at the RfD. This is expected given that the RfD was set at a level 10-fold lower than the human NOAEL for the effect. Any aldicarb exposure encountered in a given meal will be removed from the body prior to any subsequent exposure. Thus acute risk assessments for aldicarb should be based on the amount received in any individual meal and the exposures from meal to meal should not be added together over the course of a 24-hour day.

3. Detailed analysis of the pharmacokinetics of reversal of cholinesterase inhibition has shown that the very rapid reversibility of effects following exposure allows safe exposure to low levels of aldicarb (i.e., RfD).

4. In the dermal exposure risk assessment section, it was clearly demonstrated that release of aldicarb from the granule formulation is very slow and thus the amount absorbed is extremely low. Therefore, any inhibition which occurs is rapidly reversed within seconds. Furthermore, this is in line with the pharmacokinetic model for oral administration, as stated in the chapter.

5. For the overall risk assessment for aldicarb, we have clearly demonstrated that both the humans and animals are very similar (i.e., toxicity profile and rapid reversibility for RBC cholinesterase inhibition) in their response to this product; thus there should be no requirement for an interspecies 10×-fold safety factor.

In-depth risk assessment methodologies such as these, coupled with appropriate toxicological research, provide greater certainty in the risk assessment and, in the case of aldicarb, show that it can be used safely for crop protection, both for agricultural workers and for consumers.

REFERENCES

Alvarez, A. P. (1992). "Pharmacology and Toxicology of Carbamates." In "Clinical and Experimental Toxicology of Organophosphates and Carbamates" (B. Ballantyne and T. C. Marrs, eds.), pp. 40–46. Butterworth–Heinemann.

Anderson, S., Tyl, R., Gilliam, A., Tobia, A., and Rieth, J. (2000). The toxicokinetics of peripheral cholinesterase inhibition from orally administered aldicarb in adult male CD® rats. Unpublished abstract (submitted to Society of Toxicology, 2001 Meeting).

Baron, R. (1994). A carbamate insecticide: A case study of aldicarb. *Environ. Health Perspect.* **103**(Suppl. 11), xxx–xxx.

California Environmental Protection Agency (1998). "Summary of Toxicology Data for Aldicarb." Chemical Code # 000575, Tolerance # 00269, SB 950 # 130, File # T981120, Department of Pesticide Regulation, Medical Toxicology Branch, Sacramento.

Carlock, L., Chen, W., Gordon, E., Killeen, J., Manley, A., Meyer, L., Mullin, L., Pendino, K., Percy, A., Sargent, D., and Seaman, L. (1999). Regulating and assessing risks of cholinesterase-inhibiting pesticides: Divergent approaches and interpretations. *J. Toxicol. Environ. Health* **2**, 105–160.

Cohrssen, J., and Covello, V. (1989). "Risk Analysis: A Guide to Principles and Methods for Analyzing Health and Environmental Risks." United States Council on Environmental Quality, Executive Office of the President (ISBN 0-934213-20-80).

Dourson, M., Knauf, L., and Swartout, J. (1992). On reference dose and its underlying toxicity data base. *Toxicol. Ind. Health* **8**, 171–189.

Food Quality Protection Act of 1996, 104th Congress, 2nd session. Report 104-669, Part 2, pp. 1–89. U.S. Gov. Printing Office, Washington, DC.

International Agency for Research on Cancer (IARC) (1991). "Occupational Exposures in Insecticide Application, and Some Pesticides," Vol. 53. IARC, Lyon, France.

International Programme on Chemical Safety (IPCS) (1991). "Aldicarb," Environmental Health Criteria 121. World Health Organization, Geneva.

International Programme on Chemical Safety (IPCS) (1994). "Assessing Human Health Risks of Chemicals: Derivation of Guidance Values for Health-Based Exposure Limits," Environmental Health Criteria 170. World Health Organization, Geneva.

Food and Agriculture Organization–World Health Organization (FAO/WHO) (1992). Aldicarb. *In* "Joint FAO/WHO Meeting on Pesticide Residues," Rome, 21–30 September 1992.

O'Brien, R. D. (1967). "Insecticides: Action and Metabolism." Academic Press, New York.

Phillips, J., Powell, G., Scarborough, A., Barraj, L., and Petersen, B. (2000). Acute dietary risk assessment of aldicarb, a reversible carbamate insecticide. Unpublished abstract (submitted to Society of Toxicology, 2001 Meeting).

Renwick A., and Lazarus, N. (1998). Human variability and noncancer risk assessment—an analysis of the default uncertainty factor. *Regul. Toxicol. Pharmacol.* **27**, 3–20.

Rieth, J., and Starr, T. (1989). Chronic bioassays: Relevance to quantitative risk assessment of carcinogens. *Regul. Toxicol. Pharmacol.* **10**, 160–173.

Rotenberg, M., and Almog, S. (1995). Evaluation of the decarbamylation process of cholinesterase during assay of enzyme activity. *Clin. Chim. Acta* **240**, 107–116.

Swartout, J., Price, P., Dourson, M., Carlson-Lynch, H., and Keenan, R. (1998). A probabilistic framework for the reference dose. *Risk Anal.* **18**, 271–282.

Tobia, A., McCahon, P., and Carmichael, N. (2000). A safety and tolerability study of aldicarb at various dose levels in healthy male and female human volunteers. Unpublished abstract (submitted to Society of Toxicology, 2001 Meeting).

Tyl, R., Ross, W., Basham, K., Gilliam, A., Myers, C., Rieth, J., Lunchick, C., and Tobia, A. (2000). Cholinesterase activity in CD® rats following topical application of TEMIK® 15G for one week. Unpublished abstract (submitted to Society of Toxicology, 2001 Meeting).

U.S. Environmental Protection Agency (U.S. EPA) (1984). "Pesticide Assessment Guidelines: Subdivision F, Hazard Evaluation, Human and Domestic Animals." U.S. Environmental Protection Agency, Washington, DC.

U.S. Environmental Protection Agency (U.S. EPA) (1987). "Pesticide Assessment Guidelines, Subdivision U, Applicator Exposure Monitoring." NTIS PB87-133286, U.S. Environmental Protection Agency, Washington, DC.

U.S. Environmental Protection Agency (U.S. EPA) (1993). "Reference Dose (RfD): Description and Use in Health Risk Assessments." Background Document 1A, Integrated Risk Information, March 15, 1993, U.S. Environmental Protection Agency, Washington, DC.

U.S. Environmental Protection Agency (U.S. EPA) (1998). "The Pesticide Handlers Exposure Database (PHED), Version 1.1—PHED Surrogate Exposure Guide, Estimates of Worker Exposure." U.S. Environmental Protection Agency, Washington, DC.

U.S. Environmental Protection Agency (U.S. EPA) (2000).

WHO (1987).

Williams, R., Rieth, J., and Tobia, A. (2000). Non-linear mixed effects models for cholinesterase activity in humans exposed to aldicarb. Unpublished abstract (submitted to Society of Toxicology, 2001 Meeting).

Imidacloprid: A Neonicotinoid Insecticide

Larry P. Sheets
Bayer Corporation

54.1 INTRODUCTION

Imidacloprid is the principal representative of a new pesticide class, the neonicotinoid insecticides. These insecticides are designed to act on nicotinic receptors to control insect pests and, at the same time, to be relatively nontoxic to vertebrate species. This is accomplished by selecting compounds for commercial development that are highly specific for subtypes of nicotinic receptors that occur in insect tissues. The effect of neonicotinoid insecticides on the central nervous system of vertebrates is further reduced by poor penetration of the blood–brain barrier. The toxicology database supports the success of this strategy for imidacloprid, with signs of nicotinic stimulation (e.g., tremor) evident only at relatively high levels of exposure. By oral administration, imidacloprid is rapidly absorbed, metabolized in the liver, and excreted, primarily via the urine. Results from long-term dietary-exposure studies support rapid metabolism, with little evidence of cumulative toxicity and minimal effects, even at maximum-tolerated doses. Imidacloprid is not mutagenic or carcinogenic. Furthermore, it is not a primary embryotoxicant or a reproductive toxicant, nor is it teratogenic. Due to its high insecticidal potency and relatively low mammalian toxicity, imidacloprid has a very high margin of safety.

54.2 HISTORICAL OVERVIEW

54.2.1 CHEMISTRY

Imidacloprid [1-[(6-chloro-3-pyridinyl)methyl]-N-nitro-2-imidazolidinimine] is the first representative of the neonicotinoid insecticides that was registered for use and is presently the most important commercial product. The history of the neonicotinoids can be traced to the late 1970s, when chemists at Shell Chemical Company investigated the heterocyclic nitromethylenes as potential insecticides (Schroeder and Flat-

tum, 1984; Soloway et al., 1978). An excellent review of the discovery and early development of these insecticides has been compiled by Yamamoto and Casida (1999). The term "neonicotinoid" is used to distinguish these chemicals from the nicotinoids (Tomizawa and Yamamoto, 1993), with the neonicotinoids being more highly effective as insecticides and less toxic to vertebrate species. Representatives from this group are also referred to as "chloronicotinyls" to emphasize the importance of the chlorine atom for insecticidal potency.

Imidacloprid was discovered in 1984 by chemists at Nihon Bayer Agrochem who were exploring the introduction of a 3-pyridylmethyl group on the nitromethylene heterocycle structure (Shiokawa et al., 1986). The introduction of this moiety has been shown to greatly increase insecticidal activity and reduce mammalian toxicity (Kagabu et al., 1992; Zwart et al., 1992 and 1994), while retaining the many other properties that are important for commercial applications. Since the discovery of imidacloprid, several other chemical analogs with the 6-chloro-3-pyridylmethyl moiety have been developed for commercial use (Fig. 54.1). Included in this group are acetamiprid (Takahashi et al., 1992; Yamada et al., 1999), nitenpyram (Minamida et al., 1993) and, more recently, thiacloprid.

The replacement of the chloropyridinyl moiety with a chlorothiazolyl group led to the development of a "second generation" of neonicotinoid insecticides (Maienfisch et al., 1999). This substitution has been shown to further reduce potency in assays with mammalian receptors but does not appear to reduce toxicity to mammals or to reduce activity at the insect nicotinic receptor (Chao and Casida, 1997; Liu et al., 1993; Zhang et al., 2000). Compounds in this group that have been developed for commercial use include clothianidin (TI-435) and thiamethoxam (CGA 293′343; Maienfisch et al., 1999) (Fig. 54.1). Thiamethoxam is the first representative from this group that was registered for use (Wiesner and Kayser, 2000).

1123

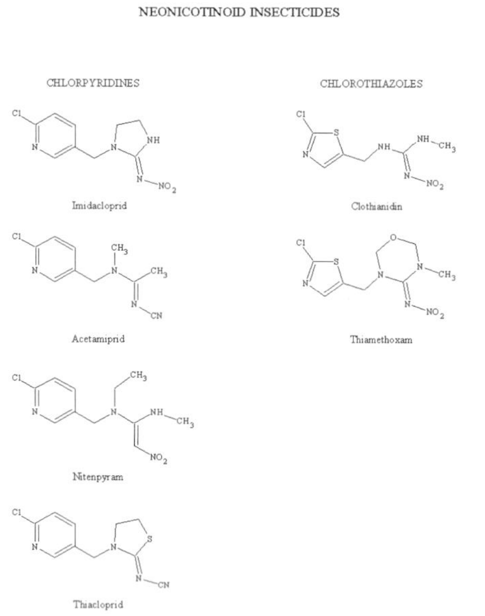

NEONICOTINOID INSECTICIDES

Figure 54.1 Neonicotinoid insecticides.

54.2.2 NICOTINIC ACTIVITY

54.2.2.1 Insects

The insecticidal activity of the neonicotinoids is attributed to actions on post-synaptic nicotinic receptors (Buckingham *et al.*, 1997; Nagata *et al.*, 1998) which, in insects, are located exclusively in the central nervous system. In insects, multiple subtypes of nicotinic receptor have been identified which express different physiological and pharmacologic properties (Gundelfinger and Schulz, 2000; Wiesner and Kayser, 2000). With respect to the neonicotinoids, it has been determined that imidacloprid acts on at least three pharmacologically distinct subtypes of nicotinic receptor in the cockroach (Buckingham *et al.*, 1997). Further characterization of the nicotinic receptors that exist in insect tissues and the relative activity of neonicotinoids on the various subtypes are very active areas of research.

The treatment of insect neuronal preparations with a neonicotinoid produces a bi-phasic response, consisting of an initial increase in the frequency of spontaneous discharge that is followed by a complete block to nerve impulse propagation (Schroeder and Flattum, 1984). Signs of intoxication in the American cockroach (*Periplaneta americana*) following exposure to imidacloprid consist of uncoordinated abdominal quivering, wing flexing, tremor, and violent whole-body shaking, followed by prostration and death (Schroeder and Flattum, 1984). Insecticidal activity is greatly enhanced by synergists that inhibit oxidative degradation (Liu and Casida, 1993), which would appear to support including a synergist in commercial formulations.

54.2.2.2 Mammals

Mammalian tissues also contain many subtypes of nicotinic receptor. The various subtypes are derived from five homologous subunits, in combinations that are formed from nine α, four β, γ, δ and ε subunits (Tomizawa *et al.*, 1999). In mammals, nicotinic receptors are located in many tissues, including autonomic ganglia, skeletal muscle (neuromuscular junction), spinal cord, and a number of brain regions. Differences in binding properties to the various receptor subtypes contribute greatly to the much lower activity of neonicotinoids in vertebrate tissues, as compared to tissues from insects (Yamamoto *et al.*, 1998). There is an extensive database for differential sensitivity with imidacloprid (Chao and Casida, 1997; Liu and Casida, 1993; Matsuda *et al.*, 1998; Methfessel, 1992; Nagata *et al.*, 1999; Tomizawa *et al.*, 1999) that has been summarized by Tomizawa and Casida (1999). The relative specificity for the nicotinic receptor in insects is used to select compounds for commercial development. The success of this strategy is reflected by very high margins of safety for these insecticides (Leicht, 1993).

The acute toxicity (defined by lethal potency) of various neonicotinoid insecticides and related analogs in mammals is most closely related to potency at the α_7 nicotinic receptor subtype, with a decreasing relationship reported sequentially at α_4, β_2, α_3, and α_1 nicotinic receptors, respectively (Tomizawa and Casida, 1999). However, acute toxicity in mammals involves complex actions at multiple receptor subtypes, with relative subtype specificity conferred by even minimal structural changes. Furthermore, the actions of neonicotinoids at these receptor subtypes involve a combination of agonist and antagonist effects (Nagata *et al.*, 1998). Given this combination of actions, known or expected differences in relative specific activity at each nicotinic receptor subtype, and expected differences in distribution to target tissues, the toxic effects *in vivo* would likely vary among representative compounds. However, there has been no systematic assessment of toxicity *in vivo*, with tests conducted under appropriately standardized conditions.

54.3 METABOLISM AND TOXICOKINETICS

The information available on the metabolism and toxicokinetics of imidacloprid in the rat is described in additional detail elsewhere (Thyssen and Machemer, 1999). Briefly, there are two major routes of metabolism in mammals. The first involves oxidative cleavage to imidazolidine and 6-chloronicotinic acid. The imidazolidine moiety is then excreted via the urine. The nicotinic moiety is further degraded via glutathione-conjugation to a derivative of mercapturic acid and then to methyl mercaptonicotinic acid. This moiety is also conjugated with glycine to form a hippuric acid conjugate for excretion. The second substantive route in the biotransformation of imidacloprid involves the hydroxylation of the intact molecule in the imidazolidine ring, followed by the elimination of water and the formation of an unsaturated metabolite.

In the rat, there are no qualitative differences between males and females after the oral administration of a low dose of 1 mg/kg body weight or a dose of 20 mg/kg body weight. At both dose levels, the same complement of metabolites is present in both sexes, although at the higher dose of 20 mg/kg body weight, orally treated females exhibit a slightly higher renal elimination than males. More than 90% of a given dose is eliminated within 24 hours, with total excretion by 48 hours. Eighty percent of the dose is excreted via the urine, with the rest eliminated via the feces.

Imidacloprid is absorbed and widely distributed to organs within one hour following oral administration to rats. Whole-body autoradiography indicates that imidacloprid is not distributed to fatty tissues, to tissues in the central nervous system (CNS), or to the mineral components of bone. These results indicate that there is low potential for accumulation and poor penetration of the blood–brain barrier, at least to dose levels of up to 20 mg/kg body weight. Poor penetration of the blood–brain barrier has also been reported with other neonicotinoids (Yamamoto *et al.*, 1995). This property reduces their access to receptors in the CNS, such that centrally mediated effects would not be expected at low levels of exposure.

54.4 MAMMALIAN TOXICOLOGY

The peer-reviewed literature includes very little information on the toxicity of imidacloprid or other neonicotinoid insecticides in mammals. Work that has been published has generally dealt with a determination of acute lethal potency (e.g., LD50) for a series of structural analogs, without further assessment. One such study reported the presence of tremor in mice that had been treated with an acute oral dose of imidacloprid or one of several other neonicotinoids (Chao and Casida, 1997). This finding provides evidence of nicotinic stimulation at near-lethal or lethal dose levels. A second source is a book edited by Yamamoto and Casida (1999), with chapters that discuss mammalian toxicology data for imidacloprid (Thyssen and Machemer, 1999), nitenpyram (Akayama and Minamida, 1999), and thiamethoxam (Maienfisch *et al.*, 1999). Finally, there is a published comparison of the findings of neurotoxicity studies that were conducted in industry laboratories with commercial products (Sheets, 2001). This work is summarized in Section 54.11.4, following a review of the findings with imidacloprid.

The general absence of published information on the toxicology of imidacloprid and other neonicotinoids in mammals contrasts with the extensive database that has been generated by industry laboratories to support the registration of commercial products. The remainder of this chapter is largely devoted to a review of the toxicology studies that constitute the database that Bayer has generated for imidacloprid. These studies were performed in accordance with regulatory guidelines, including those of the U.S. EPA (FIFRA), the OECD, and the Japanese MAFF, and in compliance with the associated Good Laboratory Practice (GLP) requirements. The compound tested in these studies was technical-grade imidacloprid, with a purity of 94–98% active ingredient. For extended periods of exposure, imidacloprid was generally mixed in the diet and provided for *ad libitum* consumption. Animals were acquired from commercial vendors as purpose-bred animals and were housed under standardized conditions that meet or exceed accepted standards for animal care.

54.5 ACUTE TOXICITY

An overview of the results for acute toxicity studies that have been conducted with imidacloprid is provided in Table 54.1. Acute exposure to imidacloprid was determined to produce minimal evidence of toxicity by dermal and inhalation routes of exposure and moderate acute toxicity by oral administration. Imidacloprid is not an irritant and does not produce evidence of dermal sensitization.

To assess acute oral toxicity, technical-grade imidacloprid was administered as an aqueous suspension to fasted, young-adult Wistar rats (5/sex/dose). Doses of 50 mg/kg in males and 100 mg/kg in females produced no evidence of exposure. By comparison, higher doses of up to 315 mg/kg in males or females produced clinical signs, without causing mortality. At dose levels greater than 315 mg/kg, the incidence of mortality increased rather abruptly, with 20% mortality in both sexes at a dose of 400 mg/kg and 100% mortality at 500 mg/kg body weight. Clinical signs that were evident following treatment included tremor, gait incoordination, and evidence of decreased motility and activity, as well as nasal and urine staining. Signs of intoxication were evident within 15–40 minutes following oral administration and, with few exceptions (e.g., stains), were reversible within eight to 24 hours following treatment. This outcome is consistent with the rapid distribution and metabolism profile that was summarized in Section 54.3. Treatment-related deaths generally occurred within three to seven hours following treatment.

Table 54.1
Acute Toxicity Studies with Imidacloprid[a]

Animal species	Route of exposure	LD$_{50}$/LC$_{50}$ (mg/kg BW/mg/m^3 air)
Mouse	Oral	131–168
Rat	Oral	424–475
Rat	Dermal	>5000
Rat	Inhalation AE 4h	>69[b]
Rat	Inhalation dust 4h	>5323[c]
Rabbit	Dermal	Not an irritant
Rabbit	Eye	Not an irritant
Guinea pig	Dermal	Negative for sensitization[d]

[a]LD$_{50}$ and LC$_{50}$ values represent the results for both sexes.
[b]Aerodynamic droplet size <5 μM; 100%; max conc.
[c]Aerodynamic particle size <5 μM; 4–11%.
[d]Magnusson and Kligman Test.

54.6 SUBCHRONIC TOXICITY

54.6.1 RAT

Imidacloprid was administered through the diet for a period of 13 weeks to young-adult Wistar rats (10/sex/dietary level) to examine cumulative toxicity, with sustained exposure, and to establish dietary levels for the chronic toxicity/carcinogenicity study. In this study, the test substance was provided for *ad libitum* consumption at concentrations of 150, 600, or 2400 ppm, which corresponded to average daily doses of 14, 61, or 300 mg/kg body weight for males and 20, 83, or 422 mg/kg body weight for females. Satellite groups of control and high-dose animals (10/sex/level) were retained for four weeks after the 13-week period of exposure to assess reversibility. Measures of cholinesterase activity (brain, plasma, and erythrocyte) were included to verify the expected absence of inhibition.

Clinical signs associated with treatment were not evident in males or females at any dietary level. Body weight and food consumption were reduced at the 600 ppm (males only) and 2400 ppm (both sexes) dietary levels. The average body weight for high-dose males and females was approximately 15% less than control. The liver was the principal target organ, with hypertrophy of hepatocytes and sporadic cell necrosis in high-dose males only. Liver pathology was mild at termination of the study and was fully reversible within the recovery period. Other effects in high-dose males and females included elevated serum alkaline phosphatase and alanine aminotransferase (ALAT) activities and a slight increase in blood clotting time. There was no inhibition of cholinesterase activity at any dietary level. The NOEL (no-observed-effect level) for this study was 14 mg/kg/day in males and 83 mg/kg/day in females.

54.6.2 DOG

Toxicity was examined in a nonrodent species by administering imidacloprid through the diet for a period of 13 weeks to young-adult, pure-bred beagle dogs (4/sex/dietary level) at dietary concentrations of 200, 600, or 1800/1200 ppm.

The 1800 ppm dietary level produced a sharp reduction in weight gain, relative to controls. Body weight was regained after week 4, upon reducing the high dose to 1200 ppm. Tremor was evident in males and females in the 600 ppm and 1800/1200 ppm dietary groups. The tremor was more severe and occurred at a higher incidence in high-dose animals, relative to the next lower dose. However, it was noted that tremor was not observed at comparable dietary levels in other dog studies, including the one-year dietary study (see Section 54.7.4). There was no evidence of tissue damage by clinical chemistry, gross necropsy examination, tissue weight, or microscopic examination at any dietary level. The NOEL for this study was 200 ppm in both sexes.

54.7 CHRONIC TOXICITY AND CARCINOGENICITY

54.7.1 RAT

A combined chronic toxicity/carcinogenicity study was performed, with imidacloprid administered through the diet for a period of two years to Wistar rats (50/sex/dietary level). An additional set of animals (10/sex/level) was reserved for interim examination after twelve months. The test substance was provided for *ad libitum* consumption at concentrations of 100, 300, 900, or 1800 ppm, which corresponded to average daily doses of 5.7, 17, 51, or 103 mg/kg body weight for males and 7.6, 25, 73, or 144 mg/kg body weight for females.

Treatment-related clinical signs were not evident in either sex, and there was no effect on survival at any dietary level. Body weight was reduced by 12% in both sexes at the 1800 ppm dietary level and by 5–8% in males and females at the 900 ppm dietary level, and was not affected at lower levels of exposure. At 1800 ppm, serum alkaline phosphatase, creatine kinase, and aspartate aminotransferase (ASAT) activities were elevated and cholesterol was reduced. Microscopic lesions were also apparent in the thyroid at this dietary level, with mineralization of the colloid, fewer colloid aggregation cites, and parafollicular hyperplasia sites. These lesions were ascribed to an enhancement of biological aging processes and were not accompanied by a change in thyroid function (e.g., plasma T3, T4, and TSH levels were normal). Mineralization of the colloid in the thyroid follicles was also evident in males at 300 ppm and in both sexes at 900 ppm. There was no change in liver morphology and no inhibition of cholinesterase activity (brain, plasma, or erythrocyte) at any level. The NOEL in this study was 5.7 mg/kg/day. There was also no evidence of carcinogenicity.

54.7.2 MOUSE

To further assess oncogenic potential, imidacloprid was administered through the diet for a period of 24 months to B6C3F1 mice (50/sex/dietary level), at concentrations of 100, 330, 1000, or 2000 ppm. An additional set of animals (10/sex/level) was reserved for interim examination after twelve months. These dietary concentrations resulted in average daily doses of 20, 66, 208, or 414 mg/kg body weight for males and 30, 104, 274, or 424 mg/kg body weight for females.

There were no clinical signs associated with treatment and no effect on survival at any dietary level. Males and females that received the 2000 ppm dietary level had a marked decrease in body weight gain, relative to controls, with correspondingly lower food and water consumption. The difference in body weight reached 29% less than controls, indicating that this level exceeded an MTD. Liver changes were also evident at 2000 ppm but not at lower dietary levels. These consisted of low-grade periacinary hepatocyte hypertrophy, which was considered to represent metabolic adaptation to this xenobiotic. Effects that were evident at 1000 ppm consisted of reduced food consumption (females only) and reduced body weight, relative to controls, for males and females (up to 10% and 5%, respectively). There were no changes in serum chemistry, tissue weight, or tissue morphology (by gross and microscopic examination) associated with treatment at any dietary level. The number, type, distribution, and time of occurrence of tumors provided no evidence that imidacloprid has carcinogenic potential. The overall NOEL in this study was 330 ppm in males and females.

54.7.3 CLASSIFICATION FOR CARCINOGENICITY

Based on the collective results of the chronic toxicity and carcinogenicity studies in the rat and mouse, the U.S. EPA has classified imidacloprid in category "E." This classification indicates that the database for imidacloprid supports evidence of noncarcinogenicity for humans.

54.7.4 DOG

To evaluate chronic toxicity in a nonrodent species, imidacloprid was administered through the diet for a period of 52 weeks to young-adult, pure-bred beagle dogs (4/sex/dietary level). The test substance was provided for *ad libitum* consumption at concentrations of 200, 500, or 1250 ppm. The 1250 ppm dietary concentration was increased to 2500 ppm from week 17 onwards. These levels corresponded to daily doses of 6.1, 15, and 41/72 mg/kg/day.

The 1250 ppm dietary level was associated with a slight, but transient, fall in food consumption in both sexes. A similarly transient effect was evident when the dietary concentration was increased to 2500 ppm during week 17. The tremor that was evident in the subchronic dog study, at dietary concentrations of 600 ppm or greater (see Section 54.7.2), was not evident here at any dietary concentration. Effects at the highest dietary level included a slight increase in plasma cholesterol (females only) and a slight increase in hepatic cytochrome P-450 activity (both sexes). The induction of cytochrome P-450 enzymes was associated with a slight increase in liver weight. Thus, the liver was the principal target organ. The chronic NOEL in the dog was 15 mg/kg/day.

54.8 MUTAGENICITY

Imidacloprid has been evaluated for mutagenicity using a full complement of *in vitro* and *in vivo* tests that is required for registration. The results from this database indicate that imidacloprid is not mutagenic (Table 54.2). Briefly, the *in vitro* point mutation tests were negative. This includes the results of chromosomal aberration tests conducted *in vitro*, which were negative at non-cytotoxic concentrations and showed only slightly positive effects at cytotoxic concentrations. *In vivo* chromosomal aberration tests were also all negative. Finally, the mitotic

recombination test that is conducted in yeast, the rec assay with *Bacillus subtilis*, and the unscheduled DNA synthesis (UDS) test were also all negative.

54.9 DEVELOPMENTAL TOXICITY

54.9.1 RAT

The potential for imidacloprid to produce developmental toxicity, including teratogenicity, was examined in the rat. In this study, mated female Wistar rats (25/dose level) were treated daily, by gavage, on gestation days 6 through 15, with doses of 10, 30, or 100 mg/kg body weight per day. On day 21 postcoitum, the fetuses were delivered by cesarean section and examined for development, including skeletal alterations.

The highest dosage of 100 mg/kg/day produced signs of maternal toxicity and a delay in embryo development. The offspring of the high-dose dams had wavy ribs as a reversible finding. While an increased incidence of wavy ribs, relative to controls, was ascribed to treatment, it was noted that the incidence was within the range of historical controls. No fetal malformations were evident at any dose level. The maternal NOEL was 10 mg/kg body weight per day and the fetal NOEL was 30 mg/kg body weight per day. These results indicate that imidacloprid is not a primary embryotoxicant and is not teratogenic.

54.9.2 RABBIT

The potential for imidacloprid to produce developmental toxicity was also examined in the rabbit. In this study, mated Chinchilla rabbits (16/dose level) were treated by gavage on gestation days 6 through 18, with daily doses of 8, 24, or 72 mg/kg body weight. Cesarean section and examination of embryo and fetal development, including fetal skeletal alterations, were conducted on day 28 postcoitum.

The highest dosage of 72 mg/kg/day produced severe maternal toxicity, including some deaths. Abortions and complete resorptions, delayed ossification, and reduced fetal weights were also evident at this dose level. The next lower dose produced decreased food consumption and reduced body weight gain, relative to controls, but no effects on the fetus. Thus, embryotoxicity was only evident at a maternally-toxic dose. As with the rat, no fetal malformations were evident at any dose level. The maternal NOEL was 8 mg/kg body weight per day and the fetal NOEL was 24 mg/kg body weight per day. These results indicate that imidacloprid is not a primary embryotoxicant and is not teratogenic.

54.10 REPRODUCTIVE TOXICITY

The potential effects of imidacloprid on reproduction and development were examined in a two-generation, two-litter study

Table 54.2
Mutagenicity Studies with Imidacloprid

Point mutation	
Salmonella microsome (AMES) test	Negative
Reverse mutation test *E. Coli*	Negative
HPRT Chinese hamster ovary (CHO)	Negative
Chromosomal aberration in vitro	
Cytogenetics human lymphocytes	Slightly positive
	(At cytotoxic concentrations only)
Sister chromatid exchange (SCE)	Slightly positive
Chinese hamster ovary (CHO)	(At cytotoxic concentrations only)
Chromosomal aberration in vivo	
Micronucleus mouse bone marrow	Negative
Sister chromatid exchange	
Chinese hamster bone marrow	Negative
Cytogenetics	
Chinese hamster bone marrow	Negative
Cytogenetics	
Mouse spermatogonia	Negative
Other genotoxicity tests	
Mitotic recombination yeast	Negative
Rec assay (*B. subtilis*)	Negative
Unscheduled DNA synthesis	
Rat hepatocytes	Negative

in Wistar rats (30/sex/dietary level in the parental generation). In this study, technical-grade imidacloprid was mixed in the diet for *ad libitum* consumption, at dietary concentrations of 100, 250, and 700 ppm. The treated feed was provided during a prepairing period of 84 days and throughout pairing, gestation, and lactation for breeding of the F1A and F1B litters. Following weaning of the F1B litters on day 21 postpartum, the F1-generation parental animals were selected. The diets were fed for 105 days prior to pairing and throughout pairing, gestation, and lactation periods for breeding of the F2A and F2B litters. This study included assessments of gonadal function, estrus cycle, mating behavior, conception, parturition, lactation, weaning, and the growth and development of the offspring of multiple generations, as well as neonatal morbidity, mortality, and behavior.

Maternal toxicity was evident at the high dose as a decrease in body weight gain and food consumption, relative to controls. A pronounced reduction in body weight gain and food consumption, relative to controls, occurred during lactation. These effects coincided with the large increase in dietary exposure that occurs during lactation, when food consumption increases rather dramatically to support the offspring. Liver enzymes (cytochrome P-450, *O*-demethylase, and *N*-demethylase) were also induced in high-dose maternal animals. In the offspring, toxicity was evident at the high dose as a marked decrease in body weight gain, relative to controls, before weaning on postnatal day 21. There were no effects on reproduction or development at any dietary level. More specifically, there was no

effect of treatment on mating indices, fertility, gestation, conception, litter size, or mortality, at any dietary level. There was also no evidence of pathology, in the form of malformations, gross lesions, a change in tissue weight, or histopathology, at any exposure level. The NOEL in this study was 6.7 mg/kg body weight per day for the adult and 12.5 mg/kg body weight per day for the offspring.

54.11 NEUROTOXICITY

54.11.1 GENERAL

The toxicology database for imidacloprid includes acute and subchronic neurotoxicity screening studies that were performed in accordance with the U.S. EPA (FIFRA) guidelines. These studies were conducted using young-adult male and female rats, following an acute oral dose, administered by gavage, or with 13 weeks of dietary exposure. Both studies included a functional observational battery (FOB) and a computer-automated test (figure-eight maze) to measure spontaneous activity, including habituation. At term (on day 14 after the acute dose or during week 14 of dietary exposure), a subset of the animals (6/sex/dose level) was anesthetized and perfused using an aldehyde fixative, and representative skeletal muscle and neural tissues were collected for microscopic examination.

54.11.2 ACUTE NEUROTOXICITY

To evaluate acute neurotoxicity, Sprague-Dawley rats (12/sex/dose level) received a single oral dose of imidacloprid, administered by gavage as an aqueous suspension at doses of 42, 151, or 307 mg/kg body weight in males and 20, 42, 151, or 307 mg/kg body weight in females. Animals were evaluated using the FOB and the figure-eight maze one week prior to treatment, again at the time of peak neurobehavioral signs, which was approximately four hours following treatment, and on days 7 and 14 following treatment.

The only evidence of systemic toxicity at 42 mg/kg was a slight decrease in the activity of females in the figure-eight maze. Additional effects that were evident at 150 mg/kg included tremor (one female), a slight decrease in body temperature, and red nasal stain. The highest dose produced severe acute toxicity, including lethality (two males and eight females). These deaths occurred within four hours to 24 hours following treatment. At the 4-hour observation period, tremor was apparent in all animals that were still alive and was more severe, relative to the next lower dose. Body temperature was also reduced an average 2.0°C and 5.5°C in males and females, respectively. Additional effects at this lethal dose included evidence of motor incoordination (e.g., incoordinated gait and impaired aerial righting), autonomic signs (e.g., perianal and urine stains), and CNS depression (e.g., minimal activity and a diminished response to stimuli).

Clinical signs following acute exposure generally resolved in surviving animals within eight hours to 24 hours following treatment. Urine stain was the only effect that persisted for up to four days after treatment. All findings in the FOB and the figure-eight maze had resolved by day 7, which was the first test occasion following the day 0 time-point. Neuropathology was not evident at the highest dose level. The NOEL was 42 mg/kg for males and 20 mg/kg for females.

54.11.3 SUBCHRONIC NEUROTOXICITY

To assess neurotoxicity with a sustained exposure, imidacloprid was administered via the diet for 13 weeks to young-adult Fischer-344 rats (12/sex/dietary level), at dietary concentrations of 150, 1000, and 3000 ppm. These dietary levels resulted in average daily exposures of 9.3, 63, and 196 mg/kg for males and 10.5, 69, and 213 mg/kg for females. The FOB and automated test of activity were performed one week prior to the initiation of treatment and during weeks 4, 8, and 13 of exposure.

There was little evidence of toxicity in this study at any dietary concentration. Effects at dietary levels of 1000 ppm and 3000 ppm were generally limited to decreased food consumption and an associated decrease in body weight gain, relative to controls. The difference in body weight for high-dose males and females averaged 15% and 8% less than control, respectively. Toxicity was not evident by cage-side observation or the automated test of motor activity, at any dietary level. On the last test occasion (week 13), there was a modest increase in the incidence of high-dose males, relative to controls, with a slightly

uncoordinated righting response that was ascribed to treatment. There was no evidence of neuropathology at the high dose. The NOEL for this study was 9.3 mg/kg body weight per day for males and 10.5 mg/kg body weight per day for females.

54.11.4 COMPARISON WITH OTHER NEONICOTINOIDS

The results from the neurotoxicity studies with imidacloprid compare closely with the findings of the acute and subchronic neurotoxicity studies that were conducted in industry laboratories with acetamiprid, clothianidin, thiacloprid, and thiamethoxam (Sheets, 2001). Comparisons involving clothianidin and thiacloprid are facilitated by the fact that those studies were conducted under comparable conditions and in the same laboratory as the studies with imidacloprid.

For each of these compounds, the time of peak effects ranged from two hours to six hours following administration by gavage. The most consistent finding at a low dose was decreased activity, which was evident by observation and in the automated test devices. By comparison, the most common effects at higher dose levels were tremor, impaired pupillary function (either dilated or pin-point pupils), incoordinated gait, and hypothermia. In studies that included a lethal dose, deaths occurred within four hours to 24 hours following treatment. Except for some residual staining, recovery generally occurred within eight hours to 24 hours following treatment. Neuropathology was not evident with any of these compounds.

The results from subchronic neurotoxicity studies with acetamiprid, clothianidin, thiacloprid, and thiamethoxam are also comparable with the findings with imidacloprid. Each compound produced minimal effects, other than decreased body weight and food consumption, at higher dose levels, and little or no overt evidence of an effect on the nervous system. Typically, there were no clinical signs, FOB findings, or effects on spontaneous activity in the automated devices, and little evidence of cumulative toxicity at any dietary level. Finally, none of these compounds produced neuropathology at the highest dietary level.

54.11.5 DEVELOPMENTAL NEUROTOXICITY

There is little information in the published literature to assist in determining the potential for imidacloprid, or any other neonicotinoid insecticide, to affect the developing nervous system. While the results from the developmental toxicity and multigeneration reproduction toxicology studies with imidacloprid provide no indication of developmental neurotoxicity, these studies are relatively limited in such assessment.

A much more rigorous assessment of effects on the developing nervous system is provided by studies that are conducted according to the U.S. EPA guideline for a developmental neurotoxicity study (U.S. EPA, OPPTS 870.6300). This study design includes a complement of automated tests of cognition, auditory startle habituation, motor activity ontogeny, and an extensive neuropathology assessment. A developmental neurotoxicity study has recently been completed with imidacloprid. Publication of this work is planned.

REFERENCES

Akayama, A., and Minamida, I. (1999). Discovery of a new systemic insecticide, nitenpyram and its insecticidal properties. *In* "Nicotinoid Insecticides and the Nicotinic Acetylcholine Receptor" (I. Yamamoto and J. E. Casida, eds.), pp. 127–148. Springer-Verlag, Tokyo.

Buckingham, S. D., Lapied, B., Le Corronc, H., Grolleau, F., and Sattelle, D. B. (1997). Imidacloprid actions on insect neuronal acetylcholine receptors. *J. Exp. Biol.* **200**, 2685–2692.

Chao, S. L., and Casida, J. E. (1997). Interaction of imidacloprid metabolites and analogs with the nicotinic acetylcholine receptor of mouse brain in relation to toxicity. *Pest. Biochem. Physiol.* **58**, 77–88.

Gundelfinger, E. D., and Schulz, R. (2000). Insect nicotinic acetylcholine receptors: Genes, structure, physiology and pharmacological properties. *In* "Handbook of Experimental Pharmacology, Vol. 144, Neuronal Nicotine Receptors" (F. Clementi, D. Fornasari, and C. Gotti, eds.), pp. 497–521. Springer-Verlag, Tokyo.

Kagabu, S., Moriya, K., Shibuya, K., Hattori, Y., Tsuboi, S., and Shiokawa, K. (1992). 1-(6-Halonicotinyl)-2-nitromethylene-imidazolidines as potential new insecticides. *Biosci. Biotech. Biochem.* **56**(2), 362–363.

Leicht, W. (1993). Imidacloprid: A chloronicotinyl insecticide. *Pestic. Outlook* **4**(3), 17–21.

Liu, M.-Y., and Casida, J. E. (1993). High affinity binding of [³H]Imidacloprid in the insect acetylcholine receptor. *Pestic. Biochem. Physiol.* **46**, 40–46.

Liu, M.-Y., Lanford, J., and Casida, J. E. (1993). Relevance of [³H]Imidacloprid binding site in house fly head acetylcholine receptor to insecticidal activity of 2-nitromethylene- and 2-nitroimino-imidazolidines. *Pestic. Biochem. Physiol.* **46**, 200–206.

Maienfisch, P., Brandl, F., Kobel, W., Rindlisbacher, A., and Senn, R. (1999). CGA 293′343: A novel, broad-spectrum neonicotinoid insecticide. *In* "Nicotinoid Insecticides and the Nicotinic Acetylcholine Receptor" (I. Yamamoto and J. E. Casida, eds.), pp. 177–209. Springer-Verlag, Tokyo.

Matsuda, K., Buckingham, S. D., Freeman, J. C., Squire, M. D., Baylis, H. A., and Sattelle, D. B. (1998). Effects of the alpha subunit on imidacloprid sensitivity of recombinant nicotinic acetylcholine receptors. *Brit. J. Pharmacol.* **123**, 518–524.

Methfessel, C. (1992). Effect of imidacloprid on the nicotinergic acetylcholine receptors of rat muscle. *Pflanzenschutz Nachrichten Bayer* **45**, 369–380.

Minamida, I., Iwanaga, K., Tabuchi, T., Aoki, I., Fusaka, T., Ishizuka, H., and Okauchi, T. (1993). Synthesis and insecticidal activity of acyclic nitroethene compounds containing a heteroarylmethylamino group. *J. Pesticide Sci.* **18**, 41.

Nagata, K., Aoyama, E., Ikeda, T., and Shono, T. (1999). Effects of nitenpyram on the neuronal nicotinic acetylcholine receptor-channel in rat phaeochromocytoma PC12 cells. *J. Pesticide Sci.* **24**, 143–148.

Nagata, K., Song, J. H., Shono, T., and Narahashi, T. (1998). Modulation of the neuronal nicotinic acetylcholine receptor-channel by the nitromethylene heterocycle Imidacloprid. *J. Pharmacol. Exper. Ther.* **285**, 731–738.

Schroeder, M. E., and Flattum R. F. (1984). The mode of action and neurotoxic properties of the nitromethylene heterocycle insecticides. *Pest. Biochem. Physiol.* **22**, 148–160.

Sheets, L. P. (2001). Neonicotinoid Insecticides. *In* "Neurotoxicology Handbook" (E. J. Massaro, ed.), Vol. 1. Humana Press, Totowa, NJ. In press.

Shiokawa, K., Tsuboi, S., Kagabu, S., and Moriya, K. (1986). *Jpn. Kokai Tokkyo Koho JP* 61-267575.

Soloway, S. B., Henry, A. C., Kollmeyer, W. D., Padgett, W. M., Powell, J. E., Roman, S. A., Tieman, C. H., Corey, R. A., and Horne, C. A. (1978). Nitromethylene insecticides. *Adv. Pestic. Sci.* **4**, 206–217.

Takahashi, H., Mitsui, J., Takakusa, N., Matsuda, M., Yoneda, H., Suzuki, J., Ishimitsu, K., and Kishmoto, T. (1992). NI-25, a new type of systemic and broad spectrum insecticide. *In* "Brighton Crop Protection Conferences B Pest and Diseases," Vol. 1, pp. 89–96.

Thyssen, J., and Machemer, L. (1999). Imidacloprid: Toxicology and metabolism. *In* "Nicotinoid Insecticides and the Nicotinic Acetylcholine Receptor" (I. Yamamoto and J. E. Casida, eds.), pp. 213–222. Springer-Verlag, Tokyo.

Tomizawa, M., and Casida, J. E. (1999). Minor structural changes in nicotinoid insecticides confer differential subtype selectivity for mammalian nicotinic acetylcholine receptors. *Br. J. Pharmacol.* **127**, 115–122.

Tomizawa, M., Latli, B., and Casida, J. E. (1999). Structure and function of insect nicotinic acetylcholine receptors studied with nicotinoid insecticide affinity probes. *In* "Nicotinoid Insecticides and the Nicotinic Acetylcholine Receptor" (I. Yamamoto and J. E. Casida, eds.), pp. 271–292. Springer-Verlag, Tokyo.

Tomizawa, M., Otsuka, H., Miyamoto, T., and Yamamoto, I. (1995). Pharmacological effects of Imidacloprid and its related compounds on the nicotinic acetylcholine receptor with its ion channel from the Torpedo electric organ. *J. Pesticide Sci.* **20**, 49–56.

Tomizawa, M., and Yamamoto, I. (1993). Structure-activity relationships of nicotinoids and Imidacloprid analogs. *J. Pesticide Sci.* **18**, 91–98.

Wiesner, P., and Kayser, H. (2000). Characterization of nicotinic acetylcholine receptors from the insects *Aphis craccivora*, *Myzus persicae*, and *Locusta migratoria* by radioligand binding assays: Relation to thiamethoxam action. *J. Biochem. Mol. Toxicol.* **14**, 221–230.

Yamada, T., Takashi, H., and Hatano, R. (1999). A novel insecticide, Acetamiprid. *In* "Nicotinoid Insecticides and the Nicotinic Acetylcholine Receptor" (I. Yamamoto and J. E. Casida, eds.), pp. 149–176. Springer-Verlag, Tokyo.

Yamamoto, I., and Casida, J. E. (1999). "Nicotinoid Insecticides and the Nicotinic Acetylcholine Receptor." Springer-Verlag, Tokyo.

Yamamoto, I., Tomizawa, M., Saito, T., Miyamoto, T., Walcott, E. C., and Sumikawa, K. (1998). Structural factors contributing to insecticidal and selective actions of neonicotinoids. *Arch. Insect Biochem. Physiol.* **37**, 24–32.

Yamamoto, I., Yabuta, G., Tomizawa, M., Saito, T., Miyamoto, T., and Kagabu, S. (1995). Molecular mechanism for selective toxicity of nicotinoids and neonicotinoids. *J. Pesticide Sci.* **20**, 33–40.

Zhang, A., Kayser, H., Maienfisch, P., and Casida, J. E. (2000). Insect nicotinic acetylcholine receptor: Conserved neonicotinoid specificity of [³H]Imidacloprid binding site. *J. Neurochem.* **75**, 1294–1303.

Zwart, R., Oortgiesen, M., and Vijverberg, H. P. M. (1992). The nitromethylene heterocycle 1-(pyridin-3-yl-methyl)-2-nitromethylene-imidazolidine distinguishes mammalian from insect nicotinic receptor subtypes. *Eur. J. Pharmacol.* **228**, 165–169.

Zwart, R., Oortgiesen, M., and Vijverberg, H. P. M. (1994). Nitromethylene heterocycles: Selective agonists of nicotinic receptors in locust neurons compared to mouse N1E-115 and BC3H1 cells. *Pestic. Biochem. Physiol.* **48**, 202–213.

CHAPTER

55

Interactions with the gamma-Aminobutyric Acid A-Receptor: Polychlorocycloalkanes and Recent Congeners

Gerald T. Brooks
University of Portsmouth

55.1 INTRODUCTION

Chlorinated insecticides have been with us for 60 years. With the exception of lindane (gamma-hexachlorocyclohexane, HCH) and endosulfan, which are relatively biodegradable and still find extensive uses, most have already been phased out or are being phased out. Their insecticidal properties were discovered at a time when the study of biochemical toxicology was in its infancy. However, the metabolism of dichlorodiphenyl-trichloroethane (DDT) was soon discovered after resistance to it appeared in 1947 and the similarities between the actions of DDT and the natural pyrethrins and cross-resistance to them in insects provided the stimulus that soon led to recognition of DDT action on the sodium channel of nerve membrane. The history of lindane and the cyclodiene-related group (collectively polychlorocycloalkanes, PCCAs) is more complex, partly because of the variety of commercially viable insecticides that arose from the early discoveries.

Lindane was soon found to be biodegradable but the strongly residual nature of the cyclodiene insecticides and the discovery that aldrin was converted into its stable epoxide, dieldrin, led to the view that these insecticides were inert. Moreover, apart from lindane, there were no other insecticide classes with recognized similar toxic action at the time and the mode of action was completely unknown and would not be revealed until more than 30 years later (ca. 1982)! A comprehensive account of the salient toxicology of these compounds was given in the first edition of this handbook (Smith, 1991). The present account summarizes research on the cyclodiene and related insecticides, which led to an appreciation of their structure–toxicity relationships and in the end to an understanding of their mode of action as noncompetitive antagonists acting in the chloride ion channel of the gamma-aminobutyric acid A (GABA)-receptor. Developments

subsequent to this discovery make research in this area a subject of continuing fascination.

For uniformity, the chemical nomenclature used follows that in the first edition. Other systems are in use, for which see Bedford (1974) and Brooks (1974). Simple acronyms and common names will be used wherever possible for chemical compounds as the full chemical names become cumbersome, especially for some of the skeletal rearrangement products so common in this series.

55.2 DISCOVERY OF POLYCHLOROCYCLOALKANE METABOLISM AS A FACTOR IN TOXICITY

55.2.1 BACKGROUND

According to the account of Lauger *et al.* (1944), DDT was the first molecule rationally designed as an insecticide, based on the known fumigant properties of chlorobenzene and the anesthetic properties of highly lipophilic chloroform. In contrast, the insecticidal properties of technical-HCH (t-HCH) (Bender, 1935) and the first cyclodiene insecticides (Hyman, 1949; Kearns *et al.*, 1945) were discovered as a result of the commercial interest in new uses for readily available chlorine and for hydrocarbons such as benzene and cyclopentadiene, chlorinated hydrocarbons being of general interest, for example, as dielectrics and fire retardants. Thus, Bender added benzene to liquid chlorine in a field and noticed that the product killed insects. Hyman sought new uses for cyclopentadiene; hexachlorocyclopentadiene ("hex") was known to be stable and, at first surprisingly, was found to react easily with cyclopentadiene in a Diels–Alder reaction, which led to chlordene, and later with norbornadiene (NB) to give aldrin. The addition of two chlorines to chlordene gave the chlordane isomers, with greatly increased insecticidal potency, whereas allylic chlorination gave heptachlor. A variant of the synthesis of aldrin, in which hexachloronorbornadiene (HCNB) reacted with cyclopentadiene, gave the isomeric isodrin and both compounds underwent chemical epoxidation to their crystalline epoxides, dieldrin and endrin, respectively.

These heavily chlorinated insecticides were at that time considered to be rather inert, whereas t-HCH was long known to be readily dechlorinated to trichlorobenzenes, etc., which was its practical use. The potent insecticidal activity of lindane (gamma-HCH; **1**, Fig. 55.1) was not established until 1943, 10 years after Bender's original observation, because lindane comprised only 10–15% of t-HCH and was readily lost during purification, which resulted mainly in crystalline, but inactive alpha- and beta-HCH (Slade, 1945). It is unfortunate that due to the high potency of lindane, t-HCH could be used directly and extensively as a practical insecticide, resulting in contamination of the environment with the remaining inactive isomers; lindane itself is relatively biodegradable and continues to be a valuable insecticide.

All of these discoveries predate modern biochemical toxicology. Indeed, resistance to modern insecticides, beginning with DDT in 1947, afforded the initial stimulus for research in this area, which subsequently became known as insect, or insecticide, toxicology and developed in parallel with but somewhat behind mammalian toxicology. One major mechanism of insect resistance to DDT was eventually found to involve its enzymatic dehydrochlorination to DDE (Sternburg *et al.*, 1954). When it was discovered that certain nontoxic DDT analogs and some other compounds suppressed resistance when co-applied with DDT, studies of the mechanisms of this synergistic effect became an important aspect of insect toxicology and synergists later became standard tools for the detection of metabolic detoxication. Natural pyrethrins were well known to be strongly synergized by various inactive methylenedioxyphenyl derivatives (e.g., piperonyl butoxide: PBO) but, as esters, these insecticides were considered likely to to be hydrolyzed *in vivo* and the mechanism of the synergistic effect was not understood. Insect resistance to the cyclodienes became evident in the early 1950s, but from research conducted on housefly resistance after 1957 (Brooks, 1960) it appeared not to involve enzymatic detoxication, in contrast to the situation with DDT. Meanwhile, Ryan and Engel (1957) found that carbon monoxide inhibited the C_{21}-hydroxylation of 17-hydroxyprogesterone by microsomes from the vertebrate adrenal cortex and showed this inhibition to be light reversible; in Klingenberg (1958) reported that rat liver microsomes contained a similar pigment, subsequently called cytochrome P450 (CyP450) (Estabrook *et al.*, 1963), that appeared to be important in the metabolism of steroids and drugs, and, in 1965, this pigment was shown to be present in microsomal preparations from insects (Lewis, 1967; Ray, 1967).

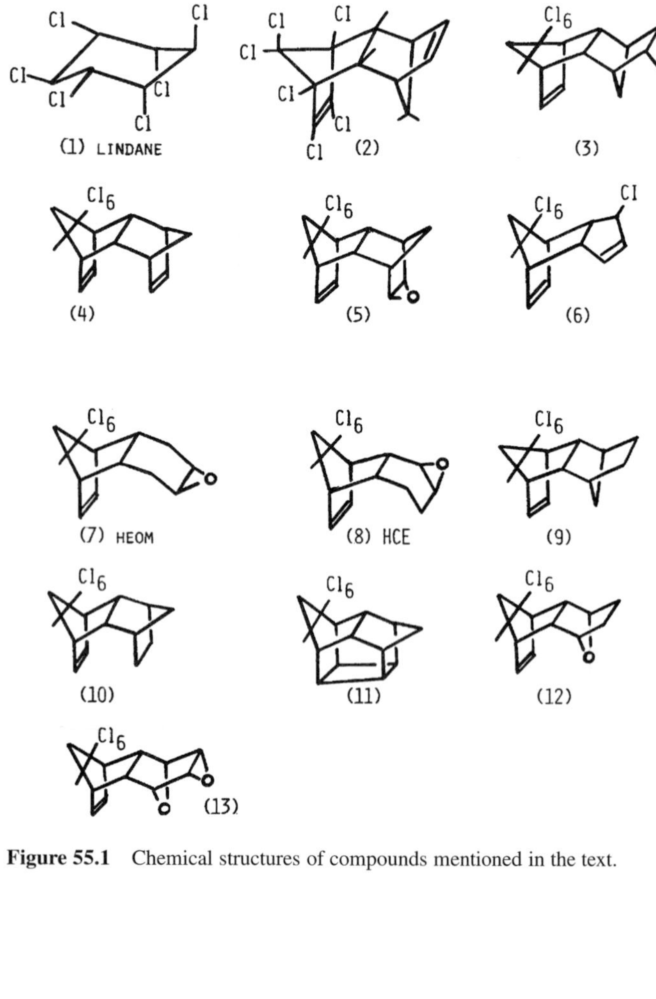

55.2.2 LINDANE, ALDRIN, DIELDRIN, ISODRIN, AND ENDRIN AND ANALOGS

A new age dawned in insect toxicology in 1960, when Sun and Johnson published the results of synergism experiments with several classes of organophosphorus insecticides and some cyclodienes (Sun and Johnson, 1960). The latter showed small factors of either antagonism (for aldrin, **2**, Fig. 55.1) or synergism (for dieldrin, **3**; isodrin, **4**; and endrin, **5**) when used in combination with the methylenedioxyphenyl (MDP) synergist sesoxane (sesamex), representative of the well-known pyrethrin synergist structures. They suggested that their results could be explained by the inhibition of metabolic oxidations *in vivo*, showed that sesoxane inhibited the epoxidation of aldrin *in vivo*, and postulated that the long-known synergism of pyrethrins by methylenedioxyphenyl compounds resulted, in fact, from inhibition of their oxidative detoxication. The small factors of antagonism for aldrin and heptachlor (**6**, Fig. 55.1) suggested that epoxidation, their only reported biotransformation at that time, was a bioactivation (toxication) reaction, so that the precursors were possibly propesticides (in current terminology).

At this time, numerous nonepoxide cyclodiene analogs were found to be synergized by sesoxane (Brooks and Harrison, 1963, 1964a), indicating that they had intrinsic toxicity of their own, although they may be pharmacokinetically less efficient

Figure 55.1 Chemical structures of compounds mentioned in the text.

than the epoxides. Also, epoxidation generally produces another toxicant, so that the level of toxic material in the tissues is maintained, whereas it is attenuated if the conversion is a detoxication reaction. Remarkably, considering the small structural change involved, removal of the unchlorinated methanobridge from dieldrin gave the isomeric cyclohexane-derived epoxides HEOM and HCE (**7** and **8**, Fig. 55.1), which were inactive (HEOM) and poorly toxic (HCE). With sesoxane, however, HCE became as toxic as dieldrin to houseflies, whereas HEOM toxicity was not improved. HCE was then found to be hydroxylated by mixed-function oxidases (MFOs) *in vivo*, mostly with epoxide ring retention, whereas HEOM suffered only addition of water to the epoxide ring, which was found to be an enzymic process, not inhibited by sesoxane (Brooks, 1966). The relative efficiencies of these pathways (Fig. 55.2) *in vitro* are shown in Table 55.1, from which it is evident that, for HCE, oxidation is the main route in microsomes from several species; liver microsomes from birds and the rat hydroxylated HEOM to some extent, whereas those from rabbit and pig liver and houseflies hydrated the epoxide ring too rapidly for oxidation to be observed. Similar products and their conjugates are formed *in vivo* (Chipman and Walker, 1979), and the availability of two routes, one blockable by MFO-inhibiting synergists *in vivo* in insects, offered the possibility of selective toxicity in favor of vertebrates, which have epoxide ring hydration available as an escape route. Because the hydration of HEOM could not be significantly inhibited *in vivo*, its intrinsic toxicity was not demonstrable by the use of any known synergist. However, HEOM had the same toxicity as DDT to tsetse flies and was toxic to some species of mosquitoes, which appeared not to hydrate the epoxide ring efficiently, thus establishing that HEOM *was* intrinsically toxic (Brooks *et al.*, 1981).

These observations verified the Sun–Johnson hypothesis regarding, the action of MDP synergists, completely altered the perspective regarding the "inertness" of cyclodienes, and provided the first firm evidence for the existence of epoxide hydro-

lases (EHs), which Boyland (1950) had suggested to mediate the ultimate metabolism of aromatic hydrocarbons via labile, nonisolable epoxides. Also, sesoxane was found to stabilize certain of the metabolically labile cyclodienes in both dieldrin-resistant (R-) and dieldrin-susceptible (S-) houseflies but it synergized them only in S-flies, supporting the view that resistance did not involve metabolic detoxication (Brooks and Harrison, 1964b).

Korte and Arent (1965) reported that dieldrin-treated rabbits excreted *trans*-6,7-dihydroxy-6,7-dihydroaldrin (*t*-DDA; **1**, Fig. 55.3) in their urine, indicating the epoxide ring opening of dieldrin to occur *in vivo*. Dieldrin and the heptachlor epoxides were subsequently found to be hydrated slowly in microsomal preparations from the livers of rabbits and pigs (Brooks and Harrison, 1969b; Brooks *et al.*, 1970). This challenged the hitherto prevailing view that cyclodienes would accumulate indefinitely in the tissues of treated animals, a challenge reinforced by the pharmacokinetic studies of Ludwig *et al.* (1964) and Robinson *et al.* [cited in Brooks (1969)] on mammals, birds, and marine organisms. The continual improvement in techniques for preparing microsomes from liver and other animal tissues afforded opportunities for the rapid examination of the likely phase 1 metabolites and stimulated interspecies comparisons of cyclodiene metabolism (Craven *et al.*, 1976;

Table 55.1
Oxidation Versus Hydration of HCE and Hydration of HEOM by Microsomes from Vertebrate Liver and Houseflies

	Pigeon	Quail	Rat	Housefly	Rabbit	Pig
HCE[a]						
Oxidation[b]	1.0	0.7[c]	1.3	1.3	2.0	1.0
Hydration[b]	0	0.02[c]	0.03	0	0.33	1.0
HEOM[d]						
Hydration rate[e]	0.005	0.06	5.74	37.0	46.0	100

[a] Vertebrate liver and housefly abdomen microsomes (+NADPH); incubations for birds 90 min at 42°C; others 30 min at 37°C.
[b] Conversion of epoxide (HCE), percent/min at pH 7.4.
[c] 11,000 g supernatant.
[d] Incubations with pig liver and housefly microsomes at 30°C for 30 min (pH 8.4), with rabbit and rat liver microsomes at 37°C (pH 7.4), and bird liver microsomes (El Zorgani *et al.*, 1970) at 42°C (pH 7.4).
[e] Relative to pig liver (100 is equivalent to 31 μg HEOM-diol formed/mg microsomal protein/min).

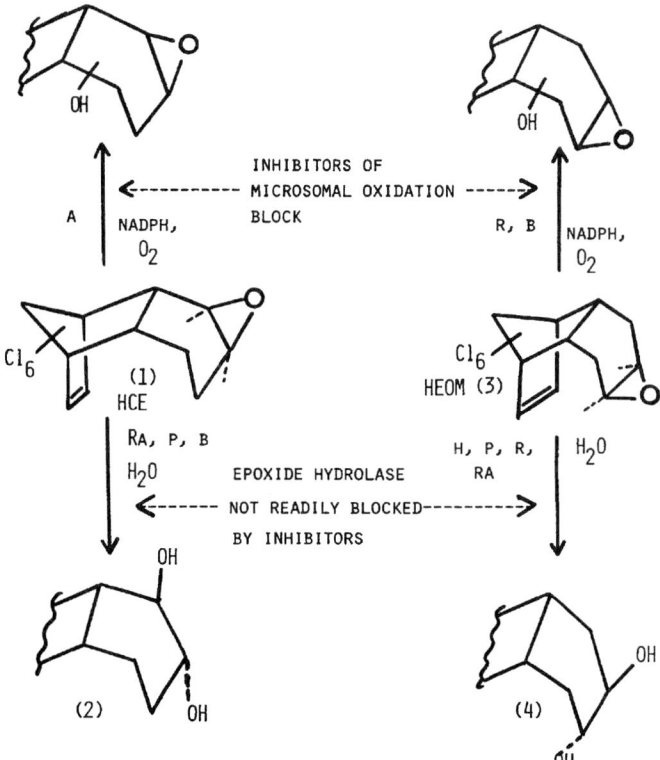

Figure 55.2 Alternative phase I metabolic pathways for HCE and HEOM and the effect of inhibitors. Epoxide ring hydration (**1** gives **2** and **3** gives **4**) is enzymic and only one enantiomer of HCE is hydrated: A, all species examined; B, some birds; H, housefly; P, pig; R, rat; Ra, rabbit. Pathways *in vitro* and *in vivo* for housefly; for mammals and birds, results are for liver homogenates and microsomes but similar products and their conjugates are formed *in vivo*.

El Zorgani *et al.*, 1970; Slade *et al.*, 1975). In contrast to alpha- and especially beta-HCH, lindane proved to be quite biodegradable, and its complex metabolism in insects and vertebrates via dehydrochlorination and oxidation to chlorinated phenols and their conjugates is well documented (Brooks, 1974; Smith, 1991; Ullman, 1972).

In contrast to the conversion of aldrin and isodrin into their stable 6,7-epoxides, dieldrin and endrin (Giannotti *et al.*, 1957; Kunze and Laug, 1953), 6,7-dihydroaldrin (**9**, Fig. 55.1) and 6,7-dihydroisodrin (**10**) lacking the olefinic double bond, are monohydroxylated in the 6-(7-)position by microsomal oxidases (Brooks, 1966; Brooks and Harrison, 1969a) and *in vivo* in houseflies. The synergism of these dihydro-compounds by sesoxane in this insect indicates that this is a detoxication, in contrast to the epoxidation reactions. This result also suggests that the dihydro-compounds are intrinsically toxic, although they act more slowly than the epoxides. Notably, these dihydro-compounds have the same synergized toxicity as photoisodrin (**11**), the complete cage rearrangement product of isodrin, which is as polar as endrin (based on R_F values) and acts more rapidly than the dihydro-compounds. Also, the 5,8-oxirane (**12**), which has a "built-in" epoxide function, is similar in toxicity to dieldrin when synergized and acts more rapidly than the other dihydro-compounds discussed (Brooks, 1966; Brooks and Harrison, 1963), again supporting the view that such compounds are intrinsically active and that epoxidation (or an appropriate increase in polarity) improves the pharmacokinetic properties of these molecules, besides maintaining the total level of toxicant in the tissues. This does not, however, rule out a possibly more efficient binding of the epoxides at the site of action.

Insect poisoning by commercial cyclodienes was not at first recognized to be reversible because their persistence in the tissues led to eventual death due to desiccation and starvation, without any recovery. Housefly poisoning by HCE was noted to be reversible, however, and even insects poisoned with HCE/sesoxane combinations would occasionally recover after prolonged periods of knockdown, although their wing musculature appeared to be permanently damaged. A further complication arose when 6,7-dihydroxydihydroaldrin (aldrin-*trans*-diol; *t*-DDA; **1**, Fig. 55.3) (Wang *et al.*, 1971) and subsequently the corresponding *cis*-DDA (Burt, 1973) were found to be rapidly neuroactive when applied to isolated nerve ganglia of the American cockroach (*Periplaneta americana*), in contrast to dieldrin, which acted significantly more slowly. Wang *et al.* (1971) then suggested that the slow action of dieldrin was related to a requirement for its conversion into *trans*-DDA, as the active neurotoxicant liberated at the site of action by dieldrin hydration. Small amounts of these diols were later reported to be dieldrin metabolites in this insect (Nelson and Matsumura, 1973). However, *t*-DDA caused prostration only slowly when injected into cockroaches, quite different from the rapid action of dieldrin *in vivo*.

The bioactivation hypothesis was further supported by the neuroactivity of *t*-DDA observed on frog nerve–muscle preparations (Akkermans *et al.*, 1974, 1975). The findings for cock-

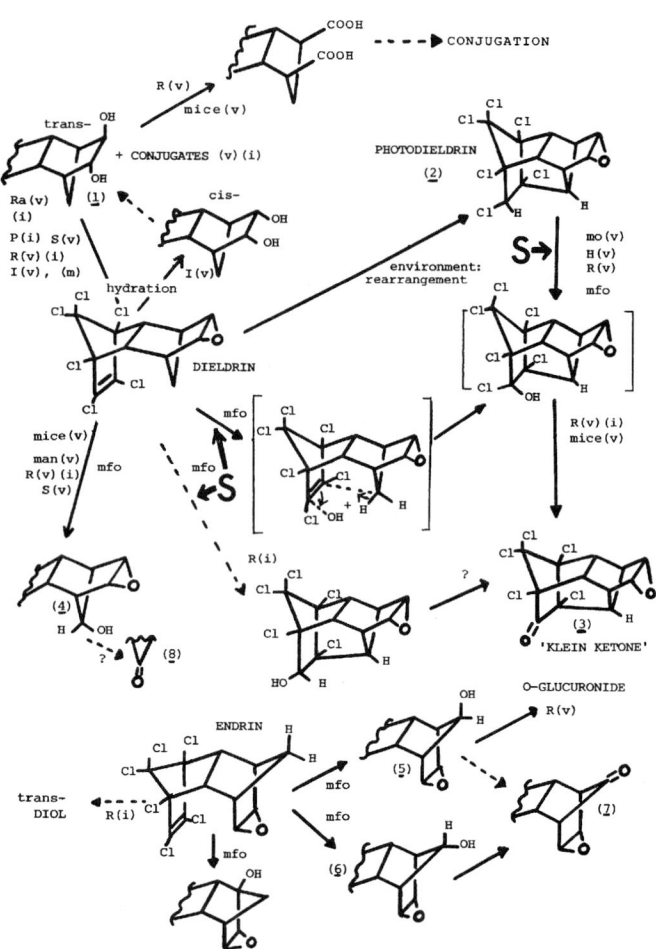

Figure 55.3 Biotransformation routes of dieldrin, photodieldrin, and endrin. Wavy line indicates only partial ring structure shown. H, housefly; I, some insects; mo, mosquito; m, microorganisms; P, pig; Ra, rabbit; R, rat; S, sheep; v, *in vivo*; i, *in vitro*; S →, sesoxane inhibits. See text for references.

roach were confirmed (Schroeder *et al.*, 1977; Shankland and Schroeder, 1973), but, based on the less intense neuroactive effect of the diols and their very slow action *in vivo*, the diols were concluded to be detoxification products in the cockroach. Both diols are produced as metabolites of dieldrin by rats and mice and appear to be detoxification products in these mammals. These pharmacokinetic studies raise questions about possible internal barriers to the penetration of such molecules and their metabolites to critical sites in the nervous system. Similar problems are apparent throughout the series and are difficult to resolve experimentally. Moreover, a particular metabolite might be a bioactivation product in one species but a detoxification product in another.

The tendency for molecular rearrangements in the environment (e.g., from exposure to sunlight) and *in vivo* has complicated investigations on residues and metabolites. Photoconversion products are frequently more toxic than the parent insecticides and may themselves be further metabolized; for example, photodieldrin (PD; **2**, Fig. 55.3) is oxidatively dechlorinated to the pentachloroketone (**3**, Fig. 55.3; "Klein's ketone";

Klein *et al.*, 1970) in rats and insects (Baldwin and Robinson, 1969; Baldwin *et al.*, 1972; Khan *et al.*, 1970; Matthews and Matsumura, 1969); PD has a much shorter half-life (2–3 days) than dieldrin (10–13 days) in rat adipose tissue but is two- to four-fold more toxic to rodents and insects (Table 55.2). Dieldrin-treated rats excrete 9-hydroxy-dieldrin (9-HD; **4**, Fig. 55.3) in the feces and the pentachloroketone in the urine (Richardson *et al.*, 1968), and these are considered to arise by alternative modes of attack from beneath the ring system (Fig. 55.3). The same pentachloroketone (**3**) was produced, along with varying amounts of 9-HD and *cis*- and *trans*-DDA, in American cockroaches, German cockroaches (*Blattella germanica*), and houseflies (Nelson and Matsumura, 1973).

The pentachloroketone (**3**) was reported to be more toxic than photodieldrin to mosquitoes and houseflies (Khan *et al.*, 1970) but less toxic and slower acting than PD to the German cockroach (Kadous and Matsumura, 1982; Reddy and Khan, 1977) indicating that PD itself is the active toxicant in this insect. PD acted four-fold more rapidly (LD$_{50}$, 0.01 μg/insect) than dieldrin (LD$_{50}$, 0.05 μg/insect) and two-fold more rapidly than the pentachloroketone (LD$_{50}$, 0.13 μg/insect) observations that suggest it has pharmacokinetic properties more favorable for toxicity than the other compounds. 9-HD (**4**) appeared to be more toxic (LD$_{50}$, 0.02 μg/insect) than dieldrin to the German cockroach and may contribute to dieldrin's toxicity in this insect; the *cis*- and *trans*-DDAs appeared to be relatively nontoxic when injected. From other experiments on the American cockroach, it seems clear that these metabolites can enter the nerve cord from the insect body and are also produced in small amounts by metabolism in the nerve itself.

Isodrin was found to be epoxidized to endrin (Fig. 55.3) in houseflies (Brooks, 1960) and subsequently by liver microsomes from rats and rabbits, as a result of mixed-function oxidase (MFO) action (Nakatsugawa *et al.*, 1965; Wong and Terriere, 1965). Endrin incubated with pig or rat liver microsomes in the presence of reduced nicotinamide adenine dinucleotide phosphate (NADPH) gave a monohydroxy-derivative, formation of which was inhibited by sesoxane, indicating MFO involvement (Brooks, 1969). It soon became clear from mammalian studies that the inversion of the unchlorinated norbornene nucleus in isodrin and endrin (as compared with aldrin and dieldrin) exposes this ring to enzymatic hydroxylation *in vivo* and greatly increases the rate of elimination of these compounds from mammalian tissues, in contrast to their behavior in insect tissues. Endrin is generally more toxic to vertebrates and less toxic to some insects than dieldrin; whereas the latter undergoes 9-hydroxylation *syn* to the epoxide ring and 9-HD (**4**, Fig. 55.3) is eliminated by conjugation in mammals, endrin is both *syn*- (slowly) and *anti*- (rapidly) hydroxylated; the *anti*-derivative (**5**, Fig. 55.3) is rapidly conjugated and excreted but the *syn*-isomer (**6**, Fig. 55.3) is further oxidized to 9-keto-endrin (9-KEN, also called 12-keto-endrin; **7**, Fig. 55.3), a remarkable example of the profound influence of stereochemistry on metabolic pathways.

Bridge-end (tertiary) hydroxylation also occurs and endrin *trans*-diol is a minor metabolite. 9-KEN is some five-fold more

toxic than endrin to rats and appears to be the ultimate toxic metabolite of endrin (Bedford *et al.*, 1975a; Hutson *et al.*, 1975). Species differences are evident, since Kadous and Matsumura (1982) reported the order of endrin metabolite toxicity to male German cockroaches as 5-OH > *anti*-9-OH > 9-keto-, whereas the order on topical application was 9-keto ~ *syn*-9-OH > endrin ≫ *anti*-9-OH to houseflies and 9-*syn*-OH > 9-keto-> endrin ≫ *anti*-9-OH to blowflies (Brooks and Mace, 1987). Also in this report, *syn*-9-hydroxydieldrin (9-HD; **4**) was essentially nontoxic to houseflies and blowflies, whereas the order 9-oxadieldrin (9-OD; **13**, Fig. 55.1) ~ dieldrin > 9-ketodieldrin (9-KD; **8**, Fig. 55.3) and 9-oxadieldrin (9-OD) ~ 9-KD > dieldrin, respectively, was found for houseflies and blowflies. Toxic 9-KD is apparently not formed from 9-HD *in vivo*, possibly because, in contrast to the situation with endrin, steric hindrance prevents enzymic attack on the hydroxyl group. Each set of toxicities lies within a narrow range and the toxicities of 9-KD and 9-OD might be expected to be similar, because 9-OD is an isostere of 9-KD, in which −C=O has been replaced by the more compact 5,8-bridged oxirane structure. These results show that several of the oxidative metabolites of these insecticides retain insect toxicity and may contribute to the toxic effect of the parent insecticides.

55.2.3 HEPTACHLOR, CHLORDENE, DIHYDROHEPTACHLOR, CHLORDANE, AND ISOBENZAN

Further chlorination of the feebly toxic chlordene, the Diels–Alder adduct of "hex" and cyclopentadiene, gave heptachlor, the dihydroheptachlor isomers (Table 55.3 and Fig. 55.4), and the chlordane isomers (Fig. 55.5). The nontoxic adduct of "hex" and *cis*-2-butene-1,4-diol, namely 5,6-bis(hydroxymethyl)-hexachloronorbornene-2-ene, is the precursor to which isobenzan, endosulfan (Fig. 55.6), bromocyclen (Bromodan®), and chlorbicyclen (Alodan®) (Fig. 55.7; **20** and **21**, respectively) are related. The last two compounds were once used to control animal ectoparasites because of their low mammalian toxicity; endosulfan is still used extensively today, whereas isobenzan was discontinued in 1965.

A preparation of heptachlor is mentioned in the original Hyman patent (Hyman, 1949) on chlordane. Numerous investigations from 1951 demonstrated the formation of heptachlor *exo*-epoxide, m.p. 160°C (HE160; Fig. 55.4); the less insecticidal *endo*-epoxide, m.p. 90°C (HE190) is not formed *in vivo* but can be obtained indirectly by chemical synthesis. The biotransformations of chlordene and heptachlor involve allylic hydroxylation for chlordene, hydrolysis of allylic chlorine for heptachlor, epoxidation (Miles *et al.*, 1969), and epoxide ring hydration (Brooks, 1966; Fig. 55.4). Microorganisms can degrade heptachlor by removing the allylic chlorine, either reductively or by hydrolysis, so that the degradation routes for chlordene can then be followed (Miles *et al.*, 1969); in some soils, the production of 1-hydroxychlordene (**1**, Fig. 55.4) is comparable to HE160 production. The hydroxylated metabolites appear to

Table 55.2
Toxicity Data for Some Polychlorocyclohexane Insecticides and Their Transformation Products

Compound	Rodent acute oral LD$_{50}$[a] (mg/kg)	Topical 24-h LD$_{50}$[b] housefly (μg/g)
Lindane	90–190	1.5
Aldrin	38–60	1.5
6,7-Dihydroaldrin		40 (3.0)
5,8-Oxadihydroaldrin		30 (1.5)
Dieldrin	47	1.0
	77 (m)	
HCE	>400	90 (2.0)
	200–400 (m)	
HEOM		>500
Photodieldrin	10	0.12
	7 (m)	
Didechlorodieldrin (DD)	0.9	0.2
	1.4	
9-Hydroxydieldrin (9-HD)	>400 (m)	750
trans-Dihydroaldrin-diol (t-DDA)	1,250 (m)	>750
Isodrin	12–17	3.0
6,7-Dihydroisodrin		39 (4.0)
Photoisodrin	>2,000	15 (3.0)
Endrin	5.6	2.0
	29 (m)	
9-Keto-endrin	1.0	0.95
anti-9-Hydroxy-endrin (AHEN)	2.5–5.5	>100
syn-9-Hydroxy-endrin	1.2	1.2
Heptachlor epoxide (HE160)	60	1.0
Heptachlor epoxide (HE90)		6.0
1-Hydroxychlordene	2,400–4,600	Inactive
Chlordene		50 (20)
Chlordene exo-epoxide		35 (4.0)
1-Hydroxy-chlordene exo-epoxide		Inactive
trans-Chlordane	1,100	11
cis-Chlordane	500–600	4.0
alpha-Endosulfan	76	5.0
beta-Endosulfan	240	9.0
Endosulfan sulfate	76	9.5
Endosulfan diol	>15,000	>500
Endosulfan ether	>15,000	>500
alpha-Hydroxy-endosulfan ether	1,750	>500
Endosulfan lactone	306 (m)	>500
Isobenzan	3–10	1.0
	6.0 (m)	
Bromocyclen (Bromodan®)	13,000	11.5
Chlorbicyclen (Alodan®)	15,000	15.5
Mirex	600–>3,000	
Chlordecone	125	
Toxaphene (technical)	90–270	
Toxaphene (component B)	75 (m; ip)	

[a] For rat unless marked (m) for mouse.

[b] Parenthetic values in housefly column are toxicities measured with sesoxane (5 μg), preapplied before the insecticide to inhibit microsomal oxidases.
Data from Brooks and Harrison (1964a), Buchel et al. (1966a, 1966b), Jager (1970), Khan et al. (1970), Korte (1967), Maier-Bode (1968), Miles et al. (1969), and Bedford et al. (1975a), Smith (1991).

be detoxification products in mammals. This is difficult to prove in insects, however.

Chlordene (**2**, Fig. 55.4) and its *exo*-epoxide (**3**, Fig. 55.4) have a weak housefly toxicity, which is synergized 10-fold by sesoxane, suggesting that the biotransformations observed in microsomal preparations are detoxications (Brooks, 1966; Brooks and Harrison, 1964a, 1967a, b). Is heptachlor much more toxic than chlordene because the allylic chlorine inhibits hydroxylation in this position and also ensures that heptachlor is converted into the metabolically stable epoxide ?—a question reminiscent of the aldrin/dieldrin situation. The view that heptachlor is intrinsically toxic is supported by the toxicity (Table 55.3) of the alpha- and beta-dihydroheptachlor isomers (Fig. 55.4), formed by the addition of hydrogen chloride to the double bond of chlordene. Their housefly toxicity also is synergized by sesoxane, which suggests that metabolic hydroxylation, which for them replaces the epoxidation of heptachlor, results in detoxication. Beta-dihydroheptachlor (beta-DH; Fig. 55.4; **2**, Table 55.3) is particularly interesting because of its low mammalian toxicity (Buchel *et al.*, 1966a, 1966b). In the presence of NADPH, pig liver microsomes converted alpha-, beta-, and gamma-DH into a variety of hydroxylation products, which are illustrated for beta-DH in Fig. 55.4. These were chlorohydrins, obtained by simple hydroxylation of the cyclopentane rings; alcohols, formed by elimination of the single chlorine atom on the cyclopentane ring; dihydroxy-compounds; and a ketone (e.g., 2-keto-dihydrochlordene from beta-DH, which may afford the corresponding alcohol via a keto-reductase reaction). The 2-OH-dihydrochlordene excreted by rats fed beta-DH (Korte, 1967) may arise in this way. Similar metabolites were produced in housefly microsomes, although no dihydroxy-compounds were detected. Sesoxane inhibited the hydroxylations, which doubtless explains the synergism against houseflies observed *in vivo* (Table 55.3).

The metabolism of the two chlordane isomers, alpha- (= *trans*-1,2-dichlorodihydrochlordene) and beta- (= *cis*-1,2-dichlorodihydrochlordene), is complex (Fig. 55.5). Either isomer might give heptachlor by dehydrochlorination and hence HE160 and all the metabolites arising therefrom. In fact, the metabolites in rats include 1-*exo*,2-dichlorochlordene (**1**, Fig. 55.5), oxychlordane (**2**), 1-*exo*-hydroxy-2-chlorochlordene (**3**), 1-*exo*-hydroxy-2-chloro-2,3-epoxychlordene (**4**), 1-*exo*-hydroxy, 2-*endo*-chlorodihydrochlordene (chlordene chlorohydrin), 1,2-*trans*-dihydroxydihydrochlordene, and the metabolites of heptachlor (Brimfield and Street, 1979; Brimfield *et al.*, 1978; Tashiro and Matsumura, 1977). A similar series of compounds was excreted in the form of unidentified conjugates in the urine of rabbits treated with these chlordane isomers (Balba and Saha, 1978).

These biotransformations demonstrate the remarkable versatility of the drug-metabolizing enzymes. In particular, the formation in rats of oxychlordane (Fig. 55.5), analogous to heptachlor epoxide and said to be more toxic than *trans*-chlordane (Street and Blau, 1972), is a bioactivation due to the unexpected formation of a stable epoxide *in vivo*, presumably following an enzymatic desaturation that introduced a 2,3-double bond. There was no evidence for epoxide formation from either *cis*- or *trans*-chlordane in houseflies, however. Notably, *trans*-chlordane was three-fold less toxic than *cis*-chlordane to this insect, and neither isomer was synergized by sesoxane (Brooks

Table 55.3
Toxicities of Dihydroheptachlor and Chlordane Isomers to Housefly and Mouse

Compound	A	B	C	D	Housefly LD$_{50}$ (μg/fly)[a]	Housefly LD$_{50}$ (μg/fly with sesoxane)[a]	Mouse acute oral LD$_{50}$ (mg/kg)
(**1**) α-	Cl	H	H	H	0.26	0.015	1,285
(**2**) β-	H	Cl	H	H	0.16	0.015	>9,000
(**3**) γ-	H	H	Cl	H	1.8	0.07	>6,000
(**4**)[b]	Cl	H	Cl	H	0.22	0.22	1,100
(**5**)[b]	Cl	Cl	H	H	0.08	0.08	500–600
(**6**)	H	Cl	Cl	H	0.04	—	>600
(**7**)[b]	Cl	H	H	Cl	0.04	—	31
Alodan		—			0.31	0.05	15,000[c]
Dieldrin		—			0.02	0.02	75—100

[a] Topical application; sesoxane applied (5 μg/20 mg fly) before insecticide.
[b] **4**, *trans*-chlordane; **5**, *cis*-chlordane; **7**, δ-chlordane.
[c] LD$_{50}$ for rat.
Data compiled from Brooks and Harrison (1964a, 1967b) and Buchel *et al.* (1966a, b).

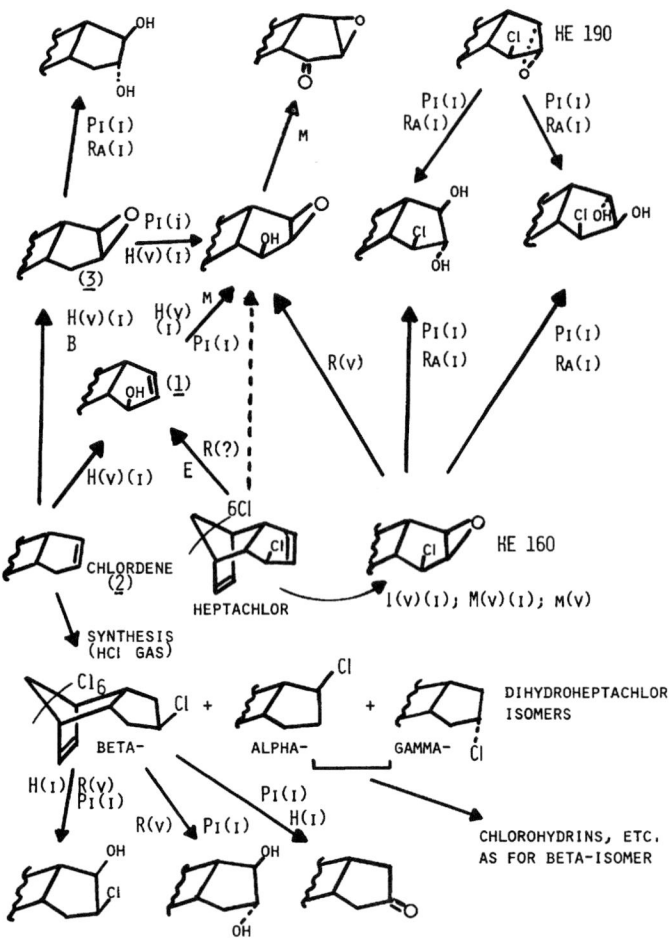

Figure 55.4 Biotransformations of chlordene, heptachlor, and the dihydroheptachlor isomers. B, bacteria; H, housefly; I, some insects; M, mammals generally; Pi, pig; R, rat; m, microorganisms; Ra, rabbit; E, abiotic conversion; v, *in vivo*; i, *in vitro*. All structures contain the fully chlorinated norbornene moiety.

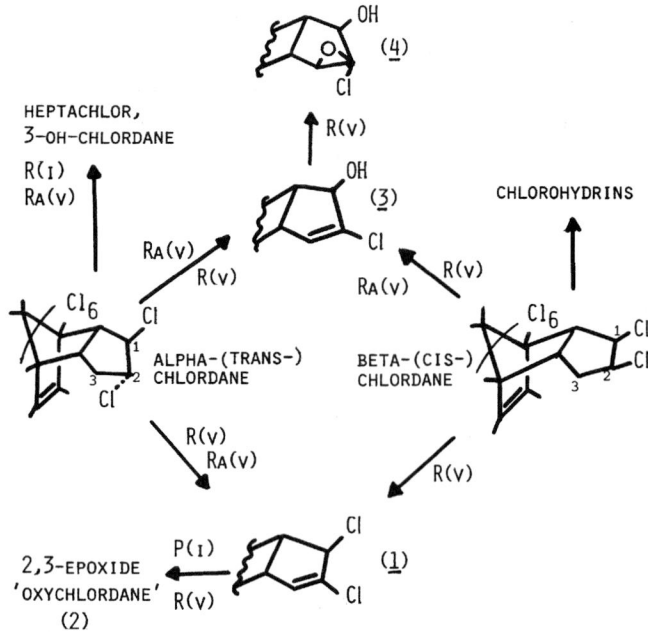

Figure 55.5 Biotransformations of the *cis*- and *trans*-chlordane isomers. Abbreviations as in Fig. 55.3. All structures contain the fully chlorinated norbornene moiety.

and Harrison, 1964a), indicating that intrinsic toxicities were being measured. Alpha- and beta-DH were as toxic as heptachlor when synergized; synergized gamma-DH was four-fold less toxic than synergized alpha- and beta-DH and as toxic as *cis*-chlordane (Table 55.3). This suggests that the 2-*endo*-chlorine atoms in *trans*-chlordane and gamma-DH contribute less to toxicity than the *exo*-chlorines present in alpha- and beta-DH and *cis*-chlordane. Moreover, an additional chlorine introduced into the 2-*exo*-position of gamma-DH (Table 55.3) increases its toxicity more than 40-fold, so that the resulting *gem*-dichloro-compound is as toxic as beta-DH having the single *exo*-chlorine in this position.

Does this extra *exo*-chlorine simply reduce the possibilities for metabolic detoxification that are more likely for gamma-DH (*exo*-side of the ring exposed to enzymatic attack) and *trans*-chlordane, or do *exo*-chlorines increase the affinity of these molecules for a critical binding site in the nervous system? That synergized gamma-DH is as toxic as *cis*-chlordane (unaffected by sesoxane) may suggest that metabolism is the only factor involved and that the *exo*- or *endo*-disposition of the chlorines is immaterial. There is also the interesting question of the

role of symmetry; the most insecticidal compounds in this series are beta-DH, the 2,2-*gem*-dichloro-analog (gamma-DH), and 1-*exo*, 3-*exo*-dichlorodihydrochlordene (delta-chlordane; Table 55.4), all having a plane of symmetry, in contrast to the other molecules discussed, for which the enantiomers may differ in toxicity (see later discussion on the heptachlor epoxide enantiomers in Section 55.3.1).

Production of isobenzan (Telodrin® ceased in 1965 (Jager, 1970), but this molecule (Fig. 55.6) remains of theoretical interest as a cyclic ether analog of gamma-chlordane, which, like the latter, has high insect and mammalian toxicity. Enzymatic attack on the chlorinated cyclic ether structure of isobenzan analogous to the biotransformations noted for the chlordane isomers results in hydrophilic metabolites such as derivatives of the gamma-hydroxy-acid (**1**, Fig. 55.6), which afforded the lactone (**2**) and alcohol (**3**) on hydrolysis. Alternatively, these might arise directly by oxidative or hydrolytic elimination of chlorine atoms from the cyclopentane ring. Of particular interest because they illustrate the variety of structures having toxicity in this series is the mixture of two interconvertible isomeric ketones (**14** and **15**, Fig. 55.7), with high insect and mammalian toxicity (housefly LD$_{50}$, 0.5 μg/g; rat LD$_{50}$, 7 mg/kg), which can be obtained chemically from 5,6-bis(hydroxymethyl)-HCNB ("endosulfan-diol"). Transannular dehydrochlorination affords an even more toxic cage ketone (**16**, Fig. 55.7; housefly LD$_{50}$, 0.25 μg/g; rat acute oral LD$_{50}$, 1.0 mg/kg). These analogs of isobenzan are more compact versions of the various cage molecules formed from dieldrin and provide further evidence that the dichloroethylene moiety of cyclodienes can be replaced by other polar moieties without loss of toxicity and with increased toxicity in some cases.

Table 55.4
Insect Toxicity of Aldrin and Dieldrin Relatives, Including Some Molecules with Fewer Chlorine Atoms

X = Y = carbon, except for compounds (3) and (4)

Chemical	Chlorination in aldrin analog						HF[a]	GR[b]
	1	2	3	4	10-*syn*	10-*anti*		
(1)	---------	- - -		6-Cl	-------	------ (aldrin)	0.55	2.0
(2)	---------	- - -		6-Cl	- - - ---------	6,7-epoxide: dieldrin	1.0	1.0
(3)	---------	- - -		6-Cl	- - - ---------	6,7-N=N—	3.6	5.3
(4)	---------	- - -		6-Cl	- - - ---------	6,7-N=N(→ O)—	4.45	2.1
(5)	1	H	H	4	10s	10a	2.1	9.3
(6)	1	H	H	4	10s	10a (6,7-epoxide: DD)	3.8	8.0
(7)	1	H	H	4	H	H	0.03	0.8
(8)	1	2	3	4	H	10a	0.08	0.65
(9)	1	2	3	4	10s	H	0.02	Inactive

[a] Housefly toxicity compared with dieldrin (1.0) by direct spray.
[b] German cockroach toxicity compared with dieldrin (1.0) by exposure to dry films on paper.
Data compiled from Soloway (1965).

55.2.4 ENDOSULFAN (THIODAN)

Technical endosulfan is a 7:3 mixture of the alpha- (m.p. 109°C) and beta- (m.p. 213°C) isomers, the former (Fig. 55.6) having an "extended," dieldrin-like structure (see also Section 55.4.3) and the latter having a cagelike structure resembling endrin stereochemically. The alpha-isomer is more toxic than the beta-isomer to mammals and houseflies; both are oxidized *in vivo* to endosulfan sulfate (**4**, Fig. 55.6), which resembles beta-endosulfan stereochemically and has similar toxicity to alpha-endosulfan, so that this conversion is analogous to the aldrin-to-dieldrin one. The cyclic sulfite (and sulfate) ester structures completely alter the behavior of the endosulfans, which disappear quite rapidly from living tissue, partly by hydrolysis to the parent nontoxic endosulfan-diol and metabolites similar to those formed from isobenzan. The sulfate is formed faster from the alpha- than from the beta-isomer in houseflies and is as toxic as beta-endosulfan to these insects (Barnes and Ware, 1965); cyclodiene-resistant flies eliminated these isomers more rapidly than normal (S-) flies, but the tissues contained only the toxic sulfate, which also appears in the body fat of mammals but disappears rapidly when exposure ceases. Endosulfan-treated locusts excreted the sulfate, endosulfan ether, alpha-hydroxy-endosulfan ether (**3**, Fig. 55.6), and the corresponding lactone (**2**). Endosulfan-treated mice stored the sulfate transiently in their fat and excreted endosulfan, the sulfate, and the parent diol in feces (Maier-Bode, 1968). It is evident that endosulfan is a relatively nonpersistent compound in mammals (Dorough *et al.*, 1978) and has generally favorable environmental properties, apart from high fish toxicity, which requires caution in aquatic situations. With the exception of the toxic sulfate, metabolites of endosulfan isomers are undoubtedly detoxication products.

55.2.5 TOXAPHENE, MIREX, CHLORDECONE (KEPONE)

Toxaphene (camphechlor) is a complex mixture of some 177 compounds obtained by chlorinating camphene to a 67–69% chlorine content (Pollock and Kilgore, 1980; Saleh *et al.*, 1979). The identified compounds are actually chlorinated bornanes arising from the Wagner–Meerwein rearrangement of the camphene skeleton, among which the octachloronorbornanes; 2,2,5-*endo*, 6-*exo*-8,8,9,10-octachloro-norbornane (**17**, Fig. 55.7) and 2,2,5-*endo*,6-*exo*-8,9,9,10-octa-chloronorbornane (**18**, Fig. 55.7), are highly potent, with mouse ip LD_{50} values of 2–3 mg/kg (Turner *et al.*, 1977). The less toxic 2,2,5-*endo*,6-*exo*,8,9,10-heptachloronorbornane (**19**; compound B; LD_{50}, 75 mg/kg) was potentiated eight-fold by PBO administered prior to the insecticide, suggesting the possibility of oxidative detoxication mechanisms for this compound. Experiments with rat liver preparations confirmed metabolism by MFO, and the formation of glutathione and glucuronide conjugates (Chandurkar and Matsumura, 1979) could be demonstrated (see Smith, 1991).

The positioning of the added chlorine substituents in compound B seems to be critical; at the 3-*exo*-position and in the 10-chloromethyl moiety, an additional chlorine greatly reduces mouse toxicity, as does the combination of 3-*exo*-chlorination and 5,6-dehydrochlorination, to give a vinylic chlorine atom. Notably also, the simpler (less bulky) molecules

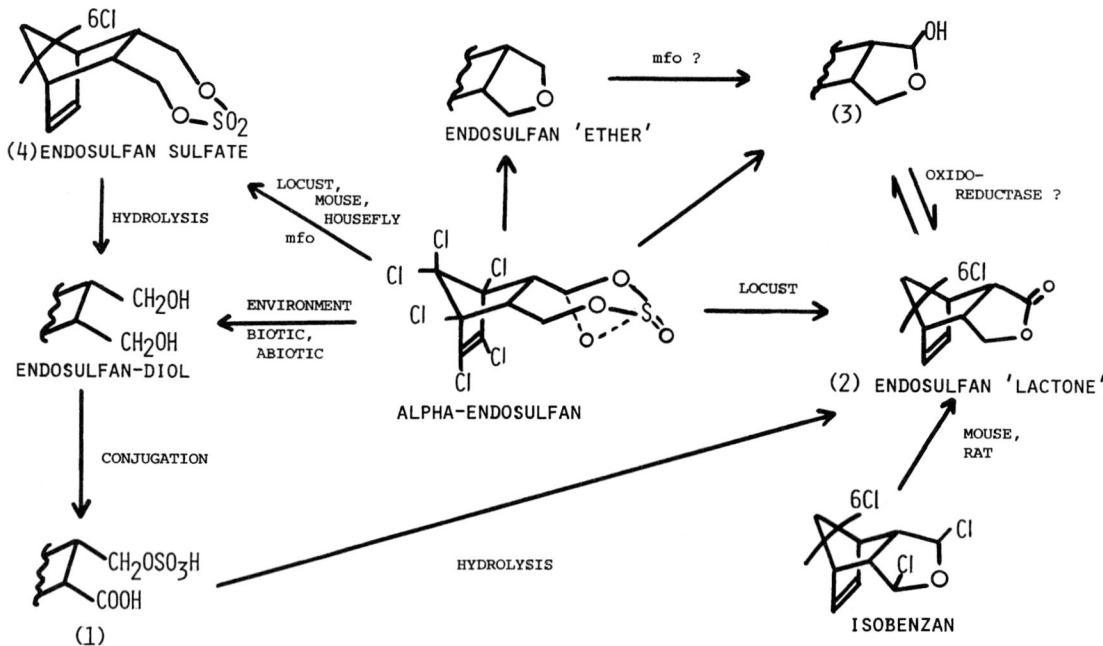

Figure 55.6   Major transformations of alpha-endosulfan and isobenzan. All structures contain the fully chlorinated norbornene moiety. Note that --O-- indicates the skewed ("*trans*") position of the second oxygen in the "twist-chair" (asymmetric) configuration of alpha-endosulfan (Schmidt *et al.*, 1997).

hexachloronorbornene-2,5-diene and heptachloronorborn-2-ene used to prepare cyclodiene insecticides lack toxicity, which only appears when halomethyl groups are introduced into the nucleus as in bromocyclen (Bromodan®; **20**, Fig. 55.7) and chlorobicyclen (Alodan®, **21**). Both are synergized 10-fold by sesoxane in houseflies (Brooks and Harrison, 1964a; Table 55.2) and are quite good insecticides with very favorable mammalian toxicity (rat acute oral LD$_{50}$s, 13000–15000 mg/kg); that is, they appear to be considerably more selective (insect versus mammal) than the most toxic components of toxaphene.

Mirex (**22**, Fig. 55.7) is the fully chlorinated cage molecule, formed by the self-condensation of two molecules of "hex," and might be expected to be rather resistant to enzymatic attack. Animal tissue levels plateau only slowly on exposure and decrease very slowly when exposure ceases. One chlorine atom is reductively replaced in the environment to give photomirex (8-monohydro-mirex), which appears to behave like mirex in the rat (Chu *et al.*, 1979; Hallett *et al.*, 1978). Reductive dechlorination can occur *in vivo*; 2,8-dihydromirex and 5,10-dihydromirex have been identified as rat metabolites. Whereas 2,8-dihydromirex does not appear to be further metabolized, 5,10-dihydromirex appears to be converted into more polar metabolites, which appear in rat urine (Yarbrough *et al.*, 1983). Mirex has low mammalian toxicity (rat oral LD$_{50}$ ranging from 600 to > 3000 mg/kg) and its signs of poisoning differ from those produced by the less chlorinated cyclodienes.

The metabolism of mirex in houseflies is equally slow, and Shankland (1982) compared its slow insecticidal action with the delayed onset of dieldrin poisoning discussed earlier. The onset of poisoning following topical application of lethal doses of mirex to the American cockroach occurred only after 3 days. Moreover, when isolated sixth abdominal ganglia were irrigated with suspensions of 5×10^{-4} M mirex for 4 h, there was no change in the patterns of spontaneous activity or elicited postganglionic responses. Ganglia excised from symptomatic cockroaches showed, however, spontaneous after-discharge behavior characteristic of poisoning following dieldrin treatment. Hemicholinium-3, which depletes Ach stars, eliminated the neuroactivity in giant fibers, but the ganglia remained responsive to nicotine, as is found in dieldrin poisoning. Because mirex appears to be highly resistant to biotransformation, Shankland concluded that the delayed action was unlikely to involve a requirement for bioactivation and must arise from the intrinsic properties of this highly chlorinated molecule, such as slow penetration through diffusion barriers in the insect central nervous system.

Chlordecone (Kepone, **23**, Fig. 55.7) differs from mirex in having a carbonyl group, which is probably responsible for its moderately rapid clearance from animal tissues. In humans and pigs, this is via the alcohol (chlordecol), and a cytosolic keto-reductase, which can effect this reduction, has been found in gerbil and human liver (Molowa *et al.*, 1986). Bloomquist and Shankland (1983) found that chlordecone produced the same signs of poisoning as mirex in the American cockroach and concluded that chlordecone has the same mode of action as dieldrin, although, like mirex, it acts more slowly. From experiments on the displacement of [^{3}H] picrotoxinin (PTX) binding by mirex and chlordecone from American cockroach head membranes, Tanaka *et al.* (1984) concluded that chlordecone interacts with the PTX-binding site, as expected, whereas mirex was much less potent in this respect; moreover, dieldrin-resistant

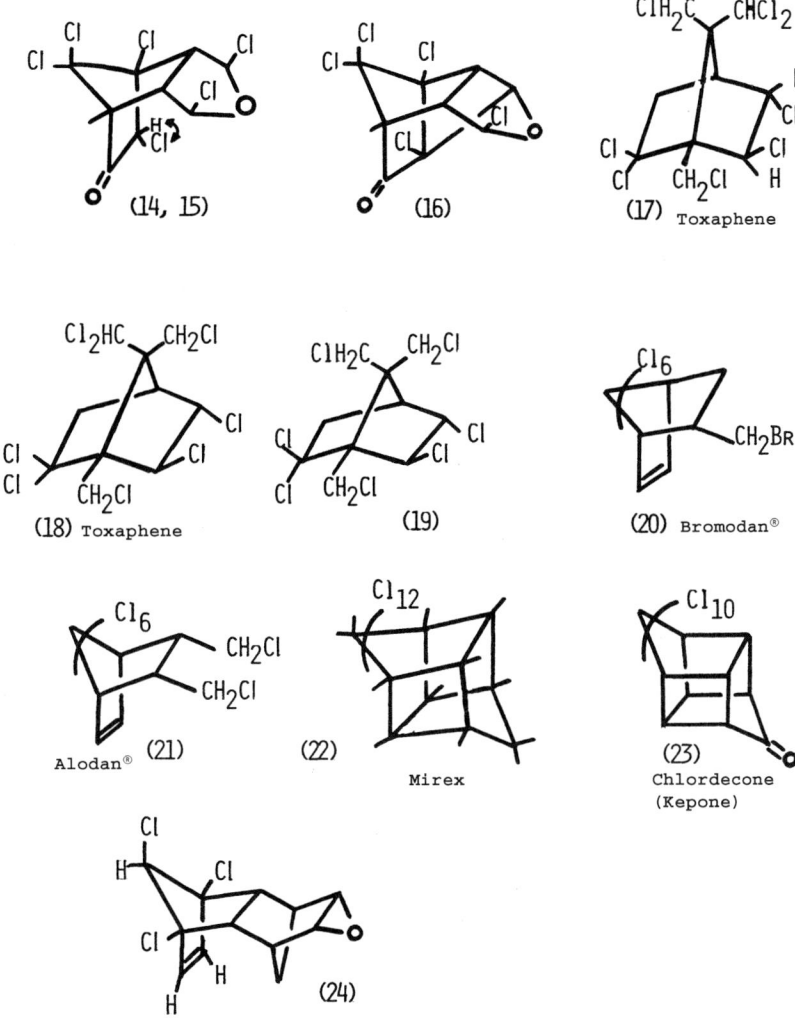

Figure 55.7   Chemical structures of compounds mentioned in the text.

German cockroaches were resistant to chlordecone but not to mirex. Chlordecone is also known to have inhibitory effects on neurotransmitter uptake in mammals and such an action may also contribute to its insect toxicity.

55.3 STRUCTURE–TOXICITY RELATIONSHIP AND MODE OF ACTION

55.3.1 FULLY CHLORINATED CYCLODIENES: SUBSTITUTED HEXACHLORONORBORNENES (HCNB)

Soloway (1965) published a comprehensive review on the structure–activity relationships of cyclodiene insecticides at a time when information on their metabolism was just beginning to appear, so his review makes only passing reference to the possible influence of metabolism but provides a great deal of information about toxicity trends in numerous series of cyclodiene analogs. Initially, he emphasized the similarity between heptachlor epoxide HE160/*cis*-chlordane and HE90/*trans*-chlordane (Figs. 55.4 and 55.5), each pair having two similarly oriented electronegative atoms (i.e., oxygen and chlorine), with toxicity greater in the first (*exo,exo*) orientation than in the second (*exo,endo*) orientation of these substituents. Delta-chlordane (Table 55.3) with 1-*exo*,3-*exo* chlorine substituents is a highly insecticidal symmetrical variant of the orientation found in the HE160/*cis*-chlordane pair.

Interestingly, delta-chlordane is an analog of alodan in which the two side-chain chlorines have become fixed in the *exo*-positions by the extra carbon atom of the cyclopentane ring and their insect toxicities are of the same order when alodan is synergized by sesoxane (Table 55.3). The second (3-*exo*) chlorine in delta-chlordane has a severe effect on mammalian toxicity, because this molecule has a much higher rodent toxicity than either alodan, alpha- (**1**, Table 55.4) or beta-dihydroheptachlor (**2**) (DH), or the chlordane isomers (**4**, **5**). As noted already, the order of housefly toxicity of the DH-isomers is beta-DH > alpha-

DH > gamma-DH; beta-DH has an *exo*-chlorine and is also symmetrical, alpha-DH has an *exo*-chlorine but is asymmetrical, whereas gamma-DH has an *endo*-chlorine, which, being "hidden" beneath the ring system, may be less accessible to a critical binding site and also leaves the *exo*-face of the ring more exposed to metabolic attack from the *exo*-side (compare the metabolism of endrin in Section 55.2.2).

Soloway presented insect toxicity data for many derivatives of HCNB of the chlordane, isobenzan, endosulfan, aldrin, and isodrin series, together with lindane, which already appeared to have the same mode of action (Busvine, 1964). He concluded that high insecticidal activity required the presence of two electronegative centers within a narrow range of distance and direction with respect to one another and placed on or across the plane of symmetry defined by the CCl₂-bridge. Many cyclodienes fulfill these requirements but some, such as dihydroaldrin, dihydroisodrin, and photoisodrin (**9**, **10**, and **11**, respectively, Fig. 55.1) (only one electronegative center) and bromodan (**20**, Fig. 55.7), alpha-DH, *exo*-chlordene epoxide (Fig. 55.4), and HCE (**8**, Fig. 55.1) (asymmetrical), do not, yet are indicated to have high intrinsic toxicities when their metabolism is suppressed *in vivo*. Evidently, the involvement of a second electronegative center such as an epoxide ring in binding to the site of action may increase the affinity of the molecule for this site, by hydrogen bonding, for example. Thus, lack of a second electronegative center may explain the earlier noted slow action of the dihydro-compounds, which, in the absence of an inhibitor of metabolic oxidations, may afford them increased opportunity for both detoxication and binding to inert storage sites. Notably, the cage molecule photoisodrin is more polar than the related dihydroisodrin and dihydroaldrin and acts rapidly, especially when synergized; it may have the more favorable pharmacokinetic properties of the more rapidly acting epoxides, although apparently lacking their second electronegative center (Brooks, 1973; Brooks and Harrison, 1963).

There is limited information about the relative toxicities of enantiomeric forms of chiral cyclodienes, which are obviously of interest in this context. The epoxide hydrolases of pig liver microsomes selectively hydrate the same enantiomers of chlordene epoxide, HCE and HE90 (Brooks *et al.*, 1968). The isolated residual epoxides appeared to have the same order of toxicity to houseflies as their respective racemates, which are not detectably hydrated by this insect (Brooks *et al.*, 1970). Miyazaki *et al.* (1978, 1979, 1980) synthesized the pure enantiomers of chlordene, chlordene *exo*-epoxide, HE160, 2-chloroheptachlor (Fig. 55.8), and 3-chloroheptachlor and found that their toxicities to the German cockroach (topical LD₅₀, μg/g) were in the order (+)-chlordene (148) > racemic chlordene (>300) > (−)-chlordene (inactive); (−)-chlordene epoxide (74) > racemic chlordene epoxide (158) > (+)-epoxide (inactive); racemic heptachlor (2.64) > (+)-heptachlor (3.38) > (−)-heptachlor (5.32); (+)-HE160 (1.29) > racemate (1.82) > (−)-HE160 (2.98); (+)-2-chloroheptachlor (20) > racemate (50) > (−)-2-chloroheptachlor (100); 3-chloroheptachlor (enantiomers and racemate inactive).

Miyazaki *et al.* concluded that (−)-chlordene is intrinsically nontoxic to the German cockroach, observing that the corresponding (+)-epoxide (nontoxic) formed *in vivo* is metabolized to the expected oxidative and hydrolytic products (Brooks and Harrison, 1965) at about the same rate as the toxic (−)-epoxide from observably toxic (+)-chlordene. However, they also considered (+)-chlordene to be intrinsically inactive, therefore requiring bioactivation by conversion into the toxic (−)-epoxide *in vivo*. Unfortunately, these experiments did not include a synergist to suppress oxidative metabolism. Experiments with houseflies showed that both chlordene and dihydrochlordene had low but measurable toxicities to that insect, which were synergized by sesoxane (Brooks, 1966; Brooks and Harrison, 1964a); in fact, synergized chlordene was only five-fold less toxic than synergized chlordene *exo*-epoxide. The role of epoxidation in the toxicities of the heptachlor enantiomers (or those of 2-chloroheptachlor) has not been reported. The (+)- to (−)-heptachlor toxicity ratio for German cockroach was 1.56; for (+)- to (−)-HE160 it was 2.3 and for (+)- to (−)-2-chloroheptachlor it was 5.0, with the more toxic (+)-antipodes

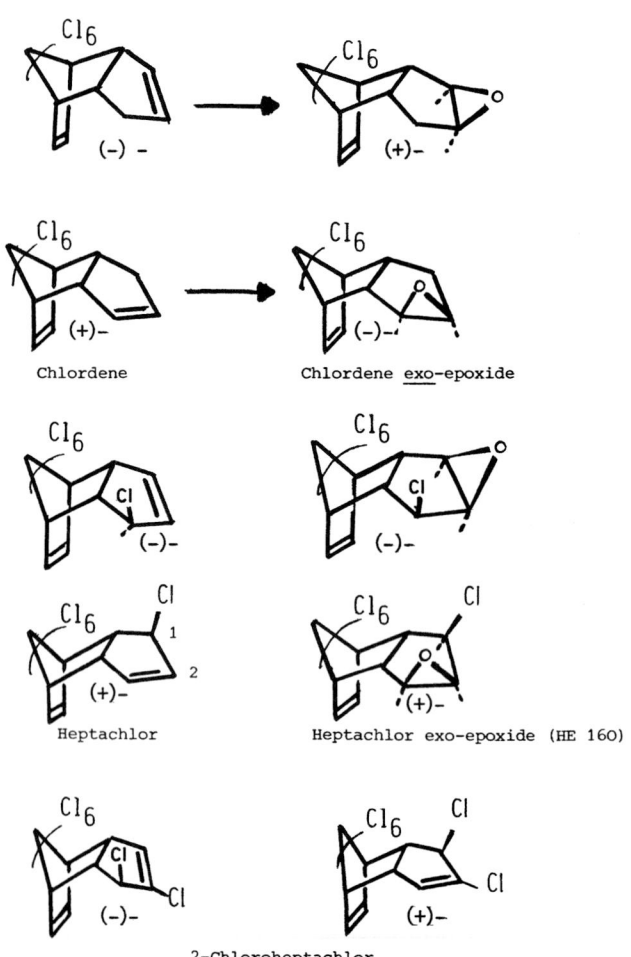

Figure 55.8 Absolute stereochemical configuration of the enantiomers of chlordene, chlordene epoxide, heptachlor, heptachlor epoxide (HE160), and 2-chloroheptachlor as established by Miyazaki *et al.* (1978, 1979, 1980).

and toxic (−)-chlordene epoxide all having the same absolute stereochemistry (Fig. 55.8).

Apart from (+)-chlordene epoxide and the antipodes of 3-chloroheptachlor, the other antipodes are clearly all active but the ratio of 2.3 for the HE160 antipodes is likely to be the safest measure of comparative intrinsic toxicities in this series because the known stability of this epoxide should avoid or minimize the complication of metabolism *in vivo*. Thus, although one absolute configuration of HE160 is favored, both are toxic, which might be expected if the critical binding site is in a symmetrical (or nearly symmetrical) cylinder of about the same diameter as the molecules discussed, so that either antipode can interact reasonably well with such a site in the bore of the structure, now known to be the chloride ionophore of the GABA$_A$-receptor (Section 55.4).

Notably, alpha-DH must exist in enantiomeric forms, which, if superimposed, give a symmetrical "composite" molecule that resembles both delta-chlordane and isobenzan (its oxygen isostere). Likewise, superimposition of the enantiomers of both HE160 and HE90 gives "composites" that are similar to both delta-chlordane and isobenzan. Such symmetrical molecules might be expected to interact particularly well with a close-fitting cylindrical binding site.

55.3.2 COMPOUNDS WITH FEWER, OR NO CHLORINE ATOMS

55.3.2.1 Reductive Dechlorination of Cyclodienes

Early information (Soloway, 1965) indicated that the unchlorinated methano-bridge of aldrin could be replaced by 9-*syn*-Cl−CH− and that of isodrin by −CH$_2$CH$_2$− or spirocyclopropane, but the overall molecular length could not exceed that delineated by dieldrin or alpha-endosulfan. There were, however, interesting indications that some of the chlorine atoms in the hexachloronorbornene moiety could be replaced by hydrogen (Table 55.4). Species differences were evident; an aldrin analog (**7**, Table 55.4) having only the two one- and four-bridge chlorines was reported to be nearly as toxic as dieldrin to the German cockroach, although nontoxic to other insects tested. In aldrin, the methano-bridge chlorine atom *anti* to the chlorinated double bond was found to be more important for toxicity than the syn-chlorine (compare **8** and **9**, Table 55.4), and replacement of the two ethylenic chlorines in dieldrin by hydrogen to give didechloro-dieldrin (DD; **6**, Table 55.4) increased housefly toxicity four-fold and toxicity to the German cockroach eight-fold; the latter insect appears to be particularly sensitive to these compounds. The high toxicity of diazaaldrin and its N-oxide (**3** and **4**, Table 55.4) should also be noted.

Of interest was the possibility that if the increase in toxicity effected by replacement of the ethylenic chlorines in dieldrin proved to be a general phenomenon for cyclodiene insecticides, it might be possible to combine the change to a tetrachloronorbornene moiety with a more labile epoxide ring or other labile system (e.g., cyclic sulfite as in endosulfan) to produce useful insecticides having both oxidative and hydrolytic

detoxication routes that would be more selective and environmentally acceptable. Selective dechlorination of several series of cyclodienes was undertaken to test this possibility (Brooks, 1975, 1977, 1980, 1985; Brooks and Mace, 1987; Brooks et al., 1981). It transpired that the effect of dechlorination was not uniform but depended on the structure of the molecule as a whole. The most consistent observation for all series was the greater importance of the *anti*- versus the *syn*-chlorine atom in the pentachloronorbornene moiety, as noted for aldrin by Soloway (1965). These two changes for dieldrin were combined to give the 1,4,*anti*-10-trichloro-analog of dieldrin (DSD; **24**, Fig. 55.7), which approached dieldrin in toxicity to houseflies and blowflies and was 7–20-fold more toxic than its 10-*syn*-chloro-isomer with the chlorine atom adjacent to the double bond. Thus, the pentagonal arrangement of chlorine atoms evident in lindane and in the cyclodienes derived from HCNB (Busvine, 1964) is not sacrosanct for cyclodienes.

55.3.2.2 Structural Convergence of Cyclodienes and Their Dechlorinated Analog with Other Cage Convulsants Acting at the Chloride Ionophore

Further information arose from comparisons with the naturally occurring convulsant picrotoxinin (PTX; Fig. 55.9), which Hathway et al. (1965) found to have effects similar to those of dieldrin and isobenzan on ammonia metabolism in rat brain. PTX antagonizes the action of GABA by blocking the chloride ion channel associated with its receptor (Kadous et al., 1983; Takeuchi and Takeuchi, 1966, 1972). Evidence was then reported that cyclodienes and lindane compete with PTX at a commmon binding site in cockroach brain (Matsumura and Ghiasuddin, 1983; Tanaka et al., 1984), and this was the site of convulsant action of these compounds, a proposal supported by the similarity in the neurophysiological effects of of the cyclodienes and PTX and the cross-resistance to PTX shown by cyclodiene-resistant cockroaches. The structural similarities among PTX, HE160, and lindane led Ozoe and Matsumura (1986) to elaborate the two electronegative center hypothesis of Soloway (1965) in a series of PTX analogs that emphasized the importance of the bulky *trans*-substituent on the lactone ring as a third requirement for interaction with the PTX binding site.

This is the point of convergence (Fig. 55.9) with the cyclodienes (B) and lindane (C), for which the 10-*anti*-chlorine and the central axial chlorine (or the central equatorial chlorine), respectively, appear to provide the appropriate bulky substituent (Brooks and Mace, 1987) and the highly toxic cage compounds such as *t*-butylbicyclophosphorothionate (TBPS) and *t*-butylbicycloorthobenzoate (TBOB), in which the *t*-butyl-moiety is the necessary bulky substituent (Casida et al., 1985; Palmer and Casida, 1985). The highly insecticidal orthobenzoate EBOB (Fig. 55.10) proved to be the best ligand for the insect GABA-receptor chloride ionophore, and [^{3}H]-EBOB has been used subsequently in binding displacement studies with numerous putative channel blockers at the PTX binding site. Attempts to simplify the orthobenzoate ring system of these potent

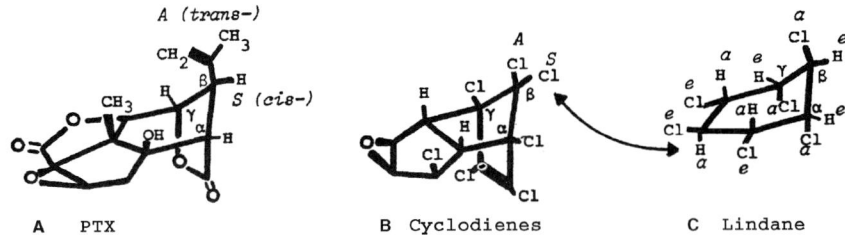

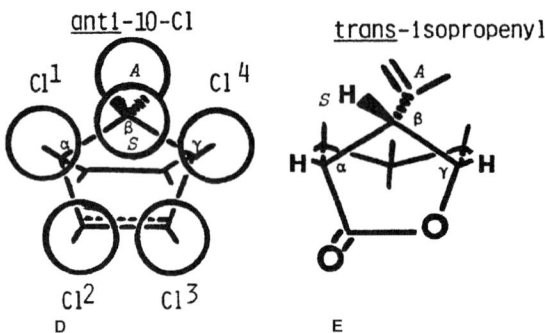

Figure 55.9 Structures of (A) picrotoxinin (PTX) with its bulky beta-isopropenyl group *trans-* (or *anti-*) to the lactone ring; (B) heptachlor epoxide; (C) lindane, showing the aaaeee configuration of chlorine atoms essential for toxicity. A, *anti-*; S, *syn-*; a, axial; e, equatorial substituents. D shows the highly chlorinated face of a cyclodiene insecticide, as in heptachlor epoxide (B above), and E, the lactone ring system as in PTX, both viewed from the right ("end-on" position). In the corresponding view of lindane (C viewed from below), note that the chlorine equivalent to the *syn-*10-chlorine of fully chlorinated cyclodienes is replaced by a hydrogen (double arrow). However, the electrostatically more favored superimposition of lindane on PTX (Calder *et al.*, 1993) is C viewed from the right, in which the three-axial chlorines of lindane are together equivalent to the *trans-*bulky isopropenyl substituent and lactone ring of PTX.

cage convulsants and the search for structural changes to confer selective toxicity in favor of mammals versus insects produced numerous insecticidal dithianes, oxathianes, and their sulfoxides and sulfones (Palmer and Casida, 1995; Wacher *et al.*, 1992).

Figure 55.10 further shows the convergence of structural changes between partly (Brooks and Mace, 1987) and totally (Ozoe *et al.*, 1990) dechlorinated alpha-endosulfan (**1**, Fig. 55.10) (which surprisingly retains measurable housefly toxicity (LD$_{50}$, ca. 43 μg/g; 20-fold less toxic than alpha-endosulfan, when co-applied with sesoxane), the toxic *t*-butyl trioxabicyclooctanes (TBOs) such as **2** (Fig. 55.10) (Palmer and Casida, 1985), and the dithianes described by Elliott *et al.* (1990). Although the 1,3-dioxan (not shown but analogous to structure **7**) corresponding to **2** (Fig. 55.10) is weakly insecticidal (Palmer and Casida, 1995), the hybrid molecule (**3**) of deschloro-alpha-endosulfan (**1**) and that 1,3-dioxan was more toxic than fully dechlorinated alpha-endosulfan (**1**), indicating that extra rigidity conferred on the 1,3-dioxan structure can improve insecticidal activity. In the hybrid molecule (**3**), the norbornene moiety appears to provide the bulky substituent (compare *t*-butyl in **2**), while possibly increasing the conformational rigidity of the dioxan moiety. Furthermore, Ozoe *et al.* (1993) showed that the extended structure **4**

(Fig. 55.10) is highly insecticidal and that compound **5** has intermediate toxicity, which is entirely lost by any chlorination in the norbornene nucleus. Thus, the dioxan (**5**) loses its housefly toxicity (LD$_{50}$, 5.5 μg/g) completely when one- or two-bridge chlorines are introduced and there is evidently a crossover point between the two structural types, because the fully chlorinated but not extended dioxan (**6**) has the same toxicity, which is much reduced in various partially dechlorinated analogs (see Section 55.4.3 for further discussion).

Bridge bis-chlorination of fully dechlorinated alpha-endosulfan (Fig. 55.10) greatly reduces its housefly toxicity (Ozoe *et al.*, 1993), but the 10-*anti*-chlorine analog retains measurable toxicity and several dechlorinated analogs having this Cl atom in combination with one ethylenic chlorine and the two bridge-end chlorines are highly toxic, showing that the additional chlorines are required for binding this shortened molecule in the critical site (Brooks and Mace, 1987), implying the requirement for a minimum of four chlorines for high toxicity. Nevertheless, at least one of the bridge-end chlorines in cyclodienes can be replaced, because a dieldrin analog (**25**, Fig. 55.11), which has one bridge-end carbon atom replaced by nitrogen, has appreciable insect toxicity (Gladstone and Wong, 1977).

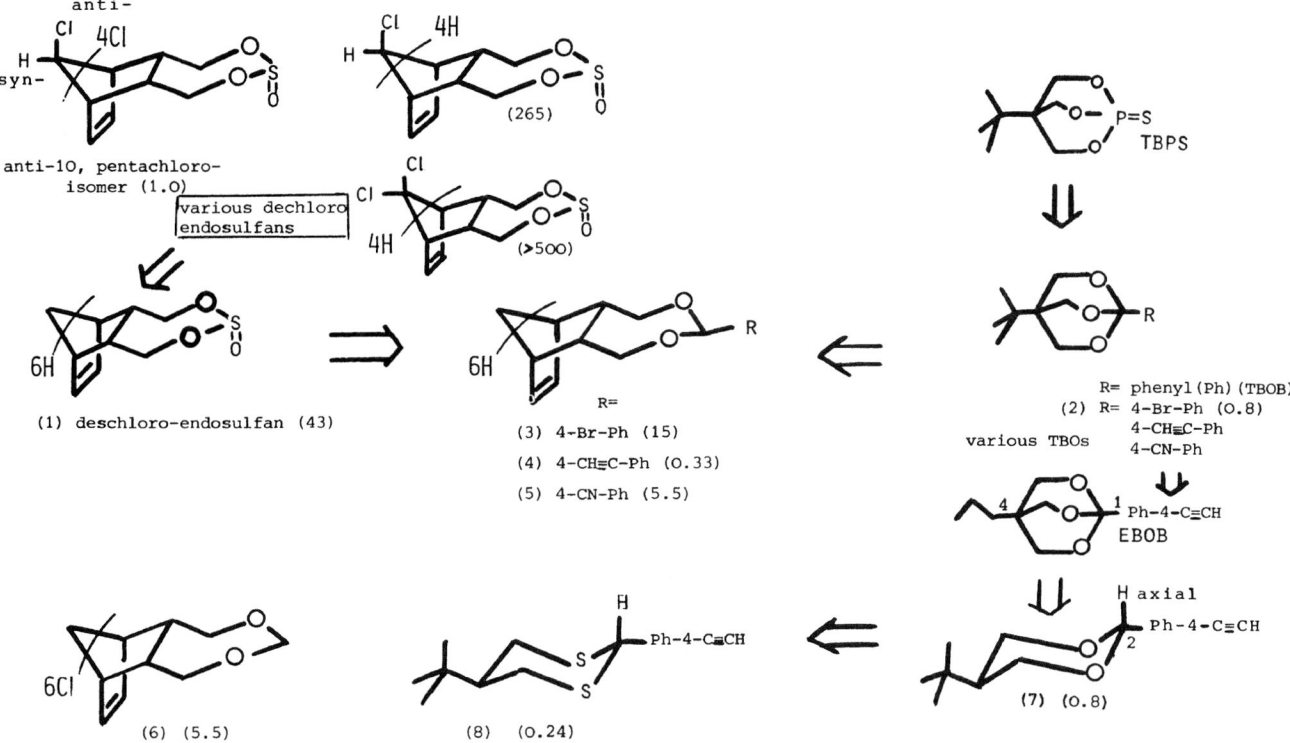

Figure 55.10 Convergence between exploration of reductively dechlorinated alpha-endosulfan analog (norbornene type) (Brooks and Mace, 1987; Ozoe *et al.*, 1990, 1993), the trioxabicyclooctane-derived cage convulsants, and the more recent dioxans and dithianes (Pulman *et al.*, 1996). The bracketed number following a chemical number or structure is the housefly topical LD_{50} (µg/g; measured in the presence of sesoxane or piperonyl butoxide).

Many trioxabicyclooctanes are highly toxic to both mammals and insects but remarkable selectivity can be conferred on some structures by appropriate derivatization; thus, the trimethylsilyl-derivative (**26**, Fig. 55.11) of the 4-*n*-butyl analog of EBOB (Fig. 55.10) is highly toxic to houseflies (LD_{50}, 0.43 µg/g) but poorly toxic to mice (LD_{50}, > 400 mg/kg). This derivative appears to be oxidatively reconverted into its toxic ethynyl precursor in houseflies, whereas in the mouse this oxidative bioactivation is much less important (Palmer *et al.*, 1991b).

Because all the compounds mentioned and some other classes of cage convulsants are believed to act at the PTX binding site, a considerable array of compact molecules is now available with which to delineate this site. A 4-ethynylphenyl-substituent in the 2-position of 5-*t*-butyl-1,3-dioxane (**7**, Fig. 55.10) or 1,3-dithiane (**8**, Fig. 55.10) was found to be more effective than a 4-bromophenyl-substituent; the *trans*-(linear) ethynylphenyl dithiane (**8**) was somewhat more toxic to houseflies than the analogous *trans*-dioxane (**7**) and *cis*- (angular) isomers were generally equally toxic to or less toxic than *trans*-isomers (Palmer and Casida, 1995; Pulman *et al.*, 1996). With the possibility of oxidation at sulfur *in vivo*, which may enforce additional conformational rigidity and also increase binding propensity, the situation becomes more complex (see Section 55.4.3).

55.3.3 LINKS BETWEEN POLYCHLOROCYCLOALKANE AND RECENT HETEROCYCLICS APPARENTLY ACTING AT THE CHLORIDE IONOPHORE

Recently, arylpyrazoles, such as fipronil (**27**, Fig. 55.11), and various 5-alkyl-2-arylpyrimidines (**28**) and 1,3-thiazines (**29**) (Pulman *et al.*, 1996), in which the planar heterocyclic ring replaces the spacers formed by the TBO and 1,3-dioxane and dithiane structures, have been added to the list of chloride ionophore blockers. Insecticidal activity was also found in triazoles (**30**, **31**) (Boddy *et al.*, 1996; Von Keyserlingk and Willis, 1992) and pyrimidinones (**32**) (Whittle *et al.*, 1995) and a spirosultam (**33**) (Bloomquist *et al.*, 1993), demonstrating the diversity of structures that probably act at this site.

Cole *et al.* (1994) examined the inhibition of [³H]-alpha-endosulfan binding in housefly head membranes by lindane and several cyclodienes and concluded that these insecticides are the only GABA-receptor ionophore blockers that consistently inhibit the binding in these membranes not only of the earlier used ligands such as [³⁵S]-TBPS and [³H]-EBOB but also of [³H]-alpha-endosulfan. However, a representative dithiane, EBOB, fipronil, and other pyrazoles were less effective in inhibiting [³H]-alpha-endosulfan binding than the chlorinated insecticides, from which it appeared that the latter compete

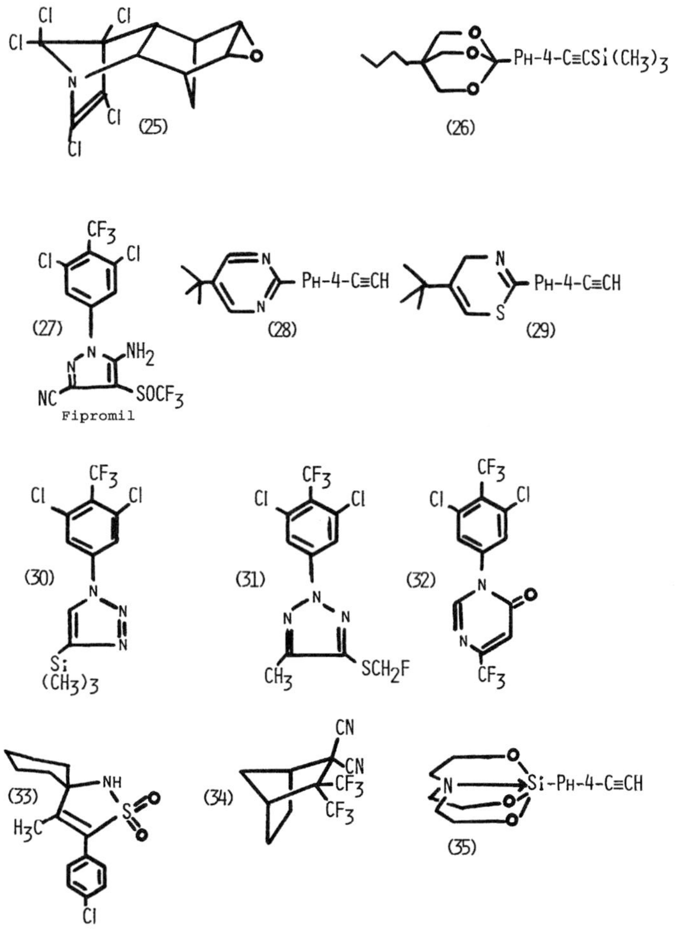

Figure 55.11   Chemical structures of compounds mentioned in the text (**25–35**).

directly for the endosulfan site, whereas the others bind with different inhibition kinetics or at a site more closely coupled to the EBOB than to the endosulfan binding domain. Notably, the channel activator avermectin B_a did not inhibit endosulfan binding.

An even more suitable ligand for the chlorinated insecticides is [^{3}H]-BIDN (**34**, Fig. 55.12) (Holyoke *et al.*, 1994), a simple norbornene derivative, which has high insect and mammalian toxicity (Kölbl *et al.*, 1981; Middleton and Bingham, 1982). Several putative affinity probes for the binding site have also been described (Casida and Pulman, 1994).

When aryl pyrazoles synthesized as herbicides were found to be insecticidal, their convulsive activity was not immediately recognised to result from GABA-antagonism (Klis *et al.*, 1991). Cole *et al.* (1993) reported subsequently that several compounds, including fipronil (**27**, Fig. 55.11) (Colliot *et al.*, 1992; Hatton *et al.*, 1988), which has become a commercially successful insecticide, blocked the GABA-gated chloride ionophore with higher potency for a site in housefly than in mouse brain, offering the possibility of selective toxicity. Fipronil has relatively low acute mammalian toxicity (Section 55.4.3). It inhibits [^{3}H]-EBOB binding to housefly head membranes and dieldrin-resistant flies show some resistance to it (Cole *et al.*,

1993; Colliot *et al.*, 1992), providing a clue to its mode of action.

The cyclodiene insecticides and lindane were found to be potent displacers of [^{35}S]-TBPS binding to GABA-receptors in rat brain and inhibitors of GABA-dependent ^{36}Cl ion flux into rat brain microsacs, from which it was suggested that these PCCAs act as noncompetitive blockers of GABA$_A$-receptors (Abalis *et al.*, 1985; Gant *et al.*, 1987; Lawrence and Casida, 1984). Potency in these assays correlates with toxicity (Casida *et al.*, 1988) but TBPS is not a potent insecticide and [^{35}S]-TBPS is unsuitable as a radioligand for insect studies; it appears that the structural features required for binding at the housefly GABA-receptor are different from those for the mammalian one and [^{3}H]-EBOB, a highly potent insecticide, was ultimately designed as a superior ligand for insect binding studies (Deng *et al.*, 1991) and generally provides a good correlation between its displacement by PCCAs and their housefly toxicities. By use of this ligand, it was concluded that PCCA, PTX, dithiane-related compounds, and phenylpyrazoles all have the same mode of insecticidal action, a view supported by the up to 27-fold cross-resistance to EBOB shown by dieldrin-resistant houseflies (Cole *et al.*, 1993).

Moreover, the naturally occurring insecticide avermectin B_{1a} and derived moxidectin (Fisher, 1997), which behave as GABA-agonists, stimulating rather than inhibiting chloride ion influx, are potent noncompetitive inhibitors of EBOB binding. This implies that avermectin action involves the chloride ionophore but that it is bound at a site different from that involving EBOB and PCCA; nor, in contrast to EBOB, is there cross-resistance to dieldrin, so that the channel modification that confers dieldrin resistance does not apparently involve the avermectin binding site (Deng *et al.*, 1991). Based on ligand binding studies, Deng *et al.* (1993) proposed four partly associated sites in the housefly GABA chloride ionophore that are relevant to insecticidal action: site A, interacting with EBOB and its isosteres; B with TBPS and isosteres; C with phenylpyrazoles; and D with avermectins. Action at sites A and C gives similar signs of poisoning and cross-resistance to dieldrin; PCCA and some TBPS isosteres may act at both A and B. The avermectin site D is coupled in some way with A and C but not to the TBPS site B, which is also distinct from the phenylpyrazole site C. Thus, the reduced affinity for [^{3}H]-EBOB binding observed in dieldrin-resistant houseflies is due to its reduced affinity for the PCCA binding site, and the cross-resistance noted for TBOs, lindane, toxaphene, cyclodienes, dithianes, arylsilatranes (**35**, Fig. 55.11), and PTX suggests that the structural modifications in the EBOB binding site are involved in resistance to all these insecticides (Hawkinson and Casida, 1993) but fortunately do not confer resistance to avermectins, which have very high toxicity against agricultural and household insect pests, phytophagous mites, and plant and animal nematodes.

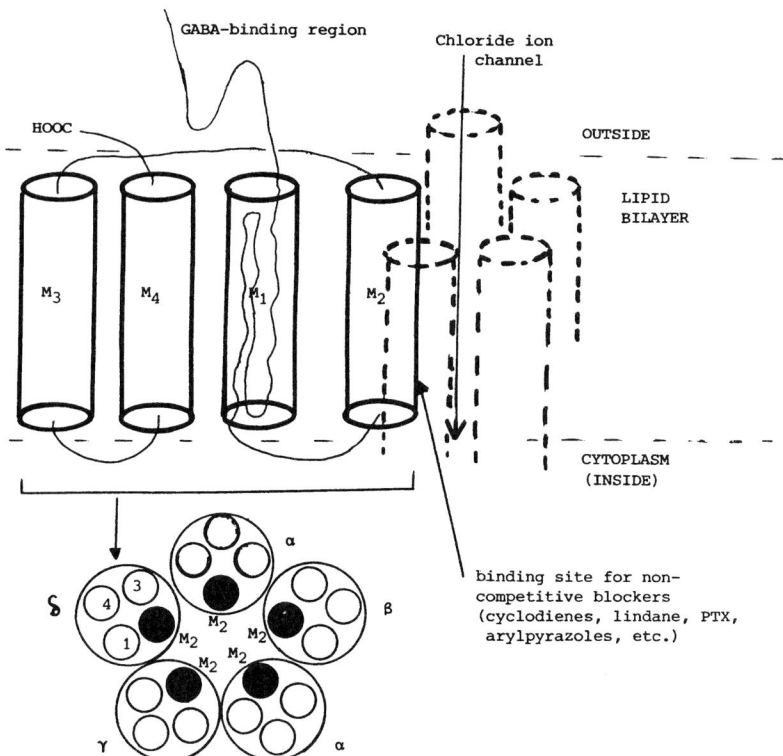

Figure 55.12 Schematic representation of the GABA$_A$-receptor of mammalian brain, showing five *trans*-membrane glycoprotein subunits, each with their four *trans*-membrane helices (M$_1$–M$_4$), of which the M$_2$ segments (shown as cylinders, and black circles in the plan view) are believed to form the pore of the integral chloride ion channel (MacDonald and Olsen, 1994). A modified subunit carrying cyclodiene resistance in *Drosophila* (Rdl) shows homology with the mammalian brain beta-subunit (ffrench-Constant *et al.*, 1991).

55.4 MOLECULAR MECHANISM OF ACTION

55.4.1 TOPOGRAPHY OF THE GAMMA-AMINOBUTYRIC ACID A-RECEPTOR

GABA is the principal neurotransmitter of the mammalian and insect central nervous system (CNS) and the insect neuromuscular junction. In mammals, baclofen-sensitive GABA$_B$-receptors are coupled to calcium and potassium channels and the action of GABA is mediated by G-proteins. In contrast, GABA$_A$-receptors, of interest here, are members of the super family of ligand-gated ion channels that contain a chloride ionophore (Schofield *et al.*, 1987). Simplistically, an inhibitory GABA-ergic nerve terminal abutting on the presynaptic terminal of another nerve that releases a neurotransmitter (e.g., acetylcholine, ACh) releases GABA when stimulated. GABA then diffuses to the presynaptic terminal of the other nerve, where it binds to a GABA$_A$-receptor, causing entry of chloride ions and resulting in hyperpolarization of the terminal and inhibition of release of the other neurotransmitter. Thus, postsynaptic stimulation of the other nerve by its transmitter (e.g., ACh) is reduced. This inhibitory mechanism explains the apparent cholinergic effects of dieldrin and lindane on Ameri-

can cockroach ganglia (Shankland and Schroeder, 1973; Uchida *et al.*, 1978), because disinhibition (blockade of a presynaptic chloride ionophore) of the presynaptic terminal of a cholinergic nerve should result in uninhibited ACh release and consequent hyperstimulation of the postsynaptic terminal, as is observed. The same basic mechanism for disinhibition may, of course, affect nerve terminals involving neurotransmitters other than ACh (Joy, 1982) with a variety of possible effects, depending on the species and on differing nerve architecture.

The GABA$_A$-receptor of human brain consists of four or five 50–60 kDa glycoprotein subunits, each of which contains four (M$_1$–M$_4$) hydrophobic domains (alpha-helices) that traverse the membrane (Fig. 55.12) (MacDonald and Olsen, 1994; Schofield *et al.*, 1987) and contribute to and stabilize the walls of the chloride ionophore. The five M$_2$-domains are believed to be arranged so as to form the 5.6-Å-diameter lumen of the channel, with the side chains of their threonines and serines forming hydrophilic rings that contribute to the induction of ion flow.

55.4.2 MOLECULAR BIOLOGY OF CYCLODIENE RESISTANCE

Recently, a cyclodiene resistance-conferring gene, Rdl, from the fruit fly, *Drosophila melanogaster*, has been cloned and shows homology with the mammalian brain beta-subunit (ffrench-Constant *et al.*, 1991). Dieldrin resistance was subsequently found to be associated with the point mutation alanine 302 to serine (Ala^{302}–Ser) within the M$_2$ membrane-spanning domain, near the site conferring charge selectivity in the closely related nicotinic ACh-receptor (ffrench-Constant *et al.*, 1993a, b).

Homooligomeric, wild-type Rdl-receptors expressed in Xenopus oocytes showed the expected electrophysiological properties of GABA-receptors; channels containing the Ala^{302}–Ser mutation, when similarly expressed, were identical with the wild-type ones but had consistently lower sensitivity to dieldrin and PTX, sensitivity to these being reduced about 100-fold. Notably, Lee *et al.* (1995) reported no detectable specific [^{3}H]-EBOB binding in resistant *D. melanogaster* strains carrying the Ala^{302}-replacement, despite high specific binding to membranes from susceptible flies, indicating the involvement of Ala^{302} in EBOB binding to GABA-receptors containing Rdl subunits. Similar results were found for the dieldrin resistance mutation Ala^{302}–glycine found in *Drosophila simulans* (ffrench-Constant *et al.*, 1993a, b). Furthermore, EBOB blocks chloride ion currents generated by Rdl homomultimers expressed in insect cells and the Ala^{302}–Ser replacement reduces sensitivity to this block 10-fold (Lee *et al.*, 1995).

Examination of the Rdl gene from three different insect orders has revealed that in all cases Ala^{302} is replaced by either a serine or a glycine (less effectively), indicating that this mechanism is universal. The change confers reduced sensitivity to PTX, lindane, and TBPS, lower channel conductances, extended channel open times and shorter closed times, and a markedly reduced rate of GABA-induced receptor desensitization. From a simple model to represent binding and allosteric changes, it has been suggested that the preceding mutations are the only ones that can directly weaken cyclodiene binding to the desensitized (antagonist favored) conformation of the receptor and simultaneously destabilize the antagonist-favored conformation through an allosteric mechanism, resulting in a powerful dual-resistance mechanism (ffrench-Constant *et al.*, 1995; Zhang *et al.*, 1994). In this model, the antagonist associates with the open channel but binds much more tightly when the channel next changes into the desensitized (closed) state, so that this configuration is stabilized.

If homomultimers are present *in vivo*, which may not, however, be the case (Zhang *et al.*, 1995), the preceding mutation could lead to a resistant ion channel with a ring of up to five serines replacing the five alanines in the wild-type Rdl ion channel, which would greatly increase the polarity of this region (5-CH$_2$OH replacing 5-CH$_3$) and considerably alter its affinity for the various toxicants under discussion; even one or two added hydroxyl groups introduced here in a heteromultimer might have a significant effect and also reduce the energy barriers for ion permeation by participating in hydrogen bonding with water (Leonard *et al.*, 1988). Analogies with the nACh receptor are evident and the closed configuration of the mutated chloride channel may remain somewhat ion permeable (Zhang *et al.*, 1994; Revah *et al.*, 1991).

55.4.3 MOLECULAR TOXICOLOGY OF NONCOMPETITIVE CHLORIDE IONOPHORE BLOCKERS

The localization of Ala^{302} to the PTX/cyclodiene binding site in Rdl prompts some further consideration of the information on the structure–toxicity relationships outlined in earlier sections. The cylinder formed by the amino-acid sequences Leu^{303}, Ala^{302}, Val^{301} in five adjacent M$_2$ domains (helices) provides a quasi-centrosymmetrical lipophilic pocket into which cyclodiene insecticides and other noncompetitive chloride ionophore blockers (NCBs) might fit. The molecular dimensions of cyclodienes, taking into account the known range of allowable molecular substituents in these rather compact molecules, are sufficient to block a 5.6-Å pore. If the pore is more or less centrosymmetrical, a cyclodiene molecule could fill the pocket and interact with all of its walls simultaneously because similar binding sites are presented around the lumen even if the arrangement is not a homomultimer. This would explain the observed toxicity of *both* enantiomeric forms of asymmetric molecules such as heptachlor epoxide; the forms may differ somewhat in toxicity, however, if the channel is not completely symmetrical, as is found (Miyazaki *et al.*, 1980). Symmetrical molecules should be particularly effective, because they may be able to offer a symmetrically distributed electronegative center (or centers) to similar binding sites on opposite sides of the channel, as in the case of delta-chlordane and isobenzan, each having two symmetrically substituted chlorines on their five-membered rings. These molecules may be viewed as symmetrical composites of the enantiomeric forms of alpha-DH and heptachlor epoxide (HE160), respectively, as suggested in Section 55.3.1

In a hypothetical model (Fig. 55.13) in which the HCNB moiety of cyclodienes is presumed bound at the synaptic end of the lipophilic pocket so that its *gem*-dichloro-bridge is presented to the channel wall, then the second electronegative center in, for example, dieldrin, is directed toward the cytoplasmic end of the pocket with its epoxide ring and unchlorinated methano-bridge fixed in an inward direction toward the channel lumen. This "cytoplasmic" end of the molecule is then close to the critical ring of Ala^{302}-methyl groups around the channel lumen, which when replaced by –CH$_2$OH groups inhibits the binding of NCBs. Dieldrin and alpha-endosulfan (extended molecules) appear to provide the limiting acceptable molecular "lengths," as noted earlier, whereas isobenzan, endrin, and beta-endosulfan are more compact. On this model, it might be argued also that the *anti*-10-chlorine atom (Fig. 55.9 and Table 55.4) of the dichloromethano-bridge of cyclodienes is better accommodated in the lipophilic pocket than the *syn*-10-chlorine, which may interfere sterically with the large side-chain alkyl groups of the ring of Leu^{303}s that lie at the synaptic end of the pocket, making this *syn*-chlorine universally unfavorable for toxicity.

The same argument might explain the four-fold increase in dieldrin toxicity effected by removal of the ethylenic chlorines (in DD, Table 55.4), because these chlorines might also interfere sterically in this region. This increase in toxicity is not uni-

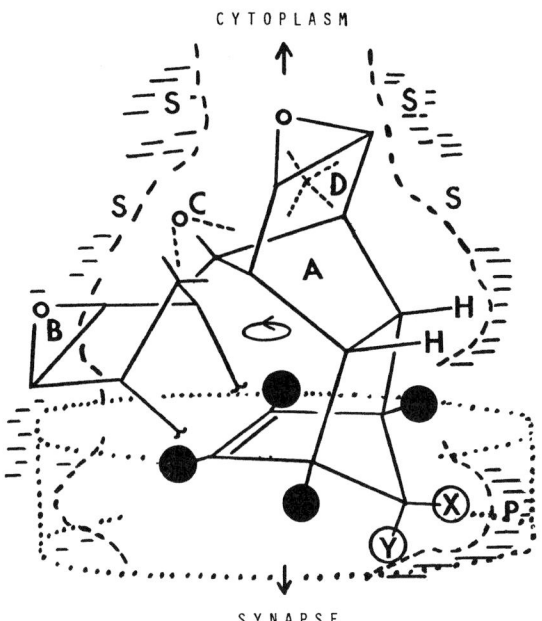

CYTOPLASM

SYNAPSE

Figure 55.13 Dieldrin (A) is oriented in a hypothetical binding site in or near the chloride ion channel lumen (in the region of Leu^{303}?) with chlorine X (10-*anti*-chlorine) located in a subsite P that accommodates a bulky substituent. Its epoxide ring then penetrates a three-dimensional region S near Ala^{302}, which may interact, especially in the closed channel configuration, with the electronegative moieties of various cyclodienes when similarly oriented. If, however, Y (the 10-*syn*-chlorine) is presented to P, then the epoxide ring cannot so readily interact with zone S (dieldrin orientation B). C indicates the approximate position of the epoxide ring of endrin and also of the sulfur of beta-endosulfan, when *either* X *or* Y in these molecules is bound to subsite P; D is the approximate position of the endrin methano-bridge when its 10-*anti*-chlorine is located in P, corresponding to dieldrin orientation A. In this model, the dotted cylinder is the region containing a ring of leucine side chains. Note that a substituted benzene ring and some other extensions are permissible in the arrowed directions when the bridging system is unchlorinated (see Fig. 55.10 and related discussion, Section 55.4.3).

versal for cyclodienes, however, and the *syn*-chlorine atom is still present in DD, so that its adverse effect on toxicity is more than offset by removal of the ethylenic chlorine atoms. Further reductive replacement of the *syn*-10-chlorine atom in DD to give the trichloro-derivative DSD (**24**, Fig. 55.7) reduces toxicity to the level of dieldrin again (Brooks and Mace, 1987). The *syn*-10-chloro-isomer of DSD is significantly less toxic than DSD or dieldrin, again indicating the greater importance of the 10-*anti*-chlorine for toxicity. The difference in toxicities between *syn*- and *anti*-10-monodechloro-isomers is less marked for endrin and beta-endosulfan (the endrin-like isomer) but remains evident for alpha-endosulfan.

This observation was discussed (Brooks, 1992) in connection with the insect cross-resistance spectrum for lindane/cyclodienes first noted by Busvine (1964), in which lindane, isobenzan, endrin, and the endosulfan isomers retain measurable toxicity to dieldrin-resistant insects (Brooks and Harrison, 1964a; Busvine, 1964). The first three molecules and beta-endosulfan are rather compact compared with dieldrin and alpha-endosulfan; the latter has been considered to be extended

and dieldrin-like (Fig. 55.6), but recent structural studies indicate a more complex situation (see later).

If the 10-*anti*-chlorine of dieldrin (X in Fig. 55.13) corresponds to the bulky *anti*-substituent found in PTX and must be presented to an appropriate lipophilic pocket in a binding subsite (P, Fig. 55.13) so as to place the epoxide ring in a correct position (in the region of S) with respect to the remainder of the binding site, then the 10-*syn*-chlorine (Y in Fig. 55.13), if similarly presented, cannot place the epoxide ring in the same position. If this latter position is modified in resistance to prevent interaction with the epoxide ring, dieldrin can no longer bind; however, *either* bridge-chlorine of endrin or beta-endosulfan can be offered to the bulky substituent binding subsite (P) such that the epoxide ring or sulfite moiety will still be placed in approximately their original positions (near to C), still able to interact with the critical site (S), on account of the more compact "cage" shape of these molecules.

Consequently, these molecules may still be able to interact to some extent with the binding site that has been modified to exclude binding with dieldrin. On this model, alpha-endosulfan is anomalous in retaining effectiveness, because the same arguments apply as to dieldrin yet this molecule was actually somewhat more toxic than beta-endosulfan to dieldrin-resistant houseflies (Brooks and Harrison, 1964a). Two further observations may be significant, however. First, endosulfan sulfate (**4**, Fig. 55.6) formed *in vivo* from both endosulfan isomers may be the critical toxicant; it has the same structural (cage) configuration as beta-endosulfan (Forman *et al.*, 1965) and is formed faster from alpha- than from beta-endosulfan in some living organisms. Second, alpha-endosulfan has recently been reported (Schmidt *et al.*, 1997) to exist in the asymmetrical "twist-chair" conformation, in which the C—O bonds are "*trans*," not parallel as usually depicted (Fig. 55.6). Molecular models suggest that this twisted configuration may be more flexible, allowing the S=O moiety to occupy several spatial positions between the extremes represented by beta-endosulfan and the extended alpha-structure shown in Fig. 55.6. Consequently, the alpha-isomer might be expected to be intrinsically at least as effective as the beta-isomer in terms of their interactions with the resistance-modified binding site, regardless of possible oxidation to the sulfate *in vivo*. In the case of endrin, the 9-keto-(12-keto-) metabolite is presumed to be the ultimate toxicant in mammals (Hutson *et al.*, 1975) and may contribute to endrin toxicity in insects (Kadous and Matsumura, 1982); notably, this oxidation places a second, additional, electronegative center at D, near to the upper subsite S (Fig. 55.13), which may improve binding potency toward the resistance-modified binding site.

Lindane resembles a very compact cyclodiene and might bind without conflict with a subsite modified for dieldrin resistance or in more than one orientation, and similar arguments apply to isobenzan. Interestingly, isobenzan may be regarded as a "composite" of the HE160 enantiomers, in which an "in plane" oxygen replaces the epoxide rings. Dieldrin resistance normally confers total resistance to HE160 (Brooks and Harrison, 1964a; Busvine, 1964) so the more compact placement of oxygen in isobenzan, combined with a possible increase in binding affinity associated with the symmetrical chlorine substituents, appears to overcome both dieldrin and HE160 resistance to some extent. Notably, diaza-aldrin (**3**, Table 55.4), in which the unchlorinated double bond is replaced by —N=N— and which is probably converted into its N-oxide (**4**, Table 55.4) *in vivo*, is much more toxic than dieldrin to some insects (Busvine, 1964; Soloway, 1965) but dieldrin-resistant insects are immune to it. Using the TBPS binding assay in rat brain membranes, it has recently been confirmed that this molecule inhibits the binding competitively and therefore interacts directly with the PTX binding site (Ozoe *et al.*, 1995).

Other modifications of the dichloroethylene moiety of dieldrin are acceptable to the binding site, as in photodieldrin (converted *in vivo* into Klein's ketone, however; Fig. 55.3) and the ketone analogs (**14**, **15**, **16**, Fig. 55.7) derived from isobenzan. From the analogy with PTX, the dichloroethylene moiety, unchlorinated double bond, and ketone derivatives in these various analogs may correspond to the lactone system of PTX. In lindane, the best superimposition with PTX/cyclodienes is apparently that in which two of the axial chlorines substitute for the lactone ring of PTX and the third axial chlorine provides the equivalent of the bulky *trans*-isopropenyl group of PTX or *anti*-10-chlorine of cyclodienes. This last configuration of lindane is favored electrostatically (Calder *et al.*, 1993), although in it the bridge-end chlorines, which complete the pentagonal arrangement of chlorine atoms seen in cyclodienes (Brooks and Mace, 1987), are replaced by hydrogens. Replacement of the bridge-end chlorines by hydrogen reduces the toxicity of some cyclodienes (Soloway, 1965) and, notably, whether bulky alkyl groups in the alpha- and beta-positions of gamma-butyrolactones (cf. PTX) stabilize the open or closed states of the ionophore and hence induce anticonvulsant or convulsant activity depends markedly on the stereochemistry of these substituents relative to the carbonyl group (Holland *et al.*, 1995; Klunk *et al.*, 1983; Peterson *et al.*, 1994). However, the replacement of one bridge-end carbon atom of dieldrin by nitrogen (available for hydrogen bonding) gives azadieldrin (**25**, Fig. 55.11) without great loss in toxicity compared with dieldrin (Gladstone and Wong, 1977), another indication that some modification in this region of cyclodienes is possible.

The preceding discussion indicates that numerous modifications of the HCNB moiety retain binding capacity to the critical site. In this context, it may be noted that BIDN (**34**, Fig. 55.11), in which the simple norbornene nucleus carries two strongly electron-withdrawing substituents (*gem*-di-CN and *gem*-di-CF$_3$), is highly toxic to both mammals and insects (Kölbl *et al.*, 1981). The allowable length compatible with toxicity of the fully chlorinated cyclodienes appears to be restricted, however (see earlier). TBPS has approximately the same molecular length as cyclodienes such as dieldrin, but there is the question of how the binding of cyclodienes to the critical site relates to that of the extended unchlorinated molecule EBOB or similar molecules in which an aromatic substituent replaces the bulky 4-alkyl group (Palmer *et al.*, 1991a). Superimposition of cyclodienes, aryl-TBOs, aryldithianes, aryl-silatranes (**35**, Fig. 55.11), and PTX by CoMFA (comparative

molecular field analysis) (Calder *et al.*, 1993) supports the view that all act at the same or overlapping sites. Interesting additional information is available from work on the molecular hybrids of dechlorinated alpha-endosulfan (Fig. 55.10) (Ozoe *et al.*, 1993) and insecticidal dioxans (Palmer and Casida, 1995) mentioned previously (Section 55.3.2.2).

In this series (Ozoe *et al.*, 1993), the fully chlorinated molecule (**6**, Fig. 55.10) cannot be extended but has the same housefly toxicity as the unchlorinated extended molecule (**5**, Fig. 55.10) related to the compounds reported by Casida. The latter molecule cannot be chlorinated; a single bridge chlorine abolishes its housefly toxicity. Assuming that the hybrid molecule (**5**) is a rigid form of the corresponding dioxan in which the unchlorinated norbornene moiety serves as the bulky substituent (e.g., *t*-butyl) (Ozoe *et al.*, 1990) and occupies a spatial region equivalent to that occupied by the HCNB moiety of cyclodienes, it is evident that the combination of substituted phenyl, dioxan, and norbornene moieties can bind to the receptor and afford potentially excellent insect toxicity, as found in 5-*t*-butyl-2-(4-ethynylphenyl)-1,3-dioxane (**7**, Fig. 55.10). However, chlorination may disrupt this binding in the corresponding deschoro-alpha-endosulfan analog with a 4-cyanophenyl substituent by forcing the "extended" molecule into a position it cannot occupy in the ion channel for steric reasons.

Thus, the compact unchlorinated norbornene moiety may not by itself have sufficient binding potency in the lipophilic pocket bounded by the Leu[301], Ala[302], and Val[303] rings, but an added aromatic ring with an appropriate 4-substituent (particularly ethynyl), which, according to this model, binds additionally in a region of the channel pore beyond Ala[302] and near to Val[301] and Arg[300], may greatly reinforce the interaction. Conversely, the bulky, fully chlorinated cyclodiene interacts well with the closed configuration of the spherical pocket, but extension is impossible in this case because the added benzene ring in the extended HCNB moiety would be forced into steric hindrance with the valine isopropyl groups and the narrow cytoplasmic end of the channel; this contains the large guanidinyl side chains of Arg[300] and might admit only "sticklike" structures such as the ethynyl moiety.

Support is given to this hypothesis by the application (Akamatsu *et al.*, 1997) of CoMFA analysis to compare alpha-endosulfan analogs (their series 2) with the hybrid extended norbornene derivatives (series 1) (Ozoe *et al.*, 1993; Fig. 55.10) analogous to the 1,3-dioxanes reported by Casida (Fig. 55.10). When the simple cyclodienes were closely superimposed on the extended molecules with a 2-(4-cyanophenyl) substituent, the housefly toxicity of some of the extended molecules was not well predicted until, in the superposition, the extended molecules were rotated 15° clockwise about their common bond on the norbornene ring junction (C4a–C8a in Table 55.4). This rotation enabled the separate correlation equations for the two series derived by CoMFA on the basis of close superimposition to be combined satisfactorily into a single equation representing the housefly toxicities of both series. The two series compared could not, however, be brought together in the same way when the measure of biological activity was the displacement of [^{35}S]-TBPS binding from rat brain membranes. In compound **5** (Fig. 55.10), the previous rotation turns the aromatic ring toward the center of the ion channel as modeled in Fig. 55.13, away from a region sterically forbidden according to CoMFA, and incidentally may "rock" the unchlorinated norbornene moiety into closer contact with the lipophilic pocket than it can achieve when chlorinated. Conversely, chlorination of the norbornene moiety of these extended molecules would have the reverse effect, forcing the aromatic ring toward the channel wall, into sterically forbidden space.

The extending group in TBOs need not necessarily be aromatic, because short alkyl chains with a terminal ethynyl group give insecticidal activity, especially when synergized (Smith *et al.*, 1993) as do 4-ethynylcyclohexyl groups in TBOs and dithianes (Weston *et al.*, 1995). A further interesting feature of the dithianes is their conversion into sulfoxides and sulfones, which doubtless occurs *in vivo*; the equatorial (*trans*- with respect to *t*-butyl; *linear*) 5-*t*-butyl-2-(4-Br-phenyl)-1,3-dithiane (**8**, Fig. 55.10; two-substituent is equatorial 4-Br-Ph) is twofold more toxic than the *cis*- (2-axial; *angular*) isomer, and the corresponding 4-ethynylphenyl-isomers have equal toxicity when synergized; for each isomer, conversion into the isomeric monosulfoxides and monosulfone progressively increases toxicity (Palmer and Casida, 1992).

The not dissimilar toxicities of the *trans*- (linear) and *cis*- (angular) dithianes is intriguing. If, in the pore model (Fig. 55.13), the bulky *t*-butyl substituent is placed in the lipophilic pocket as for the other bulky substituents discussed previously, then the sulfoxides and sulfones from the isomeric dithianes occupy rather different positions in this lipophilic site; only in the linear isomer do these moieties occupy positions near the two ester oxygens of alpha-endosulfan and the epoxide ring of dieldrin, toward the cytoplasmic end of the channel and near to Ala[302]. For the angular isomer, the SO (or SO$_2$) moieties are placed at the synaptic end of the lipophilic pocket and lie toward the channel center, in this case, the aromatic ring overlies the trioxabicyclooctane ring of TBOs and its 4-substituent reaches only the aromatic ring of the linear isomer, so that the position of this part of the angular molecule is foreshortened in the cytoplasmic direction relative to the linear one. All of the molecules discussed can be superimposed, and with the cyclodiene molecules oriented in this way, the sulfite moiety of beta-endosulfan (and the SO$_2$ of endosulfan sulfate) lies in the region occupied by the aromatic ring of the angular dithiane isomer. It should be noted, however, that the possibility of *cis*- to *trans*-rearrangement exists for the dithianes *in vivo* (Pulman *et al.*, 1996), in which case, the *cis*-isomers would merely be precursors of the linear (*trans*-) molecules, which are more readily accommodated in the model.

Among the heterocyclic compounds of recent interest that are believed to act by blocking the GABA-gated chloride ionophore, the experimental spirosultam LY 219048 (**33**, Fig. 55.11) contains an obvious lipophilic bulky substituent in the form of the cyclohexane ring, in analogy with the compounds discussed previously. Probably because this ring may be susceptible to metabolic attack, the compound is not very toxic

to insects but its toxicity to mice is similar to that of endrin (Bloomquist *et al.*, 1993). Other insecticidal compounds such as the phenylpyrazoles (e.g., fipronil; **27**, Fig. 55.11) have little obvious structural similarity to the compounds discussed in previous sections yet inhibit [^{3}H]-EBOB binding to housefly head membranes and are believed to act at the PCCA/PTX binding site (Cole *et al.*, 1993). Some other compounds containing the common 2,6-dichloro-4-trifluoromethylphenyl moiety combined with a pyrimidinone (e.g., **32**, Fig. 55.11) and other small heterocyclic rings were described by Whittle *et al.* (1995) but these lacked the broad-spectrum insecticidal activity shown by fipronil, which was introduced in 1993 (Colliot *et al.*, 1992) and now has a wide range of applications for crop protection by foliar, soil or seed treatment. Its mammalian toxicity is generally moderate (rat acute oral LD$_{50}$, 97 mg/kg; mouse acute oral LD$_{50}$, 95 mg/kg) and it is readily converted into degradation products, including the corresponding sulfone, in the environment (Tomlin, 1997).

The substitution pattern in the phenyl and heterocyclic rings of these compounds places these ring planes at right angles (Whittle *et al.*, 1995) so that the molecules are "space filling" in these two planes and are relatively rigid, with the pyrazole ring skewed with respect to the benzene ring because of the pyramidal linking nitrogen. The substituents ($-NH_2$, $-CN$, $-SOCF_3$) are attached to double bonds and are fixed in the plane of the pyrazole ring, although they can rotate about their attaching bonds, which may be particularly important for the critical $-SOCF_3$ group. This group confers insect (housefly LD$_{50}$, 0.3 µg/g) and vertebrate (mouse ip LD$_{50}$, 30 mg/kg) toxicity, even in the analogous molecule lacking both the $-NH_2$ and $-CN$ substituents, which, however, clearly optimize the binding properties of fipronil. In these molecules, the sulfur atom requires bioactivation through sulfoxide/sulfone formation to confer toxicity.

How do the phenylpyrazoles bind to the chloride ionophore in relation to the other molecules discussed previously? They inhibit EBOB binding in housefly head membranes noncompetitively, which may involve irreversible or slowly reversible inhibition or action at an allosteric but coupled site (Cole *et al.*, 1993). Whittle *et al.* (1995) explored a series of compounds, including pyrimidinone **32** (Fig. 55.11) on the basis of their commonality of dipole direction with phenylpyrazoles; the positive end of the dipole lies toward the benzene ring in active compounds. If this ring, with its strongly electron-withdrawing $-CF_3$ moiety, is placed in the channel pore binding site so that the $-CF_3$ is in a similar position to that occupied by the 4-ethynyl group of EBOB, according to the model discussed earlier, that is, in the region of Arg[300], then the benzene ring with its chlorine atoms and the pyrazole ring with its substituents are well placed to bind with channel components in this quasi-centrosymmetrical ionophore and, notably, the $-SOCF_3$ moiety is then placed near to Ala[302] in a region occupied by the endosulfan ester oxygens, the oxygens of TBOs, the oxygens or sulfurs of dioxans and oxidized *trans*- (linear) dithianes, and the second electronegative center (e.g., the epoxide ring of dieldrin) of cyclodienes, when these molecules are located in the lipophilic pocket bounded by Leu[303].

These molecules might penetrate the chloride ionophore from either the extracellular (synaptic) mouth or the cytoplasmic mouth or by first penetrating the lipid bilayer and then entering the channel laterally. Current understanding of the nACh-receptor (nAChR) ionophore, which has analogies with the GABA$_A$ ionophore, may be relevant. According to Unwin (1995), the M$_2$ cylinders (alpha-helices) (Fig. 55.12) are kinked inward in the region of a ring of leucines when the ionophore is closed; in the open configuration, the cylinders are twisted laterally, moving the leucine side chains away from the pore. By analogy, a cyclodiene (for example) may enter a similar open conformation in the chloride ionophore and then become tightly bound when the pore reverts to the closed conformation, as suggested by ffrench-Constant *et al.* (1995).

Nakanishi *et al.* (1997) provide an interesting discussion on the question of mode of channel entry, based on research on philanthotoxins (PhTXs) binding to the nAChR. In particular, they noted that an *n*-butyl side chain introduced into the hydrophilic polyamine chain of PhTX-433 increases potency eight-fold. The *n*-butyl moiety is so placed as to reach the area of Leu[251] when the molecule is inserted linearly into the AChR ionophore from the cytoplasmic end, and the authors speculate that the increased potency might result from additional hydrophobic binding between the *n*-butyl side chain and the alkyl groups of Leu[251]; potency decreases below that of the parent PhTX-433 when this side chain is placed in other positions along the polyamine chain. Hydrophobic binding must also have a significant role in the interaction of the cage convulsants with the chloride ionophore. Here we recall that the hybrid (unchlorinated) molecule **4** (Fig. 55.10) combines the bulky norbornene (hydrophobic binding) and dioxan moieties with the additional binding capacity evidently conferred by the benzene ring with its electronegative 4-ethynyl substituent; it is more toxic (when oxidative metabolism is inhibited) than many fully chlorinated cyclodienes. No doubt work with the affinity probes currently under development (Casida and Pulman, 1994) will resolve some of these questions regarding the exact location of binding subsites in the chloride ionophore.

55.5 CONCLUSIONS

Some 45 years after serious toxicological research on the PCCA insecticides began, there is now a broad understanding of their mode of action and, due to rapid progress in the application of molecular biology, the tantalizing mechanism of insect resistance to them has been illuminated. Furthermore, new structural classes of chemicals have now emerged that appear to act in the same way. Although many chemicals found to interact with the picrotoxinin binding site in the GABA$_A$-receptor chloride ionophore are highly toxic to both mammals and insects, binding studies with radioligands have indicated differences between their GABA-receptors that offer the prospect of selective insect toxicity involving this target.

The commercially successful insecticide fipronil appears to fulfill these expectations and other new chemicals are likely to follow. There is also the possibility of "building in" selectivity by using the "propesticide" approach, which exploits differences between insects and nontarget organisms in their biotransformation routes for chemically derivatized toxicants and has been applied successfully to alleviate the mammalian toxicity of other classes of insecticides.

Meanwhile, many questions remain to be answered that are of fundamental importance in understanding the molecular action of neurotransmitters and insecticides on ion channels. The intense interest in this subject, stimulated by rapid advances in molecular biology, will ensure a prominent use for the PCCA insecticides and the newer chemicals with related actions, as tools in these explorations.

REFERENCES

Abalis, I. M., Eldefrawi, M. E., and Eldefrawi, A. T. (1985). High affinity stereospecific binding of cyclodiene insecticides and gamma-hexachlorocyclohexane to gamma-aminobutyric acid receptors. *Pestic. Biochem. Physiol.* **24**, 95–102.

Akamatsu, M., Ozoe, Y., Fujita, T., Mochida, K., Nakamura, T., and Matsumura, F. (1997). Sites of action of noncompetitive GABA antagonists in houseflies and rats: Three dimensional QSAR analysis. *Pestic. Sci.* **49**, 319–332.

Akkermans, L. M. A., van den Bercken, J., van der Zalm, J. M., and van Stranten, H. W. M. (1974). Effects of dieldril and some of its metabolite on synaptic transmission in the frog motor end plate. *Pestic. Biochem. Physiol.* **4**, 313–324.

Akkermans, L. M. A., van den Bercken, J., and van der Zalm, J. M. (1975a). Effects of aldrin-transdiol on neuromuscular facilitation and depression. *Eur. J. Pharmacol.* **31**, 166–175.

Akkermans, L. M. A., van den Bercken, J., and Versluijs-Helder, M. (1975b). Excitatory and depressant effects of dieldrin and aldrin-transdiol on the spinal cord of the toad (*Xenopus laevis*). *Eur. J. Pharmacol.* **34**, 133–142.

Balba, H. M., and Saha, J. G. (1978). Studies on the distribution, excretion and metabolism of alpha- and gamma-isomers of [^{14}C] chlordane in rabbits. *J. Environ. Sci. Health*, **B13**, 211–233.

Baldwin, M. K. (1971). "The Metabolism of the Chlorinated Insecticides Aldrin, Dieldrin, Endrin and Isodrin." Ph.D. Thesis, University of Surrey, Guildford, UK.

Baldwin, M. K., and Robinson, J. (1969). Metabolism in the rat of the photoisomerisation product of dieldrin. *Nature* (*London*) **224**, 283–284.

Baldwin, M. K., Robinson, J., and Parke, D. V. (1972). A comparison of the metabolism of HEOD (Dieldrin) in the CF1 mouse with that in the CFE rat. *Food Cosmet. Toxicol.* **10**, 333–351.

Barnes, W., and Ware, G. W. (1965). The absorption and metabolism of C^{14}-endosulfan in the housefly. *J. Econ. Entomol.* **58**, 286–291.

Bedford, C. T. (1974). Von Baeyer/IUPAC names and abbreviated chemical names of metabolites and artifacts of aldrin (HHDN), dieldrin (HEOD) and endrin. *Pestic. Sci.* **5**, 473–489.

Bedford, C. T., Harrod, R. K., Hoadley, E. C., and Hutson, D. H. (1975a). The metabolic fate of endrin in the rabbit. *Xenobiotica*, **5**, 485–500.

Bedford, C. T., Hutson, D. A., and Natoff, I. L. (1975b). The acute toxicity of endrin and its metabolites to rats. *Toxicol. Appl. Pharmacol.* **33**, 115–121.

Bender, H. (1935). Benzene hexachloride and other chlorinated carbocyclics. U.S. Patent 2010841.

Bloomquist, J. R., and Shankland, D. L. (1983). The mode of action and neurotoxicity of mirex, chlordecone and four hydrogenated mirex analogues. *Pestic. Biochem. Physiol.* **19**, 235–242.

Bloomquist, J. R., Jackson, J. L., Karr, L. L., Ferguson, H. J., and Gajewski, R. P. (1993). Spirosultam LY 219048: A new chemical class of insecticide acting upon the GABA receptor/chloride ionophore complex. *Pestic. Sci.* **39**, 195–202.

Boddy, K. L., Briggs, G. G., Harrison, R. P., Jones, T. H., O'Mahony, M. J., Marlow, I. D., Roberts, B. G., Bardsley, R., and Reid, J. (1996). The synthesis and insecticidal activity of 2-aryl-1,2,3-triazoles. *Pestic. Sci.* **48**, 189–196.

Brimfield, A. A., and Street, J. C. (1979). Mammalian biotransformation of chlordane: *in vivo* and primary hepatic comparisons. *Ann. N.Y. Acad. Sci.* **320**, 247–256.

Brimfield, A. A., Street, J. C., Futsell, J., and Chatfield, D. A. (1978). Identification of products arising from the metabolism of *cis*- and *trans*-chlordane in rat liver microsomes *in vitro*: Outline of possible metabolic pathway. *Pestic. Biochem. Physiol.* **9**, 84–95.

Brooks, G. T. (1960). Mechanisms of resistance of the adult housefly (*M. domestica*) to cyclodiene insecticides. *Nature* (*London*) **186**, 96–98.

Brooks, G. T. (1966). Progress in metabolic studies of the cyclodiene insecticides and its relevance to structure–activity correlations. *World Rev. of Pest Control* **5**, 62–84.

Brooks, G. T. (1969). The metabolism of diene-organochlorine (cyclodiene) insecticides, *Residue Rev.* **27**, 81–138.

Brooks, G. T. (1973). The design of insecticidal chlorohydrocarbon derivatives. *In* "Drug Design" (E. J. Ariens, ed.), Vol. 4, pp. 379–444. Academic Press, New York.

Brooks, G. T. (1974). "Chlorinated Insecticides," Vol. 1, pp. 87–98. CRC Press, Cleveland.

Brooks, G. T. (1975). The insect toxicities of biodegradable derivatives of chlorinated norbornenes. *In* "Proceedings of the Eight British Insecticide and Fungicide Conference," Vol. 2, pp. 381–387. British Crop Protection Council, Farnham, Surrey, UK.

Brooks, G. T. (1977). Action and inaction of certain non-anticholinesterase insecticides. *In* "Proceedings of the 1977 British Crop Protection Conference—Pests and Diseases," Vol. 3, pp. 731–740. British Crop Protection Council, Farnham, Surrey, UK.

Brooks, G. T. (1980). The preparation of some reductively dechlorinated analogues of dieldrin, endosulfan and isobenzan. *J. Pestic. Sci.* (*Tokyo*) **5**, 565–574.

Brooks, G. T. (1985). The preparation of reductively dechlorinated analogues of endrin and some other cyclodiene insecticides. *J. Pestic. Sci.* (*Tokyo*) **10**, 241–245.

Brooks, G. T. (1992). Progress in structure–activity studies on cage convulsants and related GABA receptor chloride ionophore antagonists. *In* "Insecticides: Mechanism of Action and Resistance" (D. Otto and B. Weber, eds.), pp. 237–242. Intercept, Andover, UK.

Brooks, G. T., and Harrison, A. (1963). Relations between structure, metabolism and toxicity of the "cyclodiene" insecticides. *Nature* (*London*) **198**, 1169–1171.

Brooks, G. T., and Harrison, A. (1964a). The effect of pyrethrin synergists, especially sesamex, on the insecticidal potency of hexachlorocyclopentadiene derivatives ("cyclodiene" insecticides) in the adult housefly, *M. domestica* L. *Biochem. Pharmacol.* **13**, 827–840.

Brooks, G. T., and Harrison, A. (1964b). The metabolism of some cyclodiene insecticides in relation to dieldrin resistance in the adult housefly, *M. domestica* L. *J. Insect Physiol.* **10**, 633–641.

Brooks, G. T., and Harrison, A. (1965). Structure–activity relationships among insecticidal compounds derived from chlordene. *Nature* (*London*) **205**, 1031–1032.

Brooks, G. T., and Harrison, A. (1967a). The metabolism of dihydrochlordene and related compounds by housefly (*M. domestica* L.) and pig liver microsomes. *Life Sci.* **6**, 681–689.

Brooks, G. T., and Harrison, A. (1967b). The toxicity of alpha-dihydroheptachlor and related compounds to the housefly (*M. domestica* L.) and their metabolism by housefly and pig liver microsomes. *Life Sci.* **6**, 1439–1448.

Brooks, G. T., and Harrison, A. (1969a). The oxidative metabolism of aldrin and dihydroaldrin by houseflies, housefly microsomes and pig liver microsomes and the effect inhibitors. *Biochem. Pharmacol.* **18**, 557–568.

Brooks, G. T., and Harrison, A. (1969b). Hydration of HEOD (dieldrin) and the heptachlor epoxides by microsomes from the livers of pigs and rabbits. *Bull. Environ. Contam. Toxicol.* **4**, 352–361.

Brooks, G. T., and Mace, D. W. (1987). Toxicity and mode of action of reductively dechlorinated cyclodiene insecticide analogues on houseflies (*M. domestica* L.) and other diptera. *Pestic. Sci.* **21**, 129–142.

Brooks, G. T., Barlow, F., Hadaway, A. B., and Harris, A. G. (1981). The toxicities of some analogues of dieldrin, endosulfan and isobenzan to blood-sucking diptera, especially tsetse flies. *Pestic. Sci.* **12**, 475–484.

Brooks, G. T., Harrison, A., and Lewis, S. E. (1970). Cyclodiene epoxide ring hydration by microsomes from mammalian liver and houseflies. *Biochem. Pharmacol.* **19**, 255–273.

Brooks, G. T., Lewis, S. E., and Harrison, A. (1968). Selective metabolism of cyclodiene enantiomers by pig liver microsomal enzymes. *Nature* (*London*) **220**, 1034–1035.

Buchel, K. H., Ginsberg, A. E., and Fischer, R. (1966a). Synthese and struktur von heptachlor-methano-tetrahydrindanen. *Chem. Ber.* **99**, 405–415.

Buchel, K. H., Ginsberg, A. E., and Fischer, R. (1966b). Synthese und struktur von isomeren des chlordans. *Chem. Ber.* **99**, 421–430.

Burt, P. E. (1973). "Mode of Action of Insecticides." Rothamsted Experimental Station Annual Report, p. 171.

Busvine, J. R. (1964). The insecticidal potency of gamma-BHC and the chlorinated cyclodiene compounds and the significance of resistance to them. *Bull. Entomol. Res.* **55**, 271–288.

Calder, J. A., Wyatt, J. A., Frenkel, D. A., and Casida, J. E. (1993). CoMFA validation of the superposition of six classes of compounds which block GABA receptors non-competitively. *J. Comput.-Aided Mol. Des.* **7**, 45–60.

Casida, J. E., and Pulman, D. A. (1994). Recent advances in heterocyclic insecticides acting as GABA antagonists. *In* "Advances in the Chemistry of Insect Control III" (G. G. Briggs, ed.), pp. 36–51. Royal Society of Chemistry, Cambridge.

Casida, J. E., Palmer, C. J., and Cole, L. (1985). Bicycloorthocarboxylate convulsants: Potent GABA$_A$ receptor antagonists. *Mol. Pharmacol.* **28**, 246–253.

Casida, J. E., Nicholson, R. A., and Palmer, C. J. (1988). Trioxabicyclooctanes as probes for the convulsant site of the GABA-gated chloride channel in mammals and arthropods. *In* "Neurotox 88, Molecular basis of drug and pesticide action" (G. G. Lunt, ed.), Elsevier Science Publishers, Amsterdam, 125–144.

Chandurkar, P. S., and Matsumura, F. (1979). Metabolism of toxaphene components in rats. *Arch. Environ. Contam. Toxicol.* **8**, 1–24.

Chipman, J. K., and Walker, C. H. (1979). The metabolism of dieldrin and two of its analogues: the relationship between rates of microsomal metabolism and rates of excretion of metabolites in the male rat. *Biochem. Pharmacol.* **28**, 1337–1345.

Chu, I., Villeneuve, D. C., Secours, V., Becking, G. C., Viau, A., and Benoit, F. (1979). The absorption, distribution and excretion of photomirex in the rat. *Drug. Metab. Dispos.* **7**, 24–27.

Cole, L. M., Nicholson, R. A., and Casida, J. E. (1993). Action of phenylpyrazole insecticides at the GABA-gated chloride channel. *Pestic. Biochem. Physiol.* **46**, 47–54.

Cole, L. M., Saleh, M. A. and Casida, J. E. (1994). House fly head GABA-gated chloride channel: [^{3}H]-endosulfan binding in relation to polychlorocycloalkane insecticide action. *Pestic. Sci.* **42**, 59–63.

Colliot, F., Kukorowski, K. A., Hawkins, D. W., and Roberts, D. A. (1992). Fipronil: a new soil and foliar broad spectrum insecticide. *British Crop Protection Conference-Pests and Diseases*, British Crop Protection Council, Farnham, UK **1**, 29–34.

Craven, A. C. C., Brooks, G. T., and Walker, C. H. (1976). The inhibition of HEOM epoxide hydrase in mammalian liver microsomes and insect pupal homogenates. *Pestic. Biochem. Physiol.* **6**, 132–141.

Deng, Y., Palmer, C. J., and Casida, J. E. (1991). Housefly brain gamma-aminobutyric acid-gated chloride channel: Target for multiple classes of insecticides. *Pestic. Biochem. Physiol.* **41**, 60–65.

Deng, Y., Palmer, C. J., and Casida, J. E. (1993). Housefly head GABA-gated chloride channel: four putative binding sites differentiated by [3H] EBOB and [35S] TBPS. *Pestic. Biochem. Physiol.* **47**, 98–112.

Dorough, H. W., Huhtanen, K., Marshall, T. C. M., and Bryant, H. E. (1978). Fate of endosulfan in rats and toxicological considerations of apolar metabolites. *Pestic. Biochem. Physiol.* **8**, 241–252.

Elliott *et al.* (1990).

Elliott, M., Pulman, D. A., Larkin, J. P., and Casida, J. E. (1992). Insecticidal 1,3-dithianes. *J. Agric. Food Chem.* **40**, 147–151.

El Zorgani, G. A., Walker, C. H., and Hassall, K. A. (1970). Species differences in the *in vivo* metabolism of HEOM, a chlorinated cyclodiene epoxide. *Life Sci.* **9**, 415–420.

Estabrook, R. W., Cooper, D. Y., and Rosenthal, O. (1963). The light-reversible carbon monoxide inhibition of the steroid C-21 hydroxylation system of the adrenal cortex. *Biochem. Z.* **338**, 741–755.

ffrench-Constant, R. H., Steichen, J. C., and Ode, P. J. (1993b). Cyclodiene insecticide resistance in *Drosophila melanogaster* (Meigen) is associated with a temperature-sensitive phenotype. *Pestic. Biochem. Physiol.* **46**, 73–77.

ffrench-Constant, R. H., Steichen, J. C., Rocheleau, T. A., Aronstein, K., and Roush, R. T. (1993b). A single amino-acid substitution in a gamma-butyric acid subtype A receptor locus is associated with cyclodiene insecticide resistance in *Drosophila* populations. *Proc. Natl. Acad. Sci. U.S.A.* **90**, 1957–1961.

ffrench-Constant, R. H., Rocheleau, T. A., Steichen, J. C., and Chalmers, A. E. (1993a). A point mutation in a *Drosophila* GABA receptor confers insecticide resistance. *Nature (London)* **363**, 449–451.

ffrench-Constant, R. H., Zhang, H.-G., and Jackson, M. B. (1995). Biophysical analysis of a single amino-acid replacement in the resistance to dieldrin gamma-aminobutyric acid receptor: Novel dual mechanism for cyclodiene insecticide resistance. *In* "Molecular Action of Insecticides on Ion Channels," ACS Symposium Series 591 (J. Marshall Clark, ed.), pp. 192–204. Am. Chem. Soc., Washington, DC.

Fisher, M. H. (1997). Structure–activity relationships of the avermectins and milbemycins. *In* "Phytochemicals for Pest Control," ACS Symposium Series 658 (P. A. Hedin, R. M. Hollingworth, E. P. Masler, J. Miyamoto, and D. G. Thompson, eds.), Am. Chem. Soc., Washington, DC. pp. 220–238.

Forman, S. E., Durbetaki, A. J., Cohen, M. V., and Olofson, R. A. (1965). Conformational Equilibria in Cyclic Sulfites and Sulfates: the Configurations and Conformations of the Two Isomeric Thiodans. *J. Org. Chem.* **30**, 169–175.

Gant, D., Eldefrawi, F., and Eldefrawi, A. T. (1987). Cyclodienes inhibit GABA$_A$-receptor-regulated chloride transport. *Toxicol. Appl. Pharmacol.* **88**, 313–321.

Giannotti, O., Metcalf, R. L., and March, R. B. (1957). The mode of action of aldrin and dieldrin in *Periplaneta americana* (L.). *Ann. Entomol. Soc. Am.* **49**, 588–592.

Gladstone, C. M., and Wong, J. L. (1977). Azadiene chemistry 4. Insecticidal activities and chemical reactivities of azadieldrin and azaaldrin. Comparison with aldrin and dieldrin. *J. Agric. Food Chem.* **25**, 489–493.

Hallett, D. J., Khera, K. S., Stoltz, D. R., Chu, I., and Villeneuve, D. C. (1978). Photomirex: Synthesis and assessment of acute toxicity, tissue distribution and mutagenicity. *J. Agric. Food Chem.* **26**, 288–291.

Hathway, D. E., and Mallinson, A. (1964). Effect of telodrin on the liberation and utilisation of ammonia in rat brain. *Biochem. J.* **90**, 51–60.

Hathway, D. E., Mallinson, A., and Akintonwa, D. A. A. (1965). Effects of dieldrin, picrotoxin and telodrin on the metabolism of ammonia in brain. *Biochem. J.* **94**, 676–686.

Hatton, L. R., Hawkins, D. W., Pearson, C. J., and Roberts, D. A. (1988). Derivatives of N-phenylpyrazoles. European Patent 295,117.

Hawkinson, J. E., and Casida, J. E. (1993). Insecticide binding sites on gamma-aminobutyric acid receptors of insects and mammals. *In* "Pest Control with Environmental Safety," ACS Symposium Series 524 (S. O. Duke, J. J. Menn, and J. R. Plimmer, eds.), pp. 126–143. Am. Chem. Soc., Washington, DC.

Holland, K. D., Mathews, G. C., Bolos-Sy, A. M., Tucker, J. B., Reddy, P. A., Covey, D. F., Ferrendeli, J. A., and Rothman, S. M. (1995). Dual modula-tion of the gamma-aminobutyric acid type A receptor/ionophore by alkyl-substituted gamma-butyrolactones. *Mol. Pharmacol.* **47**, 1217–1223.

Holyoke, C. W., Rauh, J. J., Kleier, D. A., Schnee, M. A., Cordova, D., Benner, E. A., Watson, M. K., Bai, D., Howard, M. H., and Sattelle, D. B. (1994). "Advances in the Chemistry of Insecticides." Royal Society of Chemistry, Cambridge.

Hutson, D. H., Baldwin, M. K., and Hoadley, E. C. (1975). Detoxication and bioactivation of endrin in the rat. *Xenobiotica* **5**, 697–714.

Hyman, J. (1949). Improvements in, or related to method of forming halogenated organic compounds and the products resulting therefrom. British Patent 618432.

Jager, K. W. (1970). "Aldrin, Dieldrin, Endrin and Telodrin: An Epidemiological and Toxicological Study of Long-Term Occupational Exposure." Elsevier, Amsterdam.

Joy, R. M. (1982). Mode of action of lindane, dieldrin and related insecticides in the central nervous system. *Neurobehav. Toxicol. Teratol.* **4**, 813–823.

Kadous, A. A., and Matsumura, F. (1982). Toxicity of metabolites of dieldrin, photodieldrin and endrin in the cockroach. *Arch. Environ. Contam. Toxicol.* **11**, 635–643.

Kadous, A. A., Ghiasuddin, S. M., Matumura, F., Scott, J. G., and Tanaka, K. (1983). Differences in the picrotoxin receptor between the cyclodiene resistant and susceptible strains of the German Cockroach. *Pestic. Biochem. Physiol.* **19**, 157–166.

Kearns, C. W., Ingle, L., and Metcalf, R. L. (1945). New chlorinated hydrocarbon insecticides. *J. Econ. Entomol.* **38**, 661–668.

Khan, M. A. Q., Sutherland, D. J., Rosen, J. D., and Carey, W. F. (1970). Effect of sesamex on the toxicity and metabolism of cyclodienes and their photoisomers in the housefly. *J. Econ. Entomol.* **63**, 470–475.

Klein, A. K., Dailey, R. E., Walton, M. S., Beck, V., and Link, J. D. (1970). Metabolites isolated from urine of rats fed 14C-photodieldrin. *J. Agric. Food Chem.* **18**, 705–708.

Klingenberg, M. (1958). Pigments of rat liver microsomes. *Arch. Biochem. Biophys.* **75**, 376–386.

Klis, S. F. L., Nijman, N. J., Vijverberg, H. P. M., and van den Bercken, J. (1991). Phenylpyrazoles, a new class of pesticide: Effects on neuromuscular transmission and acetyl choline responses. *Pestic. Sci.* **33**, 213–222.

Klunk *et al.* (1982).

Klunk, W. E., Kalman, B. L., Ferrendelli, J. A., and Covey, D. F. (1983). Computer assisted modelling of the picrotoxinin and gamma-butyrolactone receptor site. **23**, 511–518.

Kölbl, H., Gompper, Behrenz, W., Hammann, I., Homeyer, B., and Hermann, G. (1981). "Agents for Pest Control." DE 3141 119 A1, Bayer AG.

Korte, F. (1967). Metabolism of 14C-labelled insecticides in microorganisms, insects and mammals. *Botyu kagaku* **32**, 46–59.

Korte, F., and Arent, H. (1965). Metabolism of insecticides. IX. Isolation and identification of dieldrin metabolites from the urine of rabbits after oral administration of dieldrin-14C. *Life Sci.* **4**, 2017–2026.

Kunze, F. M., and Laug, E. P. (1953). Toxicants in tissues of rats on diets containing dieldrin, aldrin, endrin and isodrin. *Fed. Proc.* **12**, 339.

Lauger, D., Martin, H., and Muller, P. (1944). Uber konstitution und toxische wirkung von naturlichen und neuen synthetischen insektentotenden stoffen. *Helv. Chim. Acta* **27**, 892.

Lawrence, J., and Casida, J. E. (1984). Interactions of lindane, toxaphene and cyclodienes with brain specific *t*-butylbicyclophosphorothionate receptor. *Life Sci.* **35**, 171–178.

Lee, H. J., Zhang, H.-G., Jackson, M. B., and ffrench-Constant, R. H. (1995). Binding and physiology of 4'-ethynyl-4-*n*-propylbicycloorthobenzoate (EBOB) in cyclodiene-resistant *Drosophila*. *Pestic. Biochem. Physiol.* **51**, 30–37.

Leonard, R. J., Labarca, C. G., Charnet, P., Davidson, N., and Lester, H. A. (1988). Evidence that the M$_2$ membrane spanning region lines the ion channel pore of the nicotinic receptor. *Science* **242**, 1578–1581.

Lewis, S. E. (1967). Effect of carbon monoxide on metabolism of insecticides *in vivo*. *Nature (London)* **215**, 1408–1409.

Ludwig, G., Weis, J., and Korte, F. (1964). Excretion and distribution of aldrin-14C and its metabolites after oral administration for a long period of time. *Life Sci.* **3**, 123–130.

MacDonald, R. L., and Olsen, R. W. (1994). GABA$_a$-receptor channels. *Ann. Rev. Neurosci.* **17**, 569–602.

Maier-Bode, H. (1968). Properties, effect, residues and analytics of the insecticide endosulfan. *Residue Rev.* **22**, 1–44.

Matsumura, F., and Ghiasuddin, S. M. (1983). Evidence for similarities between cyclodiene type insecticides and picrotoxinin in their action mechanisms. *J. Environ. Sci. Health, B* **18**, 1–14.

Matthews, H. B., and Matsumura, F. (1969). Metabolic fate of dieldrin in the rat. *J. Agric. Food Chem.* **17**, 845–852.

Middleton, W. J., and Bingham, E. M. (1982). Fluorine containing 1,1-dicyanoethylenes: Their preparation, Diels–Alder reaction and derived norbornenes and norbornanes. *J. Fluorine Chem.* **20**, 397–418.

Miles, J. R. W., Tu, C. M., and Harris, C. R. (1969). Metabolism of heptachlor and its degradation products by soil microrganisms. *J. Econ. Entomol.* **62**, 1334–1338.

Miyazaki, A., Hotta, T., Marumo, S., and Sakai, M. (1978). Synthesis and absolute stereochemistry and biological activity of optically active cyclodiene insecticides. *J. Agric. Food Chem.* **26**, 975–977.

Miyazaki, A., Sakai, M., and Marumo, S. (1979). Comparative metabolism of enantiomers of chlordene and chlordene epoxide in German cockroaches, in relation to their remarkably different insecticidal activity. *J. Agric. Food Chem.* **27**, 1403–1405.

Miyazaki, A., Sakai, M., and Marumo, S. (1980). Synthesis and biological activity of optically active heptachlor, 2-chloroheptachlor and 3-chloroheptachlor. *J. Agric. Food Chem.* **28**, 1310–1311.

Molowa, D. T., Wrighton, S. A., Blank, R. V., and Guzelian, P. S. (1986). Characterization of a unique aldo-keto-reductase responsible for the reduction of chlordecone in the liver of gerbil and man. *J. Toxicol. Environ. Health* **17**, 375–384.

Nakanishi, K., Huang, D., Monde, K., Tokiwa, Y., Fang, K., Liu, Y., Jiang, H., Huang, X., Matile, S., Usherwood, P. N. R., and Berova, N. (1997). Philanthotoxins and the nicotinic acetylcholine receptor. *In* "Phytochemicals for Pest Control," ACS Symposium Series 658 (P. A. Hedin, R. M. Hollingworth, E. P. Masler, J. Miyamoto, and D. G. Thompson, eds.), pp. 339–353. Am. Chem. Soc., Washington, DC.

Nakatsugawa, T., Ishida, M., and Dahm, P. A. (1965). Microsomal epoxidation of cyclodiene insecticides. *Biochem. Pharmacol.* **14**, 1853–1865.

Nelson, J. O., and Matsumura, F. (1973). Dieldrin (HEOD) metabolism in cockroaches and houseflies. *Arch. Environ. Contam. Toxicol.* **1**, 224–244.

Ozoe, Y., and Matsumura, F. (1986). Structural requirements for bridged bicyclic compounds acting on picrotoxinin receptor. *J. Agric. Food Chem.* **34**, 126–134.

Ozoe, Y., Matsumoto, K., Mochida, K., Nakamura, T., and Matsumura, F. (1995). Nitrogen analogues of aldrin as non-competitive antagonists of GABA$_A$-receptor. *J. Pestic. Sci. (Tokyo)* **20**, 317–319.

Ozoe, Y., Sawada, Y., Mochida, K., Nakamura, T., and Matsumura, F. (1990). Structure–activity relationships in a new series of insecticidally active dioxatricycloalkenes derived by structural comparison of the GABA antagonists bicycloorthocarboxylates and endosulfan. *J. Agric. Food Chem.* **38**, 1264–1268.

Ozoe, Y., Takayama, T., Sawada, Y., Mochida, K., Nakamura, T., and Matsumura, F. (1993). Synthesis and structure–activity relationships of a series of insecticidal dioxatricyclododecenes acting as the noncompetitive antagonists of GABA$_A$ receptors. **41**, 2135–2141.

Palmer, C. J., and Casida, J. E. (1985). 1,4-Disubstituted 2,6,7-trioxabicyclo [2.2.2] octanes: a new class of insecticides. *J. Agric. Food Chem.* **33**, 967–980.

Palmer, C. J., and Casida, J. E. (1992). Insecticidal 1,3-dithianes and 1,3-dithiane 1,1-dioxides. *J. Agric. Food Chem.* **40**, 492–496.

Palmer, C. J., and Casida, J. E. (1995). Insecticidal 1,3-oxathianes and their oxides. *J. Agric. Food Chem.* **43**, 498–502.

Palmer, C. J., Cole, L. M., Larkin, J. P., Smith, I. H., and Casida, J. E. (1991a). (4-ethynylphenyl)-4-substituted -2,6,7-trioxabicyclo[2.2.2] octanes: Effect of 4-substituent on toxicity to houseflies and mice and potency at the GABA-gated chloride channel. *J. Agric. Food Chem.* **39**, 1329–1334.

Palmer, C. J., Cole, L. M., Smith, I. H., Moss, M. D. V., and Casida, J. E. (1991b). Silylated 1-(4-ethynylphenyl)-2,6,7-trioxabicyclo[2.2.1] octanes: Structural features and mechanisms of proinsecticidal action and selective toxicity. *J. Agric. Food Chem.* **39**, 1335–1341.

Peterson, E. M., Kun Xu, Holland, K. D., McKeon, A. C., Rothman, S. M., Ferrendelli, J. A., and Covey, D. F. (1994). Alpha-spirocyclopentyl and alpha-spirocyclopropyl-gamma-butyrolactones: Conformationally constrained derivatives of anticonvulsant and convulsant alpha, alpha-disubstituted gamma-butyrolactones. *J. Med. Chem.* **37**, 275–286.

Pollock, G. A., and Kilgore, W. W. (1980). Toxicities and descriptions of some toxaphene fractions: Isolation and identification of a highly toxic component. *J. Toxicol. Environ. Health* **6**, 115–125.

Pulman, D. A., Smith, I. H., Larkin, J. P., and Casida, J. E. (1996). Heterocyclic insecticides acting at the GABA-gated chloride channel: 5-Alkyl-2-arylpyrimidines and 1,3-thiazines. *Pestic. Sci.* **46**, 237–245.

Ray, J. W. (1967). The epoxidation of aldrin by housefly microsomes and its inhibition by carbon dioxide. *Biochem. Pharmacol.* **16**, 99–107.

Reddy, G., and Khan, M. A. Q. (1977). Metabolism of [^{14}C]-photodieldrin in house flies. *J. Agric. Food Chem.* **25**, 25–28.

Revah, F., Bertrand, D., Galzi, J. L., Devillers-Theiry, A., Mulle, C., Hussy, N., Bertrand, S., Ballivet, M., and Changeux, J. P. (1991). Mutations in the channel domain alter desensitisation of a neuronal nicotine receptor. *Nature (London)* **353**, 846–849.

Richardson, A., Baldwin, M. K., and Robinson, J. (1968). Metabolites of dieldrin in the urine and faeces of rats. *Chem. Ind. (London)* 588–590.

Ryan, K. J., and Engel, L. L. (1957). Hydroxylation of steroids at carbon-21. *J. Biol. Chem.* **225**, 103–114.

Saleh, M. A., Skinner, R. F., and Casida, J. E. (1979). Comparative metabolism of 2,2,5-endo,6-exo,8,9,10-heptachloronorbornene and toxaphene in six mammalian species and chickens. *J. Agric. Food Chem.* **27**, 731–737.

Schmidt, W. F., Hapeman, C. J., Fettinger, J. C., Rice, C. P., and Bilboulian, S. (1997). Structure and asymmetry in the isomeric conversion of beta- to alpha-endosulfan. *J. Agric. Food Chem.* **45**, 1023–1026.

Schofield, P. R., Darlison, M. G., Fujita, N., Burt, D. R., Stephenson, F. A., Rodriguez, H., Rhee, L. M., Ramachandran, J., Reale, V., Glencorse, T. A., Seeburg, P. H., and Barnard, E. A. (1987). Sequence and functional expression of the GABA$_A$-receptor shows a ligand-gated receptor super-family. *Nature (London)* **328**, 221–227.

Schroeder, M. E., Shankland, D. E., and Hollingworth, R. M. (1977). The effects of dieldrin and isomeric diols on synaptic transmission in the American cockroach and their relevance to the dieldrin poisoning syndrome. *Pestic. Biochem. Physiol.* **7**, 403–415.

Shankland, D. L. (1982) Neurotoxic action of chlorinated hydrocarbon insecticides. *Neurobehav. Toxicol. Teratol.* **4**, 805–811.

Shankland, D. L., and Schroeder, M. E. (1973). Pharmacological evidence for a discrete neurotoxic action of dieldrin (HEOD) in the American cockroach, *Perplaneta americana* (L.). *Pestic. Biochem. Physiol.* **3**, 77–86.

Slade, R. E. (1945). The gamma-isomer of hexachlorocyclohexane (gammexane). *Chem. Ind. (London)* **40**, 314–319.

Slade, M., Brooks, G. T., Hetnarski, H., and Wilkinson, C. F. (1975). Inhibition of the enzymatic hydration of the epoxide HEOM in insects. *Pestic. Biochem. Physiol.* **5**, 35–46.

Smith, A. G. (1991). Chlorinated hydrocarbon insecticides. *In* "Handbook of Pesticide Toxicology" (W. J. Hayes, Jr., E. R. Laws, Jr., eds.), Vol. 2, pp. 731–915. Academic Press, New York.

Smith, I. H., Budd, T. C., Sills, J. H., and Casida, J. E. (1993). Insecticidal 1-(alkynyl alkyl)-3-cyano-2,6,7-trioxabicyclo[2.2.1] octanes. *J. Agric. Food Chem.* **41**, 1114–1117.

Soloway, S. B. (1965). Correlation between biological activity and molecular structure of the cyclodiene insecticides. *Adv. Pest Control Res.* **6**, 85–126.

Sternburg, J., Kearns, C. W., and Moorefield, H. (1954). DDT-dehydrochlorinase, an enzyme found in DDT-resistant flies. *J. Agric. Food Chem.* **2**, 1125.

Street, J. C., and Blau, S. E. (1972). Oxychlordane. Accumulation in rat adipose tissue on feeding chlordane isomers or technical chlordane. *J. Agric. Food Chem.* **20**, 395–397.

Sun, Y. P., and Johnson, E. R. (1960). Synergistic and antagonistic actions of insecticide—synergist combinations and their mode of action. *J. Agric. Food Chem.* **8**, 261–266.

Takeuchi, A., and Takeuchi, N. (1966). On the permeability of the presynaptic terminal of the crayfish neuromuscular junction during synaptic inhibition and the action of GABA. *J. Physiol.* **183**, 433–449.

Takeuchi, A., and Takeuchi, N. (1972). Actions of transmitter substances on the neuromuscular functions of vertebrates and invertebrates. *Adv. Biophys.* **3**, 45–95.

Tanaka, K., Scott, J. G., and Matsumura, F. (1984). Picrotoxinin receptor in the central nervous system of the American cockroach: Its role in the action of cyclodiene-type molecules. *Pestic. Biochem. Physiol.* **22**, 117–127.

Tashiro, S., and Matsumura, F. (1977). Metabolic routes of *cis*- and *trans*-chlordane in rats. *J. Agric. Food Chem.* **25**, 872–880.

Tomlin, C. D. S., ed. (1997). "Pesticidehonval," 4th ed., PPC, 545–547. British Crop Protection Council, Farnham, Surrey, UK.

Turner, W. V., Engel, J. L., and Casida, J. E. (1977). Toxaphene components and related compounds: preparation and toxicity of some hepta-, octa- and nonachloronorbornanes, hexa- and heptachlorobornenes, and a hexachlorobornadiene. *J. Agric. Food Chem.* **25**, 1394–1401.

Uchida, M., Fujita, T., Kurihara, N., and Nakajima, M. (1978). Toxicities of gamma-BHC and related compounds. *In* "Pesticide and Venom Neurotoxicity" (D. L. Shankland, R. M. Hollingworth, and T. Smyth, Jr., eds.), pp. 133–151. Plenum, New York.

Ullman and Wong *et al.* (1972).

Unwin, N. (1995). Acetylcholine receptor channel imaged in the open state *Nature (London)* **373**, 37–43.

Von Keyserlingk, H. C., and Willis, R. J. (1992). The Gaba-activated chloride channel in insects as target for insecticide action—A physiological study. *In* "Insecticides: Mechansim of Action and Resistance" (D. Otto and B. Weber, eds.), pp. 205–236. Intercept, Andover, UK.

Wacher, V. J., Toia, R. F., and Casida, J. E. (1992). 2-Aryl-5-tert-butyl-1,3-dithianes and their S-oxidation products: Structure–activity relationships of potent insecticides acting at the GABA-gated chloride channel. *J. Agric. Food Chem.* **40**, 497–505.

Wang, C. M., Narahashi, T., and Yamada, M. (1971). The neurotoxic action of dieldrin and its derivatives in the cockroach. *Pestic. Biochem. Physiol.* **1**, 84–91.

Weil, E. D., Colson, J. G., Hoch, P. E., and Gruber, R. H. (1969). Toxic chlorinated methanoisobenzofuran derivatives. *J. Heterocyc. Chem.* **6**, 643–649.

Weston, J. B., Larkin, J. P., Pulman, D. A., Holden, I., and Casida, J. E. (1995). Insecticidal isomers of 4-tert-butyl-1-(4-ethynylcyclohexyl)-2,6,7-trioxabicyclo[2.2.1] octane and 5-tert-butyl-2-(4-ethynylcyclohexyl)-1,3-dithiane. *Pestic. Sci.* **44**, 69–74.

Whittle, A. J., Fitzjohn, S., Mullier, G., Pearson, D. P. J., Perrior, T. R., Taylor, R., and Salmon, R. (1995). The use of computer-generated electrostatic surface maps for the design of new GABA-ergic insecticides. *Pestic. Sci.* **44**, 29–31.

Wong and Terriere (1965).

Yarbrough, J. D., Grimley, J. M., Karl, P. I., Chambers, J. E., Case, R. S., and Alley, E. G. (1983). Tissue disposition, metabolism and excretion of cis- and trans-5,10-dihydrogen mirex. *Drug Metab. Dispos.* **11**, 611–614.

Zhang, H.-G., ffrench-Constant, R. H., and Jackson, M. B. (1994). A unique amino acid of the *Drosophila* GABA-receptor with influence on drug sensitivity by two mechanisms. *J. Physiol.* **479**, 65–75.

Zhang, H.-G., Lee, H.-J., Rocheleau, T., ffrench-Constant, R. H., and Jackson, M. B. (1995). Subunit composition determines picrotoxinin and biculline sensitivity of *Drosophila* GABA-receptors. *Mol. Pharmacol.* **48**, 835–840.

The Avermectins: Insecticidal and Antiparasitic Agents

Jim Stevens and Charles B. Breckenridge
Syngente Crop Protection

56.1 INTRODUCTION

The avermectins are macrocyclic lactones isolated from the fermentation broth of the soil actinomycete, *Streptomyces avermitilis*. Included in this avermectin group are abamectin and emamectin benzoate, which are used as insecticides, and ivermectin, which is sold for parasite control in human and veterinary medicine. Because the avermectins act as $GABA_A$ receptor agonists in vertebrates, their general safety for use as pest control agents in mammals depends on an intact blood–brain barrier in juvenile and adult animals and an intact blood–placental barrier *in utero*. Inherent in the integrity of these barriers is the substance P-glycoprotein. Intact P-glycoprotein barriers are present in human adults (male and female, pregnant and nonpregnant), newborns, and children. This fact is supported by significant clinical evidence from in excess of 50 million people; a genetically varied population throughout the world, including thousands of pregnant women, have been administered therapeutic doses (0.15–0.20 mg/kg) of ivermectin. However, there is also experimental evidence that certain laboratory animals, such as genetically polymorphic CF-1 mice and rat pups early postnatally, do not possess intact P-glycoprotein blood–brain barriers. Unfortunately, in the process of establishing the hazard profile for the mectins, both of these models were used. This has resulted in very low NOELs (no observed effect levels) based on neurotoxicity in the CF-1 polymorphic mouse. The World Health Organization's JMPR and the U.S. Environmental Protection Agency have concluded that the CF-1 polymorphic mouse is not an appropriate model for human risk assessment for the avermectins; the JMPR has recognized the flawed nature of the rat pup model for testing of these avermectins. However, a consistent understanding of the inappropriateness of applying results from standard animal models used for toxicity testing to human risk assessment is yet to be fully appreciated.

56.2 CHEMISTRY AND FORMULATIONS

Abamectin belongs to a general class of closely related macrocyclic lactones either produced directly by the actinomycete *Streptomyces avermitilis* or generated through semisynthetic modifications (Fisher and Mrozik, 1989). The structure for the natural avermectins is given in Fig. 56.1. The basic structural motif of the avermectins is evident in the natural product avermectin B1a, which is the principal constituent of the insecticide abamectin. As used in pesticides, abamectin consists of 80% or more of avermectin B_{1a} and 20% or less of avermectin B_{1b} and is called avermectin B_1 (Fisher and Mrozik, 1989). Their structures are shown in Fig. 56.2.

Chemical modification of avermectin B1a has yielded a number of semisynthetic materials. Emamectin (4″-epimethylamino-4″-deoxyavermectin B1a) benzoate is shown in Fig. 56.3. Emamectin and ivermectin differ from avermectin B_1 by having only a single bond at the $C_{22}C_{23}$ position (instead of a double bond). The major manufacturers, trade names, and formulations for abamectin, emamectin benzoate, and ivermectin are given in Table 56.1.

56.3 USES

Abamectin and emamectin benzoate (Novartis) are used as insecticides and ivermectin (Merck) is sold for parasite control in human and veterinary medicine. Abamectin and emamectin migrate into treated leaves, exhibit oral activity against insect pests, and display rapid breakdown in sunlight; all of these features favor their use in integrated pest management (Bloomquist, 1999). Abamectin is used primarily to control mites, and emamectin benzoate has been designed primarily for control of lepidopterian species in vegetable, cotton, and tobacco.

Ivermectin has found great favor in both the pharmaceutical and the veterinary product marketplaces. In human medicine,

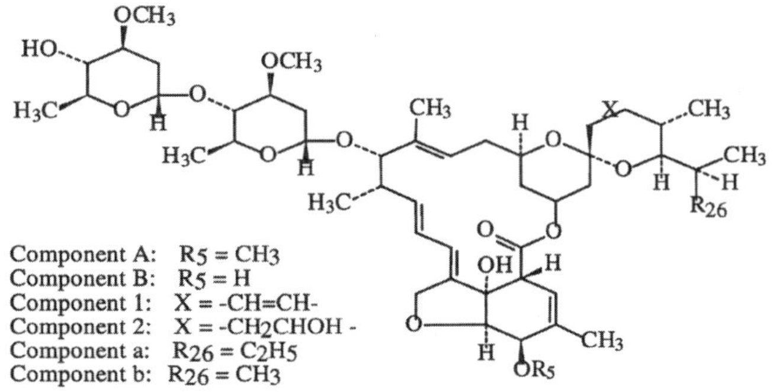

Figure 56.1 Structure of the natural avermectins.

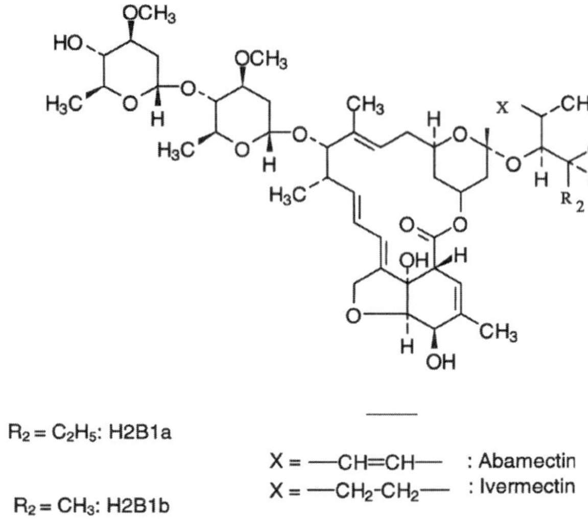

Component A: R5 = CH3
Component B: R5 = H
Component 1: X = -CH=CH-
Component 2: X = -CH2CHOH -
Component a: R26 = C2H5
Component b: R26 = CH3

Figure 56.2 Structures of ivermectin and abamectin.

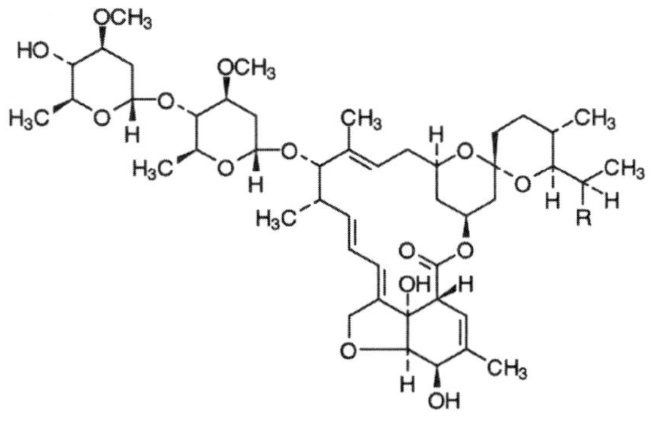

R2 = C2H5: H2B1a

R2 = CH3: H2B1b

X = —CH=CH— : Abamectin
X = —CH2-CH2— : Ivermectin

Figure 56.3 Structure of emamectin benzoate.

Table 56.1

Chemical Structures, Trade Names, Major Manufactures, and Formulations for the Avermectins

Chemical	Trade names	Major manufactures	Formulation	
Abamectin	Agri-mek	Novartis		0.15 lb/gal
	Zephyr			0.15 lb/gal
Emamectin	Proclaim	Novartis	5% granule	
benzoate	Denim			0.16 lb/gal
Ivermectin	Ivomec	Merck & Co.		Tablets
	Mectizan			Injectables
	Stromectal			

ivermectin has been used as an anthelmintic in the treatment of infection of intestinal threadworm, river blindness (onchocerciasis), and lymphatic filariasis. Its uses in veterinary medicine have been as anthelmintic and antiparasitic agents, including treatment of heartworm, hookworm, threadworm, and whipworm (FAO/WHO, 1992; 1993; Greene *et al.*, 1989).

56.3.1 MODE OF ACTION OF THE AVERMECTINS

The avermectins were first demonstrated to possess anthelmintic activity in 1979 (Burg *et al.*, 1979). The avermectins act as chloride channel-blocking insecticides, causing hyperexcitability and convulsions. Arena *et al.* (1995) demonstrated that in insects stimulation of glutamate (inhibitory) chloride channels is the most sensitive target site for the avermectins. The glutamate-gated chloride channels of insect and nematode skeletal muscle are especially important as they mediate avermectin-induced muscle paralysis in these organisms. These effects are mediated via a specific, high-affinity (10^{-10} M) binding site (Turner and Schaeffer, 1989).

In vertebrates, the effects occur via poisoning of the central nervous system (CNS) through reactions at the receptor for the inhibitory neurotransmitter γ-aminobutyric acid (GABA); see Fig. 56.4. The avermectins open the GABA$_A$ receptor chloride channel by binding to the GABA recognition site (receptor protein) and act as partial agonists (Abalis *et al.*, 1986). Chloride ions then flow into the postsynaptic neuron. This chloride permeability increase can significantly hyperpolarize (make more negative) the membrane potential, which has a dampening effect on nerve impulse firing. There is also a reversible dose-dependent increase in chloride ion permeability in response to very low doses of avermectins.

In GABA-insensitive neurons with no inhibitory innervation, the avermectins induce an irreversible increase in chloride ion conductance through interacting with voltage-dependent chloride channels. Avermectin intoxication in mammals begins with hyperexcitability, tremors, and incoordination and later develops into ataxia and coma-like sedation. This is similar to the mode of action of ethanol and barbiturates (Eldefawi and

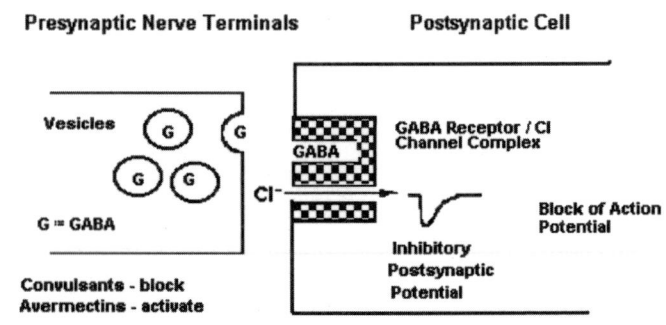

Figure 56.4 Depiction of the mechanism of action for the avermectins in the brain (after Bloomquist, 1999).

Eldefawi, 1987) and benzodiazepine sedatives (Williams and Yarbrough, 1979). However, the avermectins are less specific in their action and can affect a variety of other ligand- and voltage-gated chloride channels. The general safety of the avermectins depends on the presence of an intact P-glycoprotein blood–brain barrier.

56.3.2 IMPORTANCE OF THE P-GLYCOPROTEIN BLOOD–BRAIN BARRIER

In mammals, the circulatory system is the most important transport system in the body. The microvasculature, which includes an estimated 40 billion capillaries in the human, serves as a site of substance exchange and is vital for the transportation of chemicals throughout the body (Aigner *et al.*, 1997). These capillaries consist of a single layer of endothelial cells (continuous, discontinuous, and fenestrated) surrounded by a basement membrane. The capillaries with continuous endothelial cells are only present in a few organs, including the intestine, bile duct, liver, pancreas, kidney, adrenal, testes, placenta, and brain (Thiebaut *et al.*, 1987). In addition to this structural feature, two other pathways exist at some sites in the brain and the placenta for the further elimination of xenobiotics and intracellular metabolites. These pathways are (1) biotransformation and (2) direct transport by transmembrane pumps such as P-glycoprotein (Fisher and Sikic, 1995; Gottesman and Pastan, 1993).

P-glycoproteins are large-membrane proteins (150–180 kDa) consisting of two identical subunits each with a single adenosine 5′-triphosphate (ATP)–binding site and several transmembrane domains (Juliano and Ling, 1976). They are highly expressed in endothelial cells at areas that have a barrier function (e.g., the blood–brain barrier and the blood–placental barrier). P-glycoprotein barriers have also been identified in the adrenal gland, colon, testes, and the gravid uterus (Tiirikainen and Krusius, 1991). In addition, its localization along the apical surfaces of the intestines, proximal tubule of the kidney, and the bile ducts of the liver imply that P-glycoprotein is probably involved in secretory functions in humans.

P-glycoprotein is a member of a highly conserved multigene family with isoforms identified in a wide variety of mammalian species, including humans, rats, mice, hamsters, pigs, guinea pigs, rhesus monkeys, orangutans, cows, and chickens (Saunders, 1977). Further, P-glycoprotein has been identified in fruit flies (Wu *et al.*, 1991) and in tobacco hornworms and budworms (Lanning *et al.*, 1996). In addition, P-glycoprotein has been found in mussels and sponges (Kurelec and Pivcevic, 1991), in yeast (McGrath and Varshavsky, 1989), in parasites (Descoteaux *et al.*, 1992), and in nematodes (Lincke *et al.*, 1992). The fact that P-glycoprotein is conserved across phylogenic lines suggests that it is an ancient protein associated with fundamental cellular functions.

56.3.2.1 Implications of an Incomplete P-glycoprotein Blood–Brain Barrier in Hazard Testing

Unlike other transporters, P-glycoprotein transports a variety of chemically unrelated compounds. These compounds are commonly large lipophilic molecules that contain at least one aromatic ring and a positively charged nitrogen atom. Initially, P-glycoprotein interactions were thought to be limited to only the natural products such as anthracyclines, vinca alkaloids, actinomycin D, epipodophyllotoxins, taxol, and taxotere. However, it is now known that P-glycoprotein also transports steroid hormones, peptide antibiotics, immunosuppressive agents, and calcium channel blockers (Ueda *et al.*, 1997). Recently, pesticides have also been demonstrated to interact with P-glycoprotein. Such agents include abamectin (Didier and Loor, 1996), ivermectin (Schinkel *et al.*, 1995), 2-acetylaminofluorene and pentachlorophenol (Toomey and Epel, 1995), thiodicarb, and chlorpyrifos (Lanning *et al.*, 1996).

P-glycoprotein is encoded as three isoforms. Mouse P-glycoproteins are known as mdr1a (also called mdr3 or Pgy1), mdr1b (also called mdr1 or Pgy2), and mdr2 (Pgy3) (Borst *et al.*, 1993). The isoform mdr1a is primarily found in the intestinal brush border epithelium, the microvessel endothelial cells in the brain and testis, and the microvillus border of the trophoblast and Hofbauer cells of the placenta (MacFarland *et al.*, 1994; Nakamura *et al.*, 1997). The isoform mdr1b has been reported in the adrenal gland, kidney, and gravid uterus. Both mdr1a and mdr1b play roles in the multidrug resistance phenotype and are able to pump xenobiotics out of the cells. The isoforms mdr1a and mdr1b of the mouse are comparable to the human MDR1 gene in this regard (Mauad *et al.*, 1994). The isoform mdr2 has been shown necessary for bile production and is probably the phosphatidyl choline transporter. Mouse mdr2 is comparable to the human MDR3 (also called MDR2) gene and does not confer multidrug resistance to cells.

P-glycoprotein transport processes have been conserved across species, probably because such a transporter system is essential for adaptation and survival (Saunders, 1977). It is therefore probably not surprising that a population genotypically recessive for P-glycoprotein has not been identified. However, it has been possible to develop a "knockout" mouse for the mdr1a gene (Schinkel *et al.*, 1994; 1995). In addition, polymorphism for mdr1a P-glycoprotein gene expression has been reported for the CF-1 mouse (Umbenhauer *et al.*, 1997) and the collie dog (Lankas *et al.*, 1997).

56.3.2.2 Impact of an Incomplete P-glycoprotein Blood–Brain Barrier in Animal Model

Animals with a recessive mdr1a $(-/-)$ genotype do not have an intact blood–brain or blood–placental barrier because they are deficient in P-glycoprotein expression. Studies using knockout mice homozygous for disruption of mdr1a (Schinkel *et al.*, 1994; 1995) have clearly demonstrated that the presence/absence of P-glycoprotein is a major determinant of drug entry in the brain. Studies with CF-1 mice polymorphic for

P-glycoprotein (Umbenhauer *et al.*, 1997) have shown this same response.

Mice with disrupted P-glycoprotein and CF-1 mice without P-glycoprotein were shown to be significantly more susceptible to the effects of neurotoxicants. Brain levels of ivermectin in the knockout mice that do not express P-glycoprotein [mdr1a (−/−) genotype] were elevated approximately 90-fold over the wild type [mdr1a (+/+) genotype] and sensitivity to ivermectin was increased (Schinkel *et al.*, 1994; 1995).

Further, CF-1 mice show a unique developmental response to avermectins due to the polymorphic nature of the P-glyco-protein gene. These mdr1a (−/−) animals could be present in a population of CF-1 mice in a range from 0 to 100%, depending on the genotype of the parental animals (Umbenhauer *et al.*, 1997). Therefore, experiments carried out with P-glycoprotein substrates in the heterogeneous population of the CF-1 mouse must be interpreted with caution and may be unsuitable for risk assessment.

Besides the CF-1 mouse model, there are other unique features noted in the standard hazard testing models. The Sprague–Dawley rat pup does not establish a complete P-glycoprotein blood–brain barrier until appropriately 3 weeks postpartum, making it highly vulnerable to neurotoxic effects (Lankas *et al.*, 1989).

56.4 HAZARD IDENTIFICATION AND DOSE RESPONSE

As previously indicated, in vertebrates, the avermectins increase membrane permeability to chloride ions and act as $GABA_A$ agonists; this is similar to the mode of action of the benzodiazepine sedatives (Turner and Schaeffer, 1989). Their toxicity follows this mode of action in overdose scenarios or in animal models with compromised mdr1a P-glycoprotein barriers. The acute toxicology profiles for ivermectin and abamectin (EPA, 1999a; Lankas and Gordon, 1989) and emamectin benzoate (EPA, 1999b) are shown in Table 56.2.

Table 56.2

Acute Oral Toxicity Studies on Ivermectin, Abamectin (Lankas and Gordon, 1989; EPA, 1999a), and Emamectin Benzoate (EPA, 1999b)

Species	LD50 (mg/kg)		
	Ivermectin	Abamectin	Emamectin
SD rat	50	11	76–88
SD rat, neonato[a]	2	1.5	—
CD-1 mouse	—	220	107–120
CF-1 mouse[b]	25	14–24	22–31
Beagle dogs	80	—	—
Rhesus monkeys	> 24	> 24	—

[a]P-glycoprotein-deficient blood–brain barrier is seen in neonatal rats (Lankas *et al.*, 1989).
[b]CF-1 mice tested were polymorphic for P-glycoprotein (Umbenhauer *et al.*, 1997).

Table 56.3

Acute Toxicity and Plasma Concentrations of Ivermectin and Abamectin (Lankas and Gordon, 1989)

	Monkey		Humans
	Ivermectin	Abamectin	Ivermectin
Therapeutic dose			0.2 mg/kg
Peak plasma levels	—	—	20 ng/ml
Minimum effect level	2 mg/kg	2 mg/kg	—
Peak plasma levels	110 ng/ml	76 ng/ml	
Signs of toxicity	Emesis	Emesis	
Toxic effect level	8 mg/kg	8 mg/kg	6.6–8.6 mg/kg[a]
Peak plasma levels	270 ng/ml	150 ng/ml	Unknown
Signs of toxicity	Emesis	Emesis	Emesis, mydriasis, sedation
Overdose level	24 mg/kg	24 mg/kg	
Peak plasma levels	680 ng/ml	390 ng/ml	
Signs of toxicity	Emesis, mydriasis, sedation	Emesis, mydriasis, sedation	

[a]Overdose in humans.

These three avermectin-derived materials responded quite similarly in the different laboratory models. A comparison of the response of ivermectin and abamectin in the monkey as well as the response noted in the human with ivermectin is presented in Table 56.3.

Signs of overdosing noted at 24 mg/kg of ivermectin or abamectin in the monkey were the same as observed in the human overdose at approximately 9 mg/kg. These signs were essentially identical to those observed in 10 adults who accidentally ingested tablets or solutions intended for veterinarian use (Greene, 1991).

Subchronic dietary exposure to the three avermectins in the rat, mouse, and dog yielded similar results, as shown in Table 56.4. Although there are slight differences between the NOELs for abamectin and emamectin in the CD-1 mouse (probably the result of dose selection), the responses noted in the rat and dog were similar for the three avermectins. The aver-

Table 56.4

90-Day Dietary Toxicity Studies with Ivermectin (FAO/WHO, 1994), Abamectin (EPA, 1999a), and Emamectin Benzoate (EPA, 1999b)

	Exposure (mg/kg/day)					
	Ivermectin		Abamectin		Emamectin	
Study	mg/kg		mg/kg		mg/kg	
SD rat	0.8	0.4	1.4	0.4	2.5	0.5
CD mouse	NS[a]	NS	8	4	5.4	0.5
Beagle dog	2.0	0.5	> 1.0	0.5	0.5	0.25

[a]No study available.

Table 56.5
Chronic Dietary Toxicity Studies with Ivermectin (FAO/WHO, 1994), Abamectin (EPA, 1999a), and Emamectin Benzoate (EPA, 1999b)

Study	Exposure (mg/kg/day)					
	Ivermectin		Abamectin		Emamectin	
	mg/kg		mg/kg		mg/kg	
SD rat (105 weaks)[a]	0.8	0.4	2.0	1.5	2.5	0.25
CD-1 mouse (18 months)	—	—	8	4	5.0 (M) 7.5 (F)	2.5
Beagle dog (12 months)	1.0	0.5	0.5	0.25	0.5	0.25

[a]Rat studies with ivermectin and abamectin were only 53 weeks in duration.

mectins are equally well tolerated following chronic dietary administration, as shown in Table 56.5.

The NOELs found in the chronic dog and mouse oncogenicity studies were comparable for ivermectin, abamectin, and emamectin. The NOEL in the chronic rat study was higher for abamectin than for emamectin or ivermectin. This apparent difference between abamectin and emamectin was most likely due to differences in dose selection between the studies.

The avermectins are not genotoxic as has been demonstrated in a variety of standard tests for mutagenicity, clastogenicity, and unscheduled deoxyribonucleic acid (DNA) synthesis, as presented in Table 56.6. The maternotoxicity and developmental/fetotoxicity NOELs and LOELs for these three avermectins are shown in Table 56.7.

In the CF-1 mouse, SD rat, and rabbit developmental toxicity studies with ivermectin, cleft palate and clubbed feet (rabbit only) were observed at maternally toxic doses (Lankas and

Table 56.6
Genotoxicity Studies with Ivermectin (FAO/WHO, 1994), Abamectin (EPA, 1999a), and Emamectin Benzoate (EPA, 1999b)

	Tests	Mectin		
		Ivermectin	Abamectin	Emamectin
Mutation	Ames (+/− activation)	Negative	Negative	Negative
	Mouse lymphoma	Negative	—	—
	V-79 Chinese hamster lung (+/− activation)	—	Negative	Negative
Clastogenicity	Mouse bone marrow *in vivo*	—	Negative	Negative
	Chinese hamster ovary *in vitro*	—	—	Negative
Other	Alkaline elution/rat hepatocyte	—	Negative	Negative
	Unscheduled DNA synthesis in human fibroblasts	Negative	—	—

Gordon, 1989). Similar findings were noted in the CF-1 mouse and rabbit studies with abamectin. Neither of these effects was noted with emamectin (EPA, 1999b). Sedation was observed in overdosed rabbit dams. Severe neurotoxicity (tremors, convulsion, and coma) was observed in some of the polymorphic CF-1 mice with a compromised blood–brain barrier and blood–placental barrier (Umbenhauer *et al.*, 1997). These effects were also observed with ivermectin administered to the mrd1a knockout mouse (Schinkel *et al.*, 1994; 1995). Furthermore, the incidence of cleft palate correlated with the maternal mortality in a CF-1 mouse study (Lankas *et al.*, 1997). The incidence of cleft palate was also linked to the polymorphism of mdr1a in the CF-1 mouse (Umbenhauer *et al.*, 1997).

Developmental toxicity studies have also been conducted with the 8,9-Z-isomer of abamectin in the CF-1 mouse to further evaluate the phenomenon of the linkage of developmental toxicity to the blood–placental barrier (Table 56.8). The NOEL for maternal and developmental toxicity was 0.1 mg/kg/day and 0.05 mg/kg/day, respectively. In young adult CF-1 mice, which were genotyped for their P-glycoprotein expression, the brain concentrations of the isomer 8 h after treatment were 60 times higher in (−/−) males and females than in the (+/+) male and female CF-1 mice. Brain concentrations of the delta-8,9-isomer of avermectin B1a in (−/−) CF-1 fetuses were higher than in (−/+) fetuses, which, in turn, were higher than in (+/+) fetuses. To study the development of P-glycoprotein in the placenta in the CF-1 mouse, normal homozygous (+/+) female

Table 56.7
Developmental Toxicity Studies with Ivermectin (FAO/WHO, 1994), Abamectin (EPA, 1999a), and Emamectin Benzoate (EPA, 1999b)

	Dose (mg/kg/day)					
	Ivermectin		Abamectin		Emamectin	
Study	LOEL	NOEL	LOEL	NOEL	LOEL	NOEL
Maternotoxicity						
CF-1 mouse[a,b]	0.2	0.1	0.075	0.05	—	—
Rabbit	6.0	3.0	2.0	1.0	6.0	3.0
SD rat	10.0	5.0	2.0	1.6	4.0	2.0
Fetotoxicity						
CF-1 mouse[a]	—	0.8[c]	0.4	0.2	—	—
Rabbit	3.0	1.5	2.0	1.0	—	6.0[c]
SD rat	—	10.0[c]	2.0	1.6	8.0[d]	4.0
Developmental						
CF-1 mouse[a]	0.4	0.2	0.4	0.2	—	—
Rabbit	3.0	1.5	2.0	1.0	—	6.0[c]
SD rat	10.0	5.0	2.0[d]	1.6	8.0[d]	4.0

[a]CF-1 animals tested were polymorphic for P-glycoprotein (Umbenhauer *et al.*, 1997).

[b]Not evaluated with emamectin benzoate.

[c]No adverse effects at the highest dose tested.

[d]No cleft palates seen at the highest dose tested.

Table 56.8
Genotyping Study of CF-1 Mice Treated with Δ8,9-isomer (Wise *et al.*, 1997)

	Control		5 mg/kg		
	+/− F; +/− M	+/− F; +/− M	+/− F; +/+ M	+/− F; +/+ M	+/− F; +/+ M
Number of fetuses examined	108	105	141	125	127
Number of fetuses with cleft palate	1	0	0	18	80
Number of litters examined	8	9	12	12	12
Number of litters with cleft palate	1	0	0	6	11
Pups with −/− genotype	19	50	NF[b]	NF	31
Pups with +/− genotype	15	NF	NF	41	29
Pups with +/+ genotype	32	NF	39	31	NF
−/− with cleft palate	0%	0%	NF	NF	97%
+/− with cleft palate	0%	NF	NF	39%	45%
+/+ with cleft palate	0%	NF	0%	0%	NF

[a] Genotype for P-glycoprotein: +, functional gene; −, defective gene.
[b] NF, genotype not found.

and homozygous (+/+) males were mated and the concentration of P-glycoprotein was measured in the placenta (Lankas *et al.*, 1989).

The human population is known to be homozygous positive for this gene. The human fetus is therefore protected *in utero* due to a good placental–blood barrier with proper expression of P-glycoprotein (MacFarland *et al.*, 1994; Nakamura *et al.*, 1997). Furthermore, this protein has been identified in the capillaries of the brain of the human fetus as early as the third trimester (28 weeks) (Van Kalken *et al.*, 1992). The level of expression at 28 weeks is already the same as that of an adult.

Ivermectin has been extensively used worldwide at the high doses administered to humans (in monitored clinical trials as well as in more general therapeutic applications) (FAO/WHO, 1991). If a subpopulation of humans without P-glycoprotein existed, it would have been readily identified. Because humans and other primates have not been shown to have subpopulations deficient in P-glycoprotein, the CF-1 mouse developmental toxicity data are not particularly relevant for use in human risk assessments to the avermectins (FAO/WHO, 1997).

The critical levels and effects for multigeneration reproduction studies with the avermectins are shown in Table 56.9. The LOEL (lowest observed effect level) and NOEL values for ivermectin and abamectin were quite similar; the LOEL and NOEL for emamectin benzoate were somewhat higher. Early postpartum rat pup mortality has been observed with all three avermectins (EPA, 1999a; 1999b; Lankas *et al.*, 1989).

Lankas *et al.* (1989) observed a significant increase in mortality between days 7 and 14 postpartum in treated dams nursing treated and control pups. In contrast, the mortality, growth, and development of treated and control pups nursing from con-

Table 56.9
Multigeneration Reproductive Toxicity Studies in SD Rats with the Avermectins (EPA, 1999a; 1999b; Lankas and Gordon, 1989)

	Ivermectin		Abamectin		Emamectin	
	LOEL	NOEL	LOEL	NOEL	LOEL	NOEL
Mg/kg/day	0.4	0.2	0.4	0.12	3.6	0.6
Effect	Neonatal mortality		Neonatal mortality		Clinical signs	

trol dams were similar. Because toxicity was only observed in control and treated pups cross-fostered to treated dams, it was concluded that neonatal toxicity of ivermectin in rats was a function of postnatal lactation exposure only and not due to *in utero* exposure. Further, these investigators administered purified, tritium-labeled avermectin B_{1a} (ivermectin B_{1a}) and sampled plasma and milk from dams treated orally with 2.5 mg/kg/day of radiolabeled ivermectin B_{1a} for 61 days. The pattern for pup mortality, milk concentration, pup liver, plasma, and brain concentration of ivermectin, and percentage of adult levels for P-glycoprotein in the pup brain barrier are presented in Table 56.10.

In contrast to rodents, the blood–brain barrier is formed prenatally in many species, including humans (Betz and Goldstein, 1981; Bohr and Mollgard, 1974; Jette *et al.*, 1995; Lankas *et al.*, 1989; Saunders, 1977; Van Kalken *et al.*, 1992). Furthermore, the blood–placental barrier is also intact in human infants at birth (MacFarland *et al.*, 1994; Nakamura *et al.*, 1997).

Rats also differ from humans by having an increased utilization of fats at the time of parturition (Amano, 1967; Chiu *et al.*,

Table 56.10
Pup Mortality, Milk and Pup Tissue Toxicokinetics, and Brain P-Glycoprotein Level Following a Daily Dose of 2.5 mg/kg/day of Tritiated Ivermectin for 61 Days (Lankas *et al.*, 1989)

Day dose (mg/kg)	Pup mortality	Maternal milk level (μg/g)	Pup plasma level (μg/g)	Pup liver level (μg/g)	Pup brain level (μg/g)	Rat pup brain p-gp level (%)[b]
Day 1	−0.22/day[a]	—	0.094	1.640	0.100	
Day 2						6.5
Day 4		2.324	0.276	3.918	0.251	
Day 5	19.3/day					5.7
Day 6		1.482	0.804	6.106	0.318	
Day 7						
Day 8	16.9/day					4.4
Day 10		1.052	0.893	6.648	0.264	
Day 11						6.9
Day 14						19
Day 15	0.86/day					
Day 17						37
Day 20						89

[a]Corrected for background by subtracting the pup mortality observed in the control group.
[b]Cukierski (1995); P-glycoprotein expressed as percent of adult level.

1986; Scow *et al.*, 1964). This results in a greater release of lipophilic compounds such as abamectin and ivermectin from body fat into milk. In addition, rat milk has a much higher fat content than human milk and this leads to an increased transfer of lipophilic xenobiotic compounds to the neonatal animal compared to what would be anticipated in nursing humans. Ogbuokiri *et al.* (1993) reported that after a single oral dose up to 12 mg ivermectin administered to lactating women who were not breastfeeding the peak concentration in plasma was seen at 4 h posttreatment. The peak concentration in milk occurred at the same time point, but was 2–3 times lower than what was seen in plasma. These findings contrast with those found in rats where the concentration of ivermectin observed in rat milk was about threefold higher than that in plasma. Based on the uniqueness of the time profile of P-glycoprotein development and milk concentration of lipophilic toxicants in rats, it can be safely concluded that these pup deaths cannot be extrapolated to humans.

56.5 HUMANS: EXPERIENCE WITH IVERMECTIN

Ivermectin has been used clinically for over a decade for the control of *Onchocerca volvulus* and other parasites in veterinary and human medicine (FAO/WHO, 1993). Onchoceriasis is endemic in large areas of Africa and Latin America. It is estimated that nearly 20 million people are infected and another 85 million are at risk. Large and diverse populations have been treated with ivermectin in Africa (Burnham, 1993; Chijioke and Okonkwo, 1992; Chippaux *et al.*, 1993; De Sole *et al.*, 1989a; 1989b; Doumbo *et al.*, 1992; Gardon *et al.*, 1997;

Ogunba and Gemade, 1992; Pacque *et al.*, 1990; 1991; Whitworth *et al.*, 1991), Polynesia (Cartel *et al.*, 1992), and Latin America (Collins *et al.*, 1992).

Typical human doses range from 0.1 to 0.2 mg/kg (FAO/WHO, 1993). The major effect noted following the administration of ivermectin is a severe inflammatory response, called the Mazzotti reaction. The Mazzotti reaction is secondary to the efficacy of ivermectin in killing the microfiliae, which dislodge from their site of infestation and are subsequently transported in the blood and body fluids (Ackerman *et al.*, 1990). This acute exacerbated immune response can be characterized by pruritis, erythema, edema, vesicle formation, papule formation, and scaling. Adenitis, fever, and hypotension may occur, and severe inflammatory changes may be noted in both the anterior and the posterior segments of the eye.

The World Health Organization reviewed reports on the response to treatment for over 26,000 patients administered ivermectin for parasite control (FAO/WHO, 1993). Single oral doses up to 0.2 mg/kg (bw) produced no major effects except for those resulting from the eradication of the parasite infestation (the Mazzotti reaction). The effects observed in over 200,000 patients treated with ivermectin are summarized in Table 56.11.

Although the primary effect noted following the administration of ivermectin was the Mazzotti reaction, there were two cases of serious neurological response in two patients out a population of 17,877 treated with ivermectin (Gardon *et al.*, 1997). Headache was a common side effect noted, but no association between headache and treatment was observed in a double-blind study on 7148 people conducted by Burnham (Burnham, 1993). During the first year of treatment, pain, edema, itch-

Table 56.11
Observations from Patients Treated with Ivermectin

Population treated	Incidence of	Dose (μg/kg)	Main effects observed	Reference
14,911	52 (0.35%)	130–200	37 (0.25%) cases of severe symptomatic postural hypotension 13 (0.09%) cases of severe fever 2 (0.01%) cases of dyspnea	De Sole *et al.* (1989a)
118,925	835 (0.7%)	150	230 (0.19%) cases of headache 210 (0.17%) cases of general pains 150 (0.12%) cases of pruritis 120 (0.10%) cases of edema 80 (0.06%) cases of fever 20 (0.02%) cases of dizziness 15 (0.01%) cases of vomiting 10 (0.01%) cases of diarrhea	Ogunba and Gemade (1992)
7,566	992 (13.1%)	150–200	Primarily Mazzotti reaction 460 cases of headache	Ogunba and Gemade (1992)
50,929	93 (1.83%)	150–200	49 cases of severe symptomatic postural hypotension 34 cases of severe fever 3 cases of severe dyspnea 3 cases of severe pain	Chijioke and Okonkwo (1992)
7,699	100 (1.3%)	150	Primarily Mazzotti reaction	De Sole *et al.* (1989b)

ing, and rash were found statistically associated with treatment. These reactions diminished in the second year and disappeared by the third year. Hence, in this large human study, patients treated with ivermectin did not exhibit any of the expected neurological side effects that would have occurred if the blood–brain barrier had been compromised.

The populations treated have included not only adults, but also children of all ages and, inadvertently, pregnant women. Epidemiological follow-up of more than 1000 pregnant women treated with ivermectin (primarily in the first trimester) did not yield any indication of an increase in the incidence of miscarriage, stillbirths, or congenital malformations (Burnham, 1993; Chippaux *et al.*, 1993; Pacque *et al.*, 1990). Based on this extensive human database, there should be little concern that neurotoxicity or birth defects might occur in humans exposed to the avermectins at doses less than 0.2 mg/kg.

56.6 RISK CHARACTERIZATION

Previous joint meetings in 1992 (FAO/WHO, 1992) and 1994 (FAO/WHO, 1994) had established the acceptable daily intake (ADI) for abamectin at 0.0002 mg/kg bw using the NOEL (pup toxicity) of 0.12 mg/kg/day derived from the multigeneration reproduction study conducted in Sprague–Dawley rats to which a 500-fold uncertainty factor was applied (Table 56.12). This 500× factor was based on the standard 10× for interspecies differences and 10× for interindividual differences plus an extra 5× due to concern over the teratogenicity of the abamectin's

delta-8,9-isomer in the CF-1 strain of mouse. In 1997, the World Health Organization's JMPR reexamined the basis for setting the ADI for abamectin and declared that the CF-1 mouse was not suitable for human risk assessment because of its heterozygous (+/−) or homozygous (−/−) genetics for P-glycoprotein (FAO/WHO, 1997; Lankas *et al.*, 1997; Umbenhauer *et al.*, 1997). This same rationale, that is, the absence of P-glycoprotein blood–brain barrier in rat pups, postnatally (Betz and Goldstein, 1981; Lankas *et al.*, 1989; Terao *et al.*, 1996), led the JMPR to readjusted the ADI for abamectin to 0.002 mg/day (bw) by reducing the uncertainty factor from 500- to 50-fold for the ADI from the rat multigeneration study.

The EPA also declared that the CF-1 mouse was unsuitable for human risk assessment but failed to consider the compromised unprotected postpartum period unique to rat pups and a 100-fold uncertainty factor was applied to the NOEL for the multigeneration reproduction study conducted with abamectin (EPA, 1999a). Temporary tolerances were also set for emamectin benzoate in 1999 (EPA, 1999b); unfortunately, the EPA appears to have not applied the same criteria with regard to the inappropriateness of the CF-1 mouse, polymorphic to P-glycoprotein, for human risk assessment. Not only was the NOEL for a 15-day neurotoxicity study in the CF-1 mouse used, but 300-fold uncertainty factor was also applied to the NOEL derived from this study in order to calculate the reference dose (RfD).

Under appropriate testing conditions, these avermectins are not developmental toxins or reproductive toxins; neither are the

Table 56.12
Chronic ADI/RfD Values Established for the Avermectins

Avermectin	Organization	Study/ incidence used	Uncertainty factor	ADI or RfD mg/kg/day
Ivermectin	JECFA (FAO/WHO, 1992)	Developmental toxicity (CF-1 mouse)	10—intraspecies 10—interspecies	0.001
Abamectin	JMPR (FAO/WHO, 1994)	Multigeneration reproduction (SD rat)	10—intraspecies 10—interspecies 5—teratogenic concerns	0.0002
	JMPR (FAO/WHO, 1997)	Multigeneration reproduction (SD rat)	10—intraspecies 5—interspecies	0.002
	EPA, 1999a	Multigeneration reproduction (SD rat)	10—intraspecies 10—interspecies	0.0012
Emamectin benzoate	EPA, 1999b	15-day neurotoxicity study (CF-1 mouse)	10—intraspecies 10—interspecies 3—short duration of study used	0.00025

genotoxic or carcinogenic. Further, the hazard profiles for the three avermectins evaluated are qualitatively and often quantitatively similar. Because of these facts, it would appear to be appropriate to use critical values from the avermectin used extensively clinically for the risk characterization of this class of chemical. Therefore, for acute risk characterization, a clinical dose of 0.2 mg/kg could be used as the NOEL (FAO/WHO, 1993). Conservatively, a $10\times$ interindividual uncertainty factor could be applied, as well as the $3\times$-uncertainty factor proposed by the EPA, that is, $30\times$, for an acute RfD of 0.0067 mg/kg.

Likewise, using the common mechanism approach for the avermectins, the chronic RfD based on the NOEL for the 1-year dog study (the most sensitive species in the chronic studies) would be suitable. The NOEL for the dog with ivermectin and abamectin (Lankas and Gordon, 1989) and emamectin benzoate (EPA, 1999b), that is, 0.5, 0.25, and 0.25 mg/kg/day, respectively, should be used instead of relying on the data from studies of shorter duration. The chronic RfD of emamectin, based on either study, would be 0.25 mg/kg/day divided by $100\times$ and $3\times$, or 0.00083 mg/kg/day, which is essentially the same as the JMPR ADI for abamectin (FAO/WHO, 1997).

56.7 CONCLUSIONS

The use of inappropriate animal models for characterizing human risk unfortunately is not well recognized. The hazard assessment of the avermectins provides a better understanding of just two instances in which our surrogate models for humans fail. First, CF-1 mice are more sensitive to the avermectins due to its heterozygous expression of P-glycoprotein. Second, the increased postnatal pup mortality in rats is due to a lack of expression of P-glycoprotein at birth and a high milk concentration of lipophilic toxicants unique to this species. The clinical use of ivermectin as well as special studies provides reassur-

ance that humans are homozygous positive (unimodal) for the P-glycoprotein gene. Further, humans express P-glycoprotein fully at birth. Therefore, as long as animal models continue to be used to characterize potential risks to the human population, it will be critical to appreciate the appropriateness or inappropriateness of the genetics that drive the biological responses in animal surrogates.

REFERENCES

Ackerman, S. J., Kephart, G. M., Francis, H., Awadzi, K., Gleich, G. J., and Ottesen, E. A. (1990). Eosinophil degranulation: An immunologic determinant in the pathogenesis of the Mazzotti reaction in human onchoceriasis. *J. Immunol.* **144**, 3961–3969.

Abalis, I. M., Eldefawi, A. T., and Eldefawi, M. E. (1986). Actions of avermectin B1a on the gamma-aminobutyric acid A receptor and chloride channels in rat brain. *J. Biochem. Toxicol.* **1**, 69–82.

Aigner, A., Wolf, S., and Gassen, H. G. (1997). Transport and detoxication: Principles, approaches, and perspectives for research on the blood–brain barrier. *Angew. Chem., Int. Ed. Engl.* **36**, 24–41.

Amano Y. (1967). Changes of the levels of blood glucose during pregnancy in the rat. *Jpn. J. Pharmacol.* **17**, 105–114.

Arena, J. P., Lui, K. K., Paress, P. S., Frazier, E. G., Cully, D. F., Mrozik, H., and Schaeffer, J. M. (1995). The mechanism of action of avermectins in *Caenorhabditis elegans*: Correlation between activation of glutamate-sensitive chloride current, membrane binding, and biological activity. *J. Parasitol.* **82**, 286–291.

Betz, L., and Goldstein, G. W. (1981). Developmental changes in metabolism and transport properties of capillaries isolated from rat brain. *J. Physiol.* **312**, 365–376.

Bloomquist, J. R. (1999). "Insecticides: Chemistries and Characteristics." Virginia Polytechnic Institute and State University, Blacksburg, VA. Available at http://ipmworld.umn.edu/chapters/bloomq.htm.

Bohr, V., and Mollgard, K. (1974). Tight junctions in human fetal choroid plexus visualized by freeze etching. *Brain Res.* **81**, 314–318.

Borst, P., Schinkel, A. H., Smit, J. J. M., Wagennar, E., van Deemter, L., Smith, A. J., Eijdems, E. W. H. M., Baas, F., and Zaman, G. J. R. (1993). Classical and novel forms of multidrug resistance and the physiological functions of P-glycoproteins in mammals. *Pharmacol. Ther.* **60**, 289–299.

Burg, R. W., Miller, B. M., Baker, E. E., Burnbaum, J., Currie, S. A., Hartman, R., Kong, Y.-L., Monaghan, R. L., Olson, G., Putter, I., Tunac, J. B., Wallick, H., Stapley, E. O., Oiwa, R., and Omura, S. (1979). Avermectins, new family of potent anthelmintic agents; producing organism and fermentation. *Antimicrob. Agents Chemother.* **15**, 361–367.

Burnham, G. M. (1993). Adverse reactions to invermectin treatment for onchocerciasis: Results of a placebo-controlled, double-blind trial in Malawi. *Trans. R. Soc. Trop. Med. Hyg.* **87**, 313–317.

Cartel, J. L., Nguyen, N. L., Moulia-Pelat, J. P., Plichart, R., Martin, P. M. V., and Spiegel, A. (1992). Mass chemoprophylaxis of lymphatic filariasis with a single dose of ivermectin in a Polynesian community with a high *Wuchereria bancrofti* infection rate. *Trans. R. Soc. Trop. Med. Hyg.* **86**, 537–540.

Chijioke, C. P., and Okonkwo, P. O. (1992). Adverse events following mass ivermectin therapy for onchocerciasis. *Trans. R. Soc. Trop. Med. Hyg.* **86**, 284–286.

Chippaux, J. P., Gardon-Wendel, N., Gardon, J., and Ernould, J. C. (1993). Absence of any adverse effects of inadvertent ivermectin treatment during pregnancy. *Trans. R. Soc. Trop. Med. Hyg.* **87**, 118.

Chiu, S. H., Sestokas, E., Taub, R., Buhs, R. P., Gleen, M., Sestokas, R., Vandenheuval, W. J., Arison, B. H., and Jacob, T. A. (1986). Metabolic disposition of ivermectin in tissues of cattle, sheep, and rats. *Drug Metab. Dispos.* **14**, 590–600.

Collins, R. C., Gonzales-Peralta, C., Castro, J., Zea-Flores, G., Cupp, M. S., Richards, F. O., Jr., and Cupp, E. W. (1992). Ivermectin: Reduction in prevalence and infection intensity of *Onchocerca volvulus* following biannual treatments in five Guatemalan communities. *Am. J. Trop. Med. Hyg.* **47**, 156–169.

Cukierski, M. A. (1995). "Exploratory study of P-glycoprotein development in Rat Fetuses and Pups." Unpublished report, Merck Project Number TT #94-739-0, Merck & Co., West Point, PA.

Descoteaux, S., Ayala, P., Orozco, E., and Samuelson, J. (1992). Primary sequences of two P-glycoprotein genes of *Entamoeba histolytica*. *Mol. Biochem. Parasitol.* **54**, 201–212.

De Sole, G., Awadzi, K., Remme, J., Dadzie, K. Y., Giese, J., Karam, M. F. M., and Opuku, N. O. (1989a). A community trial of ivermectin in the onchocerciasis focus of Asubende, Ghana. II. Adverse reactions. *Trop. Med. Parasitol.* **40**, 375–382.

De Sole, G., Remme, J., Awadzi, K., Accorsi, S., Alley, E. S., Ba, O., Dadzie, K. Y., Giese, J., Karam, M., and Keita, F. M. (1989b). Adverse reactions after large-scale treatment of onchocerciasis with ivermectin: Combined results from eight community trials. *Bull. World Health Org.* **67**, 707–719.

Didier, A., and Loor, F. (1996). The abamectin derivative ivermectin is a potent P-glycoprotein inhibitor. *Anti-Cancer Drugs* **7**, 745–751.

Doumbo, O., Soula, G., Kodio, B., and Perrenoud, M. (1992). Invermectine et Grossesses en Traitement de Masse au Mali. *Bull. Soc. Pathol. Exp.* **88**, 247–251.

Eldefawi, A. T., and Eldefawi, M. E. (1987). Receptors for g-aminobutyric acid and voltage-dependent chloride channels as targets for drugs and toxicants. *FASEB J.* **1**, 262–271.

Endicott, J. A., and Ling, V. (1989). The biochemistry of P-glycoprotein mediated multidrug resistance. *Annu. Rev. Biochem.* **58**, 137–171.

FAO/WHO (1991). "Pharmaceuticals: Ivermectin." Available at http://www.inchem.org/documents/pims/pharm/ivermect.htm.

FAO/WHO (1992). "Toxicological Evaluation of Certain Veterinary Drug Residues in Food." Report of the 36th meeting of the Joint FAO/WHO Expert Committee on Food Additives (JECFA), WHO Food Additive Series 27, pp. 10–18.

FAO/WHO (1993). "Toxicological Evaluation of Certain Veterinary Drug Residues in Food." Report of the 40th Meeting of the Joint FAO/WHO Expert Committee on Food Additives (JECFA), WHO Food Additive Series 31, pp. 23–36.

FAO/WHO (1994). Pesticide Residues in Food—1994. "Report of the Joint Meeting of the FAO Panel of Experts on Pesticide Residues in Food and the Environment and the WHO Expert Group on Pesticide Residues." FAO Plant Production and Protection Paper 127, pp. 15–17.

FAO/WHO (1997). Pesticide Residues in Food—1997. "Joint Meeting of the FAO Panel of Experts on Pesticide Residues in Food and the Environment and the WHO Expert Group on Pesticide Residues." September 22–October 1, 1997, pp. 22–34.

Fisher, G. A., and Sikic, B. I. (1995). Clinical studies with modulators of multidrug resistance. *Drug Resist. Clin. Oncol. Hematol.* **9**, 363–382.

Fisher, M. H., and Mrozik, H. (1989). Chemistry. *In* "Ivermectin and Abamectin" (W. C. Campbell, Ed.), pp. 1–23. Springer-Verlag. New York.

Gardon, J., Gardon-Wendel, N., Ngangue, D., Kamgno, J., Chippaux, J. P., and Boussinesq, M. (1997). Serious reactions after mass treatment of onchocerciasis with ivermectin in an area endemic for Loa loa infection. *Lancet* **350**, 18–22.

Gottesman, M. M., and Pastan, I. (1993). Biochemistry of multidrug resistance mediated by the multidrug transporter. *Annu. Rev. Biochem.* **62**, 385–427.

Greene, B. M. (1991). Expert report on the safety of ivermectin. *In* "Ivermectin—Report to JECFA," Vol. 1. Unpublished Report, MSD Research Laboratories, Lauterbach, Germany.

Greene, B. M., Brown, K. R., and Taylor, H. R. (1989). Use of ivermectin in humans. *In* "Ivermectin and Abamectin" (W. C. Campbell, Ed.), pp. 311–323. Springer-Verlag, New York.

Jette, L., Murphy, G. F., Leclerc, J. M., and Beliveau, R. (1995). Interaction of drugs with P-glycoprotein in brain capillaries. *Biochem. Pharmacol.* **50**, 1701–1709.

Juliano, R. L., and Ling, V. (1976). A surface glycoprotein modulating drug permeability in Chinese hamster ovary cell mutants. *Biochim. Biophys. Acta* **455**, 152–162.

Kurelec, B., and Pivcevic, B. (1991). Evidence for a multi-xenobiotic resistance mechanism in the mussel *Mytilus galloprovincialis*. *Aquat. Toxicol.* **19**, 291–302.

Lankas, G. R., and Gordon, L. R. (1989). Toxicology. *In* "Ivermectin and Abamectin" (W. C. Campbell, Ed.), pp. 89–112. Springer-Verlag, New York.

Lankas, G. R., Cartwright, M. E., and Umbenhauer, D. (1997). P-glycoprotein deficiency in a subpopulation of CF-1 mice enhances avermectin-induced neurotoxicity. *Toxicol. Appl. Pharmacol.* **143**, 357–365.

Lankas, G. R., Minsker, D. H., and Robertson, R. T. (1989). Effects of ivermectin on reproduction and neonatal toxicity in rats. *Food Chem. Toxicol.* **27**, 523–529.

Lanning, C. L., Fine, R. L., Corcoran, J. J., Ayad, H. A., Rose, R. L., and Abou-Donia, M. B. (1996). Tobacco budworm P-glycoprotein: Biochemical characterization and its involvement in pesticide resistance. *Biochim. Biophys. Acta* **1291**, 155–162.

Lincke, C. R. I., van Groenigen, M., and Borst, P. (1992). The P-glycoprotein gene family of *Caenorhabditis elegans*: Cloning and characterization of genomic and complementary DNA sequences. *J. Mol. Biol.* **228**, 701–711.

MacFarland, A., Abramovich, D. R., Ewen, S. W. B., and Pearson, C. K. (1994). Stage-specific distribution of P-glycoprotein in first-trimester and full-term human placenta *Histochem. J.* **26**, 417–423.

Mauad, T. H, van Nieuwkerk, C. M. J., Dingemans, K. P., Smit, J. J. M., van den Bergh Weerman, M. A., Verkruisen, R. P., Groen, A. K., Oude Elferink, R. P. J., van der Valk, M. A., Borst, P., and Offerhaus, G. J. A. (1994). Mice with homozygous disruption of the mdr2 P-glycoprotein gene: A novel animal model for studies of nonsuppurative inflammatory cholangitis and hepatocarcino-genesis. *Am. J. Pathol.* **145**, 1237–1245.

McGrath, J.P., and Varshavsky, A. (1989). The yeast STE6 gene encodes a homologue of the mammalian multidrug resistance P-glycoprotein. *Nature* **340**, 400–404.

Nakamura, Y., Ikeda, S.-I., Furukawa, T., Sumizawa, T., Tani, A., Akiyama, S.-I., Nagata, Y. (1997). Function of P-glycoprotein expressed in placenta and mole. *Biochem. Biophys. Res. Comun.* **235**, 849–853.

Ogbuokiri, J. E., Ozumba, B. C., and Okonkwo, P. O. (1993). Ivermectin levels in human breast milk. *Eur. J. Clin. Pharmacol.* **45**, 389–390.

Ogunba, R. O. and Gemade, F. I. I. (1992). Preliminary observations on the distribution of ivermectin in Nigeria for control of river blindness. *Ann. Trop. Med. Parasitol.* **86**, 649–655.

Pacque, M., Munoz, B., Greene, B. M., and Taylor, H. R. (1991). Community-based treatment of onchocerciasis with ivermectin: Safety, efficacy, and acceptability of yearly treatment. *J. Infect. Dis.* **163**, 381–385.

Pacque, M., Munoz, B., Poetschke, G., Foose, J., Greene, B. M., and Taylor, H. R. (1990). Pregnancy outcome after inadvertent ivermectin treatment during community-based distribution. *Lancet* **338**, 486–489.

Saunders, N. R. (1977). Ontogeny of the blood–brain barrier. *Exp. Eye Res. Suppl.* 523–550.

Schinkel, A. H., Smit, J. J. M., van Tellingen, O., Beijnen, J. H., Wagennar, E., van Deemter, L., Mol, C. A. A. M., van der Valk, M. A., Robanus-Maandag, E. C., te Riele, H. P. J., Berns, A. J. M., and Borst, P. (1994). Disruption of the mouse mdr1a P-glycoprotein gene leads to a deficiency in the blood–brain barrier and to increased sensitivity of drugs. *Cell* **77**, 491–502.

Schinkel, A. H., Wagennar, E., van Deemter, L., Mol, C. A. A. M., and Borst, P. (1995). Absence of the mdr1a P-glycoprotein in mice affects tissue distribution and pharmacokinetics of dexamethasone, digoxin and cyclosporin A. *J. Clin. Invest.* **96**, 1698–1705.

Scow, R. O., Chernick, S. S., and Brinley, M. S. (1964). Hyperliperdemia and ketosis in the pregnant rat. *Am. J. Physiol.* **206**, 796–804.

Terao, T., Hisanaga, E., Sai, Y., Tamai, I., and Tsuji, A. (1996). Active secretion of drugs from the small intestinal epithelium in rats by P-glycoprotein functioning as an absorption barrier. *J. Pharm. Pharmacol.* **48**, 1083–1089.

Thiebaut, F., Tsuruo, T., Hamada, H., Gottesman, M. M., Pastan, I., and Willingham, M. C. (1987). Cellular localization of the multidrug-resistance gene product P-glycoprotein in normal human tissues. *Proc. Natl. Acad. Sci. U.S.A.* **84**, 7735–7738.

Tiirikainen, M., and Krusius, T. (1991). Multidrug resistance. *Ann. Med.* **23**, 509–520.

Toomey, B. H., and Epel, D. (1995). A multi-xenobiotic transporter in *Urechis caupo* embryos: Protection from pesticides? *Marine Environ. Res.* **39**, 299–300.

Turner, M. J., and Schaeffer, J. M. (1989). Mode of action of ivermectin. *In* "Ivermectin and Abamectin" (W. C. Campbell. Ed.), pp. 73–87. Springer-Verlag, New York.

Ueda, K., Taguchi, Y., and Morishoma, M. (1997). How does P-glycoprotein recognize its substrate? *Cancer Biol.* **8**, 151–159.

Umbenhauer, D. R., Lankas, G. R., Pippert, T. R., Wise, D., Cartwright, M. E., Hall, S. J., and Beare, C. M. (1997). Identification of a P-glycoprotein-deficient subpopulation in the CF-1 mouse strain using a restriction fragment length polymorphism. *Toxicol. Appl. Pharmacol.* **146**, 88–94.

U.S. Environmental Protection Agency (EPA) (1999a). Avermectin; pesticide tolerance for emergency exemptions: Final rule. *Fed. Reg.* **64**, 16843–16850.

U.S. Environmental Protection Agency (EPA) (1999b). Emamectin benzoate; pesticide tolerance: Final rule. *Fed. Reg.* **64**, 27192–27200.

Van Kalken, C. K., Giaccone, G., van der Valk, P., Kuiper, C. M., Hadisaputro, M. M. N., Bosma, S. A. A., Scheper, R. J., Meijer, C. J. L. M., and Pineda, H. M. (1992). Multidrug resistance gene (P-glycoprotein) expression in the human fetus. *Am. J. Pathol.* **141**, 963–1072.

Whitworth, J. A. G., Morgan, D., Maude, G. H., Downham, M .D., and Taylor, D. W. (1991). A community trial of ivermectin for onchocerciasis in Sierra Leone: Adverse reactions after the first five treatments rounds. *Trans. R. Soc. Trop. Med. Hyg.* **85**, 501–505.

Williams, M., and Yarbrough, G. G. (1979). Enhancement of the *in vitro* binding and some of the pharmacological properties of diazepam by a novel antihelmintic agent, avermectin B_{1b}. *Eur. J. Pharmacol.* **56**, 1273–1276.

Wise, L. D., Lankas, G. R., Umbenhauer, D. R, Pippert, T. R, and Cartwright, M. E. (1997). CF-1 mouse sensitivity to abamectin-induced cleft palate correlates with fetal/placental P-glycoprotein genotype. *Teratology* **55**, 41.

Wu, C. T., Budding, M., Griffin, M. S., and Croop, J. M. (1991). Isolation and characterization of *Drosophila* multidrug resistance gene homologs. *Mol. Cell. Biol.* **11**, 3940–3948.

Inhibitors and Uncouplers of Mitochondrial Oxidative Phosphorylation

Robert M. Hollingworth
Michigan State University

57.1 INTRODUCTION TO OXIDATIVE PHOSPHORYLATION: FUNCTIONS AND DYSFUNCTIONS

57.1.1 GENERAL CONCEPTS

Oxidative phosphorylation (oxphos) is the primary process by which the energy derived from the catabolism of carbohydrates, fats, and proteins is used to synthesize ATP in virtually every cell of eukaryotic organisms. Since ATP is the universal source of chemical energy in the cell, any events that significantly disrupt its production or enhance its degradation will have widespread, multiple, and possibly severe physiological consequences. It is therefore not surprising that the complex, specialized machinery of oxphos is the target for a large variety of natural and synthetic toxicants, among which are a number of pesticides. Compounds that have a primary action on oxphos have a long history of use to control pests. Today, compounds that disrupt oxphos in the target species are widely used as fungicides and have important uses as insecticides and acaricides. They are of much lower significance as herbicides.

Naturally occurring oxphos poisons such as rotenone have been used by native peoples for centuries. Oxphos was also the target of some of the earliest synthetic organic pesticides such as 2,4-dinitro-o-cresol which was in use to control tussock moth caterpillars in the 1890s. In last two decades, a large number of newer pesticides have been discovered that affect oxphos and many are now on market with others in the later stages of development. One problem in covering these new materials is that there is little detailed, publicly available toxicological information available, partly because of their newness and partly because of their safer nature. Many of these newer compounds have very favorable toxicological characteristics and may never generate the intense toxicological scrutiny given to some of their predecessors. On the other hand, many older compounds

in this class with a more extensive toxicological literature have been, or are in the process of being, replaced because they present risks that, by current standards, are unacceptable (e.g., arsenicals, dinitrophenols, and some uses of organotins). In other cases (e.g., rotenone) they have become limited in use because of their low intrinsic activity compared to their modern counterparts. Many of these older compounds were covered in depth in the first edition of this handbook and, because of their declining importance, are given less attention here.

Finally, several older compounds affecting mitochondria that continue to be widely used are covered in other chapters of this edition [e.g., pentachlorophenol (Chapter 65), the bipiridyl herbicides such as paraquat (Chapter 70), and the fumigant phosphine and the metal phosphides that generate it (Chapter 86).

Pesticides (or their active metabolites) can be divided into several broad classes according to the potency and specificity with which they affect oxphos and related mitochondrial functions:

1. Compounds which are potent disrupters of oxphos *in vitro* and the consequences of oxphos disruption can plausibly explain many or all of their toxic effects. This chapter focuses primarily on these compounds.

2. Compounds which are of low potency in affecting mitochondria but which may achieve sufficient concentration *in vivo* at high doses to impact oxphos. There is a continuum between compounds in classes 1 and 2.

3. Compounds for which other specific targets are primary in causing toxicity (e.g., neurotoxic insecticides), but for which oxphos is a possible secondary target which could be involved in some types of adverse responses.

4. Compounds which are generally reactive and have multiple sites of action, one of which is likely to be oxphos. Many older fungicides, and most fumigants, are multisite inhibitors, with a relatively nonspecific mode of action. They probably impact oxphos and respiration as part of their primary actions but also have many other deleterious effects on cell functions. Examples include methyl isothiocyanate and its generators (dazomet and metam-sodium), thiophosgene generators (captan, captafol, folpet), electrophilic alkylating agents (chloropicrin, ethylene dibromide, and methyl bromide), the carbon disulfide generator, sodium tetrathiocarbonate, sulfhydryl reactive compounds (acrolein, chlorothalonil, dithianon, quintozene, and some dithiocarbamate fungicides such as maneb, mancozeb, zineb, ziram), fungicidal cationic surfactants which act as general membrane disruptants (dodine, guazatine, and iminoctadine), and metal salts and derivatives (e.g., copper-, arsenic-, and mercury-containing pesticides).

5. Compounds which have no direct effect on oxphos but which can affect oxphos indirectly through the consequences of their primary action. These compounds include lipid, nucleic acidic, or protein biosynthesis inhibitors, and extramitochondrial generators of reactive oxygen species which impact oxphos functions as well as other cellular events.

Generally much less is known about the specific role of mitochondria in the toxic action of the groups 2 through 5 than those in group 1. In particular, data obtained by incubating mitochondria with relatively high concentrations of pesticides *in vitro* may demonstrate effects on oxphos, but establishing that these have significance *in vivo* is much more difficult and often is not attempted. Nevertheless such actions may be toxicologically significant and this is considered briefly in Section 57.2.

The criterion for inclusion in this chapter is that a compound must be known to have its most important primary toxic effect on oxphos in vertebrates or, if this unclear, the compound has a primary effect on mitochondrial oxphos in target species with a probability of similar action in vertebrates. Most of the sites at which these newer pesticides act are highly conserved across all eukaryotes, and frequently it has been shown that there is little difference in the sensitivity of the target system in a fungus or insect compared to that in a vertebrate. It is not unreasonable therefore to assume initially that these and vital oxphos sites in nontarget species are likely to be important in generating at least some of their toxic effects in non-Karget species also.

The data regarding the general properties, uses, and toxicological profiles of individual compounds are drawn from a variety of sources. Many are cited individually as each compound is described. However, two sources contributed to many of the compound descriptions, *The Pesticide Manual* (Tomlin, 2000) and *The Farm Chemicals Handbook* (Meister, 2000), and these are acknowledged here as a general resource for these data.

57.1.2 THE MITOCHONDRION AND THE MACHINERY OF OXIDATIVE PHOSPHORYLATION

Mitochondria are organelles that occur in virtually every eukaryotic cell. Much of the earliest work in understanding mitochondrial functions focused on their central role in cel-

lular energetics and, particularly, the production of ATP by oxphos. This process is now quite well understood. The mitochondrion is bounded by two membranes. The outer one is relatively permeable and allows free exchange of small molecular weight solutes with the external cellular environment. The inner membrane is not readily permeable to ions, is highly specialized, and is unusual in that it contains large amounts of the phosopholipid, cardiolipin, but little cholesterol. The control of its permeability is the key to energy conservation during oxphos. The individual catalytic components responsible for oxphos are located in and span across the inner membrane. Also spanning the inner membrane are a number of proteins which act as translocators for ions and for the precursors and products of oxphos such as tricarboxylic acid cycle substrates, and inorganic phosphate, ADP and ATP. Within the inner membrane is a matrix which contains a number of enzymes responsible for feeding the products of intermediary metabolism of carbohydrates, fats, and proteins to oxphos such as the tricarboxylic acid cycle, fatty acid oxidation, and the enzymes of the urea cycle which is responsible for elimination of wastes from the cell. The mitochondrial DNA which codes for a number of subunits of components of the respiratory chain is also located in this matrix. In addition to oxphos the mitochondrion has a number of other significant cellular functions including an important role in Ca^{2+} regulation within the cell, thermoregulation in some situations, and as a regulator of apoptosis and cell death.

Despite these common roles, mitochondria vary widely in number, form, and activity between different tissues. These differences in functional significance and sensitivity to disruption play an important role in determining which tissues are likely to be injured by exposure to mitochondrial poisons.

Information on the structure, functions, and bioenergetics of mitochondria are presented in greater detail in several books (Ernster, 1992; Nicholls and Ferguson, 1992; Scheffler, 1999; Tyler, 1992).

57.1.3 OXIDATIVE PHOSPHORYLATION

Oxidative phosphorylation (Fig. 57.1) consists of two closely coupled processes; electron transport and the phosphorylation

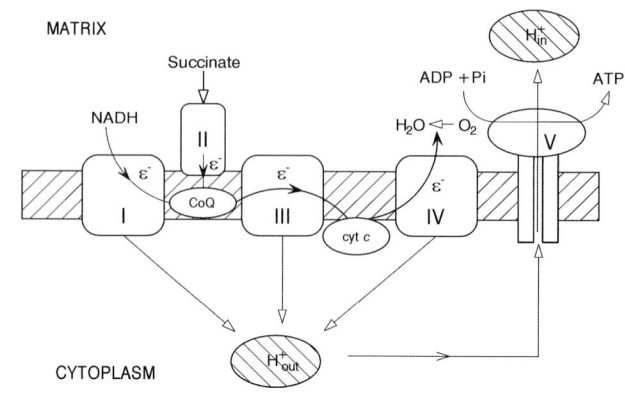

Figure 57.1 Schematic overview of mitochondrial oxidative phosphorylation.

of ADP. In electron transport, the oxidation of intermediates from carbohydrates, fats, and proteins creates NADH and reduced flavoproteins. These reduced carriers are reoxidized by the transfer of electrons down a chain of redox carriers culminating in the reduction of molecular oxygen and its incorporation into water. As the electrons pass from a higher energy state to a lower one, the free energy change at three points is sufficient to drive the pumping of protons outward across the inner mitochondrial membrane which is proton-impermeable. This creates an energy gradient across the membrane, termed the proton electrochemical gradient ($\Delta\tilde{\mu}_{H+}$) or, when expressed in electrical potential units, the proton-motive force (Δp). This consists of both an electrical component, the mitochondrial membrane potential ($\Delta\Psi_m$) due to the charge separation, and a chemical component (ΔpH) due to the unequal distribution of protons across the membrane. In mitochondria most of Δp (typically about 200–220 mV) can be attributed to $\Delta\Psi_m$ (typically about 150–180 mV) (Nicholls and Budd, 2000). The value of ΔpH is usually in the range of 0.5–1.0 pH units.

The passage of these protons back across the inner membrane discharges the electrochemical gradient and occurs primarily by passage through channels in the membrane-spanning mitochondrial ATP synthase. The passage of protons through this enzyme drives the phosphorylation of ADP to ATP. The proton gradient is also used to power other transport processes across the membrane such as ionic regulation and amino acid uptake.

The profound importance of oxphos can be judged, not only from the severe toxicological effects of compounds that disrupt it, but also from the fact that a normally active human synthesizes (and utilizes) approximately 40 kg of ATP daily. Under conditions of high muscular activity, this rate may increase by 10 to 20 fold. In addition to muscular tissues, the nervous system is also a heavy user of ATP. The human brain, which contributes 2% to the body weight, produces 20% of the ATP, mainly to power ion pumps. Since there are no appreciable other energy storage forms and ATP has a half life in cells of only a few seconds, continual resynthesis is crucial. An interruption of ATP biosynthesis of only a few minutes leads to permanent brain damage.

Oxphos is the major, but not the sole, source of ATP synthesis in the cell. Glycolysis provides less than 10% of the ATP under conditions of full oxidation of glucose. However, since glycolysis produces ATP much more rapidly than oxphos, it is the major short term source of energy for skeletal muscle contraction in vertebrates. This cannot continue long since it incurs an "oxygen debt" due to the large amounts of lactic acid produced by glycolysis under anaerobic conditions, which must be reoxidized later by lactate dehydrogenase in well oxygenated tissues. When mitochondria are compromised and cannot transfer electrons to oxygen, this reoxidation cannot occur, glycolysis will slow, and lactate will accumulate in the tissues. Under extreme circumstances this can cause lactic acidosis, a potentially life-threatening condition.

Finally it is worth noting that mitochondria tend to congregate in the cell around areas with a high rate of ATP utilization which is consumed very rapidly after synthesis. As shown by Aw and Jones (1985) there is a gradient of ATP away from the mitochondrion. In a condition in which ATP synthesis is partially compromised it is reasonable to assume that those functions furthest from the mitochondria will suffer the greatest deficit in ATP availability.

Knowledge of the structure and mechanism of the components of oxphos has shown remarkable advances in the last decade and has recently been reviewed by Saraste (1999) and Scheffler (1999).

57.1.3.1 Electron Transport

The mitochondrial electron transport chain is illustrated in Fig. 57.2. The primary source of electrons is NADH which donates them to the chain through mitochondrial complex I (NADH : ubiquinone oxidoreductase). In sequence these electrons pass to complex III (ubiquinol : cytochrome c oxidoreductase) and then to complex IV (cytochrome oxidase) in which molecular oxygen is reduced and protonated to form water. In this process ubiquinone (Q) and cytochrome c act as mobile electron carriers within the inner mitochondrial membrane or the intermembrane space. A second, and significant, route by which electrons feed into the chain is by enzymes such as succinate dehydrogenase which reduce FAD. This passes electrons into the chain through complex II (succinate : ubiquinone oxidoreductase). Glycerol-3-phospate dehydrogenase (involved in shuttling extramitochondrial NADH across the impermeable inner membrane) and β-hydroxybutyrate dehydrogenase (not shown in Fig. 57.2) are similar FAD-linked enzymes located in the inner membrane with significance in some mitochondria.

During the passage of electrons down this chain, protons are pumped outward across the inner membrane by complexes I, III, and IV. Thus substrates which yield NADH ultimately activate all three proton pumps whereas those that yield FADH only activate pumps in complexes III and IV, yielding proportionally less energy and ATP.

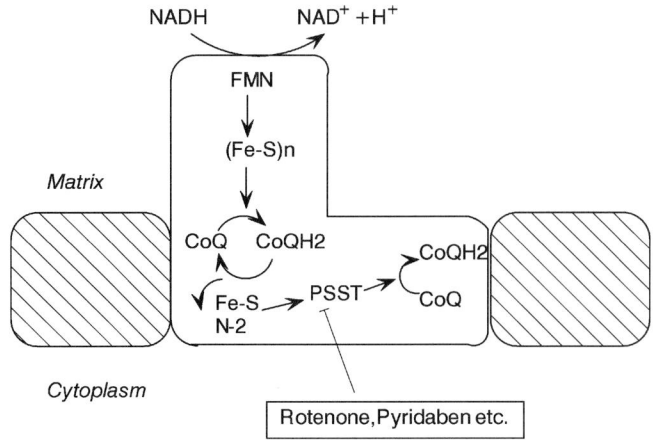

Figure 57.2 Major elements of mitochondrial complex I (NADH : ubiquinone oxidoreductase) and the site of action of inhibitors.

Complex I (NADH : Ubiquinone Oxidoreductase) This is the largest and least well understood of the four complexes forming the respiratory chain. In vertebrates it consist of at least 42 polypeptide subunits which are thought to be arranged in an L-shaped configuration (Fig. 57.2). The shorter arm of the "L" extends into the matrix and is the locus of the NADH binding site. The longer arm is integrated into the inner membrane and contains the ubiquinone binding site or sites. Current models propose the presence of two Q binding sites acting in a Q cycle analogous to that established for complex III and invoke a ubisemiquinone radical ion as an intermediate resulting from a one electron transfer to ubiquinone (e.g., see Degli Esposti and Ghelli, 1994). In between these binding sites is a series of electron acceptors and donors including a flavoprotein and several (perhaps seven) iron–sulfur centers whose exact relationship remains to be determined. Four protons are translocated across the membrane for the reduction of each ubiquinone molecule to ubiquinol. The iron–sulfur complex designated N2 is believed to be the final carrier that passes electrons to ubiquinone. This is the region at which most of the known potent inhibitors act, including rotenone and a series of newer acaricide–insecticides such as pyri daben.

Complex II (Succinate : Ubiquinone Oxidoreductase) In contrast to complex I, complex II is relatively simple consisting of only four subunits (Fig. 57.3). Although no high resolution structure for this complex is yet available, the structure of the closely related fumurate reductase of *E. coli* has recently been resolved at 3.3 angstroms (Iverson *et al.*, 1999). Despite its apparent simplicity, important features of the structure and mechanism of internal electron transfer of complex II remain to be established. Two of the four subunits extend into the matrix. One of these carries the catalytic site for the conversion of succinate to fumarate. The two electrons released in this oxidation are collected by an FAD cofactor and passed on through three iron–sulfur clusters in the second unit. Together, these two units

represent the enzyme succinate dehydrogenase. The other two subunits act as membrane anchors for the succinate dehydrogenase. They share a *b*-type cytochrome of unknown function. Two quinone binding sites are present, one near the inner face and the other near the outer face of the membrane in an arrangement reminiscent to that of complex III, although in the case of complex II no protons are pumped outward as occurs in the Q cycle of complex III. Complex II is the locus of action for a group of fungicides collectively termed carboxamides.

Complex III (Ubiquinol : Cytochrome *c* Oxidoreductase) Complex III (which is often termed cytochrome *c* reductase or the bc_1 complex) consists of 11 peptide subunits in vertebrates. The understanding of its structure has been remarkably advanced by high resolution x-ray crystallography (Iwata *et al.*, 1998; Xia *et al.*, 1997), including definition of the binding sites of the (E)-β-methoxyacrylate inhibitor, myxothiazol, and antimycin A (Iwata *et al.*, 1998). However, some details of electron flow through the complex and the proton pumping mechanism are still unknown. Much of the complex protrudes into the matrix. The electron transfer chain from ubiguinol involves, in sequence, an iron–sulfur complex (named after Rieske), cytochrome *b*, and cytochrome c_1, arranged as shown diagrammatically in Fig. 57.4. The reaction is completed by the transfer of an electron from cytochrome c_1 to the mobile carrier, cytochrome *c*. During these electron transfers, four protons are transferred from the matrix to the cytoplasmic side of the inner membrane. Two reaction centers for ubiquinone are present. One designated Q_i (or Q_N) is located toward the matrix (inner, negative) face of the inner membrane, while the other (Q_o or Q_P) is located near the cytoplasmic (outer, positive) face. Together they are postulated to operate in the "Q cycle" in which the electron pair received from ubiquinol is split, one being passed on to the Rieske iron–sulfur center and thence to cytochromes c_1. The other electron is passed back to ubiquinone via cytochrome *b* yielding ubiquinol. A point of toxicological significance is that during the operations of the Q cycle, ubisemiquinone radical ions (Q^-) are created as partial reaction products. By interactions with molecular oxygen, these can act as a source for reactive oxygen species (ROS) such as superoxide, hydroxyl radicals, hydrogen peroxide, and peroxynitrile radicals which may cause lipid peroxidation and other damaging cellular oxidations. Most inhibitors interact with either the Q_o site (e.g., myxothiazol) or the Q_i site (e.g., antimycin A). This complex is inhibited by a few insecticides, but, more significantly, it is the site of action of some very important new fungicides strobilurins that bind at the myxothiazol site.

Complex IV Cytochromes Oxidase The final complex in the respiratory chain is cytochrome *c* oxidase, otherwise know as cytochrome oxidase. During the action of complex IV, cytochrome *c* is reoxidized and the electrons from the respiratory chain are used to reduce molecular oxygen resulting in the formation of water. During this process two protons are pumped outward from the matrix for each atom of oxygen reduced. The complex structure of the 13 subunit bovine cytochrome

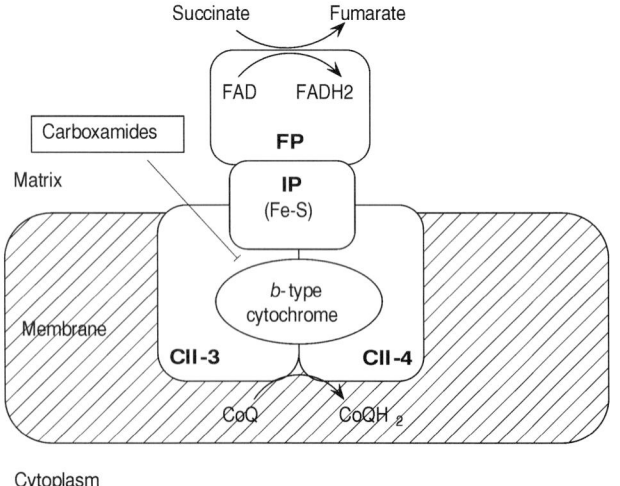

Figure 57.3 Major elements of mitochondrial complex II (succinate : ubiquinone oxidoreductase) and the site of action of inhibitors.

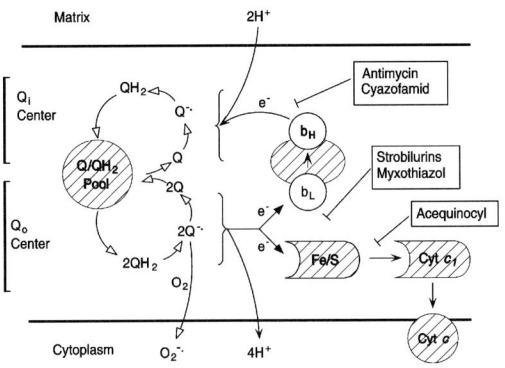

Figure 57.4 Major elements of mitochondrial complex III (ubiquinol : cytochrome c oxidoreductase) and the site of action of inhibitors.

oxidase has been determined with high resolution (Tsukihara *et al.*, 1996). It contains two hemes (cytochrome a and cytochrome a_3), two copper centers, and two centers in which magnesium and zinc respectively are coordinated and which are probably involved in stabilizing the complex rather than in its redox reactions. The terminal cytochrome a_3 operates in conjunction with one of the copper atoms to cleave molecular oxygen. A point of toxicological significance (Scheffler, 1999) is that during the reduction of oxygen by complex IV, reactive partially oxidized species such as the superoxide radical are formed. Leakage of such ROS from complex IV could contribute to oxidative stress in the cell, although leakage of electrons from higher potential sites earlier in the respiratory chain is perhaps a more general source of ROS. Much more detail might be given on the intricate operations of this oxidase, but since it is not known to be an important site of action for current pesticides, the reader is referred to Scheffler (1999) for additional discussion. Two exceptions to this generalization regarding lack of pesticidal significance are hydrogen cyanide, which is still used as a fumigant, and a second fumigant, phosphine (generated from such precursors as aluminum phosphide), which is also known to inhibit cytochrome oxidase.

Phosphine is discussed elsewhere in this work (Chapter 86) and complex IV is not considered further in this chapter.

57.1.4 THE SYNTHESIS OF ATP

57.1.4.1 Complex V (ATP Synthase)

The linked processes of discharge of the electrochemical gradient and the synthesis of ATP is carried out by complex V (ATP synthase). This remarkable structure (considerably simplified in Fig. 57.5) has been shown to be a molecular-sized motor consisting of three major components (Abrahams *et al.*, 1994; Boyer, 1997; Stock *et al.*, 1999; see Scheffler, 1999 and Saraste, 1999 for overviews). A rotor system consisting of 9–12 "c" subunits is embedded in the inner membrane. Although the mechanism of operation of the rotor system is still debated, it is likely that protons pass through the rotor and at the same time cause it to spin at rates up to 100 or more revolutions per second. This membrane-located portion of the complex is the F_0 component of the ATP synthase. Attached to the rotor is an axle (γ subunit) which is eccentric or bent and which contacts the third component, a head consisting of six subunits (alternating α and β) which is attached to the inner side of the membrane (not shown in diagram). As the rotor spins and turns the axle, the axle alternately squeezes and relaxes the β units causing a configurational change that drives the combination of ADP and inorganic phosphate to synthesize ATP. As the β unit relaxes, its binding site opens to accept ADP and Pi. As the unit is squeezed by the rotating axle, ATP is expelled. Thus three ATP molecules are synthesized for each full rotation of the axle. The head portion of the complex is the F_1 component of the synthase. At least three, but perhaps four, protons are needed to drive the synthesis of one ATP molecule, paralleling the stoichiometry of three to four "c" subunits for each ATP catalytic site.

Since the ATP synthase machinery (as with the electron transport chain) is reversible, it can hydrolyze ATP back to ADP under appropriate circumstances, at the same time pumping protons back out of the matrix. When operating in this mode it is often referred to as the mitochondrial Mg-dependent ATPase or F_1F_0-ATPase. The isolated F_1 portion of the complex can also act as an ATPase but without the capability to translocate protons.

Several groups of chemicals inhibit this machinery, primarily by interference with the rotary mechanism (F_0 component). These include antibiotics such as oligomycin, carbodiimides or carbodiimide generators such as the pesticide diafenthiuron, and the organotin biocides.

The existence of this proton circuit comprising the pumping of protons out of the matrix by the respiratory chain and their reentry through the ATP synthase means that in healthy mitochondria with an intact inner membrane there is a close coupling between the consumption of ATP and the rate of respiration. As ATP is consumed, ADP builds up, the rate of ATP synthase rises, protons reenter the matrix, the value of the electrochemical gradient tends to decline, and electron flow through

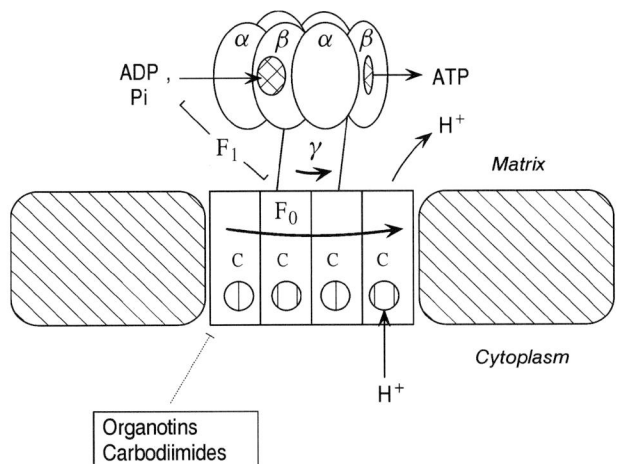

Figure 57.5 Major elements of mitochondrial complex V (ATP synthase) and the site of action of inhibitors.

the respiratory chain increases to maintain it. Substrate oxidation and ADP phosphorylation are therefore coupled together and respond rapidly and efficiently to the varying energy demands of the cell.

57.1.5 SIGNIFICANCE OF QUINONE BINDING SITES FOR PESTICIDE ACTION

It is notable that most of the pesticides that inhibit mitochondrial electron transport do so by binding in or around the ubiquinone binding sites of complexes I, II, or III. Complex IV, which contains no quinone binding site, is inhibited only by compounds which complex the metal redox centers such as cyanide or azide. The nature of these quinone binding sites and their roles as targets for pesticides and other inhibitors have been reviewed by Rich (1996), Rich and Fisher (1999), and Berry *et al.* (1999). The abounding variety of natural and synthetic inhibitors that act on these site in complexes I and III indicates that structural requirements for inhibitors are not highly restrictive. As pointed out by Degli Esposti (1998) and Miyoshi (1998), the main requirements for many inhibitors of complex I are a cyclic head attached to a lipophilic chain that approximates the structure of ubiquinone.

57.1.6 MECHANISMS BY WHICH CHEMICALS DISRUPT OXPHOS

Pesticides may act in several different ways to disrupt oxphos and hence cause damage to cells and tissues. First, they may inhibit the operations of the electron transport chain and the pumping of protons across the inner membrane so that the electrochemical potential gradient is not maintained. Second, they may prevent this gradient from being coupled to the synthesis of ATP. This uncoupling action generally occurs through by a compound's ability to increase the permeability of the inner membrane to protons, or other ions, and to discharge the energy stored in the gradient wastefully. This mechanism is shown in its simplest form in Fig. 57.6, where a lipophilic weak acid shuttles protons across the membrane from the outer side to the inner side, driven only by the simple physicochemical processes of association at the lower pH on the outer side of the membrane, dissociation at the more alkaline inner face, and diffusion along its chemical and electrical potential gradients. The net result is for such a compound to act as a shuttle which continually and rapidly transports protons back across the membrane and thereby discharges the electrochemical gradient formed by the activity of the electron transport chain.

The third mechanism for interference with oxphos is to block the machinery of the ATP synthase and bring it to a halt. A fourth mechanism by which pesticides may interfere with mitochondrial functions and lead to tissue injury is by diverting electrons from the electron transport chain which wastes energy unproductively and can create ROS such as superoxide anion radicals and hydroxyl radicals leading to oxidative damage to the mitochondrion and other cellular constituents in the process

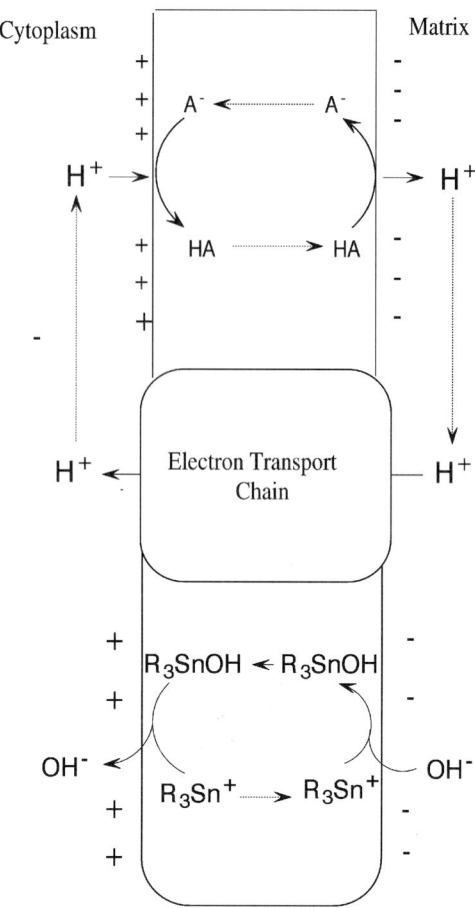

Figure 57.6 Basic mechanism of action of protonophoric uncouplers (HA) and suggested mechanism of uncoupling by triorganotin pesticides (R_3SnOH).

often termed "oxidative stress" (e.g., see Kowaltkowski and Vercesi, 1999). Oxphos can also be impacted by compounds that inhibit the transport mechanisms that convey ATP precursors (ADP and inorganic phosphate) into the matrix and ATP itself out into the cytoplasm. Finally, arsenical compounds that yield arsenate ions *in vivo* have a special mechanism termed arsenolysis that prevents ATP biosynthesis.

The first three of these mechanisms by which pesticides disrupt oxidative phosphorylation have somewhat different effects on cellular energetics and integrity depending on the degree to which the ATPase activity of complex V is stimulated, and whether the mitochondrial membrane potential ($\Delta\Psi_m$) can be preserved. These ideas are well reviewed by Nicholls and Budd (2000) and Wallace and Starkov (2000).

57.1.6.1 Uncoupling of Oxphos

Uncouplers, generally acting as protonophores, discharge the electrochemical gradient which prevents further synthesis of ATP and the operation of other processes linked to this energy gradient such as ion pumping and the production of ROS. In addition the loss of the gradient also causes complex V (ATP synthase) to run in reverse as an ATPase which rapidly eliminates residual ATP from the cell. Even though glycolysis may continue to provide some ATP in the uncoupled cell, this too is subject to the rapid ATPase activity. In almost all cells this represents an energy catastrophe and the consequences are rapid and drastic.

57.1.6.2 Inhibition of Electron Transport

Whether acting at complexes I, II, III, or IV, electron transport inhibitors have essentially the same effect in that electron flow through the chain is prevented. Inhibition of the respiratory chain reduces or eliminates its ability to pump protons and to maintain $\Delta \tilde{\mu}_{H+}$, ATP synthesis, and related reactions. Although both complexes I and II can independently reduce ubiquinone, the inhibition of either complex alone eventually blocks the respiratory chain through feedback effects on the citric acid cycle which provides NADH for complex I and succinate for complex II. As $\Delta \tilde{\mu}_{H+}$ falls, the action of complex V tends to reverse which destroys extramitochondrial ATP, but in so doing pumps protons back out from the matrix side and so tends to maintain the $\Delta \tilde{\mu}_{H+}$ value close to that of uninhibited mitochondria. However, in contrast to uncouplers, the permeability of the inner membrane to protons is not increased, so that the protons now being pumped from the matrix cannot readily return and ATP is eliminated from the cell more slowly than is the case with uncouplers. Glycolysis may then, at least in the short term, be able to maintain a level of ATP in the cell that prevents catastrophic consequences depending on the relative kinetics of ATP synthesis and destruction. In the longer term, ATP synthesis may be unsustainable and again drastic effects on cellular integrity result. Since there is reserve capacity in some elements of the respiratory chain, a fairly high percentage inhibition of activity may be necessary before electron transport is limited [e.g., in brain mitochondria, complex I activity can be inhibited by 70 to 75% before it becomes the limiting factor in electron transport through the chain of respiratory carriers (Davey and Clark, 1996), and in human osteosarcoma-derived cells, it can be inhibited by 35–40% before respiration declines (Barrientos and Moraes, 1999)].

57.1.6.3 Inhibition of ATP Synthase

In addition to preventing the synthesis of ATP from the electrochemical gradient, inhibitors of ATP synthase also block the ATPase activity of this complex. This allows glycolysis to continue to provide ATP to the cell. Since electron transport is not eliminated and $\Delta \tilde{\mu}_{H+}$ is not discharged (it may in fact be somewhat increased), the mitochondrial membrane potential is maintained so that other processes driven by this potential such as ion transport across the inner membrane and the generation of ROS continue unabated. The length of time for which the cell can maintain its integrity under these circumstances will depend on the balance between its capability to produce ATP by glycolysis and its rate of ATP consumption. Different cell types vary considerably in this regard (Nicholls and Budd, 2000), but even those with a vigorous glycolytic capability are likely to fail eventually in the face of continued ATP synthase inhibition.

57.1.6.4 Redox Cycling and Generation of ROS

An additional group of compounds that can severely impact oxphos and mitochondrial integrity are those which have redox potentials within the span of that of the electron transport chain. In the simplest mode this allows them to accept electrons from carriers in the chain (e.g., complex I or complex III), thus diverting electron flow from the useful conservation of energy. Such alternative acceptors are likely to be particularly dangerous if they can be reoxidized efficiently, for example, by reaction with oxygen or tissue thiols, or by returning the electrons to the electron transport chain at a point of lower redox potential (e.g., complex IV). In either case this establishes a futile redox cycle in which the compound continually diverts electrons from the chain and bypasses some or all of the energy conservation sites (Fig. 57.7; compound). In the case of those compound that are reoxidized by oxygen or tissue thiols, the additional production of reactive free radicals, particularly the superoxide anion radical and other ROS, presents a second threat to the integrity and efficiency of oxphos and general cellular integrity (compounds B and C). Depending on the kinetics of their reduction and reoxidation, they may greatly increase oxygen consumption and discharge the electrochemical gradient and generate heat. This resembles the effects of uncouplers, since the respiratory chain continues to accept electrons from NADH, but this is not coupled to the generation of ATP.

Few pesticides are known to be capable of this type of mitochondrial toxicity, but paraquat and related herbicides (see Chapter 70) are highly efficient electron acceptors which generate large amounts of ROS as a primary mechanism of action. Naphthoquinones and nitrosamines which can be formed as pesticide metabolites are also known to be capable of redox cycling. The acaricide acequinocyl (Section 57.5.2.2) is a naphthoquinone derivative, but it is has not been reported to be involved in redox cycling reactions with mitochondria. Several other pesticides (e.g., anthraquinone, dithianon, and quinoclamine) are naphthoquinones and might be involved in such cycling. If it were to occur, this would severely impact oxidative phosphorylation and mitochondrial functions in a

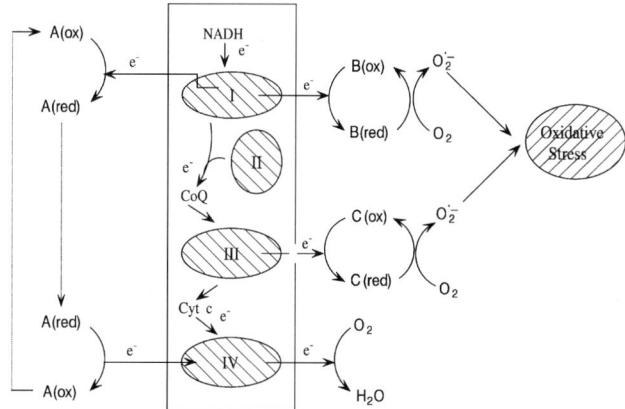

Figure 57.7 Diagrammatic representation of redox cycling and the generation of reactive oxygen species by the electron transport chain.

manner similar to that shown with menadione (Henry et al., 1995) and adriamycin. This type of action is reviewed in greater detail by Wallace and Starkov (2000).

57.1.6.5 Inhibition of ADP/ATP Exchange

In support of oxphos, the adenine nucleotide transporter (ANT), that conveys ADP into the matrix and ATP outward from it across the impermeable inner membrane, is critical to maintain the synthesis and supply of ATP to the cell. Inhibitors of this transport system are known and have toxic effects. Bongkrekic acid and atractylosides block the ANT, acting specifically at the ATP and ADP binding sites, respectively (Fiore et al., 1998). Recently, a new fungicide, MON 65500 (N-allyl-4,5-dimethyl-2-(trimethylsilyl)thiophene-3-carboxamide) with the proposed common name of silthiofam (Beale et al., 1998), has been shown to block the ATP transporter in fungal mitochondria as its primary fungicidal action (Joseph-Horne et al., 2000). It is unclear whether it has the same capability in vertebrate mitochondria, but since this compound shows very low toxicity to many other fungi and to vertebrates (the acute oral LD_{50} for the rat is >5000 mg/kg), it maybe relatively selective for the ANT of the target species.

57.1.6.6 Arsenolysis

Arsenates (lead or calcium) and arsenites were once widely used as pesticides. Their acute toxicity, concerns regarding their carcinogenicity and environmental accumulation, and lack of high efficacy have led to their general demise in this use. Their mechanisms of toxicity are multiple, but one effect, specific to the arsenate ion, involves effects on oxphos. In this case arsenate is able to replace phosphate during conversion of ADP to ATP. The resulting ADP–arsenate ester is unstable and rapidly hydrolyzes to ADP and arsenate (Moore et al., 1983). Thus, although the mitochondrial electrochemical gradient is discharged and ADP is consumed, no energy conservation occurs. Although loosely referred to as uncoupling, since the consequences parallel those of uncoupling in increasing respiration and the wastage of energy as heat, this is not really accurate. Respiration and phosphorylation remain coupled and effectively transfer energy from substrates to an esterified ADP product. The biochemical perturbation arises from the instability of this product. The stimulation of mitochondrial respiration by arsenate is also distinguishable from that caused by uncouplers since it is blocked by the ATP synthase inhibitor oligomycin (Welle and Slater, 1967).

57.1.7 TOXICOLOGIC CONSEQUENCES OF DISRUPTING OXIDATIVE PHOSPHORYLATION

57.1.7.1 General Effects

The mitochondrion is an extremely intricate machine. The disruption of oxphos leads to a web of complex interrelated consequences. A few examples of these interlocking processes, which often involve positive and negative feedback circuits, include the fact that the membrane potential is responsible for driving ATP synthesis but also is directly involved in regulating ion accumulation such a Ca^{2+}, in driving the reduction of NADPH by NADH, and in generating ROS through components of the electron transport chain. These ROS, unless effectively neutralized, are capable of destroying critical components of the electron transport chain (e.g., see Zhang et al., 1990). The presence of increased levels of ROS also leads to damage to the mitochondrial inner membrane which, in turn, impacts both calcium regulation and the ability of the mitochondrion to maintain the electrochemical gradient across it. At another level, the NADPH produced by mitachondrial is essential for the reduction of glutathione as an important antagonist of ROS-induced cellular injury. Calcium dysregulation also leads to the increased generation of ROS and finally may trigger events which lead to apoptosis. The many interactions between these events can be hard to fully comprehend but they are reviewed by Jabs (1999) and Nicholls and Budd (2000).

Beyond the direct impact on the mitochondrion itself, the failure of ATP biosynthesis leads to many problems for the cell. Fatty acid, nucleic acid, protein, and sterol biosynthesis all require large amounts ATP and are likely to fail rapidly in an energy-compromised cell. Thus, a severe reduction in the availability of energy to the cell can lead to a variety of effects these range from a blockage in cell division, to impaired maintenance of the cellular cytoskeleton and intracellular transport due to effects on ATP-dependent tubulin polymerization, to dysfunction in ionic regulation through effects on ion pumps that are ATP-dependent, and beyond.

However, a reduction in ATP-dependent cellular functions is not the only deleterious effect of a compromised oxphos. As noted, the electron transport chain has the capability of producing large amounts of ROS, particularly free radicals [see Nicholls and Budd (2000) for an excellent review]. Even when operating in a healthy cell, up to 2% of the oxygen consumed by the respiratory chain is converted to superoxide radicals and thence to other ROS through the "leakage" from the electron transport chain (Boveris, 1984; Kowaltkowski and Vercesi, 1999). The superoxide is produced when electrons are transferred from intermediate sites such as flavoproteins, Fe–S complexes, or ubiquisemiquinone radicals directly to oxygen rather than passed down the usual carriers to cytochrome oxidase. This electron leakage may arise in several locations including a site upstream of the rotenone inhibition site in complex I (Cadenas et al., 1977; Hensley et al., 1998; Herrero and Barja, 1997). A variety of studies have shown that the partial inhibition of complex I increases the level of ROS, free radical production, and subsequent lipid peroxidation in submitochondrial particles (Hasegawa et al., 1990; Takeshige and Minakami, 1979; Turrens and Boveris, 1980), isolated mitochondria (Hensley et al., 1998; Pitkanen and Robinson, 1996), and cells in culture (Barrientos and Moraes, 1999). The critical role of ROS in the lethal action of rotenone, a strong complex I inhibitor, in cultured cells was demonstrated by Seaton et al. (1997) who showed that a variety of antioxidants and free radical scavengers antagonized the ability of rotenone to induce apoptosis in rat PC12 cells. This enhanced oxidative stress induced by partial inhibition of complex I, rather than ATP depletion, has been cited as the critical event in rotenone's ability to cause apoptosis (Seaton et al., 1998), and in support of the hypothesis that a deficiency in complex I activity (either genetic or chemically induced) is a cause of the oxidative cell death in the dopaminergic tracts of the substantia nigra that underlies Parkinson's disease. Barrientos and Moraes (1999) provide a particularly illuminating and complete analysis and comparison of the two potential causes of cell death caused by partial inhibition of complex I. Using rotenone and other tools, they assessed the relationship between complex I inhibition, respiration, ROS production, lipid peroxidation, the membrane potential, and the occurrence of apoptosis. Their conclusion is that the key event in causing apoptosis is an increased production of ROS rather than a decrease in ATP levels in the cells.

Complex III also generates large amounts of ROS under appropriate circumstances. The site of electron transfer here is probably at the Q_o site (Fig. 57.4) where the highly reactive ubisemiquinone radical can transfer an electron to molecular oxygen, creating a superoxide anion. Different types of complex III inhibitors have different effects on this ROS generation. Antimycin-A type inhibitors increase superoxide production by blocking the normal pathway for electron transfer from Q_o to Q_i. On the other hand, myxathiazol (and by extension other structurally related commercial fungicides based on strobilurin) decrease ROS production by preventing the formation of the ubisemiquinone radical.

The complex and often contradictory results regarding the generation of ROS by mitochondria and the effects of inhibitors, including pesticides such as rotenone and the carboxamide fungicide, carboxin, on this process are reviewed by McLennan and Degli Esposti (2000). Under different experimental conditions such inhibitors may either increase or decrease the production of ROS. On the other hand, mitochondrial uncouplers, which reduce the mitochondrial membrane potential that drives ROS production, generally decrease the rate of ROS production by mitochondria.

An effective complex of antioxidative defenses is needed to prevent significant injury to the cell. When these defenses, such as superoxide dismutase, peroxidases, and tissue thiols, such as GSH, are inactivated or depleted, the general phenomenon of oxidative stress can occur which is characterized by lipid oxidation, membrane destruction, and DNA and protein oxidations (Kowaltkowski and Vercesi, 1999).

57.1.7.2 Apoptosis and Necrosis

A wave of recent interest in the machinery of a poptosis (programmed cell death) has done much to shed light on the complex web of events which follows interference with oxidative phoshorylation, and at the same time has highlighted the central role of the mitochondrion in controlling apoptosis as well as in cellular energetics. Apoptosis may be regarded as the orderly destruction and resorption of cells (whether during organ development or due to cellular injury) which occur constantly in

the body and is characterized by blebbing of the plasma membrane, shrinkage of the cell, condensation of the chromatin and digestion of the DNA in a "ladderlike" fashion, cell shrinkage, controlled digestion of the plasma membrane to form small apoptotic bodies, and resorption of these by neighboring cells without an inflammatory response. This stands in contrast to cellular necrosis (accidental cell death) in which more drastic damage to cellular functions and bioenergetics leads to a catastrophic collapse of all cellular functions, swelling of mitochondria and the cell in general, and rupture of the cell membrane with release of its contents and the concomitant possibility of an inflammatory response. In fact these two processes probably lie at the extreme ends of a continuum of modes of cell death. While necrosis is always a pathological event, apoptosis has important physiological functions such as the shaping of tissues and organs and the removal of injured cells. Inhibition of apoptosis can lead to anatomical malformations, autoimmune disease, and cancer. On the other hand excessive apoptosis removes healthy, vital cells and may be involved in degenerative diseases such as Parkinsonism (Kroemer et al., 1998) and immunotoxicity.

One critical determinant of whether apoptosis or necrosis occurs in an injured cell is the status of cellular energetics as defined by levels of ATP. Key events in apoptosis depend on the availability of a minimal level of ATP. If the ATP level drops too far, apoptosis cannot occur and necrosis is the likely result. Thus compounds that cause apoptosis are often found to cause necrosis when present at higher concentrations. Clearly, compounds which affect ATP levels may lead to either type of cell death and resulting organ injury. A detailed discussion of the biochemistry of apoptosis and the possible role of mitochondria and oxphos lies beyond the scope of this chapter and can be obtained from recent reviews (Brown et al., 1999; Hengartner, 2000; Jabs, 1999; Kroemer et al., 1998; Robertson and Orrenius, 2000). However, an outline of what is known is provided here to help to illuminate the critical role of mitochondria and oxidative phosphorylation in this process.

Apoptosis may be initiated by humoral factors acting on cellular receptors or by actions within the mitochondrion. In the latter case, the key event is thought to be the opening of a very large pore, the permeability transition pore, spanning both the outer and inner mitochondrial membranes, in a process termed the mitochondrial permeability transition. This immediately causes drastic changes in mitochondrial function including discharge of the potential across the inner membrane, which drives ATP biosynthesis and ionic regulation, and the loss of the soluble cytochrome c and other apoptogenic factors from the mitochondrion. The appearance of cytochrome c in the cytoplasm activates a series of cysteine proteases (caspases) which in turn activate endonucleases that begin to digest the nuclear material. The mitochondrial permeability transition can be trigged by internal calcium dysregulation. This may result from a series of causes (often interlinked) such as loss of the ATP necessary for intracellular calcium regulation, the generation of reactive oxygen species in amounts that damage mitochondrial membranes, and changes in the status of antioxidative mechanisms (e.g., cellular sulfhydryl groups) which protect against the mitochondrion's constant production of free radicals.

The mitochondrial permeability transition is thought to be created by the interaction of at least three proteins which have other functions in mitochondrial activity (Crompton *et al.*, 1999): the ANT, the voltage-dependent anion channel (also termed porin) which is a large voltage-dependent pore in the outer mitochondrial membrane that upon opening allows solutes up to 5000 Daltons to enter the mitochondrion, and cyclophilin D, a soluble protein in the matrix which may be involved in protein folding through catalysis of *cis-trans* isomerization of prolyl peptide bonds. The manner in which these come together to form the transition pore and the possible presence of other components remain to be established. Inhibitors of the normal functions of these components (e.g., bongkrekic acid for ANT or cyclosporin A for cyclophilin D) antagonize apoptosis.

The pesticides described in this chapter may be involved in the apoptotic process in several ways [e.g., rotenone may exert an anticancer action at high doses by encouraging apoptosis of tumor-initiated cells through its effects on the bioenergetics of the cell (Section 57.3.2.1)]. Organotins cause the apoptosis of thymus cells and consequent loss of cellular immunity, probably by directly triggering the mitochondrial permeability transition (Section 57.6.2.1). More speculatively, diafenthiuron reacts with and changes the characteristics of porin in some species, although it not clear whether this action has any implications for apoptosis (Section 57.6.2.2). Obviously, there is much more to learn about the relationship between oxphos disruption by pesticides and both the mechanisms and toxicological significance of cellular apoptosis and necrosis.

57.2 OXIDATIVE PHOSPHORYLATION AS A TARGET FOR PESTICIDE ACTION AND ITS RELEVANCE FOR TOXICITY

57.2.1 GENERAL CONSIDERATIONS

Somewhere in the range of 40 to 50 pesticide active ingredients, acting either as respiratory inhibitors or uncouplers, have effects on mitochondrial oxphos *in vitro* at nanomolar to micromolar concentrations. Taken in conjunction with signs of poisoning and other evidence, it seems reasonable to suppose that their acute toxicity and many, though perhaps not all, of their chronic toxic effects arise by these disruption of mitochondrial energetics. These compounds are the main focus of this chapter and are discussed in detail in Sections 57.3 through 57.7. However, they represent only a part of the total spectrum of the interactions of pesticides with oxphos. It is probable that other pesticides interact with oxphos in vertebrates with some specificity but with relatively low potency, and that others interact with multiple cellular targets, among which is oxphos, but they are not specific to this site in their biochemical mechanisms of cellular disruption. Examples of the latter

group are sulfhydryl reactive compounds and general membrane disruptants. Although mitochondria may be involved in their toxicity, other sites may be equally or more important and it is often difficult to determine which are the primary and critical biochemical injuries and which are secondary or noncritical. In the former group (specific for oxphos, but weakly active) are a number of compounds, particularly fungicides and herbicides, which tend to have their pesticidal actions on physiological systems that are not present in animals including photosynthesis, essential amino acid biosynthesis, and cell wall biosynthesis. These often have very low acute toxicities to vertebrates. At oral doses of 1000–5000 mg/kg, and assuming reasonably efficient uptake, internal concentrations in the cells of nontarget species might reach 1 mM or higher. Many pesticides can be shown to perturb mitochondrial functions at such concentrations *in vitro*. However, only rarely has research been conducted to investigate the occurrence and significance of such low potency mitochondrial actions in the toxicology of relatively safe compounds *in vivo*.

Fairly typical results that show the frequency with which pesticides in general exert such low potency effects on mitochondria are provided in a pair of papers by Yamano and Morita (1993, 1995). They examined the effects of 48 common pesticides of varied structures on respiration in isolated rat liver mitochondria. These compounds were not chosen because of any known ability to interact with mitochondria. Of the 48 compounds, 42% (20) were found to impact oxphos at concentrations of 1 mM or lower. Half of these were uncouplers and half were electron transport inhibitors. However, it is significant to note that only 1 (the obsolete herbicide trichlamide, acting as an uncoupler) was active at a concentration as low as 1 μM, and only 1 more (the insecticide amitraz acting as an inhibitor) was active at 10 μM. There was no obvious correlation between the ability of these compounds to disrupt oxphos and their toxicities to isolated rat hepatocytes at 1 mM. Thus, although the ability to alter oxphos *in vitro* is a rather common property of pesticides, this often occurs at relatively high concentrations that may or may not have toxicological significance *in vivo*.

A similar conclusion can be drawn from a study of the *in vitro* effect of 47 structurally and functionally varied pesticidal chemicals and metabolites on rat liver mitochondrial energetics by Abo-Khatwa and Hollingworth (1974). Eight of the compounds chosen were already known to be active as uncouplers or inhibitors of oxidative phosphorylation and gave appropriate results. Of the other 39 compounds, only 10 (26%) had appreciable effects on oxidation or phosphorylation at concentrations below 100 μM. Of the others, 41% had threshold activities at 0.1 to 1.0 mm and 33% were inactive even at 1 mM. Thus again, many varied pesticides had the capability to interact with mitochondria, but few showed high potency.

Read *et al.* (1998) have also published data on the action of a 164 chemicals on oxphos functions in beef heart submitochondrial particles (SMPs fragments of the inner mitochondrial membrane). Of these compounds, approximately 50 have pesticidal uses, including all classes of pesticidal activity and a wide range of structural types. Twelve of these 50 are compounds widely recognized to have potent effects on mitochondrial respiration that can explain most, if not all, of their toxic effects (e.g., dinitrophenols and other phenolic uncouplers, and organotins). All of these known oxphos-perturbing compounds had EC_{50} values of 3 ppm (roughly 10 μM) or less. The most active compounds were rotenone and fentin hydroxide with EC_{50} values of 10 and 33 nM, respectively. Among the 37 compounds which are not generally recognized to act through oxphos effects, 46% had EC_{50} values of 100 μM or higher, and 32% had EC_{50} values between 10 and 100 μM. The remaining 8 compounds with EC_{50} values below 10 μM were all highly lipophilic neurotoxicants. In general, the potency of these compounds against SMPs was higher than in the studies of Yamano and Morita (1993, 1995) with intact mitochondria, perhaps because penetration barriers are removed during the disruption of mitochondria to form the SMPs.

In the study by Read et al. (1998), the correlation of potency in causing oxphos effects with whole organism toxicity (using log transformations) is surprisingly good (e.g., an r^2 value of 0.763 was obtained in correlating the EC_{50} on SMPs with toxicity to fish for 104 varied chemicals, and a value of 0.859 was obtained for a subset of 19 neurotoxic insecticides). However, it is unlikely that these compounds have their toxic action primarily by effects on oxphos rather than the nervous system, More likely, their high lipophilicity bestows the ability to concentrate in lipid bilayer membranes which is a prerequisite for both neurological and mitochondrial actions.

57.2.2 SPECIFIC HERBICIDES AND OXPHOS IN VERTEBRATES

There are a number of examples of compounds that act as herbicides by affecting specific plant functions and that are of unknown mode of action in vertebrates, but which have been shown to interfere with oxphos in vertebrate mitochondria in vitro. These compounds include the chlorophenoxy herbicides (2,4-D, 2,4,5-T, and MCPA) that act in plants as hormone (auxin) mimics and that are weak uncouplers in rat liver mitochondria in vitro (Abo-Khatwa and Hollingworth, 1974; Zychlinski and Zolnierowicz, 1990). At 1–10 mM, 2,4-D decreased ATP, glutathione, and NADH level in rat hepatocytes (Palmeira et al., 1994a), inhibited complexes II and III strongly, and uncoupled mitochondria at 0.5 mM in isolated rat liver mitochondria. However, 2,4-D is 1000-fold less potent as an uncoupler than the dinitrophenolic compound dinoseb (Palmeira et al., 1994b). Nevertheless, signs of poisoning in humans include several such as hyperventilation, tachycardia, and pyrexia and sweating that are typically seen with uncouplers (Flanagan et al., 1990).

The phenylcarbamate herbicide, terbutol, and its N-demethyl metabolite were toxic to rat hepatocytes at 1 mM in vitro. Cytotoxicity was accompanied by loss of ATP and free sulfhydryl groups, including glutathione. These herbicides also impaired the respiration of rat liver mitochondria in vitro (Suzuki et al., 1997). However, the relationship of these observation to the in vivo toxicity of terbutol is unknown.

The pyridazinone herbicide chloridazon is a photosynthetic electron transport inhibitor in plants (Tomlin, 2000). It has a low acute toxicity to vertebrates (acute oral LD_{50} of at least 800 mg/kg in rats) and the symptoms of poisoning bear a close resemblance to those of a mitochondrial uncoupler, including apathy, dyspnea, hyperventilation, death in clonic convulsions, and very rapid rigor mortis. However, its effects on rat liver mitochondria were complex and hard to interpret involving an inhibition of succinate oxidation, an increase in respiration with glutamate as substrate, and an increase in ATPase activity, but with an increase in the efficiency of respiratory control with both substrates (Guzy et al., 2000; Mlynarcikova et al., 1999). Mitochondrial disruption may therefore play a central role in its acute toxicity to vertebrates, but the mechanism is unclear.

In each of these cases, even though the herbicides are only weakly active on oxphos, this may be the major biochemical target in vertebrates, but clear proof is lacking.

57.2.3 SECONDARY EFFECTS OF COMPOUNDS ACTING ON OTHER TARGETS IN VERTEBRATES: NEUROTOXICANTS

There are many reports in the literature of pesticides that are known to be potent neurotoxicants in vertebrates also affecting mitochondrial functions in vitro. This usually occurs at relatively high concentrations compared to those needed to affect ion channels enzyme and receptors in the vertebrate nervous system. These reports include several organophosphate anticholinesterases (Carlson and Ehrich, 1999; Holmuhamedov et al., 1996; Moreno and Madeira, 1990; Sitkiewicz et al., 1980), organochlorines such as DDT (Moreno and Madeira, 1991), and pyrethroids (Gassner et al., 1997; Read et al., 1998) which affect sodium channels, the DDT metabolite DDE which is not neurotoxic (Ferreira et al., 1997), and the organochlorines chlordane, dieldrin, endosulfan, and heptachlor, which act on GABA-gated chloride channels (Kannan et al., 2000; Meguro et al., 1990; Mishra and Shukla, 1995). Such effects could well explain the cytotoxicity of these compounds in vitro (e.g., the apoptotic effects found by Kannan et al. with endosulfan in a human leukemic cell line at 10–200 μM), but their acute toxicity in vivo is much more likely to result from specific neurological effects at lower concentrations.

For example, the formamidine insecticide/acaricides (chlordimeform and amitraz) have been shown to affect oxphos by acting as uncouplers at 10–100 μM concentrations in vitro (Abo-Khatwa and Hollingworth, 1973, 1974; Yamano and Morita, 1993). However, it is probable that their acute toxic effects in vivo in vertebrates are related to their effects as α-adrenergic agonists (e.g., see Costa et al., 1989; Hsu et al., 1988) and local anesthetics (e.g., see Pfister et al., 1978) rather than to their mitochondrial actions.

Another example is provided by the organochlorine insecticide chlordane. This inhibits respiration (states 3 and 4) in isolated rat liver mitochondria at 50–100 μM (Ogata et al., 1989) but quite high doses *in vivo* (100 mg/kg daily for four days) caused no major changes in functions of liver mitochondria in rats (Ogata and Izushi, 1991). Similarly, the anticholinesterase insecticide parathion at 0.1–1.0 mM caused several effects on oxphos in rat liver mitochondria including inhibition of complex II and ATP synthase and partial inhibition of the Pi transporter (Moreno and Madeira, 1990), and parathion and methyl parathion alter the fluidity of the mitochondrial membrane *in vitro* at 0.05 mM (Antunes-Madeira *et al.*, 1994; Lopes *et al.*, 1997). However, methyl parathion has been reported to have no effect on liver mitochondria *in vivo* in rats (Mihara *et al.*, 1981). Nor did chronic exposure to several structurally related organophospates in rats cause diminished mitochondrial activity and ATP production in the brain (Fukushima *et al.*, 1997). While it is not possible to rigorously exclude the possibility that some toxic effects of organophosphorus insecticides result from their effects on oxphos rather than from their very potent ability to inhibit acetylcholinesterase, the claim that oxphos effects may play an important role in their toxicity based on such *in vitro* assays (e.g., see Sitkiewicz *et al.*, 1980) is quite speculative.

On the other hand, endrin, an organochlorine insecticide, acts as a blocker of GABA-gated chloride channels which clearly accounts for many of its acute toxic effects. Endrin induced the formation of reactive oxygen species in isolated rat peritoneal macrophages and in hepatic mitochondria and microsomes at submicromolar concentrations, and it decreased microsomal membrane fluidity *in vitro* (Bagchi and Stohs, 1993). Interestingly, the same effects were observed *in vivo* in rats when endrin was given orally at a sublethal dose (4.5 mg/kg) (Bagchi *et al.*, 1993). Thus it would be a mistake to routinely dismiss the mitochondrial effects of potent neurotoxicants observed *in vitro* as likely to be relatively unimportant *in vivo*.

While it certainly does not explain all the results, one underlying reason for the reports of large number of pesticides that affect mitochondrial oxphos at high concentration *in vitro* may be that many of these pesticides are significantly lipophilic, and, at relatively high concentrations *in vitro*, can affect mitochondria through the simple disordering of the membrane integrity that is critical for mitochondrial functions and survival. Such effects on membrane structure, fluidity, and integrity have been shown to lead to a changed membrane environment for the components of oxphos and consequent alterations in their activity, membrane leakage, and uncoupling, and to the increased generation of ROS and oxidative stress (e.g., see Antunes-Madeira and Madeira, 1979; Stolze and Nohl, 1994).

Examples of studies showing various types of changes in membrane ordering and fluidity by pesticides, generally at quite high concentrations (10 μM to 1 mM) compared to their most potent known effect on target receptors or enzymes, include chlorinated hydrocarbons, e.g., Moreno and Madeira (1991) with DDT, Ferreira *et al.* (1997) with its nontoxic metabolite, DDE, Antunes-Madeira and Madeira (1979) with aldrin, and Bagchi *et al.* (1993) and Bagchi and Stohs (1993), with en-

drin. Similar studies with organophosphates include malathion (Antunes-Madeira and Madeira, 1979), parathion (Antunes-Madeira *et al.*, 1994), and methyl parathion (Lopes *et al.*, 1997). Lipophilic organotins such as tributyl- and triphenyltin also are well known to have general membrane disruptive effect (e.g., causing disruption of erythrocyte membranes at concentrations as low as 5 μM) (Gray *et al.*, 1987).

A final factor that makes interpretation of some *in vitro* results with mitochondria difficult is that many discrepancies can be found between different reports of such weakly active compounds on mitochondria. In their survey of a range of pyrethroid insecticides Yamano and Morita (1993, 1995) found no consistent pattern of effects on rat liver mitochondrial respiration and none had an effect at a concentration less than 100 μM. On the other hand, Gassner *et al.* (1997), also using rat liver mitochondria, reported that the pyrethroids permethrin and cyhalothrin inhibit mitochondrial complex I with IC_{50} values near 10 μM. Similarly, in their studies with bovine heart submitochondrial particles, Read *et al.* (1998) found that permethrin was one of the more potent inhibitors, active at less than 1 μM. By contrast, permethrin is reported to have no effect on rat liver mitochondria at 1 mM by Yamano and Morita (1993).

The numerous contradictions in the published reports of the effects of DDT on oxphos are reviewed by Moreno and Madeira (1991). It has been described by different authors as either a stimulator or an inhibitor of oxphos and related mitochondrial ATPase activity. Organophosphate insecticides were generally found to have no consistent effect on mitochondrial respiration at 1 mM (Yamano and Morita, 1993, 1995) but other authors have reported varied effects at much lower concentrations. The phenoxyacetic acid herbicide MCPA is reported to act like oligomycin in increasing the mitochondrial membrane potential through inhibition of mitochondrial ATP synthase in rat hepatocytes exposed at 2.5 mM (Camatini *et al.*, 1996) whereas Zychlinski and Zolnierowicz (1990) concluded that MCPA and related herbicides are weak uncouplers for rat hepatic mitochondria *in vitro*, an action that would tend to discharge the membrane potential. Variations between the biological preparations and techniques in these studies, and the fact that some compounds have biphasic or multiple effect on oxphos as their concentration is increased, may underlie some of these discrepancies, but others are not easily explained, and considerable caution is appropriate in interpreting the results from any single study, particularly in terms of possible toxic effects *in vivo*.

In closing this section, it is worth noting the report that a formulation of Tordon herbicide (a mixture of picloram and 2,4-D) inhibited mitochondrial complex I *in vitro* (Pereira *et al.*, 1994). Subsequent investigation revealed that all the mitochondrial effects were due to a surfactant in the formulation and not to the active pesticidal ingredients either singly or in combination (Oakes and Pollak, 1999). This nicely illustrates the dangers of using commercial formulations in such studies *in vitro* and the ability of detergents to damage mitochondrial membranes.

57.3 INHIBITORS OF COMPLEX I

57.3.1 INTRODUCTION

Until recently, the only pesticide thought to act primarily through the inhibition of complex I was rotenone. Although this is a familiar compound to toxicologists and biochemists, it currently has only minor uses as an insecticide because of its relatively low level of activity and short duration of action. Its extremely high toxicity to fish underlies its continuing use as a piscicide, but this, too, is a negative factor for its widespread use against insects. In the last decade, a number of new pesticides that act on complex I with powerful acaricidal activity and some insecticidal actions have been developed and several are now used worldwide. These compounds, fenazaquin, fenpyroximate pyridaben, pyrimidifen, and tebufenpyrad, have the broad structural commonality of being lipophilic nitrogen heterocycles. The properties, mechanism of action, and toxicology of these compounds have been reviewed by Hollingworth and Ahammadsahib (1995).

Because these compounds have the capability to inhibit complex I in vertebrates as well as in invertebrates with high potency, they generally possess a higher degree of acute toxicity to mammals than most modern pesticides. They also resemble rotenone in having very high toxicities to aquatic species in most cases.

The structure–activity relations of several groups of complex I inhibitors, including rotenone and the lipophilic heterocyclic pesticides, has been reviewed by Miyoshi (1998) with the broad conclusion that necessary structural features for the agrochemical inhibitors are a heterocyclic ring with two nitrogens and a hydrophobic tail structure. Akagi *et al.* (1996) modeled the three-dimensional conformations of tebufenpyrad, fenpyroximate, and pyridaben (see Fig, 57.8 for structures) and concluded that a common structure featuring a lone electron pair in the heterocyclic ring and a hydrophobic extension with a terminal *tert*-Bu-substituted phenyl group existed among these compounds. The active conformations were nonplanar with the heterocyclic group and the hydrophobic tail held at about a 90° angle. This is also believed to be the active configuration of rotenone (Miyoshi, 1998).

The emergence of these inhibitors has provided new tools to investigate the nature of the rotenone binding domain in complex I and its relationship to the binding sites for other complex I inhibitors and to the coenzyme Q reduction site(s). These results tend to be to confusing and there remains substantial disagreement regarding the number and relationship of binding sites for inhibitors in this region. The reader is referred to reviews by Degli Esposti (1998), Lümmen (1998, 1999), Ohnishi *et al.* (1999), and Okun *et al.* (1999) for additional details. However, the conclusion seems to be generally accepted that these lipophilic nitrogen heterocycles bind at, or very close to, a high affinity rotenone binding site, which, in turn is located close to the site where coenzyme Q is reduced (see Fig. 57.2). Two (or even three) Q binding sites may be present and it has been proposed that different types of inhibitors bind preferentially to

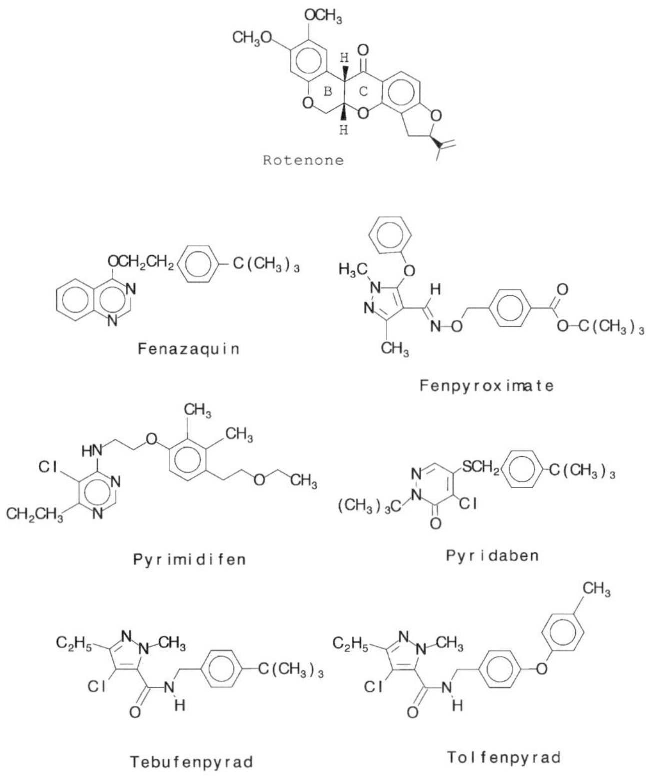

Figure 57.8 Pesticides that act as inhibitors of complex I.

these different Q binding sites or can otherwise be divided into classes based on the kinetics of their interactions with complex I (Degli Esposti, 1998; Degli Esposti and Ghelli, 1994; Friedrich *et al.*, 1994; Lümmen, 1999) but the specific details vary among these models and in some cases are contradictory. As few as one binding site near the Q reduction site (Lümmen, 1999) to as many as three (Degli Esposti, 1998) have been proposed. The case for two sites corresponding to the putative two quinone binding sites is reviewed by Degli Esposti and Ghelli (1999). These results are analyzed by Lümmen (1999) and the reasons for the apparent disparity in results are discussed. However, it is clear that complex I is indeed complex and the specific binding loci of these inhibitors remain to be established definitively. The culmination of these studies is the identification, using a photoaffinity label derived from the acaricide pyridaben, of the 23 kDa PSST subunit of complex I as the high affinity binding site for this compound and probably also for rotenone and several other complex I inhibitors (Schuler *et al.*, 1999). This subunit is believed to link electron transfer from the terminal iron–sulfur cluster, N2, to the ubiquinone reduction site (Fig. 57.2).

57.3.2 PROPERTIES OF SPECIFIC COMPOUNDS

57.3.2.1 Rotenone

(2*R*,6a*S*,12a*S*)-1,2,6,6a,12,12a-hexahydro-2-isoprenyl-8,9-dimethoxychromeno[3,4-*b*]furo[2,3-*h*]chromen-6-one (Fig. 57.8) has CAS Reg. No. 83-79-4.

Rotenone occurs in a large number of leguminous plants, but for commercial use, it has primarily been derived from the roots of *Derris* species (*D. elliptica*, *D. longicarpa*, and *D. mallaccensis*) from Southeast Asia and *Lonchocarpus* species (*L. urucu*, *L. nicou*, and *L. utilis*) from South America. The commercial material derived from *Lonchocarpus* is termed cubé, barbasco, nekoe, or timbo, while that from *Derris* is called derris root or tuba root. The root and its extracts contain a variety of compounds related to rotenone which are collectively termed rotenoids. Cubé root from Peru, which is currently the only commercial source of rotenone in the United States, may be used as a ground powder (5–20% total rotenoids) or further extracted with organic solvents. Additional purification and the addition of stabilizers to prevent oxidation and microbial contamination may follow. High quality commercial cubé resin typically contains 80–90% total rotenoids. In addition to rotenone itself, these rotenoids include deguelin, rotenolone, sumatrol, tephrosin, and toxicarol. They have variable but lesser insecticidal activity than rotenone. In cubé, rotenone itself constitutes approximately 40% of these rotenoids with deguelin being the second most common constituent at about 20%. These two components are the most active inhibitors of mitochondrial complex I in cubé resin (Fang and Casida, 1998) and are responsible for virtually all of its acute toxicity to insects, fish, mammals and cells in culture (Fang and Casida, 1997; Fang *et al.*, 1997). A large number of minor components of cubé resin have also been identified and their biological potencies assessed (Fang and Casida, 1997, 1999a, 1999b). The composition, origins, and toxicology of rotenoids have been extensively reviewed (Metcalf, 1955; Negherbon, 1959; Fukami and Nakajima, 1971; Haley, 1978; Gosselin *et al.*, 1984; Ray, 1991). The reader is referred to these sources for coverage of much of the earlier work on rotenone and its toxicology. The discussion below focuses primarily on more recent results.

General Properties   Pure natural rotenone consists of colorless dimorphic crystals, m.p. 163°C or 181°C depending on form, v.p. $<1 \times 10^{-3}$ Pa (20°C), w.s. 0.142 ppm, log P4.16. As described by Miyoshi (1998), rotenone has three chiral centers (Fig. 57.8). The naturally occurring compound has the 6aS, 12aS, 5′R configuration. The three-dimensional structure of this isomer of rotenone, revealed by x-ray crystallographic analysis, shows an "L" shaped molecule, strongly bent at the joining of the B and C rings. This molecular feature is critical for high inhibitory activity against complex I. The detailed structural features of the rotenone molecule necessary to inhibit complex I have been investigated and reviewed by Ueno *et al.* (1996). The structure–toxicity relationships of rotenoids are reviewed further by Miyoshi (1998).

Uses   Rotenone has been employed in commercial agriculture since at least 1848 when it was used as an insecticide in plantations in British Malaya, but its insecticidal properties were known much earlier to native people in several parts of the world (Haley, 1978). It was introduced as a commercial insecticide in the United States at the turn of the 20th century

and was once used widely. It now has very limited significance as an insecticide and acaricide in commercial agriculture, although it remains useful in organic production systems, in home and garden products, and for ectoparasite control (e.g., fleas and ticks) on pets. Rotenone is often combined with other insecticides such as pyrethrins or with synergists such as piperonyl butoxide which inhibit microsomal oxidative reactions and thereby enhance its rather low insecticidal activity and broaden it spectrum of action. Rotenone-containing materials have long been used by indigenous people as fish poisons. Due to its high toxicity to fish, rotenone continues to be used as a piscicide to remove unwanted species from bodies of water and to conduct fish surveys. In the 10 years from 1988 to 1997, 94,739 kg of rotenone were used in fish control projects in North America (Finlayson *et al.*, 2000). These uses are increasingly controversial because of concerns regarding the breadth of their environmental impact, possible human exposure through drinking water or consumption of treated fish, and even animal rights issues (Finlayson *et al.*, 2000). Trade names include Chem Fish, Fish-tox, Noxfish, Peru Cube Powder, Prentox, Rotenone Powder, and Synpren-Fish.

Toxicology Profile   The primary data sources are Haley (1978), Gosselin *et al.* (1984), Ray (1991), and Cal EPA (1997). Most of the studies described used technical (85–90% pure) or analytical grade rotenone (95–99% pure). In a few cases the purity is unstated.

Acute Toxicity   The acute toxicity of rotenone to mammals is unusually variable (Ray, 1991; Table 57.1) and is strongly dependent on the formulation and route of exposure. When formulated as an emulsifiable concentrate, the acute toxicity may be very high (EPA toxicity class I), while other formulations such as dusts are much less toxic (EPA class III). In rats and dogs, the dust formulation is more toxic by inhalation than by oral dosing. Another significant factor governing both the oral and the respiratory toxicity is the particle size with smaller particles being more toxic. The critical factor underlying these variations in acute toxicity is probably the effect of formulation and particle size on the rate of uptake because rotenone has a very high intrinsic toxicity to vertebrates (e.g., the LD$_{50}$ after intraperitoneal administration to mice is only 1.6 mg/kg) (Haley, 1978). Acute poisoning symptoms include emesis and, at higher doses, increased respiration, muscle tremors, and, ultimately, respiratory and behavioral depression, convulsions, and respiratory failure. Severe hypoglycemia is observed in dogs and rabbits.

Irritation/Sensitization   Local effects caused by exposure to rotenone include mild skin irritation and stronger eye irritation which may be due to components in the plant extract other than rotenone itself (Gosselin *et al.*, 1984; Haley, 1978).

Subchronic Toxicity   In a 6 month oral dosing study in dogs, the lowest observed effect level (LOEL) was found at 2 mg/kg/day with endpoints including hematological changes,

Table 57.1
Acute Toxicity of Pesticides Acting as Inhibitors of Mitochondrial Complex I to Selected Nontarget Species

| Compound | LD$_{50}$ (mg/kg) | | | | Acute dermal | LC$_{50}$ (mg/l) Inhalation | LC$_{50}$ (ppb) (24–96 h) | |
| | Acute oral | | | | | | | |
	Rat (M; F)	Mouse(M)	Quail	Duck	Rat or rabbit	Rat	Fish[a]	*Daphnia*
Rotenone	132–1500	350	1680[b]	>2000	>5000	0.02	1.9–75	26
Fenazaquin	134; 138	2449	1747	>2000	>5000	1.9	3.8–34	4.1
Fenpyroximate	480; 245	520	>2000	>2000	>2000	0.33	79–290	204
Pyridaben	1100; 570	424	>2250	>2500	>2000	0.64	1.1–8.3	0.59
Pyrimidifen	148; 115	245	—	445	>2000	—	93	—
Tebufenpyrad	595; 997	224	>2000	>2000	>2000	2.66	18–95	48

[a] Range of values from several species, most commonly including the rainbow trout and bluegill.
[b] Pheasant.

emesis, diarrhea, and decreased body weight. Gastrointestinal lesions were found at 10 mg/kg/day.

Chronic Toxicity In a 2-year dietary study in rats, lowered body weight was seen with rotenone at 37.5 ppm and an increased incidence of adrenal gland angiectisis and hemorrhage was noted at 75 ppm (3.8 mg/kg/day).

Carcinogenicity The evidence regarding rotenone's potential carcinogenicity is conflicting and convoluted. In earlier work, a dietary study with Osborne–Mendel rats given cubé powder at concentrations from 50 to 1000 ppm showed no increase in tumors (Hansen *et al.*, 1965). A similar result was obtained in a 28-month feeding study with dogs. The cubé powder contained 5.8% rotenone and 12% other extractives with 82% inert material. In a lifetime dietary study with tubatoxin (90% rotenone) in two strains of mice, Innes *et al.* (1969) found no adverse effects, but only a single, low dose (3 ppm) was used. Neither of these studies would be considered adequate to assess carcinogenicity by current standards.

In a series of reports that caused particular concern in the regulatory community in the United States, Gosálves and his co-workers (see Gosálvez, 1983 for a review), claimed that rotenone, given either intraperitoneally (1.7 mg/kg/day for 42 days) or orally (13.5 mg/kg/day for 45 days), greatly increased the number of fibroadenomas of the mammary gland in female albino and Wistar rats. Only one adenocarcinoma was observed, but some of the tumors were transplantable. The fibroadenomas were encapsulated and contained numerous malformed mitochondria which were deficient in respiratory control and oxphos. Gosálves subsequently suggested that these positive results, at least in part, were due to the tumor-enhancing effect of deficiencies in his diets, particularly a low level of riboflavin.

These results precipitated extensive additional research. Freudenthal *et al.* (1981) carried out several studies. Rotenone was administered subchronically (42 days) at 1.7 or 3.0 mg/kg/day either by gavage to Wistar rats or intraperitoneally to Sprague–Dawley rats and the animals were maintained for 14 to 18 months. The intraperitoneal study paralleled the conditions used by Gosálves *et al.* but in a different strain of rats. A dietary study with Syrian golden hamsters, lasting 18 months with rotenone concentrations from 125 to 1000 ppm, was also conducted. Gross and microscopical examination of the tissues revealed no significant increases in neoplasms of any kind in the rat studies, but an increase in adrenal cortical adenomas was recorded in females in the gavage study. Three adrenal cortical carcinomas were also observed in the hamsters at the highest dosage, but it was concluded that it was questionable whether these were related to the rotenone treatment. No other increases in neoplastic lesions were seen. Evaluation of the hamster study was made more difficult by high mortality in all treatments, possibly due to *E. coli* infection.

Subsequently, Abdo *et al.* (1988) reported on two National Toxicology Program lifetime dietary studies, one in F344/N rats at rotenone concentrations of 38 and 75 ppm and the other in B6C3F1 mice at 600 and 1200 ppm. In the mice of both sexes and female rats, no significant adverse effects were seen. However, in male rats a small increase in adenomas of the parathyroid gland was seen at 75 ppm. This increase in a rare benign tumor was not statistically significant but it was notable in being far above the incidence in historical controls and was judged to probably be related to the rotenone treatment.

Finally, Greenman *et al.* (1993) attempted to repeat the experimental conditions used by Gosálves and colleagues exactly with intraperitoneal administration of rotenone for 42 days to female Wistar rats. No evidence of increased tumors, mammary or otherwise, was observed. In this paper he states that Gosálves had been unable to repeat previous mammary tumor results when the study was rerun with higher dietary levels of riboflavin. Since the difference in dietary riboflavin in Gosálves *et al.*'s original work and in the Greenman study is only about twofold, it seems unlikely to account for the radically different results on mammary tumorigenesis that they observed.

The most reasonable conclusion to be reached from this suite of studies is that the weight of evidence suggests that rotenone is not an animal carcinogen but that the issue is still not fully resolved.

The chronic feeding study with cubé powder in rats of Hansen *et al.* (1965) gave an unexpected result. At the highest dietary doses (500 and 1000 ppm) a very clear decrease in the incidence of mammary tumor below that found in the control animals was seen. A decrease in pituitary adenomas was also observed in these high dose animals. A similar effect was observed in the carcinogenicity study in B6C3F1 mice conducted by Abdo *et al.* (1988) in which rotenone at 1200 ppm reduced the background incidence of hepatocellular carcinoma and neoplasms of the subcutaneous tissues well below that of the controls in males and increased their survival time. Cunningham *et al.* (1995) investigated rotenone's high dose antitumorigenic effect in B6C3F1 male mice further and observed a dose-dependent decrease in hepatocellular proliferation. They attributed the antitumor action to rotenone's ability to block cell turnover which is in known to be an action that correlates with decreased tumor development. Rotenone has a well-established ability to decrease growth and division in a number of cell types *in vitro* (see below). In a further study to establish the biochemical mechanism for this antiproliferative effect, Wang *et al.* (1999) concluded that rotenone probably acted through two complementary mechanisms. The first is to cause an increase in apoptosis which removes DNA-damaged liver cells before they can progress to a carcinogenic condition, and the second is to decrease the energy status of the cells which favors a lower rate of basal hepatocyte proliferation. Both effects, in turn, result from the inihibition of electron transport. A previous study in B6C3F1 mice by Isenberg *et al.* (1997) using diethylnitrosamine to initiate DNA injury and a peroxisome proliferator to promote the development of these preneoplastic loci to focal lesions showed that rotenone antagonized the growth of the focal lesions. These authors arrived at the same conclusion as Wang *et al.* (1999) regarding a dual mechanism for this effect based on increased apoptosis and reduced proliferation.

A number of other studies have also clearly demonstrated that rotenone antagonizes the proliferation of tumor cells. Figueras and Gosalvez (1973) found that rotenone injected intraperitoneally in mice at 3 mg/kg/day completely prevented the proliferation of a massive dose of Ehrlich ascites tumor cells. Mean time to death was increased by 110% compared to controls and, even so, death in the rotenone-treated animals was due to the toxic effects of the rotenone rather than tumor formation.

Further confirming the anticancer activity of rotenoids, Gerhäuser *et al.* (1995, 1997) discovered that four rotenoids from *Mundulea sericae* reduced the formation of chemically induced preneoplastic lesions in cultured mammary glands exposed to 7,12-dimethylbenz(a)anthracene and inhibited the development of papillomas in the two-stage mouse skin model. Subsequently, the effect of deguelin was studied *in vivo* in the two-stage (7,12-dimethylbenz(a)anthracene/phorbol ester) mouse skin model and on rat mammary tumors induced by *N*-methylnitrosourea. A strong anticancer effect was seen in each case (Udeani *et al.*, 1997).

This general antiproliferative action was related to the ability of rotenoids to inhibit the expression of phorbol ester-induced ornithine decarboxylase (ODC) in mouse cells. ODC is involved in the regulation of cell proliferation and tumor promotion and is utilized as a biomarker for cancer chemopre-

ventive agents. In turn, the rotenoid effect on ODC induction was attributed to an observed rapid decrease in cellular ATP levels due to complex I inhibition. The alternative hypothesis that rotenoids could have their anticancer activity by inhibiting tubulin polymerization was rejected since deguelin is inactive in this regard, and activity correlated with complex I inhibitory activity rather than antimitotic capability among several other compounds.

Rowlands and Casida (1998) confirmed this anticancer action using MCF-7 human breast cancer cells. Rotenoids such as rotenone and deguelin were also shown to decrease the mitogen-induced expression of ODC and to decrease the phorbol ester-induced production of reactive oxygen species in the cells. These authors concluded that the inhibition of complex I by rotenoids probably decreased the production of phorbol ester-induced reactive oxygen species which, in turn, regulate the expression of ODC activity. This concept was supported by the observation that two potent complex I inhibitors, the pesticides pyridaben and fenazaquin, caused an identical effect on ROS and ODC levels. This work was extended to include 29 rotenone analogs (Fang and Casida, 1998, 1999a) and 8 flavonoids and stilbenes (Fang and Casida, 1999b) isolated from cubé insecticide. With these compounds, the ability to inhibit complex I from bovine heart was well correlated with their ability to decrease phorbol ester-induced ODC activity in the human cancer cells and their cytotoxicity to MCF-7 and Hepa1clc7 cells, thus confirming an intimate connection between these different biological activities.

Mutagenicity/Genotoxicity A large number of studies on rotenone's capability to cause mutations or chromosomal effects have been conducted and are reviewed by Cal EPA (1997). Most of these results have been negative, but mutations were reported in an *in vitro* mouse lymphoma cell study, and increased sister chromatid exchange was observed in a study with Chinese hamster ovary cells. Recently, Guadaño *et al.* (1998) examined the effect of rotenone on sister chromatid exchange, chromosomal aberrations, and micronuclei formation in cultured human lymphocytes. An increase in micronuclei was observed which was tentatively attributed to the well-known effects of rotenone on microtubule aggregation and spindle formation (Section 57.3.2.1). The weight of this evidence clearly suggests that rotenone is not genotoxic.

Reproductive Toxicity In a two-generation dietary study in rats, the LOEL was found to be 37.5 ppm (1.88 mg/kg/day). Effects at this dose included reduced weight gain of both the pups and adults. Live litter sizes were reduced at 75 ppm. A reproduction study in hamster was conducted with 500 or 1000 ppm rotenone in the diet for 3 months. At 500 ppm, poor litter survival and maternal deaths occurred. At 1000 ppm, reduced testicular size and infertility were observed.

Developmental Toxicity/Teratogenicity The status of rotenone as a teratogen is inconclusive. Several types of developmental effects have been observed in studies with rats and mice, but generally at a dose that caused at least some minimal adverse effects in the mothers. In the rat, increased skeletal deformities including unossified sternebrae, renal pelvic cavitation, and distended ureters were seen in the offspring when 6 mg rotenone/kg/day was administered by gavage during pregnancy, but the same and lower doses also caused maternal effects such as lowered weight gain and several clinical signs (Cal EPA, 1997). Skeletal abnormalities in the form of supernumerary ribs were also seen in a teratology study in rats dosed orally with 5 mg rotenone/kg/day on days 6 to 15 of pregnancy, but again some maternal toxicity (reduced weight gain) was evident at this dose, and a dose of 10 mg/kg caused significant maternal lethality (Khera *et al.*, 1982). On the other hand, in an oral feeding study in rats during pregnancy, Spencer and Sing (1982) found an adverse effect on the fetuses at 100 ppm in the form of reduced fetal survival whereas the first maternal toxicity was observed only at higher doses of 400 ppm. The reason for the discrepancy between these studies is unclear.

In the mouse, a LOEL dose of 24 mg/kg/day was fetotoxic and caused resorptions and decreased litter size. However, maternal toxicity, including mortality, was observed at the same dose. In an additional study in mice, no adverse developmental or toxic effects were seen at 15 mg/kg/day.

Neurotoxicity Some of the earliest investigations of the toxic effects of rotenone demonstrated that it has the ability to block nerve transmission (Fukami, 1976), but there is no reason to suppose that this occurs other than by its effects as a respiratory inhibitor. As already discussed, because of its high respiratory activity, the nervous system in general is an important target tissue for compounds which affect oxphos. However, recent studies with rotenone and other complex I inhibitors have raised significant questions regarding their capability to cause specific neurodegenerative diseases, particularly parkinsonism (Betarbet *et al.*, 2000; Hollingworth and Ahammadsahib, 1995). A number of epidemiological studies have identified exposure to pesticides in general as a significant risk factor for the development of parkinsonism (e.g., see Gorell *et al.*, 1998; Menegon *et al.*, 1998), but specific causative agents have not been identified. At the same time, a relationship between the inhibition of complex I and the degeneration of dopaminergic tracts in the substantia nigra, which is a hallmark of parkinsonism, was brought to the fore by studies of the complex I inhibitor MPP$^+$ in connection with the contamination of a street drug in San Francisco (reviewed by Tipton and Singer, 1993). MPP$^+$ (which is not a pesticide) is specifically taken up and concentrated in dopaminergic neurons by the dopamine uptake system in sufficient quantities to inhibit complex I. It thus might be unusual or unique in its ability to cause destructive effects on these neurons in the substantia nigra since most complex I inhibitors are not likely to be concentrated in this way. This conclusion was supported by the work of Ferrante *et al.* (1997) who observed that when rotenone, a complex I inhibitor that does not interact with the dopamine transporter, was infused intravenously into rats for 7–9 days at 10–18 mg/kg/day, lesions in the striatum and globus pallida were observed but

no specific neurodegeneration in the substantia nigra occurred. Systemic toxicity (cardiovascular effects) was also observed at these doses.

However, other studies with rotenone in rats have shown that, under specific circumstances, it can cause loss of dopaminergic neurons in the substantia nigra and induce a condition that closely resembles parkinsonism [e.g., Heikkila *et al.* (1985) injected rotenone into the left median forebrain of rats and saw an extensive loss of dopaminergic functions in the neostriatum]. More specifically, recent work by Betarbet *et al.* (2000) has shown that the continuous intravenous infusion of rotenone in rats (2–3 mg/kg/day for 1–5 weeks) caused no systemic toxicity or generalized neuropathology but selectively destroyed dopaminergic tracts in the substantia nigra even though complex I was inhibited uniformly in the brain by about 75%, as judged by binding of tritiated dihydrorotenone. This treatment also induced the development of Lewy-like cellular inclusions and behavioral deficits which replicated those in parkinsonism. When administered at higher doses that cause systemic toxicity, rotenone caused more generalized neuronal lesions. The reason no comparable dopaminergic pathology was seen in the substantia nigra in the study of Ferrante *et al.* (1997) which was also conducted at higher rotenone doses causing systemic toxicity remains to be explained.

Rotenone, as a highly lipophilic molecule, probably distributes readily throughout the nervous system and into cells. Neuronal cell death may be caused through the generation of reactive oxygen species that occurs on the partial inhibition of complex I. Free radical generation leading to apoptosis has been observed with low concentrations of rotenone in cultured neuronal dopaminergic cells (Betarbet *et al.*, 2000; Hartley *et al.*, 1994). It is significant in this regard to note that the degree of inhibition of complex I (75%) observed in their study does not inhibit overall electron transport in brain mitochondria because complex I is present in excess (Davey and Clark, 1996). Also, not all nerve cells were affected to the same degree (e.g., although dopaminergic neurons were destroyed in the striatum, GABAergic and cholinergic ones were not). The reason for the high sensitivity of the dopaminergic cells is unclear, but there is direct evidence that dopaminergic neurons have an unusually high sensitivity to disturbances of energy metabolism (Marey-Semper *et al.*, 1993), and it has been suggested that this could be because they are already under oxidative stress because of their metabolism of dopamine and its precursors. These are catechols that form quinones which can take part in redox cycling reactions.

It is important to keep in mind that in such studies, rotenone is being used as a convenient inhibitor of complex I to develop an animal model for parkinsonism. The results by no means implicate it as a likely cause of Parkinson's disease in human populations. No evidence for parkinsonism-like signs or neurodegenerative pathology has been reported in several subchronic and chronic dietary studies with rotenone in animals at a variety of dose levels (Cal EPA, 1997). The dietary or dermal routes of exposure obviously correspond much more closely to the typical human experience with rotenone than the intravenous infusion method used by Betarbet *et al.* (2000). This mode of administration bypasses several of the normal physical and metabolic barriers that protect the brain against poisoning. Also, many other compounds besides rotenone to which humans may be exposed, both pesticidal and naturally occurring, can inhibit complex I (Degli Esposti, 1998). They too would need to be considered if the theory that complex I inhibition underlies parkisonism is correct. Further, if the key event in the induction of Parkinson's disease is the generation of reactive oxygen species in dopaminergic neurons, many other types of compounds that generate free radicals such as inhibitors of complex III and redox cycling agents, or compounds that interfere with the normal protective radical scavenging mechanisms, might also cause this type of neurodegeneration. The available evidence and patterns of use do not suggest that rotenone is likely to be a significant primary or general cause of Parkinson's disease in human populations.

Hormonal Actions   There is little indication from the available toxicology data that rotenone has endocrine disruptive effects. In a specific study to examine possible estrogenic actions in the positive rat mammary tumorigenesis studies of Gonsalves et al., Olson and Sheehan (1979) found that rotenone did not act as an estrogen or estrogen antagonist either *in vitro* or *in vivo*.

Human Toxicology   Rotenone appears to be moderately toxic to humans. The oral lethal dose has been estimated to be 300–500 mg/kg, but toxicity is likely to be strongly formulation-dependent, and the presence of other bioactive components such as the synergist piperonyl butoxide in the commercial mixture might considerably influence its potency. In practice, human poisoning is extremely rare probably because of the low rotenone content of many commercial products, its frequently poor uptake from the gastrointrestinal tract, and its rapid emetic action (Gosselin *et al.*, 1984; Ray, 1991).

The signs, symptoms, and treatment of poisoning by rotenone are discussed by Ray (1991) and Reigart and Roberts (1999). These include numbness at sites of exposure, nausea, vomiting, and tremors (Haley, 1978). Neither fatalities nor systemic poisoning has been reported in the occupational use of rotenone. Numbness of the oral mucous membrane has been reported in workers or volunteers who were exposed to derris orally. Dermatitis and respiratory irritation, sometimes severe, have also been reported in those exposed occupationally under conditions of poor hygiene, but it is unclear whether these effects are due to rotenone or other constituents of the crude plant extracts. The one human death reported involved a child who consumed about 10 ml of an oily rotenone extract, giving an estimated exposure of 40 mg/kg. After vomiting, she gradually lost consciousness and died of respiratory arrest with postmortem evidence of anoxic damage to heart, lungs, and brain (DeWilde *et al.*, 1986). The ingestion of rotenone-containing roots was apparently a common means of committing suicide among inhabitants of New Ireland (Ray, 1991).

No antidotes for rotenone poisoning are known and decontamination followed by supportive therapy, if necessary, is indicated. Since menadione (vitamin K3) has been shown to bypass the rotenone inhibition site in complex I and to antagonize rotenone-induced respiratory depression and decreased blood pressure in rabbits (Santi and Toth, 1965), its use in human therapy has been proposed (Gosselin *et al.*, 1984).

Biochemical Mechanism of Action   The ability of rotenone to inhibit respiration and glutamate oxidation was first described by Fukami (1956, reviewed in Fukami 1976) using insect tissues. The extension of this work to show potent inhibition of rat liver mitochondrial respiration and the localization of rotenone's site of action in or near complex I was described in a series of papers by Lindahl and Oberg (1961). A large number of subsequent papers, reviewed by Haley (1978) and (Singer and Ramsay, 1992, 1994), have confirmed the view that the primary site of action for rotenone is the inhibition of respiration by interaction with complex I. Two binding sites have been identified for rotenone within complex I, a high affinity site and a lower affinity one, both of which must be occupied for full inhibition of electron flow through the complex (Singer and Ramsay, 1992, 1994). The recent studies with a photoaffinity label for the putative rotenone binding site already described also reveal a high affinity and a lower affinity binding site (Schuler *et al.*, 1999). These authors concluded that the 23 kDa PSST subunit of complex I plays a key role in high affinity binding.

Rotenone inhibits cellular growth and division in many biological systems with inhibitory effects on cell division observed at 10–100 nM concentrations in a number of types of isolated cells [Ray, 1991; see Haley (1978) for earlier work]. At least two possible mechanisms for this antimitotic action have been described: a slowing of progression through the cell cycle due to rotenone's effects on respiration and ATP availability, and a direct effect on microtubule assembly and spindle formation which arrests cell division in mitosis and resembles the effects of colchicine in disrupting spindle formation (Brinkley *et al.*, 1974; Barham and Brinkley, 1976a, 1976b). Rotenone inhibited the rate of polymerization of rat brain tubulin *in vitro* with an IC_{50} of 0.46 μM, a potency about fivefold higher than that of colchicine (Hoebeke and van Nijen, 1975), and, at a fairly high concentration (12 μM), it inhibited the polymerization of tubulin from bovine brain *in vitro*. Rotenone antagonized the binding of ^{3}H-colchicine to bovine brain tubulin over the concentration range of 0.1 to 10 μM (Brinkley *et al.*, 1974), indicating an ability to bind directly to a site on the tubulin molecule. Although tubulin polymerization is an ATP-dependent process and in whole cells, failure to assemble tubulin could arise by an indirect action on ATP levels, Figueras and Gosalvez (1973) showed that the effect of rotenone on microtubule assembly does not arise through ATP deficiency but through direct binding to tubulin. Meisner and Sorfensen (1966) also observed that rotenone specifically arrests the cell cycle in metaphase by inhibition of spindle formation and concluded that this was probably due to binding to tubulin rather than a direct effect on cell bioenergetics. Recently, Barrientos and Moraes (1999) found that the rotenone concentration needed to impact microtubule assembly in a human osteosarcoma-derived cell lines was fivefold higher than that which inhibited complex I by 100% (10^{-7} M) and concluded that the two effects occur at nonoverlapping concentrations.

The mechanism of cytotoxicity of rotenone has been studied in some detail. The depletion of ATP and inhibition other cellular functions driven by the mitochondrial membrane potential is potentially deleterious, although cells in culture treated with rotenone can frequently maintain adequate ATP for basic survival and cell division through glycolysis if glucose is provided. A second biochemical effect underlying rotenone's cytotoxicity may be an increase in superoxide and other ROS in the cell due to its inhibitory actions on complex I, as described in Section 57.1.7.1. This situation is quite complex since under some circumstances rotenone may also reduce the production of ROS (e.g., see the discussion of the role of rotenone as an anticancer agent and the induction of ODC above). This varied effect on ROS is discussed in detail by McLennan and Degli Esposti (2000).

Absorption, Metabolism, and Elimination In mammals, rotenone is rapidly metabolized by oxidation, involving both ring hydroxylation and O-demethylation, and then eliminated (Ray, 1991). After an oral dose of ^{14}C-rotenone in rats, most of the label was excreted in the feces and elimination was complete in 48–72 hr. No parent compound was excreted. Evidence was obtained for enterohepatic recycling of compounds excreted in the bile (Cal EPA, 1997). The metabolism of rotenone has been reviewed by Yamamoto (1969) and further studies were conducted by Yamamoto *et al.* (1971). *In vitro*, rotenone is subject to a variety of cytochrome P-450-catalyzed oxidations in vertebrate and insect tissues oxidation occurs (e.g., at both the methyl group and the double bond of the isopropenyl group, and at the carbon atom adjacent to the keto group between the B and C rings to yield a pair of enantiomers, rotenolones I and II) (Fig. 57.8). Rotenoids are also subject to oxidative O-demethylation (Unai *et al.*, 1973). In each case the metabolic product is less active as a complex I inhibitor. However, some oxidations do not eliminate toxicity. The 8'-hydroxy metabolite produced by oxidation of the methyl group of the isopropenyl side chain has an intraperitoneal toxicity to mice equal to that of rotenone, and rotenolone I also possesses considerable toxicity (Yamamoto, 1969). In fish, oxidative metabolism by liver microsomes also produces rotenolones and the products from the oxidation of the isopropenyl double bond (Erickson *et al.*, 1992). The comparative metabolism of rotenone in mammals, fish, and insects was investigated by Fukami *et al.* (1969) in relationship to its differential toxicity between these groups.

Environmental Fate and Toxicity Rotenone is only slightly toxic to birds (Table 57.1). However it is highly toxic to many aquatic species, including fish (Table 57.1), probably because of the rapid uptake of this lipophilic compound and the presence of a sensitive and critical target site. Extensive additional data on the toxicity of rotenone to fish and other aquatic species are provided by Haley (1978). The generally high toxicity of rotenone to aquatic organisms includes many other species such as frogs and leeches (lethal effects at 100 ppb) and oysters (reduced shell growth at 10 ppb). Gingerich studied the uptake, metabolism, and elimination of rotenone in rainbow trout (Gingerich, 1986) and bluegill sunfish (Gingerich and Rach, 1985). In the bluegill, metabolism was quite rapid with only 20% of the radioactivity in the body being in the form of rotenone. The biological concentration factor (BCF) for total radioactivity in the whole body was 125, but because of the extensive metabolism, the BCF for rotenone was only 26. Six metabolites were found, with one being major. The half-life for the first and major phase of elimination was 25.8 hr and 80% of the radioactivity was lost in 3 days during the depuration period. Rainbow trout cleared rotenone more slowly with an elimination half-life of 68.5 hr and 85% of the radioactivity in the tissues was unchanged rotenone. An exception was the liver where rotenone represented less than 40% of the radioactivity present. The major route of excretion was through hepatobiliary excretion of polar metabolites.

The high sensitivity of rotenone to photodecomposition (Cheng *et al.*, 1972) and oxidation limits its residual activity in the field and residues rapidly dissipate with a half life of 1–3 days under typical conditions. The speed of degradation depends on such predictable factors as the intensity of sunlight and the water temperature, e.g., the half life for rotenone in water varies from 10.3 days at 5°C to 13.9 hr at 25°C (Gilderhus *et al.*, 1986; Finlayson *et al.*, 2000, pp. 191–192). Rotenone binds strongly to soils with an estimated K_{oc} of 10,000 ml/g (Augustijn-Beckers *et al.*, 1994). Because of its rapid degradation after use in aquatic systems, the immediate impacts of rotenone's use in fish management programs on nontarget species are likely to be short-lived (Finlayson *et al.*, 2000), but even so, due to the initial impact, reductions in some benthic aquatic invertebrate populations may still be appreciable as long as five years after use (Mangum and Madrigal, 1999). It's use in a small pond study led to the immediate loss of the zooplankton population which did not return to normal until 8 months later (Beal and Anderson, 1993).

57.3.2.2 Lipophilic Nitrogen Heterocycles

A group of novel acaricides, some also having insecticidal activity, that have their primary toxic action by inhibition of respiration in complex I was discovered in the 1980s and is now widely used. All are lipophilic compounds (log *P* values range from 4.6 to 6.4) with nitrogen-containing heterocyclic (specifically pyrazole, pyrimidine, or pyridazine) ring systems. Their properties and mechanism of action have been reviewed by Hollingworth and Ahammadsahib (1995), Degli Esposti (1998), and Lümmen (1998).

Fenazaquin: General Propertics and Uses 4-*Tert*-butyl-phenethylquinazolin-4-yl ether (Fig. 57.8), with CAS Reg. No. 120928-09-8, was discovered by DowElanco Co. and is described by Longhurst *et al.* (1992).

It exists as colorless crystals, m.p. 78–80°C, v.p. 3.4×10^{-6} Pa (25°C), w.s. 0.22 ppm (25°C), log $P5.51$.

Fenazaquin (EL-436) is an acaricide on a wide range of crops under the trade names of Boramae, Demitan, Magister, Magus, Matador, Pride, and Totem.

Toxicology Profile The primary source of data is Anonymous (1993a).

Acute Toxicity Fenazaquin has a relatively low acute oral toxicity to mice but it is much more toxic to rats (Table 57.1). The toxicity to guinea pigs lies between these two extremes with an LD$_{50}$ at 812 mg/kg. The dermal and inhalation toxicity are also moderate to low.

Irritation/Sensitization Fenazaquin causes slight eye irritation in rabbits but it is not a skin irritant or sensitizer.

Subchronic Toxicity In 90-day dietary or gavage studies in rats, no notable toxicity was seen other than deceased food intake and weight gain at 30 mg/kg/day. The same was true in 90-day dietary studies at 50 mg/kg/day in hamsters and 15 mg/kg/day in dogs and in a one year dietary study in dogs at 12 mg/kg/day. A 21-day dermal study in rabbits was equally devoid of toxicological finding at 1000 mg/kg/day.

Chronic Toxicity A two-year oral study in rats at doses up to 18 (M) or 25 (F) mg/kg/day revealed a moderate decrease in serum cholesterol and triglycerides. Treatment-related focal hepatocellular abnormalities were seen but no neoplasms were found. The no observed effect level (NOEL) was about 0.5 mg/kg/day. A second 18-month gavage study in Syrian golden hamsters revealed no specific toxicity other than a reduction in body weight at the highest dose, 35 mg/kg/day. A significant decrease in amyloidosis (a common disease in aging hamsters) was compound-related. The mechanism of this effect is unknown. The LOEL was 15 mg/kg/day.

Carcinogenicity Results were negative in the above rat and hamster studies.

Mutagenicity/Genotoxicity No genotoxicity was observed in standard battery of seven assays with microbial and mammalian systems.

Reproductive Toxicity No reproductive effects were observed in a multigenerational study in rats at doses as high as 25 mg/kg/day.

Developmental Toxicity/Teratotogenicity No developmental toxicity or teratogenicity was observed in rats at the highest dose tested (40 mg/kg/day). In rabbits a marginal increase in early resorptions was found at the highest dose (60 mg/kg/day).

Biochemical Mechanism of Action Fenazaquin was shown to be a strong inhibitor of respiration in complex I of rat liver mitochondria and purified bovine heart complex I with IC$_{50}$ values in the range 20–50 nM by Hollingworth *et al.* (1994). Okun *et al.* (1999) confirmed this result using bovine submitochondrial particles. In a study using ^{3}H-fenazaquin, Wood *et al.* (1996) showed high affinity binding to electron transport particles from bovine heart mitochondria. A variety of inhibitors of complex I competed with fenazaquin in this assay, including rotenoids and pyridaben, and their potency as inhibitors of complex I correlated well with their ability to displace fenazaquin from its binding site. However, subsequent studies with a photoaffinity analog of fenazaquin labeled a protein (probably subunit d) in the stalk region of ATP synthase. Since fenazaquin does not inhibit the oligomycin-sensitive mitochondrial Mg^{2+}-ATPase activity in mitochondria (Gadelhak and Hollingworth, unpublished), the relevance of this binding site for the toxic action of fenazaquin is dubious. Probably this is a low affinity site and the labeling arises from the high concentration of the photoaffinity label used in the study.

Fenazaquin is a peroxisome proliferator in mice and rats *in vivo* (Stott, 1996) but, as is typical of these compounds (Roberts, 1999), it is much less potent in hamsters. Studies with primary cultured hepatocytes from several species showed that fenazaquin caused a sevenfold increase in the activity of the peroxisome indicator enzyme, acyl coA oxidase, in mice, and a threefold increase in rats, but no change in hamster and human hepatocytes. In mouse hepatocytes an inhibition of gap junctional intercellular communication and significant oxidative stress were observed, but this was not seen with hepatocytes from the other species. As already noted, chronic feeding studies did not show an increased incidence of tumors (either of the liver or any other organ) in rats and hamsters. However, it is worth noting that the decrease in cholesterol and triglycerides and increase in hepatocellular focal abnormalities seen in the chronic study in rats are typical of the actions of a peroxisome proliferator (Roberts, 1999). Because of these species differences, Stott concluded that the hamster and rat, rather than the mouse, were the most appropriate models for human cancer risk assessment with fenazaquin.

Fenazaquin inhibits complex I and blocks the induction of ornithine decarboxylase by several agents in human breast cancer cells *in vitro*. In this regard, fenazaquin's action parallels that of rotenone, and the block of ornithine decarboxylase correlates with anticancer activity. It is postulated that both the block of the decarboxylase and the anticancer action arise from a common cause (i.e., a reduction in the production of reactive oxygen species by the mitochondrial respiratory chain) (Rowlands and Casida, 1998). This hypothesis is discussed further in relationship to rotenone (Section 57.3.2.1).

Absorption, Metabolism, and Elimination After an oral dose in rats, fenazaquin was rapidly absorbed with a peak plasma level appearing in 8 hr, almost quantitatively and rapidly metabolized, and eliminated primarily in the feces (80%) with significant amounts also in the urine (20%). Similar results were obtained with goats. Initial metabolites in rats and goats were formed by three reactions; cleavage of the ether linkage, oxidation of the *tert*-butyl group to an alcohol and then a carboxylic acid, and oxidation of the quinazoline ring between the two nitrogen atoms.

Environmental Fate and Toxicity   Fenazaquin has a low acute toxicity to birds (Table 57.1). The LC_{50} value in 5-day feeding studies in mallard ducks and bobwhite quail were >5000 ppm and the dietary NOEL in a one-generation reproduction study was 287 ppm.

Fenazaquin does have a very high toxicity to fish and other aquatic species (Table 57.1). The no-effect concentration in a 63-day early life stage study in rainbow trout was extremely low, (0.96 ppb). Aquatic invertebrates are equally sensitive, with a no-effect concentration of 1.4 ppm for *Daphnia* growth and reproduction in a 3-week study. Shell growth is inhibited in the Eastern oyster at 5.4 ppb, and the acute LC_{50} for brown shrimp is 15 ppb (Anonymous, 1993a). A mean BCF of 500–520 was found in trout but on depuration, 80% of the radioactivity was eliminated in 24 hr. Based on this result, Perkins *et al.* (1992) concluded that fenazaquin is unlikely to represent a bioaccumulation threat in fish. An aquatic microcosm study was used to simulate drift and runoff after application at 5 times the highest recommended use rate. No adverse effects were seen on aquatic life.

Fenazaquin is rapidly and strongly adsorbed onto soil particles with K_d values ranging from 54 to 687 and K_{oc} values from 18,700 to 41,200. The half-life for photolysis on the soil surface is 15 days under the summer sun at 40° latitude and 25°C, and the aerobic half-life in soils varies from 33 to 114 days with degradation mainly depending on microbial activity. It therefore has a low potential for leaching and accumulation in soils (Anonymous, 1993a). The half-life for photolysis in water is about 15 days under the same conditions as the soil photolysis. Fenazaquin is extremely stable to hydrolysis at neutral and alkaline pH (half-life is over a year) but it is hydrolyzed much more rapidly under acidic conditions. It is resistant to degradation by microbial action. In an aqueous microcosm study fenazaquin had a half-life in the water of 1 to 2 days as it partitioned onto solids where its half-life was about 5 months (Perkins *et al.*, 1992).

Fenpyroximate: General Properties and Uses   *Tert*-butyl (E)-α-(1,3-dimethyl-5-phenoxypyrazol-4-ylmethyleneaminooxy)-*p*-toluate (Fig. 57.8), CAS Reg. No. 134098-61-6, was discovered by Nihon Nohyaku Co and is described by Konno *et al.* (1990). The development of fenpyroximate has been reviewed by Hamaguchi *et al.* (1995).

It exists as white crystals, m.p. 101–102°C, v.p. 7.4 $\times$ 10^{-6} Pa (25°C), w.s. 14.6 ppb (20°C), log P 5.01. Fenpyroximate can exist as E (*trans*) and Z (*cis*) geometrical isomers. The commercial insecticide is the E-form. In solution, fenpyroximate is readily degraded by photolysis to the Z-isomer with a half-life of 1.5 hr under conditions replicating those of sunlight. The Z-isomer then degrades with a half-life of 10.5 hr (Swanson *et al.*, 1995).

Fenpyroximate (NNI-850, HOE 555-02A) is a widely used acaricide. Trade names include Acaben, Akari, Danitron, Dintron, Dynamite, Meteor, Naja, Ortus, Pamanrin, and Sequel.

Toxicology Profile   The toxicological properties of fenpyroximate have been reviewed (FAO/WHO, 1996; U.S. EPA, 1999a) based almost entirely on unpublished studies submitted for registration. These are the source of much of the information below. An earlier summary of toxicity studies on fenpyroximate has also been published (Anonymous, 1992a).

Acute Toxicity   Fenpyroximate is moderately toxic after oral dosing in rodents but is somewhat more toxic by inhalation (Table 57.1). Signs of acute toxicity include hypoactivity and hypopnea. At necropsy, irritation of the gastrointestinal tract after oral dosing, and of the respiratory system after inhalation, was observed.

Irritation/Sensitization   Fenpyroximate is not a skin irritant. It is a mild to moderate eye irritant and a moderate dermal sensitizer. Occular and dermal irritation have been noted among workers manufacturing fenpyroximate.

Subchronic Toxicity   In mice fed fenpyroximate at levels as high as 2000 ppm (175 mg/kg/day) for four weeks the only effects observed were several changes in hematological parameters and reduced food consumption and body weight gain. At 100 ppm (7.4 mg/kg/day) results in rats were similar with minimal liver hypertrophy and decreased white blood cell counts and plasma protein levels. At 500 ppm females had lowered acetyl- and butyrylcholinesterase levels in the blood. A subchronic oral feeding study with dogs caused some mortality at 50 mg/kg/day after appetite and body weight loss. Organ weight changes and signs of histopathological changes in the liver and kidney were also seen at this dose. Slight bradycardia and increased diarrhea were recorded at lower doses down to 10 mg/kg/day, the LOEL.

Chronic Toxicity   Non-neoplastic effects seen in chronic toxicity studies in rats at the highest dose tested (150 ppm; 6.9 mg/kg/day) included depressed growth, gastric ulceration, and pancreatic lobular degeneration in males and interstitial proliferation of the ovary and distention of the uterus in females. Pituitary neoplasia which compressed the brain was observed in males. There was a high incidence of pituitary adenoma in all treatment groups which nevertheless fell within the historical control range. In a lifetime feeding study in mice with doses as high as 72 mg/kg/day, no adverse effects were observed except reduced weight gain which was first noted at 10 mg/kg/day. In dogs, the results were quite similar to those in the subchronic study.

Carcinogenicity   Studies were negative in lifetime dietary studies in mice and rats and it was concluded that there was no evidence of compound-related carcinogenicity.

Mutagenicity/Genotoxicity   Results were uniformly negative in a battery of *in vitro* and *in vivo* tests including point mutations in *S. typhimurium* and *E. coli*, mutation in Chinese hamster lung cells, chromosomal aberrations in human lymphocytes *in vitro*, micronucleus formation *in vivo* in CD-1 mice, DNA repair in *Bacillus subtilis,* and unscheduled DNA synthesis in rat hepatocytes.

Reproductive Toxicity   No negative effects were observed in reproductive performance in rats in a two-generation study. Reduced weight gain in both the parents and offspring occurred at the highest dose tested (100 ppm; 8.6 mg/kg/day).

Developmental Toxicity/Teratogenicity   No evidence of teratogenocity or fetotoxicity was observed in rats and rabbits at doses that were not also maternally toxic. An increase in the number of thoracic ribs was observed at the highest dose, 25 mg/kg/day, in rats. An increase in incidence of retinal folds in rabbits at 5 mg/kg/day fell within the historical control range.

Neurotoxicity   No evidence of delayed neurotoxicity was observed in hens at two oral doses of 5000 mg/kg given 21 days apart.

Biochemical Mechanism of Action   A variety of studies show that fenpyroximate is a powerful inhibitor of mitochondrial respiration, acting specifically at complex I. This was first described by Motoba *et al.* (1992) who obtained an IC_{50} for complex I from the mite (*Tetranychus*) *in vitro* of 80 nM compared to 400 nM for that from rat liver. Fenpyroximate *in vivo* depleted ATP in mites and caused malformation of the mitochondria, particularly in peripheral nerves. Friedrich *et al.* (1994) confirmed that fenpyroximate is a high potency inhibitor of vertebrate complex I and assigned it to the same inhibitor class as piericidin A. Okun *et al.* (1999), using a bovine mitochondrial preparation, characterized the relative potencies of several complex I-inhibiting acaricides as pyrimidifen > fenazaquin > fenpyroximate > rotenone. The I_{50} values in this study ranged from 2 to 20 nM. Degli Esposti (1998) obtained a similar result with an IC_{50} of 4.6 nM for beef heart submitochondrial particles, making fenpyroximate slightly more active than rotenone. Jewess (1994) reported that fenpyroximate strongly inhibits NADH oxidation in blowfly flight muscle mitochondria and displaces ^{3}H-dihydrorotenone from its specific binding site on complex I in blowfly muscle submitochondrial particles.

The high specificity of fenpyroximate as a miticide is not based primarily on differences in target site sensitivity since it inhibits the mitochondrial complex I from rat liver and from spider mites with less than a 10-fold difference in potency (Motoba *et al.*, 1992). The main mechanism of selectivity has been shown to depend on differential rates of metabolic detoxification, particularly through removal of the t-Bu group yielding the free carboxylic acid analog. This metabolite is inactive as a complex I inhibitor. This apparent hydrolysis is largely catalyzed by cytochrome P-450 through hydroxylation of the t-Bu

group followed by intramolecular ester cleavage. Oxidative ester cleavage was rapid in the several mammals, fish, and insects tested but it did not occur in mites (Motoba *et al.*, 2000).

Absorption, Metabolism, and Elimination   Fenpyroximate is well absorbed, extensively metabolized, and rapidly excreted in rats after an oral dose, primarily (70–90%) in the feces (FAO/WHO, 1996; Nishizawa *et al.*, 1993). The elimination half-life was 6–9 hr at 2 mg/kg and 35–49 hr at 400 mg/kg. Considerable biliary excretion occurred (approximately 50% in 48 hr). Multiple sites of metabolism were identified including oxidation of the *tert*-butyl group and pyrazole methyl group, ester and oxime ether hydrolysis, aryl hydroxylation, *N*-demethylation, and *E/Z* isomerization. The uptake of fenpyroximate after dermal application in rats was very low.

Environmental Fate and Toxicity   Fenpyroximate has a very low toxicity to birds, and it is less toxic to fish and *Daphnia* than most of the other members of this group of pesticides, but it is still potent enough to be classified as highly toxic by the U.S. Environmental Protection Agency (Table 57.1). It is moderately persistent in soils with a half-life of 26–50 days where it is degraded primarily by microbial action (Izawa *et al.*, 1993).

Pyridaben: General Properties and Uses   2-*Tert*-butyl-5-(4-*tert*-butylbenzylthio)-4-chloropyridazin-3(2H)-one (Fig. 57.8), CAS Reg. No. 96489-71-3, was discovered by Nissan Chemical Industries and is described by Hirata *et al.* (1988). The development of pyridaben is discussed by Hirata *et al.* (1995).

It exists as white crystals, m.p. 111–112°C, v.p. 2.5 × 10^{-4} Pa (20°C), w.s. 12 ppb (24°C), log P6.37. It is relatively stable to heat and hydrolysis but sensitive to photolytic decomposition with a half-life of about 30 min at pH 7.

Pyridaben (NC-129, BAS 3001) is widely used as an acaricide with a long residual action and as an insecticide mainly against sucking insects. Trade names include Nexter, Oracle, Poseidon, Pyramite, Sanmite, and Starling.

Toxicology Profile   The general sources of data are U.S. EPA (1997a, 1998a, 2000a). Another useful source is the detailed summary of the regulatory toxicological studies of pyridaben provided by Igarashi and Sakamoto (1994).

Acute Toxicity   Pyridaben shows moderate to low acute toxicity to mammals (Table 57.1). The intraperitoneal LD_{50} was 68 mg/kg in male rats (Igarashi and Sakamoto, 1994). The dermal toxicity is low but toxicity by the inhalation route is quite high. With sublethal doses in mice and rats, clinical signs included decreased food consumption, diarrhea, hypothermia, bradycardia, bradypnea, decreased spontaneous motor activity, abnormal gait, prostration, eye closing, amd piloerection. At near lethal or lethal doses (300 mg/kg or more) depression of the central nervous and cardiovascular systems were stronger, but no change occurred in motor functions, including coordination, muscle strength, and neuromuscular transmission, or in sensory functions. Early gastric lavage was effective in presenting poisoning in rats and loperamide was efficacious in reducing the diarrhea that occurred at low doses.

Irritation/Sensitization Pyridaben caused slight and readily reversible eye irritation in rabbits, but it was not a skin irritant or sensitizer in guinea pigs in either the maximization test or the modified Buelher test. However, moderate to severe skin reactions were seen in a dermal exposure study when pyridaben was applied to pregnant Himalayan rabbits at 70 mg/kg/day over 2 weeks.

Subchronic/Chronic Toxicity In subchronic and chronic feeding studies with mice, rats, and dogs, toxicological observations were unremarkable with endpoints being decreased food intake and weight gain, and sporadic changes in clinical chemistry or organ weights. The most sensitive endpoint was in the dog with an LOEL in a one-year dietary study of 0.5 mg/kg/day based on increased clinical signs (emesis, salivation) and decreased body weight.

Carcinogenicity Pyridaben was not oncogenic in typical lifetime feeding studies in the rat and mouse. It is classified by the U.S. Environmental Protection Agency as a Group E compound (no evidence for carcinogenicity to humans).

Mutagenicity/Genotoxicity Pyridaben was negative in a battery of microbial and mammalian tests (Ames *Salmonella* assay, Chinese hamster V79 cell point mutation assay, Chinese hamster lung cell cytogenetic damage *in vitro*, micronucleus assay in mice *in vivo*, the rec-assay in *Bacillus subtilis*, and DNA damage and repair test in *E. coli*).

Reproductive Toxicity No adverse reproductive effects were observed in a multigenerational study in rats at dietary doses up to 80 ppm.

Developmental Toxicity/Teratogenicity Delayed ossification was seen in rats and rabbits after oral administration to pregnant animals during organogenesis, but this was believed to be a secondary result of maternal stress. Fetal and placental weights were decreased in rats at 30 mg/kg/day and abortions occurred in rabbits at the highest dose (15 mg/kg/day). In both species these events occurred only at doses that were clearly maternally toxic. No evidence for teratogenicity was seen.

Neurotoxicity Pyridaben caused only a low degree of acute neurotoxicity in a standard battery of neurobehavioral tests when given at a single oral dose of 200 mg/kg in males. Effects included piloerection, hypoactiviy, tremors, and lowered body temperature, but these were sporadic and transient. In a longer term (90 day) study in rats, no neurotoxicity or neuropathology was seen at oral doses up to 27 mg/kg/day, but plasma cholinesterase activity was reduced in females.

Biochemical Mechanism of Action Pyridaben inhibited respiration in insects *in vivo* and blocked respiration at complex I in several mitochondrial preparations *in vitro* (Hollingworth *et al.*, 1994). The inhibitory potency was extremely high with IC_{50} values of 0.8 nM for isolated beef heart complex I and 4.0 nM for rat liver mitochondria. The very high activity of pyridaben as an inhibitor of complex I has been confirmed by Degli Esposti (1998). As already described in the Introduction (Section 57.3.1), using photoaffinity label methodology, the binding site for pyridaben in bovine heart submitochondrial particles has been shown to be the PSST subunit of complex I (Schuler *et al.*, 1999).

Like fenazaquin (Section 57.3.2.2) and rotenone (Section 57.2.2), pyridaben also blocks complex I and the induction of ornithine decarboxylase in human breast cancer cells *in vitro*, an action that correlates with antiproliferative and anticancer activity (Rowlands and Casida, 1998).

Oxidation of the sulfur group in pyridaben yields the corresponding sulfoxide and sulfone. Compared to pyridaben, these compounds have a reduced ability to inhibit complex I and reduced toxicity to vertebrates. However, they show an increased toxicity to mammalian cells *in vitro*. This may indicate a second mechanism of toxicity for pyridaben in which sulfur oxidation activates the molecule to become reactive with nucleophiles such as tissue thiols (Schuler and Casida, 1998). The occurrence and possible toxicological significance of such an action *in vivo* are unknown.

Absorption, Metabolism, and Elimination An oral dose of pyridaben in rats was absorbed fairly well (38–46% of the dose), rapidly and completely metabolized, and eliminated mainly in the feces (80–97%) within 96 hr. Nearly 20% of the excreted residue in the feces was the parent compound. A large number of metabolites (20–30) were detected in the urine and feces with none predominant. They arose primarily from oxidation of the two *tert*-Bu groups and glutathione conjugation with the pyridazinone ring, probably following oxidation of the sulfur atom (Hirata *et al.*, 1995). Considerable biliary excretion occurred (22–30% in 24 hr) and there was evidence of enterohepatic circulation of these metabolites.

Environmental Fate and Toxicity Pyridaben has a low acute toxicity to birds, but it is extremely toxic to aquatic species (Fig. 57.8). Its persistence in soil is relatively brief due to rapid microbial degradation (e.g., the half-life under aerobic conditions is reported to be less than 3 weeks). In natural water in the dark, the half-life is about 10 days, due mainly to microbial action since pyridaben is stable to hydrolysis over the pH range 5–9. The half-life including aqueous photolysis is about 30 min at pH 7 (Tomlin, 2000).

Pyrimidifen: General Properties and Uses 5-Chloro-*N*-{2-[4-(2-ethoxyethyl)-2,3-dimethylphenoxy]ethyl}-6-ethylpyrimidin-4-amine (Fig. 57.8), CAS Reg. No. 105779-78-0, was discovered by Ube Industries with joint development by the Sankyo Company.

It exists as a white crystal, m.p. 69–71°C, v.p. 1.6×10^{-7} Pa (25°C), w.s. 2.17 ppm (25°C), log P4.59. It is stable to hydrolysis over a broad pH range.

Pyrimidifen (E-787, SU-8801, SU-9118) is used as an acaricide and insecticide under the trade name Miteclean.

Toxicology Profile   The general data source is Anonymous (1999b).

Acute Toxicity   Pyrimidifen has a higher acute oral toxicity to mammals and birds than most other members of this group (Table 57.1). Signs of poisoning in rats include apathy, decreased respiration, abnormal gait, and decreased urinary output.

Irritation/Sensitization   Pyrimidifen causes slight eye irritation but no dermal irritation or sensitization.

Subchronic Toxicity   In a 90-day dietary study in rats, toxicological effects were rather nonspecific including decreased weight gain, some changes in blood chemistry, and changes in organ weights. An increase in liver weight was seen in females at 0.69 mg/kg/day, the lowest dose tested. Similar results were seen in mice and the LOEL was established at 17.7 mg/kg/day. In dogs the LOEL was 0.5 mg/kg/day based on observations of diarrhea. Increased salivation and reduced body weight gain were seen at the highest dose, 4.5 mg/kg/day.

Chronic Toxicity   In a 2-year study in rats, dietary levels at 100 ppm (3.9 mg/kg/day) increased the incidence of benign adrenal pheochromocytoma. Increased weight and discoloration of the kidney and lipofuscin deposition in the tubules were also seen. The signs of toxicity in parallel long-term feeding studies in dogs and mice were unremarkable.

Carcinogenicity   Long-term feeding studies in rats, mice, and dogs proved negative for carcinogenicity.

Mutagenicity/Genotoxicity   Pyrimidifen gave negative results in the Ames assay and a bacterial DNA repair test (Rec-assay). It did not cause chromosome aberrations in the Chinese hamster lung fibroblast assay.

Reproductive Toxicity   None was seen in a two-generation study in rats at doses of 7.6–9.5 mg/kg/day.

Developmental Toxicity/Teratogenicity   Some minor skeletal abnormalities were found when pyrimidifen was fed to pregnant rats and rabbits at 20–25 mg/kg/day, but these doses also caused maternal toxicity and it was concluded that pyrimidifen is not teratogenic.

Biochemical Mechanism of Action   Pyrimidifen is an extremely potent inhibitor of complex I in bovine submitochondrial particles (I_{50} of 2 nM) and competes with high affinity for a binding domain that is in common with fenazaquin, fenpyroximate, and rotenone (Okun *et al.*, 1999).

Tebufenpyrad: General Properties and Uses N-(4-tert-butylbenzyl)-4-chloro-3-ethyl-1-methylpyrazole-5-carboxamide (Fig. 57.8), CAS Reg. No. 119168-77-3, was discovered by Mitsubishi Kasei Corporation and was developed in partnership with the American Cyanamid Co. It is described by Kyomura *et al.* (1990) and Inoue and Fukuchi (1994). The structural conformation of tebufenpyrad has been determined by x-ray crystallography (Osano *et al.*, 1991). The synthesis and structure–acaricidal activity relations of tebufenpyrad and related compounds are described by Okada *et al.* (1991). A closely related compound, tolfenpyrad (OMI-88; CAS Reg. No. 129558-76-5; Fig. 57.8), with stronger insecticidal activity than tebufenpyrad and reasonable mammalian safety is currently under development in Japan (Okada *et al.*, 1999).

General Properties   Tekufenpyrael exists as white crystals, m.p. 61–62°C, v.p. 1×10^{-5} Pa (25°C), w.s. 2.8 ppm (25°C), log P4.61–5.04. It is stable to aqueous hydrolysis with a half-life over 28 days at pH 5–9.

Uses   Tebufenpyrad (MK-239, SAN-831, AC 801,757) is used primarily as an acaricide but it also has activity against sucking insects. Trade names include Comanché, Masaï, Oscar, and Pyranica.

Toxicology Profile   The general sources of the data are Anonymous (1993b) and Mitsubishi Chemical Industries (1995).

Acute Toxicity   Tebufenpyrad shows moderate acute toxicity to mammals (Table 57.1). The toxicity to rabbits is higher with an acute oral LD_{50} between 40 and 100 mg/kg. By the dermal and inhalation routes its toxicity is low. Clinical signs of poisoning include slowed respiration, decreased locomotor activity, and prostration. Increased salivation is also seen after respiratory exposure. In an attempt to test therapeutic strategies, rabbits dosed orally at 100 mg/kg (LD_{100}) were given dimorpholamine intravenously at 3 or 6 mg/kg intravenously when respiration had decreased to 50% of normal. This treatment improved respiratory function significantly but it is not stated whether mortality was decreased.

Irritation/Sensitization   Tebufenpyrad caused slight, reversible eye irritation in rabbits, but it was not a skin irritant or sensitizer.

Subchronic Toxicity   A uniform picture emerges for 90-day dietary or gavage studies in rats, mice, and dogs. The only effects consistently observed were decreased weight gain and increased liver weight at the highest doses [about 28 mg/kg/day in the rat, 160 (M) to 220 (F) mg/kg/day in mice, and 10 mg/kg/day in dogs]. Some liver hypertrophy was seen in rats, and vomiting and diarrhea occurred in dogs.

Chronic Toxicity   Longer term exposures in these animals caused essentially the same responses as in the 90-day studies, but at somewhat lower doses. The NOELs in both rats

(24-month dietary exposure) and dogs (12-month oral dosing) were found at 1 mg/kg/day. Chronic gastritis was observed in the dogs at the highest dose (20 mg/kg/day). The NOEL in an 18-month dietary study in mice was 4 mg/kg/day.

Carcinogenicity   No evidence of carcinogenicity was seen in the lifetime dietary studies in mice and rats.

Mutagenicity/Genotoxicity   Tebufenpyrad is not mutagenic or clastogenic in a typical battery of bacterial and mammalian tests including the Ames *Salmonella*, Chinese hamster ovary cell, chromosomal aberrations in lymphocytes, mouse micronucleus, and unscheduled DNA synthesis assays.

Reproductive Toxicity   No serious adverse reproductive effects were observed in a two-generation dietary study in rats. A decrease in pup weight gain was recorded at the highest dose, 16 mg/kg/day, which was the LOEL for the study.

Developmental Toxicity/Teratogenicity   No developmental or teratogenic effects were observed when tebufenpyrad was given orally during organogenesis to rats at 150 mg/kg/day or to rabbits at 40 mg/kg/day, the highest doses tested. The NOEL for maternal effects was about 15 mg/kg/day in each study.

Biochemical Mechanism of Action   Like the other compounds in this group, tebufenpyrad is a powerful and specific inhibitor of complex I with an I_{50} value of 6 nM for bovine heart submitochondrial particles (Degli Esposti, 1998) and 2 nM for mitochondria from housefly flight muscle (Lümmen, 1998).

Absorption, Metabolism, and Elimination   Tebufenpyrad is rapidly metabolized and cleared after an oral dose in rats. The metabolism of tebufenpyrad in rats *in vitro* and *in vivo* was investigated by Ogawa and Ihashi (1993). Hydroxylations of the ethyl and t-Bu groups were the predominant reactions both *in vitro*, using an S-9 liver fraction, and *in vivo*. Subsequent oxidation of these initial alcohols to carboxylic acids and conjugation of the alcohols with sulfate occurred *in vivo*. Little cleavage of the amide bond was observed.

Environmental Fate and Toxicity   Tebufenpyrad is relatively safe to birds (Table 57.1). In 8-day feeding studies in mallard ducks and quail, the LC_{50} was >5000 ppm in both species. Like the other members of this group it is highly toxic to fish and to *Daphnia* (Table 57.1). Other aquatic invertebrates are also highly sensitive to tebufenpyrad (e.g., the LC_{50} for mysid shrimps is 22 ppb and the EC_{50} for the inhibition of shell growth in the Eastern oyster is 62 ppb). The 22-day no-effect concentration for reproduction in *Daphnia* is very low at 2.4 ppb. The uptake, metabolism, and excretion of tebufenpyrad by carp have been studied by Saito *et al.* (1994). The BCF at steady state, which was reached within about 4 days of exposure, was 864. However, less than 4% of the radioactivity in the body was unchanged tebufenpyrad, so the BCF for the parent is only 29. The major metabolites were formed by sequential oxidation of the

tert-butyl group to the alcohol and then to the carboxylic acid and their subsequent conjugation with sulfate and glucuronic acid residues. The half-life for elimination during the depuration phase was about 12 hr with 98% of the radioactivity cleared within 7 days. Thus, although tebufenpyrad is lipophilic, is readily taken up from water, and might be expected to show a high level of bioaccumulation, it is also rapidly metabolized and cleared which greatly decreases the degree of accumulation. The acylation of the amide nitrogen between the two rings in analogs of tebufenpyrad produces compounds that are improved as acaricides and also show much lower toxicity to fish, perhaps due to differential rates of metabolic deacylation to release the active compound in these organisms (Obata *et al.*, 1999).

Tebufenpyrad binds firmly to soil organic matter with K_{oc} values from 1380 to 4930. Together with its low water solubility, this indicates a very low potential for leaching. It has a moderate persistence in aerobic soils with a half-life of about 1 to 2 months.

57.4 INHIBITORS OF COMPLEX II

57.4.1 INTRODUCTION

Relatively few pesticides are thought to have their primary toxic action through effects on complex II. Important pesticides that do act in this way are fungicides in the carboxamide (carboxanilide) group. These have been reviewed by Kulka and von Schmeling (1995). In some cases the information regarding these compounds that is available in the open literature or toxicological databases is quite minimal. Based on this rather limited information, they seem to have virtually no notable adverse effects and they have attracted minimal toxicological interest beyond the studies required by regulatory authorities to obtain approval for use.

57.4.2 PROPERTIES OF SPECIFIC COMPOUNDS

57.4.2.1 Carboxamides

The forerunner of the group is the fungicide carboxin which was discovered in the mid-1960s (Kulka and von Schmeling, 1995). A relatively large number of carboxamides have subsequently been used as agricultural fungicides, but several of these are not now produced commercially [e.g., benodanil, mebenil, methfuroxam, metsulfovax, and pyracarbolid; Tomlin (2000)]. On the other hand, new members are still being added to the group (e.g., thifluzamide and furametpyr were both first registered for use as pesticides in the 1990s). The carboxamides are systemic fungicides with both protectant and curative actions which are used in seed treatments and in foliar and soil treatments, primarily to control Basidiomycetes. They are often used in mixtures with other fungicides or insecticides. They generally have low or very low toxicities to terrestrial vertebrates and aquatic species, earthworms, and insects. Their chronic toxicity is equally unremarkable. The lack of recorded incidents of human poisoning appears to substantiate their safety under practical conditions of use. However, the toxicological information available in the open literature is quite limited for most of these compounds. They are rapidly metabolized and eliminated by mammals. It is interesting to note that fungicides within the carboxin group have proved effective as potential therapeutic agents for the human immunodeficiency virus (HIV-1) by inhibiting the viral reverse transcriptase (Bader *et al.*, 1991). Considerable work has followed from this discovery but this lies outside the scope of the chapter.

Succinate-ubiquinone oxidoreductase was shown to be the target for carboxin and oxycarboxin in fungi 30 years ago (Mathre, 1971; White, 1971). The extensive work on this topic is reviewed in detail by White and Georgopoulos (1992) and Schewe and Lyr (1995). Despite the statement by Schewe and Lyr (1995) that mammalian mitochondria "show a sensitivity to carboxins comparable to those of sensitive fungi," a view that is also supported by the work of Mowery *et al.* (1976, 1977), other results indicate that complex II from vertebrate mitochondria is often significantly less sensitive to inhibition by carboxamides than that of target fungi (Mathre, 1971; Motoba *et al.*, 1988; Shimizu *et al.*, 1992). It appears that results vary with the type of preparation, the electron acceptor used in the assay, and the structure of the carboxamide tested. The complex II from non-target fungal and plant mitochondria is generally found to be markedly less sensitive than that of target fungi. This allows for the use of these compounds in plant protection without phytotoxicity (Schewe and Lyr, 1995; Shimizu *et al.*, 1992).

The precise binding site for the carboxamides is not known. Solubilized succinic dehydrogenase from bovine heart or fungal mitochondria, consisting of the FP and IP subunits (Fig. 57.3), is not inhibited by carboxin and other carboxanilides (Mowery *et al.*, 1976; Schewe and Lyr, 1995; Shimizu *et al.*, 1992), so the binding site probably lies within the membrane-associated anchor portion of the complex. Inhibition arises from a disruption of the transfer of electrons from the iron–sulfur center to ubiquinone, a situation analogous to the acaricide–insecticides that inhibit complex I (Section 57.3.1). This is in accord with photoaffinity labeling studies that indicate that carboxamides bind to a site associated with the ubiquinone-binding proteins of complex II (CII-3 and CII-4, Fig. 57.3) and not to the flavoprotein-containing or iron–sulfur proteins (White and Georgopoulos, 1992). A recent study by Matsson *et al.* (1998) using carboxamide-resistant mutants of *Paracoccus denitrificans* concluded that the key mutation is in one of these two membrane-located anchor polypeptides at a location adjacent to the Fe–S cluster. It was suggested that this may form part of the carboxamide binding site.

On other hand, in the fungus *Ustilago maydis*, a study of resistance to carboxin showed that it is associated with a point mutation in the gene encoding the third iron–sulfur cluster in the IP subunit (Keon *et al.*, 1994). These authors concluded that carboxamides are probably interposed between this high poten-

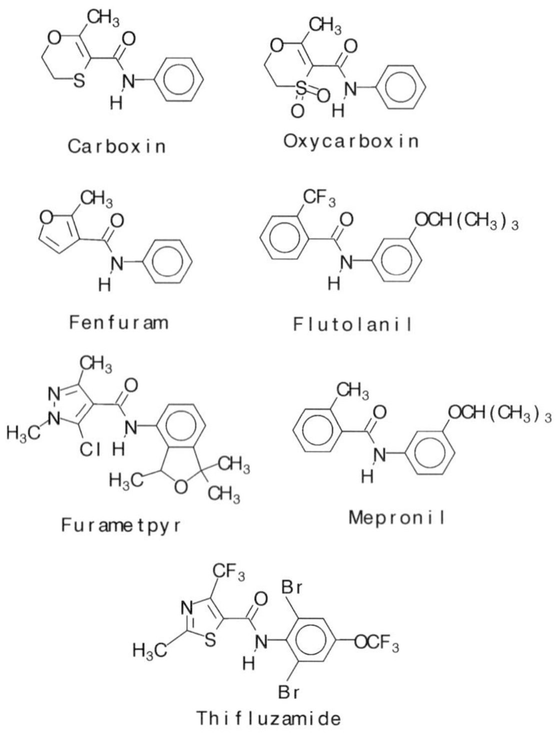

Figure 57.9   Pesticides that act as inhibitors of complex II.

tial iron–sulfur center and the ubiquinone binding proteins and thereby hinder electron transfer between them. This resistance mutation may then cause a conformational change in the IP subunit that allows it to continue to feed electrons to the ubiquinone site even in the presence of the carboxin. An identical result was found by Skinner *et al.* (1998) in a different organism. They concluded that this mutation affecting carboxin sensitivity may not be occurring within the carboxin binding domain but at an allosteric site that controls the access of carboxin to its binding site. Inhibitor access is restricted in the resistant form leading to a decrease in target site sensitivity. Clearly, multiple mutations may lead to carboxin resistance (Georgopoulos, 1995) and these appear to operate by different mechanisms. The exact nature of the inhibition of complex II by carboxamides therefore still awaits clarification and depends on the development of a more detailed knowledge of the structure and mechanism of the complex.

Carboxin: General Properties and Uses   5,6-Dihydro-2-methyl-1,4-oxathiin-3-carboxanilide (Fig. 57.9), CAS Reg. No. 5234-68-4, was discovered by Uniroyal Chemical Co. and is described by von Schmeling and Kulka (1966).

It exists as white crystals (dimorphic), m.p. 92–93°C or 98–100°C (depending on form), v.p. 2.5×10^{-5} Pa (25°C), w.s. 199 ppm (25°C), log P2.2, HLC 3×10^{-5} Pa m^3 mol^{-1}. It is stable to hydrolysis from pH 5 to 9.

Carboxin is a systemic fungicide used as a seed treatment and to prevent seedling diseases of cereals and many other crops. It is often formulated in combination with other fungicides or insecticides. Common trade names include Cerevax, Enhance, Hiltavax, Kemikar, Kisvax, Oxatin, and Vitavax.

Toxicology Profile   The primary sources of data are U.S. EPA (1989a) and Cal EPA (1994), which provide an extensive overview of the toxicology and fate of carboxin based on unpublished studies submitted for pesticide registration, and the HSDB (2000).

Acute Toxicity   Carboxin has a very low acute toxicity to terrestrial vertebrates by all routes of exposure (Table 57.2).

Irritation/Sensitization   Carboxin is not a skin irritant but it can cause serious eye irritation.

Subchronic Toxicity   A 90-day feeding study in rats at doses up to 1000 mg/kg body weight/day (20,000 ppm in the diet) revealed no gross pathological changes. Increased blood urea nitrogen and decreased hemoglobin were seen, but only in females at the highest dose. The LOEL was 30 mg/kg/day and involved microscopic inflammatory degenerative renal changes including cortical tubular degeneration. Fibrosis of the kidney medulla was observed at 100 mg/kg/day. In a parallel study with mice, female mortality was seen at the highest dose (912 mg/kg/day). No gross pathology was seen, but microscopic liver centrilobular hypertrophy was observed at higher doses (about 400 mg/kg/day and higher).

Chronic Toxicity   In a 2-year dietary studies in rats, a result similar to the 90-day study was obtained with chronic nephritis and degeneration of tubular cells observed at 200 ppm in males and 300 ppm in females (Cal EPA, 1994). No serious adverse effects were detected in a 1-year feeding study in dogs at the highest dose tested, 7500 ppm.

Carcinogenicity   In mice, no carcinogenic responses were recorded in dietary studies with doses as high as 751 (M) and 912 (F) mg/kg/day although decreased survival and liver hypertrophy were seen at the highest doses. An increase in pulmonary and alveolar–bronchiolar adenomas in males at the highest dose was judged probably not to be compound-related (U.S. EPA, 1989a). Results were also negative in a 2-year studies in rats with dietary levels up to 600 ppm. Because of the equivocal positive effect in male mice, carboxin was placed by the U.S. Environmental Protection Agency in carcinogen group D (not classifiable as to human carcinogenicity).

Mutagenicity/Genotoxicity   Carboxin is nonmutagenic or very weakly mutagenic in several bacterial and fungal cell systems (Adhikari and Grover, 1989; de Bertoldi *et al.*, 1980; Grover *et al.*, 1990; Moriya *et al.*, 1983; U.S. EPA, 1989a) and in the SOS microplate assay using *E. coli* (Venkat *et al.*, 1995). It was reported to cause dose-dependent clastogenic activity with a variety of chromosomal aberrations in rat bone marrow cells after *in vivo* administration at doses of 191 and 382 mg/kg, and in studies with plants (Adhikari and Grover, 1988, 1989).

However, in other similar tests with rats, the clastogenic response was negative at doses as high as 2000 mg/kg (Cal EPA, 1994). In studies with Chinese hamster ovary cells *in vitro* an increase in chromosomal aberrations was seen with metabolic activation, although false positives in this test are common (Cal EPA, 1994). Carboxin also caused unscheduled DNA repair in primary rat hepatocytes over the concentration range of 5.1 to 103 μg/ml (U.S. EPA, 1989a). The evidence regarding the genotoxicity of carboxin is therefore mixed, but a significant possibility does exist that carboxin has genotoxic effects.

Reproductive Toxicity   No treatment-related effects on reproductive performance were observed at 5–30 mg/kg/day in a three-generation study in rats, but moderate growth suppression was seen in nursing pups at 30 mg/kg/day (U.S. EPA, 1989a). A subsequent two-generation study (Cal EPA, 1994) confirmed this result but at 200 ppm (M) and 300 ppm (F) it also revealed the nephrotoxicity typically seen in rats with this compound.

Developmental Toxicity/Teratogenicity   In a developmental study in pregnant rats at 175 (but not 90) mg/kg/day, carboxin caused decreased fetal weight but this dose also caused decreased weight gain in the dams. No specific teratogenicity was observed. Rabbits dosed at 375 and 750 mg/kg/day during gestation had increased abortions but maternal toxicity was also observed. No developmental effects or fetal malformations were detected. Carboxin therefore does not appear to be a developmental toxicant or teratogen.

Human Toxicology   The only published example of human poisoning by carboxin involves a 7-year-old boy who ate several handfuls of carboxin-treated wheat seed. Symptoms included vomiting and headache which developed within 1 hr but were rapidly resolved after administration of an emetic. The amount of carboxin consumed is unclear (U.S. EPA, 1989a).

Biochemical Mechanism of Action   Carboxin is a strong inhibitor of succinic deydrogenase from a target fungus, *Ustilago maydis* (Mathre, 1971). With *Rhizoctonia solani* mitochondrial succinate dehydrogenase, carboxin has an I_{50} of 0.32 μM. White and Thorn (1975) obtained an I_{50} value of 0.5 μM in the same system. Reports of its activity against vertebrate mitochondrial complex II are varied. Mathre (1971) and Shimizu *et al.* (1992) report that carboxin is at least 10- to 20-fold more active against the sensitive fungal enzyme than complex II in mitochondria from rodent liver for which IC_{50} values were >30 μM. On the other hand Mowery *et al.* (1976, 1977) found that using various complex II preparation from bovine heart, carboxin was a potent inhibitor with I_{50} values below 1 μM. It is possible that differences both between the species and the types of complex II preparations studied can explain these discrepancies. Carboxin is also reported to inhibit oxidative metabolism and, specifically, succinate dehydrogenase in mitochondria from rat liver and bone but no estimate of its potency is given (Gosselin *et al.*, 1984).

Table 57.2
Acute Toxicity of Pesticides Acting as Inhibitors of Mitochondrial Complex II to Selected Nontarget Species

| | LD$_{50}$ (mg/kg) | | | | LC$_{50}$ (mg/l) | LC$_{50}$ (ppb) | |
| | Acute oral | | | | Acute dermal | Inhalation | (24–96 hr) | |
Compound	Rat (M; F)	Mouse (M)	Quail	Duck	Rat or rabbit	Rat	Fish[a]	*Daphnia*
Carboxin	3820	4150	24,000[b]	—	>4000	>20	1200–2300	84,400
Fenfuram	12,900	2450[c]	—	—	4500	>10.3	11,000	—
Flutolanil	>10,000	>10,000	>2000	>2000	>5000	>5.98	2300–5400	50,000[d]
Furametpyr	640; 590	660	—	—	>2000	—	1650	—
Mepronil	>10,000; >10,000	>10,000	>8000[b]	—	>10,000	>1.32	8600–10,000	>10,000
Oxycarboxin	5816; 1632	—	—	1250	>5000	>2.0	19,900–28,100	69,100
Thifluzamide	>5000	—	—	—	>5000	—	1200–2900	1600

[a] Range of values from several species, most commonly including the rainbow trout and carp.
[b] Data for hen.
[c] Data for cat.
[d] Six hr exposure.

Absorption, Metabolism, and Elimination When carboxin was fed to rats and rabbits by gavage at 235 mg/kg, approximately 40% of dose was excreted in the feces by rats mostly as unchanged carboxin, but only 10% was excreted through the fecal route in rabbits (Waring, 1973). In the urine, excretion was almost complete in 24 hr. Some parent compound was excreted in the urine unchanged, particularly by rats. Major metabolites were the products of *para* and *ortho* hydroxylation of the phenyl moiety followed by glucuronidation (Waring, 1973). Excretion of carboxin sulfoxide was not seen although some other sulfoxidized metabolites were identified. In dogs, oxidation to the sulfoxide occurred and this was excreted in the urine along with the parent compound (Gosselin *et al.*, 1984).

Environmental Fate and Toxicity Carboxin's toxicity to birds is very low (Table 57.2). In 8-day feeding studies with birds, the LC$_{50}$ was greater than >4640 ppm in the feed with mallard ducks and >10,000 ppm with bobwhite quail. Carboxin has a low acute toxicity to aquatic species including fish and invertebrates such as *Daphnia* (Table 57.2) and juvenile crayfish (LC$_{50}$ of 217 ppm). A bioconcentration factor of 34 has been calculated for carboxin which suggests little risk of accumulation by aquatic species.

Carboxin is converted to its sulfoxide *in vivo* and in water and soils, but further oxidation to the sulfone (oxycarboxin, see below) is extremely slow. Carboxin's half-life in soils is 1–3 days (Balasubramanya and Patil, 1980; Chin *et al.*, 1970, Wauchope *et al.*, 1992). The range of K_{oc} values (80–259) indicates a medium to high mobility in soil and significant leaching is observed in laboratory tests (U.S. EPA, 1989a).

Fenfuram: General Properties and Uses 2-Methylfuran-3-carboxanilide (Fig. 57.9), CAS Reg. No. 24691-80-3, was discovered by Shell Research Ltd. and developed by Aventis CropScience.

It exists as colorless to light brown crystals, m.p. 109–110°C, v.p. approximately 2×10^{-5} Pa (20°C), w.s. 100 ppm

(20°C). It is very stable to heat and to hydrolysis except under strongly acid or alkaline conditions.

Fenfuram is a systemic fungicide used in seed treatments for cereals under the trade name Pano-ram.

Toxicology Profile Published data regarding the toxicology of fenfuram are very limited. The primary source of data is Tomlin (2000).

Acute Toxicity Fenfuram has a low acute toxicity to vertebrates (Table 57.2). The intraperitoneal LD$_{50}$ in rats is 1490 m/kg.

Subchronic/Chronic Toxicity In a 90-day dietary study in dogs a NOEL of 300 mg/kg/day was observed. In a 2-year feeding study in rats, the NOEL was 10 mg/kg/day.

Mutagenicity Fenfuram was negative in the Ames assay.

Absorption, Metabolism, and Elimination After an oral dose, rats eliminated 83% in 16 hr, primarily in the urine.

Biochemical Mechanism of Action Fenfuram inhibits succinate oxidation in mitochondria from the target species, *Ustilago maydis,* with an I$_{50}$ value of 4.2 μM (White and Thorn, 1975).

Environmental Fate and Toxicity Fenfuram's toxicity to fish appears to be very low (Table 57.2). The half-life for fenfuram in soil is about 42 days and the K_{oc} value is about 300, indicating reasonably firm binding to soil organic matter (Augustijn-Beckers *et al.*, 1994).

Flutolanil: General Properties and Uses α, α, α-Trifluoro-3'-isopropoxy-*o*—toluanilide (Fig. 57.9), CAS Reg. No. 66332-96-5, was discovered by Nihon Nohyaku Co. Ltd. and is described by Araki and Yabutani (1981) and Araki (1985). Its development is reviewed by Kurono (1985) and Araki and Yabutani (1993).

It is exists as white crystals, m.p. 104–105°C, v.p. 6.5 × 10^{-6} Pa (25°C) (Tomlin, 2000), also widely cited as 1.8 × 10^{-3} Pa (20°C) (e.g., see Araki, 1985), w.s. 9.6 ppm (20°C), log P3.7. It is stable to heat (5 hr at 100°C) and in solution at pH 3–9. Flutolanil is relatively resistant to photodegradation (Tsao and Eto, 1991).

Flutolanil (NNF-136) is a systemic fungicide with both protective and curative actions on a wide range crops turf and ornamentals through foliar, seed, or soil application. Trade names include Folistar, Iota, Monarch, Moncut, Prostar, Protar, and Symphonie.

Toxicology Profile   The primary sources of data are Araki (1985) and the U.S. Environmental Protection Agency's IRIS (Integrated Risk Information System) data base (http://www.epa.gov/ngispgm3/iris). The toxicology of flutolanil has been reviewed in Japanese (Anonymous, 1988).

Acute Toxicity   Flutolanil has a very low acute toxicity to terrestrial vertebrates (Table 57.2).

Irritation/Sensitization   Flutolanil is nonirritating to the eyes and skin.

Subchronic Toxicity   Ninety-day feeding studies in rats and dogs gave LOELs of 200 and 400 mg/kg/day, respectively. The major finding was liver enlargement.

Chronic Toxicity   A 2-year feeding study in dogs had an LOEL of 250 mg/kg/day with emesis, salivation, soft stools, and lowered body weight gain as the major observations.

Carcinogenicity   Flutolanil was not oncogenic in a 2-year feeding study. The U.S. Environmental Protection Agency's category is Class E (evidence of noncarcinogenicity for humans).

Mutagencity/Genotoxicity   Flutolanil is not mutagenic in several standard tests (Ames assay, Rec DNA repair assay).

Reproductive Toxicity   In a three-generation reproduction and teratology study in rats, even at 10,000 ppm (662–1002 mg/kg/day) in the diet, no compound-related clinical signs of toxicity, mortality, or differences in food consumption were observed. No effect was seen on pregnancy or litter size but increased fetal mortality did occur, though only at a dietary level of 1000 ppm. Increased liver weight was found in all three generations. At both the 1000 and 10,000 ppm doses, reproductive toxicity was observed in the form of reduction in pup and, subsequently, in adult body weights in both sexes. Possible enlargement of the renal pelvis was seen in the high dose group.

Developmental Toxicity/Teratogenesis   A teratology study in rabbits had a LOEL of 200 mg/kg/day with an endpoint of increased resorptions. However, maternal toxicity was also seen at this dose. No teratogenic effects were seen.

Biochemical Mechanism of Action   Flutolanil was shown to inhibit growth of the fungal pathogen *Rhizoctonia solani* and to inhibit its succinate dehydrogenase complex 100% at 2 ppm *in vivo*, a concentration that also decreased ATP production by 50% (Hirooka *et al.*, 1990). At a concentration of 10 μM *in vitro*, flutolanil inhibited succinate dehydrogenase activity in mitochondria from target fungi by 80–90%, but only 15% inhibition was seen with the comparable enzyme from rat liver mitochondria (Motoba *et al.*, 1988). Yamano and Morita (1995) tested flutolanil against rat liver hepatocytes, mitochondria, and microsomes *in vitro* at 1 mM. No cytotoxicity or lipid peroxidation were observed and tissue sulfhydryl levels were not significantly affected. However, mitochondrial respiration was inhibited with a threshold (20% inhibition) at 0.1 mM.

Absorption, Metabolism, and Elimination   Flutolanil is rapidly metabolized and excreted in rats, mainly through oxidative removal of the isopropyl group and subsequent conjugation of the phenol (Murakami *et al.*, 1983).

Environmental Fate and Toxicity   Flutolanil has a low acute toxicity to birds (Table 57.2). It also has a very low acute toxicity to most aquatic species (Table 57.2). It has a low potential for bioconcentration from water by fish. A bioconcentration factor of 20 in carp, with a plateau reached after 1 day of exposure, and a moderately high clearance rate (half-life of 5.8 days) have been reported by Tsuda *et al.* (1992). Flutolanil undergoes firm binding to soil colloids and has a low leaching potential. Degradation in soils is primarily by microbial action but is relatively slow with half-lives in both flooded and upland soils in the range of 160 to 320 days.

Furametpyr: General Properties and Uses   (*RS*)-5-chloro-*N*-(1,3-dihydro-1,1,3-trimethylisobenzofuran-4-yl)-1,3-dimethylpyrazole-4-carboxamide (Fig. 57.9), CAS Reg. No. 123572-88-3, was discovered by Sumitomo Chemical Co. and is described by Oguri (1997).

It exists as colorless to light brown crystals, m.p 150°C, v.p. 4.7 × 10^{-6} Pa (25°), w.s. 225 ppm (25°C), log P2.36, HLC 7 × 10^{-6} Pa m^3 mol^{-1}. Furametpyr consists of a mixture of two optical isomers.

Furametpyr (S-658) is a systemic fungicide for the control of leaf sheath blight of rice under the trade name Limber.

Toxicological Profile   Available data are very limited. The primary source is Oguri (1997).

Acute Toxicity   The acute oral toxicity of furametpyr to mammals is higher than that of other members of the group, but it is still relatively modest (Table 57.2).

Irritation/Sensitization   Furmetapyr causes slight eye irritation and skin sensitization but no skin irritation.

Subchronic/Chronic Toxicity   No data seem to have been published regarding furametpyr's chronic or other toxic actions.

Biochemical Mechanism of Action   Furametpyr inhibits succinate but not NADH oxidation in mitochondria from the fungus *Rhizoctonia solani* (Oguri, 1997).

Environmental Fate and Toxicity   No data were found regarding furametpyr's toxicity to birds, but its toxicity to fish is low.

Mepronil: General Properties and Uses   3′-Isopropoxy-*o*-toluanilide (Fig. 57.9), CAS Reg. No. 55814-41-0, was discovered by Kumiai Chemical Industry Co. Ltd. and is described by Kawada *et al.* (1985). Mepronil's development is discussed by Doi (1981).

It exists as white crystals, m.p. 92–93°C, v.p. 5.6×10^{-5} Pa (20°C), w.s. 12.7 ppm (20°C), log P 3.66. It is stable to hydrolysis over the range of pH 5 to 9 and relatively stable to photolysis with 34–62% destruction by sunlight after 80 days exposure (Yumita and Yamamoto, 1982).

Mepronil (KCO-1) is a systemic fungicide with protective and curative actions in a broad range of crops against basidomycete fungi through seed treatment, soil, and foliar applications. Trade names include Basitac.

Toxicology Profile   The primary source of data is Doi (1981).

Acute Toxicity   The acute toxicity of mepronil to vertebrates is very low (Table 57.2). Even by intraperitoneal injection, the acute LD_{50} in rats and mice is over 5000 mg/kg.

Irritation/Sensitization   Mepronil is nonirritating to eyes and skin.

Subchronic/Chronic Toxicity   NOELs in 2-year feeding studies ranged from 5.9 mg/kg/day for male rats to 72.9 mg/kg/day in females. Results with mice gave NOELs of 13.7 and 17.8 mg/kg/day in males and females, respectively.

Mutagenicity/Genotoxicity   Mepronil is not mutagenic in standard tests.

Teratogenicity   Mepronil is not teratogenic in the rat or rabbit.

Biochemical Mechanism of Action   A series of substituted benzanilides, including mepronil, was shown to inhibit succinate dehydrogenase activity with considerable potency in isolated fungal mitochondria (Motoba *et al.*, 1988; White, 1987). Shimizu *et al.* (1992) also demonstrated that mepronil inhibited succinate oxidation in mitochondria isolated from the mycelia of the fungus *Rhizoctonia solani* with an I_{50} value of 0.25 μM. The oxidation of NADH was not inhibited. Mitochondria from other fungi, plants, and from rat and mouse liver were much less sensitive with I_{50} values for the vertebrate enzyme in the range of 50–100 μM. Yamano and Morita (1995) tested mepronil against rat liver hepatocytes, mitochondria, and microsomes *in vitro* at 1 mM. No cytotoxicity or lipid peroxidation were observed and tissue sulfhydryl levels were not

significantly affected. However, mitochondrial respiration was inhibited with a threshold (20% inhibition) at 0.1 mM.

Environmental Fate and Toxicity   Mepronil has a very low acute toxicity to birds and aquatic vertebrates and invertebrates (Table 57.2). The reported half-life for mepronil in flooded soils ranges from 46 to 51 days.

Oxycarboxin: General Properties and Uses   5,6-Dihydro-2-methyl-1,4-oxathiin-3-carboxanilide 4,4-dioxide (Fig. 57.9), CAS Reg. No. 5259-88-1, was discovered by Uniroyal Chemical Co. and is described by von Schmeling and Kulka (1966).

It exists as white crystals, m.p. 128–130°C, v.p. $<5.6 \times 10^{-6}$ Pa (25°C), w.s. 1400 ppm (25°C), log P 0.772, HLC $<1 \times 10$–6 Pa m^3 mol^{-1}. It is stable to heat but slowly hydrolyzed (half life of several weeks) at neutral pH and room temperature.

Oxycarboxin is a systemic fungicide with curative action, mainly used in foliar applications on turf and ornamentals but also used on some food crops. Trade names include Carbexsin, Carboject, Oxykisvax, and Plantvax.

Toxicology Profile   The primary sources of data are HSDB (2000) and Cal DFA (1987a).

Acute Toxicity   Oxycarboxin has a low acute toxicity to vertebrates (Table 57.2).

Irritation/Sensitization   Oycarboxin is a mild eye irritant but not a skin irritant.

Chronic Toxicity   In 2-year dietary studies a NOEL for rats was observed at 15 mg/kg/day based on minor thyroid changes and for dogs the NOEL was 75 mg/kg/day.

Mutagenicity/Genotoxicity   Oxycarboxin was not mutagenic in yeast and fungal assays (de Bertoldi *et al.*, 1980) or in the Ames assay (Moriya *et al.*, 1983).

Reproductive Toxicity   In a three-generation study in rats, no adverse reproductive effects were recorded at doses that were not toxic to the parents.

Biochemical Mechanism of Action   Oxycarboxin inhibits oxidative metabolism and specifically succinate dehydrogenase activity in both fungal (Mathre, 1971; White and Thorn, 1975) and vertebrate (Gosselin *et al.*, 1984) mitochondria, but the potency was much higher against the enzyme from the target species (*Rhizoctonia solani*, $I_{50} = 6.8$ μM; *Ustilago maydis*, $I_{50} = 8.0$ μM) than vertebrates (rat and mouse liver, $I_{50} = 50$–100 μM) (Shimizu *et al.*, 1992). It is less potent than carboxin as an inhibitor of complex II in both fungi and vertebrates (Mathre, 1971; Shimizu *et al.*, 1992; White and Thorn, 1975).

Environmental Fate and Toxicity   Oxycarboxin's acute toxicity to birds is relatively low (Table 57.2). In 8-day dietary studies, it also showed low toxicity to birds; bobwhite quail had an LC_{50} of >10,000 ppm and mallard ducks had an LC_{50} of >4640 ppm. Oxycarboxin has a notably low acute toxicity for fish and other aquatic species (Table 57.2).

The half-life of oxycarboxin in soil is 2–8 weeks with the most prominent metabolites resulting from the opening of the oxathiin ring. The corresponding aniline is also produced by amide hydrolysis. Its low log P value and high water solubility (K_d values ranging from 74 to 98) suggest that leaching in soil could occur quite readily and that bioconcentration in fish is unlikely to occur.

Thifluzamide: General Properties and Uses $2',6'$-Dibromo-2-methyl-$4'$-trifluoromethoxy-4-trifluoromethyl-1,3-thiazole-5-carboxanilide (Fig. 57.9), CAS Reg. No. 130000-40-7, was discovered by Monsanto and developed by Rohm & Haas. It is described by (O'Reilly *et al.*, 1992).

It exists as a white to light brown powder, m.p. 178–179°C, w.s. 1.6 ppm (20°C), log P4.1 and is stable to hydrolysis over the range pH 5–9.

Thifluzamide (MON 24000) is used as a seed and foliar fungicide on a wide range of crops and turfgrass under the trade name of Greatam.

Toxicology Profile   The primary source of data is O'Reilly *et al.* (1992).

Acute Toxicity   Thifluzamide shows a low acute toxicity to vertebrates, (Table 57.2).

Irritation/Sensitization   Thifluzamide is moderately irritating to the eyes and slightly irritating to skin.

Mutagenicity/Genotoxicity   Thiflizamide gave negative results in the Ames and mouse micronucleus assays.

Biochemical Mechanism of Action   Thifluzamide is a very potent inhibitor of succinate dehydrogenase from mitochondria isolated from *Rhizoctonia solani* with an I_{50} value of about 20 nM compared to 180 nM for carboxin (Phillips and Rejda-Heath, 1993).

Environmental Fate and Toxicity   Data are unavailable for the acute toxicity to birds, but in short term studies with bobwhite quail and mallard ducks, thifluzamide was practically nontoxic with LC_{50} values >5620 ppm in the diet. Its toxicity to aquatic organisms is also low (Table 57.2).

57.5 INHIBITORS OF COMPLEX III

57.5.1 INTRODUCTION

Until recently, very few pesticides had complex III as their primary site of action and none had broad usage. This has now changed with the introduction of a new class of broad-spectrum fungicides colloquially termed the "strobilurins" after the naturally occurring strobilurins from mushrooms that acted as their model. These are rapidly becoming a major component in fungal pathogen management programs worldwide. Remarkably, several other new fungicides, which are not in the strobilurin family, also have their toxic effect in target species through inhibition of complex III. Two compounds with activity as insecticides or acaricides also fall within this class.

At least three groups of inhibitors of complex III have been identified (Jordan *et al.*, 1999a; von Jagow and Link, 1986). The first group displaces ubiquinone from the Q_o binding on the low potential heme of cytochrome *b* located on the outer face of the inner mitochondrial membrane (Fig. 57.4; b, c). Several natural products including myxothiazol and the strobilurins bind at this site. A second group of inhibitors, the hydroxyquinones, acts at the Rieske iron sulfur center rather than cytochrome *b* (Fig. 60.45 bh). The third group, typified by antimycin A, displaces coenzyme Q from the Q_i binding site located toward the inner face of the inner mitochondrial membrane by binding to the high potential heme of cytochrome *b* (Fig. 60.45–66). The mechanism of operation of complex III and the molecular nature of the interactions of these inhibitors with the quinone binding sites have been reviewed by Berry *et al.* (1999). Pesticides are now in use that affect each of these three sites. Like most recently developed pesticides, they appear to have toxicological properties that indicate a high degree of safety to terrestrial species. A greater degree of risk may exist for aquatic organisms in some cases.

57.5.2 PROPERTIES OF SPECIFIC COMPOUNDS

57.5.2.1 Strobilurin Analogs

The strobilurins are an extremely important, new, and expanding group of fungicides which were developed from the naturally occurring strobilurins and oudemansins (Fig. 57.10). These natural compounds, which contain the key methyl (E)-β-methoxyacrylate grouping, are produced by fungi in the genera *Strobilurus* and *Oudemansiella*. They are fungicidal but too photounstable to be useful in agriculture. The discovery, development, and general properties of the commercial strobilurin fungicides have been reviewed by Beautement *et al.* (1991), Leroux (1996), Sauter *et al.* (1996, 1999), and Clough and Godfrey (1998). Important synthetic strobilurin fungicides include azoystrobin (Zeneca), pyraclostrobin (BASF), kresoxim-methyl (BASF), picoxystrobin (Zeneca), trifloxystrobin (Novartis), and metominostrobin (Shionogi). In the near future more strobilurins are likely to be developed including compounds with acaricidal (e.g., fluacrypyrim; Nippon Soda) as well as fungicidal activity. As a group, their toxicological properties appear to be near ideal with a high potency against pathogenic fungi but presenting little risk to most other organisms. Both natural and synthetic strobilurins have their primary toxic effect by inhibition of mitochondrial respiration in complex III (Becker

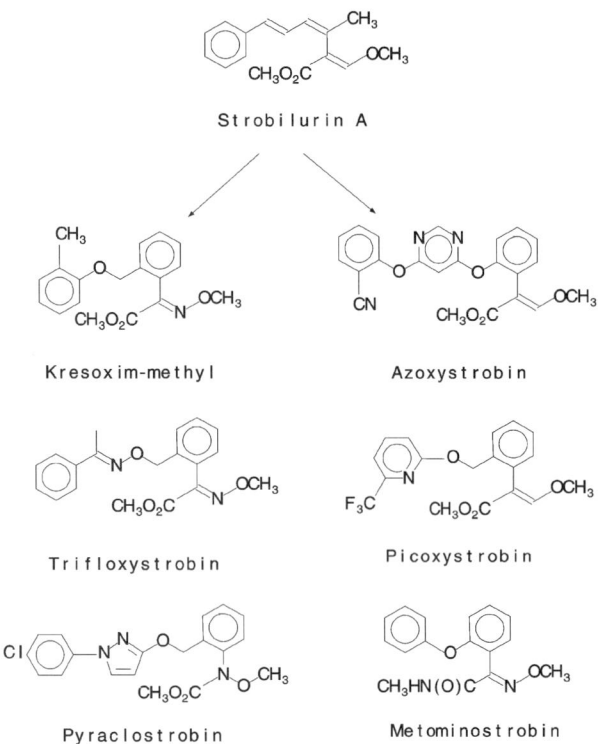

Figure 57.10   Pesticides that act as inhibitors of complex III—Strobilurin and the fungicides derived from it.

et al., 1981). The specific binding site has been shown to be within the Q_o domain (Fig. 57.4).

Available toxicology data indicate a high to very high degree of safety to mammals and birds and several strobilurins have been classified as reduced risk pesticides by the U.S. Environmental Protection Agency. Their acute toxicity is shown in Table 57.3. This high degree of safety probably does not arise primarily from an insensitivity of the site of action in higher organisms since the mitochondrial complex III of fungi, yeast, maize, insects, and rats is strongly inhibited by a range of strobilurin analogs *in vitro*. Only minor species selectivity is evident except that the plant enzyme is significantly less sensitive than the others (Röhl and Sauter, 1994; Sauter *et al.*, 1996). The major factor in their safety appears to be differential uptake and biotransformation, particularly the rapid hydrolysis of the ester group in higher organisms which deactivates the compound as a respiratory inhibitor (Köhle *et al.*, 1994). This view is supported by their generally high toxicity to aquatic species, both vertebrate and invertebrate, in standard bioassays which probably results from the rapid rate of uptake of these lipophilic compounds from water and their high intrinsic activity as respiratory inhibitors. The recent development of acaricidal analogs of strobilurins again indicates that this group of compounds is capable of inhibiting complex III across a broad range of organisms.

Because of their recent and continuing development, most of the toxicological information regarding these compounds must be drawn from the results of standard toxicology tests submitted

to regulatory authorities prior to registration. In these studies, the strobilurins generally show no, or only weak, evidence of mutagenicity, carcinogenicity, neurotoxicity, reproductive toxicity, or teratogenicity. An exception is kresoxim-methyl which has shown hepatic carcinogenic effects in rats at high dietary levels. Irritancy to skin and eye is either absent or mild in most cases. Trifloxystrobin is a strong dermal sensitizer but the other strobilurins do not share this characteristic.

Azoxystrobin: General Properties and Uses   Methyl (*E*)-2-{2-[6-(2-cyanophenoxy)pyrimidin-4-yloxy]phenyl}-3-methoxyacrylate (Fig. 57.10), CAS Reg. No. 131860-33-8, was discovered by Zeneca Agrochemicals and is described by Godwin *et al.* (1992).

It exists as a white powder, m.p. 116°C, v.p. 1.1×10^{-10} Pa (25°C), w.s. 6 ppm (20°C), log *P* 2.5, HLC 7.3×10^{-9} Pa m^3 mol^{-1}. It is table to hydrolysis. A half-life of 11–17 days was obtained in an aqueous photolytic study.

Azoxystrobin (ICIA5504) is a very broad spectrum fungicide with systemic activity and both protectant and curative actions used on a broad range of crops including fruits, vegetables, small grains, and turf grass. Trade names include Abound, Amistar, Bankit, Heritage, Ortiva, Priori, and Quadris. In 1999 axozystrobin was the leading proprietary fungicide in the world with sales of $415 million (Godwin *et al.*, 2000).

Toxicology Profile   The primary data sources is the U.S. EPA (1997b, 1997c).

Acute Toxicity   Azoxystrobin has a very low acute and chronic toxicity to mammals (Table 57.3).

Irritation/Sensitization   Azoxystrobin is a slight to moderate eye irritant and a slight skin irritant. It is not a dermal sensitizer.

Subchronic Toxicity   Sustained dietary exposure to azoxystrobin in vertebrates causes minimal toxicity. In 90-day dietary studies the LOEL was 211 mg/kg/day for rats and 250 mg/kg/day for dogs.

Chronic Toxicity   In a 2-year dietary study in mice the LOEL was found at 2000 ppm (272 (M) or 363 (F) mg/kg/day) marked by decreased weight gain and food utilization. In a 2-year dietary study in rats at a dose of 82 mg/kg/day, biliary toxicity was observed in males (but not females). No significant adverse effects were observed in dogs fed at 200 mg/kg/day in the diet for 1 year. At doses of 25 mg/kg/day and above, liver changes (increased weight and serum liver enzymes) were seen, but no histopathology was evident and the response was judged to be adaptive rather than toxic.

Carcinogenicity   Standard lifetime dietary studies with rats (1500 ppm) and mice (2000 ppm) revealed no compound-related increase in tumors. The U.S. Environmental Protection Agency considered azoxystrobin "not likely to be a human carcinogen."

Table 57.3
Acute Toxicity of Pesticides Acting as Inhibitors of Mitochondrial Complex III to Selected Nontarget Species

| Compound | LD_{50} (mg/kg) | | | | Acute dermal | LC_{50} (mg/l) Inhalation | LC_{50} (ppb) (24–96 hr) | |
| | Acute oral | | | | | | | |
	Rat (M; F)	Mouse (M)	Quail	Duck	Rat or rabbit	Rat	Fish[a]	Daphnia
Strobilurin analogs								
Azoxystrobin	>5000, >5000	>5000	>2000	>2000	>2000	0.96	470–1600	259
Kresoxim-methyl	>5000	—	>2150	—	>2000	>5.6	190–499	186
Metominostrobin	776; 708	1778	—	—	>2000	>1.88	17,500–22,500	14,000–22,300
Picoxystrobin	>5000	—	—	—	>2000	>2.12	65–75	18
Pyraclostrobin	>5000	—	>2000	—	>2000	>0.31 <1.07	6.2–77	15.7
Trifloxystrobin	>5000	—	>2000	>2250	>2000	>4.65	14–78	25
Other pesticides								
Acequinocyl	>5000	>5000	>2000	>2000	>2000	>0.84	>33,000	16
Cyazofamid	>5000	—	—	—	>2000	—	>70,500	—
Famoxadone	>5000	>5000	>2250	—	>2000	>5.3	11–49	12
Fenamidone	>5000; 2028	—	>2000	—	>2000	>2.1	740	—
Hydramethylnon	817; 1502	—	1828	>2510	>5000	2.9	90–1700	1140

[a]Range of values from several species, most commonly including the rainbow trout and bluegill.

Mutagenicity/Genotoxicity   Evidence regarding the genotoxicity of azoxystrobin is mixed. Negative results were obtained in the Ames, mouse micronucleus, and unscheduled DNA synthesis assays in rats, but the compound was weakly positive for forward mutations in the mouse lymphoma cell assay and for chromosomal aberrations in human lymphocytes *in vitro*. Since no clastogenic effects were seen *in vivo*, azoxystrobin was determined not to be genotoxic.

Reproductive Toxicity   No adverse reproductive effects were observed in a multigenerational study in rats. The NOEL for toxicity was found at 300 ppm (32 mg/kg/day) based on liver changes and body weight reductions in the parents. Biliary toxicity, again confined to adult males, was observed at 200 ppm in the form of hyperplasia and inflammation of the lining of the bile duct and hepatic proliferative cholangitis.

Developmental Toxicity/Teratogenicity   No developmental effects were seen in rabbits at doses as high as 500 mg/kg/day. In rats, no developmental effects were seen at doses that were not also maternally toxic. No evidence of teratogenicity was noted in either study.

Neurotoxicity   None was seen with a single dose of 200 mg/kg in rats or with subchronic dosage at 38.5 mg/kg/day.

Biochemical Mechanism of Action   The inhibitory effect on complex III is typical of other strobilurins and is specifically described by Wiggins and Jager (1994).

Absorption, Metabolism, and Elimination   After an oral dose, azoxystrobin is well absorbed in the rat. It is extensively metabolized and rapidly excreted, particularly in the feces, with the primary metabolic route being ester hydrolysis. Glutathione-S-transferase-catalyzed conjugations with glutathione also occur at several sites in the molecule *in vitro* with the major site of attack being the pyrimidine ring, but these conjugates were not observed *in vivo* (Turner and Joseph, 1998). Percutaneous absorption is minimal.

Environmental Fate and Toxicity   This aspect of azoxystrobin's properties has been reviewed by Pilling *et al.* (1996) and U.S. EPA (1997b). It has a very low toxicity to birds, but it is highly toxic to both freshwater fish and invertebrates (Table 57.3). Feeding bobwhite quail and mallard ducks for 8 days with azoxystrobin in the diet gave LC_{50} values over 5200 mg/kg/day in each case, and a chronic reproduction study in mallards had a LOEC at 3000 ppm. Its toxicity to estuarine and marine invertebrates is variable from moderate to very high based on studies with mysid shrimps (acute LC_{50} of 56 ppb) and pacific oyster larvae (acute LC_{50} of 1300 ppb). The chronic effects on aquatic invertebrates are also potent. An early life-stage chronic toxicity test in the fathead minnow gave a LOEC of 193 ppb, and a life-cycle toxicity study in *Daphnia* had a LOEC of 84 ppb.

In aerobic and anaerobic soil metabolism studies in the laboratory, a half-life of 72 to164 days was obtained, indicating a moderate degree of persistence. However, in field studies, azoxystrobin is degraded quite rapidly in soils with a half-life of 1 to 5 weeks. Both photodegradation and, to a lesser degree, microbial metabolism are involved in its dissipation since the compound is relatively stable to hydrolysis. The half-life for photolysis in soils is in the range of 11 to 15 days. With a typical K_{oc} of about 500 (range 300 to 1690) and K_d values in the range of 1.5 to 23 ml/g, depending on nature of the soil, azoxystrobin has a low to moderate potential for mobility in soil, but little movement down the soil profile was seen in field studies.

Kresoxim-Methyl: General Properties and Uses   Methyl (E)-2-methoxyimino-[2-(o-tolyloxymethyl)phenyl] acetate (Fig. 57.10), CAS Reg. No. 143390-89-0, was discovered by BASF AG and is described by Ammermann *et al.* (1992). Its development and structure–activity relations are reviewed by Sauter *et al.* (1996).

It exists as white crystals, m.p. 97–102°C, v.p. 2.3 × 10^{-6} Pa (20°C), w.s. 2 ppm (20°C), log P3.4, HLC 3.6 × 10^{-4} Pa m^3 mol^{-1}. It is slowly hydrolyzed in water at pH 7 (half-life 34 days) but much faster at pH 9 (half-life 7 hr).

Kresoxim-methyl (BAS 490F) is a long-lasting broad spectrum fungicide with protective and curative capabilities used on fruit, cereals, and greenhouse ornamentals. Trade names include Alliage, Candit, Cygnus, Discus, Mantra, Mentor, Sovran, and Stroby.

Toxicology Profile   The primary sources of data are U.S. EPA (1998b), FAO/WHO (1998), and Cal EPA (1999).

Acute Toxicity   Kresoxim-methyl has a very low acute toxicity to mammals (Table 57.3). No clinical signs of poisoning were observed in rats at doses of 5000 mg/kg.

Irritation/Sensitization   Kresoxim-methyl is not a dermal irritant or sensitizer, but it causes slight eye irritation.

Subchronic Toxicity   In 90-day dietary studies, azoxystrobin caused minimal toxicity at high doses. In mice the only effect seen at dietary levels up to 8000 ppm [1900 (M) and 2600 (F) mg/kg/day] was an adaptive increase in liver weight. In rats, the LOEL was 580 mg/kg/day based on decreased weight gain and changes in clinical chemistry parameters. In dogs, the LOEL was found at 25,000 ppm (770 mg/kg/day) based on vomiting and reduced body weight. Dermal application in rats at 1000 mg/kg/day for 21 days caused no observable effects.

Chronic Toxicity   In chronic studies, LOEL values in 1 to 2 year feeding studies in mice, rats, and dogs were about 350, 440, and 735 mg/kg/day, respectively. Effects noted include decreased food intake and body weight gain and the occurrence of microscopic liver and biliary alterations in rats. Histopathological examination revealed alterations in liver (amyloidosis) and kidney (renal papilliary necrosis) in mice. No notable adverse effects were seen in dogs.

Carcinogenicity   Liver carcinoma was observed in the lifetime rat feeding study in both sexes at 8000 ppm [370 (M) and 500 (F) mg/kg/day]. The findings included increased hepatocellular carcinoma and neoplastic changes in the biliary system. An extensive series of mechanistic studies in rats clearly indicate that kresoxim-methyl at this dose does not cause an increase in liver cell foci but does cause reversible hepatocellular proliferation. It therefore appears that it acts as a tumor promoter rather than an initiator, and it may therefore have a threshold for its tumorigenic action. It certainly appears that kresoxim-methyl is not genotoxic (below). Considerable discussion of this issue is provided in Cal EPA (1999). No carcinogenic response was seen in parallel lifetime feeding studies in mice. Kresoxim-methyl has been given an interim carcinogen classification of category C (possible human carcinogen) by the U.S. Environmental Protection Agency.

Mutagenicity/Genotoxicity   Kresoxim-methyl was uniformly negative in an extensive battery of standard tests for mutagenic and clastogenic activity using microbial and mammalian cells *in vitro* and *in vivo* studies with mammals.

Reproductive Toxicity   No effects on reproduction were observed in rats in a two-generation study with doses up to 1000 ppm in the diet. At 4000 ppm, reduced weight gain in pups was observed but this dose was also maternotoxic.

Developmental Toxicity/Teratogenicity   In the two-generation reproductive toxicity study in rats, decreased pinna unfolding occurred at 4000 ppm. An increase in incomplete vertebral ossification was found in rats at a dose of 1000 mg/kg/day during gestation which was not toxic to the mothers. No developmental or teratogenic effects were observed in rabbits given doses up to 1000 mg/kg/day.

Neurotoxicity   A single dose of 2000 mg/kg failed to induce any behavioral changes or neuropathology in rats. Subchronic (90-day) feeding studies at doses up to 16,000 ppm also proved negative for neurotoxicity.

Biochemical Mechanism of Action   Using cytochrome redshift analysis, Röhl (1994) showed that kresoxim-methyl binds to the bc_1 complex of yeast mitochondria with high affinity ($K_d = 70$ nM) and a single binding site. Röhl and Sauter (1994) showed that differences in the sensitivities of complex III from a broad range of species [yeast, *Botrytis cinerea*, corn (maize), house fly, and rat] to kresoxim-methyl and related strobilurins were relatively small, though the rat enzyme tended to be less sensitive than that from *Botrytis*. In the case of kresoxim-methyl this interspecific difference in I$_{50}$ values was about 10-fold. The corn enzyme was the least sensitive overall. Although, as these authors stress, the quantitative comparison of I$_{50}$ values obtained with different enzyme preparations must be treated with caution, this suggests that much of the very high selective toxicity of kresoxim-methyl must reside in pharmacokinetic factors. This was confirmed by Sauter *et al.* (1995) who conclude that rapid degradation by hydrolysis is a critical factor governing the low toxicity of this compound to vertebrates.

Absorption, Metabolism, and Elimination   Kresoxim-methyl is poorly absorbed after an oral dose in rats with 50% uptake at 50 mg/kg and 25% at 500 mg/kg. The absorbed material is quickly eliminated in urine (20 to 30%) and feces (70 to 80%) with extensive metabolism. Peak plasma levels were reached in 0.5 to 1 hr and 8 hr at the low and high dose, respectively. Plasma half-lives range from 16.9 to 30.5 hr, depending on the dose. Ester hydrolysis is the first major metabolic step, but there are multiple sites of biotransformation on the molecule and 34 metabolites were identified from rats. Ester hydrolysis by plasma from rats and mice was very rapid (half-life of 2 to 5 min). The metabolism of kresoxim-methyl by hepatocytes from a range of vertebrate species is described and compared to its metabolism by these species *in vivo* by Salmon and Kohl (1996).

Environmental Fate and Toxicity   Kresoxim-methyl has a low toxicity to birds. It is highly toxic to aquatic vertebrates and invertebrates in standard laboratory tests (Table 57.3), but studies in more complex ecosystems indicate that it is not hazardous to aquatic organisms, when used as recommended, due to its rapid breakdown.

Kresoxim-methyl is rapidly degraded in soils with a half-life of 1–2 days. The primary metabolite is the free acid. Its moderate soil absorption (K_{oc} 219–372) suggests the possibility of significant mobility in soil.

Metominostrobin: General   Properties   and   Uses
(E)-2-methoxyimino-N-methyl-2-(2-phenoxyphenyl)acetamide (Fig. 57.10), CAS Reg. No. 133408-50-1, was discovered by Shionogi Co. Ltd. and is described by Furuta (1999). Structure–fungicidal activity relationships in this series are described by Kataoka *et al.* (1998).

It exists as a white crystalline powder, m.p. 87–89°C, v.p. 1.8×10^{-5} Pa (25°C), w.s. 128 ppm (20°C), log P2.32. Metominostrobin exists as geometrical isomers at the oxime moiety. The E-isomer is 5- to 20-fold more fungicidal than the Z-isomer and the commercial product consists only of the E-form (Kataoka *et al.*, 1998).

Metominostrobin (SSF-126) is registered in several Asian countries as a systemic long-lasting preventative and curative agent against rice blast under the trade name of Oribright.

Toxicology Profile   The primary source of data is Furuta (1999).

Acute Toxicity   The acute toxicity to rats and mice is somewhat higher than with other strobilurin fungicides but it is still quite low (Table 57.3).

Irritation/Sensitization   The formulated material causes slight eye irritation, but it is not a skin irritant or sensitizer.

Mutagenicity/Genotoxicity   Metominostrobin was negative in a battery of four genotoxicity tests involving mutagenic and clastogenic endpoints in bacteria and mammals.

Biochemical Mechanism of Action   Metominostrobin differs from the other members of this class in two ways. First it was not developed using the natural strobilurins as a model but through an independent lead from screening synthetic chemicals (Kataoka *et al.*, 1998). It thus represents an example of convergent evolution in chemical discovery. It is also differs from other stobilurins in being an amide rather than an ester. Despite these differences, its mode of action is the same as that of the other strobilurins involving inhibition of respiration by binding to the cytochrome bc_1 complex (Furuta, 1999; Mizutani *et al.*, 1996). It is proposed that, as part of its action, the inhibition of complex III induces the production of cytotoxic superoxide radical anions in target fungi (Furuta, 1999).

Environmental Fate and Toxicity   Data on the acute toxicity to birds were not found, but in an 8-day dietary study in mallard ducks the LC_{50} value was >5200 ppm, indicating a low degree of sensitivity to this compound. The low toxicity to aquatic species in standard tests is very notable compared to that of the other strobilurins so far disclosed (Table 57.3). The half-life in aerobic soil is 98 days, indicating a moderate level of environmental persistence.

Picoxystrobin: General Properties and Uses   Methyl (E)-2-{2-[6-(trifluoromethyl)pyridin-2-yloxymethyl]-phenyl}-3-methoxyacrylate (Fig. 57.10), CAS Reg. No. 117428-22-5, was discovered by Zeneca Agrochemicals and is described by Godwin *et al.* (2000).

It exists as a solid, m.p. 75°C, v.p. 5.5×10^{-6} Pa (20°C), log P3.6, w.s. 3.1 ppm (20°C). Picoxystrobin is degraded fairly rapidly in water with a half-life of 7–15 days.

Picoxystrobin (ZEN 90160) is being developed as a broad spectrum fungicide with preventative and curative actions specifically intended for use on cereals.

Toxicology Profile   The primary source of data is Godwin *et al.* (2000). Only an outline of the toxicology data for picoxystrobin is currently available.

Acute Toxicity   Picoxystrobin has a very low acute toxicity to the rat by the oral, dermal, and inhalation routes (Table 57.3).

Irritation/Sensitization   Picoxystrobin is not a skin or eye irritant or a dermal sensitizer.

Carcinogenicity   No evidence of carcinogencity was seen in lifetime feeding studies in rats and mice.

Genotoxicity   No genotoxicity was observed in a standard battery of tests.

Reproductive Toxicity   No reproductive toxicity was observed in a multigenerational study in rats.

Developmental Toxicity/Teratogenicity   No adverse effects were observed in developmental studies in the rabbit and rat.

Absorption, Metabolism, and Elimination   Studies in rats showed that picoxystrobin is well absorbed, extensively metabolized, and rapidly eliminated. Dermal absorption is low.

Environmental Fate and Toxicity No acute toxicity data for birds were found, but short-term and subchronic feeding studies with birds revealed low toxicity (e.g., it had a 21-week NOEL of 1350 mg/kg/day in mallard ducks). Picoxystrobin is highly toxic to aquatic species in laboratory bioassays (Table 57.3). However, studies under normal use conditions in the field indicated a low level of risk to aquatic species in practice. The BCF in fish is 290, indicating a low to moderate bioaccumulation capability. Picoxystrobin degrades rapidly in the soil with a half-life of 3–35 days under field conditions. It is quite firmly bound to soil components (K_{oc} 790–1200), indicating a low potential for leaching.

Pyraclostrobin: General Properties and Uses

Methyl N-(2-{[1-(4-chlorophenyl)-$1H$-pyrazol-3-yl]oxymethyl}phenyl)-N-methoxycarbamate (Fig. 57.10), CAS Reg. No. 175013-18-0, was discovered by BASF Corp. and is described by Ammermann *et al.* (2000).

It exists as white to light beige crystals, m.p. 64–65°C, v.p. 2.6×10^{-8} Pa (20°C), log P 3.99, w.s. 1.99 ppm (20°C), HLC 5.3×10^{-6} Pa m^3 mol^{-1}. It is stable to hydrolysis at pH 5–7 (half-life >30 days) but is quite rapidly photolyzed with a half-life less than 2 hr.

Pyraclostrobin (BAS 500 F) is a very broad spectrum fungicide with preventative and curative properties and a long residual action. It affects all stages of fungal growth and has uses on fruits, vegetables, small grains, and grasses. Trade names include Cabrio EG and Headline.

Toxicology Profile Primary sources of data are Ammermann *et al.* (2000) and Cal EPA (2001).

Acute Toxicity Pyraclostrobin has a very low oral toxicity to mammals though it is somewhat more toxic by inhalation (Table 57.3).

Irritation/Sensitization Pyraclostrobin causes slight eye and moderate skin irritation. It is not a dermal sensitizer.

Subchronic Toxicity Hyperplasia of the duodenal mucosa and increases in liver and spleen weights were observed in rats fed pyraclostrobin at 500 ppm and above in a 90-day dietary study. Histological findings at doses as low as 150 ppm (11.7 mg/kg/day) included hepatocellular hypertrophy, extramedullary hematopoiesis, distension of the sinusoids, and histocytosis of the spleen. These effects were the basis for setting the LOEL. In a 90-day dietary study in dogs, hypertrophy of the duodenal mucosa was seen at 450 ppm (13.3 mg/kg/day). Reduced boy weights and changes in blood chemistry also were seen at this dose. Mice, in a 90-day feeding study, also showed thickening of the duodenal mucosa together with erosion or ulcers in the glandular stomach and a decrease in lipid vacuolization in the adrenal cortex. Females were more sensitive than males with adrenal effects occurring at 50 ppm (12.9 mg/kg/day).

Chronic Toxicity No major adverse effects were seen in either rats or dogs in typical chronic dietary studies. In the 2-year study in rats, changes in liver-derived serum enzymes and a slight decrease in body weight were observed at 200 ppm. In a second study to determine carcinogenicity, hepatocelluar necrosis was thought to be treatment-related in rats at 200 ppm. In dogs the LOEL was obtained at 400 ppm (11 mg/kg/day) based on increased diarrhea and lowered weight gains.

Carcinogenicity No evidence for carcinogenicity was obtained in long-term rat and mouse dietary studies.

Mutagenicity/Genotoxicity Pyraclostrobin was not mutagenic or clastogenic in a battery of five typical tests in microbial and mammalian systems.

Reproductive Toxicity No results of toxicological concern were seen in rats in a two-generation dietary study with doses up to 300 ppm.

Developmental Toxicity/Teratogenicity Developmental toxicity studies were negative in the rat and rabbit. Early resorptions were seen in rabbits at higher doses (5 mg/kg/day or greater) but these doses also elicited maternal toxicity. No teratogenic effects were observed.

Neurotoxicity No evidence for neurotoxicity was discovered in a battery of neurobehavioral and neuropathological assays in rats at acute oral doses up to 1000 mg/kg, or in a 90-day test at 50 mg/kg/day (males) or 112 mg/kg/day (females).

Biochemical Mechanism of Action Pyraclostrobin inhibits complex III from yeast and fungus with IC$_{50}$ values of 20–29 nM (Ammermann *et al.*, 2000).

Absorption, Metabolism, and Elimination Only about 50% of an oral dose of either 5 or 50 mg/kg pyraclostrobin was absorbed in rats. The absorbed dose was rapidly metabolized and eliminated in the bile (33% of the dose) and urine (10–15% of the dose). Major routes of metabolism involved demethoxylation and hydroxylation of the pyrazole and other ring systems followed by glucuronidation. No sign of tissue bioaccumulation was observed.

Environmental Fate and Toxicity Pyraclostrobin has a low toxicity to birds, but it shows an extremely high level of toxicity to fish and other aquatic species in laboratory tests (Table 57.3). The toxicity to estuarine and marine invertebrates is equally high. Mysid shrimps have a 96-hr LC$_{50}$ of 4.2 ppb and the EC$_{50}$ for the inhibition of shell deposition in oysters is 12.5 ppb. However, it is claimed that in practice, risk to aquatic species is likely to be minimal due to the low levels of exposure. Pyraclostrobin is rapidly degraded in aerobic soils (the half-lives in the field range from 2 to 37 days). It is immobile in soil (K_{oc} 6000–16,000 ml/g) and therefore unlikely to leach.

Trifloxystrobin: General Properties and Uses Methyl (E)-methoxyimino-{(E)-α-[1-(α, α, α-trifluoro-m-tolyl)ethyl-idene-aminooxy]-o-tolyl} acetate (Fig. 57.10), CAS Reg. No. 141517-21-7, was discovered by Novartis Crop Protection, Inc. and is described by Margot *et al.* (1998).

It exists as a white powder, m.p. 73°c, v.p. 3.4×10^{-6} Pa (25°C), w.s. 0.61 ppm (25°C), log P 4.5, HLC 2.3×10^{-3} Pa m^3 mol^{-1}. Trifloxystrobin has two oxime linkages, each showing geometrical isomerism. The commercial compound is the E, E-isomer. The hydrolysis half-life is 11.4 weeks at pH 7 and 27 hr at pH 9. It is stable at pH 5.

Trifloxystrobin (CGA-279202) is a very broad spectrum foliar fungicide registered for use on fruits, vegetables, turf, and ornamentals. Trade names include Compass, Flint, and Stratego.

Toxicology Profile The primary sources of data are Margot *et al.* (1998), U.S. EPA (1999b), Anonymous (2000a), and Cal EPA (2000a).

Acute Toxicity Trifloxystrobin shows a very low acute toxicity to mammals and birds (Table 57.3).

Irritation/Sensitization Trifloxystrobin is a strong dermal sensitizer in the maximization test in guinea pigs but not in the Beuhler test. It is a mild eye and skin irritant.

Subchronic Toxicity In 90-day feeding studies, no remarkable findings were made in mice at 500 ppm but microscopic abnormalities in liver and spleen were observed at 7000 ppm (1275–1650 mg/kg/day). Blood chemistry and organ weights were affected in dogs at 500 mg/kg /day. In rats, pancreatic hypertrophy was the most sensitive endpoint, seen at 2000 ppm (130 mg/kg/day).

Chronic Toxicity In chronic dietary studies, mice fed 1000 ppm in diet for 18 months developed hepatocellular hypertrophy and focal liver necrosis. Rats showed reduced weight gain at 750 ppm and this was associated with a decrease in tumor incidence which was attributed to the decreased body weight. In a 1-year study in dogs, clinical signs, increased liver weights, and hepatocellular hypertrophy were noted at 50 mg/kg/day.

Carcinogenicity Trifloxystrobin is regarded by the U.S. Environmental Protection Agency as "unlikely to be a human carcinogen" based on negative studies in rats and mice.

Mutagenicity/Genotoxicity No adverse effects were observed in a standard battery of tests for clastogenicity and DNA repair. An increased mutation rate was observed in Chinese Hamster V79 cells, but trifloxystrobin was negative for mutagenicity in the Ames *Salmonella* test.

Reproductive Toxicity In a two-generation study in rats, no reproductive effects were observed at the highest dose, 1500 ppm.

Developmental Toxicity/Teratogenicity In a 2-year dietary study in rats, the most sensitive effect was a reduction in pup weight gain at 750 ppm. Teratology studies in with dietary exposure of pregnant rats and rabbits gave no indication of higher sensitivity to trifloxystrobin *in utero* compared to maternal effects. The only effect noted was enlargement of the thymus gland in rats at 1000 mg/kg.

Neurotoxicity No neurotoxicity was observed in rats at single oral dose of 2000 mg/kg in a functional observation test battery.

Biochemical Mechanism of Action Like other strobilurins, trifloxystrobin inhibits respiration at complex III (Margot *et al.*, 1998).

Absorption, Metabolism, and Elimination In rats, goats, and poultry, trifloxystrobin was poorly absorbed from the gastrointestinal tract and much was excreted in the feces unchanged. In rats, the absorbed compound was rapidly cleared (tissue half-life of 13 to 42 hr) with extensive metabolism, particularly through hydrolysis of the ester group. Other significant metabolic routes were O-demethylation of the methoxyimino group and oxidation of the methyl side chain to the corresponding alcohol and carboxylic acid. Percutaneous absorption is very slight.

Environmental Fate and Toxicity Trifloxystrobin has a low acute toxicity to birds (Table 57.3). Prolonged dietary exposure at levels of 320 ppm (bobwhite quail) or 500 ppm had no effects on health or reproduction. It is extremely toxic to fish and several kinds of aquatic invertebrates. The LC$_{50}$ to mysid shrimp is 9 ppb (Anonymous, 2000a). Bioconcentration in fish is limited, probably due to rapid metabolism and depuration. Trifloxystrobin is rapidly degraded in surface water by microbial action with a half-life of a few hours. The photolysis half-life in water is 31.5 hr with the initial reaction being E to Z isomerization. Trifloxystrobin binds firmly to soil particles (log K_{oc} 1642–3745 in five soils) and its half-life in soils in field studies ranges from a 1.9 to 16 (mean 5.4) days, indicating a low environmental persistence and leaching potential (Anonymous, 2000a).

57.5.2.2 Other Pesticidal Inhibitors of Complex III

Cyazofamid, famoxadone, and fenamidone are three other recent fungicides which inhibit mitochondrial respiration at complex III but that fall outside the strobilurin chemical class. Famoxadone and fenamidone, having obvious structural similarities and a similar spectrum of fungicidal activity, form a subclass of their own. They act at the same general biochemical site as the strobilurins. Cyazofamid is in a separate structural class and inhibits complex III at a different site than the compounds so far discussed. Two pesticides acting on invertebrates, acequinoyl (an acaricide) and hydramethylnon (an insecticide), are also thought to have their primary pesticidal actions as complex III inhibitors.

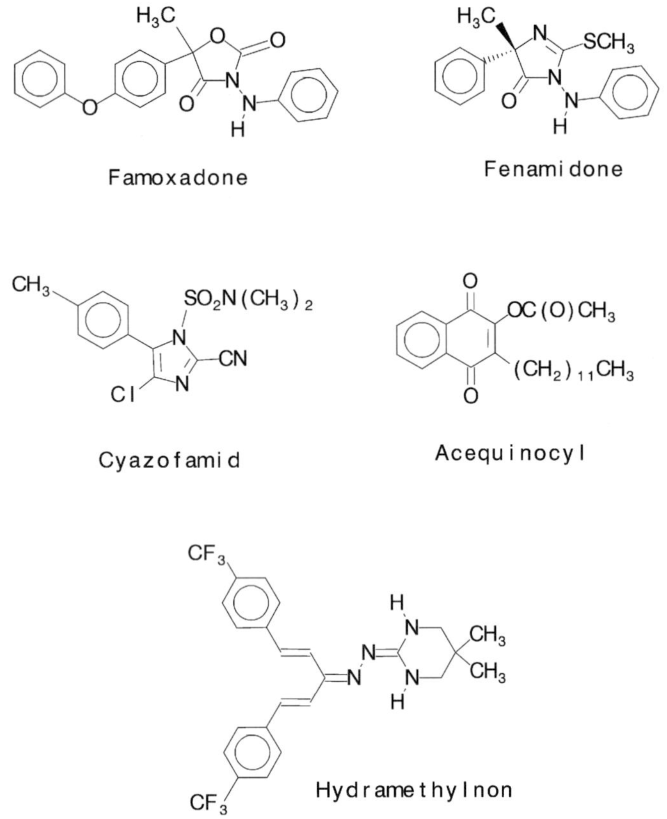

Famoxadone

Fenamidone

Cyazofamid

Acequinocyl

Hydramethylnon

Figure 57.11 Pesticides that act as inhibitors of complex III—Other inhibitors.

Cyazofamid: General Properties and Uses 4-Chloro-2-cyano-N,N-dimethyl-5-p-tolylimidazole-1-sulfonamide (Fig. 57.11), CAS Reg. No. 120116-88-3, was discovered by Ishihara Sangyo Kaisha, Ltd. and is described by Mitani et al. (1998).

It exists as an ivory powder, m.p. 153°C, v.p. <1.3×10^{-5} Pa, w.s. 0.12 ppm (20°C, pH 5), log P3.2 (25°C).

Cyazofamid (IKF-916) is a new systemic foliar and soil fungicide. Trade names include Docious, Mildust, and Ranman.

Toxicology Profile The primary source of data, which are so far very limited, is Mitani et al. (1998).

Acute Toxicity Cyazofamid appears to have a low acute toxicity to vertebrates (Table 57.3).

Irritation/Sensitization Data are not available.

Subchronic/Chronic Toxicity Cyazofamid caused no toxic effects in dogs fed at 1000 mg/kg/day in a 90-day study.

Mutagenicity/Genotoxicity Cyazofamid is negative in the Ames bacterial mutagenesis test.

Biochemical Mechanism of Action Cyazofamid is reported to inhibit complex III but at the Q_i site (antimycin site) which

differs from that of other recent fungicidal inhibitors of complex III which act at the Q_o site (Fig. 57.4). It is claimed to be specific in its inhibitory action to mitochondria from oomycete fungi (Mitani et al., 1998).

Environmental Fate and Toxicity Too few data are yet available on cyazofamid's acute effects on birds and fish to judge its level of toxicity to these organisms, but limited data for fish (carp) indicate a very low level of toxicity (Table 57.3). With a K_{oc} value of 490–6300 and a half-life in soil of 4–5 days, cyazofamid binds firmly to soils and undergoes rapid environmental degradation (Mitani et al., 1998).

Famoxadone: General Properties and Uses 3-Anilino-5-methyl-5-(4-phenoxyphenyl)-1,3-oxazolidine-2,4-dione (Fig. 57.11), CAS Reg. No. 131807-57-3, was discovered by DuPont Agricultural Products and is described by Joshi and Sternberg (1996). Its discovery, development, and structure–activity relations are discussed by Sternberg et al. (2001).

It exists as a pale cream powder, m.p. 140–142°C, v.p. 6.4×10^{-7} Pa (20°C), w.s. 52 ppb (20°C), log P4.65 (pH 7), HLC 4.6×10^{-3} Pa m^3 mol^{-1} (20°C). The hydrolytic half-life is 2 days at pH 7. Hydrolysis is more rapid under alkaline conditions and slower at acidic pH (Jernberg and Lee, 1999). Famoxadone exists as a pair of optical isomers. The S-isomer is significantly more fungitoxic than the R-isomer.

Famoxadone (DPX-JE874) is a new broad spectrum fungicide for vegetables, fruits, and cereals. It has both preventative and curative capability. Trade names include Charisma and Famoxate.

Toxicology Profile The primary source of data is Anonymous (2000b).

Acute Toxicity Famoxadone is practically nontoxic to mammals by all routes of exposure (Table 57.3).

Irritation/Sensitization Famoxadone is a minimal skin and eye irritant. It does not cause dermal sensitization.

Subchronic Toxicity NOELs of 40, 200, and 350 ppm were obtained in 90-day dietary studies in dogs, rats, and mice, respectively.

Chronic Toxicity The long-term (1–2 year) dietary NOELs were also 200 ppm in rats and 40 ppm in dogs. A NOEL of 700 ppm was established in mice. A NOEL of 100 mg/kg/day was observed when famoxadone was given to monkeys by gavage for 1 year. Effects seen in these studies at higher doses (LOELs) included hepatotoxicity in rats and mice and hemolysis in rats and monkeys. Lens opacities were seen in dogs fed 300 ppm for 1 year.

Carcinogenicity No carcinogenic response was observed in long-term feeding studies in rats and mice.

Mutagenicity/Genotoxicity Famoxadone was positive for chromosomal aberrations in an *in vitro* test, but negative in bacterial and mammalian mutation and unscheduled DNA synthesis tests *in vitro*, in a mouse micronucleus test, and in an unscheduled DNA synthesis tests *in vivo*. The weight of evidence therefore suggest that famoxadone is not genotoxic.

Reproductive Toxicity No reproductive effects were seen in a two-generation study in rats at doses below those causing maternal toxicity. Pup weight was decreased at 800 ppm.

Developmental Toxicity/Teratogenicity No teratogenic or developmental effects were seen in rats or rabbits at the highest doses tested (1000 mg/kg/day).

Neurotoxicity No neurotoxic effects were observed in rats with dietary exposure at 800 ppm for 90 days.

Biochemical Mechanism of Action Studies establishing that famoxadone is an extremely potent Inhibitor of mitochondrial electron transport acting at complex III in mitochondria from fungi, plants, and mammals are reviewed by Jordan *et al.* (1999a, b). The site of inhibition is cytochrome *b* within the Q_0 domain which prevents the transfer of electrons from cytochrome *b* to cytochrome c_1 (Fig. 57.4). The site appears to be close to, but not fully identical with, the binding sites on cytochrome *b* of myxothiazol on the one hand and the strobilurins on the other. However, field isolates of the fungus *Mycosphaerella fijiensis* having a point mutation in the target site that caused resistance to strobilurin fungicides also showed cross-resistance to famoxadone (Sierotzki *et al.*, 2000).

Famoxodone shows little selectivity at the target site level since I_{50} values for electron transport in rat and beef heart submitochondrial particles are in the range of 10–20 nM. These are somewhat lower than the I_{50} values for several comparable preparations from fungi. The $S(-)$ isomer is approximately 100-fold more active as an inhibitor than the $R(+)$ isomer and 25- to 30-fold more active in disease control (Jordan *et al.*, 1999a). Famoxadone is notably more potent as an inhibitor of complex III from rat heart and fungal mitochondria than azoxystrobin and kresoxim-methyl (Anonymous, 2000b).

Absorption, Metabolism, and Elimination After an oral dose famoxadone is poorly absorbed and rapidly excreted in mammals, mainly in the feces. Hydroxylation of the two phenyl rings at the *para* position is the major routes of metabolism (Lee *et al.*, 1999).

Environmental Fate and Toxicity Famoxadone has a low acute toxicity to birds (Table 57.3). Dietary studies in mallard ducks and quail (probably over 8 days) also indicated a low toxicity with LC_{50} values > 5620 ppm. In standard laboratory assays, the acute toxicity to aquatic species is very high, including both vertebrates and invertebrates (Table 57.3). *Daphnia*, oysters, and mysid shrimp all have 48–96 hr EC_{50}s of 1.4 to 12 ppb. It is believed that these potentially negative effects are likely to be minimized in practice by the rapid breakdown of famoxadone in water and other environmental media and its strong binding to particulates (Jernberg and Lee, 1999).

With an average K_{oc} of 3740 ml/g and a half-life in soils ranging from 6 to 12 days (Jernberg and Lee, 1999), famoxadone degrades rapidly and is unlikely to leach into groundwater. The half-life in the water phase of natural systems is less than 0.5 hr.

Fenamidone: General Properties and Uses *S*-5-methyl-2-methylthio-5-phenyl-3-phenylamino-3,5-dihydro-4H-imidazol-4-one (Fig. 57.11), CAS Reg. No. 161326-34-7, was discovered by Rhône-Poulenc Agro. and is described by Mercer *et al.* (1998).

It exists as a white woolly powder, m.p. 137°C, v.p. 3.4 × 10^{-7} Pa (25°C), w.s. 7.8 ppm (20°C), log *P* 2.8. Only the *S*-isomer is active and the commercial product is stereospecific for this isomer.

Fenamidone (RPA 407213) is a potent fungicide from a new chemical class primarily active against downy mildews. It has both curative and protective actions. Trade names include Fenomen and Reason.

Toxicology Profile The primary sources of data are Mercer *et al.* (1998) and Anonymous (1999b).

Acute Toxicity Fenamidone has a low to very low acute toxicity to mammals (Table 57.3).

Irritation/Sensitization Fenamidone is not a skin or eye irritant nor is it a dermal sensitizer.

Mutagenicity/Genotoxicity Fenamidone is negative in the Ames and mouse micronucleus assays.

Developmental Toxicity/Teratogenicity Fenamidone is non-teratogenic in rats and rabbits.

Biochemical Mechanism of Action Fenamidone inhibits electron transport in complex III. The exact site of action within the complex is unknown. With the *S*-enantiomer, the I_{50} value for the inhibition of respiration in mushroom mitochondria is 0.56 μM. The *R*-enantiomer is much less active (Mercer *et al.*, 1998).

Environmental Fate and Toxicity The acute toxicity of fenamidone to birds is low (Table 57.3) and 8-day dietary studies with bobwhite quail and mallard ducks also reveal a very low toxicity with an LC_{50} > 5200 ppm (Mercer *et al.*, 1998). The toxicity to fish is high (Table 57.3) but it is claimed that fenamidone's impact on aquatic species is likely to be low when it is used according to the label (Anonymous, 1999b). The soil half-life is short (<10 days). Fenamidone is bound to soil fairly strongly (K_{oc} > 400) and leaching is unlikely.

Acequinocyl: General Properties and Uses 3-Dodecyl-2-hydroxy-1,4-naphthoquinone acetate (Fig. 57.11), CAS Reg. No. 57960-19-7, was discovered by DuPont and is under development by Agro-Kanesho Co. Ltd. and Tomen Agro. It is described by Kinoshita *et al.* (1999) and Wakasa and Watanabe (1999).

It exists as a fine yellow powder, m.p. 60°C, v.p. 5.18 × 10^{-5} Pa (40°C), w.s. 6.7 ppb (25°C), log $P > 6.2$. Hydrolysis half-life (pH 7, 25°C) is 53 hr. Acequinocyl is less stable at higher pH (half-life is 76 min at pH 9) and more stable under acidic conditions (half-life is 86 days at pH 4).

Acequinocyl is a highly lipophilic naphthoquinone derivative. Similar compounds (2-alkyl-3-hydroxy-1,4-naphthoquinones) have been known for a considerable time to have a variety of pesticidal activities including antibacterial, acaricidal, antimalarial, fungicidal, and insecticidal actions (e.g., see Jacobsen and Pedersen, 1986). Acequinocyl was patented as a pesticide by E. I du Pont de Nemours & Co. (Bellina and Fost, 1977), but it was not immediately developed. Closely related compounds, showing good activity against sucking insects and mites, have recently been described based on 2-alkyl-3-hydroxy-1,4-naphthoquinone derivatives with unsaturated, branched alkyl chains that were isolated from a Chilean plant, *Calceolaria andina* (Khambay *et al.*, 1997). These, too, are under evaluation as commercial pesticides.

Acequinocyl (DPX-3792, AKD-2023, TM-413) is a specific acaricide currently under development in many countries (Kinoshita *et al.*, 1999) under the trade name Kanemite.

Toxicology Profile The primary source of data is Wakasa and Watanabe (1999).

Acute Toxicity Acequinocyl shows an extremely low level of acute toxicity to vertebrates (Table 57.3).

Irritation/Sensitization It has very slight activity as a dermal and eye irritant and is not a dermal sensitizer.

Carcinogenicity It showed no evidence of carcinogenicity in rats and mice in chronic dietary studies.

Mutagenicity/Genotoxicity Acequinocyl was negative in a range of standard tests (Ames *Salmonella* assay, DNA repair, chromosomal aberrations).

Reproductive Toxicity No notable reproductive toxicity was observed in rats in a multigenerational study.

Developmental Toxicity/Teratogenicity Acequinocyl caused no adverse effects in rats and rabbits in studies of developmental toxicity.

Biochemical Mechanism of Action The de-acetylated metabolite of acequinocyl, 2-hydroxy-3-dodecyl-1,4-naphthoquinone, strongly inhibits respiration in complex III of insect mitochondria (Koura *et al.*, 1998). Compounds in this class have long been known to be complex III inhibitors in vertebrate systems (von Jagow and Link, 1986). Structurally they resemble ubiquinone and they bind at the Q_o center, probably competing with ubiquinone for this site. They differ from the strobilurin like inhibitors by acting to prevent electron transfer to cytochrome c_1 and the consequent reoxidation of the Rieske iron–sulfur center (Fig. 57.4). Their inhibitory potency depends on their lipophilicity and the optimal alkyl chain length is reached with the undecyl group.

Acequinocyl itself is initially inactive as a respiratory inhibitor using mitochondria *in vitro*, but inhibition develops slowly with time (Koura *et al.*, 1998). The hydrolytic conversion of acequinocyl to the deacetylated metabolite has been shown to occur in isolated mitochondria (Koura *et al.*, 1998; Rich, 1996) and it seems very likely that this metabolite is the active toxicant and that acequinocyl is a propesticide. It has no significant effects on complex I. As described in Section 57.1.6.4, some naphthoquinones can act as electron acceptors from the mitochondrial electron transport chain leading to redox cycling and serious oxidative stress. It is not known whether this occurs with acequinocyl or its active metabolite, but this effect was not seen with the closely related naphthoquinones developed by Khambay (Khambay, 1998).

Environmental Fate and Toxicity Acequinocyl has a low acute toxicity to birds and its toxicity to fish is extremely low (Table 57.3). In a striking contrast, its toxicity to *Daphnia* is extremely high (Wakasa and Watanabe, 1999). The bioconcentration factor in fish (carp) is moderate (170–387) despite acequinocyl's lipophilicity. Acequinocyl is rapidly degraded by soil microorganism with a soil half-life of less than 3 days. Because of its very high lipophilicity and the correspondingly high K_{oc} value that ranges from 33,900 to 123,000, it is firmly bound to soil organic matter and has a very low leaching potential.

Hydramethylnon: General Properties and Uses 5,5-Dimethylperhydropyrimidin-2-one 4-trifluoromethyl-α-(4-trifluoromethylstyryl) cinnamylidenehydrazone (Fig. 57.11), CAS Reg. No. 67485-29-4, was discovered by American Cyanamid Co. and is described by Lovell (1979).

It exists as yellow to tan crystals, m.p. 189–191°C, v.p. 3.7 × 10^{-6} Pa (25°C), w.s. 7 to 9 ppb (25°C), log P 4.45 (U.S. EPA, 1998c) [also reported as 2.31 (Tomlin, 2000)], HLC 0.78 Pa m^3 mol^{-1} (25°C). It is relatively stable to hydrolysis over the pH range 5 to 9.

Hydramethylnon (AC 217,300) is the sole member of the class of amidinohydrazine insecticides. It is used as a slow acting bait for the agricultural and household control of ants, cockroaches, and termites. Trade names include Amdro, Combat, Maxforce, and Siege.

Toxicology Profile The primary data sources are U.S. EPA (1998c) and Cal EPA (2000b).

Acute Toxicity As shown in Table 57.3, hydramethylnon has a low or moderate toxicity for terrestrial vertebrates. The acute clinical signs of poisoning in rats include hyopactivity, diuresis, ataxia, anorexia, epistaxis, chromodacryorrhea, and salivation.

Irritation/Sensitization Hydramethylnon is a moderate eye irritant but it is not a skin irritant or sensitizer.

Subchronic/Chronic Toxicity Decreased food consumption and wasting leading to death were seen in dogs fed at 6 mg/kg/day for 3 months. Similar but less severe effects were also seen in rats in a 90-day feeding study. In chronic dietary studies, rats developed glomerulonephrosis at 25–50 ppm. Testicular atrophy was observed at 50 ppm and higher doses which was not accompanied by any general decrease in body weight.

Carcinogenicity Hydramethylnon is classified by the U.S. Environmental Protection Agency as a group C carcinogen (possible human carcinogen) due to an increase in lung adenomas and carcinomas in female mice dosed at 4.45 mg/kg/day. Much discussion has ensued regarding the possible confounding effects of Sendai virus infections on this diagnosis (Cal EPA, 2000b). No carcinogenic responses was observed in male mice or rats of either sex.

Mutagenicity/Genotoxicity Hydramethylnon was negative in a typical battery of five tests involving mutation in microorganisms and chromosomal aberrations and dominant lethality in mammals.

Reproductive Toxicity Testicular atrophy was seen in a number of subchronic and chronic feeding studies with rats, mice, and dogs. Histopathologic findings included aspermia hypospermia, interstitial cell hyperplasia of Leydig cells, and germinal cell degeneration. This led to decreased male reproductive success in a two-generation study in rats (LOEL of 3.32 mg/kg/day). Hydramethylnon is therefore a general reproductive toxicant that specifically targets germinal cells of the testis.

Developmental Toxicity/Teratogenicity Hydramethylnon caused no developmental effects in rats and rabbits at doses that did not also cause maternal toxicity.

Immunotoxicity When Amdro was fed to calves at 113.5 g/calf/day, leukopenia was evident after 2 weeks with decreased numbers of lymphocytes and eosinophils. However, no evidence was seen for a depression of cellular immunity (Evans *et al.*, 1984).

Biochemical Mechanism of Action Hydramethylnon inhibits respiration in insects *in vivo*, resulting in behavioral depression and eventual paralysis similar to that caused by rotenone and antimycin A. It also depresses respiration in Chinese hamster ovary cells *in vitro* with a 24-hr LC_{50} of about 1 μM. It inhibits respiration at micromolar concentrations in isolated rat liver mitochondria acting specifically at complex III (Hollingshaus, 1987). Inhibition is slow in developing and the specific binding location within the complex is not known. Hydramethylnon is reported to have a disordering effect on model lipid bilayer membranes (Hollingshaus, 1987) but the role of such effects in its inhibitory actions on complex III are unclear. In its slowly developing inhibitory action on mitochondrial respiration *in vitro* and its ability to disrupt membrane structure, as well as in aspects of its structure, hydramethylnon resembles some alkylguanidines and biguanidines used in the treatment of diabetes mellitus and as antimicrobial agents (Schäfer, 1981).

Absorption, Metabolism, and Elimination After oral administration in rats, hydramethylnon is rapidly eliminated, almost entirely as the unchanged compound in the feces. Absorbed material was metabolized relatively slowly. Dermal absorption is very limited.

Environmental Fate and Toxicity Hydramethylnon's acute toxicity to birds is moderate to low (Table 57.3). Its acute toxicity to aquatic species is quite variable. It is of relatively low toxicity to some fish and Daphnia (Table 57.3) but it is highly toxic to other fish species (e.g., channel catfish have a 96-hr LC_{50} value of 90 ppb). Because of its limited use patterns, strong binding to soil components, and rapid photodegradation it is unlikely that hydramethylnon presents a significant threat to any aquatic species in practice. It shows some tendency to bioconcentrate in fish (BCF is 1300 for the whole body) and depuration is relatively slow with a half-life of about 14 days.

Hydramethylnon is rapidly degraded in the environment by photolysis (the half-life in water is less than or about 1 hr). The half-life in soil is 3–55 days in field studies but degradation is biphasic with a much slower second phase. Hydramethylnon binds tightly to soil (K_d values of 1039–1782 ml/g) and it is unlikely to leach into groundwater.

57.6 INHIBITORS OF ATP SYNTHASE

57.6.1 INTRODUCTION

In view of the large and exquisitely complex machinery that is responsible for the synthesis of ATP from ADP and inorganic phosphate, and its critical role in cellular bioenergetics, it is perhaps surprising that no large number of poisons are known that act at this site. Only two groups of pesticides are strong inhibitors of this complex with evidence that this inhibition plays an important role in their toxic actions. These are the organotins and diafenthiuron, an insecticide that generates a reactive carbodiimide inhibitor. The inclusion of the organotin pesticides in this section is a matter of convenience rather than an indication that complex V is known to be the major target for their toxic effects. In fact, they have several effects on mitochondria and oxphos in addition to inhibiting complex V, and they have a number of potent effects on nonmitochondrial biochemistry also. It is often unclear which of these effects, if any, predominates under given conditions *in vivo* and thus could be regarded as the most significant biochemical lesion underlying an adverse response.

Several other pesticides show considerable activity against this site *in vitro*, but the evidence that it is their primary site action *in vivo* is lacking. These compounds include two chlorinated diphenyl sulfone acaricides, chlorfenson and tetradifon. These are reported to be potent (submicromolar or low micromolar) inhibitors of ATP synthase from mites, fish, and mammals *in vitro* (Bustamente and Pedersen, 1973; Cutcomp *et al.*, 1972) although they were less active in other reports (Abo-Khatwa and Hollingworth, 1974; Kadir and Knowles, 1991). Kadir and Knowles (1991), in a limited study, found that a number of other specific halogenated acaricides including chloropropylate, bromopropylate, flubenzimine, chlorfenson, and propargite inhibited oligomycin-sensitive Mg^{2+}-ATPase from the bulb mite *in vitro* with a potency greater than that of the organotin cyhexatin. Of these compounds, only tetradifon, bromopropylate, and propargite are still use (Tomlin, 2000). There appears to be no evidence regarding the possible occurrence and significance of this inhibition of complex V *in vivo* either in mites or vertebrates, but it may be considered as a plausible target site for these compounds.

57.6.2 ORGANOTIN PESTICIDES

57.6.2.1 History and Uses

Since the 1950s, organotins have been widely and increasingly used as pesticides with multiple applications as fungicides, acaricides, molluscicides, wood preservatives, disinfectants, rodent repellants, and antifouling agents. All pesticidal organtins are trisubstituted with aromatic or aliphatic groups such as phenyl or butyl moieties. The less toxic dialkyl and monoalkyltins have important industrial uses as stabilizers and catalysts in plastic production (Fent, 1996a) but are not employed as pesticides. Trimethyl and triethyltins are too toxic to both plants and vertebrates to be utilized as pesticides. However, organotins with longer alkyl chains (tributyltin, fenbutatin-oxide), aromatic rings [triphenyltin (fentin)], or alicyclic groups (azocyclotin, cyhexatin) have proved to be effective for a variety of pesticidal purposes. Each of these triorganotins may occur in several forms which vary in the fourth group coordinated with the tin atom (e.g., they can exist and be utilized as hydroxides, chlorides, acetates, or as other forms).

As reviewed by Fent (1996a) many of these compounds have been plagued by problems with chronic toxicity which have led to the cancellation and limitation of uses. Most notably, the use of tributyltins (and some triphenyltins) as antifouling agents in paints for ships' hulls became widespread in the 1970s. This has led to significant environmental effects on aquatic species in and around harbors and coastal areas due to the leaching of the tin compounds from the paint. Because they have long half-lives in sediments, are lipophilic, which leads to ready bioaccumulation by biota, and many aquatic species are highly sensitivity to their toxicological effects, population reductions have been widely observed. This is particularly notable with mollusks, which may be severely affected at concentrations below 10 ppb. Because of these impacts, restrictions were placed on this use of tributyltin by many nations in the 1980s (Fent, 1996a). However, these measures have not been universally effective in reducing organotin levels or their biological adverse effects, and a complete international ban on this use of organotin biocides is now being debated and would take effect in 2003. Much less is known regarding the occurrence and toxicological impact of organotins in wastewater and sewage sludge, although tributyl- and triphenyltin can be detected in sludge in the concentration range of 0.1 to 1.0 ppm (Fent, 1996b), and this merits additional study (Fent, 1996a, 1996b).

57.6.2.2 Chemical Properties

The chemistry of bioactive organotins has been reviewed in detail by Fent (1996a). Organotins have ionic character and tend to dissociate in water, releasing the corresponding substituted tin cation. The pKa of tributyltin hydroxide is approximately 6.4, meaning that at physiological pH it is predominantly but not wholly in the form of the undissociated hydroxide. Other pesticidal organotins hydroxides have similar pKa values in the 5.0 to 6.5 range. Forms other than the hydroxide, such as tin oxides, acetates, or chlorides, tend to hydrolyze to form the corresponding hydroxide in aqueous solutions, but the rate varies depending on the solution conditions. The aqueous speciation of tributyl- and triphenyltins and its relationship to *n*-octanol partition coefficients have been studied by Amold *et al.* (1997) who developed a simple model of the effects of pH and salt concentration on their partitioning behavior.

The speciation of these compounds therefore is complex depending on the starting compound, pH, temperature, and the presence of counterions in solution (e.g., in seawater with its high chloride ion level, the formation of the organotin chlorides is favored). In turn speciation governs water solubility, lipophilicity and thus partitioning into lipoprotein membranes, rates of uptake into living organisms, and strength of binding to soil colloids. Tributyl- and triphenyltins have a water solubility minimum in the pH range 6 to 8, and solubility decreases with increasing salinity, so that the solubility in seawater is only 40% of that in distilled water at pH 7 to 8 (Inaba *et al.*, 1995).

The undissociated organotin molecule, which is generally more lipophilic than the corresponding cation, will be more effective in each of the processes above (e.g., the octanol : water partition coefficient of tributyltin chloride increases from 3.25 at pH 6.0 to 3.9 at pH 8.0 as ionization is suppressed, and its bioaccumulation by, and toxicity to, water fleas and carp increases correspondingly). Similar results showing an increase in bioaccumulation by several aquatic organisms with increasing water pH have been reported with triphenyltin (Fent, 1996a; Looser *et al.*, 1998). It is worth noting that the organotin cations themselves are relatively lipophilic, so that uptake into living organisms does not cease at lower pHs (Looser *et al.*, 1998), and their lipophilicity will tend to increase with the increasing carbon atom content of the attached groups.

Because of their more or less ready conversion in solution to a mixture of the hydroxide and cationic forms, any differences in toxicological effects between organotins sharing the same organic substituents but with a different fourth coordinated group (e.g., tributyltin hydroxide and tributytin chloride) will tend to be small. The major difference will arise primarily from the effect of the fourth subsituent on their lipophilicity and initial bioavailability.

Other than undergoing hydrolytic conversion to the hydroxide form, pesticidal organotins are relatively unreactive. The conclusion that triorganic tins are only weakly interactive with sulfhydryl groups (Aldridge and Cremer, 1955), has been disputed by Byington and his colleagues (e.g., see Wulf and Byington, 1975). Under some circumstances organotin cations have the capability to coordinate with proteins, particularly those with sulfhydryl groups [e.g., triethyltin forms a pentacoordinate complex with hemoglobin through its cysteine13α and histidine 20α (Taketa *et al.*, 1980)]. A significant observation is that, like arsenite, the organotins bind much more avidly to vicinal dithiol groups than monothiols (Stridh *et al.*, 1999b). This also true of dialktltins (Aldridge, 1976). In at least two cases, dithiothreitol, a dithiol, has been found to be active in antagonizing organotin inhibition of enzymes while monothiols such as glutathione were inactive (Nebbia *et al.*, 1999; Rao *et al.*, 1987). The inhibition of several key enzymes by organotins has been attributed to sulfhydryl binding (see below).

57.6.2.3 General Toxicology

The literature addressing the toxicology and environmental impact of tributyltins and, to a lesser degree, triphenyltins, is substantial. Much less attention has been paid to the organotins that are primarily of interest in agriculture, such as cyhexatin, and, particularly, azocyclotin and fenbutatin-oxide. Since the tributyltins have already been reviewed in depth on a number of recent occasions (Benya, 1997; Boyer, 1989; Meador, 2000; Tanabe, 1999) they are not included here specifically, but reference is made to those aspects of their toxicology that can throw additional light on the other members of the group. Reviews of the general toxicology of tin compounds include Hall and Pinkney (1985) focusing on their aquatic toxicology and Fent (1996a) focusing on their general and ecotoxicology. The toxicity of organotins has a strong tendency to follow the order trisubstituted > disubstituted > monosubstituted and this sequence is also the general pathway of metabolism for pesticidal organotins in both vertebrates and the environment. However, some disubstituted tin metabolites do show high toxicity which must be considered in evaluation of the overall safety of the parent trisubstituted compound.

In experimental animals, organotins have a general ability to cause cytotoxicity in many tissues and organs including skin, intestine, kidney, liver, lung, and brain. The impacted organ systems tend to be those most directly exposed by the route of administration. These results are similar to observations with human exposures in which dermal, hepatotoxic, nephrotoxic, and neurological effects have been recorded. These broadly toxic actions *in vivo* are paralleled *in vitro* by the high toxicity of trisubstituted organotins to isolated cells from many sources.

Evidence of cytotoxicity may be observed at aqueous concentrations in the general range of 10 nM to 1 μM (Fent, 1996a).

The toxicology of individual compounds is presented below, but it is clear that many organotin pesticides as a group present several specific toxicological hazards at relatively low doses.

1. They have endocrine modulatory characteristics as indicated by their effects on male reproduction in mammals (reduced testicular size, reduced spermatazoon production) and their ability to cause sex alterations in mollusks. In this case, female mollusks develop male characteristics, a process termed imposex. Their potency in the latter effect is very high with masculinization of females occurring at a water concentration of just a few ppt. The biochemical mechanism(s) for these effects is not known with certainty, but there are a large number of studies relating to the imposex phenomenon, which are briefly reviewed here.

Changes in androgen/estrogen levels in mollusks undergoing organotin-induced imposex have been observed in several studies (e.g., see Bettin *et al.*, 1996; Morcillo *et al.*, 1998; Spooner *et al.*, 1991). The role of aromatases, which are cytochrome P-450-catalyzed enzymes responsible for the conversion of testosterone to estradiol, in controlling the androgen/estrogen ratio has been studied. Evidence has been presented both in favor (Bettin *et al.*, 1996; Morcillo *et al.*, 1998) and against (Morcillo and Porte, 1999) the hypothesis that estradiol levels are decreased and testosterone levels increased specifically because organotins inhibit aromatase action *in vivo*. Other possibilities to explain imposex include an effect on the enzymes that degrade sex hormones and excretory transport systems (Ronis and Mason, 1996), and a direct stimulatory effect on androgen receptors. In this regard, Yamabe *et al.* (2000) examined the effect of tributyl- and triphenyltin on androgen-dependent transcription and cell proliferation in human prostate cancer cells. Stimulation of androgen-dependent gene transcription and cell proliferation occurred at concentrations of triphenyltin as low as 1 nM. They concluded that trisubstituted organotins activate androgen-receptor-mediated transcription but act at a target site other than the hormone-binding site of the receptor. Whether such direct androgen receptor effects occur in mollusks is unknown.

2. Many organotins are clearly immunotoxic, both *in vitro* and *in vivo,* in a range of vertebrate species including mammals and fish (Boyer, 1989; Fent, 1996a). In rats, atrophy of the thymus is observed, antibody responses are reduced, and resistance to disease is diminished (Snoeij *et al.*, 1989). In fish, and several marine invertebrates, decreased phagocytic activity and resistance to microbial pathogens were observed at environmentally relevant concentrations of tributyltin (Cooper *et al.*, 1995; Wishkovsky *et al.*, 1989). Many studies have shown that tributyltins cause thymus atrophy and T-cell immunodeficiency *in vivo* (reviewed in Benya, 1997). This, at least in part, is related to the ability of organotins to initiate apoptosis in thymocytes which has been reported in many studies both *in vitro*, at low micromolar concentrations are effective (e.g., see Aw *et al.*, 1990; Bollo *et al.*, 1996; Oyama *et al.*, 1991; Raffray and Cohen, 1991), and *in vivo* (see Boyer, 1989; Nishida *et al.*, 1990). Tributyltin is significantly more potent than triphenyltin in this thymolytic action (Aw *et al.*, 1990). Both the T-cell-dependent humoral and cellular immune responses are inhibited.

In addition to effects on T-cells, organotins also have deleterious effects on human B lymphocytes derived from tonsil tissue, including the induction of apoptosis at *in vitro* concentrations of 100 nM (De Santiago and Aguilar-Santelises, 1999). Tributyltin has been shown to inhibit the tumor killing activity of human natural killer lymphocytes at submicromolar concentrations *in vitro* (Whalen *et al.*, 1999), and triphenyltin is only slightly less potent than tributyltin in this action (Whalen *et al.*, 2000). If this effect also occurs *in vivo* it would be expected to increase sensitivity to viruses and tumor formation. In fact, triphenyltin is a tumorigen (Section 57.6.2.6), and dietary tributyltin is suspected of increasing susceptibility to infections and causing deaths in several mammalian wildlife species (Kannan *et al.*, 1997, 1998). In a comparative study, triphenyltin and cyhexatin were most active in decreasing spleen weight in mice dosed orally, while tributylin oxide and fenburatin-oxide were least active (Pieper and Casida, 1976).

3. Pesticidal organotins as a group are generally not genotoxic, although some have been shown to be clastogenic (or co-clastogenic) *in vitro* and *in vivo* (Sasaki *et al.*, 1993; U.S. EPA, 1999c; Yamada and Sasaki, 1993), nor have they been found to be carcinogenic. Fentin is the exception to this rule.

4. They tend to be strong skin and eye irritants. Skin contact may cause local burns and dermatitis with pruritus and pustular outbreaks. Contact with concentrated materials on the eye can cause acute conjunctivitis and corneal opacity that can be irreversible. Their respiratory toxicity tends to be high and, after inhalation, severe irritation of the airways and the pulmonary tissues may occur. By the oral route, inflammation of the gastric mucose and ulceration can occur.

5. The aquatic toxicology of most organotins gives particular cause for concern (Fent, 1996a; Tanabe, 1999). Not only are they highly toxic by acute exposure with LC_{50} values around 1–10 ppb, but they have cumulative properties which means that, on more prolonged exposure, toxic endpoints can be seen at ppt concentrations. Additionally, their endocrine disruptive and immunotoxic effects occur in aquatic species also. As already described, these have given rise to well-documented, significant, and widespread impacts on aquatic species and communities which are very slow to reverse because of the persistence of these compounds in sediments and because of their continued input into the aquatic environment. Much less seems to have been done to study their potential impact on terrestrial nontarget organisms.

57.6.2.4 Human Toxicology

The signs, symptoms, and treatment of organotin poisoning are discussed by Reigart and Roberts (1999). Absorption of

organotins, either through the skin or gastrointestinal tract, is generally limited and relatively few poisonings and no deaths have been reported as a result of occupational exposure to organotin pesticides. The primary effects are on the central nervous system and include headache, nausea, vomiting, dizziness, mental disturbances, photophobia, and, sometimes, convulsions. Epigastric pain and elevation of blood sugar have been observed. There are no specific antidotes and treatment involves decontamination and supportive therapies.

A number of studies of human illnesses, some of them serious, after occupational exposure or suicide attempts have been reported. Since they all involve triphenyltin acetate, they will be discussed in the section on fentin (Section 57.6.2.6). The irritant properties of organotins also cause illnesses. Inhalation exposure to latex paint containing bis(tributyltin) oxide used on internal walls caused mucous membrane irritation (Wax and Dockstader, 1995), and contact dermatitis among painters has been attributed to this compound in paints (Goh, 1985). Additional examples of human pathology arising from organotin exposure are provided by Boyer (1989).

The general public is exposed to organotin pesticides through the diet. Organotin residues in fish for human consumption occur at typical levels of 0.01–1.0 ppm, primarily as tributyl- and triphenyltin. Levels in shellfish may be higher. Generally consumption is below current acceptable daily intakes (ADIs) set with immunotoxicity as the endpoint (Cardwell *et al.*, 1999; Fent, 1996a). However the margins of safety below the AOI are not large and ADIs are subject to revision in the light of new knowledge. Consequently, high levels of consumption of fish and mollusks from contaminated areas may be of some toxicological concern. A recent study of blood levels of butyltins in residents of Michigan gave a peak value of 100 ng/ml. It was concluded that these levels were below those needed to affect human natural killer lymphocytes, a sensitive endpoint, but that sporadic incidences of higher exposure were possible that could have toxicological impacts (Kannan *et al.*, 1999).

57.6.2.5 Biochemical Mechanisms of Toxicity

Pesticidal organotins have several potential biochemical mechanisms of toxicity which may vary in relative importance between different compounds or be evident at different concentrations *in vitro*. These have been reviewed by Boyer (1989) and Fent (1996a). Since there may be overlaps in the potencies with which individual organotin compounds cause these different effects, it is generally difficult to determine which is the critical biochemical lesion for a given response and, in some cases, it seems reasonable to suppose that several relevant biochemical effects may occur concurrently.

1. Organotins inhibit mitochondrial ATP synthase (complex V), often with considerable potency. Tricyclohexyltin has been reported to inhibit mitochondrial oligomycin-sensitive Mg^{2+}-ATPase from several nonmammalian sources with I_{50} values of 0.1–100 nM (Desaiah *et al.*, 1973; Mehrotra *et al.*, 1985; Pieper and Casida,

1965). This exceeds the sensitivity shown by typical mammalian enzymes (1–10 μM; Aldridge, 1976) and would help explain the selective toxicity of miticidal organotins such as cyhexatin and azocyclotin for invertebrates. In general agreement with these results, triphenyl-, tricyclohexyl-, and tribenzyltin derivatives were found to inhibit ATP synthase activity at low micromolar concentrations but they did not inhibit electron transport or cause uncoupling in rat and plant mitochondria (Chandra et al., 1989).

Orangotins inhibit ATPase activity in mitochondria only when the entire F_0F_1 complex is present. The dissociated F_1 component also has ATPase activity, but this is not susceptible to inhibition by oligomycin or organotins, and inhibition of proton conductivity persists even after its removal (Gould, 1976; Papa et al., 1982). This indicates that the triorganotins inhibit ATP synthase by interaction with the membrane-bound F_0 component. Studies by Matsuno-Yagi and Hatefi (1993a, 1993b) confirm that inhibition occurs in the F_0 segment of the complex and suggest that it may be due to freezing the ATPase structure in such a way as to inhibit the rotary motion required for rapid proton flux and ATP synthesis. However, the site of action of triorganotins is different from that of other F_0 inhibitors such as oligomycin and dicyclohexylcarbodiimide (Papa et al., 1982; Matsuno-Yagi and Hatefi, 1993a). The inhibitory potency toward ATP synthase tends to increase with the increasing size (and lipophilicity) of the organic substituents (Aldridge et al., 1977).

2. Since both the hydroxide and chloride forms of triorganic tins are lipophilic and dissociable, they can locate within the lipoprotein inner mitochondrial membrane and, in the presence of chloride ions, shuttle OH^- ions outward in exchange for inward-moving Cl^- ions. This tends to destroy the pH gradient created by the electron transport chain and represents a form of uncoupling, which increases mitochondrial respiratory rates and causes mitochondrial swelling (Selwyn, 1976; Wulf and Byington, 1975). However, this effect does not approach that of 2,4-DNP in the degree of stimulation of respiration (Aldridge et al., 1977). The Cl^-/OH^- exchange diminishes the chemical portion of the protonmotive force (Δp) that is created by the differential pH, but it is electroneutral and does not alter the more important electrical portion of the mitochondrial membrane potential ($\Delta\Psi_m$). The potency of organotins in this effect peaks when the organic substituents are propyl groups and decreases as the size of the substituents increases further (Aldridge et al., 1977).

A variant of this mechanism has been proposed by Bragadin and Marton (1997, Fig. 60.6). They provide evidence that trialkyltins enter the mitochondrial inner membrane as the tin cation, depending on their lipophilicities. The cations are driven to the inner membrane face by the membrane potential where they pick up a hydroxyl ion to form the hydroxide. This is followed by the outward diffusion of the hydroxide to the outer membrane face where, at the lower pH there, it dissociates again. This tin cation/tin hydroxide cycling is no longer an electoneutral process and results in the discharge of

the membrane potential as well as the proton gradient. In this context, it is notable that tributyltin acts as a mitochondrial uncoupler even in a chloride-free medium which proves that a mechanism other than Cl^-/OH^- exchange is operating (Bragadin et al., 2000).

3. Mitochondrial swelling is observed even in the absence of chloride ion in the medium which indicates an additional and independent mechanism from that related to Cl^-/OH^- exchange. Potency here is somewhat lower than for the first two effects but increases rapidly with the size of the organic substituents (Aldridge et al., 1977). Bragadin and Marton (1997) and Bragadin et al. (2000) conclude that, in this case, organotins are causing the opening of the mitochondrial permeability transition pore. In turn this leads to rapid and severe swelling. In the case of fentin, the opening of the pore has been attributed to a special mechanism involving the interaction of the organotin with sulfhydryl groups since it is antagonized by sulfhydryl agents but not by cyclosporin A, a compound which reverses the effects of many compounds which induce the permeability transition (Zazueta et al., 1994).

These three actions on mitochondria have been reviewed by Aldridge (1976) and Selwyn (1976). Their relative contributions vary with structure [e.g., for short chain trialkyltins tins the most potent action is the facilitation of Cl^-/OH^- exchange, whereas for the compounds with longer chains or aryl substituents which are used as pesticides, the potency is approximately the same for all three effects (Aldridge et al., 1977)]. Because of this, with pesticidal tributyl and triphenyltins, no respiratory stimulation attributable to the Cl^-/OH^- exchange is seen because it is overridden by the inhibitory effects on ATP synthase. Little further elaboration of these conclusions has been made in the last 25 years, and it is not clear which (if any) of these mitochondrial actions predominates as the ultimate cause of toxic effects in vivo.

4. Organotins inhibit other ATPases such as Na^+/K^+-ATPase and Ca^{2+}-ATPase (Mehrotra et al., 1985; Sahib and Desaiah, 1986). Inhibition of the latter enzyme, which occurs with appoteeny comparable to the inhibition of the mitochondrial Mg^{2+}-ATPase, could contiribute to the ability of organotins to disrupt calcium regulation within cells. The potency in the inhibition of the Na^+/K^+-ATPase is generally lower.

5. Organotins are lipophilic and amphipathic and can act as detergents with general membrane-disruptant properties at concentrations a low as 1–10 μM. Tributyltin disrupts the erythrocyte membrane structure causing hemolysis at about 5 μM (Gray et al., 1987) and studies with planar bilayer lipid membranes (Radecka et al., 1999) reveal that the membrane depolarization was greatest with trialkyltins and was directly related to their lipophilicity. Langner et al. (1998) compared tetra-, tri-, and diphenyltin chlorides for their actions on lipid bilayer membranes made from phosphatidylcholine and for their hemolytic potencies. Tetraphenyltin had little interaction with the model membrane, diphenyltin located toward its center, and triphenyltin oriented more to the surface in the headgroup region. The order of hemolytic potencies was tri > di > tetra, and these differences in potency were explained on the basis of the different locations of these compounds within the bilayer membrane.

6. Membrane permeability and calcium regulation are affected in cells *in vitro* leading to an influx of calcium, a decrease in transmembrane potential, activation of NF-kappa B, and efflux of cellular proteins including cytochrome *c* and tumor necrosis factor-α (Aw *et al.*, 1990; Marinovich *et al.*, 1996b; Oyama *et al.*, 1991; Stridh *et al.*, 1999a; Zazueta *et al.*, 1994). These events underlie the well-established ability of organotins to cause apoptosis in some cell types (e.g., thymocytes) at concentrations lower than those which cause necrosis (Aw *et al.*, 1990; Raffray and Cohen, 1991). An apoptotic response was observed in cultured mouse thymocytes at a concentrations of triphenyltin acetate as low as 12 nM (Bollo *et al.*, 1996). Interestingly, the increase in membrane permeability does not seem to involve the typical activation of the mitochondrial membrane permeability transition (Stridh *et al.*, 1999b; Zazueta *et al.*, 1994). Current knowledge regarding the mechanism by which organotins induce apoptosis has been reviewed by Robertson and Orrenius (2000) but much remains to be learned about this complex web of events.

7. Tributyl and triphenyltins cause microtubule disassembly and disruption of the mitotic spindle and other elements of the cytoskeleton (Chow and Orrenius, 1994; Jensen *et al.*, 1991; Marinovich *et al.*, 1996b). This effect increases with increasing lipophilicity of the tin compound (Jensen *et al.*, 1991) and may involve thiol group modification by the organotins (Chow and Orrenius, 1994). The mechanism of this effect is unclear since triphenyltin did not have a direct effect on actin polymerization in a cell-free system and it may occur indirectly through effects on the cellular environment (Marinovich *et al.*, 1996a).

8. Triorganotins inhibit several important sulfhydryl-dependant enzymes which has been attributed to their coordination with protein sufhydryls and other functional groups. These enzymes include Na^+,K^+-ATPase (Rao *et al.*, 1987), caspases involved in apoptosis (Stridh *et al.*, 1999b), glutathione *S*-aryltransferase (Henry and Byington, 1976), hemoglobin (Santroni *et al.*, 1997; Taketa *et al.*, 1980), and cytochrome P450-dependent monooxygenases (Fent, 1996a; Nebbia *et al.*, 1999).

9. Organotins appear to be able to decrease the activity of cytochrome P-450-dependent monoxygenase systems in several ways, including both direct interactions with the enzyme proteins and indirect effects through modulation of their synthesis and degradation. Rosenberg *et al.* (1981) in a study of the effects of tricyclohexyltin and tributyltin on heme biosynthesis in rats discovered that they increase heme degradation and decrease its synthesis. The major effect is an enhancement in degradation of heme through the induction of the activity of heme oxygenase (Fent and Stegeman, 1993; Rosenberg and Kappas, 1989). This oxygenase is the rate-limiting enzyme in heme degradation and its activity was increased at a subcutaneous dose of cyhexatin as low as 1.9 mg/kg. This is reflected in a decrease in level and activity of cytochrome P-450 isoforms. The level of inhibition of monooxygenase activity was more than 50% at a dose of 15 mg/kg. The maximal effect occurred at 48 to 72 hr after dosing and the response was prolonged for at least 10 days. The sensitivity to this action seems to vary among species and, perhaps, among organotin agents. No effect was seen on P-450 activity in rabbits and lambs after the sublethal administration of fentin acetate (Nebbia *et al.*, 1997), but the effect has been confirmed in a number of species [e.g., with tributyltin in fish by Fent and Stegeman (1993) and in the dogwhelk by Spooner *et al.* (1991)].

Organotins (tributyl, tricyclohexyl, and triphenyl) also act directly to decrease the level of cytochrome P-450 and increase the level of its inactive P-420 form *in vitro* in microsomes from both mammals and fish. Corresponding losses occur in oxidative activity. This destructive effect is greatest on the β-naphthoflavone-inducible CYP1A family (Fent and Bucheli, 1994; Fent *et al.*, 1998; Kim *et al.*, 1998; Rosenberg and Drummond, 1983; Rosenberg *et al.*, 1981). Fent *et al.* (1998) also reported that the P-450 reducing enzyme, NAD(P)H : cytochrome *c* reductase, was significantly inhibited in fish exposed to triphenyltin *in vivo*. The effect on P-450 may occur through interaction with sulfhydryl and/or histidine residues (Fent and Bucheli, 1994; Nebbia *et al.*, 1999). Studies with fish hepatoma cells by Brüschweiler *et al.* (1996) indicated that the effect of organotins on P-450 levels and activity occurs by a direct interaction with the apoprotein and not through an effect on the synthesis of the protein. However, inhibition occurs only at relatively high concentrations (0.1 to 1.0 mM) and its significance *in vivo* is unclear. In one case it was concluded that the concentration needed to inactivate P-450 *in vitro* in liver microsomes from marine mammals was more than 10-fold higher than the levels occurring in the liver *in vivo* (Kim *et al.*, 1998) and Fent *et al.* (1998) concluded that inactivation of the CYP1A in the scup, a marine fish, occurred at doses *in vivo* that would be reached only under conditions of very high contamination with triphenyltin, but that inhibition on NAD(P)H cytochrome *c* reductase occurred at doses that are more environmentally realistic.

The potential toxicological implications of cytochrome P-450 inactivation are considerable but not fully investigated. The possible role of aromatase inhibition in causing imposex has already been described. Cytochrome P-450 monooxygenases are also key enzymes in the biotransformations (both activative and inactivative) of xenobiotics, and self-synergism of organotins seems possible since their degradation occurs primarily through P-450-catalyzed oxidations.

10. Enzymes of xenobiotic biotransformation in addtion to monooxygenase are also affected by organotins *in vitro* and *in vivo*. In particular, organotins are very effective inhibitors of glutathione-*S*-transferases (Henry and Byington, 1976). The inhibitory potency may be high. Triphenylltin inhibited a glutathione-*S*-transferase from the chicken with an IC_{50} value of 100 nM (Thomson *et al.*, 1998). Triphenyltin was also a strong inhibitor of transferase activity in fish *in vitro* (George and Buchanan, 1990). Inhibition also occurs *in vivo*. The effect on glutathione-*S*-transferase in the liver after subchronic oral exposure to triphenyltin acetate in rabbits was biphasic with an increase at 15 ppm in the diet but a significant decrease at 150 ppm (Di Simplicio *et al.*, 2000), but it remains to be shown that the inhibition of these enzymes has important physiological consequences. They are an important element in the degradation of electrophilic xenobiotics, and their inhibition could lead to enhanced sensitivity to such agents, but also they play a role in some biosynthetic processes in the cell [e.g., in the conversions of prostaglandins (Thomson *et al.*, 1998)].

57.6.2.6 Properties of Specific Compounds

Azocyclotin: General Properties and Uses Tri(cyclohexyl)-1*H*-1,2,4-triazol-1-yltin (Fig. 57.12), CAS Reg. No. 41083-11-8, was discovered by Bayer AG and is described by Kolbe (1977).

It exists as colorless crystals, decomposing at 219°C, v.p. 6×10^{-11} Pa (25°C), w.s. 0.12 ppm (20°C), log *P* 5.3, HLC 7×10^{-2} Pa m^3 mol^{-1} (20°C), pKa 5.36. In living systems or under alkaline conditions, azocyclotin is readily hydrolyzed to yield tricycohexyltin hydroxide, a related organotin acaricide (Section 57.6.2.6). Chemical hydrolysis is slow at neutral pH (half-life of 81 hr at pH 7) but faster under alkaline conditions (half-life of 8 hr at pH 9).

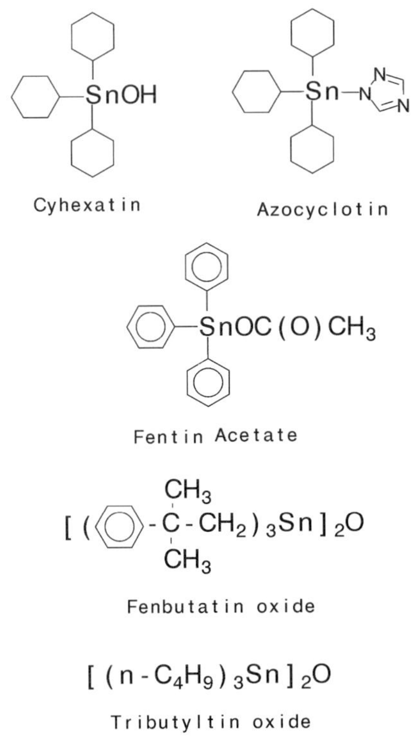

Cyhexatin   Azocyclotin

Fentin Acetate

Fenbutatin oxide

Tributyltin oxide

Figure 57.12 Pesticides that act as inhibitors of complex V—Organotins.

Azocyclotin (BAY BUE 1452) is an acaricide used on cotton, fruits, and ornamentals under the trade name of Peropal.

Toxicology Profile The toxicology of azocyclotin has been reviewed on several occasions by the Joint FAO/WHO Meeting on Pesticide Residues (e.g., see FAO/WHO, 1982, 1990a). These are the primary data sources for the results presented below. Since azocyclotin is readily converted to tricyclohexyltin hydroxide (cyhexatin) there should be considerable similarities in their toxicological properties.

Acute Toxicity Azocyclotin's acute toxicity to terrestrial vertebrates generally lies in the range of 100–400 mg/kg (Table 57.4). The acute oral LD$_{50}$ to the guinea pig is 261 mg/kg and falls within this range (Kolbe, 1977). Symptoms in rats, mice, and guinea pigs began about an hour after oral dosing and persisted for up to 14 days. They were characterized by generalized depression of health, drowsiness and lethargy, and loss of weight, with breathing disorders and diarrhea at higher doses. Azocyclotin's toxicity by inhalation is particularly high.

Irritation/Sensitization Azocyclotin is a strong dermal and a corrosive eye irritant.

Subchronic Toxicity When rats were dosed orally for 30 days at 20 mg/kg day, a variety of effects were observed and some deaths occurred. Particular changes of note were leucopenia and decreased thymus weight. The latter effect was also seen at 2 mg/kg day. Changes in the weight and function of other organs were also noted including the liver. There was no evidence of the brain edema that is seen with triethyltin. No histopathology was seen in any organ. In dogs, 500 ppm in the diet for 90 days caused no notable effects other than anemia. Inhalation studies over 3 weeks in rats caused weight decreases in the thymus and liver with an LOEL at about 0.001 mg/l, a level which again indicates the high toxicity of azocyclotin by this route of exposure.

Chronic Toxicity In chronic dietary studies in rats and mice, no effects other than growth retardation were seen at levels as high 50 ppm. Dogs tolerated even higher doses without serious consequences.

Carcinogenicity No evidence of carcinogenicity was seen in the chronic dietary studies.

Mutagenicity/Genotoxicity Azocyclotin was uniformly negative in a standard battery of *in vitro* tests for mutagenicity and chromosomal effects.

Reproductive Toxicity A three-generation reproductive study was conducted in rates. At the highest dietary concentration, 50 ppm, body weight depression in the pups during lactation and in the parents were the only effects of note.

Table 57.4
Acute Toxicity of Pesticides Acting as Inhibitors of Mitochondrial Complex V (ATP Synthase) to Selected Species

| | LD$_{50}$ (mg/kg) | | | | Acute dermal | LC$_{50}$ (mg/l) | LC$_{50}$ (ppb) | |
| | Acute oral | | | | | Acute inhalation | (24–96 hr) | |
Compound	Rat (M; F)	G. pig	Quail	Duck	Rat or rabbit	Rat	Fish[a]	*Daphnia*
Azocyclotin	209, 363	261	144	250–375[b]	>5000	0.02	4–100	40
Cyhexatin	540	780	—	654[b]	>2000	—	60–550	—
Fenbutatin-oxide	4400	1450[c]	2510	—	>2000	0.072–0.23	4.8–270	31–80
Fentin acetate	81–298	20	77	—	2000	0.044	320	0.32–32
Fentin hydroxide	171, 110	27	—	—	1600	0.060	42–110	16.5
Diafenthiuron	2068	—	>1500	>1500	>2000	0.56	0.7–3.8	<500
Tetradifon	>14,700	—	—	—	>10,000	>3.0	880–2100	>2000

[a]Range of values from several species, most commonly including the rainbow trout and carp.
[b]Data for chickens.
[c]Data for mice.

Developmental Toxicity/Teratogenicity In a study with dietary administration to rabbits during gestation, azocyclotin caused gastrointestinal upsets and decreased weight gain in the does at 0.3 mg/kg/day. Minimal fetotoxicity was seen at 1.0 mg/kg/day, the highest dose tested, but no teratogenic effects were observed. At a higher dose (3 mg/kg/day) in a preliminary study, stomach ulceration, abortions, and deaths occurred. Even at a dose of 30 mg/kg/day in a third study, no teratogenesis was observed although this dose was highly toxic and even lethal to the dams. In a dermal study in rabbits at doses up to 300 mg/kg/day, skin irritation was commonly seen together with reduced feed intake, emaciation, and increased resorptions and abortions at the high dose but no teratogenicity was observed.

Immunotoxicity The decreases in thymus weights and leucopenia seen in rats raise suspicions of immunotoxicity which is often seen with other organotins, but no specific studies appear to have been conducted with azocyclotin.

Biochemical Mechanism of Action No studies seem to have been published regarding biochemical actions of azocyclotin, but since it is converted to cyhexatin, observations with this compound are likely to apply to azocyclotin also.

Absorption, Metabolism, and Excretion Azocyclotin was poorly absorbed after an oral dose in rats and the absorbed dose was cleared relatively slowly from the body, primarily in the feces. Only a very low proportion of the dose was voided in the urine. A special study on liver effects in rats showed that a single dose of 25 mg/kg caused a decrease in some, but not all, cytochrome P-450-catalyzed oxidations which lasted several days (FAO/WHO, 1982).

Environmental Fate and Toxicity Azocyclotin is extremely toxic to the reference aquatic species (Table 57.4). Its persistence in soil varies from a few days to several weeks. In an aquatic microcosm it was rapidly hydrolyzed to cyhexatin (Kordel and Stein, 1997). In the aquatic microcosm, azocyclotin, when applied pre-adsorbed onto soil, reduced zooplankton populations at concentrations as low as 45 ppt and severe effects on population structures were seen at 135 ppt (Fliedner *et al.*, 1997).

Cyhexatin: General Properties and Uses Tricyclohexyltin hydroxide (Fig. 57.12), CAS Reg. No. 13121-70-5, was discovered by Dow Chemical Co. and is described by Alison *et al.* (1968).

It exists as colorless crystals, m.p. 195–198°C, v.p. <10^{-8} Pa (20°C), w.s. <1 ppm (25°C). It is stable to aqueous hydrolysis under slightly acid to alkaline conditions.

Cyhexatin (Dowco 213, TD-2383) is used as a contact acaricide on a wide range of crops. Trade names include Acarstin, Aracnol, Metaran, Mitacid, Oxotin, Pennstyl, Plictran, and Triran. Because of concerns about its potential teratogenicity in rabbits after both oral and dermal administration, cyhexatin was withdrawn from use in a number of countries in the late 1980s.

Toxicology Profile The toxicology of cyhexatin has been reviewed several times by the FAO/WHO Joint Meeting on Pesticide Residues (see FAO/WHO, 1990b, 1992a, 1995). These reviews are the major data source for the results presented below. Additional data are available from Cal DFA (1987a, b).

Acute Toxicity Cyhexatin has moderate acute toxicity for vertebrates by the oral route and a low dermal toxicity (Table 57.4). Relatively small differences in acute oral LD$_{50}$ and inconsistent results were obtained in comparing technical and micronized cyhexatin in rats (FAO/WHO, 1995). Clinical signs of poisoning at 50 mg/kg included anorexia, diarrhea, and Central Nervous System (CNS) depression. After intrarumenal doses of 500 and 750 mg/kg in sheep, severe cardiovascular and respiratory pathology was observed at autopsy (Johnson *et al.*, 1975).

Irritation/Sensitization Cyhexatin is an eye and skin irritant.

Subchronic Toxicity The only subchronic studies reported were in rabbits at oral and dermal doses of 3 mg/kg/day for 13 days. Reduced weight gain and skin irritation in the dermal study were the only effects reported.

Chronic Toxicity A 12-month dietary study in dogs used doses from 0.25 to 0.75 mg/kg/day. Only marginal effects relating to organ weight were observed at the highest dose. In a 2-year dietary study in rats at 1, 3, or 6 mg/kg/day, decreased weight gain was seen at 3 and 6 mg/kg/day. Bile duct hyperplasia was observed at all does. Other high dose effects were liver hepatocellular alterations, degenerative myopathy, and radiculomyelopathy of the spinal cord. In a study with B6C3F1 mice using the same exposure protocol, no consistent adverse effects were observed.

Carcinogenicity No evidence for carcinogenicity was obtained from the long-term dietary studies with cyhexatin in mice and rats.

Mutagenicity/Genotoxicity Cyhexatin was negative in the Ames assay (Moriya *et al.*, 1983). Additional studies in the Ames assay, a Chinese hamster ovary cell forward mutation assay, a mouse bone marrow micronucleus test, and an unscheduled DNA repair assay in rat hepatocytes all proved negative (Cal EPA, 1997). In an additional study (Hrelai *et al.*, 1994) cyhexatin gave weakly positive results in inducing sister chromatid exchange in human peripheral blood lymphocytes *in vitro*, but it was inactive in inducing chromosomal aberrations in mouse bone marrow cells *in vivo*. Cyhexatin was also negative in a study of the ability of pesticides to increase the unwinding rate of DNA in rat hepatocytes *in vivo* (Grilli *et al.*, 1991). The weight of evidence suuggests that cyhexatin is not genotoxic.

Reproductive Toxicity A two-generation reproduction study in rats revealed no reproductive toxicity apart from reduced pup weight even though the highest dose (6 mg/kg/day) caused several forms of maternal toxicity including decreased body weight and biliary hyperplasia. A second dietary study in rats utilized 10 (0.7 mg/kg/day), 30, or 100 ppm of micronized cyhexatin and incorporated a teratology component in the study. At 30 and/or 100 ppm a number of effects were seen including reduced food intake, lower body weights, litter size, pup weight and survival, and sternal ossification defects. An increase in cleft plate and thoracic blood vessel malformations was detected at 30 ppm but this was not dose-related since it was not seen at 100 ppm. Overall it was concluded that there was no evidence of the induction of developmental abnormalities. A subsequent study of the effects of dietary restriction on reproduction and development in rats suggested that many, but not all, of these reproductive effects were probably related to reduced food intake because of the unpalatability of the diet. The decreased pup survival seen at 30 ppm was considered to be a compound-related effect and was used as the LOEL.

Because of the unpalatability of diets containing cyhexatin (and other organotins) reduced food intake and consequently reduced weight gain can complicate the interpretation of dietary studies in experimental animals. To examine this effect further, a pair feeding study in rats was run in which food availability to control animals was matched with that consumed *ad libitum* by the treated groups. This reproductive toxicity study was continued for one generation at the single dietary cyhexatin concentration of 30 ppm. The only adverse effect of note was reduced weight gain in the pups. Since this effect was decreased but still evident with pair feeding, it was concluded that it is, at least in part, a compound-related effect.

Developmental Toxicity/Teratogenicity This area of the toxicology of cyhexatin is controversial. Based on positive studies in rabbits, the compound was withdrawn from many markets. However, the multiple studies conducted on its developmental effects and teratogenicity in rabbits present conflicting results. Between 1990 and 1995 the FAO/WHO JMPR received the results of eight teratology studies of cyhexatin in rabbits conducted under reasonably similar conditions (FAO/WHO, 1990b, 1992a, 1995). In terms of teratology, there were two negative oral and two negative dermal studies compared to three positive oral and one positive dermal one. The panel could not reconcile the results from these studies. After considering the weight of evidence and the possible existence of artifacts and uncertainties in some of the positive studies, they concluded that cyhexatin is not teratogenic in rabbits (FAO/WHO, 1995). Teratology studies in rats were uniformly negative.

FAO/WHO (1990b) reported the results of four studies that examined the teratology of cyhexatin in rabbits after oral administration during gestation. Two studies found teratogenic effects in the form of hydrocephalus with a LOEL of 0.75 mg/kg/day in one study and 3.0 mg/kg/day in the other. Dilated cerebral ventricles were seen in a few other animals. Embryo and fetal toxicity were observed at 0.75 and1.0 mg/kg/day, respectively. These values are all clearly below the doses causing maternal toxicity. In the other two studies, which appear equally valid, no adverse effects were observed at these doses. The possibilities that the hydrocephalus resulted from infection rather than the treatment or was due to poor mixing and nonhomogeneity of the diets were raised by the review panel, but evidence for either of these explanations is far from conclusive.

In a teratology study employing dermal application in rabbits with doses up to 3 mg/kg on days 6 through 18 of gestation, an increase in folded retinas was observed but no clear dose–response relationship emerged and fixation artifacts were suspected. Several instances of hydrocephalus were observed at the highest dose. Skin irritation was also noted at the highest dose, but no systemic toxicity or embryotoxcity was observed. In a subsequent study with a similar protocol, the only adverse effect observed was skin irritation.

A further study in rabbits (FAO/WHO, 1992a) compared two samples of cyhexatin from different manufacturing sites with different particle sizes to a very high purity sample (99.7%) for their embryotoxicity and teratology. Oral doses of 0.75, 1.5, and 3 mg/kg/day were administered during gestation. In general the severity of effects was greater with the smaller particle size and included lowered food intake and weight gains, pre- and postimplantation losses, fetotoxicity, and reduced litter size. A high incidence of folded lenses was observed at all doses. These were further evaluated later and the possibility of fixation artifacts was again raised since the folding was slight and there was no clear dose–response relationship in their occurrence (FAO/WHO, 1995). Some rib malformations and a small increase in dilation of brain ventricles occurred at 3 mg/kg/day at a rate above that seen in historical controls. There was no evidence of hydrocephaly. Other than particle size effects there were no obvious and consistent differences between the samples.

One further study was reported (FAO/WHO, 1995) with dermal doses of 0.5, 1.0, and 3.0 mg/kg/day. No evidence of teratology or maternal toxicity was obtained.

In rats, oral doses of 0.5 to 5.0 mg/kg/day resulted in no maternal toxicity or teratogenicity. An increase in the variability of the number of verterbrae at the highest dose was interpreted as evidence of fetotoxicity. An additional study revealed no notable adverse effects at 10 mg/kg/day but in neither of these studies was a dose given that was sufficient to cause maternal toxicity (Cal EPA, 1997).

Immunotoxicity No studies specifically addressing the immunotoxicity of cyhexatin were located.

Human Toxicology No cases of human poisoning by cyhexatin were found. Medical surveillance by ELF Atochem (France) of workers in plants manufacturing organotin compounds, including cyhexatin, revealed no adverse effects on hematological, clinical chemical, or immunological parameters. The urinary tin levels of these workers were no higher than those of unexposed control populations.

A study of occupational exposure in workers mixing and spraying Plictran 50W in orchard systems in Michigan determined that dermal exposure ranged from 0.7 to 7 mg/day. Very little exposure occurred through inhalation. Protective clothing and respirators were used. Fruit thinners and pickers had dermal exposures of 21 mg/day when working on the day of spraying and 0.83 mg/kg with a 14-day postapplication interval. In a second study conducted in Europe, dermal exposure in mixer/loader/applicators ranged from 0.8 to 19 mg/day. Blood tin level increased by up to 20-fold after exposure and peaked at 20.5 μg/l in one individual. The levels had not returned to normal 2 days after exposure ended.

Biochemical Mechanism of Action Cyhexatin behaves as a typical inhibitor of mitochondrial respiration acting at complex V. It inhibits Mg^{2+}-dependent ATPase activity in mitochondria from mouse liver and housefly thoraces *in vitro* with similar I_{50} values of about 700 nM (Ahmad and Knowles, 1972). Desaiah *et al.* (1973) found that cyhexatin inhibits oligomycin-sensitive Mg^{2+}-dependent ATPase (complex V) from spider mites and fish brain with subnanomolar potencies. In a study with beef heart mitochondria, Mehrotra *et al.*

(1985) concluded that cyhexatin inhibited oligomycin-sensitive Mg^{2+}-dependent ATPase with an I_{50} value of 10–20 nM. It also inhibited Ca^{2+}-dependent ATPase in mitochondria with a similar potency. The authors concluded that it was likely to interfere with both ATP biosynthesis and Ca^{2+} transport in mitochondria. Other ATPases also are inhibited *in vitro* such as the Na^+, K^+-ATPase of rat brain synaptosomes with an IC_{50} value of 2 μM. This inhibition was completely antagonized by preincubation of the synaptosomes with the dithiol dithiothreitol, but not with the monothiols, glutathione or cysteine (Rao *et al.*, 1987). The toxicological significance of this observation is unclear. Both the basal and isoproterenol-stimulated Ca^{2+}-ATPase from the cardiac sarcoplasmic reticulum was inhibited with high potency (IC_{50} of 25 nM; Sahib and Desaiah, 1986). This inhibition also occurred in rats *in vivo* and a decrease in the uptake of Ca^{2+} was seen. Since Ca^{2+} uptake by the sarcoplasmic reticulum mediates cardiac relaxation, this inhibitory action on Ca^{2+} flux could lead to cardiac dysfunction (Sahib and Desaiah, 1987). In totality, these results show that cyhexatin potently inhibits several types of ATPases with differing but potentially vital roles in cellular activities. In another study by this group, Kodaventi *et al.* (1989) report that cyhexatin inhibits calmodulin-activated adenylate cyclase solubilized from subcellular fractions of rat brain with a threshold at 50 nM. All these types of inhibition may well have consequences for animals exposed to cyhexatin, but their absolute and relative importance is unclear, and it remains difficult to connect *in vitro* biochemical findings with *in vivo* toxicology for this and other triorganotins.

Cyhexatin has several other potentially important biochemical actions besides the inhibition of complex V and other ATPases. These were included in the discussion of the general biochemical mechanisms of action of organotins (Section 57.6.2.5). Cyhexatin inhibited 5-HT uptake by blood platelets from rats *in vitro* and moderately in platelets taken from rats 30 min after the intraperitoneal administration of cyhexatin at 5 mg/kg (Johnson and Knowles, 1983), but the toxicological significance of this action is unclear.

Absorption, Metabolism, and Elimination A large number of pharmacokinetic studies on cyhexatin have been presented (FAO/WHO, 1992a, 1995). They show that the compound is poorly absorbed in mice, rats, and rabbits after oral dosing, and in rabbits after dermal application. The bioavailability after an oral dose was much higher in rabbits than rats. In rats, blood tin levels peaked at 3–4 hr after a single oral dose of cyhexatin and then declined to levels near those of controls over 24 hr. The micronized product often gave higher blood levels than technical cyhexatin (and also higher toxicity) but the results were not uniform among species and routes of administration. In pregnant rabbits given 3 mg/kg/day over the course of gestation, the half-life of tin in the maternal blood was about 8 hr. The disposition of cyhexatin in rats was slow with an elimination half-life after chronic dosing was terminated of 10 days for most tissues, but 40 days for brain and muscle. Initial residues were cyhexatin but this was subsequently converted to dicyclohexyltin. The major route of elimination of both oral and dermal doses in rats and rabbits was the urine, but the fecal route also contributed significantly to clearance.

The typical pathway of metabolism in mammals involves sequential conversion to dicyclohexyltin oxide, cyclohexylstannoic acid, and inorganic tin. The initial attack on cyhexatin involves microsomal oxidase attack to form the 2-, 3-, and 4-hydroxycyclohexyl analogs. The 2-hydroxy metabolite is readily converted to dicyclohexyltin (Kimmel *et al.*, 1980).

Environmental Fate and Toxicity Cyhexatin's acute toxicity (Table 57.4) and dietary toxicity to birds is moderate to low with 8-day dietary LC_{50} values of 3189 ppm for mallard ducks and 520 ppm for bobwhite quail. No reproductive impairment was observed in bobwhite quail fed 5 or 20 ppm prior to egg laying and through the egg laying cycle (Fink, 1975).

Cyhexatin is generally much more toxic to aquatic species than terrestrial ones (Table 57.4). Devries *et al.* (1991) conducted a comparative study of the effects of several organotins on the development of rainbow trout fry. Trout were continually exposed for 110 days to these compounds, beginning at the yolk sac stage. Of the triorganotins, cyhexatin chloride was more toxic than either tributyl or triphenyltin chlorides. It caused 100% mortality of fry within 1 week at a concentration of 3 nM and only a few trout survived exposure at 0.6 nM (0.24 ppb) for the full 110 days. Thymus atrophy, seen in mammals with many triorganotins, was not observed, but evidence of immunotoxic effects was obtained even at the lowest concentration tested, as indicated by decreased resistance to a bacterial challenge with *Aeromonas hydrophila*.

In the environment, cyhexatin binds firmly to soils and is converted to di- and monocyclohexyl tins and inorganic tin with half life of about 10 days (Muller and Bosshardt, 1987). This, and its low water solubility, indicate that it has a low potential to leach from soils. It's degradation is enhanced faster by exposure to UV light on soils or in water. In aquatic systems it is mainly adsorbed on sediments. The half-life for degradation in an aquatic microcosm study was 68 days (Kordel and Stein, 1997).

Fenbutatin-Oxide: General Properties and Uses Bis[tris(2-methyl-2-phenylpropyl)tin] oxide (Fig. 57.12), CAS Reg. No. 13356-08-6, was discovered by Shell Chemical Co.

It exists as colorless crystals, m.p. 145°C, v.p. 8.5×10^{-8} Pa (20°C), w.s. 12.7 ppb (20°C), log *P* 5.2. Fenbutatin-oxide hydrolyzes very slowly and reversibly in aqueous solution to the corresponding monotin hydroxide. At pH 5–9, less than 10% conversion occurred in 30 days at 25°C. Fenbutatin-oxide is also very stable to heat, light, and oxidation.

Fenbutatin-oxide (SD 14114) is a long-lasting nonsystemic acaricide. It also controls some sucking insects. Common trade names include Lexitin, Novran, Osadan, Torque, and Vendex.

Toxicology Overview The toxicology of fenbutatin-oxide has been reviewed by the Joint FAO/WHO Meeting on Pesticide Residues (FAO/WHO, 1993) and by the U.S. EPA (1994).

These reports are the primary data sources for the overview below.

Acute Toxicity Fenbutatin-oxide has a low acute toxicity to terrestrial vertebrates (Table 57.4). Toxicity by inhalation is considerably higher than by the oral and dermal routes. Inhalation exposure produced necrosis of bronchiolar and renal tubule epithelia, lung congestion, and edema. An intraperitoneal LD_{50} of 33 mg/kg in the rat (FAO/WHO, 1993) suggests that fenbutatin-oxide has a high intrinsic toxicity if it is absorbed systemically.

Irritation/Sensitization As with other organotins it is somewhat irritating to skin and a severe eye irritant but it is not a dermal sensitizer.

Subchronic Toxicity No specific target organ was evident in subchronic and chronic dietary studies. A 3-week dermal application study in rabbits at doses up to 5 mg/kg/day caused no systemic activity but severe local skin irritation and edema occurred. An initial range-finding study in rats showed reductions in food intake, body weight, and some organ weights and changes at dietary concentrations of 300 ppm and above. However, a pair-feeding study established that this was due to unpalatability of the diet rather than systemic toxicity.

Chronic toxicity Emesis and diarrhea were common but otherwise no major adverse effects were seen in a 2-year dietary study in dogs in which doses up to 60 mg/kg/day were administered by capsule. No adverse effects except reduced weight gains due to diet unpalatability were recorded in 2-year dietary studies in rats and mice with fenbutatin-oxide at levels up to 600 ppm. In a lifetime feeding study, female rats showed a decrease in the number of leucocytes at higher exposure levels with an LOEL at 15 mg/kg/day.

Carcinogenicity Fenbutatin-oxide is classified as a group E carcinogen (evidence of noncarcinogenicity in humans) by the U.S. Environmental Protection Agency since none of the chronic studies above revealed evidence of carcinogenicity.

Mutagenicity/Genotoxicity No evidence of genotoxicity was obtained in an extensive battery of *in vitro* and *in vivo* tests. Additional studies by Moriya *et al.* (1983) also gave negative results.

Reproductive Toxicity In a multigeneration study in rats, a LOEL was set at 17 to 20 mg/kg/day based on reduced pup body weight. Parental effects in the form of reduced food intake and weight occurred at the same dose. A special study on the effects of a single high oral dose of febutatin-oxide on the reproductive tract of male rabbits proved negative, even at toxic doses that casued lethality, emaciation, and lesions of the gastric mucosa.

Developmental Toxicity/Teratogenicity In standard studies with oral dosing in pregnant females, an increase in abortions and resorptions was observed in rabbits at an oral dose of 5 mg/kg/day. This was accompanied by anorexia and gastric lesions in the does. A similar study in rats demonstrated maternal toxicity at 30 mg/kg/day, but no reproductive endpoints or treatment-related malformations were seen.

Neurotoxicity   Because of the brain edema known to be caused by triethyltin, a study was performed in rats with fenbutatin-oxide at a dose of 1000 mg/kg. No evidence of brain pathology was seen although triethyltin bromide, as a positive control, caused the anticipated lesions. No effect was seen on EEG patterns in dogs dosed orally with 30 mg/kg/day for 14 days.

Immunotoxicity   Results of a 7-day feeding study in mice tentatively indicated that fenbutatin-oxide has a lower potential to cause immunotoxicity than other organotins.

Biochemical Mechanism of Action   Few investigations have been conducted with fenbutatin-oxide at the biochemical level. In one study, Machera *et al.* (1996) exposed nauplii of the brine shrimp *Artemia* to fenbutatin-oxide for 24 hr and found that Mg^{2+}-ATPase activity in whole tissues was inhibited by 66% at a water concentration of 25 ppb. The Na^+/K^+-ATPase activity was also inhibited but to a lower degree. Studies on platelets conducted by Johnson and Knowles (1983) and Knowles and Johnson (1996) showed that fenbutatin-oxide inhibited 5-hydroxytryptamine uptake by, and enhanced its release from, rat platelets at 10 μM *in vitro* and after intraperitoneal treatment at 2.5 mg/kg. This was attributed to its effects on ATP production. No effect was seen on the aggregation of rat platelets *in vitro* at 10 μM.

Absorption, Metabolism, and Elimination   Fenbutatin-oxide was very poorly absorbed after oral dosing. In rats, 99% of single or repeated oral doses was excreted in the feces, almost entirely as unchanged fenbutatin-oxide. Metabolites identified both in animals and soil include β, β-dimethylphenethylstannoic acid and the bis-dealkylation product, 1,3-dihydroxy-1,1,3,3-tetrakis(2-methyl-2-phenylpropyl)distannoxane. This metabolite showed no appreciable toxicity to rats in a subchronic study at levels of dietary exposure up to 300 ppm and it did not cause brain edema in rats after oral dosing at 100 mg/kg (FAO/WHO, 1993).

Environmental Fate and Toxicity   The acute toxicity to birds appears to be very low (Table 57.4). Similarly, the dietary 8-day LC_{50} for bobwhite quail is >5620 ppm in the diet. Avian reproduction studies in mallard ducks and bobwhite quail showed no adverse effect at dietary doses up to 150 ppm. By contrast, fenbutatin-oxide is very highly toxic to both vertebrate and invertebrate aquatic species (Table 57.4). An LC_{50} value as low as 1.7 ppb was obtained with rainbow trout and most LC_{50} values for fish and aquatic invertebrates are below 50 ppb. A developmental study in rainbow trout showed that growth and survival of juveniles was impaired at concentrations above 0.31 ppb, and

a life-cycle study in *Daphnia* showed that survival is impaired at concentrations greater than 16 ppb. Additional tests on estuarine and marine organisms also established the very high aquatic toxicity of fenbutatin-oxide with LC_{50} values of 2.8 ppb for mysid shrimps and 0.4 ppb for eastern oyster larvae. Machera *et al.* (1996) obtained an LC_{50} of 50 ppb for brine shrimp nauplii using a 55% formulation of fenbutatin-oxide. Fenbutatin-oxide has a rather high BCF of 490–730 in bluegill sunfish, which in view of its high log P value and resistance to metabolism is not surprising. The true BCF factor is probably higher since the concentration of fenbutatin-oxide did not reach an equilibrium during the course of this study (U.S. EPA, 1994). Depuration was slow with only 50–75% of the tissue residues being cleared in 14 days.

Despite its high aquatic toxicity in laboratory tests, the impact of fenbutatin-oxide in actual use may be lower than predicted since it binds very strongly to soil and sediments which limits its availability in the water phase of natural aquatic systems. Binding to soil also results in minimal mobility in the soil and a low potential to leach. K_d values range from 1282 to 2333, depending on soil type. Both hydrolytic and photolytic degradation are very slow with half-lives over 100 days in typical laboratory studies. Microbial metabolism in the soil under both aerobic and anaerobic conditions is also extremely slow with half-lives of months to years. As a result, fenbutatin-oxide is persistent in soils with a half-life estimated to be slightly less than 1 year based on field measurements (Grey *et al.*, 1995). Other estimates of its half-life under varying field and environmental conditions range from 271 to 1367 days (U.S. EPA, 1994). This stability gives fenbutatin-oxide the capability to accumulate under conditions of repeated use.

Fentin: General Properties and Uses   Triphenyltin is used as a pesticide in any of three forms, as the hydroxide (CAS Reg. No. 76-87-9), as the acetate (CAS Reg. No. 900-95-8), or, to a lesser extent, as the chloride (CAS Reg. No. 639-58-7) (Fig. 57.12). It was discovered by Hoechst (acetate) and N.V. Philips-Duphar (hydroxide) and is described by van der Kerk and Luijten (1954). A comprehensive monograph on the chemistry, biological properties, toxicology, and environmental fate of triphenyltins is provided by Bock (1981). Fentin hydroxide was first registered in the United States in 1971. In 1985 the U.S. Environmental Protection Agency instituted a Special Review based on its potential developmental toxicity to mixers, loaders, and applicators. This and other toxicological issues were resolved in a recent Reregistration Eligibility Decision (U.S. EPA, 1999c) which included a number of steps to reduce exposure.

The hydroxide exists as colorless crystals with m.p. 118–120°C, v.p. 6.5×10^{-6} Pa (20°C), w.s. about 1 ppm (pH 7, 20°C), log P3.43, pKa 5.20. The acetate exists as colorless crystals with m.p. 121–123°C, w.s. about 19 ppm (pH 5, 20°C), v.p. 1.9×10^{-3} Pa (60°), log P3.1–3.4. The chloride exists as colorless crystals, m.p. 106–107°C. The acetate and chloride are quite readily hydrolyzed to the hydroxide (e.g., the half-life of the acetate in water at pH 7 is <3 hr). On gentle heating, the hydroxide is dehydrated to bis(triphenyltin) oxide. Ultraviolet irradiation gradually dearylates triphenyltins to inorganic tin.

The principal use of all forms of fentin is as nonsystemic foliar fungicides with additional activity as antifeeding agents for some insects. Fentin acetate and chloride also control algae and snails in rice and fish ponds and fentin compounds are used as antifouling agents on marine vessels. Common trade names include Brestan H, Du-Ter, Flo-Tin, Haitin, Photon, Pro-Tex, SuperTin, Suzu H, and Tubotin (hydroxide), Aquatin and Tinmate (chloride), and Brestan, Phytex, Radar, Suzu, Triacetane, and Trimastan (acetate).

Toxicology Profile Fentin hydroxide has been very extensively tested for toxicity in experimental animals and a variety of adverse effects have been displayed, although an unexplained lack of reproducibility between some studies is apparent. A wealth of older toxicology results dating back to the 19th century are provided by Bock (1981) but generally are not included here. The primary data sources are FAO/WHO (1992b) and U.S. EPA (1999c) which report a large number of unpublished studies conducted in the 1980s.

Acute Toxicity Fentin hydroxide is generally of moderate to high acute toxicity to terrestrial vertebrates by the oral and dermal routes, but it has a much higher toxicity by inhalation (Table 57.4). Results from different studies tend to be rather variable. A value for the dermal LD_{50} as low as 127 mg/kg has been reported for the rabbit although the value for rat is 1600 mg/kg (FAO/WHO, 1992b). Fentin acetate has a roughly similar acute toxicity which is reasonable since it is rapidly converted to the hydroxide *in vivo*. Sensitivity seems to vary considerably among different mammalian species [e.g., the oral LD_{50} values for mice vary from 81 to 245 mg/kg, but for male guinea pigs the LD_{50} is only 25 mg/kg (FAO/WHO, 1992b)]. For the rabbit a value of 80 mg/kg has been recorded. Reports also vary for the acute dermal toxicity with a value for the rat >2000 mg/kg, but only 350 mg/kg for the mouse (FAO/WHO, 1992b). Like fentin hydroxide, the acetate is very toxic by inhalation (Table 57.4). Its intrinsic toxicity is very high as revealed by an intraperitoneal LD_{50} value of 3.6 mg/kg for male rats. Fentin chloride is extremely toxic with an acute oral LD_{50} to the mouse of 18 mg/kg. Signs of intoxication are typical of triorganotins and include anorexia, emesis, tremors, diarrhea, drowsiness, and ataxia.

Irritation/Sensitization As with other organotins, fentin hydroxide is a severe eye irritant. Skin irritation is mild to moderate and it is not a dermal sensitizer. Fentin acetate has similar properties but did give a positive Buehler test for skin sensitization in guinea pigs (FAO/WHO, 1992b).

Subchronic Toxicity In subchronic feeding studies in rats, multiple hematologic and blood chemistry changes were observed at higher doses of 7 to 8 mg/kg/day, The most sensitive endpoint was a decrease in IgG antibodies observed at the lowest dose tested, 0.75 mg/kg/day. These levels were still depressed after a 4-week recovery period. A similar result was obtained in a mouse subchronic feeding study with decreased levels of immunoglobulin antibodies seen at the lowest dose, 0.75 mg/kg/day, more extensive antibody effects and decreased adrenal weights at 3.8 mg/kg/day, and decreased ovary weights and hemoglobin at 19.5 mg/kg/day. In a parallel study in guinea pigs, decreased leucocyte counts were observed at the lowest dose tested, 0.1 mg/kg/day. In a subchronic dermal studies in Wistar rats only skin irritation without systemic toxicity was seen at 10 mg/kg/day, but several effects on biochemical parameters in the blood and clinical signs (piloerection, mydriasis, dyspnea) and some deaths were seen at 20 mg/kg/day. A second dermal study using Charles River rats failed to reveal any systemic toxicity at 20 mg/kg/day. A 13-week subchronic inhalation study in rats had an LOEL at 0.002 mg/l. Adverse effects at this very low exposure level included reductions in white blood cells, lung and respiratory irritation and edema, and death, particularly in males.

Additional 70-day subchronic dietary studies have been conducted with rabbits and lambs at concentrations from 15 to 150 ppm (Dacasto *et al.*, 1994). In both species, decreased body weight and decreased relative thymus weight were recorded. In the rabbit, the major lesions were found in the thymus and lymph nodes. Lambs showed similar but less severe lesions.This immunosuppressive activity echoes that seen in rodents, but the lamb and rabbit are much less sensitive.

Chronic Toxicity A 1-year feeding study in dogs showed no major effects at the highest dose, about 0.6 mg/kg/day. However, a lifetime study in mice had an endpoint based on a decreased leucocyte count at 0.25 mg/kg/day. In a chronic dietary study in rats, decreases in immunoglobulins and increased deaths were seen at doses as low as 0.3–0.4 mg/kg/day and decreased immunoglobulins were also found in a parallel mouse study with doses as low as 0.85 mg/kg/day. These were the lowest doses tested and no NOEL was established.

Mutagenicity/Genotoxicity Fentins (both as the acetate and hydroxide) are generally negative in standard genotoxicity tests, but fentin hydroxide gave a positive result for chromosomal aberrations after metabolic activation in human lymphocytes (Moriya *et al.*, 1983). A similar positive result with activation is reported by FAO/WHO (1992b). Positive result were also obtained in two mouse lymphoma mutation assays. These positives were tentatively interpreted by FAO/WHO (1992b) in terms of the toxicity of fentin to the lymphocytes rather than as a specific clastogenic action. In any case, the results of clastogenicity studies *in vivo* have been negative.

Carcinogenicity Fentin hydroxide caused pituitary and testicular (Leydig cell) tumors in rats 1–2 mg/kg/day and hepatocellular adenomas and carcinomas in mice at about 15 mg/kg/day in standard long-term dietary studies. Two previous chronic dietary studies at comparable dose rates in mice, and one in rats, had proved negative for carcinogenicity (FAO/WHO, 1992b).

Fentin hydroxide was classified as a B2 carcinogen (probable human carcinogen) by the U.S. Environmental Protection Agency. A Q_1^* value of 18.3 $(mg/kg/day)^{-1}$ was calculated.

Reproductive Toxicity   Fentin hydroxide causes reproductive toxicity. Decreases in litter size, pup weight, and the relative sizes of the spleen and thymus of weanlings were observed in rats in a multigenerational feeding study at a dose (0.9 mg/kg/day) that did not cause maternal toxicity. A study of the effects of fentin hydroxide on male fertility in rats when given orally at 20 mg/kg/day for 25 days showed a reduction in spermatazoa count that was reversed after a 70-day recovery period.

Ema *et al.* (1997) observed that an oral dose of triphenyltin chloride of either 4.7 or 6.3 mg/kg given to female rats on days 0 to 3 of pregnancy induces implantation failures by enhancing preimplantation embryonic loss. No subsequent adverse effects were seen at these doses on the fetuses where implantation was successful. By using a pair-feeding approach, they concluded that this was not due to the decreased food consumption commonly seen in studies with organotins (Harazano *et al.*, 1998). In further exploring the mechanism for this effect, Ema *et al.* (1999) found that oral doses that caused early implantation losses also suppressed uterine decidualization as indicated by greatly decreased uterine weights. At these doses, fentin chloride also significantly reduced serum levels of progesterone, which is required for decidualization. Ema *et al.* therefore conclude that fentin in some way interferes with progesterone biosyntheses which decreases the receptivity of the uterus and leads to implantation failures.

Developmental Toxicity/Mutagenicity   In dietary studies with pregnant rabbits, fentin hydroxide caused both fetotoxicity and teratogenicity. These were detected in the form of decreased implantations and increased resorptions, decreased fetal weight, and various malformations including poorly ossified skeletal elements at an LOEL of 1 mg/kg/day. Fetotoxicity, but only relatively minor effects on ossification, were seen at 8 mg/kg/day in several studies in rats. Hamsters at 12 mg/kg/day showed decreased pup weight and various malformations including skeletal and other minor anomalies. In every case, these doses also caused maternal toxicity in the form of reduced feeding and weight gain and sometimes more severe toxic effects. A dermal study in rats gave negative results at the highest dose tested, 3 mg/kg/day. Reports of occasional hydronephrosis, hydrocephalus, omphalocele, and hydroureter in some previous studies led to the establishment of a special study of the induction of these effects in rats. However, no evidence for such irreversible structural effects was seen at 8 mg/kg/day which was clearly toxic to the darns.

Immunotoxicity   There is strong evidence for immunotoxicity. Lymphocytes and immunoglobulins were decreased after subchronic or chronic dietary administration of fentin in guinea pigs, mice, and rats at low doses. In specific tests for immunotoxicity, decreases in spleen weights, leucocytes, lymphocytes,

and antibody immunogloblins, and lymphoid depletion in the thymus and spleen were observed in mice. Effects on the spleen were seen with doses as low as 1.2 mg/kg/day in mice. Similar, but less extensive, effects were observed in rats beginning at a dose of 3.4 mg/kg/day. Ishaaya *et al.* (1976) showed that fentin acetate fed to mice for 4 days at dietary levels of 30 to 300 ppm caused a dose-related decrease in spleen weight and in the number of blood leucocytes.

A review of the literature on this topic (FAO/WHO, 1992b) indicates that short-term (up to 13 weeks) exposure to fentins caused immunosuppression marked by lymphopenia and lymphocyte depletion in the spleen and thymus resulting in altered cellular and humoral immunity, but these effects are transient and tend to diminish on longer exposure. Some tests of immune function show no response to organotins. Overall it appears that fentins display weak immunosuppressive actions and that these appear at doses that reduce levels of circulating lymphocytes and the weight of the lymphoid organs.

Endocrine Effects   Fentin hydroxide appears to be an endocrine disrupter. It causes testicular and pituitary tumors in rats and changes in both adrenal and ovary weights in mice. Embryo implantation losses caused by fentins may involve decreased progesterone levels (Ema *et al.*, 1999). Fentins also induce masculinization of female mollusks (imposex) as describe later. Further mechanistic studies are needed to determine its status in this respect.

Human Toxicology   According to U.S. EPA (1999c) there have been very few, if any, well documented cases of human poisoning by triphenyltin hydroxide in the United States.

However, FAO/WHO (1992b) provides several examples of fentin poisoning. Two cases involved occupational inhalation of Brestan 60 (60% fentin acetate with 15% maneb) during preparation of spray solutions by farmers. Signs of poisoning were nausea, dizziness, transient loss of consciousness, convulsions, persistent headache, photophobia, and impaired liver functions. Recovery occurred after 10–15 days (Manzo and Richelmi, 1981). A further example of human poisoning by triphenyltin acetate with neurological signs involved a 36-year-old male who developed dizziness and generalized paroxysmal abnormalities with slowed EEG rhythms after dermal exposure. Skin injury was also reported (Colosio *et al.*, 1991).

Wu *et al.* (1990) described a case based on a suicide attempt by a 23-year-old male who consumed a fentin acetate-containing molluscicidal preparation (amount unstated). Abdominal pains, diarrhea, vomiting, severe ataxia, and coma resulted. The patient also showed neurological effects including a reversible sensorimotor polyneuropathy that developed 2 months after exposure. A full recovery was attained in 3.5 months. This diagnosis has been questioned by Cavanaugh (1995) on the basis of the long delay in the appearance of some neurological symptoms and the lack of previous evidence for triphenyltin-induced neurotoxicity in humans. In the same issue, Wu *et al.* defended their diagnosis. Subsequently, a second case of human poisoning by fentin acetate with substantial neurological involvement has been reported by Lin *et al.* (1998). In this case, the patient, an 18-year-old female who intentionally consumed about 33 g of a 45% triphenyltin acetate formulation, felt weakness and nausea 3 days later despite previous gastric lavage and treatment with activated chrcoal. After hospitalization, she lost full consciousness for 9 days, showing sponteous involuntary movement of the hands, facial twitching, and emotional instability. Diplopia, drowsines, giddiness and vertigo, bidirectional nystagmus, confusion, and disorientation also developed. An EEG showed mild cortical dysfunction wihout seizures. Scans by MRI and Tc-99m HMPAO brain SPECT to assess regional blood flow were unremarkable. Thus fentin may cause cellular dysfunction in the brain without evident structural damage. Leucopenia was noted on the sixth day and liver impairment occurred on the ninth day. Borderline delayed peripheral neuropathy developed on day 53. Recovery of normal neurological functions took 1 year. Further examples of fentin poisoning with neurological involvement, in addition to those cited by FAO/WHO above, have been reported by Lin and Hsueh (1993) involving exposure by ingestion; included irritability, blurred vision, headache, and disturbances of consciousness as well as reversible acute nephropathy (proximal tubule necrosis) and hepatitis.

Biochemical Mechanism of Action   Fentin compounds inhibit mitochondrial ATPase activity with considerable potency. Pieper and Casida (1965) found an I_{50} value of 100 nM for the inhibition of ATPase by triphenyltin chloride in a housefly thoracic particulate preparation. With triphenyltin hydroxide, Ahmad and Knowles (1972) calculated an I_{50} values slightly below 1 μM for Mg^{2+}-stimulated ATPase activity in both mouse liver and housefly thoracic mitochondria.

Several other mechanistic studies with fentin were outlined in Section 57.6.2.5. The effects of organotins on cytochrome P-450 and its toxicological implications were described. Enough work has been conducted with fentins in this regard to indicate that they are relatively potent in this action. Further studies that shed additional light on the mechanisms of toxicity of fentin are presenterd below.

Zazueta *et al.* (1994) studied the effect of fentin on membrane permeability and calcium regulation in mitochondria from rat kidney. At low micromolar concentrations it induced a rapid increase in permeability with a fall in membrane potential and a loss of calcium and matrix proteins as it induced the mitochondrial pemeability transition. This was not due to a general detergent effect since it was efficiently reversed by sulfhydryl reagents. This opening of the permeability transition pore was not reversed by cyclosporin A, but EDTA was effective. Several potential mechanisms for this effect are considered including a role for fentin in enhancing calcium cycling across the membrane, but the authors suggest that the most likely is the binding of fentin to sulfhydryl groups that trigger the transition pore to open. Tributyltin causes similar effects (Stridh *et al.*, 1999b).

In a recent study of the effect of phenyltins on human NK (natural killer) cells *in vitro*, Whalen *et al.* (2000) found that 1 μM triphenyltin almost eliminated their tumor killing capability without reducing their general viability. Over 24 hr fentin decreased the ability of NK cells to bind to tumor cells, but this is a secondary effect since a dramatic decrease in NK cell killing efficiency was seen within 1 hr of exposure to tin compounds when cell binding was still unaffected. The order of potency among phenyltins was triphenyl>diphenyl>monophenyl, but triphenyltin was slightly less active than tributyltin. Since NK cells are a primary defense against tumor and virus-infected cells, a decrease in their efficiency *in vivo* could lead to enhanced sensitivity to tumor formation and viral infections.

Absorption, Metabolism and Elimination   Clearance of an oral dose of triphenyltin hydroxide in rats was primarily by the biliary route. In different studies 80–100% of the dose was recovered in the feces with much being in the form of the parent compound, indicating limited uptake, averaging 40% of the dose. Successive oxidative removal of the phenyl groups eventually produces inorganic tin. Because of slow clearance, on repeated dosing cumulation of residues occurs in tissues giving levels up to sevenfold above those found with a single dose. The significance of cytochrome P-450 oxidations in the degradation of fentin is underlined by the observation of Ohhira *et al.* (2000) that when mice are administered SKF-525A, a P-450 inhibitor, together with fentin, the levels of fentin in the tissues are increased about threefold after 24 hr and the amount of metabolites is reduced. Because of the elevated tissue levels of fentin, hyperglycemia was observed in the SKF-525A-treated animals but not in the controls. In hamsters, oxidative dearylation of fentin is slower, the levels in the tissues, including the pancreas, reach a higher level than in rats, and hamsters show a hyperglycemic response to trifentin without manipulation of P-450 activities (Ohhira *et al.*, 2000).

Fentin hydroxide binds strongly to the skin making dermal absorption studies difficult. Little of the dermal dose is absorbed in 10 hr, but slow uptake may continue for some time from reservoirs held in the skin (U.S. EPA, 1999c).

Environmental Fate and Toxicity   Fentin hydroxide has a moderate to high acute toxicity to birds (Table 57.4). It is very highly toxic to aquatic species in general. In a study of the effects of organotins on the development of rainbow trout fry by Devries *et al.* (1991) fentin chloride caused acute mortality at 15 nM. The no-effect concentration on juvenile development was very low at 0.12 nM (0.05 ppb). Diphenyltin was about 100-fold less active. Thymus atrophy, seen with fentin in mammals, was not observed in the fish, but evidence of immunotoxic effects was obtained even at the lowest effect level as indicated by decreased resistance to a bacterial challenge.

As noted previously, fentin has a very strong capability to cause the imposex phenomenon in mollusks by its action as a xenoandrogen. Its potency in this regard in the rock shell (*Thais clavigera*) was about the same as that of tributyltin (Horiguchi *et al.*, 1997). As usual, di- and monophenyltins were much less active. Fentin induced imposex in the female ramshorn snail (*Marisa cornuarietis*) with an EC_{10} after exposure for 4 months of 12.3 ppt. Fecundity was reduced at an even lower concentration (5.4 ppb) with a complete lack of spawning at 163 ppt (Schulte-Oehlmann *et al.*, 2000).

Fentin hydroxide binds very strongly to soils (K_{oc} values range from 1900 to 54,000 ml/g; U.S. EPA, 1999c) and to humic substances in water (Looser *et al.*, 1998). It is resistant to both hydrolysis and photolysis. Estimates of the half-life for its degradation in soil range from 21 to about 140 days. A BCF of 3700 for whole body accumulation in fish indicates a significant capability for bioaccumulation. Larvae of the fish (*Thymallus thymallus*) showed a similar BCF value of 2200 (Looser *et al.*, 1998). It is also bioconcentrated by aquatic invertebrtaes with BCF factors ranging from 190 for *Daphnia* to 680 for *Chironomus*. Uptake was higher at pH 8 than pH 5, as expected from the dissociation of the hydroxide at acidic pH, but uptake seemed to occur even with the triphenyltin cation.

57.6.3 OTHER INHIBITORS OF COMPLEX V

57.6.3.1 Diafenthiuron

1-*Tert*-butyl-3-(2,6-diisopropyl-4-phenoxyphenyl)thiourea (Fig. 57.13), CAS Reg. No. 80060-09-9, was discovered by Ciba-Geigy Corp. and is described by Streibert *et al.* (1988). Its development and properties are described by Drabek *et al.* (1990).

General Properties It exists as a white powder, m.p. 150°C, v.p. 2.2×10^{-7} Pa (20°C), solubility in water 0.06 ppm (25°C), log P 5.76, HLC 1.28×10^{-2} Pa m^3 mol^{-1}. It is converted by ultraviolet light to the corresponding carbodiimide CGA 140400 (Drabek *et al.*, 1990).

Uses Diafenthiuron (CGA 106,603) is used as an insecticide, particularly against whiteflies and aphids, and as an acaricide. Trade names include Pegasus and Polo.

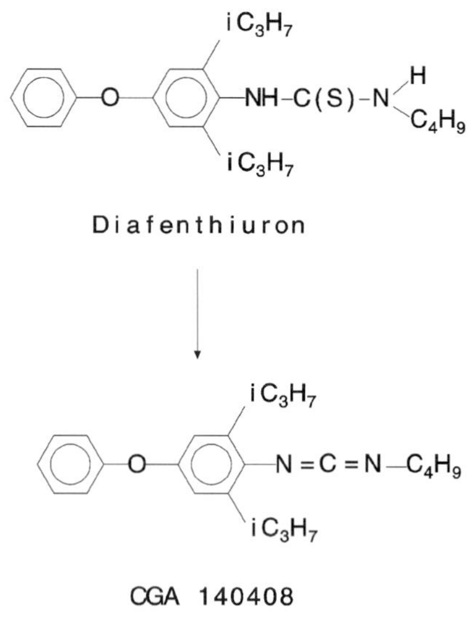

Figure 57.13 Pesticides that act as inhibitors of complex V—Diafenthiuron and its active metabolite.

Toxicology Profile The sources of data are Streibert *et al.* (1988) and Anonymous (1992b). Only limited data are available.

Acute Toxicity The acute toxicity of diafenthiuron to terrestrial vertebrates is low (Table 57.4). The target tissue in rats fed large doses of diafenthiuron is the lung where it increased lung weight associated with an increased incidence of alveolar foam cells. At high lethal doses given intraperitoneally, mice die within 4–24 hr with symptoms of lethargy, respiratory distress, and intermittent tonic contractions of the limb extensors, but at lower doses only lethargy, anorexia, and dehydration are seen and death may be delayed for many days (Petroske and Casida, 1995).

Irritation/Sensitization Diafenthiuron is only slightly irritating to the skin or eye and it is not a dermal sensitizer.

Chronic Toxicity Reversible edema of the pancreas was observed in dogs in a 1-year study. Chronic feeding studies in mice caused proliferative lesions (focal hyperplasia, adenoma, and carcinomas) which were considered to be secondary to the cytotoxicity caused by the high dose and not predictive of carcinogenicity in humans.

Carcinogenicity No additional results on the carcinogenicity of diafenthiuron were found.

Mutagenicity/Genotoxicity Diafenthiuron has not been found to be mutagenic in a suite of standard tests.

Reproductive Toxicity Diafenthiuron was not found to be a reproductive toxicant.

Developmental Toxicity/Teratogenicity Diafenthiuron was negative in studies of teratogenicity.

Biochemical Mechanism of Action Diafenthiuron is a propesticide. The active metabolite is the corresponding carbodiimide (CGA 140,408) which is produced on the leaf surface by sunlight and by oxidative metabolism in living organisms (Petroske and Casida, 1995; Ruder and Kayser, 1992; Ruder *et al.*, 1991). This conversion is shown in Fig. 57.13. CGA 140,408 is stabilized against nucleophilic attack through steric shielding of the highly reactive carbodiimide center by the surrounding bulky and hydrophobic alkyl groups. It does react with water slowly, producing the urea analog, and with carboxylic acid groups in fatty acids and some amino acids. This reactivity is central to its mechanism of action since the carbodiimide reacts covalently with a critical aspartate residue in the F_0 portion of mitochondrial ATP synthase, thus blocking ATP biosynthesis (Ruder and Kayser, 1993). This parallels the action of the well-known ATP synthesis inhibitor, dicyclohexylcarbodiimide (DCCD). This compound has been shown to react with a specific aspartate residue in the "*c*" subunit of the F_0 component (Fig. 57.5). Only 1 "*c*" subunit of the 9–12 present in each F_0

unit needs to be derivatized in order to fully block ATP synthase activity. It is postulated that this carboxylic acid group is intimately concerned with proton transport through the F_0 system by protonation on the cytoplasmic face and subsquent deprotonation toward the matrix side (Fillingame, 1992).

Additional evidence that the carbodiimide is the active agent and the site of action in insects is ATP synthase was derived by Ruder and his colleagues (Ruder *et al.*, 1991; Ruder and Kayser, 1992, 1993) and is reviewed by Hollingworth and Gadelhak (1998). This includes the observation that although both compounds are ATPase inhibitors *in vivo*, only the carbodiimide is an active inhibitor *in vitro*, that the carbodiimide acts more rapidly and potently in insects than its parent, and that in insects the toxicity of diafenthiuron is antagonized by piperonyl butoxide, a microsomal monooxygenase inhibitor. After *in vivo* exposure, diafenthiuron caused a significant decrease in ATP levels in the nervous system of locusts, the apparent target tissue in insect, and the severity of poisoning correlated well with the degree of inhibition ATP synthase in this tissue.

Vetebrate mitochondrial ATP synthase is also sensitive to inhibition by the carbodiimide both *in vitro* and *in vivo*, but piperonyl butoxide does not antagonize the acute toxicity of diafenthiuron in mice (Petroske and Casida, 1995). Even so, these authors concluded that the levels of the carbodiimide produced in mice *in vivo* were sufficient to cause severe inhibition of ATPase activity, as judged by the sensitivity of the enzyme *in vitro*. They also observed that whereas the intraperitoneal LD_{50} in mice for diafenthiuron was 15 mg/kg, that of the carbodiimide was only 0.3 mg/kg, although the same symptomatology was observed. This again supports the activation hypothesis.

In insects, but not in rats or plants, the carbodiimide metabolite also reacts with porin (the voltage dependent anion channel) of the outer mitochondrial membrane (Ruder and Kayser, 1993; Wiesner *et al.*, 1996). The toxicological significance of this reaction is unclear, in part because the functions of porin are unclear. The open porin channel is large, nonselective, and appears to allow a range of solutes to enter the mitochondrion which may then be taken up through the inner membrane. It also is an attachment site for several cytoplasmic enzymes such as hexokinase (Crompton *et al.*, 1999). Finally, as already described, it is probably a critical component of the mitochondrial permeability transition pore that is central to the role of mitochondria in apotosis. The reaction with carbodiimides does not change the conductance of this channel, but it does alter its voltage dependence, leading to a shift moring the open the closed state (Wiesner *et al.*, 1996).

It also seems reasonable to suppose that the extensive production of a carbodiimide *in vivo,* even one of reduced reactivity, would lead to the alkylation of other cellular macromolecules, as is true for DCCD (e.g., see Solioz, 1984). If so, it has not been reported except for the finding of derivatized fatty acids as metabolites *in vivo*. However, Petroske and Casida (1995) concluded that although the rapid acute toxicity to mice at high doses of diafenthiuron could be explained by the inhibition of ATP synthase, the delayed toxicity seen at lower doses was not related to such inhibition since this enzyme had already

recovered well before death occurred. Other sites of action may therefore be significant in the causation of this type of toxicity.

It has been suggested that diafenthiuron and its carbodiimide may act in insects by stimulating biogenic amine (octopamine) receptors (Kadir and Knowles, 1991). This capability often correlates with activity on α_2-adrenergic receptors in vertebrates. However, the octopaminergic action of these compounds could not be confirmed in subsequent studies (Hollingworth and Gadelhak, 1998).

Metabolic Fate Diafenthiuron is rapidly metabolized and excreted mainly in the feces as urea and fatty acid derivatives formed from the carbodiimide intermediate. In mice treated with diafenthiuron intraperitoneally, the carbodiimide was found in several tissues. It was also proposed that a thiourea sulfoxide was formed, leading to the production of the corresponding formamidine after desulfoxidation (Petroske and Casida, 1995).

Environmental Fate and Toxicity In birds, 8-day feeding studies indicated low toxicity with LC_{50} values >1500 mg/kg in bobwhite quail and mallard ducks. Diafenthiuron is strongly absorbed on soils and degradation is rapid varies from (half-life <1 hr to 1.4 days). It is much more toxic to fish in standard tests than to terrestrial vertebrates (Table 57.4). However, it is claimed that the rapid degradation of diafenthiuron in the field means that there is very little practical hazard to aquatic species (Anonymous, 1992b).

57.7 MITOCHONDRIAL UNCOUPLERS

57.7.1 INTRODUCTION

Mitochondrial uncouplers are a group of relatively simple but very effective toxicants. They act by discharging the proton gradient across the inner mitochondrial membrane and bypassing the concomitant phosphorylation of ADP to ATP. Thus the potential energy represented by the proton-motive force, Δp, is dissipated as heat and ATP synthesis ceases. Even worse from the point of view of cellular disruption is that as Δp is lowered, the ATP synthase (complex V) operates in reverse to hydrolyze ATP. Thus even the ATP created by the continuation of glycolysis is rapidly destroyed with dire implications for cellular survival. The mitochondrion has become a machine for destroying rather than synthesizing ATP.

The mechanism by which typical uncouplers achieve this effect is by acting as protonophores which shuttle protons across the impermeable inner mitochondrial membrane along their electrical and chemical gradients (McLaughlin and Dilger, 1980; Wallace and Starkov, 2000). This is a purely physicochemical process. The requirements for a molecule to be an effective uncoupler are only that it should be a lipophilic weak acid. In the simplest form of this mechanism, shown in Fig. 57.6, the uncoupler (generically shown as HA) tends to locate within the phospholipid bilayer membrane because of its lipophilic nature. At the matrix face of the membrane it encounters an elevated pH and, as a weak acid, will tend to dissociate and release a proton to the matrix. The resulting anion (A^-) passes back to the cytoplasmic face of the membrane along its concentration gradient and according to the charge differential across the membrane. The most powerful uncouplers have anions that are also lipophilic. Molecular features encouraging this are the presence of aromatic systems in the molecule conjugated with the acidic center which allow dispersion of the negative charge across the molecule, and shielding of the negative charge by bulky, lipophilic neighboring groups. At the cytoplasmic face, the anion (A^-) encounters a more acidic environment, tends to become protonated, and, again according to its chemical gradient within the membrane, will diffuse back across to the matrix face where the proton is discharged. A proton is translocated across the membrane in each turn of this cycle. Additional, more complex variations on this basic theme are possible and are described by Wallace and Starkov (2000). Other mechanisms of achieving uncoupling exist such as redox cycling (as reviewed in Section 57.1.6.4). Organotin pesticides which have both respiratoy uncoupling and inhibitory properties are covered in Section 57.6.2.

A protonophoric uncoupler thus acts as a catalyst which creates a proton short circuit across the inner membrane. It is not consumed as it uncouples, nor is a binding site required for its action. Indeed, protonophoric uncouplers are capable of discharging ion gradients and increasing the conductivity of simple artificial phospoholipid bilayer membranes (Bakker et al., 1973; Cunarro and Weiner, 1975). This means that uncouplers generally show, at most, very modest selectivity between mitochondria from different organisms, and useful selective toxicity is likely to be achieved primarily through differences in the pharmacokinetics of uncouplers between target and nontarget species.

"Uncoupling" refers to the fact that in the uncoupled state, the rate of oxidation of substrates and passage of electrons down the transport chain to oxygen is no longer tightly coupled to and controlled by the rate of synthesis of ATP. Respiration is uncoupled from phosphorylation. In this condition, the electron transport chain is free to run at its maximum rate which is typically several-fold faster than in the coupled state. Thus, in the presence of uncouplers, substrates are oxidized and oxygen is consumed at a much higher rate than in the normal cell. The large amounts of energy released in this process are not conserved and are wasted as heat.

The implications of the above mechanism of action are confirmed by the signs and symptoms of poisoning caused by typical uncouplers in both experimental animals and humans. These include fatigue, nausea and vomiting, hyperactivity, flushed skin, sweating, fever (particularly in larger animals including humans), dehydration and thirst, dyspnea, deep and rapid respiration, tachycardia, cyanosis, asphyxial convulsions, and coma. The very rapid onset of rigor mortis after death is an indicator for this mode of poisoning. For some uncouplers, but not others, edema and spongy degeneration of the white matter of the brain and spinal cord are induced as ATP-dependent ion pumps are disrupted and osmotic effects cause swelling of the myelin sheath (e.g., see bromethalin and chlorfenapyr, Section 57.7.2.3). Most of these signs and symptoms can be readily related to mitochondrial uncoupling action which causes decreased ATP levels, increased respiratory chain activity and oxygen consumption, the generation of heat, failed ionic regulation and consequent osmotic swelling, and, over time, the consumption of energy reserves within the body. Considerable weight loss is seen under conditions of chronic but sublethal exposure, and it is interesting that in the 1930s, the uncoupler 2,4-dinitrophenol (2,4-DNP) was quite widely employed as a weight reduction drug. Although effective in such a use, the several severe side effects, including peripheral neuritis, liver injury, and the induction of cataracts in perhaps 1% of those taking this therapy, led fairly rapidly to its discontinuation (Gasiewicz, 1991; Kurt et al., 1986).

In a study of the activities of a broad range of uncouplers in mice, Ilivicky and Casida (1969) found that they produced very similar signs of poisoning of the type described above, and these signs could readily be distinguished from those of mitochondrial respiratory inhibitors or nonmitochondrial poisons. There was a rough but persuasive correlation between the ability of these varied compounds to uncouple mitochondria in vitro and their toxicities to mice when administered intraperitoneally. Toxicity also correlated well with the degree of uncoupling of the mitochondria in brain in vivo but less well with the degree of uncoupling of liver mitochondria. Brain mitochondria were generally somewhat more sensitive to the action of these uncouplers than liver mitochondria when tested in vitro. On the basis of this work it seems reasonable to conclude that pesticidal compounds that are strong uncouplers in vitro cause most or all of their acute toxic effects in vivo through uncoupling, and that the nervous system is a particularly sensitive target for their actions.

Most uncouplers are also inhibitors of the respiratory chain at somewhat higher concentrations than those needed for uncoupling, and a biphasic effect on respiration is typical with stimulation turning to inhibition as the concentration is increased. This inibition of respiration probably arises because uncouplers also inhibit specific steps in the respiratory chain at concentrations higher than those that cause uncoupling. There are probably compounds with the reverse properties (i.e., they are weaker as uncouplers than inhibitors, but the uncoupling phase will not seen in this case because respiratory inhibition predominates). Probable examples of this are some 2,6-dinitro-4-alkylphenols which clearly are potential uncouplers but which generally are found to be respiratory inhibitors with mitochondria in vitro (Ilivicky and Casida, 1969). The ability of the isomeric 2-alkyl-4,6-dinitrophenols, which are potent uncouplers in vitro, to also inhibit respiratory complexes I and III (and also photosystem II in the photosynthetic apparatus) at higher concentrations has been studied by Saitoh et al. (1992) and Singer and Ramsay (1994). All three of these electron transport components have Q binding sites for which these phenols compete. The structural analogy between these phenols and Q was stressed by Singer and Ramsay (1994), particularly the branching pattern in the alkyl chain that mimics the initial isoprenyl group in Q. In mitochondria, alpha branching of the alkyl group with a chain length of four or five carbon atoms gave optimal inhibition of respiration with I_{50} values between 0.1 and 1 μM. Saitoh *et al.* (1992) suggested that the function of the alpha branch was to hold the alkyl chain perpendicular to the plain of the phenyl ring.

57.7.2 PROPERTIES OF SPECIFIC COMPOUNDS

57.7.2.1 Dinitrophenols

The toxicology of dinitrophenols has been reviewed by Gosselin *et al.* (1984) and Gasiewicz (1991).

Status and Uses These compounds were reviewed in considerable detail in the first edition of this handbook (Gasiewicz, 1991). Dinitrophenol derivatives were used as insecticides as early as 1892 but it was not until the 1930s that their value as herbicides was discovered. At one time, a considerable number of dinitrophenol derivatives were registered for use in the United States with a broad range of pesticidal activities including herbicidal, acaricidal, insecticidal, and fungicidal applications. These were typically 2,4-DNP derivatives with an added alkyl chain ortho to the hydroxy group and included such pesticides as binapacryl, DNOC, dinocap, dinobuton, dinoseb, dinocturon, and dinoterb. Both the free phenols and various metallic or amine salt forms have been used. In a number of cases the phenolic group was esterified with an acidic group which tends to decrease their phytotoxicity and mammalian toxicity and to increase formulation options. Such dinitrophenolic esters are regarded as propesticides and the 2,4-dinitrophenolic component is liberated more or less rapidly *in vivo* to carry out its toxic uncoupling actions.

As a result of their adverse toxicology, particularly their high acute toxicity and tendency to cause birth defects and chronic reproductive effects, and the advent of more desirable and selective pesticides, the dinitrophenols have been largely superceded in the United States and many developed countries, and only a few registered uses for these compounds now remain (e.g., in the United States only 2,4-DNP and dinocap are still registered for pesticidal use). However, other compounds in this class such as DNOC, dinocap, dinoterb, and dinobuton are still in use in some countries (Tomlin, 2000).

Because of this steep decline in use and the fact that no important new or changed views of their toxicology have appeared in the last decade, the section here is limited to specific information on dinocap and an overview of the general properties of these pesticides. For more extensive coverage of the properties, and toxicology of other individual dinitrophenolic pesticides, the reader is referred to the previous edition of this handbook (Gasiewicz, 1991).

Overview of Toxicology The dinitrophenolic pesticides are all derivatives of 2,4-DNP, a compound which itself has minor uses as a fungicide in fabric and leather preservation, but which is more familiar as the archetype uncoupler of mitochondrial oxidative phosphorylation. Pesticidal analogs typically have an additional alkyl substituent in the ring "ortho" to the hydroxy moiety which increases the lipophilicity of the molecule and thereby considerably increases uncoupling activity and toxicity compared to 2,4-DNP itself in both vertebrates and insects (Ilivicky and Casida, 1969; Miyoshi *et al.*, 1987; Miyoshi and Fujita, 1988). However, all these compounds cause their major toxicological actions in the same way as 2,4-DNP. The variations in lipophilicity and in the form of the phenol employed (free acid, alkali metal salt, alkoxyamine salt, or esterified) lead to variations in the rate of absorption and this impacts the toxicity of the different pesticidal dinitrophenol derivatives. Also, in the phenolic ester forms, the rate at which the ester is hydrolyzed *in vivo* also will impact the speed of action and ultimate toxicity of these propesticides.

In general the dinitrophenolic pesticides tend to have relatively high acute toxicities by the standard of modern pesticides and lack sufficient selective toxicity due to the universality of uncoupling as a process which is deleterious to all multicellular organisms. The hazardous nature of some of these compounds has resulted in numerous examples of human poisoning and some deaths in addition to those observed during the use of these compounds as slimming agents. These adverse responses are particularly frequent with the more acutely toxic analogs such as DNOC (Gasiewicz, 1991). Other specific toxicological actions including the induction of cataracts by some members of the group (Gasiewicz, 1991) and the clear ability of others [e.g., dinocap (Section 57.7.2.1) and dinoseb (U.S. EPA, 1989c)] to act as teratogens, has raised particular concern over worker exposure and has led to severe regulatory actions. In general, these compounds do not appear to be general genotoxicants though there are scattered literature reports of positive tests for genotoxicity with dinitrophenolic pesticides. The dinitrophenols as a class do not appear to be carcinogenic.

Human Toxicology and Therapy The signs, symptoms and treatment of dinitrophenol poisoning are reviewed by Hallenbeck and Cunningham-Burns (1985), Gasiewicz (1991), and Reigart and Roberts (1999). In addition to the generalized signs of poisoning described above (Section 57.7.1), in which a range of neurotoxic effects are prominent, renal failure may occur rapidly with high doses. Hepatotoxicity marked by jaundice is also a possible sequel. Exposure by inhalation can lead to tightness of the chest and pulmonary edema in addition to systemic effects. The onset of symptoms is often rapid after exposure but can be delayed for 1–2 days. The toxic effects tend to be more severe at elevated environmental temperatures (Gasiewicz, 1991). Death may arise from hyperthermia, or respiratory or cardiovascular failure, and can occur within 24–48 hours. After exposure ceases, recovery tends to be protracted because of the relatively slow rate of clearance of many dinitrophenolic pesticides. Half-lives in human blood may be in the range of 5 to 7 days (Gasiewicz, 1991). The bright yellow

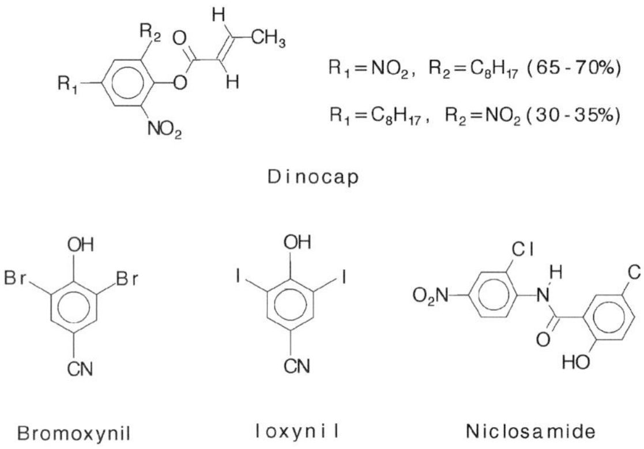

Figure 57.14   Uncouplers of oxidative phosphorylation—Phenols.

color of these compounds leading to staining of sites of exposure (skin, hair, or clothing), and the urine and sclerae, is an important (but not absolutely definitive) indicator of exposure. Decontamination of sites of exposure and supportive treatment (control of fever by physical means, fluid, electrolyte, and energy replacement, and oxygen administration) are indicated. Salicylate antipyretics are contraindicated since these too can act as uncouplers and there is evidence that they may exacerbate dinitrophenolic poisoning in experimental animals. Other antipyretics are ineffective since the hyperthermia is a general tissue response rather than a disorder of central temperature regulation. Forced diuresis has been recommended for some phenolic uncouplers (Gasiewicz, 1991). No specific antidotes are available.

Dinocap: General Properties and Uses   Dinocap is a complex mixture of 2,6-dinitro-4-octylphenyl and 2,4-dinitro-6-octylphenyl crotonates where the octyl moiety is a mixture of 1-methylheptyl, 1-ethylhexyl, and 1-propylpentyl isomers (Fig. 57.14). The commercial material has about a 2 : 1 ratio of 6-octyl to 4-octyl isomers. The CAS Reg. No. is 131-72-6 (6-octyl, 1-methylheptyl single isomer) or 39300-45-3 (mixed isomers). It was discovered by Rohm & Haas Co. The chemical composition of dinocap is described by Kirby and Hunter (1965) and Kurtz *et al.* (1970). A series of samples of the technical product produced around 1970 were analyzed by Kurtz *et al.* They contained 72–77% 2,4- and 2,6-dinitrooctylphenyl crotonates, 4–7% mixed dinitrooctylphenols, 0.5–1% mononitrooctylphenols, 1–4% crotonic acid, 2–6% octenes (used in the synthesis of the crotonates), several unknown constituents at less than 1% each, and 6–13% nonvolatiles which was mainly complex polymeric material without pesticidal activity. The samples averaged 83% as active ingredients (crotonates and phenols). Total 6-octyl isomers constituted 68% of the active ingredients and 4-octyl isomers were the remaining 32%. Of this 68% as 6-alkyl components, 26% had 1-methylheptyl chains and the other 42% had either 1-ethylhexyl or 1-propylpentyl (ratios not determined). The complexity of this mixture of isomeric esters and free phenols creates a considerable challenge for analytical chemists in assessing environmental residues of dinocap (Heimlich *et al.*, 1995).

Dinacap exists as a dark brown liquid, b.p. 138–140°C at 0.05 mm Hg, v.p. 7.5×10^{-8} Pa (25°C), log P 4.54, w.s. 4 ppm. Estimated half-lives for hydrolysis to the phenol are 3.5 years, 129 days, and 12.9 days at pHs 7, 8, and 9, respectively (HSDB, 2000).

Dinocap is a foliar fungicide with acaricidal activity. It was first used in the 1930s. Trade names include Caprane, Crotonate, Crotothane, Karathane, Mildane, Mildex, and Sialite.

Toxicology Overview   A Special Review of all pesticide products containing dinocap was initiated in 1985 by the U.S. Environmental Protection Agency, primarily in response to studies with rabbits that revealed birth defects and chronic reproductive effects. This was completed in 1989 and the conclusion were reviewed (U.S. EPA, 1989b). Measures to reduced applicator exposure and warnings on the label regarding its potential teratogenicity were required for continued registration. The toxicology of dinocap from a regulatory standpoint has also been reviewed on several occasions by the FAO/WHO Joint Meeting on Pesticide Residues [e.g., see (1990c, 1999a)]. A brief addendum to the major report in FAO/WHO (1999a) is provided in FAO/WHO (1999b). These reports and the review by Gasiewicz (1991) lead to the conclusions below. Most studies were performed on technical dinocap mixture. Some recent studies have used purer materials (90–95%), and, in some cases, the single 6- and 4-(1-methylheptyl) isomers have been employed. These differences in isomer mix and purity may have led to differences in the toxic effects observed, since it appears that specific isomers or impurities are responsible for at least some toxic effects.

Acute Toxicity   This varies considerably with species (Table 57.5; FAO/WHO, 1990c). Rats and rabbits are relatively insensitive (acute oral LD50s vary from 510 to 3100 mg/kg in a range of reports) whereas mice and dogs are approximately 10-fold more sensitive (acute oral LD_{50}s ranging from 50–265 mg/kg). The intravenous LD_{50} in rats is only 2.5 mg/kg, illustrating the high intrinsic toxicity of dinocap. The acute oral toxicities provided in FAO/WHO (1999a) are several-fold lower than those in Table 57.5 (mainly from Larson *et al.*, 1959), at least in part because dinocap of higher purity was utilized. Clinical signs of poisoning are typical of those already described for dinitrophenolic uncouplers in general.

Irritation/Sensitization   Dinocap is an irritant to the eye, skin, and mucous membranes and a dermal sensitizer in both test animals and humans (FAO/WHO, 1999a; Gasiewicz, 1991).

Subchronic Toxicity   In 90-day dietary studies, pathological changes including hepatic necrosis were observed in dogs (6.25 mg/kg/day) and rabbits (30 mg/kg/day). Degenerative changes were also seen in the gastrointestinal tract and kidney in the rabbits. In a 28-day dietary study in mice, hepatocellular necrosis was similarly observed but only at doses (500 ppm and higher) that also caused deaths.

Table 57.5
Acute Toxicity of Pesticides Acting as Mitochondrial Uncouplers to Selected Nontarget Species

| Compound | LD$_{50}$ (mg/kg) | | | | Acute dermal | LC$_{50}$ (mg/l) Acute inhalation | LC$_{50}$ (ppb) (24–96 hr) | |
| | Acute oral | | | | | | | |
	Rat (M; F)	Mouse	Quail	Duck	Rat or rabbit	Rat	Fish[a]	*Daphnia*
2,4-Dinitrophenol	30–71	72	—	—	—	—	—	—
Dinobuton	140	2540	150[b]	—	>5000	—	—	—
Dinocap	980; 1190	180	—	—	>4700	3.0	15–33	75[c]
Dinoterb	62	25	—	—	150[d]	—	3.4	—
DNOC	25–40	16–47	15.7	23	200–1000	—	450–6000	5700
Bromoxynil	81; 93	110–160	100–193	200	>3660	0.27	63–5000	19,220[e]
Bromoxynil octanoate	400; 238	—	148	2050	>2000(M); 1310(F)	0.81	53–150	96
Ioxynil	110	200–230	30[f]	1200	>2000	0.4	3300–8500	3900
Ioxynil octanoate	190–390	—	1000[f]	1200	>912; 1240[g]	—	4000	—
Niclosamide	>5000	1500	60[h]	>1000	>1000	20	13–230	200
Pentachlorophenol	146; 175	74–177	—	380	320	0.2	32–205	—
TFM	160; 141	—	—	—	>2000	—	0.6–37	—
Bromethalin	10.7; 9.1	5.0	4.6–11	—	2000	0.024	38–598	2–5
Chlorfenapyr	441; 1152	55	34	10	>2000	1.9	7.4–500	6.1
Fluazinam	>5000	>5000	1782	>4190	>2000	0.47	110–150	190
Sulfluramid	5000	—	473	—	>2000	>4.4	>10,000	210–390
LPOS	154; 154	—	42	81	>2000	0.21	4200–49,000	67,000

[a] Range of values from several species, most commonly including the rainbow trout and bluegill.
[b] Data for hen.
[c] Data for the sideswimmer (*Gammarus fasciatus*).
[d] Data for guinea pig.
[e] Data vary widely with source; see text.
[f] Data for pheasant.
[g] Data for mouse.
[h] Species unknown.

Chronic Toxicity At a sublethal dose (150 ppm), weight reductions and atrophy of the testes was seen in an 18-month feeding study in CD-1 mice but no hepatotoxicity was noted in this case. In a 2-year dietary study in rats, doses of 125 mg/kg/day caused reduced growth and survival and spleen enlargement in males. The significance of the cataracts reported in a dietary study in white Peking ducklings at doses of 50–2500 ppm (Larson *et al.*, 1959) is difficult to ascertain since this action was inconsistent and not clearly dose-dependent (Gasiewicz, 1991).

In a 2-year dietary study in dogs, retinal atrophy was seen at 60 ppm. However, this is not considered relevant for human risk assessment since it occurs secondarily to damage to the tapetum lucidum which is absent in humans. No retinal effects were seen in rats and mice which also lack this structure (FAO/WHO, 1999a).

Carcinogenicity Dinocap was not carcinogenic in lifetime feeding studies in rats at dietary concentrations up to 2000 ppm, or in mice at dietary concentrations up to 200 ppm (about 35 mg/kg/day).

Mutagenicity/Genotoxicity Dinocap showed no evidence of genotoxicity in a typical battery of tests *in vitro* and *in vivo*. However, in one study, a positive result was obtained in the Ames *Salmonella* assay (Moriya *et al.*, 1983).

Reproductive Toxicity No specific reproductive toxicity was seen in rats in a multigenerational dietary study at concentrations up to 1000 ppm which were reduced to 400 ppm in the second generation due to high mortality in pups (FAO/WHO, 1999a). In another study in rats, decreased growth rates and survival of offspring in the second generation were recorded at dietary doses of 104–126 mg/kg/day (Fraczek, 1979 in Gasiewicz, 1991).

Developmental Toxicity/Teratogenicity Based on a substantial series of developmental toxicity studies, the U.S. Environmental Protection Agency (U.S. EPA, 1989b) and the FAO/WHO JMPR panel (FAO/WHO, 1999a) both concluded that dinocap is teratogenic in animals, particularly in mice, and that it therefore poses a risk of teratogenicity to humans.

In an initial exploratory study, Gray *et al.* (1986) assessed the teratogenicity of technical dinocap (84% active ingredients) in CD-1 mice. Cleft palate, extreme abdominal distension (ballooning) and twisting of the neck and tilting of the head (torticollis) were observed in the offspring when mice were dosed orally during pregnancy at 25 mg/kg/day. This dose also caused high postnatal mortality but was not toxic to the mothers. Torticollis was also seen at a lower incidence at 12 mg/kg/day and caused a variety of locomotor aberrations including repeated circling and rolling over. These behavioral effects were tentatively attributed to a reduction in the formation of otoliths in the inner ear.

By contrast, teratogenicity was lacking in a parallel study in Sprague–Dawley rats at doses as high as 150 mg/kg/day, although an increase in the incidence of supernumerary ribs was observed at this dose (FAO/WHO, 1999a). In hamsters, only slightly retarded growth was observed which occurred at or near maternally toxic doses of 50 mg/kg/day or higher.

The lack of clear teratogenic effects in rats and hamsters was confirmed by Rogers et al. (1988) who noted significant differences in the ratios of adult to developmental toxicities (A/D ratios) between the species tested. For mice, an A/D ratio of about 8.6 was calculated compared to the hamster and rat with A/D ratios of 1 or less, indicating that developmental toxicity only occurred in the presence of maternal toxicity.

In a follow-up study in mice using a standardized experimental protocol for assessing developmental toxicity, Rogers et al. (1986) observed developmental effects after oral administration at the lowest dose of 5 mg/kg/day. Significant maternal toxicity only occurred at 80 mg/kg/day. A low incidence of cleft palate in mice at 5 mg/kg/day increased to an incidence of 75% at 40 mg/kg/day. Reduced fetal weight and moderate to severe hydronephrosis was also recorded beginning at 5 mg/kg/day. Increases in supernumerary ribs appeared at 20 mg/kg/day and a few examples of exencephaly and umbilical hernias were also observed in mice at higher doses. Otolith development was not studied in this protocol. Clearly dinocap causes multiple types of teratogenic effects in mice.

A further investigation of the unusual behavioral effects seen in weanling mice including a study of the effect of prenatal exposure to dinocap on the swimming ability in the offspring, head-tilting (torticollis), and reductions in otolith development was conducted by Gray et al. (1988). Considerable difficulties in swimming were observed in mice with torticollis and even in some animals without this postural abnormality. The authors confirmed that the behavioral deficits arise because of a partial or complete failure to develop otoliths and concluded that the otolith status is the most sensitive endpoint in detecting this type of teratogenesis. In a special study with CD-1 mice conducted by Rogers et al. (1989), the reduction in fetal otolith formation was found to be dose-dependent with a threshold at 10 mg/kg/day. Maternal toxicity was not observed until the dose reached 60 mg/kg/day. By contrast, otoliths were affected in the Syrian golden hamster only at 100 mg/kg/day, a dose that also caused severe maternal and fetal toxicity. This again demonstrates the relatively high sensitivity of mice to the teratogenic actions of dinocap. The induction of effects on otolith production has rarely been reported before in teratogenicity studies,

but as Rogers et al. point out, it would not be observed directly in standard testing protocols. No mechanism has been proposed by which dinocap might affect otolith development.

Interestingly, Rogers et al. (1987) discovered that two major ingredients of dinocap, the individual isomers 2,6-dinitro-4-(1-methylheptyl)phenyl crotonate and 2, 4-dinitro-6-(1-methylheptyl)phenyl crotonate (each at 95% purity) were not active as teratogens in mice either alone or in combination. At the same dose (25 mg/kg/day) technical dinocap gave the typical range of teratogenic effects seen in other studies. The technical dinocap had 84% active ingredients but the impurities were not characterized. Presumably the composition of this sample resembles that described by Kurtz et al. (1970) quite closely. This raises a critical question regarding the nature of the teratogenic agent(s) in this mixture and the possible role of other alkyl chain isomers or minor impurities in the technical material. This significant question does not appear to have been resolved. However, the positive teratogenic respone in CD-1 mice was confirmed in all essential details by an additional study conducted by the registrant using a higher purity sample of dinocap [94.4% compared to 84% in the studies of Gray et al. (1986) and Rogers et al. (1986)]. The LOEL for developmental effects in this study was 10 mg/kg/day (FAO/WHO, 1999a). Unfortunately, the detailed compostion of the purified material is not provided in this publication.

Similar teratogenic effects including cleft palate and decreased otolith production were seen in CD-1 mice after dermal exposure to a formulated version of dinocap (Karathane LC XF) at 25 mg active ingredient/kg/day. This dose caused no maternal toxicity (FAO/WHO, 1999a).

In rabbits, teratogenicity studies revealed an increased incidence of skeletal malformations such as vertebral asymmetry and malformed ribs at 48 mg/kg/day, but this dose also caused obvious maternal toxicity. In a previous study (Costlow et al., 1986; FAO/WHO, 1990c), hydrocephaly and neural tube defects were found in rabbits at doses of 3 mg/kg/day and higher. Such effects were completely lacking in the second study, perhaps because the purity of the dinocap had been increased from 84% to 95.4% (FAO/WHO, 1999a). Costlow et al. (1986) found no developmental or teratogenic effects in rabbits when dinocap was applied demally.

The mouse teratogenicity data were used by the FAO/WHO JMPR panel to set an ADI of 0.008 mg/kg using an elevated 500-fold safety factor since malformations were seen after both dermal and oral exposures and in three test species (FAO/WHO, 1999a).

Immunotoxicity An assessment of the immunotoxicity of dinocap in female C57BL/6J mice administered by gavage for 7 to 12 days revealed adverse effects at doses of 25 mg/kg/day. These effects included decreased thymus weight, increased spleen weight, a reduction in the proliferative responses of lymphocytes to concanavalin A and phytohemaglutinin, and a suppression of the IgM and IgG plaque-forming response to sheep red blood cells. Using cultured mouse thymocytes, dinocap at 10 μg/ml also caused a depression in the proliferative and mitogen-stimulated responses with no evidence of cytotoxicity, Although adverse immunological effects were seen in this study, it was concluded that these were relatively modest and only seen at high doses *in vivo* (Smialowicz *et al.*, 1992).

Human Toxicology   No serious human poisonings by dinocap appear to have been reported (FAO/WHO, 1990c, 1999a), although Gasiewicz (1991) cites a single case of dinocap poisoning in an agricultural worker which was marked by allergic dermatitis, dyspnea, and thirst, Nine days after these symptoms an outbreak of vesicles over the entire body followed. Complete recovery was attained in 1 month after cortisone treatment. The level of exposure is undefined but it must have been considerable in view of the symptoms described. The estimated daily human intakes of dinocap produced by several dietary models represent 0–2% of the ADI which indicates a very low degree of risk to the general population through food consumption (FAO/WHO, 1999b). A study of worker exposure to dinocap in California estimated joint dermal and inhalation exposures ranging from 0.028 to 0.49 mg/kg/day depending on the type of protective clothing worn (Wang, 1988).

Biochemical Mechanism of Action   It is reasonable to assume that dinocap requires hydrolysis to release the free phenol in order to cause uncoupling and that this occurs rapidly *in vivo* [e.g., Ilivicky and Casida (1969) found strong uncoupling of brain and liver mitochondria *in vivo* within 30 minutes of administering a toxic intraperitoneal dose of dinocap to mice]. By comparison with 2,4-DNP, the predominant phenolic isomer of dinocap, 2,4-dinitro-6-octylphenol, is likely to be a strong uncoupler [e.g., Hemker (1962) found that one phenolic component of dinocap had an uncoupling activity 7- to 25-fold higher than that of 2,4-DNP in rat liver mitochondria]. Similarly, Ilivicky and Casida (1969) concluded that 6-sec-butyl-2,4-DNP is an uncoupler with an activity about 50-fold greater than that of 2,4-DNP. However, there may be complications in this apparently simple story. As pointed out by Corbett *et al.* (1984), the 4-alkyl-2,6-dinitrophenol components of the dinocap chemical mixture may act as respiratory inhibitors rather than uncouplers. Ilivicky and Casida (1969), studying the related sec-butyl analogs of 2,4-DNP, found that the 4-alkyl-2,6-dinitro analog was not an uncoupler at any concentration, but acted as a strong inhibitor of oxphos with appreciable activity at 0.1 μM. In mice, it caused an entirely different suite of poisoning signs than uncouplers that were characterized by ataxia and, sometimes, convulsions, but no immediate rigor mortis after death. As discussed in the Introduction to this section, even the 2,4-dinitro-6-alkyl components of the mixture can inhibit respiration if concentrations rise further beyond those that cause uncoupling. The effects of dinocap *in vivo* may therefore tend to lie in balance between respiratory uncoupling and inhibition, depending on the relative contents of the 4- and 6-alkyl phenolic forms, their relative rates of release by ester hydrolysis and removal by further metabolism, and the concentrations that they achieve in the tissues. In the case of the dinocap, the signs of poisoning in animals clearly

indicate that uncoupling predominates in most situations. However, there may be exceptions. It is interesting to note in this context that: (1) Larson *et al.* (1959) observed that dinocap caused an increase in respiration rates typical of an uncoupler after oral adminsitration in female rats but no increase in male rats, whereas 2,4-DNP stimulated respiration in both sexes, and (2), that whereas the 6-octyl isomers of dinocap are better as acaricides, the 4-octyl isomers are superior as fungicides (Tomlin, 2000).

Absorption, Metabolism, and Excretion   Dinocap [as the purified 2,4,-dinitro-6-(1-methylheptyl) isomer] was well absorbed (60–70%) after a single oral dose of 25 mg/kg in mice and reached peak plasma concentration at 2 to 6 hr after dosing. The half-life for plasma clearance was about 6 hr. After dermal application at 25 mg/kg, the peak plasma concentration was about 25% of that with the oral dose and was reached after 6 to 8 hr, but the clearance rate was the same. This indicates a rapid but incomplete (25% in 4 hr) absorption through the skin. A study of the penetration of dinocap through isolated mouse and human skin samples indicated a more rapid penetration in the mouse, which is typical, but it did not model the *in vivo* data closely and the results are therefore of dubious relevance quantitatively (FAO/WHO, 1999a).

These pharmacokinetic results after oral dosing in mice were quite similar to those obtained in previous studies in rabbits, using the same single isomer of dinocap (FAO/WHO, 1990c). This is extensively metabolized and excreted in rabbits with biphasic elimination kinetics, giving half-lives of about 3 and 44 hr after oral dosing. The elimination half-lives after dermal dosing were more variable but were approximately 10-fold higher than those determined orally. Total absorption was 60–69% of the dose orally and 4 to 9% dermally. A dermal penetration study in rhesus monkeys also indicated incomplete absorption with 5–20% of the dose recovered in the excreta depending on the application conditions (FAO/WHO, 1999a).

The metabolic fate of the 1-methylheptyl component of dinocap in rats and mice is reviewed in detail in FAO/WHO (1999a). After an oral dose of 100 mg/kg, rats eliminated 30% of the dose in the urine in 24 hr. After an oral dose of 25 m/kg mice, eliminated 58% in the 24 hr urine. At least 12 metabolites were identified in each species. Of the metabolites found in rat, 85% were also found in the mouse, and 70% of those found in the mouse were also found in rat. Dinocap was metabolized by extensive initial hydrolysis, oxidation of the two terminal carbon atoms of the side chain, and β-oxidative chain shortening. Sulfate conjugation products of the phenol were found in mice and products of nitroreduction followed by *N*-acetylation in rats.

Environmental Fate and Toxicity   Dinocap is moderately toxic to birds but its toxicity to fish and aquatic invertebrates is extremely high (Table 57.5). It binds strongly in soils with a high clay and organic matter content with an estimated K_{oc} value of 44,000. It therefore has a low potential to move into groundwater. In soil it is degraded both by microbial and photochemical actions with a field half-life of 4–6 days (HSDB, 2000).

57.7.2.2 Other Phenolic Pesticides with Uncoupling Activity

A number of other phenolic pesticides have uncoupling activity which plays a significant part in their toxicity. Since it is only necessary to develop a weak acid with lipophilic properties to obtain an active uncoupler, a variety of phenolic structures with a combination of electron withdrawing and lipophilic groups fit within this category. These compounds include nitrophenols such as the sodium salt of *p*-nitrophenol itself, which, in combination with sodium nitroguicaolate, has uses as a plant growth regulator under the trade name of Atonik, and 3-trifluoromethyl-4-nitrophenol, a compound with limited uses as a specific lampreycide in the Great Lakes region of the United States. Further information on its uses and toxicology is available from a recent U.S. Environmental Protection Agency publication (U.S. EPA, 1999d). A detailed survey of the toxicological properties of *p*-nitrophenol is also available in U.S. EPA (1998e).

Several halophenols such as pentachlorophenol and herbicides in the bromoxynil family are also powerful uncouplers. Since the 1930s, pentachlorophenol has been used in huge amounts for the preservation of wood products against fungal and insect pests, as a nonselective herbicide, as a cotton defoliant, as a molluscicide, and as a wide spectrum fungicide and bactericide. In the United States it now retains only its use in wood preservation. It is used both as the free phenol and its sodium salt. The compound is covered in detail in Chapter 65. Halogenated salicylanilides such as niclosamide, a widely used common anthelmintic and molluscicide, also have strong uncoupling properties. Acute toxicity data for some of these other phenolic uncouplers are included in Table 57.5 for comparative purposes. The more economically important ones are described in further detail below.

Bromoxynil: General Properties and Uses   3,5-Dibromo-4-hydroxybenzonitrile (Fig. 57.14), CAS Reg. No. 1689-84-5, was developed by Amchem Products Inc. and May & Baker Ltd. The herbicidal activity of bromoxynil and the closely related herbicide ioxynil were described independently by Carpenter and Heywood (1963) of May & Baker, and by Wain (1963) of Wye College, while they were also under study by Amchem. The chemistry, acute toxicity, and biological properties of bromoxynil have been reviewed by Carpenter *et al.* (1964) and its development has been described by Heywood (1966).

Bromoxynil is also utilized as its octanoate ester (CAS Reg. No. 1689-99-2) and its potassium salt (CAS Reg. No. 2961-68-4). Use has also been made of the heptanoate ester. The esters are propesticides which are readily converted to bromxoynil *in vivo* by esterase activity. Bromoxynil has also been used as its butyrate ester but this was voluntarily withdrawn from the U.S. market in 1989 due to concerns regarding its developmental toxicity (U.S. EPA, 1998d).

Bromoxynil is an active metabolite of the herbicide bromofenoxim (3,5-dibromo-4-hydroxybenzaldehyde 2,4-dinitrophenyloxime, CAS Reg. No. 13181-17-4) which is metabolized in mammals to a mixture of 2,4-DNP and bromoxynil, both active as mitochondrial uncouplers. This compound (trade name Faneron) now appears to no longer be marketed (Tomlin, 2000).

Bromoxynil is a white crystalline solid, m.p. 194–195°C, v.p. 6.3×10^{-6} Pa (20°C), w.s. 130 ppm (20–25°C), log P2.8 (unionized phenol), HLC 1.34×10^{-5} Pa m^3 mol^{-1}, pKa 3.9–4.2. The octanoate ester is a waxy cream solid, m.p. 45–46°C, v.p. 1.9×10^{-4} Pa (25°C), w.s. 3 ppm (25°C) (Tomlin, 2000) [also cited as 80 ppm (25°C) by Wauchope *et al.* (1992)], log P5.4. The hydrolysis half-lives at pH 5, 7, and 9 are 34.1, 11.5, and 1.7 days, respectively. The properties of the heptanoate are very similar. The potassium salt has a water solubility of 61,000 ppm (20–25°C).

Bromoxynil and its esters are widely used as selective contact herbicides for postemergent control of broad-leaved weeds. They are often included in mixtures with other herbicides to broaden the spectrum of control. Common trade names include Brominal, Bromotril, Buctril, Certrol, Combine, Connect, Emblem, Labuctril, Merit, Pardner, Sabre, Terset, Toplan, and Torch. An estimated 2.5 to 3 million pounds of all forms of the active ingredient are used annually in the United Sates (U.S. EPA, 1998d).

Toxicology Profile   The primary sources of data are Cal EPA (1995) and U.S. EPA (1998d). The U.S. Environmental Protection Agency (U.S. EPA, 1998d) concluded that there are no important toxicological differences between bromoxynil and its esters since the esters are rapidly cleaved to the free phenol *in vivo*. However, this conclusion has been questioned by the California Environmental Protection Agency (Cal EPA, 1995) based on differences in their pharmacokinetics, toxicological effects, and potencies.

Acute Toxicity   There are several sources of data for these values [e.g., Carpenter *et al.* (1964), Ahrens (1994), U.S. EPA (1998d), and Tomlin (2000)]. While they are in reasonable agreement in most cases, they are rarely identical and there are a few instances where the values offered appear to be incompatible. These are noted below. The data in Table 57.5 include the range of values recorded in these sources where they are reasonably close.

Bromoxynil is highly toxic to mammals and birds (Table 57.5). The data for the acute oral toxicity to the rat are from U.S. EPA (1998d). Alternative values for the acute oral LD$_{50}$ in rats range from 190 mg/kg (Carpenter *et al.*, 1964) up to 440 mg/kg (Ahrens, 1994). The acute oral LD$_{50}$ values for guinea pigs, cats, and rabbits are 63, 75, and 260 mg/kg, respectively (Carpenter *et al.*, 1964). The acute toxicity of the potassium salt of bromoxylin is not notably different from that of the free phenol (Tomlin, 2000).

The octanoate ester has a lower acute oral toxicity to rats than the phenol but tends to have a greater acute dermal toxicity since it is absorbed more readily. Its acute oral LD$_{50}$ to rabbits is 325 mg/kg, only slightly more than that of the phenol at 260 mg/kg (Tomlin, 2000).

Irritation/Sensitization The phenol is a moderate eye irritant but not a skin irritant or sensitizer. The octanoate is a mild skin and eye irritant and also acts as a skin sensitizer.

Subchronic Toxicity In subchronic (90 day) dietary studies in rats, very high mortality was observed at 1456 ppm [168 mg/kg/day (M) and 250 mg/kg/day (F)]. At the next lower dose (58 or 76 mg/kg//day) decreased body weight and changed clinical blood chemistry were observed. In a similar study with mice, hepatoxocity in the form of hepatocellular hypertrophy, degeneration, and vacuolization was seen with a LOEL of 13 mg/kg/day for males and 39 mg/kg/day for females. In dogs, doses of 16 mg/kg/day caused mortality. At lower doses, diarrhea, panting, salivation, an unsteady gait, and hematological effects were recorded. The LOEL was 1 to 5 mg/kg/day.

Parallel subchronic studies with the octanoate ester revealed a possible increase in necrosis of thymic lymphocytes and cardiac myofibers in rats at a dietary concentration of 1100 ppm [91 mg/kg/day (M), 111 mg/kg/day (F)]. A subchronic dietary study of the octanoate in dogs gave results qualitatively similar to those with the free phenol.

Chronic Toxicity In a 1-year study in dogs with the phenol, results similar to those in the subchronic study were obtained with a LOEL/NOEL of 1.5 mg/kg/day. No gross or histopathological changes were seen. This study has been used by the U.S. Environmental Protection Agency to set the reference dose (ADI) for bromoxynil at 0.015 mg/kg/day. A 2-year study in Fischer 344 rats gave no toxicological endpoints at the highest dose administered (5 mg/kg/day). Using Sprague–Dawley rats and higher doses, spongiosis hepatitis was seen in males at 8.2 mg/kg/day together with foci of cellular alteration at 28 mg/kg/day. No other notable toxic effects were seen in either sex. Lifetime feeding studies in CD-1 mice resulted in a variety of signs of hepatotoxicity at 12–14 mg/kg/day and an increase in neoplasms at 46–53 mg/kg/day.

Carcinogenicity Bromoxynil did not act as a carcinogen in the long-term rat studies. However, it was positive for liver tumors in two chronic dietary studies in mice. In Swiss white mice, males showed a dose-resulted increase in incidence of liver adenomas and carcinomas (approximately 50% of each type at higher doses). The effect was statistically significant at 13 mg/kg/day. The CD-1 mice showed a similar increase in hepatocellular adenomas and carcinomas. This was observed in both sexes but the effect was much more severe in males with an increase occurring at the lowest dose administered (3.1 mg/kg/day). Based on these results, and the positive results in some genotoxicity tests, the U.S. Environmental Protection Agency has classified bromoxynil as a Class C (possible human) carcinogen with a Q_1^* value of 0.103 $(mg/kg/day)^{-1}$ (U.S. EPA, 1998d).

Mutagenicity/Genotoxicity Bromoxynil gave primarily negative results in a series of 10 *in vitro* and *in vivo* tests for mutations and chromosomal effects. However, it was positive in a DNA repair test in *E. coli* and in a forward mutation test in mouse lymphoma cells. It also caused chromosomal aberrations in Chinese hamster ovary cells *in vitro*. The latter two response were seen only with metabolic activation. The octanoate was negative in a smaller array of assays.

Developmental Toxicity/Teratogenicity Rats demonstrated reduced ossification and an increased incidence of supernumerary ribs at an oral dose 12.5 mg/kg/day which was not toxic maternally. Similar responses were seen in rats in another oral studies at 5 mg/kg/day and in a dermal study at 50 mg/kg/day. Studies with rabbits gave the same effects with a LOEL of 15 mg/kg/day for the increased incidence of supernumerary ribs. In mice the same result was obtained but only in the presence of maternal toxicity. Other malformations, some severe, and increased resorptions were observed in all these studies but only at higher doses with clear maternal toxicity. The octanoate ester gave generally similar results with a LOEL for increased supernumerary ribs in a dermal study in rats of 15 mg/kg/day; however, a dermal study in rabbits was negative for developmental toxicity although significant skin irritation was observed.

Developmental toxicity studies with mice, using the free phenol, and in rats, using both the phenol and the octanoate, have also been described by Rogers *et al.* (1991). The only developmental effect observed was an increased incidence of supernumerary ribs. This occurred with the phenol in mice at 32 and 96 mg/kg/day and with both the phenol and the octanoate in rats at an equimolar dose of 15 or 22 mg/kg/day. In each case the extra ribs were seen only at doses that were also maternally toxic. The difficulties in interpreting the observation of supernumerary ribs in developmental toxicity studies are discussed by Chernoff (1990) and Chernoff *et al.* (1991) in the context of these studies with bromoxynil. Supernumerary ribs are seen in control animals and an elevated incidence is often observed in reproductive toxicology studies. This increase may be related to maternal toxicity, particularly in mice. The extra ribs tend to disappear during subsequent development in rats but not mice The authors conclude that their significance as an indicator of developmental toxicity and the extrapolation of results to other species remains problematical.

Based on these indications of teratogenicity, the U.S. Environmental Protection Agency has maintained a 10-fold additional safety factor for bromoxynil to protect females of reproductive age (U.S. EPA, 1998d).

Reproductive Toxicity No adverse effects on reproductive performance were observed with bromoxynil in a two-generation study in rats at doses up to 21 mg/kg/day. Decreased body weight gain during lactation and delayed eye opening were seen as developmental endpoints at this dose but this also caused lowered weight gain in the parents. A dermal study with bromoxynil octanoate in rats did not result in reproductive or developmental effects at doses that were not also systemically toxic to the parents. Significant skin irritation did occur at 100 mg/kg/day.

Endocrine Effects   Van den Berg *et al.* (1991) investigated the potential of a number of halogenated compounds to lower plasma thyroid hormone level through competiton with hormone transporters. Bromoxylin was a strong competitor for the thyroxine binding site of transthyretin and reduced the levels of both thyroxine (T4) and triiodothyronine (T3) in the plasma of rats. The interpretation of this observation in terms of human risk is complex and the effects on transporter binding and thyroxine levels at least may not be clinically significant (Brucker-Davis, 1998).

Human Toxicology   Only a very limited number of instances of human poisoning by bromoxynil have been reported (U.S. EPA, 1998d). Eye and skin illnesses predominated in California's Pesticide Illness Surveillance Program from 1982 to 1993 and these averaged about one per year for bromoxynil. Four workers in a manufacturing plant making both bromoxynil and ionoxynil developed typical symptoms of uncoupler poisoning including excessive perspiration, thirst, fever, emesis, myalgia, and weight loss. This was attributed to an increase in the production levels of the herbicides without adequate increases in ventilation which created excessive exposure to fine dusts. The effects reversed rapidly after exposure ceased (Conso *et al.*, 1977). Based on current data, no significant concerns were expressed by U.S. Environmental Protection Agency regarding dietary risks to human populations from anticipated bromoxynil residues in food and water (U.S. EPA, 1998d).

Biochemical Mechanism of Action   Bromoxynil's primary toxic effects in plants are produced through the inhibition of photosynthesis in photosystem II with uncoupling of photophophorylation as a second possible contributing effect (Ahrens, 1994). It is a fairly potent mitochondrial uncoupler *in vitro* (Parker, 1965) with a UC$_{50}$ value in rat liver mitochondria of 3.2–5 µM, an activity which is about 5- to 10-fold higher than that of 2,4-DNP. The signs and symptoms of acute poisoning in vertebrates (including humans) are in reasonable accord with uncoupling being the primary mechanism of toxic action.

Absorption, Metabolism, and Elimination   A study with the octanoate ester in rats showed that after an oral dose, uptake was moderate. Peak plasma levels were attained 7 to 10 hr after dosing. Most of the dose was eliminated within 7 days, primarily in the urine. The ester was rapidly and completely converted to the free phenol and excreted in the urine either as the phenol or its conjugates. The heptanoate is also converted to the phenol rapidly and completely *in vivo*. Dermal uptake studies in rats show an absorption in 24 hr of 11 to18% for the octanoate depending on concentration, and about 3% for the phenol. A toxicokinetic study with bromoxynil itself was conducted in rats by Stahler *et al.* (1991).

Environmental Fate and Toxicity   Among the bird species tested, the pheasant appears to be the most sensitive to bromoxynil with an acute oral LD$_{50}$ of 50 mg/kg (Table 57.5). Hens are less sensitive with an LD$_{50}$ of 240 mg/kg (Carpenter *et al.*, 1964). Although bromoxynil octanoate has about the same acute toxicity as the phenol to quail it is much less toxic to mallards (Table 57.5). Short-term feeding studies in birds with both bromoxynil and its octanoate ester revealed only slight toxicity with LC$_{50}$ values above 1000 ppm in the diet in all cases. In an avian reproduction study in mallard ducks a NOEL of 102 ppm was determined with adverse effects including a lower number of eggs laid, fewer live embryos, and regression of the ovary. Bobwhite quail were less sensitive than the mallards. Reported values for the toxicity of the phenol (and its potassium salt) to fish vary widely from an LC$_{50}$ of 63 ppb for catfish to 4000 ppb for the bluegill sunfish and 5000 ppb for harlequin fish which seem to be unusually resistant to chemicals in this class. The values reported by Ahrens (1994) and Tomlin (2000) are generally much lower (50–500 ppb) than those in U.S. EPA (1998d) (2000–4000 ppb). The LC$_{50}$ for *Daphnia* is given as 12,500 ppb in Tomlin (2000) and 19,200 ppb in U.S. EPA (1998d) but as 110 ppb in Ahrens (1994). The reason for these large differences is unclear. Carpenter *et al.* (1964) note that the toxicity of bromoxynil to fish is very dependent on the hardness of the water, presumably because of decreased solubility of the calcium salt. In soft water the LC$_{50}$ to harlequin fish was 5000 ppb. In hard water the LC$_{50}$ rose to 63,000 ppb.

The octanoate is uniformly more toxic to aquatic species than bromoxynil phenol, probably because its notably higher lipophilicity leads to faster uptake (Table 57.5). The high aquatic toxicity of the octanoate is also supported by data for other estuarine and marine organisms (e.g., it has an LC$_{50}$ for mysid shrimps of 65 ppb and an EC$_{50}$ for the inhibition of shell formation in the Eastern oyster of 155 ppm). The BCF for the octanoate in bluegill sunfish was 230-fold and depuration occurred in 14 days which indicates a limited capability for bioconcentration. Decreased juvenile survival was seen in a chronic exposure study with fathead minnows at concentrations as low as 18 ppb for the octanoate, and life-cycle studies with *Daphnia magna* indicated that survival, reproduction, and growth were diminished at 5–6 ppb. Despite this high toxicity, the U.S. Environmental Protection Agency concluded that under normal conditions, the risk to birds and aquatic vertebrate from use of the octanoate ester is likely to be low and to be moderate for aquatic invertebrates (U.S. EPA, 1998d).

Bromoxynil octanoate hydrolyzes rapidly in the environment. Half-lives of 1 to 14 days have been recorded in the field and 2 days in a laboratory study which are in general agreement with a previous study in three soil types (Ingram and Pullin, 1974). Both the octanoate and the resulting phenol are also subject to significant microbial and photolytic degradation. Nolte *et al.* (1995) found that in the dark under simulated groundwater conditions, bomoxynil was very stable with less than 10% degradation in 1 month. The octanoate was rapidly hydrolyzed to the phenol under these conditions. However, exposure to sunlight degraded bromoxynil rapidly with significant loss in

4 hr. Millet *et al.* (1998) have calculated photolytic half-lives for bromoxynil in water that range from 0.12 days in summer to 4 days in winter at a 50° latitude. The photolytic half-life of the octanoate on soil was 2.6 days. Microbial metabolic reactions include hydrolysis of the ester and nitrile groups and debromination. The debromination of bromoxynil in simulated groundwater conditions occurs by halide exchange reactions in which chlorine replaces the bromine atoms (Grass *et al.*, 2000).

The phenol has the physicochemical characteristics that would allow leaching to groundwater under favorable circumstances but its rapid degradation in the soil makes this less likely and this is borne out by the extreme rarity of detections of bromoxynil in surveys of well water in the United States (U.S. EPA, 1998d). It is detected more frequently in surface waters due to runoff (1.1% of samples), generally at sub-ppb levels, but its persistence there is low with a half-life of <12 hr. The octanoate has characteristics [$K_d = 190–300$ ml/g, K_{oc} estimated as 10,000 (Wauchope *et al.*, 1992)] that suggest strong binding to soils and low leaching capability. However, other estimates of these values [$K_d = 7.0$ and $K_{oc} = 1003$ (U.S. EPA, 1998d)] indicate a greater degree of soil mobility.

Ioxynil: General Properties and Uses 4-Hydroxy-3,5-diiodobenzonitrile (Fig. 57.14) has CAS Reg. No. 1689-83-4. Like its close relative, bromoxynil, ioxynil is also used in several forms, as the free phenol, as the sodium salt (CAS Reg. No. 2961-62-8), or in esterified forms, particularly as the octanoate (CAS Reg. No. 3861-47-0). Water- and oil-soluble salts of the phenol are also utilized in combinations with amines such as dimethylamine and triethanolamine.

Ioxinyl was developed by May & Baker Ltd. and Amchem Products Inc. and is described by Carpenter and Heywood (1963) and Wain (1963). The chemistry, acute toxicity, and biological properties of ioxynil have been reviewed by Carpenter *et al.* (1964), and its development was described by Heywood (1966). Ioxynil has also been referred to under the common name bantrol (HSDB, 2000).

The free phenol is a colorless solid, m.p. 212–213°C, v.p. $<1 \times 10^{-3}$ Pa (20°C) [estimated as 1.9×10^{-5} Pa (25°C)], w.s. 50 ppm (20°C, pH unstated) and 130 ppm (25°C), log P 3.43 (25°C, unionized phenol), 0.90 at pH 6.5, pKa 3.96, HLC 5.5×10^{-10} atm m^3 mole^{-1}. The 1-octanol/water partiton coefficient and pKa value were determined by Chamberlain *et al.* (1996). The octanoate ester is a white solid, m.p. 59–60°C, v.p. 3.7×10^{-3} Pa (105°C), practically insoluble in water. It is easily hydrolyzed to release ioxynil under alkaline conditions. The alkali metal salts are readily soluble in water (e.g., the sodium salt has a solubility of 14% at 20–25°C).

Ioxynil and its derivatives are selective contact postemergent herbicides. They are often combined with other herbicides, particularly chlorophenoxy compounds and sometimes with bromoxynil, to extend the herbicidal range. Trade names for the various forms of ioxynil include Actril, Actrilawn, Bentrol, Belgran, Certrol, Cipotril, Dantril, Iotox, Iotril, Oxytril, Sanoxynil, Totril, Toxynil, and Trevespan.

Toxicology Profile Published information on the toxicology of ioxynil is incomplete. The toxicology of ioxynil was previously reviewed in the first edition of this Handbook (Stevens and Sumner, 1991). The other primary sources of data are HSDB (2000) and Ahrens (1994). The biological properties of ioxynil including aspects of its toxicology and the occurrence of occupational poisoning have been reviewed (Anonymous, 1991).

Acute Toxicity Ioxynil is a highly toxic compound to mammals with a potency broadly equivalent to that of bromoxynil (Table 57.5). Ioxynil is also highly toxic by acute oral exposure to cats, guinea pigs, and rabbits (LD$_{50}$ values 75, 76, and 180 mg/kg, respectively; Carpenter *et al.*, 1964). The value for the inhalation toxicity to rats in Table 57.5 is from Ahrens (1994). It appears to be more in accord with the other data than that in Tomlin (2000) of >3 mg/l. The octanoate ester is somewhat less toxic than the phenol to rats. It has moderate toxicity by the dermal route. The sodium salt generally has similar toxicity to that of the free phenol, although a surprisingly high acute percutaneous LD$_{50}$ in rats for the formulated salt of 210 mg/kg has been cited (Tomlin, 2000).

Irritation/Sensitization Ioxynil is a mild eye and skin irritant, but it is not a skin sensitizer.

Subchronic Toxicity In a 90-day feeding study in rats, ioxynil caused no adverse effects at dietary concentrations as high as 111 ppm (about 5.4 mg/kg/day) (Hayes, 1982). Dogs given ioxynil octanoate at 4.5 mg/kg/day for 3 months also showed no adverse effects (Ahrens, 1994). In a 30-week dietary study in dogs, weight loss and anemia were observed with a NOEL of 10 mg/kg/day.

Chronic Toxicity In an 18-month dietary study in mice, liver and thyroid hypertrophy were observed at 30 and 100 ppm (approximately 5 and 15 mg/kg/day). A 24-month dietary study in rats also revealed thyroid toxicity at the same dietary concentrations. The NOEL was found at 10 ppm (0.5 mg/kg.day). Concern regarding the thyrotoxic and possible teratogenic effects of ioxynil led to regulatory review and the cancellation of many domestic uses of ioxynil in the UK (Flanagan *et al.*, 1990; Ogilvie and Ramsden, 1988).

Carcinogenicity No data were found.

Mutagenicity/Genotoxicity Ioxynil was nonmutagenic in an extensive battery of tests for mutations, chromosomal aberrations, and DNA damage and repair using both bacterial and mammalian systems. In additional studies, Carere *et al.* (1978) and Moriya *et al.* (1983) also obtained negative results with ioxynil in the Ames *Salmonella* assay.

Reproductive Toxicity Ioxynil was negative for reproductive toxicity in a study in rats.

Developmental Toxicity/Teratogenicity According to WHO/IPCS/ILO (1993) "animal tests show that this substance possibly causes malformations in human babies." Both the phenol and the octanoate carry the European Community's Hazard Rating R63 "possible risk of harm to the unborn child" (Tomlin, 2000). No details of the studies underlying these designations were found. Studies in experimental animals were positive for teratogenicity. The NOEL was set at 5 mg/kg/day for rats and 15 mg/kg/day for rabbits (Ahrens, 1994).

Hormonal Effects Because of the occurrence of thyroid hyperplasia in animal studies with ioxynil, and its structural similarities to 3,5,3'-triiodo-L-thyronine, Ogilvie and Ramsden (1988) examined its binding *in vitro* to human plasma proteins in order to evaluate its possible effects on the synthesis, transport, and metabolism of thyroid hormones. Ioxynil bound significantly to both hormone binding sites on the thyroxine binding prealbumin but not to the thyroxin binding globulin or albumin. It was concluded that ioxynil is unlikely to interfere with hormone transport by the globulin *in vivo,* and it is not a general mimic of thyroxine since many compounds with a variety of structures bind to the prealbumin. However, it could displace triiodothyronine from its binding to the prealbumin and accumulate in the cerebrospinal fluid where the prealbumin is concentrated. These results did not clearly explain the effects of ioxynil on the thyroid *in vivo.*

Human Toxicology There are a number of examples of human poisoning by ioxynil either through exposure during its manufacture or use, or through suicide attempts. In a few cases, ingestion of ioxynil alone has been reported, but more commonly exposure is in conjunction with other herbicides, particularly chlorophenoxy compounds. As described below, the ingestion of 2 to 3 g of ioxynil by an adult can lead to death in less than an hour. The ingestion of 18 g by an adult led to death in 15 hr even with hospital care. Blood concentrations in fatal cases have ranged from 0.04 to 0.67 g/l (Flanagan *et al.,* 1990).

After acute exposure, ioxynil, generally in conjunction with chlorophenoxy herbicides, may cause dizziness, hyperthermia, sweating, gastrointestinal disturbances and vomiting, tachycardia and possible cardiac arrest, pulmonary edema, weakness, increased respiration, acidosis and renal failure arising from dehydration, weight loss, myalgias of the legs, euphoria, agitation, syncope, coma, and death. No antidotes are known. Treatment after decontamination is supportive and symptomatic. Activated charcoal (25 to100 g in adults) given as a slurry may be helpful. As with other uncouplers, salicylates are contraindicated. Further discussion of treatment and monitoring options is given in HSDB (2000).

Smysl *et al.* (1977) report a fatal example of ioxynil intoxication in which a 54-year-old man who had previously undergone gastrectomy mistakenly swallowed an 11.3% solution of ioxynil. He died 45 minutes later. Autopsy revealed hyperemia of all organs, and edema of the lungs and brain.

The estimated amount of ioxynil consumed was 2–3 g (i.e., approximately 30–40 mg/kg). Ioxynil was present in the serum at 13.2 ppm. Alcohol was also present at a concentration of 0.135%.

A report of nonfatal intoxications in workers manufacturing both bromoxynil and ioxynil (Conso *et al.,* 1977) has already been described (Section 57.7.2.2).

Dickey *et al.* (1988) report a case of poisoning in a 37-year-old woman who ingested 190 ml of a mixture of two herbicides, ioxynil (35 g/l) and MCPP (105 g/l), a chlorophenoxy plant hormone mimic. Symptoms included metabolic acidosis, tachycardia, pupillary constriction, and pyrexia. Seventeen hr after ingesting the herbicide, the patient developed fever, muscle rigidity, and cardiac asystole, and died 1 hour later. The authors considered it unusual that this patient suffered no loss of consciousness prior to death since coma is commonly reported as an early event in such poisonings. Moderate pulmonary and cerebral edema and early necrosis of the liver and renal tubules were recorded at autopsy. Most of the signs of poisoning appear to be typical of those caused by oxphos uncouplers which is reasonable since the blood level of MCPP 10 hr before death was 515 mg/l whereas that of ioxynil was 317 mg/l, and ioxynil has an acute toxicity to mammals that is several times higher than that of MCPP. In addition, chlorophenoxy herbicides themselves have weak uncoupling activity. The reported amount of ioxynil ingested (6.7 g) would represent a dose of about 50 mg/kg for a person weighing 130–140 pounds.

In a study of occupational poisoning by a three-component herbicide mixture containing ioxynil, isoproturon (a urea herbicide), and MCPP, Gibaud (1983) concluded that only ioxynil was responsible for the toxic actions of the product, and the effects resembled those of other well-established phenolic uncouplers.

Flanagan *et al.* (1990) review 11 similar cases of poisoning by ioxynil. Ten also involved co-exposure to chlorophenoxy herbicides. Seven of the 11 patients died. Signs and symptoms were typical of uncoupling, but chlorophenoxy herbicides also cause many of these effects. Of the 3 patients who died after admission to hospital, in each case fatal cardiac arrest occurred 5 to 8 hr after admission. Alkaline diuresis was found to enhance clearance of the chlorophenoxy compounds but was ineffective in speeding the elimination of ioxynil.

Biochemical Mechanism of Action Ioxynil behaves as a typical phenolic uncoupler in studies with rat liver mitochondria. Respiration is increased at lower concentrations and inhibition occurs at higher concentrations. It is a reasonably potent uncoupler (UC$_{50}$ of 1 μM) making it about threefold more active than bromoxynil and 30-fold more active than 2,4-DNP (Parker, 1965). It also acted as a typical protonophoric uncoupler in mung bean mitochondria with activity at 4 μM compared to 0.5 μM for dinoseb (Moreland and Novitzky, 1988).

Absorption, Metabolism, and Elimination Ioxynil is absorbed through the skin and eyes, causing local pain and redness.

Environmental Fate and Toxicity The acute toxicity of ioxynil to birds is variable (Table 57.5). As with bromoxynil, pheasants are very susceptible whereas mallards appear to be remarkably resistant (Ahrens, 1994). The value for hens lies in between with an acute oral LD_{50} of 200 mg/kg (Carpenter et al., 1964). The octanoate has quite low toxicity to birds, even for pheasants which are very sensitive to the free phenol (Table 57.5). Both the free phenol and the octanoate have relatively low toxicities to aquatic species, although data are limited (Table 57.5). This stands in notable contrast to the often very high toxicity of its relative, bromoxynil, to aquatic forms. The estimated BCF value of 3 for ioxynil indicates a very low probability of bioconcentration from water by aquatic organisms.

The estimated K_{oc} of 75 suggests ioxynil binds only weakly to soil colloids and will have a high mobility in the soil. It degrades rapidly in aerobic soil, primarily by microbial action, with a half-life of 9–10 days. Initial steps in degradation involve the hydrolysis of the cyano group to yield the benzamide and benzoic acid (Hsu and Camper, 1975). Deiodination also occurs, probably by halogen exchange with bromine and chlorine (Grass et al., 2000). The half-life for atmospheric photodegradation, primarily through reaction with photochemically derived hydroxyl radicals, is about 74 days. The degradation of ioxynil in natural water samples in the dark, approximating the conditions of groundwater, is slow with 10% degradation requiring over 1 month (Nolte et al., 1995). However, photodegradation increases the rate of loss markedly. Millet et al. (1998) report calculated half-lives for photolysis in water ranging from 0.10 day in summer to 3 days in winter at a 50° latitude. Ioxynil is occasionally detected in surface water runoff sources in areas of use in Europe (HSDB, 2000) but only at extremely low concentrations (0.01 to 0.1 ppb).

Ioxynil has a relatively low toxicity to aquatic species (Table 57.5) which presents a contrast to some results with bromoxynil in fish. Carpenter et al. (1964) note that the toxicity of ioxynil to fish, like that of bromoxynil, is very dependent on the hardness of the water, presumably because of decreased solubility of the calcium salt. In soft water the LC_{50} to harlequin fish was 3300 ppb. In hard water the LC_{50} increased to 74,000 ppb.

Niclosamide: General Properties and Uses 2′,5-Dichloro-4′-nitrosalicylanilide (Fig. 57.14) has CAS Reg. No. 50-65-7. Niclosamide is utilized either as the free acid or as its salt with 2-aminoethanol (CAS Reg. No. 1420-04-8). The common name of the salt is clonitralid or niclosamide-olamine. It was discovered by Bayer AG and is described by Gönnert and Schraufstätter (1958). The development and properties of niclosamide are reviewed by Gönnert (1962) and Schraufstätter (1962). The chemistry, uses, and toxicology of niclosamide are described in detail by Andrews et al. (1983) and by Knowles (1991) in the previous edition of this handbook. There have been no important changes in our understanding of niclosamide's toxicology in the last decade, so coverage here provides a briefer outline and focuses predominantly on more recent or additional data. Niclosamide is just one of several currently available

salicylanilides that are used clinically as anthelmintics and fasciolicides including closantel, oxyclozamide, rafoxamide, and resortantel. The chemistry, mode of action, pharmacokinetics, and toxicity of these compounds have recently been reviewed by Swan (1999).

Niclosamide exists as yellowish grey crystals, m.p. 230°C, v.p. $<1 \times 10^{-3}$ Pa (20°C), w.s. 1.6 ppm (pH 6.4, 20°C)/110ppm (pH 9.1, 20°C), log P4.7 (1.0 at pH 9.6).

Clonitralid exists as yellow crystals, m.p. 216°C, v.p. 1.3×10^{-6} Pa (25°C), w.s. 230 ppm (20°C).

Niclosamide is hydrolyzed only slowly at physiological pH (half-life about 7 days at pH 6.9) but it is susceptible to photolysis (e.g., a 60–80% loss was observed after 16 hr exposure of an aqueous solution to sunlight), but results seem to be very variable and formulated material may be much more stable (Andrews et al., 1983).

Niclosamide (BAY 25648) and its salt are used as a molluscicides in the control of snails that vector schistosomiasis, in human and veterinary practice as nematicides and as anthelmintics/cestocides in the treatment of internal parasites, particularly tapeworms, and as lampreycides (often in combination with 3-trifluoromethyl-4-nitrophenol). Trade names include Bayluscide, Cestocid, Fenasal, Mansonil, Niclocide, Phenesal, and Yomesan.

Toxicology Profile The primary source of data is U.S. EPA (1999d). Older toxicology results have been extensively reviewed by Andrews et al. (1983) and Knowles (1991) and much of that work is not included here. The data presented below are in complete agreement with these previous studies regarding the unremarkable toxicology of niclosamide in experimental animals even at high doses. The level of genotoxicity of niclosamide seems to be a matter of some dispute, but since chronic exposure studies to assess its carcinogenicity have been conducted in both rats and mice with negative results, the issue does not seem to be a crucial one. One data gap is that no multigenerational study for reproductive toxicity was found.

Acute Toxicity The acute toxicity of niclosamide to a variety of mammalian species is low by all normal routes of exposure. This is true both for free niclosamide (Table 57.5) and its ethanolamine salt (Andrews et al., 1983). It is much more toxic by intravenous administration with an LD_{50} in rats of 7.5 mg/kg (Vega et al., 1988), which demonstrates the high intrinsic toxicity of the molecule. Signs of acute poisoning include vomiting, hypopnea, convulsions, and sedation (Andrews et al., 1983).

Irritation/Sensitization Niclosamide is a strong eye irritant, but not a skin irritant. It is a moderate dermal sensitizer.

Subchronic Toxicity In a 90-day dietary study in rats, no treatment-related effects were seen at doses up to 500 mg/kg/day. In a similar study in dogs with doses up to 25 mg/kg/day, no notable specific adverse effects were observed either. In hamsters the only response noted with dietary concentrations up to 726 mg/kg/day was reduced weight gain.

Chronic Toxicity   A series of older chronic dietary studies in rats and dogs is summarized by Andrews *et al.* (1983). Rats appear to tolerate at least 1000 mg niclosamide/kg/day and dogs tolerate100 mg/kg/day without evidence of adverse effects.

Carcinogenicity   In 1978 the National Cancer Institute conducted an 18-month dietary study in Osborne–Mendel rats and B6C3F1 mice using clonitralid at doses up to 1421 mg/kg/day (rat) or 78 mg/kg/day (mouse). This study was flawed because of inadequate survival among the male mice, but there was no evidence of carcinogenicity in female mice or in rats of either sex (U.S. EPA, 1999d). No evidence of carcinogenicity was seen in the other chronic studies reviewed by Andrews *et al.* (1983).

Mutagenicity/Genotoxicity   Niclosamide was negative for forward mutations in a mouse lymphoma cell assay *in vitro* and for chromosomal effects in mouse bone marrow cells *in vivo* (U.S. EPA, 1999d). In contrast, in a similar study of the induction of chromosome aberrations and sister chromatid exchange in mouse bone marrow cells *in vivo*, Giri *et al.* (1996) reported that niclosamide gave positive responses. After an intraperitoneal dose of 25 mg/kg, both indices of genotoxicity were significantly increased compared to controls. A similar oral dose had no effects on sister chromatid exchange but did increase chromosomal aberrations. Niclosamide also gave some positive results in a study on the induction of chromosomal aberrations in human peripheral lymphocytes both *in vivo* and *in vitro* (Ostrosky-Wegman *et al.*, 1986). Results differed considerably between individuals. Three of five patients showed an increase in chromosomal aberrations after niclosamide treatment but no evidence for sister chromatid exchange was observed. The *in vitro* results with human lymphocytes from several individuals also revealed substantial variability in responses for both clastogenicity and sister chromatid exchange. A metabolic activation (hepatic S9) system was necessary for most positive results *in vitro*. The results of additional studies on the genotoxicity of niclosamide are outlined by Espinosa-Aguirre *et al.* (1991).

When clonitralid was tested in a dominant lethal assays in mice at levels that caused minor symptoms of intoxication, no evidence of mutagenicity was seen in the progeny (Andrews *et al.*, 1983). A negative result was also obtained in a modified Ames assay (MacPhee and Podger, 1977) with or without activation, but a formulated sample of niclosamide was used in this study. Subsequent studies using versions of the Ames *Salmonella* mutation assay and technical niclosamide gave negative results when conducted without the inclusion of a metabolic activation (liver S9) system, but when the activation system was included, a weak positive result was obtained (Andrews *et al.*, 1983). The positive mutagenic outcome with activation was confirmed in a series of studies by Espinosa-Aguirre *et al.* (1989, 1991) and Cortinas de Nava *et al.* (1983). The role of metabolic activation in these positive resonses was studied

further by Espinosa-Aguirre *et al.* (1991). The hydrolysis products of niclosamide were either inactive (5-chlorosalicylic acid) or only weakly active (2-chloro-4-nitroaniline) in the Ames assay. Based on the use of *Salmonella* mutants with enhanced or diminished nitroreductase and *N*-acetylase activity, reduction of the nitro group and subsequent acetylation was considered to be the key reaction sequence leading to the formation of mutagens. Nitroreduction is an important metabolic pathway for niclosamide in mammals including humans (Andrews *et al.*, 1983; Knowles, 1991), and its *N*-acetylamino metabolite has been detected in human urine after oral dosing with niclosamide (Duhm *et al.*, 1961), which elevates the significance of its probable mutagenic activity. A direct test of the potency of this metabolite in mutagenesis assays would be valuable.

Mice treated orally with five daily doses of niclosamide also produced Ames-active mutagens in the urine and the mutagenic activity was somewhat increased by the addition of β-glucuronidase (Cortinas de Nava *et al.*, 1983; Vega *et al.*, 1988). The amount of mutagen production was dose-dependant over the range of doses utilized from 30 to 100 mg/kg. Sperm malformations were also seen at doses of 60 mg/kg and higher but the relationship of this effect to the appearance of urinary mutagens is speculative.

The evidence suggesting that niclosamide is converted to one or more genotoxic products by vertebrate tisssues is therefore strong. However, as already mentioned, there appears to be no evidence that niclosamide is carcinogenic in rats and mice *in vivo*.

Reproductive Toxicity   No information on reproductive toxicity seems to be available from typical regulatory guideline studies. Vega *et al.* (1988) observed an increase in abnormal sperm morphology in two strains of mice after five daily oral doses of niclosamide at 30–120 mg/kg. No effects on testis weight or sperm count were seen and the implications for reproductive success were not assessed.

Developmental Toxicity/Teratogenicity   A study of pregnant rabbits at oral doses of niclosamide up to 180 mg/kg/day revealed no maternal toxicity. Peritoneal hemorrhage was an effect seen in some fetuses but this was regarded as only equivocally related to the treatment. This study was considered to have several significant flaws by U.S. EPA (1999d). Awad (1995) conducted a developmental study with niclosamide in Wistar rats at a single dose of 80 mg/kg/day. An increase in the incidence of skeletal malformations in fetuses and evidence of fetotoxicity were claimed, but the results are marginal and it appears that the increase in malformations was not statistically significant. The dose administered was only 2% of the LD_{50} (4000 mg/kg) in these rats. Previous studies in rats and rabbits revealed no developmental toxicity (Andrews *et al.*, 1983). Overall it appears very unlikely that niclosamide is a developmental toxicant in mammals.

Human Toxicology   Niclosamide is used as an oral medication for intestinal parasites, particularly tapeworms, in both human and veterinary practice. A dose of 2 g per peron is typically given. Transient gastrointestinal upsets, abdominal discomfort, anorexia, diarrhea, drowsiness, and dizziness have been observed occasionally as adverse effects, but there appear to be no recorded incidents of serious poisoning, long lasting side-effects, or death due to the use of niclosamide either in its clinical or pesticidal uses. Severe dermatitis has been reported in a few cases in using a 25% EC formulation of niclosamide, but this was probably due to other chemicals in the formulation. Further information on human responses to niclosamide is provided by Andrews *et al.* (1983), Knowles (1991), and HSDB (2000).

Biochemical Mechanism of Toxicity   Niclosamide and closely related salicylanilides are very strong uncouplers (Gönnert *et al.*, 1963; Ilivicky and Casida, 1969; Williamson and Metcalf, 1967) with the most potent compounds showing activity on isolated mammalian and insect mitochondria at concentrations as low as 1 nM. Niclosamide is active as an uncoupler at 10–100 nM which almost 1000-fold more active than 2,4-DNP. Typically of uncouplers, niclosamide stimulates mitochondrial respiration at lower concentrations but inhibits respiration as the concentration is increased (Gönnert and Schraufstätter, 1958). Niclosamide stimulated succinate-based oxygen consumption in snail tissues with a maximal effect at the remarkably low concentration of 0.1 nM (Ishak *et al.*, 1970). At higher concentrations, respiration was again inhibited. Many other studies with tissues and mitochondria from target and nontarget species fully support the concept that uncoupling occurs at low concentrations followed by inhibition at higher ones and that effects on oxphos are likely to be a major factor underlying the toxicity of niclosamide (Andrews *et al.*, 1983).

Absorption, Metabolism, and Excretion   After an oral dose of niclosamide in rats, two-thirds of the dose passed out in the feces and one-third was absorbed and then excreted in the urine after nitroreduction. The amide bond does not appear to be hydrolyzed to any great extent. Studies in human volunteers also showed limited uptake of niclosamide from the gastrointestinal tract after oral dosing. Only 2–25% was eliminated in the urine over 4 days. Considerable variations in pharmacokinetics between individual were noted. It was concluded that uptake is limited and metabolism of the absorbed dose is rapid, primarily occurring by nitroreduction followed by *N*-acetylation (Andrews *et al.*, 1983; Duhm *et al.*, 1961).

Niclosamide is poorly absorbed after dermal application also. A study in rats and minipigs found that only 2% and 16% respectively of a dermal application had been absorbed in 1 week (Brennan *et al.*, 1991).

Environmental Fate and Toxicity   This topic is reviewed by Andrews *et al.* (1983) and in outline by Tomlin (2000). The toxicity to birds is very varied with one species (unstated) having an acute oral LD_{50} as low as 60 mg/kg while for others it is over 2000 mg/kg (U.S. EPA, 1999d; Table 57.5). In a short-term avian dietary study (species unstated), the LC_{50} was

over 5419 ppm, indicating a very low level of toxicity. The acute toxicity of niclosamide to fish is high to very high (Table 57.5) which necessitates care in its use in aquatic systems. The sea lamprey is highly sensitive with an LC_{50} of 49 ppb which assures niclosamide's efficacy as a lampreycide. The toxicity to aquatic invertebrates is very varied. Crayfish and some aquatic insects are relatively tolerant of niclosamide, *Daphnia* are quite sensitive, and snails are highly sensitive (LC_{50} values of 49–63 ppb) in keeping with its molluscicidal uses. In practical use for snail control, a concentration of 600–1000 ppb for 8 hr or 333 ppb for 24 hr is recommended. Consequently significant fish toxicity is likely to occur during its use in anti-schistosomiasis programs (Andrews *et al.*, 1983). The uptake and metabolism of niclosamide has been studied in rainbow trout by Lech and his colleagues (e.g., see Statham and Lech, 1975). Limited bioconcentration was observed and depuration was essentially complete in 48 to 72 hr. Residues were strongly concentrated in the bile. A glucuronyl conjugate of niclosamide was identified as the major biliary metabolite.

Niclosamide tends to be more toxic as the pH and water hardness decrease. It is only moderately bound to soil organic matter and soil microbial decomposition is slow (Gönnert and Schraufstätter, 1958). However, rapid degradation with a half-life of 0.3 days was reported in rice paddies in association with its use as a molluscide (Calumpang *et al.*, 1995). The behavior of niclosamide in aquatic systems has been studied in detail by Monkiedje *et al.* (1995). They found that hydrolysis occurred at pH values above 7, but little photolysis was seen in water. Under field conditions its half-life in ponds was 3.4 days.

57.7.2.3 Amine Uncouplers

When connected to an appropriate combination of strong electron-withdrawing and lipophilic groups (R, R'), secondary amines (R-NH-R') act as lipophilic weak acids and thus fit the definition of uncouplers. The structural and physicochemical requirements for potent diarylamine uncouplers have been determined by Guo *et al.* (1991a, b). They concluded that like phenolic uncouplers, the best diarylamine uncouplers are lipophilic weak acids that can locate within the mitochondrial membrane and act as protonophores, although some differences between these two groups were also noted in shielding effects by bulky groups around the amine moiety. A number of these amine uncouplers are used as pesticides including a rodenticide (bromethalin), a fungicide (fluazinam), and an insecticide (chlorfenapyr). Sulfluramid, a minor insecticide, also fits within the definition of this amine uncoupler group, but is considered separately for other reasons.

Bromethalin: General Properties and Uses α, α, α-Trifluoro-*N*-methyl-4,6-dinitro-*N*-(2,4,6-tribromophenyl)-*o*-toluidine (Fig. 57.15), CAS Reg. No. 63333-65-7, was discovered by Eli Lilly & Co. and is described by Dreikorn *et al.* (1979). Its development and properties are reviewed by Dreikorn and O'Doherty (1984).

It exists as white crystals, m.p. 150–151°C, v.p. 1.3×10^{-5} Pa (25°C), w.s. <10 ppb, log P 4.26. Bromethalin is not

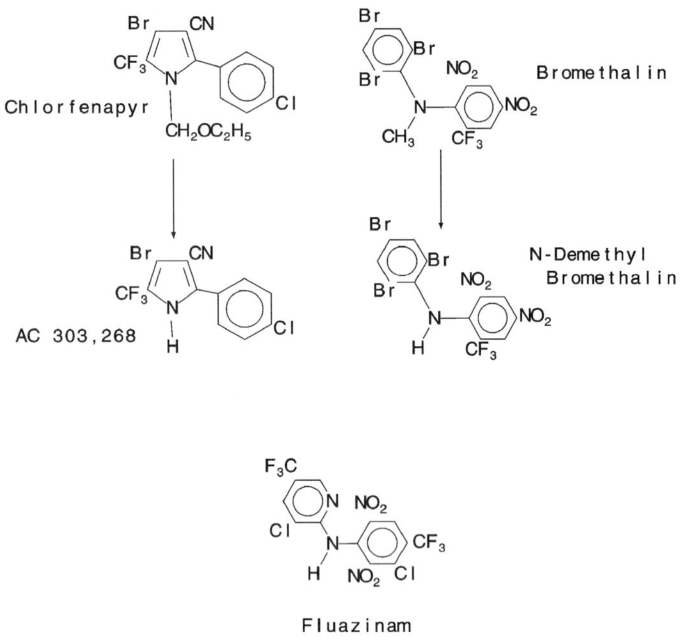

Figure 57.15 Uncouplers of oxidative phosphorylation—Secondary amines.

subject to hydrolysis, but it is very sensitive to photodegradation.

Bromethalin (EL-614) is a rodenticide used in baits. Trade names include Assault, Trounce, and Vengeance.

Toxicology Profile The primary source of data is U.S. EPA (1998f).

Acute Toxicity As a commercial rodenticide, bromethalin necessarily shows a high toxicity to rodents (Table 57.5; values from U.S. EPA, 1998f). It is also highly toxic to other vertebrates such as dogs and cats with acute oral LD_{50} values of 4.8 and 18 mg/kg, respectively. Van Lier and Cherry (1988) provide lower acute oral LD_{50} values (i.e., 2.0 mg/kg for the rat, 1.8 mg/kg for the cat, and 5.3 mg/kg for the mouse). LD_{50} values for the monkey (species unstated) and rabbit are 5.0 and 13.0 mg/kg, respectively. A notable exception to the high acute toxicity of bromethalin is the guinea pig for which the acute oral LD_{50} is over 1000 mg/kg (van Lier and Cherry, 1988). Bromethalin's acute toxicity by dermal application is low, but its inhalation toxicity is very high (Table 57.5).

At lower toxic doses, signs of acute poisoning in rodents (Dorman *et al.*, 1992a; van Lier and Cherry, 1988), dogs (Dorman *et al.*, 1990a, 1990b), and cats (Dorman *et al.*, 1992b) include slowly developing ataxia, hypothermia, hindlimb paralysis, loss of responses to sensory stimulation, labored respiration, depression, coma, and death generally due to respiratory arrest and often with terminal clonic convulsions. Focal motor seizures also occurred in cats. At higher doses in rodents (van Lier and Cherry, 1988) and dogs (Dorman *et al.*, 1990a) the clinical signs develop more rapidly over 4 to 24 hr and involve a stronger component of neuroexcitation including hyperexcitation, tremors, and generalized seizures.

Pathological examinations in the above studies gave very similar results across different mammalian species. They revealed generalized spongy degeneration and edema of the white matter of the brain, spinal cord, and optic nerve. This is caused by the separation of the myelin lamellae at the interperiod lines and the collection of fluid between the lamellae (edema) with progression to disruption of the lamellae and coalescence of the vacuoles into larger watery areas (spongy changes). Swelling of astrocytes and oligodendroglial cells also occurs. No inflammatory or macrophage response is seen, axonal degeneration is lacking, and the neural pathology is slowly reversible in surviving animals. Lipid peroxidation can be observed in the brain (Dorman *et al.*, 1992b).

Many of the clinical signs and lethal consequences from bromethalin toxicosis are likely to arise from pressure effects on neuronal conduction due to extensive brain and spinal column swelling. The brain water content in rats may increase by as much as 15% during severe acute poisoning. The cerebrospinal fluid pressure is also increased by almost 400% (van Lier and Cherry, 1988). The corticosteroid dexamethasone was effective in reducing this increase in cerebrospinal fluid pressure in rats as was the intravenous infusion of urea or 25% mannitol as hyperosmotic diuretic agents.

The electroencephlographic changes in dogs dosed with bromethalin at 6.25 mg/kg orally have been described by Dorman *et al.* (1991). Abnormal changes included spike and spike-wave patterns, high voltage slow wave activity, photoconvulsive or photoparoxysmal irritative responses, and voltage depression in all leads.

The administration of a commercial extract of *Gingko biloba* to rats by gavage antagonized lipid peroxidation and the development of edema in the brains of rats treated with a toxic oral dose of bromethalin (1 mg/kg) and reduced the severity of the signs of poisoning. This preparation was chosen because of evidence that it ameliorated similar neurological effects caused by triethyltin (Dorman *et al.*, 1992a). Other possible treatments for poisoning were examined by Dorman *et al.* (1990c). The repeated administration of a charcoal–sorbitol mixture immediately after dosing was effective but, contrary to the experience of van Lier and Cherry (1988) in rats, the administration of furosemide, mannitol, and dexamethasone in various combinations upon the appearance of clinical signs in dogs did not decrease the severity of poisoning.

A number of case of poisoning by bromethalin in nontarget species including domestic cats have been reported (Martin and Johnson, 1989).

Irritation/Sensitization Bromethalin is an eye irritant, but it is not a skin irritant or sensitizer.

Subchronic Toxicity The LOEL for bromethalin was 0.125 mg/kg/day in 90-day gavage studies in both rats and dogs. The most sensitive endpoint was spongy degeneration of the white matter of the brain, optic nerve, and spinal column. No other effects were observed in rats. Severe neurological signs and deaths occurred in dogs given 0.2 mg/kg/day subchronically.

Chronic Toxicity No chronic exposure studies appear to have been performed with bromethalin since they are not required for the registration of this compound for nonfood use as a rodenticide (U.S. EPA, 1998f).

Mutagenicity/Genotoxicity Bromethalin was not mutagenic in a battery of tests. No tests for clastogenicity were reported.

Carcinogenicity See *Chronic Toxicity* is observed.

Reproductive Toxicity See *Chronic Toxicity* is observed.

Developmental Toxicity/Teratogenicity No developmental toxicity was observed in standard studies in rats and rabbits at doses up to 0.5 mg/kg/day. Severe maternal toxicity and some deaths occurred at the highest dose.

Neurotoxicity The critical effects of bromethalin on the white matter of the central nervous system have been described. No delayed neurotoxicity was observed in hens given two high oral doses of bromethalin.

Human Toxicology One possible example of human poisoning by bromethalin has been described by Buller et al. (1996). In this case a 28-year-old male was found unconscious with evidence of consumption of rat poison. Two open packets, one containing bromethalin (0.01%) and the other diphacinone (an anticoagulant) were nearby. On tactile stimulation, tremors and strong myoclonic contractions were seen. Clinical laboratory results were normal. After decontamination and 2 days of supportive and symptomatic therapy, recovery was near complete and the patient was discharged. No estimate was provided of the amount of rodenticide consumed. Bromethalin does cause neurological signs in experimental animals, but its specific role in this incident is uncertain. The very low concentration of active ingredient does not seem to be congruent with severe poisoning. A person of 70 kg would need to consume 700 g of a 0.01% bait to achieve a dose of 1 mg/kg. Also, the signs of poisoning that are described are of limited comparability to those in experimental animals poisoned by bromethalin where spontaneous tremors and convulsions are seen primarily at high lethal doses. The nature of the treatment administered to resolve this poisoning was not described.

Biochemical Mechanism of Action Bromethalin is a propesticide which must be converted by *N*-demethylation to the corresponding free diphenylamine to initiate toxicity (van Lier and Cherry, 1988; Fig. 57.15). Unlike bromethalin itself, the activation product is a strong uncoupler of brain and liver mitochondria from rats (van Lier and Cherry, 1988)) with similar UC_{50} values of 600 and 870 nM, respectively. *N*-demethylbromethalin was even more active as an uncoupler against mouse liver mitochondria. Based on comparative phamacokinetic studies in the rat, van Lier and Cherry concluded that bromethalin is converted rapidly and almost quantitatively to *N*-demethyl bromethalin. Inducers of microsomal

cytochrome P-450 monooxygenases (3-methylcholanthrene and Aroclor 1254) caused an increase in toxicity when given to mice 1 to 3 days prior to an oral challenge dose of bromethalin at the LD_{50}. Phenobarbital, on the other hand, which induces a different suite of P-450 isoforms, antagonized its toxicity. A microsomal oxidation inhibitor, SKF-525A, given 1 hour before bromethalin antagonized its toxicity as expected if oxidative activation is occurring. On the other hand, SKF-525A increased the toxicity of *N*-demethyl bromethalin, suggesting that this is detoxified by microsomal oxygenase action. The delay in toxicity caused by this necessary metabolic activation probably contributes to the effective rodenticidal action of bromethalin since it tends to minimize bait-shyness.

The characteristic swelling and vacuolization of the white matter of the brain and spinal cord has been attributed to the failure of the pumps responsible for ion regulation in the myelin sheath due to the uncoupling activity of the activation product. In turn, this causes ions to accumulate followed by osmotic entry of water, swelling, and splitting of the myelin layers to form vacuoles (Dorman et al., 1992b; van Lier and Cherry, 1988).

Both in its structure and in its toxicological effects, bromethalin closely resembles fentrifanil, an experimental diarylamine acaricide. This compound is a potent direct-acting uncoupler of oxphos (Nizamani and Hollingworth, 1980) and causes vacuolization of myelin and edema of the white matter of the central nervous system (Lock et al., 1981) which appears to be identical to that caused by bromethalin. These and other chemically induced myelinopathies are reviewed in detail by van Gemert and Killeen (1998).

Absorption, Metabolism, and Elimination After oral dosing in rats, bromoethalin was taken up rapidly with a half-life for absorption into the plasma of 2.7 hr. Clearance from the plasma after dosing ceased was slower with a half-life of about 5.6 days (van Lier and Cherry, 1988) *N*-demethylbromethalin was the major metabolite.

Environmental Fate and Toxicity Birds are highly sensitive to the acute toxic effects of bromethalin (Table 57.5). In 8-day feeding studies with birds the LC_{50}s were 210 ppm for bobwhite quail and 620 ppm for mallard ducks, indicating a moderate to high toxicity. Bromethalin is also extremely toxic to aquatic vertebrates and invertebrates (Table 57.5), but because of its use patterns and formulations it is unlikely to present a significant risk in practice. It is rather persistent with an average half-life in aerobic soils of 178 days.

Chlorfenapyr: General Properties and Uses 4-Bromo-2-(4-chlorophenyl)-1-ethoxymethyl-5-trifluoromethylpyrrole-3-carbonitrile (Fig. 57.15), CAS Reg. No. 122453-73-0, was discovered by American Cyanamid and is described by Lovell et al. (1990). Its development and properties ar reviewed by Addor et al. (1992).

It exists as light yellow crystals, m.p. 100–101°C, v.p. $<1.3 \times 10^{-5}$ Pa (25°C), w.s. 0.14 ppm (25°C), log P4.83.

Chlorfenapyr (AC 303,630, MK-242) is a new broad spectrum insecticide and acaricide. It was developed by structural modification of a microbial natural product, dioxapyrrolomycin, as described by Addor *et al.* (1992). A general review of chlorfenapyr's properties, mechanism of action, and structure–activity relations is provided by Hunt and Treacy (1997). Although it is now widely used as an insecticide in many countries, concerns over its relatively long environmental persistence and potential for acute lethal and reproductive toxicity in birds and possible aquatic toxicity have made it a controversial compound in the United States (Williams, 1999) and so far have limited its registration to nonagricultural uses. Trade names include Alert, Citrex, Intrepid, Phantom, Pirate, Stalker, and Sunfire.

Toxicology Profile   The primary data source is U.S. EPA (1997d).

Acute Toxicity   The acute toxicity to rats is remarkably low for a compound that ultimately acts as a powerful uncoupler but the toxicity to mice and other vertebrates is considerably higher (Table 57.5).

Irritation/Sensitization   Chlorfenapyr is a moderate but reversible eye irritant, but not a skin irritant. It does not cause dermal sensitization in guinea pigs.

Subchronic Toxicity   In a 90-day dietary toxicity study in rats, the LOEL was found to be 48 mg/kg/day based on reduced body weight and liver weight increases. At higher doses (97.5 mg/kg/day) males exhibited decreased activity, ataxia, anorexia, and chromodacryorrhea, and multiple alterations were seen in blood chemistry. In a similar study in mice, an LOEL for chlorfenapyr was found at 14.8 mg/kg/day in males and 40 mg/kg/day in females with an endpoint of hepatocellular hypertrophy. Spongiform encephalopathy was noted in the brain and the myelin of the spinal cord in both sexes at 63–76 mg/kg/day, a dose that was lethal to some animals. In dogs, no remarkable adverse effects other than lowered weight gains were seen in either a 90-day or a 1-year dietary study with doses up to 10.1 mg/kg/day. A 28-day dermal study in rabbits showed first adverse efects at 400 mg/kg involving liver alterations (particularly vacuolization which increased in severity at 1000 mg/kg) and blood chemistry changes.

Chronic Toxicity   A 1-year dietary study in dogs revealed only decreased body weigh at the highest dose (8.7 mg/kg/day). In an 18-month dietary study in mice, neuropathology in the form of extensive vacuolization of the white matter of the brain and spinal cord was again observed along with skin ulceration at 16.6 (M) to 21.9 (F) mg/kg/day. A 2-year study in rats revealed liver toxicity in the form of non-neoplastic hepatocellular enlargement at 15 (M) and 18.6 (F) mg/kg/day in the diet.

Carcinogenicity   No carcinogenic response was seen in the mouse chronic study, but in the study in rats, an increased incidence of malignant histiocytic sarcoma and testicular interstitial cell tumors was discovered in males fed 30.8 mg chlorfenapyr/kg/day for 2 years. Some increase in liver adenomas and/or carcinomas was observed in females but the results were inconsistent. A significant increase in endometrial stromal polyps was also observed. As a result of the rat study, the carcinogenicity of chlorfenapyr was classified by the U.S. Environmental Protection Agency as "cannot be determined, suggestive."

Mutagenicity/Genotoxicity   Chlorfenapyr is not mutagenic or clastogenic in a standard battery of assays including mutations in bacterial and mammalian cells, a micronucleus test in mice *in vivo*, and chromosomal aberration and DNA repair assays in mammalian cells *in vitro*.

Reproductive Toxicity   In a two-generation study in rats, the only reproductive adverse effect observed with chlorfenapyr was reduced weight gain in the pups which occurred at 22 mg/kg/day. This dose also caused lower weight gains in the parents.

Developmental Toxicity/Teratogenicity   No evidence for developmental toxicity was found in studies with pregnant rats at doses up to 225 mg/kg/day and rabbits at doses up to 30 mg/kg/day.

Neurotoxicity   The neurotoxic effects of chlorfenapyr have also given cause for concern. In an acute test, rats given 180 mg/kg showed no notable neurobehaviorial response beyond lethargy and no neuropathology. In a 1-year dietary study in rats, myelin sheath swelling was recorded after 13 weeks at 28–37 mg/kg/day. At 52 weeks, the myelinopathic process was more generalized and severe and was seen at a dose of 13.6 mg/kg/day. Only males were affected. The effect had disappeared after a recovery period of 16 weeks. As already described, similar effects were observed in dietary studies with mice.

Biochemical Mechanism of Action   Chlorfenapyr shows virtually no uncoupling activity but removal of the *N*-ethoxymethyl group through microsomal oxidation (Fig. 57.15) releases the corresponding free pyrrole (AC 303,268) which is a lipophilic weak acid with very strong uncoupling activity (Black *et al.*, 1994). Inhibition of this oxidative activation reaction in insects *in vivo* with piperonyl butoxide antagonizes the toxicity of chlorfenapyr (Treacy *et al.*, 1994). AC 302,268 has an acute toxicity higher than that of chlorfenapyr in both vertebrates and insects (e.g., the acute oral LD$_{50}$ for the rat is 29 mg/kg). Upon injection into insects it cause an almost immediate and massive stimulation of respiration whereas the parent chlorfenapyr does so only after a significant delay (Black *et al.*, 1994). All these observations support the idea that chlorfenapyr is a proinsecticide and requires metabolic conversion to the active uncoupler, AC 303,268, before it exerts a toxic action. AC 303,268, and its further degradation products, is a common metabolites of chlorfenapyr found in studies with vertebrates (below).

Absorption, Metabolism, and Elimination An oral dose of chlorfenapyr was poorly absorbed in rats and over 80% was eliminated in the feces. The absorbed dose was rapidly cleared in the urine. Urinary metabolites included products of N-alkoxy side chain oxidation and removal (e.g., AC 303,268) and ring hydroxylation products and their conjugates. Similar results were obtained with goats and hens. In fish and soil, debromination is observed as an additional metabolic route (U.S. EPA, 1997d).

Environmental Fate and Toxicity The acute toxicity of chlorfenapyr to birds is high to very high (Table 57.5). The subchronic toxicity to birds is also very high (e.g., in mallard ducks, chlorfenapyr at 2.5 ppm in the diet reduced adult body weights and decreased egg-laying and hatch rates by about 40–60%). Risk assessments by the U.S. Environmental Protection Agency suggested a substantial reproductive risk to birds from some uses of chlorfenapyr and indicated the need for the development of mitigation strategies (U.S. EPA, 1997d). Although these results suggest that there is a considerable potential for the use of chlorfenapyr to cause acute and reproductive toxicity in wild birds, there appear to be no reports of detectable impacts on birds or other wildlife when these have been closely monitored in areas where chlorfenapyr has been used (e.g., see Williams, 1999). Chlorfenapyr is also very highly toxic to fish and aquatic invertebrates (Table 57.5) which raises additional questions regarding its potential environmental impact and risk mitigation strategies.

Chlorfenapyr binds firmly to soil with a K_{oc} value about 11,500 ml/g. This and its low water solubility indicate a low leaching potential but also imply possible environmental movement by surface runoff attached to soil colloids. Chlorfenapyr has a rather long half-life of 1.4 years in aerobic soils which suggests a capacity for some environmental accumulation with repeated use, possibly to toxic levels (U.S. EPA, 1997d).

Fluazinam: General Properties and Uses 3-Chloro-N-(3-chloro-5-trifluoromethyl-2-pyridyl)-α, α, α-trifluoro-2,6-dinitro-p-toluidine (Fig. 57.15), CAS Reg. No. 79622-59-6, was discovered by Ishihara Sangyo Kaisha, Ltd. and is described by Anema *et al.* (1992).

It exists as yellow crystals, m.p. 115–117°C, v.p. 1.5 × 10^{-3} Pa (25°C), w.s. 0.157 ppm (pH 7, 25°C), log P 3.56.

Fluazinam (ASC-66825, IKF-1216) is a broad spectrum fungicide with additional acaricidal properties which is used on fruits, vegetables, and turfgrass. Trade names include Altima, Frowncide, Legacy, Shirlan, and Shogun.

Toxicology Profile The general source of data is U.S. EPA (2000b).

Acute Toxicity Fluazinam has a very low acute toxicity to terrestrial vertebrates by the oral and dermal routes but is somewhat more toxic by inhalation (Table 57.5).

Irritation/Sensitization Fluazinam is irritating to the skin and very irritating to the eye. It is a weak dermal sensitizer.

Subchronic Toxicity At the LOEL (41 mg/kg/day) in a 13-week study, male rats showed hepatocellular hypertrophy and chronic sinusodial inflammation. In a subchronic dietary study in dogs, the LOEL was 100 mg/kg/day based on ocular changes and bile duct hyperplasia sometimes with cholangiofibrosis.

Chronic Toxicity In a chronic feeding study in dogs the LOEL was 10 mg/kg/ day based on nonspecific toxicity. No ocular effects were seen. At the highest doses (100 and 1000 ppm) in a chronic feeding study in mice, macroscopic and microscopic lesions were produced in a number of tissues, particularly the liver and testes. In a chronic dietary study in rats, a LOEL was obtained at 100 ppm (about 4.3 mg/kg/day) based on a number of effects including macroscopic and microscopic lesions in multiple organs. A second study in rats also revealed lesions in the liver and testes as notable toxic endpoints. In a parallel study in mice, using dietary concentrations from 1000 to 7000 ppm, it was noted that an impurity in the technical material caused vacuolization in the brain and spinal cord, an effect seen with some other potent uncouplers (Section 57.7.2.3).

Carcinogenicity No evidence of carcinogenicity was found in a 2-year rat dietary study. In mice, some increases in hepatocellular adenomas were seen at 3000 ppm, but this was not dose-dependent and no carcinomas were found. It was concluded that fluazinam is not a carcinogen in mice (U.S. EPA, 2000b).

Mutagenicity/Genotoxicity No genotoxic effects were observed in a battery of tests including two mutation tests in bacteria, a chromosome aberrations test in mammalian cells, a mouse micronucleus test, and a DNA repair test in bacteria.

Reproductive Toxicity In a two-generation reproduction study in rats, the dietary NOEL for reproductive effects was 100 ppm (10.1 mg/kg/day) which was well above the NOEL for parental toxicity (20 ppm).

Developmental Toxicity/Teratogenicity In both rats and rabbits, developmental effects were seen only at doses higher than those that were maternally toxic.

Neurotoxicity No neurotoxic effects were seen in rats with an acute oral doses up to 2000 mg/kg, or in a subchronic study with doses up to 233 mg/kg/day.

Hormonal Actions No evidence for adverse effects related to the disruption of estrogen actions was seen in any mammalian or avian study.

Human Toxicology   There has been a history of skin irritation and sensitization associated with the repeated application of fluazinam in agricultural uses (Adams, 1997; Bruynzeel *et al.*, 1995; van Ginkel and Sabapathy, 1995).

Biochemical Mechanism of Action   Fluazinam is a lipophilic weak acid with strong uncoupling activity on mitochondria *in vitro* (Brandt *et al.*, 1992; Guo *et al.*, 1991c; Hollingworth and Gadelhak, 1998). A detailed analysis of the relationship between physicochemical characteristics, structure, and uncoupling activity for fluazinam and its analogs is provided by Guo *et al.* (1991a, b). Fluazinam bears a structural resemblance to the active metabolite of bromethalin, but it differs greatly from this compound in its very low acute toxicity, primarily because it reacts readily with cellular thiols such as glutathione through the chlorine substituent in the phenyl ring (Clarke *et al.*, 1998; Guo *et al.*, 1991a; Hollingworth and Gadelhak, 1998). Analyses of the quantitative structure–activity relationships for the toxicity of fluazinam analogs to several fungi have led to the conclusion that, in addition to uncoupling effects, reactivity with sulfhydryl groups may contribute to the toxicity of fluazinam in some cases (Akagi *et al.*, 1995, 1996b). Sulfhydryl (or other nucleophilic) reactions are probably also involved in the skin irritation and sensitization seen with fluazinam which resembles that caused by 1-chloro-2,4-dinitrobenzene, a well-known sulfhydryl-reactive compound.

Absorption, Metabolism, and Excretion   After an oral dose in rats, rapid and complete elimination occurred, primarily in the feces. Metabolites included products of nitro reduction, and glutathione and glucuronide conjugation (U.S. EPA, 2000b).

Environmental Fate and Toxicity   Fluazinam has a low acute toxicity to birds, but it is much more toxic to fish and aquatic invertebrates (Table 57.5). It binds strongly to soil with K_d values from 143 to 820. In the soil, it has a half-life of 33–62 days (Tomlin, 2000).

57.7.2.4 Perfluorooctanesulfonic Acid and Derivatives

The insecticidal properties of this chemical class were discovered serendipitously. Perfluororalkanecarboxylic acid and perfluoroalkanesulfonic acid derivatives have numerous industrial uses as surfactants (e.g., in conditioning paper products, fabric stain-proofing, and antifoaming agents). While investigating slow-acting insecticides for the control of fire ants, Vander Meer *et al.* (1985, 1986) included perfluorooctanesulfonamide surfactants as formulation aids. Control formulations made in this way, and lacking an apparent active ingredient, also showed excellent delayed toxicity to the ants. Subsequent studies of a variety of related fluorinated alkylsulfonamides showed that optimum insecticidal activity is found with an eight carbon chain leading to the development of sulfluramid as a slow-acting insecticide. The free perfluorooctanesulfonic acid was also found to have good insecticidal properties (Vander Meer

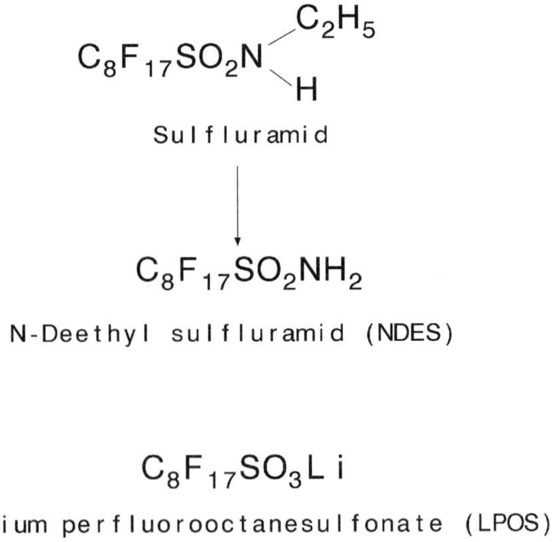

Figure 57.16   Pefluorooctanesulfonyl pesticides.

et al., 1985) and the lithium salt of this acid was recently registered for limited use in the United States (U.S. EPA, 1999e).

Sulfluramid: General Properties and Uses   *N*-ethylperfluorooctane-1-sulfonamide (Fig. 57.16), CAS Reg. No. 4151-50-2, was discovered by Vander Meer *et al.* (1985), developed by Griffin Chemical Co., and described and reviewed by Vander Meer *et al.* (1987). Structure–activity relationships for this group of compounds as insecticides are presented by Vander Meer *et al.* (1985, 1987).

It exists as colorless crystals, m.p. 96°C, v.p. 5.7×10^{-5} Pa (25°C), practically insoluble in water, log P 3.1, >6.8 (unionized form), pKa 9.5 (methanol). The technical material is a mixture of isomers, with approximately 70–90% linear and 10–30% branched perfluorooctane chains.

Sulfluramid (GX 071) is primarily a stomach poison and is used in bait formulations to control cockroaches, ants, termites, and wasps under the trade names of Alstar, Finitron, Mirex-S, Transflur, and Volcano. Sulfluramid-impregnated cardboard is used for termite control under the name FirstLine.

Toxicology Profile   The primary source of data is U.S. EPA (1989d).

Acute Toxicity   Sulfluramid has a low acute toxicity to vertebrates by all routes of exposure (Table 57.5), although there is some confusion regarding the exact LD$_{50}$. Values in the literature range from 500 to >5000 mg/kg. Signs of poisoning in rats (Vander Meer *et al.*, 1986) include decreased food consumption, weight loss, and emaciation. Transient lethargy, depression, and dyspnea were observed in sheep given sulfluramid orally at 15 mg/kg (Vitayavirasuk and Bowen, 1999).

Irritation/Sensitization   Sulfluramid is not an eye irritant but it does cause mild skin irritation.

Subchronic Toxicity In dogs, pale mucous membranes, tachypnea, weight loss, diarrhea, and lethargy were observed after high doses for 2 weeks (Schnellmann, 1990). In 90-day dietary exposure studies, NOELs ranged from 10 ppm for rats to 100 ppm for dogs (F).

Chronic Toxicity No results of chronic toxicity testing, including carcinogenicity studies, were found, probably because sulfluramid is not registered for food uses.

Carcinogenicity See *Chronic Toxicity*.

Mutagenicity/Genotoxicity Sulfluramid gave negative results in limited genotoxicity testing (Ames mutagenicity and Chinese hamster ovary sister chromatid exchange assays).

Reproductive Toxicity As a result of the observation that the oral administration of sulfluramid caused transient sterility in dogs, Stump *et al.* (1997) studied the effect of oral doses (0.3 to 3.0 mg/kg/day) in pregnant New Zealand White rabbits. Neonatal mortality was seen at each dose, but no treatment-related effects were seen on sexual maturation or testicular function in the offspring and no histopathological findings in the reproductive organs were noted.

Developmental Toxicity/Teratogenicity No results were found in this area.

Biochemical Mechanism of Action Sulfluramid is readily metabolized to its *N*-deethylated analog, perfluorooctanesulfonamide (NDES). Studies *in vitro* with kidney proximal tubules (Schnellmann, 1990) showed that sulfluramid caused an increase in respiratory rate over the range of 10–100 μM and cellular necrosis at higher concentrations. NDES was several-fold more potent than sulfluramid in these actions. Further investigation with renal mitochondria indicated that NDES is a moderately active mitochondrial uncoupler causing a 50% increase in state 4 respiration at 5 μM through its action as an ionophore (Schnellmann and Manning, 1990). Although the parent sulfluramid also stimulated state 4 respiration in mitochondria, the authors concluded that this was because of its conversion to its *N*-deethyl metabolite by the mitochondria and that it did not itself act as a protonophore. An uncoupling activity is possible since in these compounds the sulfonamide group is weakly acidic. Sulfluramid has a pKa of 9.5 in methanol whereas NDES has a pKa of 9 these values should be about 2 units lower in water. They have high log *P* values. In addition, a special mechanism of uncoupling may be occurring with the desethyl analog. It has been shown that fatty acids can act as protonophoric uncouplers since the anionic form can be transported back across the mitochondrial inner membrane by a specific transporter system (Wallace and Starkov, 2000). As a fatty acid analog, NDES may bind to this transporter, thus facilitating its transfer across the membrane and promoting its uncoupling potency. The specific protonophoric action of sulfluramid, and, more actively, NDES, leading to mitochon-

drial uncoupling has been confirmed by Starkov *et al.* (2001) and Gadelhak and Hollingworth (unpublished).

Studies with cockroaches show that both sulfluramid and NDES cause a strong increase in respiratory rates *in vivo*, but sulfluramid does so only after a 30–60 min delay, whereas NDES has an almost immediate effect (Hollingworth and Gadelhak, 1998). The respiratory rate increase caused by sulfluramid, but not by NDES, is inhibited by pretreatment of the insects with the microsomal monooxygenase inhibitor piperonyl butoxide. This fully supports the idea that sulfluramid is a propesticde that must be converted to NDES which then acts as an uncoupler.

In addition, perfluorooctanesulfonic acid and its derivatives are extremely powerful surfactum (e.g., see Kissa, 2001; Shinoda *et al.*, 1972) and the ability to disrupt membrane integrity must also be considered as a possible contributory mechanism to their effects on mitochondria.

Human Toxicology In a study of workers in a pesticide packaging plant in Brazil, Machado-Neto *et al.* (1999) measured dermal exposure to sulfluramid. It was concluded that this level of exposure was well within safety limits based on a NOEL (rat, 90-day, oral) of 10 mg/kg/day and a 10-fold safety factor. Even with a 100-fold safety factor, these exposure would have been regarded as acceptable.

Absorption, Metabolism, and Elimination Sulfluramid is converted to its *N*-deethyl analog *in vitro* (Schnellmann and Manning, 1990) and *in vivo* in rats and dogs (Arrendale *et al.*, 1989; Manning *et al.*, 1991) and sheep (Vitayavirasuk and Bowen, 1999). Manning *et al.* (1991) found that sulfluramid is absorbed slowly and incompletely from the gastrointestinal tract in rats but the absorbed dose is rapidly *N*-deethylated. The half-life for clearing sulfluramid from the blood was 16 to 20 hr, depending on the vehicle used for administration. NDES had a much longer half-life for clearance of 103 to 107 hr. Grossman *et al.* (1992) also studied the distribution and elimination of sulfluramid in rats dosed for 56 days in their diet at 75 mg/kg. No mortality was observed. NDES was present at all times in the blood and tissues, but sulfluramid itself could not be detected. The clearance half-life from the blood for NDES at the end of the exposure was 10.8 days. The rate and extent of any further conversion of either sulfluramid or NDES to perfluorooctanesulfonic acid were not assessed in these studies and are unclear, but the slow clearance of NDES suggests that such a conversion cannot be rapid if it occurs at all. The free acid also has insecticidal properties and significant mammalian toxicity (Section 57.7.2.4).

Environmental Fate and Toxicity Limited data suggest that sulfluramid has moderate oral toxicity to birds (Table 57.5). The data from 8-day dietary studies in birds tend to confirm this with LC50 values of 460 ppm for bobwhite quail and 165 ppm for mallard ducks. Its toxicity to fish is very low with LC50 values for several species greater than 8000 to 10,000 ppm, but it is considerably more toxic to *Daphnia* (Table 57.5).

The fate of sulfluramid in the environment is unclear, but, despite its high chemical stability, eventually it may degrade to perfluorooctanesulfonic acid. The environmental properties of this compound are outlined in below.

Lithium Perfluorooctanesulfonate (LPOS): General Properties and Uses   The structure of LPOS is shown in Fig. 57.16. It has CAS Reg. No. 29457-72-5. It was discovered by Vander Meer *et al.* (1985) and developed by S. C. Johnson & Sons. It readily dissociates in water to yield perfluorooctanesulfonic acid (PFOS). Since the toxicological properties of the two compounds should be very similar they are treated jointly in this discussion. Perfluorooctanesulfonic acid is an extremely strong acid and under virtually all biological and environmental conditions it will exist solely in the form of the dissociated sulfonate anion. For simplicity, both the acid and its anion are here referred to as PFOS.

LPOS is an off-white powder, decomp. 308°. PFOS has a v.p. of 3.3×10^{-4} Pa (20°C). Its w.s. varies from 519 ppm in pure water to 5 ppm in unfiltered sea water, HLC 7.2×10^{-9} atm m^3 mole^{-1} in pure water.

LPOS is registered in the United States for outdoor residential nonfood use only, particularly in bait stations for wasps and hornets. The trade name is Sulfotine. Derivatives of PFOS have also been widely used as stable surfactants in surface coatings to repel soil, oil, and water from paper and fabrics [e.g., in Scotchgard®, in paints and adhesive, in fire-retardant foams, and in a variety of other industrial and domestic applications (U.S. EPA, 2000c)]. Almost 6.5 million pounds were produced in 2000. The amount of this material used for insect control is minor.

Toxicology Profile   The primary sources of data for LPOS are U.S. EPA (1999e) and Cal EPA (2000c), and for PFOS it is U.S. EPA (2000c).

Acute Toxicity   LPOS has a moderate acute toxic for mammals by the oral and inhalation routes and a low dermal toxicity. The acute oral LD$_{50}$ of PFOS to rats is 251 mg/kg.

Irritation/Sensitization   LPOS is a severe but reversible eye irritant and a slight skin irritant.

Subchronic Toxicity   LPOS administered for 90 days in the drinking water decreased body weight, suppressed hematopoiesis, decreased serum triglycerides, and caused hepatic vacuolization in females with LOELs in the range of 0.3 to 3.0 mg/kg/day. Anorexia and convulsions were reported after lethal subchronic doses of PFOS in rats. In parallel with the LPOS study, these signs were accompanied by hepatotoxicity (increased liver enzymes, hepatic vacuolization, and hypertrophy), gastrointestinal effects, and hematologic abnormalities at doses of 2 mg/kg/day or more.

In Rhesus monkeys after repeat oral dosing with PFOS, signs of poisoning included emesis, diarrhea, anorexia, hypoactivity, prostration, convulsions, and death. Atrophy of the salivary glands and pancreas, a marked decrease in serum cholesterol, and lipid depletion in the adrenals were also reported. No monkeys survived beyond 3 weeks at 10 mg/kg/day or beyond 7 weeks at 4.5 mg/kg/day. Many of these responses were also seen in Cynomolgus monkeys given doses of the potassium salt of PFOS for 26 weeks. At the LOEL, 0.75 mg/kg/day, morbidity, decreased body weight, and lowered cholesterol were noted (Seacat *et al.*, 2001). Hormonal effects included lowered triiodothyronine levels, increased thyroid-stimulating hormone, and lowered estradiol levels in males. Hepatocellular hypertrophy and lipid vacuolization, but no evidence of peroxisomal proliferation, were seen. The microscopic changes in the liver completely reversed after 27 weeks of recovery. It was concluded that adverse effects in this study occurred only at serum levels greater than 100 ppm and were reversible.

Chronic Toxicity   No data were found regarding chronic toxicity and carcinogenicity since LPOS is not registered for food uses (U.S. EPA, 1999e).

Carcinogenicity   See *Chronic Toxicity*.

Mutagenicity/Genotoxicity   Neither LPOS nor PFOS is genotoxic in standard tests for mutation (Ames and Chinese hamster ovary cell assay), for chromosomal effects (mouse micronucleus and Chinese hamster ovary cell assays), or for DNA damage and repair (unscheduled DNA synthesis in rat primary hepatocytes).

Reproductive Toxicity   In a two-generation reproductive study in rats, dietary PFOS had an LOEL of 0.4 mg/kg/day for second generation offspring based on reductions in body weight. Reversible delays in reflex and physical development raised concerns regarding the potential for developmental neurotoxicity. Considerable mortality was seen in first generation offspring at higher dietary PFOS doses (1.6 and 3.2 mg/kg/day).

Developmental Toxicity/Teratogenicity   No increased fetal sensitivity compared to the maternal parent was observed in developmental studies in pregnant rats and rabbits. LPOS was not teratogenic in rabbits but at oral doses of 4 mg/kg/day during days 7 through 19 of gestation it did cause increased abortions, postimplantation losses, premature deliveries, and growth retardation (Henwood *et al.*, 1994a; U.S. EPA, 1999e). In rats, teratogenicity (cleft palate, edema, decreased bone ossification) and embryolethality were observed, but only at a dose (12 mg/kg/day) that also caused severe maternal toxicity and some maternal mortality (Henwood *et al.*, 1994b; U.S. EPA, 1999e). Parallel studies with PFOS (U.S. EPA, 2000c) showed similar effects in rats exposed at 5 mg/kg./day. In rabbits exposed to PFOS during gestation, reductions in fetal weight and increases in delayed ossification were seen at doses of 2.5 mg/kg/day and higher.

Absorption, Metabolism, and Elimination   PFOS is firmly bound to liver proteins and resists clearance in male rats and mice. Clearance is also delayed by enterohepatic circulation of the acid, perhaps conjugated as the glucuronide (Vitayavirasuk and Bowen, 1999). The administration of cholestyramine has been shown to speed the elimination of both perfluorooctanecarboxylic acid and PFOS by binding these compounds in the gut leading to enhanced fecal elimination (Johnson *et al.*, 1984). In Cynomolgus monkeys the serum half-life of PFOS was 193–224 days (Seacat *et al.*, 2001).

Biochemical Mechanism of Action   The biochemical mechanism underlying the acute toxicity of LPOS is unknown. It is not a conventional uncoupler because it is a very strong acid and could not act as a transmembrane protonophore in the typical uncoupler model. Despite this, it caused a rapid and strong increase in respiration in cockroaches immediately after injection (Hollingworth and Gadelhak, 1998) although it has a rather weak ability to increase respiratory rates in mitochondria *in vitro*. The unfluorinated analog of PFOS, octanesulfonic acid, was completely inactive in causing these effects. The strong surfactant properties of PFOS may cause general membrane disruption. The lack of strong uncoupling activity and the production of a nonspecific ion permeability in mitochondrial membranes have also been reported by Starkov *et al.* (2001).

Like its more extensively studied analog, perfluorooctanoic acid, PFOS is a peroxisome proliferator in rodents (Haughom and Spydevold, 1992; Hosokawa and Satoh, 1993; Sohlenius *et al.*, 1993). This probably occurs because these compounds resemble long chain fatty acids and induce the peroxisomal enzymes responsible for fatty acid catabolism, but these perfluorinated analogs are not metabolizable. In rats, PFOS caused a pronounced reduction in cholesterol and triacylglycerols in serum coupled with a rise in the liver triacylglycerols and an increase in palmitate oxidation and carboxylesterase activity. The hypolipemic effect was attributed to reduced production of cholesteryl esters and enhanced oxidation of fatty acids in the liver which led to impaired production of lipoprotein particles. In the mouse, a typical induction of the enzyme involved in fatty acid oxidation, peroxisomal catalase, and the ω-hydroxylation of lauric acid were observed. PFOS was found to act as a typical peroxisome proliferator in subchronic feeding studies in Cynomolgus monkeys (Seacat *et al.*, 2001). Also like perfluorooctanoic acid, PFOS has been shown to inhibit intercellular communication via gap junctions in rat liver epithelial cells *in vitro* (Upham *et al.*, 1998). This action correlates well with the ability to act as a tumor promoter. Perfluorooctanoic acid is a known hepatocarcinogen and, because of its parallel actions as a peroxisome proliferator and inhibitor of gap junctions, it is reasonable to speculate that PFOS may act similarly. The role of peroxisome proliferation in carcinogenesis remains controversial, particularly in regard to the extrapolation of results in rodents to humans who appear to be much less sensitive to this effect. Comprehensive reviews of this topic are provided in an IARC Technical Report (IARC, 1995) and by Cattley *et al.* (1998) and Roberts (1999).

Human Toxicology   In routine screening, PFOS was detected in the serum of fluorochemical manufacturing workers with a mean value of approximately 2 ppm (Olsen *et al.*, 1999). PFOS levels less than 6 ppm did not cause any changes in serum hepatic enzymes, cholesterol, or lipoproteins and no evidence of health effects were observed. In tests of blood bank samples from the United States, PFOS was identified at concentrations in the general range of 10–100 ppb in serum with mean levels of 30–54 ppb (Hansen *et al.*, 2001; U.S. EPA, 2000c) indicating general human exposure to PFOS and/or its derivatives. Because of these observations, coupled with the widespread industrial and domestic use of perfluorooctanesulfonyl surfactants, their long environmental persistence, and indications of the resultant bioaccumulation of PFOS in humans and the environment, their manufacturer, the 3M Company, has recently decided to phase out their production by the end of 2002 (U.S. EPA, 2000c).

Absorption, Metabolism, and Excretion   PFOS is well absorbed after an oral dose and distributes primarily in the serum and liver. It is not metabolized. Elimination is slow and occurs through both the urine and feces. A limited study with retired manufacturing workers indicated an elimination half-life of approximately 4 years (U.S. EPA, 2000c).

Environmental Fate and Toxicity   LPOS is highly toxic to birds on acute exposure, but it is only slightly to moderately toxic to fish and the toxicity to *Daphnia* is low. PFOS is an extremely stable compound in the environment with little propensity for degradation chemically, photochemically, or microbiologically (U.S. EPA, 2000c). Because of the extensive industrial use of PFOS derivatives, it can be detected in low amounts in wildlife worldwide including the Arctic and remote Pacific Ocean locations (Giesy and Kannan, 2001). The levels found were typically in the range of 10–500 ng/g tissue, but up to 3680 ng/g was detected in the livers of mink in the midwestern United States. The highest levels were found in more industrialized areas. These authors present evidence that PFOS can bioaccumulate within food chains (e.g., mink fed fish containing PFOS at 120 ng/g wet weight accumulated about 2600 ng/g in their liver). So far, no toxic effects have been ascribed to the widespread occurrence of this compound in fish, birds, and marine mammals, and the concentrations detected appear to be less than those known to cause adverse effects. The mechanisms of degradation of the various perfluorooctanesulfonyl compounds to PFOS, and the routes of global transport and biological accumulation, remain to be established. Because of its low Henry's Law constant value, PFOS is unlikely to volatilize from water to air.

57.8 ABBREVIATIONS

2,4-DNP	2,4-dinitrophenol
ADI	Acceptable daily intake

BCF	Biological concentration (bioconcentration) factor
CAS Reg. No.	Chemical Abstracts Service Registry Number
DCCD	Dicyclohexylcarbodiimide
EC_{50}	Concentration that causes an effect at 50% of the maximum level
F	Female
HLC	Henry's law constant
I_{50}	Concentration needed to cause 50% inhibition of a process
JMPR	Joint Meeting of the FAO Panel of Experts on Pesticide Residues in Food and the Environment and the WHO Core Assessment Group on Pesticide Residues
K_d	Equilibrium constant for binding to soil
K_{oc}	Equilibrium constant for binding to soil, adjusted for organic matter content
GABA	Gamma-aminobutyric acid
LC_{50}	Concentration lethal to 50% of the population
LD_{50}	Dose lethal to 50% of the popualtion
LOEC	Lowest concentration causing an observable effect
LOEL	Lowest observable (adverse) effect level
$\log P$	Logarithm of the 1-octanol:water partition coefficient
LPOS	Lithium perfluorooctanesulfonate
M	Male
mg/kg	Milligrams of compound per kilogram of body weight
m.p.	Melting point
NDES	N-deethyl sulfluramid (perfluorooctanesulfonamide)
NOEL	No observable (adverse) effect level
ODC	Ornithine decarboxylase
Oxphos	Oxidative phosphorylation
PFOS	Perfluorooctanesulfonic acid
pKa	Negative logarithm of the dissociation constant (Ka)
ppb	Parts per billion
ppm	Part per million
ppt	Parts per trillion
Q	Coenzyme Q (ubiquinone)
Q_1^*	Unit cancer potency factor from the USEPA cancer risk model
ROS	Reactive oxygen species
SmP	submitochondrial particle
UC_{50}	Concentration causing 50% uncoupling of respiration
v.p.	Vapor pressure
w.s.	Water solubility

ACKNOWLEDGEMENTS

I would like to recognize the assistance of Dr. Jerry Baron and those colleagues from agrochemical companies who provided information on individual pesticides, Dr. Satoru Miyazaki for his assistance in the translation of documents from Japanese, and Dr. Kurunthachalam Kannan for helphul discussions on the environmental effects of organotins and perfluoroctanesulfonic acid and its derivatives.

REFERENCES

Abdo, K. M., Eustis, S. L., Hasemen, J., Huff, J. E., Peters, A., and Persing, R. (1988). Toxicity and carcinogenicity of rotenone given in the feed of F344/N rats and B6C3F1 mice for up to two years. *Drug Chem. Toxicol.* **11**, 225–235.

Abo-Khatwa, N., and Hollingworth, R. M. (1973). Chlordimeform: Uncoupling activity against rat liver mitochondria *in vitro*. *Pestic. Biochem. Physiol.* **3**, 358–369.

Abo-Khatwa, N., and Hollingworth, R. M. (1974). Pesticidal chemicals affecting some energy-linked functions of rat liver mitochondria *in vitro*. *Bull. Environ. Contam. Toxicol.* **12**, 446–454.

Abrahams, J. P., Leslie, A. G. W., Lutter, R., and Walker, J. E. (1994). Structure at 2.8 angstrom resolution of F₁-ATPase from bovine heart mitochondria. *Nature (London)* **370**, 621–628.

Adams, R. M. (1997). Reflecting on developments in occupational dermatitis. *Clin. Dermatol.* **15**, 473–447.

Addor, R. W., Babcock, T. J., Black, B. C., Brown, D. C., Diehl, R. E., Furch, J. A., Kameswaran, V., Kamhi, V. M., Kremer, K. A., Kuhn, D. G., Lovell, J. B., Lowen, G. T., Miller, T. P., Peevey, R. M., Siddens, J. K., Treacy, M. F., Trotto, S. H., and Wright, D. P. (1992). Insecticidal pyrroles—Discovery and overview. *ACS Sympos. Ser.* **504**, 283–297.

Adhikari, N., and Grover, I. S. (1988). Genotoxic effects of some systemic pesticides: *In vivo* chromosomal aberrations in bone marrow cells from rats. *Environ. Mol. Mutagen.* **12**, 235–242.

Adhikari, N., and Grover, I. S. (1989). Comparative mutagenesis of vitavax. *Environ. Mol. Mutagen.* **14**(Suppl. 15), 5.

Ahmad, S., and Knowles, C. O. (1972). Biochemical mode of action of tricyclohexyltin. *Comp. Gen. Pharmacol.* **3**, 125–133.

Ahrens, W. H. (1994). "Herbicide Handbook." 7th ed. Weed Science Society of America, Champaign, IL.

Akagi, T., Mitani, S., Komyoji, T., and Nagatani, K. (1995). Quantitative structure–activity relationships of fluazinam and related fungicidal *N*-phenylpyridinamines: Preventive activity against *Botrytis cinerea*. *J. Pestic. Sci.* **20**, 279–290.

Akagi, T., Takahashi, Y., and Sasaki, S.-I. (1996a). Exhaustive conformational searches for superimposition of acaricidal compounds. *Quant. Struct.–Activity Relat.* **15**, 290–295.

Akagi, T., Mitani, S., Komyoji, T., and Nagatani, K. (1996b). Quantitative structure–activity relationships of fluazinam and related fungicidal *N*-phenylpyridinamines: Preventive activity against *Sphaerotheca fulginea*, *Pyricularia oryzae* and *Rhizoctonia solani*. *J. Pestic. Sci.* **21**, 23–29.

Aldridge, W. N. (1976). The influence of organotin compounds on mitochondrial functions. *In* "Organotin Compounds: New Chemistry and Applications" (J. J. Zuckerman, ed.), Advances in Chemistry Ser. 157, pp. 186–196. American Chemical Society, Washington, DC.

Aldridge, W. N., and Cremer, J. E. (1955). The biochemistry of organotin compounds: Diethyltin chloride and triethyltin sulfate. *Biochem. J.* **61**, 406–418.

Aldridge, W. N., and Cremer, J. E. (1956). Studies on the reactivity of organotins. *Biochem. J.* **68**, 685–692.

Aldridge, W. N., Street, B. W., and Skilleter, D. N. (1977). Oxidative phosphorylation. Halide-dependent and halide-independent effects of triorganotin and triorganolead compounds on mitochondrial functions. *Biochem. J.* **168**, 353–364.

Alison, W. E., Doty, A. E., Hardy, J. L., Kenaga, E. E., and Whitney, W. K. (1968). Laboratory evaluations of Plictran® miticide against two-spotted spider mites. *J. Econ. Entomol.* **61**, 1254–1257.

Ammermann, E., Lorenz, G., Schelberger, K., Wenderoth B., Sauter, H., and Rentzea, C. (1992). BAS 490 F—A broad spectrum fungicide with a new mode of action. *Proc. Brighton Plant Prot. Conf. Pests Diseases* **1**, 403–410.

Ammermann, E., Lorenz, G., Schelberger, K., Mueller, B., Kirstgen, R., and Sauter, H. (2000). BAS 500 F—The new broad-spectrum strobilurin fungicide. *Proc. BCPC Conf. Pests Diseases 2000* **2**, 541–548.

Amold *et al.* (1997).

Andrews, P., Thyssen, J., and Lorke, D. (1983) . The biology and toxicology of molluscicides: Bayluscide. *Pharmacol. Therap.* **19**, 245–295.

Anema, B. P., Bouwman, J. J., Komyoji, T., and Suzuki, K. (1992). Fluazinam, a novel fungicide for use against *Phytophthora infestans* in potatoes. *Proc. Brighton Crop Protect. Conf. Pests Diseases* **2**, 663–668.

Anonymous (1988). An outline of toxicity tests using flutolanil. *J. Pestic. Sci.* **13**, 153–156 [In Japanese].

Anonymous (1991). Ioxynil. *J. Pestic. Sci.* **16**, 349–354 [In Japanese].

Anonymous (1992a). "Polo/Pegasus Technical Product Information." Ciba-Geigy Ltd., Basel.

Anonymous (1992b). Summary of toxicity studies on pesticides: Fenpyroximate. *J. Pestic. Sci.* **17**, S261–S267 [In Japanese].

Anonymous (1993a). "Fenazaquin: A Profile," Agricultural Products Research, DowElanco European Area, Letcombe Regis, UK.

Anonymous (1993b). "Masaï Acaricide," Technical Bulletin FHT-D313-3M-9301, American Cyanamid Co., Princeton, NJ.

Anonymous (1999a). Summary of toxicity studies on pyrimidifen. *J. Pestic. Sci.* **24**, 241–244.

Anonymous (1999b). "Fenomen Technical Brochure." Rhône-Poulenc Agro, Lyon.

Anonymous (2000a). "Evaluation of the New Active Trifloxystrobin in the Product Flint Fungicide." National Registration Authority for Agricultural and Veterinary Chemicals, Canberra, Australia.

Anonymous (2000b). "Famoxate® Technical Bulletin." DuPont Crop Protection, Newark, DE.

Antunes-Madeira, M. C., and Madeira, V. M. C. (1979). Interaction of insecticides with lipid membranes. *Biochim. Biophys. Acta* **550**, 384–392.

Antunes-Madeira, M. C., Videira, R. A., and Madeira, V. M. (1994). Effects of parathion on membrane organization and its implications for the mechanisms of toxicity. *Biochim. Biophys. Acta* **1190**, 149–154.

Araki, F. (1985). Moncut (flutolanil), a new systemic fungicide. *Jpn. Pestic. Info.* **47**, 23–25.

Araki, F., and Yabutani, K. (1981). α,α,α-Trifluoro-3′-isopropoxy-*o*-toluanilide (NNF-136), a new fungicide for the control of diseases caused by basidiomycetes. *Proc. Brighton Plant Prot. Conf. Pests Diseases* **1**, 3–9.

Araki, F., and Yabutani, K. (1993). Development of a systemic fungicide, flutolanil. *J. Pestic. Sci.* **18**, S69–S77 [In Japanese].

Arnold, C. G., Weidenhaupt, A. David, M. M., Mueller, S. R., Haderlein, S. B., and Schwarzenbach, R. P. (1997). Aqueous speciation and 1-octanol-water partitionning of tributyl- and triphenyltin: Effect of PH and ion composition. *Environ. Sci. Technol.* **31**, 2596–2602.

Arrendale, R. F., Stewart, J. T., Manning, R., and Vitayavirasuk, B. (1989). Determination of GX-071 and its major metabolite in rat blood by cold on-column injection capillary GC/ECD. *J. Agric. Food Chem.* **37**, 1130–1135.

Augustijn-Beckers, P. W. M., Hornsby, A. G., and Wauchope, R. D. (1994). The SCS/ARS/CES pesticide properties database for environmental decision-making. II. Additional compounds. *Rev. Environ. Contam. Toxicol.* **137**, 1–82.

Aw, T. Y., and Jones, D. P. (1985). ATP concentration gradients in cytosol of liver cells during hypoxia. *Am. J. Physiol.* **249**, 385–392.

Aw, T .Y., Nicotera, P., Manzo, L., and Orrenius, S. (1990). Tributyltin stimulates apoptosis in rat thymocytes. *Arch. Biochem. Biophys.* **283**, 46–50.

Awad, O. M. (1995). Assessment of the developmental toxicity of *in utero* exposure of Wistar rats to ametryne and niclosamide. *Pestic. Biochem. Physiol.* **53**, 1–9.

Bader, J. P., McMahon, J. B., Schultz, R. J., Narayanan, V. L., Pierce, J. B., Harrison, W. A., Weislow, O. S., Midelfort, C. F., Stinson, S. F., and Boyd, M. R. (1991). Oxathiin carboxaniide, a potent inhibitor of human immunodeficiency virus reproduction. *Proc. Natl. Acad. Sci. U.S.A.* **88**, 6740–6744.

Bagchi, M., and Stohs, S. J. (1993). *In vitro* induction of reactive oxygen species by 2,3,7,8-tetrachlorodibenzo-*p*-dioxin, endrin, and lindane in rat peritoneal macrophages, and hepatic mitochondria and microsomes. *Free Radic. Biol. Med.* **14**, 11–18.

Bagchi, M., Hassoun, E. A., Bagchi, D., and Stohs, S. J. (1993). Production of reactive oxygen species by peritoneal macrophages and hepatic mitochondria and microsomes from endrin-treated rats. *Free Radic. Biol. Med.* **14**, 149–155.

Bakker, E. P., van den Heuvel, E. J., Weichmann, A. H. C. A., and van Dam, K. (1973). A comparison between uncouplers of oxidative phosphorylation in mitochondria and in different artificial membrane systems. *Biochem. Biophys. Acta* **292**, 78–87.

Balasubramanya, R. H., and Patil, R. B. (1980). Degradation of carboxin and oxycarboxin in different soils. *Plant Soil* **57**, 195–201.

Barham, S. S., and Brinkley, B. R. (1976a). Action of rotenone and related respiratory inhibitors on mammalian cell division. 1. Cell kinetics and biochemical aspects. *Cytobios* **15**, 85–96.

Barham, S. S., and Brinkley, B. R. (1976b). Action of rotenone and related respiratory inhibitors on mammalian cell division. Ultrastructural studies. *Cytobios* **15**, 97–109.

Barrientos, A., and Moraes, C. T. (1999). Titrating the effects of mitochondrial complex I impairment in the cell physiology. *J. Biol. Chem.* **274**, 16188–16197.

Beal, D. L., and Anderson, R. V. (1993). Response of zooplankton to rotenone in a small pond. *Bull Environ. Contam. Toxicol.* **51**, 551–556.

Beale, R. E., Phillion, D. P., Headrick, J. M., O'Reilly, P., and Cox, J. (1998). MON65500: A unique fungicide for the control of take-all in wheat. *Proc. 1998 Brighton Crop Protect. Conf. Pest Diseases* **2**, 343–350.

Beautement, K., Clough, J. M., de Fraine, P. J., and Godfrey, C. R. A. (1991). Fungicidal β-methoxyacrylates: From natural products to novel synthetic agricultural fungicides. *Pestic. Sci.* **31**, 499–519.

Becker, W. F., von Jagow, G., Anke, T., and Steglich, W. (1981). Oudemansin, strobilurin A, strobilurin B and myxothiazole: New inhibitors of the bc_1 segment of the respiratory chain with an (E)-β-methoxyacrylate system as common structural elements. *FEBS Lett.* **132**, 329–333.

Bellina, R. F., and Fost, D. L. (1977). Acaricidal and aphicidal 2-higher alkyl-3-hydroxy-1,4-naphthoquinone carboxylic acid esters. German Patent 2,641,343 (*Chem. Abst.* **87**, 117721).

Benya, T. J. (1997). Bis(tributyltin) oxide toxicology. *Drug Metab. Rev.* **29**, 1189–1284.

Bernardi, P., Colonna, R., Costantini, P., Eriksson, O., Fontaine, E., Ichas, F., Massari, S., Nicolli, A., Petronilli, V., and Scorrano, L. (1998). The mitochondrial permeability transition. *Biofactors* **8**, 273–281.

Berry, E. A., Zhang, Z., Huang, L.-S., and Kim, S.-H. (1999). Structures of quinone-binding sites in bc complexes: functional implications. *Biochem. Soc. Trans.* **27**, 565–572.

Betarbet, R., Sherer, T. B., MacKenzie, G., Garcia-Osuna, M., Panov, A. V., and Greenamyre, J. T. (2000). Chronic systemic pesticide exposure reproduces features of Parkinson's disease. *Nature Neurosci.* **3**, 1301–1306.

Bettin, C., Oehlmann, J., and Stroben, E. (1996). TBT-induced imposex in marine neogastropods is mediated by an increasing androgen level. *Helgoland Meeresunters.* **50**, 299–317.

Black, B. C., Hollingworth, R. M., Ahammadsahib, K. I., Kukel, C.D., and Donovan, S. (1994). Insecticidal action and mitochondrial uncoupling activity of AC-303,630 and related halogenated pyrroles. *Pestic. Biochem. Physiol.* **50**, 115–128.

Bock, R. (1981). Triphenyltin compounds and their degradation products. *Res. Rev.* **79**, 1–262.

Bollo, E., Ceppa, L., Cornaglia, E., Nebbia, C., Biolatti, B., and Dacasto, M. (1996). Triphenyltin hacetate toxicity: A biocemical and ultrastructural study on mouse thymocytes. *Human Exptl. Toxicol.* **15**, 219–225.

Boveris, A. (1984). Determination of the production of superoxide radicals and hydrogen peroxide in mitochondria. *Meth. Enzymol.* **105**, 429–434.

Boyer, I. J. (1989). Toxicity of dibutyltin, tributyltin and other organotin compounds to humans and to experimental animals. *Toxicol.* **55**, 253–298.

Boyer, P. D. (1997). The ATP synthase—A splendid molecular machine. *Annu. Rev. Biochem.* **66**, 717–749.

Bragadin, M., and Marton, D. (1997). A proposal for a new mechanism of interaction of trialkyltin (TAT) compounds with mitochondria. *J. Inorg. Biochem.* **68**, 75–78.

Bragadin, M., Marton, D., Toninello, A., and Viola, E. R. (2000). Tributyltin and mitochondria: New evidence in favor of an uncoupling mechanism. *Inorg. Chem. Commun.* **3**, 255–258.

Brandt, U., Schubert, J., Geck, P., and von Jagow, G. (1992). Uncoupling activity and physicochemical properties of derivatives of fluazinam. *Biochim. Biophys. Acta* **1101**, 41–47.

Brennan, P., Johnson, D., Rider, S., Cone, N., Goldman, M., Buckpitt, A., and Chung, H. (1991). Dermal absorption of niclosamide in rats and minipigs. *Biopharmac. Drug Dispo.* **12**, 547–556.

Brinkley, B. R., Barham, S. S., Barranco, S. C., and Fuller, G. M. (1974). Rotenone inhibition of spindle microtubule assembly in mammalian cells. *Exp. Cell Res.* **85**, 41–46.

Brown, C. C., Nicholls, D.C., and Cooper, C. E. (1999). "Mitochondria and Cell Death." Princeton Univ. Press, Princeton, NJ.

Brucker-Davis, F. (1998). Effects of environmental synthetic chemicals on thyroid function. *Thyroid* **8**, 827–856.

Brüschweiler, B. J., Würgler, F. E., and Fent, K. (1996). Inhibition of cytochrome P4501A by organotins in fish hepatoma cells PLHC-1. *Environ. Toxicol. Chem.* **15**, 728–735.

Bruynzeel, D. P., Tafelkruijer, J., and Wilks, M. F. (1995). Contact dermatitis due to a new fungicide used in the tulip bulb industry. *Contact Dermatit.* **33**, 8-11. (Also see *Contact Dermatit.* **35**, 70 (1996) for an erratum correction.)

Buller, G., Heard, J., and Gorman, S. (1996). Possible bromethalin-induced toxicity in a human case report. *J. Toxicol. Clin. Toxicol.* **34**, 572–573.

Bustamente, E., and Pedersen, P. L. (1973). Tetradifon: An oligomycin-like inhibitor of energy-linked activities of rat liver mitochondria. *Biochem. Biophys. Res. Commun.* **51**, 292–298.

Cadenas, E., Boveris, A., Ragan, C. I., and Stoppani, A. O. M., (1977). Production of superoxide radicals and hydrogen peroxide by NADH-ubiquinone reductase and ubiquinol-cytochrome *c* reductase from beef heart mitochondria. *Arch. Biochem. Biophys.* **180**, 248– 257.

Cal DFA (1987a). "Summary of Toxicology Data: Oxycarboxin." California Department of Food and Agriculture, Medical Toxicology Branch (now listed under California Environmental Protection Agency), Sacramento, CA.

Cal DFA (1987b). "Summary of Toxicology Data: Cyhexatin (Plictran)." California Department of Food and Agriculture, Medical Toxicology Branch (now located in the California Environmental Protection Agency), Sacramento, CA.

Cal EPA (1994). "Summary of Toxicology Data: Carboxin." California Environmental Protection Agency, Department of Pesticide Regulation, Medical Toxicology Branch, Sacramento, CA.

Cal EPA (1995). "Bromoxynil Octanoate, Bromoxynil: Summary of Toxicology Data." Department of Pesticide Registration, California Environmental Protection Agency, Sacramento, CA.

Cal EPA (1997). "Summary of Toxicology Data: Rotenone." Department of Pesticide Regulation, California Environmental Protection Agency, Sacramento, CA.

Cal EPA (1999). "Summary of Toxicology Data: Kresoxim-Methyl." California Environmental Protection Agency, Department of Pesticide Regulation, Sacramento, CA.

Cal EPA (2000a). "Summary of Toxicology Data: Trifloxystrobin." California Environmental Protection Agency, Department of Pesticide Regulation, Sacramento, CA.

Cal EPA (2000b). "Summary of Toxicology Data: Hydramethylnon." California Environmental Protection Agency, Department of Pesticide Regulation, Sacramento, CA.

Cal EPA (2000c). "Summary of Toxicology Data: Lithium (Perfluoro Octane) Sulfonate." California Environmental Protection Agency, Department of Pesticide Regulation, Sacramento, CA.

Cal EPA (2001). "Summary of Toxicology Data: Pyraclostrobin." California Environmental Protection Agency, Department of Pesticide Regulation, Sacramento, CA.

Calumpang, S. M. F., Median, M. J. B., Tejada, A. W., and Medina, J. R. (1995). Environmental impact of two molluscicides, niclosamide and metaldehyde, in a rice paddy ecosystem. *Bull. Environ. Contam. Toxicol.* **55**, 494–451.

Camatini, M., Colombo, A., Bonfanti, P., Doldi, M., Urani, C., Dibisceglia, M., and Nagelkerke, J. F. (1996). *In vitro* biological systems as models to evaluate the toxicity of pesticides. *Intern. J. Environ. Anal. Chem.* **65**, 153–167.

Cardwell, R. D., Keithly, J. C., and Simmonds, J. (1999). Tributyltin in U.S. market-bought seafood and assessment of human health risks. *Human Ecolog. Risk Assess.* **5**, 317–335.

Carere, A., Ortali, V. A., Cardamone, G., Torracca, A. M, and Raschetti, R. (1978). Microbial mutagenicity studies of pesticides *in vitro*. *Mutat. Res.* **57**, 277–286.

Carlson, K., and Ehrich, M. (1999). Organophosphorus compound-induced modification of SH-SY5Y human neuroblastoma mitochondrial transmembrane potential. *Toxicol. Appl. Pharmacol.* **160**, 33–42.

Carpenter, K., and Heywood, B. J. (1963). Herbicidal action of 3:5-dihalogeno-4-hydroxybenzonitriles. *Nature (London)* **200**, 28–29.

Carpenter, K., Cottrell, H. J., De Silva, W. H., and Heywood, B. J. (1964). Chemistry and biological properties of two new herbicides—Ioxynil and bromoxynil. *Weed Res.* **4**, 175–195.

Cattley, R. C., DeLuca, J., Elcombe, C., Fenner-Crisp, P., Lake, B. G., Marsman, D. S., Pastoor, T. A., Popp, J. A., Robinson, D. E., Schwetz, B., Tugwood, J., and Wahli, W. (1998). Do peroxisome proliferating compounds pose a hepatocarcinogenic hazard to humans? *Regul. Toxicol. Pharmacol.* **27**, 47–60.

Cavanaugh, J. B. (1995). Suspected triphenyltin poisoning. *J. Neurol. Neurosurg. Psychiatry* **59**, 661–662.

Chamberlain, K., Evans, A. A., and Bromilow, R. H. (1996). 1-octanol/water partition coefficient (Kow) and pKa for ionisable pesticides measured by a pH-metric method. *Pestic. Sci.* **47**, 265–271.

Chandra, S., Polya, G. M., James, B. D., and Magee, R. J. (1989). Inhibition of oxidative phosphorylation by organotin thiocarbamates. *Chem. Biol. Interact.* **71**, 21–36.

Cheng, H. I., Yamamoto, I., and Casida, J. E. (1972). Rotenone photodecomposition. *J. Agric. Food Chem.* **20**, 850–856.

Chernoff, N. (1990). Studies on maternal toxicity, formation of supernumerary ribs, and evidence for embryonic repair of xenobiotic-induced injury. *Teratology* **42**, 18A.

Chernoff, N., Roger, J. M., Turner, C. I., and Francis, B. M. (1991). Significance of supernumerary ribs in rodent developmental toxicity studies: Postnatal persistence in rats and mice. *Fundam. Appl. Toxicol.* **17**, 448–453.

Cherry, L. D., Gunnoe, M. D., and van Lier, R. B. L. (1982). The metabolism of bromethalin and its effects on oxidative phosphorylation and cerebrospinal fluid pressure. *Toxicologist* **2**, 108.

Chin, W. T., Stone, G. M., and Smith, A. E. (1970). Degradation of carboxin (Vitavax) in water and soil. *J. Agr. Food Chem.* **18**, 731–732.

Chow, S. C., and Orrenius, S. (1994). Rapid cytoskeleton modification in thymocytes induced by the immunotoxicant tributyltin. *Toxicol. Appl. Pharmacol.* **127**, 19–26.

Clarke, E. D., Greenhow, D. T., and Adams, D. (1998). Metabolism-related assays and their application to agrochemical research: Reactivity of pesticides with glutathione and glutathione transferases. *Pestic. Sci.* **54**, 385–393.

Clough, J. M., and Godfrey, C. R. A. (1998). The strobilurin fungicides. *In* "Fungicidal Activity: Chemical and Biological Approaches to Plant Protection" (D. Hutson and J. Miyamoto, eds.), pp. 109–148. Wiley, Chichester, UK.

Colosio, C., Tomasini, M., Cairoli, S., Foa, V., Minoia, C., Marinovich, M., and Galli, C. L. (1991). Occupational triphenyltin acetate poisoning: a case report. *Br. J. Ind. Med.* **48**, 136–139.

Conso, F., Neel. P., Pouzelet, C., Efthymiou, M. L., Gervais, P., and Gaultier, M. (1977). Acute human toxicity of halogenated hyroxybenzonitrile derivatives (iozynil, bromoxynil). *Arch. Mal. Prof. Med. Trav. Secur. Soc.* **38**, 674–677 [In French].

Cooper, E. L., Arizza, V., Cammarata, M., Pellerito, L., and Parrinello, N. (1995). Tributyltin affects phagocytic activity of *Ciona intestinalis* hemocytes. *Comp. Biochem. Physiol.* **112C**, 285–289.

Corbett, J. R., Wright, K., and Baillie, A. C. (1984). "The Biochemical Mode of Action of Pesticides," 2nd ed. Academic Press, London.

Cortinas de Nava, C., Espinosa, J., Garcia, L., Zapata, A. M., and Martinez, E. (1983). Mutagenicity of antiamebic and anthelmintic drugs in the *Salmonella typhimurium* microsomal test system. *Mutat. Res.* **117**, 79–91.

Costa, L. G., Wu, D. S., Olibet, G., and Murphy, S. D. (1989). Formamidine pesticides and α_2−adrenoceptors: Studies with amitraz and chlodimeform in rats. *Neurotoxicol. Teratol.* **11**, 405–411.

Costlow, R. D., Lutz, M. F., Kane, W. W., Hurt, S. S., and O'Hara, G. P. (1986). Dinocap: Developmental toxicity studies in rabbits. *Toxicologist* **6**, 85.

Crompton, M., Virji, S., Doyle, V., Johnson, N., and Ward, J. M. (1999). The mitochondrial permeability transition pore. *In* "Mitochondria and Cell Death" (C. C., Brown, D. C. Nicholls, and C. E. Cooper, eds.). Princeton Univ. Press, Princeton, NJ.

Cunarro, J., and Weiner, W. M. (1975). Mechanism of action of agents that uncouple oxidative phosphorylation: Direct correlation between proton-carrying and respiratory-releasing properties using rat liver mitochondria. *Biochem. Biophys. Acta* **387**, 234–240.

Cunningham, M. L., Soliman, M. S., Badr, M. Z., and Matthews, H. B. (1995). Rotenone, an anticarcinogen, inhibits cellular proliferation but not peroxisome proliferation in mouse liver. *Cancer Lett.* **95**, 93–97.

Cutcomp, L. K., Desaiah, D., and Koch, R. B. (1972). The *in vitro* sensitivity of fish brain ATPases to organochlorine acaricides. *Life Sci.* **11**, 1123–1133.

Dacasto, M., Valenza, F., Nebbia, C., Ovanni, R. G., Cornaglia, E., and Soffietti, M. G. (1994). Pathological findings in rabbits and sheep following the subacute administration of triphenyltin acetate. *Vet. Human Toxicol.* **36**, 300–304.

Davey, G. P., and Clark, J. B. (1996). Threshold effects and control of oxidative phosphorylation in nonsynaptic rat brain mitochondria. *J. Neurochem.* **66**, 1617–1624.

de Bertoldi, M., Griselli, M., Giovannetti, M., and Barale, R. (1980). Mutagenicity of pesticides evaluated by means of gene-conversion in *Saccharomyces cerevisiae* and *Aspergillus nidulans*. *Environ. Mutagen.* **2**, 359–370.

Degli Esposti, M. (1998). Inhibitors of NADH-ubiquinone reductase: An overview. *Biochim. Biophys. Acta* **1364**, 222–235.

Degli Esposti, M., and Ghelli, A. (1994). The mechanism of proton and electron transport in mitochondrial complex I. *Biochim. Biophys. Acta* **1187**, 116–120.

Degli Esposti, M., and Ghelli, A. (1999). Ubiquinone and inhibitor sites in complex I: One, two or three? *Biochem. Soc. Trans.* **27**, 606–609.

Desaiah, D., Cutkomp, L. K., and Koch, R. B. (1973). Inhibition of spider mite ATPases by Plictran and three organochlorine acaricides. *Life Sci.* **13**, 1693–1703.

De Santiago, A., and Aguilar-Santelises, M. (1999). Organotin compounds decrease *in vitro* survival, proliferation and differentiation of normal human B lymphocytes. *Human Expt. Toxicol.* **18**, 619–624.

Devries, H., Penninks, A. H., Snoeij, N. J., and Seinen, W. (1991). Comparative toxicity of organotin compounds to rainbow trout (*Oncorhynchus mykiss*) yolk-sac fry. *Sci. Tot. Environ.* **103**, 229–243.

DeWilde, A. R., Heyndrickx, A., and Carnton, D. (1986). A case of fatal rotenone poisoning in a child. *J. Forensic Sci.* **31**, 1492–1498.

Dickey, W., McAleer, J. J. A., and Callender, M. E. (1988). Delayed sudden death after ingestion of MCPP and ioxynil: An unusual presentation of hormonal weedkiller intoxication. *Postgrad. Med. J.* **64**, 681–682.

Di Simplicio, P., Dacasto, M., Carletti, M., Giannerini, F., and Nebbia, C. (2000). Changes in hepatic and renal glutathione-dependent enzyme activities in rabbits and lambs subchronically treated with triphenyltin acetate. *Vet. Human. Toxicol.* **42**, 159–162.

Doi, S. (1981). Basitac® (Mepronil). *Jpn Pestic. Inf.* **38**, 17–20.

Dorman, D. C., Simon, J., Harlin, K. A., and Buck, W. B. (1990a). Diagnosis of bromethalin toxicosis in the dog. *J. Vet. Diagn. Invest.* **2**, 123–128.

Dorman, D. C., Parker, A. J., and Buck, W. B. (1990b). Bromethalin toxicosis in the dog. 1. Clinical effects. *J. Amer. Anim. Hosp. Assn.* **26**, 589–594.

Dorman, D. C., Parker, A. J., and Buck, W. B. (1990c). Bromethalin toxicosis in the dog. 2. Selected treatments for the toxic syndrome. *J. Amer. Anim. Hosp. Assn.* **26**, 595–598.

Dorman, D. C., Parker, A. J., and Buck, W. B. (1991). Electroencephalographic changes associated with bromethalin toxicosis in the dog. *Vet. Hum. Toxicol.* **33**, 9–11.

Dorman, D. C., Cote, L. M. and Buck, W. B. (1992a). Effects of an extract of *Gingko biloba* on bromethalin-induced cerebral lipid peroxidation and edema in rats. *Am. J. Vet. Res.* **53**, 138–142.

Dorman, D. C., Zachary, J. F., and Buck, W. B. (1992b). Neuropathologic findings of bromethalin toxicosis in the cat. *Vet. Pathol.* **29**, 139–144.

Drabek, J., Böger, M., Ehrenfreund, J., Stamm, E., Steinemann, A., Alder, A., and Burckhardt, U. (1990). New thioureas as insecticides. *In* "Recent Advances in the Chemistry of Insect Control II" (L. Crombie, ed.), pp. 170–183. Royal Society of Chemistry, Cambridge, UK.

Dreikorn, B. A., and O'Doherty, G. O. P. (1984). The discovery and development of bromethalin, an acute rodenticide with a unique mode of action. *ACS Sympos. Ser.* **255**, 45–63.

Dreikorn, B. A., O'Daugherty, G. O. P., Clinton, A. J., and Kramer, K. E. (1979). EL-614, a novel acute rodenticide. *Proc. Brit. Crop Protect. Conf. Pest Diseases* **2**, 491–498.

Duhm, B., Maul, W., Medenwald, H., Patzschke, K., and Wegner, L. A. (1961). Radioactive research with a new molluscicide. *Z. Naturfors.* **16B**, 509–515 [In German].

Ema, M., Miyawaki, E., Harazano, A., and Ogawa, Y. (1997). Effects of triphenyltin chloride on implantations and pregnancy in rats. *Reprod. Toxicol.* **11**, 201–206.

Ema, M., Miyawaki, E., and Kawashima, K. (1999). Suppression of uterine decidualization as a cause of implantation failure induced by triphenyltin chloride in rats. *Arch. Toxicol.* **73**, 175–179.

Erecinska, M., and Wilson, D. F. (1981). "Inhibitors of Mitochondrial Function." Pergamon, Oxford.

Erickson, D. A., Laib, F. E., and Lech, J. J. (1992). Biotransformation of rotenone by hepatic microsomes following pretreatment of rainbow trout with inducers of cytochrome P450. *Pestic Biochem. Physiol.* **42**, 140–150.

Ernster, L. (1992). "Molecular Mechanisms in Bioenergetics." Elsevier Science, Amsterdam.

Espinosa-Aguirre, J. J., Santos, J. R., and Cortinas de Nava, C. (1989). Influence of the UVR repair system on the mutagenicity of antiparasitic drugs. *Mutat. Res.* **222**, 161–166.

Espinosa-Aguirre, J. J., Reyes, R. E., and Cortinas de Nava, C. (1991). Mutagenic activity of 2-chloro-4-nitroaniline and 5-chlorosalicylic acid in *Salmonella typhimurium*: Two possible metabolites of niclosamide. *Mutat. Res.* **264**, 139–145.

Esposti, M. D., and Ghelli, A. (1994). The mechanism of proton and electron transport in mitochondrial complex I. *Biochim. Biophys. Acta Bioenerg.* **1187**, 116–120.

Evans, D. L., Jacobsen, K. L., and Miller, D. M. (1984). Hematological and immunological responses of Holstein calves to a fire ant toxicant. *Am. J. Vet. Res.* **45**, 1023–1027.

Fang, N., and Casida, J. E. (1997). Novel bioactive cubé insecticide constituents: isolation and preparation of 13-*homo*-13-oxa-6a,12a-dehydrorotenoids. *J. Org. Chem.* **62**, 350–353.

Fang, N., and Casida, J. E. (1998). Anticancer action of cubé insecticide: Correlation for rotenoid constituents between inhibition of NADH : ubiquinone oxidoreductase and induced ornithine decarboxylase activities. *Proc. Natl. Acad. Sci. U.S.A.* **95**, 3380–3384.

Fang, N., and Casida, J. E. (1999a). Cube resin insecticide: Identification and biological activity of 29 rotenoid constituents. *J. Agric. Food Chem.* **47**, 2130–2136.

Fang, N., and Casida, J. E. (1999b). New bioactive flavonoids and stilbenes in cubé resin insecticide. *J. Nat. Prod.* **62**, 205–210.

Fang, N., Rowlands, J. C., and Casida, J. E. (1997). Anomalous structure-activity relationships of 13-homo-13-oxarotenoids and 13-homo-13- oxadehydrorotenoids. *Chem. Res. Toxicol.* **10**, 853–858.

FAO/WHO (1982). Azocyclotin. *In* "Pesticide Residues in Food—1981 Evaluations." FAO Plant Production and Protection Pap. 42, Food and Agriculture Organization of the United Nations, Rome.

FAO/WHO (1990a). Azocyclotin. *In* "Pesticide Residues in Foods—1989. Evaluations 1989, Part II—Toxicology." FAO Plant Production and Protection Pap. 100/2, pp. 23–26. Food and Agriculture Organization of the United Nations, Rome.

FAO/WHO (1990b). Cyhexatin. *In* "Pesticide Residues in Foods—1989. Evaluations 1989, Part II—Toxicology." FAO Plant Production and Protection Pap. 100/2, pp. 27–38. Food and Agriculture Organization of the United Nations, Rome.

FAO/WHO (1990c). Dinocap. *In* "Pesticide Residues in Food—1989: Evaluations 1989, Part II—Toxicology." FAO Plant Production and Protection Pap. 100/2, pp. 75–94. Food and Agricultural Organization of the United Nations, Rome.

FAO/WHO (1992a). Cyhexatin. *In* "Pesticide Residues in Food—1991. Evaluations 1991, Part II—Toxicology." WHO/PCS/92.52, pp. 129–143. World Health Organization, Geneva.

FAO/WHO (1992b). Fentin. *In* "Pesticide Residues in Food—1991. Evaluations 1991, Part II—Toxicology." WHO/PCS/92.52, pp. 73–208. World Health Organization, Geneva.

FAO/WHO (1993). Fenbutatin-oxide. *In* "Pesticide Residues in Food—1992. Evaluations 1992, Part II—Toxicology," WHO/PCS/93.34, pp. 193–210. World Health Organization, Geneva.

FAO/WHO (1995). Cyhexatin (addendum). *In* "Pesticide Residues in Food—1994. Evaluations 1994, Part II—Toxicology." WHO/PCS/95.2, pp. 65–75. World Health Organization, Geneva.

FAO/WHO (1996). Fenpyroximate. *In* "Pesticide Residues in Food—1995. Part II: Toxicological and Environmental Evaluations." WHO/PCS/96.48, pp. 105–122. World Health Organization, Geneva, Switzerland.

FAO/WHO (1998). Kresoxim-methyl. *In* "Pesticide Residues in Foods—1998. Evaluations Part II. Toxicological." WHO/PCS/99-8, pp. 179–201. World Health Organization, Geneva, Switzerland.

FAO/WHO (1999a). Dinocap. *In* "Pesticide Residues in Food—1998: Evaluations 1998, Part II—Toxicological." WHO/PCS/99.18, pp. 89–105. World Health Organization, Geneva.

FAO/WHO (1999b). Dinocap. *In* "Pesticide Residues in Food—1999: Report 1999." FAO Plant Production and Protection Pap. 153, pp. 69–73. World Health Organization, Rome.

Fent, K. (1996a). Ecotoxicology of organotin compounds. *Crit. Revs. Toxicol.* **26**, 1–117.

Fent, K. (1996b). Organotin compounds in municipal wastewater and sewage sludge: Contamination, fate in treatment process and ecotoxicological consequences. *Sci. Total Environ.* **185**, 151–159.

Fent, K., and Bucheli, T. D. (1994). Inhibition of hepatic microsomal monooxygenase system by organotins *in vitro* in freshwater fish. *Aquat. Toxicol.* **28**, 107–126.

Fent, K., and Stegeman, J. J. (1993). Effects of tributyltin *in vivo* on hepatic cytochrome P450 forms in marine fish. *Aquatic. Toxicol.* **24**, 219–240.

Fent, K., Woodin, B. R., and Stegeman, J. J. (1998). Effects of triphenyltin and other organotins on hepatic monooxygenase system in fish. *Comp. Biochem. Physiol. C* **121**, 277–288.

Ferrante, R. J., Schulz, J. B., Kowall, N. W., and Beal, M. F. (1997). Systemic administration of rotenone produces selective damage of the striatum and globus pallidus, but not the substantia nigra. *Brain Res.* **753**, 157–162.

Ferreira, F. M., Madeira, V. M., and Moreno, A. J. (1997). Interactions of 2,2-bis(*p*-chlorophenyl)-1,1-dichloroethylene with mitochondrial oxidative phosphorylation. *Biochem. Pharmacol.* **53**, 299–308.

Figueras, M. J., and Gosalvez, M. (1973). Inhibition of the growth of Ehrlich ascites tumors by treatment with the respiratory inhibitor rotenone. *Eur. J. Cancer.* **9**, 529–531.

Fillingame, R. H. (1992). H$^+$ transport and coupling by the F$_0$ sector of the ATP synthase: Insights into the molecular mechanism and function. *J. Bioenerg. Biomembr.* **24**, 485–491.

Fink, R. J. (1975). The effect of tricyclohexyltin hydroxide on the reproductive capability of bobwhite quail. *Toxicol. Appl. Pharmacol.* **33**, 189.

Finlayson, B. J., Schnick, R. A., Cailteux, R. L., DeMong, L., Horton, W. D., McClay, W., Thompson. C. W., and Tichacek, G. J. (2000). "Rotenone Use in Fisheries Management: Administrative and Technical Guidelines Manual." American Fisheries Society, Bethesda, MD.

Fiore, C., Trezeguet, V., Le Saux, A., Roux, P., Schwimmer,.C., Dianoux, A.-C., Noel, F., Lauquin, G. J.-M., Brandolin, G., and Vignais, P. V. (1998). The

mitochondrial ADP/ATP carrier: Structural, physiological and pathological aspects. *Biochimie* **80**, 137–150.

Flanagan, R. J., Meredith, T. J., Ruprah, M., Onyon, L. J., and Liddle, A. (1990). Alkaline diuresis for acute poisoning with chlorophenoxy herbicides and ioxynil. *Lancet* **335**, 454–458.

Fliedner, A., Remde, A., Niemann, R., Schafers, C., and Stein, B. (1997). Effects of the organotin pesticide azocyclotin in aquatic microcosms. *Chemosphere* **35**, 209–222.

Fraczek (1979).

Freudenthal, R. I., Thake, D. C., and Baron, R. L. (1981). "Carcinogenic Potential of Rotenone: Subchronic Oral and Peritoneal Administration to Rats and Chronic Dietary Administration to Syrian Golden Hamsters." EPA 600/S1-81-037, U.S. Environmental Protection Agency, Washington, DC.

Friedrich, T., van Heek, P., Leif, H., Ohnishi, T., Forche, E., Kunze, B., Jansen, R., Trowitzsch-Kienast, W., Höfle, G., Reichenbach, H., and Weiss, H. (1994). Two binding sites of inhibitors in NADH : ubiquinone oxidoreductase (complex I). Relationship of one site with the ubiquinone-binding site of bacterial glucose : ubiquinone oxidoreductase. *Eur. J. Biochem.* **219**, 691–698.

Fukami, H., and Nakajima, M. (1971). Rotenone and the rotenoids. *In* "Naturally Occurring Insecticides" (M. Jacobson and D. G. Crosby, eds.), pp. 71–97, Dekker, New York.

Fukami, J. (1956). Effect of some insecticides on the respiration of insect organs, with special reference on the effects of rotenone. *Botyu-Kagaku* **21**, 122–130.

Fukami, J. (1976). Insecticide as inhibit of respiration. *In* "Insecticide Biochemistry and Physiology" (C. F. Wilkinson, ed.), pp. 353–396, Plenum, New York.

Fukami, J., Shishido, T., Fukunaga, K., and Casida, J. E. (1969). Oxidative metabolism of rotenone in mammals, fish, and insects and its relation to selective toxicity. *J. Agric. Food Chem.* **17**, 1217–1226.

Fukushima, T., Hojo, N., Isobe, A., Shiwaku, K., and Yamane, Y. (1997). Effects of organophosphorous compounds on fatty acid compositions and oxidative phosphorylation system in the brain of rats. *Exp. Toxicol. Pathol.* **49**, 381–386.

Furuta, T. (1999). Oribright® (metominostrobin)—A new fungicide for rice blast control. *Agrochems. Jpn.* **74**, 20–21.

Gasiewicz, T. A. (1991). Nitro compounds and related phenolic pesticides. *In* "Handbook of Pesticide Toxicology" (W. J. Hayes, Jr. and E. R. Laws, Jr., eds.), Vol. 3, pp. 1191–1269. Academic Press, San Diego.

Gassner, B., Wuthrich, A., Scholtysik, G., and Solioz, M. (1997). The pyrethroids permethrin and cyhalothrin are potent inhibitors of the mitochondrial complex I. *J. Pharmacol. Exp. Therap.* **281**, 855–860.

George, S. G., and Buchanan, G. (1990). Isolation, properties and induction of plaice liver cytosolic glutathione-*S*-transferases. *Fish Physiol. Biochem.* **8**, 437–449.

Georgopoulos, S. G. (1995). The genetics of fungicide resistance. *In* "Modern Selective Fungicides—Properties, Applications, Mechanisms of Action," 2nd ed. (H. Lyr, ed.), pp. 39–52. Gustav Fischer Verlag, Jena.

Gerhäuser, C., Mar, W., Lee, S. K., Suh, N., Luo, Y., Kosmeder, J., Luyengi, L., Fong, H. H. S., Kinghorn, A. D., Moriarty, R. M., Mehta, R. G., Constantinou, A., Moon, R. C., and Pezzuto, J. M. (1995). Rotenoids mediate potent cancer chemopreventive activity through transcriptional regulation of ornithine decarboxylase. *Nature Med.* **1**, 260–265.

Gerhäuser, C., Lee, S. K., Kosmeder, J. W., Moriarty, R. M., Hamel, E., Mehta, R. G., Moon, R. C., and Pezzuto, J. M. (1997). Regulation of ornithine decarboxylase induction by deguelin, a natural product cancer chemopreventive agent. *Cancer Res.* **57**, 3429–3435.

Gibaud, G. (1983). "A Case of Occupational Poisoning in an Agricultural Environment. Use of an Herbicide Containing Ioxynil. Parallel with Other Substances Acting on Cellular Respiration." Université Pierre et Marie Curie, Faculté de médecine Broussais–Hôtel-Dieu, Paris, France [In French].

Giesy, J. P., and Kannan, K. (2001). Global distribution of perfluoroctane sulfonate in wildlife. *Environ Sci. Technol.* **35**, 1339–1342.

Gilderhus, P. A., Allen, J. L., and Dawson, V. K. (1986). Persistence of rotenone in ponds at different temperatures. *N. Am. J. Fisher. Manag.* **6**, 129–130.

Gingerich, W. H. (1986). Tissue distribution and elimination of rotenone in rainbow trout. *Aquat. Toxicol.* **8**, 27–40.

Gingerich, W. H., and Rach, J. J. (1985). Uptake, biotransformation and elimination of rotenone by bluegills (*Lepomis macrochirus*). *Aquat. Toxicol.* **6**, 179–196.

Giri, A. K., Adhikari, N., and Khan, K. A. (1996). Comparative genotoxicity of six salicylic acid derivatives in bone marow cells of mice. *Mutat Res. Genet. Toxicol.* **370**, 1–9.

Godwin, J. R., Anthony, V. M., Clough, J. M., and Godfrey, C. R. A. (1992). ICIA5504: A novel, broad spectrum, systemic β-methoxyacrylate fungicide. *Proc. Brighton Crop Prot. Conf. Pest Diseases* **1**, 435–442.

Godwin, J. R., Bartlett, D. W., Clough, J. M., Godfrey, C. R. A., Harrison, E. G., and Maund, S. (2000). Picoxystrobin: A new strobilurin fungicide for use on cereals. *Proc. BCPC. Conf. Pest Diseases 2000* **2**, 533–540.

Goh, C. L. (1985). Irritant dermatitis from tri-*n*-butyl tin oxide in paint. *Contact Dermatitis* **12**, 161–163.

Gönnert, R. (1962). Bayluscide, a new compound for controlling medically important freshwater snails. *Pflanzenshutz-Nachrichten Bayer (Engl. Ed.)* **15**, 4–25.

Gönnert, R., and Schraufstätter, E. (1958). A new molluscicide: Molluscicide Bayer 73. *Proc. Int. Conf. Trop. Med. Malar.* **2**, 197–202.

Gönnert, R., Johannis, J., Schraufstätter, E., and Strufe, R. (1963). Constitution and cestocidal activity of Yomesan. *Medizin Chem.* **7**, 540–567 [In German].

Gorell, J. M., Johnson, C. C., Rybicki, B. A., Peterson, E. L., and Richardson, R. J. (1998). The risk of Parkinson's disease with exposure to pesticides, farming, well water, and rural living. *Neurology* **50**, 1346–1350.

Gosálvez, M. (1983). Carcinogensis with the insecticide rotenone. *Life Sci.* **32**, 809–816.

Gosselin, R. E., Smith, R. P., and Hodge, H. C. (1984). "Clinical Toxicology of Commercial Products," 5th ed., pp. 366–367. Williams and Wilkins, Baltimore.

Gould, J. M. 1976). Inhibition by triphenyltin chloride of a tightly-bound membrane component involved in photophosphorylation. *Eur. J. Biohehm.* **62**, 567–575.

Grass, B., Mayer, H., Nolte, J., Preuss, G., and Zullei-Seibert, N. (2000). Studies on the metabolism of hydroxybenzonitrile herbicides: I. Mass spectrometric identification. *Pest. Manag. Sci.* **56**, 49–59.

Gray, B. H., Porvaznik, M., Flemming, C., and Lee, L.H. (1987). Tri-*n*-butyltin: a membrane toxicant. *Toxicology* **47**, 35–54.

Gray, L. E., Jr., Rogers, J. M., Kavlock, R. J., Ostby, J. S., Ferrell, J. M., and Gray, K. L. (1986). Prenatal exposure to the fungicide dinocap causes behavioral torticollis, ballooning and cleft palate in mice. *Teratogen. Carcinogen. Mutagen.* **6**, 33–43.

Gray, L. E., Jr., Rogers, J. M., Ostby, J. S., Kavlock R. J., and Ferrell, J. M. (1988). Prenatal dinocap exposure alters swimming behavior in mice due to complete otolith agenesis in the inner ear. *Toxicol. Appl. Pharmacol.* **92**, 266–273.

Greenman, D. L., Allaben, W. T., Burger, G. T., and Kodell, R. L. (1993). Bioassay for carcinogenicity of rotenone in female Wistar rats. *Fund. Appl. Tox.* **20**, 383–390.

Grey, A., Dutton, A. J., and Eadsforth, C. V. (1995). Fenbutatin oxide, fate in soil after extensive commercial use in Italy and Spain. *Pestic. Sci.* **43**, 295–302.

Grilli, S., Ancora, G., Rani, P., Valenti, A., Mazzullo, M., and Colacci, A. (1991). In vivo unwinding fluorimetric assay of the damage induced by fenarimol and DNOC in rat liver DNA. *J. Toxicol. Environ. Helath* **34**, 485–494.

Grossman, M. R., Mispagel, M. E., and Bowen, J. M. (1992). Distribution and tissue elimination in rats during and after prolonged dietary exposure to a highly fluorinated sulfonamide pesticide. *J. Agric. Food Chem.* **40**, 2502–2509.

Grover, I. S., Dhingra, A. K., Adhikari, N., and Ladhar, S. S. (1990). Genotoxicity of pesticides and plant systems. *Prog. Clin. Biol. Res.* **340E**, 91–106.

Guadaño, A., González-Coloma, A., and de la Peña, E. (1998). Genotoxicity of the insecticide rotenone in cultured human lymphocytes. *Mutat. Res.* **414**, 1–7.

Guo, Z.-J., Miyoshi, H., Komyoji, T., Haga, T., and Fujita, T. (1991a). Uncoupling activity of a newly developed fungicide, fluazinam (3-chloro-N-(3-chloro-2,6-dinitro-4-trifluoromethylphenyl)-5-trifluoromethyl-2-pyridinamines). *Biochim. Biophys. Acta* **1056**, 89–92.

Guo, Z.-J., Miyoshi, H., Komyoji, T., Haga, T., and Fujita, T. (1991b). Quantitative analysis with physicochemical substituent and molecular parameters of uncoupling activity of substituted diarylamines. *Biochim. Biophys. Acta* **1059**, 91–98.

Guo, Z.-J., Miyoshi, H., Nagatani, K., Komyoji, T., Haga, T., and Fujita, T. (1991c). Correlation of the acid dissociation constants of some multisubstituted diphenylpyridiylamines and phenylpyridylamines. *J. Org. Chem.* **56**, 3692–3700.

Guzy, J., Barnova, E., Chavkova, Z., Dubayova, K., Tomeckova, V., Marekova, M., Kusnir, J., and Mlynarcikova, H. (2000). The effect of chloridazone on the energetic metabolism in rat liver mitochondria. *J. Trace Microprobe Techniques* **18**, 241–244.

Haley, T. J. (1978). A review of the literature of rotenone 1,2,12,12a-tetrahydro-8,9-dimethoxy-2-(1-methylethynyl)-1-benzopyrano[3,5-b]furo[2,3-h][1]benzopyran-6-(6h)-one. *J. Environ. Pathol. Toxicol.* **1**, 315–337.

Hall, L. W., Jr., and Pinkney, A. E. (1985). Acute and sublethal effects of organotin compounds on aquatic biota: An interpretative literature evaluation. *Crit. Rev. Toxicol.* **14**, 159–209.

Hallenbeck, W. H., and Cunningham-Burns (1985). "Pesticides and Human Health." Springer-Verlag, New York.

Hamaguchi, H., Kajihara, O., and Katoh, M. (1995). Development of a new acaricide, fenpyroximate. *J. Pestic. Sci.* **20**, 173–175, 203–212 [In Japanese].

Hansen, K. J., Clemen, L. A., Ellefson, M. E., and Johnson, H. O. (2001). Compound-specific, quantitative characterization of organic fluorochemicals in biological matrices. *Environ. Sci. Technol.*, to appear.

Hansen, W. H., Davis, K. J., and Fitzhugh, O. G. (1965). Chronic toxicity of cubé *Toxicol. Appl. Pharmacol.* **7**, 535–542.

Harazano, A., Ema, M., and Kawashima, K. (1998). Evaluation of malnutrition as a cause of tributyltin-induced pregnancy failure in rats. *Bull. Environ. Contam. Toxicol.* **61**, 224–230.

Hartley, A., Stone, J. M., Heron, C., Cooper, J. M., and Schapira, A. H. V. (1994). Complex I inhibitors induce does-dependent apoptosis in PC12 cells: Relevance to Parkinson's disease. *J. Neurochem.* **63**, 1987–1991.

Hasegawa, E., Takeshige, K., Oishi, T., Murai, Y., and Minakami, S. (1990). 1-Methyl-4-phenylpyridinium (MPP$^+$) induces NADH-dependent superoxide formation and enhances NADH-dependent lipid peroxidation in bovine heart submitochondrial particles. *Biochem. Biophys. Res. Commun.* **170**, 1049–1055.

Haughom, B., and Spydevold, O. (1992). The mechanism underlying the hypolipemic effect of perfluorooctanoic acid (PFOA), perfluorooctane sulphonic acid (PFOS) and clofibric acid. *Biochim. Biophys. Acta* **1128**, 65–72.

Hayes, W. J., Jr. (1982). "Pesticides Studied in Man," pp. 520–567. Williams & Wilkins, Baltimore.

Heikkila, R. E., Nicklas, J. W., Vyas, I., and Duvoisin, R. C. (1985). Dopaminergic toxicity of rotenone and the 1-methyl-4-phenylpyridinium ion (MPP$^+$) after their stereotaxic administration to rats: implications for the mechanism of 1-methyl-4-phenyl-1,2,3,6-tetrahydropyridine (MPTP) toxicity. *Neurosci. Lett.* **62**, 389–394.

Heimlich, F., Davies, A. N., Kuckuk, R., Linscheid, M., Mayer, H., and Nolte, J. (1995). Identification of dinocap in water using GC/IR and GC/MS. *Fresenius J. Analyt. Chem.* **352**, 743–747.

Hemker, H. C. (1962). Lipid solubility as a factor influencing the activity of uncoupling phenols. *Biochim. Biophys. Acta* **63**, 46–54.

Hengartner, M. O. (2000). The biochemistry of apoptosis. *Science* **407**, 770–776.

Henry, R. A., and Byington, K. H. (1976). Inhibition of glutathione-*S*-aryltransferase from rat liver by organogermanium, lead and tin compounds. *Biochem. Pharmacol.* **25**, 2291–2295.

Henry, T. R., Solem, L. E., and Wallace, K. B. (1995). Channel-specific induction of the cyclosporine A-sensitive mitochondrial permeability transition by menadione. *J. Toxicol. Environ. Health* **45**, 489–504.

Hensley, K., Pye, Q. N., Maidt, M. L., Stewart, C. A., Robinson, K. A., Jaffrey, F., and Floyd, R. A. (1998). Interaction of α-phenyl-*N-tert*-butyl nitrone and alternative electron acceptors with complex I indicates a substrate reduction site upstream from the rotenone binding site. *J. Neurochem.* **71**, 2549–2557.

Henwood, S. M., McKee-Pesik, P., Costello, A. C., and Osimitz, T. G. (1994a). Developmental toxicity study with lithium perfluorooctane sulfonate in rabbits. *Teratology* **49**, 398.

Henwood, S. M., McKee-Pesik, P., Costello, A. C., and Osimitz, T. G. (1994b). Developmental toxicity study with lithium perfluorooctane sulfonate in rats. *Teratology* **49**, 398.

Herrero, A., and Barja, G. (1997). ADP-regulation of mitochondrial free radical production is different with complex I- or complex II-linked substrate: Implications for the exercise paradox and brain hypermetabolism. *J. Biomembr. Bioenerget.* **20**, 241–249.

Heywood, B. J. (1966). Hydroxybenzonitrile herbicides. *Chem. Ind.* **47**, 1946–1952.

Hirata, K., Kudo, M., Miyake, T., Kawamura, Y., and Ogura, T. (1988). NC-129—A new acaricide. *Proc. Brit. Crop Prot. Conf. Pests Diseases* **1**, 41–48.

Hirata, K., Kawamura, Y., Kudo, M., and Igarashi, H. (1995). Development of a new acaricide, pyridaben. *J. Pestic. Sci.* **20**, 177–179, 213–221 [In Japanese].

Hirooka, T., Kasahara, H., Miyagi, Y., and Kunoh, H. (1990). Effects of the systemic fungicide flutolanil on morphology of *Rhizoctonia solani* following inhibition of succinate oxidation. *J. Pestic. Sci.* **15**, 47–53.

Hoebeke, J., and van Nijen, G. (1975). Quantitative turbidometric assay for potency evaluation of colchicine-like drugs. *Life Sci.* **17**, 591–596.

Hollingshaus, J. G. (1987). Inhibition of mitochondrial electron transport by hydramethylnon a new amidinohydrazone insecticide. *Pestic. Biochem. Physiol.* **27**, 61–70.

Hollingworth, R. M., and Ahammadsahib, K. I. (1995). Inhibitors of respiratory complex I: Mechanisms, pesticidal actions and toxicology. *Rev. Pestic. Toxicol.* **3**, 277–302.

Hollingworth R. M., and Gadelhak, G. G. (1998). Mechanisms of action and toxicity of new pesticides that disrupt oxidative phosphorylation. *Revs. Toxicol.* **2**, 253–266.

Hollingworth, R. M., Ahammadsahib, K. I., Gadelhak, G., and McLaughlin, J. L. (1994). New inhibitors of complex I of the mitochondrial electron transport chain with activity as pesticides. *Biochem. Soc. Trans.* **22**, 230–233.

Holmuhamedov, E. L., Kholmoukhamedova, G. L., and Baimuradov, T. B. (1996). Non-cholinergic toxicity of organophosphates in mammals: Interaction of ethaphos with mitochondrial functions. *J. Appl. Toxicol.* **16**, 475–481.

Horiguchi, T., Shiraishi, H., Shimizu, M., and Morita, M. (1997). Effects of triphenyltin chloride and five other organotin compounds on the development of imposex in the rock shell, *Thais claviger. Environ. Pollut.* **95**, 85–91.

Hosokawa, M., and Satoh, T. (1993). Differences in the induction of carboxylesterase isozymes in rat liver microsomes by perfluorinated fatty acids. *Xenobiotics* **23**, 1125–1133.

Hrelai, P., Vigagni, F., Maffei, F., Morotti, M., Colacci, A., Perocco, P., Grilli, S., and Cantelli-Forti, G. (1994). Genetic safety evaluation of pesticides in different short-term tests. *Mutat. Res.* **321**, 219–228.

HSDB (2000). Hazardous Substances Data Bank, U.S. National Library of Medicine, http://toxnet.nlm.nih.gov.

Hsu, J. M. C., and Camper, N. D. (1975). Degradation of ioxynil to CO_2 in soil. *Pestic. Biochem. Physiol.* **5**, 47–51.

Hsu, W. H., Smith, B. E., and Hollingworth, R. M. (1988). The bradycardic and mydriatic effects of chlordimeform and its demethylated analogs in the rat: Antagonism by idazoxan but not prazosin. *Life Sci.* **43**, 1897–1904.

Hunt, D. A., and Treacy, M. F. (1997). Pyrrole insecticides: A new class of agriculturally important insecticides functioning as uncouplers of oxidative phosphorylation. *In* "Insecticides with Novel Modes of Action" (I. Ishaaya and D. Degheele, eds.), pp. 138–151. Springer-Verlag, Berlin.

IARC (1995). "Peroxisome Proliferation and its Role in Carcinogenesis." IARC Technical Rep. 24, International Agency for Research on Cancer, Lyon, France.

Igarashi, H., and Sakamoto, S. (1994). Summary of toxicity studies with pyridaben. *J. Pestic. Sci.* **19**, S243–S251.

Ilivicky, J., and Casida, J. E. (1969). Uncoupling action of 2,4-dinitrophenols, 2-trifluoromethylbenzimidazoles and certain other pesticide chemicals upon mitochondria from different sources and its relation to toxicity. *Biochem. Pharmacol.* **18**, 1389–1401.

Inaba, K., Shiraishi, H., and Soma, Y. (1995). Effects of salinity, pH and temperature on aqueous solubility of four organotin compounds. *Water Res.* **29**, 1415–1417.

Ingram, G. H., and Pullin, E. M. (1974). Persistence of bromoxynil in three soil types. *Pestic. Sci.* **5**, 287–291.

Innes, J. R. M., Ulland, B. M., Valerio, M. G., Petrucelli, L., Fishbein, L., Hart, E. R., Pallotta, A. J., Bates, R. R., Falk, H. L., Gart, J. J., Klein, M., Mitchell, I., and Peters, J. (1969). Bioassay of pesticides and industrial chemicals for tumorigenicity in mice: A preliminary note. *J. Natl. Cancer Inst.* **42**, 1101–1114.

Inoue, K., and Fukuchi, T. (1994). Pyranica® (tebufenpyrad, MK-239), a new miticide. *Agrochem. Japan* **64**, 12–14.

Isenberg, J. S. , Kolaja, K. L., Ayoubi, S. A., Watkins, J. B., III, and Klaunig, J. E. (1997). Inhibition of WY-14,643 induced hepatic lesion growth in mice by rotenone. *Carcinogenesis* **18**, 1511–1519.

Ishaaya, I, Engel, J. L., and Casida, J. E. (1976). Dietary triorganotins affect lymphatic tissues and blood composition of mice. *Pestic. Biochem. Physiol.* **6**, 270–279.

Ishak, M. M., Sharaf, A. A., Mohamed, A. M., and Mousa, A. H. (1970). Studies on the mode of action of some molluscicides on the snail, *Biomphalaria alexandrina*. 1. Effect of Bayluscide, sodium pentachlorophenate, and copper sulfate on succinate, glutamate and reduced TMPD oxidation. *Comp. Gen. Pharmacol.* **1**, 201–208.

Iverson, T. M., Luna-Chavez, C., Cecchini, G., and Rees, D. C. (1999). Structure of the *Escherichia coli* fumarate reductase respiratory complex. *Science* **284**, 1961–1966.

Iwata, S., Lee, J. W., Okada, K., Lee, J. K., Iwata, M., Rasmussen, B., Link, T. A., Ramaswamy, S., and Jap, B. K. (1998). Complete structure of the 11-subunit bovine mitochondrial cytochrome bc_1 complex. *Science* **281**, 64–71.

Izawa, Y., Hirano, A., Funayama, S., and Uchida, M. (1993). Degradation of fenpyroximate in upland soils under laboratory conditions. *J. Pestic. Sci.* **18**, 67–75.

Jabs, T. (1999). Reactive oxygen intermediates as mediators of programmed cell death in plants and animals. *Biochem. Pharmacol.* **57**, 231–245.

Jacobsen, N., and Pedersen, L. K. (1986). Activity of 2-(1-alkenyl)-3-hydroxy-1.4-naphthoquinines and related compounds against *Musca domestica*. *Pestic. Sci.* **17**, 511–516.

Jensen, K. G., Onfelt, A., Wallin, M., Lidums, V., and Andersen, O. (1991). Effects of organotin compounds on mitosis, spindle structure, toxicity and *in vitro* microtubule assembly. *Mutagenesis* **6**, 409–416.

Jernberg, K. M., and Lee, P. W. (1999). Fate of Famoxamate in the environment. *Pestic. Sci.* **55**, 587–589.

Jewess, P. J. (1994). Insecticides and acaricides which act at the rotenone binding site of mitochondrial NADH : ubiquinone reductase; competitive displacement studies using a ^{3}H-labelled rotenone analog. *Biochem. Soc. Trans.* **22**, 247–251.

Johnson, J. D., Gibson, S. J., and Ober, R. E. (1984). Cholestyramine-enhanced fecal elimination of ^{14}C in rats after administration of ammonium ^{14}C-perfluorooctanoate and potassium ^{14}C-perfluorooctanesulphonate. *Fundam. Appl. Toxicol.* **4**, 972–976.

Johnson, J. H., Younger, R. L., Witzel, D. A., and Radeleff, R. D. (1975). Acute toxicity of tricyclohexyltin hydroxide to livestock. *Toxicol. Appl. Pharmacol.* **31**, 66–71.

Johnson, T. L., and Knowles, C. O. (1983). Effects of organotins on rat platelets. *Toxicology* **29**, 39–48.

Jordan, D. B., Livingston, R. S., Bisaha, J. J., Duncan, K. E., Pember, S. O., Picollelli, M. A., Schwartz, R. S., Sternberg, J. A., and Tang, X.-S. (1999a). Mode of action of famoxadone. *Pestic. Sci.* **55**, 105–118.

Jordan, D. B., Livingston, R. S., Bisaha, J. J., Duncan, K. E., Pember, S. O., Picollelli, M. A., Schwartz, R. S., Sternberg, J. A., and Tang, X.-S. (1999b).

Oxazolidinones: A new chemical class of fungicides and inhibitors of mitochondrial cytochrome bc_1 function. *Pestic. Sci.* **55**, 197–218.

Joseph-Horne, T., Heppner, C., Headrick, J., and Holloman, D. W. (2000). Identification and characterization of the mode of action of MON 65500: A novel inhibitor of ATP export from mitochondria of the wheat "take-all" fungus, *Gaeumannomyces graminis* var. *tritici. Pestic. Biochem. Physiol.* **67**, 168–186.

Joshi, M. M., and Sternberg, J. A. (1996). DPX-JE874: A broad-spectrum fungicide with a new mode of action. *Proc. Brighton Crop Protect. Conf. Pests Diseases* **1**, 21–26.

Kadir, H. A., and Knowles, C. O. (1991). Inhibition of ATP dephosphorylation by acaricides with emphasis on the anti-ATPase activity of the carbodiimide metabolite of diafenthiuron. *J. Econ. Entomol.* **84**, 801–805.

Kannan, K., Senthilkumar, K., Loganathan, B. G., Takahashi, S., Odell, D. K., and Tanabe, S. (1997). Elevated accumulation of tributyltin and its breakdown products in Botttlenose Dolphins (*Tursiops truncatus*) found stranded along the U.S. Atlantic and Gulf Coasts. *Environ. Sci. Technol.* **31**, 296–301.

Kannan, K., Guruge, K. S., Thomas, N. J., Tanabe, S., and Giesy, J. P. (1998). Butyltin residues in southern sea otters (*Enhydra lutris nereis*) found dead along California coastal waters. *Environ. Sci. Technol.* **32**, 1169–1175.

Kannan, K., Senthilkumar, K., and Giesy, J. P. (1999). Occurrence of butyltin compounds in human blood. *Environ. Sci. Technol.* **33**, 1776–1779.

Kannan, K., Holcombe, R. F., Jain, S. K., Alvarez-Hernandez, X., Chervenak, R., Wolf, R. E., and Glass, J. (2000). Evidence for the induction of apoptosis by endosulfan in a human T-cell leukemic line. *Molec. Cell. Biochem.* **205**, 53–66.

Kataoka, T., Hayase, Y., Masuko, M., Niikawa, M., Ichinari, M., Takenaka, H., Tanimoto, N., Hayashi, Y., and Takeda, R. (1998). Synthesis and fungicidal activities of phenoxyphenyl alkoxyiminoacetamide derivatives, *J. Pestic. Sci.* **23**, 96–106.

Kawada, S., Sakamoto, A., and Shimazaki, I. (1985). Development of a new fungicide, mepronil. *J. Pestic. Sci.* **10**, 315–324 [In Japanese].

Keon, J. P. R., Broomfield, P. L. E., White, G. A., and Hargreaves, J. A. (1994). A mutant form of the succinate dehydrogenase iron-sulphur protein subunit confers resistance to carboxin in the maize smut pathogen *Ustilago maydis. Biochem. Soc. Trans.* **22**, 234–237.

Khambay, B. P. S. (1998). Aspects of the development of naphthoqinones as pesticides. *Abst. Pap. Amer. Chem. Soc.* **206**, AGRO-028.

Khambay, B. P. S., Batty, D., Beddie, D. G., Denholm, I., and Cahill, M. R. (1997). A new group of plant-derived naphthoquinone pesticides. *Pestic. Sci.* **50**, 291–296.

Khera, K. S., Whalen, C., and Angers, G. (1982). Teratogenicity study on pyrethrum and rotenone (natural origin) and ronnel to pregnant rats. *J. Toxicol. Environ. Health* **10**, 111–119.

Kim, G. B., Nakata, H., and Tamabe, S. (1998). In vitro inhibition of hepatic cytochrome P450 and enzyme activity by butyltin compounds in marine mammals. *Environ. Pollut.* **99**, 255–261.

Kimmel, E. C., Casida, J. E., and Fish, R. H. (1980). Bioorganic chemistry. Microsomal monooxygenase and mammalian metabolism of cyclohexyltin compounds including the miticide cyhexatin. *J. Agric. Food Chem.* **28**, 117–122.

Kinoshita, S., Koura, Y., Kariya, H., Ohsaki, N., and Watanabe, T. (1999). AKD-2023: A novel miticide. Biological activity and mode of action. *Pestic. Sci.* **55**, 659–660.

Kirby A. H. M., and Hunter, L. D. (1965). Identification of dinitro-octylphenols in certain commercial fungicides. *Nature (London)* **208**, 189–190.

Kissa, E. (2001). "Fluorinated Surfactants and Repellents," 2nd ed. Marcel Dekker, New York.

Knowles, C. O. (1991). Miscellaneous pesticides. In "Handbook of Pesticide Toxicology" (W. J. Hayes, Jr. and E. J. Laws, Jr., eds.), Vol. 3, pp. 1471–1526. Academic Press, San Diego.

Knowles, C. O., and Johnson, T. L. (1996). Influence of organotins on rat platelet aggregation mechanisms. *Environ. Res.* **39**, 172–179.

Kodaventi, P. R., Mehrotra, B. D., Chetty, S. C., and Desaiah, D. (1989). Inhibition of calmodulin-activated adenylate cyclase in rat brain by selected insecticides. *Neurotoxicology* **10**, 219–228.

Köhle, H., Gold, R. E., and Ammermann, E. (1994). Biokinetic properties of BAS 490 F and some related compounds. *Biochem. Soc. Trans.* **22**, 65S.

Kolbe, W. (1977). Studies on the occurrence of fruit tree red spider mite *Panonychus ulmi* (1943-1977), and its control with ®Peropal. *Pflanzenschutz-Nachr. (Engl. Ed.)* **30**, 325–338.

Konno, T., Kuriyama, K., Hamaguchi, H., and Kajihara, O. (1990). Fenpyroximate (NNI 850), a new acaricide. *Proc. Brighton Crop Prot. Conf. Pests Diseases* **1**, 71–78.

Kordel, W., and Stein, B. (1997). Fate of the organotin pesticide azocyclotin in aquatic microcosms. *Chemosphere* **35**, 191–207.

Koura, Y., Kinoshita, S., Takasuka, K., Koura, S., Osaki, N., Matsumoto, S., and Miyoshi, H. (1998). Respiratory inhibition of acaricide AKD-2023 and its deacetyl metabolite. *J. Pestic. Sci.* **23**, 18–21.

Kowaltkowski, A. J., and Vercesi, A. E. (1999). Mitochondrial damage induced by conditions of oxidative stress. *Free Rad. Biol. Med.* **26**, 463–471.

Kroemer, G., Dallaporta, B., and Resche-Rigon, M. (1998). The mitochondrial death/life regulator in apoptosis and necrosis. *Annu. Rev. Physiol.* **60**, 619–642.

Kuhn, D. G., Addor, R. W., Diehl, R. E., Furch, J. A., Kamhi, V. M., Henegar, K. E., Kremer, K. A., Lowen, G. T., Black, B. C., Miller, T. P., and Treacy, M. F. (1993). Insecticidal pyrroles. *ACS Sympos. Ser.* **524**. 219–232.

Kulka, M., and von Schmeling, B. (1995). Carboxin fungicides and related compounds. In "Modern Selective Fungicides—Properties, Applications, Mechanisms of Action." 2nd ed. (H. Lyr, Ed.), pp. 133–147. Gustav Fischer Verlag, Jena.

Kurono, H. (1985). Steps to Moncut, a new systemic fungicide. *Jpn. Pestic. Inf.* **46**, 6–10.

Kurt, T. L., Anderson, R., Petty, C., Bost, R., Reed, G., and Holland, J. (1986). Dinitrophenol in weight loss: The poison center and public health safety. *Vet. Human Toxicol.* **28**, 574–575.

Kurtz, C. P., Baum, H., and Swittenbak, C. (1970). Gas chromatographic determination of total active ingredient content of Karathane Technical and Karathane WD. I. Development of the method. *J. Assoc. Offic. Anal. Chemists* **53**, 887–895.

Kyomura, N., Fukuchi, T., Kohyama, Y., and Motojima, S. (1990). Biological characteristics of a new acaricide MK-239. *Proc. Brighton Crop Prot. Conf. Pests Diseases* **1**, 55–62.

Langner, M., Gabrielska, J., Kleszczynska, H., and Pruchnik, H. (1998). Effect of triphenyltin compounds on lipid bilayer organization. *Appl. Organometal. Chem.* **12**, 99–107.

Larson, P. S., Finnegan, J. K., Smith, R. B., Jr., Haag, H. B., Hennigar, G. R., and Patterson, W. M. (1959). Acute and chronic toxicity studies on 2,4-dinitro-6-(1-metylheptyl)phenyl crotonate (Karathane). *Arch. Int. Pharmacodyn. Therap.* **119**, 31–42.

Larson, P. S., Finnegan, J. K., Smith, R. B., Jr., Haag, H. B., Hennigar, G. R., and Patterson, W. M. (1959). Acute and chronic toxicity studies on 2,4-dinitro-6-(1-methylheptyl)phenyl crotonate (Karathane). *Arch. Int. Pharmacodyn. Therap.* **119**, 31–42.

Lee, P. W. , Lee, D. Y., Brown, A. M., and Jernberg, K. M. (1999). Comparative metabolism of famoxadone in fish, plants and animals. *Pestic. Sci.* **55**, 589–594.

Leroux, P. (1996). Recent developments in the mode of action of fungicides. *Pestic. Sci.* **47**, 191–197.

Lin, J. L., and Hsueh, S. (1993). Acute nephropathy of organotin compounds. *Amer. J. Nephrol.* **13**, 124–128.

Lin, T. J., Hung, D. Z., Kao, C. H., Hu, W. H., and Yang, D. Y. (1998). Unique cerebral dysfunction following tripheyltin acetate poisoning. *Human Exptl. Toxicol.* **17**, 403–405.

Lindahl, P. E., and Oberg, K. E. (1961). Effect of rotenone on respiration and its point of attack. *Exptl. Cell Res.* **23**, 228–237.

Lock, E. A., Scales, M. D. C., and Little, R. A. (1981). Observations on 2′-chloro-2,4-dinitro-5′,6-di(trifluoromethyl)diphenylamine-induced edema in the white matter of the central nervous system. *Toxicol. Appl. Pharmacol.* **60**, 121–130.

Longhurst, C., Bacci, L., Buendia, J., Hatton, C. J., Petitprez, J., and Tsakonas, P. (1992). Fenazaquin, a novel acaricide for the management of spider mites in a variety of crops. *Proc. Brighton Crop Prot. Conf. Pests Diseases* **1**, 51–58.

Looser, P. W., Bertschi, S., and Fent., K. (1998). Bioconcentration and bioavailability of organotin compounds: Influence of pH and humic substances. *Appl. Organometal. Chem.* **12**, 601–611.

Lopes, V. I. C. F., Antunes-Madeira, M. C., and Madeira, V. M. C. (1997). Effects of methyl parathion on membrane fluidity and its implications for the mechanisms of toxicity. *Toxicol. In Vitro* **11**, 337–345.

Lovell, J. B. (1979). Amidinohydrazones—A new class of insecticides. *Proc. Brit. Crop Prot. Conf. Pests Diseases* **2**, 575–582.

Lovell, J. B., Wright, D. P., Jr., Gard, I. E., Miller, T. P., Treacy, M. F., and Addor, R. W. (1990). AC 303,630—An insecticide–acaricide from a novel class of chemistry. *Proc. Brighton Crop Protect. Conf. Pests Diseases* **1**, 37–42.

Lümmen, P. (1998). Complex I inhibitors as insecticides and acaricides. *Biochim. Biophys. Acta* **1364**, 287–296.

Lümmen, P. (1999). Biochemical aspects of *N*-heterocyclic complex-I inhibitors with insecticidal activity. *Biochem. Soc. Trans.* **27**, 602–606.

Machado-Neto, J. G., Queiroz, M. E., Carvalho, D., and Bassini, A. J. (1999). Risk of intoxication with sulfluramid in a packing plant of Mirex-S. *Bull. Environ. Contam. Toxicol.* **62**, 515–519.

Machera, K., Cotou, E., and Anastassiadou, P. (1996). Fenbutatin acute toxicity on *Artemia* nauplii: Effects of sublethal concentrations on ATPase activity. *Bull. Environ. Contam. Toxicol.* **56**, 159–164.

MacPhee, D. G., and Podger, D. M. (1977). Mutagenicity tests on anthelmintics: Microsomal activation of viprynium embonate to a mutagen. *Mutat. Res.* **48**, 307–312.

Mangum, F. A., and Madrigal, J. L. (1999). Rotenone effects on aquatic macroinvertebrates of the Strawberry River, Utah: A five year summary. *J. Freshwater Ecol.* **14**, 125–135.

Manning, R. O., Bruckner, J. V., Mispagel, M. E., and Bowen, J. M. (1991). Metabolism and disposition of sulfluramid, a unique polyfluorinated insecticide, in the rat. *Drug Metab. Dispos.* **19**, 205–211.

Manzo, L., and Richelmi, P. (1981). Poisoning by triphenyltin acetate. Report of two cases and determination of tin in blood and urine by neutron activation analysis. *Clin. Toxicol.* **18**, 1343–1353.

Marey-Semper, I., Gelman, M., and Lévi-Strauss, M. (1993). The high sensitivity to rotenone of striatal dopamine uptake suggest the existence of a constitutive metabolic deficiency in dopaminergic neurons from the substantia nigra. *Eur. J. Neurosci.* **5**, 1029–1034.

Margot, P., Huggenberger, F., Amrein, J., and Weiss, B. (1998). CGA 279202: A new broad-spectrum strobilurin fungicide. *Proc. Brighton Plant Prot. Conf. Pest Diseases* **2**, 375–382.

Marinovich, M., Guizzetti, M., Grazi, E., Trombetts, G., and Galli, C. L. (1996a). F-actin levels but not actin polymerization are affected by triphenyltin in HL-60 cells. *Environ. Toxicol. Pharnacol.* **1**, 13–12.

Marinovich, M., Viviani, B., Corsini, E., Ghilardi, F., and Galli, C. L. (1996b). NF-kappa B activation by triphenyltin triggers apoptosis in HL-60 cells. *Exp. Cell Res.* **226**, 98–104.

Martin, T., and Johnson, B. (1989). A suspected case of bromethalin toxicity in a domestic cat. *Vet. Human. Toxicol.* **31**, 239–240.

Mathre, D. E. (1971). Mode of action of oxathiin systemic fungicides. III. Effect on mitochondrial activities. *Pestic. Biochem. Physiol.* **1**, 216–224.

Matsson, M., Ackrell., B. A. C., Cochran, B., and Hederstedt, L. (1998). Carboxin resistance in *Paracoccus denitrificans* conferred by a mutation in the membrane-anchor domain of succinate-quinone reductase (complex II). *Arch. Microbiol.* **170**, 27–37.

Matsuno-Yagi, A., and Hatefi, Y. (1993a). Studies on the mechanism of oxidative phosphorylation. Different effects of F_0 inhibitors on unisite and multisite ATP hydrolysis by bovine submitochondrial particles. *J. Biol. Chem.* **268**, 1539–1545.

Matsuno-Yagi, A., and Hatefi, Y. (1993b). Studies on the mechanism of oxidative phosphorylation. ATP synthesis by submitochondrial particles inhibited at F_0 by venturicidin and organtin compounds. *J. Biol. Chem.* **268**, 6168–6173.

McLaughlin, S. G., and Dilger, J. P. (1980). Transport of protons across membranes by weak acids. *Physiol. Rev.* **60**, 825–863.

McLennan, H. R., and Degli Esposti, M. (2000). The contribution of mitochondrial respiratory complexes to the production of reactive oxygen species. *J. Bioenerget. Biomembr.* **32**, 153–162.

Meador, J. P. (2000). Predicting the fate and effects of tributyltin in marine systems. *Rev. Environ. Contam. Toxicol.* **166**, 1–48.

Meguro, T., Izushi, F., and Ogata, M. (1990). Effect of heptachlor on hepatic mitochondrial oxidative phosphorylation in rat. *Ind. Health* **28**, 151–157.

Mehrotra, B. D., Prasada Rao, K. S., and Desaiah, D. (1985). Effect of plictran on beef heart mitochondrial ATPases. *Toxicol. Lett.* **26**, 25–30.

Meisner, H. M., and Sorfensen, L. (1966). Metaphase arrest of Chinese hamster cells with rotenone. *Exp. Cell Res.* **42**, 291–295.

Meister, R. T., ed. (2000). "Farm Chemicals Handbook 2000." Meister, Willoughby, OH.

Menegon, A., Board, P. G., Blackburn, A. C., Mellick, G. D., and Le Couteur, D. G. (1998). Parkinson's disease, pesticides, and glutathione transferase polymorphisms. *Lancet* **352**, 1344–1346.

Mercer, R. T., Lacroix, G., Gouot, J. M., and Latorse, M. P. (1998). RPA 407213: A novel fungicide for the control of downy mildews, late blight and other diseases on a range of crops. *Proc. Brighton Crop Protect. Conf. Pests Diseases* **2**, 319–326.

Metcalf, R. L. (1955). "Organic Insecticides," Wiley Interscience, New York.

Mihara, K., Isobe, N., Ohkawa, H., and Miyamoto, J. (1981). Effects of organophosphorus insecticides on mitochondrial and microsomal functions in the liver of rat with special emphasis on fenitrothion toxicity. *J. Pestic. Sci.* **6**, 307–316.

Millet, M., Palm, W. U., and Zetzsch, C. (1998). Abiotic degradation of halobenzonitriles: Investigation of the photolysis in solution. *Ecotoxicol. Environ. Saf.* **41**, 44–50.

Mishra, R., and Shukla, S. P. (1995). Effects of endosulfan on bioenergetic properties of skeletal muscle mitochondria from the freshwater crayfish (*Clarias Batrachus*). *Comp. Gen. Physiol.* **112C**, 153–161.

Mitani, S., Araki, S., and Matsuo, N. (1998). IKF-916—A novel systemic fungicide for the control of oomycete plant diseases. *Proc. Brighton Crop Protect. Conf. Pests Diseases* **2**, 351–358.

Mitsubishi Chemical Industries (1995). Summary of toxicity studies on pesticides: Tebufenpyrad. *J. Pestic. Sci.* **20**, 553–557 [In Japanese].

Miyoshi, H. (1998). Structure–activity relationships of some complex I inhibitors. *Biochim. Biophys. Acta* **1364**, 236–244.

Miyoshi, H., and Fujita, T. (1988). Quantitative analyses of the uncoupling activity of substituted phenols with mitochondria from flight muscles of house flies. *Biochim. Biophys. Acta* **935**, 312–321.

Miyoshi, H., Nishioka, T., and Fujita, T. (1987). Quantitative relationship between protonophoric and uncoupling activities of substituted phenols. *Biochim. Biophys. Acta* **891**, 194–204.

Mizutani, A., Miki, N., Yukioka, H., and Masuko, M. (1996). Mechanism of action of a novel alkoxyiminoacetamide fungicide SSF-126. In "Modern Fungicides and Antifungal Compounds" (H. Lyr, P. E. Russell, and H. D. Sisler, eds.), pp. 93–99. Intercept, Andover, UK.

Mlynarcikova, H., Legath, J., Guzy, J., Kovalkovicova, N., and Ivanko, S. (1999). Effect of chloridazon on the animal organism. *Gen. Physiol. Biophys.* **18**, 99–104.

Monkiedje, A., Englande, A. J., and Wall, J. H. (1995). Assessment of the physicochemical propereties of *Phytolacca dodecandra* (Endod-S) and niclosamide under laboratory and field conditions. *J. Environ. Sci. Health B* **30**, 73–94.

Moore, S. A., Moennich, D. M., and Gresser, E. J. (1983). Synthesis and hydrolysis of ADP-phosphate by beef heart submitochondrial particles. *J. Biol. Chem.* **247**, 6970–6977.

Morcillo, Y., and Porte, C. (1999). Evidence of endocrine disruption in the imposer-affected gastropod *Bolinus brandaris*. *Environ. Res.* **81**, 349–354.

Morcillo, Y, Ronis, M. J. J., and Porte, C. (1998). Effects of tributyltin on the phase I testosterone metabolism and steroid titres of the clam *Ruditapes decussata*. *Aquat. Toxicol.* **42**, 1–13.

Moreland, D. E., and Novitzky, W. P. (1988). Effects of inhibitors and herbicides on the membrane potential of mung bean mitochondria. *Pestic. Biochem. Physiol.* **31**, 247–260.

Moreno, A. J., and Madeira, V. M. (1990). Interference of parathion with mitochondrial bioenergetics. *Biochim. Biophys. Acta* **1015**, 361–367.

Moreno, A. J., and Madeira, V. M. (1991). Mitochondrial bioenergetics as affected by DDT. *Biochim. Biophys. Acta* **1060**, 166–174.

Moriya, M., Ohta, T., Watanabe, K., Miyazawa, T., Kato, K., and Shirasu, Y. (1983). Further mutagenicity studies on pesticides in bacterial reversion assay systems. *Mutat. Res.* **116**, 185–216.

Motoba, K., Uchida, M., and Tada, E. (1988). Mode of antifungal action and selectivity of flutolanil. *Agric. Biol. Chem.* **52**, 1445–1449.

Motoba, K., Suzuki, T., and Uchida, M. (1992). Effect of a new acaricide, fenpyroximate, on energy metabolism and mitochondrial morphology in adult *Tetranychus urticae* (two-spotted spider mite). *Pestic. Biochem. Physiol.* **4**, 37–44.

Motoba, K., Nishizawa, H., Suzuki, T., Hamaguchi, H., Uchida, M., and Funayama, S. (2000). Species-specific detoxification metabolism of fenpyroximate, a potent acaricide. *Pestic. Biochem. Physiol.* **67**, 73–84.

Mowery, P. C., Ackrell, A. C., and Singer, T. P. (1976). Carboxins: Powerful selective inhibitors of succinate oxidation in animal tissues. *Biochem. Biophys. Res. Commun.* **71**, 354–361.

Mowery, P. C., Steenkamp, D. J., Ackrell, A. C., Singer, T. P., and White, G. A. (1977). Inhibition of mammalian succinate dehydrogenase by carboxins. *Arch. Biochem. Biophys.* **178**, 495–506.

Muller, M. D., and Bosshardt, H. P. (1987). Degradation and residues of cyclohexyltin compounds in orchard soil following field application of cyhexatin. *Bull. Environ. Contam. Toxicol.* **38**, 627–633.

Murakami, N., Uchida, M., Yabutani, K., Okada, M., and Aizawa, H. (1983). Metabolism of flutolanil in rats. *J. Pestic. Sci.* **8**, 483–491.

Nebbia, C., Dacasto, M., Ceppa, L., Gennaro Soffietti, M., Spinelli, R., Bergo, V., and Di Simplicio, P. (1997). The comparative effects of subchronic administration of triphenyltin acetate (TPTA) on the hepatic and renal drug-metabolizing enzymes in rabbits and lambs. *Vet. Res. Commun.* **21**, 117–125.

Nebbia, C., Ceppa, L., Dacasto, M., and Carletti, M. (1999). Triphenyltin acetate-mediated *in vitro* inactivation of rat liver cytochrome P-450. *J. Toxicol. Environ. Health A* **56**, 433–447.

Negherbon, W. O. (1959). "Handbook of Toxicology. III. Insecticides: A Compendium." Wright Air Development Center (WADC) Technical Rep. 55-16, pp. 661–672, Wright-Patterson Air Force Base, OH.

Nicholls, D. C., and Budd, S. L. (2000). Mitochondria and neuronal survival. *Physiol. Rev.* **80**, 315–360.

Nicholls, D. G., and Ferguson, S. J. (1992). "Bioenergetics 2." Academic Press, London.

Nishida, H., Matsui, H., Sugiura, H., Kitagaki, K., Fuchigami, M., Inagaki, N., Nagai, H., and Koda, A. (1990). The immunotoxicity of triphenyltin chloride in mice. *J. Pharmacobio-Dynam.* **13**, 543–548.

Nishizawa, H., Motoba, K., Suzuki, T., Ohsima, T., Hamaguchi, H., and Uchida, M. (1993). Metabolism of fenpyroximate in rats. *J. Pestic. Sci.* **18**, 59–66.

Nizamani, S. M., and Hollingworth, R. M. (1980). Fentrifanil: A diarylamine acaricide with potent uncoupling activity. *Biochem. Biophys. Res. Commun.* **96**, 704–710.

Nolte, J., Heimlich, F., Grass, B., Zullei-Seibert, N., and Preuss, G. (1995). Studies on the behavior of dihalogenated hydroxybenzonitriles in water. *Fresenius J. Anal. Chem.* **351**, 88–91.

Oakes, D. J., and Pollak, J. K. (1999). Effects of a herbicide formulation, Tordon 75D®, and its individual components on the oxidative functions of mitochondria. *Toxicology* **136**, 41–52.

Obata, T., Fujii, K., Funaki, E., Tsutsumiuti, K., Ohoka, A., Suizu, S., and Kanetsuki, Y. (1999). Synthesis and selective bioactivity of new pyrazolecarboxamide derivatives. *J. Pestic. Sci.* **24**, 35–37.

Ogata, M., and Izushi, F. (1991). Effects of chlordane on parameters of liver and muscle toxicity in man and experimental animals. *Toxicol. Lett.* **56**, 327–337.

Ogata, M., Izushi, F., Eto, K., Sakai, R., Bunji, I., and Noguchi, N. (1989). Effect of chlordane on hepatic mitochondrial respiration. *Toxicol. Lett.* **48**, 67–74.

Ogawa, K., and Ihashi, Y. (1993). Identification of metabolites of the acaricide, tebufenpyrad, formed in *in vivo* and *in vitro* systems of rats. *J. Pestic. Sci.* **19**, 169–179.

Ogilvie, L. M., and Ramsden, D. B. (1988). Ioxynil and 3,5,3′-triiodothyronine: Comparison of binding to human plasma proteins. *Toxicol. Lett.* **44**, 281–287.

Oguri, Y. (1997). Limber® (furametpyr, S-658)—A new systemic fungicide. *Agrochems. Jpn.* **70**, 15–18.

Ohhira, S., and Matsui, H., (1996). Comparative study on the metabolism of triphenyltin in hamsters and rats after a single oral treatment with triphenyltin chloride. *Toxicol. Lett.* **85**, 3–8.

Ohhira, S., Matsui, H., and Watanabe, K. (2000). Effects of pretreatment with SKF-525A on triphenyltin metabolism and toxicity in mice. *Toxicol. Lett.* **117**, 145–150.

Ohnishi, T., Magnitsky, S., Toulokhonova, L., Yano, T., Yagi, T., Burbaev, D. S., and Vinogradov, A. D. (1999). EPR studies of the possible binding sites of the cluster N2, semiquinones, and specific inhibitors of the NADH : quinone oxidoreductase (complex I). *Biochem. Soc. Trans.* **27**, 586–590.

Okada I., Okui, S., Takahashi, Y. and Fukuchi, T. (1991). Synthesis and acaricidal activity of pyrazole-5-carboxamide derivatives. *J. Pestic. Sci.* **16**, 623–629.

Okada, I., Okui, S., Fukuchi, T., and Yoshiya, K. (1999). Synthesis and insecticidal activity of *N*-(tolyloxybenzyl)-pyrazolecarboxamide derivatives. *J. Pestic. Sci.* **24**, 393–396.

Okun, J. G., Lümmen, P., and Brandt, U. (1999). Three classes of inhibitors share a common binding domain in mitochondrial complex I (NADH : ubiquinone oxidoreductase). *J. Biol. Chem.* **274**, 2625–2630.

Olsen, G. W., Burris, J. M., Mandel, J. H., and Zobel, L. R. (1999). Serum perfluorooctane sulfonate and hepatic and lipid chemistry tests in fluorochemical production employees. *J. Occup. Env. Med.* **41**, 799–806.

Olson, M. E., and Sheehan, D. M. (1979). Failure of rotenone to interfere with 17-β-estradiol action in the rat uterus. *Cancer Res.* **39**, 4438–4440.

O'Reilly, P., Kobayashi, S., Yamane, S., Phillips, W. G., Raymond P., and Castanho, B. (1992). MON 24000: A novel fungicide with broad-spectrum disease control. *Proc. Brighton Crop Protect. Conf. Pests Diseases* **1**, 427–434.

Osano, Y. T., Okada, I., Okui, S., and Matsuzaki, T. (1991). Crystal-structure of an acaricide, *N*-(4-t-butylbenzyl)-4-chloro-3-ethyl-1-methylpyrazole-5-carboxamide. *Anal. Sci.* **7**, 181–182.

Ostrosky-Wegman, P., Garcia, G., Montero, R., Perez Romero, B., Alvarez Chacon, R., and Cortinas de Nava, C. (1986). Susceptibility to genotoxic effects of niclosamide in human peripheral lymphocytes exposed *in vitro* and *in vivo*. *Mutat. Res.* **173**, 81–87.

Oyama, Y., Chikahisa, L., Tomiyoshi, F., and Hayashi, H. (1991). Cytotoxic actions of triphenyltin on mouse thymocytes: A flow-cytometric study using fluorescent dyes for membrane potential and intracellular Ca^{2+}. *Japan. J. Pharmacol.* **57**, 419–424.

Palmeira, C. M., Moreno, A. J., and Madeira, V. M. C. (1994a). Metabolic alterations in hepatocytes promoted by the herbicides paraquat, dinoseb and 2,4-D. *Arch. Toxicol.* **68**, 24–31.

Palmeira, C. M., Moreno, A. J., and Madeira, V. M. (1994b). Interactions of herbicides 2,4-D and dinoseb with liver mitochondrial bioenergetics. *Toxicol. Appl. Pharmacol.* **127**, 50–57.

Papa, S., Guerrieri, F., de Gomez-Puyou, M. T., Barranco, J., and Gomez-Puyou, A. (1982). *Eur. J. Biochem.* **128**, 1–7.

Parker, V. H. (1965). Uncouplers of rat-liver mitochondrial oxidative phosphorylation. *Biochem. J.* **97**, 658–662.

Pereira, L. F., Campello, A. P., and Silveira, O. (1994). Effect of Tordon 2,4-D 64/240 triethanolamine BR on the energy metabolism of rat liver mitochondria. *J. Appl. Toxicol.* **14**, 21–26.

Perkins, J. M., Chen, W. L., and Briant, R. E. (1992). Uptake and elimination of fenazaquin by rainbow trout in relation to predicted environmental concentrations. *Proc. Brit. Crop Protect. Conf. Pests Diseases* **2**, 877–882.

Petroske, E., and Casida, J. E. (1995). Diafenthiuron action: Carbodiimide formation and ATPase inhibition. *Pestic. Biochem. Physiol.* **53**, 60–74.

Pfister, W., Chinn, C., Noland, V., and Yim, G. K. W. (1978). Similar pharmacological actions of chlordimeform and local anesthetics. *Pestic. Biochem. Physiol.* **9**, 148–156.

Phillips, W. G., and Rejda-Heath, J. M. (1993). Thiazole carboxanilide fungicides. A new structure-activity relationship for succinate dehydrogenase inhibitors. *Pestic. Sci.* **38**, 1–7.

Pieper, G. R., and Casida, J. E. (1965). Housefly adenosine triphosphatases and their inhibition by insecticidal organotins. *J. Econ. Entomol.* **58**, 392–400.

Pilling, E. D., Earl, M., and Joseph, R. S. I. (1996). Azoxystrobin: Fate and effects in the terrestrial environment. *Proc. Brighton Crop Protect. Conf. Pests Diseases* **1**, 315–322.

Pitkanen, S., and Robinson, B. H. (1996). Mitochondrial complex I deficiency leads to increased production of superoxide radicals and induction of superoxide dismutase. *J. Clin. Invest.* **98**, 345–351.

Radecka, H., Zielinska, D., and Radecki, J. (1999). Interaction of organic derivatives of tin (IV) and lead (IV) with model lipid membranes. *Sci. Total Environ.* **234**, 147–153.

Raffray, M., and Cohen, G. M. (1991). Bis(tri-*n*-butyltin)oxide induces programmed cell death (apoptosis) in immature rat thymocytes. *Arch. Toxicol.* **65**, 135–139.

Rao, K. S., Chetty, S. C., and Desaiah, D. (1987). Effects of tricyclohexylhydroxytin on the kinetics of adenosine triphosphtase system and protection by thiol reagents. *J. Biochem. Toxicol.* **2**, 125–140.

Ray, R. E. (1991). Pesticides derived from plants and other organisms. In "Handbook of Pesticide Toxicology" (W. J. Hayes, Jr., and E. R. Laws, Jr., eds.), Vol. 2, pp. 585–636. Academic Press, San Diego.

Read, H. W., Harkin, J. M., and Gustavson, K. E. (1998). Environmental applications with submitochondrial particles. In "Microscale Testing in Aquatic Toxicology: Advances, Techniques, and Practice" (P. G. Wells, K. Lee, and C. Blaise, eds.), pp. 31–52. CRC Press, Boca Raton, FL.

Reigart, J. R., and Roberts, J. R. (1999). "Recognition and Management of Pesticide Poisonings," 5th ed. EPA Document 735-R-98-003, United States Environmental Protection Agency, Washington, DC.

Rich, P. R. (1996). Quinone binding sites of membrane proteins as targets for inhibitors. *Pestic. Sci.* **47**, 287–296.

Rich, P. R., and Fisher, N. (1999). Generic features of quinone-binding sites. *Biochem. Soc. Trans.* **27**, 561–565.

Roberts, R. A. (1999). Peroxisome proliferators: Mechanisms of adverse effects in rodents and molecular basis for species differences. *Arch. Toxicol.* **73**, 413–418.

Robertson, J. D., and Orrenius, S. (2000). Molecular mechanisms of apoptosis induced by cytotoxic chemicals. *Crit. Rev. Toxicol.* **30**, 609–627.

Rogers, J. M., Carver, B., Gray, L. E., Jr., Gray, J. A., and Kavlock, R. J. (1986). Teratogenic effects of the fungicide dinocap in the mouse. *Teratogen. Carcinogen. Mutagen.* **6**, 375–381.

Rogers, J. M., Gray, L. E., Jr., Carver, B. D., and Kavlock, R. J. (1987). Developmental toxicity of dinocap in the mouse is not due to two isomers of the major active ingredient. *Teratogen. Carcinogen. Mutagen.* **7**, 341–346.

Rogers, J. M., Barbee, B., Burkhead, L. M., Rushin, E. A., and Kavlock, R. J. (1988). The mouse teratogen dinocap has lower A/D ratios and is not teratogenic in the rat and hamster. *Teratology* **37**, 553–559.

Rogers, J. M., Burkhead, L. M., and Barbee, B. D. (1989). Effects of dinocap on otolith development: Evaluation of mouse and hamster fetuses at term. *Teratology* **39**, 515–523.

Rogers, J. M., Francis, B. M., Barbee, B. D., and Chernoff, N. (1991). Developmental toxicity of bromoxynil in mice and rats. *Fundam. Appl. Toxicol.* **17**, 442–447.

Röhl, F. (1994). Binding of BAS 490 F to bc_1-complex from yeast. *Biochem. Soc. Trans.* **22**, 64S.

Röhl, F., and Sauter, H. (1994). Species dependence of mitochondrial respiration inhibition by strobilurin analogs. *Biochem. Soc. Trans.* **22**, 63S.

Ronis, M. J. J., and Mason, A. Z. (1996). The metabolism of testosterone by the periwinkle (*Littorina littorea*) in vitro and in vivo: Effects of tributyl tin. *Mar. Environ. Res.* **42**, 161–166.

Rosenberg, D. W., and Drummond, G. S. (1983). Direct in vitro effects of bist(tri-*N*-butyltin)oxide on hepatic cytochrome P450. *Biochem. Pharmacol.* **32**, 3823–3829.

Rosenberg, D. W., and Kappas, A. (1989). Action of orally administered organotin on heme metabolism and cytochrome P-450 content and function in intestinal epithelium. *Biochem. Pharmacol.* **38**, 1155–1161.

Rosenberg, D. W., Drummond, G. S., and Kappas, A. (1981). The influence of organometals on heme metabolism: In vivo and in vitro studies with organotins. *Mol. Pharmacol.* **12**, 1150–1158.

Rowlands, J. C., and Casida, J. E. (1998). NADH-ubiquinone oxidoreductase inhibitors block induction of ornithine decarboxylase activity in MCF-7 human breast cancer cells. *Pharmacol. Toxicol.* **83**, 214–219.

Ruder, F. J., and Kayser, H. (1992). The carbodiimide product of diafenthiuron reacts covalently with two mitochondrial proteins, the F_0-proteolipid and porin, and inhibits mitochondrial ATPase in vitro. *Pestic. Biochem. Physiol.* **42**, 248–261.

Ruder, F. J., and Kayser, H. (1993). The carbodiimide product of diafenthiuron inhibits mitochondria in vivo. *Pestic. Biochem. Physiol.* **46**, 96–106.

Ruder, F. J., Guyer, W., Benson, J. A., and Kayser, H. (1991). The thiourea insecticide/acaricide diafenthiuron has a novel mode of action: Inhibition of mitochondrial respiration by its carbodiimide product. *Pestic. Biochem. Physiol.* **41**, 207–219.

Sahib, K .I. A., and Desaiah, D. (1986). Tricyclohexyltin hydroxide effects on cationic and substrate activation kinetics of β-adrenergic-stimulated calcium ATPase. *J. Biochem. Toxicol.* **1**, 55–66.

Sahib, K. I., and Desaiah, D. (1987). Inhibition of β-adrenergic stimulated calcium pump of cardiac sarcoplasmic reticulum by tricyclohexyltin hydroxide. *Cell. Biochem. Funct.* **5**, 149–154.

Saito, H., Hirano, M., and Shigeoka, T. (1994). Uptake, distribution, metabolism and excretion of tebufenpyrad by carp, *Cyprinus carpio*. *J. Pestic. Sci.* **19**, 93–101.

Saitoh, I., Miyoshi, H., Shimizu, R., and Iwamura, H. (1992). Comparison of structure of quinone redox site in the mitochondrial cytochrome-bc_1 complex and photosystem II (Q_B site). *Europ. J. Biochem.* **209**, 73–79.

Salmon, F., and Kohl, W. (1996). Use of fresh and cryopreserved hepatocytes to study the metabolism of pesticides in food-producing animals and rats. *Xenobiotica* **26**, 803–811.

Santi, R., and Toth, C .E. (1965). Toxicology of rotenone. *Il Farmaco* **20**, 270–279.

Santroni, A. M., Fedeli, D., Gabbianelli, R., Zolese, G., and Falcioni, G. (1997). Effect of organotin compounds on trout hemoglobin. *Biochem. Biophys. Res. Commun.* **238**, 301–304.

Saraste, H. (1999). Oxidative phosphorylation at the *fin de siécle*. *Science* **283**, 1488–1454.

Sasaki, Y. F., Yamada, H., Sugiyama, C., and Kinae, N. (1993). Increasing effect of tri-n-butyl and triphenyltins on the frequency of chemically induced chromosome aberrations in cultured Chinese hamster cells. *Mutat. Res.* **300**, 5–14.

Sauter, H., Ammermann, E., Benoit, R., Brand, S., Gold, R. E., Grammenos, W., Köhle, H., Lorenz, G., Müller, B., Röhl, F., Schirmer, U., Speakman, J. B., Wenderoth, B., and Wingert, H. (1995). Mitochondrial respiration as a target for antifungals: lessons from research on strobilurins. In "Antifungal Agents—Discovery and Mode of Action" (D. K. Dixon, L. G. Copping, and D. W. Hollomon, eds.), pp. 173–191. BIOS Scientific, Oxford.

Sauter, H., Ammermann, E., and Röhl, F. (1996). Strobilurins—From natural products to a new class of fungicides. In "Crop Protection Agents from Nature" (L. G. Copping, ed.), pp. 50–81. Royal Society of Chemistry, Cambridge, UK.

Sauter, H., Steglich, W., and Anke, T. (1999). Strobilurins: Evolution of a new class of active substances. *Angew. Chem. Internat.* **38**, 1328–1349.

Schäfer, G. (1981). Guanidines and biguanidines. In "Inhibitors of Mitochondrial Functions" (M. Erecinska and D. F. Wilson, eds.), pp. 165–185. Pergamon Press, Oxford.

Scheffler, I. E. (1999). "Mitochondria." Wiley-Liss, New York.

Schewe, T., and Lyr, H. (1995). Mechanism of action of carboxin fungicides and related compounds. In "Modern Selective Fungicides—Properties, Applications, Mechanisms of Action." 2nd ed. (H. Lyr, ed.), pp. 149–161. Gustav Fischer Verlag, Jena.

Schewe, T., Rapaport, S., Böhme, G., and Kunz, W. (1973). Concerning the site of action of the systemic fungicide carboxin on the respirator chain. *Acta Biol. Med. Germ.* **31**, 73–86 [In German].

Schnellmann, R. G. (1990). The cellular effects of a unique pesticide sulfluramid (*N*-ethylperfluorooctanesulfonamide) on rabbit renal proximal tubules. *Toxicol. In vitro* **4**, 71–74.

Schnellmann, R. G., and Manning, R. O. (1990). Perfluorooctane sulfonamide: a structurally novel uncoupler of oxidative phosphorylation. *Biochim. Biophys. Acta* **1016**, 344–348.

Schraufstätter, E. (1962). Chemical development of Bayluscide. *Pflanzenshutz-Nachrichten Bayer (Engl. Ed.)* **15**, 25–33.

Schuler, F., and Casida, J. E. (1998). "Pyridaben Acaricide–Insecticide: Mechanistic Studies on the Sulfur Oxidation Products." Abst. Pap. 216th Amer. Chem. Soc. Mtg., AGRO 111.

Schuler, F., Yano, T., Di Bernado, S., Yagi, T., Yankovskaya, V., Singer, T. P., and Casida, J. E. (1999). NADH-quinone oxidoreductase: PSST subunit couples electron transfer from iron-sulfur cluster N2 to quinone. *Proc. Natl. Acad. Sci. U.S.A.* **96**, 4149–4153.

Schulte-Oehlmann, U., Tillmann, M., Markert, B., Oehlmann, J., Watermann, B., and Scherf, S. (2000). Effects of endocrine disruptors on prosobranch snails (Mollusca : Gastropoda) in the laboratory. Part II. Triphenyltin as a xeno-androgen. *Exotoxicol.* **9**, 399–412.

Seacat, A. M., Butenhoff, J. L., Hansen, K. J., Olssen, G. W., and Thomford, P. J. (2001). Toxicity of potassium perfluorooctanesulfonate in Cynomolgus monkeys after twenty-six weeks of oral dosing and one year of recover. *Toxicolog. Sci.* **60C1**, suppl., 1348.

Seaton, T. A., Cooper, J. M., and Schapira, A. H. (1997). Free radical scavengers protect dopaminergic cell lines from apoptosis induced by complex I inhibitors. *Brain Res.* **777**, 110–118.

Seaton, T. A., Cooper, J. M., and Schapira, A. H. (1998). Cyclosporin inhibition of apoptosis induced by mitochondrial complex I toxins. *Brain Res.* **809**, 12–17.

Selwyn, M. J. (1976). Triorganotin compounds as ionophores and inhibitors of ion translocating ATPases. *In* "Organotin Compounds: New Chemistry and Applications." (J. J. Zuckerman, ed.). Advances in Chemistry Ser. 157, pp. 204–226. American Chemical Society, Washington, DC.

Shimizu, T., Nakao, T., Suda, Y., and Abe, H. (1992). Mechanism of action and selectivity of a fungicide, mepronil. *J. Pestic. Sci.* **17**, 39–46.

Shinoda, K., Hato, M., and Hayashi, T. (1972). The physicochemical properties of aqueous solutions of fluorinated surfactants. *J. Phys. Chem.* **76**, 909–914.

Sierotzki, H., Parisi, S., Steinfeld, U., Tenzer, I., Poirey, S., and Gisi, U. (2000). Mode of resistance to respiration inhibitors at the cytochrome bc_1 enzyme complex of *Mycosphaerella fijiensis* field isolates. *Pest. Manag. Sci.* **56**, 833–841.

Singer, T. P., and Ramsay, R. R. (1992). NADH-ubiquinone oxidoreductase. *In* "Molecular Mechanisms in Bioenergetics" (L. Ernster, ed.), pp. 145–162. Elsevier, New York.

Singer, T. P., and Ramsay, R. R. (1994). The reaction sites of rotenone and ubiquinone with mitochondrial NADH dehydrogenase. *Biochim. Biophys. Acta* **1187**, 198–202.

Sitkiewicz, D., Skonieczna, M., Krzywicka, K., Dziedzic, E., Staniszewska, K., and Bicz, W. (1980). Effects of organophosphorus insecticides on the oxidative processes in rat brain synaptosomes. *J. Neurochem.* **34**, 619–626.

Skinner, W., Bailey, A., Renwick, A., Keon, J., Gurr, S., and Hargreaves, J. (1998). A single amino-acid substitution in the iron-sulphur protein subunit of succinate dehydrogenase determines resistance to carboxin in *Mycosphaerella graminicola*. *Curr. Genet.* **34**, 393–398.

Skonieczna, M., Sitkiewicz, D., and Bicz, W. (1980). Modification of oxidative phosphorylation in brain mitochondria during development and aging by the oxygen analog of Ronnel. *Pestic. Biochem. Physiol.* **14**, 314–318.

Skulachev, V. P. (1999). Mitochondrial physiology and pathology: concepts of programmed cell death of organelles, cells and organisms. *Molec. Aspects Med.* **20**, 139–184.

Smialowicz, R. J., Luebke, R. W., and Riddle, M. M. (1992). Assessment of the immunotoxic potential of the fungicide dinocap in mice. *Toxicology* **75**, 235–247.

Smysl, B., Smyslova, O., and Kosatik, A. (1977). Acute fatal ioxynil poisoning. *Arch. Toxicol.* **37**, 241–245 [In German].

Snoeij, N. J., Penninks, A. H., and Seinen, W. (1989). Thymus atrophy and immunosuppression induced by organotin compounds. *Arch. Toxicol.* **13**, 171–174.

Sohlenius, A. K., Eriksson, A. M., Hogstrom, C., Kimland, M., and DePierre, J. W. (1993). Perfluorooctane sulfonic acid is a potent inducer of peroxisomal fatty acid beta-oxidation and other activities known to be affected by peroxisome proliferators in mouse liver. *Pharmacol. Toxicol.* **72**, 90–93.

Solioz, M. (1984). Dicyclohexylcarbodiimide as a probe for proton translocating enzymes. *Trends Biochem. Sci.* **9**, 309–312.

Spencer, F., and and Sing, L.-T. (1982). Reproductive responses to rotenone during decidualized pseudogestation and gestation in rats. *Bull. Environ. Contam. Toxicol.* **28**, 360–368.

Spooner, N, Gibbs, P. E., Bryan, G. W., and Goad, L. J. (1991). The effect of tributyltin upon steroid titres in the female dogwhelk, *Nucella lapillus*, and the development of imposex. *Mar. Environ. Res.* **32**, 37–49.

Stahler, M., Gericke, S., and Beitz, H. (1991). Results of the toxicokinetics of bromoxynil in rats. *Z. Gesamte Hyg.* **37**, 56–58 [In German].

Starkov, A., Butenhoff, J. L., Seacat, A. M., and Wallace, K. B. (2001). Structural determination of mitochondrial dysfunction caused by *in vitro* exposure to selected perfluorooctanyl compounds. *Toxicol. Sci.* **60C1**, suppl., 346–349.

Statham, C. N., and Lech, J. J. (1975). Metabolism of $2',5$-dichloro-$4'$-nitrosalicylanilide (Bayer 73) in rainbow trout (*Salmo gairdneri*). *J. Fish. Res. Bd. Can.* **32**, 515–522.

Sternberg, J. A., Geffken, D., Adams, J. B., Jr., Pöstages, R., Sternberg, C. G., Campbell, C. L., and Moberg, W. K. (2001). Famoxadone: the discovery and optimization of a new agricultural fungicide. *Pest Manag. Sci.* **57**, 143–152.

Stevens, J. T., and Sumner, D. D. (1991). Herbicides. *In* "Handbook of Pesticide Toxicology" (W. J. Hayes, Jr. and E. J. Laws, Jr., eds.), Vol. 3, pp. 1317–1408. Academic Press, San Diego.

Stock, D., Leslie, A. G. W., and Walker, J. E. (1999). Molecular architecture of the rotary motor in ATP synthase. *Science* **286**, 1700–1705.

Stockdale, M., Dawson, A. P., and Selwyn, M. J. (1970). Effect of trialkytin and triphenyltin compounds on respiration. *Eur. J. Biochem.* **15**, 342–351.

Stolze, K., and Nohl, H. (1994). Effect of xenobiotics on the respiratory activity of rat heart mitochondria and the concomitant formation of superoxide radicals. *Environ. Toxicol. Chem.* **13**, 499–502.

Stott, W. T. (1996). Regulatory implications of peroxisome proliferation: An industrial perspective. *Ann N. Y. Acad. Sci.* **804**, 641–648.

Streibert, H. P., Drabek, J., and Rindlisbacher, A. (1988). CGA 106630—A new type of acaricide/insecticide for the control of the sucking pest complex in cotton and other crops. *Proc. Brighton Plant Prot. Conf. Pests Diseases* **1**, 25–32.

Stridh, H., Gigliotti, D., Orrenius, S., and Cotgreave, I. (1999a). The role of calcium in pre- and postmitochondrial events in tributytin-induced T-cell apoptosis. *Biochem. Biophys. Res. Commun.* **266**, 460–465.

Stridh, H., Orrenius, S., and Hampton, M. B. (1999b). Caspase involvement in the induction of apoptosis by the environmental toxicants tributyltin and triphenyltin. *Toxicol. Appl. Pharmacol.* **156**, 141–146.

Stump, D. G., Nemec, M. D., Holson, J. F., Piccirillo, V. J., and Mares, J. T. (1997). Study of the effects of sulfluramid on pre- and postnatal development, maturation and fertility in the rabbit. *Toxicologist* **36**, 357.

Suzuki, T., Yaguchi, K., Suga, T., and Nakagawa, Y. (1997). Cytotoxic effects of 2,6-di-*tert*-butyl-4-methylphenyl *N*-methylcarbamate (terbutol) herbicide on hepatocyte and mitochondria isolated from male rats. *Env. Toxicol. Pharmacol.* **3**, 167–173.

Swan, G. E. (1999). The pharmacology of halogenated salicylanilides and their anthelmintic use in animals. *J. South Afric. Vet. Assn.* **70**, 61–70.

Swanson, M. B., Ivancic, W. A., Saxena, A. M., Allton, J. D., and O'Brien, G. K. (1995). Direct photolysis of fenpyroximate in a buffered aqueous solution under a xenon lamp. *J. Agric. Food Chem.* **43**, 513–518.

Sweet, S., Duivenvoorden, W., and Singh, G. (1998). Mitochondria as a critical target for toxicity. *In Vitro Molec. Toxicol.* **11**, 73–81.

Takeshige, K., and Minakami, S., (1979). NADH- and NADPH-dependent formation of superoxide anions by bovine heart submitochondrial particles and NADH-ubiquinone reductase preparation. *Biochem. J.* **180**, 129–135.

Taketa, F., Siebenlist, K., Kasten-Jolly, J., and Palosaari, N. (1980). Interaction of triethyltin with cat hemoglobin: identification of binding sites and effects on hemoglobin function. *Arch. Biochem. Biophys.* **203**, 466–472.

Tanabe, S. (1999). Butyltin contamination in marine mammals—A review. *Marine Poll. Bull.* **39**, 62–72.

Terada, H. (1981). The interaction of highly active uncouplers with mitochondria. *Biochim. Biophys. Acta* **639**, 225–242.

Thomson, A. M., Meyer, D. J., and Hayes, J. D. (1998). Sequence, catalytic properties and expression of chicken glutathione-dependent prostglandin D-2 synthase, a novel class Sigma glutathione-S -transferase. *Biochem. J.* **333**, 317–325.

Tipton, K. F., and Singer, T. P. (1993). Advances in our understanding of the mechanism of the neurotoxicity of MPTP and related compounds. *J. Neurochem.* **61**, 1191–1206.

Tomlin, C. D. S. (2000). "The Pesticide Manual," 12th ed. British Crop Protection Council, Farnham, Surrey, UK.

Treacy, M., Miller, T., Black, B., Gard, I., Hunt, D., and Hollingworth, R. M. (1994). Uncoupling activity and pesticidal properties of pyrroles. *Biochem. Soc. Trans.* **22**, 244–247.

Tsao, R., and Eto, M. (1991). Photolysis of flutolanil fungicide and the effects of some photosensitizers. *Agric. Biol. Chem.* **55**, 763–768.

Tsuda, T., Aoki, S., Kojima, M., and Harada, H. (1990). The influence of pH on the accumulation of tri-n-butyltin chloride and triphenyltin chloride in carp. *Comp. Biochem. Physiol. C* **95**, 151–153.

Tsuda, T., Aoki, S., Kojima, M., and Fujita, T. (1992). Accumulation and excretion of pesticides used in golf courses by carp (*Cyprinus carpio*) and willow shiner (*Gnathopogon caerulescens*). *Comp. Biochem. Physiol.* **101C**, 63–66.

Tsukihara, T., Aoyama, H., Yamashita, K., Tomizaki, T., Yamaguchi, H., Shinzawa-Itoh, K., Nakashima, R., Yaono, R., Yoshikawa, S., Yamashita, E., and Shinazawa-Itoh, K. (1996). The whole structure of the 13-subunit oxidized cytochrome oxidase at 2.8 angstroms. *Science* **272**, 1136–1144.

Turner, J., and Joseph, R. (1998). "In Vitro Reactivity of Azoxstrobin with Glutathione and Glutathione Transferase." Abst. 9th Internat. Congr. Pestic. Chem., No. 5C-002.

Turrens, J. F., and Boveris, A. (1980). Generation of superoxide anion by the NADH dehydrogenase of bovine heart mitochondria. *Biochem. J.* **191**, 421–427.

Tyler, D. (1992). "The Mitochondrion in Health and Disease." VCH, New York.

Udeani, G. O., Gerhauser, C., Thomas, C. F., Moon, R. C., Kosmeder, J. W., Kinghorn, A. D., Moriarty, R. M., and Pezzuto, J. M. (1997). Cancer chemopreventive activity mediated by deguelin, a naturally occurring rotenoid. *Cancer Res.* **57**, 3424–3428.

Ueno, H., Miyoshi, H., Inoue, M., Niidome, Y., and Iwamura, H. (1996). Structural factors of rotenone required for inhibition of various NADH-ubiquinone oxidoreductases. *Biochim. Biophys. Acta* **1276**, 195–202.

Unai, T., Cheng, H.-M., Yamamoto, I., and Casida, J. E. (1973). Chemical and biological O-demethylation of rotenone derivatives. *Agr. Biol. Chem.* **37**, 1937–1944

Upham, B. L., Deocampo, N. D., Wurl, B., and Trosko, J. E. (1998). Inhibition of gap junctional intercellular communication by perfluorinated fatty acids is dependent on the chain length of the fluorinated tail. *Int. J. Cancer* **78**, 491–495.

U.S. EPA (1989a). Carboxin. *In* "Drinking Water Health Advisory. Pesticides," pp. 151–164. Lewis, Brighton, MI.

U.S. EPA (1989b). Dinocap: Notice of intent to cancel registrations; conclusion of Special Review. *Fed. Reg.* **54**(23), 5908–5920.

U.S. EPA (1989c). Dinoseb. *In* "Drinking Water Health Advisory. Pesticides," pp. 323–334. Lewis, Chelsea, MI.

U.S. EPA (1989d). "EPA Pesticide Fact Sheet 3/89: Sulfluramid (GX-071)." U.S. Environmental Protection Agency, Washington, DC.

U.S. EPA (1994). "Reregistration Eligibility Decision (RED): Fenbutatin-Oxide." EPA 738-R-94-024, U.S. Environmental Protection Agency, Washington, DC.

U.S. EPA (1997a). BASF Corporation; Pesticide tolerance petition filing. *Fed. Reg.* **62**, 11450–11453.

U.S. EPA (1997b). "Pesticide Fact Sheet: Azoxystrobin." Office of Prevention, Pesticide and Toxic Substances, U.S. Environmental Protection Agency, Publication 7501C, Washington, DC.

U.S. EPA (1997c). Zeneca Ag products; Pesticide tolerance petition filing. *Fed. Reg.* **62**, 11441–11447.

U.S. EPA (1997d). "Chlorfenapyr-129093: Health Effects Division Risk Characterization for Use of the New Chemical Chlorfenapyr in/on Cotton (5F4456)." U.S. Environmental Protection Agency, Washington, DC.

U.S. EPA (1998a). Pyridaben (Sanmite) pesticide tolerances for emergency exemptions 9/98. *Fed. Reg.* **63**, 53294–53301.

U.S. EPA (1998b). "Pesticide Fact Sheet: Kresoxim-Methyl." Office of Pesticide Programs, U.S. Environmental Protection Agency, Washington, DC.

U.S. EPA (1998c). "Reregistration Eligibility Decision (RED): Hydramethylnon." Document 738-R-98-023, U.S. Environmental Protection Agency, Washington, DC.

U.S. EPA (1998d). "Reregistration Eligibility Decision (RED). Bromoxynil." EPA738-R-98-013, U.S. Environmental Protection Agency, Washington, DC.

U.S. EPA (1998e). "Reregistration Eligibility Decision (RED). Paranitophenol." EPA 738-R-97-016, U.S. Environmental Protection Agency, Washington, DC.

U.S. EPA (1998f). "Reregistration Eligibility Decision: Rodenticide Cluster:" 738-R-98-007, United States Environmental Protection Agency, Washington, DC.

U.S. EPA (1999a). Notice of filing of pesticide petitions. *Fed. Reg.* **64**, 8090–8102.

U.S. EPA (1999b). "Pesticide Fact Sheet: Trifloxystrobin." Office of Pesticide Programs, U.S. Environmental Protection Agency, Washington, DC.

U.S. EPA (1999c). "Reregistration Eligibility Decision (RED): Triphenyltin Hydroxide (TPTH)." EPA 738-R-99-010, U.S. Environmental Protection Agency, Washington, DC.

U.S. EPA (1999d). "Reregistration Eligibility Decision (RED): 3-Trifluoro-Methyl-4-Nitro-Phenol and Niclosamide." EPA 738-R-99-007, U.S. Environmental Protection Agency, Washington, DC.

U.S. EPA (1999e). "New Pesticide Fact Sheet: Lithium Perfluorooctane Sulfonate (LPOS). EPA-730-F-99-009, U.S. Environmental Protection Agency, Washington, DC.

U.S. EPA (2000a). Pyridaben; Pesticide tolerance. *Fed. Reg.* **65**, 43704–43713.

U.S. EPA (2000b). Notice of filing pesticide petitions to establish and to extend tolerances for certain pesticide chemicals in or on food. *Fed. Reg.* **65**, 76253–76258.

U.S. EPA (2000c). Perfluorooctyl sulfonates; proposed significant new use rule. *Fed. Reg.* **65**, 62319–62333.

van den Berg, K. J., van Raaij, J. A. G. M., Bragt, P. C., and Notten, W. R. F. (1991). Interactions of halogenated industrial chemicals with transthyretin and effects on thyroid-hormone levels *in vivo. Arch. Toxicol.* **65**, 15–19.

van der Kerk, G. J. M., and Luijten, J. G. A. (1954). Investigations on organotin compounds. III. The biocidal properties of organotin compounds. *J. Appl. Chem.* **4**, 314–322.

Vander Meer, R. K., Lofgren, C. S., and Williams, D. F. (1985). Fluoroaliphatic sulfones: A new class of delayed-action insecticides for control of *Solenopsis invicata* (Hymenoptera : Formicidae). *J. Econ. Entomol.* **78**, 1190–1197.

Vander Meer, R. K., Lofgren, C. S., and Williams, D. F. (1986). Control of *Solenopsis invicta* with delayed-action fluorinated toxicants. *Pestic. Sci.* **17**, 449–455.

Vander Meer, R. K., Lofgren, C. S., and Williams, D. F. (1987). Fluorinated sulfonamides—A new class of delayed-action toxicants for fire ant control. *ACS Sympos. Ser.* **355**, 226–240.

van Gemert, M., and Killeen, J. (1998). Chemically induced myelinopathies. *Internat. J. Toxicol.* **17**, 231–275.

van Ginkel, C. J., and Sabapathy, N. N. (1995). Allergic contact dermatitis from the newly introduced fungicide fluazinam. *Contact Dermat.* **32**, 160–162.

van Lier, R .B., and Cherry, L. D. (1988). The toxicity and mechanism of action of bromethalin: A new single-feeding rodenticide. *Fund Appl. Tox.* **11**, 664–672.

Vega, S. G., Guzman, P., Garcia, L., Espinosa, J., and Cortinas de Nava, C. (1988). Sperm shape abnormality and urine mutagenicity in mice treated with niclosamide. *Mutat Res.* **204**, 269–276.

Venkat, J. A., Shami, S., Davis, K., Nayak, M., Plimmer, J. R., Pfeil, R., and Nair, P. P. (1995). Relative genotoxic activities of pesticides evaluated by a modified SOS microplate assay. *Environ. Mol. Mutagen.* **25**, 67–76.

Vitayavirasuk, B., and Bowen, J. M. (1999). Pharmacokinetics of sulfluramid and its metabolite desethylsulfluramid after intravenous and intraruminal administration of sulfluramid to sheep. *Pestic. Sci.* **55**, 719–725.

von Jagow, G., and Link, T. A. (1986). Use of specific inhibitors on the mitochondrial bc_1 complex. *Methods Enzymol.* **126**, 253–271.

von Schmeling, B., and Kulka, M. (1966). Systemic fungicidal activity of 1,4-oxathiin derivatives. *Science* **152**, 659–660.

Wain, R. L. (1963). 3:5-Dihalogeno-4-hydroxybenzonitriles: New herbicides with molluscicidal activity. *Nature (London)* **200**, 28.

Wakasa, F., and Watanabe, S. (1999). Kanemite® (acequinocyl, AKD-2023)—A new acaricide for control of various species of mites. *Agrochems. Jpn.* **75**, 17–20.

Wallace, K. B., and Starkov, A. A. (2000). Mitochondrial targets of drug toxicity. *Annu. Rev. Pharmacol. Toxicol.* **40**, 353–388.

Wang, C., Youssef, J., Saran, B., Rothberg, P. G., Cunningham, M. L., Molteni, A., and Badr, M. (1999). Diminished energy metabolism and enhanced apoptosis in livers of B6C3F1 mice treated with the antihepatocarcinogen rotenone. *Mol. Cell. Biochem.* **201**, 25–32.

Wang, G. M. (1988). Regulatory decision-making and the need for and use of exposure data on pesticides detemined to be teratogenic in test animals. *Teratol. Carcinogen. Mutagen.* **8**, 117–126.

Waring, R. H. (1973). The metabolism of Vitavax by rats and rabbits. *Xenobiotics* **3**, 65–71.

Wauchope, R. D., Buttler, T. M., Hornsby, A. G., Augustijn-Beckers, P. W. M., and Burt, J. P. (1992). The SCS/ARS/CES pesticide properties database for environmental decision-making. *Rev. Environ. Contam. Toxicol.* **123**, 1–155.

Wax, P. M., and Dockstader, L. (1995). Tributyltin use in interior paints: a continuing health hazard. *J. Toxicol. Clin. Toxicol.* **33**, 239–241.

Weisner, P., Popp, B, Schmid, A., Benz, R., and Kayser, H. (1996). Isolation of mitochondrial porin of the fly *Protophormia*: Porin modification by the pesticide CGA 140'408 studied in lipid bilayer membranes. *Biochem. Biophys. Acta* **1282**, 216–224.

Welle, H. F., and Slater, E. C., (1967). Uncoupling of respiratory-chain phosphorylation by arsenate. *Biochim. Biophys. Acta* **143**, 1–17.

Whalen, M. M., Longanathan, B. G., and Kannan, K. (1999). Immunotoxicity of environmentally relevant concentrations of butyltins on human natural killer cells *in vitro. Environ. Res.* **81**, 108–116.

Whalen, M. M., Hariharan, S., and Longanathan, B. G. (2000). Phenyltin inhibition of the cytotoxic functions of human natural killer cells. *Environ. Res.* **84**, 162–169.

White, G. A. (1971). A potent effect of 1.4-oxathiin systemic fungicides on succinate oxidation by a particulate preparation from *Ustilago maydis. Biochem. Biophys. Res. Commun.* **44**, 1212–1219.

White, G. A. (1987). Substituted benzanilides: Structural variation and inhibition of complex II activity in mitochondria from a wild-type strain and a carboxin-selected mutant strain of *Ustilago maydis. Pestic. Biochem. Physiol.* **27**, 249–260.

White, G. A., and Georgopoulos, S. G. (1992). Target sites of carboxamides. *In* "Target Sites of Fungicide Action" (W. Köller, ed.), pp. 1–29. CRC Press, Boca Raton, FL.

White, G. A., and Thorn, G. D. (1975). Structure–activity relationships of carboxamide fungicides and the succinic dehydrogenase complex of *Cryptococcus laurentii* and *Ustilago maydis. Pestic. Biochem. Physiol.* **5**, 380–395.

WHO/IPCS/ILO (1993). "International Chemical Safety Cards: Ioxynil." ICSC No. 0900, World Health Organization, Geneva.

Wiesner, P., Popp, B., Schmid, A., Benz, R., and Kayser, H. (1996). Isolation of a mitochondrial porin of the fly Protophormia: Porin modification by the pesticide CGA 140'408 studied in lipid bilayer membranes. *Biochem. Biophys. Acta* **1282**, 216–224.

Wiggins, T. E., and Jager, B. J. (1994). Mode of action of the new methoxy-acrylate antifungal agent ICIA5504. *Biochem. Soc. Trans.* **22**, 68S.

Williams, W. (1999). Pirate fear. *Sci. Amer.* **281**, 26–30.

Williamson, R. L., and Metcalf, R. L. (1967). Salicylanilides: A new group of active uncouplers of oxidative phosphorylation. *Science* **158**, 1694–1695.

Wishkovsky, A., Mathews, E. S., and Weeks, B. A. (1989). Effect of tributyltin on chemiluminescent response of phagocytes from three species of estuarine fish. *Arch. Environ. Contam. Toxicol.* **18**, 825–831.

Wood, E., Latli, B., and Casida, J. E. (1996). Fenazaquin acaricide specific binding sites in NADH : Ubiquinone oxidoreductase and apparently the ATP synthase stalk. *Pestic. Biochem. Physiol.* **54**, 135–145.

Wu, R. M., Chang, Y. C., and Chiu, H. C. (1990). Acute triphenyltin intoxication: A case report. *J. Neurol. Neurosurg. Psychiatry* **53**, 356–357.

Wulf, R. G., and Byington, K. H. (1975). On the structure-activity relationships and mechanism of organotin induced, non energy dependent swelling of liver mitochondria. *Arch. Biochem. Biophys.* **167**, 176–185.

Xia, D., Yu, C.-A., Kim, H., Xia, J.-Z ., Kachurin, A. M., Zhang, L., Yu, L., Deisenhofer, J., Yu, C. A., and Xian, J. Z. (1997). Crystal structure of the cytochrome bc_1 complex from bovine heart mitochondria. *Science* **277**, 60–66.

Yamabe, Y., Hoshino, A., Imura, N., Suzuki, T., and Himeno, S. (2000). Enhancement of androgen-dependent transcription and cell proliferation by tributyltin and triphenyltin in human prostate cancer cells. *Toxicol. Appl. Pharmacol.* **169**, 177–184.

Yamada, H., and Sasaki, Y. F. (1993). Organotins are co-clastogens in a whole mammalian system. *Mutat. Res.* **301**, 195–200.

Yamamoto, I. (1969). Mode of action of natural insecticides. *Resid. Rev.* **25**, 161–174.

Yamamoto, I., Unai, T., Ohkawa, H., and Casida, J. E. (1971). Stereochemical considerations in the formation and biological activity of the rotenone metabolites. *Pestic. Biochem. Physiol.* **1**, 143–150.

Yamano, T., and Morita, S. (1993). Effects of pesticides on isolated rat hepatocytes, mitochondria, and microsomes. *Arch. Environ. Contam. Toxicol.* **25**, 271–278.

Yamano, T., and Morita, S. (1995). Effects of pesticides on isolated rat hepatocytes, mitochondria, and microsomes. II. *Arch. Environ. Contam. Toxicol.* **28**, 1–7.

Yumita, T., and Yamamoto, I. (1982). Photodegradation of mepronil. *J. Pestic. Sci.* **7**, 125–132.

Zazueta, C., Reyes-Vivas, H., Bravo, C., Pichardo, J., Corona, N., and Chavez, E. (1994). Triphenyltin as inductor of mitochondrial membrane permeability transition. *J. Bioenerg. Biomembr.* **26**, 457–462.

Zhang, Y., Marcillat, O., Giulivi, C., Enster, L., and Davies, K. J. (1990). The oxidative inactivation of mitochondrial electron transport chain coponents and ATPase. *J. Biol. Chem.* **265**, 1633–1636.

Zychlinski, L., and Zolnierowicz, S. (1990). Comparison of uncoupling activities of chlorophenoxy herbicides in rat liver mitochondria. *Toxicol. Lett.* **52**, 25–34.

CHAPTER

58

Pyrethroid Chemistry and Metabolism

Hideo Kaneko and Junshi Miyamoto
Sumitomo Chemical Co., Ltd.

Natural pyrethrins, the insecticidal ingredient occurring in the flowers of *Tanacetum cinerariaefolium* (also known as *Chrysanthemum cinerariaefolium* or *Pyrethrum cinerariaefolium*), have been used widely for human and animal health protection by controlling indoor pest insects such as cockroaches, houseflies, and mosquitoes. Natural pyrethrins consist of six compounds (pyrethrin I and II; jasmolin I and II; and cinerin I and II). The investigation of the chemical structures of natural pyrethrins was started in 1920s and their absolute stereochemistry was completed, and elucidated in the early 1970s (Chamberlain *et al.*, 1998). Along with the investigations, extensive efforts on modification of chemical structures have been made in many laboratories to improve chemical properties in terms of stability in the environment (air, light, and heat) as well as better biological performance (higher selective toxicity). From these investigations, many synthetic pyrethroids have been elaborated and worldwide used for agricultural and sanitary purposes. They can be classified into the so-called first- and second-generation pyrethroids. The characteristic feature of the first-generation pyrethroids, which are esters of chrysanthemic acid and alcohols having furan ring and terminal side chain moieties, is to be highly sensitive to light, air, and temperature. Therefore, these pyrethroids have been used mainly for control of indoor pests. On the other hand, the second-generation pyrethroids, which commonly have 3-phenoxybenzyl alcohol derivatives in the alcohol moiety, have excellent insecticidal activity as well as sufficient stability in outdoor conditions by replacement of photolabile moieties with dichlorovinyl, dibromovinyl substituent and aromatic rings. Thus the second-generation pyrethroids are used worldwide for agricultural pests.

Many *in vivo* and *in vitro* metabolism studies of synthetic pyrethroid insecticides including their chiral and geometrical isomers have been carried out in mammals for safety assessment. However, all detailed metabolism data have not been published. In these cases, the reports of joint World Health Organization–Food and Agricultural Organization (WHO/FAO) expert meetings on pesticide residues and of the International

Programme on Chemical Safety (IPCS), Environmental Health Criteria (WHO), were referred to. This chapter deals with metabolism of more than 20 pyrethroid insecticides in laboratory animals and human beings in alphabetical order, being focused mainly on *in vivo* metabolism. The positions labeled with ^{3}H or ^{14}C are stated as the acid or alcohol moiety unless specified, because the acid or alcohol moiety does not undergo further degradation to a smaller pieces. Data on nomenclature and physical chemistry are mainly cited from *A World Compendium, The Pesticide Manual*, 11th edition (Tomlin, 1997), and *Metabolic Pathways of Agrochemicals, Part 2, Insecticides and Fungicides* (Roberts and Hutson, 1999). In addition, there are several excellent reviews about mammalian metabolism of pyrethroids; however, the book *The Pyrethroid Insecticides* (Leahey, 1985) was mainly referred to.

58.1 ALLETHRIN (BIOALLETHRIN, *d*-ALLETHRIN, *S*-BIOALLETHRIN)

Chemical Name (*RS*)-3-allyl-2-methyl-4-oxocyclopent-2-enyl (1*RS*)-*cis-trans*-2,2-dimethyl-3-(2-methylprop-1-enyl) cyclopropanecarboxylate.

Synonyms Allethrin (BSI, ISO, JMAF, ESA) is the common name in use. The trade name is Pynamin. *d*-Allethrin (trade name Pynamin Forte) is an ester of (1*R*)-*cis-trans*-chrysanthemic acid and (*RS*)-allethrolone. Bioallethrin is an ester of (1*R*)-*trans*-chrysanthemic acid and (*RS*)-allethrolone. *S*-Bioallethrin is an ester of (1*R*)-*trans*-chrysanthemic acid and (*S*)-allethrolone. The CAS registry number are 584-79-2 (allethrin, bioallethrin) and 28434-00-6 (*S*-bioallethrin).

Physical and Chemical Properties (*d*-Allethrin) The empirical formula is $C_{19}H_{26}O_3$; molecular weight is 302.4. Its form is a yellow to amber viscous liquid; its specific gravity is 1.01 at 20°C; log K_{ow} = 4.96. It is practically insoluble in

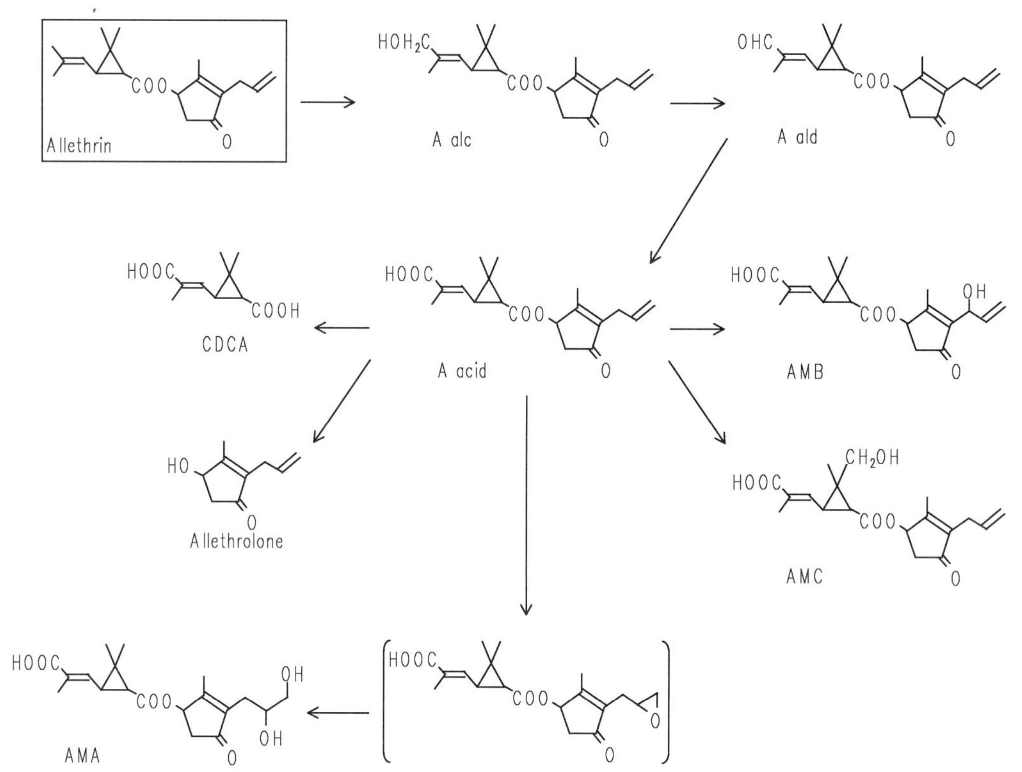

Figure 58.1 Metabolic pathways of allethrin in animals.

water, but is soluble in most organic solvents. It is unstable to UV light and is hydrolyzed in alkaline media.

Metabolism When allethrin labeled with ^{14}C in the acid moiety or with ^{3}H or ^{14}C in the alcohol moiety was orally administered to rats at 1–5 mg/kg, the ^{14}C and ^{3}H derived from the acid and alcohol moieties were excreted into the urine (47–51%) and feces (27–29%) within 48 hr after administration. Most of the metabolites excreted into the urine are ester linkage-cleaved products [chrysanthemic dicarboxylic acid (CDCA) and allethrolone] and ester linkage-retaining products. However, the fecal metabolites are not adequately characterized (Elliott *et al.*, 1972; IPCS, 1989).

The major metabolic reactions (Fig. 58.1) of allethrin are as follows: (1) hydrolysis of the ester linkage, (2) formation of the 2,3-diol from the allyl moiety, (3) hydroxylation at the methylene position of the allyl moiety, (4) hydroxylation at one of the *gem*-dimethyl groups, and (5) oxidation at the *trans*-methyl group of the isobutenyl moiety. In addition, epoxidation of the double bond of the acid moiety takes place *in vitro* in mouse liver microsomes (Class *et al.*, 1990).

There are some species differences in *in vitro* microsome oxidation sites of allethrin between rats and mice: rat microsomes appear to preferentially oxidize the *trans*-methyl group of the isobutenyl moiety. On the other hand, the major oxidation sites by mouse microsomes are the *trans*-methyl group of the isobutenyl group, the methylene position of the allyl group and the 7,8 double bond of the acid moiety (Class *et al.*, 1990).

58.2 BIFENTHRIN

Chemical Name 2-Methylbiphenyl-3-ylmethyl (*Z*)-(1*RS*)-*cis*-3-(2-chloro-3,3,3-trifluoroprop-1-enyl)-2,2-dimethylcyclopropanecarboxylate.

Synonyms Bifenthrin (BSI, ANSI, ISO) is the common name in use. The trade name is Talster. Code designations include FMC 54800. The CAS registry number is 82657-04-3.

Physical and Chemical Properties The empirical formula is $C_{23}H_{22}ClF_3O_2$; molecular weight is 422.9. Its form is a viscous liquid or a crystalline, or waxy solid; its specific gravity is 1.21 at 25°C; log $K_{ow} \geq 6$. It is less soluble (0.1 mg/l) in water and is soluble in most organic solvents. It is rather stable in natural daylight and water (pH 5–9).

Metabolism Male and female rats were treated with ^{14}C-bifenthrin labeled in the acid or alcohol moiety at single oral doses of 4 and 35 mg/kg. ^{14}C was rapidly excreted into feces and urine, and the excretion rates of the ^{14}C to feces and urine were 66–83% and 13–25%, respectively. Highest residues were found in the fat, with values of slightly more than 1 ppm after low-dose administration and 8 and 16 ppm in males and females, respectively, after application of the high dose. Residue levels in other organs were in most cases <0.2 ppm after low-dose administration and <1 ppm after high-dose administration (FAO/WHO, 1992).

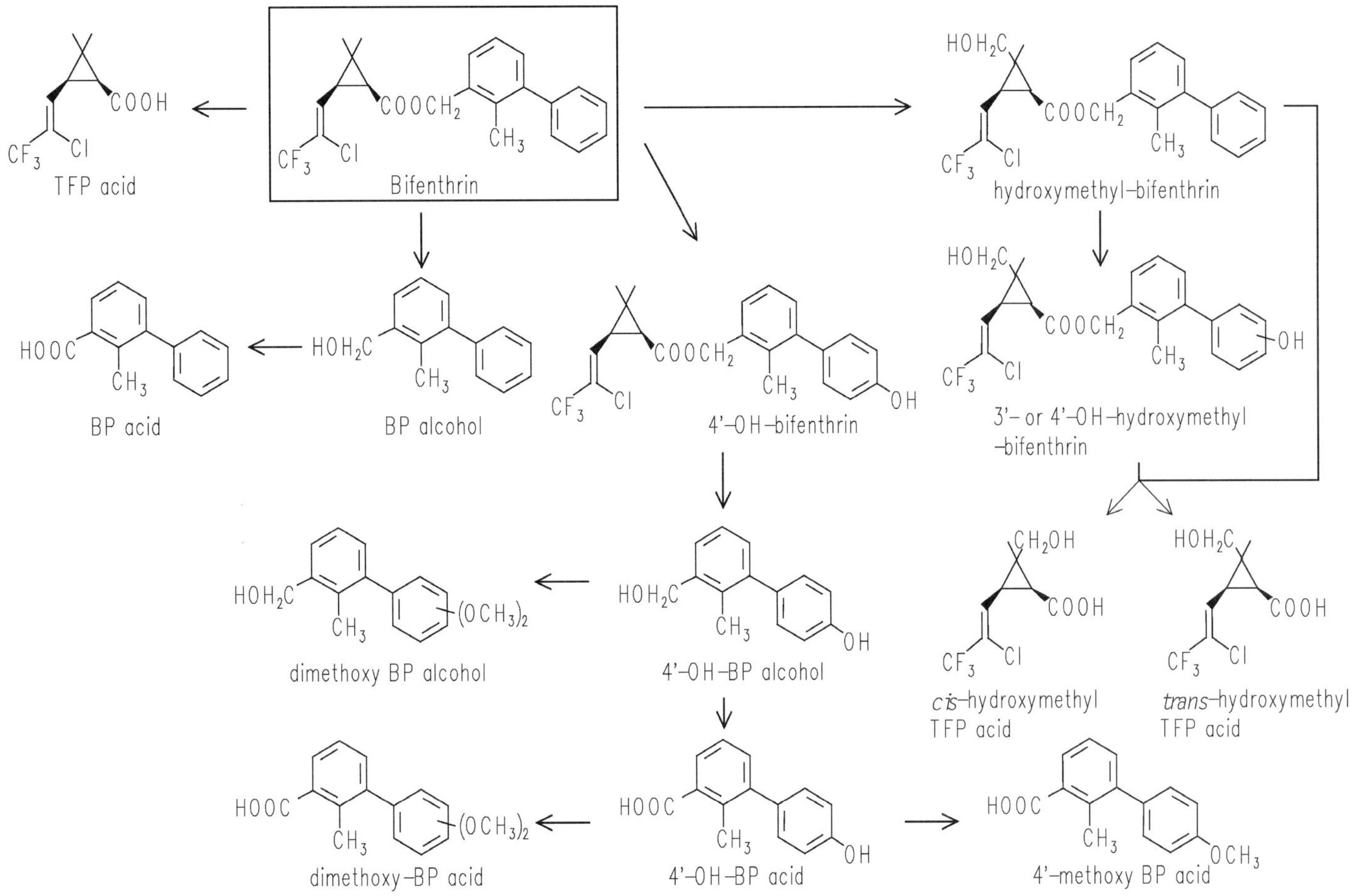

Figure 58.2 Metabolic pathways of bifenthrin in animals.

The major fecal metabolites possessed intact ester linkage hydroxylated in the acid or alcohol moiety such as hydroxymethyl-bifenthrin, 4′-OH-bifenthrin, and 3′- or 4′-OH-hydroxymethyl bifenthrin. Ester-cleaved products derived from mono- and dihydroxylated parent compounds were also detected. On the other hand, the majority of urinary metabolites were ester-cleaved products such as 4′-OH-BPacid (4′-hydroxy-2-methyl-3-phenylbenzoic acid), BPacid (2-methyl-3-phenylbenzoic acid), 4′-OH-BPalcohol (4′-hydroxy-2-methyl-3-phenylbenzyl alcohol), dimethoxy-BPacid, 4′-methoxy BPacid, dimethoxy BPalcohol, BPalcohol, TFPacid [3-(2-chloro-3,3,3-trifluoro-1-propenyl)-2,2-dimethyl-cyclopropanecarboxylic acid], cis- and trans-hydroxymethyl TFPacid. The major metabolic pathways (see Fig. 58.2) are considered to be hydrolysis of ester linkage, oxidation at the methyl group of the acid moiety and at the 3′- and 4′-positions of the phenyl group, and O-methylation. The conjugation reactions are considered to take place; however, detailed information is not available (FAO/WHO, 1992).

The tissue residues were examined after oral administration of ^{14}C-bifenthrin at 0.5 mg/kg/day for 70 days. The peak ^{14}C concentrations on an average were 9.6 ppm in fat, 1.7 ppm in skin, 0.4 ppm in liver, 0.3 ppm in kidney, 1.7 ppm in ovaries, 3.2 ppm in sciatic nerve, 0.06 ppm in whole blood, and 0.06 ppm in plasma. Analyses were extended for an additional 85 days following cessation of dosing (depuration phase). Half-lives of 51 days (fat), 50 days (skin), 19 days (liver), 28 days (kidney), and 40 days (ovaries and sciatic nerve) were estimated from ^{14}C-depuration. Analysis of the fat revealed that the parent chemical accounted for a majority (65–85%) of the ^{14}C-residues in fat.

58.3 CYCLOPROTHRIN

Chemical Name (RS)-α-Cyano-3-phenoxybenzyl (RS)-2,2-dichloro-1-(4-ethoxyphenyl) cyclopropanecarboxylate.

Synonyms Cycloprothrin (BSI, ISO) is the common name in use. The trade name is Cyclosaal. Code designations include GH-414 and NK-8116. The CAS registry number is 63935-38-6.

Physical and Chemical Properties The empirical formula is $C_{26}H_{21}Cl_2NO_4$; molecular weight is 482.4. Its form is a yellow to brown viscous liquid; its specific gravity is 1.256 at 25°C; $\log K_{ow} = 4.19$. It is less soluble (0.091 mg/l) in water at 25°C, but is soluble in most organic solvents.

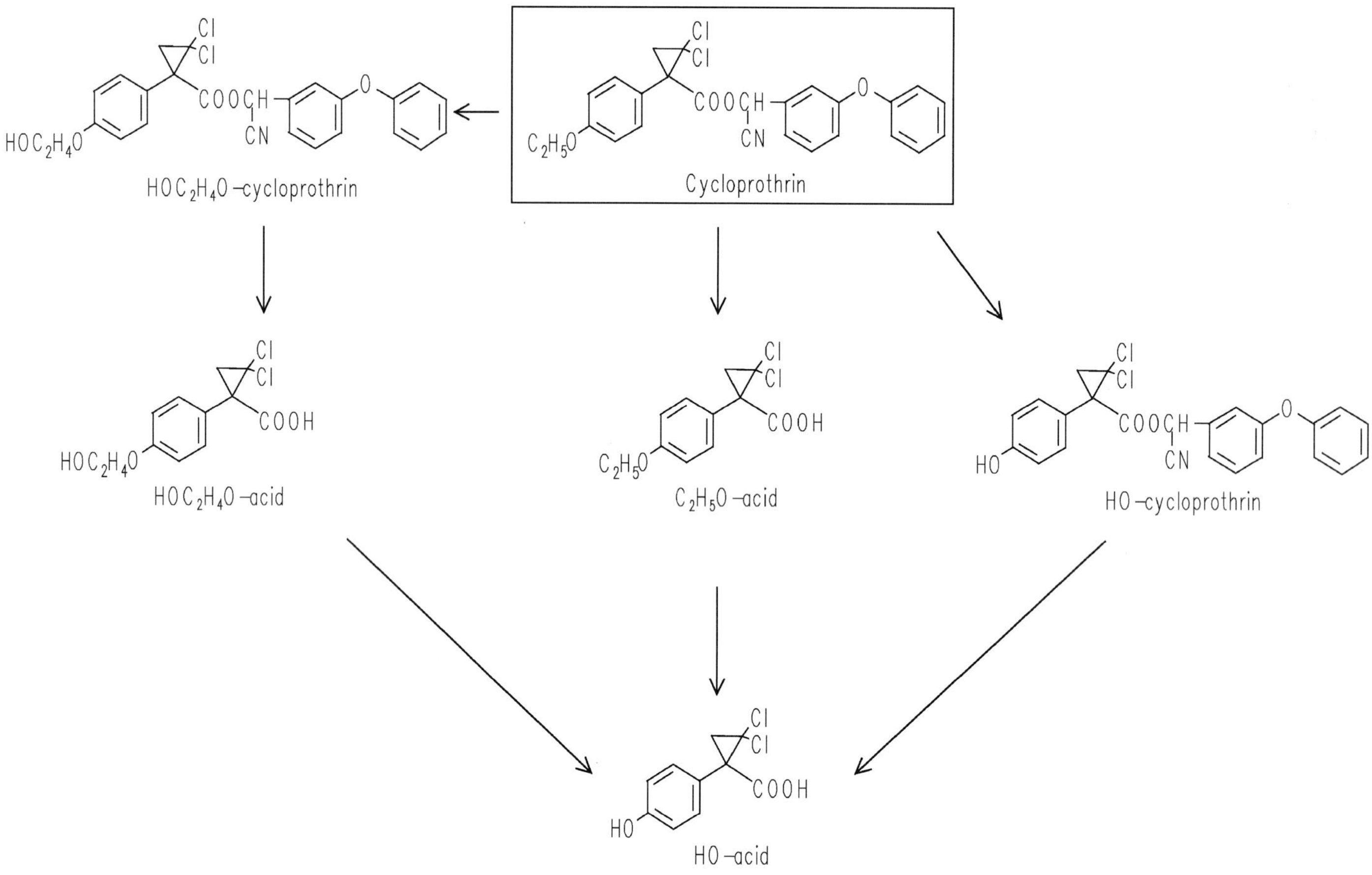

Figure 58.3 Metabolic pathways of cycloprothrin in animals.

Metabolism On single or consecutive (once a day for 7 days) oral administration of cycloprothrin labeled with ^{14}C in the acid moiety to male rats at 50 mg/kg/day, the ^{14}C was rapidly and almost completely eliminated into urine (36%) and feces (63%) within 7 days after administration. [14]C tissue residue levels reached maximum 3 hr after single oral administration and thereafter decreased with time. [14]C tissue residue levels after repeated administration were about 3.6 times higher compared with those of a single oral dose. [14]C residue levels were relatively high in the fat and skin and ^{14}C depletion from these tissues was slower than from other tissues (Seguchi *et al.*, 1991).

HO-acid was a predominant metabolite in urine and feces, accounting for 39% of the dose. In addition, HO-cycloprothrin, C_2H_5O-acid, and HOC_2H_4O-acid were also found in the feces and urine as minor metabolites. The major metabolic pathways of cycloprothrin (Fig. 58.3) are cleavage of the ester linkage and oxidation at the ethoxy position of the acid moiety (Seguchi *et al.*, 1991). Although metabolism of the alcohol moiety is not available, it can be predicted on the basis of metabolism of pyrethroids having the same alcohol moiety such as fenvalerate and fenpropathrin.

58.4 CYFLUTHRIN

Chemical Name (*RS*)-α-Cyano-4-fluoro-3-phenoxybenzyl (1*RS*)-*cis-trans*-3-(2,2-dichlorovinyl)-2,2-dimethylcyclopropanecarboxylate.

Synonyms Cyfluthrin (BSI, ISO, BAN) is the common name in use. Trade names are Baythroid, Baygon aerosol, and Solfac. Code designations include Bay FCR 1272. The CAS registry number is 68359-37-5.

Physical and Chemical Properties The empirical formula is $C_{22}H_{18}Cl_2FNO_3$; molecular weight is 434.3. Its form is a colorless crystal; its specific gravity is 1.28 at 20°C; log $K_{ow} = 6$. It is less soluble (0.002–0.003mg/l) in water at 20°C, but is soluble in most organic solvents. It is rather stable at room temperature and in acidic water, but is unstable in alkaline water.

Metabolism The acid moiety of cyfluthrin is the same as those of permethrin and cypermethrin; accordingly, metabolism of the acid moiety was not investigated, because the acid moiety should undergo the same metabolic fate after ester hydrolysis. [14]C derived from the alcohol moiety was rapidly and com-

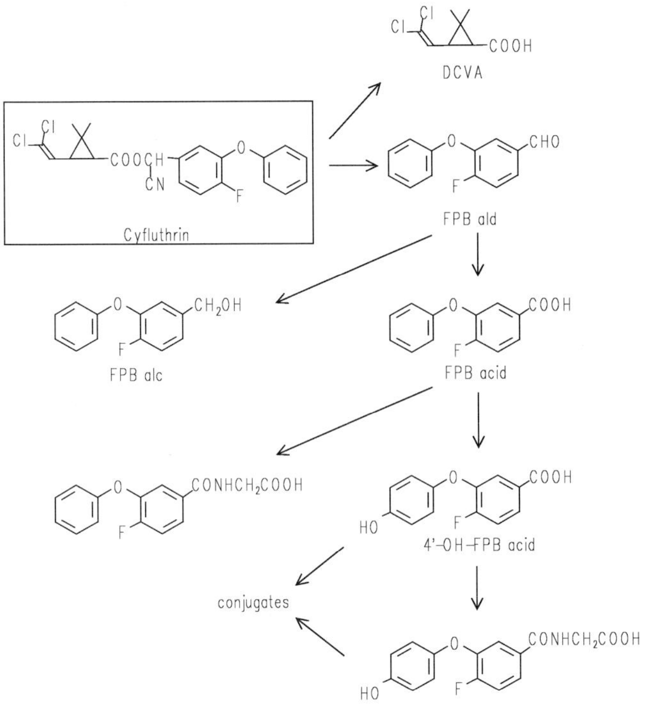

Figure 58.4 Metabolic pathways of cyfluthrin in animals.

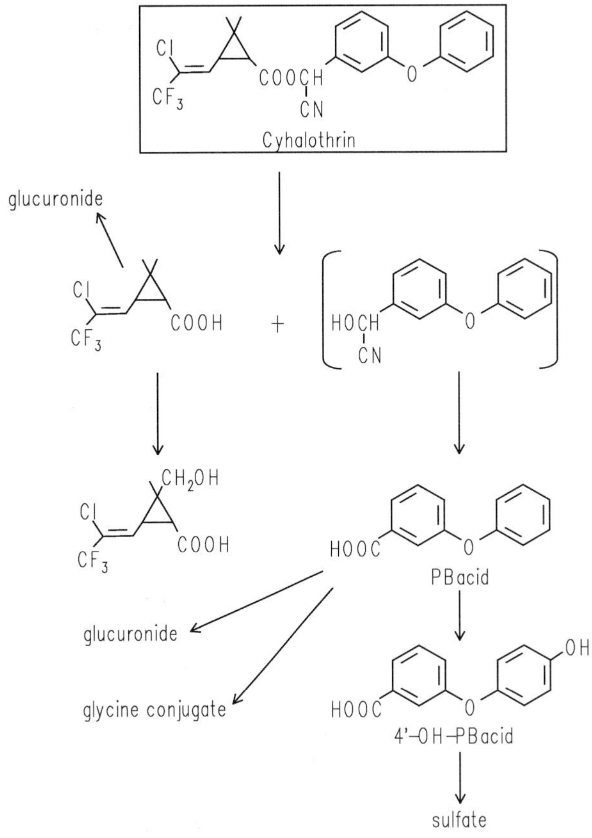

Figure 58.5 Metabolic pathways of cyhalothrin in animals.

pletely excreted into urine and feces after single oral administration of ^{14}C-alcohol-labeled preparation to rats at 0.5 and 10 mg/kg, 55–70 and 25–35% of the dose being excreted into urine and feces, respectively. Excretion of ^{14}C into bile was about 34%. The fat and sciatic nerve showed relatively higher ^{14}C tissues residues (FAO/WHO, 1986).

Major metabolic pathways (Fig. 58.4) are ester cleavage and oxidation at the 4′ position of the alcohol moiety. Major metabolites were 4′-OH-FPBacid [4-fluoro-3-(4′-hydroxyphenoxy)benzoic acid] and its conjugates (glucuronide or sulfate), accounting for about 40–50% of recovered urinary ^{14}C from rats given the labeled preparation at 0.5 mg/kg. Glycine conjugates of FPBacid (4-fluoro-3-phenoxybenzoic acid) and 4′-OH-FPBacid were also found as minor metabolites. The hydroxylation at the 4′-position of the alcohol moiety is major in rats for cyfluthrin as with pyrethroids having the 3-phenoxybenzyl alcohol or α-cyano-3-phenoxybenzyl alcohol, although cyfluthrin has the fluoro atom in 4-position of the benzyl ring (FAO/WHO, 1986).

The metabolism of cyfluthrin was examined in humans after exposure of nine male volunteers to aerosol (unlabeled cyfluthrin). The *cis*- and *trans*-acid metabolites and FPBacid were detected, indicating that the ester hydrolysis occurs in humans (Leng *et al.*, 1997).

58.5 CYHALOTHRIN (λ-CYHALOTHRIN)

Chemical Name (*RS*)-α-cyano-3-phenoxybenzyl (*Z*)-(1*RS*)-*cis*-3-(2-chloro-3,3,3-trifluoropropenyl)-2,2-dimethylcyclopropanecarboxylate; λ-cyhalothrin, (*RS*)-α-cyano-3-phenoxy-

benzyl (*Z*)-(1*R*)-*cis*-3-(2-chloro-3,3,3-trifluoropropenyl)-2,2-dimethylcyclopropanecarboxylate.

Synonyms Cyhalothrin (BSI, ISO, BAN) and λ-cyhalothrin are the common names in use. Trade names are Cyhalon and Grenade for cyhalothrin and Karate, Warrior, and Icon for λ-cyhalothrin. Code designations include PP563 and ICI146814 for cyhalothrin and PP321 and ICIA0321 for λ-cyhalothrin. The CAS registry numbers are 68085-85-8 for cyhalothrin and 91465-08-6 for λ-cyhalothrin.

Physical and Chemical Properties (Cyhalothrin) The empirical formula is $C_{23}H_{19}ClF_3NO_3$; molecular weight is 449.9. Its form is a yellow to brown viscous oil; its specific gravity is 1.25 at 25°C; log K_{ow} = 6.8. It is less soluble (0.004 mg/l) in water at 20°C, but is soluble in most organic solvents. It is stable to light and unstable in alkaline medium.

Metabolism Cyhalothrin was rapidly excreted into urine and feces after oral administration of ^{14}C-labeled acid or alcohol preparation to rats at 1 or 25 mg/kg, and ^{14}C was excreted into feces (40–65%) and into urine (20–40%) for 7 days. The fat showed the highest residue compared with other tissues.

Major metabolic reactions (Fig. 58.5) are ester hydrolysis and hydroxylation at the alcohol moiety. The metabolic fates of the alcohol moiety, α-cyano-3-phenoxybenzyl alcohol, was the same as those of pyrethroid insecticides having the same alcohol moiety such as fenvalerate, cypermethrin, and deltamethrin. The cyano group of the alcohol moiety of cyhalothrin is expected to undergo conversion to SCN ion. The major metabolites of the acid moiety is cyclopropylcarboxylic acid and its glucuronide and those from the alcohol moiety is PBacid, 4'-OH-PBacid and sulfate of 4'-OH-PBacid (FAO/WHO, 1984; IPCS, 1990a).

λ-Cyhalothrin is manufactured by crystallization of the more active pair of enantiomers from cyhalothrin. The comparative metabolism of λ-cyhalothrin with or without enantiomer pair A and cyhalothrin revealed that enantiomer pair A had little or no effect on the absorption, distribution tissue retention, or metabolic profiles, implying that enantiomers of cyhalothrin behave independently (IPCS, 1990a).

58.6 CYPERMETHRIN (α-, β-, θ, ζ-CYPERMETHRIN)

Chemical Name (RS)-α-Cyano-3-phenoxybenzyl (1RS)-cis-trans-3-(2,2-dichlorovinyl)-2,2-dimethylcyclopropanecarboxylate. α-Cypermethrin is a racemate comprising ((S)-(1R)-cis) and ((R)-(1S)-cis). β-Cypermethrin is a mixture comprising two enantiomeric pairs in the ratio of about 2 : 3. θ-Cypermethrin is a mixture of enantiomers ((S)-(1R)-trans) and ((R)-(1S)-trans) in the ratio of 1 : 1. ζ-Cypermethrin is a mixture comprising ((S)-(1RS)-cis-trans).

Synonyms Cypermethrin (BSI, ISO, ANSI, BAN) is the common name in use. Trade names are Agrothrin, Arrivo, Cymbush, Cymperator, Cynoff, Ripcord, and several other names. Code designations include NRDC149, PP383, FMC30980, WL43467, and LE79-600. The CAS registry number is 52315-07-8.

Physical and Chemical Properties The empirical formula is $C_{22}H_{19}Cl_2NO_3$; molecular weight is 416.3. Its form is a yellow-brown viscous semisolid; its specific gravity is 1.23 at 20°C; $\log K_{ow} = 6.6$. It is less soluble (0.004 mg/l) in water at 20°C, but is soluble in most organic solvents. It is relatively stable to light in weakly acidic water, but is unstable in alkaline medium.

Metabolism On single oral administration of each of [14]C-(1RS)- trans- and (1RS)- cis-cypermethrin labeled in the benzyl ring, the cyclopropane ring, or the CN group to male and female rats at 1–5 mg/kg, ^{14}C from the acid and alcohol moieties was rapidly and almost completely excreted into the urine and feces. The ^{14}C from the CN group was relatively slowly excreted in the urine and feces, the total recovery being 50–67%. The tissue residues of rats treated with the acid- or alcohol-labeled preparations were generally very low except for the fat (ca. 1 ppm). In contrast, the CN-labeled preparation showed relatively high residue levels, especially in the stomach (contents), intestines, and skin (Crawford et al., 1981a).

The major metabolic reactions (Fig. 58.6) of trans- and cis-cypermethrin were cleavage of ester linkage, oxidation at the trans- and cis-methyl cyclopropane ring and at 4'-position of the phenoxy group, and conversion of the CN group to SCN ion. The following minor species differences were observed: (1) oxidation at 5- and 6-positions of the alcohol moiety was observed in mice but not in rats; (2) ester metabolites such as 2'-OH-, 5-OH-, and trans-OH,4'-OH-cypermethrin were detected in feces of mice but not of rats. The remarkable species difference in metabolites was the PBacid–taurine conjugate, which was the predominant metabolite in mice, but it was not detected in rats. The ester linkage of cis-cypermethrin seems to be more stable than that of the corresponding trans isomer, based on the nature of urinary and fecal metabolites and excretion rate (Crawford et al., 1981b; Edwards et al., 1990; Hutson and Casida, 1978; Hutson et al., 1981).

There are, additionally, species differences of conjugation reactions of the alcohol moiety in other species; PBacid–glycine is predominant in sheep, cat, gerbil, and ferret; PBacid–taurine in ferret; PBacid–glycylvaline in mallard duck; and PBacid–glucuronide and/or 4'-OH-PBacid–glucuronide in hamster, guinea-pig, marmoset, and rabbit. The rat was unique in utilizing sulfuric acid for conjugation of 3-phenoxybenzyl moiety among animal species tested (Huckle et al., 1981).

Metabolism of cypermethrin (cis : trans = 1 : 1) in humans was investigated after oral administration to six male volunteers at 3.3 mg per person. The four metabolites from the acid and alcohol moieties were analyzed in urine. The amount of cis- and trans-Cl₂CA was approximately equal to that of PBacid and 4'-OH-PBacid. The ratio of trans- to cis-Cl₂CA was on average 2 : 1, implying that ester hydrolysis is the major metabolic pathway and that the trans isomer was more rapidly hydrolyzed than the cis isomer, as is the case with rats. On the other hand, dermal application of cypermethrin (cis : trans = 56 : 44) led to formation of the different ratio of metabolites (the ratio of trans- to cis-Cl₂CA is 1 : 1.2) from oral administration (Woollen et al., 1992).

58.7 CYPHENOTHRIN

Chemical Name (RS)-α-Cyano-3-phenoxybenzyl (1R)-cis-trans-2,2-dimethyl-3-(2-methylprop-1-enyl)cyclopropanecarboxylate.

Synonyms Cyphenothrin (BSI, ISO) is the common name in use. The trade name is Gokilaht. Code designations include S-2703 Forte. The CAS registry number is 39515-40-7.

Physical and Chemical Properties The empirical formula is $C_{24}H_{25}NO_3$; molecular weight is 375.5. Its form is a viscous yellow liquid; its specific gravity is 1.08 at 25°C; $\log K_{ow} = 6.2$. It is less soluble (<0.01 mg/l) in water at 25°C, but is soluble in most organic solvents. It is stable under normal storage conditions.

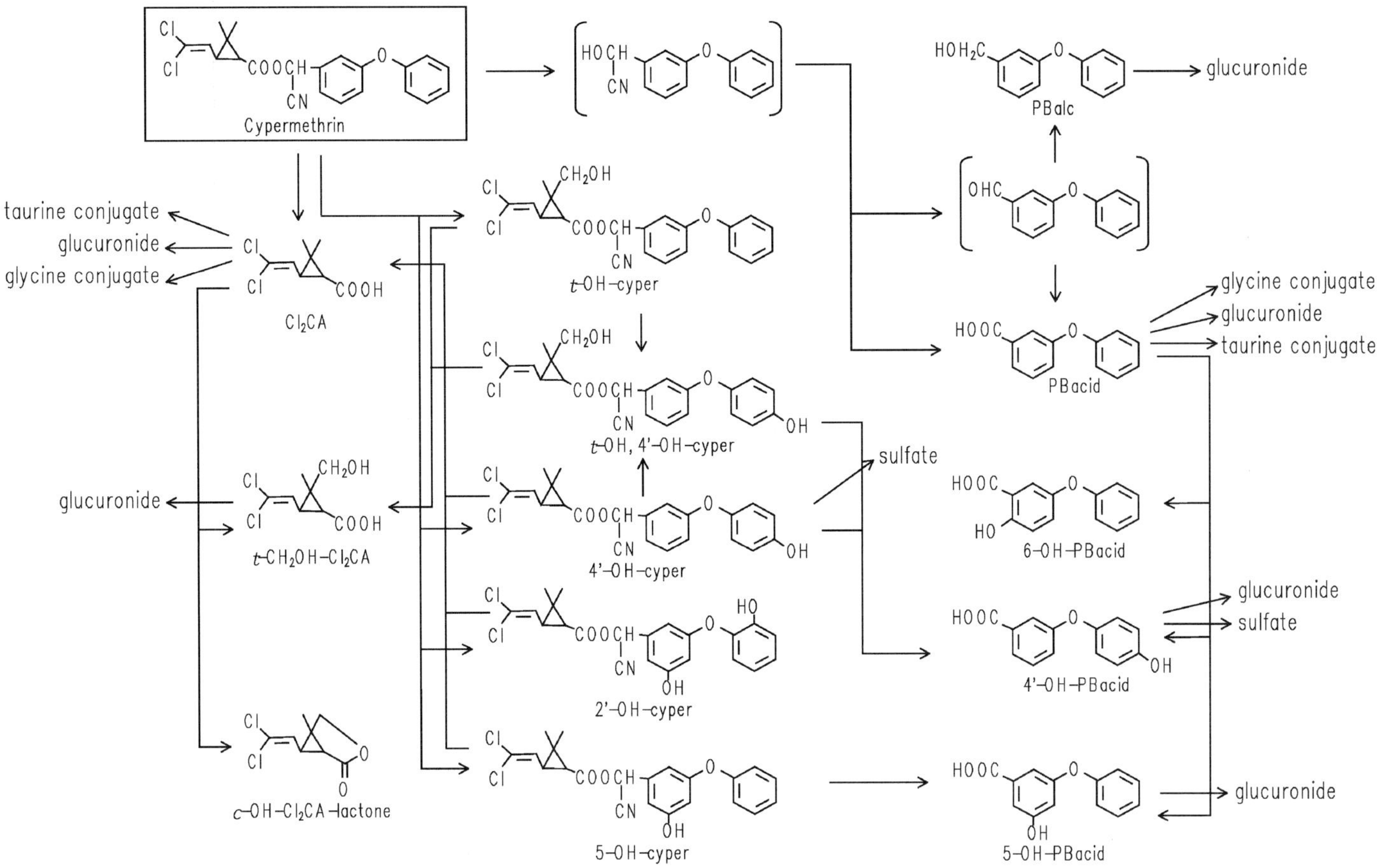

Figure 58.6 Metabolic pathways of cypermethrin in animals.

Metabolism Single oral or subcutaneous administration of [14]C-*trans*- or *cis*-cyphenothrin labeled in the acid or alcohol moiety to rats at 2–4 mg/kg resulted in almost complete elimination of the ^{14}C from the animal body. Major excretion routes with the acid- or alcohol- (except for the CN group) labeled preparation were the urine and feces. The total recovery of the ^{14}C within 7 days after administration of these labeled preparations was more than 93% in urine and feces. On the other hand, the ^{14}C derived from the CN group was more slowly excreted. In addition, 4–6% of the ^{14}C was expired as [14]CO$_2$. The total ^{14}C recovery was 60–80% for the *trans* and *cis* isomers. The three labeled preparations of the *trans* and *cis* isomers showed more urinary excretion of the ^{14}C with subcutaneous than with oral administration (Kaneko *et al.*, 1984c).

[14]C tissue residue levels 7 days after single oral or subcutaneous administration of each of the ^{14}C-labeled preparations of *trans*- and *cis*-cyphenothrin were measured. With the acid- and alcohol-labeled preparations of the *trans* and *cis* isomers, the tisssue residue levels were generally very low. On the other hand, the CN-labeled preparation showed relatively higher tissue residues than other labeled preparations.

Both the *trans* and *cis* isomers underwent the following major metabolic reactions (Fig. 58.7): (1) oxidation at the 2′- and 4′-phenoxy positions of the alcohol moiety; (2) oxidation at the isobutenyl and the *gem*-dimethyl groups of the acid moiety; (3) cleavage of ester linkage; (4) conversion of the CN ion to SCN ion and CO$_2$; and (5) conjugation of the resulting carboxylic acids and phenols with glucuronic acid, sulfuric acid, and glycine.

In vivo and *in vitro* comparative metabolism studies of phenothrin and cyphenothrin showed the following results: (1) The *trans* isomers of cyphenothrin and phenothrin were hydrolyzed more rapidly *in vitro* (liver homogenates) and *in vivo* than the corresponding *cis* isomers, and *cis*-cyphenothrin was hydrolyzed to a larger extent than *cis*-phenothrin. (2) Plasma esterases showed a different substrate specificity from the liver esterases and hydrolyzed the *trans* and *cis* isomers of cyphenothrin and phenothrin to nearly the same extents. From the results of the *in vivo* and *in vitro* studies, the CN group introduced into the molecule did not affect the biodegradability of *trans*-cyphenothrin, but rather made *cis*-cyphenothrin more biodegradable than *cis*-phenothrin. These *in vivo* metabolic profiles (ester hydrolysis rate, excretion pattern into urine and feces) may be mainly determined by activity and/or substrate specificity of the liver esterases (Kaneko *et al.*, 1984c).

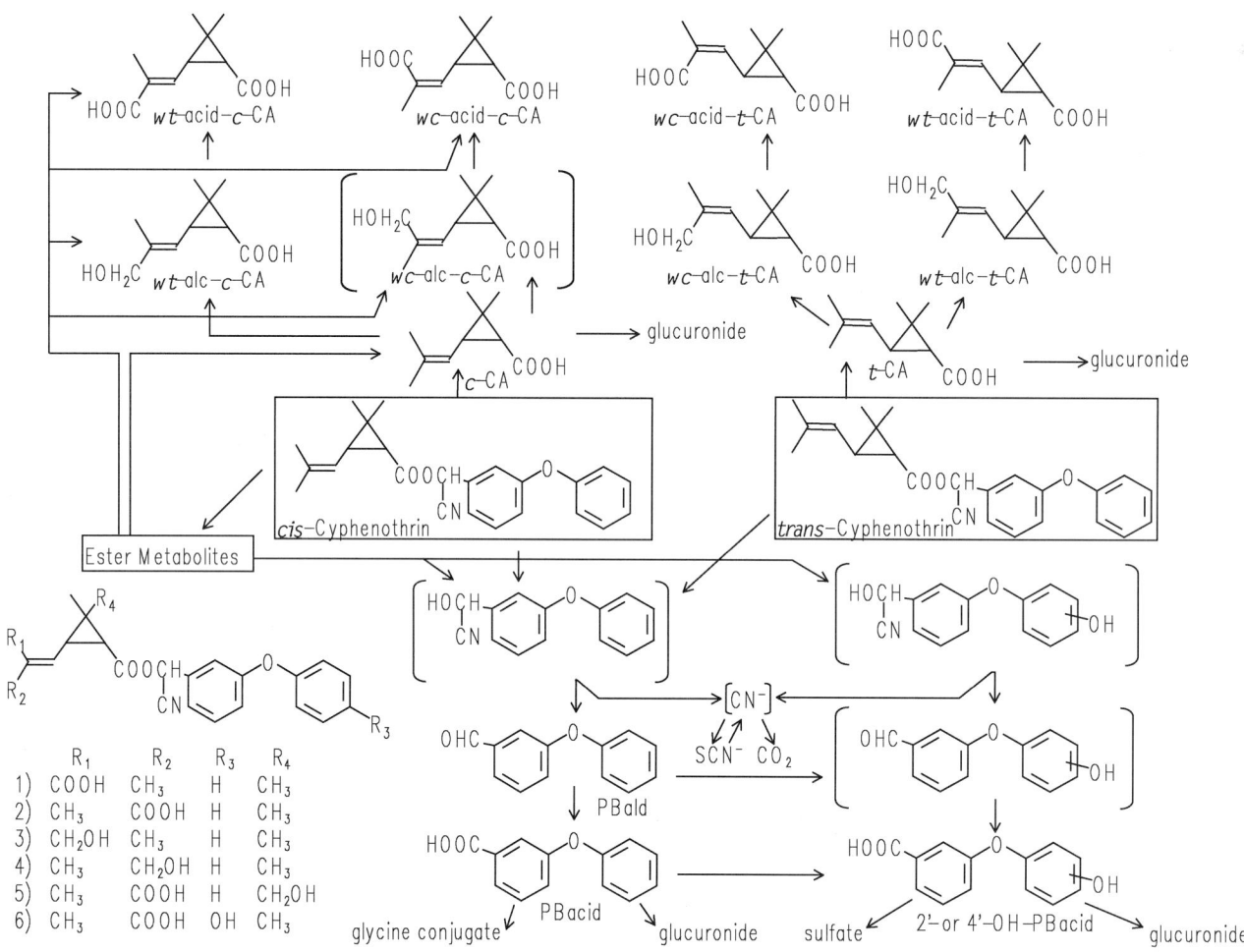

Figure 58.7 Metabolic pathways of cyphenothrin in animals.

58.8 DELTAMETHRIN

Chemical Name (S)-α-Cyano-3-phenoxybenzyl (1R)-cis-3-(2,2-dibromovinyl)-2,2-dimethylcyclopropanecarboxylate.

Synonyms Deltamethrin (BSI, ISO) is the common name in use. Trade names are Decis, Butox, K-Othrine, Kordon, and Sadethrin. Code designations include NRDC 161, AEF 032640, and RU 22974. The CAS registry number is 52918-63-5.

Physical and Chemical Properties The empirical formula is $C_{22}H_{19}Br_2NO_3$; molecular weight is 505.2. Its form is a colorless crystal; its specific gravity (bulk density) 0.55 at 25°C; log K_{ow} = 4.6. It is less soluble (< 0.0002 mg/l) in water at 25°C, but is soluble in most organic solvents. It is stable to air and in acidic conditions, but rather unstable in alkaline medium.

Metabolism On oral administration to rats at 0.60–1.64 mg/kg, the acid and alcohol moieties of deltamethrin were almost completely eliminated from the body within 2–4 days. On the other hand, the CN group was eliminated more slowly than

the acid and alcohol moieties, the total recovery during 8 days being 79% of the dosed radiocarbon (43 and 36% in the urine and feces, respectively). ^{14}C tissue residues with deltamethrin preparation labeled in the acid moiety or in the alcohol moiety were generally very low whereas the fat showed somewhat higher residue levels (0.1–0.2 ppm). The ^{14}C derived from the CN group showed relatively high residue levels, especially in skin and stomach. Essentially all the ^{14}C in the stomach was SCN ion (Ruzo *et al.*, 1978).

The major metabolic reactions (Fig. 58.8) of deltamethrin in rats are oxidation at the *trans*-methyl relative to the carbonyl group of the acid moiety and 2'-, 4'-, and 5-positions of the alcohol moiety, cleavage of ester linkage, conversion of the CN group to SCN ion and 2-iminothiazolidine-4-carboxylic acid (ITCA), and conjugation of these carboxylic acid and phenol derivatives with sulfuric acid, glycine, and/or glucuronic acid.

Although the major metabolic pathways in mice are similar to those in rats, there are the following species differences in metabolism: (1) amino acid conjugation reactions of the alcohol moiety (rat, glycine; mouse, taurine); (2) rats produced more phenolic metabolites than mice; and (3) mice produce *trans*-

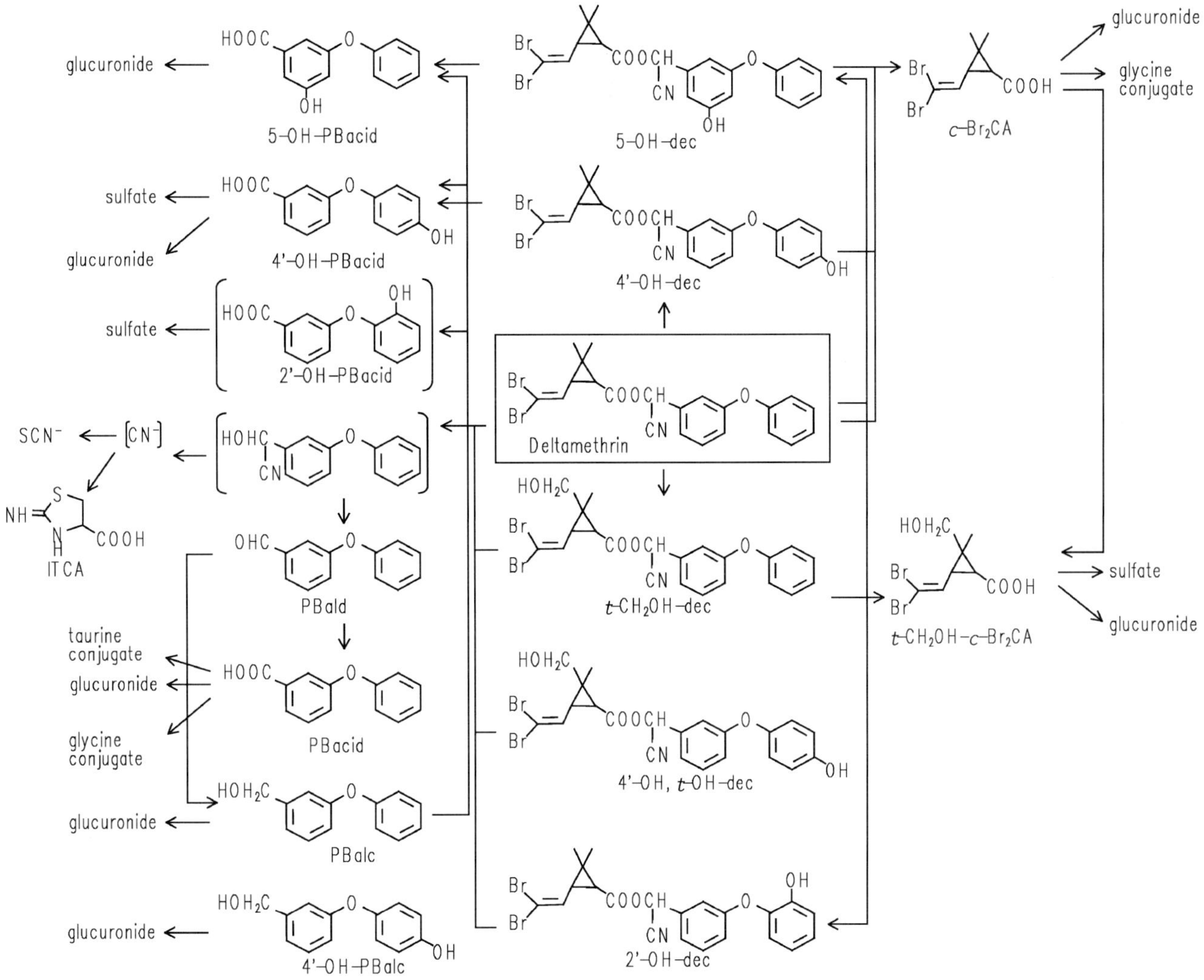

Figure 58.8 Metabolic pathways of deltamethrin in animals.

hydroxymethyl cyclopropanecarboxylic acid to a larger extent than rats (Ruzo *et al.*, 1978, 1979).

A human metabolism study of deltamethrin was carried out in three volunteers after a single oral dose of 3 mg of ^{14}C-deltamethrin per person. The ^{14}C was more rapidly excreted into urine (51–59%) than into feces (10–26%), total excretion of ^{14}C being 64–77% of the dose for 96 hr (IPCS, 1990b).

58.9 EMPENTHRIN

Chemical Name (*E*)-(*RS*)-1-Ethynyl-2-methylpent-2-enyl (1*RS*)-*cis-trans*-2,2-dimethyl-3-(2-methylprop-1-enyl)cyclopropanecarboxylate.

Synonyms Empenthrin (BSI, ISO) is the common name in use. The trade name is Vaporthrin. Code designations include S-2852 Forte. The CAS registry number is 54406-48-3.

Physical and Chemical Properties The empirical formula is $C_{18}H_{26}O_2$; molecular weight is 274.4. Its form is a yellow liquid; its specific gravity is 0.927 at 20°C; log K_{ow} = 5(est). It is less soluble (0.111 mg/l) in water at 25°C, but is soluble in most organic solvents. It is stable under normal conditions.

Metabolism When single oral administration of (1*R*)-*cis*- or (1*R*)-*trans*-empenthrin labeled with ^{14}C in the alcohol moiety was given to rats at 3–600 mg/kg (female), 97–106% of the dosed ^{14}C was rapidly eliminated into urine and feces within 7 days after administration. Monitoring of the expired air indicated that less than 1.1% of the dose was excreted as ^{14}CO$_2$. Urinary, fecal, and exhaled ^{14}C excretion accounted for 22–41, 60–74, and 1–2% of the dose, respectively (Isobe *et al.*, 1992).

^{14}C tissue levels reached maxima at 1–8 hr after administration of the *cis* or *trans* isomer at 3 mg/kg and decreased thereafter. Liver and kidney tissues showed higher ^{14}C concentrations than other tissues. No notable sex-related difference

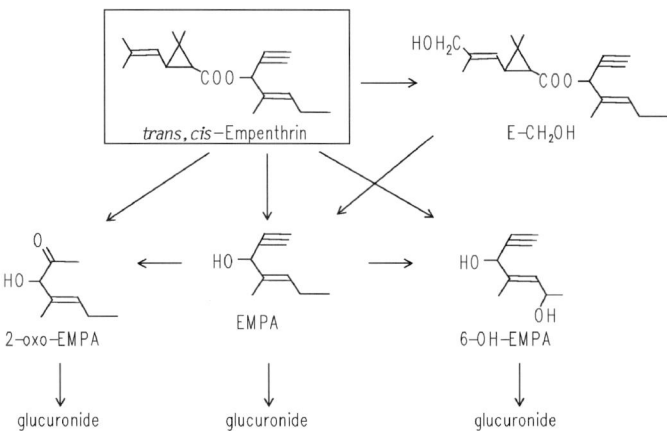

Figure 58.9 Metabolic pathways of empenthrin in animals.

was observed in distribution or excretion of the radioactivity. ^{14}C tissue residues were lower in rats receiving the *trans* isomer than in those receiving the *cis* isomer.

The parent compound accounted for 7–13 and 17–26% of the dose in the feces of rats receiving the *cis* and *trans* isomers, respectively. The major metabolites were 1-ethynyl-2-methylpent-2-enol (EMPA), 6-OH-EMPA, and 2-oxo-EMPA and their glucuronides. An ester-retaining metabolite by *E*-methyl hydroxylation at the isobutenyl group in the acid moiety was also found.

Major metabolic reactions (Fig. 58.9) in rats were cleavage of the ester linkage and glucuronide formation of the resulting alcohol derivatives; as a minor pathway, oxidation of the methylene group in the alcohol moiety, and hydration of the triple bond in the alcohol moiety were found. In addition, the oxidation at the methyl group of the isobutenyl group occurred (Isobe *et al.*, 1992).

58.10 ETOFENPROX

Chemical Name 2-(4-Ethoxyphenyl)-2-methylpropyl 3-phenoxybenzyl ether.

Synonyms Etofenprox (ISO, BSI, INN) is the common name in use. Code designations include MTI-500. The trade name is Trebon. The CAS registry number is 80844-07-01.

Physical and Chemical Properties The empirical formula is $C_{25}H_{28}O_3$; molecular weight is 376.5. Its form is a white crystal; its specific gravity is 1.157 at 23°C; log K_{ow} = 7.05. It is less soluble (<0.001 mg/l) in water at 25°C, but is soluble in most organic solvents. It is stable to light and in acidic and alkaline medium.

Metabolism The metabolism of etofenprox has been studied in rats and dogs.

On single oral administration of ^{14}C-etofenprox (a 1 : 1 mixture of [1-^{14}C-propyl]-etofenprox and [α-^{14}C-benzyl]-etofenprox to both sexes of rats at 30 or 180 mg/kg, ^{14}C excretion

rates in feces and urine were 87–90 and 7–9%, respectively, of the dosed ^{14}C 5 days after administration. No ^{14}C was found in expired air. Plasma ^{14}C reached peak levels after 3–5 hr. ^{14}C excreted into bile was found to account for 10–30% and unchanged etofenprox was not found in the bile. ^{14}C tissue concentration was the highest in fat, as unchanged parent compound. When ^{14}C-etofenprox was administered to pregnant rats (gestation day 10 to day 16) at 30 mg/kg/day, the ^{14}C was transferred to the fetus through the placenta; however, their levels were low compared to other tissues of mother animals. Etofenprox was secreted in milk as the unchanged compound (FAO/WHO, 1993).

The major fecal metabolites were deethylated etofenprox (DE) and 4'-OH-etofenprox (4'OH). The major biotransformation routes (Fig. 58.10) involve *O*-deethylation of the ethoxyphenyl moiety and hydroxylation of the phenoxybenzyl moiety followed by conjugation with glucuronide or sulfate. Oxidation of the α-CH_2 group followed by hydrolysis represents an additional route.

On single oral administration of ^{14}C-etofenprox (a 1 : 1 mixture of [1-^{14}C-propyl]-etofenprox and [α-^{14}C-benzyl]-etofenprox to beagle dogs of each sex at 30 mg/kg, total excretion in feces was 90 and 6% of the dosed ^{14}C in urine over 5 days after administration. Based on the results of metabolites in excreta, the total estimated gastrointestinal absorption was 14–51%. Tissue concentrations were highest in liver. The results indicate a lower gastrointestinal absorption rate in dogs than in rats. The major biotransformation routes were the same as in rats (FAO/WHO, 1993).

58.11 FENPROPATHRIN

Chemical Name (*RS*)-α-Cyano-3-phenoxybenzyl 2,2,3,3-tetramethylcyclopropanecarboxylate.

Synonyms Fenpropathrin (BSI, ISO, ANSI) is the common name in use. Trade names are Rody, Danitol, Meothrin, Ortho, and Danitol. Code designations include S-3206. The CAS registry number is 64257-84-7.

Physical and Chemical Properties The empirical formula is $C_{22}H_{23}NO_3$; molecular weight is 349.4. Its form is a yellow-brown solid; its specific gravity is 1.15 at 25°C; log K_{ow} = 6. It is less soluble (0.0141 mg/l) in water at 25°C, but is soluble in most organic solvents. It is stable to light, but is unstable in alkaline medium.

Metabolism Single oral administration of ^{14}C-acid- and ^{14}C-alcohol-labeled-fenpropathrin preparations to rats at 2.4–26.8 mg/kg resulted in almost complete elimination of the ^{14}C from the animal body within 7 days. Major excretion routes of ^{14}C-acid and ^{14}C-alcohol preparations were the urine and feces. The ^{14}C recoveries with the acid and alcohol preparations were 96–102% (urine, 27–44%; feces, 58–70%) and 96–98% (urine, 26–43%; feces, 54–71%), respectively. The ^{14}C excretion pattern

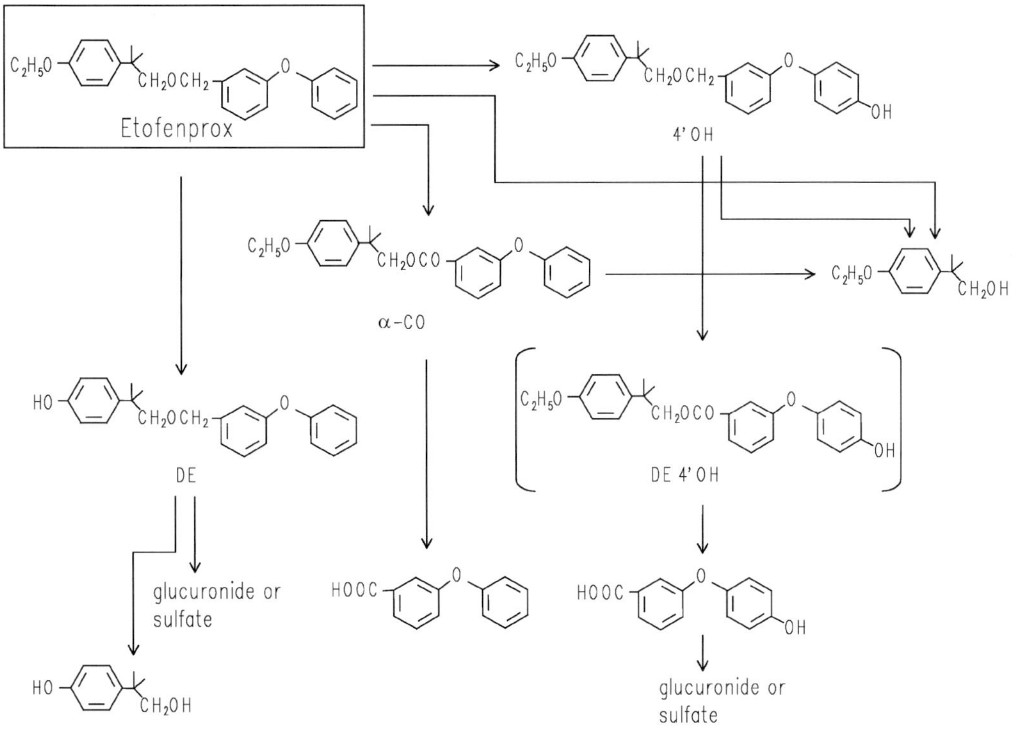

Figure 58.10 Metabolic pathways of etofenprox in animals.

into the urine and feces was very similar between both labeled preparations (Kaneko *et al.*, 1987).

With ^{14}C-acid and -alcohol preparations, the tissue residue levels 7 days after single oral administration of each of the ^{14}C-labeled fenpropathrin preparations were generally very low. However, the fat showed slightly higher residue level for both labeled preparations compared with other tissues (Kaneko *et al.*, 1987).

Fenpropathrin was rapidly metabolized in rats via cleavage of the ester linkage, oxidation at both or one methyl group of the acid moiety and at the 4′-position of the alcohol moiety, and conjugation with sulfuric acid, glucuronic acid, and amino acid (Fig. 58.11). The CN group is presumed to undergo the same metabolic reaction, conversion of the CN group to SCN ion, as those observed in pyrethroid insecticides having α-cyano-3-phenoxybenzyl alcohol such as cyphenothrin, deltamethrin, and fenvalerate. The major urinary metabolites were sulfate of 4′-OH-PBacid from the alcohol moiety and free and glucuronides of 2,2,3,3-tetramethylcyclopropanecarboxylic acid (TMPA) and its hydroxymethyl derivatives from the acid moiety. The major fecal metabolites retained ester linkage with oxidation at the 4′-position of the alcohol and the *trans*-methyl group (Crawford and Hutson, 1977; Kaneko *et al.*, 1987).

58.12 FENVALERATE (ESFENVALERATE)

Chemical Name (*RS*)-α-cyano-3-phenoxybenzyl (*RS*)-2-(4-chlorophenyl)-3-methylbutyrate; esfenvalerate is (*S*)-α-cyano-3-phenoxybenzy (*S*)-2-(4-chlorophenyl)-3-methylbutyrate.

Synonyms Fenvalerate (BSI, ISO, ESA) is the common name in use. Trade names are Sumicidin, Pydrin, and several other names. Code designations include S-5602 and WL43775. Esfenvalerate (BSI, ISO) is an insecticidally active isomer of four isomers of fenvalerate and is the common name in use. Trade names are Sumi-alpha and Asana. Code designations include S-5602Aα, DPX-YB656, and S-1844. The CAS registry numbers are 51630-58-1 for fenvalerate and 66230-04-4 for esfenvalerate.

Physical and Chemical Properties (Fenvalerate) The empirical formula is $C_{25}H_{22}ClNO_3$; molecular weight is 419.9. Its form is a viscous yellow or brown liquid and sometimes partly crystalline at room temperature; its specific gravity is 1.17 at 25°C; log $K_{ow} = 6.2$. It is less soluble (< 0.01 mg/l) in water at 25°C, but is readily soluble in most organic solvents. It is relatively stable in acidic media, but unstable in alkaline medium.

Metabolism Single oral administration of the ^{14}C preparations of fenvalerate and its (2*S*) isomer labeled in the acid or alcohol moiety to both sexes of rats and mice at 6.7–8.4 mg/kg resulted in almost complete elimination of the ^{14}C from the animal body. Major excretion routes for the ^{14}C in both animal species were the urine and feces. The total recovery of the ^{14}C 6 or 7 days after administration was 93–102% in rats and mice. In contrast, the ^{14}C from the ^{14}CN-preparation of fenvalerate and its (2*S*) isomer was more slowly excreted than other ^{14}C preparations, and mainly into the urine and feces. Additionally approximately 6–14% of the ^{14}C was expired as ^{14}CO$_2$ in the two species. The total recovery of the ^{14}C was 75–81% in

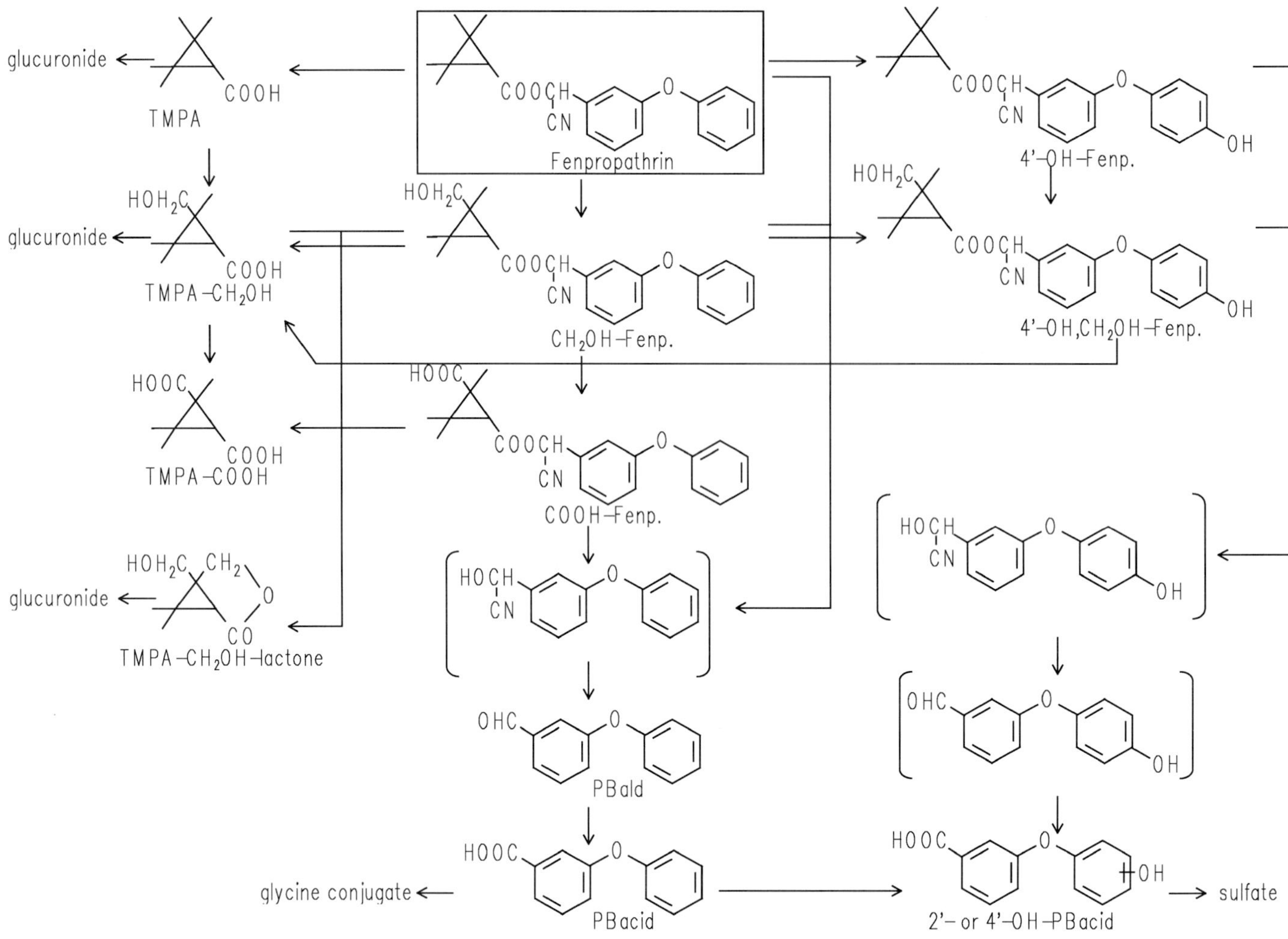

Figure 58.11 Metabolic pathways of fenpropathrin in animals.

rats and 88–89% in mice (Kaneko *et al.*, 1981a; Ohkawa *et al.*, 1979).

Single oral administration of ^{14}C-acid- and ^{14}C-alcohol (ring)-fenvalerate to beagle dogs resulted in rapid ^{14}C elimination from the animal bodies. Major ^{14}C excretion routes were the urine and feces. The ^{14}C recovery was 87% (55.5 and 31.6% in the feces and urine) and 79% (42.3 and 36.8% in the feces and urine) 3 days after oral administration of the acid- and alcohol-labeled preparations, respectively (Kaneko *et al.*, 1984a).

^{14}C tissue residue levels 6 or 7 days after administration of ^{14}C-labeled preparations to both sexes of rats and mice were determined. With the preparations of fenvalerate and its (2S) isomer labeled in the acid and alcohol moieties except for the CN group, the residue level in the fat was relatively higher in rats and mice, whereas the residue levels in other tissues, including blood, hair, liver, kidney, and skin, were low. However, administration of the CN-labeled preparations resulted in somewhat higher tissue residues, in general, compared with other labeled preparations. Higher residues were especially found in the hair, skin, stomach, blood, and fat, and it was found

that most of these residues was due to retention of SCN ion. The ^{14}C levels in these tissues were lower in mice than in rats.

Fenvalerate underwent the following major metabolic reactions (Fig. 61.12); hydroxylation at 4′-phenoxy position of the alcohol moiety and C-2 and C-3 positions of the acid moiety, cleavage of the ester linkage, conversion of the CN group to SCN ion and CO_2, and conjugation of the resulting carboxylic acids, phenols, and alcohols with glucuronic acid, sulfuric acid, and/or glycine.

With the alcohol moiety, the following apparent species differences were observed between dogs and rodents such as rats and mice: (1) hydroxylation at both the 2′- and 4′-positions of the alcohol moiety occurred in rats and mice, but only at the 4′-position in dogs; (2) PBalc and 4′-OH-PBalc from the alcohol moiety were obtained from dogs to a considerable extent, but were not detected in rats or mice; (3) PBacid–glycine was found to a larger extent in dogs than in rats or mice. There were also the following remarkable species differences, particularly in the major conjugates of the alcohol moiety: PBacid–glycine was predominant in dogs, 4′-OH-PBacid–sulfate in rats, and

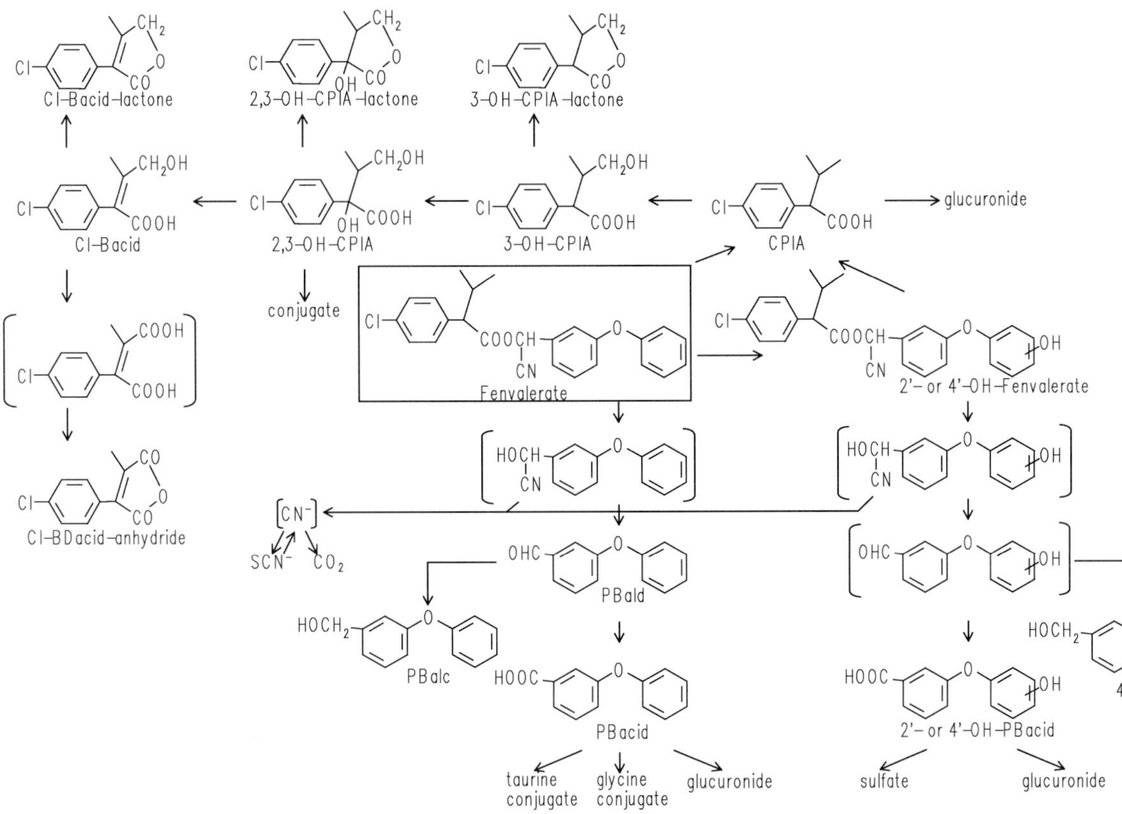

Figure 58.12 Metabolic pathways of fenvalerate in animals.

PBacid–taurine in mice (Kaneko *et al.*, 1981a; Ohkawa *et al.*, 1979).

A comparative metabolism study of the four optical isomers of fenvalerate was carried out. The ^{14}C-labeled preparations of the four isomers labeled in the acid moiety were administered to rats and mice, out of the four isomers, only the $(2R, \alpha S)$ isomer produced cholesterol ester conjugate, which is an ester of the acid moiety 2-(4-chlorophenyl)isovaleric acid (CPIA) of the $(2R, \alpha S)$ isomer and cholesterol. This metabolite was found in relatively larger amounts in spleen, lymph node, adrenal, and liver tissues than other tissues. This conjugate was demonstrated to be formed by transesterification reaction, not by any of three known pathways of cholesterol ester biosynthesis (acyl-coA: cholesterol o-acyltransferase (ACAT), lecithin: cholesterol o-acyltransferase (LCAT), and cholesterol esterase), and to be a causative agent of granulomatous changes which were caused by long-term or subacute administration of fenvalerate, but not by esfenvalerate (Kaneko *et al.*, 1986a, 1988; Miyamoto *et al.*, 1986; Okuno *et al.*, 1986). In addition, a comparative metabolism study of fenvalerate and esfenvalerate was carried out and the results showed that there was no significant differences in metabolism between fenvalerate and esfenvalerate except for formation of a cholesterol ester conjugate from fenvalerate and that the other three isomers of fenvalerate did not seem to affect the absorption, excretion, distribution (including placentral transfer), and biotransformation of esfenvalerate (Isobe *et al.*, 1990; Shiba *et al.*, 1990).

58.13 FLUCYTHRINATE

Chemical Name (RS)-α-Cyano-3-phenoxybenzyl (S)-2-(4-difluoromethoxyphenyl)-3-methylbutyrate.

Synonyms Flucythrinate (BSI, ISO, ANSI) is the common name in use. Trade names are Cybolt, Cythrin, Fluent, and Pay-Off. Code designations include AC 222705 and CL222705. The CAS registry number is 70124-77-5.

Physical and Chemical Properties The empirical formula is $C_{26}H_{23}F_2NO_4$; molecular weight is 451.4. Its form is a dark amber viscous liquid; its specific gravity is 1.189 at 22°C; $\log K_{ow} = 6.8$. It is less soluble (0.5 mg/l) in water at 21°C, but is soluble in most organic solvents. It is unstable in alkaline conditions.

Metabolism Flucythrinate is the same as fenvalerate in terms of chemical structure except for substitution of the benzene ring of the acid moiety: chlorine atom for fenvalerate and the difluoromethoxy group for flucythrinate. When ^{14}C-preparations of flucythrinate labeled in the acid or alcohol moiety were administered to rats at 19.7 mg/kg, ^{14}C was excreted into urine (20–30%) and feces (70–73%).

The major metabolic reactions (Fig. 58.13) are cleavage of ester linkage and oxidation at the *gem*-dimethyl groups of the acid moiety and the $4'$-position of the alcohol moi-

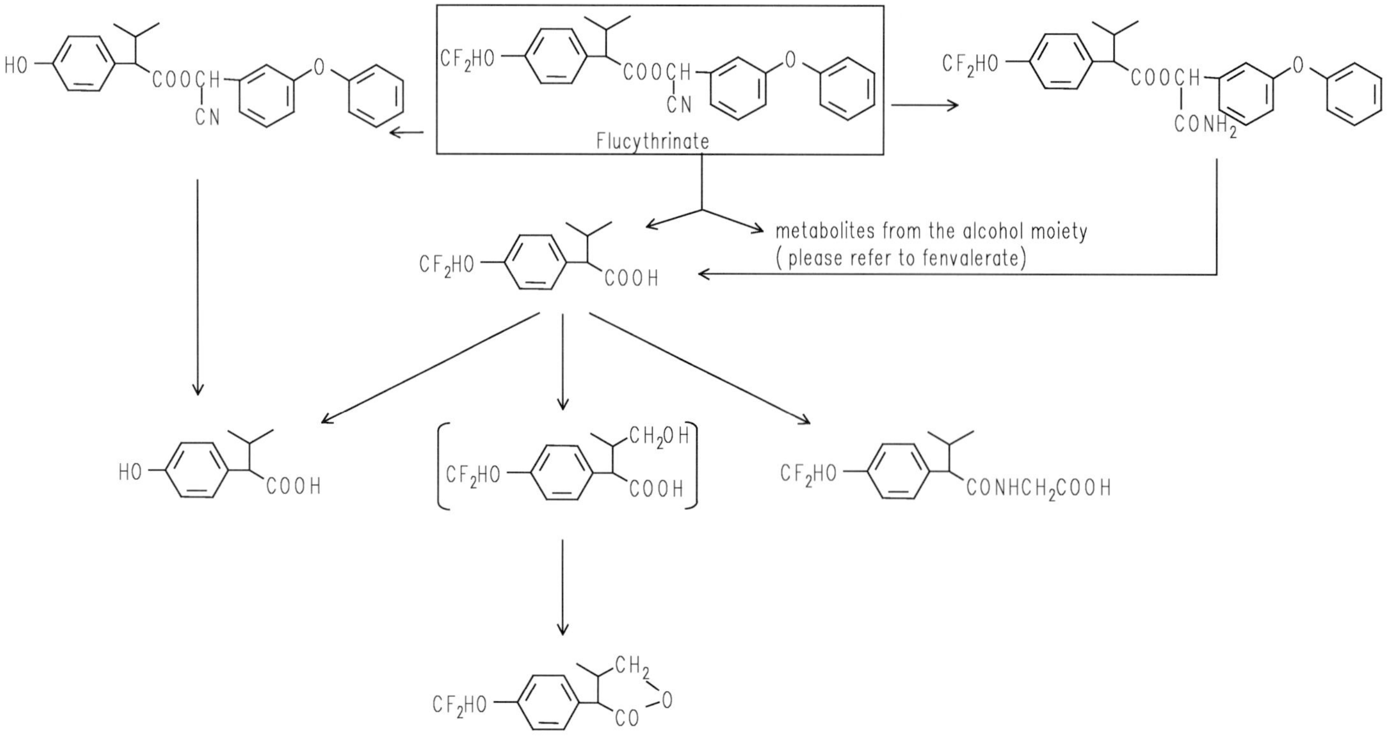

Figure 58.13 Metabolic pathways of flucythrinate in animals.

ety. In addition, de-difluoromethylation takes place. The major metabolites from the alcohol moiety are the same as those from fenvalerate and the major metabolite from the acid moiety is 2-(4-difluoromethoxyphenyl)-3-methylbutyric acid (FAO/WHO, 1985).

58.14 FLUMETHRIN

Chemical Name (RS)-α-Cyano-4-fluoro-3-phenoxybenzyl 3-(β,4-dichlorostyryl)-2,2-dimethylcyclopropanecarboxylate.

Synonyms Flumethrin (BAN) is the common name in use. Trade names are Bayticol and Bayvarol. Code designations include BAY VI6045, and BAY Vq1950. The CAS registry number is 69770-45-2.

Physical and Chemical Properties The empirical formula is $C_{28}H_{22}Cl_2FNO_3$; molecular weight is 510.4. Its form is a yellowish and highly viscous oil; log $K_{ow} = 6.2$. It is less soluble (0.001 mg/l) in water at 20°C, but is soluble in most organic solvents.

Metabolism When ^{14}C-flumethrin labeled in the acid moiety was administered to rats at 1–5 mg/kg, absorption was rapid, but incomplete. The maximum ^{14}C levels in plasma were obtained in about 8 hr after administration.

The major urinary metabolites are 3-(2-chloro-2-(4-chloro-phenyl)ethenyl)-2,2-dimethylcyclopropanecarboxylic acid (flumethrin acid) and its glucuronide from the acid moiety, and

4-fluoro-3-phenoxybenzoic acid (FPBacid), 4′-OH-FPBacid, and their glycine conjugates from the alcohol moiety. The major fecal metabolites were unchanged flumethrin and flumethrin acid.

The major metabolic reactions (Fig. 61.14) of flumethrin are ester hydrolysis and oxidation of the 4′-position of the alcohol moiety (FAO/WHO, 1996).

58.15 τ-FLUVALINATE (FLUVALINATE)

Chemical Name (RS)-α-Cyano-3-phenoxybenzyl N-(2-chloro-α,α,α-trifluoro-p-tolyl)-D-valine; fluvalinate is (RS)-α-cyano-3-phenoxybenzy N-(2-chloro-α,α,α-trifluoro-p-tolyl)-DL-valine.

Synonyms τ-Fluvalinate (BSI, ISO) is the common name in use. Trade names are Mavrik and Klartan. Code designations include SAN5271. The CAS registry numbers are 102851-06-9 for τ-fluvalinate and 69409-94-5 for fluvalinate.

Physical and Chemical Properties The empirical formula is $C_{26}H_{22}ClF_3N_2O_3$; molecular weight is 502.93. Its form is a viscous amber oil; its specific gravity is 1.26 at 25°C; log $K_{ow} = 4.26$ or 6.4. It is less soluble (<0.001 mg/l) in water at 25°C, but is soluble in most organic solvents. It is unstable to light and in alkaline medium.

Metabolism The metabolism of fluvalinate has been extensively studied with the ^{14}C-preparation labeled in the acid moi-

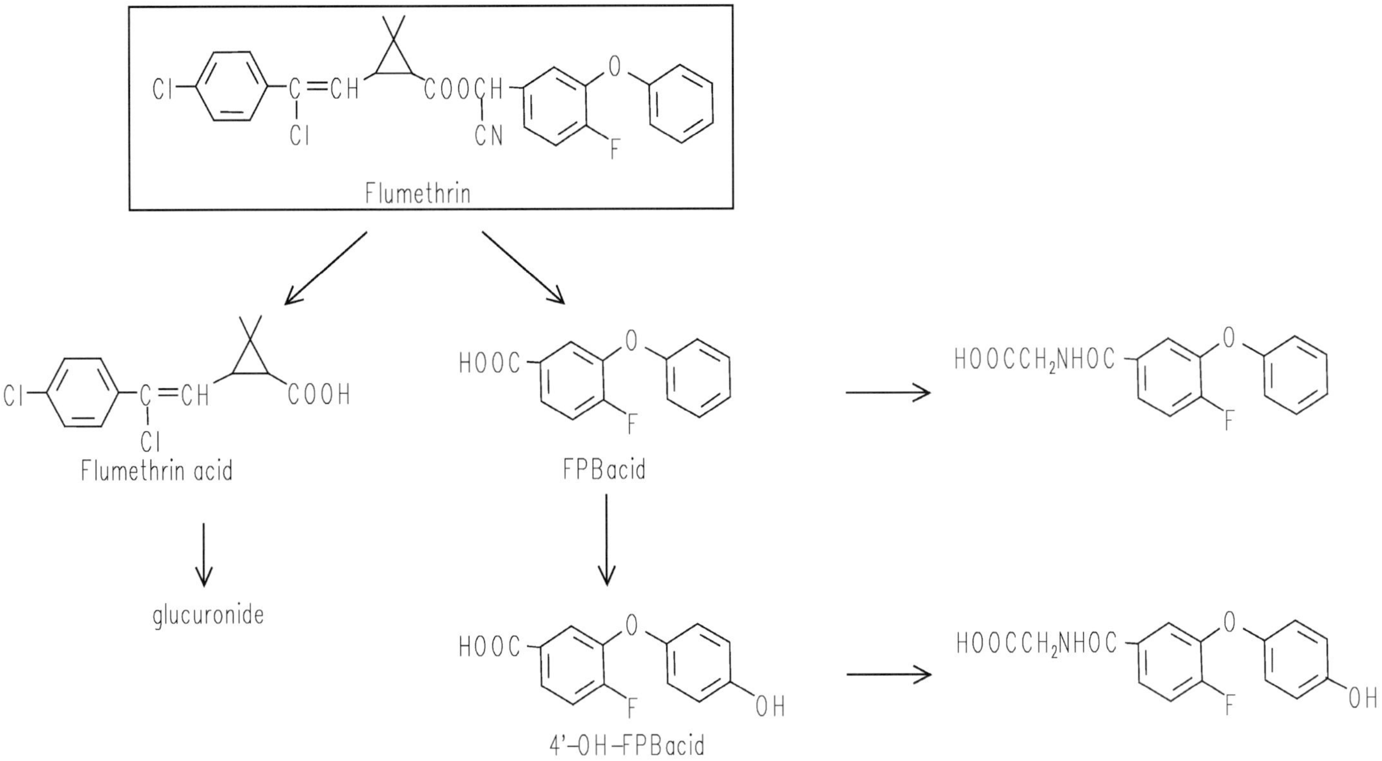

Figure 58.14 Metabolic pathways of flumethrin in animals.

ety. When fluvalinate labeled with ^{14}C in the acid moiety was administered to rats at 1 mg/kg, ^{14}C was rapidly excreted into urine (9–19%) and feces (75–88%) within 4 days after administration. The major ^{14}C component (45% of the fecal ^{14}C) was the parent compound. Liver showed relatively higher ^{14}C tissue residue than other tissues, indicating that the ^{14}C tissue residues from fluvalinate are somewhat different from those of other pyrethroids having the same alcohol moiety. The major metabolic pathways (Fig. 58.15) are cleavage of ester linkage and oxidation at the acid and alcohol moieties. Ester hydrolysis leads to formation of anilino acid. The anilino acid is further conjugated with amino acids (glycine, serine, threonine, and valine), bile acids (cholic, taurochoric, and taurochenodeoxycholic), and glycerols (oleoyl- and linoleoylglycerol). In addition, an amide derivative of anilino acid was found. These conjugation reactions of anilino acid with bile acid (cholic acid, taurocholic acid, and taurochenodeoxycholic acid) and with glycerol and monoglycerides have rarely been reported as conjugates with xenobiotics (Quistad et al., 1982, 1983).

The major urinary metabolites are anilino acid, its hydroxymethyl derivative, its glycine conjugate, haloaniline, and sulfate conjugate of hydroxyhaloaniline. On the other hand, the major fecal metabolites are anilino acid, its amide derivative, and several conjugates of anilino acid with several endogenous components. An unexpected difference between fluvalinate and other pyrethroids is the minimal amount of hydroxylation at the 4′-position of the alcohol moiety. Thus 4′-hydroxy-

fluvalinate is a very minor fecal metabolite, whereas the amount of 4′-hydroxylated parent compound is significant for other pyrethroids, that is, 4′-hydroxy-deltamethrin and 4′-hydroxy-cypermethrin (Quistad et al., 1982, 1983).

When ^{14}C-fluvalinate labeled in the alcohol moiety was orally administered to rats, the alcohol moiety showed metabolic fates similar to those of pyrethroids having α-cyano-3-phenoxybenzyl alcohol (Staiger and Quistad, 1984).

When ^{14}C-acid-fluvalinate was administered to rhesus monkeys at 1 mg/kg, the ^{14}C was excreted into urine (37%) and feces (55%) within 5 days after administration. The major metabolites found were anilino acid as its hydroxymethyl derivatives and glucuronide. There are several species differences between rats and monkeys: (1) glucuronide conjugation of anilino acid is a major metabolic pathway in rhesus monkeys, whereas little or no glucuronides are detected in rats; (2) conjugation with bile acids is a significant reaction in rats, but it is only a very minor process in rhesus monkeys; and (3) conjugation with glycerol and monoglycerides occurs in rats, but is not detected in rhesus monkeys (Quistad and Selim, 1983).

58.16 IMIPROTHRIN

Chemical Name 2,5-Dioxo-3-(2-prop-2-ynyl)imidazolidin-1-ylmethyl (1R)-cis,trans-2,2-dimethyl-3-(2-methylprop-1-enyl)cyclopropanecarboxylate.

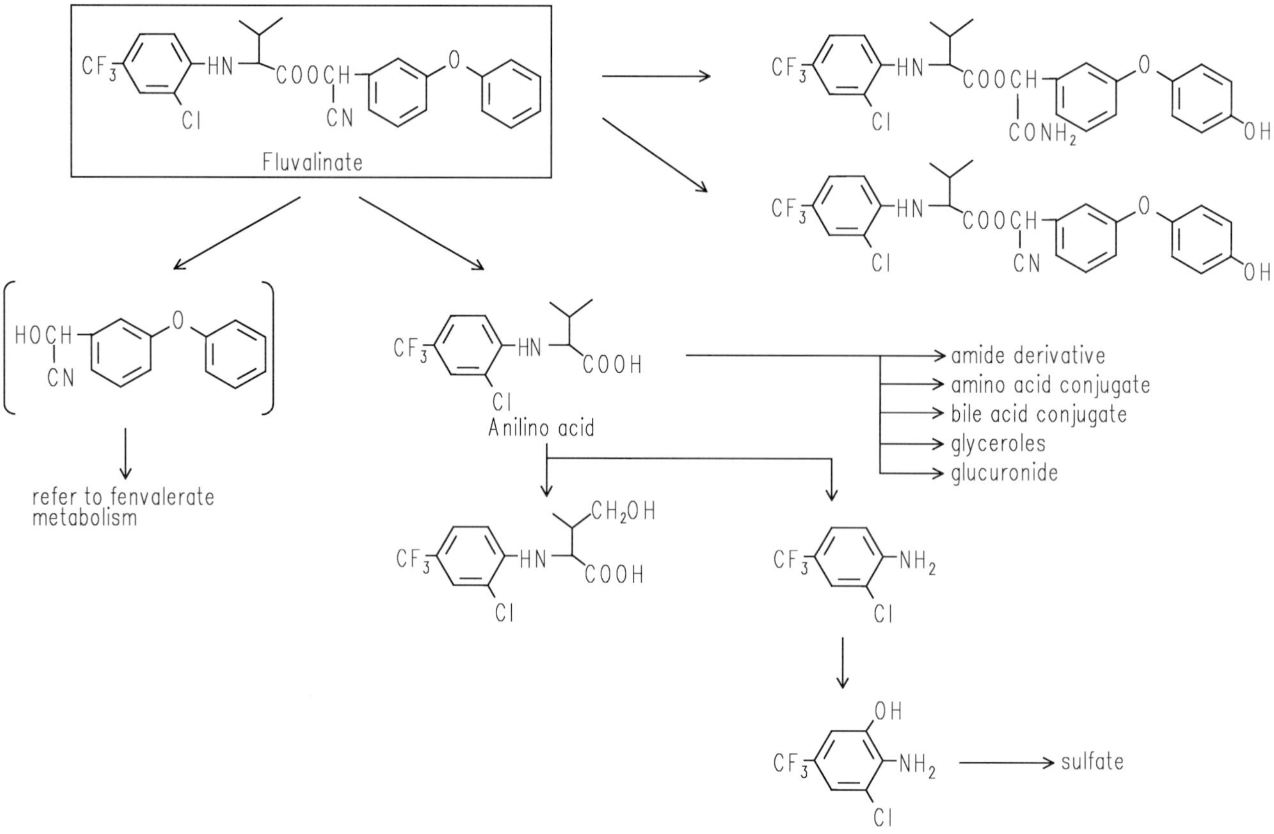

Figure 58.15 Metabolic pathways of fluvalinate in animals.

Synonyms Imiprothrin (BSI, ISO) is the common name in use. Code designations include S-4056F and S-41311. The trade name is Pralle. The CAS registry number is 72963-72-5.

Physical and Chemical Properties The empirical formula is $C_{17}H_{22}N_2O_4$; molecular weight is 318.4. Its form is a viscous liquid; its specific gravity is 1.1 at 20°C; log $K_{ow} = 2.9$. It is less soluble (93.5 mg/l) in water at 25°C, but is soluble in most organic solvents.

Metabolism When ^{14}C-(1R)-trans- or (1R)-cis-imiprothrin labeled in the alcohol moiety was administered orally to rats at 1 or 200 mg/kg, the ^{14}C was rapidly and almost completely eliminated from rats within 7 days after administration (98–103% of the dosed ^{14}C). The urinary ^{14}C-excretion was 83–97%, whereas the fecal excretion was 16% or less. The urinary excretion of ^{14}C for the *trans* isomer was slightly larger (89–97%) than that for the *cis* isomer (83–91%). ^{14}C-excretion into the expired air was less than 3%. ^{14}C tissue residues on the 7th day after administration were generally low in all of the dosed group. There were no marked sex-related differences in the rate of ^{14}C-excretion and the ^{14}C-tissue residues between either treatment group (Saito *et al.*, 1996).

The major metabolic reactions (Fig. 58.16) of *trans*- and *cis*-imiprothrin in rats are (1) cleavage of the ester linkage,

(2) cleavage of the imidomethylene linkage, (3) hydroxylation of the imidazolidine ring, (4) dealkylation of the 2-propynyl group, and (5) oxidation at the *trans*-methyl group in the isobutenyl side chain (Saito *et al.*, 1995). The major urinary metabolites were 2,4-dioxo-1-(2-propynyl)-imidazolidine (PGH), PGH-OH, and hydantoin (HYD) from the *trans* isomer and these ester-cleaved metabolites and metabolites with intact ester linkage from the *cis* isomer.

58.17 KADETHRIN (RU15525)

Chemical Name 5-benzyl-3-furylmethyl (E)-(1R)-cis-2,2-dimethyl-3-(2-oxothiolan-3-ylidenemethyl) cyclopropane-carboxylate.

Synonyms Kadethrin (kadethrine) is the common name in use and is also the trade name. Code designations include RU 15525. The CAS registry number is 58769-20-3.

Physical and Chemical Properties The empirical formula is $C_{23}H_{24}O_4S$; molecular weight is 396.5. Its form is a yellow-brown viscous oil; log $K_{ow} = 5.4$. It is practically insoluble in water, but is soluble in most organic solvents. It is unstable to light and in alkaline medium.

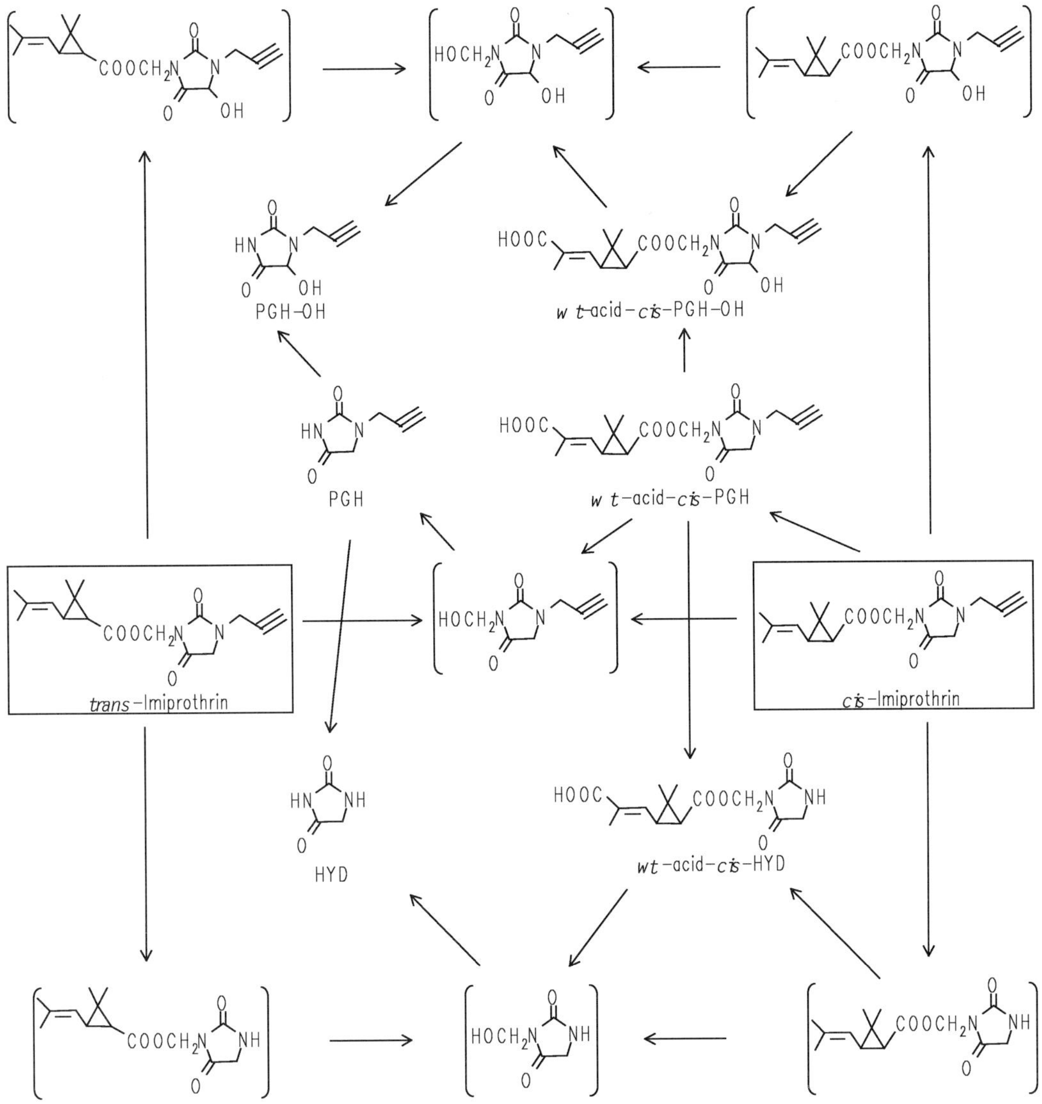

Figure 58.16 Metabolic pathways of imiprothrin in animals.

Metabolism The acid moiety of kadethrin is unique in terms of chemical structure and the alcohol moiety is the same as that of resmethrin. The metabolism of kadethrin has been studied after oral administration of ^{14}C-labeled preparations in the acid or alcohol moiety to rats. The ^{14}C from the acid and alcohol moieties was rapidly and completely excreted into urine and feces (Ohsawa and Casida, 1980).

The major metabolic reactions (Fig. 58.17) are cleavage of the ester linkage and oxidation at the acid and alcohol moieties. The alcohol moiety after ester hydrolysis is further metabolized as shown in the studies with resmethrin (Miyamoto *et al.*, 1971). The acid moiety initially undergoes hydrolysis of the thiolactone ring, and the resulting mercaptan derivative is oxidized directly to a sulfonic acid or is first methylated before oxidation to a methyl sulfoxide and then a methyl sulfone. Hydroxylation reactions and thiolactone hydrolysis also occur on the intact molecule (Ohsawa and Casida, 1980).

58.18 PERMETHRIN

Chemical Name 3-Phenoxybenzyl (1*RS*)-*cis-trans*-3-(2,2-dichlorovinyl)-2,2-dimethylcyclopropanecarboxylate.

Synonyms Permethrin (BSI, ISO, ANSI, ESA, BAN) is the common name in use. There are many trade names, such as Adion, Ambush, Assithrin, Cliper, Coopex, Corsair, Dragnet, Dragon, and Eksmin. Code designations include S-3151, PP 557, FMC 33297, NRDC143, WL43479, and LE79-519. The CAS registry number is 52645-53-1.

Physical and Chemical Properties The empirical formula is $C_{21}H_{20}Cl_2O_3$; molecular weight is 391.3. Its form is a pale yellow-brown liquid; its specific gravity is 1.19–1.27 at 20°C; log $K_{ow} = 6.1$. It is less soluble (ca. 0.2 mg/l) in water at 20°C, but is soluble in most organic solvents. It is more stable in acid medium than in alkaline medium.

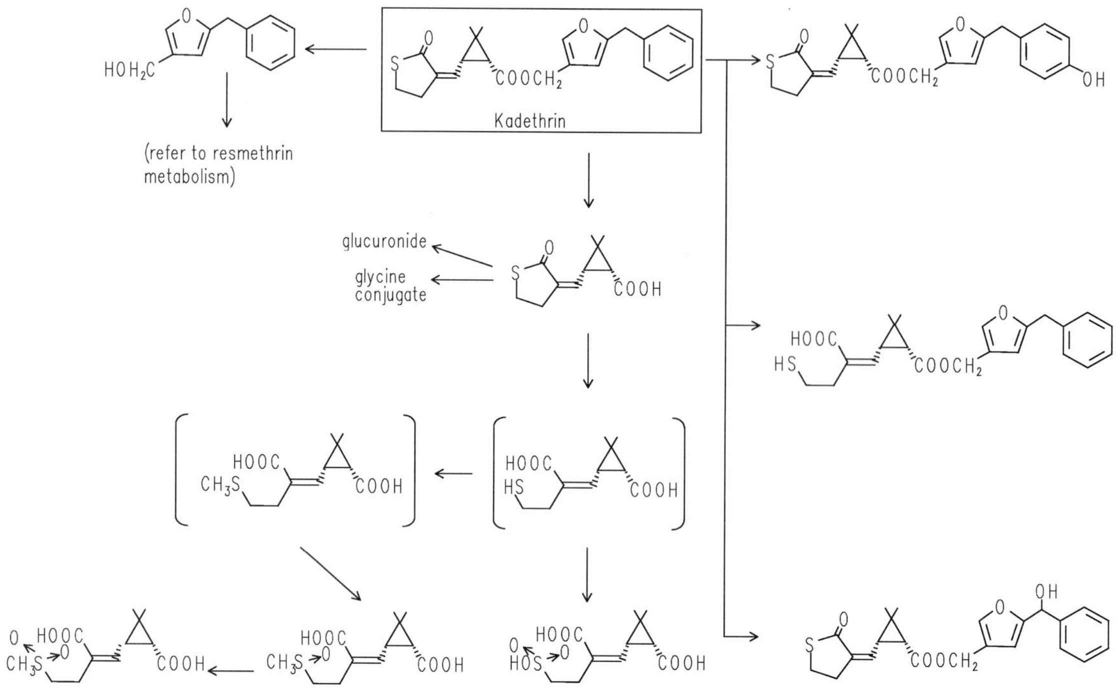

Figure 58.17 Metabolic pathways of kadethrin in animals.

Metabolism The metabolism of permethrin has been studied in detail in a wide variety of animals *in vivo* and *in vitro* (rats, cows, hens, and goats). However, the *in vivo* metabolism data relating to mammalian toxicology are limited to rats.

When the four ^{14}C-preparations of (1RS)-*trans*-, (1R)-*trans*-, (1RS)-*cis*, and (1R)-*cis*-permethrin labeled in the alcohol and acid moieties were administered orally to male rats at 1.6–4.8 mg/kg, the compounds were rapidly metabolized and the ^{14}C from the acid and alcohol moiety was almost completely eliminated from the body within a few days. The ^{14}C from the *cis* isomer was excreted into the urine and feces almost equally, whereas more than 80% of the dosed ^{14}C from the *trans* isomer appeared in the urine. The ^{14}C tissue residues were very low although the fat with the *cis* isomer showed relatively higher residue levels (Elliott *et al.*, 1976; Gaughan *et al.*, 1977).

The major metabolic reactions (Fig. 58.18) of both permethrin isomers were oxidation at the *trans* and *cis* positions of the *gem*-dimethyl group of the acid moiety and at the 2'- and 4'-positions of the alcohol moiety, ester cleavage, and the conjugation of the resulting carboxylic acids, alcohols, and phenols with glucuronic acid, glycine, and sulfuric acid. The *cis* isomer is more stable than the *trans* isomer, and the *cis* isomer yielded four fecal ester metabolites which resulted from hydroxylation at the 2'- and 4'-positions of the phenoxy group, at the *trans*-methyl group, and at both of the two latter sites. The ester-cleaved metabolites were extensively excreted into the urine, whereas the metabolites retaining ester linkage were found only in the feces. There were no significant differences in metabolism between the (1RS)-isomers and (1R)-isomers (Elliott *et al.*, 1976; Gaughan *et al.*, 1977).

Rat and mouse liver microsomes hydrolyzed the *trans* isomers more rapidly than the *cis* isomers, however, mouse microsomes oxidized the *cis* isomers more extensively than rat microsomes. The preferential oxidation sites of the alcohol moiety are the 4'-position for rats and the 2'-, 4'-, and 6-positions for mice (Shono *et al.*, 1979; Soderlund and Casida, 1977).

58.19 PHENOTHRIN (*d*-PHENOTHRIN)

Chemical Name 3-phenoxybenzyl (1RS)-*cis-trans*-2,2-dimethyl-3-(2-methylprop-1-enyl)cyclopropanecarboxylate.

d-Phenothrin is a mixture of two isomers [((1R)-*cis*) and ((1R)-*trans*)].

Synonyms Phenothrin (BSI, ISO, BAN) is the common name in use. The trade name is Sumithrin for *d*-phenothrin. Code designations include S-2539 for phenothrin and S-2539 Forte for *d*-phenothrin. The CAS registry number is 26002-80-2.

Physical and Chemical Properties The empirical formula is $C_{23}H_{26}O_3$; molecular weight is 350.5. Its form is a pale yellow to yellow-brown liquid; its specific gravity is 1.06 at 20°C; log $K_{ow} = 7.4$. It is less soluble (0.01 mg/l) in water at 25°C, but is soluble in most organic solvents. It is unstable to light and in alkaline medium.

Metabolism The metabolism of phenothrin was studied in rats after single oral or dermal application of *trans*- and *cis*-phenothrin labeled with ^{14}C in the alcohol moiety at several

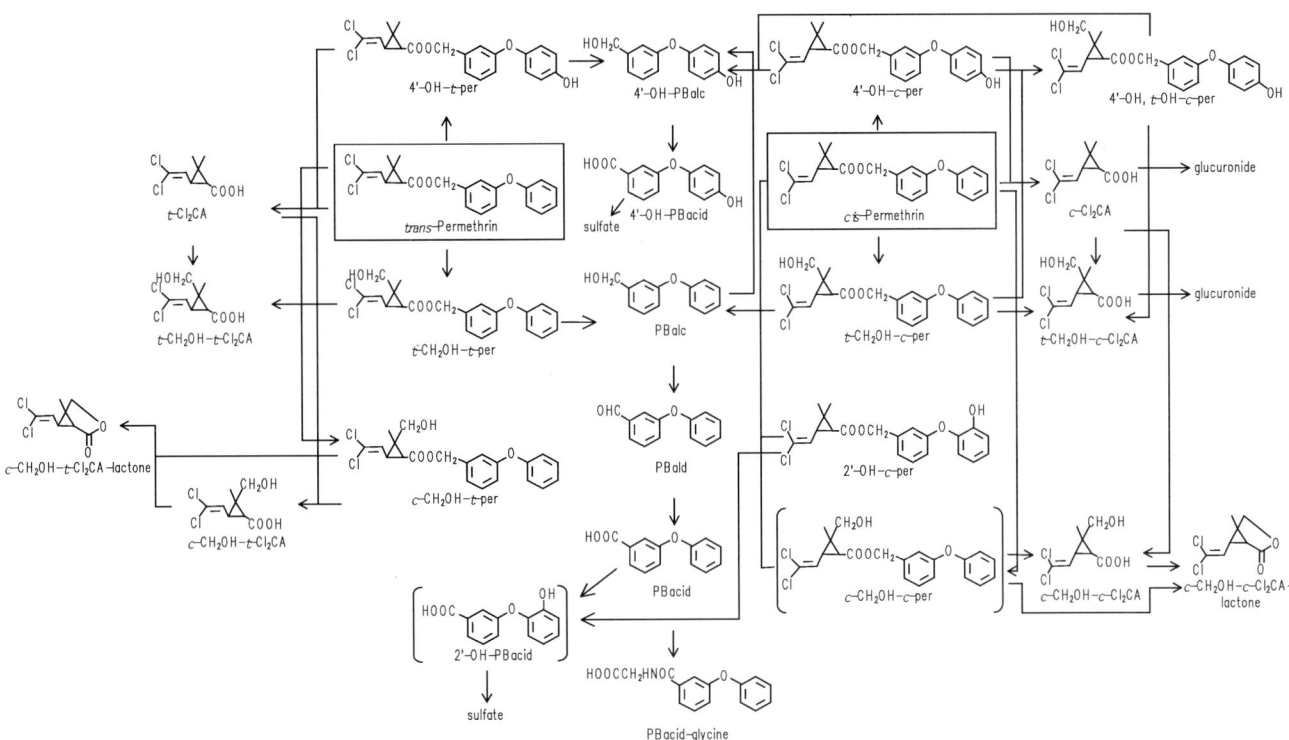

Figure 58.18   Metabolic pathways of permethrin in animals.

doses (Kaneko *et al.*, 1981b; Miyamoto *et al.*, 1974; Suzuki *et al.*, 1976). The major excretion route of ^{14}C was urine for the *trans* isomers, whereas it was feces for the *cis* isomers. The residue levels of ^{14}C were generally very low except in fat, which showed slightly higher residue levels. Dermal absorption rate of ^{14}C was estimated to be 3–17% in rats, depending on the formulation used.

In addition, comparative metabolism of the six isomers [(1R)-*trans*, (1RS)-*trans*, (1S)-*trans*, (1R)-*cis*, (1RS)-*cis*, and (1S)-*cis*] of phenothrin was investigated after single oral administration of ^{14}C-labeled preparation of the six phenothrin isomers to rats and mice at 10 mg/kg (Kaneko *et al.*, 1984c). There were no significant differences in the amount of ^{14}C urinary and fecal excretion between (1R)-*trans* and (1RS)-*trans* isomers or between (1R)-*cis* and (1RS)-*cis* isomers. On the other hand, the (1S)-*trans* and (1S)-*cis* isomers showed slightly larger ^{14}C urinary excretion than the corresponding (1R)- and (1RS)-*trans* and *cis* isomers, respectively (Izumi *et al.*, 1984).

The major metabolic reactions (Fig. 58.19) of the *cis* isomer in both animals were oxidation at the *cis*- and *trans*-methyl of the isobutenyl group, at the *trans*-methyl of the *gem*-dimethyl group attached to the cyclopropane ring and the 4′-position of the alcohol moiety. Hydroxylation at the 2′-position of the alcohol moiety occurred to a smaller extent. On the other hand, with the *trans* isomer, the main metabolic reaction was cleavage of ester linkage. The hydroxylation at the 4′-position of the alcohol moiety occurred with the *trans* isomer to the same degree as that with the *cis* isomer. Moreover, small amounts of the metabolites hydroxylated at the *trans*-methyl of the isobutenyl

group and at the 2′-position of the alcohol moiety were obtained from the *trans* isomer. The species differences observed in phenothrin were as follows: (1) 4′-OH-PBacid–sulfate and PBacid–taurine were characteristic to rats and mice, respectively, as is the case with fenvalerate, deltamethrin, and cypermethrin. (2) All six phenothrin isomers underwent cleavage of the ester linkage and hydroxylation at the 4′-position of the alcohol moiety more rapidly in rats than in mice, and these facts may contribute to the higher urinary ^{14}C excretion in rats than in mice (Izumi *et al.*, 1984; Kaneko *et al.*, 1984b; Miyamoto *et al.*, 1974; Suzuki *et al.*, 1976).

With respect to metabolic reactions, the (1S)-*trans* and (1S)-*cis* isomers underwent ester cleavage to a larger extent than the other chiral isomers in both rats and mice. There were some differences in the extent of oxidation at the 4′-position of the alcohol moiety of phenothrin isomers among three *trans* isomers and among three *cis* isomers. With the *trans* isomers, there was no apparent difference in the extent of hydroxylation at the 4′-position, whereas the (1S)-*cis* isomers underwent hydroxylation to a slightly larger extent compared with the other *cis* isomers. Based on the results, it may be concluded that the (1R) and (1RS) isomers behaved in similar metabolic manners, and that the (1S) isomers received cleavage of the ester linkage slightly more readily than the corresponding (1R) and (1RS) isomers, although the (1S) isomers also received the same metabolic reactions as the (1R) and (1RS) isomers. However, purified carboxyesterase showed virtually no difference in ester hydrolysis between (1R)-*trans* and (1S)-*trans* isomers or between (1R)-*cis* and (1S)-*cis* isomers, although it hydrolyzed

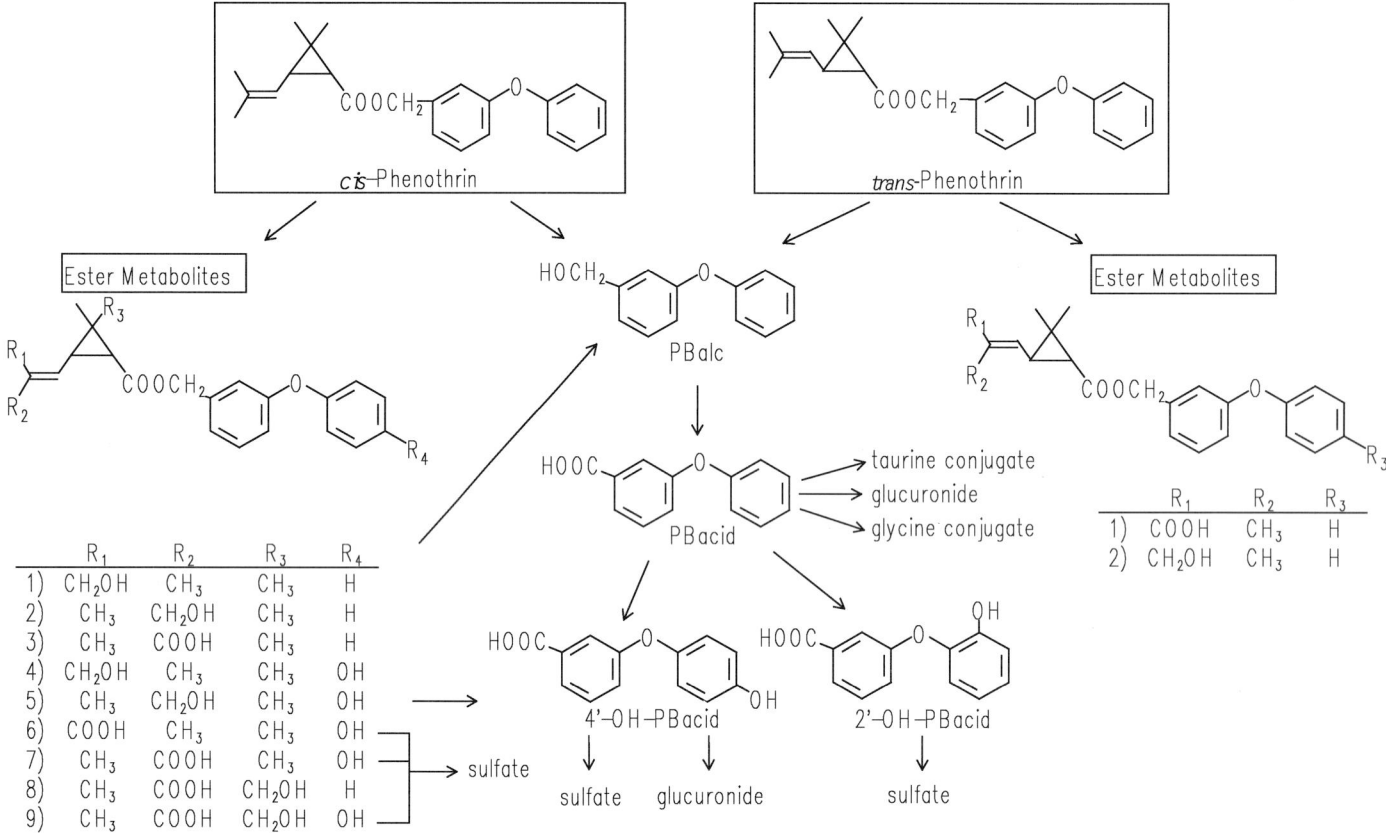

Figure 58.19   Metabolic pathways of phenothrin in animals.

the (1R)-*trans* and (1S)-*trans* isomers more rapidly than the (1R)-*cis* and (1S)-*cis* isomers, respectively (Izumi *et al.*, 1984; Suzuki and Miyamoto, 1978).

58.20 PRALLETHRIN

Chemical Name   (S)-2-Methyl-4-oxo-3-prop-2-ynylcyclopent-2-enyl   (1R)-*cis-trans*-2,2-dimethyl-3-(2-methylprop-1-enyl)cyclopropanecarboxylate.

Synonyms   Prallethrin (BSI, ISO) is the common name in use. The trade name is Etoc. Code designations include S-4068 SF. The CAS registry number is 23031-36-9.

Physical and Chemical Properties   The empirical formula is $C_{19}H_{24}O_3$; molecular weight is 300.4. Its form is a yellow to yellow-brown liquid; its specific gravity is 1.03 at 20°C; $\log K_{ow} = 4.49$. It is less soluble (8 mg/l) in water at 25°C, but is soluble in most organic solvents.

Metabolism   On single oral or subcutaneous administration of (4S,1R)-*trans*- or (4S,1R)-*cis*-prallethrin labeled with ^{14}C in the alcohol moiety to rats at 2 mg/kg, 96–104% of the dosed ^{14}C was eliminated into urine and feces within 7 days after administration. Monitoring of the expired air indicated that less than 0.1% of the dose was excreted as $^{14}CO_2$ (Shiba *et al.*, 1988).

Urinary excretion of ^{14}C with the *trans* isomer was larger (60–78%) than the *cis* isomer (17–32%), whereas ^{14}C fecal excretion with the *trans* isomer was smaller than that with the *cis* isomer. ^{14}C levels in blood and other tissues reached maximum within 3 hr after oral administration and thereafter decreased rapidly. ^{14}C tissue residues were generally very low on the 7th day after administration (Shiba *et al.*, 1988).

Nineteen metabolites were identified in urine and feces (Shiba *et al.*, 1988). Two new types of S-linked conjugation (sulfonic acid and mercapturic acid types) were additionally identified (Tomigahara *et al.*, 1994c).

The major biotransformation reactions (Fig. 58.20) of prallethrin are summarized as follows: (1) oxidation at the methyl group of the isobutenyl group in the acid moiety; (2) hydroxylation at the C-1 or the C-2 position of the propynyl group in alcohol moiety; (3) cleavage of the ester linkage; and (4) conjugation of resulting metabolites with glucuronic acid, sulfuric acid, sulfonic acid, or mercapturic acid.

58.21 PYRETHRINS

Chemical Name   The six known insecticidally active compounds in pyrethrum are esters of two acids and three alcohols. Specifically, pyrethrin I is the pyrethrolone ester of chrysanthemic acid, pyrethrin II is the pyrethrolone ester of pyrethric

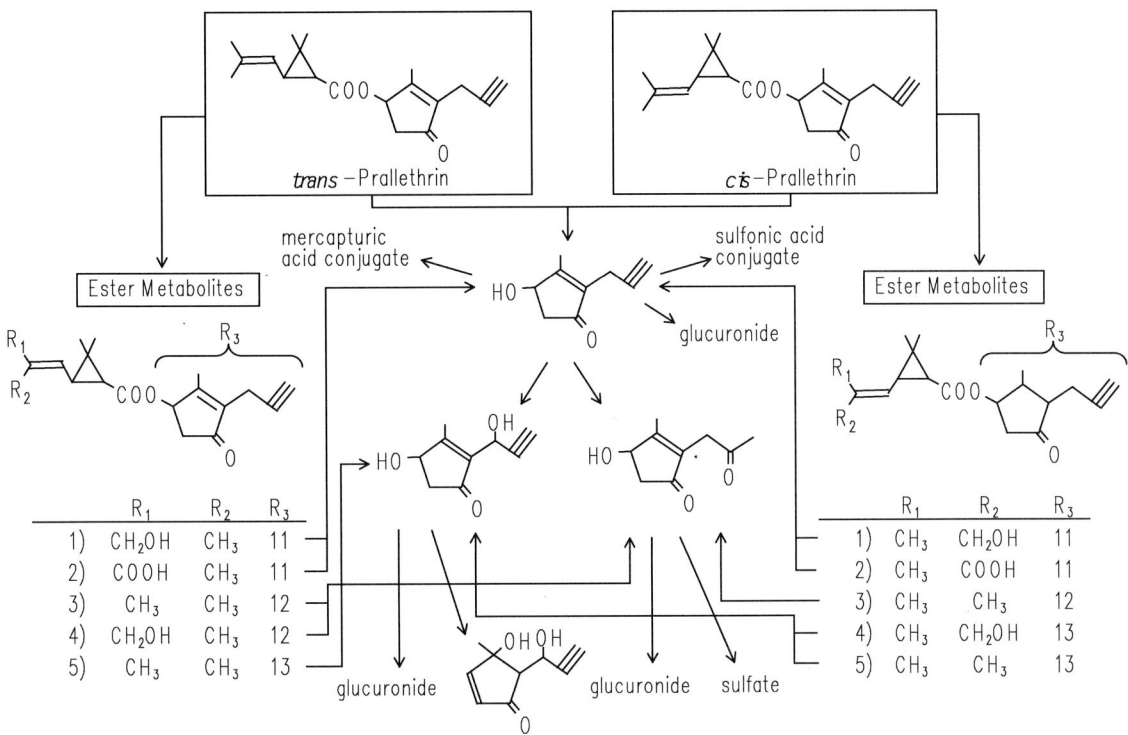

Figure 58.20   Metabolic pathways of prallethrin in animals.

acid, cinerin I is the cinerolone ester of chrysanthemic acid, cinerin II is the cinerolone ester of pyrethric acid, jasmolin I is the jasmolone ester of chrysanthemic acid, and jasmolin II is the jasmolone ester of pyrethric acid.

Synonyms   Pyrethrins (BSI, ISO, JMAF, ESA) is the common name in use. There are several trade names such as Alfadex, Evergreen, and ExciteR. The CAS registry numbers are 121-21-1 (pyrethrin I), 4466-14-2 (jasmolin I), 25402-06-6 (cinerin I), 121-29-9 (pyrethrin II), 1172-63-0 (jasmolin II), and 121-20-0 (cinerin II).

Physical and Chemical Properties   Empirical formulas and molecular weights:

Pyrethrin I	$C_{21}H_{28}O_3$	328.4
Pyrethrin II	$C_{22}H_{28}O_5$	372.4
Cinerin I	$C_{20}H_{28}O_3$	316.4
Cinerine II	$C_{21}H_{28}O_5$	360.4
Jasmolin I	$C_{21}H_{30}O_3$	330.4
Jasmolin II	$C_{22}H_{30}O_5$	374.5

Their forms may be viscous oils or tan dusts; $\log K_{ow} = 5.9$ (pyrethrin I), 4.3 (pyrethrin II). They are practically insoluble in water, but are readily soluble in most organic solvents. They are unstable to light and air.

Metabolism   On single oral administration of pyrethrin I and pyrethrin II labeled with ^{3}H or ^{14}C in the acid or alcohol moiety

to rats and mice at 1–5 mg/kg, the ^{3}H and ^{14}C from both compounds were excreted into urine and feces almost equally. The *trans*-methyl group of the isobutenyl side group of pyrethrin I is readily oxidized to hydroxymethyl derivatives, and further to the corresponding carboxylic acid derivatives through aldehydes. Hydrolyis of the methyl ester of pyrethrin II yields the same acid. This acid is further oxidized at the pentadienyl group of the alcohol moiety, which is probably initiated by epoxidation of the terminal double bond. Hydrolysis of this epoxide resulted in formation of isomeric diols, one of which is conjugated with an unidentified aromatic acid (Elliott *et al.*, 1972).

The major metabolic reactions (Fig. 58.21) of both compounds were hydrolysis of methoxycarbonyl group, oxidation at the *trans*-methyl of the isobutenyl group of the acid moiety, and epoxidation at the pentadienyl side chain to yield initially a 4,5-epoxide from which the two diol derivatives were derived (Casida *et al.*, 1971; Elliott *et al.*, 1972).

58.22 RESMETHRIN (BIORESMETHRIN, CISMETHRIN)

Chemical Name   5-benzyl-3-furylmethyl (1*RS*)-*cis-trans*-3-(2-methylprop-1-enyl)-cyclopropanecarboxylate.

Synonyms   Resmethrin (BSI, ISO, ANSI, JMAF, ESA) is the common name in use. Trade names are Chrysron and Synthrin. Code designations include SBP-1382, NRDC104, and FMC17370. Bioresmethrin and cismethrin are (1*R*)-*trans* and

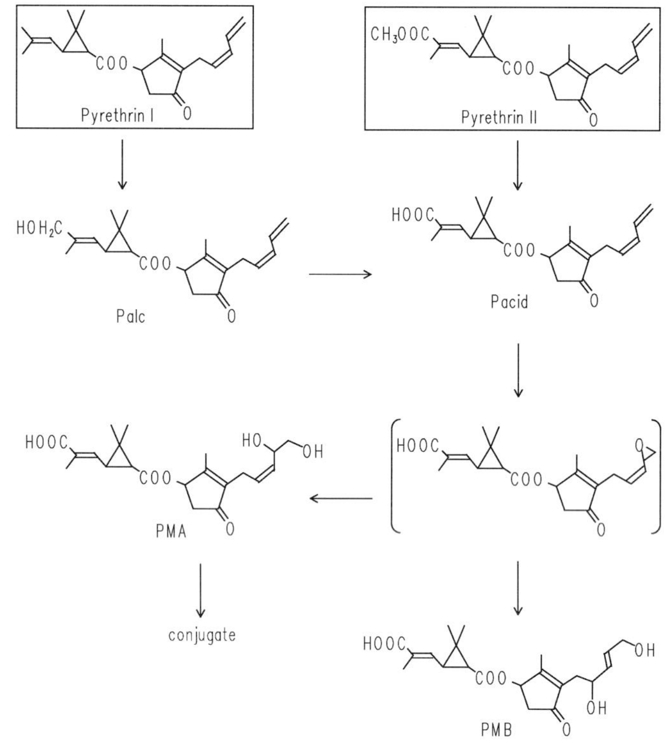

Figure 58.21 Metabolic pathways of pyrethrin in animals.

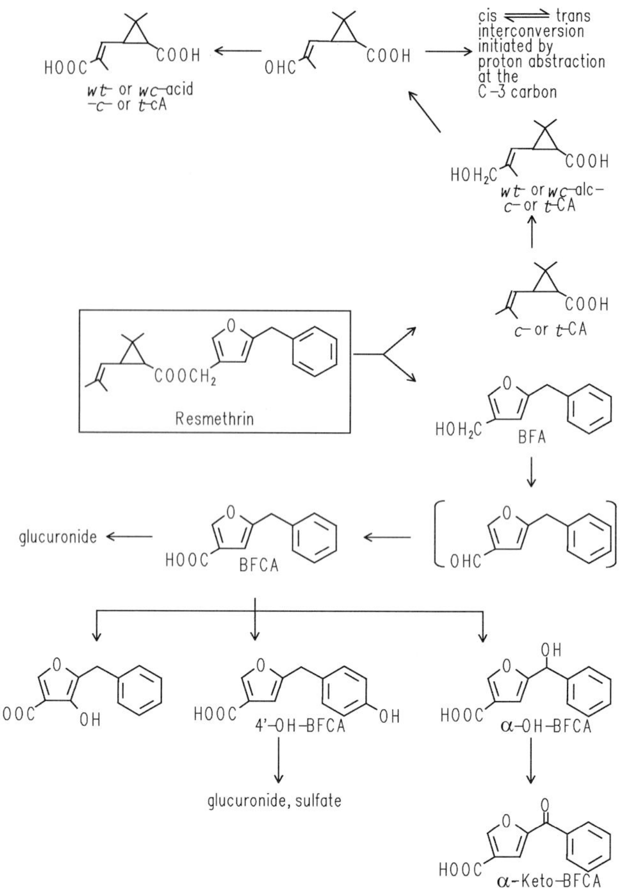

Figure 58.22 Metabolic pathways of resmethrin in animals.

(1R)-*cis* isomers of resmethrin, respectively. The CAS registry number is 10453-86-8.

Physical and Chemical Properties   The empirical formula is $C_{22}H_{26}O_3$; molecular weight is 338.4. Its form is a colorless crystal; its specific gravity is 0.958–0.968 at 20°C; log K_{ow} = 5.43. It is less soluble (0.038 mg/l) in water at 25°C, but is soluble in most organic solvents. It is unstable to air and light.

Metabolism   The metabolism of resmethrin was studied in rats after single oral administration of (1RS,*trans*)-, (1R,*trans*)-, or (1R,*cis*)-resmethrin labeled with ^{14}C in the alcohol or acid moiety (Miyamoto *et al.*, 1986; Ueda *et al.*, 1975a). In addition, *in vitro* studies with mouse and rat liver microsomes have also been carried out to elucidate metabolism of resmethrin in detail (Ueda *et al.*, 1975b). Resmethrin was rapidly metabolized and the ^{14}C from the acid moiety was more rapidly eliminated from the body than that from the alcohol moiety. The major metabolites were 5-benzyl-3-furoic acid (BFCA), 4'-OH-BFCA, and α-OH-BFCA from the alcohol moiety and hydroxymethyl and dicarboxylic acid derivatives of chrysanthemic acid from the acid moiety. Although the *trans*-methyl group of the isobutenyl group was predominantly oxidized in bioresmethrin and cismethrin, the *cis*-methyl group of cismethrin was also oxidized. In addition, epimerization at C-3 of the cyclopropane ring was found, leading to isomerized forms of dicarboxylic acid derivatives of chrysanthemic acid. Bioresmethrin was hydrolyzed

more rapidly in rat liver microsomes than cismethrin, whereas the plasma did not show this *cis–trans* specificity (White *et al.*, 1976).

The major metabolic reactions (Fig. 58.22) of resmethrin are cleavage of the ester linkage, oxidation at the *trans*- and the *cis*-methyl group of the isobutenyl group, at the 4'-position of the benzene ring, and at the benzylic position of the alcohol moiety, and conjugation of the resulting metabolites with glucuronic acid and sulfuric acid.

58.23 TETRAMETHRIN (*d*-TERAMETHRIN)

Chemical   Name   3,4,5,6-Tetrahydrophthalimidomethyl (1RS)-*cis-trans*-chrysanthemate; *d*-tetramethrin is composed of the (1R) isomers.

Synonyms   Tetramethrin (BSI, ISO, ANSI) is the common name in use. Trade names are Neo-Pynamin and Duracide for tetamethrin and Neo-Pynamin Forte, Tedion V-18, Duracide, and Tedone for *d*-tetramethrin. Code designations include SP 1103 and FMC 9260. The CAS registry numbers are 7696-12-0; 51348-90-4 for (1R)-*cis* isomer and 1166-46-7 for (1R)-*trans* isomer.

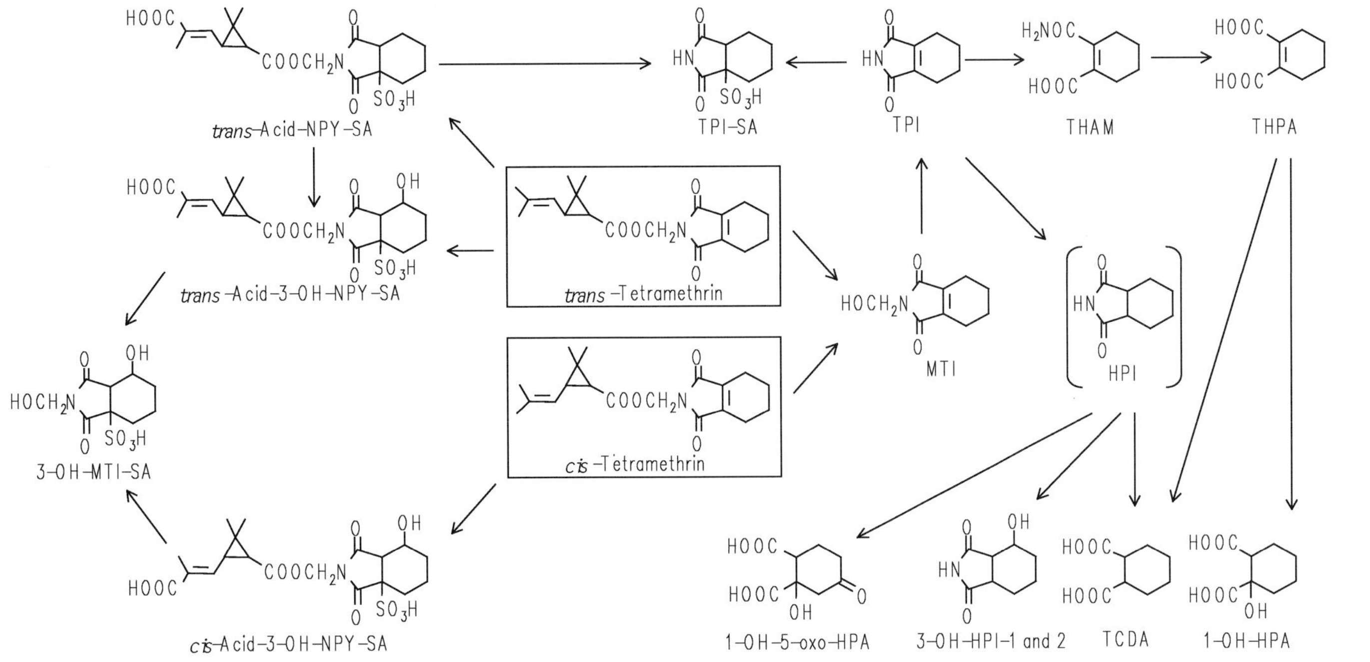

Figure 58.23 Metabolic pathways of tetramethrin in animals.

Physical and Chemical Properties (Tetramethrin) The empirical formula is $C_{19}H_{25}NO_4$; molecular weight is 331.4. Its form is a colorless crystal; its specific gravity is 1.1 at 20°C; its vapor pressure is 0.944 mPa at 30°C; log K_{ow} = 4.6. It is less soluble (1.83 mg/l) in water at 25°C, but is soluble in most organic solvents. It is unstable in strong acid and alkaline medium.

Metabolism *In vivo* and *in vitro* metabolism of this pyrethroid in rats had been reported several times in the 1960s, 1970s, 1980s, and 1990s. The metabolic fates of the alcohol moiety, the tetrahydrophthalimido group, appeared to be completed in the 1990s. On the other hand, the metabolic fate of the acid moiety was the same as that of pyrethroids having chrysanthemic acid such as resmethrin (Kaneko *et al.*, 1981c; Ueda *et al.*, 1975a).

When ^{14}C-(1*RS*)-*trans*- or ^{14}C-(1*RS*)-*cis*-tetramethrin labeled in the alcohol moiety was administered orally to rats at 2 or 250 mg/kg, the ^{14}C was almost completely eliminated from rats within 7 days after administration. ^{14}C recovery in feces and urine was 38–56 and 42–58%, respectively, with the *trans* isomer, and 66–91 and 9–31%, respectively, in feces and urine with the *cis* isomer. Fourteen metabolites were found in excreta. For both isomers the main metabolites were sulfonate derivatives in feces and alcohol derivatives and dicarboxylic acid derivatives derived from the 3,4,5,6-tetrahydrophthalimide moiety in urine. The sulfonic acid conjugates have a sulfonic acid group incorporated into the double bond of the 3,4,5,6-tetrahydrophthalimide moiety. Two of five sulfonic acid conjugates (*trans*-Acid-3-OH-NPY-SA and TPI-SA) were detected in the urine; however, their amounts were smaller than in the feces. In addition, the sulfonic acid conjugates were not detected in the bile or urine of the bile-duct-cannulated rat given ^{14}C-

alcohol-*trans*- or *cis*-tetramethrin. Therefore, it is likely that the sulfonic acid conjugates were produced in the intestinal tract (Tomigahara *et al.*, 1994b).

The major metabolic reactions (Fig. 58.23) of *trans*- and *cis*-tetramethrin in rats were as follows: (1) cleavage of ester linkage; (2) cleavage of the imide likage; (3) hydroxylation of cyclohexene or cyclohexane ring of the 3,4,5,6-tetrahydrophthalimide moiety; (4) oxidation at the methyl group of the isobutenyl moiety of the acid moiety; (5) reduction at the 1,2-double bond of the 3,4,5,6-tetrahydrophthalimide moiety; and (6) incorporation of a sulfonic acid group into the 1,2-double bond of the 3,4,5-6-tetrahydrophthalimide moiety (Kaneko *et al.*, 1981c; Miyamoto *et al.*, 1968; Tomigahara *et al.*, 1994a, b, 1996).

The ^{14}C was rapidly and almost completely excreted into the urine and feces after a single oral dose of each of the ^{14}C-(1*R*)-*trans*, (1*RS*)-*trans*, (1*R*)-*cis*, and (1*RS*)-*cis* isomers labeled in the acid moiety to pregnant rats at 300 mg/kg. The ^{14}C from both the *trans* isomers was excreted into the urine to a larger extent than the feces. There were no statistical differences in the ^{14}C excretion between both the *trans* isomers. The ^{14}C derived from both the *cis* isomers was almost completely eliminated from rat body for 7 days as with the *trans* isomers. However, significant differences were observed in the excretion of the ^{14}C into the urine and feces between the (1*R*)- and (1*RS*)-*cis* isomers. There were no appreciable differences in ^{14}C tissue residues and the nature of metabolites between the (1*R*)- and (1*RS*)-*cis* isomers, although there were significant differences in absorption in the gastrointestinal tissues between these isomers. From these findings, once entered into the bloodstream, the (1*R*)- and (1*RS*)-*cis* isomers apparently undergo the same metabolic reactions. Overall there seems to be no significant

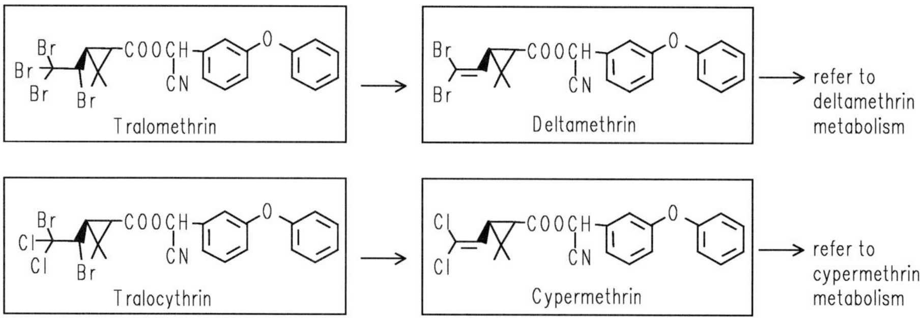

Figure 58.24

differences in the metabolic reactions between the *trans* isomers and between the *cis* isomers. The nature and amounts of the metabolites detected in the fetus with Neo-Pynamin [a mixture of (1*RS*)-isomers] and Neo-Pynamin Forte [a mixture of (1*S*)-isomers] were nearly the same, indicating that these two compounds behaved in the same way to give the same placental transfer regardless of their optical differences (Kaneko *et al.*, 1984b).

58.24 TRALOMETHTIN

Chemical Name (*S*)-α-Cyano-3-phenoxybenzyl (1*R*)-*cis*-2, 2-dimethyl-3-[(*RS*)-1,2,2,2-tetrabromoethyl] cyclopropanecarboxylate.

Synonyms Tralomethrin (BSI, ANSI, ISO) is the common name in use. Trade names are Saga, Scout, Tralox, Tracker, and Tralate. Code designations include RU 25474, NU831, and HAG 107. The CAS registry number is 66841-25-6.

Physical and Chemical Properties The empirical formula is $C_{22}H_{19}Br_4NO_3$; molecular weight is 665.0. Its form is an orange to yellow resinous solid; its specific gravity is 1.70 at 20°C; log K_{ow} is about 5. It is less soluble (0.080 mg/l) in water at 25°C, but is soluble in most organic solvents.

Metabolism A comparative metabolism study has been carried out on the fate of tralomethrin and deltamethrin in male rats after single oral administration of ^{14}C-tralomethrin and ^{14}C-deltamethrin labeled in the acid moiety, the alcohol moiety, and the CN group at 0.3–0.5 mg/kg (Cole *et al.*, 1982). Tralomethrin was not normally detected in the treated animals or their excreta because it undergoes rapid and substantially complete debromination to form deltamethrin. After formation of deltamethrin, this compound appears to undergo the same metabolic fate of deltamethrin (Fig. 58.24). Similarly, tralocythrin was rapidly converted to (1*R*, α*S*)-*cis*-cypermethrin by debromination as is the case with tralomethrin (Cole *et al.*, 1982). The debromination was mediated by tissue thiols such as glutathione (Kaneko *et al.*, 1986b; Ruzo *et al.*, 1981).

58.25 SUMMARY

All the pyrethroid insecticides investigated so far are rapidly metabolized in mammals and their metabolites are almost completely excreted in the urine and feces within several days of a single oral or subcutaneous administration except their cyano moiety. Tissue residues are generally very low, showing that they are biodegradable and nonbioaccumulative (Miyamoto *et al.*, 1995). This is due partly to rapid metabolism. The major metabolic reactions of pyrethroids are commonly oxidation of methyl groups and aromatic rings in the molecules, hydrolysis of the ester linkage, and several types of conjugation reactions. With respect to cleavage of the ester linkage, there are significant differences between geometrical *trans* and *cis* isomers. The *trans* isomers of pyrethroids having chrysanthemic acid derivatives in the acid moiety such as phenothrin and permethrin are more rapidly hydrolyzed than the corresponding *cis* isomers, and the *cis* isomers yield more metabolites retaining intact ester linkage than the *trans* isomers (Casida and Ruzo, 1980; Leahey, 1985; Miyamoto, 1976, 1981; Ruzo and Casida, 1977). With respect to oxidation, the *trans*-methyl of the isobutenyl group in chrysanthemates is oxidized preferentially to the *cis*-methyl group, and the 4′-position of the phenoxy ring in the phenoxybenzyl derivatives is more readily oxidized than all other positions. Conjugation reactions of pyrethroids include hydrophilic conjugations with glucuronic acid, sulfuric acid, and amino acids and lipophilic conjugations with cholesterol, bile acid, and triglyceride. The optical isomers of pyrethroids do not show significant differences in metabolism reactions, except that only one isomer of the four optical isomers of fenvalerate produces the cholesterol ester conjugate.

Although human data are very limited, there seems to be substantially no remarkable species difference in metabolism between laboratory animals and human beings. Ester hydrolysis and oxidation reaction seem to be major metabolic reactions in human beings for pyrethroids.

REFERENCES

Casida, J. E., and Ruzo, L. O. (1980). Metabolic chemistry of pyrethroid insecticides. *Pestic. Sci.* **11**, 257–269.

Casida, J. E., Kimmel, E. C., Elliott, M., and Janes, N. F. (1971). Oxidative metabolism of pyrethrins in mammals. *Nature* **230**, 326–327.

Chamberlain, K., Matsuo, N., Kaneko, H., and Khambay, B. P. S. (1998). Pyrethroids. *In* "Chirality in Agrochemicals" (N. Kurihara and J. Miyamoto, eds.), pp. 9–84. Wiley, New York.

Class, T. J., Ando, T., and Casida, J. E. (1990). Pyrethroid metabolism: Microsomal oxidation metabolites of (*S*)-bioallethrin and the six natural pyrethrins. *J. Agric. Food Chem.* **38**, 529–537.

Cole, K. M., Ruzo, L. O., Wood, E. J., and Casida, J. E. (1982). Pyrethroid metabolism: Comparative fate in rats of tralomethrin, tralocythrin, deltamethrin and (1*R*,α*S*)-*cis*-cypermethrin. *J. Agric. Food Chem.* **30**, 631–636.

Crawford, M., and Hutson, D. H. (1977). The metabolism of the pyrethroid insecticide (±)-α-cyano-3-phenoxybenzyl 2,2,3,3-tetramethylcyclopropanecarboxylate, WL41706, in the rats. *Pestic. Sci.* **8**, 579–599.

Crawford, M. J., Croucher, A., and Hutson, D. H. (1981a). Metabolism of *cis*- and *trans*-cypermethrin in rats. Balance and tissue retention study. *J. Agric. Food Chem.* **29**, 130–135.

Crawford, M. J., Croucher, A., and Hutson, D. H. (1981b). The metabolism of the pyrethroid insecticide cypermethrin in rats: Excreted metabolites. *Pestic. Sci.* **12**, 399–411.

Edwards, R., Millburn, P., and Hutson, D. H. (1990). Comparative metabolism and disposition of [^{14}C-benzyl]-cypermethrin in quail, rat and mouse. *Pestic. Sci.* **30**, 159–181.

Elliott, M., Janes, N. F., Kimmel, E. C., and Casida, J. E. (1972). Metabolic fate of pyrethrin I, pyrethrin II, and allethrin administered orally to rats. *J. Agric. Food Chem.* **20**, 300–313.

Elliott, M., Janes, N. F., Pulman, D. A., Gaughan, L. C., Unai, T., and Casida, J. E. (1976). Radiosynthesis and metabolism in rats of the 1R-isomers of the insecticide permethrin. *J. Agric. Food Chem.* **24**, 270–276.

Food and Agriculture Organization–World Health Organization (FAO/WHO) (1985). Flucythrinate. *In* "Pesticide Residues in Food: 1985 Evaluations. Part I. Residues." FAO Plant Production and Protection Paper, Food and Agriculture Organization of the United Nations, Rome.

FAO/WHO (1984). Cyhalothrin. *In* "Pesticide Residues in Food: 1984 Evaluations. Part II. Toxicology." FAO Plant Production and Protection Paper, Food and Agriculture Organization of the United Nations, Rome.

FAO/WHO (1986). Cyfluthrin. *In* "Pesticide Residues in Food: 1986 Evaluations. Part II. Toxicology." FAO Plant Production and Protection Paper, Food and Agriculture Organization of the United Nations, Rome.

FAO/WHO (1992). Bifenthrin. *In* "Pesticide Residues in Food: 1992 Evaluations. Part II. Toxicology." FAO Plant Production and Protection Paper, Food and Agriculture Organization of the United Nations, Rome.

FAO/WHO (1993). Etofenprox. *In* "Pesticide Residues in Food: 1993 Toxicology Evaluations." FAO Plant Production and Protection Paper, Food and Agriculture Organization of the United Nations, Geneva.

FAO/WHO (1996). Flumethrin. *In* "Pesticide Residues in Food: 1996 Toxicology Evaluations." FAO Plant Production and Protection Paper, Food and Agriculture Organization of the United Nations, Geneva.

Gaughan, L. C., Unai, T., and Casida, J. E. (1977). Permethrin metabolism in rats. *J. Agric. Food Chem.* **25**, 9–17.

Huckle, K. R., Hutson, D. H., and Millburn, P. (1981). Species differences in the metabolism of 3-phenoxybenzoic acid. *Drug Metab. Dispos.* **9**, 352–359.

Hutson, D. H., and Casida, J. E. (1978). Taurine conjugation in metabolism of 3-phenoxybenzoic acid and the pyrethroid insecticide cypermethrin in mouse. *Xenobiotica* **8**, 565–571.

Hutson, D. H., Gaughan, L. C., and Casida, J. E. (1981). Metabolism of the *cis*- and *trans*-isomers of cypermethrin in mice. *Pestic. Sci.* **12**, 385–398.

International Programme on Chemical Safety (IPCS) (1989). "Allethrins—Allethrin, *d*-Allethrin, Bioallethrin and *S*-Bioallethrin," Environmental Health Criteria 87. World Health Organization, Geneva.

IPCS (1990a). "Cyhalothrin," Environmental Health Criteria 99. World Health Organization, Geneva.

IPCS (1990b). "Deltamethrin," Environmental Health Criteria 97. World Health Organization, Geneva.

Isobe, N., Kaneko, H., Shiba, K., Saito, K., Ito, S., Kakuta, N., Saito, A., Yoshitake A., and Miyamoto, J. (1990). Metabolism of esfenvalerate in rats and

mice and effects of its isomers on metabolic fates of esfenvalerate. *J. Pestic. Sci.* **15**, 159–168.

Isobe, N., Suzuki, T., Nishikawa, J., Kaneko, H., Nakatsuka, I., and Yoshitake, A. (1992). Metabolism of empenthrin isomers in rats. *J. Pestic. Sci.* **17**, 27–37.

Izumi, T., Kaneko, H., Matsuo, M., and Miyamoto, J. (1984). Comparative metabolism of the six stereoisomers of phenothrin in rats and mice. *J. Pestic. Sci.* **9**, 259–267.

Kaneko, H., Izumi, T., Matsuo, M., and Miyamoto, J. (1984a). Metabolism of fenvalerate in dogs. *J. Pestic. Sci.* **9**, 269–274.

Kaneko, H., Izumi, T., Ueda, Y., Matsuo, M., and Miyamoto, J. (1984b). Metabolism and placental transfer of stereoisomers of tetramethrin isomers in pregnant rats. *J. Pestic. Sci.* **9**, 249–258.

Kaneko, H., Matsuo, M., and Miyamoto, J. (1984c). Comparative metabolism of stereoisomers of cyphenothrin and phenothrin isomers in rats. *J. Pestic. Sci.* **9**, 237–247.

Kaneko, H., Matsuo, M., and Miyamoto, J. (1986a). Differential metabolism of fenvalerate and granuloma formation. I. Identification of a cholesterol ester derived from a specific chiral isomer of fenvalerate. *Toxicol. Appl. Pharmacol.* **83**, 148–156.

Kaneko, H., Ohkawa, H., and Miyamoto, J. (1981a). Comparative metabolism of fenvalerate and the [2*S*,α*S*]-isomer in rats and mice. *J. Pestic. Sci.* **6**, 317–326.

Kaneko, H., Ohkawa, H., and Miyamoto, J. (1981b). Adsorption and metabolism of dermally applied phenothrin in rats. *J. Pestic. Sci.* **6**, 169–182.

Kaneko, H., Ohkawa, H., and Miyamoto, J. (1981c). Metabolism of tetramethrin isomers in rats. *J. Pestic. Sci.* **6**, 425–435.

Kaneko, H., Shiba, K., Yoshitake, A., and Miyamoto, J. (1987). Metabolism of fenpropathrin (S-3206) in rats. *J. Pestic. Sci.* **12**, 385–395.

Kaneko, H., Takamatsu, Y., Kitamura, N., Yoshitake, A., and Miyamoto, J. (1986b). *In vivo* and *in vitro* conversion of tralomethrin to deltamethrin in larvae of tobacco cutworm. *Spodoptera litura. J. Pestic. Sci.* **11**, 533–540.

Kaneko, H., Takamatsu, Y., Okuno, Y., Abiko, J., Yoshitake, A., and Miyamoto, J. (1988). Substrate specificity for formation of cholesterol ester conjugates from fenvalerate analogues and for granuloma formation. *Xenobiotica* **18**, 11–19.

Leahey, J. P. (1985). "The Pyrethroid Insecticides." Taylor & Francis, London.

Leng, G., Leng, A., Kuhn, K.-H., Lewalter, J., and Pauluhn, J. (1997). Human dose-excretion studies with the pyrethroid insecticide cyfluthrin: Urinary metabolite profile following inhalation. *Xenobiotica* **27**, 1273–1283.

Miyamoto, J. (1976). Degradation, metabolism and toxicity of synthetic pyrethroids. *Environ. Health Perspect.* **14**, 15–28.

Miyamoto, J. (1981). The chemistry, metabolism and residue analysis of synthetic pyrethroids. *Pure Appl. Chem.* **53**, 1967–2022.

Miyamoto, J., Kaneko, H., and Takamatsu, Y. (1986). Stereoselective formation of a cholesterol ester conjugate from fenvalerate by mouse microsomal carboxyesterase(s). *J. Biochem. Toxicol.* **1**, 79–94.

Miyamoto, J., Kaneko, H., Tsuji, R., and Okuno, Y. (1995). Pyrethroids, nerve poisons: How their risks to human health should be assessed. *Toxicol. Lett.* **82/83**, 933–940.

Miyamoto, J., Nishida, T., and Ueda, K. (1971). Metabolic fate of resmethrin, 5-benzyl-3-furylmethyl *dl-trans*-chrysanthemate in the rats. *Pestic. Biochem. Physiol.* **1**, 293–306.

Miyamoto, J., Sato, Y., Yamamoto, K., Endo, M., and Suzuki, S. (1968). Biochemical studies on the mode of action of pyrethroidal insecticides. Part 1. Metabolic fate of phthalthrin in mammals. *Agric. Biol. Chem.* **32**, 628–640.

Miyamoto, J., Suzuki, T., and Nakae, C. (1974). Metabolism of phenothrin or 3-phenoxybenzyl *d-trans*-chrysanthemumate in mammals. *Pestic. Biochem. Physiol.* **4**, 438–450.

Ohkawa, H., Kaneko, H., Tsuji, H., and Miyamoto, J. (1979). Metabolism of fenvalerate (Sumicidin) in rats. *J. Pestic. Sci.* **4**, 143–155.

Ohsawa, K., and Casida, J. E. (1980). Metabolism in rats of the potent knockdown pyrethroid kadethrin. *J. Agric. Food Chem.* **28**, 250–255.

Okuno, Y., Seki, T., Ito, S., Kaneko, H., Watanabe, T., Yamada, H., and Miyamoto, J. (1986). Differential metabolism of fenvalerate and granuloma formation. II. Toxicological significance of a lipophilic conjugate from fenvalerate. *Toxicol. Appl. Pharmacol.* **83**, 157–169.

Quistad, G. B., and Selim, S. (1983b). Fluvalinate metabolism by rhesus monkeys. *J. Agric. Food Chem.* **31**, 596–599.

Quistad, G. B., Staiger, L. E., Jamieson G. C., and Schooley, D. A. (1983). Fluvalinate metabolism by rats. *J. Agric. Food Chem.* **31**, 589–596.

Quistad, G. B., Staiger, L. E., and Schooley, D. A. (1982). Xenobiotic conjugation: A novel role for bile acids. *Nature* **296**, 462–464.

Roberts, T., and Hutson, D. (1999). "Metabolic Pathways of Agrochemicals. Part 2. Insecticides and Fungicides." The Royal Society of Chemistry Information Services, Cambridge.

Ruzo, L. O., and Casida, J. E. (1977). Metabolism and toxicology of pyrethroids with dihalovinyl substitutuents. *Environ. Health Perspect.* **21**, 285–292.

Ruzo, L. O., Engel, J. L., and Casida, J. E. (1979). Decamethrin metabolites from oxidative, hydrolytic and conjugative reactions in mice. *J. Agric. Food Chem.* **27**, 725–731.

Ruzo, L. O., Gaughan, L. C., and Casida, J. E. (1981). Metabolism and degradation of the pyrethroids tralomethrin and tralocythrin in insects. *Pestic. Biochem. Physiol.* **15**, 137–142.

Ruzo, L. O., Unai, T., and Casida, J. E. (1978). Decamethrin metabolism in rats. *J. Agric. Food Chem.* **26**, 918–924.

Saito, K., Kaneko, H., Tomigahara, Y., Nakatsuka, I., and Yamada, H. (1995). Metabolism of imiprothrin isomers in rats: Biotransformation and excretion. *J. Pestic. Sci.* **20**, 529–540.

Saito, K., Kaneko, H., Tomigahara, Y., Nakatsuka, I., and Yamada, H. (1996). Metabolism of imiprothrin isomers in rats: Absorption and distribution. *J. Pestic. Sci.* **21**, 49–55.

Seguchi, K., Asaka, S., Katoh, Y., and Yamaguchi, I. (1991). Metabolism of cycloprothrin in rats. *J. Pestic. Sci.* **16**, 591–598.

Shiba, K., Kakuta, N., Kaneko, H., Nakatsuka, I., Yoshitake, A., Yamada, H., and Miyamoto, J. (1988). Metabolism of the pyrethroid insecticide S-4068F in rats. *J. Pestic. Sci.* **13**, 557–569.

Shiba, K., Kaneko, H., Kakuta, N., Yoshitake, A., and Miyamoto, J. (1990). Placental transfer of esfenvalerate and fenvalerate in pregnant rats. *J. Pestic. Sci.* **15**, 169–174.

Shono, T., Ohsawa, K., and Casida, J. E. (1979). Metabolism of *trans-* and *cis-*permethrin, *trans-* and *cis-*cypermethrin and deltamethrin by microsomal enzymes. *J. Agric. Food Chem.* **27**, 316–325.

Soderlund, D. M., and Casida, J. E. (1977). Effects of pyrethroid structure on rate of hydrolysis and oxidation by mouse liver microsomal enzymes. *Pestic. Biochem. Physiol.* **7**, 391–401.

Staiger, L. E., and Quistad, G. B. (1984). Fluvalinate metabolism in rats. *J. Agric. Food Chem.* **32**, 1130–1133.

Suzuki, T., and Miyamoto, J. (1978). Purification and properties of pyrethroid carboxyesterase in rat liver microsome. *Pestic. Biochem. Physiol.* **8**, 186–198.

Suzuki, T., Ohno, N., and Miyamoto, J. (1976). New metabolites of (+)-*cis* fenothrin, 3-phenoxybenzyl (+)-*cis* chrysanthemumate, in rats. *J. Pestic. Sci.* **1**, 151–152.

Tomigahara, Y., Mori, M., Shiba, K., Isobe, N., Kaneko, H., Nakatsuka, I., and Yamada, H. (1994a). Metabolism of tetramethrin isomers in rat. I. Identification of a sulphonic acid type of conjugate and reduced metabolites. *Xenobiotica* **24**, 473–484.

Tomigahara, Y., Mori, M., Shiba, K., Isobe, N., Kaneko, H., Nakatsuka, I., and Yamada, H. (1994b). Metabolism of tetramethrin isomers in rat. II. Identification and quantitation of metabolites. *Xenobiotica* **24**, 1205–1214.

Tomigahara, Y., Onogi, M., Miki, M., Yanagi, K., Shiba, K., Kaneko, H., Nakatsuka, I., and Yamada, H. (1996). Metabolism of tetramethrin isomers in rat. III. Stereochemistry of reduced metabolites. *Xenobiotica* **26**, 201–210.

Tomigahara, Y., Shiba, K., Isobe, N., Kaneko, H., Nakatsuka, I., and Yamada, H. (1994c). Identification of two new types of S-linked conjugates of Etoc in rat. *Xenobiotica* **24**, 839–852.

Tomlin, C. D. S. (1997). "A World Compendium, The Pesticide Manual," 11th ed. British Crop Protection Council, Berks.

Ueda, K., Gaughan, L. C., and Casida, J. E. (1975a). Metabolism of (+)-*trans-* and (+)-*cis*-resmethrin in rats. *J. Agric. Food Chem.* **23**, 106–115.

Ueda, K., Gaughan, L. C., and Casida, J. E. (1975b). Metabolism of four resmethrin isomers by liver microsomes. *Pestic. Biochem. Physiol.* **5**, 280–294.

White, I. N. H., Verschoyle, R. D., Moradian, M. H., and Barnes, J. M. (1976). The relationship between brain levels of cismethrin and bioresmethrin in female rats and neurotoxic effects. *Pestic. Biochem. Physiol.* **6**, 491–500.

Woollen, B. H., Marsh, J. R., Laird, W. J. D., and Lesser, J. E. (1992). The metabolism of cypermethrin in man: Differences in urinary metabolic profiles following oral and dermal administration. *Xenobiotica* **22**, 983–991.

CHAPTER

59

Pyrethroid Insecticides: Mechanisms of Toxicity, Systemic Poisoning Syndromes, Paresthesia, and Therapy

David E. Ray

MRC Applied Neuroscience Group

59.1 MECHANISMS OF TOXICITY

The widespread use of the pyrethroids in agricultural and public health applications has acted as a stimulus for study of their mode of action in insects and also of their toxicity to nontarget organisms. Generally speaking, these two actions are similar, the molecular targets present in insects being qualitatively similar to those seen in mammals. The relative resistance of mammals to pyrethroids is attributable to a combination of their faster metabolic disposal, higher body temperature, and a lower sensitivity of the analogous target sites (Song and Narahashi, 1996b). The toxicology of the pyrethroids has been reviewed by several authors (Aldridge, 1990; Narahashi *et al.*, 1998; Soderlund and Knipple, 1995; Vijverberg and van den Bercken, 1990). Many different mechanisms of action have been proposed for the pyrethroids, which are potent agents with a wide range of actions on biological systems (Table 59.1). Any evaluation of these competing mechanisms of action must be informed by knowledge of potency, because only those effects that are only seen at the lowest concentrations are likely to have much biological significance. Unfortunately, much of the published data on pyrethroid concentrations must be used with caution, because the pyrethroids have very low water solubilities, readily partition into lipids, and show potent binding to glass and plastics. This means that it is very difficult to be certain what the true concentration is (Ray *et al.*, 1997) or to compare directly across *in vitro* systems with different physical–chemical characteristics. Furthermore, whereas actions at some of these target sites have appreciable biological consequences at less than 1% modification (Song and Narahashi, 1996b), others may require 90% modification before an effect is seen. Hence, in constructing Table 59.1, the lowest concentration needed to

produce a significant biological response has been cited, rather than the ED_{50}, which can underestimate potency.

Pyrethroids are primarily functional toxins (Narahashi *et al.*, 1998), readily causing hyperexcitation, but having little or direct cytotoxic potential in mammalian cells, although insect cells are more vulnerable to pyrethroid toxicity (Meola *et al.*, 1997). Thus, inexcitable mammalian cells are little affected by pyrethroids: A number of pyrethroids only produce growth inhibition at 10^{-5} M and no cytotoxicity at 10^{-4} M (Squiban *et al.*, 1986). In contrast, the interaction with the sodium channel shows dissociation constants on the order of 10^{-8} M (Soderlund, 1985), producing profound hyperexcitation in nerve or muscle cells. Similarly, hepatocytes in culture showed decreased viability after treatment with permethrin only at 100 ng/10^6 cells (El Tawil and Abdel Rahman, 1997), a level that is approximately 10–100 times higher than that reached in the brain of intoxicated animals. This marked resistance of inexcitable cells to pyrethroids has enabled purely *in vitro* studies to be made at pyrethroid concentrations many orders of magnitude higher than could be survived *in vivo*. Obviously, such high-concentration studies are of very limited value in any extrapolation to human toxicology.

59.1.1 ACTIONS ON SODIUM CHANNELS

Voltage-gated sodium channels are vital to the function of most excitable cells and are seen in all organisms from jellyfish upward. They are responsible for the generation of the inward sodium current that produces the action potential in most cells and are closed at normal resting potentials. Their structure and function have been recently reviewed (Conley and Brammar, 1999; Marban *et al.*, 1998). They consist of an α subunit, which

Table 59.1
Some Potential Targets of Pyrethroids in Mammals

Target	Concentration[a]	Reference
Protein phosphorylation	10^{-13} M	Enan and Matsumura (1993)
Voltage-gated sodium channels	10^{-10} M	Ghiasuddin and Soderlund (1985)
Voltage-gated chloride channels	10^{-10} M	Ray et al. (1997)
Noradrenaline release	10^{-10} M	Brooks and Clark (1987)
Membrane depolarization	10^{-8} M	Eells et al. (1992), Rekling and Theophilidis (1995)
Voltage-gated calcium channels	$<10^{-7}$ M	Hagiwara et al. (1988)
GABA-gated chloride channels	10^{-7} M	Lawrence et al. (1985)
Nicotinic receptors	10^{-7} M	Sherby et al. (1986)
Mitochondrial complex I	10^{-7} M	Gassner et al. (1997)
Lymphocyte proliferation	10^{-6} M	Diel et al. (1998)
Mitochondrial ATPase	10^{-5} M	Prasada Rao et al. (1984)
Intercellular gap junctions	10^{-5} M	Hemming et al. (1993), Tateno et al. (1993)
Chromosomal damage	10^{-4} M	Barrueco et al. (1992)

[a]Nominal pyrethroid concentration needed to produce a significant effect. Actual concentrations may, however, vary with experimental conditions.

confers pore function, resembles those of other voltage-gated ion channels, and can take several possible isoforms; and the β_1 and β_2 subunits, which may be absent in nonmammalian channels and which modify the basic function of the α subunit. There are many variant forms of the α subunit, 10 being characterized in the rat, and channels are also subject to glycosylation and phosphorylation, which further modify function. The channel is highly ion selective, favoring sodium over potassium ions by a factor of 30, yet maintains a relatively high conductance of 10–25 pS. Depolarization-driven activation [via the m-gate of Hodgkin and Huxley (1952)] is sensed by the four S4 segments in the α subunit and probably mediated by the S6 segment. Time-dependent inactivation of the channel [via the h-gate of Hodgkin and Huxley (1952)] is less well defined in molecular terms, but is probably related to the cytoplasmic domain between the S3 and S4 segments of the α subunit. Unfortunately, a standardized nomenclature for the many channel isoforms has not been accepted, and descriptions based on pharmacological properties (e.g., tetrodotoxin resistant) or tissue source (e.g., brain I, II, III) are widely used. Expression is controlled by many different genes.

The interaction of pyrethroids with the sodium channel has the effect of slowing both the activation and the inactivation properties of the sodium channel (Ginsburg and Narahashi, 1993), leading to a stable hyperexcitable state. This effect is amplified by the high level of expression of sodium channels in most excitable cells, which means that only about 0.1% of sodium channels need to be modified by a pyrethroid in order for the extra current generated to render a cell hyperexcitable (Song and Narahashi, 1996b). Although activation is slowed at the single channel level, this high density of sodium channels means that sufficient unmodified channels are always present to ensure that the activation phase of the action potential is not appreciably delayed. However, in the falling phase of the action potential, even a low proportion of modified channels can

generate enough extra current to delay inactivation. This slower rate of inactivation of pyrethroid-modified channels generates a prolonged depolarizing "tail" current that follows the normal action potential. This "tail" can trigger a second action potential if the current is both large enough and lasts for the 0.5–1 ms needed for the unmodified sodium channels to recover excitability. Hence, what would normally be a single-action potential can become converted into double or continuous discharges (Fig. 59.1). This produces a profound disruption of neuronal function. Action potential amplitude generally remains constant, the effect of pyrethroids in delaying the recruitment of open channels after depolarization (which would decrease action potential amplitude) and in delaying the closing of these same channels with time (which would increase ampli-

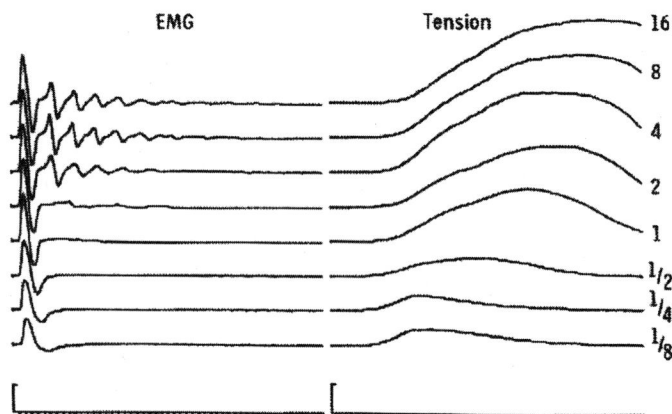

Figure 59.1 Repetitive firing in the electromyogram (EMG) and increased muscle twitch (tension) induced by deltamethrin (3 mg/kg iv) in rat muscle are only seen if sufficiently long intervals are allowed for recovery between stimuli. At the shorter intervals (lower records), the abnormal repetitive activity is completely lost and the muscle twitch also becomes normal. The interstimulus interval is indicated on the left of each record (in seconds) and the time course of the individual responses on the horizontal axis (1- and 10-ms markers).

Table 59.2
Prolongation of Sodium Channel Currents by Type I and Type II Pyrethroids

Pyrethroid (class)	System	Time constant (ms)	Reference
Control	TTX-sensitive rat cells	1.3	Song *et al.* (1996)
Tetramethrin (I)	TTX-sensitive rat cells	7.1	Song *et al.* (1996)
Fenvalerate (II)	TTX-sensitive rat cells	112	Song *et al.* (1996)
Control	TTX-resistant rat cells	1.9	Song *et al.* (1996)
Tetramethrin (I)	TTX-resistant rat cells	3.2	Song *et al.* (1996)
Fenvalerate (II)	TTX-resistant rat cells	388	Song *et al.* (1996)
Permethrin (I)	Frog nerve fiber[a]	7.3	Vijverberg and de Weille (1985)
Cismethrin (I)	Frog nerve fiber[a]	21	Vijverberg and de Weille (1985)
Fenvalerate (II)	Frog nerve fiber[a]	463	Vijverberg and de Weille (1985)
Deltamethrin (II)	Frog nerve fiber[a]	1772	Vijverberg and de Weille (1985)
Fenfluthrin (I)	Rat skeletal muscle[a]	2.3	Wright *et al.* (1988)
Cismethrin (I)	Rat skeletal muscle[a]	5.8	Wright *et al.* (1988)
Cyphenothrin (I/II)	Rat skeletal muscle[a]	9.3	Wright *et al.* (1988)
Fenvalerate (II)	Rat skeletal muscle[a]	14	Wright *et al.* (1988)
Deltamethrin (II)	Rat skeletal muscle[a]	33	Wright *et al.* (1988)

[a] Time constant of the abnormal pyrethroid-induced current.

tude), cancelling out in most systems (Ginsburg and Narahashi, 1993).

Another significant feature is that, after modification by pyrethroids, sodium channels retain many of their other normal functions, such as their selectivity for sodium ions and conductance. Their link with membrane potential is also retained, although shifted so as to increase excitability (Narahashi *et al.*, 1998). This means that, after exposure to moderate doses of pyrethroids, cells can still continue to function—but in a new and relatively stable state of abnormal hyperexcitability. In insects, this state corresponds to the incapacitating but sublethal level of effect known as "knock down." The amplitude of the sodium current continues undiminished until the level of sodium entry associated with this hyperexcitability overwhelms the capacity of the sodium pump to remove it (Narahashi, 1985). Very high concentrations of pyrethroids, or levels of hyperactivity beyond those that the cell can sustain, can thus cause depolarization and conduction block (Vijverberg and de Weille, 1985). This depolarization is more readily produced by those pyrethroids that hold the sodium channel open longest. Hence, although 2-Hz stimulation presents no difficulty for normal rat skeletal muscle, the prolonged repetitive discharges and enhanced contractions induced by deltamethrin cannot be sustained at this rate (Fig. 59.1), although they are sustained at lower frequencies.

An important characteristic of this pyrethroid-generated tail current is that the amplitude and duration are independent. The current amplitude is dependent only on the proportion of sodium channels modified and hence shows a sigmoidal relationship with pyrethroid concentration or dose. The current duration is dependent only on the pyrethroid structure, some pyrethroids, such as permethrin, holding the channel open for relatively short times and others, such as deltamethrin, holding it open for much longer (Table 59.2). Individual pyrethroids thus generate a characteristic time constant for prolongation of the sodium channel tail current that is virtually independent of dose (Brown and Narahashi, 1992). There is a continuous distribution of time constants across the range of pyrethroid structures, with type I pyrethroids producing the shorter time constants and type II pyrethroids producing the longer time constants. This holds true in both insects and amphibia, where the time constants vary from tens of milliseconds to seconds (Vijverberg and de Weille, 1985), and in mammals, where the absolute time constants are rather shorter (Table 59.2). In all cases, the threshold of hyperexcitability is reached once the decaying tail current remains above the threshold to precipitate a second abnormal action potential for as long as the time needed for excitability to return. This can be achieved by increasing either the amplitude *or* the duration of the tail current.

The different forms of the sodium channel show differential sensitivity to pyrethroids. Pyrethroids act most readily on the tetrodotoxin-resistant subtype of the sodium channel (Song and Narahashi, 1996a), which is expressed in the developing mammalian brain and in the adult dorsal root ganglia. The tetrodotoxin-resistant channels were 10 times more sensitive than tetrodotoxin-sensitive channels in the same cells (Ginsburg and Narahashi, 1993). Insect sodium channels are 100 times more sensitive than the rat brain IIa channel (Warmke *et al.*, 1997), which explains in part the resistance of mammals. The rat brain IIa form of the sodium channel is sensitive to type II, but not type I pyrethroids, an effect enhanced 20-fold by the presence of the accessory β_1 subunit (Smith and Soderlund, 1998). Channels expressing only the α subunit are capable of showing all of the the characteristics of pyrethroid modi-

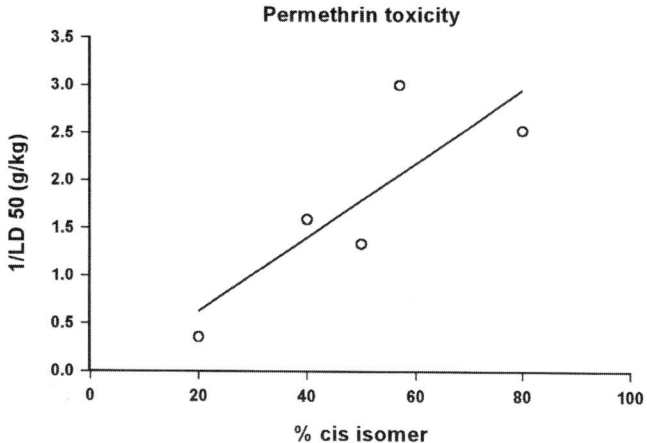

Figure 59.2 Effect of isomeric composition on the oral LD_{50} of permethrin to rats. Data taken from WHO/IPCS (1990).

fication, but require relatively high pyrethroid concentrations of 10^{-8}–10^{-7} M (Trainer *et al.*, 1997). It has been proposed that some of the regional selectivity of action of the pyrethroids parallels the distribution of sensitive sodium channel subtypes, although there are at present only limited data to support this attractive idea. Thus, striatal brain slices showed neurotransmitter release in response to type II pyrethroids that was not shown by hippocampal slices of similar capacity (Eells and Dobocovich, 1988). When these brain regions were examined *in vivo*, the striatum is the first site to show electroencephalogram (EEG) discharges and hyperexcitability (Ray, 1980), whereas the hippocampus showed only enhanced inhibition (Joy *et al.*, 1989). A similar differential was seen when the activation of early-response genes by mild pyrethroid intoxication was examined, hippocampus showing very little response, but specific cortical, thalamic, and hypothalamic areas showing marked activation (Hassouna *et al.*, 1996). Unfortunately, the distribution of the different sodium channel subtypes across these brain regions is not yet known. Peripheral nerve (SNS/PN3) sodium-channels are highly sensitive to pyrethroids, especially to type II compounds, which produce effects at 10^{-9} M (Soderlund *et al.*, 2000), and action at these channels may be relevant to the production of paresthesia. Unfortunately, all such studies are difficult to interpret at present because it has proved difficult to reproduce the high pyrethroid sensitivity of *in vivo* systems in single-channel electrophysiological experiments. Hence, it is not possible to rank the various sodium channel types in terms of absolute sensitivity, other than when they are co-expressed in the same test system.

Pyrethroid action on the sodium channel shows a marked stereospecificity that results in some isomers being far more toxic than others (Soderlund, 1985). For example, the $1R$ and $1S$ *cis* isomers bind competitively to one site, and the $1R$ and $1S$ *trans* isomers bind noncompetitively to another (Narahashi, 1986). The $1S$ forms do not modify the channel function but do block the effect of the $1R$ isomers. In whole mammals, the $1R$ isomers are thus active and the $1S$ isomers inactive and essentially nontoxic. Isomerism at the third carbon of the cyclo-

propane ring gives *cis* and *trans* isomers that show insecticidal activity (Elliott *et al.*, 1978) but differential mammalian toxicity, with the *cis* isomers being about 10 times more potent than the *trans* ones (Gray, 1985). A final chiral center is generated if a cyano substituent is added to the alcohol, giving eight possible isomers. Again, this affects potency, with only the α-S and not the α-R forms being toxic to both insects and mammals. This stereospecificity has been exploited in the synthesis of pure isomers such as deltamethrin to produce a remarkable degree of selective toxicity (Glomot, 1982). A practical consequence of this is that the toxicity of products such as permethrin, which are commonly sold as mixtures, can vary from batch to batch. Thus, the rat oral LD_{50} value of commercial permethrin varies from 430 to 8900 mg/kg (FAO/WHO, 1980). This is illustrated in Fig. 59.2, which shows that the toxicity of permethrin samples is largely determined by their *cis* isomer content.

59.1.2 OTHER ACTIONS

Many target sites other than the sodium channel may be relevant to poisoning. These are summarized in Table 59.1. To put these into context, the tissue concentration of pyrethroids in the brain during intoxication varies from 1 to 30 nmol/g tissue (Anadon *et al.*, 1996; Rickard and Brodie, 1985) in rats, although the free concentration is probably lower. The complex nature of the effects of pyrethroids on the central nervous system has led various workers to suggest that they also act via antagonism of γ-aminobutyric acid (GABA)–mediated inhibition, modulation of nicotinic cholinergic transmission, enhancement of noradrenaline release, or direct actions on calcium or chloride ion channels. However, because neurotransmitter-specific pharmacological agents offer only poor or partial protection against poisoning (see Section 59.5), it is likely that these other effects represent only secondary mechanisms of action of the pyrethroids. Indeed, most neurotransmitter release is secondary to increased sodium entry (Eells *et al.*, 1992).

Action on the voltage-dependent chloride channel has also been proposed as a target of pyrethroids (Forshaw and Ray, 1990). Voltage-sensitive chloride channels are found in brain, nerve, muscle, and salivary gland, and their function is to control cell excitability, chloride and sodium conductance having reciprocal effects on membrane excitability (Adrian and Marshall, 1976). Unlike the sodium channel, many functionally different kinds of chloride channels are seen, but the channels that have been shown to be sensitive to pyrethroids belong to the maxi chloride channel class (Franciolini and Petris, 1990). Maxi channels have not been characterized at the molecular level, but are activated by depolarization, have high conductance, are calcium-independent, and are inactivated by protein kinase C phosphorylation (Forshaw and Ray, 1993). A similar, but calcium-dependent maxi channel is unaffected by pyrethroids. Type II pyrethroids decrease chloride channel currents at low enough concentrations to be relevant to mammalian poisoning (Ray *et al.*, 1997), and reduce chloride current in vagus nerve removed from rats during poisoning (Forshaw and

Ray, 1990). The pyrethroid-induced decrease in maxi chloride channel current is brought about by a fall in open-state probability, which serves to increase excitability and therefore would synergize pyrethroid actions on the sodium channel. Of the few pyrethroids that have been tested, only those producing type II poisoning seem to affect maxi chloride channels (Ray et al., 1997). Because agents such as ivermectin and pentobarbitone, which open chloride channels, have antagonist actions on pyrethroid-evoked salivation, choreoathetosis, and repetitive firing in skeletal muscle (Forshaw et al., 2000), it seems likely that chloride channel actions contribute to most components of the type II poisoning syndrome. Indeed, an action on voltage-gated chloride channels may play a major part in the generation of the salivation and myotonia, although its role in the centrally generated signs of poisoning appears to be limited to synergizing the primary action of pyrethroids on the sodium channel.

Voltage-dependent calcium channels have been proposed as a target of pyrethroids and are good candidates in insects, with primary effects on T-type calcium currents being seen at 10^{-7} M (Duce et al., 1999). However, some mammalian calcium channels appear to be less sensitive, with tetramethrin producing 75% block of T and 30% block of L currents in neuroblastoma cells only at 10^{-5} M, and type II pyrethroids having no effect (Narahashi, 1988). In contrast, rabbit sinoatrial node cells were far more sensitive, 10^{-7} M tetramethrin (a type I pyrethroid) producing complete block of T current, but having no effect on L current until 10^{-5} M (Hagiwara et al., 1988). Unfortunately, the effect of lower concentrations was not reported. The action on voltage-gated calcium channels is interesting as one of the rare instances of a type I pyrethroid-specific effect.

At relatively high concentrations, pyrethroids can also act on GABA-gated chloride channels (Bloomquist et al., 1986), and this effect may contribute to the seizures that accompany severe type II poisoning. Several other reports have suggested a role for the $GABA_A$ receptor–ionophore complex in components of type II pyrethroid toxicity. Deltamethrin inhibits binding of ligand to the mammalian GABA complex by 50% at 10^{-7} M (Lawrence et al., 1985), and GABA-stimulated chloride flux is reduced by 72% by 10^{-6} M cis-cypermethrin (Abalis et al., 1986). As with voltage-gated chloride channels, these effects are specific for type II pyrethroids. Contrary evidence against a major GABA antagonist effect of pyrethroids is that deltamethrin does not reduce $GABA_A$-mediated hippocampal inhibition (Joy and Albertson, 1991), nor does the in vivo toxicity of deltamethrin correlate well with its potency in inhibiting GABA-induced ^{36}Cl influx (Ramadan et al., 1988). An even more marked differential is seen in invertebrates, with sodium effects at 10^{-12} M and GABA effects at 10^{-6} M (Chalmers et al., 1987). Pyrethroids, however, potentiate pentylenetetrazole convulsions by interaction with benzodiazepine binding sites (Devaud et al., 1986) at more reasonable doses, and this may indicate a potential for action via GABA. Similarly, type II pyrethroids show dose additivity with GABA antagonists in terms of acoustic startle (Crofton and Reiter, 1987). An additive effect on startle response shows that both GABA antagonists and pyrethroids induce hyperexcitable states, although

it does not prove a common mechanism. Indeed, deltamethrin also enhances tryptamine and (to a lesser extent) strychnine toxicity as well as that of the GABA antagonist pentazol (Chanh et al., 1984). A further problem for the GABA hypothesis is that the choreoathetosis, which is seen at lower doses than those that evoke seizures, has been shown to be of spinal origin (Bradbury et al., 1983). GABA is not an important neurotransmitter in the spinal cord, and Ogata et al. (1988) have shown that deltamethrin does not block the $GABA_A$-gated chloride current in dorsal root ganglia. Of pharmacological agents acting on the GABA receptor, baclofen had no therapeutic properties in deltamethrin-poisoned rats (Bradbury et al., 1983). GABA antagonists were ineffective at preventing the increased hippocampal inhibition produced by deltamethrin (Joy and Albertson, 1991). Diazepam (2 mg/kg iv) was ineffective at controlling deltamethrin choreoathetosis in rats (Cremer et al., 1980), although it does prevent the seizures associated with late-stage poisoning (Gammon et al., 1982). Diazepam was also ineffective in fenvalerate-poisoned humans (He et al., 1989). It appears that the undoubted potential of type II pyrethroids to act at the GABA receptor is of limited practical significance other than in cases of severe intoxication.

The peripheral benzodiazepine receptor has also been proposed as a target of pyrethroids, Devaud et al. (1986) finding that the proconvulsant action of low doses of both type I and type II pyrethroids were blocked by the peripheral benzodiazepine receptor antagonist PK11195. This antagonist also reduced the inhibitory effect of ivermectin on deltamethrin-evoked salivation in rats (Forshaw et al., 2000), suggesting that some component of the salivation is mediated via the peripheral benzodiazepine receptor. Competitive binding at both central and peripheral-type benzodiazepine receptors has been shown to occur in rat parotid and submandibular glands (Yamagishi and Kawaguchi, 1998).

The mechanism whereby pyrethroids interact with ion channels is not known, but type II pyrethroids stimulate protein kinase C–dependent protein phosphorylation at as low a concentration as 10^{-13} M in vitro by a direct mechanism (Enan and Matsumura, 1993). Because sodium and chloride ion channel activity is modulated by the phosphorylation state, this is likely to be a very important mechanism of action. Pyrethroids are capable of acting directly in systems with no phosphorylation capacity, but at somewhat higher concentrations (Forshaw et al., 1993).

Pyrethroids have no direct anticholinesterase activity (Ray and Cremer, 1979) and have little effect on acetylcholine sensitivity of muscle (Sherby et al., 1986), but do inhibit acetylcholine-activated calcium flux at 10^{-7} M and slow the desensitization of the nicotinic receptor (Sherby et al., 1986). This may lead to some degree of potentiation of nicotinic transmission in the central nervous system (CNS). The marked increase in neocortical blood flow seen during pyrethroid intoxication is cholinergically mediated (being blocked by atropine or lesioning the cholinergic innervation), but this probably represents an indirect effect of pyrethroids on the cholinergic system (Lister and Ray, 1988).

A more sensitive effect is the simulation of noradrenaline release from brain synaptosomes, which has an ED_{50} of only 2.9×10^{-9} M for deltamethrin, although type I pyrethroids were ineffective (Brooks and Clark, 1987). Cultured cells proved much less sensitive, requiring 10^{-5} M (Bickmeyer et al., 1994). This noradrenaline release parallels increased calcium entry and may indicate an action via voltage-sensitive calcium or sodium channels. Related effects are seen in whole animals, where deltamethrin markedly increases plasma noradrenaline (Cremer and Seville, 1982) and enhances the noradrenaline-mediated contraction of mesenteric blood vessels and cardiac contractility (Forshaw and Bradbury, 1983). It has been suggested that the calcium effects may be mediated by an action on calmodulin, but calmodulin-stimulated phosphodiesterase activity is inhibited by pyrethroids only at 10^{-6}–10^{-4} M (Rashatwar and Matsumara, 1985). Narahashi (1986) has also described a decrease in fast calcium current in neuroblastoma cells at concentrations similar to those prolonging sodium current. The significance of this is not yet clear, but it may be related to the depression of neurosecretion measured in vitro after in vivo dosing of pyrethroids (Dyball, 1982).

Other biochemical changes are the marked increases in cerebellar cyclic GMP (glutamine monophosphate) seen during type II intoxication (Aldridge et al., 1978). This effect would appear to be entirely secondary to the increased motor activity, however (Brodie, 1983), and could not be reproduced in cerebellar slices (Lock and Berry, 1981). Similarly, there are changes in the concentration of several neurotransmitters in the brain, which parallel the motor symptoms (Aldridge et al., 1978; Hudson et al., 1986) but which are probably only of secondary importance. Pyrethroids have been shown to inhibit mitochondrial Mg^{2+}-ATPase activity, but only at 2×10^{-5} M (Prasada Rao et al., 1984). Just subtoxic levels of type II pyrethroids have a tumor promoter–like activity in rat liver, although not acting as tumor initiators (Hemming et al., 1993). This action has been attributed to an inhibition of gap–junction communication, but the high pyrethroid concentrations needed to produce this effect in vitro (Table 59.1) cast doubt on the hypothesis (Hemming et al., 1993; Tateno et al., 1993).

59.2 SYSTEMIC POISONING

Fortunately, there have been relatively few reports of systemic poisoning, because use of adequate protective clothing prevents intoxication even under tropical conditions (Moretto, 1991). However, systemic poisoning can occur under conditions of misuse or inadequate user protection (He et al., 1989), and, in a study of sprayers where dermal contamination was poorly controlled, 0.3% showed signs of mild pyrethroid poisoning (Chen et al., 1991). When systemic toxicity does occur, the central signs of poisoning can be difficult to control and may be confused with intoxication by other pesticides such as anticholinesterases, which also cause salivation and hyperexcitability. Given the common formulation of pyrethroids with volatile

solvents such as xylene, symptoms of poisoning can be complicated by solvent toxicity, and solvents may also introduce additional skin effects. Mild poisoning symptoms may also be amplified by anxiety (Lessenger, 1992), which may itself be precipitated by fear or by the disconcerting paresthesia resulting from dermal contact with pyrethroids (Flannigan et al., 1985). In some low-exposure cases, poisoning may be more apparent than real. Thus, of 64 cases of self-diagnosed pyrethroid intoxication following very low level exposure to a variety of pyrethroids, 58 showed either no somatic effects or ones that were unrelated to pyrethroid exposure, and 6 showed reversible changes that were of ambiguous etiology. No CNS or PNS (peripheral nervous system) lesions were found in any of these cases (Altenkirch et al., 1996). Such cases are in marked contrast with frank occupational poisonings (He et al., 1989) and may relate more to public perception of hazard than to real toxicity.

The blood half-life of pyrethroids is on the order of tens of hours (Anadon et al., 1996; Gray et al., 1980), and intoxication by the oral route is correspondingly short lasting. Some investigators have found even shorter half-lives. Thus, cyfluthrin was found to have a plasma half-life of 19–86 min in humans (Leng and Lewalter, 1999). Inherent toxic potential can be high though, as intravenous LD_{50}s range from more than 250 to 0.5 mg/kg (Ray, 1991), but toxicity is limited in practice by rapid hydrolysis in blood and liver. Toxicity by the dermal route is further limited by low absorption through the skin and the capacity for dermal metabolic destruction of pyrethroids (Bast et al., 1997). In humans, the bioavailability of dermal pyrethroids is about 1% (Woollen et al., 1992), compared to 36% for gastric absorption. Hence, the dermal route of exposure presents relatively little risk of systemic poisoning although, in cases of very severe skin contamination, intoxication has lasted for several weeks (He et al., 1989), possibly due to a reservoir of pyrethroid bound to the epidermis. Once absorbed, pyrethroids are rapidly distributed throughout the body, their high lipophilicity and lack of exclusion by the multidrug transporter glycoprotein (Bain and LeBlanc, 1996) ensuring ready entry into the brain (Gray et al., 1980).

All of the motor signs of systemic pyrethroid intoxication are generated at the spinal level, being relatively unchanged by destruction of the brain (Bradbury et al., 1983), although other brain areas show a range of secondary responses to intoxication. Recording from central and peripheral sites shows that a modest level of hyperactivity in sensory fibers is amplified at the first synapse and becomes further amplified in polysynaptic pathways (Forshaw et al., 1987).

Animal studies have shown that the major neurotoxic hazard presented by pyrethroids to adults is acute excitation. Near-lethal doses of all classes of pyrethroids can give rise to an axonal degeneration in peripheral nerve closely resembling Wallerian degeneration (Aldridge, 1990), but this effect is inherently reversible and is only seen at dose levels that produce prolonged and severe motor signs. Central neuropathology has been described in one study of adult rats given 15 daily doses of the type II pyrethroid deltamethrin at doses just be-

Table 59.3
Signs of Pyrethroid Poisoning and Classification of Some Pyrethroids

Type I (T) poisoning[a]	Type II (CS) poisoning[a]
	Profuse watery salivation
Severe fine tremor	Coarse tremor
	Increased extensor tone
Marked reflex hyperexcitability	Moderate reflex hyperexcitability
Sympathetic activation	Sympathetic activation
	Choreoathetosis
	Seizures
Paresthesia (dermal exposure)	Paresthesia (dermal exposure)
Type I pyrethroids	Type II pyrethroids
Permethrin	Fenvalerate
Pyrethrins[b]	Cyhalothrin
Bioallethrin	Deltamethrin
Cismethrin	Cypermethrin

[a]As seen in the rat.

[b]Pyrethrins are the natural plant product, as distinct from the synthetic pyrethroids.

low the threshold for motor signs (Husain *et al.*, 1994). The animals were stated to show 40% increases in the weight of pons/medulla and hippocampus, apparently without morphological change, and also degeneration of cerebellar Purkinje cells. These findings do not appear to be internally consistent, and their significance must be considered questionable. Other workers have found no central pathology associated with the maximum survivable dose of pyrethroids (Holton *et al.*, 1997).

Despite the continuous variation in duration of the abnormal sodium current with pyrethroid structure described in Section 59.1, the effects of all pyrethroids can be described in terms of just two well-demarcated poisoning syndromes (Table 59.3) that are seen in both mammals and insects. The longer current prolongations are far more disruptive, and pyrethroids with time constants of more than about 10 ms (the normal time constant of the unmodified sodium channel being about 0.5 ms) cause incoordination, choreoathetosis, seizures, and direct effects on skeletal and cardiac muscle and salivary gland. Reflex hyperexcitability can be seen, as a dose-dependent combination of enhancement and suppression (Hijzen and Slangen, 1988; Wright *et al.*, 1988). This is called the type II, or choreoathetosis/salivation, syndrome (Aldridge, 1990). Those pyrethroids (Table 59.2) producing shorter prolongations of less than about 10 ms in mammals (Wright *et al.*, 1988) cause a less complex syndrome of simple reflex hyperexcitability and fine tremor, which is termed the type I, or tremor, syndrome, and closely resembles that produced by dichlorodiphenyltrichloroethane (DDT) (Aldridge, 1990). Pyrethroids producing intermediate time constants of about 10 ms produce a complex, mixed syndrome in which the characteristic signs of both type I and type II poisoning are superimposed (Wright *et al.*, 1988). Almost all reports of human poisoning relate to the more potent type II pyrethroids, so it is not certain how well this description of

the two syndromes applies to humans, although what has been described fits quite well with the earlier experimental animal observations.

A similar division into two classes has been made by a number of authors for systemic effects in insects (Clements and May, 1977; Gammon *et al.*, 1981; Salgado *et al.*, 1983), in amphibians (Ruigt and van den Bercken, 1986), and in mammals (Barnes and Verschoyle, 1974; Verschoyle and Aldridge, 1980; Wright *et al.*, 1988). Generally speaking, there is fairly good agreement across species (Wright *et al.*, 1988), with most noncyano substituted pyrethroids falling into group I and most of the cyano pyrethroids into group II. Some authors have objected to such a division on the grounds that qualitatively similar electrophysiological changes are produced by all active pyrethroids in both invertebrates (Leake *et al.*, 1985) and mammals (Staatz-Benson and Hosko, 1986) or because some pyrethroids show intermediate characteristics (Gammon *et al.*, 1981; Verschoyle and Aldridge, 1980). All type II pyrethroids have a cyano substituent, but not all type I pyrethroids lack one, the *trans* and *cis* isomers of flurocyphenothrin somewhat confusingly producing type I and II effects, respectively. Both pyrethroid classes have a similar range of mammalian toxicity but, for commercial pesticides, the type II pyrethroids such as deltamethrin and cypermethrin are generally more toxic than the type I pyrethroids such as permethrin. A classification of the more common pyrethroids is given in Table 59.3.

Both type I and II pyrethroids cause marked adrenal activation in rats, probably by a direct stimulation of noradrenaline release (Brooks and Clark, 1987), with the increases in blood adrenaline and noradrenaline accompanying motor signs (Cremer and Seville, 1982). The type II pyrethroid, deltamethrin, causes increased corticosteroid secretion at even lower doses (de Boer *et al.*, 1988). Hence, it is important to remember that even moderate pyrethroid poisoning occurs against a background of profound adrenal activation. Adrenal activation has been proposed as the mechanism whereby low doses of fenvalerate reduce conditioned avoidance behavior in rats (Moniz *et al.*, 1994).

59.2.1 TYPE I POISONING

The type I pyrethroids produce the simplest poisoning syndrome and produce sodium tail currents with relatively short time constants (Wright *et al.*, 1988). Poisoning closely resembles that produced by DDT and was first clearly distinguished by Verschoyle and Aldridge (1980). It involves a progressive development of fine whole-body tremor, exaggerated startle response, incoordinated twitching of the dorsal muscles, hyperexcitability, and death (Ray, 1982b). The tremor can be so severe as to double the whole-body metabolic rate in the rat at sublethal dose levels (Cremer and Seville, 1982) and can lead to prostration and death. At sublethal dose levels, respiration and blood pressure are well sustained (Ray, 1982b), but plasma noradrenaline, lactate, and, to a lesser extent, adrenaline are greatly increased (Cremer and Seville, 1982). Type I effects are generated largely by action on the central nervous system, as shown by the good correlation between brain levels of cismethrin and tremor (White *et al.*, 1976) and the induction of tremor by small quantities of cismethrin directly injected into the CNS (Gray and Rickard, 1982; Staatz *et al.*, 1982). Poisoning is associated with marked increases in both spinal (Carlton, 1977; Staatz-Benson and Hosko, 1986) and brainstem (Forshaw and Ray, 1986) excitability although not with marked effects on the higher centers. Thus, lethal doses of cismethrin do not induce cortical EEG spiking (Ray, 1982a), although supralethal doses in paralyzed, ventilated animals do (Staatz and Hosko, 1985). Also, when cismethrin is injected into the lateral ventricles, tremor is seen only when enough is given to reach the brainstem (Gray and Rickard, 1982) and, although primary increases in reflex excitability are seen in the brainstem and spinal cord, only secondary effects are seen at the cerebellar, thalamic, and cerebral cortical levels (Ray, 1982a). In addition to these central effects, there is evidence for repetitive firing in sensory nerves, which, although a small effect in one study (Staatz-Benson and Hosko, 1986), was more pronounced in others (Forshaw and Ray, 1986; Wright *et al.*, 1988). Such repetitive firing is analogous to that seen in amphibians (Vijverberg *et al.*, 1982) and probably contributes to the hyperexcitable state produced by the central actions of the type I pyrethroids.

59.2.2 TYPE II POISONING

The type II pyrethroids produce a more complex poisoning syndrome and act on a wider range of tissues. They give sodium tail currents with relatively long time constants (Wright *et al.*, 1988), which may be the reason for their ability to act on the whole range of excitable tissues. Human type II poisoning seems to be characterized by paresthesia (if via the dermal route), dizziness, nausea, listlessness, and muscular fasciculations (Chen *et al.*, 1991). More severe poisoning caused epigastric pain, nausea and vomiting (if via the oral route), hypersalivation and pulmonary edema, opisthotonos, seizures, and coma (He *et al.*, 1989).

First noted by Barnes and Verschoyle (1974), type II poisoning in rats involves progressive development of nosing and exaggerated jaw opening, similar to that seen in response to an irritant placed on the tongue; salivation, which may be profuse; increasing extensor tone in the hind limbs, causing a rolling gait; incoordination progressing to a very coarse tremor; choreoform movements of the limbs and tail often precipitated by sensory stimuli; generalized choreoathetosis (writhing spasms); tonic seizures; apnea; and death (Ray, 1982b). At lower doses, more subtle repetitive behavior is seen (Brodie and Aldridge, 1982) and learned behavior is impaired (Moniz *et al.*, 1994). In dogs, similar symptoms are seen, but salivation and upper airway hypersecretion and gastrointestinal symptoms are more prominent (Thiebault *et al.*, 1985). Unlike the type I pyrethroids, type II pyrethroids generally decrease rather than increase the startle response to sound (Crofton and Reiter, 1984), although this is a complex response and at low doses some type II pyrethroids give an increased startle (Hijzen and Slangen, 1988). The cerebral cortical response to sound is also depressed (Ray, 1980) and the latency of the visual response increased (Dyer, 1985). As in type I poisoning, plasma noradrenaline is increased by type II pyrethroids, but there is also a large increase in adrenaline and in blood glucose (Cremer and Seville, 1982; Ray and Cremer, 1979), which is not seen in type I poisoning. Type II, but not type I, pyrethroids also increase cardiac contractility both directly by action on cardiac muscle and via circulating and locally released catecholamines (Forshaw and Bradbury, 1983). They also cause repetitive firing and potentiate contraction in skeletal muscle (Forshaw and Ray, 1986). These effects are limited to a large degree by physiological compensation, which maintains blood pressure at normal levels in intact rats despite some arrhythmias, and by the inability of skeletal muscle to sustain repetitive firing for more than a few seconds at normal discharge frequencies (Fig. 59.1). Both effects are therefore of secondary importance in the normal animal. As with type I pyrethroids, the primary action is on the central nervous system, because symptoms correlate well with brain concentrations (Rickard and Brodie, 1985) and can be reproduced in part by microinjection into the CNS (Brodie, 1985; Staatz *et al.*, 1982). The former injection studies showed, however, that actions at all levels of the neuroaxis are needed to reproduce the full range of effects. Thus, although choreoathetosis can be reproduced in spinal rats (Bradbury *et al.*, 1983), other symptoms are generated at higher levels and are associated with EEG spiking at cortical and subcortical sites, which ultimately progresses to slow-wave activity and loss of consciousness not seen with type I pyrethroids (Condes Lara *et al.*, 1999; Ray, 1980). By this stage, many neurotransmitter systems have become involved, because both specific and nonspecific pharmacological interventions can control the seizures.

Although there is evidence for increased neuronal activity in both the spinal cord (Staatz-Benson and Hosko, 1986) and the brain (Ray, 1980; Staatz and Hosko, 1985), the type II pyrethroids do not produce the repetitive activity in sensory nerves seen with type I pyrethroids (Wright *et al.*, 1988). This again is analogous to the effects seen in amphibians (Vijverberg *et al.*, 1982). As might be expected, both classes of pyrethroids produce large increases in brain glucose utilization, this being most marked in motor areas (Cremer and Seville, 1985; Cremer *et al.*, 1983). Such increases seem to be secondary to increased neuronal activity and are paralleled by increased brain blood flow except in the cerebral cortex, where the flow increase is disproportionally large (Lister and Ray, 1988).

59.2.3 MIXED/INTERMEDIATE POISONING

Complex, mixed signs representing a combination of type I and type II poisoning are produced by some pyrethroids. These appear to represent a true superimposition of the I and II poisoning syndromes (Wright *et al.*, 1988) and to represent a transitional state. Evidence in support of this is given by measurement of the time constants of the sodium after-potential produced by the pyrethroids. These are short for the type I and long for the type II pyrethroids (Table 59.2). For the whole range of pyrethroids, time constants range from 5 to 1772 ms in amphibians (Vijverberg and de Weille, 1985) and from 2.3 to 33 ms in mammals (Wright *et al.*, 1988). The structures producing mixed signs fit in the middle of these ranges.

The related question of what might happen in the case of simultaneous exposure to a type I and a type II pyrethroid appears not to have been addressed in the whole animal. However, Song *et al.* (1996) used tetramethrin (a type I pyrethroid) and fenvalerate (a type II pyrethroid) and compared their actions on tetrodotoxin-resistant sodium channels in isolated neonatal rat dorsal root ganglion cells. The measure used was the degree of prolongation of the time constant, which reflects the nature of the pyrethroid effect and is more or less independent of dose. If tetramethrin was added to preparations showing a characteristic fenvalerate response, this disappeared and was replaced by a response very similar to that generated by tetramethrin alone. When the preparation was washed, it reverted to a fenvalerate response (the fenvalerate response being poorly reversible in this system). Although these data should be interpreted with some caution because both pyrethroids were used at very high nominal concentrations, the result implies that type I and II actions may be mutually exclusive.

59.3 PARESTHESIA AND LOCAL IRRITATION

In addition to systemic toxicity, pyrethroids can produce important local effects: skin contamination producing paresthesia, ingestion producing gastrointestinal irritation (Thiebault *et al.*, 1985), and inhalation upper respiratory tract irritation (Pauluhn and Machemer, 1998). The gastrointestinal irritation is rare (being limited to cases of ingestion) and has not been well studied, but is presumably a similar phenomenon to the more common dermal paresthesia. Respiratory tract irritation can be produced at comparable thresholds in rats and humans, but is rarely reported. Dermal exposures far below the threshold for systemic poisoning can lead to a local paresthesia, which is evoked by all classes (the pyrethrins and type I and II pyrethroids), with a severity roughly in proportion to their systemic toxic potential (Aldridge, 1990). Although the plant products associated with impure pyrethrum extracts can give rise to classical contact dermatitis, the pure synthetic pyrethroids produce only a simple paresthesia, not inflammation or erythema (Flannigan *et al.*, 1985). However, inflammation can be evoked by some pesticide solvents or by scratching. One case of a probable immune reaction to a pyrethroid has been described (Box and Lee, 1996). The simple paresthesia is dose dependent in severity and duration, lasting for 4–30 h after a single application. When mild, the sensation is of continuous tingling or pricking or, when more severe, burning. The effect is annoying but not disabling and does not appear to be associated with any lasting ill effects on nerve conduction (LeQuesne *et al.*, 1980). An animal model of paresthesia has been developed (Cagen *et al.*,

1984). In addition, an electrophysiological test (enhancement of the supernormal phase in two-pulse stimulation) can detect peripheral nerve hyperexcitability up to 24 h after exposure in animals (Parkin and LeQuesne, 1982). This test has also proved useful for monitoring pyrethroid effects in humans (He *et al.*, 1991).

The mechanism of paresthesia has not been studied directly, but presumably the sensation is caused by abnormal pyrethroid-induced repetitive activity in skin nerve terminals, which are exposed to higher concentrations than penetrate the rest of the body. Such an idea is supported by the observation that veratrine produces a similar response to the pyrethroids in a guinea pig model of paresthesia (McKillop *et al.*, 1987). Repetitive activity in sensory nerves is certainly seen during systemic intoxication in rats (Wright *et al.*, 1988), but the effect is much less than that seen in the central nervous system, suggesting that nerve terminals are not markedly sensitive to pyrethroids in mammals. The reversible peripheral nerve damage produced by pyrethroids is an unrelated effect, because it appears only when severe systemic poisoning is repeatedly produced (Aldridge, 1990; Rose and Dewar, 1983).

59.4 DEVELOPMENTAL NEUROTOXICITY

Neonatal rats are 4–17 times more vulnerable than adults to the acute toxicity of type I and II pyrethroids, probably due to their lesser capacity for metabolic detoxification (Cantalamessa, 1993), an observation that is consistent with neonates and adults having similar brain concentrations at different, but equitoxic, doses (Sheets *et al.*, 1994).

A number of more specific effects of exposure to pyrethroids during early development have been described in rats or mice. Cypermethrin at 4% of the LD_{50} over postnatal days 10–16 caused an increase in the renal D_1 receptor density in rats, which persisted at least until day 9 (Cantalamessa *et al.*, 1998). The pyrethroids permethrin and deltamethrin [in addition to DDT, polychlorinated biphenyls (PCBs), nicotine, and paraquat] have also been reported to induce permanent changes in behavior and neurochemistry of adult mice when administered directly to the neonate (Eriksson and Fredriksson, 1991; Eriksson *et al.*, 1990a, b, 1992; Fredriksson *et al.*, 1993; Talts *et al.*, 1998). These effects were seen at dose levels that are not acutely toxic. It should be noted that, at much higher doses, DDT acts directly on sodium channels in the same way as type I pyrethroids (Woolley, 1982), but that the other agents have very different mechanisms of action. It was proposed that the pyrethroid effects resulted from exposure at a critical period of rapid brain growth, during which the developing motor and sensory systems are believed to be especially vulnerable to chemical insult (Eriksson *et al.*, 1990a, 1992). Indeed, neonatal rats are known to be sensitive to neuroactive pharmaceuticals such as haloperidol, postnatal exposure to which causes similarly enduring changes in dopamine receptor–mediated behavior that persist into adulthood (Cuomo *et al.*, 1983; Rosengarten and Friedhoff, 1979; Thiel *et al.*, 1989). However, in these cases, the dose required to produce developmental effects in the neonate is close to that producing acute effects in the adult. It has been proposed that the lasting effects of neonatal treatment of mice with bioallethrin and deltamethrin (a decrease in muscarinic receptor density and a decrease in open-field habituation) are a result of an induced lack of appropriate cholinergic inhibitory capacity in the neonate (Eriksson *et al.*, 1992; Rekling and Theophilidis, 1995). However, the acute increases in receptor density (4 or 7% of control) produced by DDT or type I pyrethroids (Ahlbom *et al.*, 1994; Eriksson *et al.*, 1992) are only modest. They appear to be too small to account for any subsequent maldevelopment, given the large receptor reserve shown by many receptors (Bencherif *et al.*, 1995; Ek and Antonsson, 1993; Feuerstein *et al.*, 1994; Zhu, 1993), including central cholinergic systems—unless the changes were concentrated in a specific subpopulation. These positive results also contrast with a lack of effect of longer term, higher dose dietary administration of pyrethroids in rat multigeneration studies conducted for regulatory purposes (Deshmukh, 1992; Gomes *et al.*, 1991), except where the dose level is so high as to produce maternal toxicity (Abdelkhalik *et al.*, 1993). Unpublished work in my own laboratory has reproduced the lasting change in muscarinic receptor density produced by low doses of DDT reported by Eriksson *et al.* in mice, but not that produced by pyrethroids.

The overall physiological significance of this pyrethroid-induced muscarinic receptor deficit clearly needs further investigation. It is interesting that a major type of sodium channel is found in the developing rat brain with a peak density level in brainstem on postnatal days 10–21 and with a higher binding affinity for saxitoxin than in the adult (Xia and Haddad, 1994). This could be a potential site for low-dose pyrethroid and DDT developmental neurotoxicity. However, it appears than that a clarification of the question of the reproducibility and applicability of the effects seen in mice to other species will be needed before any more general conclusions can be drawn with regard to the potential developmental toxicity of pyrethroids in humans.

A different effect is the delayed development of the blood–brain barrier in rat pups given cypermethrin. Adult rats were unaffected at these or higher doses (Gupta *et al.*, 1999). The minimum dose needed to produce this effect was only 2% of the adult LD_{50}, but represented 20% of the neonatal LD_{50} (Cantalamessa, 1993), so it is possible that the effect was relatively nonspecific. Vascular damage and delayed neuronal development were also reported in neonatal rats given 0.7 mg/kg/day deltamethrin ip for 5 days (Patro *et al.*, 1997). This dose produced a marked decrease in pup body weight though, so it is likely in this case that the effects were also nonspecific in origin.

59.5 THERAPY FOR PYRETHROID POISONING

The most commonly encountered sign of pyrethroid poisoning is dermal paresthesia. This can be treated by lavage of the contaminated skin with oil (Malley *et al.*, 1985), as pyrethroids bind avidly to skin and cannot be removed by soap and water. Vitamin E cream has been found particularly effective for treating paresthesia in clinical trials (Flannigan *et al.*, 1985; Malley *et al.*, 1985) and also in some (Song and Narahashi, 1995), but not all (Oortgiesen *et al.*, 1990) *in vitro* preparations. The vitamin E was effective if applied to the skin from 29 h before to 15 min after the pyrethroid, and protection lasted for more than 5 h. The concentration required to give greater protection than that of the corn oil solvent alone was very high (50%) and so the specificity of vitamin E protection is unclear. Similarly, in humans, considerable relief can be obtained by use of presumably inert preparations such as corn oil or Vaseline as well as vitamin E (Tucker *et al.*, 1983). It is not clear how vitamin E produces this effect, but it may in part be due to sequestration of lipophilic pyrethroids into the vitamin E (Song and Narahashi, 1995) or to a more specific membrane-stabilizing action. Topical treatment with local anesthetic has been described in humans and in animals (FAO/WHO, 1982; Malley *et al.*, 1985), but the loss of sensation may be more inconvenient than the paresthesia itself.

Systemic poisoning has proved rather more difficult to deal with although, because pyrethroids produce no morphological damage and are rapidly removed from the body, only symptomatic treatment is needed. Two approaches are possible: attempting to antagonize the primary ion channel effects of the pyrethroids or controlling the secondary consequences mediated by specific chemical neurotransmitters. Pyrethroids do not, however, seem to single out a particular neurotransmission system: Both type I (Staatz *et al.*, 1982) and type II (Chugh *et al.*, 1991) pyrethroids act on multiple neurotransmitter systems. Thus, micromolar concentrations of type II pyrethroids evoke release of both dopamine and acetylcholine from brain slices via a sodium channel–dependent mechanism (Eells and Dobocovich, 1988). Both type I and type II pyrethroids can act as proconvulsants (Chanh *et al.*, 1984; Devaud *et al.*, 1986) via GABA-ergic and glutamatergic systems. However, diazepam is only poorly effective against systemic pyrethroids in rats (Staatz *et al.*, 1982), effective only against the terminal seizures of the type II syndrome in another study (Cremer *et al.*, 1980), and only moderately effective in the dog (Thiebault *et al.*, 1985). Even the salivation characteristic of type II poisoning, although undoubtedly cholinergically mediated and controllable by atropine in animals (Ray and Cremer, 1979) and in humans (He *et al.*, 1989), is also controlled very effectively by the chloride ion channel agonist ivermectin (Forshaw *et al.*, 2000), which has no anticholinergic actions.

Consequently, the most successful attempts at therapy have been based on ion channel or membrane-stabilizing drugs. An ideal therapeutic agent would antagonize the abnormal, pyrethroid-evoked sodium current but leave the normal one unchanged. In a survey of the relative ability of a range of drugs to antagonize the pyrethroid-evoked and normal sodium currents in neuroblastoma cells (Oortgiesen *et al.*, 1990), it was found that tetracaine and lidocaine were particularly effective. Lidocaine was also effective at antagonizing pyrethroid effects in intact rat hippocampus (Joy *et al.*, 1990) and modestly effective against motor signs (Bradbury *et al.*, 1983), but local anesthetics are not practical for systemic therapy because of their cardiotoxicity. Phenytoin, phenobarbitone, and valproate were found to act equally on the pyrethroid-evoked and normal sodium currents (Oortgiesen *et al.*, 1990); diazepam, mephenesin, and urethane had less action on the abnormal pyrethroid-evoked current than on the normal one. Hence, although urethane was found to be very effective *in vivo* (increasing the deltamethrin LD_{50} by 348%), this was only at a dose close to that producing anesthesia (LeClercq *et al.*, 1986), a dose at which urethane is also a lung carcinogen. Similarly, mephenesin was only effective against type I poisoning at doses producing marked muscle relaxation but, surprisingly, was effective against type II poisoning at rather lower doses. Mephenesin is also one of very few agents capable of antagonizing ongoing pyrethroid poisoning (Bradbury *et al.*, 1983). The longer lasting mephenesin derivative, methocarbimol, antagonized the motor signs of both type I and type II pyrethroids (Hiromori *et al.*, 1986), although this also required use of the maximum tolerated dose.

A novel approach has been to attempt to develop therapy targeted at the voltage-gated chloride channel, a site of action for type II (although not type I) pyrethroids (Ray *et al.*, 1997). The chloride channel agonist ivermectin was effective at restoring the membrane conductance of vagus nerve taken from rats given an LD_{50} dose of deltamethrin (Forshaw and Ray, 1990). Ivermectin also controlled deltamethrin-induced salivation and repetitive discharges in muscle (Forshaw *et al.*, 2000). Unfortunately, the central actions of ivermectin are severely limited by multidrug receptor pump activity at the blood–brain barrier, which largely excludes ivermectin, but not pyrethroids, from the brain (Schinkel *et al.*, 1996). However, pentobarbitone is another effective chloride channel agonist, which increases both channel open probability and channel number in neuroblastoma cells, and does penetrate the blood–brain barrier. Pentobarbitone was effective against all the type II motor signs caused by deltamethrin at only 25% of the anesthetic dose. An equisedative dose of phenobarbitone (which does not act on chloride channels) was ineffective against type II signs, other than the terminal seizures (Forshaw *et al.*, 2000), which suggests that pentobarbitone was not just acting as a membrane stabilizer, but had some more specific action—probably on the chloride channels. This anomalous action of pentobarbitone suggests that a combination of a local-anesthetic-type sodium channel blocker and a chloride channel agonist would provide an effective treatment for type II pyrethroid poisoning. Although phenobarbitone has been tried and found ineffective as a type II pyrethroid antidote in humans (He *et al.*, 1989), pentobarbitone does not appear to have been tested clinically.

Because type II poisoning involves a combined action on the central nervous system, adrenals, autonomic system, and muscle, multidrug therapy may be needed. Thus, mephenesin proved effective at blocking all type II motor and cardiovascular effects produced by deltamethrin, but had no effect on the salivation or the increased neocortical blood flow, and only a modest effect on the (presumably adrenergic) increase in blood glucose (Bradbury *et al.*, 1983). Combined drug therapies have proved only moderately effective so far: A combination of clomethiazole (membrane stabilizer), diazepam (against seizures), and atropine (against salivation) increased the LD_{50} of deltamethrin by 24% (LeClercq *et al.*, 1986) in rats. However, because pyrethroids show very steep dose–response curves, even a modest shift such as this can have a dramatic consequence: The combination of methocarbimol and atropine prevented all deaths at LD_{80} doses of pyrethroids in rats (Hiromori *et al.*, 1986).

REFERENCES

Abalis, I. M., Eldefrawi, M. E., and Eldefrawi, A. T. (1986). Effects of insecticides on GABA-induced chloride influx into rat brain microsacs. *J. Toxicol. Environ. Health* **18**, 13–23.

Abdelkhalik, M. M., Hanafy, M. S. M., and Abdelaziz, M. I. (1993). Studies on the teratogenic effects of deltamethrin in rats. *Deutsche Tierarztliche Wochenschrift* **100**, 142–143.

Adrian, R. H., and Marshall, M. V. (1976). Action potentials reconstructed in normal and myotonic muscle fibres. *J. Physiol.* **258**, 125–143.

Ahlbom, J., Fredriksson, A., and Eriksson, P. (1994). Neonatal exposure to a type I pyrethroid (bioallethrin) induces dose–response changes in brain muscarinic receptors and behaviour in neonatal and adult mice. *Brain Res.* **645**, 318–324.

Aldridge, W. N. (1990). An assessment of the toxicological properties of pyrethroids and their neurotoxicity. *Crit. Rev. Toxicol.* **21**, 89–104.

Aldridge, W. N., Clothier, B., Forshaw, P., Johnson, M. K., Parker, V. H., Price, R. J., Skilleter, D. N., Verschoyle, R. D., and Stevens, C. (1978). The effect of DDT and the pyrethroids cismethrin and decamethrin on acetylcholine and cyclic nucleotide content of rat brain. *Biochem. Pharmacol.* **27**, 1703–1706.

Altenkirch, H., Hopmann, D., Brockmeier, B., and Walter, G. (1996). Neurological investigations in 23 cases of pyrethroid intoxication reported to the German Federal Health Office. *Neurotoxicology* **17**, 645–651.

Anadon, A., Martinez Larranaga, M. R., Fernandez Cruz, M. L., Diaz, M. J., Fernandez, M. C., and Martinez, M. A. (1996). Toxicokinetics of deltamethrin and its 4'-HO-metabolite in the rat. *Toxicol. Appl. Pharmacol.* **141**, 8–16.

Bain, L. J., and LeBlanc, G. A. (1996). Interaction of structurally diverse pesticides with the human MDR1 gene product P-glycoprotein. *Toxicol. Appl. Pharmacol.* **141**, 288–298.

Barnes, J. M., and Verschoyle, R. D. (1974). Toxicity of new pyrethroid insecticide. *Nature* **248**, 711.

Barrueco, C., Herrera, A., Caballo, C., and Delapena, E. (1992). Cytogenetic effects of permethrin in cultured human-lymphocytes. *Mutagenesis* **7**, 433–437.

Bast, G. E., Taeschner, D., and Kampffmeyer, H. G. (1997). Permethrin absorption not detected in single-pass perfused rabbit ear, and absorption with oxidation of 3-phenoxybenzyl alcohol. *Arch. Toxicol.* **71**, 179–186.

Bencherif, M., Fowler, K., Lukas, R. J., and Lippiello, P. M. (1995). Mechanism of upregulation of neuronal nicotinic acetyl choline receptors in clonal cell lines and primary cultures of fetal rat brain. *J. Pharmacol. Exp. Ther.* **275**, 987–994.

Bickmeyer, U., Weinsberg, F., and Wiegand, H. (1994). Effects of deltamethrin on catecholamine secretion of bovine chromaffin cells. *Arch. Toxicol.* **68**, 532–534.

Bloomquist, J. R., Adams, P. M., and Soderlund, D. M. (1986). Inhibition of gamma-aminobutyric acid–stimulated chloride flux in mouse brain vesicles by polychloroalkane and pyrethroid insecticides, *Neurotoxicology* **7**, 11–20.

Box, S. A., and Lee, M. R. (1996). A systemic reaction following exposure to a pyrethroid insecticide: *Hum. Exp. Toxicol.* **15**, 389–390.

Bradbury, J. E., Forshaw, P. J., Gray, A. J., and Ray, D. E. (1983). The action of mephenesin and other agents on the effects produced by two neurotoxic pyrethroids in the intact and spinal rat. *Neuropharmacology* **22**, 907–914.

Brodie, M. E. (1983). Correlations between cerebellar cyclic GMP and motor effects induced by deltamethrin: Independence of olivo-cerebellar tract. *Neurotoxicology* **4**, 1–12.

Brodie, M. E. (1985). Deltamethrin infusion into different sites in the neuraxis of freely-moving rats. *Neurobehav. Toxicol Teratol.* **7**, 51–55.

Brodie, M. E., and Aldridge, W. N. (1982). Elevated cerebellar cyclic GMP levels during the deltamethrin-induced motor syndrome. *Neurobehav. Toxicol. Teratol.* **4**, 109–113.

Brooks, M. W., and Clark, J. M. (1987). Enhancement of norepinephrine release from rat brain synaptosomes by alpha cyano pyrethroids. *Pestic. Biochem. Physiol.* **28**, 127–139.

Brown, L. D., and Narahashi, T. (1992). Modulation of nerve membrane sodium-channel activation by deltamethrin. *Brain Res.* **584**, 71–76.

Cagen, S. Z., Malley, L. A., Parker, C. M., Gardiner, T. H., Van Gelder, G. A., and Jud, V. A. (1984). Pyrethroid-mediated skin sensory stimulation characterised by a new behavioural paradigm. *Toxicol. Appl. Pharmacol.* **76**, 270–279.

Cantalamessa, F. (1993). Acute toxicity of 2 pyrethroids, permethrin and cypermethrin, in neonatal and adult-rats. *Arch. Toxicol.* **67**, 510–513.

Cantalamessa, F., Barili, P., Cavagna, R., Sabbatini, M., Tenore, G., and Amenta, F. (1998). Influence of neonatal treatment with the pyrethroid insecticide cypermethrin on the development of dopamine receptors in the rat kidney. *Mech. Ageing Dev.* **103**, 165–178.

Carlton, M. (1977). Some effects of cismethrin on the rabbit nervous system. *Pestic. Sci.* **8**, 700–712.

Chalmers, A. E., Miller, T. A., and Olsen, R.. W. (1987). Deltamethrin: A neurophysiological study of the sites of action. *Pestic. Biochem. Physiol.* **27**, 36–41.

Chanh, P. H., Navarro-Delmasure, C., Chanh, A. P. H., Cheav, S. L., Ziade, F., and Samaha, F. (1984). Pharmacological effects of deltamethrin on the central nervous system. *Drug Res.* **34**, 175–181.

Chen, S. Y., Zhang, Z. W., He, F. S., Yao, P. P., Wu, Y. Q., Sun, J. X., Liu, L. H., and Li, Q. G. (1991). An epidemiologic-study on occupational acute pyrethroid poisoning in cotton farmers. *Br. J. Ind. Med.* **48**, 77–81.

Chugh, Y., Sankaranarayanan, A., and Sharma, P. L. (1991). Effect of fenvalerate and endosulfan on behavioral despair and forced locomotor-activity in albino mice. *Asia Pacific J. Pharmacol.* **6**, 31–35.

Clements, A. N., and May, T. E. (1977). The actions of pyrethroids upon the peripheral nervous system and associated organs in the locust. *Pestic. Sci.* **8**, 661–680.

Condes Lara, M., Graff Guerrero, A., and Vega Riveroll, L. (1999). Effects of cypermethrin on the electroencephalographic activity of the rat: A model of chemically induced seizures. *Neurotoxicol. Teratol.* **21**, 293–298.

Conley, E. C., and Brammar, W. J. (1999). "The Ion Channel Facts Book." Academic Press, San Diego.

Cremer, J. E., and Seville, M. P. (1982). Comparative effects of two pyrethroids, deltamethrin and cismethrin, on plasma catecholamines and on blood glucose and lactate. *Toxicol. Appl. Pharmacol.* **66**, 124–133.

Cremer, J. E., and Seville, M. P. (1985). Changes in regional cerebral blood flow and glucose metabolism associated with symptoms of pyrethroid toxicity. *Neurotoxicology* **6**, 1–12.

Cremer, J. E., Cunningham, V. J., Ray, D. E., and Sarna, G. S. (1980). Regional changes in brain glucose utilization in rats given a pyrethroid insecticide. *Brain Res.* **194**, 278–282.

Cremer, J. E., Cunningham, V. J., and Seville, M. P. (1983). Relationships between extraction and metabolism of glucose, blood flow, and tissue blood volume in regions of rat brain. *J. Cereb. Blood Flow Metab.* **3**, 291–302.

Crofton, K. M., and Reiter, L. W. (1984). Effects of two pyrethroid insecticides on motor activity and the acoustic startle response in the rat. *Toxicol. Appl. Pharmacol.* **75**, 318–328.

Crofton, K. M., and Reiter, L. W. (1987). Pyrethroid insecticides and the gamma-aminobutyric acid A receptor complex: Motor activity and the acoustic startle response in the rat. *J. Pharmacol. Exp. Ther.* **243**, 946–954.

Cuomo, V., Cattabeni, F., and Racagni, G. (1983). The influence of early postnatal treatment with haloperidol on the effects induced by small doses of apomorphine on locomotion of adult rats. *Neuropharmacology* **22**, 1137–1139.

de Boer, S. F., van der Gugten, J., Slangen, J. L., and Hijzen, T. H. (1988). Changes in plasma corticosterone and catecholamine contents induced by low doses of deltamethrin in rats. *Toxicology* **49**, 263–270.

Deshmukh, P. B. (1992). 3-Generation reproductive studies of a synthetic pyrethroid—cyhalothrin. *Toxicol. Lett.* **64**, 779–781.

Devaud, L. L., Szot, P., and Murray, T. F. (1986). PK 11195 antagonism of pyrethroid-induced proconvulsant activity. *Eur. J. Pharmacol.* **121**, 269–273.

Diel, F., Detscher, M., Schock, B., and Ennis, M. (1998). *In vitro* effects of the pyrethroid S-bioallethrin on lymphocytes and basophils from atopic and nonatopic subjects. *Allergy* **53**, 1052–1059.

Duce, I. R., Khan, T. R., Green, A. C., Thompson, A. J., Warburton, S. P. M., and Wong, J. (1999). Calcium channels in insects. *In* "Progress in Neuropharmacology and Neurotoxicology of pesticides and Drugs" (J. D. Beadle, ed.), pp. 56–66. Royal Soc. Chem., Cambridge.

Dyball, R. E. J. (1982). Inhibition by decamethrin and resmethrin of hormone release from the isolated rat neurohypophysis—A model mammalian neurosecretory system. *Pestic. Biochem. Physiol* **17**, 42–47.

Dyer, R. S. (1985). The use of sensory evoked potentials in toxicology. *J. Appl. Toxicol.* **5**, 24–40.

Eells, J. T., and Dobocovich, M. L. (1988). Pyrethroid insecticides evoke neurotransmitter release from rabbit striatal slices. *J. Pharmacol. Exp. Ther.* **246**, 514–521.

Eells, J. T., Bandettini, P. A., Holman, P. A., and Propp, J. M. (1992). Pyrethroid insecticide–induced alterations in mammalian synaptic membrane-potential. *J. Pharmacol. Exp. Ther.* **262**, 1173–1181.

Ek, B., and Antonsson, B. M. (1993). Studies of muscarinic receptor reserve linked to phosphoinositide hydrolysis in parotid gland and cerebral cortex. *Acta Physiol. Scand.* **147**, 289–295.

Elliott, M., Farnham, A. W., Janes, N. F., and Soderlund, D. M. (1978). Insecticidal activity of the pyrethrins and related compounds. XI. Relative potencies of isomeric cyano-substituted 3-phenoxybenzyl esters. *Pestic. Sci.* **9**, 112–116.

El Tawil, O. S., and Abdel Rahman, M. S. (1997). Effect of cypermethrin on isolated male and female rat hepatocytes. *J. Toxicol. Environ. Health* **52**, 461–474.

Enan, E., and Matsumura, F. (1993). Activation of phosphoinositide protein-kinase-c pathway in rat-brain tissue by pyrethroids. *Biochem. Pharmacol.* **45**, 703–710.

Eriksson, P., and Fredriksson, A. (1991). Neurotoxic effects of two different pyrethroids, bioallethrin and deltamethrin, on immature and adult mice: Changes in behavioral and muscarinic receptor variables. *Toxicol. Appl. Pharmacol.* **108**, 78–85.

Eriksson, P., Ahlbom, J., and Fredriksson, A. (1992). Exposure to DDT during a defined period in neonatal life induces permanent changes in brain muscarinic receptors and behaviour in adult mice. *Brain Res.* **582**, 277–281.

Eriksson, P., Archer, T., and Fredriksson, A. (1990a). Altered behaviour in adult mice exposed to a single oral dose of DDT and its fatty acid conjugate as neonates. *Brain Res.* **514**, 141–142.

Eriksson, P., Nilsson-Hakansson, L., Nordberg, A., Aspberg, A., and Fredriksson, A. (1990b). Neonatal exposure to DDT and its fatty acid conjugate—Effects on cholinergic and behavioural variables in adult mouse. *Neurotoxicology* **11**, 345–354.

Feuerstein, T. J., Saauermann, W., Allgaier, C., Agneter, E., and Singer, E. A. (1994). New insight into receptor theory as provided by an artificial partial agonist made-to-measure. *Naunyn-Schmiedeberg's Arch. Pharmacol.* **350**, 1–9.

Flannigan, S. A., Tucker, S. B., Key, M. M., Ross, C. E., Fairchild, E. J., Grimes, B. A., and Harrist, R. B. (1985). Synthetic pyrethroid insecticides: A dermatological evaluation. *Br. J. Ind. Med.* **42**, 363–372.

Food and Agriculture Organization/World Health Organization (FAO/WHO) (1980). "FAO Plant Production and Protection." Paper 20 (Supplement), Food and Agriculture Organization, Rome.

Food and Agriculture Organization/World Health Organization (FAO/WHO) (1982). "FAO Plant Production and Protection." Paper 42 (Monographs), Food and Agriculture Organization, Rome.

Forshaw, P. J., and Bradbury, J. E. (1983). Pharmacological effects of pyrethroids on the cardiovascular system of the rat. *Eur. J. Pharmacol.* **91**, 207–213.

Forshaw, P. J., and Ray, D. E. (1986). The effects of two pyrethroids, cismethrin and deltamethrin, on skeletal muscle and the trigeminal reflex system in the rat. *Pestic. Biochem. Physiol.* **25**, 143–151.

Forshaw, P. J., and Ray, D. E. (1990). A novel action of deltamethrin on membrane resistance in mammalian skeletal-muscle and non-myelinated nerve-fibers. *Neuropharmacology* **29**, 75–81.

Forshaw, P. J., and Ray, D. E. (1993). A voltage-dependent chloride channel in NIEl15 neuroblastoma-cells is inactivated by protein-kinase-c and also by the pyrethroid deltamethrin. *J. Physiol.* **467**, 252.

Forshaw, P. J., Lister, T., and Ray, D. E. (1987). The effects of 2 types of pyrethroid on rat skeletal-muscle. *Eur. J. Pharmacol.* **134**, 89–96.

Forshaw, P. J., Lister, T., and Ray, D. E. (1993). Inhibition of a neuronal voltage-dependent chloride channel by the type-ii pyrethroid, deltamethrin. *Neuropharmacology* **32**, 105–111.

Forshaw, P. J., Lister, T., and Ray, D. E. (2000). The role of voltage-gated chloride channels in type II pyrethroid insecticide poisoning. *Toxicol. Appl. Pharmacol.* **163**, 1–8.

Franciolini, F., and Petris, A. (1990). Chloride channels of biological membranes. *Biochim. Biophys. Acta* **1031**, 247–259.

Fredriksson, A., Fredriksson, M., and Eriksson, P. (1993). Neonatal exposure to paraquat or MPTP induces permanent changes in striatum dopamine and behaviour in adult mice. *Toxicol. Appl. Pharmacol.* **122**, 258–264.

Gammon, D. W., Brown, M. A., and Casida, J. E. (1981). Two classes of pyrethroid action in the cockroach. *Pestic. Biochem. Physiol.* **15**, 181–191.

Gammon, D. W., Lawrence, L. J., and Casida, I. E. (1982). Pyrethroid toxicology: Protective effects of diazepam and phenobarbitol in the mouse and cockroach. *Toxicol. Appl. Pharmacol.* **66**, 290–296.

Gassner, B., Wuthrich, A., Scholtysik, G., and Solioz, M. (1997). The pyrethroids permethrin and cyhalothrin are potent inhibitors of the mitochondrial complex I, *J. Pharmacol. Exp. Ther.* **281**, 855–860.

Ghiasuddin, S. M., and Soderlund, D.M. (1985). Pyrethroid insecticides—potent, stereospecific enhancers of mouse-brain sodium-channel activation. *Pestic. Biochem. Pnysiol.* **24**, 200–206.

Ginsburg, K. S., and Narahashi, T. (1993). Differential sensitivity of tetrodotoxin-sensitive and tetrodotoxin-resistant sodium-channels to the insecticide allethrin in rat dorsal-root ganglion neurons. *Brain Res.* **627**, 239–248.

Glomot, R. (1982). Toxicity of deltamethrin to higher vertebrates. *In* "Deltamethrin" (R. Lhoste, ed.), Roussel Uclaf, Marseilles.

Gomes, M. D., Bernardi, M. M., and Spinosa, H. D. (1991). Pyrethroid insecticides and pregnancy—Effect on physical and behavioral-development of rats. *Vet. Hum. Toxicol.* **33**, 315–317.

Gray, A. J. (1985). Pyrethroid structure–toxicity relationships in mammals. *Neurotoxicology* **3**, 25–35.

Gray, A. J., and Rickard, J. (1982). Toxicity of pyrethroids to rats after direct injection into the central nervous system. *Neurotoxicology* **6**, 127–138.

Gray, A. J., Connors, T. A., Hoellinger, H., and Nam, N. H. (1980). The relationship between the pharmacokinetics of intravenous cismethrin and biotesmethrin and their mammalian toxicity. *Pestic. Biochem. Physiol.* **13**, 281–293.

Gupta, A., Agarwal, R., and Shukla, G. S. (1999). Functional impairment of blood–brain barrier following pesticide exposure during early development in rats. *Hum. Exp. Toxicol.* **18**, 174–179.

Hagiwara, N., Irisawa, H., and Kameyama, M. (1988). Contribution of 2 types of calcium currents to the pacemaker potentials of rabbit sino-atrial node cells. *J. Physiol.* **395**, 233–253.

Hassouna, I., Wickert, H., El Elaimy, I., Zimmermann, M., and Herdegen, T. (1996). Systemic application of pyrethroid insecticides evokes differential expression of c-Fos and c-Jun proteins in rat brain. *Neurotoxicology* **17**, 415–431.

He, F. S., Deng, H., Ji, X., Zhang, Z. W., Sun, J. X., and Yao, P. P. (1991). Changes of nerve excitability and urinary deltamethrin in sprayers. *Int. Arch. Occup. Environ. Health* **62**, 587–590.

He, F. S., Wang, S. G., Liu, L. H., Chen, S. Y., Zhang, Z. W., and Sun, J. X. (1989). Clinical manifestations and diagnosis of acute pyrethroid poisoning. *Arch. Toxicol.* **63**, 54–58.

Hemming, H., Flodstrom, S., and Warngard, L. (1993). Enhancement of altered hepatic foci in rat-liver and inhibition of intercellular communication in-vitro by the pyrethroid insecticides fenvalerate, flucythrinate and cypermethrin. *Carcinogenesis* **14**, 2531–2535.

Hijzen, T. H., and Slangen, J. L. (1988). Effects of type I and type II pyrethroids on the startle response in rats. *Toxicol. Lett.* **40**, 141–152.

Hiromori, T., Nakanishi, T., Kawaguchi, S., Sako, H., Suzuki, T., and Miyamoto, J. (1986). Therapeutic effects of methocarbamol on acute intoxication by pyrethroids in rats. *J. Pestic. Sci.* **11**, 9–14.

Hodgkin, A. L., and Huxley, A. F. (1952). A quantitative description of membrane current and its application to conduction and excitation in nerve. *J. Physiol.* **117**, 500–544.

Holton, J. L., Nolan, C. C., Burr, S. A., Ray, D. E., and Cavanagh, J. B. (1997). Increasing or decreasing nervous activity modulates the severity of the gliovascular lesions of 1,3-dinitrobenzene in the rat: Effects of the tremorgenic pyrethroid, bifenthrin, and of anaesthesia. *Acta Neuropathol.* **93**, 159–165.

Hudson, P. M., Tilson, H. A., Chen, P. H., and Hong, J. S. (1986). Neurobehavioral effects of permethrin are associated with alterations in regional levels of biogenic amine metabolites and amino acid neurotransmitters. *Neurotoxicology* **7**, 143–153.

Husain, R., Malaviya, M., and Seth, P. K. (1994). Effect of deltamethrin on regional brain polyamines and behavior in young rats. *Pharmacol. Toxicol.* **74**, 211–215.

Joy, R. M., and Albertson, T. E. (1991). Interactions of GABA-A antagonists with deltamethrin, diazepam, pentobarbital, and SKF100330A in the rat dentate gyrus. *Toxicol. Appl. Pharmacol.* **109**, 251–262.

Joy, R. M., Albertson, T. E., and Ray, D. E. (1989). Type-I and type-II pyrethroids increase inhibition in the hippocampal dentate gyrus of the rat *Toxicol. Appl. Pharmacol.* **98**, 398–412.

Joy, R. M., Lister, T., Ray, D. E., and Seville, M. P. (1990). Characteristics of the prolonged inhibition produced by a range of pyrethroids in the rat hippocampus. *Toxicol. Appl. Pharmacol.* **103**, 528–538.

Lawrence, L. J., Gee, K. N., and Yamamura, H. I. (1985). Interactions of pyrethroid insecticides with chloride ionophore-associated binding sites. *Neurotoxicology* **6**, 87–98.

Leake, L. D., Buckley, D. S., Ford, M. G., and Salt, D. N. (1985). Comparative effects of pyrethroids on neurones of target and non-target organisms. *Neurotoxicology* **6**, 99–116.

LeClercq, M., Cotonat, J., and Foulhoux, P. (1986). Recherche d'un antagonisme a l'intoxication par la deltamethrine. *J. Toxicol. Clin. Exp.* **6**, 85–93.

Leng, G., and Lewalter, J. (1999). Role of individual susceptibility in risk assessment of pesticides. *Occup. Environ. Med.* **56**, 449–453.

LeQuesne, P. M., Maxwell, I. C., and Butterworth, S. T. G. (1980). Transient facial symptoms following exposure to synthetic pyrethroids: A clinical and electrophysiological assessment. *Neurotoxicology* **2**, 1–11.

Lessenger, J. E. (1992). 5 office workers inadvertently exposed to cypermethrin. *J. Toxicol. Environ. Health* **35**, 261–267.

Lister, T., and Ray, D. E. (1988). The role of basal forebrain in the primary cholinergic vasodilation in rat neocortex produced by systemic administration of cismethrin. *Brain Res.* **450**, 364–368.

Lock, E. A., and Berry, P. N. (1981). Biochemical change in the rat cerebellum following cypermethrin administration. *Toxicol. Appl. Pharmacol.* **59**, 508–514.

Malley, L. A., Cagen, S. Z., Parker, C. M., Gardiner, G. A., Van Gelder, G. A., and Rose, C. P. (1985). The effect of vitamin E and other amelioratory agents on the fenvalerate-mediated skin sensation. *Toxicol. Lett.* **29**, 51–58.

Marban, E., Yamagishi, T., and Tomaselli, G. F. (1998). Structure and function of voltage-gated sodium channels. *J. Physiol.* **508**, 647–657.

McKillop, C. M., Brock, J. A. C., Oliver, G. J. A., and Rhodes, C. (1987). A quantitative assessment of pyrethroid-induced paraesthesia in the guinea-pig flank model. *Toxicol. Lett.* **36**, 1–7.

Meola, S., Meola, R., Barhoumi, R., Miles, J. M., and Burghardt, R. C. (1997). Laser cytometric analysis of permethrin toxicity in insect and mammalian epithelial cells. *Toxic Substance Mech.* **16**, 237–249.

Moniz, A. C., Bernardi, M. M., and Spinosa, H. S. (1994). Effects of a pyrethroid type-II pesticide on conditioned behaviors of rats. *Vet. Hum. Toxicol.* **36**, 120–124.

Moretto, A. (1991). Indoor spraying with the pyrethroid insecticide lambda-cyhalothrin—Effects on spraymen and inhabitants of sprayed houses. *Bull. World Health Org.* **69**, 591–594.

Narahashi, T. (1985). Nerve membrane ionic channels as the primary target of pyrethroids. *Neurotoxicology* **6**, 3–22.

Narahashi, T. (1986). Mechanisms of action of pyrethroids on sodium and calcium channel gating. *In* "Neuropharmacology of Pesticide Action" (M. G. Ford, G. G. Lunt, R. C. Reay, and P. N. R. Usherwood, eds.), pp. 36–40. Ellis Horwood, Chichester.

Narahashi, T. (1988). Molecular and cellular approaches to neurotoxicology: Past, present and future. *In* "Neurotox '88: Molecular Basis of Drug and Pesticide Action" (G. G. Lunt, ed.), pp. 269–288. Excerpta Medica, Amsterdam.

Narahashi, T., Ginsburg, K. S., Nagata, K., Song, J. H., and Tatebayashi, H. (1998). Ion channels as targets for insecticides. *Neurotoxicology* **19**, 581–590.

Ogata, N., Vogel, S. M., and Narahashi, T. (1988). Lindane but not deltamethrin blocks a component of GABA-activated chloride channels. *FASEB J.* **2**, 2895–2900.

Oortgiesen, M., van Kleef, R. G. D. M., and Vijverberg, H. P. M. (1990). Block of deltamethrin-modified sodium current in cultured mouse neuroblastoma cells: Local anaesthetics as potential antidotes. *Brain Res.* **518**, 11–18.

Parkin, P. J., and LeQuesne, P, M. (1982). Effect of a synthetic pyrethroid deltamethrin on excitability changes following a nerve impulse. *J. Neurol. Neurosurg. Psych.* **45**, 337–342.

Patro, N., Mishra, S. K., Chattopadhyay, M., and Patro, I. K. (1997). Neurotoxicological effects of deltamethrin on the postnatal development of cerebellum of rat. *J. Biosci.* **22**, 117–130.

Pauluhn, J., and Machemer, L. H. (1998). Assessment of pyrethroid-induced paraesthesias: Comparison of animal model and human data. *Toxicol. Lett.* **96**, 361–368.

Prasada Rao, K. S., Chetty, C. S., and Desaiah, D. (1984). *In vitro* effects of pyrethroid on rat brain and liver ATPase activities. *J. Toxicol. Environ. Health* **14**, 257–265.

Ramadan, A. A., Bakry, N. M., Marei, A. S. M., Eldefrawi, A. T., and Eldefrawi, M. E. (1988). Action of pyrethroids on GABA-A receptor function. *Pestic. Biochem. Physiol.* **32**, 97–105.

Rashatwar, S. S., and Matsumara, F. (1985). Interaction of DDT and pyrethroids with calmodulin and its significance in the expression of enzyme activities of phosphodiesterase. *Biochem. Pharmacol.* **34**, 1689–1694.

Ray, D. E. (1980). An EEG investigation of decamethrin-induced choreoathetosis in the rat. *Exp. Brain Res.* **38**, 221–227.

Ray, D. E. (1982a). Changes in brain blood flow associated with deltamethrin induced choreoathetosis in the rat. *Exp. Brain Res.* **45**, 269–276.

Ray, D. E. (1982b). The contrasting actions of two pyrethroids (deltamethrin and cismethrin) in the rat. *Neurobehav. Toxicol. Teratol.* **4**, 801–804.

Ray, D. E. (1991). Pesticides derived from plants and living organisms. *In* "Handbook of Pesticide Toxicology" (W. J. Hayes and E. R. Laws, eds.), pp. 585–636. Academic Press, San Diego.

Ray, D. E., and Cremer, J. E. (1979). The action of decamethrin (a synthetic pyrethroid) in the rat. *Pestic. Biochem. Physiol.* **10**, 333–340.

Ray, D. E., Sutharsan, S., and Forshaw, P. J. (1997). Actions of pyrethroid insecticides on voltage-gated chloride channels in neuroblastoma cells. *Neurotoxicology* **18**, 755–760.

Rekling, J. C., and Theophilidis, G. (1995). Effects of the pyrethroid insecticide, deltamethrin, on respiratory modulated hypoglossal motoneurons in a brain-stem slice from newborn mice. *Neurosci. Lett.* **198**, 189–192.

Rickard, J., and Brodie, M. E. (1985). Correlation of blood and brain levels of the neurotoxic pyrethroid deltamethrin with the onset of symptoms in rats. *Pestic. Biochem. Physiol.* **23**, 143–156.

Rose, G. P., and Dewar, A. J. (1983). Intoxication with four synthetic pyrethroids fails to show any correlation between neuromuscular dysfunction and neurobiochemical abnormalities in rats. *Arch. Toxicol.* **53**, 297–316.

Rosengarten, H., and Friedhoff, A. J. (1979). Enduring changes in dopamine receptor cells of pups from drug administration to pregnant and nursing rats. *Science* **203**, 1133–1135.

Ruigt, G. S. F., and van den Bercken, J. (1986). Action of pyrethroids on a nerve–muscle preparation of the clawed frog, *Xenopus laevis*. *Pestic. Biochem. Physiol.* **25**, 176–187.

Salgado, V. L., Irving, S. N., and Miller, T. A. (1983). The importance of nerve tenninal depolarization in pyrethroid poisoning of insects. *Pestic. Biochem. Physiol.* **20**, 169–182.

Schinkel, A. H., Wagenaar, E., Mol, C. A. A. M., and Van Deemter, L. (1996). P-glycoprotein in the blood–brain barrier of mice influences the brain penetration and pharmacological activity of many drugs. *J. Clin. Invest.* **97**, 2517–2524.

Sheets, L. P., Doherty, J. D., Law, M. W., Reiter, L. W., and Crofton, K. M. (1994). Age-dependent differences in the susceptibility of rats to deltamethrin. *Toxicol. Appl. Pharmacol.* **126**, 186–190.

Sherby, S. M., Eldefrawi, A. T., Deshpande, S. S., Albuquerque, E. X., and Eldefrawi, M. E. (1986). Effects of pyrethroids on nicotinic acetylcholine receptor binding and function. *Pestic. Biochem. Physiol.* **26**, 107–115.

Smith, T. J., and Soderlund, D. M. (1998). Action of the pyrethroid insecticide cypermethrin on rat brain IIa sodium channels expressed in *Xenopus* oocytes. *Neurotoxicology* **19**, 823–832.

Soderlund, D. M. (1985). Pyrethroid–receptor interactions: Stereospecific binding and effects on sodium channels in mouse brain preparation. *Neurotoxicology* **6**, 35–46.

Soderlund, D. M., and Knipple, D. C. (1995). Actions of insecticides on sodium-channels—Multiple-target sites and site-specific resistance. *Am. Chem. Soc. Symp. Ser.* **591**, 97–108.

Soderlund, D. M. *et al.* (2000). Differential sensitivity of sodium channel auxiliary subunit gene from the house fly (Musca domestica). *Neurotoxicology* **21**, 127–137.

Song, J. H., and Narahashi, T. (1995). Selective block of tetramethrin-modified sodium channels by (+/−)-alpha-tocopherol (vitamin E). *J. Pharmacol. Exp. Ther.* **275**, 1402–1411.

Song, J. H., and Narahashi, T. (1996a). Differential effects of the pyrethroid tetramethrin on tetrodotoxin-sensitive and tetrodotoxin-resistant single sodium channels. *Brain Res.* **712**, 258–264.

Song, J. H., and Narahashi, T. (1996b). Modulation of sodium channels of rat cerebellar Purkinje neurons by the pyrethroid tetramethrin. *J. Pharmacol. Exp. Ther.* **277**, 445–453.

Song, J. H., Nagata, K., Tatebayashi, H., and Narahashi, T. (1996). Interactions of tetramethrin, fenvalerate and DDT at the sodium channel in rat dorsal root ganglion neurons. *Brain Res.* **708**, 29–37.

Squiban, A., Marano, F., and Ronot, X. (1986). The action of deltamethrine, a pyrethrinoid. *Biol. Cell* **57**, A51.

Staatz, G., and Hosko, N. H. (1985). Effect of pyrethroid insecticides on EEG activity of conscious, immobilized rats. *Pestic. Biochem. Physiol.* **24**, 231–239.

Staatz, C. G., Bloom, A. S., and Lech, J. J. (1982). A pharmacological study of pyrethroid neurotoxicity in mice. *Pestic. Biochem. Physiol.* **17**, 287–292.

Staatz-Benson, C. G., and Hosko, M. J. (1986). Interaction of pyrethroids with mammalian spinal neurons. *Pestic. Biochem. Physiol.* **25**, 19–30.

Talts, U., Fredriksson, A., and Eriksson, P. (1998). Changes in behavior and muscarinic receptor density after neonatal and adult exposure to bioallethrin. *Neurobiol. Aging* **19**, 545–552.

Tateno, C., Ito, S., Tanaka, M., and Yoshitake, A. (1993). Effects of pyrethroid insecticides on gap junctional intercellular communications in balb/c3t3 cells by dye-transfer assay. *Cell Biol. Toxicol.* **9**, 215–221.

Thiebault, J. J., Bost, J., and Foulhoux, P. (1985). Experimental intoxication by deltamethrin in the dog and its treatment. *Collect. Med. Leg. Toxicol. Med.* **131**, 47–62 (in French).

Thiel, R., Chahoud, I, Schwabe, R., and Neubert, D. (1989). Device for monitoring locomotor activity of 120 animals: Motility of offspring of dams exposed to haloperidol. *Neurotoxicology* **10**, 621–628.

Trainer, V. L., McPhee, J. C., Boutelet Bochan, H., Baker, C., Scheuer, T., Babin, D., Demoute, J P., Guedin, D., and Catterall, W. A. (1997). High affinity binding of pyrethroids to the alpha subunit of brain sodium channels. *Mol. Pharmacol.* **51**, 651–657.

Tucker, S. B., Flannigan, S, A., and Smolenaky, M. H. (1983). Comparison of therapeutic agents for synthetic pyrethroid exposure. *Contact Dermatitis* **9**, 316.

Verschoyle, R. D., and Aldridge, W. N. (1980). Structure–activity relationships of some pyrethroids in rats. *Arch. Toxicol.* **45**, 325–329.

Vijverberg, H. P. M., and de Weille, J. R. (1985). The interaction of pyrethroids with voltage-dependent Na channels. *Neurotoxicology* **6**, 23–34.

Vijverberg, H. P. M., and van den Bercken, J. (1990). Neurotoxicological effects and the mode of action of pyrethroid insecticides. *Crit. Rev. Toxicol.* **21**, 105–126.

Vijverberg, H. P. M., Ruigi, G. S. F., and van den Bercken, J. (1982). Structure-related effects of pyrethroid insecticides on the lateral-line sense organ and on peripheral nerves of the clawed frog, *Xenopus laevis. Pestic. Biochem. Physiol.* **18**, 315–324.

Warmke, J. W., Reenan, R. A. G., Wang, P. Y., Qian, S., Arena, J. P., Wang, J. X., Wunderler, D., Liu, K., Kaczorowski, G. J., Vander Ploeg, L. H. T., Ganetzky, B., and Cohen, C. I. (1997). Functional expression of *Drosophila* para sodium channels—Modulation by the membrane protein TipE and toxin pharmacology. *J. Gen. Physiol.* **110**, 119–133.

White, I. N. H., Verschoyle, R. D., Moradian, M. H., and Barnes, J. M. (1976). The relationship between brain levels of cismethrin and bioresmethrin in female rats and neurotoxic effects. *Pestic. Biochem. Physiol.* **6**, 491–500.

WHO/IPCS (1990). "Environmental Health Criteria 94: Permethrin." World Health Organization, Geneva.

Woollen, B. H., Marsh, J. R., Laird, W. J. D., and Lesser, J. E. (1992). The metabolism of cypermethrin in man—differences in urinary metabolite profiles following oral and dermal administration. *Xenobiatica* **22**, 983–991.

Woolley, D. E. (1982). Neurotoxicity of DDT and possible mechanisms of action. *In* "Mechanisms of Actions of Neurotoxic Substances" (K. N. Prasad and A. Vernadulkis, eds.), pp. 95–141. Raven Press, New York.

Wright, C. D. P., Forshaw, P. J., and Ray, D. E. (1988). Classification of the actions of 10 pyrethroid insecticides in the rat, using the trigeminal reflex and skeletal-muscle as test systems. *Pestic. Biochem. Physiol.* **30**, 79–86.

Xia, Y., and Haddad, G. G. (1994). Postnatal development of voltage-sensitive Na^+ channels in rat brain. *J. Comp. Neural.* **345**, 279–287.

Yamagishi, H., and Kawaguchi, M. (1998). Characterization of central- and peripheral-type benzodiazepine receptors in rat salivary glands. *Biochem. Pharmacol.* **55**, 209–214.

Zhu, B.-T. (1993). The competitive and noncompetitive antagonism of receptor-mediated drug actions in the presence of spare receptors. *J. Pharmacol. Toxicol. Meth.* **29**, 85–91.

DDT and its Analogs

Andrew G. Smith
Medical Research Council Toxicology Unit, United Kingdom

60.1 INTRODUCTION

Chlorinated insecticides have had a "bad press" over the last few decades. Their use has declined dramatically. Even the few uses worldwide and the few countries this applies to are under tremendous environmental pressure to cease completely. It is difficult for us now to accept that in their time the chlorinated insecticides were of outstanding importance for human health. As with penicillin, it was wartime that showed their tremendous utility. For the first time, pests could be confidently controlled and importantly irradicated. It is estimated that DDT alone was responsible for the saving of tens of millions of human lives. Many areas of the world are now free of such pests as malaria purely as the result of DDT use in the postwar period. That is not to say that our present concerns of environmental toxicity of these chemicals are not perfectly valid. Clearly, the large-scale administration of these persistent chemical had significant costs for wildlife and are undesirable. Whether there are any costs for chronic human health through environmental exposure is a very difficult issue. In the last 10 years or so DDT, its analogs, and other chemicals have been considered as insidious endocrine disruptors causing cancer and reproductive disorders but on the whole, DDT and its analogs have apparently been extremely safe for humans. It would seem prudent to retain their use, in a tightly controlled manner, as an important reserve weapon in the fight against insect pests. It is not always easy to substitute with newer insecticides that are more expensive and have their own undesirable effects. This chapter describes aspects of the known toxicity of DDT and its analogs such as methoxychlor. Although much of the work reported is now some years old (WHO, 1979), it is extremely important and very pertinent to today's discussions and arguments on the hazards of environmental exposures (Smith, 2000).

60.2 DDT

DDT came to widespread attention because it dramatically controlled typhus and malaria in time of war. When it became available for civilian use, it controlled flies and other pests that annoy large numbers of people and may transmit disease, and

it increased the production of important crops. Knowledge that traces of it are stored in essentially everyone in the world has kept DDT in the spotlight. Later it was implicated in the injury of a wide variety of wildlife. Under these circumstances, it is no wonder that DDT probably has been studied more thoroughly than any other pesticide and is used to illustrate many principles and concepts in toxicology including very important topics such as human exposure levels and effects on domestic and wild animals. In the following discussion, details of storage and excretion of DDT in humans are covered as well as toxic actions in humans and experimental animals.

DDT was first synthesized by Zeidler (1874) who called it dimonochlorophenyltricholoräthan. However, it was put to no use until its insecticidal properties were demonstrated by Paul Müller in 1939. The first sample sent to the United States arrived in September 1942. Results of the tests were so encouraging that manufacture was given high priority both in the U.S. and UK. At first, the entire production was used for the protection of troops against malaria, typhus, or certain other vector-borne diseases, or against biting flies or other insects, that are merely pests (Hayes, 1982). As the supply increased, DDT was used in the United States for control of malaria in war areas, that is, in the vicinity of military installations, ports, and transportation centers. As a result of this effort, mosquito transmission of malaria was brought to an end in the United States in 1953, even though military personnel and other infected persons from the tropics continued to reintroduce the disease extensively as late as 1972 and in diminishing numbers thereafter.

The revolution in the control of malaria and typhus among allied troops and among certain civilian populations during World War II was accomplished with relatively little DDT. Far greater amounts were required for the control of agricultural and forest pests that became possible after the compound was released in the United States for commercial use on August 31, 1945. Civilian use in other countries became possible a little later with tremendous effect. An informative account of its discovery and early use, especially in Europe, can be found in West and Campbell (1946).

60.2.1 IDENTITY, PROPERTIES, AND USES

p,p'-DDT is 1,1'-(2,2,2-trichloroethylidene)-bis(4-chlorobenzene). Common nomenclatures that have been used are 1,1,1-trichloro-2,2-bis(p-chlorophenyl)ethane, 1,1,1-trichloro-2,2-bis(4-chlorophenyl)ethane, and 1,1-bis(4-chlorophenyl)-2,2,2-trichloroethane. Because the older terminology has been used widely in the past and continues to be so, especially since many abbreviations are based on it (e.g., p,p'-DDT and o,p'-DDT), the o and p nomenclature will be used for referring to DDT in its abbreviated form.

DDT is universally accepted as the common name of the insecticide. As approved by BSI, DDT refers to the technical product, and there is historical justification for that practice because DDT is an acronym for *d*ichloro*d*iphenyl*t*richloroethane. p,p'-DDT was approved by BSI as a separate term. Zeidler (1874) called the compound di-monochlorophenyltrichloräthan. When used as a drug, DDT was known in the United Kingdom as dicophane (BP), in Sweden as klorfenoton, and in the United States as chlorphenothane (USP).

DDT was sold under a variety of trade names, including Anofex®, Cesarex®, Didimac®, Digmar®, Diniocide®, Genitox®, Guesarol®, Gyron®, Ixodex®, Neocid®, and Zerdane®. Code designations for DDT include IMS-16 and ENT-1,506. The CAS registry number for p,p'-DDT is 50-29-3. DDT has the empirical formula $C_4H_9Cl_5$ and a molecular weight of 354.49. Pure p,p'-DDT is a white, tasteless, almost odorless crystal-line solid melting at 108.5 to 109.0°C. Technical DDT is a waxy solid. A typical example of technical DDT had the following composition: p,p'-DDT, 77.1%; o,p'-DDT, 14.9%; p,p'-DDD, 0.3%; o,p'-DDT, 14.9%; p,p'-DDD, 0.3%; o,p'-DDD, 0.1%; p,p'-DDE, 4.0%; o,p'-DDE, 0.1%; and unidentified compounds, 3.5%. The vapor pressure of DDT is 1.5×10^{-7} mm Hg at 20°C. DDT is highly soluble in a polar organic solvents: solubility per 100 ml acetone, 58 gm; ethanol, 2 gm; benzene, 106 gm; carbon tetrachloride, 45 gm; cyclohexanone, 116 gm; ethyl ether, 28 gm; petroleum ethers and kerosene, 4–10 gm. It is practically insoluble in water.

The structure of p,p'-DDT and the structures of several of its analogs are compared in Table 60.1. The table is confined to compounds that have occurred in commercial DDT and analogs that have had some use as insecticides. It must be emphasized that even the commercially available insecticidal analogs have strikingly different properties. Especially remarkable are the slow metabolism and marked storage of DDT and its metabolite DDE and the rapid metabolisms and negligible storage of methoxychlor. Table 60.1 does not include the wide range of compounds that have been synthesized and studied in connection with structure-activity relationships, often with the hope of emphasizing the good properties of DDT and reducing its undesirable properties. For a more extensive consideration of analogs, see Metcalf (1973). Further information of related chemicals will be found in Section 60.2.3.5.

60.2.2 FORMULATIONS AND PRODUCTION

Technical DDT has been formulated in almost every conceivable form including solutions in xylene or petroleum distillates, emulsifiable concentrates, water-wettable powders, granules, aerosols, smoke candles, charges for vaporizers, and lotions. Aerosols and other household formulations were combined with synergized pyrethrins. Production and use of DDT in the United States and other countries have been discussed previously (Hayes, 1991; Smith, 1991).

Before 1945, all of the DDT produced in the United States was used or allocated by the military services for medical and public health uses. Early in 1945, it became available for extensive experimental work in agriculture, and it was commercially available in limited quantities early in the autumn of the same year. The results were so spectacular that use increased until 1959. In response to a demand for exports, production continued to increase until about 1963. Even before 1963, some restrictions were placed on its use, mainly to minimize residues in food and in the feed of animals that produced milk and meat. Among the first of these restrictions was that on its use in the dairy cattle industry. Another important factor reducing the use of DDT was the increasing resistance of pests. One of the first species to be affected was the housefly; because of its abundance and widespread distribution, its resistance was bound to be noticed by the public generally. Although many pests of public importance have been resistant to DDT in some or all of their range, resistance among vectors of malaria has been minimal. Because malaria control constitutes such a large segment of vector control, the use of DDT for vector control remained stable, while its use in agriculture continued to decline, especially in temperate climates.

Prophetically when Sweden banned DDT from January 1, 1970, they pointed out that "the need for insecticides is rather small in Sweden compared to that in many other countries" and that the ban of this and certain other chlorinated hydrocarbon insecticides could be used as a tool to explore scientific problems about their movement (Hayes, 1969). In order to respond to ecologists who considered that the widespread occurrence of DDT in the environment was inherently bad and was the direct cause of injury to certain fish and birds, government agencies of some other countries attempted to justify restrictions on the use of DDT by its alleged threat to human health. This did not prevent the same agencies from providing that DDT might be used, if needed, to combat any future threat from vector-borne disease within their boundaries. To this day the hazard of DDT and DDE to humans is still a highly debatable matter. Although many countries severely restrict or ban the use of DDT, it is still used for both agriculture and vector control, in some tropical countries. It is possible that complete abolishment of its use worldwide in vector control might have significant repercussions. Information apparently is not available on how much of the agricultural use involves food protection or how much loss of food production would result if use of DDT were discontinued. How much of the use of DDT is in public health is still also unknown, but the picture with malaria control is clear. In 1971,

Table 60.1
Structure of p,p'-DDT and a Few of Its Analogs that Have Had Commercial Use

Name	Chemical name[a]	R_1	R_2	R_3
DDT	1,1,1-trichloro-2,2-bis(4-chlorophenyl)ethane	Cl	H	CCl_3
Bulan[®][b]	2-nitro-1,1-bis(4-chlorophenyl)butane	Cl	H	$CH(NO_2)CH_2CH_3$
Chlorfenethol (DMC)	1,1-bis(4-chlorophenyl)ethanol	Cl	OH	CH_3
Chlorobenzilate	ethyl 4,4′-dichlorobenzilate	Cl	OH	$COOCH_2CH_3$
Chloropropylate	isopropyl 4,4′-dichlorobenzilate	Cl	OH	$COOCH(CH_3)_2$
DFDT	1,1,1-trichloro-2,2-bis(4-flurophenyl)ethanol	F	H	CCl_3
Dicofol (Kelthane[®])	2,2,2-trichloro-1,1-bis(4-chlorophenyl)ethanol	Cl	OH	CCl_3
Ethylan (Perthane[®])	1,1-dichloro-2,2-bis(4-ethylphenyl)ethane	CH_2CH_3	H	$CHCl_2$
Methoxychlor	1,1,1-trichloro-2,2-bis(4-methoxyphenyl)ethane	OCH_3	H	CCl_3
Prolan[®][b]	2-nitro-1,1-bis(4-chlorophenyl)propane	Cl	H	$CH(NO_2)CH_3$
TDE[c]	1,1-dichloro-2,2-bis(4-chlorophenyl)ethane	Cl	H	$CHCl_2$

[a] Chemical names: The names used here are those which are commonly encountered.
[b] A mixture of Prolan and Bulan (1 : 2) has been sold in the past as Dilan[®].
[c] As an insecticide, this compound has had the approved name of TDE; as a metabolite of DDT it usually is called DDD. It has been sold under thename Rhothane[®]; as a drug, the o,p'-isomer is called mitotane.

WHO calculated that substitution of malathion or propoxur for DDT would increase the cost of malaria control approximately 3.4- and 8.5 fold, respectively, and this increase could not be supported in some countries without a decrease in the coverage of control programs (WHO, 1971). Despite these increased costs, DDT use has been mainly overtaken by other pesticides. However, a proposal for its complete ban is still a controversial matter (Curtis and Lines, 1999; Attaran *et al.*, 2000; Roberts *et al.*, 2000).

60.2.3 TOXICITY TO LABORATORY ANIMALS

60.2.3.1 Symptomatology

The description of DDT intoxication in animals given by Domenjoz (1944) remains one of the best. The first perceptible effect is abnormal susceptibility to fear, with violent reaction to normally subthreshold stimuli. There is definite motor unrest and increased frequency of spontaneous movements. As poisoning increases, hyperirritability like that seen in strychnine poisoning develops, but convulsions do not appear at this time. A fine tremor, recognizable at first only as a terror reaction, is later present as an intention tremor in connection with voluntary movement, and then intermittently without observable cause. Finally it is present as a coarse tremor without interruption even for several days. Spontaneous movement is limited, and food intake stops so that surviving animals lose weight. In the later stages, especially in some species, there are attacks of epileptiform, tonic-clonic convulsions with opisthotonos. All the signs are strengthened by external stimuli and become manifest at first through external stimuli. In all stages, the animals show normal position and labyrinth reflexes. The picture of poisoning in mammals recalls the disturbances of movement and tone that are known in human pathology as the amyostatic syndrome. Symptoms appear several hours after oral administration of the compound, and death may follow after 24–72 hr. The latent period after intravenous administration at about the LD 50 level is approximately 5 min; signs of poisoning reach a maximal level in about 30 min, and survivors are symptom-free in 18–24 hr. Animals that survive recover completely.

In addition to the features of poisoning already mentioned, Cameron and Burgess (1945) noticed that as rats, guinea pigs, and rabbits become sick they become cold to the touch and show ruffled fur. Some show diarrhea. Muscular tremors were preceded by muscular weakness which occurred first in the back and later in the hind legs. The front legs were relatively spared so that animals showing marked weakness of the hindquarters could still drag themselves about. However, several authors have found that the tremor characteristic of DDT poisoning generally starts in the muscles of the face, including the eyelids, and spreads caudally with variable severity until all the muscles are affected. Furthermore, although weakness of hindquarters has been seen, it was not a common finding.

Although there is a general similarity in the clinical effects of DDT in all vertebrate species, some characteristic differences exist. Cats show greater extensor rigidity and opisthotonos than other laboratory animals. The stiffness appears first in the distal part of the extremities and later extends to the proximal part and to the trunk. Poisoned cats show marked pilomotor activity. Convulsions are also prominent in dogs, as is ataxia. Tremors

Table 60.2
Comparison of Acute LD 50 to Laboratory Animals[a]

Species	Formulation[b]	S.c. (mg/kg)	I.v. (mg/kg)	I.p. (mg/kg)	Oral (mg/kg)	Dermal (mg/kg)
Rat	w/p	<2000			500–2500	1000
	o	200–1500	47	80–200	113–450	250–3000
Mouse	w/p	1000–1500			300–1600	375
	o	300			100–800	250–500
Guinea pig	w/p				2000	1500
	o	900		150	250–560	1000
Rabbit	w/p				275	375
	o	250–3200	30–41	<2100	300–1770	300–2820
Dog	w/p					
	o		68		>300	
Cat	w/p				100–410	
	o	>650	32			
Monkey	w/p					
	o		55			

[a]Modified from Hayes (1959).
[b]w/p suspension in water or as powder. o, solution in oil.

are so pronounced in rats that it may be difficult to detect clonic convulsions in them.

Poisoning produced by repeated doses of DDT differs from that produced by a single dose only insofar as the animal may be gradually debilitated, especially by malnutrition. If food intake is maintained, tremor may last for weeks or even, intermittently, for months. If the animals survive a short time after dosing stops, recovery is complete. However, food intake may be interfered with in at least two ways. Tremor and more severe signs may interfere mechanically with eating. Animals offered food containing high concentrations of DDT often eat little or nothing and lose weight rapidly. This seems to be due to taste, not an effect on appetite, as the same animals will show excellent appetites when offered the same kind of food containing no DDT just after refusing the major portion of their daily ration of contaminated food. Animals that have suffered severe weight loss as a result of DDT poisoning may die partly as a result of general debility. Even though severely ill, animals that survive a few days after the last of many doses of DDT go on to recovery.

Table 60.2 summarizes the acute toxicity of DDT to common laboratory animals. It may be concluded that dissolved DDT is absorbed by all routes, although DDT powder is absorbed through the skin to only a negligible degree. Remarkably it is frequently impossible to put enough DDT dust on the skin of animals to kill them, so that a LD 50 value for this formulation cannot be determined with precision by the dermal route. Although formulation is important in determining the toxicity of DDT by other routes, the difference is not so great as it is in connection with skin exposure. In round figures, DDT is about 4 times more toxic when given intravenously than when given orally and about 40 times more toxic intravenously than dermally. In general, DDT, like some other lipophilic chemicals, appears more toxic orally as a solution in vegetable oil or ani-

mal fat than when given in some petroleum fractions. Acute oral LD 50 values of DDT metabolites commonly found in tissues or excreta are less toxic than the most absorbable preparations of the parent compounds.

At an oral dosage of 150 mg/kg, p,p'-DDT produces severe illness in rats and kills about half of them, but o,p' DDT at the same dosage produces no illness, even thought the concentrations of the two compounds in the brain at various intervals after dosing are about the same. At a dosage of 3000 mg/kg, o,p' DDT produces mild to moderate illness, and the concentration in the brain is 5–9 times the concentration of p,p'-DDT necessary to produce similar symptoms. Thus, p,p'-DDT appears to be inherently more toxic than the o,p' isomer (Dale et al., 1966).

Rats tolerate higher tissue levels of DDA than of DDT. Eighteen hours after intravenous injection of DDA at a rate of 100 mg/kg, tissue levels still were higher than are usually found in animals fatally poisoned by DDT (Judah, 1949). DDA produces somewhat less injury than DDT to the liver but, especially at high intravenous dosages, produces greater damage to the kidney (Lillie et al., 1947). This is consistent with the finding of Spicer et al. (1947) that, following administration of DDT, DDA constitutes a higher proportion of DDT-related compounds in the kidney (25%) than in any other tissue, being 12% in the liver, 10% in the brain, and even less in other tissues.

Young animals eat more than adults in relationship to their body weight. For this and other reasons, young animals often are more susceptible than adults to poison in food. However, there is no evidence that DDT is more toxic to young animals of any species, including humans, and in the rat the young are less susceptible to a single dose (Table 60.3). They are about equally susceptible to repeated doses. According to Henderson and Woolley (1969), the relative insusceptibility of the young

Table 60.3
Effect of Age on the Toxicity of DDT to Rats

Number of doses	Age[a]	LD 50 (mg/kg)[b]	Reference
1	Newborn	>4000	Lu *et al.* (1965)
1	Newborn	2356	Harrison (1975)
1	10 days	728	Henderson and Woolley (1969)
1	14–16 days	437	Lu *et al.* (1965)
1	weaning	355	Lu *et al.* (1965)
1	2 months	250	Henderson and Woolley (1969)
1	2 months	152	Mitjavila *et al.* (1981a)
1	3–4 months	194	Lu *et al.* (1965)
1	middle-aged	235	Lu *et al.* (1965)
1	adult	225	Harrison (1975)
4	reweaning	279	Lu *et al.* (1965)
4	adult	285	Lu *et al.* (1965)

[a]Data from more than one strain of rat.
[b]Total intake of one or more doses.

is associated with relatively poor absorption of DDT by their central nervous systems and by lesser inherent susceptibility of the young brain to DDT already absorbed by it. Further study by the same authors (Henderson and Woolley, 1970) showed that fatal poisoning of both 10- and 60-day-old rats involves hyperexcitability and intense tremor followed by prostration and eventual respiratory failure. However, in the adult rat, DDT causes convulsions, an increase in respiration and heart rate, and a lethal increase in body temperature prior to death, but the body temperature of the immature rat decreases during acute intoxication by DDT. The authors suggested that, whereas DDT is a direct depressant of respiration in both young and old rats, the additional toxic responses manifested by seizures and hyperthermia account for the increased lethality of DDT in mature animals. No acute LD 50 could be established for hamsters (Agthe *et al.*, 1970), which also seem resistant to chronic effects of DDT (Table 60.4).

There is virtually no sex difference in the acute toxicity of DDT to rats; the LD 50 is 113 and 118 in males and females, respectively (Gaines, 1960). A similar situation is observed with mice (Agthe *et al.*, 1970). When DDT is fed to rats at ordinary dietary levels, the two sexes store it equally. However, at higher dosages, females store more of the compound; the difference is explained mainly by the lesser activity of the liver microsomal enzymes in female rats and only in part by relatively higher food intake of the females.

60.2.3.2 Response to Repeated Doses

The effects of repeated doses of DDT are summarized in Table 60.4. The 90-dose oral LD 50 of technical DDT in rats is 46.0 mg/kg/day (Gaines, 1969). The chronicity index is 5.4. Thus the compound has only a moderate tendency to cause cumulative effects, and this limited tendency is fully explained by the accumulation of DDT itself in tissues as a result of contin-

uing intake. In fact, this accumulation, which is strictly dosage dependent, is detectable at all measurable levels of intake.

If storage is considered undesirable *per se,* then DDT is without a no-injurious-effect level. However, the same may be said for all compounds that are absorbed, for the presence of all of them in the bodies of exposed organisms-perhaps at very low levels and for relatively short periods-may be assumed; failure to demonstrate low levels of storage does not depend on physiology but only on limitations of the analytical techniques employed.

A number of papers have reported no-effect levels for DDT within parameters other than storage, namely rat, 0.05 mg/kg/day; dog, 8mg/kg/day; and monkey, 2.2–5.54 mg/kg/day (see Smith, 1991). There remain reports of effects in animals at the lowest dosages investigated. For example, decreased serum albumin and increased β- and α-globulins in the blood of rats and rabbits maintained on a dosage of 0.2 mg/kg/day for 3–11 months were reported by Kagan *et al.* (1969).

In summary, the lowest dosages that have been studied in animals are of the same order of magnitude as those encountered by people who made or formulated DDT and, therefore, hundreds of times greater than the dosages encountered by ordinary people. The animal studies have continued long after a steady state of storage has been achieved. The results permit the conclusion that bioaccumulation sufficient to produce neurotoxicity or other clinical effects, including a reduction of the life span, can occur only at dosage levels substantially higher than those encountered by the most heavily exposed workers, let alone those exposed environmentally. DDT dosages encountered by workers produce in some groups of mice and rats a small but detectable increase of the liver changes (hypertrophy, margination, and lipospheres) characteristic of rodents at much higher doses (Smith, 1991). The same changes occur in low incidence in control mice and rats but not in other animals.

Table 60.4
Effect on Various Species of Prolonged Oral Administration of DDT

Range (mg/kg/day)	Dosage Method and concentration (ppm)	Species,[a] number, and sex	Maximum duration	Results	References
41–80	800 ppm in diet	rat	2 yr	increased mortality, typical liver changes, and liver carcinomas	Fitzhugh and Nelson (1947)[b]
	46 mg/kg, then 140 ppm in diet	mouse 36 M, 36 F	1.5 yr	hepatomas in 51 and 21% of M and F compared with 18 and 0.6% of controls	Innes et al. (1969)
	1000 ppm in diet	hamster 25 M, 30 F	1.9 yr	no liver tumors and survival slightly less than controls	Agthe et al. (1970)
	1000 ppm in diet	hamster 30 M, 30 F	1.5 yr	no liver tumors but decreased serum cholinesterase	Graillot et al. (1975)
	1000 ppm in diet	hamster 35 M, 36 F	2.4 yr	no liver tumors and survival as controls	Rossi et al. (1983)
	3200 ppm in diet	dog 10	4 yr	100% mortality; liver damage, no tumors	Lehman (1951, 1952, 1965)
	5000 ppm in diet	monkey 1M	10 wk	100% mortality	Durham et al. (1963)
	50 mg/kg/day	monkey 6	14 wk	100% mortality; no hematologic effects	Cranmer et al. (1972)
21–40	400 ppm in diet	rat 24 M, 12 F	2 yr	increased mortality, typical liver changes	Fitzhugh and Nelson (1947)[b]
	500 ppm in diet	rat 37 M, 35 F	2.9 yr	liver tumors in 45%	Rossi et al. (1977)
	500 ppm in diet	rat 38 M, 38 F	2.3 yr	liver tumors in 18% F	Cabral et al. (1982b)
	250 ppm in diet	mouse 103 M, 90 F	2 gen	risk of liver tumor increased 3.7- and 18.5-fold in M and F, respectively	Tomatis et al. (1972)
	250 ppm in diet	mouse 31 M, 121 F	2 gen	liver tumors in 48 and 59% of M and F	Terracini et al. (1973)
	500 ppm in diet	hamster 39 M, 40 F	1.7 yr	no liver tumors and survival as controls	Cabral et al. (1982a)
	2000 ppm in diet	dog 4	4 yr	25% mortality; minor liver damage but no tumors	Lehman (1951, 1952, 1965)
11–20	100 ppm in diet	mouse 100 M, 100 F	2 yr	hepatomas increased in F of one strain but no increase in hepatocarcinomas	Fitzhugh (1970)
	100 ppm in diet	mouse 30 M, 30 F	2 yr	risk of liver tumors increased 4.4-fold	Walker et al. (1973)
	100 ppm in diet	mouse 30 M, 3 F	2 yr	risk of liver tumors increased 3.3- and 4.2-fold in M and F	Thorpe and Walker (1973)
6–10	50 ppm in diet	mouse 127 M, 104 F	2 gen	risk of liver tumors increased 2.45- and 3.46-fold in M and F, respectively	Tomatis et al. (1972)
	50 ppm in diet	mouse 30 M, 30 F	2 yr	risk of liver tumors increased 2.9-fold	Walker et al. (1973)
	400 ppm in diet	dog 2	4 yr	no effect	Lehman (1951, 1952, 1965)
2.6–5	20 ppm in diet	mouse 48 M, 128 F	2 gen	no increase in tumors	Terracini et al. (1973)

(continues)

Table 60.4

(*continued*)

Range (mg/kg/day)	Dosage Method and concentration (ppm)	Species,[a] number, and sex	Maximum duration	Results	References
	200 ppm in diet	monkey	7.5 yr	no effects	Durham *et al.* (1963)
1.26–2.5	10 ppm in diet	mouse 104 M, 124 F	2 gen	risk of liver tumors increased 2.26- and 2.46-fold in M and F, respectively	Tomatis *et al.* (1972)
0.63–1.26	25 ppm in diet	rat	2 yr	no clinical effect; M survived longer than controls	Treon and Cleveland (1955)
0.31–0.63	10 ppm in diet	rat	2 yr	typical liver changes; no effect on reproduction	Fitzhugh (1948)
	12.5 ppm in diet	rat	2 yr	no effect	Treon and Cleveland (1955)
	2.8–3.0 ppm in diet	mouse 683	5 gen	tumors in 28.7%, including lung carcinomas, lymphomas, and leukemias	Tarján and Kemeny (1969)
0.16–0.31	2 ppm in diet	mouse 124 M, 111 F	2 gen	risk of liver tumor doubled in M, unchanged in F	Tomatis *et al.* (1972)
	2 ppm in diet	mouse 58 M, 135 F	2 gen	no increase in tumors	Terracini *et al.* (1973)
0.08–0.16	2.5 ppm in diet	rat	2 yr	no effect	Treon and Cleveland (1955)

[a] Various strains of rats were used: Osborne–Mendel (Fitzhugh and Nelson, 1947), Carworth (Treon and Cleveland, 1955), Wistar (Rossi *et al.*, 1977), MRC-Porton (Cabral *et al.*, 1982b). Mouse strains used were (C57BL/6 × C3H/An)F1 and (C57BL/6 × AKR)F1 (Innes *et al.*, 1969), CFI (Tomatis *et al.*, 1972; Thorpe and Walker, 1973; Walker *et al.*, 1973), BALB/cJ andC₃HeB/FeJ (Fitzhugh, 1970), BALB/c (Tarján and Kemeny, 1969; Terracini *et al.*, 1973).
[b] Slides reexamined by Reuber (1978).

60.2.3.3 Absorption

Most DDT dust is of such large particle size that any that is inhaled is deposited in the upper respiratory tract and eventually is swallowed. Toxicity data indicate that respiratory exposure to DDT is of no special importance. The absorption of DDT from the gastrointestinal tract is slow. Whereas intravenous injection at the rate of 50 mg/kg produces convulsions in rats in 20 min, convulsions occur only after 2 hr when DDT is administered orally at a rate two or more times the LD 50 value. The onset of convulsions is delayed for about 6 hr when DDT is given to rats orally at approximately the LD 50 value (Dale *et al.*, 1963). DDT dissolved in animal or vegetable fats is absorbed from the gastrointestinal tract about 1.5–10 times more effectively than is undissolved DDT (e.g., Keller and Yeary, 1980; Palin *et al.*, 1982), but large doses of the compound in the gastrointestinal tract are poorly absorbed from nonabsorbable solvents. At high dosage levels, less [¹⁴C]DDT is absorbed and stored in organs following oral than following intraperitoneal administration, and a higher proportion is excreted in the feces than after intraperitoneal administration (40 versus 0.9%) (Bishara *et al.*, 1972). However, in connection with small repeated doses, the kind of solvent used made little difference; apparently the occurrence of bile in the intestine and the presence of some fat in the diet are sufficient to promote absorption of the compound.

Rothe *et al.* (1957) reported that after giving radioactive DDT by stomach tube as an emulsion of a peanut oil solution they recovered 41–57% of it in lymph. Less than 0.1% was found in the urine, 7.4–37.1% was in the feces or in the intestinal contents, and 19–67% of the activity was found in the carcass. Of the administered DDT not found in feces and intestinal contents, 47–65% was found in the lymph. Fifty percent of the DDT-derived material found in the lymph was absorbed in the first 2.5–7 hr, and 95% was absorbed by 18 hr. Because the lymphatic duct in the rat is not a single vessel, Rothe *et al.* (1957) were unable to exclude the possibility that some or all of the DDT that they later recovered from the carcasses of their animals had been transported to the general circulation by collateral lymph vessels rather than by the hepatoportal system. They gave indirect evidence for supposing that little or no DDT is absorbed from the gastrointestinal system by the blood, and this has been confirmed by Palin *et al.* (1982). Most of the DDT absorbed into the lymph is carried in the lipid core of chylomicrons and thence into the plasma proteins (Pocock and Vost, 1974; Sieber *et al.*, 1974). *p,p'*-DDT is taken up at a rate which is different from those of its metabolites and *o,p'*-DDT (Sieber, 1976) and which does not strictly parallel differences in lipid solubility.

As already stated, dermal absorption of DDT is very limited.

60.2.3.4 Distribution and Storage

The distribution and storage of DDT in animals can be summarized as below. Original references can be found in Smith (1991).

1. DDT is stored in all tissues the highest concentrations of DDT usually being found in adipose tissue. Rats store DDT in their fat at all measurable dietary levels including trace concentrations.

2. Following repeated doses, storage in the fat increases rapidly at first and then more gradually until a peak or plateau is reached. Repeated doses at a moderate rate could result in greater total storage of DDT in the fat than a single dose at the highest rate that can be tolerated or even a single dose at a rate that frequently is fatal. The equilibrium storage of DDT in each tissue varies directly with the daily dosage. However (with the apparent exception of the dog), storage in the fat and perhaps in other tissues is less extensive in relation to dosage at higher dietary levels.

3. The rat apparently tends to lose a part of the DDT it has stored in fat at the peak level reached in about 6 months, even though it continued on the same diet.

4. There is a measurable difference between the storage patterns of different species; that of the dog differs most.

5. At higher dosage levels but not at ordinary residue levels, the female rat consistently stores more DDT in its fat than the male when fed the same diet. The difference is accounted for only in part by the greater food intake of the female and must depend partly on more rapid biotransformation in the male. Other species show little or no sex difference.

6. The amount of DDT stored in the tissues is gradually reduced if exposure to the compound is discontinued or diminished.

Other observations regarding storage include the finding that rats whose brains contain DDT at a concentration of 25 ppm or less (wet weight) usually survive, whereas higher levels tend to be fatal regardless of whether absorption followed one or many doses. Of samples that may be collected *in vivo,* the concentration of DDT in serum most accurately reflects its concentration in the brain, the critical tissue.

Adams *et al.* (1974) observed that about the same concentrations of DDT and related compounds are stored by male rats and by females that reproduce successfully. The lower storage in mated females probably is accounted for by transfer to the young via the placenta and the milk. However, other factors may be involved.

When DDT, some of its analogs, and several other chlorinated hydrocarbon insecticides were fed to male and female rats for four generations, there was little variation in storage of the materials from one generation to another and no evidence of a continuing increase in succeeding generations (Adams *et al.,* 1974). The concentrations of DDT in the blood and other tissues of the fetus are lower than those in corresponding tissues of the mother (Dedek and Schmidt, 1972).

DDE constituted about 4% of technical DDT. Most species convert some of the DDT they ingest to DDE. Finally, most species, including humans, store DDE more tenaciously than they do DDT, the greater part of which is metabolized by a different pathway from that of DDA and excreted more rapidly.

The result is that DDE, expressed as a percentage of total DDT-related compounds, increases in individuals after DDT intake decreases and increases in successive steps of the food chain. The Rhesus monkey apparently is an exception. Monkeys store DDE when it is fed to them. However, when feeding is stopped, the rate of loss of DDE stored in fat is more rapid than that of DDT (Durham *et al.,* 1963). Whether it is relative inability to form DDE, unusual ability to excrete it, or a combination of both that accounts for the fact that little or no DDE can be found in monkeys fed DDT is not entirely clear.

60.2.3.5 Metabolism

The chemical nature of the chief metabolite excreted in the urine was first elucidated by White and Sweeney (1945). 2,2-bis(4-chlorophenyl) acetic acid (DDA) was isolated from the urine of rabbits chronically administered DDT. Later work by many authors confirmed that DDA isomers are the major urinary metabolites of p,p'-DDT and o,p'-DDT in all mammals, including humans, but the nature of all excreted metabolites still may not have been elucidated fully.

The ability of phenobarbital and especially diphenylhydantoin to promote the excretion of DDT was discovered in humans (Davies *et al.,* 1969) and later confirmed in animals (Alary *et al.,* 1971; Cranmer, 1970; Fries *et al.,* 1971). This is of course consistent with our current knowledge of the induction of drug metabolizing enzymes.

That portion of the metabolism of DDT that leads to DDA in rats was explored by Peterson and Robinson (1964), who gave evidence for the sequence of changes leading to DDA involving reduction to 1,1-dichloro-2, 2-bis(4-chlorophenyl)ethane (DDD) followed by dehydrochlorination to 1-chloro-2,2-bis(4-chlorophenyl)ethane (DDMU), which was apparently converted to 2,2-bis-(4-chlorophenyl)ethanol (DDOH) via 2,2-bis(4-chlorophenyl)ethane (DDNU); see Fig. 60.1. The compound identified as a "probable" intermediate aldehyde between p,p'-DDA was later synthesized and shown to be highly labile (McKinney *et al.,* 1969; Peterson and Robinson, 1964), confirming that it is unlikely to accumulate in tissues in measurable amounts. Kujawa *et al.* (1985) obtained evidence for its formation from p,p' DDD by rat liver homogenates and its presence in the urine of rats injected with DDD. Two additional metabolites, bis(p-chloro-phenyl)methane (DDM) and bis(p-chlorophenyl) methyl ketone (DBP), were identified in chicks (Abou-Donia and Menzel, 1968). Not only was DBP found to result from the metabolism of DDA with DDM as an intermediate, but DBP was the only metabolite of DDE administered.

Organ perfusion studies indicated that the liver is capable of biotransformation of DDT, DDE, DD, DDMU, and other possible metabolites (Datta and Nelson, 1970). Cultures of human embryonic lung cells are capable of metabolizing DDT to DDA via DDD (North and Menzer, 1973). On the other hand perfusion of rat, guinea pig, pig and human skin samples has shown poor percutaneous passage of DDT ($<1\%$) and no evidence for cutaneous metabolism (Moir *et al.,* 1994).

When DDA was discovered, it was postulated that DDE was a step in its formation (White and Sweeney, 1945); however,

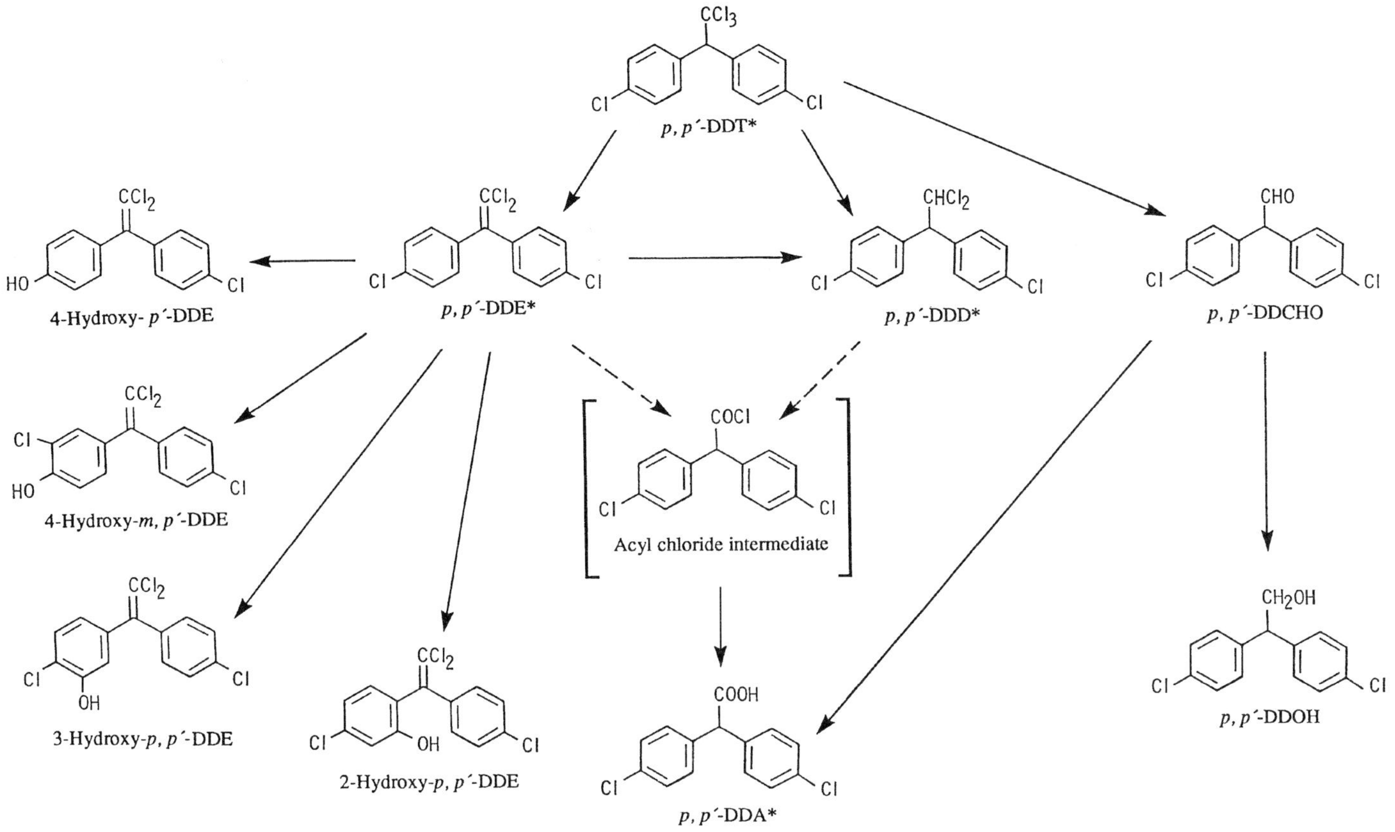

Figure 60.1 Metabolites of p,p'-DDT and the postulated route of metabolism in the rat. The metabolites indicated by an asterisk have been found in humans.

rats which produced both DDE and DDA from DDT were said by Peterson and Robinson (1964) to be incapable of forming DDA when fed preformed DDE. This finding was contradicted by Datta (1970) and by Datta and Nelson (1970), who claimed that ^{14}C-labeled p,p' DDE was converted by rats to 1-chloro-2,2-bis(4-chlorophenyl)ethene (p,p'-DDMU), which then underwent further metabolism to p,p'-DDA. Datta suggested that the predominance of detoxication via DDE or DDD may depend on physiological response or the amount of toxicant used. DDE is stored in tissue as first demonstrated in connection with human fat (Mattson *et al.*, 1953; Pearce *et al.*, 1952). In fact DDE is stored more tenaciously than DDT.

The way in which DDE is lost from storage remained something of a mystery. In humans (Cueto and Biros, 1967), seals, and guillemots (Jansson *et al.*, 1975) part of it is excreted unchanged, but the fact that its elimination is promoted by inducers of drug metabolism enzymes strongly suggests that much undergoes metabolism, conjugation, or both. That metabolism does occur was first demonstrated by identification of two hydroxylated derivatives of DDE in the feces of wild seals and guillemots and in the bile of seals (Jansson *et al.*, 1975). When p,p'-DDE was fed to rats, the same metabolites and one other were isolated from the feces, accounting for about 5% of the dose (Sundström *et al.*, 1975). Later, a fourth hydroxylated derivative was identified in the feces of rats fed p,p'-DDE. The metabolites are m-hydroxy-p,p'-DDE [1,10-dichloro-2-

(p-chloro-m-hydroxyphenyl)-2,2(p-chlorophenyl)ethylene, the major metabolite], o-hydroxy-p,p'-DDE, p-hydroxy-m,p'-DDE (the product of an NIH shift), and p-hydroxy-p'-DDE. A scheme involving m,p-epoxy-p,p'-DDE and o,m'-epoxy-p,p'-DDE was proposed for the formation of these metabolites as well as a fifth metabolite (Sundström, 1977). In mice, feeding DDE increased the hepatic levels of radioactivity from [14C]DDE and decreased that in the urine and feces (Gold and Brunk, 1986). The only metabolite identified was the o-hydroxylated product.

DDE is metabolized not only to easily excretable phenols but also to m-methylsulfone-p,p'-DDE. In the blubber of seals from the Baltic, this compound was found in a concentration of 4 ppm along with DDE (138 ppm), DDD (10 ppm), DDT (78 ppm), and various polychlorinated biphenyls (PCBs) and their metabolites (150 ppm) (Jenson and Jansson, 1976). Sulfur-containing metabolites of halogenated aliphatic and aromatic chemicals usually arise by initial conjugation with glutathione. The possibility of glutathione-derived conjugates of DDT requires further attention.

In vitro the reductive dechlorination of p,p'-DDT to DDD can occur with a cytochrome P-450 system, especially under anaerobic conditions (Esaac and Matsumura, 1980; Hassall, 1971; Zaidi, 1987). A one-electron reduction of DDT to the 1,1-dichloro-2,2-bis(p-chlorophenyl)ethyl radical seems to occur, followed by abstraction of a hydrogen atom, possibly from lipid, to give DDD (Kelner *et al.*, 1986). The reduction of DDT to DDD is stimulated by thiols in an unknown manner. The formation of an intermediate radical explains binding to microsomal lipid, especially under anaerobic conditions (Baker and Van Dyke, 1984). DDD, on the other hand, needs aerobic conditions for binding, implying that further metabolism is required. Other studies with mouse liver microsomes have shown the formation of 2,2-bis(*p*-chlorophenyl)-1,2-ethanediol (DDNU-diol) from DDNU, suggesting that a reactive epoxide intermediate might be formed (Planche *et al.*, 1979). When synthesized, however, the ethylene oxide (DDNU-oxide) was not mutagenic.

Gold and colleagues examined the metabolism of DDT metabolites in mice *in vivo*. The results seem to be a little different from that previously accepted for rats. It is thought that DDMU can undergo epoxidation; the resulting mutagenic epoxide is hydrolyzed and oxidized to 2-hydroxy-2,2-bis(4-chlorophenyl)acetic acid (αOH-DDA), which is excreted in the urine (Gold *et al.*, 1981; Gold and Brunk, 1982). Another route of metabolism of DDT in both the mouse and hamster (Gold and Brunk, 1982, 1983, 1984) seems to be the formation of DDA by a route involving hydroxylation on the C-1 side chain carbon of DDD. Loss of HC1 gives an intermediate acyl chloride, 2,2-bis(4-chlorophenyl)acetyl chloride (C1-DDA), capable of reacting with cellular proteins, DNA, etc., or losing water to give DDA.

Since this work, the metabolism of DDT in rats has been reexamined (Fawcett *et al.*, 1981, 1987) and seems to be similar to that described above for hamsters and mice. The conversion of *p,p'*-DDD to *p,p'*-DDA occurs primarily by hydroxylation leading to C1-DDA, which on hydrolysis gives DDA. This acyl chloride may also be formed from DDE via an epoxidation route. Although DDMU is converted to DDA (Gold and Brunk, 1984; Fawcett *et al.*, 1987), there is now considerable doubt as to whether it is an important intermediate in DDT metabolism. In addition, there is evidence to suggest that DDOH is a reduction product of DDCHO formed directly from DDT and not a precursor. A current scheme for the metabolism of *p,p'*-DDT in rats is shown in Fig. 60.1 and is still probably incomplete. For instance, the role of DDOH still appears to be uncertain (Kujawa *et al.*, 1985).

The interconversions of *o,p'*-DDT and *p,p'* DDT have been reported (Abou-Donia and Menzel, 1968; French and Jeffries, 1969; Klein *et al.*, 1965), but there is considerable doubt as to whether these occur *in vivo* (Cranmer *et al.*, 1972).

Compared to *p,p'*-DDT, the more rapid excretion of *o,p'*-DDT is explained at least in part by the observed ring hydroxylation of the parent compound in rats (Feil *et al.*, 1973) and chickens (Feil *et al.*, 1975) and of its metabolite *o,p'*-DDD in rats (Reif and Sinsheimer, 1975) and humans (Reif *et al.*, 1974) (see Fig. 60.2).

At least 13 metabolites were detected in rats. Ring hydroxylation, which has not been observed with *p,p'*-DDT or *p,p'*-DDD (but has been seen with *p,p'*-DDE), occurs in all species but with species differences. For example, *o,p'*-DDE and three hydroxylated *o,p'*-DDEs were found in the exc-

reta of chickens but not in the excreta of rats. In two patients with adrenal carcinoma for which they were receiving *o,p'*-DDD at a rate of 2000 mg/day, as much as 46–56% of the daily intake was recovered in the urine. Just over half of the recovered material was in the form of *o,p'*-DDA, but the remainder was in the form of hydroxylated derivatives, mainly *m*-hydroxy-, *p*-hydroxy-, *m*-hydroxy-*p*-methoxy-, and *p*-hydroxy-*m*-methoxy-*o,p'*-DDA. All hydroxylation had occurred on the ring that had its chlorine in the *o* position (Reif *et al.*, 1974). When the metabolism of a single 100-mg oral dose of *o,p'*-[^{14}C]DDD was studied in rats, averages of 7.1 and 87.8% of the activity were recovered in the urine and feces, respectively, within 8 days (Reif and Sinsheimer, 1975). The high recovery indicated rapid excretion with little storage.

o,p'-DDD is specifically toxic for the adrenal cortex in a number of species including humans. *In vitro* studies suggest that this is due to its activation in adrenal mitochondria to a metabolite which binds covalently. Unlike the situation in liver, a metabolite more polar than DDA is also produced (Martz and Straw, 1977, 1980; Pohland and Counsell, 1985). More recently, Lund *et al.* (1988) showed that 3-methysulfonyl-*p,p'*-DDE is selectively covalently bound and toxic to the adrenal zona fasciculata of mice. A single dose of 3-methylsulfonyl-*p,p'*-DDE to mouse dams caused high binding in the adrenals of suckling pups with extensive vacuolation and necrosis of the zona fasciculata. Slight degenerative changes were seen in fetal adrenals after dosing mothers with 50 mg/kg (Jonnsson *et al.*, 1992). The binding and damage probably results from cytochrome P450 activation (CYP11B) in adrenal mitochondria (Jonnsson *et al.*, 1991, 1995). A similar cytochrome P450-mediated activation may account for the covalent binding of *o,p'*-DDD in mouse lung (Lund *et al.*, 1986, 1989) and may be related to the acyl chloride formation already reported for *p,p'*-DDT in rats and mice (Fig. 60.1). Cytochrome P450-mediated activation to the acyl chloride has also been proposed as partly accounting for the toxicity of DDD to isolated rabbit Clara cells and human bronchial epithelial cells (Nichols *et al.*, 1995).

Of the compounds shown in Figs. 60.1 and 60.2 only DDT, DDD, DDE, and DDA commonly are reported in the tissues or excreta of animals, including humans. Conjugates of DDOH with fatty acids in the livers and spleens of rats given DDT have been reported (Leighty *et al.*, 1980) and can be removed *in vivo* by treatment with bile salts, heparin, or lecithin (Leighty, 1981).

Although microorganisms, plants, insects, and birds produce many of the same metabolites found in mammals, there are interesting differences. Nearly 20 derivatives (including mammalian metabolites) have been identified, and the chemical structures of others are still unknown. Some aspects of nonmammalian, as well as mammalian, metabolism have been reviewed (Fishbein, 1974; Klein and Korte, 1970; Korte, 1979; Menzie, 1969; Schroeder and Dorozalska, 1975). The metabolism of microorganisms and plants, as well as that of domestic animals, may influence the composition of DDT-derived residues in human food, but there is no evidence that

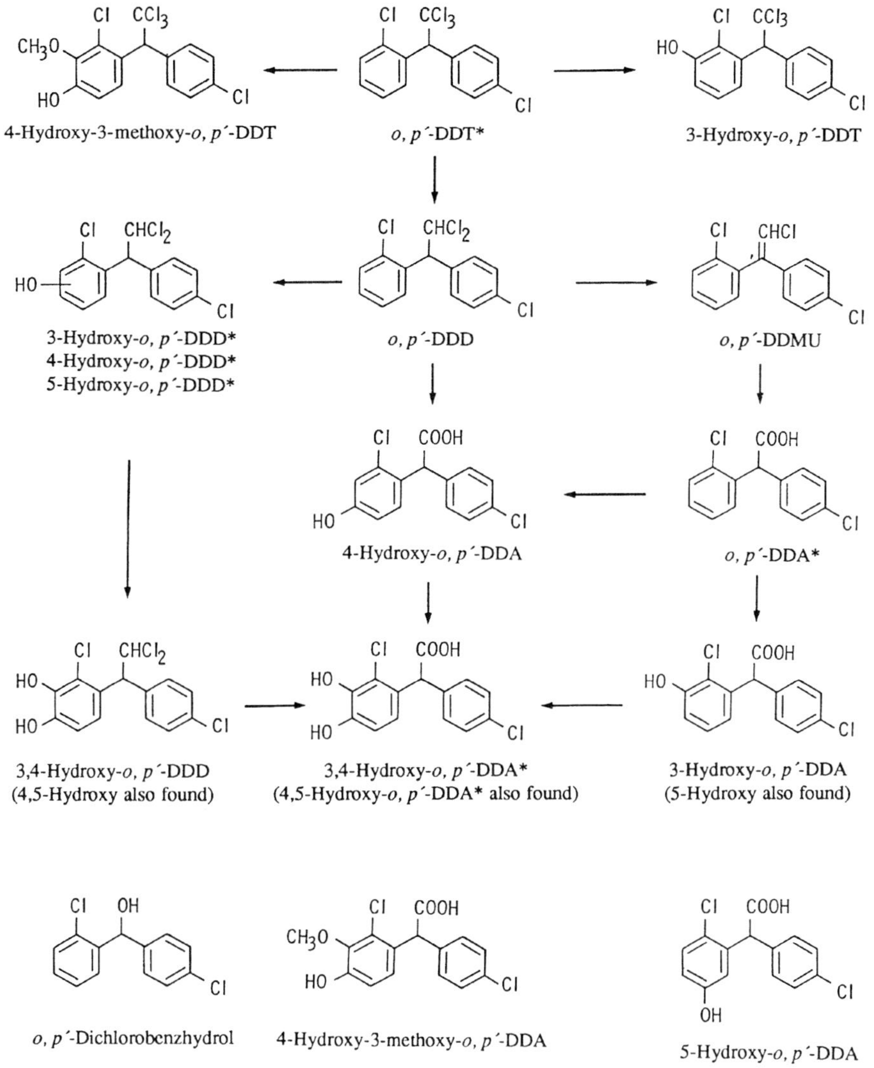

Figure 60.2 Metabolism of o,p'-DDT in the rat. Compounds indicated by an asterisk have been found in humans, including those humans treated with large doses of o,p'-DDD. In rats, glycine and serine conjugates of o,p'-DDA have been found in the urine, and the aspartic acid conjugate of o,p'-DDA has been found in the feces.

these residues contain a significant amount of any compound not formed from DDT by human metabolism.

60.2.3.6 Excretion

When large doses of DDT are ingested, some of the compound is unabsorbed. Only traces of unaltered DDT may be found in the feces when exposure is by any route other than oral. However, true fecal excretion of DDT metabolites was established irrespective of the route of administration (Hayes, 1965), although either DDT metabolites are not excreted by humans in the feces to any important degree, or they are excreted in one or more forms different from those demonstrated in rats. The bile appears to be the principal source of DDT metabolites in the feces of rats. When the bile duct was cannulated before intravenous injection of radioactive DDT, 65% of the dose was recovered in the bile, 2% in the urine, and only 0.3% in the feces (Jensen *et al.*, 1957). The different routes of excretion

are not unrelated. Burns *et al.* (1957) found that there was an increase in urinary excretion of radioactive material following ligation of the bile duct in rats fed radioactive DDT. This supports the finding by Jensen and his colleagues that most of the metabolites in bile are DDA or closely related to it. Although an enterohepatic circulation of the metabolites of DDT has not been proved directly, it seems likely that such a circulation exists. The difference between the excretion of DDT and its metabolites in rats and the slower excretion in birds seems to be the reduced ability of birds to further metabolize DDE (Fawcett *et al.*, 1981). The excretion of DDE in rats is dependent on dose and probably involves induction of drug-metabolizing systems (Ando, 1982). The excretion of DDT in milk was first published by Woodard *et al.* (1945) in connection with a dog fed at the rate of 80 mg/kg/day. Within a short time, excretion of DDT in milk was reported in rats, goats, and cows, and in 1951 it was demonstrated in women (Laug *et al.*, 1951). Telford and

Guthrie (1945) reported that rats fed a diet containing 1000 ppm produced milk toxic to their young. Following these early studies, the presence of DDT was demonstrated repeatedly in the milk of cows. Cows fed substantial, not nontoxic, residues of DDT commonly excrete 10% or more of the total dose in their milk (Hayes, 1959).

The proportion of the mother's DDT intake that could be recovered from her milk varied from 12.6 to 30.2% and averaged 24.6% in rats receiving the compound from their diet at an average rate of 32.4 mg/kg/day. Under these circumstances, the dosage of the young was somewhat less than half of that of their mothers on a milligram per kilogram basis. The oral dosage of 32.4 mg/kg/day was well tolerated by both dams and pups, as was also true of an intraperitoneal dosage of 100 mg/kg/day. An intraperitoneal dosage of 200 mg/kg/day killed some dams, but most of the pups of other dams survived. All of the pups of these mothers experienced reduced milk intake and reduced weight gain. The concentration of DDT in the brains of these pups was much lower than in pups killed by oral administration of the compound, indicating that the young of mothers receiving massive dosages of DDT suffer malnutrition but not poisoning (Hayes, 1976).

Wilson *et al.* (1946) showed that DDT was secreted from the skin of a cow maintained on an oral dosage of about 53 mg/kg/day.

Because DDA is the main form in which DDT is excreted, it might be expected that, following its direct administration, DDA would be excreted relatively efficiently. During the first several days after oral dosing, rabbits excreted DDA in the urine approximately 15 times faster than animals given DDT at an equivalent dosage. Although the rate of DDA excretion associated with DDT increased more rapidly, so that the values differed by a factor of only 5 after day 20 of feeding (Smith *et al.*, 1946).

60.2.3.7 Biochemical Effects

The main mechanism of action of DDT is its effect on membranes in the nervous system, especially axonal membranes. The effect on axons may be related to inhibition of Na^+-, K^+-, and Mg^{2+}-adenosine triphosphatase derived from a nerve ending fraction of rabbit brain that is inhibited by DDT. A similar enzyme that binds DDT was isolated from the synapses of rat brain (Bratowski and Matsumura, 1972). There has been considerable interest in a Ca-ATPase which may regulate calcium levels at the axon surface (Ghiasuddin and Matsumura, 1979), and DDT is known to cause prolonged opening of the ion gates of the sodium channel perhaps by affecting phosphorylation in the α-subunit protein (Ishikawa *et al.*, 1989). Song *et al.* (1996) showed that DDT appeared to interact with sodium channels of rat dorsal, not ganlion neurons, in the same manner as type I and type II pyrethroids. At a supralethal dosage of 600 mg/kg, DDT caused in rats a marked decrease in the concentration of cortical and striatal acetylcholine and of brain stem 3-methoxy-6-hydroxphenylglycol and 5-hydroxyindoleacetic acid (Hrdina *et al.*, 1973; Hudson *et al.*, 1985; Tilson *et al.*,

1986). *p*-Chlorophenylalanine blocked all of the neurotoxic signs of poisoning, and other inhibitors blocked one or another but not all of the effects. It was suggested that changes in the metabolism of 5-hydroxytryptamine and norepinephrine may be responsible for DDT-induced hypothermia and acetylcholine may be related to tremors and convulsions (Hrdina *et al.*, 1973). Although spinal α-adrenoceptors have been proposed as modulating DDT-induced tremor (Herr and Tilson, 1987), attenuation of DDT-induced motor dysfunction requires blockade of α-adrenoceptors in regions other than solely the spinal cord (Herr *et al.*, 1989). At a lower dose of DDT (180 mg/kg), but one which still induced convulsive tremor, acetylcholine and cyclic GMP were increased in the cerebellum (Aldridge *et al.*, 1978). In adult rats and mice there is a decrease in the cholinergic muscarinic receptors of rat brain (Eriksson *et al.*, 1984), particularly in the cerebellum (Fonseca *et al.*, 1986). The palmitic acid conjugate of DDOH can also have this effect (Eriksson and Nordberg, 1986). Disturbances of brain lipid metabolism have been observed in monkeys after chronic exposure to DDT (Sanyal *et al.*, 1986). Khaikina and Shilina (1971) reported that administration of DDT to rats at only one-fifth of the LD 50 for 20 days increased by 188% the amount of 5-hydroxyindoleacetic acid excreted in their urine. This indicated a change in the metabolism of serotonin, but it probably does not support a serotonin deficiency as a DDT mode of action (Chung *et al.*, 1981).

It is evident that many of the side effects of DDT are the result of its induction of drug metabolizing enzymes. Oral administration of o,p'-DDT to dogs at a rate of 50 mg/kg/day stimulates the microsomal enzymes of the liver. These changes in the liver are initially accompanied by an increase in the size of the adrenals and of the cells of the zone faciculata; these cells become vacuolated and devoid of acidophilic cytoplasm, and their nuclei become hyperchromatic and often peripheral in position. Synthesis of cortocosteroids by the adrenal is not blocked (Copeland and Cranmer, 1974). Thus, the effect of a substantial dosage of o,p'-DDT is quite different from that of o,p'-DDD, although part of the metabolism of o,p'-DDT must be by that route.

The tissue level of p,p'-DDE necessary to induce liver microsomal enzymes is lower in the rat than in the quail (and possibly in other birds). Thus Bunyan *et al.* (1972), using residues in the heart as an index, found a maximal increase in cytochrome P-450 per weight of liver and a maximal activity of aniline hydroxylase activity at tissue levels of approximately 3 ppm DDE in rats and 40 ppm DDE in quail. However, at any given dietary level, higher tissue levels were reached by quail than by rats, so the dosage responses of the two were similar. These authors concluded that DDE is more important that DDT in inducing microsomal enzymes, but in humans the opposite appears to be true. The significance of the induction of hepatic enzymes and any correlation with the potential hepatocarcinogenicity of DDT can be found elsewhere in this chapter and is particularly discussed in Smith (1991). In the female rat multiple bi-daily doses of DDT induced hepatic CYP2B and 3A proteins but not CYP1A1 or 1E1 (Li *et al.*, 1995) and caused elevated hydroxylation at 16 and 6 β of testosterone. DDT, DDE, and DDD all induced CYP2B and 3A in male rat liver to not disimilar degrees despite marked differences in bio retention (Nims *et al.*, 1998).

In squirrel monkeys (and presumably in other species) only 2 days on a vitamin C-deficient diet impairs both the induction of o-demethylase and the stimulation of the glucuronic acid system by DDT (5 mg/monkey/day) (Chadwick *et al.*, 1971). In guinea pigs, maintenance of induction of microsomal enzymes requires a higher dietary level of vitamin C than does prevention of scurvy (Wagstaff and Street, 1971).

Since lipids are associated with the function of microsomal enzymes and DDT induces these enzymes, it might have been expected that DDT and essential fatty acids would interact. Tinsley and Lowry (1972) found that the growth of female rats receiving p,p'-DDT at a dietary level of 150 ppm was depressed if they received a diet deficient in essential fatty acids but was slightly stimulated if they received the same diet supplemented with these acids. It was suggested that DDT influenced essential fatty acid metabolism by increasing the demand for them. Sampson *et al.* (1980) found that DDT did not exacerbate aspects of essential fatty acid deficiency but did alter lipid metabolism in an unexplained way. Exposure of rats to DDT by the intratracheal route has shown lung lipid metabolic changes but the significance is unclear (Narayan *et al.*, 1990a, b).

In contrast, a variety of diets (containing fats that may occur in the human diet and that were in approximately the same proportion as fats in typical human food in the United States) had little or no influence on the storage of DDT and a wide range of pesticides fed to rats for four generations in combination at rates only 200 times those found in food in the United States (Adams *et al.*, 1974). Fat mobilization can cause rapid release of stored DDT, but this does not seem to be associated with any major toxic effect assessed pathologically or biochemically (Mitjavila *et al.*, 1981b).

DDT has been shown *in vitro* and sometimes *in vivo* to influence some enzymes of intermediary metabolism and other miscellaneous enzymes. For instance, DDT and a variety of analogs have been shown to affect isolated rat liver mitochondria but the significance of this *in vivo* is uncertain (Ohyama *et al.*, 1982). Whether this is linked to the effects caused by 3-methyl sulfonyl-p,p'-DDE in adrenal mitochondria is not known.

The hyperglycemia observed during much of the early part of acute poisoning may be associated with an increase in four gluconeogenic enzymes (pyruvate carboxylase, phosphoenolpyruvate carboxykinase, fructose-1,6-diphosphatase, and glucose-6-phosphatase) (Kacew and Singhal, 1973). Increase in these enzymes in the renal cortex of rats have been observed after a single dose at a rate as low as 100 mg/kg or greater or following 45 daily doses at rates of 5 or 25 mg/kg/day. The changes are not mediated through release of corticosteroids from the adrenal glands. The fact that 100 mg/kg is the smallest single dosage that produced a statistically significant change in these enzymes indicates that their alteration is a complication rather than a cause of poisoning. High concentrations of DDT inhibit phosphatidase, muscle phosphatases, carbon an-

hydrase, and oxaloacetic carboxylase and increase the activity of cytochrome oxidase and succinic dehydrogenase. However, none of these changes with the possible exception of inhibition of carbonic anhydrase appear to have any connection with the toxic action of DDT or even with its side effects (Hayes, 1959). Neal *et al.* (1944) reported a small but consistent increase in the volume of urine excreted in 24 hr when dogs were dosed orally or by insufflation at the rate of 100 mg/kg/day. The possibility that increased urinary output is related to the inhibition of carbonic anhydrase (Torda and Wolff, 1949) may deserve attention, but data from volunteers receiving 3.5 or 35 mg/person/day indicated no increase in urinary volume compared with controls (Hayes *et al.*, 1971). Many enzymes including plasma amylase, aldylase, glutamic pyruvic transaminase, and isocitric dehydrogenase were not changed in squirrel monkeys given dosages from 0.05 to 50 mg/kg/day, the latter of which proved fatal within 14 weeks (Cranmer *et al.*, 1972).

60.2.3.8 Effects on the Nervous System

The major toxic action of DDT is clearly on the nervous system, probably by slowing down closing of "gates" in axon sodium channels (Dubois and Bergman, 1977; Hong *et al.*, 1986; Woolley, 1982, 1985), and it requires an intact organism for full expression. For other biochemical mechanisms related to the nervous system see Section 60.2.3.7. The fact that DDT causes a myotonic response in muscle and substitution of a train of spikes for the normal diphasic electroneurogram (Eyzaguire and Lilienthal, 1949) is in marked contrast to the absence of detectable injury or, in fact, any response in other isolated tissues.

In spite of the importance of the nervous system, a detailed review of early literature indicates that although the presence of some specialized nervous function may be necessary for the manifestation of DDT poisoning, the mere occurrence of specialized nervous fibers in certain protozoa or the occurrence of a rather complex nervous system in mollusks is not sufficient to render these forms susceptible. Just as there is little explanation still for the effect of DDT in susceptible species, the fact that certain species and even entire phyla are inherently resistant to the compound is still not entirely understood.

A review (Hayes, 1959) of literature on the effects of DDT on the nervous system showed that all major parts, both central and peripheral, are affected. Whereas effects on specific portions, notably the cerebellum and the motor cortex, have been viewed as of greatest importance, it probably is more accurate to emphasize the interaction of functions, all modified to some degree.

Farkas *et al.* (1968) found that electrocardiogram wave frequency showed considerable increase in resting rats that had received 20 mg/kg/day as a result of dietary intake. Rats that had received 5mg/kg/day did not exhibit this change while at rest, but even these exhibited abnormalities when exposed to a rhythmic light stimulus. Electrical activity may become abnormal only a minute or two after administration of a large dose of DDT. Four stages culminating in generalized seizure were described by Joy (1973). Phenobarbital, but not diphenylhydantoin or trimethadione, was effective in stopping seizures.

The most characteristic effect of DDT in contrast to dieldrin, for example, is the production of tremor. Sufficient dosages of DDT produce tremor even at ambient temperatures that approach body heat. However, dosages of DDT that produce no other clinical effect make rats more sensitive to low temperatures. This sensitivity may be demonstrated by having the rats swim to exhaustion in cool water. The ability of the rat to keep afloat is more dependent on coordination than on physical strength. DDT appreciably reduces the swimming time (Hayes, 1982; Smith, 1991).

Like tremor, the coldness of the skin and ruffling of the fur seen in acute poisoning probably represent an indication of disturbed thermal regulation. Apparently, it was not until the work of Hrdina *et al.* (1975) that an increase of almost 3°C in body temperature was reported in rats following a fatal (600 mg/kg) oral dosage of DDT.

The central nervous systems of mice and hamsters are equally sensitive, the concentration of DDT in their brains at death being similar (Gingel and Wallcave, 1974). However, after an oral dosage of 500 mg/kg, the DDT concentration of the mouse brain was twice that of the hamster. This cannot be explained by a difference in absorption, metabolism, or excretion but apparently is due to a difference in permeability of the blood-brain barriers of the two species. When animals received DDT at a dietary level of 205 ppm for 6 weeks, the residues in fat and liver were seven to eight times higher in the mouse, a fact only partially explained by the greater food intake of mice relative to body weight. Although urinary excretion of [^{14}C] DDT was similar in previously unexposed hamsters and mice, this excretion was stimulated in the hamster but little affected in the mouse by previous dietary exposure to DDT.

Careful studies have shown that neurotoxic actions of DDT following oral dosing of rats are significantly affected by the volume of the dosing solution. Not surprisingly this is probably the consequence of higher partitioning of DDT in oil and greater gut motility but it illustrates the importance of pharmacokinetic knowledge in comparative studies (McDaniel and Moser, 1997). Both DDT and DDE interact similarly with model and native membranes, causing disordering effects in cholesterol rich membranes, such as brain microsomes (Antunes-Madeira *et al.*, 1993; Antunes-Madeira and Madeira, 1993). Whether these effects have any bearing on neurotoxicity *in vivo* is unknown.

60.2.3.9 Cause of Death

Death from DDT poisoning is usually the result of respiratory arrest. The heart continues to beat to the end and in some instances continues a little while after respiration stops. Deichmann *et al.* (1950) found that the onset of hyperirritability was accompanied by an increase in the frequency and amplitude of respiration. Later, with the occurrence of tremors, the depth of respiration frequently returned to a more normal level, but the rate remained high. In some animals respiration stopped suddenly after a deep inspiration during a tonic convulsion. In other animals the rate and amplitude decreased progressively and finally ceased without any terminal spasm. Animals that die of respiratory failure caused by DDT do so after a relatively long period of muscular activity that leaves them exhausted.

It was shown by Phillips and Gilman (1946) and Phillips *et al.* (1946) that the hearts of dogs given large intravenous doses of DDT were sensitized to epinephrine. This was true not only of injected epinephrine but also of the compound released by the adrenal glands during a seizure. Stimulated in this way, the sensitized hearts of dogs developed an irreversible, fatal ventricular fibrillation. However, the hearts of monkeys were able to recover from fibrillation and resume normal rhythm. It is not clear how important sensitization of the myocardium is when DDT is administered by other routes, but ventricular fibrillation may be the cause of death in animals that die suddenly soon after onset of poisoning.

Thus, DDT not only sensitizes the myocardium in a way similar to that of halogenated hydrocarbon solvents but also, through its action on the central nervous system, produces the stimulus that increases the likelihood of fibrillation.

There is no evidence that repeated, tolerated doses of DDT sensitize the heart (Jeyaratnam and Forshaw, 1974). Rats were fed DDT at a dietary level of 200 ppm (about 10 mg/kg/day) for 8 months, during which they received weekly intraperitoneal doses of vasopressin which causes a temporary myocardial ischemia. Electrocardiograms showed no significant increase in cardiac arrhythmias in the DDT-fed rats compared with controls. Intravenous noradrenaline given at the end of the 8-month period did not produce a greater incidence of arrhythmias in the DDT-fed rats.

60.2.3.10 Mutation and Carcinogenesis

DDT has been tested in a number of ways for possible mutational effect. Much of this work has been reviewed in detail together with most of the carcinogenicity studies shown in Table 60.4 (Coulston, 1985). For example, Shirasu *et al.* (1976) listed DDT as a negative chemical in microbial mutagenicity screening studies including metabolic activation systems with both DDT and DDE (McCann and Ames, 1976; Shirasu *et al.*, 1977).

At a dosage of 105 mg/kg DDT produced no increase of dominant lethals in mice (Epstein and Shafner, 1968). However, concentrations of 10 ppm or greater produced chromosome breaks and exchange figures in a marsupial somatic cell line (Palmer *et al.*, 1972). A slight mutagenic effect in mammals has been reported by Markarian (1966). Deletions plus gaps were reported to be more common in the chromosomes of mice that had received DDT. On the whole, *in vitro* tests of the mutagenicity of DDT have given only negative or dubious results (Coulston, 1985).

An unconventional test for mutagenicity involved examination of explants of pulmonary tissue from embryonic mice whose dams had been fed dietary concentrations of 10 and 50 ppm DDT (Shabad *et al.*, 1972). An increase of diffuse hyperplasia and focal proliferation was observed, but a dosage–response relationship was not clear. Some of the embryos were allowed to live and the experiment was repeated in subsequent generations. There was no continuing progression of the reported changes in succeeding generation.

The question of whether DDT is carcinogenic really seems to be restricted, experimentally, to its action in the liver of some rodents. Some of the positive findings shown in Table 60.4 have not been found in other studies (National Cancer Institute, 1978a). However, there is still the evidence that DDT can act as a promoter of liver carcinogenesis initiated by aflatoxin and of other chemicals *in vitro* and *in vivo* (Peraino *et al.*, 1975; Rojanapo *et al.*, 1987; Schulte-Hermann, 1985; Sugie *et al.*, 1987; Williams and Numoto, 1984).

DDT causes inhibition of intercellular communication in cultured rat liver epithelial cells and in hamster cell lines (Flodstrom *et al.*, 1990; Tsushimoto *et al.*, 1983; Wärngård *et al.*, 1989; Williams *et al.*, 1981). This could be protected against by extracts of green tea (Sigler and Ruch, 1993). Using freeze-fracture analysis of hepatocytes from rats exposed *in vivo* to DDT Sugie *et al.* (1987) showed that both gap junction size and number were reduced. Tateno *et al.* (1994) provided evidence that in these *in vivo* experiements with rats changes in connexin 32 and connexin 26 expression might be responsible. Additional studies with the rat "oval" cell line WB-F344, which does not express connexin 32 but rather connexin 43 predominantly, showed not a decreased expression but a decrease in the phosphorylated form (Ruch *et al.*, 1994). Subsequent investigations suggest this is due to endocytosis of gap junctions and lysosomal connexin 43 P2 degradation (Guan and Ruch, 1996).

Some evidence suggests that *o,p'*-DDT can support the growth of an estrogen-responsive tumor (Robison *et al.*, 1985a).

The significance of the effects of DDT and other chlorinated hydrocarbon insecticides on the liver in relation to hepatocarcinogenicity have been discussed in detail previously (Smith, 1991) and will not be discussed here.

60.2.3.11 Other Miscellaneous Effects on Organs and Tissues

Many early reports reviewed by Hayes (1959) indicate that large doses of DDT may have no effect on the blood or they may produce a moderate leukocytosis and a decrease in hemoglobin, with or without a decrease in the concentration of red cells. The leukocytosis probably is secondary to stimulation of the sympathetic nervous system, while the loss of hemoglobin may be nutritional in origin. A later study with squirrel monkeys did not confirm the early results (Cranmer *et al.*, 1972). A range of hematologic parameters remained unchanged in squirrel monkeys dosed orally at rates of 0, 0.05, 0.5, 5, and 50 mg/kg/day, even though the highest dosage was fatal within 14 weeks.

Average protein-bound iodine levels of 5.42 and 6.93 μg/%, respectively, were reported in the sera of 42 workers occupationally exposed to chlorinated hydrocarbon insecticides and 51 workers not so exposed. The differences were statistically significant even though all values fell within the normal range of 4–8 μg/% (Wassermann *et al.*, 1971). It was not recorded whether the workers involved were from the same factory as

those with 10 or more years of occupational exposure whose plasma DDT levels were reported that after a single large dose (100 mg/kg) to rats thyroidal ^{131}I release was completely inhibited for more than 12 hr. The view of Clifford and Weil (1972) was that there was no evidence that occupational exposure to DDT has had any effect on human endocrine organs.

What at first appeared to be an immunological response to DDT in guinea pigs really involved a quite different, predictable effect. Animals sensitized to diphtheria toxoid were less susceptible to anaphylaxis in response to a challenge dose of the toxoid if they were pretreated with DDT at a dosage of only 10–20 mg/kg/day (Gabliks *et al.*, 1973, 1975). Direct measurement of antitoxin production indicated little or no difference between protected and unprotected animals. Furthermore, some protection was given by DDT administered for only 3 days prior to the induction of anaphylaxis. Further study showed that DDT treatment reduced the histamine levels in the lungs of both immunized and nonimmunized animals. The number of detectable mast cells was also reduced; this was true whether the count was made in tissues from guinea pigs dosed systemically with DDT or in lungs and mesenteries from untreated animals exposed to DDT *in vitro* at concentrations ranging from 10 to 45 ppm. These results indicated that the protection offered by DDT was the result of a reduction of the amount of histamine available for sudden release in response to a challenge dose of toxoid (Askari and Gablicks, 1973). Regardless of exposure to DDT, immunization leads to an increase in detectable mast cells (Gabliks *et al.*, 1975). Banerjee *et al.* (1996) have compared DDT with some of its metabolites in suppressing aspects of humoral and cellular immune response in rats: DDE and DDD but not DDA appeared to play a role. DDT has been reported to cause acute renal failure in rats after intravenous infusion (Koschier *et al.*, 1980).

60.2.3.12 Effects on Reproduction

In recent years the possibility that environmental levels of DDT isomers and metabolites might have effects on human reproductive function and carcinogenesis in breast and testes has become a major issue. It was shown very early that DDT produces a striking inhibition of testicular growth and secondary sexual characteristics of cockerels when injected subcutaneously in dosages as high as 300 mg/kg/day (Burlington and Linderman, 1950). Changes in the testis involve the tubules and not the interstitial tissues, and they have been attributed to an estrogen-like action of DDT. Before the problem of residues became evident, DDT was used extensively for control of lice and common mites on chickens without any adverse effects on egg production or other aspects of reproduction. It must be emphasized that many rats would be killed the first day if they were given the dosage of DDT that has been shown to affect the testis of cockerels. The report that under special conditions DDT has a gonadotoxic effect is of questionable significance in view of the results of multigeneration tests in rats, mice, and dogs (Rybakova, 1968). Dean *et al.* (1980) were unable to demonstrate any changes in either serum androgens or testicular synthesis of testosterone in young rats after exposure to DDT despite significant induction of metabolism of testosterone by isolated hepatic microsomes. However, more recent evidence supports the view that DDT and its metabolite DDE can disrupt male reproductive development and act as antiandrogens by binding androgen receptors in a nonproductive manner (Kelce *et al.*, 1995, 1998). DDE, like vinclozolin and flutamide, changed the expression of androgen receptor regulated genes, such as the prostatic mRNA prostatein C3, in castrated-tetosterone treated male rats (Kelce *et al.*, 1997). Exposure of male rats to DDE *in utero* and by lactation showed that by some parameters Long–Evans rats were more sensitive than Sprague–Dawley, e.g., ano-genital distance, but DDE had no effects on testes, epididymus, seminal vesicles, or vental prostate weights (You *et al.*, 1998). Effects were minimal at maternal doses <10 mg/kg/day. Confirmation that Long–Evans rats were more sensitive to DDE than some other strains was reported from studies designed to detect antiandrogen endocrine disrupters and appeared to act centrally rather than peripherally (O'Connor *et al.*, 1999). The effects of p,p'-DDE on the development of the rat prostate was confirmed with Holtzman rats exposed *in utero* or by lactation (Loeffler and Peterson, 1999) without changes in serum androgen concentrations. This suggests effects on androgen signalling pathways within the prostate. Some evidence for a partial interaction with the antiandrogenic effects of TCDD was suggested from dual dosing experiments. The significance of these studies with regard to human male development is really not clear given the considerably greater experimental exposures.

Intraperitoneal injection of as little as 5 mg/kg of technical DDT or 1 mg/kg of o,p'-DDT causes a significant increase in weight of the uterus of normal immature female rats or of ovariectomized adult females (Welch *et al.*, 1969). A very much smaller stimulation is caused by p,p'-DDT. Treatment of rats with DDT, especially o,p'-DDT, inhibited uptake of the hormone by the uterus *in vivo,* possibly by competition for binding sites. Isomers of DDD and DDE do not influence uterine weight or the binding of estradiol (Welch *et al.*, 1969). It seems unlikely that metabolic activities of o,p'-DDT is necessary as is true of activation of o,p'-methoxychlor (Kupfer and Bulger, 1979). The action of o,p'-DDT on the uterus seems to be as a long-acting agonistic estrogen interacting with the same receptor as 17β-estradiol (Galand *et al.*, 1987; Ireland *et al.*, 1980; Robison *et al.*, 1984). However, some differences from estradiol have been recorded (Robison *et al.*, 1985b). The lesser enantiomer of o,p'-DDT seems to be the active isomer (McBain, 1987). The binding and estrogenic activity of DDT analogs in rats is only about 1/10,000 as great as that of diethylstilbestrol (Nelson, 1973), an important point when considering potential effects of trace levels relative to endogenous oestrogens. o,p'-DDT inhibited DNA synthesis in cultured bovine oviductal and uterine cells to a greater degree than methoxchlor, especially uterine epithelial and stromal cells (Tiemann *et al.*, 1996). However, at lower concentrations both o,p'-DDT and methoxchlor stimulated DNA synthesis.

A considerably smaller dosage of o,p'-DDT resulting from a dietary level of 10 ppm for 2–9 months had no effect on reproduction in ewes (Wrenn *et al.*, 1971a). In a similar way, dietary levels of o,p'-DDT as high as 40 ppm, giving a dosage level of about 2.1 mg/kg/day in rats, failed to interfere with reproduction and lactation in these animals, although dosage was continued through two pregnancies (Wrenn *et al.*, 1971b).

The report (Heinriks *et al.*, 1971) that o,p'-DDT significantly advances puberty, induces persistent vaginal estrus after a period of normal estrus cycles, and causes other reproductive abnormalities in female rats would at first appear inconsistent with the lack of effect of technical DDT or o,p'-DDT on reproduction cited above. The same is true of other effects of o,p'-DDT subcutaneously on the second, third, and fourth days of life (counting the day of birth as zero). Because rat pups on the third day weighed about 12 gm or less each, it follows that the subcutaneous dosage was about 83.3 mg/kg/day or more, that is, about 40 times greater than the highest oral dosage of o,p'-isomer fed to breeding rats and more than 10^5 times greater than human dietary exposure.

Ottoboni (1969) found that female rats reproduced normally when fed DDT for two generations at dietary levels as high as 200 ppm (about 10 mg/kg/day except during lactation, when intake is increased about threefold). In fact, at a dietary level of 20 ppm, the dams had a significantly longer reproductive life span (14.5 months) than their littermate controls (8.9 months); the number of females becoming pregnant after the age of 17 months and the number of successful pregnancies after that age were significantly different in the two groups (Ottoboni, 1972).

In a study focused mainly on DDT in milk, the full ability of rats to reproduce at a dietary level of 200 ppm was confirmed, and the ability of dams injected intraperitoneally at levels as high as 100 mg/kg/day to rear their young was demonstrated (Hayes, 1976).

A six-generation test of reproduction in mice showed no effect of DDT at a dietary level of 25 ppm on fertility, gestation, viability, lactation, and survival (Keplinger *et al.*, 1970). A level of 100 ppm produced a slight reduction in lactation, and survival in some generations but not all, and the effect was not progressive. A level of 250 ppm was distinctly injurious to reproduction. The dietary concentrations used determine dosages of 3.33, 13.3, and 33.2 mg/kg/day in nonpregnant, nonlactating, adult, female mice. The intake is much higher in both young and lactating mice.

Four female dogs of unstated age that previously had received DDT at the rate of 12 mg/kg/day, 5 days/week, for 14 months were bred when they went into heat (Deichmann *et al.*, 1971). The males involved had been fed aldrin (0.15 mg/kg/day) plus DDT (60 mg/kg/day) for 14 months prior to breeding but not during breeding. Two of the females went into heat but failed to become pregnant, and one failed to come into heat during 12 months after feeding stopped. Four of six pups born to the fourth female died within 1 week of birth; the other two were weaned successfully even though only two posterior mammae of the mother were functional. A three-generation study failed to confirm any of the injuries suggested by the study of four dogs. In the three-generation study, male and female dogs were fed technical DDT from weaning at rates of

0,1, 5, and 10 mg/kg day. Observations were made on 135 adult females, 63 adult males, and 650 pups. There were no statistically significant differences among controls and DDT-treated dogs in length of gestation, fertility, success of pregnancy, litter size, or lactation ability of the dams; in viability at birth, survival to weaning, sex distribution, and growth of pups; or in morbidity, mortality, organ/body weight ratios, or gross histological abnormalities in all the animals studied. The only clear difference was that DDT-treated females had their first estrus 2 or 3 months earlier than the control dogs. There was a slight increase in liver/body weight ratio in some DDT-treated animals but the difference was not statistically significant, not dosage related, and not associated with any histological change (Ottoboni *et al.*, 1977).

When *p,p'*-DDT was administered to pregnant mice at a rate of 1 mg/kg on days 10, 12, and 17 of gestation, it was not teratogenic but did alter the gonads and decrease the fertility of the young, especially the females (McLachlan and Dixon, 1972). A single dose at the rate of 15 mg/kg or repeated doses of 2.5 mg/kg/day given during pregnancy may be embryotoxic but not teratogenic to mice (Schmidt, 1973). DDT was shown to be more toxic than methoxychlor to preimplantation mouse embryos in culture (Alm *et al.*, 1996).

Teratogenic effects of DDT have not been seen in studies of reproduction, including those for two generations in rats, six generations in mice, and three generations in dogs (Smith, 1991). Because of the estrogenic properties of large doses of DDT, the compound was considered as a possible cause of abortion in dairy cattle, but no evidence for a relationship was found (Macklin and Ribelin, 1971). A similar conclusion was reached regarding human abortions (O'Leary *et al.*, 1970).

60.2.3.13 Behavioral Effects

Behavioral changes may be demonstrated in animals receiving DDT daily at rates too low to produce illness. Khairy (1959) detected ataxia in the form of changes in gait in rats that had been fed DDT at dietary levels of 100 ppm or more for 21 days. The results were recorded in terms of the tangent, that is, the ratio of the width and length of step. At a dosage of about 5 mg/kg/day the ratio was less than normal, a change attributed to an exaggeration of the stretch reflex. At dosages of about 10, 20, and 30 mg/kg/day, the ratio was progressively increased above normal as a result of broadening of the gait and shortening of the steps. These same dosage levels did not affect problem-solving behavior or speed of locomotion. The experimental animals were found to be generally less reactive to stress than normal ones. The acoustic startle response of rats is significantly increased after a 12.5 mg/kg dose of *p,p'*-DDT but can be attenuated by phenytoin and an adrenergic receptor antagonist, phenoxybenzamine (Herr and Tilson, 1987; Herr *et al.*, 1987; Saito *et al.*, 1986; Tilson *et al.*, 1985, 1985), which also decreased DDT-induced myoclonus (Hwang and Van Woert, 1978). See also Section 60.2.3.8.

60.2.3.14 Pathology

Morphological changes are inadequate to account for death from DDT poisoning. Changes that occur in the liver have been discussed previously (Smith, 1991). Mild to moderate morphological changes have been reported in the kidneys of animals that had received massive single doses or repeated doses; examples are fatty degeneration, necrosis, and calcification (Lillie *et al.*, 1947; Stohlman and Lillie, 1948) or slight brown pigmentation of the convoluted tubular epithelium (Fitzhugh and Nelson, 1947). However, it sometimes has happened that a complete absence of change in the kidney has been reported in connection with other studies carried out in the same laboratories (Lillie and Smith, 1944; Nelson *et al.*, 1944).

60.2.3.15 Treatment of Poisoning in Animals

The more successful studies of treatment of animals poisoned by DDT involve the nervous system. A full discussion of this can be found in Smith (1991). In essence sodium phenobarbitol affords little help in rats but in dogs and cats, to a lesser extent monkeys, it protected against tremors and death (Phillips and Gilman, 1946).

More recently, Tilson *et al.* (1985, 1986) have reported that phenytoin attenuates the tremor produced in rats by DDT and permethrin but not by lindane and chlordecone.

Vaz and his colleagues (1945) were apparently the first to note the antidotal effect of calcium in DDT poisoning. Dogs were given DDT orally as a 10% oily solution at a daily dosage of 100 mg/kg until signs of intoxication appeared. The same dosage could then be repeated to produce intense symptomatology from which the animals would recover spontaneously in 12–24 hr. For the actual tests, a larger challenge dosage of DDT (150–200 mg/kg) was used. Each dose of calcium gluconate (30 ml of a 10% solution) was injected intravenously into dogs weighing 8–18 kg. Dogs that were injected with calcium gluconate daily for 4 days and challenged with a large dose of DDT on the fourth day developed no symptoms or only slight ones. Dogs receiving a single dose of calcium gluconate showed symptoms of short duration and survived following a dosage of DDT large enough to kill two controls.

Koster (1947) studied cats poisoned by the intravenous injection of a soya lecithin–corn oil emulsion of DDT. A comparison was made of several aspects of intoxication, including number of convulsions, general severity (tremors, prostration, dyspnea), duration, and mortality. Both calcium gluconate and sodium gluconate reduced mortality but not severity. Gluconic acid increased the survival time and reduced mortality but did not reduce convulsions or severity. Calcium chloride reduced convulsions but not mortality or tremors. The lifesaving capacity of calcium gluconate at a rate of 40 mg/kg was confirmed by Judah (1949), even though he found normal blood calcium values in most poisoned but unmedicated animals. One animal showed a high calcium value, and Cameron and Burgess (1945) reported a similar result. Calcium has, then, an antidotal action against DDT in intact animals of several species. The hypothesis has been advanced that certain neurotoxins, including DDT, act by delaying the restoration of calcium ions to a surface complex following breaking of the chelate linkage of calcium ions to surface polar groups by an initial exciting impulse (Gordon and Welsh, 1948). This action of the neurotoxin is conceived as depending largely on its physical rather than on its chemical properties. The hypothesis is still helpful in explaining the fact that a wide variety of chemically unrelated compounds produce repetitive responses in excitable tissue and also the fact that many compounds that show a high toxicity for arthropods and mammals are fat-soluble and chemically relatively inert. On the other hand, calcium may help to offset the effects of DDT on calcium-dependent ATPases, especially in the neuronal axons (see Section 60.2.3.7).

Having observed the effect of DDT on the metabolism of glucose and glycogen, Laüger and colleagues (1945a, b) investigated the use of glucose as an antidote. All of the 10 dogs given 2000 mg of DDT per kilogram of body weight orally in the form of an oil solution died within 8–24 hr. Five of the 10 dogs treated with one or more 20-ml doses of 20% glucose survived the same dosage of DDT.

Koster (1947) found that glucose given before or after a LD 33 dosage reduced convulsions and mortality and, when given before the poison, reduced tremors, prostration, and dyspnea in cats, but was ineffective against a LD 95 dosage except to increase the time of survival.

60.2.4 TOXICITY TO HUMANS

60.2.4.1 Experimental Oral Exposure

Table 60.5 summarizes the effects of one or a few oral doses of DDT. The results are consistent with those in accidents reported by Garrett (1947) and Hsieh (1954) in which it was possible to estimate accurately the amount ingested. It may be concluded that a single dose of 10 mg/kg produces illness in some but not all subjects even though no vomiting occurs. Smaller doses generally produce no illness. Persons who were made sick by 10 mg/kg did not show convulsions, but convulsions have occurred in accidents when the dosage level was 16 mg/kg or greater (Hsieh, 1954). Rarely, a dosage as high as 20 mg/kg may be taken without apparent effect (MacCormack, 1945). Dosages at least as high as 285 mg/kg have been taken accidentally without fatal result (Garrett, 1947). However, large doses lead to prompt vomiting so the amount actually retained cannot be determined accurately.

In acute poisoning a slight decrease in hemoglobin and a moderate leukocytosis without any constant deviation in the differential white count have been observed in volunteers (Velbinger, 1947a, b). These findings are considered secondary to the neurological effects.

In the course of tests with volunteers, dilute colloidal aqueous suspensions of DDT are apparently odorless and tasteless (Domenjoz, 1944; Hoffman and Lendle, 1948). Saturated alcoholic solutions of DDT have a weak aromatic taste, or rather odor. Some people find these solutions slightly anesthetic to the tongue (Hoffman and Lendle, 1948). The taste of DDT in vegetable oil is so slight that many persons cannot identify capsules containing 0, 3.5, and 35 mg of DDT when they are presented separately but can arrange them in proper order when one of each is available for comparison.

The possible clinical effects of many repeated doses of DDT were first explored by Fennah (1945). Because of his interest in predicting the results of indiscriminate use, he expressed the exposures in terms of environmental levels rather than in dosage units. The exposures were clearly higher than those ordinarily encountered. In one test, lasting a total of 11.5 months, Fennah daily inhaled 100 mg of pure DDT and drank water dusted at the rate of 3240 mg/m². Much of the inhaled dust must have been deposited in the upper respiratory tract and swallowed. Later, for 1 month, Fennah ate food all of which had been sprayed at the rate of 2160 mg/m² after it had been served. No ill effect of any kind was observed. However, it must be said that these days we would examine more closely possible subtle chronic effects.

Some studies of DDT in volunteers have been designed to explore the details of storage and excretion of the compounds in humans and to search for possible effects of doses considered to be safe. In the first of these studies, men were given 0, 3.5, and 35 mg/person/day (Hayes, 1969). These administered dosages plus DDT measured in the men's food resulted in dosage levels of 0.0021–0.0034, 0.038–0.063, and 0.36–0.61 mg/kg/day, respectively, the exact value depending on the weight of each individual. Six volunteers received the highest dosage of technical DDT for 12 months, and three received it for 18 months. A smaller number of men ingested the lower dosage of technical DDT or one of the dosages of p,p'-DDT for 12–18 months. No volunteer complained of any symptom or showed any signs of illness that did not have an easily recognizable cause clearly unrelated to the exposure of DDT. At intervals, the men were given a systems review, physical examination, and a variety of laboratory tests. Particular attention was given to the neurological examination and liver function tests, because the major effects of DDT in animals involve the nervous system and the liver.

The same result was obtained in a second study in which the same dosages were given for 21 months and the volunteers were observed for a minimum of 27 additional months (Hayes et al., 1971). In the first study, the storage of DDT was proportional to dosage, but there was a then unexplained difference in the storage of the p,p'-isomer and of technical DDT. Following dosing for 12 months, the pure material was stored in fat at an average concentration of 340 ppm, but the technical material was stored at an average of only 234 ppm. The difference was statistically significant for the 3.5 mg/person/day dosages given for 3–6 and for 7–18 months. The difference was significant for the 35 mg/person/day doses after 7–18 months of dosing but not after only 3–6 months. Men who ate p,p'-DDT showed a definite increase in the absolute amount of DDE stored. After 6 months at a dosage of 35 mg/person/day, eight men showed an average DDE fat storage of 32.6 ± 7.0 ppm as compared to 12.3 ± 1.5 ppm for the same individuals upon entering the investigation. There was a further increase of DDE storage as

Table 60.5
Summary of the Effects of One or a Few Oral Doses of DDT on Volunteers

Dose (mg) and formulation	Result	Reference
250 × 9, suspension	no effect	Domenjoz (1944)
15,00 butter solution	no effect, but mice killed when fed 6 and 12 hr after dose	MacCormack (1945)
500, oil solution	no clinical effect	Neal et al. (1946)
770, oil solution	no clinical effect; DDA measured in urine	Neal et al. (1946)
250, suspension	none except slight disturbance of sensitivity of mouth	Velbinger (1947a, b)
250, oil solution	variable hyperesthia of mouth	Velbinger (1947a, b)
500, oil solution	variable hyperesthia of mouth	Velbinger (1947a, b)
750, oil solution	disturbance of sensitivity of lower part of face; uncertain gait; peak reaction (6 hr after ingestion) characterized by malaise, cold moist skin, and hypersensitivity to contact; reflexes normal	Velbinger (1947a, b)
1000, oil solution	same as above; no joint pains, fatigue, fear or difficulty in seeing or hearing	Velbinger (1947a, b)
1500, oil solution	prickling of tongue and around mouth and nose beginning 2.5 hr after dose; disturbance of equilibrium; dizziness; confusion; tremor of extremities; peak reaction (10 hr after ingestion) characterized by great malaise, headache, and fatigue; delayed vomiting; almost complete recovery in 24 hr	Velbinger (1947a, b)

exposure progressed. However, DDT was stored in so much greater concentration that the relative storage of DDE decreased sharply. Thus, after 6 months at a dosage of 35 mg/person/day, eight men stored only 14% of their total DDT-derived material in the form of DDE as compared to 65% for the same persons at the beginning of the investigation.

The storage of DDE by men who ate technical DDT presented a different picture. Until 18 months after exposure, there was no clear evidence that these men stored any more DDE after exposure than they did before. However, at 18 months the only three samples available showed DDE concentrations ranging from 28 to 85 ppm, all substantially above general population levels. Thus, both the total amount stored and the rate at which DDT converted to DDE served to distinguish the metabolism of p,p'-DDT and technical DDT in humans (Hayes et al., 1956). This was true even though later study showed that the concentration of DDE in serum increased immediately in persons ingesting technical DDT at rates of 10 and 20 mg/person/day. Of course, daily values were subject to considerable variation, but the upward slopes of the graphs recording the results were apparent in 60 days or less and apparently the graphs were straight throughout the 50 month feeding period. Under the same conditions, the level of DDT in serum increased within 1 day and continued to increase in a curvilinear fashion for 5 months (Apple et al., 1970). A similar rapid increase reaching its maximum in 30 hr after a single exposure has been observed in workers (Apple et al., 1970). The more rapid excretion of o,p'-DDT was demonstrated by Morgan and Roan (1972).

In a second study in which the volunteers received 0, 3.5, and 35 mg/person/day, the storage of DDT was again proportional to dosage with the real but very gradual accumulation

of DDE (Hayes, 1969, 1982; Smith, 1991). A steady state of storage was approached later in the second study (18.8–21.5 months) than in the earlier one (about 12 months). The second study was superior in that more men were observed for a longer period but inferior in that dosing was less regular. Because of the latter difficulty, it seems impossible to decide whether 12 months or 21.5 months is a more valid estimate of the time necessary for people to approach a steady state of storage when intake is uninterrupted and unvarying in amount. It is interesting that the storage levels eventually reached at the same dosage in the two studies were statistically indistinguishable in most instances. In the one instance in which a statistical difference existed, the greater storage by men in the second study may have been explained by the fact that some of them inadvertently received higher doses than intended. DDT was lost slowly from storage in fat after dosing was stopped. The concentration remaining following 25.5 months of recovery was from 32 to 35% of the maximum stored for those who had received 35 mg/person/day but was 66% for those who had received only 3.5 mg/person/day, indicating slower loss at lower storage levels (Hayes et al., 1971).

Morgan and Roan (1971) fed volunteers not only technical DDT but also p,p'-DDD. They found that DDE is stored more tenaciously than the other compounds in humans, the order being p,p'-DDE > p,p'-DDT > o,p'-DDT ≥ p,p'-DDD. The slow metabolism of DDT to DDE was confirmed. It was noted that p,p'-DDT is lost from storage in adipose tissue much more slowly in humans than in the monkey, dog, or rat.

Less than 18% of p,p'-DDE is carried in human erythrocytes. In plasma of ordinary fat content, less than 1% of all DDT-related compounds is carried by the chylomicrons. p,p'-

DDT and p,p'-DDE are found mainly in the triglyceride-rich, low-density, and very low-density lipoproteins. Following continuous electrophoresis, these compounds are found mainly in association with plasma albumin and α-globulins (Morgan and Roan, 1972).

DDA is the main urinary metabolite of DDT. In humans, it was found first in a volunteer by Neal *et al.* (1946), who reported that, following ingestion of 770 mg of p,p'-DDT, excretion rose sharply to 4.0 mg/day during the second 24-hr period, decreased rapidly on the third and fourth days, decreased gradually thereafter, but was still above baseline on day 14. Later studies in volunteers who received smaller but repeated doses confirmed the very rapid rise in excretion of DDA (Hayes *et al.*, 1971; Roan *et al.*, 1971) and showed that a steady state of excretion was reached after about 6–8 months. During a 56-week period of continued dosing after equilibrium was fully established, the concentration of DDA associated with technical DDT at the rate of 35 mg/person/day varied from 0.18 to 9.21 ppm and averaged 2.98 ppm; corresponding values for p,p'-DDT were 0.40–6.27 ppm with a mean of 1.88 ppm. Thus technical DDT, as compared to p,p'-DDT, was excreted more effectively and stored less.

During the latter half of the dosing period, it was possible in the two groups receiving recrystallized and technical DDT at the rate of 35 mg/person/day to account for an average of 13 and 16%, respectively, of the daily dose in terms of urinary DDA. The excretion of DDA was relatively constant in each individual, but marked differences were observed between men receiving the same dose (Hayes, 1969; Smith, 1991).

60.2.4.2 Experimental Dermal Exposure

Depending on dosage, oral administration of DDT to volunteers has produced either no illness or brief poisoning entirely similar to that seen in experimental animals. The oral dosage necessary to produce any clinical effect was almost always 10 mg/kg or more. It is a strange coincidence that, in two studies involving only three subjects in all, experimental dermal exposure to DDT was followed by fatigue, aching of the limbs, anxiety or irritability, and other subjective complaints. Recovery was delayed a month or more (Case, 1945; Wigglesworth, 1945). In neither study was there an independent control. Although the dosage was unmeasured, the amounts of DDT absorbed must have been much smaller than those involved in the oral studies. One of the studies involved self-experimentation by one man. A somewhat more severe test on six volunteers produced no toxic or irritant effect at all (Dangerfield, 1946). In view of all other experiments and extensive practical experience, it is probable that the illnesses reported by Wigglesworth and Case were unrelated to DDT.

With the exceptions just mentioned, dermal exposure to DDT has been associated with no illness and usually no irritation (Cameron and Burgess, 1945; Chin and T'Ant, 1946; Dangerfield, 1946; Domenjoz, 1944; Draize *et al.*, 1944; Fennah, 1945; Haag *et al.*, 1948; Wasicky and Unti, 1944). In fact, Hoffman and Lendle (1948) reported that even subcutaneous

injection of colloidal suspensions of DDT in saline in concentration up to 30 ppm caused no irritation. Zein-el-Dine (1946) reported that DDT-impregnated clothing caused a slight, transient dermatitis, but the method of impregnation was not stated and the absence of solvent was not guaranteed. Other more thorough studies of DDT-impregnated clothing have found it nonirritating (Cameron and Burgess, 1945; Domenjoz, 1944).

Chin and T'Ant (1946) applied smallpads impregnated with different formulations of DDT to the inner surface of the forearm of 32 volunteers whose cutaneous sensation had previously been measured for a period of 5 weeks. Pads impregnated with all the elements of the formulation except DDT were applied to the corresponding position on the other arm as a control. Powdered DDT and 5% solutions of DDT showed little effect. Ten percent and 20% solutions in olive oil and petroleum showed no remarkable effect on sensation of pain, cold, or heat but reduced tactile sensation in most cases so that the minimal pressure that could arouse this sensation was 1–2.5 gm/cm^2 higher than in the control.

60.2.4.3 Experimental Respiratory Exposure

Neal *et al.* (1944) reported almost continuous daily exposure to aerosols sufficient to leave a white deposit of DDT on the nasal vibrissae of the volunteers. This exposure produced moderate irritation of the nose, throat, and eyes. Except for this irritation during exposure, there were no symptoms, and laboratory tests and physical examination, including neurological evaluation, failed to reveal any significant changes. The studies by Fennah (1945) that involved both respiratory and oral exposure, produced no detectable ill effect, as discussed above. Stammers and Whitfield (1947) reported tests in which volunteers were exposed to DDT dispersed into the air either by volatilizing units or by continuously or intermittently operated aerosol dispensers. In some instances, a slight odor and some dryness of the throat were noticed, but otherwise the results were negative.

60.2.4.4 Therapeutic Use

The early use of DDT for treating human body lice, head lice, and scabies was reviewed by Simmons (1959). Obviously, these uses offered a possibility of dermal absorption, but such absorption of dry DDT is very limited. Persons who had DDT blown into their clothing as they wore it must have inhaled some of the compound, and this was especially true of persons who used hand or power equipment to apply the dust to hundreds of people per day in mass delousing stations set up to control typhus (West and Campbell, 1946). However, the dosages absorbed cannot have been so large as in some instances in which DDT has been administered by mouth. Even smaller absorbed dosages for the general population were involved in the use of DDT for the control of other vector-borne diseases, especially malaria. These facts must not lead us to forget the tremendous contribution that DDT has made to human health through control of the vectors of typhus, malaria, plague, and several lesser diseases (Coulston, 1985; Hayes, 1991; Spindler, 1983).

DDT has been used on an experimental basis at oral dosage rates varying from 0.3 to 3 mg/kg/day for periods up to 7 months in an attempt to decrease serum bilirubin levels in selected patients with jaundice (Thompson *et al.*, 1969). No side effects were observed. No improvement was noted in patients with jaundice based on cirrhosis who had no demonstrated liver enzyme deficiency. However, in a patient with familial, nonhemolytic, unconjugated jaundice based on a deficiency of glucuronyltransferase, treatment with DDT rapidly reduced the plasma bilirubin level to the normal range and relieved the patient of nausea and malaise from which he had suffered intermittently. The liver function tests as well as other laboratory findings remained normal. The improvement was maintained during the 6 months when DDT was administered and had persisted for 7 additional months at the time the report was written. In this case, a dosage of 1.5 mg/kg/day produced a steady rise in plasma levels of p,p'-DDT from an initial level of 0.005 ppm to a maximum of 1.33 ppm at the end of treatment. At this time, the concentration in body fat was 203 ppm. Plasma levels fell slowly after dosing was stopped (Thompson *et al.*, 1969). The highest daily intake in this series was six times greater than the highest level administered in earlier studies of volunteers and about 7500 times greater than the DDT intake of the general population at that time and even more than would be expected these days. The highest value for p,p'-DDT in serum observed in the entire series was 1.330 ppm, compared to 0.996 ppm, the highest value reported by Laws *et al.* (1967) for formulation-plant workers. A lesser induction of the microsomal enzymes has been observed in workers also (Kolmodin *et al.*, 1969; Poland *et al.*, 1970).

Rappolt (1970) used a single dose of 5000 mg of DDT to promote the metabolism of phenobarbital, of which his three patients had taken an overdose. The treatment appeared useful. Neither Rappolt (1970) nor Thompson *et al.* (1969) encountered any side effects of DDT. However, in addition to whatever action it may have had in promoting the metabolism of phenobarbital, the DDT administered by Rappolt must have acted largely as a pharmaceutical antidote for the barbituate. The largest dose previously administered intentionally was 1500 mg, which caused moderate poisoning in a volunteer, who, of course, had received no barbiturate (Table 60.5).

60.2.4.5 Accidental and Intentional Poisoning

The earliest symptom of poisoning by DDT is hyperesthesia of the mouth and lower part of the face (Hayes, 1982). This is followed by paresthesia of the same area and of the tongue and then by dizziness, an objective disturbance of equilibrium, paresthesia and tremor of the extremities, confusion, malaise, headache, fatigue, and delayed vomiting. The vomiting is probably of central origin and not due to local irritation. Convulsions occur only in severe poisoning. Onset may be as soon as 30 min after ingestion of a large dose or as late as 6 hr after smaller but still toxic doses. Recovery from mild poisoning usually is essentially complete in 24 hr, but recovery from severe poisoning requires several days. In two instances, there was some residual weakness and ataxia of the hands 5 weeks after ingestion.

Involvement of the liver has been mentioned in only a small proportion of cases of accidental poisoning by DDT. In three men who ate pancakes made with DDT and who ingested 5000–6000 mg each, slight jaundice appeared after 4–5 days and lasted 3–4 days (Naevested, 1947). Hepatic involvement and convulsions were reported in an unsuccessful attempt at suicide by ingesting DDT and lindane (Eskenasy, 1972).

Cases of individual and suicidal poisoning in which effects were clearly caused by DDT ingestion are summarized in Table 60.6. The signs and symptoms of poisoning were entirely consistent with those observed in volunteers, except that the spectrum of effects was broader because some of the accidental and suicidal doses were very high. A few persons apparently have been killed by uncomplicated DDT poisoning, but none of these cases was reported in detail. Death has been caused much more frequently by the ingestion of solutions of DDT, but in most of these instances the signs and symptoms were predominantly or exclusively those of poisoning by the solvent (Hayes, 1959). This does not mean that the toxicity of the solvent always predominates. For example, the recurrent convulsions in a case reported by Cunningham and Hill (1952), though more characteristic of poisoning by one of the cyclodienes, was certainly not typical of solvent poisoning. A 2-year-old child drank an unknown quantity of fly spray of which 5% was DDT, but the nature of the other active ingredients or the solvent was unknown. About 1 hr after consumption the child became unconscious and had a generalized, sustained convulsion. Convulsions were present when the child was hospitalized 2 hr after taking the poison, but the fits were controlled by barbiturates and other sedatives. Convulsions reoccurred on day 4 and again on day 21 but were stopped each time following renewal of treatment. On day 12, it was noted that the patient was deaf. Hearing began to improve about day 24 and was normal, as were other neurological and psychic findings, when the patient was seen about 2.5 months after the accident.

Clinical effects of one toxicant may be modified by combining it with another. For example, one would not expect prolonged illness from DDT at a rate of 27 mg/kg. However, when DDT and lindane were ingested in a suicidal attempt at dosages thought to be 27 and 18 mg/kg respectively, clinical remission of convulsions and of liver involvement was delayed until day 20, and the EEG did not return to normal until day 39 (Eskenasy, 1972).

What little is known about the effect of DDT on the human heart fails to show whether cardiac arrhythmia might be a possible cause of death in acute poisoning, as is true in some species of laboratory animals. Palpitations, tachycardia, and "irregular heart action" have been noted in some but not all cases of acute poisoning (Hsieh, 1954; Mackeras and West, 1946; Naevested, 1947).

There do not seem to be any accidents or suicides involving respiratory or dermal exposure leading to recognized signs and symptoms of DDT poisoning. This is true even though sufficient respiratory exposure to aerosols or sufficient dermal exposure to solutions can cause poisoning in animals, and the difference is certainly one of dosage.

60.2.4.6 Use Experience

Despite its bad press and concern over its environmental impact the safety record for humans in the use of DDT is phenomenally good considering the huge quantitites distributed [Coulston, 1985; Food and Agriculture Organization/World Health Organization (FAO/WHO), 1985]. It has been used for mass delousing in such a way that the bodies and inner clothing of thousands of people of all ages and states of health were liberally dusted with the compound. By necessity, the applicators worked in a cloud of the material. Other applicators have sprayed the interior of hundreds of millions of homes in tropical and subtropical countries under conditions that Wolfe *et al.* (1959) showed involved extensive dermal and respiratory exposure. A smaller number of people have made or formulated DDT for many years. Extensive experience and numerous medical studies of groups of workers have been reviewed (Hayes, 1959). Dermatitis was commonly observed among workers who used DDT solutions. The rashes were clearly due to the solvent, especially kerosene. As often happens with rashes caused by petroleum distillates, they were most severe in people when they first started work and cleared in a few days unless contamination was exceptionally severe. A smaller number of workers experienced mild narcotic effects (vertigo and nausea) from solvents when working in confined spaces. Gil and Miron (1949) reported that some persons suffered temporary irritability, fatigue, and other ill-defined symptoms after exposure in the dusty atmosphere of a delousing station, but the relation of these atypical findings to DDT was not clear. With these exceptions due largely to solvents, no illnesses clearly attributable to the formulations, much less to DDT, were revealed by the early studies.

Mild moderate poisoning by DDT itself may have occurred among a group of factory workers exposed to air concentrations of 5–4200 mg/m^3, but no measurements were made of DDT in blood, fat, or urine. The workers complained of parethesia of the extremities, headache, dizziness, and some other difficulties less clearly linked to DDT (Aleksieva *et al.*, 1959). Even higher concentrations in air have been associated with tremor of the tongue and hands as well as with numerous subjective findings (Burkatzkaya *et al.*, 1961).

Ortlee (1958) carried out clinical and laboratory examinations of 40 workers, all of whom were exposed to a number of other pesticides. They had been employed at this work, with heavy exposure, for 0.4–6.5 years with slightly less exposure for as much as 8 years. Exposure was so intense that during working hours many of the men were coated with a heavy layer of concentrated DDT dust. By comparing their excretion of DDA with that of volunteers given known doses of DDT, it was possible to estimate that the average absorbed dosages of three groups of the workers with different degrees of occupational exposure were 14, 30, and 42 mg/person/day. With the exception of the excretion of DDA and the occurrence of a few cases of minor irritation of the skin and eyes, no correlation was found between any abnormality and exposure to the insecticide. Since very large doses of DDT injure the nervous system and liver of experimental animals, special attention was given to a complete neurological examination and to laboratory tests for liver function. Although a few abnormalities were revealed, none related to DDT was detected.

Laws *et al.* (1967) studied 35 men employed from 11 to 19 years in a plant that had produced DDT continuously and exclusively since 1947 and, at the time of the study, produced 2722 metric tons per month. Findings from medical history, physical examinations, routine clinical laboratory tests, and chest x-ray films did not reveal any ill effects attributable to exposure to DDT. No case of cancer or blood dyscrasia was found among the 35 heavily exposed workers in a DDT factory, nor did the medical records of 63 men who had worked there for more than 5 years reveal these diseases. Two men were employed who had a history of successfully treated cancer before they came to work, but no employee had contracted cancer during the 19 years the plant had operated; during this period, the workforce varied from 110 to 135. A study of liver function of the heavily exposed men is discussed near the end of this section.

Measurement of storage offered direct evidence of the men's heavy exposure. The overall range of storage of the sum of isomers and metabolites of DDT in the men's fat was 38–647 ppm, compared to an average of 8 ppm for the general population. Based on their storage of DDT in fat and excretion of DDA in urine, it was estimated that the average daily intake of DDT by the 20 men with high occupational exposure was 17.5–18 mg/person/day, compared to an average of 0.028 mg/person/day then found for the general population. There was significant correlation between the concentrations of total DDT-related material in the fat and serum of the workers. The concentration in fat averaged 338 times greater than that in serum, a factor about three times greater than that for people without occupational exposure. Compared to people in the general population, workers were found to store a smaller proportion of DDT-related material in the form of DDE; the difference was shown to be related chiefly to intensity rather than duration of exposure. DDE is relatively much less important and DDA much more important as excretory products in occupationally exposed men than in men of the general population. After Laws *et al.* (1967) had completed their study, it was found that the 36 most heavily exposed workers involved had fathered 58 children before they began working at the DDT factory and 93 children afterward (Wilcox, 1967).

Laws *et al.* (1973) made a detailed study of the liver function of 31 men who had made and formulated DDT and who had been the subjects of the earlier study already discussed. Judging from their excretion and storage, the men's exposure was equivalent to an oral intake of DDT at rates ranging from 3.6 to 18 mg/man/day for periods ranging from 16 to 25 years and averaging 21 years. All tests were in the normal range for total protein, albumin, total bilirubin, thymol turbidity, and retention of sufobromophthalein sodium. One man had mild elevation of alkaline phosphatase and SGPT. Another man had elevated alkaline phosphatase concentration of 14 units, while a third man had an elevated SGPT.

Comparison of the residue levels of DDE, o,p'-DDT, and p,p'-DDT in blood of factory workers exposed to DDT formulations and showing apparent tempory clinical symptoms and those without symptoms showed no significant differences. Levels were approximately 10-fold greater than those of unexposed controls (Chand *et al.*, 1991).

By far the largest number of heavily exposed workers whose health has been investigated are those associated with malaria control (WHO, 1973). In Brazil, periodic clinical examinations were made of 202 sprayers exposed to DDT for 6 or more years, 77 sprayers exposed for 13 years ending in 1959, and 406 controls. During a 3-year period, a survey of illnesses requiring medical care during the 6 months preceding each periodic medical examination failed to demonstrate any difference between exposed and control groups. A small number of analyses indicated that the concentration of DDT in the blood of sprayers was about three times higher than that of controls. In India, the blood levels of 144 sprayers were 7.5–15 times greater than those in controls and were at least as high as those reported for workers who had made and formulated DDT elsewhere (Misra *et al.*, 1984). When the sprayers were examined, no differences from controls were found except that knee reflexes were brisker, slight tremor was more often present, and a times Romberg test was more poorly performed by the sprayers. The positive results led to the selection of 20 men for re-examination by a neurologist, who concluded that the differences found initially were not real or that the tests had returned to normal within the few months between the two examinations. In any event, the signs were not dosage related, since they showed no correlation with serum levels of DDT. Subsequently cognitive functions of Indian DDT sprayers were tested and DDT levels were 8.5 times higher than those in controls and visuomotor functions were significantly depressed.

Perhaps in contrast to the above studies, the levels of DDT and its metabolites in the sera from 23 applicators in malaria control in Natal were significantly higher than in the population protected by the spraying (Bouwman *et al.*, 1991a). Although serum GGT was not statistically different from controls the mean in applicators was greater than the maximum laboratory mean level and ALT values were significantly greater in the applicators although not deemed clinically significant. Members of households which had been sprayed internally with DDT had significantly greater levels in their serum than people from non-sprayed households (sum of DDT and metabolites was 140.0 μg/l compared to 6.4μg/gl). Athough GGT levels were greater in the high DDT group this seemed to be associated with alcohol consumption (Bouwman *et al.*, 1991b).

The induction by DDT level of microsomal enzymes of human liver was demonstrated first in workers (see Section 60.2.4.4) and DDT may be more important than DDE in this regard, as indicated by the fact that Poland *et al.* (1970) observed induction in men with average serum levels of 0.573 and 0.506 ppm for DDT and DDE, respectively, while Morgan and Roan (1974) found no induction in men with corresponding values of 0.052 and 0.222 ppm.

As noted under Section 60.2.4.4 DDT has been used successfully to induce microsomal enzymes in order to promote metabolism of bilirubin in a case of congenital defect and to promote metabolism of phenobarbital in a case of overdose. DDT promotes its own metabolism in some species of laboratory animals. That the same is true in humans is indicated by the fact that storage of DDT is relatively less at higher dosages. However, the metabolism and subsequent excretion of DDT can be promoted even more by phenobarbital and especially diphenylhydontoin (see Section 60.2.3.5) and by some other drugs (McQueen *et al.*, 1972). Establishment of a reduced equilibrium appeared to require about 2 months. Within this period, the regression of the level of DDT plus DDE on duration of treatment with diphenylhydantoin was highly significant.

In addition to the studies already mentioned regarding workers with extensive storage and/or excretion of DDT as a result of truly heavy exposure to DDT, studies also have been made of a larger number of workers with lesser storage and/or excretion following lesser exposure to DDT but greater exposure to other insecticides. Continuing, meticulous study discussed by Hayes (1975) under Community Studies as well as the work of Tsutsui *et al.* (1974), Ouw and Shandar (1974), and Morgan and Lin (1978) failed to reveal effects of clinical significance among workers with prolonged, moderate exposure to a wide variety of pesticides. In a review of results for 2620 persons exposed to pesticides and 1049 persons not occupationally exposed, Morgan and Lin (1978) found that, apart from serum pesticide concentrations, the only significant and consistent charge associated with occupational exposure was a depression of serum bilirubin. This presumably was a reflection of a slight induction of liver microsomal enzymes. In addition, there was a tendency for serum alkaline phosphatase to increase with increasing concentrations of DDT plus DDE in the serum, but the differences were small in all instances and statistically significant for SGOT and LDH only. Wong *et al.* (1984) could find no significant overall cause specific mortality excess among men potentially exposed at work to DDT from 1935 to 1976. Similarly, a population of 499 persons living downstream from a defunct DDT-manufacturing plant showed no DDT-specific illnesses or ill health despite total DDT serum levels three times the national mean (Kreiss *et al.*, 1981). There was, however, a possible association between serum DDT and serum cholesterol, triglyceride, and γ-glutamyl transpeptidase levels.

A positive linear correlation has been reported for the concentrations of vitamin A and of DDT-related compounds in the serum of men with at least 5 years of occupational exposure to DDT. However, the workers' DDT levels were little higher than those of persons in the general population (see Table 7.15 in Hayes, 1975, and Table 15.11 in Smith, 1991), and their vitamin A levels were within normal limits (Keil *et al.*, 1972b).

Evidence regarding mutagenic activity of DDT and its significance in humans in uncertain. Comparing samples collected in winter and during the peak season of pesticide application, a slight increase in chromatid breaks was reported in the cultured lymphocytes of workers exposed to a wide variety of insecticides said to include DDT (Yoder *et al.*, 1973). A somewhat larger increase was reported for men exposed mainly to herbicides (You *et al.*, 1998). The paper failed to explain why exposure to DDT was claimed at a time when its use was banned. In another study lymphocytes cultured from workers with an average DDT plasma level of 0.999 ppm showed significantly more chromosomal and chromatid abberations than did cells cultured from controls with an average plasma level of 0.275 ppm (Rabello and Pereira, 1975). The difference was not significant in other comparisons in which the average plasma levels were 1.030 versus 0.380 ppm and 0.240 versus 0.030 ppm, respectively. Examination of all of the data presented by the authors suggests that a simple dosage–effect relationship was present, with a detectable effect starting somewhere between 0.2 and 0.4 ppm and increasing at levels higher than 0.4 ppm. Some chromosomal aberrations have also been observed with human lymphocyte cultures by Preston *et al.* (1981), but DDT did not cause unscheduled DNA synthesis in SV40-transformed human cells (Ahmed *et al.*, 1977).

Although there is a lot of evidence against DDT causing liver cancer in humans in Western countries, there is still the outside possibility of it acting as a promoter of potent carcinogens. Aflatoxin is a well-known human carcinogen in areas of Southeast Asia such as Thailand, where DDT and other chlorinated insecticides have been used more recently. In Denmark, Unger and Olsen (1980) found significantly higher levels of DDE in adipose tissue from terminal cancer patients than in tissue from patients who died from other causes. In the United States, DDT and DDE levels were measured in 919 subjects in 1974 and 1975 (Austin *et al.*, 1989). After 10 years there was no correlation between these levels and overall mortality or cancer mortality except a slight correlation with respiratory cancer death. Of course, increased storage often correlates with emaciation of whatever cause (Hayes, 1975). A study has been made of 1043 deaths that occurred between 1956 and 1992 among men who used DDT in an antimalarial campaign in Sardinia in the late 1940s (Cocco *et al.*, 1997). Workers had a significant increased risk for liver and biliary tract cancers and multiple myeloma. However, nonexposed workers also showed elevated incidences of cancer.

In the past decade there has been continued speculation and controversy as to whether many environmental chemicals, including chlorinated pesticides, can act as so-called "endocrine disrupters." As with all environmental exposures, this is an extremely difficult issue to develop to firm conclusions. In some studies, DDT was particularly targeted as being linked with a rising incidence of breast cancer (Wolff, 1995). Much of the evidence has been reviewed in detail by Ahlborg *et al.* (1995), but is not supportive or is inconclusive. Unger *et al.* (1984) found no relationship between breast fat tissue DDT (and DDE) and the incidence of mammary cancer. Although in the studies of Mussalo-Rauhamaa *et al.* (1990) correlation with β-hexachlorocyclohexane was found, none was observed with DDT. In contrast, elevated levels of DDT or DDE were reported in cancerous breast tissue fat compared with tissue from benign mammary disease (Falck *et al.*, 1992; Guttes *et al.*, 1998). Studies on the relationship between blood levels of DDT and/or DDE and breast cancer in the United States have been mixed. Some have shown a relationship with either blood p,p'-DDE levels and mammary cancer occurrence (Wolff *et al.*, 1993) or p,p'-DDE levels and hormone-responsive breast cancer (Dewailly *et al.*, 1994a, b).

It has been proposed that increased estrogen receptor level in breast tumors over two decades could be explained by organochlorine exposure (Dewailly *et al.*, 1997). In contrast, a number of studies have found no relationship between blood levels of DDE and risk of breast cancer (Hunter *et al.*, 1997; Kreiger *et al.*, 1994; Schecter *et al.*, 1997). The last study is of additional interest in that women in North Vietnam were examined who had generally high levels of DDT or DDE due to exposure from antimalarial use. Many of the studies up to 1994 were examined by meta-analysis and appeared to confirm the lack of association between DDE levels in tissues and breast cancer incidence (Key and Reeves, 1994). However, there are many *in vitro* investigations which purport to agree with the hypotheses (e.g., Ardies and Dees, 1998; Shekhar *et al.*, 1997) and further investigations to clarify the issue are required. Probably there will be a further concern around p,p-DDE acting as an antiandrogen (Kelce *et al.*, 1995, 1998) (see Section 60.2.3.12).

There have been reports that pancreatic cancer might be associated with exposure to DDT and ethylan. In a nested case–control mortality study among 5586 workers at a chemical plant, interviews with next of kin and co-workers and examination of work records showed that DDT exposure appeared to be associated with pancreatic cancer as identified by pathology, clinical surgical, autopsy records, or death certificates (Garabrant *et al.*, 1992). Among subjects whose mean exposure to DDT was 47 months, the risk was 7.4 times that among subjects with no exposure. DDD and ethylan exposures were also correlated. Malats *et al.* (1993) subsequently questioned the validity of the classification of pancreatic cancer. They proposed that despite the difficulties it might strengthen the findings if comparisons were made between histologically confirmed cases. Interestingly, this indeed turned out be true (Garabrant *et al.*, 1993). For those cases in which pancreatic cancer classification was based only on death certificates no association with exposure to DDT or its analogues was found. This theme has been developed further by Fryzek *et al.* (1997) looking at 66 residents of Michigan (39–70 years of age) who had been diagnosed histologically as having pancreatic cancer. Exposure was assessed by self-reporting questionnaires. In this cohort from the general population, a significant increased risk for exposure to ethylan was observed. Cases were 10.7 times more likely to report exposure to ethylan compared to controls. Nonsignificantly increased odds-ratios were for exposure to DDT and chloropropylate. Epidemiological studies of this sort with small case numbers are very difficult to perform and interpret. However, given the importance of breast and prostate cancer incidences in the United States and Europe it would seem wise to keep an open mind that DDT analogs might play a role in certain circumstances. Presumably where possible, future studies will address this issue.

Table 60.6
Summary of the Effects of the Accidental or Suicidal Ingestion of DDT

Individual dose (mg), formulation, and number of persons	Results and reference
300–4500, in food, 1 man	onset in 1 hr; vomiting; restlessness; headache; heart weak and slow; recovery next day (Muhlens, 1946)
Unknown dose, in tarts, 25 men	onset in 2–2.5 hr; all weak and giddy; 4 vomited; 2 hospitalized; 1 confused, incordinated, weak; one with palpitations and numbness of hands; recovery in 24–48 hr (Mackeras and West, 1946)
5000–6000, in pancakes, 3 men	onset 2–3 hr; throbbing headache; dizziness; incoordination; paresthesias of extremities; urge to defecate; wide nonreacting pupils; reduced vision; dysarthria; facial weakness; tremor; ataxic gait; reduced sensitivity to touch; reduced reflexes; positive Romberg; slightly low blood pressure and persistent irregular heart action; partial recovery in 2–3 days, but slight jaundice appeared 4–5 days after ingestion and lasted 3–4 days; all normal 19 days after poisoning except irregular heart action in one (Naevested, 1947)
2000, in pancakes, 2 men	no illness (Naevested, 1947)
Up to 20,000, in bread, 28 men	onset in 30–60 min in those most severely affected, men first seen 2–3 after ingestion; in spite of severe early vomiting that reduced the effective dose, severity of illness and especially intensity of numbness and paralysis of extremities proportional to amount of DDT ingested; all but 8 men recovered in 48 hr; 5 others fully recovered in 2 weeks, but 3 men still had some weakness and ataxia of their hands 5 weeks after ingestion (Garrett, 1947)
Unknown dose, in flour, about 100 women	onset about 3.5 hr after ingestion; total of about 85 cases of which 37 were hopitalized; symptoms mild and similar to those in earlier outbreaks except gastrointestinal disturbance in most severe cases included abdominal pain and diarrhoea as well as nausea; most fully recovered in 24 hr (Jude and Girard, 1949)
Unknown dose, 14 cases	symptoms in established cases similar to those reported earlier (Francone et al., 1952) with the exception of one man who was already sick when he received a dosage of 6 mg/kg, poisoning did not occur at dosages of 5.1–10.3 mg/kg. Ingestion of 16.3–120.5 mg/kg produced excessive perspiration, nausea, vomiting, convulsions, headache, increased salivation, tremors, tachycardia, and cyanosis of the lips. Onset varied from 2 to 6 hr, depending on dosage. Recovery required as much as 2 days (Hsieh, 1954).
286–1716, in meatballs, 8 cases, 11 exposed	
Unknown dose, 1 case	death 13 hr after suicidal ingestion (Committee on Pesticides, 1951)
Unknown dose, 22 unrelated cases	22 separate cases, including 15 attempted suicides; some complicated by solvents; 3 deaths (Committee on Pesticides, 1951)

60.2.4.7 Dosage Response

The clinical effects of different dosage levels of DDT in humans are summarized in Tables 7.24 in Hayes (1975) and in Tables 60.5 and 60.6, herein. The degree of storage determined by different dosage levels of DDT has been summarized in Fig. 7.4 in Levine (1991) and details regarding higher than normal dosage rates are given in Table 15.9 in Smith (1991). A clinically useful degree of induction of microsomal enzymes was obtained with a DDT dosage of 1.5 mg/kg/day for 6 months (see Section 60.2.4.4). As discussed in Section 60.2.4.6 workers who absorbed a dosage of about 0.25 mg/kg/day showed demonstrable but only slight induction (Poland et al., 1970). Workers with less exposure as indicated by lower serum levels of DDT showed no detectable induction.

60.2.4.8 Storage in Fat

The highest reported storage of DDT and related compounds remains that of a healthy worker whose fat contained DDT and DDE at concentrations of 648 and 483 ppm, respectively (Hayes et al., 1956). Laws et al. (1967) reported considerably lower storage values among the most exposed persons in a DDT manufacturing plant (see Table 15.11 of Smith, 1991). An important point is that whereas almost all investigations of workers are said to have been carried out on "heavily exposed" populations (or words to that effect), some of the groups studied had absorbed little more DDT than is absorbed by the general population—especially the general population of some tropical countries.

The first evidence that humans metabolize a part of the DDT they absorb to DDE was obtained from the analysis of fat from a worker (Mattson et al., 1953). The accumulation of DDE relative to total DDT-related compounds is best illustrated in humans. Of the total DDT stored in the fat of workers exposed to technical DDT (about 4% DDE) for 11–19 years, only 38% was in the form of DDE, and, of course, some of that DDE came from their diets including meat (Laws *et al.*, 1967). In India, where many people avoid meat but may consume milk, cheese, and eggs, 34–41% of total DDT stored by people without special exposure was DDE (Dale *et al.*, 1965). In the United States, during a time when DDT residues in food were decreasing, the proportion of total DDT in the form of DDE increased from about 60% in 1955 to about 80% in 1970; during the same interval the concentration of total DDT in body fat decreased from about 15 ppm to less than 10 ppm as recorded in Table 7.10 in Hayes (1975). By 1980, DDE constituted 86.7% of total DDT in one population (Kreiss *et al.*, 1981). Thus, a low proportion of DDE indicates a relatively high intake of preformed DDT and relatively few years for metabolism of stored DDT to DDE.

A number of factors, especially dosage, age, sex, race, and various disease states have been discussed in connection with the storage and excretion of DDT by people but only dosage has been shown to be of practical importance. DDT and related compounds are stored at much lower rates in the general population than in persons with occupational exposure. However, these relatively low levels of storage constitute one of the most important aspects of the measurable effects of pesticides on people (Dale and Quinby, 1963). Briefly, storage of total DDT in the body fat of ordinary people in the United States increased from 5.3 ppm in 1950 to about 15.6 ppm in 1955 and 1956 (see Table 15.12, Smith, 1991). Thereafter, the levels decreased gradually (Burns, 1974), albeit somewhat irregularly, to about 8 ppm in 1970 and 3 ppm in 1980. In fact, despite concerns about residues of DDT, levels have continued to fall. In annual surveys in the United States based on 898–1920 samples per year, the geometric mean levels for total DDT in adipose tissue on a lipid basis were 7.88, 7.95, 6.88, 5.89, and 5.02 ppm for fiscal years 1970, 1971, 1972, 1973, and 1974, respectively. For each year, the values were higher for older age groups and higher for black than for white people. During fiscal year 1974, the values for persons 0–14, 15–44, and 45 years old or more were 2.15, 4.91, and 6.55 ppm, respectively, for white people and 4.02, 9.18, and 11.91 ppm, respectively, for black people (Kutz *et al.*, 1977). The values would have been somewhat lower if they had been based on wet weight. It has been calculated that if exposure to DDT ceased it would take 10–20 years for DDT to disappear from a person but that DDE would persist throughout the life span (Morgan and Roan, 1977).

60.2.4.9 Storage in Blood and Other Organs

No information seems to be available on blood levels of DDT in persons poisoned by the compound. Concentrations measured in the blood or serum of workers in the past are shown in Table 15.11 of Smith (1991). The highest value for total DDT in serum reported from several countries was 2.2 ppm (with an average of 0.7371 ppm) based on gas chromatography (Laws

et al., 1967). A different situation is indicated by a report by Genina *et al.* (1969), who used a total chloride method to analyze samples of blood from controls and from persons with occupational exposure to DDT, polychloropinene, and BHC. These authors reported chloroorganic compounds as high as 38.4 ppm in the blood of warehousemen. This concentration is about 20 times the highest value found by the same authors in their control group. The factor of 20 is not remarkable, but (especially in view of the fact that polychloropinene and BHC are excreted more readily than DDT and DDE) values as high as 9 ppm in the controls are completely unexpected. Whether the difference was based on massive exposure or the crude analytical methodology employed is unclear.

The concentrations of DDT in the blood of ordinary people are shown in Table 15.13 in Smith (1991). It is of interest that although each person without special exposure to DDT has relatively constant serum levels of DDT and DDE, DDE values differ more than the DDT values from person to person (Apple *et al.*, 1970). Whether this reflects differences in metabolism or differences in past exposure is unclear. Kreiss *et al.* (1981) have shown that DDE in serum samples of a community exceptionally exposed to DDT increased with age of the individual.

Levels of DDT and its metabolites in the serum from those aged 21 years rose over a 12 month period following application of the pesticide to their homes in KwaZulu, South Africa. In contrast, levels fell in the age group 3–20 years, showing the complexity of any phamacokinetic interpretations (Bouwman *et al.*, 1994).

Surveys have demonstrated a gradual decline in the concentrations of DDT and related compounds in human fat. Presumably a similar decline has occurred in the levels of these compounds in human serum. Consumption of fish appeared to be a predictor of plasma DDE levels but most reliable were age and serum cholesterol (Laden *et al.*, 1999). When storage of DDT has been found to be greater in black people, the difference could be accounted for by greater exposure (D'Ercole *et al.*, 1976; Hayes, 1975). However, Sandifer (1974), who found that the concentrations of DDT in the sera of blacks was two to three times greater than those in whites, also found a significant correlation between total DDT and deficiency of glucose-6-phosphate dehydrogenase, a condition much more common in blacks than whites. Thus, a genetic factor in the storage of DDT appears possible, but much stronger evidence would be necessary to confirm it. Whether the high storage in blacks is strictly environmental or partly genetic, it is certain that as high or higher levels have been recorded among several groups of rural blacks in different parts of the southeastern United States (Arthur, 1976; D'Ercole *et al.*, 1976; Keil *et al.*, 1972a, b, 1973) than were reported by Kreiss *et al.* (1981) among blacks in Triana, Alabama, who had mean values of 0.096 and 0.062 ppm for total DDT in the serum of males and females, respectively.

Storage of DDT and related compounds in the organs of adults and fetuses in the general population was discussed and tabulated by Hayes (1975). Concentrations in the viscera of adults averaged 1.0 ppm, but concentrations in lymph nodes and especially bone marrow (a fatty tissue) approached the level in adipose tissue (≥ 6.0 ppm). Concentrations in some viscera of stillborn infants were similar to those in adipose tissue of the same infants and also in adults, suggesting that there had been a mobilization of DDT from fat prior to death.

Saxena *et al.* (1987) have reported that the levels of DDT in human leiomyomatous uterine tissue were significantly higher than those in normal tissue (means of 0.845 and 0.103 ppm, respectively). Whether this is related to any estrogenic actions of DDT is unknown. See also Section 60.2.4.6.

60.2.4.10 Secretion in Milk

No information is available on the secretion of DDT in the milk of women who were occupationally exposed to the compound or who were made ill by it, regardless of circumstances. The concentrations of DDT in the milk of women in various general populations are shown in Table 15.14 of Smith (1991). Values reported from Guatemala and early values from the USSR were much higher than those from other countries, and yet there was no indication of illness among babies fed such milk. The significance of DDT in milk and the dosages that different concentrations of it determine were discussed by Hayes (1975), Jenson (1983), Spindler (1983), and Coulston (1985).

Quinby *et al.* (1965a, b) noted that women apparently were in negative DDT balance during lactation, but no direct measurement of DDT intake of women participating in the study was made. Subsequently, the ingestion of DDT in food and the secretion of DDT in milk were measured in the same women, and the fact of negative balance was confirmed (Adamovic and Sokic, 1973; Adamovic *et al.*, 1978; Cocisiu *et al.*, 1976) and may be a significant factor in determining the lower levels of DDT found in women than men in the general population (Adamovic and Sokic, 1973). Jonsson *et al.* (1977) found significantly lower levels of DDT (mean of 0.008 ppm) and of DDE (mean of 0.035 ppm) than had been reported earlier for the milk of city dwellers. However, levels remained quite high (0.05–1.90 ppm) in some rural black people (Woodard *et al.*, 1976). Some evidence suggested that DDT levels are higher in milk from smokers than nonsmokers, although there may be an occupational explanation (Coulston, 1985).

In areas of KwaZulu, human milk levels of DDT and metabolites were significantly higher in women whose houses had been treated with DDT to interrupt malaria transmision (Bouwman *et al.*, 1990a, b). Primiparous mothers had significantly more than multiparous mothers. Transfer from the mother's milk to the child's blood was clearly demonstrated (Bouwman *et al.*, 1992).

Overall, despite the presence of DDT in human milk and placenta, there seems little risk to neonates in many different populations. Most evidence has shown a continuing decline in DDT levels in humans since it was banned for use in many parts of the world [e.g., Stevens *et al.* (1993) have found a marked decline in levels since 1974]. Clearly, levels would have to be very high before any advice against breast feeding could be given.

60.2.4.11 Excretion of DDT-Related Compounds

Among workers whose DDT intake was estimated to be about 35 mg/day, Ortlee (1958) found that the concentration of DDA in urine ranged from 0.12 to 7.56 ppm and averaged 1.71 ppm. Among workers whose exposure was about half as great, Laws *et al.* (1967) found concentrations from 0.01 to 2.67 ppm with a mean of 0.97 ppm. Continuous sampling of a DDT-formulating plant worker's urine showed that excretion of DDA increased promptly when exposure began on each of five consecutive workdays but often continued after exposure, sometimes reached a peak about midnight, and then decreased rapidly. On day 6, when there was no occupational exposure to DDT, the excretion of DDA continued until a very low level was reached. The highest concentration of DDA reported in this study was 0.68 ppm (Wolfe and Armstrong, 1971). The urine of people in the general population contains not only DDA but also neutral compounds including p,p'-DDT and p,p'-DDE (Cueto and Biros, 1967). Men with heavy occupational exposure to DDT excreted much more DDA but showed only a statistically insignificant increase in excretion of DDT and DDE.

The urinary excretion of DDT derived material is of such an order of magnitude that it may account for much of the excretion of absorbed DDT. The excretion of DDA by people with different kinds and degrees of exposure is presented in Table 15.15 of Smith (1991).

DDT and DDE are also excreted in the bile and higher levels than normal were found in the bile of one pest-control operator (Paschal *et al.*, 1974). Further discussion of the storage and excretion of DDT can be found in Levine (1991).

60.2.4.12 Other Laboratory Findings

In the absence of occupational DDT poisoning, there has been no opportunity to explore (as has been done with the cyclodiene insecticides) the relationship between clinical and EEG findings. In fact, the only DDT workers studied in this regard were exposed also to benzene hexahydrochloride and benzilan, so the findings might have been related to one or more of the compounds or to their interaction. Electroencephalograms were obtained from 73 of these workers exposed for periods ranging from 7 months to 20 years (Israeli and Mayersdorf, 1973; Mayersdorf and Israeli, 1974). Just over 78% of the records were normal and 21.9% were abnormal. The most severe changes involved persons exposed to the three compounds for 1–2 years; less severe changes were seen with either shorter or longer exposure. The changes were not correlated with age; the range and mean of age for those judged abnormal were almost identical with these values for persons considered normal. Some of the records showed bitemporal sharp waves with shifting lateralization combined with low voltage theta activity. Other records showed spike complexes, paroxysmal discharges composed of slow and sharp waves most pronounced anteriorly, and low-voltage rhythmic spikes posteriorly. None of the persons examined showed any abnormal clinical neurological finding. The incidence of abnormal electroencephalograms in the general population is 9.0 or 9.2%, according to other investigators cited by Israeli and Mayersdorf. Czegledi-Janko and Avar (1970) considered that at that time nonspecific EEG abnormalities occurred in 10–20% of the general population, so there is some question of whether the results are meaningful.

Clinical laboratory findings associated with DDT poisoning are not specific and it is difficult to diagnose that poisoning has occured from this agent rather than others.

60.2.4.13 Treatment of Poisoning

No useful guidance regarding treatment has been gleaned from the very few cases of DDT poisoning that have occurred. Animal studies indicate that sedatives, ionic calcium, and glucose or another ready source of energy would be useful. On the basis of experience in treating people poisoned by different convulsive poisons, it seems likely that diazepam would be beneficial.

60.3 TDE

60.3.1 IDENTITY, PROPERTIES, AND USES

TDE is 1,1-dichloro-2,2-bis(4-chloro-phenyl)ethane (Table 60.1). The common name TDE(ISO) is an acronym for *t*etra-chloro*d*iphenyl*e*thane. Except in France, it is a generally recognized name for the compound as a synthetic insecticide. For reasons that are obscure, the word DDD (an acronym for *d*ichloro*d*iphenyl*d*ichloroethane) has been used more commonly for 1,1-dichloro-2,2-bis (chlorophenyl)ethane when viewed as a metabolite of DDT or when used as a therapeutic drug, and this distinction has been retained here. Almost everything we know about the compound relevant to humans is associated with its use as a drug rather than its use as an insecticide. Nonproprietary names for the o,p'-isomer which is used as a drug include chlordithane (USSR) and mitotane (United States). A proprietary name for the insecticide has been Rhothane®. Code designations include D-3, ENT-4,225, ME-1,700, and NSC-38,721 (for o,p'-isomer only).

TDE has the empirical formula $C_{14}H_{10}Cl_4$ and a molecular weight of 320.05. The pure material forms colorless crystals melting at 109–110°C. The technical material consisted mainly of the p,p'-isomer but also contained a substantial proportion of o,p'-isomer and lesser proportions of related compounds.

The insecticidal properties of TDE were first described by Laüger *et al.* (1944). The formulations have included the technical material; wettable powders, 5%; emulsion concentrates, 25%; and dusts, 5% and 10%.

60.3.2 TOXICITY TO LABORATORY ANIMALS

The effects of TDE are similar to those of DDT, but TDE is much less toxic in the rat and in humans. Gaines (1969) found the oral LD 50 in both male and female rats to be greater than 4000 mg/kg, Lehman (1951, 1952) reported 3400 mg/kg as an oral LD 50 in rats and 1200 as a dermal value in rabbits. Rabbits

were killed quickly by dermal applications at the rate of 400 mg/kg day; they were made severely ill but did not die when treated at the rate of 200 mg/kg/day for 90 days. In rats fed for 2 years, the lowest dietary level producing gross effects was 400 ppm and the lowest level fed (100 ppm, about 5 mg/kg/day) produced tissue damage. In the rat, pathology is indistiguishable from that caused by DDT (Lehman, 1951, 1952).

60.3.2.1 Absorption, Distribution, Metabolism, and Excretion

The metabolism of p,p'-DDD has been described earlier in this chapter. Regardless of dosage form, 75% or more of o,p'-DDD is absorbed from the gastrointestinal tract (Korpachev, 1972a). Following repeated doses, storage of o,p'-DDD reached its highest point in 10–20 days and then decreased somewhat in spite of continued intake. Elimination was rapid after treatment stopped but was detectable longest in the adrenals and adipose tissues (Korpachev, 1972b). The metabolism of o,p'-DDD in the rat has been investigated thoroughly by Reif and Sinsheimer (1975); their major results are summarized in Fig. 60.3 which also records the metabolites found in humans by Reif *et al.* (1974). More recent studies to explain the covalent binding of o,p'-DDD in lung and adrenals are also described Section 60.2.

60.3.2.2 Biochemical Effects

The basis for the action of o,p'-DDD on the adrenal is not understood fully in connection with any species but it is clear that marked species differences exist (see Section 60.2). The mechanism that leads to prompt atrophy in the dog may be quite different from the mechanisms that limit the production or increase the breakdown of corticosteroids in species in which most or all of the adrenal cells stay alive.

It is clear that a reduction of steroid production accompanies atrophy of the dog. Kupfer (1967) considered: (*a*) reduced steroid production in species other than the dog, including the possibility that such reduction is secondary to inhibition of glucose-6-phosphate dehydrogenase activity in the adrenals, and (*b*) blockage of steroid action by a steroid metabolite formed under the influence of DDD. However, the existence of these effects, much less their importance, remains obscure. Hart and Straw (1971a) showed that administration of o,p'-DDD to dogs for only 2–48 hr completely blocked the normal increase in steroid production in response to ACTH *in vitro* but, paradoxically, produced a marked increase in the incorporation of labeled amino acids into protein of the slices. The same authors presented evidence that the site of action is the intramitochondrial conversion of cholesterol to pregnenolone (Hart and Straw, 1971b), specifically, ACT-activated conversion and not baseline steroid production (Hart and Straw, 1971d). A secondary site involves inhibition of intramitochondrial conversion of 11-deoxycortisol to cortisol (Hart and Straw, 1971d). Further evidence supporting the importance of the primary site was found by Komissarenko *et al.* (1972). o,p'-DDD inhibited ACTH-induced steroid production by 797% within 2 hr, and the active principle is either o,p'-DDD per se or a derivative formed in the adrenal gland of the intact dog (Hart and Straw, 1971c). o,p'-DDD applied to liver slices *in vitro* is not effective in reducing ACTH-induced steroidogenesis in the slices. However, the compound did reduce the formation of corticosteroid from progesterone or deoxycorticosterone added to homogenates made from adrenal cortices from dogs, chickens, rats, and human fetuses. These results are consistent with the view that the action of o,p'-DDD is to block 11-β-hydroxylation (Kravchenko, 1973). Furthermore, a concentration of 16 ppm produced this effect in a monolayer culture of human fetal adrenal cells (Komissarenko, 1971). Martz and Straw (1973) interpreted the decrease in adrenocortical heme and P-450 produced by o,p'-DDD in the dog as a suggestion that the compound is metabolized to a more active form, and this is supported by *in vitro* studies with isolated adrenal mitochondria (Martz and Straw, 1980; Pohland and Counsell, 1985). Whether these actions are related the covalent binding of 3-methylsulfonyl-p,p'-DDE in mouse adrenals by CYP11B has yet to be investigated (see Sections 60.2 and 60.2.3.5).

There is evidence for a peripheral action of o,p'-DDD on steroid transformation in humans also, although the site of action is different. This evidence was obtained by studying the excretion of metabolites of small injected doses of radioactive steroid before and during administration of the drug. It was concluded that 3β-hydroxy-Δ^5-steroid dehydrogenase was inhibited (Bradlow *et al.*, 1963).

Further evidence that o,p'-DDD has some inhibitory effect on the synthesis of corticosteroids in humans was provided by *in vitro* tests on adrenal tissue removed surgically from patients, some of whom had been under treatment with the drug (Touito *et al.*, 1978). Total doses prior to surgery had varied from 324 to 2280 gm and had been given over periods of 1–12 months. Compounds whose synthesis (from radioactive precursors added to incubation flasks) was inhibited in tissue from treated patients were cortisol, corticosterone, 18-hydroxycorticosterone, and aldosterone. Direct addition of o,p'-DDD to human adrenal tissue *in vitro* was without effect on synthesis of corticosteroids.

Following massive dosage (60 mg/kg, iv), all of the isomers of DDD inhibit ACTH-induced steroid production in the dog, but the inhibition reached 50% of control in only 27 min after dosing with the m,p'-isomer (Hart *et al.*, 1973). There was a marked temporal correlation between the percentage inhibition of ACTH-induced steroid production, the disruption of normal cellular structure of the innermost zones of the adrenal cortex, and the severity of the damage to mitochondria in these zones caused by the three isomers. The effectiveness of m,p'-DDT for treating metastatic adrenocortical carcinoma had already been demonstrated (Nichols *et al.*, 1961). However, in humans and dogs m,p'-DDD is less effective than o,p'-DDD (deFossey *et al.*, 1968; Reznikov, 1973). Administration of o,p'-DDD to dogs is followed by a decrease in plasma albumin and an increase in globulins, especially α_2-, β^1-, and γ-globulin (Vanyurikhina, 1972). The relation of these changes to the suppresion of adrenal function is unknown, and their clinical significance is also unknown.

Guinea pigs receiving o,p'-DDD intraperitoneally at a rate of 100, 200, or 300 mg/kg/day for 20 days showed decreases in ascorbic acid levels corresponding to dosage (Petrun' and Nikulina, 1970). It was speculated that this might interfere with synthesis of corticosteroids. Like other chlorinated hydrocarbon insecticides, o,p'-DDD stimulates hepatic microsomal oxygenation of both drugs and steroids and this may explain much of its action on corticoid metabolism in a wide range of species (Kupfer, 1967). Increased breakdown is evidenced by increased excretion of polar metabolites while nonpolar metabolites remain stable or even decrease—fainding encountered in human patients (Hellmann *et al.*, 1973). However, the demonstrated effect on corticoid metabolism fails to explain why o,p'- and m,p'-DDD are unique in their overall effects on the adrenal, including their ability to produce adrenocortical atrophy in the dog. Other powerful inducers of microsomal enzymes lack these effects. Furthermore, in some systems DDD is a relatively weak inducer compared, for example, to DDT and DDE (Gillett *et al.*, 1966). Whereas induction does occur in dogs, its interpretation is complex; for example, the induction caused by repeated doses can be suppressed by cortisol (Martz and Straw, 1972). Mikosha (1985) has proposed that inhibition of NADP reduction by malic enzyme in adrenals may play a role in o,p'-DDD action, perhaps by causing a decrease in steroid metabolism (Ojima *et al.*, 1985).

60.3.2.3 Effects on Organs and Tissues

DDD is used to control different forms of adrenal overproduction of corticoids in humans. This therapy originally was based on the demonstration that DDD (Nelson and Woodard, 1948, 1949) and especially o,p'-DDD (Cueto and Brown, 1958; Komissarenko *et al.*, 1968) cause gross atrophy of the adrenals and degeneration of the cells of its inner cortex in dogs. This is true even though it was first reported (Komissarenko *et al.*, 1970; Nelson and Woodard, 1948, 1949; Zimmerman *et al.*, 1956) that DDD produces almost no detectable damage to the adrenals of a variety of species, including humans. In the dog, o,p'-DDT produces gross atrophy of the adrenals when administered at a dosage of only 4 mg/kg/day. The dosage of technical grade DDD required to produce the same effect is 50–200 mg/kg/day (Cueto and Brown, 1958). However, in spite of its exceptional susceptibility, there is a definite threshold below which the dog does not respond. About 15% of technical DDT was o,p'-isomer, much of which is gradually metabolized to o,p'-DDD. Yet dogs remained healthy and reproduced normally in a three-generation study involving dosages of technical DDT as high as 10 mg/kg/day.

DDD has been little used for Cushing's syndrome in dogs (Lubberink *et al.*, 1971), but it is effective at lower dosages than those used in humans, and side effects are less serious and less frequent (Schechter *et al.*, 1973). It is an interesting fact that p,p'-DDE and the –OH analog of p,p'-DDD causes moderate hypertrophy of the dog adrenal and 2,2-bis(p-

chorophenyl)ethane causes moderate hyperplasia (Larson *et al.*, 1955).

The effect of DDD on thymolymphatic tissues is poorly understood. In one of the earliest studies of the compound, Lillie *et al.* (1947) reported that the spleen of all treated animals showed impressive siderosis. Much later Gawhary (1972) reported that, in rabbits, intramuscular injection of a commercial grade DDD (mainly *p,p'*-isomer) caused acute *atrophy* of the thymus and hypertrophy of the adrenal, although the *m,p'*-isomer at a dosage of 100 mg/kg/day caused *hypertrophy* of the thymus and an increase in its choline acetylase activity. Decrease in the weight of the thymus and spleen as well as the adrenal glands of rats treated with *o,p'*-DDD was reported by Hamid *et al.* (1974).

Furthermore, Cueto and Moran (1968) and Cueto (1970) showed that, at a dosage of 50 mg/kg/day for 14 days, *o,p'*-DDD caused a gradually progressive hypotensive failure in dogs injected with epinephrine or norepinephrine, while leaving unchanged the cardioaccelerator and immediate pressor response of these drugs. The hypotensive failure was associated with weakening of the contractile force of the heart and with a reduction of plasma volume. The latter may have been caused by loss of fluid from the intravascular compartment and was not caused by release of histamine. The hypotensive state could be prevented to a significant degree by pretreatment with prednisolone.

In mice, *p,p'*-TDE at a dietary level of 250 ppm moderately increased the incidence of lung tumors in both sexes (Tomatis *et al.*, 1974). DDD (*p,p'*-TDE) is toxic to isolated rabbit Clara cells and human bronchial epithelial cells by what appears to be cytochrome P450 activation to the acyl chloride (Nichols *et al.*, 1995). The *o,p'*-isomer was protective in rats treated earlier with the established carcinogen dimethylbenz[a]anthracene (DMBA) (Kravt'sova *et al.*, 1971). Leydig cell tumors were reported in the testis of rats receiving *o,p'*-DDD at the rate of 0.6 mg/kg/day for 285–348 days (Lacassagne, 1971). This report is inconsistent with other studies (Lehman, 1951, 1952), and this may indicate that a contaminant was involved or a strain variation in the response. In an NCI study (1978a) there was a possible effect of TDE in causing an increased incidence of follicular cell carcinoma or follicular cell adennoma of the thyroid in male Osborne–Mendel rats but no effects in female B6C3F1 mice.

TDE was found not to be mutagenic in *Drosophila* (Vogel, 1972). It was found mutagenic in two of three indicator organisms in host-medicated tests but not in direct tests, suggesting that a metabolite was the active agent. However, in the same series of studies, both DDT and DDA were negative (Buselmaier *et al.*, 1973).

In addition to atrophy of the zona fasciculata and zona reticularis in the dog, *o,p'*-DDD changes the ultrastructure of most cell types of the anterior pituitary of that species. The most striking feature is an increase in corticotrophocytes such as is seen following adrenalectomy, and the increase in cells is presumably associated with increased production of ACTH.

The hypothalamus also is involved (Gordienko and Kozyritsii, 1970; Gordienko and Kozyritskii, 1973). In spite of their severe nature, the changes produced in the dog adrenal are at least partially reversible (Komissarenko *et al.*, 1972). Dosage–response relationships of mitochondrial swelling and of some other details of pathology in the dog adrenal have been explored by Gordienko and Kozyritskii (1973) and by Powers *et al.* (1974), who also investigated regeneration of the gland.

Hypertrophy of the thyroid in dogs receiving 25 mg/kg and its inhibition in those receiving 50 mg/kg had been reported (Gordienko *et al.*, 1972).

60.3.3 TOXICITY TO HUMANS

60.3.3.1 Therapeutic Use

Following the demonstration that DDD caused atrophy of a part of the adrenal cortex of dogs, the compound has been used in humans in the hope of controlling excessive cortical secretion or of reducing the size of adrenal tumours. The underlying condition may be hyperplasia or adrenocortical carcinoma. Early attempts using mixed isomers and/or dosages less than 100 mg/kg/day often were ineffective, although side effects might be produced (Sheehan *et al.*, 1953). The dosage of *o,p'*-DDD has varied from 7 to 285 mg/kg/day, but a dosage of approximately 40 or more often 100 mg/kg/day for many weeks has been necessary to produce any benefit in humans (Bergenstal *et al.*, 1960; Bledsoe *et al.*, 1964; Gallagher *et al.*, 1962; Gutierrez and Crooke, 1980; Komissarenko *et al.*, 1970; Southern *et al.*, 1966a, b; Verdon *et al.*, 1962; Wallace *et al.*, 1961).

The effects of idiopathic hyperplasia may be controlled; in fact, a state of adrenal insufficiency may be produced (Canlorbe *et al.*, 1971; Helson *et al.*, 1971; Korthe-Schutz, 1977) or of adrenocortical activity secondary to a tumor that produces ACTH (Carey *et al.*, 1973). Very early attempts to use DDD for treating Cushing's syndrome often failed because the *o,p'*-isomer was not used and sometimes because the dosage was small but this was not true for what apparently was the first therapeutic use (Sheehan *et al.*, 1953). Using the *o,p'*-isomer, a favorable response is produced in about one-fourth to one-half of patients with inoperable adrenocortical carcinoma (Canlorbe *et al.*, 1971; Gutierrez and Crooke, 1980; Hoffman and Mattox, 1972; Hutter and Kahoe, 1966; Lubitz *et al.*, 1973; Montgomery and Struck, 1973). In fact an occasional cure, involving complete regression of metastases, is produced by chemotherapy including *o,p'*-DDD (Hart *et al.*, 1973; Pellerin *et al.*, 1975; Perevodchikova *et al.*, 1972; Rappalport *et al.*, 1978; Shick *et al.*, 1973). Other patients have lived for several years (Bricaire and Luton, 1977; McKierman *et al.*, 1978). More commonly, symptoms are relieved and life is prolonged only about 7–8 months or a little longer (Canlorbe *et al.*, 1971; Hoffman and Mattox, 1972; Hutter and Kahoe, 1966; Lubitz *et al.*, 1973), or even less (Hajjar *et al.*, 1975). The success of treatment often is indicated early by a reduction of steroid excretion (Hoffman and Mattox, 1972; Lubitz *et al.*, 1973), but steroid excretion may increase, decrease, or remain unchanged (Fukushima *et al.*, 1971). Removal of the tumor and *o,p'*-DDD treatment may be combined (Levy *et al.*, 1985). The success of treatment is greater in Cushing's syndrome due to adrenal hyperplasia (Weisenfeld and Goldner, 1962). An early example of what appeared to be complete cure was reported by Bar-Hay *et al.* (1964). Ten of 17 patients with this condition experienced cure or remission for 12–32 months after the drug had been withdrawn (Luton *et al.*, 1973).

The large dosage of *o,p'*-DDD necessary to produce clinical benefit often produces general lassitude, anorexia, nausea, vomiting, diarrhea, and/or dermatitis (Bochner *et al.*, 1969; Danowski *et al.*, 1964; Halmi and Lascari, 1971; Hoffman and Mattox, 1972; Hutter and Kahoe, 1966; Naruse *et al.*, 1970; Southern *et al.*, 1961; Weisenfeld and Goldner, 1962). Gynecomastia, hematuria, leukopenia, and thrombocytopenia have been reported more rarely (Luton *et al.*, 1972; Perevodchikova *et al.*, 1972). The symptoms disappear soon after administration of the drug is stopped or the dosage is reduced. Furthermore, some patients do not develop toxicity. A 10-year-old girl received 7500 mg/day for a total of 9 kg without discernible side effects (Helson *et al.*, 1971).

Even large, therapeutic doses of *o,p'*-DDD cause no histological alterations of the adrenals in humans (Wallace *et al.*, 1961). However, electron microscopy revealed degenerative changes in the mitochondria of the zona fasciculata of a patient who had received *o,p'*-DDD at the rate of about 3000 mg/day for 1 month (Temple *et al.*, 1969). Dosages in the therapeutic range (specifically those between 110 and 140 mg/kg/day) produced no detectable injury to the liver, kidney, or bone marrow even though the patients exhibited the reversible symptoms listed earlier (Bergenstal *et al.*, 1960).

Kupfer (1967) reviewed the extensive literature indicating that the effect in humans and other species, except the dog, is caused by stimulation of corticoid metabolism by massive doses of *o,p'*-DDD and not to any direct reaffect on the adrenal. Southern *et al.* (1966a, b) agreed that the effect was predominantly extra-adrenal in humans when the drug was first given but offered evidence that adrenal secretion of cortisol eventually was reduced. Even though therapeutic doses eventually have a direct effect on the adrenal, doses encountered by workers exposed to technical DDT do not (Clifford and Weil, 1972; Morgan and Roan, 1973).

Somewhat encouraging results were reported in the use of *p,p'*-DDD for treating diabetics with hyaline vasular changes and hyperpolysacharidemia (Törnblom, 1959). Apparently, there has been no attempt to use *o,p'*-DDD for this condition. *o,p'*-DDD has been used, in a much lower dosage, for treating spanomenorrhea associated with hypertrichosis (Klotz *et al.*, 1971). Menstruation was restored in 13 of 15 women with these conditions, and normal pregnancies occurred in five of them during the treatment period. The babies were normal. There was some improvement in hypertrichosis in nine and no improvement in six.

At least part of the action of *o,p'*-DDT in controlling excessive androgens involves its action on their metabolism. It was found in a study of three patients with metastatic adrenal carcinoma and one with penicious anemia that the compound decreased the conversion of labeled androgens to androsterone by about 76% and to etiocholanolone by about 80%. The main effect on androgen metabolism was consistent with induction of microsomal oxidase activity by the drug (Hellmann *et al.*, 1973).

When uptake of radioactive iodine is used for diagnosis of Cushing's syndrome, $[^{131}I]$19-iodocholesterol is the compound usually employed. DDD labeled with ^{131}I has been used for the same purpose (Skromme-Kadlubik, 1972, 1973a, b, 1974). No comparative study of the duration of storage of the two compounds appears to have been made. However, it is clear that it is possible to introduce enough radiation via ^{131}I-labeled DDD either to kill rodents or to cause atrophy of their adrenal glands, depending on the schedule of administration (Skromme-Kadlubik *et al.*, 1974). This was viewed as an indication that ^{131}I-labeled DDD might be useful for treating human adrenal carcinoma.

60.3.3.2 Analytical Findings

Studies associated with what apparently was the first attempt to use *p,p'*-DDD in treating Cushing's syndrome established that the compound is concentrated in the adrenal gland. Eleven weeks after the last course of DDD, when the concentration in adipose tissue was less than half what it had been earlier, the concentration in an adrenal biopsy was 50 ppm, wet weight. On a lipid basis, the concentrations in fat and adrenal were almost identical (Sheehan *et al.*, 1953). A patient who had received *o,p'*-DDD at the rate of 4000 mg/day for 58 days had a blood level of 6 ppm and excreted 8.3 mg of free and 39.7 mg of conjugated DDA in a 24-hr urine sample (Sinsheimer *et al.*, 1972). There is evidence for two plasma pools of *o,p'*-DDD (Slooten *et al.*, 1982).

Normal volunteers excreted increased concentrations of DDA within 24 hr of receiving *p,p'*-DDD at a rate of 5 mg/day and continued to excrete DDA at greater than predose levels for over 4 months after dosing was stopped after 81 days (Roan *et al.*, 1971).

Treatment of appropriate cases with *o,p'*-DDT usually results in a decrease in urinary steroid excretion (Gutierrez and Crooke, 1980). An unusually detailed study of the individual compounds is that of Hartwig *et al.* (1968).

In long-term administration of *o,p'*-DDD (2gm/day for 1–3 months) to patients with adrenal carcinoma or Cushing's syndrome, Ojima *et al.* (1984) found that plasma levels of pregnenolone, progesterone, cortisol, corticosterone, and some other C_{21} steroids were progressively decreased, as well as urinary excretion of 17-ketosteroids and 17-hydroxycorticosteroids. Touito *et al.* (1985), however, were unable to demonstrate any correlation between concentrations of *o,p'*-DDD in adrenals removed from patients preoperatively treated with the drug for Cushing's syndrome and inhibition of some steroid biosynthesis enzymes measured *in vitro*. There is a suggestion that *o,p'*-DDD suppresses ACTH-secreting cells in the pituitary as well as depressing steroid hormone secretion (Takamatsu *et al.*, 1981).

In some patients either *p,p'*-DDD (Törnblom, 1959) or *o,p'*-DDD (Molnar *et al.*, 1961) caused an increase in plasma cholesterol, but the opposite also may occur (Danowski *et al.*, 1964). Oddly enough, such patients are refractory to the therapeutic effects of the drug (Molnar *et al.*, 1961).

An interesting finding is that *o,p'*-DDD has a hypouricemic effect apparently by increasing the renal clearance of uric acid (Reach *et al.*, 1978; Zumoff, 1979).

The induction of microsomal enzymes by *o,p'*-DDD has been identified following their isolation from the urine of treated patients (Reif *et al.*, 1974).

Persons suffering from Cushing's syndrome can be distinguished from normal by their increased adrenal uptake of [^{131}]19-iodocholesterol. In one patient under treatment with *o,p'*-DDD, uptake of radioactive iodine was reduced but not to the normal range (Morita *et al.*, 1972). DDD is commonly found in blood and tissues from the general population. For levels of it in blood; see Table 15.13 in Smith (1991).

60.4 ETHYLAN

60.4.1 IDENTITY, PROPERTIES, AND USES

Ethylan is 1,1-dichloro-2,2-bis(4-ethylphenyl)ethane, that is, the *p,p'*-diethyl analog of DDD (Table 60.1). Ethylan is the only common name in use, but apparently it has been approved officially only in the USSR. The trade name Perthane® often is used. Code designations for ethylan include B-63,138 and Q-137. The CAS registry number is 72-56-0. Ethylan has the empirical formula $C_{18}H_{20}Cl_2$ and a molecular weight of 307.27. The pure compound is a crystalline solid with a melting point of 56–57°C. The technical product is a waxy solid with a melting point not below 40°C and with some decomposition above 52°C. The insecticide is practically insoluble in water but soluble in acetone, kerosene, and other organic solvents. Ethylan was introduced in 1950 and has been used to control pear psylla, leaf hoppers, various larvae on vegetable, and moths and carpet beetle on textiles.

60.4.2 TOXICITY TO LABORATORY ANIMALS

The oral LD 50 values for ethylan were 8170 and 9340 mg/kg in rats and mice, respectively. However, the corresponding intravenous values were only 73 and 173 mg/kg in the same species. No dermal LD 50 value could be measured; all rabbits that received a 30% solution at the rate of 3 ml/kg/day for 13 weeks survived (Finnegan *et al.*, 1955). Gaines (1960) agreed that the oral toxicity was very low (LD 50 > 4000 mg/kg).

Minimal and infrequent changes were seen in the livers of rats fed dietary levels of 2500 and 5000 ppm for 2 years. There was no effect on survival, and differences in growth rate did not correspond to dosage. Thus a dietary level of 1000 ppm might be considered a no-effect level. In contrast, the same investigators found that a dietary level of 5000 ppm was lethal to dogs within 22 weeks. Levels of 100 or 1000 ppm did not interfere with survival or growth when fed for 1 year, although the 1000 ppm level led to some atrophy of the adrenals (Finnegan *et al.*, 1955). Cortisone given at the same time as ethylan tended to block the effect of the latter on the adrenal (Bleiberg and Larson, 1957). Reznikov (1973) considered the action of *p,p'*-ethylan similar to that of *p,p'*-DDD.

60.4.2.1 Absorption, Distribution, Metabolism, and Excretion

Rats fed ethylan at a concentration of 50 ppm (about 2.5 mg/kg/day) for 6 weeks stored the compound in their fat at a concentration of 19 ppm (Finnegan *et al.*, 1955). Four generations of rats were fed a standard synthetic diet containing 20% fat to which several pesticides were added. The diets of the seven groups studied differed only in the kinds of fat (cottonseed oil, lard, etc.) they contained. The average concentration of added ethylan found by analysis in different samples of dietary fat varied from 2.01 to 2.71 ppm. No ethylan was detectable in the body fat or other tissues of the rats (Adams *et al.*, 1974). After a single dose of [^{14}C] ethylan, rats excreted 90% of the radioactivity in their feces and 5% in their urine in 2 weeks (Bleiberg and Larson, 1957).

60.4.2.2 Biochemical Effects

Ethylan reduced excretion of 17-hydroxycorticosteroids and caused adrenal atrophy in dogs (Cobey *et al.*, 1956). Dogs that had received ethylan for 10 or 14 days at a rate of 200 mg/kg/day slept 12–14 hr following anesthesia with sodium pentobarbital compared to only 6–7 hr following the same dosage of barbiturate before receiving ethylan. Similar studies with different DDD formulations revealed that increased sleeping time did not depend on the presence of adrenal atrophy, but they did not exclude the possibility that it depended on altered function of the adrenal. The increased sleeping time did not depend on reduced clearance of the barbiturate from the blood, which was not influenced by ethylan or DDD. Thus the cause remained obscure. Whatever the cause, the increase in sleeping time was peculiar to dogs and did not occur in rats treated with DDD (Nichols *et al.*, 1958). In dogs, ethylan (50 mg/kg/day for 10 days) significantly increased the glutathione reductase of the adrenal cortex but not of the liver (Komissarenko *et al.*, 1968).

60.4.2.3 Effects on Organs and Tissues

Ethylan produces adrenal cortical atrophy in the dog (Finnegan *et al.*, 1955; Larson *et al.*, 1955). No such effect was noted in the rat. Presumably the effect is virtually specific for the dog, as is true of *o,p'*-DDD, which has been more extensively studied. Dogs killed or rendered moribund by dietary level of 5000 ppm (about 105 mg/kg/day) showed marked atrophy of the adrenal cortex, the medulla was unaffected. The capsule was wrinkled, the zona glomerulosa contained cells with granular and diminished cytoplasm, and there was a focal loss of these cells. The zona fasciculata was greatly narrowed, and there was extreme vacuolization among cells in the medial two-thirds. However, fat-staining material was deficient throughout the fasiculata, especially the inner part. The zona reticularis had practically disappeared, leaving only a few cells containing lipochrome pigment. There were a few focal concentrations of lymphocytes. Atrophy was present but less severe in two of three dogs that received 1000 ppm (about 21 mg/kg/day). On the contrary, severe atrophy was produced in less than 3 weeks by an oral dosage of 200 mg/kg/day.

When ethylan was administered to mice at the highest tolerated rate for about 18 months, the results for tumorigenicity were equivocal (Innes *et al.*, 1969). Some evidence for hepatic tumor formation in female mice but not males or rats of either sex has been reported (NCI, 1979).

60.4.3 TOXICITY TO HUMANS

Ethylan was administered to nine men with metastatic carcinoma of the prostrate and to five women with metastatic carcinoma of the breast because there had been reports of a favorable effect of surgical adrenalectomy on the clinical course of some patients with these diseases and because the compound had been shown to cause adrenocortical atrophy in the dog (Taliaferro and Leone, 1957). All the patients also received ACTH either intermittently or continuously. With one exception, the dosage of ethylan varied from 50 to 150 mg/kg/day, the latter for a total of 189,000 mg within 21 days. The most intensive treatment was 200–300 mg/kg/day for a total of 96,000 mg in 6 days. The smallest dosage produced diarrhea, vomiting, and especially nausea in some patients and required cessation of treatment. In contrast, other patients, especially those who were less sick to begin with, tolerated the higher dosages, including 200–300 mg/kg/day, with no symptoms whatever. Marked thrombocytopenia and leukopenia were noted in one patient just after a 14-day course of treatment. These changes, which were attributed to ethylan, resolved promptly when treatment was stopped. There was no other evidence of hematopoietic toxicity and no evidence of hepatic, renal, neural, or other toxicity. It was not considered that the relatively brief treatments influenced the clinical course in any of the cases. However, among patients receiving 150–300 mg/kg/day in divided doses, ethylan caused a marked depression of plasma 17-hydroxycorticosteroid levels, but never below the normal range. Lower dosages had no consistent effects. No distinct benefit but nausea, vomiting, and skin rash were seen in four other patients with carcinoma who received ethylan at dosages of 1800–8000 mg/day for periods of 4–54 days (Weisenfeld and Goldner, 1962). In surveys of workers and the general population who have developed pancreatic cancer association with ethylan exposure has been reported (Garabrant *et al.*, 1992, 1993). However, those studies involved self-reporting exposure. See also Section 60.2.4.

60.5 METHOXYCHLOR

60.5.1 IDENTITY, PROPERTIES, AND USES

Methoxychlor is 1,1,1-trichloro-2,2-bis(4-methoxyphenyl) ethane or 2,2-bis(*p*-methoxyphenyl)-1,1,1-trichloroethane, that is, the *p,p′*-dimethoxy analog of *p,p′*-DDT. The structure is shown in Table 60.1. The common name, methoxychlor (BSI, ICPC, ISO), is in general use. Other nonproprietary names have included dianisyl trichloroethane, dimethoxy-DT, DMDT (an acronym for dimethoxydiphenyltrichloroethane), and methoxy DDT. One trade name is Maralate®. Code designations include OMS-466. The CAS registry number is 72-43-5.

Methoxychlor has the empirical formula $C_{16}H_{15}Cl_3O_2$ and a molecular weight of 345.65. The pure material forms colorless crystals melting at 89°C. Technical methoxychlor is a gray flaky powder containing about 88% of the *p,p′*-isomer, the remainder being mainly *o,p′*-isomer, although up to 50 other contaminants have been detected (Lamoureux and Feil, 1980; West *et al.*, 1982). The density is 1.41 at 25°C. Methoxychlor is stable to heat and ultraviolet light and resistant to oxidation; it is dehydrochlorinated by alkalies and by heavy metal catalysts. The solubilities of methoxychlor are approximately the same as those of DDT. It is readily soluble in most aromatic solvents, moderately soluble in alcohols and petroleum oils, and essentially insoluble in water.

Methoxychlor was first described by Laüger *et al.* (1944), and it was introduced about 1945. Formulations include wettable powder (25 and 50%), emulsifiable concentrate (24%), dusts (4–10%), and aerosols. Methoxychlor is effective against a wide range of insects affecting fruits, vegetables, forage crops, and livestock. The low toxicity of methoxychlor and its short biological half-life were largely responsible for its greatly expanded use following the ban on DDT in many countries.

60.5.2 TOXICITY TO LABORATORY ANIMALS

60.5.2.1 Basic Findings

In spite of its low toxicity, methoxychlor in sufficient dosage is capable of causing convulsions in the dog (Tegeris *et al.*, 1966). However, in the rat, the compound causes depression of the central nervous system (Lehman, 1951, 1952). Tremors have been noted but they are not a prominent symptom. In rabbits killed by a few doses, the only signs noted were diarrhea and anorexia (Smith *et al.*, 1946).

The acute toxicity of methoxychlor is very low; oral LD 50 values of 5000 mg/kg (Hodge *et al.*, 1950) and 6000 mg/kg (Lehman, 1951, 1952) have been reported for the rat and values of 1850 mg/kg (Domenjoz, 1946) for the mouse and 2000 mg/kg for the hamster (Cabral *et al.*, 1979a). Rats fed a dietary level of 30,000 ppm suffered a severe reduction in growth, and most of them died in less than 45 days. Those fed a dietary level of 10,000 ppm survived but gained almost no weight; paired feeding studies showed that failure of growth was due entirely to food refusal. A dietary level of 1600 ppm for 2 years caused measurable reduction of growth but produced no reduction in life span and no histological change in the tissues. Dosages of 20 mg/kg/day for 1 year or a dietary level of 200 ppm (about 10 mg/kg/day) for 2 years were both no-effect levels (Hodge *et al.*, 1950, 1952). Rabbits are relatively susceptible to methoxychlor; a dosage of 200 mg/kg/day was fatal within 15 days (Smith *et al.*, 1946).

Dogs fed the compound in their diet in such a way that they received 1000 mg/kg/day for 6 months lost weight, and many of those that received 2000, 2500, or 4000 mg/kg/day began having convulsions within 6 weeks and died within 3 additional weeks. Strangely enough, dogs that received 2500 mg/kg/day administered by gastric tube as a suspension in 1% gum tragacanth for 5 months showed no indication of injury although the amount of absorption was not clear (Tegeris *et al.*, 1966). In an earlier study lasting 1 year, the highest dosage fed to dogs (300 mg/kg/day) lost weight for a month, but later those on the two lower dosages regained their original weight (Tegeris *et al.*, 1966). A dietary level of 2500 ppm for 8–16 weeks produced no ill effects in chickens (Lillie *et al.*, 1973).

60.5.2.2 Absorption, Distribution, Metabolism, and Excretion

Mixtures containing methoxychlor appeared to pass directly from the luminal border of the rat jejunum to the intercellular spaces immediately, in addition to the usual transport through the endoplasmic reticulum toward the Golgi apparatus. Furthermore, absorption of methoxychlor was accompanied by distention of vesicles and intracellular spaces (Imai and Coulston, 1968). Storage of methoxychlor was minimal in the fat of rats that had received it for 18 weeks. No storage could be measured at a dietary level of 25 ppm, and storage decreased after the ninth week at levels of 100 and 500 ppm in spite of continued intake. Two weeks after dosing was discontinued no methoxychlor was detected (Kunze *et al.*, 1950). Storage of methoxychlor in sheep reaches a steady state in 6–8 weeks or, at certain dosage levels, actually declines after that interval in spite of continued intake perhaps due to induced metabolism. Storage loss is prompt after dosing is stopped (Reynolds *et al.*, 1975, 1976).

Following oral administration of radioactive methoxychlor to mice, 98.3% was recovered from the excreta within 24 hr. The compound was metabolized to 2-(*p*-hydroxyphenyl)-2′-(methoxyphenyl)-1,1,1-trichloroethane and 2,2-bis(*p*-hydroxyphenyl)-1,1,1-trichloroethane, which were eliminated largely in conjugated form (Kapoor *et al.*, 1970). Detailed studies have also been performed with goats (Davison *et al.*, 1982, 1983). The normally low rate of storage of methoxychlor was not influenced by simultaneous feeding of DDT or dieldrin (Street and Blau, 1966). Rat liver microsomes form both the mono and dihydroxy products as well as more polar compounds (Bulger *et al.*, 1985; Ousterhaut *et al.*, 1981). With (*R*)- and (*S*)-[monomethyl-^{2}H$_3$]methoxychlors, intramolecular deuterium effects and entantiotopic differentiation have been

observed and the demethylations appear due to CYP1B/2 and CYP2C6 isoforms (Ichinose and Kurihara, 1987; Kishimoto *et al.*, 1995; Kishimoto and Kurihara, 1996). Much of the metabolism work has been done by Kupfer and colleagues using microsomes, purified cytochrome P450 isoforms, or insect cells containing human cytochrome P450 species (Dehal and Kupfer, 1994; Kupfer and Bulger, 1987; Stresser and Kupfer, 1997, 1998a, b). In the rat, demethylation seems to occur with CYP2B isoforms which also actively hydroxylate in the *ortho* positions of methoxychlor and the mono and dimethoxy analogues. In humans, CYP2C19 and CYP1A2 seem to be responsible for demethylation. *Ortho* hydroxylation of the monodemethylated products is predominantly catalyzed by CYP3A4. On the whole bidemethylation and *ortho* hydroxylation seem to occur less readily with human samples than with rat liver. Another route of metabolism is an initial dechlorination before replacement of the methoxy groups (Davision *et al.*, 1983; Kupfer and Bulger, 1987) but this has not been greatly investigated. Phenolic products from both routes appear to be converted to activated intermediates, which may bind covalently to macromolecules (Bulger *et al.*, 1983; Kupfer *et al.*, 1986; Kupfer and Bulger, 1987). This might be related to the formation of the catechols formed by *ortho* hydroxylation (Bulger and Kupfer, 1989; Kupfer *et al.*, 1990). A scheme of methoxychlor metabolism is shown in Fig. 60.3.

60.5.2.3 Biochemical Effects

Methoxychlor induced liver microsomal enzymes in sheep, but even at a dietary level of 2500 ppm the degree of induction was less than that caused by DDT at a dietary level of 250 ppm. Methoxychlor caused no change in food consumption, body weight, liver weight, uterine weight, or estrous cycle (Cecil *et al.*, 1975). In rats, methoxychlor induced hepatic CYP2B1 and CYP3A enzymes levels, but in regimes with multiple treatment and less efficiently than DDT (Li *et al.*, 1995). Some increases in hepatic glucose-6-phospatase activity have been observed in rats given methoxychlor without showing any histological damage (Morgan and Hickenbottom, 1979), and significant decreases in lactate levels occurred even at doses <1% of the oral LD 50. Neonatal administration of methoxychlor to rats resulted in elevated levels of sex-monoamine oxidase activities in adult rats, implying changes in the brain hormone environment during development which did not become apparent until adulthood (Lamartiniere *et al.*, 1982).

Whereas massive doses of methoxychlor have an estrogenic effect in swine (Tegeris *et al.*, 1966) and perhaps other species, no such effect is detectable in chickens at a dietary level of 10 ppm (Foster, 1973) or in sheep at a dietary level of 2500 ppm (Cecil *et al.*, 1975). Even 10 ppm is a far greater residue than humans or livestock are likely to encounter.

There was no evidence that methoxychlor induced microsomal enzymes in heifers when administered at the rate of 112 mg/kg/day for 9 days, as judged by recovery of radioactivity derived from 16α, 17α-[^{14}C]dihydroxyprogestrone acetophenide (DHPA) used to synchronize estrus (Rumsey and

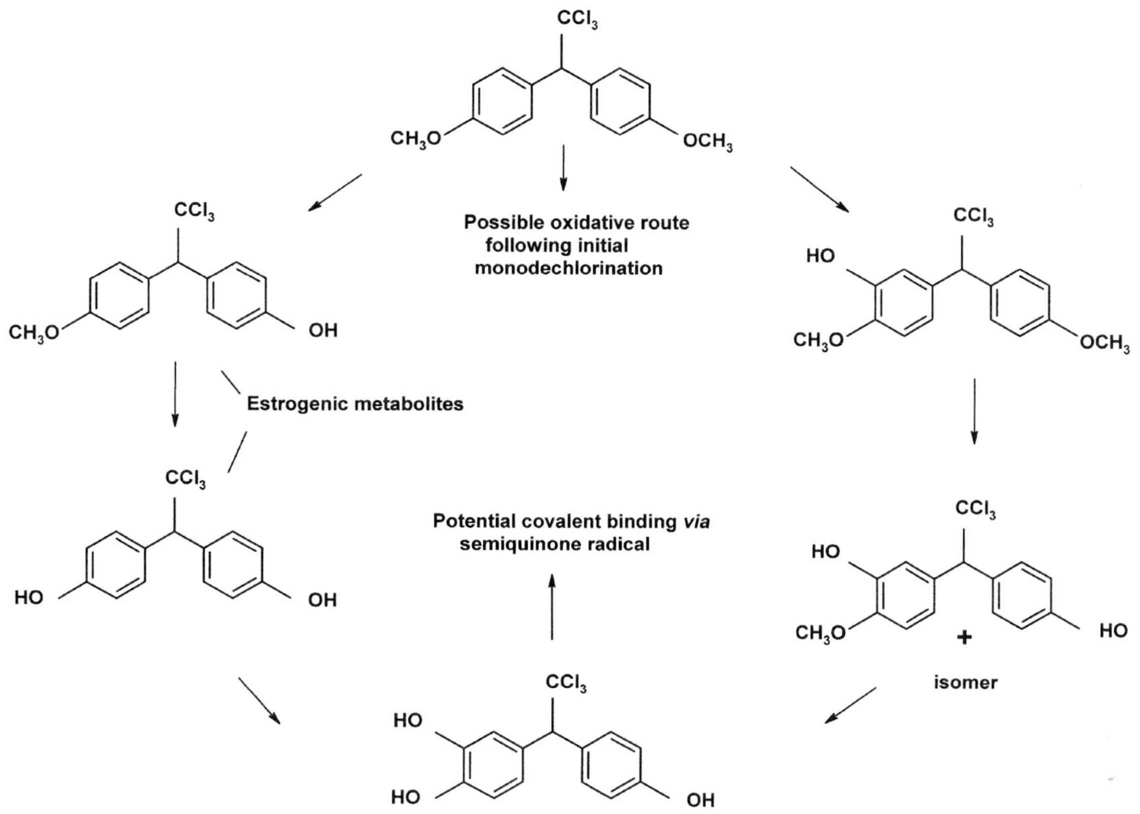

Figure 60.3 Metabolism of methoxychlor. The exact mechanisms of covalent binding are not known.

Schreiber, 1969). However, because metabolites of DHPA were not distinguished, the study cannot be considered a critical test of induction. Microsomal metabolism of methoxychlor in rat liver has been reported to result in binding to iodothyronine 5′-monodeiodinase at cysteine or lysine residues with resulting depression of iodinase activity *in vivo*. The significance of these findings on thyroid hormone metabolism and action is unknown (Zhou *et al.*, 1995).

60.5.2.4 Effects on Organs and Tissues

Of several polycyclic aromatic compounds said to be impurities in commercial methoxychlor, only one was mutagenic and in only one strain (Grant *et al.*, 1976). Mixed mutagenicity results have been more recently reported for methoxychlor (Oberly *et al.*, 1993).

Some tumors were found in rats fed for 2 years at dietary concentrations as high as 1600 ppm, but the kind and incidence did not differ from those in controls. No tumors were found in dogs that had received dietary levels up to 10,000 ppm (Hodge *et al.*, 1952). Negative results also were found in mice that received a single subcutaneous injection (10 mg/mouse) or in others given weekly skin applications (0.1 or 10 mg). However, it was concluded from identical study of other compounds regarded as carcinogens that the skin tests were not an adequate substitute for tests by other routes (Hodge *et al.*, 1966). When two strains of mice were fed technical methoxychlor at a dietary level of 750 ppm for as much as 2 years, the incidence

and malignancy of carcinoma of the testis were increased in one strain but not the other. It was suggested that the carcinogenicity was related to the estrogenic activity of methoxychlor (Reuber, 1979a). The occurrence of neoplasms of all sorts showed a very rough dosage response in male rats fed technical methoxychlor at dietary levels of 100 ppm or more and in females fed 10 ppm or more; tumors identified as carcinomas were found in both sexes but only in rats fed 2000 ppm for 2 years (Reuber, 1979b). The conclusion that methoxychlor is carcinogenic for the liver in C3H and BALB/c mice and Osborne–Mendel rats was proposed as being related to the covalent binding of activated metabolites (Kupfer and Bulger, 1987). However, anyone interested should consult the original reports, including NCI (1978b) which shows only poor evidence for carcinogenicity of methoxychlor. At a dietary level of 1000 ppm, the tumorigenic property of methoxychlor was less than additive when it was fed in combination with Aramite, DDT, and thiourea or Aramite, DDT, and aldrin (Deichmann *et al.*, 1967).

Large doses of methoxychlor (1000, 2000, or 4000 mg/kg/day) produce dosage-dependent chronic nephritis and hypertrophy of the kidneys, mammary glands, and uteri of swine (Tegeris *et al.*, 1966). In rats, Hodge *et al.* (1950) could not find characteristic liver cell changes at any dosage level. They did find striking testicular atrophy at dietary levels of 10,000 ppm or greater and this was not present in parfed controls. Similar findings were reported by Tullner and Edgcomb (1962). No atrophy was present in a dog that had received methoxychlor at 100 mg/kg/day for a month. Under certain conditions, continued massive dosage of methoxychlor produced cystic tubular nephropathy in rats (Tullner and Edgcomb, 1962).

Wistar rats given methoxychlor (100 or 200 mg/kg/day) for 760 days (males) or 14 days (females) showed inhibition of spermatogenesis and folliculogenesis (Bal, 1984). There were degenerative changes in Sertoli cells and in spermatogonia and spermatocytes, with some transformed to polynucleate cells. Cytoplasmic vacuolations were observed in the epithelium of the ductus epididymis. Atresia of the ovarian follicles was evident with pyknosis and karyorrhexis of the granulosa cells.

In rats, Lehman (1951, 1952) found that the lowest dietary level producing tissue damage was 550 ppm (about 25 mg/kg/day); the effects, which were confined to the liver, consisted mainly of a slight increase in incidence of hepatic cell adenomas. In rats and monkeys the early induction of liver enzymes and the concomitant increase in hepatic endoplasmic reticulum may be temporary, disappearing in animals treated with methoxychlor for a prolonged time (Serrone et al., 1965). In dogs, a dosage of 2500 mg/kg/day caused grossly visible congestion of the intestinal mucosa. It has also caused progressive degeneration of the mitochondria of mucosal cells of the small intestine marked in the early stages by matrical swelling and disruption of the cristae and later by disappearance of cristae and appearance of small myelin bodies. The mitochondria of these cells showed some recovery in a dog that had been returned to uncontaminated food for only 3 weeks after 12 weeks of the high dosage of methoychlor (Tegeris et al., 1968).

For other effects on organs, see the two following sections on reproduction.

60.5.2.5 Effects on Reproduction

Large doses of methoxychlor have estrogenic effects (Tullner, 1961). Methoxychlor levels of 2500 and 5000 ppm reduced mating, and only one litter was produced. However, when the same rats were returned to an uncontaminated diet, they reproduced normally. A dietary level of 1000 ppm started before mating and continued throughout lactation had no effect on reproduction in that generation, but the female pups had early vaginal opening and reduced reproduction when mature, and the reproductive behavior of mature male pups was also defective (Harris et al., 1974). The potency appeared to be 1/10000 of diethylstilboestrol. In a more recent study, male and female weanling rats were dosed with methoxychlor at 100 mg or 200 mg/day through puberty and gestation until day 15 of lactation in females (Gray et al., 1989). Although various parameters of reproductive potential were altered in both sexes, fertility was only reduced in females when mated with untreated animals. No implantations were observed in another study when female rats received the same doses of methoxychlor for 14 days before mating and during pregnancy (Bal, 1984). Preimplantation effects of methoxychlor seemed more important than postimplantation in ensuring success (Cummings and Gray, 1989).

In vitro tests showed that pure methoxychlor itself is not estrogenic, although the commercial product had some activity

and bis(4-hydroxyphenyl)trichloroethane was quite active (Bulger and Kupfer, 1977; Bulger et al., 1978a, b). The estrogenic activity of impure methoxychlor in inducing uterus growth, uterine orinithine decarboxylase and epidermal growth factor receptor, creatine kinase and peroxidase (Bulger et al., 1978b; Cummings and Metcalf, 1994; 1995; Metcalf et al., 1995) appears to be caused by the demethylated analogs (Bulger et al., 1985; Ousterhaut et al., 1981) which are also metabolites (see Section 60.5.2.2). By both *in vitro* and *in vivo* criteria, 1,1-dichloro bis(4-hydroxyphenyl)ethene is the most potent agent (Bulger et al., 1985; Cummings, 1997; Kupfer and Bulger, 1987). The estrogenic effects of methoxychlor are not restricted to those on uterine physiology and function. Both running wheel activity (estrogen controlled) and sex behavior in rats and hamsters were induced by 400 mg/kg/day (Gray et al., 1988). The actions of methoxychlor were not, however, completely identical to those of estradiol. Exposure of pregnant mice to methoxychlor has been reported to cause changes in behavior of male offspring (vom Saal et al., 1995). Methoxychlor affects the dicidual cell response of the rat uterus (Cummings and Gray, 1987, 1989), a technique mimicking the growth and development of the endometrium during pregnancy, by a mechanism that apparently occurs by interaction directly with the uterus. Other mechanisms such as embryo transport rate might also be involved (Cummings and Perreault, 1990).

Some evidence suggests that reproductive effects of methoxychlor metabolites in male rats (Bal, 1984; Tullner and Edgcomb, 1962) may be mediated, in part, by elevation of prolactin concentration and release, which in turn influences hypothalamic levels of gonadotropin-releasing hormone (Goldman et al., 1986). In studies of the effect of methoxychlor on reproductive tract development following neonatal exposure of mice, precocious vaginal opening, cornification and increased tract size, and ovarian atrophy were observed in females and reduced serum testosterone, testicular DNA content, seminal vesicles, and prostrate in males (Cooke and Eroschenko, 1990; Eroschenko and Cooke, 1990; Eroshenko et al., 1995). Changes in females were not however, completely identical to those observed with 17β-estradiol (Eroshenko, 1991). On the other hand uterine luminal proteins were identical following technical methoxychlor and 17β-estradiol administration to ovariectomised mice (Rourke et al., 1991) as were morphometric parameters (Swartz et al., 1994) although some toxicity was observed.

When rats received methoxychlor intragastrically on days 6–15 of pregnancy, dosages of 50–400 mg/kg/day reduced maternal weight gain (Khera et al., 1978). At 200 mg/kg/day, the compound decreased the number and weight of fetuses and caused delayed ossification leading to wavy ribs and other bent bones. No real teratogenesis was observed and no effects were observed *in vitro* or human and rat testicular cells when examined for single strand DNA breaks (Bjorge et al., 1996; Khera et al., 1978).

Methoxychlor prevented ovariectomy-induced bone loss in the rat (Dodge et al., 1996). Chapin et al. (1997) have dosed rats before and following birth and looked for immune and reproductive changes at doses of 0, 5, 50, or 150 mg/kg/day in a large study. Primary adult effects were reproductive and 5 mg/kg/day was not a NOAEL.

A predictable result of the rapid metabolism and excretion of methoxychlor is the fact that very little of it is excreted in the milk and is thus of low risk to humans. When the compound was fed to cows at a dietary concentration of 7000 ppm, the concentration in the milk reached slightly over 2 ppm in 91 days and remained essentially constant until feeding was stopped on day 112 (Gannon *et al.*, 1959). After dosing was stopped, the concentration in milk fell to <0.1 ppm in a week. In mice, methoxychlor fed to lactating dams did affect the reproductive tract of suckling females (Appel and Eroschenko, 1992).

In chickens, dietary levels as high as 2500 ppm (about 145 mg/kg/day) had no effect on the health of hens or their production of hatchable eggs or on the ability of cockerels to fertilize the eggs. The hens were tested for 16 weeks and the cockerels for 8 weeks (Lillie *et al.*, 1973).

In summary, methoxychlor possesses many of the estrogenic properties of 17β-estradiol probably after *in vivo* demethylation. Its fast metabolism and low potency (>1/10,000 of 17β-estradiol) do pose questions as to any risk to humans and whether all its reproductive toxicity properties are identical to estrogen requires further study. Hall *et al.* (1997) suggested that in mice methoxychlor acts as an estrogen agonist in the uterus but as antagonist in the ovary.

60.5.3 TOXICITY TO HUMANS

60.5.3.1 Experimental Exposure

Groups of volunteers were given methoxychlor at rates of 0, 0.5, 1, and 2 mg/kg/day for 8 weeks. Even the highest dosage was without detectable effect on health, clinical chemistry, or the morphology of blood, bone marrow, liver, small intestine, or testis (Stein *et al.*, 1965; Stein, 1970). The highest dosage administered by Stein was similar to 1.4 mg/kg/day, which is considered safe for occupational intake, as reflected in the threshold limit value of 10 mg/m^3. The low sensitizing property of methoxychlor has been noted (Szarmach and Poniecka, 1973).

60.5.3.2 Use Experience

There apparently has been no confirmed case of poisoning, occupational or otherwise, involving methoxychlor. However, atypical cases associated with methoxychlor have been reported.

A 21-year-old man first noticed symptoms 8–9 hr after spraying several fruit trees with a formulation diluted from a mixture containing methoxychlor (15%) and malathion (7.5%) (Harell *et al.*, 1978). The entire task took only 15–20 min, and afterward a shower was taken. The first symptoms were blurring of vision and gradual onset of nausea. Next morning, the man began vomiting and developed severe diarrhea. He sought

medical help 24 hr after exposure and was admitted to hospital about 36 hr after exposure. He was then dehydrated and suffering severe abdominal cramps and continuing diarrhea. On day 3 after exposure, jaundice was noted and continuous bilateral tinnitus began. On day 4, the patient was completely deaf and slightly dizzy. On day 5, rapidly progressive renal failure required hemodialysis. Soon afterward, peripheral sensory and motor neuropathy appeared, including hypoesthesias, paresthesias, persistent leg and foot pain, bilateral footdrop, and difficulty in moving the extremities. A generalized rash appeared. In spite of marked recovery, the patient still had profound, bilateral, sensorineural hearing loss, tinnitus, and moderate neuropathy of the legs and arms when he was reevaluated over 6 years later (Harell *et al.*, 1978). Clearly, the delay in onset and the character of the illness were not consistent with poisoning by methoxychlor, malathion, or a combination of them, regardless of dosage. No thought seems to have been given to other possible causes, whether toxic or otherwise.

A 49-year-old man who was exposed to a dust of methoxychlor and captan developed aplastic anemia a few weeks later and died within 6 months. He had also had light exposure to methoxychlor during the previous 2 years without symptoms (Ziem, 1982).

60.5.3.3 Laboratory Findings

Most investigators have not found methoxychlor in human tissue. Apparently, the first exceptions were Griffith and Blanke (1975) who reported finding the compound infrequently and in unstated concentrations in blood taken at autopsy under the medical examiner system of Virginia. Under the circumstances of collection, the possibility of occupational exposure of the deceased could not be excluded.

The reported persistence of methoxychlor for at least 7 days on the hands of a worker (Kazen *et al.*, 1974) is interesting in view of the rapid metabolism of the compound once it is absorbed. However, it must be said that with modern analytical sensitivities, methoxychlor or metabolite residues might be found more frequently.

60.5.3.4 Treatment of Poisoning

In the unlikely event that treatment is required, it must be symptomatic.

60.6 CHLOROBENZILATE

60.6.1 IDENTITY, PROPERTIES, AND USES

The IUPAC name for chlorobenzilate (BS1, ISO, JMAF) is ethyl 4,4'-dichlorobenzilate. Other names are 4,4'-chlorobenzilic acid ethyl ester, ethyl 2-hydroxy-2,2-bis(3-chlorophenyl) acetate, and ethyl 4,4'-dichlorodiphenyl glycollate. For the structure see Table 60.1. Among many proprietary names have been G23992, Acaraben®, Benz O-chlor®, Benzilan®, and

Kop-Mite®. The CAS registry number is 510-15-6. Chlorobenzilate has the empirical formula $C_{16}H_{14}Cl_2O_3$ and a molecular weight of 325.20. It is a colorless solid melting at 37–37°C. It is very soluble in acetone and hexane but virtually insoluble in water. Impurities in the technical product, which is about 95% pure, can be dichlorobenzophenon, the ethyl ether of chlorobenzilate, and 4,4-dichlorobenzil. Chlorobenzilate was introduced as a technical product in 1952. It has been used mainly as a miticide on citrus crops or to control mites in beehives.

60.6.2 TOXICITY TO LABORATORY ANIMALS

The acute oral LD 50 to mice, rats (Horn *et al.*, 1955), and hamsters (Cabral *et al.*, 1979b) is about 700 mg/kg. Symptoms in rats and mice include depressed motor activity and rapid wheezing respiration. Dogs tolerated daily oral doses of 64 mg/kg for 35 weeks and rats 500 ppm in the diet for 2 years (Horn *et al.*, 1955). After daily chlorobenzilate doses of 12.8 mg/kg to dogs, 5 days/week for 35 weeks, approximately 40% of the total dose was excreted unchanged or a urinary metabolites. No significant storage in fat of dogs or rats was reported (Horn *et al.*, 1955). Knowles and Ahmad (1971) described the conversion of chlorobenzilate by rat liver homogenates to *p,p′*-dichlorobenzilic acid, *p,p′*-dichlorbenzophenone, *p,p′*-dichlorobenzyhydrol, and *p*-chlorobenzoic acid.

In carcinogenicity studies chlorobenzilate induced hepatocellular carcinomas in mice, but the evidence in rats is uncertain (NCI, 1978c). Some testicular atrophy was observed in rats.

60.6.3 TOXICITY TO HUMANS

A case of a pesticide sprayer poisoned by chlorobenzilate has been described (Ravindran, 1978). Symptoms included ataxia, delirium, fever, and muscle pains.

Chlorobenzilate was detected in the urine of some workers employed in Florida citrus groves. Exposed workers had levels ranging from 0.07 to 6.2 mg/liter. It should be noted that the methodology employed involved oxidation to *p,p′*-dichlorobenzophenone and would not distinguish between the parent chemical and some of its metabolites. (Levy *et al.*, 1981).

60.7 DICOFOL

60.7.1 IDENTITY, PROPERTIES, AND USES

The IUPAC name is 2,2,2-trichloro-1, 1-bis (4-chlorophenyl)-2,2,2-trichloroethanol, or 1,1-bis(*p*-chlorophenyl)-2,2,2-trichloroethanol, or 4,4-dichloro-*α*-trichloro-methylbenzhydrol. For the structure see Table 60.1 Dicofol (BSI, ISO) is also called Kelthane (JMAF). Proprietary names include Acarin®, Decofol®, Hifol®, Kelthane®, and Mitigan®. Dicofol has the empirical formula $C_{14}H_9Cl_5O$ and a molecular weight of 370.50. The pure substance is colorless and melts at

78.5–70.5°C. It is soluble in most organic solvents but practically insoluble in water. Dicofol was introduced as a commercial chemical in 1955. Like chlorobenzilate, dicofol is used mainly as a miticide for citrus fruits, nuts, cotton, and beans. It still appears to be used in some countries. The technical product is a brown viscous oil with a d^{25} of 1.45. The active compounds are 80% 1,1-bis(4-chlorophenyl)-2,2,2-trichloroethanol and 20% 1-(2-chlorophenyl)-1-(4-chloropenyl)-2,2,2-trichloroethanol (the *o,p′*-isomer). The other major impurity is 1,1,1,2-tetrachloro-2,2-bis(4-chlorophenyl)ethane (Baum *et al.*, 1976). Dicofol can be produced as water-dispersable powders, as emulsions, and in a dust.

60.7.2 TOXICITY TO LABORATORY ANIMALS

In rats and rabbits the acute oral LD 50 for technical grade dicofol seems to range from 575 to 2000 mg/kg (Ben-Dyke *et al.*, 1970; Brown *et al.*, 1969; Smith *et al.*, 1959). Dogs seem to be much less sensitive (Smith *et al.*, 1959). Rats fed dicofol for up to 2 years showed no effects on survival at levels below 1000 ppm but growth was impaired (Smith *et al.*, 1959). The maximum tolerable dose for mice in a subchronic study was 500 ppm (Sato *et al.*, 1987). Dogs fed 300 ppm showed no effect after 1 year, but some deaths occurred at 900 ppm.

Dicofol seems to be metabolized in rats to 4,4′-dichlorobenzophenone, which is stored in fat and muscle as well as being excreted in the feces (Brown *et al.*, 1969). DDE was also found, but there is doubt as to whether this was due to metabolism of dicofol or to contamination of the technical product employed. Water-soluble metabolites have been detected in the urine of mice give radiolabelled dicofol. Nearly 50% of the administered doses was excreted in the urine within 24 hr. Part may be glucuronides of 4,4′-dichlorobenzhydrol (Tabata *et al.*, 1979). Brown and Casida (1987) showed that *in vivo* mice convert dicofol to dichlorobenzophenone and dichlorobenzhydrol and that DDE originates from the impurity *α*-C1-DDT.

There is little published work on the specific toxic effects of dicofol in experimental animals. Some small adverse effects associated with reproduction in rats and mice have been reported (Brown, 1972; Trifonova and Gladenko, 1980). In a comparative study, 98% dicofol, the technical product Kelthane, and DDT were given to male rats in equimolar amounts. Dicofol produced dosage-related increases in microsomal protein, cytochrome P-450, and the specific activities of cytochrome reductase, ethoxycoumarin *o*-deethylase, aminopyrine *N*-demethylase, and glutathione *S*-transferase at a potency equivalent to that of Kelthane, DDT, or phenobarbital (Narloch *et al.*, 1987). Some evidence has been obtained for its hepatocarcinogenicity in male B6C3F1 mice but not in rats (NCI, 1978d).

60.7.3 TOXICITY TO HUMANS

Only one case of possible human poisoning by dicofol seems to have been reported, and this was in combination with trichlorfon (Zolotnikova and Somov, 1978). Greenhouse workers reportedly suffered frequently from allergic dermatitis. A detailed study of the protection of workers in Florida citrus groves from contamination by dicofol has been reported (Nigg *et al.*, 1986). Dicofol has cytokinetic and cytogenetic effects on human lymphoid cells *in vitro* (Sobti *et al.*, 1983).

REFERENCES

Abou-Donia, M. B., and Menzel, D. B. (1968). The metabolism *in vivo* of 1,1,1-trichloro-2,2-bis(*p*-chlorophenyl)ethane (DDT), 1,1-dichloro-2,2-bis(*p*-chlorophenyl)ethane (DDE) in the chick by embryonic injection and dietary ingestion. *Biochem. Pharmacol.* **17**, 2143–2146.

Adamovic, V. M., and Sokic, B. (1973). Lower level phenomena of DDT cumulation in female abdominal fatty tissue. *Arh. Hig. Rada Toksicol.* **24**, 303–306 (in Russian).

Adamovic, V. M., Sokic, B., and Jonanovic-Similganski, M. (1978). Some observation concerning the ratio of the intake of organochlorine insecticides through food and amounts excreted in the milk of breast-feeding mothers. *Bull. Environ. Contam. Toxicol.* **20**, 280–285.

Adams, M., Coon, F. B., and Poling, C. E. (1974). Insecticides in the tissues of four generations or rats fed different dietary fats containing a mixture of chlorinated hydrocarbon insecticides. *J. Agric. Food Chem.* **22**, 69–75.

Agthe, C., Garcida, H., Shubik, P., Tomatis, L., and Wenyon, E. (1970). Study of the potential carcinogenicity of DDT in the Syrian golden hamster. *Proc. Soc. Exp. Biol. Med.* **134**, 113–116.

Ahlborg, U. K., Lipworth, L., Titus-Ernstoff, L., Hsieh, C.-C., Hanberg, A., Baron, J., Trichopoulos, D., and Adami, R.-O. (1995) Organochlorine compounds in relation to breast cancer, endometrial cancer and endometriosis: An assessment of the biological and epidemiological evidence. *Crit. Rev. Toxicol.* **25**, 463–531.

Ahmed, F. E., Hart, R. W., and Lewis, N. J. (1977). Pesticide induced damage and its repair in cultured human cells. *Mutat. Res.* **42**, 161–173.

Alary, J. G., Guay, P., and Brodeur, J. (1971). Effect of phenobarbital on the metabolisms of DDT in the rat and in the bovine. *Toxicol. Appl. Pharmacol.* **18**, 457–468.

Aldridge, W. N., Clothier, B., Forshaw, P., Johnson, M. K., Parker, V. H., Price, R. J., Skilleter, D. N., Verschoyle, R. D., and Stevens, C. (1978). The effect of DDT and pyrethroids cismethrin and decamethrin on the acetyl choline and cyclic nucleotide content of rat brain. *Biochem. Pharmacol.* **27**, 1703–1706.

Aleksieva, T., Vasilev, G., and Spasovski, M. (1959). Study of the toxic effects of DDT. *J. Hyg., Epidemiol., Microbiol. Immunol.* **5**, 8–15 (in Russian).

Alm, H., Tiemann, U., and Torner, H. (1996). Influence of organochlorine pesticides on development of mouse embryos *in vitro*. *Reprod. Toxicol.* **10**, 321–326.

Ando, M. (1982). Dose-dependent excretion of DDE (1,1-dichloro-2,2-bis(*p*-chlorophenyl)ethylene) in rats. *Arch. Toxicol.* **49**, 139–147.

Antunes-Madeira, M. C., Almeida, L. M., and Madeira, V. M. (1993). Depth-dependent effects of DDT and lindane on the fluidity of native membranes and extracted lipids. Implications for mechanisms of toxicity. *Bull. Environ. Contam. Toxicol.* **51**, 787–794.

Antunes-Madeira, M. C., and Madeira, V. M. (1993). Effects of DDE on the fluidity of model and native membranes: implications for the mechanisms of toxicity. *Biochim. Biophys. Acta.* **1149**, 86–92.

Appel, R. J., and Eroschenko, V. P. (1992). Passage of methoxychlor on milk and reproductive organs of nursing female mice. I. Light and scanning elctron microscopic observations. *Reprod. Toxicol.* **6**, 223.

Apple G., Morgan, D. P., and Roan, C. C. (1970). Determiants of serum DDT and DDE concentrations. *Bull. Environ. Contam. Toxicol.* **5**, 16–23.

Ardies, C. M., and Dees, C. (1998). Xenoestrogens significantly enhance risk of breast cancer during growth and adolescence. *Med. Hypotheses.* **50**, 457–464.

Arthur, R. D. (1976). "The Prevalence of and Types of Pesticides in the Air of the Mississippi Delta and the Blood Serum of the General Population of Mississippi." Final Report (E-32) from the Department of Biochemistry, Mississippi State University to the Epidemiological Studies Program, Technical Services Division, U.S. Environ. Prot. Agency, Washington, DC.

Askari, E. M., and Gablicks (1973). DDT and immunological responses. II. Altered histamine levels and anaphylactic shock in guinea pigs. *Arch. Environ. Health* **26**, 309–312.

Attaran, A., Roberts, D. R., Curtis, C. F., and Kilama, W. L. (2000). Balancing risks on the backs of the poor. *Nature Medicine* **6**, 729–731.

Austin, H., Keil, E., and Cole, P. (1989). A prospective follow-up study of cancer mortality in relation to serum DDT. *Am. J. Public Health* **79**, 43–46.

Baker, M. T., and Van Dyke, R. A. (1984). Metabolism-dependent binding of the chlorinated insecticide DDT and its metabolite DDD to microsomal protein and lipid. *Biochem. Pharmacol.* **33**, 255–260.

Bal, H. S. (1984). Effect of methoxychlor on reproductive systems of the rat. *Proc. Soc. Exp. Biol. Med.* **176**, 187–196.

Banerjee, B. D., Ray, A., and Pasha, S. T. (1996). A comparative evaluation of immunotoxicity of DDT and its metabolites in rats. *Indian J. Exp. Biol.* **34**, 517–522.

Bar-Hay, J., Benderly, A., and Rumney, G. (1964). Treatment of a case of non tumourous Cushing's syndrome with *o,p′*-DDD. *Pediatrics* **33**, 239–244.

Baum, H., Black, R. F., and Kurtz, C. P. (1976). Dicofol: Collaborative study of the hydrolysable chlorine method. *J. Assoc. Off. Anal. Chem.* **59**, 1109–1112.

Ben-Dyke, R., Sanderson, D. M., and Noakes, D. N. (1970). Acute toxicity data for pesticides. *World Rev. Pestic. Control* **9**, 119–127.

Bergenstal, D. M., Hertz, R., Lipsett, M. B., and Moy, R. H. (1960). Chemotherapy of adrenocortical cancer with *o,p′*-DDD. *Ann. Intern. Med.* **53**, 672–682.

Bishara, R. H., Born, G. S., and Christian, J. E. (1972). Radiotracer distribution and excretion study of chlorophenothane in rats. *J. Pharm. Sci.* **61**, 1912–1916.

Bjorge, C., Brunborg, G., Wiger, R., Holme, J. A., Scholz, T., Dybing, E., and Soderlund, E. J. (1996). A comparative study of chemically induced DNA damage in isolated human and rat testicular cells. *Reprod. Toxicol.* **10**, 509–519.

Bledsoe, T., Roland, D. P., Hey, R. L., and Liddle, G. W. (1964). An effect of *o,p′*-DDD on extra-adrenal metabolism of cortisol in man. *J. Clin. Endocrinol. Metab.* **24**, 1303–1311.

Bleiberg, M. J., and Larson, P. S. (1957). Studies on the adrenocortical effects and metabolism of 2,2-bis-(*p*-ethyphenyl)-1,1-dichloroethane (Perthane). *J. Pharmacol. Exp. Ther.* **119**, 133–134.

Bochner, F., Lloyd, H. M., Roeser, H. P., and Thomas, M. J. (1969). Effects of *o,p′*-DDD and aminogluthehimide on metastatic adrenocortical carcinoma. *Med. J. Aust.* **1**, 809–812.

Bouwman, H., Cooppan, R. M., Reinecke, A. J., and Becker, P. J. (1990a). Levels of DDT and metabolites in breast milk from Kwa-Zulu mothers after DDT application for malarial control. *Bull. WHO*, **68**, 761–768.

Bouwman, H., Reinecke, A. J., Cooppan, R. M., and Becker, P. J. (1990b). Factors affecting levels of DDT and metabolites in human breast milk from KwaZulu. *J. Toxicol. Environ. Health.* **13**, 93–115.

Bouwman, H., Cooppan, R. M., Botha, M. J., and Becker, P. J. (1991a). Serum levels of DDT and liver function of malaria control personnel. *S. Afr. Med. J.* **79**, 326–329.

Bouwman, J., Cooppan, R. M., Becker, P. J., and Ngxongo, S. (1991b). Malaria control and levels of DDT in serum of two populations in Kwazulu. *J. Toxicol. Environ. Health* **33**, 141–155.

Bouwman, H., Becker, P. J., Cooppan, R. M., and Reinecke, A. J. (1992). Transfer of DDT used in malaria control to infants via breast milk. *Bull. WHO* **70**, 241–250.

Bouwman, H., Becker, P. J., and Schute, C. H. J. (1994). Malaria control and longitudinal changes in levels of DDT and its metabolites in human serum from KwaZulu. *Bull. WHO* **72**, 921–930.

Bradlow, H. L., Fukushima, D. K., Zumoff, B., Hellman, L., and Gallagher, T. F. (1963). A peripheral action of o,p' DDD on steroid biotransforation. *J. Clin. Endocrinol. Metab.* **23**, 918–922.

Bratowski, T. A., and Matsumura, F. (1972). Properties of a brain adenosine triphosphatase sensitive to DDT. *J. Econ. Entomol.* **65**, 1238–1245.

Bricaire, H., and Luton, J. P. (1977). Does o,p'-DDD possess antimitotic action? Reflections on its use in the treatment of suprarenal adenocarinomas. *Nouv. Presse Med.* **6**, 3650 (in French).

Brown, J. R. (1972). The effect of dietary kelthane on mouse and rat reproduction. *Pestic. Chem. Proc. Int. IUPAC Congr. Pestic. Chem. Wnd. 1971* **6**, 531–548.

Brown, J. R., Hughes, H., and Viriyanondha, S. (1969). Storage, distribution and metabolism of 1,1-bis(4-chlorophenyl)-2,2,2-trichloroethanol. *Toxicol. Appl. Pharmacol.* **15**, 30–37.

Brown, M. A., and Casida, J. E. (1987). Metabolism of a dicofol impurity α-chloro-DDT, but not dicofol or dechlorodicofol, to DDE in mice and a liver microsomal system. *Xenobiotics* **17**, 1169–1174.

Bulger, W. H., and Kupfer, D. (1977). The *in vivo* and *in vitro* estrogenic activity of methoxychlor and its bis-phenolic analog 2,2bis(BPHT) in the rat. *Pharmacologist* **19**, 199.

Bulger, W. H., and Kupfer, D. (1989). Characterstics of monooxygenase-medicated covalent binding of methoxychlor in human and rat liver microsomes. *Drug Metab. Disp.* **17**, 487–494.

Bulger, W. H., Muccitelli, R. M., and Kupfer, D. (1978a). Studies on the *in vivo* and *in vitro* estrogenic activities of methoxychlor and its metabolites. Role of hepatic non-oxygenase in methoxychlor activation. *Biochem. Pharmacol.* **27**, 2417–2423.

Bulger, W. H., Muccitelli, R. M., and Kupfer, D. (1978b). Interactions of methoxychlor, methoxychlor base-soluble contaminant, and 2,2-bis(p-hydroxyphenyl)-1,1,1-trichloroethane with rat uterine estrogen receptor. *J. Toxicol. Environ. Health* **4**, 881–893.

Bulger, W. H., Temple, J. E., and Kupfer, D. (1983). Covalent binding of [^{14}C]methoxychlor metabolite(s) to rat liver microsomal components. *Toxicol. Appl. Pharmacol.* **63**, 367–374.

Bulger, W. H., Feil, V., and Kupfer, D. (1985). Role of hepatic monoxy-genases in generating estrogenic metabolites from methoxychlor and from identified contaminants. *Mol. Pharmacol.* **27**, 115–124.

Bunyan, P. J., Townshend, M. G., and Taylor, A. (1972). Pesticide induced changes in hepatic microsomal enzyme systems: Some effects of 1,1-di(p-chlorophenyl)-2,2-dichloroethylene (DDE) in the rat and Japanese quail. *Chem.-Biol. Interact.* **5**, 13–26.

Burkatzkaya, E. N., Voitenko, G. A., and Krasniuk, E. P. (1961). Working conditions and health status of workers at DDT production plants. *Gig. Sanit.* **26**, 24–29 (in Russian).

Burlington, H., and Linderman, V. F. (1950). Effect of DDT on testes and secondary sex characteristics of White Leghorn cockerels. *Proc. Soc. Exp. Biol. Med.* **74**, 48–51.

Burns, E. C., Dahm, P. A., and Lindquist, D. A. (1957). Secretion of DDT metabolites in the bile of rats. *J. Pharmacol. Exp. Ther.* **121**, 55–62.

Burns, J. E. (1974). Organochlorine pesticide and polychlorinated biphenyl residues in biopsied human adipose tissue—Texas 1969–72. *Pestic. Monit. J.* **7**, 122–126.

Buselmaier, W., Röhrborn, G., and Propping, P. (1973). Comparative investigations on the mutagenicity of pesticides in mammalian test systems. *Mutat. Res.* **21**, 25–26.

Cabral, J. R. P., Raitano, F., Mollner, T., Bronczyk, S., and Shubik, P. (1979a). Acute toxicity of pesticides in hamsters. *Toxicol. Appl. Pharmacol.* **48**, A192.

Cabral, J. R. P., Hall, R. K., Bronczyk, S.A. and Shubik, P. (1979b). A carcinogenicity study of the pesticide dieldrin in hamsters. *Cancer Lett.* **6**, 241–246.

Cabral, J. R. P., Hall, R. K., Rossi, L., Bronczyk, S. A., and Shubik, P. (1982a). Lack of carcinogenicity of DDT in hamsters. *Tumori* **68**, 5–10.

Cabral, J. R. P., Hall, R. K., Rossi, L., Bronczyk, S. A., and Shubik, P. (1982b). Effects of long-term intake of DDT in rats. *Tumori* **68**, 11–17.

Cameron, G.R., and Burgess, F. (1945). The toxicity of 2,2-bis(p-chlorophenyl)-1,1,1-trichloroethane (DDT). *Br. Med. J.* **1**, 865–871.

Canlorbe, P., Bader, J. C., and Job, J. C. (1971). Diagnostic problems arising from a virilizing tumor of the adrenal cortex (case report–literature review). *Sem. Hop.* **47**, 2255–2270 (in French).

Carey, R. M., Orth, D. N., and Hartmann, W. H. (1973). Malignant melanoma with ectopic production of adrenocorticotrophic hormone: Palliative treatment with inhibitors of adrenal steroid biosynthesis. *J. Clin. Endocrinol. Metab.* **36**, 482–487.

Case, R. A. M. (1945). Toxic effects of 2,2-bis(p-chlorophenyl)-1,1,1-trichloroethane (DDT) in man. *Bri. Med. J.* **2**, 842–845.

Cecil, H. C., Harris, S. J., Bitman, J., and Reynolds, P. (1975). Estrogenic effects and liver microsomal enzyme activity of technical methoxychlor and technical 1,1-trichloro-2,2-bis(p-chlorophenyl)ethane in sheep. *J. Agrc. Food Chem.* **23**, 401–403.

Chadwick, R. W., Cranmer, M. F., and Peoples, A. J. (1971). Metabolic alterations in the squirrel monkey induced by DDT administration and ascorbic acid deficiency. *Toxicol. Appl. Pharmacol.* **20**, 308–318.

Chand, B., Sankaranarayan, T., Yadava, R. L., and Narasimham, M. V. (1991). Residues of DDT and its metabolite in blood of exposed factory workers and their correlation with ill health symptoms. *J. Commun. Dis.* **23**, 245–247.

Chapin, R. E., Harris, M. W., Davis, B. J., Ward, S. M., Wilson, R. E., Mauney, M. A., Lockhart, A. C., Smialowicz, R. J., Mower, V. C., Burka, L. T., and Collins, B. J. (1997). The effects of perinatal/juvenile methoxychlor exposure on adult rat nervous, immune and reproductive system function. *Fund. Appl. Toxicol.* **40**, 138–157.

Chin, Y., and T'Ant, C. (1946). The effect of DDT on cutaneous sensation in man. *Science* **103**, 654.

Chung, Hwang, E., and Van Woert, M. H. (1981). p,p'-DDT-induced alterations in brain serotonin metabolism. *Neurotoxicology* **2**, 649–657.

Clifford, N. J., and Weil, J. (1972). Cortisol metabolism in persons occupationally exposed to DDT. *Arch. Environ. Health* **24**, 145–147.

Cobey, F. A., Taliaferro, I., and Haag, H. B. (1956). Effect of DDD and some of its derivatives on plasma 17-OH-corticosteroids in the dog. *Science* **123**, 140–141.

Cocco, P., Blair, A., Congia, P., Saba, G., Flore, C., Ecca, M. R., and Palmas, C. (1997). Proportional mortality of dichloro-diphenyl-trichloroethane (DDT) workers: A preliminary report. *Arch. Environ. Health.* **52**, 299–303.

Cocisiu, M., Aizicovici, H., Nistor, C., Unterman, H. W., Barbuta, R., and Gugles, E. (1976). Variation of the DDT and HCH contents of maternal milk in connection with food intake. *Igiena* **25**, 105–108 (in Romanian).

Committee on Pesticides (1951). American Medical Association Council on Pharmacy and Chemistry report on pharmacologie and toxicologic aspects of DDT (chlorphenothane U.S.P.). *J. Am. Med. Assoc.* **145**, 728–733.

Cooke, P. S., and Eroschenko, V. P. (1990). Inhibitory effects of technical-grade methoxychlor on development of neonatal mouse reproductive organs. *Biol. Reprod.* **42**, 585.

Copeland, M. F., and Cranmer, M. F. (1974). Effects of o,p'-DDT on the adrenal gland and hepatic microsomal enzyme system of the beagle dog. *Toxicol. Appl. Pharmacol.* **27**, 1–10.

Coulston, F. (1985). Reconsideration of the dilemma of DDT for the establishment of an acceptable daily intake. *Regul. Toxicol. Pharmacol.* **5**, 332–383.

Cranmer, M. F. (1970). Effect of diphenylhydantion on storage of DDT in the rat. *Toxicol. Appl. Pharmacol.* **17**, 315.

Cranmer, M. F. (1972). Absence of conversion of o,p'-DDT in the rat. *Bull. Environ. Contam. Toxicol.* **7**, 121–124.

Cranmer, M. F., Peoples, A., and Chadwick, R. (1972). Biochemical effects of repeated administration of p,p'-DDT on the squirrel monkey. *Toxicol. Appl. Pharmacol.* **21**, 98–101.

Cueto, C. (1970). Cardiovascular effects of o,p'-DDD. *Ind. Med. Surg.* **39**, 31–32.

Cueto, C., Jr., and Biros, F. J. (1967). Chlorinated insecticides and related materials in human urine. *Toxicol. Appl. Pharmacol.* **10**, 261–269.

Cueto C., and Brown, J. H. U. (1958). Biological studies on an adrenocorticolytic agent and the isolation of the active components. *Endocrinology* **62**, 334–339.

Cueto, C., and Moran, N. C. (1968). The circulatory effects of catecholamines and oubain in glucocorticoid-deficient animals. *J. Pharmacol. Exp. Ther.* **164**, 31–44.

Cummings, A. M. (1997). Methoxychlor as a model for environmental estrogens. *Crit.Rev. Toxiol.* **27**, 367–379.

Cummings, A. M., and Gray, L. E. (1987). Methoxychlor affects the decidual cell response of the uterus but not other progestational parameters in female rats. *Toxicol. Appl. Pharmacol.* **90**, 330–336.

Cummings, A. M., and Gray, L. E. (1989). Antifertility effect of methoxychlor in female rats: Dose and time dependent blockade of pregnancy. *Toxicol. Appl. Pharmacol.* **94**, 454.

Cummings, A. M., and Metcalf, J. M. (1994). Mechanisms of the stimulation of rat uterine peroxidase activity by methoxychlor. *Reprod. Toxicol.* **8**, 477.

Cummings, A. M., and Metcalf, J. M. (1995). Methoxychlor regulates rat uterine-estrogen induced protein. *Toxicol. Appl. Pharmacol.* **130**, 154–160.

Cummings, A. M., and Perreault, S. D. (1990). Methoxychlor accelerates embryo transport through the rat reproductive tract. *Toxicol. Appl. Pharmacol.* **102**, 110.

Cunningham, R. E., and Hill, F. S. (1952). Convulsions and deafness following ingestion of DDT. *Pediatrics* **9**, 745–747.

Curtis, C. F., and Lines, J. D. (1999). Should DDT be banned by International treaty. *Parisitology Today* **16**, 119–121.

Czegledi-Janko, G., and Avar, P. (1970). Occupational exposure to lindane: Clinical and laboratory findings. *Br. J. Ind. Med.* **27**, 283–286.

Dale, W. E., and Quinby, G. E. (1963). Chlorinated insecticides in the body fat of people in the United States. *Science* **142**, 593–595.

Dale, W. E., Gaines, T. B., Hayes, W. J., and Pearce, G. W. (1963). Poisoning by DDT: Relation between clinical signs and concentration in rat brain. *Science* **142**, 593–595.

Dale, W. E., Copeland, M. F., and Hayes, W. J., Jr. (1965). Chlorinated insecticides in the body fat of people in India. *Bull. WHO* **33**, 471–477.

Dale, W. E., Copeland, M. F., Pearce, G. W., and Miles, J. W. (1966). Concentration of o,p'-DDT in rat brain at various intervals after dosing. *Arch. Int. Pharmacodyn. Ther.* **162**, 40–43.

Dangerfield, W. G. (1946). Toxicity of DDT to man. *Br. Med. J.* **1**, 27.

Danowski, T. S., Sarver, H. E., Moses, C., and Boness, J. V. (1964). o,p'-DDD therapy in hushing's syndrome and in obesity with cushingoid changes. *Am. J. Med.* **37**, 235–250.

Datta, P. R. (1970). In vitro detoxification of p,p'-DDE to p,p'-DDA in rats. *Ind. Med. Surg.* **39**, 190–194.

Datta, P. R., and Nelson, M. F. (1970). p,p' DDT detoxication by isolated perfused rat liver and kidney. *Ind. Med. Surg.* **39**, 195–198.

Davies, J. E., Edmundson, W. F., Carter, C. H., and Barquet, A. (1969). Effect of anticonvulsant drugs on dichophane (D.D.T.) residues in man. *Lancet* **2**, 7–9.

Davison, K. L., Feil, V. J., and Lamoureux, C. H. (1982). Methoxychlor metabolism in goats. *J. Agric. Food Chem.* **30**, 130–137.

Davision, K. L., Lamoureux, C. H., and Feil, V. J. (1983). Methoxychlor metabolism in goats. 2. Metabolites in bile and movement through skin. *J. Agric. Food Chem.* **312**, 164–166.

Dean, M. E., Smeaton, T. C., and Stock, B. H. (1980). The influence of fetal and neonatal exposure to dichlorodiphenyltrichloroethane (DDT) on the testosterone status of neonatal male rat. *Toxicol. Appl. Pharmacol.* **53**, 315–322.

Dedek, W., and Schmidt, R. (1972). Studies on transplacental transport metabolism of ³H and ¹⁴C-labelled DDT in pregnant mice under hunger stress. *Pharmazie* **27**, 294–297.

deFossey, B. M., Lutton, S. P., and Bricaire, H. (1968). Our experience of o,p'-DDD in the treatment of hypercorticisms. *Ann. Endocrinal.* **29**, 93–102 (in French).

Dehal, S. S., and Kupfer, D. (1994) Metabolism of the proestrogenic pesticide methoxychlor by hepatic P450 monoxy-genases in rats and humans. Dual pathways involving novel *ortho* ring hydroxylation by CYPB *Drug Metab. Disp.* **22**, 937–945.

Deichmann, W. B., Witherup, S., and Kitzmiller, K. V. (1950). "The Toxicity of DDT. I. Experimental Observations." Kettering Lab., Cincinnati, OH.

Deichmann, W. B., Keplinger, M. L., Sala, F., and Glass, E. (1967). Synergism among oral carcinogens. IV. The simultaneous feeding of four tumorigens to rats. *Toxicol. Appl. Pharmacol.* **11**, 88–103.

Deichmann, W. B., MacDonald, W. E., Beasley, A. G., and Cubit, D. (1971). Subnormal reproduction in beagle dogs induced by DDT and aldrin. *Ind. Med. Surg.* **40**, 10–20.

D'Ercole, A. J., Arthur, R. D., Cain, J. D., and Barrentine, B. F. (1976). Insecticide exposure of mothers and newborns in a rural agricultural area. *Pediatrics* **57**, 869–874.

Dewailly, E., Ayotte, P., Brisson, J., and Dodin, S. (1994a). Breast cancer and organochlorines. *Lancet* **344**, 1707–1708.

Dewailly, E., Dodin, S., Verreault, R., Ayotte, P., Sauvé, L., Morin, J., and Brisson, J. (1994b). High organochlorine body burden in women with estrogen receptor-positive breast cancer. *J. Nat. Cancer Inst.* **86**, 232–234.

Dewailly, E., Ayotte, P., and Dodin, S. (1997). Could the rising levels of estrogen receptor in breast cancer be due to estrogenic pollutants? *J. Nat. Cancer Inst.* **89**, 888–889.

Dodge, J. A., Glasebrook, A. L., Magee, D. E., Phillips, D. E., Sato, M., Short, L. L., and Bryant, H. U. (1996). Environmental estrogens: effects on cholesterol lowering and bone in the ovariectomized rat. *J. Steroid Biochem. Mol. Biol.* **59**, 155–161.

Domenjoz, R. (1944). Experimental investigation with a new insecticide (Neocide Geigy): A contribution to the theory of action of contact poison. *Schweiz. Med. Wochenschr.* **74**, 952–958 (in German).

Domenjoz, R. (1946). On the biological action of DDT-derivative. *Arch. Int. Pharmacodyn.* **73**, 128–146 (in German).

Draize, J. G., Nelson, A. A., and Calvery, H. O. (1944). The percutaneous absorption of DDT (2,2-bis-(p-chloropheyl)-1,1,1-trichloroethane) in laboratory animals. *J. Pharmacol. Exp. Ther.* **82**, 159–166.

Dubois, J. M., and Bergman, C. (1977). Asymmetrical currents and sodium currents in Ravier nodes exposed to DDT. *Nature (London)* **266**, 741–742.

Durham, W. F., Ortega, P., and Hayes, W. J., Jr. (1963). The effect of various dietary levels of DDT on liver function cell morphology, and DDT storage in the rhesus monkey. *Arch. Int. Pharmacodyn. Ther.* **141**, 111–129.

Edmundson, W. F., Davies, J. E., Nachman, G. A., and Roeth, R. L. (1969). p,p'-DDT and p,p'-DDE in blood samples of occupationally exposed workers. *Public Health Rep.* **84**, 53–58.

Epstein, S. S., and Shafner, H. (1968). Chemical mutagens in the human environment. *Nature (London)* **219**, 385–387.

Eriksson, P., and Nordberg, A. (1986). The effects of DDT, DDOH-palmitic acid, and a chlorinated paraffin on muscarinic receptors and the sodium-dependent choline uptake in the central nervous system of immature mice. *Toxicol. Appl. Pharmacol.* **85**, 121–127.

Eriksson, P., Flakeborn, Y., Nordberg, A., and Slanina, P. (1984). Effects of DDT on muscarine and nicotine-like binding sites in CNS of immature and adult mice. *Toxicol. Lett.* **22**, 329–334.

Eroshenko, V. P. (1991). Ultrastruture of vagina and uterus in young mice after methoxychlor exposure. *Reprod. Toxicol.* **5**, 427.

Eroschenko, V. P., and Cooke, P. S. (1990). Morphological and biochemical alterations in reproductive tracts of neonatal female mice treated with the pesticide methoxychlor. *Biol. Reprod.* **42**, 573.

Eroshenko, V. P., Abuel-Atta, A. A., and Grober, M. S. (1995). Neonatal exposures to technical methoxychlor alters ovaries in adult mice. *Reprod. Toxicol.* **9**, 379.

Esaac, E. G., and Matsumura, F. (1980). Mechanisms of reductive dechlorination of DDT by rat liver microsomes. *Pestic. Biochem. Physiol.* **10**, 81–93.

Eskenasy, J. J. (1972). Status epilepticus by dichlorodiphenyltrichloroethane and hexachlorcyclohexane poisoning. *Rev. Roum. Neurol.* **9**, 435–442 (in Romanian).

Eyzaguire, C., and Lilienthal, J. L., Jr. (1949). Veratrinic effects of pentamethylenetretrazol (Metraxol) and 2,2-bis(p-chlorophenyl)-1,1,1-trichloroethane (DDT) on mammalian neuromuscular function. *Proc. Soc. Exp. Biol. Med.* **70**, 272–275.

Exon, J. H., Kerkvliet, N. I., and Talcott, P. A. (1987). Immunotoxicity of carcinogenic pesticides and related chemicals. *Environ. Sci. Health* **5**, 73–120.

Falck, F., Ricci, A., Wolff, M. S., Deckers, P. (1992). Pesticides and polychlorinated biphenyl residues in human breast lipids and their relation to breast cancer. *Arch. Environ. Health* **47**, 143–146.

Farkas, I., Desi, I., and Klemeny, T. (1968). The effect of DDT in the diet on the resting and loading electrocorticogram record. *Toxicol. Appl. Pharmacol.* **12**, 518–525.

Fawcett, S. C., Bunyan, P. J., Huson, L. W., King, L. J., and Stanley, P. I. (1981). Excretion of radioactivity following the intraperitoneal administration of ^{14}C-DDT, ^{14}C-DDE and ^{14}C-DMU to the rat and Japanese quail. *Bull. Environ. Contam. Toxicol.* **27**, 386–392.

Fawcett, S. C., King, L. F., Bunyan, P. J., and Stanley, P. I. (1987). The metabolism of ^{14}C-DDT, ^{14}C-DDD, ^{14}C-DDMU in rats and Japanese quail. *Xenobiotica* **17**, 525–538.

Feil, V. J., Lamoureux, C. H., Styrvoky, E., Zaylskie, R. G., Thacker, E. J., and Holman, G. M. (1973). Metabolism of o,p′-DDT in rats. *J. Agric. Food Chem.* **21**, 1072–1078.

Feil, V. J., Lamoureux, C. H., and Zaylskie, R. G. (1975). Metabolism of o,p′-DDT in chickens. *J. Agric. Food Chem.* **23**, 382–388.

Fennah, R. G. (1945). Preliminary tests with DDT against insect pests of food crops in the Lesser Antilles. *Trop. Agric.* **22**, 126–132.

Finnegan, J. K., Hennigar, G. R., Smith, R. B., Jr., Larson, P. S., and Haag, H. B. (1955). Acute and chronic toxicity studies on 2,2-bis-p-ethylphenyl-1,1-dichloroethane (Perthane). *Arch. Int. Pharmacodyn. Ther.* **103**, 404–418.

Fishbein, L. F. (1974). Chromatographic and biological aspects of DDT and its metabolites. *J. Chrmatogr.* **98**, 177–251.

Fitzhugh, O. G. (1948). Use of DDT insecticides on food products. *Ind. Eng. Chem.* **40**, 704–705.

Fitzhugh, O. G. (1970). A summary of a carcinogenic study of DDT in mice from Food and Drug Administration, USA. *In* "FAO/WHO 1969 Evaluations of Some Pesticide Residues in Foods," pp. 61–64. World Health Organization, Geneva.

Fitzhugh, O. G., and Nelson, A. A. (1947). The chronic oral toxicity of DDT (2,2-bis-p-chlorophenyl-1,1,1-triclorophenyl-1,1,1-trichloroethane). *J. Pharmacol. Exp. Ther.* **89**, 18–30.

Flodstrom, S., Hemming, H., Warngard, L., and Ahlborg, U. G. (1990). Promotion of altered hepatic foci development in rat liver, cytochrome P450 enzyme induction and inhibition of cell–cell communiction by DDT and some structurally related organohalogen pesticides. *Carcinogenesis* **11**, 1413–1417.

Fonseca, M. I., Aguilar, J. S., Lozpez, C., Garcia Fernandez, J. C., and De Robertis, E. (1986). Regional effect of organochlorine insecticides on cholinergic muscarine receptors of rat brain. *Toxicol. Appl. Pharmacol.* **84**, 192–195.

Food and Agriculture Organization/World Health Organization (FAO/WHO) (1985). "Pesticide Residues, Rome, 24 September–30 October 1984." FAO Plant Prod. Prot. Paper No. 62, Food Agric. Organ./World Health Organ., Rome.

Foster, T. S. (1973). Evaluation of the possible estrogenic activity of methoxychlor in the chicken by means of feeding trials. *Bull. Environ. Contam. Toxicol.* **9**, 234–242.

Francone, M. P., Mariani, F. H., and Demare, C. (1952). Clinical picture of intoxication by DDT. *Rev. Assoc. Med. Argent.* **6**, 56–59 (in Spanish).

French, M. C., and Jeffries, D. J. (1969). Degradation and disappearance of ortho, para isomer of technical DDT in living and dead avian tissues. *Science* **165**, 914–916.

Fries, G. F., Marrow, G. S., Jr., Lester, J. W., and Gordon, C. H. (1971). Effects of microsomal enzyme inducing drugs on DDT and dieldrin elimination from cows. *J. Dairy Sci.* **54**, 364–368.

Fryzek, J. P., Garabrant, D. H., Harlow, S. D., Severson, R. K., Gillespie, B. W., Schenk, M., and Schottenfeld, D. (1997). A case-control study of self-reported exposures to pesticides and pancreas cancer in Southeastern Michigan. *Int. J. Cancer.* **72**, 62–67.

Fukushima, D. K., Bradlow, H. L., and Hellman, L. (1971). Effects of o,p′-DDD on cortisol and 6 beta-hydroxycortisol secretion and metabolism in man. *J. Clin. Endorinol. Metab.* **32**, 192–200.

Gabliks, J., Askari, E. M., and Yolen, N. (1973). DDT and immunological responses. I. Serum antibodies and anaphylactic shock in guinea pigs. *Arch. Environ. Health* **26**, 305–308.

Gabliks, J., Al-Zubaidy, T., and Askari, E. (1975). DDT and immunological responses. 3. Reduced anaphylaxis and mast cell populations in rats fed DDT, *Arch. Environ. Health* **30**, 81–84.

Gaines, T. B. (1960). The acute toxicity of pesticides to rats. *Toxicol. Appl. Pharmacol.* **2**, 88–99.

Gaines, T. B. (1969) Acute toxicity of pesticides. *Toxicol. Appl. Pharmacol.* **14**, 515–534.

Galand, P., Mairesse, N., Degraef, C., and Rooryck, J. (1987). o,p-DDT(1,1,1-trichloro-2(p-chlorophenyl)-2-(o-chlorophenyl)ethane is a purely estrogenic agonist in the rat uterus *in vivo* and *in vitro*. *Biochem. Pharmacol.* **36**, 397–400.

Gallagher, T. F., Fukushima, D. K., and Hellmann, L. (1962). The effect of ortho, para' DDD on steroid hormone metabolites in adrenocortical carcinoma. *Metab. Clin. Exp.* **11**, 1155–1161.

Gannon, N., Link, R. R., and Decker, G. C. (1959). Insecticide residues in the milk of dairy cows fed insecticides in their daily ration. *J. Agric. Food Chem.* **7**, 829–832.

Garabrant, D. H., Held, J., Langholz, B., Peters, J. M., and Mack, T. M. (1992). DDT and related compounds and risk of pancreatic cancer. *J. Natl. Cancer Inst.* **84**, 764–771.

Garabrant, D. H., Held, J., and Homa, D. (1993). Response: DDT and pancreatic cancer. *J. Natl. Cancer Inst.* **85**, 328–329.

Garrett, R. M. (1947). Toxicity of DDT for man. *J. Med. Assoc. State Ala.* **17**, 74–76.

Gawhary, A. S. (1972). The effects of 2,2-bis(para-chloro-phenyl) 1,1-dichloroethane (DDD) on choline acetylase of the thymus gland. *Biochem. Pharmacol.* **21**, 887–890.

Genina, S. A., Svetlaja, E. N., and Komarova, L. I. (1969). Blood levels of organic chlorine pesticides and some hematological indicators in people employed in applying pesticides from the air. *In* "The Hygiene of Application and Toxicology of Pesticides and the Clinical Features of Pesticide Poisoning. A Collection of Papers," Issue No. 7, pp. 492–496. Vniigintoks, Kiev (in Russian).

Ghiasuddin, S. M., and Matsumura, F. (1979). DDT inhibition of Ca-ATPase of the peripheral nerves of the American lobster. *Pestic. Biochem. Physiol.* **10**, 151–161.

Gil, G. P., and Miron, B. F. (1949). Investigations of intoxication by DDT in man. *Med. Colon.* **14**, 459–470 (in French).

Gillett, J. W., Chan, T. M., and Terriere, L. C. (1966). Interactions between DDT analogs and microsomal epoxidase systems. *J. Agric. Food Chem.* **14**, 540–545.

Gingel, R., and Wallcave, L. (1974). Species differences in the acute toxicity and tissue distribution of DDT in mice and hamsters. *Toxicol. Appl. Pharmacol.* **28**, 385–394.

Gold, B., and Brunk, G. (1982). Metabolism of 1,1,1-trichloro-2,2-bis(p-chlorophenyl)ethane and 1,1-dichloro-2,2-bis(p-chlorophenyl)ethane in the mouse. *Chem.–Biol. Interact.* **41**, 327–339.

Gold, B., and Brunk, G. (1983). Metabolism of 1,1,1-trichloro-2,2-bis(p-chlorophenyl)ethane, and 1-chloro-2,2-bis(p-chlorophenyl)ethane in the hamster. *Cancer Res.* **43**, 2644–2647.

Gold, B., and Brunk, G. (1984). A mechanistic study of the metabolism of 1,1-dichloro-2,2-bis(p-chlorophenyl)ethane (DDD) to 2,2-bis(p-chlorophenyl)acetic acid (DDA). *Biochem. Pharmacol.* **33**, 979–982.

Gold, B., and Brunk, G. (1986). The effect of subchronic feeding of 1,1-dichloro-2,2-bis(4′-clorophenyl)ethane (DDE) on its metabolism in mice. *Carcinogenesis (London)* **7**, 1149–1153.

Gold, B., Leuchen, T., Brunk, G., and Gingell, R. (1981). Metabolism of a DDT metabolite via chloroepoxide. *Chem.–Biol. Interact.* **35**, 159–176.

Goldman, J. M., Cooper, R. L., Rehnerg, G. L., Hein, J. F., McElroy, W. K., and Gray, L. E. (1986). Effect of low subchronic doses of methoxychlor on the rat hypothalamic-pituitary reproductive axis. *Toxicol. Appl. Pharmacol.* **86**, 474–483.

Gordienko, V. M., and Kozyritsii, V. G. (1970). The effect of o,p′-dichlorodiphenyldichloroethane on the ultrastructure of cells of the anterior lobe of the hypophysis in dogs. *Arkh. Anat., Gistol. Embriol.* **58**, 49–57 (in Russian).

Gordienko, V. M., Bogomolets, Y. O., and Kozyritskii, V. G. (1972). Electron microscopic study of the dog thyroid gland followin administration of different doses of *o,p′*-DDD. *Tsitol. Genet.* **6**, 392–394 (in Russian).

Gordienko, V. M., and Kozyritskii, V. G. (1973). Alterations in the ultrastructure of the adrenal cortex of the dog after short-term and long-term administration of *o,p′*-DDD. *Arkh. Anat. Gistol. Embriol.* **65**, 90–95 (in Russian).

Gordon, H. T., and Welsh, J. H. (1948). The role of ions in axon surface reactions to toxic organic compounds. *J. Cell. Comp. Physiol.* **31**, 395–420.

Graillot, C., Gak, J.-C., Lancret, C., and Truhanut, R. (1975). Investigations on the states and mechanisms of toxic action or organochlorine insecticides. II. Study on the long-term toxic effects of DDT in the hamster. *Eur. J. Toxicol.* **8**, 353–359 (in French).

Grant, E. L., Mitchell, R. H., West, P. R., Mazuch, L., and Ashwood-Smith, M. J. (1976). Muatagenicity and putative carcinogenicty tests of several polycyclic aromatic compounds associated with impurities of the insecticide methoxychlor. *Mutat. Res.* **40**, 225–228.

Gray, L. E., Ostby, J. S., Ferrell, J. M., Sigmon, E. R, and Goldman, J. M. (1988). Methoxychlor induces estrogen-like alterations of behaviour and the reproduction tract in the female rat and hamster: effects on sex behaviour, running wheel activity and uterine morphology. *Toxicol. Appl. Pharmacol.* **96**, 525.

Gray, L. E., Ostby, J., Ferrell, J., Rehnberg, G., Linder, R., Cooper, R., Goldman, J., Slott, V., and Laskey, J. (1989). A dose response analysis of methoxychlor-induced alterations of reproductive development and function in the rat. *Fundam. Appl. Toxicol.* **12**, 92–108.

Griffith, E. D., Jr., and Blanke, R. V. (1975). Pesticides in people. Blood organochlorine pesticide levels in Virginia residents. *Pestic. Monit. J.* **8**, 219–224.

Guan, X., and Ruch, R. J. (1996). Gap junction endocytosis and lysomomal degradation of connexin-43-P2 in WB-F344 rat liver epithelial cell treated with DDT and lindane. *Carcinogenesis* **17**, 1791–1798.

Gutierrez, M. L., and Crooke, S. T. (1980). Mitotane (*o,p′*-DDD). *Cancer Treat. Rev.* **7**, 49–55.

Guttes, S., Failing, K., Newmann, K., Neinstein, J., Georgii, S., and Brunn, H. (1998). Chlororganic pesticides and polychlorinated biphenyls in breast tissue of women with benign and malignant breast disease. *Arch. Environ. Contam. Toxicol.* **35**, 140–147.

Haag, H. B., Finnegan, J. K., Olarson, P. S., Dreyfuss, M. L., Main, R. J., and Riese, W. (1948). Comparative chronic toxicity for warm-blooded animals of 2,2-bis(*p*-chlorophenyl)-1,1,1-trichlorethane (DDT) and 2,2-bis(*p*-chlorophenyl-1,1-dichloroethane (DDD). *Ind. Med. Surg.* **17**, 477–484.

Hajjar, R. A., Hicke, R. C., and Samoan, N. A. (1975). Adrenal corticol carcinoma: a study of 32 patients. *Cancer (Philadelphia)* **35**, 549–554.

Hall, D. L., Payne, L. A., Putnam, J. M., and Huet-Hudson, Y. M. (1997). Effect of methoxychlor on implantation and embryo development in the mouse. *Reprod. Toxicol.* **11**, 703–708.

Halmi, K. A., and Lascari, A. D. (1971). Conversion of virilization to feminization in a young girl with adrenal cortical carcinoma. *Cancer (Philadelphia)* **27**, 931–935.

Hamid, J., Sayeed, A., and MacFarlane, H. (1974). The effect of 1-(*o*-chlorophenyl)-1-(*p*-chlorophenyl)-2,2-dichloroethane (*o,p′*-DDD) on the immune response in malnutrition. *Bri. J. Exp. Pathol.* **55**, 94–100.

Harell, M., Shea, J. J., and Emmett, R. R. (1978). Bilateral sudden deafness following combined insecticide poisoning. *Laryngoscope* **88**, 1348–1351.

Harris, S. J., Cecil, H. C., and Bitman, J. (1974). Effect of several dietary levels of technical methoxychlor on reproduction in rats. *J. Agric. Food Chem.* **22**, 969–973.

Harrison, J. H., Mahoney, E. M., and Bennett, A. H. (1973). Tumors of the adrenal cortex. *Cancer (Philadelphia)* **32**, 1227–1235.

Harrison, R. D. (1975). Comparative toxicity of some selected pesticides in neonatal and adult rats. *Toxicol. Appl. Pharmacol.* **32**, 443–446.

Hart, M. M., and Straw, J. A. (1971a). Effects of 1-(*o*-chlorophenyl)-1-(*p*-chlorophenyl)-2,2-dichloroethane and puromycin on adrenocorticotropic hormone-induced steroidogenesis and on amino acid incorporation in slices of dog adrenal cortex. *Biochem. Pharmacol.* **20**, 257–263.

Hart, M. M., and Straw, J. A. (1971b). Studies on the site of action of *o,p′*-DDD in the dog adrenal cortex. I. Inhibition of ACTH-mediated pregnenolone synthesis. *Steroids* **17**, 559–574.

Hart, M. M., and Straw, J. A. (1971c). Effect of 1-(*o*-chlorophenyl)-1-(*p*-chlorophenyl)-1-(*p*-chlorophenyl)-2,2-dichloroethane. *Biochem. Pharmacol.* **20**, 1679–1688.

Hart, M. M., and Straw, J. A. (1971d). Effect of 1-(*o*-chlorophenyl)-1-(*p*-chlorophenyl)-2,2-dichloroethane *in vivo* on baseline and adrenocorticotrophic hormone-induced steroid production in dog adrenal slices. *Biochem. Pharmacol.* **20**, 1689–1691.

Hart, M. M., Regan, R. L., and Adamson, R. H. (1973). The effect of isomers of DDD on the ATH-induced steroid output, histology, and ultrastructure of the dog adrenal cortex. *Toxicol. Appl. Pharmacol.* **24**, 101–113.

Hartwig, W., Massalski, W., Kasperlik-Zaluska, A., Migdalska, B., Szamatowics, M., and Jakowiki, J. (1968). Hormonally active carcinoma of the adrenal cortex treated with *o,p′*-DDD. *Endokrynol. Pol.* **19**, 57–69 (in Polish).

Hassall, K. A. (1971). Reductive dechlorination of DDT: The effect of some physical and chemical agents on DDE production by pigeon liver preparations. *Pestic. Biochem. Physiol.* **1**, 259–266.

Hayes, W. J. (1959). Pharmacology and toxicology of DDT. *In* "DDT: The Insecticide Dichlorodiphenyl-Trichloroethane and Its Significance" (P. Müller, ed.), Vol. 2, pp. 9–247. Birkhauser, Basel.

Hayes, W. J. (1965). Review of the metabolism of chlorinated hydrocarbon insecticides especially in mammals. *Annu. Rev. Pharmacol.* **5**, 27–52.

Hayes, W. J. (1969). Sweden bans DDT. *Arch. Environ. Health* **18**, 872.

Hayes, W. J. (1975). "Toxicology of Pesticides." Williams & Wilkins, Baltimore.

Hayes, W. J. (1976). Dosage relationships associated with DDT in milk. *Toxicol. Appl. Pharmacol.* **38**, 19–28.

Hayes, W. J. (1982). "Pesticides Study in Man." Willimas & Wilkins, Baltimore.

Hayes, W. J. (1991). Introduction. *In* "Handbook of Pesticide Toxicology," pp. 1–37. Academic Press, San Diego.

Hayes, W. J., Durham, W. F., and Cueto, C., Jr. (1956). The effect of known repeated oral doses of chlorophenothane (DDT) in man. *J. Am. Med. Assoc.* **162**, 890–897.

Hayes, W. J., Dale, W. E., and Pirkle, C. I. (1971). Evidence of safety of long-term, high, oral doses of DDT for man. *Arch. Environ. Health* **22**, 119–135.

Heinriks, W. J., Gellert, R. J., Bakke, J. L., and Lawrence, N. L. (1971). DDT administered to neonatal rats induces persistent estrus syndrome. *Science* **173**, 642–643.

Hellmann, L., Bradlow, H. L., and Zumoff, B. (1973). Decreased conversion of androgens to normal 17-ketosteroid metabolites as a result of treatment with *o,p′*-DDD. *J. Clin. Endocrinol. Metab.* **36**, 801–803.

Helson, L., Wollner, N., Murphy, L., and Schwartz, M. K. (1971). Metastatic adrenal cortical carcinoma: Biochemical changes accompanying clinial regression during therapy with *o,p′*-DDD. *Clin. Chem.* **17**, 1191–1193.

Henderson, G. L., and Woolley, D. E. (1969). Tissue concentrations of DDT: Correlation with neurotoxicity in young and adult rats. *Proc. West. Pharmacol. Soc.* **12**, 58–62.

Henderson, G. L., and Woolley, D. E. (1970). Mechanisms of neurotoxic action of 1,1,1-trichloro-2,2-bis-(*p*-chlorophenyl)-ethane (DDT) in immature and adult rats. *J. Pharmacol. Exp. Ther.* **175**, 60–68.

Herr, D. W., and Tilson, H. A. (1987). Modulation of *p,p′* DDT-induced tremor by catecholaminergic agents. *Toxicol. Appl. Pharmacol.* **91**, 149–158.

Herr, D. W., Gallus, A., and Tilson, H. A. (1987). Pharmacological modification of tremor and enhanced acoustic startle by chlordecone and *p,p′*-DDT. *Psychopharmacology* **91**, 320–325.

Herr, D. W., Mailman, R. B., and Tilson, H. A. (1989). Blockade of only spinal *α*-adrenoceptors is insufficient to attenuate DDT-indued alterations in motor function. *Toxicol. Appl. Pharmacol.* **101**, 11–26.

Hodge, H. C., Maynard, E. A., Thomas, J. F., Blanchet, J. J., Jr., Wilt, W. G., Jr., and Mason, K. E. (1950). Short-term oral toxicity tests of methoxyclor (2,2-di(*p*-methoxyphenyl)-1,1,1-trichloroethane) in rats and dogs. *J. Pharmacol. Exp. Ther.* **99**, 140–148.

Hodge, H. C., Maynard, E. A., and Blanchet, H. J., Jr. (1952). Chronic oral toxicity tests of methoxychlor (2,2-di-(p-methoxyphenyl)-1.1,1-trichloroethane) in rats and dogs. *J. Pharmacol. Exp. Ther.* **104**, 60–66.

Hodge, H. C., Maynard, E. A., Downs, W. L., Ashton, J. K., and Salerno, L. L. (1966). Tests on mice for evaluating carcinogenicity. *Toxicol. Appl. Pharmacol.* **9**, 583–596.

Hoffman, I., and Lendle, L. (1948). The mode of action of a new insecticide. *Naunyn-Schmiedebergs Arch. Exp. Pathol. Pharmakol.* **205**, 223–242 (in German).

Hoffman, D. L., and Mattox, V. R. (1972). Treatment of adrenocortical carcinoma with o,p'-DDD. *Med. Clin. North Am.* **56**, 999–1012.

Hong, J. S., Herr, D. W., Hudson, P. M., and Tilson, H. A. (1986). Neurochemical effects of DDT in rat brain in vivo. *Arch. Toxicol. Suppl.* **9**, 14–26.

Horn, H. J., Bruce, R. B., and Paynter, O. E. (1955). Toxicology of chlorobenzilate. *J. Agric. Food Chem.* **3**, 752–756.

Hrdina, P. D., Singhal, R. L., Peters, D. A. V., and Ling, G. M. (1973). Some neurochemical alterations during acute DDT poisoning. *Toxicol. Appl. Pharmacol.* **25**, 276–288.

Hrdina, P. D., Singhal, R. L., and Ling, G. M. (1975). DDT and related hydrocarbon insecticides: Pharmacological basis of their toxicity in mammals. *Adv. Pharmacol. Chemother.* **12**, 31–88.

Hsieh, H. C. (1954). DDT intoxication in a family in southern Taiwan. *Arch. Ind. Hyg. Occup. Med.* **10**, 334–346.

Hudson, P. M., Chen, P. H., Tilson, H. A., and Hong, J. S. (1985). Effects of p,p-DDT on the rat brain concentrations of biogenic amine and amino acid neurotransmitters and their association with p,p'-DDT-induced tremor and hyperthermia. *J. Neurochem.* **45**, 1349–1355.

Hunter, D. J., Hankinson, S. E., Laden, F., Colditz, G. A., Manson, J. E., Willett, W., Speizer, F. E., and Wolff, M. S. (1997). Plasma organochlorine levels and the risk of breast cancer. *N. Engl. J. Med.* **337**, 1253–1258.

Hutter, A. M., and Kahoe, D. E. (1966). Adrenal cortical carcinoma. II. Results of treatment with o,p'-DDD in 138 patients. *Am. J. Med.* **41**, 581–592.

Hwang, E. C., and van Woert, M. H. (1978). p,p'-DDT-induced neurotoxic syndrome: Experimental myoclonus. *Neurology* **28**, 1020–1025.

Ichinose, R., and Kurihara, N. (1987). Intramolecular deuterium isotope effect and enantiotopic differentiation in oxidative demethylation of chiral (monomethyl-d3)methoxychlor in rat liver microsomes. *Biochem. Pharmacol.* **36**, 3761–3766.

Imai, H., and Coulston, F. (1968). Ultrastructural studies of absorption of methoxychlor in the jejunal mucosa of the rat. *Toxicol. Appl. Pharmacol.* **8**, 135–158.

Innes, J. R., Ulland, B. M., Wallerio, M. G., Petrielli, L., Fishbein, L., Hart, E. R., Pallotta, A. J., Bates, R. R., Falk, H. L., Gart, J. J., Klein, M., Mitchell, I., and Peters, J. (1969). Bioassay of pesticides and industrial chemicals for tumorigenicity in mice: A preliminary note. *J. Natl. Cancer Inst. (US)* **42**, 1101–1114.

Ireland, J. S., Mukku, V. R., Robison, A. K., and Stancel, G. M. (1980). Stimulation of uterine deoxyribonucleic acid synthesis by 1,1,1-trichloro-2-(o-chlorophenyl)ethane (o,p'-DDT). *Biochem. Pharmacol.* **29**, 1469–1474.

Ishikawa, Y., Charalambous, P., and Matsumura, F. (1989). Modification by pyrethroids and DDT of phosphorylation activities of rat brain sodium channel. *Biochem. Pharmacol.* **38**, 2449–2457.

Israeli, R., and Mayersdorf, A. (1973). Pathological changes in the EEG during work with halogen-containing insecticides. *Zentralbl. Arbeitsmed Arbeitsschutz* **23**, 340–343 (in German).

Jansson, B., Jensen, S., Olsson, M., Renberg, L., Sundström, G., and Vaz, R. (1975). Identification by GC-MS of phenolic metabolits of PCB and p,p'-DDE isolated from Baltic guillemot and seal. *Ambio* **4**, 93–97.

Jensen, J. A., Cueto, C., Dale, W. E., Rothe, C. F., Parce, G. W., and Mattson, A. M. (1957). Metabolism of insecticides. DDT metabolites in feces and bile of rats. *J. Agric. Food Chem.* **5**, 919–925.

Jenson, J. A. (1983). Chemical contaminants in human milk. *Residue Rev.* **89**, 1–128.

Jenson, S., and Jansson, B. (1976). Anthropogenic substances in seal from the Baltic: Methyl sulfone metabolites of PCB and DDE. *Ambio* **5**, 257–260.

Jeyaratnam, J., and Forshaw, J. (1974). A study of the cardiac effects of DDT in laboratory animals. *Bull. WHO* **51**, 531–535.

Jonnsson, C. J., Rodriguez-Martinez, H., Lund, B. O., Bergman, A., and Brandt, I. (1991). Adrenocortical toxicity of 3-methylsulfonyl-DDE in mice. II. Mictochondrial changes following ecologically relevant doses. *Fundam. Appl. Toxicol.* **16**, 365–374.

Jonnsson, C. J., Lund, B. O., Bergman A., and Brandt, I. (1992). Adrenocortical toxicity of 3-methylsulphonyl-DDE; 3: Studies in fetal and suckling mice. *Reprod. Toxicol.* **6**, 233–240.

Jonnsson, C. J., Rodriguez-Martinez, H., and Brandt, I. (1995). Transplacental toxicity of 3-methylsulphonyl-DDE in the developing adrenal cortex in mice. *Reprod. Toxicol.* **9**, 257–264.

Jonsson, V., Liu, G. J. K., Armbruster, J., Kettlehut, L. L., and Drucker, B. (1977). Chlorohydrocarbon pesticide residues in human milk in Greater St. Louis, Missouri, 1977. *Am. J. Clin. Nutr.* **30**, 1106–1109.

Judah, J. D. (1949). Studies on the metabolism and mode of faction of DDT. *Br. J. Pharmacol. Chemother.* **4**, 120–131.

Jude, A., and Girard, P. (1949). Toxicity of DDT intoxication by accidental ingestion. *Ann. Med. Leg.* **29**, 209–213 (in French).

Joy, R. M. (1973). Electrical correlates of preconvulsive and convulsive doses of chlorinated hydrocarbon insecticides in the CNS. *Neuropharmacology* **12**, 63–76.

Kacew, S., and Singhal, R. L. (1973). Adaptive response of hepatic carbohydrate metabolism to oral administration of p,p'-1,1,1-trichloro-2,2-bis-(p-chlorophenyl)ethane in rats. *Biochem. Pharmacol.* **22**, 47–57.

Kagan, Y. S., Rodionov, G. A., Woronina, L. Y., Velichko, L. S., Kulagin, O. M., and Peremitina, A. D. (1969). Effect of DDT on the functional and morphological condition of the liver. *Vrach. Delo* **12**, 101–105 (in Russian).

Kapoor, J. P., Metcalf, R. L., Nystrom, R. F., and Sangha, G. J. K. (1970). Comparative metabolims of methoxychlor, methiochlor and DDT in mouse, insects and in a model ecosystem. *J. Agric. Food Chem.* **18**, 1145–1152.

Kazen, C., Bloomer, A., Welch, R., Oudbier, A., and Price, H. (1974). Persistence of pesticides on the hands of some occupationally exposed people. *Arch. Environ. Health* **29**, 315–318.

Keil, J. E., Weston, W., III, Loadholt, C. B., Sandifer, S. H., and Colcolough, J. J. (1972a). DDT and DDE residues in blood from children, South Carolina—1970. *Pestic. Monit. J.* **6**, 1–3.

Keil, J. E., Sandifer, S. H., Finklea, J. H., and Priester, L. E. (1972b). Serum vitamin A elevation in DDT exposed volunteers. *Bull. Environ. Contam. Toxicol.* **8**, 317–320.

Keil, J. E., Loadholt, C. B., Sandifer, S. H., Weston, W., III, Gadsden, R. H., and Hames, C. G. (1973). Sera DDT elevation in black components of two southeastern communities: Genetics or environment? *In* "Pesticides and the Environment: A Continuing Controversy" (W. B. Diechman, ed.), pp. 203–213. Intercontinental Medical Book Corp., New York.

Kelce, W. R., Stone, C. R., Laws, S. C., Gray, L. E., and Wilson, E. M. (1995). Persistent DDT metabolite p,p'-DDE is a potent androgen receptor antagonist. *Nature* **375**, 581–585.

Kelce, W. R., Lambright, C. R., Gray, L. E., and Roberts, K. P. (1997). Vinclozolin and p,p-DDE alter androgen-dependent gene expression: *in vivo* confirmation of an androgen receptor-mediated mechanism. *Toxicol. Appl. Pharmacol.* **142**, 192–200.

Kelce, W. R., Gray, L. E., and Wilson, E. M. (1998). Antiandrogens as environmental endocrine disruptors. *Reprod. Fertil. Dev.* **10**, 105–111.

Keller, W. C., and Yeary, R. A. (1980). A comparison of the effects of mineral oil, vegetable oil and sodium sulfate on the intestinal absorption of DDT in rodents. *Clin. Toxicol.* **16**, 223–231.

Kelner, M. J., McLenithan, J. C., and Anders, M. W. (1986). Thiol stimulation of the cytochrome P-450-dependent reduction of 1,1,1-trichloro-2,2-bis(p-chlorophenyl)ethane (DDD). *Biochem. Pharmacol.* **35**, 1805–1807.

Keplinger, M. L., Diechmann, W. B., and Sala, F. (1970). Effects of combination of pesticides on reproduction in mice. *In* "Pesticides Symposia" (W. B. Deichmann, J. L. Radomski, and R. A. Penalver, eds.), pp. 125–138. Halos and Associates, Miami, FL.

Key, T., and Reeves, G. (1994). Organochlorines in the environment and breast cancer: The data so far produced provide reassurance rather than anxiety. *Br. Med. J.* **308**, 1520–1521.

Khaikina, B. I., and Shilina, V. F. (1971). The effect on serotonin metabolism of some organochlorine pesticides. *Farmakil. Toksikol. (Moscow)* **34**, 357–359 (in Russian).

Khairy, M. (1959). Changes in behaviour associated with a nervous system poison (DDT). *Q. J. Exp. Physiol.* **11**, 91–94.

Khera, K. S., Whalen, C., and Tivett, G. (1978). Teratogenicity studies on linuron, malathion, and methoxychlor in rats. *Toxicol. Appl. Pharmacol.* **45**, 435–444.

Kishimoto, D., and Kurihara, N. (1996). Effect of cytochrome P450 antibodies on the oxidative demethylation of methoxychlor catalysed by rat liver meirosomal cytochrome P450 enzymes: Isozyme specificity and alteration of enantiotopic selectivity. *Pestic. Biochem. Physiol.* **51**, 44–52.

Kishimoto, D., Oku, A., and Kurihara, N. (1995). Enantiotopic selectivity of cytochrome P450 catalysed oxidative demethylation of methoxychlor: Alteration of selectivity depending on isozymes and substrate concentrations. *Pestic. Biochem. Physiol.* **51**, 12–19.

Klein, A. K., Laug, E. P., Datta, P. R., and Mendel, J. L. (1965). Evidence for the conversion of o,p'-DDT (1,1,1-trichloro-2-o-chlorophenyl-2-p-chlorophenylethane) to p,p'-DDT (1,1,1-trichloro-2,2-bis(p-chlorophenyl)ethane) in rats. *J. Am. Chem. Soc.* **87**, 2520–2522.

Klein, W., and Korte, F. (1970). Metabolism of chlorinated hydrocarbons. *In* "Chemistry of Plant Protection and Pest Control Agents" (R. Wegler, ed.), Vol. 1, pp. 199–218. Springer-Verlag, Berlin (in German).

Klotz, H. P., Thibaut, E., and Russo, F. (1971). Weak doses of o,p'-DDD in the spanomenorrhea with hypertrichosis. *Ann. Endocrinol.* **32**, 763–767 (in French).

Knowles, C. O., and Ahmad, S. (1971). Comparative metabolism of chlorobenzilate, chloropropylate and bromopropylate acaricides by rat hepatic enzymes. *Can. J. Physiol. Pharmacol.* **49**, 590–597.

Kolmodin, B., Azarnoff, D. L., and Sjöqvist, F. (1969). Effect of environmental factors on drug metabolism: Decreased plasma half-life of antipyrine in workers exposed to chlorinated hydrocarbon insecticides. *Clin. Pharmacol. Ther.* **10**, 638–642.

Komissarenko, V. P. (1971). Effect of o,p'-DDD (clodithane) on secretion and metabolism of corticosteroids in chickens. *Fiziol. Zh. Kiev* **17**, 435–441 (in Russian).

Komissarenko, V. P., Reznikov, A. G., Gordienko, V. M., and Zak, K. P. (1968). Effect of o,p'-DDD on the morphology and function of adrenal cortex in dogs. *Endocrinol. Exp.* **2**, 21–28 (in Russian).

Komissarenko, V. P., Reziniková, A. G., and Gordienko, V. M. (1970). An experimental study of the action of o,p'-DDD on the functioning and structure of the adrenal cortex. *Vopr. Endokrinol. Obmena Veschestv. Sb.* **1**, 5–10 (in Russian).

Komissarenko, V. P., Gordiyenko, V. M., and Reznikov, A. G. (1972). Restorative processes in the adrenal cortex of dogs following administration of TDE. *Probl. Endokrinol.* **18**, 74–81 (in Russian).

Komissarenko, V. P., Chelnakova, I. S., and Mikosha, A. S. (1978). The activity of glutathione reductase in the adrenal glands and the liver of dogs following the administration of o,p'-DDD, Perthane and ACTH. *Probl. Endokrinol.* **24**, 95–98 (in Russian).

Korpachev, V. U. (1972a). Dependence of o,p'-DDD absorption on dose and drug form. *Farm. Zh.* **27**, 64–66 (in Russian).

Korpachev, V. U. (1972b). Accumulation and elimination of o,p'-DDD in organs and tissues of guinea pigs and dogs. *Fiziol. Zh.* **18**, 585–590 (in Russian).

Korte, F. (1979). Transformation of p,p'-DDT in the environment. *In* "Environmental Health Criteria 9. DDT and Its Derivatives." United Nations Environmental Programme and the World Health Organization, Geneva.

Korthe-Schutz, S., Levine, L. S., Roth, J. A., Saenger, P., and New, M. I. (1977). Virilizing adrenal tumor in a child suppressed with dexamethasone for three years. Effect of o,p'-DDD on serum and urinary androgens. *J. Clin. Endocrinol. Metab.* **44**, 433–439.

Koschier F. J., Gigliotti, P. J., and Hong, S. K. (1980). The effect of bis(p-chlorophenyl)acetic acid on the renal function of the rat. *J. Environ. Pathol. Toxicol.* **4**, 209–217.

Koster, R. (1947). Differentiation of gluconate, glucose, calcium, insulin effect on DDT poisoning in cats. *Fed. Proc., Fed. Am. Soc. Exp. Biol.* **6**, 346.

Kravchenko, V. I. (1973). The effect of o,p'-DDD on the formulation of corticosteroids by the adrenal tissue *in vitro*. *Probl. Endokrinol.* **19**, 76–79 (in Russian).

Kravt'sova, O. L., Korenevskyy, L. I., and Reznikov, O. H. (1971). The influence of o,p'-DDD on the development of DMBA-induced mammary gland tumours and adrenal cortex function in rats. *Dopov. Akad. Nauk. Ukr. RSR. Ser. B* **30**(3), 943–945 (in Russian).

Kreiger, N., Wolff, M. S., Hiatt, R. A., Rivera, M., Vogelman, J., and Orentreich, N. (1994). Breast cancer and serum organochlorines: A prospective study among white, black, and asian women. *J. Natl. Cancer Inst.* **86**, 589–599.

Kreiss, K., Zack, M. M., Kimbrough, R. D., and Needham, L. C. (1981). Cross-sectional study of a community with exceptional exposure to DDT. *J. Am. Med. Assoc.* **245**, 1926–1930.

Kujawa, M., Macholz, R., and Knoll, R. (1985). Enzymic degradation of DDT. Part 5. Direct transformation of DDD (dichlorodiphenyldichloro-ethane) to an aldehyde. *Nahrung* **29**, 517–522.

Kunze, F. M., Laug, E. P., and Prickett, C. S. (1950). The storage of methoxychlor in the fat of the rat. *Proc. Soc. Exp. Biol. Med.* **75**, 415–416.

Kupfer, D. (1967). Effects of some pesticides and related compounds on steroid function and metabolism. *Residue Rev.* **19**, 11–30.

Kupfer, D., and Bulger, W. H. (1979). A novel *in vitro* method for demonstrating proestrogens. Metabolism of methoxychlor and o,p'-DDT by liver micrososmes in the presence of uteri and effects on intracellular distribution of estrogen receptors. *Life Sci.* **25**, 975–984.

Kupfer, D., and Bulger, W. H. (1987). Biochemical toxicology of methoxychlor and related chlorinated hydrocarbons. *Rev. Biochem. Toxicol.* **8**, 183–215.

Kupfer, D., Bulger, W. H., and Nanni, F. (1986). Characteristics of the active oxygen in covalent binding of the pesticide methoxychlor to hepatic microsomal proteins. *Biochem. Pharmacol.* **35**, 2775–2780.

Kupfer, D., Bulger, W. H., and Theoharides, A. D. (1990). Metabolism of methoxychlor by hepatic P450 monooxygenases in rat and humans. 1. Characterisation of a novel catechol metabolite. *Chem. Res. Toxicol.* **3**, 8–16.

Kutz, F. W., Yobs, A. R., Strassman, S. C., and Viar, F., Jr. (1977). Effects of reducing DDT usage on total DDT storage in humans. *Pestic. Monit. J.* **11**, 61–63.

Lacassagne, A. (1971). Critical review of experimental tumours of Leydig cells, more particularly in the rat. *Bull. Cancer* **58**, 235–276 (in French).

Laden, F., Neas, L. M., Spiegelman, D., Hankinson, S. E., Willett, W. C., Wolff, M. S., and Hunter, D. J. (1999). Predictors of plasma concentrations of DDE and PCBs in a group of US women. *Environ. Health Perspect.* **107**, 75–81.

Lamartiniere, C. A., Luther, M. A., Lucier, G. W., and Illsley, N. P. (1982). Altered imprinting of rat liver monoamine oxidase by o,p'-DDT and methoxychlor. *Biochem. Pharmacol.* **31**, 647–651.

Lamoureux, C. H., and Feil, V. J. (1980). Gas chromatographic and mass spectrometric characterization of impurities in technical methoxychlor. *J. Assoc. Off. Anal. Chem.* **63**, 1007–1037.

Larson, P. S., Hennigar, G. R., Finnegan, J. K., Smith, R. B., Jr., and Haag, H. B. (1955). Observations on the relation of chemical structure to the production of adrenal cortical atrophy or hypertrophy in the dog by derivatives of 2,2-bis(p-chlorophenyl)-1,1-dichloroethane (DDD, TDE). *J. Pharmacol. Exp. Ther.* **115**, 408–412.

Laug, E. P., Kunze, F. M., and Prickett, C. S. (1951). Occurrence of DDT in human fat and milk. *Arch. Ind. Hyg. Ocup. Med.* **3**, 245–246.

Laüger, P., Martin, H., and Müller, P. (1944). Constitution and toxic effects of natural and synthetic insecticides. *Helv. Chim. Acta* **27**, 892–928 (in German).

Laüger, P., Pulver, R., and Montigel, C. (1945a). Mode of action of 4,4′-dichlorodiphenyl-trichloromethyl-methane (DDT-Geigy) in warm-blooded organisms. *Experientia* **1**, 120–121 (in German).

Laüger, P., Pulver, R., and Montigel, C. (1945b). Mode of action of 4,4′-dichlorodiphenyl-trichoromethyl-methane (DDT) in warm-blooded organism. *Hel. Physiol. Pharmacol. Acta* **3**, 405–415 (in German).

Laws, E. R., Jr., Curley, A., and Bios, F. J. (1967). Men with intensive occupational exposure to DDT. A clinical and chemical study. *Arch. Environ. Health* **15**, 766–775.

Laws, E. R., Maddrey, W. D., Curley, A., and Burse, V. W. (1973). Long-term occupational exposure to DDT. *Arch. Environ. Health* **27**, 318–321.

Lehman, A. J. (1951). Chemicals in foods: A report to the Association of Food and Drug Officials on current developments. Part II. Pesticides. Section I: Introduction. *Q. Bull. Assoc. Food Drug Off.* **15**(I), 122–125.

Lehman, A. J. (1952). Chemicals in foods: A report to the Association of Food and Drug officials on current developments. Pat II. Pesticides. Section II. Dermal toxicity. Section III. Subacute and chronic toxicity. Section IV. Biochemistry. Section V. Pathology. *Q. Bull. Assoc. Food Drug Off.* **16**(II), 3–9; (III), 47–53; (IV), 85–91; (V), 126–132.

Lehman, A. J. (1965). "Summaries of Pesticide Toxicity." Assoc. Food Drug Off. U.S., Topeka, KS.

Leighty, E. G. (1981). Decreased retention of fatty acid conjugated DDT metabolites in rats given injections of heparin, bile salts or leirthin. *Res. Commun. Chem. Pathol. Pharmacol.* **31**, 69–76.

Leighty, E. G., Fentiman, A. F., and Thompson, R. M. (1980). Conjugation of fatty acids to DDT in the rat: Possible mechanism for retention. *Toxicology* **15**, 77–82.

Levine, R. (1991). Recognised and possble effects of pesticides in humans. *In* "Handbook Pesticide Toxicology," pp. 275–360. Academic Press, San Diego.

Levy, K. A., Brady, S. E., and Pfaffenberger, C. D. (1981). Chlorobenzilate residues in citrus-workers. *Bull. Environ. Contam. Toxicol.* **27**, 235–238.

Levy, J. M, Lutz, P., Wagner, C., Sauer, P., Seiller, F., Fiscbach, M., Segura, N., and Sauvage, P. (1985). Favorable outcome of a recurring malignant adrenocortical tumor under *o,p′*-DDD therapy. *Ann. Pediatr.* **32**, 541–544 (in French).

Li, H. C., Dehal, S. S., and Kupfer, D. (1995). Induction of the hepatic CYP2B and CYP3A enzymes by the proestrogenic pesticide methoxychlor and by DDT in the rat. Effects on methoxychlor metabolism. *J. Biochem. Toxicol.* **10**, 51–61.

Lillie, R. D., and Smith, M. I. (1944). Pathology of experimental poisoning in cats, rabbits, and rats with 2,2-bis-(*para*-chlorophenyl)-1,1,1-trichlorethane. *Public Health Rep.* **59**, 979–984.

Lillie, R. D., Smith, M. I., and Stohlman, E. F. (1947). Pathologic action of DDT and certain of its analogs and derivatives. *Arch. Pathol.* **43**, 127–142.

Lillie, R. J., Cecil, H. C., and Bitman, J. (1973). Methoxychlor in chicken breeder diets. *Poult. Sci.* **52**, 1134–1138.

Loeffler, I. K., and Peterson, R. E. (1999). Interactive effects of TCDD and *p,p′*-DDE on male reproductive tract development in *in utero* and lactationally exposed rats. *Toxicol. Sci.* **154**, 28–39.

Lu, F. C., Jessup, D. C., and Lavalle, A. (1965). Toxicity of pesticides in young versus adult rats. *Food Cosmet. Toxicol.* **3**, 591–596.

Lubberink, A. A. M. E., Rijnberk, A., Der Kinderen, P. J., and Thijssen, J. H. H. (1971). Hyperfunction of the adrenal cortex: A review. *Aust. Vet. J.* **47**, 504–509.

Lubitz, J. A., Feeman, L., and Okum, R. (1973). Mitotane use in inoperable adrenal cortical carcinoma. *J. Am. Med. Assoc.* **233**, 1109–1112.

Lund, B., Klasson-Wehler, F., and Brandt, I. (1986). *o,p′*-DDD in the mouse lung: Selective uptake, covalent binding and effect on drug metabolism. *Chem.–Biol. Interat.* **60**, 129–141.

Lund, B., Bergman, A., and Brandt, I. (1988). Metabolic activation of a DDT-metabolite, 3-methylsufonyl-DDE, in the adrenal *zona fasciculata* in mice. *Chem.–Biol. Interact.* **65**, 24–40.

Lund, B. O., Ghantous, H., Bergman, A., and Brandt, I. (1989). Covalent binding of four DDD isomers in the mouse lung: Lack of structure specificity. *Pharmacol. Toxicity* **65**, 282–286.

Luton, J. P., Valcke, J. C., Remy, J. M., Mathieu de Fossey, B., and Bricaire, H. (1972). Gynecomastia after long-term treatment of Cushing's disease with *o,p′*-DDT. *Ann. Endocrinol.* **33**, 290–293 (in French).

Luton, J. P., Remy, J. M., Valcke, J. C., Laudat, P., and Bricaire, H. (1973). Cure or remission of Cushing's disease by prolonged therapeuti use of *o,p′*-DDD (with reference to 17 observations). *Ann. Endocrinol.* **34**, 351–376 (in French.

MacCormack, J. D. (1945). Infestation and DDT. *Ir. J. Med. Sci.* **6**, 627–634.

Mackeras, I. M., and West, R. F. K. (1946). "DDT" poisoning in man. *Med. J. Ast.* **1**, 400–401.

Macklin, A. W., and Ribelin, W. E. (1971). The relation of pesticides to abortion in dairy cattle. *J. Am. Vet. Med. Assoc.* **159**, 1743–1748.

Malats, N., Read, F. X., and Porta, M. (1993). DDT and pancreatic cancer. *J. Natl. Cancer Inst.* **85**, 328.

Markarian, D. S. (1966). Cytogenetic effect of some chlorine-containing organic insecticides on mouse bone-marrow cell nuclei. *Genetika* **1**, 132–137.

Martz, F., and Straw, J. A. (1972). Effects of mitotane (*o,p′*-DDD) on hepatic drug metabolism in dogs. *Fed. Proc. Fed. Am. Soc. Exp. Biol.* **31**, 581.

Martz, F., and Straw, J. A. (1973). Mitoane decreases adrenal cortical heme and P450. *Fed. Proc., Fed. Am. Soc. Exp. Biol.* **32**, 734.

Martz, F., and Straw, J. A. (1977). The *in vitro* metabolism of 1-(*o*-chlorophenyl)-1,1-dichloroethane(*o,p*-DDD) by dog adrenal mitochondria and metabolite covalent binding to mitochondrial macromolecules. A possible mechanism for the adrenocorticolytic effect. *Drug. Metabl. Dispos.* **5**, 482–486.

Martz, F., and Straw, J. A. (1980). Metabolism and covalent binding of 1-(*o*-chlorophenyl)-2,2-dichloroethane (*o,p*-DDD). Correlation between adrenoccorticolytic activity and metabolic activation be adrenocortial mitrochondria. *Drug Metab. Dispos.* **8**, 127–130.

Mattson, A. M., Spillane, J. T., Baker, C., and Pearce, G. W. (1953). Determination of DDT and related substanes in human fat. *Anal. Chem.* **25**, 1065–1070.

Mayersdorf, A., and Israeli, R. (1974). Toxic effects of chlorinated hydrocarbon insecticides on the human electroencephalogram. *Arch. Environ. Health* **28**, 159–163.

McBain, W. A. (1987). The leveo enantiomer of *o,p′*-DDT inhibits the binding of β-estradiol to the estrogen receptor. *Life Sci.* **40**, 215–221.

McCann, J., and Ames, B. N. (1976). Detection of carcinogens as mutagens in the *Salmonella*/microsome test: Assay of 300 chemicals: Discussion. *Proc. Natl. Acad. Sci. U.S.A.* **73**, 950–954.

McDaniel, K. L., and Moser, V. C. (1997). The influence of dosing volume on the toxicity of *p,p′*-DDT. *Neurotoxicology* **18**, 1071–1077.

McKierman, P., Doyle, D. A., Duffy, G. J., Towers, R. P., Duff, F. A., and O'Donovan, D. K. (1978). Brief report. *o,p′*-DDD and adrenal carcinoma. *Ir. J. Med. Sci.* **147**, 437–440.

McKinney, J. D., Boozier, E. L., Hopkins, H. P., and Suggs, J. E. (1969). Synthesis and reactions of a proposed DDT metabolite, 2,2′bis(*p*-chlorophenyl)acetaldehyde. *Experientia* **25**, 897–898.

McLachlan, J. A., and Dixon, R. L. (1972). Gonadal function in mice exposed prenatally to *p,p′*-DDT. *Toxicol. Appl. Pharmacol.* **22**, 327.

McQueen, E. G., Owen, D., and Ferry, D. G. (1972). Effect of phenytoin and other drugs in reducing serum DDT levels. *N. Z. Med. J.* **75**, 208–211.

Menzie, C. M. (1969). "Metabolism of Pesticides." Spec. Sci. Rep., Wild. No. 127. U. S. Govt. Printing Office, Washington, DC.

Metcalf, R. L. (1973). A century of DDT. *J. Agric. Chem.* **21**, 511–519.

Metcalf, J. L., Laws, S. C., and Cummings, A. M. (1995). Methoxychlor mimics the action of 17β-estradiol on induction of uterine epidermal growth factor receptors in immature female rats. *Biol. Reprod. Suppl.* **52**, 97.

Mikosha, V. A. (1985). Effect of chloditan on activity of malate enzymes in adrenal glands. *Vopr. Med. Him.* **31**, 61–64.

Misra, U. K., Nag, D., and Murti, C. R. (1984). A study of cognitive functions in DDT sprayers. *Indian Health* **22**, 199–206.

Mitjavila, S., Carrera, G., Boigegrain, R.-A., and Derache, R. (1981a). I. Evaluation of the toxic risk of DDT in the rat: During accumulation. *Arch. Environ. Contam. Toxicol.* **10**, 459–469.

Mitjavila, S., Carrera, G., and Fernandez, Y. (1981b). II. Evaluation of the toxic risk of accumulated DDT in the rat: During fat mobilization. *Arch. Environ. Contam. Toxicol.* **10**, 471–481.

Moir, D., Marwood, T. M., and Moody, R. P. (1994). *In vitro* cutaneous metabolism of DDT in human and animal skins. *Bull. Environ. Contam. Toxicol.* **52**, 474–478.

Molnar, G. D., Nunn, S. L., and Tauxe, W. N. (1961). The effect of *o,p′*-DDD therapy on plasma cholesterol in adrenal carcinoma. *Proc. Staff Meet. Mayo Clin.* **36**, 618–620.

Montgomery, J. A., and Struck, R. F. (1973). The relation of the metabolism of anticancer agents to their activity. *Fortschr. Arzneimittelforsch.* **17**, 32–304 (in German).

Morgan, D. P., and Lin, I. L. (1978). Blood organochlorine pesticide concentrations, clinical hematology and biochemistry in workers ocupationally exposed to pesticides. *Arch. Environ. Contam. Toxicol.* **7**, 423–447.

Morgan, D. P., and Roan, C. C. (1971). Absorption, storage, and metabolic conversion of ingested DDT and metabolism in man. *Arch. Environ. Health* **22**, 301–308.

Morgan, D. P., and Roan, C. C. (1972). Loss of DDT from storage in human body fat. *Nature (London)* **238**, 221–223.

Morgan, D. P., and Roan, C. C. (1973). Adrenorcortical function in persons occupationally exposed to pesticides. *J. Occp. Med.* **15**, 26–28.

Morgan, D. P., and Roan, C. C. (1974). Liver function in workers having hydrocarbon pesticides. *Arch. Environ. Health* **29**, 14–17.

Morgan, D. P., and Roan, C. C. (1977). The metabolism of DDT in man. *Essays Toxicol.* **5**, 39.

Morgan, J. M., and Hickenbottom, J. P. (1979). Comparisons of selected parameters for monitoring methoxychlor hepatotoxicity. *Bull. Environ. Contam. Toxicol.* **23**, 275–280.

Morita, R., Lieberman, L. M., Beierwaltes, W. H., Conn, J. W., Ansari, A. N., and Nishiyama, H. (1972). Percent uptake of ^{131}I radioactivity in the adrenal from radioiodinated cholesterol. *J. Clin. Endocrinol. Metab.* **34**, 36–43.

Muhlens, K. (1946). Significance of dichlor-diphenyl-trichlor methylmethane preparations as an arthropod poison in plagues, with regard to one experience. *Dtsch. Med. Wochenschr.* **71**, 164–169 (in German).

Mussalo-Rauhamaa, Häsänen, Pyysalo, H., Antervo, K., Kauppila, R., and Pantzar, P. (1990). Occurrence of beta-hexachlorocyclohexane in breast cancer patients. *Cancer* **66**, 2124–2128.

Naevested, R. (1947). Poisoning by DDT powder as well as other poisons. *Tidsskr. Nor. Laefeforen.* **67**, 261–263 (in Norwegian).

Narayan, S., Dani, H. M., and Misra, U. K. (1990a). Changes in lipid profiles of liver microsomes of rats following intratracheal administration of DDT or endosulfan. *J. Environ. Sci. Health B* **25**, 243–257.

Narayan, S., Dani, H. M., and Misra, U. K. (1990b). Lung subcellular fractions and surfactant lipid metabolism of rats exposed with DDT or endosulfan intratracheally. *J. Environ. Sci. Health B* **25**, 259–272.

Narloch, B. A., Lawton, M. P., Moody, D. E., Hammock, B. D., and Shull, L. R. (1987). The effects of dicofol on induction of hepatic microsomal metabolism in rats. *Pestic. Biochem. Physiol.* **28**, 362–370.

Naruse, R., Sasaki, T., Yamoka, T., Matsuoka, K., Negoro, Y., Itasaka, Y., Urushibata, K., Chin, T., Kaot, K., Kako, K., Goto, Y., Equichi, Y., Yogo H., Tomita, A., and Asai, M. (1970). Clinical use of *o,p'*-DDD in adrenal cortex cancer. *Horumon to Rinsho* **18**, 241–244 (in Japanese).

National Cancer Institute (NCI) (1978a). "Bioassay of DDT, TDE, and *p,p'*-DDE for Possible Carcinogenicity." Carcinogenesis Tech. Rep. Ser. No. 131, DHEW Publ. No. (NIH) 78-1325. U.S. Govt. Printing Office, Washington, DC.

National Cancer Institute (NCI) (1978b). "Bioassay of Methoxychlor for Possible Carcinogenicity." Tech. Rep. Ser. No. 35, DHEW Publ. No. (NIH) 78-835, U.S. Govt. Printing Office, Washington, DC.

National Cancer Institute (NCI) (1978c). "Bioassay of Chlorobenzilate for Possible Carcinogenicity." Tech. Rep. Ser. No. 75, DHEW Publ. No. (NIH) 78-1325, U.S. Govt. Printing Office, Washington, DC.

National Cancer Institute (NCI) (1978d). "Bioassay of Dicofol for Possible Carcinogenicity." Tech. Rep. Ser. No. 90, DHEW Publ. No. (NIH) 78-1340, U.S. Govt. Printing Office, Washington, DC.

National Cancer Institute (NCI) (1979). "Bioassay of *p,p'*-ethyl-DDD for Possible Carcinogenicity." Carcinogenesis Tech. Rep. Ser., DHEW Publ. No. (NIH) 79-1712, U.S. Govt. Printing Office, Washington, DC.

Neal, P. A., von Oettingen, W. F., Smith, W. W., Malmo, R. B., Dunn, R. C., Moran, E., Sweeney, T. R., Armstrong, D. W., and White, W. C. (1944). Toxicity and potential dangers of aerosols, mists, and dusting powders containing DDT. *Public Health Rep. Suppl.* **177**, 1–32.

Neal, P. A., Sweeney, T. R., Spicer, S. S., and von Oettingen, W. F. (1946). The excretion of DDT (2,2-bis-(*p*-chlorophenyl)-1,1-tichloroethane) in man, together with clinical observations. *Public Health Rep.* **61**, 403–409.

Nelson, J. A. (1973). Effects of DDT analogs and polychlorinated biphenyls (PCB) mixtures on ^{3}H-estradiol binding to rat uterine receptor. *Fed. Proc., Fed. Am. Soc. Exp. Biol.* **32**, 236.

Nelson, A. A., and Woodard, G. (1948). Adrenal cortical atrophy and liver damage produced in dogs by feeding 2,2-bis-(parachlorophenyl)-1,1-dichloroethane (DDD). *Fed. Proc., Fed. Am. Soc. Exp. Bio.* **7**, 277.

Nelson, A. A., and Woodard, G. (1949). Severe adrenal cortical atrophy (cytotoxic and hepatic damage produced in dogs by feeding 2,2-bis-(parachlorophenyl)-1,1-dichloroethane (DDD or TDE). *Arch. Pathol.* **48**, 387–394.

Nelson, A. A., Draize, H., Woodard, G., Fitzhugh, O. G., Smith, R. B., and Calvery, H. O. (1944). Histopathological changes following administration of DDT in several species of animals. *Public Health Rep.* **59**, 1009–1020.

Nichols, J., Kaye, S., and Larson, P. S. (1958). Barbiturate potentiating action of DDD and Pethane. *Proc. Soc. Exp. Biol. Med.* **98**, 239–242.

Nichols, J., Prestley, W. E., and Nichols, F. (1961). Effects of *m,p'*-DDT in a case of adrenal cortical carcinoma. *Curr. Ther. Res.* **3**, 266–271.

Nichols, W. K., Terry, C. M., Cutler, N. S., Appleton, M. L., Hestihi, P. K., and Yost, G. S. (1995). Oxidation at C-1 controls the cytotoxicity of 1,1-dichloro-2,2-bis(p-chlorophenyl)ethane by rabbit and human lung cells. *Drug Metab. Dispos.* **23**, 595–599.

Nigg, H. N., Stamper, J. H., and Queen, R. M. (1986). Dicofol exposure to Florida citrus applicators: Effects of protective clothing. *Arch. Environ. Contam. Toxicol.* **15**, 121–134.

Nims, R. W., Lubet, R. A., Fox, S. D., Jones, C. R., Thomas, P. E., Reddy, A. B., and Kocarek, T. A. (1998). Comparative pharmacodyanics of CY2B induction by DDT, DDE, and DDD in male rat liver and cultured rat hepatocytes. *J. Toxicol. Environ. Health* **53**, 455–477.

North, H. H., and Menzer, R. E. (1973). Metabolism of DDT in human embryonic lung cell cultures. *J. Agric. Food. Chem.* **21**, 509–510.

Oberly, T. J., Mihaelis, K. C., Rexroat, M. A., Bewsey, B. J., and Garriot, M. L. (1993). A comparison of the CHO/HGPRT+/− mutation assays using suspension treatment and soft agar cloning: Results for 10 chemicals. *Cell Biol. Toxicol.* **9**, 243.

O'Connor, J. C., Frame, S. R., Davis, L. G., and Cook, J. C. (1999). Detection of the environmental antiandrogen *p,p'*-DDE in CD and Long-Evans rats using a Tier 1 screening battery and a Hershberger assay. *Toxicol. Sci.* **51**, 44–53.

Ohyama, T., Takahashi, T., and Ogawa, H. (1982). Effects of dichlorodiphenyltrichloroethane and its analogues on rat liver mitochondria. *Biochem. Pharmacol.* **31**, 397–404.

Ojima, M., Saito, M., and Fukushima, S. (1984). Effect of an insecticide (*o,p'*-DDD) on human adrenal synthesis. *Nippon Naibunpi Gakkai Zasshi* **60**, 852–871 (in Japanese).

Ojima, M., Saitoh, M., Itoh, N., Kusano, Y., Fukuchi, S., and Naganuma, H. (1985). Effect of *o,p'*-DDD on adrenal steroidogenesis and hepatic steroid metabolism. *Nippon Naibunpi Gakkai Zasshi* **61**, 168–178.

O'Leary, J. A., Davies, J. E., and Feldman, M. (1970). Spontaneous abortion and human pesticide residues of DDT and DDE. *Am. J. Obstet. Gynecol.* **108**, 1291–1292.

Ortlee, M. F. (1958). Study of men with prolonged intensive occupational exposure to DDT. *Arch. Ind. Health* **18**, 433–440.

Ottoboni, A. (1969). Effect of DDT on reproduction in the rat. *Toxicol. Appl. Pharmacol.* **14**, 74–81.

Ottoboni, A. (1972). Effect of DDT on the reproductive lifespan in the female rat. *Toxicol. Appl. Pharmacol.* **22**, 497–502.

Ottoboni, A., Bissell, G. D., and Hexter, A. C. (1977). Effects of DDT on reproduction in multiple generations of beagle dogs. *Arch. Environ. Contam. Toxicol.* **6**, 83–101.

Ousterhaut, Struck, R. F., and Nelson, J. A. (1981). Estrogenic activities of methoxychlor metabolites. *Biochem. Pharmacol.* **30**, 2869–2871.

Ouw, K. H., and Shandar, A. G. (1974). A health survey of Wee Waa residents during 1973 aerial spraying season. *Med. J. Aust.* **2**, 871–873.

Palin, K. J., Wilson, C. G., Davis, S. S., and Phillips, A. J. (1982). The effects of oils on the lymphatic absorption of DDT. *J. Pharm. Pharmacol.* **34**, 707–710.

Palmer, K. A., Green, S., and Legator, M. S. (1972). Cytogenic effects of DDT and derivatives of DDT in a cultured mammalian cell line. *Toxicol. Appl. Pharmacol.* **22**, 355–364.

Paschal, E. H., Roan, C. C., and Morgan, D. P. (1974). Evidence of excretion of chlorinated hydrocardon metabolites by the human liver. *Bull. Environ. Contamin. Toxicol.* **12**, 547–554.

Pearce, G. W., Mattson, A. M., and Hayes, W. J., Jr. (1952). Examination of human fat for presence of DDT. *Science* **116**, 254–256.

Pellerin, D., Harouchi, A., and Soulier, Y. (1975). Corticosuprarenal tumors of children, concerning 10 cases. *Ann. Chir. Infant.* **16**, 155–179 (in French).

Peraino, C., Fry, R. J. M., Staffeldt, E., and Christopher, J. P. (1975). Comparative enhancing effects of phenobarbital, amobarbital, diphenylhydantoin, and dichlorodiphenyltrichloroethane on 2-acetylaminofluorene-induced hepatic tumorigenesis in the rat. *Cancer Res.* **35**, 2884–2890.

Perevodchikova, N. I., Platinsky, L. V., and Kerstsman, V. I. (1972). The treatment of inoperable forms of malignant tumors of the adrenal cortex with o,p'-DDD. *Vopr. Onkol.* **18**, 24–29 (in Russian).

Peterson, J. E., and Robinson, W. H. (1964). Metabolic products of p,p'—DDT in the rat. *Toxicol. Appl. Pharmacol.* **6**, 321–327.

Petrun', N. M., and Nikulina, G. G. (1970). The effect of chronic administration of different doses of o,p'-DDD on the ratio of ascorbic and dehydroascorbic acid in the adrenals and some other organs of guinea-pigs. *Vopr. Endokrinol. Obmena Veschestv* **1**, 19–22 (in Russian).

Phillips, F. S., and Gilman, A. (1946). Studies on the pharmacology of DDT (2,2-bis-(parachlorophenyl)-1,1,1-trichloroethane). I. The acute toxicity of DDT following intravenous injection in mammals with observations on the treatment of acute DDT poisoning. *J. Pharmacol. Exp. Ther.* **86**, 213–221.

Phillips, F. S., Gilman, A., and Crescitelli, F. N. (1946). Studies on the pharmacology of DDT (2,2-bis-parachlorophenyl)-1,1,1-trichloroethane). I. The sensistization of the myocardium to sympathetic stimulation during acute DDT intoxication. *J. Pharmacol. Exp. Ther.* **86**, 222–228.

Planche, G., Croisy, A., Malaveille, C., Tomatis, O., and Bartsch, H. (1979). Metabolic and mutagenicity studies on DDT and 15 derivatives. Detection of 1,1-bis(p-chlorophenyl)-2,2-dichloroethane and 1,1-bis(p-chloropshenyl)-2,2,2-trichlorophenyl acetate (Kelthane acetate) as mutagens in *Salmonella typhimurium* and of 1,1-bis(p-chlorophenyl)ethylene oxide, a likely metabolite, as an alkylating agent. *Chem.–Biol. Interact.* **25**, 157–175.

Pocock, D. E., and Vost, A. (1974). DDT absorption and chylomicron transport in rat. *Lipids* **9**, 374–381.

Pohland, R. C., and Counsell, R. E. (1985). *In vitro* and *in vivo* metabolism of a radioiodinated analog of 1-(2-chlorophenyl)-1-(4-chlorophenyl)-2,2-dichloroethane. *Drug. Metab. Dispos.* **13**, 113–115.

Poland, A., Smith, D., Kuntzman, R., Jacobson, M., and Conney, A. H. (1970). Effect of intensive occupational exposure to DDT on phenylbutazone and cortisol metabolism in human subjects. *Clin. Pharmacol. Ther.* **11**, 724–732.

Powers, J. M., Hennigar, G. R., Grooms, G., and Nichols, J. (1974). Adrenalcortical degeneration and regeneration following administration of DDT. *Am. J. Pathol.* **75**, 181–194.

Preston, R. J., Au, W., Bender, M. A., Brewen, J. G., Carrano, A. V., Heddle, J. A., McFee, A. F., Wolff, S., and Wassom, J. S. (1981). Mammalian *in vivo* and *in vitro* cytogenic assays: A report of the U.S., EPA Gene-Tox Program. *Mutat. Res.* **87**, 143–188.

Quinby, G. E., Hayes, W. J., Jr., Armstrong, J. F., and Durham, W. F. (1965a). DDT storage in the US population. *J. Am. Med. Assoc.* **191**, 109–113.

Quinby, G. E., Armstrong, J. F., and Durham, W. F. (1965b). DDT in human milk. *Nature (London)* **207**, 726–728.

Rabello, M. N., and Pereira, C. A. B. (1975). Cytogenic study on individuals occupationally exposed to DDT. *Mutat. Res.* **28**, 449–454.

Rappalport, R., Schweisguth, O., Cachin, O., and Perin, D. (1978). Malignant suprarenaloma with metastases. Extraction and treatment by o,p'-DDD following recovery. *Arch. Fr. Pediatr.* **35**, 551–554.

Rappolt, R. T. (1970). Use of oral DDT in three human babiturate intoxications: CNS arousal and/or hepatic enzyme induction by reciprocal detoxicants. *Ind. Med. Surg.* **39**, 319.

Ravindran, M. (1978). Toxic encephalopathy from chlorobenzilate poisoning: Report of case. *Clin. Encephalogr.* **9**, 170–172.

Reach, G., Elki, F., Parry, C., Corrol, P., and Milliez, P. (1978). Increased urate excretion after o,p'-DDD. *Lancet* **1**, 1269.

Reif, V. D., and Sinsheimer, J. E. (1975). Metabolism of 1-(o-chlorophenyl)-1-(p-chlorophenyl)-2,2-dichloro-ethane (o,p'-DDD) in rats. *Drug Metab. Dispos.* **3**, 15–25.

Reif, V. D., Sinsheimer, J. E., Ward, J. C., and Schteingart, D. E. (1974). Aromatic hydroxylation and alkyl oxidation in metabolism of mitotane (o,p'-DDD) in humans. *J. Pharm. Sci.* **63**, 1730–1736.

Reuber, M.D. (1978). Carcinomas of the liver in Osborne–Mendel rats ingesting DDT. *Tumor* **64**, 571–577.

Reuber, M. D. (1979a). Interstitial cell carcinomas of the testis in Balb/c male mice ingesting methoxychlor. *J. Cancer Res. Clin. Oncol.* **93**, 173–179.

Reuber, M. D. (1979b). Carcinomas of the liver in Osborne–Mendel rats ingesting methoxychlor. *Life Sci.* **24**, 1367–1371.

Reynolds, P. J., Lindahl, I. L., Cecil, H. C., and Bitman, J. (1975). DDT and methoxychlor accumulation and depletion in sheep. *J. Anim. Sci.* **41**, 274.

Reynolds, P. J., Lindahl, I. L., Cecil, H. C., and Bitman, J. (1976). A comparison of DDT and methoxychlor accumulation and depletion in sheep. *Bull. Environ. Contam. Toxicol.* **16**, 240–247.

Reznikov, A. G. (1973). Experimental data on adrenocorticolytic activity of m,p'-DDD and p,p'-Perthane. *Probl. Endokrinol.* **19**, 71–74 (in Russian).

Roan, C., Morgan, D., and Paschal, E. H. (1971). Urinary excretion of DDA following ingestion of DDT and DDT metabolites in man. *Arch. Environ. Health* **22**, 309–315.

Roberts, D. R., Manguin, S., and Mouchet, J. (2000). DDT house spraying and re-emerging malaria. *Lancet* **356**, 330–332.

Robison, A. K., Mukku, V. R., Spalding, D. M., and Stancel, G. M. (1984). The estrogenic activity of DDT: The *in vitro* induction of an estrogenic-inducible protein by o,p'-DDT. *Toxicol. Appl. Pharmacol.* **76**, 537–543.

Robison, A. K., Sirbasku, D. A., and Stancel, G. M. (1985a). DDT supports the growth of an estrogen-responsive tumor. *Toxicol. Lett.* **27**, 109–113.

Robison, A. K., Schmidt, W. A., and Stancel, G. M. (1985b). Estrogenic activity of DDT: Estrogen-receptor profiles and the responses of individual uterine cell types following o,p'-DDT administration. *J. Toxicol. Environ. Health* **16**, 493–508.

Rojanapo, W., Tepsuwan, A., Kupradinum, P., and Chutimataewin, S. (1987). Modulation of heaptocarcinogenicity of aflatoxin B_1 by the chlorinated insecticide, DDT. *In* "Eicosanoids, Lipid Peroxidation and Cancer" (S. K. Nigam, D. C. H. McBrien, and T. F. Slater, eds.), pp. 327–338. Springer-Verlag, Berlin.

Rossi, L., Ravera, M., Repetti, G., and Santi, L. (1977). Long-term administration of DDT or phenobarbital-Na inWistar rats. *Int. J. Cancer* **19**, 179–185.

Rossi, L., Barbieri, O., Sanguineti, M., Cabral, J. R. P., Bruzzi, P., and Santi, L. (1983). Carcinogenicity study with technical-grade dichlorophenyltrichloroethane and 1,1-dichloro-2,2-bis(p-chlorophenyl)ethylene in hamsters. *Cancer Res.* **43**, 776–781.

Rothe, C. F., Mattson, A. M., Nueslein, R. M., and Hayes, W. J., Jr. (1957). Metabolism of chlorophenothane (DDT): Intestinal lymphatic absorption. *Arch. Ind. Health* **16**, 82–86.

Rourke, A. W., Enroschenko, V. P., and Washburn, L. J. (1991). Protein secretions in mouse uterus after methoxychlor or estradiol exposure. *Reprod. Toxicol.* **5**, 111–114.

Ruch, R. J., Bonney, W. J., Sigler, K., Guan, X., Matesic, D., Schafer, L. D., Dupont, E., and Trosko, J. E. (1994). Loss of gap junctions from DDT-treated rat liver epithelial cells. *Carcinogenesis* **15**, 301–306.

Rumsey, T. S., and Schreiber, E. C. (1969). Excretion of radiocarbon of C-14-labeled 16-*alpha*-dihydroxyprogesterone acetophenide (DHPA) by beef heifers. *J. Agric. Food Chem.* **17**, 1210–1212.

Rybakova, M. N. (1968). The effect of certain pesticides on the hypophysis and its gonadotrophic function. *Gig. Sanit.* **33**, 27–31 (in Russian).

Saito, I., Kawamura, N., Uno, K., Hisanaga, N., Takeucki, Y., Ono, Y., Iwata, M., Gotoh, M., Okutani, H., Matsumoto, T., Fukaya, Y., Yoshitomi, S., and Ohno, Y. (1986). Relationship between chlordane and its metabolites in blood of pest control operators and spraymen. *Int. Arch. Occup. Environ. Health* **58**, 91–97.

Saitoh, K., Shaw, S., and Tilson, H. A. (1986). Noradrenergic influence on the prepulse inhibition of acoustic startle. *Toxicol. Lett.* **34**, 209–216.

Sampson, D. A., Pitas, R. E., and Jensen, R. G. (1980). Effect of chronic ingestion of DDT on physiological and biochemical aspects of fatty acid deficiency. *Lipids* **15**, 815–822.

Sandifer, S. H. (1974). Industrial and agricultural chemicals. *Pediatrics* **53**, 843–844.

Sanyal, S., Agarwal, N. J., and Subrahmanyam, D. (1986). Effect of acute sublethal and chronic administration of DDT (chlorophenotane) on brain lipid metabolism of rhesus monkeys. *Toxicol. Lett.* **34**, 47–54.

Sato, H., Toyoda, K., Furukawa, F., Hasegawa, R., Takahashi, M., and Hayashi, Y. (1987). Subchronic oral toxicity test of dicofol (1,1-bis(*p*-chlorophenyl)-2,2,2-trichloroethanol) as the basis for the design of a long-term carcinogenicity study in B6C3F1 mice. *Eisei Shikensho Hokoku* **105**, 42–45 (in Japanese).

Saxena, S. P., Hare, C., Farooq, A., Murugesan, K., Buckshee, K., and Chandra, J. (1987). DDT and its metabolites in leiomyomatous and normal human uterine tissue. *Arch. Toxicol.* **59**, 453–455.

Schechter, R. D., Stabenfeldt, G. H., Gribble, D. H., and Ling, G. V. (1973). Treatment of Chushing's syndrome in the dog with adrenocorticolytic agent (*o,p'*-DDD). *J. Am. Vet. Med. Assoc.* **162**, 629–639.

Schecter, A., Toniolo, P., Dai, L. C., Thuy, L. T. B., Wolff, M. S. (1997). Blood levels of DDT and breast cancer risk among women living in the North Vietnam. *Arch. Environ. Contam Toxicol.* **33**, 453.

Schmidt, R. (1973). Effect of 1,1,1-trichloro-2,2-bis(*p*-chlorophenyl)ethane (DDT) on the prenatal development of the mouse (under consideration of distribution of tritium-labeled and carbon-14 labeled DDT in pregnant mice). *Biol. Rundsch.* **11**, 316–317 (in German).

Schroeder, G., and Dorozalska, A. (1975). Degradation of DDT and its analogues. *Wiad. Chem.* **29**, 553–565.

Schulte-Hermann, R. (1985). Tumor promotion in liver. *Arch. Toxicol.* **57**, 147–158.

Serrone, D. M., Stein, A. A., and Coulston, F. (1965). Biochemical and electron microscopic changes observed in rats and monkeys medicated orally with methoxychlor. *Toxicol. Appl. Pharmacol.* **7**, 497.

Shabad, L. M., Kolenichenko, T. S., and Nikonova, T. V. (1972). On a possible blastomogenicity of DDT. *Vopr. Pitan.* **30**, 63–66 (in Russian).

Sheehan, H. L., Summers, V. K., and Nichols, J. (1953). DDD therapy in Cushing's syndrome. *Lancet* **1**, 312–314.

Shekhar, P. V. M., Werdell, J., and Basrur, V. S. (1997). Environmental estrogen stimulation of growth and estrogen receptor function in preneoplastic and cancerous human breast cell lines. *J. Natl. Cancer Inst.* **89**, 1774–1782.

Shick, M. (1973). Survival with adrenal carcinoma. *J. Am. Med. Assoc.* **224**, 1763.

Shirasu, Y., Moriya, M., Kato, K., Furuhashi, A., and Kada, T. (1976). Mutagenicity screening of pesticides in the microbial system. *Mutat. Res.* **40**, 19–30.

Shirasu, Y. Moriya, M., Kato, K., Lienard, F., Tezuka, H., Teramoto, S., and Kada, T. (1977). Mutagenicity screening of pesticides and modification products: A basis of carcinogenicity evaluation. *Cold Spring Harbor Conf. Cell Proliferation* **4**, 267–285.

Sieber, S. M. (1976). The lymphatic absorption of *p,p'*-DDT and some structurally-related compounds in the rat. *Pharmacology* **14**, 443–454.

Sieber, S. M., Cohn, V. H., and Wynn, W. T. (1974). The entry of foreign compounds into the thoracic duct lymph of rat. *Xenobiotica* **4**, 265–284.

Sigler, K., and Ruch, R. J. (1993). Enhancement of gap junctional intercellular communication in tumor promer-treated cells by components of green tea. *Cancer Lett.* **69**, 15–19.

Simmons, S. W. (1959). The use of DDT insecticides in human medicine. *In* "DDT: The Insecticide Dichlorodiphenyl-tricloroethane and Its Significance" (P. Müller, ed.), Vol. 2, pp. 251–502. Birhauser, Basel.

Sinsheimer, J. E., Guilford, J., Bobrin, L. D., and Schteingart, D. E. (1972). Identification of *o,p'*-dichloro-diphenylacetic acid as a urinary metabolite of 1-(*o*-chlorophenyl)-I-(*p*-chlorophenyl)-2,2-dichloroethane. *J. Pharm. Sci.* **61**, 314–316.

Skromme-Kadlubik, G., Alvarez-Cervera, J., and Cortes-Marmolejo, F. (1972). Studies of suprarenal scinitgraphy in humans using ^{131}I-DDD. *J. Nucl. Med.* **13**, 282–284.

Skromme-Kadlubik, G., Alvarez-Cervera, J., and Cortes-Marmolejo, F. (1973a). Human suprarenal gammagrams using DDD labeled with I-131. *Arch. Inst. Cardiol. Mex.* **43**, 245–248.

Skromme-Kadlubik, G., Alvarez-Cervera, J., and Cortes-Marmolejo, F. (1973b). Adrenal scanning with dichloro-diphenyl-dichloroethane ^{131}(DDD-^{131}I)—A clinical report on 100 subjects. *Int. J. Nucl. Med. Biol.* **2**, 83–96.

Skromme-Kadlubik, G., Ferez, A., and Celis, C. (1974). Selective atrophy of adrnal cortex by dichloro-diphenyl dichloroethane I-131 (DDD-I-131). *Arch. Inst. Cardiol. Mex.* **44**, 869–873.

Slooten, H. V., Seters, A. P. V., Smeenk, D., and Moolengar, A. J. (1982). *o,p'*-DDD (mitotane) levels in plasma and tissues during chemotherapy and at autopsy. *Cancer Chemother. Pharmacol.* **9**, 85–88.

Smith, A. G. (1991). Chlorinated hydrocarbon insecticides. *In* "Handbook of Pesticide Toxicology," pp. 731–915. Academic Press, San Diego.

Smith, A. G. (2000). How toxic is DDT? *Lancet* **356**, 267–268.

Smith, M. I., and Stohlman, E. F. (1944). The pharmacologic action of 2,2-bis-(*p*-chloropenyl)-1,1,1-trichloroethane and its estimation in the tissues and body fluids. *Public Health Rep.* **59**, 984–993.

Smith, M. I., and Stohlman, E. F. (1945). Further studies on the pharmacologic action of 2,2-bis(*p*-chlorophenyl)-1,1,1-trichloroethane (DDT). *Public Health Rep.* **60**, 289–301.

Smith, M. I., Bauer, H., Stohlman, E. F., and Lillie, R. D. (1946). The pharmacologic action of certain analogues and derivatives of DDT. *J. Pharmacol.* **88**, 359–365.

Smith, R. B., Larson, P. S., Finnegan, J. K., Haag, H. B., Henningar, R. G., and Cobey, F. (1959). Toxicological studies on 2,2-bis(chlorophenyl)-2,2,2-trichloroethanol (Kelthane). *Toxicol. Appl. Pharmacol.* **1**, 119–134.

Sobti, R. C., Krishan, A., and Davies, J. (1983). Cytokinetic and cytogenetic effects of agricultural chemicals on human lymphoid cells *in vitro*. II. Organochlorine pesticides. *Arch. Toxicol.* **52**, 221–231.

Song, J. H., Nagata, K., Tatebayashi, H., and Narahashi, T. (1996). Interactions of tetramethrin, fenvalerate and DDT at the sodium channel in rat dorsal root ganglion neurons. *Brain Res.* **708**, 29–37.

Southern, A. L., Weisenfield, S., Laufer, A., and Goldner, M. G. (1961). Effect of *o,p'*-DDD in a patient with Cushing's syndrome. *J. Clin. Endocrinol. Metab.* **21**, 201–208.

Southern, A. L., Tochimoto, S., Isurugi, K., Gorcher, G. G., Krikum, E., and Stypulkowski, W. (1966a). The effect of 2,2-bis-(2-chlorophenyl-4-chlorophenyl)-1,1,1-dichloroethane (*o,p'*-DDD) on the metabolism of infused cortisol-7-H. *Steroids* **7**, 11–29.

Southern, A. L., Tochimoto, S., Strom, L., Ratuschni, A., Rass, H., and Gorcher, G. (1966b). Remission in Cushing's syndrome with *o,p'*-DDD. *J. Clin. Endocrinol. Metab.* **26**, 268–278.

Speizer, F. W., and Wolff, M. S. (1997). Plasma organochlorine levels and the risk of breast cancer. *New Engl. J. Med.* **337**, 1253–1258.

Spicer, S. S., Sweeney, T. R., von Oettingen, W. F., Lillie, R. D., and Neal, P. A. (1947). Toxicological observations on goats fed large doses of DDT. *Vet. Med. (Prauge)* **42**, 289–293.

Spindler, M. (1983). DDT: Health aspects in relation to man and risk/benefit assessment based thereupon. *Residue Rev.* **90**, 1–34.

Stammers, F. M. G., and Whitfield, F. G. S. (1947). Toxicity of DDT to man and animals. *Bull. Entomol. Res.* **38**, 1–73.

Stein, A. A. (1970). Comparative toxicology of methoxychlor. *In* "Pesticides Symposia" (W. B. B. Diechmann, J. L. Radomski, and R. A. Penalver, eds.). Halos and Associates, Miami, FL.

Stein, A. A., Serrone, D. M., and Coulston, F. (1965). Safety evaluation of methoxychlor in human volunteers. *Toxicol. Appl. Pharmacol.* **7**, 499.

Stevens, M. F., Ebell, G. F., and Psaila-Savona, P. (1993). Organochlorine pesticides in Western Australian nursing mothers. *Med. J. Aust.* **158**, 238–241.

Stohlman, E. F., and Lillie, R. D. (1948). The effect of DDT on the blood sugar and of glucose administration on the acute and chronic poisoning of DDT in rabbits. *J. Pharmacol. Exp. Ther.* **93**, 351–361.

Street, J. C., and Blau, A. D. (1966). Insecticide interactions affecting residue accumulation in animal tissues. *Toxicol. Appl. Pharmacol.* **8**, 497–504.

Stresser, D. M., and Kupfer, D. (1997). Catalytic characteristics of CYP3A4: requirement for a phenolic function in *ortho* hydroxylation of estradiol and mono-*o*-demethylated methoxychlor. *Biochemistry* **36**, 2203–2210.

Stresser, D. M., and Kupfer, D. (1998a). Human cytochrome P450-catalysed conversion of the proestrogenic pesticide methoxychlor into an estrogen. Role of CYP2A and CYP1A2 in *O*-demethylation. *Drug Metab. Disp.* **26**, 868–874.

Stresser, D. M., and Kupfer, D. (1998b). Prosubstrates of CYP3A4, the major human hepatic cytochrome P450: Transformation into substrates by other P450 isoforms. *Biochem. Pharmacol.* **55**, 1861–1871.

Sugie, S., Mori, H., and Takahashi, M. (1987). Efffect of *in vivo* exposure to the liver tumor promoters phenobarbital or DDT on the gap junctions of rat hepatocytes: A quantitative freeze fracture analysis. *Carcinogenesis* **8**, 45–51.

Sundström, G. (1977). Metabolic hydroxylation of the aromatic rings of 1,1-dichloro-2,2-bis(4-chlorophenyl)ethylene (*p*,*p*-DDE) by the rat. *J. Agric. Food Chem.* **25**, 18–21.

Sundström, G., Jansson, B., and Jenson, S. (1975). Structure of phenolic metabolites of *p*,*p*′-DDE in rat, wild seal and guillemot. *Nature (London)* **255**, 627–628.

Swartz, W. J., Wink, C., and Johnson, W. D. (1994). Response of adult marine uterine epithelium to 50% methoxychlor. *Reprod. Toxicol.* **7**, 599.

Szarmach, H., and Poniecka, H. (1973). Contact allergy in agriculture. *Przegl. Dermatol.* **60**, 479–484 (in Polish).

Tabata, K., Mijata, T., and Saito, T. (1979). Water soluble metabolites of dicofol in mouse urine. *Appl. Entomol. Zool.* **14**, 490–493.

Takamatsu, J., Kitazawa, A., Nakata, K., and Furukawa, K. (1981). Does mitotane reduce endogenous ACTH secretion? *N. Engl. J. Med.* **305**, 957.

Taliaferro, I., and Leone, L. (1957). Inhibitory effect of Pethane (2,2-bis-[paraethylphenyl]-1,1-dichloroetane) on adrenocortical function in human subjects. *N. Engl. J. Med.* **257**, 855–860.

Tarján, R., and Kemeny, T. (1969). Multigeneration studies on DDT in mice. *Food Cosmet. Toxicol.* **7**, 215–222.

Tateno, C., Ito, S., Tanaka, M., Oyamada, M., and Yoshitake, A. (1994). Effects of DDT on hepatic gap junctional intercellular communication in rats. *Carcinogenesis* **15**, 517–521.

Tegeris, A. S., Earl, F. L., Smaley, H. E., and Curtis, J. M. (1966). Methoxychlor toxicity. Comparative studies in the dog and swine. *Arch. Environ. Health* **13**, 776–787.

Tegeris, A. S., VanderWeide, G. C., and Curtis, J. M. (1968). Progressive utrastructural changes in the mucosal epithelium of the small intestine of beagle dogs fed methoxychlor. *Exp. Mol. Pathol.* **8**, 243–257.

Telford, H. S., and Guthrie, J. E. (1945). Transmission of the toxicity of DDT through the milk of white rats and goats. *Science* **102**, 647.

Temple, T. E., Jones, D. J., Liddle, G. W., and Dexter, R. N. (1969). Treatment of Cushing's disease: Correction of hypercortisolism by *o*,*p*′-DDD without induction of aldosterone deficiency. *N. Engl. J. Med.* **281**, 801–805.

Terracini, B., Testa, M. C., Cabral, J. R., and Day, N. (1973). The effects of long-term feeding of DDT to BALB/c mice. *Int. J. Cancer* **11**, 747–764.

Thompson, R. P. H., Pilcher, C. W. T., Robinson, J., Stathers, G. M., McLean, A. E. M., and Williams, R. (1969). Treatment of unconjugated jaundice with dicophane. *Lancet* **2**, 4–6.

Thorpe, E., and Walker, A. I. T. (1973). The toxicology of dieldrin (HEIOD). II. Comparative long-term oral toxicity studies in mice with dieldrin, DDT, phenobarbitone, β-BHC and γ-BHC. *Food Cosmet. Toxicol.* **11**, 433–442.

Tiemann, U., Schneider, F., and Tuchsherer, A. (1996). Effects of organochlorine pesticides on DNA synthesis of cultured oviductal and uterine cells and on estrogen receptor of uterine tissue from heifers. *Arch. Toxicol.* **70**, 490–496.

Tilson, H. A., Hong, J. S., and Mactutus, C. F. (1985). Effects of 5,5-diphenylhydantoin (phenytoin) on neurobehavioral toxicity of organochlorine insecticides and permethrin. *J. Pharmacol. Exp. Ther.* **233**, 285–289.

Tilson, H. A., Hudson, P. M., and Hong, S. (1986). 5,5-Diphenylhydantoin antagonizes neurochemical and behaviour effects of *p*,*p*′-DDT but not of chlordecone. *J. Neurochem.* **47**, 1870–1878.

Tinsley, I. J., and Lowry, R. R. (1972). An interaction of DDT in the metabolism of essential fatty acids. *Lipids* **7**, 182–185.

Tomatis, L., Turusov, V., Day, N., and Charles, R. T. (1972). The effect of long-term exposure to DDT on CR-1 mice. *Int. J. Cancer* **10**, 489–506.

Tomatis, L., Turusov, V., Charles, R. T., and Boicchi, M. (1974). Effect of long-term exposure to 1,1-dichloro-2,2-bis(*p*-chlorophenyl)ethylene, to 1,1-dichloro-2,2-bis(*p*-chlorophenyl)ethane, and to the two chemicals combined on CF-1 mice. *J. Natl. Cancer Inst.* **52**, 883–891.

Torda, C., and Wolff, H. G. (1949). Effect of convulsant and anticonvulsant agents on the activity of carbonic anhydrase. *J. Pharmacol. Exp. Ther.* **95**, 444–447.

Törnblom, N. (1959). Administration of DDD (2,2-bis(parachlorophenyl)-1,1-dichloroethane) to diabetics with hyaline vascular changes and hperpolysaccharidemia. *Acta Ned. Scand.* **16**, 23–27.

Touito, Y., Bogdan, A., and Luton, J. P. (1978). Changes in corticosteroid synthesis of the human adrenal cortex *in vitro*, induced by treatment with *o*,*p*′-DDD for Cushing's syndrome: Evidence for the sites of action of the drug. *J. Steroid Biochem.* **9**, 1217–1224.

Touito, Y., Moolenaar, A. J., Bogdan, A., Auzeby, A., and Luton, J. P. (1985). *o*,*p*′-DDD (mitotane) treatment for Cushing's syndrome: Adrenal drug concentration and inhibition *in vitro* of steroid synthesis. *Eur. J. Clin. Pharmacol.* **29**, 483–487.

Treon, J. F., and Cleveland, F. P. (1955). Toxicity of certain chlorinated hydrocarbon insecticides for laboratory animals with special reference to aldrin and dieldrin. *J. Agric. Food. Chem.* **3**, 402–408.

Trifonova, T. K., and Gladenko, I. N. (1980). Determination of gonado- and embyotoxicity of pesticides. *Veterinariya (Kiev)* **6**, 58–59 (in Russian).

Tsushimoto, G., Chang, C. C., Trosko, J. E., and Matsumura, F. (1983). Cytotoxic, mutagenic, and cell–cell communication inhibitory properties of DDT, lindane, and chlordane on Chinese hamster cells *in vitro*. *Arch. Environ. Contam. Toxicol.* **12**, 721–730.

Tsutsui, J., Kato, T., and Nishikawa, T. (1974). Results of health survey on persons engaging in pesticide application in Suzuka area, Mie Pefecture. *J. Jpn. Assoc. Rural Med.* **23**, 518–521 (in Japanese).

Tullner, W. W. (1961). Uterotrophic action of the insecticide methoxychlor. *Science* **133**, 647–648.

Tullner, W. W., and Edgcomb, J. H. (1962). Cystic tubular nephropathy and decrease in testicular weight in rats following oral methoxychlor treatment. *J. Pharmacol. Exp. Ther.* **138**, 126–130.

Unger, M., and Olsen, J. (1980). Organochlorine compounds in the adipose tissue of diseased people with and without cancer. *Environ. Res.* **23**, 257–263.

Unger, M., Keaer, H., Blichert-Toft, M., Olsen, J., and Clausen, J. (1984). Organochlorine compounds in human breast fat from deceased with and without breast cancer and in a biopsy material from newly diagnosed patients undergoing breast surgery. *Environ. Res.* **334**, 24–28.

Vanyurikhina, L. T. (1972). Effect of adrenal cortex function inhibitor clodithane (*o*,*p*′-DDD) on blood serum proteins. *Fiziol. Zh. (Kiev 1955–1977)* **18**, 591–595 (in Russian).

Vaz, A., Pereira, R. S., and Malheiro, D. M. (1945). Calcium in prevention and treatment of experimental DDT poisoning. *Science* **101**, 434–436.

Velbinger, H. H. (1947a). Question of "DDT"-toxicity for humans. *Dtsch. Gesundheitswes.* **2**, 355–358 (in German).

Velbinger, H. H. (1947b). Contribution on the toxicology of DDT-active substances of dichlorodiphenyltrichloromethylmethane. *Pharmazie* **2**, 268–274 (in German).

Verdon, T. A., Bruton, J., Hrman, R. H., and Beisel, W. R. (1962). Clinical and chemical response of functioning adrenal cortical carcinoma to *ortho,para*-DDD. *Metab. Clin. Exp.* **11**, 226–234.

Vogel, E. (1972). Mutagenicity studies with DDT and its metabolites DDE, DDD, DDOM and DDA *in Dropsophila melanogaster. Mutat. Res.* **16**, 157–164.

vom Saal, F. S., Nagel, S. G., Palanza, P., Boechler, M., Parmigiani, S., and Welshons, W. V. (1995). Estrogenic pesticides: Binding relative to estradiol in MCF-7 cells and exposure during fetal life on subsequent territorial behaviour in male mice. *Toxicol. Lett.* **77**, 343–350.

Wagstaff, D. J., and Street, J. C. (1971). Ascorbic acid deficiency and induction of hepatic microsomal hydroxylative enzymes by organochlorine pesticides. *Toxicol. Appl. Pharmacol.* **19**, 10–19.

Walker, A. I. T., Thorpe, E., and Stevenson, D. E. (1973). The toxicology of dieldrin (HEOD). I. Long-term oral toxicity studies in mice. *Food Cosmet. Toxicol.* **11**, 415–432.

Wallace, Z. E., Silverstein, J. N., Villadolid, L. S., and Weisenfeld, S. (1961). Cushing's syndrome due to adrenocortical hyperplasia. *N. Engl. J. Med.* **265**, 1088–1093.

Wärngård, L., Heming, H. J., Flodström, S., Duddy, S. K., and Kass, G. E. N. (1989). Mechanistic studies on the DDT-induced inhibition of intercellular communication. *Carcinogenesis (London)* **10**, 471–476.

Wasicky, R. and Unti, O. (1944). Dichloro-diphenyl trichloroethane (DDT) does not control culicine larvae. *Arh. Hig.* **9**, 87–102.

Wassermann, M., Wassermann, D., Kedar, E., and Djavaherian, M. (1971). Immunological and detoxication interactions in p,p'-DDT fed rabbits. *Bull. Environ. Contam. Toxicol.* **6**, 426–534.

Weisenfeld, S., and Goldner, M. G. (1962). Treatment of advanced malignancy and Cushing's syndrome with DDD. *Cancer Chemother. Rep.* **16**, 335–339.

Welch, R. M., Levin, W., and Conney, A. H. (1969). Estrogenic action of DDT and its analogs. *Toxicol. Appl. Pharmacol.* **14**, 358–367.

Welsh, J. H., and Gordon, H. T. (1946). The mode of action of DDT. *Fed. Proc., Fed. Am. Soc. Exp. Biol.* **5**, 1.

West, T. F., and Campbell, G. A. (1946). "DDT. The Synthetic Insecticide." Chapman and Hall, London.

West, P. R., Chaudhary, S. K., Branton, G. R., and Mitchell, R. H. (1982). High-performance liquid chromatographic analysis of impurities and degradation products of methoxychlor. *J. Assoc. Off. Anal. Chem.* **65**, 1457–1470.

White, W. C., and Sweeney, T. R. (1945). The metabolism of 2,2-bis(p-chlorophenyl)-1,1,1-trichlorophenyl)-acetic acid; its isolation, identification, and synthesis. *Public Health Rep.* **60**, 66–71.

Wigglesworth, V. B. (1945). A case of DDT poisoning in man. *Br. Med. J.* **1**, 517.

Wilcox, A. R. (1967). "USPH Investigation-DDT Health Effects." Inter-office correspondence to M. V. Anthony, Stauffer Chemical Co.

Williams, G. M., and Numoto, S. (1984). Promotion of mouse liver neoplasms by the organochlorine pesticides chlordane and heptachlor in comparison to dichlorodiphenyltrichloroethane. *Carcinogenesis (London)* **5**, 1689–1696.

Williams, G. M., Telang, S., and Tong, C. (1981). Inhibition of intercellular communication between liver cells by the liver tumor promoter 1,1,1-trichloro-2,2-bis(p-chlorophenyl)ethane. *Cancer Lett.* **11**, 339–344.

Wilson, H. F., Allen, N. N., Bohstedt, G., Betheil, J., and Lardy, H. A. (1946). Feeding experiments with DDT-treated pea vine silage with special reference to dairy cows, sheep, and laboratory animals. *J. Econ. Entomol.* **39**, 801–806.

Wolfe, H. R., and Armstrong, J. F. (1971). Exposure of formulating plant workers to DDT. *Arch. Environ. Health* **23**, 169–176.

Wolfe, H. R., Walker, K. C., Elliott, J. W., and Durham, W. F. (1959). Evaluation of the health hazards involved in house spraying with DDT. *Bull. WHO* **20**, 1–14.

Wolff, M. S., Toniolo, P. G., Lee, E. W., Rivera, M., and Dublin, N. (1993). Blood levels of organochlorine residues and risk of breast cancer. *J. Natl. Cancer Inst.* **85**, 648–652.

Wolff, M. S. (1995). Pesticides-how research has succeeded and failed in informing policy: DDT and the link with breast cancer. *Environ. Health Perspect.* **103**, 87–91.

Wong, O., Brocker, W., Davis, H. V., and Nagle, G. S. (1984). Mortality of workers potentially exposed to organic and inorganic brominated chemicals, DBCP, TRIS, PBB and DDT. *Br. J. Ind. Med.* **41**, 15–24.

Woodard, G., Ofner, R. R., and Montgomery, C. M. (1945). Accumulation of DDT in body fat and its appearance in the milk of dogs. *Science* **102**, 177–178.

Woodard, B. T., Ferguson, B. B., and Wilson, D. J. (1976). DDT levels in milk of rural indigent blacks. *Am. J. Dis. Child.* **130**, 400–403.

Woolley, D. E. (1982). Neurotoxicity of DDT and possible mechanisms of action. *In* "Mechanisms of Action of Neurotoxic Substances" (K. Pradad and A. Vernadakis, eds.), pp. 95–141. Raven, New York.

Woolley, D. E. (1985). Application of neurophysiological techniques to toxicological problems: An overview. *Fundam. Appl. Toxicol.* **5**, 1–8.

World Health Organization (WHO) (1971). "The place of DDT in operations against malaria and other vector borne diseases. *In* "Official Records of the World Health Organization, No 190, Executive Board Forty-Seventh Session. Part II. Report on the Proposed Program and Budget Estimates for 1971," Appendix 14, pp. 176–182. World Health Organ., Geneva.

World Health Organization (WHO) (1973). "Safe Use of Pesticides. Twentieth Report of the WHO Expert Committee on Insecticides," Tech. Rep. Ser. No 513, World Health Organ., Geneva.

World Health Organization (WHO) (1979). "Environmental Health Criteria 9. DDT and Its Derivatives," United National Environment Programme and the World Health Organization, Geneva.

Wrenn, T. R., Randall, J., Weyant, R., Fries, G. F., and Bitman, J. (1971a). Influence of dietary o,p'-DDT on reproduction and lactation of ewes. *J. Anim. Sci.* **33**, 1288–1292.

Wrenn, T. R., Weyant, J. R., Fries, G. F., and Bitman, J. (1971b). Effect of several dietary levels of o,p'-DDT on reproduction and lactation in the rat. *Bull. Environ. Contam. Toxicol.* **6**, 471–479.

Yoder, J. M., Watson, M., and Benson, W. W. (1973). Lympocyte chromosome analysis of agricultural workers during extensive occupational exposure to pesticides. *Mutat. Res.* **21**, 335–340.

You, L., Casanova, M., Archibque-Engle, S., Madhabananda, S., Fan, L., and Heck, H d'A. (1998). Impaired male sexual development in perinatal Sprague–Dawley and Long–Evans Hooded rats exposed *in utero* and lactationally to p,p'-DDE. *Toxicol. Sci.* **45**, 162–173.

Zaidi, S. S. A. (1987). Possible role of rat liver NADPH cytochrome P-450 reductase in the detoxication of DDT to DDD. *Bull. Environ. Contamin. Toxicol.* **39**, 327–333.

Zeidler, O. (1874). Compounds of chloral with bromo- and chlorobenzene. *Ber. Dtsch. Chem. Ges.* **7**, 1180–1181 (in German).

Zein-el-Dine, K. (1946). The insecticide DDT. *J. Egypt. Med. Assoc.* **29**, 38–54.

Zhou, L. X., Dehal, S. S., Kupfer, D., Morell, S., McKenzie, B. A., Eccleston, E. D., and Holtzman, J. L. (1995). Cytochrome P450 catalysed covalent binding of methoxychlor to rat, hepatic, microsomal iodothyronine $5'$-monodeiodinase, type I. Does exposure to methoxychlor disrupt thyroid hormone metabolism? *Arch. Biochem. Biophys.* **322**, 390–394.

Ziem, G. (1982). Aplastic anaemia after methoxychlor exposure. *Lancet* **2**, 1349.

Zimmerman, B., Bloch, H. S., Williams, W. L., Hitchcock, C. R., and Hoeischer, B. (1956). Effects of DDT (1,1, dichloro-2,2-bis(p-chloro-phenyl)-ethane) on human adrenal. Attempt to use adrenal destructive agent in treatment of disseminated mammary and prostatic cancer. *Cancer (Philadelphia)* **9**, 940–948.

Zolotnikova, G. P., and Somov, B. A. (1978). On the role of pesticides in the occurrence of occupational dermatitis in workers of hothouses. *Vestn. Dermatol. Venerol.* **4**, 76–79 (in Russian).

Zumoff, B. (1979). The hypouricemic effect of o,p-DDD. *Am. J. Med. Sci.* **278**, 145–147.

Inorganic and Organometal Pesticides

Thomas W. Clarkson
University of Rochester

There are at least 18 elements that characterize one or more inorganic pesticides. Of these elements, 10 (chromium, copper, zinc, phosphorus, sulfur, tin, arsenic, selenium, fluorine, and chlorine) have been shown to be essential for normal growth. In these instances, the toxic effects clearly do not depend on the element *per se* but on the specific properties of one form of the element or one of its compounds, or merely on an inordinately high dosage. The other eight elements (barium, cadmium, mercury, thallium, lead, bismuth, antimony, and boron) have not been shown to be essential to growth of animals, although there is evidence that some may be. In any event, experience has shown that toxicity is not an argument against essentiality. Some highly toxic elements such as iron, selenium, arsenic, and fluorine certainly are essential to normal development.

In the following sections, representative inorganic pesticides are arranged with reference to the periodic classification of the elements. In some instances this has involved sequential consideration of the members of a periodic group, such as the halides. In other instances, a series of elements, such as the heavy metals, have been considered in the order of their atomic numbers. This arrangement of the elements helps to explain the chemistry and toxicology of.their compounds.

A final section deals with boron because the compounds involved are not important either as pesticides or as toxicants for mammals, or for both reasons.

The organometals and organometalloids are described along with the corresponding inorganic compounds. Such organic forms involve a stable covalent bond between the metal and carbon atoms, such as in methyl mercury compounds, and should be distinguished from compounds with ionic linkages to the organic moiety, such as in mercuric acetate, which are classified as inorganic compounds of the metal or metalloid. The organic species generally differ from the inorganic species in terms of kinetics, absorption, distribution, and excretion. The nature of their toxic effects may also differ markedly except for those organic species that are rapidly metabolized to the inorganic form in the body.

61.1 BARIUM

Barium is an alkaline earth metal in the same group as magnesium, calcium, strontium, and radium. Its valence is 2. All water- and acid-soluble compounds of this element are poisonous. The intravenous LD 50 values of three of these compounds expressed as Ba^{2+} in two strains of mice ranged from 8.12 to 23.31 mg/kg, the toxicity being approximately the same as that of magnesium and greater than that of strontium (Syed and Hosain, 1972).

61.1.1 BARIUM CARBONATE

61.1.1.1 Identity, Properties, and Uses

Chemical Name　Barium carbonate.

Structure　$BaCO_3$.

Synonyms　Barium carbonate occurs in nature as the mineral witherite. A code designation for commercial barium carbonate is C.L-77,099. The CAS registry no. is 513-77-9.

Physical and Chemical Properties　Barium carbonate has the empirical formula $CBaO_3$ and a molecular weight of 197.37. It is a tasteless, odorless, heavy white powder with a density of 4.2865. At about 1300°C it decomposes into BaO and CO_2. Its vapor pressure is negligible. Barium carbonate is almost insoluble in water. It is slightly soluble (1:1000) in water saturated with carbon dioxide, soluble in dilute hydrochloric or nitric acid or in acetic acid, and soluble in solutions of ammonium chloride nitrate.

Formulations and Uses　Barium carbonate is a rat poison. It also is used in ceramics, paints, enamels, rubber, and certain plastics. The technical product is 98–99% pure. Rodenticidal baits contain 20–25% of the compound.

61.1.1.2 Toxicity to Laboratory Animals

Basic Findings The oral LD 50 of a suspension of barium carbonate for wild Norway rats is 1480 mg/kg. The animals survive 1–8.5 days (Dieke and Richter, 1946). Strain differences in LD 50 values have been reported in mice (Syed and Hosain, 1972).

Apparently no study has been made of the effects of repeated doses of barium carbonate. However, the much more soluble and somewhat more toxic barium chloride has been studied. Rabbits given subcutaneous doses at rates as high as 10 mg/kg per day showed no clinical effects. Rabbits given two daily doses at the rate of 10 mg/kg developed weakness, urination, defecation, difficult breathing, bradycardia, extrasystoles, and other signs lasting 2–4 hr following each dose (Fazekas, 1968).

Absorption, Distribution, Metabolism, and Excretion Barium carbonate is highly insoluble in water. It is partially solubilized by acid in the stomach. The only real danger of the rodenticide is through ingestion. Various barium compounds can cause pneumoconiosis, but no form of poisoning by barium has been of much significance in industry.

Information is lacking on the gastrointestinal absorption of barium carbonate. Barium given orally as barium chloride is absorbed about 10 times (63–84%) more in younger rats than in mature animals (7%) (Taylor et al., 1962). Mature dogs also absorb about 7% (Cuddihy and Griffith, 1972).

Several animal studies suggest that barium is incorporated into the bone matrix in a fashion similar to calcium (Bauer et al., 1956; Bligh and Taylor, 1963; Dencker et al., 1976; Taylor et al., 1962). The uptake into bone decreases with age of the animal.

Study of rats injected intraperitoneally with ^{140}Ba indicated that excretion was most rapid during the first 4 hr and reached 7% in the urine and 20% in the feces in 24 hr (Bauer et al., 1956).

Experiments in dogs showed that barium can be actively reabsorbed by the kidney tubules. Its clearance was correlated with calcium clearance. Protein binding of barium averaged 54% and was of the same order of magnitude as that of other alkaline earths. The data did not exclude a common transport mechanism with calcium (Rahill and Walser, 1965).

Mode of Action Barium stimulates striated, cardiac, and smooth muscle, regardless of innervation. It is antagonistic to all muscle depressants, no matter whether they act primarily on nerve or muscle. Initial stimulation of contraction leads to vasoconstriction through direct action on arterial muscle, peristalsis through action on smooth muscle, tremors and cramps through action on the skeletal muscles, and various arrhythmias through action on the heart. If the dose is sufficient, stimulation is followed by weakness and eventually by paralysis of the different kinds of muscle. Some effects such as hypertension, violent tremors, and convulsions are uncommon following ingestion of barium carbonate. They are more likely to follow absorption of more soluble barium compounds. If death does

occur, it is caused by failure of muscular contraction leading to respiratory failure or cardiovascular collapse (Sollmann, 1957).

Several studies on animals exposed to barium compounds by parenteral routes indicate that barium decreases serum potassium concentrations. These experiments support findings from a human case study that hypokalemia is an important effect of acute barium toxicity [Agency for Toxic Substances and Disease Registry (ATSDR), 1992a].

61.1.1.3 Toxicity to Humans

Experimental Exposure A solution of ^{140}BaCl$_2$ was injected intramuscularly into five children and intravenously into two adults, all with normal skeletal metabolism. Three of the children and one adult also received ^{45}CaCl$_2$ in the same injection. The pattern of excretion of calcium was similar, but both the initial and final rates were slower. Bone took up barium more rapidly than calcium under the same conditions, but, because of the more rapid excretion of barium, less of it was available to the bone. However, skeletal metabolism of the two elements was closely similar.

Therapeutic Use Barium carbonate has no therapeutic uses.

Accidental Poisoning Apparently the major accident involving barium carbonate was one in which 85 British soldiers were poisoned by eating pastry made from flour accidentally contaminated by the compound intended for use as rat poison. The clinical picture was basically the same in all patients. In spite of some individual variation, three poorly defined stages could be recognized: (1) an acute gastroenteritis with mild sensory disturbance, (2) loss of deep reflexes and the onset of muscle paralysis, and (3) progressive muscular paralysis.

Often improvement in all affected systems began 3–4 hr after onset, and recovery was complete within 24–36 hr. Only a few of the most severely affected patients proceeded to the third stage. In these few, general muscle paralysis began on the second day of the illness and lasted for a further 24 hr. There was complete muscle paralysis of arms and legs, and in one case the paralysis affected the muscles of respiration, but function of the diaphragm was sufficiently spared that the patient survived. Even these dangerously ill patients remained mentally clear, and recovery was surprisingly rapid; by the fourth day all affected muscles had regained their full power. There were no deaths.

Many of the patients with severe early diarrhea recovered much more rapidly than those with delayed bowel action (Morton, 1945).

The clinical findings in other outbreaks were generally similar. Additional signs and symptoms included thirst, sweating, blurred vision, a desire to urinate, and a moderately increased blood pressure (Dean, 1950; Lewi and Bar-Khayim, 1964). Electrocardiographic changes considered characteristic of hypokalemia have also been reported (Diengott et al., 1964). Chronic effects in humans have not been well studied. All epidemiological studies have suffered from numerous limitations

(Brenniman and Levy, 1985; Brenniman *et al.*, 1979; Elwood *et al.*, 1974; Schroeder and Kraemer, 1974).

Dosage Response When barium carbonate was mistakenly used as X-ray contrast medium, six patients survived 133 g each (about 1900 mg/kg) but another died after only 53 g. The author cited earlier reports indicating that as little as 4 g (about 57 mg/kg) has proved fatal (Dean, 1950). However, such incidents must be rare, for in one large outbreak with no deaths among 85 cases, it was estimated, on the basis of analysis of the contaminated food, that the most severe cases received about 15 g of barium carbonate (about 214 mg/kg). This rate is less than the LD 50 for the rat but sufficient to kill some rats. It seems likely that vomiting is important in protecting people who ingest barium carbonate.

Although the calculation must be viewed with caution, one might (by taking the ratio of the LD 50 values into account) conclude that a dosage of 28 mg/kg/day for barium carbonate is equivalent to what many years ago was a usual but often toxic dosage of 1.7 mg/kg/day for barium chloride.

The permissible occupational intake of soluble barium salts (as Ba^{2+}) is 0.07 mg/kg/day.

Laboratory Findings Hypokalemia may occur in severe poisoning. Apparently there is no report of the concentration of barium in a case of poisoning.

Following a single substantial dose, barium is deposited in bone (Bauer *et al.*, 1957). However, under practical conditions it does not act as a bone seeker. The concentration in normal human bone ash is only 7 ppm compared to average concentrations of 2.3–28 ppm in the ash of different organs (Snowden and Stitch, 1957; Snowden, 1958). Tipton and Cook (1963) reported that (except for skin, lung, and intestine, which may be environmentally exposed) the median value for barium in tissue ash did not exceed 7 ppm in the United States. Much higher concentrations of barium usually are found in Africa, the Near East, and the Far East (Tipton *et al.*, 1965). On a wet weight basis, the concentration of barium in normal plasma does not exceed 0.44 ppm (Gofman *et al.*, 1964).

Treatment of Poisoning Emptying of the stomach by vomiting or gastric lavage should be followed by sodium or magnesium sulfate (30 g). These compounds act not only as purgatives but as detoxifying antidotes because they precipitate the toxic barium ion as insoluble barium sulfate. On the basis of both experimental studies and clinical experience, Lydtin *et al.* (1965) recommended that magnesium sulfate and calcium chloride be administered intravenously as early as possible in barium intoxication. They found this treatment effective even when administered several hours after intake of the poison.

The fluid and salt balance should be followed with particular attention to potassium and replacement therapy carried out as required. Be sure to have a respirator available. It may be lifesaving.

61.2 CHROMIUM

Chromium is a metal somewhat like iron and separated from it in the periodic table only by manganese. Chromium has valences of 2, 3, and 6, but only hexavalent chromium compounds (chromates) are important as pesticides. They are also the most toxic.

Chromium in its trivalent state is an essential element. It is thought to be a necessary part of the glucose tolerance factor of the liver and required for certain other aspects of carbohydrate metabolism (Mertz, 1967).

61.2.1 SODIUM DICHROMATE

61.2.1.1 Identity, Properties, and Uses

Chemical Name Sodium dichromate.

Structure $Na_2Cr_2O_7 \cdot 2H_2O$.

Synonyms Other names for the compound are bichromate of soda and sodium bichromate. The CAS registry no. is 10588-01-9.

Physical and Chemical Properties Anhydrous sodium dichromate has the empirical formula $Cr_2Na_2O_7$ and a molecular weight of 261.96. The dihydrate forms reddish to bright orange elongated prismatic crystals with a density of 2.348 at 25°C. The anhydrous salt melts at 356.7°C and begins to decompose at about 400°C. It is very soluble in water.

Use Sodium dichromate is used as a defoliant of cotton and other plants and as a wood preservative.

61.2.1.2 Toxicity to Laboratory Animals

Basic Findings The lethal intravenous dosages of sodium dichromate for several species are in the range 37–417 mg/kg. The toxicity of the potassium salt is of the same order of magnitude and its lethal oral dosage for the dog is 2829 mg/kg (Spector, 1955). Although one report (Schroeder, 1973) indicated that prolonged administration of 5 ppm hexavalent chromium in drinking water produced a slight decrease in growth, other studies indicate that concentrations up to 10,000 ppm may be given without ill effect (Gross and Heller, 1946; MacKenzie *et al.*, 1958).

The National Toxicology Testing Program (NTP, 1996a, b) found no adverse effects in rats given potassium dichromate in feed for 9 weeks at a dosage rate of about 2 mg Cr/kg/day. An evaluation of animal toxicity data (ATSDR, 2000) indicates few adverse effects from chromium VI compounds have been detected at oral dosage rates below 1 mg Cr/kg/day even for long-term exposures.

Absorption, Distribution, Metabolism, and Excretion Little information is available on the kinetics of disposition of chromium compounds in experimental animals. Chromate is absorbed by the lung (Baetjer *et al.*, 1959), gastrointestinal tract (MacKenzie *et al.*, 1959; Ogawa, 1976), and skin (Wahlberg, 1965). It can also be absorbed from skin injured by it, and when the burn covers as much as 10% of the body surface the absorption may be sufficient to cause fatal poisoning.

Highest tissues levels are found in kidney and liver (MacKenzie *et al.*, 1958). In rats and hamsters fed chromium compounds, fecal excretion of chromium was in the range 97–99% of the administered dose. Urinary excretion of chromium varied from 0.6 to 1.4% of the dose whether given as chromium III or VI (Donaldson and Barreras, 1966; Henderson *et al.*, 1979; Sayato *et al.*, 1980).

Effects on Organs and Tissues   Acute poisoning may produce death rapidly through shock or after several days through renal tubular damage and uremia. In most cases, the primary effect of acute exposure is kidney failure (Evan and Dail, 1974; Mathur *et al.*, 1977). Berry *et al.* (1978) noted that chromium was localized within the proximal renal tubules specifically within the lysosomes. It was retained throughout the study period of 8 months and was eliminated only when the entire cytoplasm underwent necrosis. Kirschbaum *et al.* (1981) have postulated that the initial effect is on specific elements of the microfilamentous system that is responsible for directing intracellular flow of reabsorbed solutes. The liver and other organs may be involved but generally to a lesser degree.

No evidence of carcinogenicity was found in mice given potassium chromate (mg Cr/kg/day) in drinking water for three generations (Borneff *et al.*, 1968).

61.2.1.3 Toxicity to Humans

Use Experience   Significant injury to the liver, gastrointestinal system, and blood has been reported rarely in connection with industrial exposure. However, many cases of industrial injury to the skin and to the nasal and respiratory mucous membranes have been produced by hexavalent chromium compounds (Browning, 1969). A small part of this involved chromates intended for use in pesticides. Contact dermatitis was reported in men who handled timber treated with chromium (Behrbohm, 1957).

Occupational exposure to a variety of chromium VI compounds has been associated with an increased risk of bronchiogenic and nasal cancers (for a review, see ATSDR, 2000). There is now sufficient evidence to classify chromium VI as a human carcinogen according to the definitions of the International Agency for Research on Cancer (IARC, 1980).

There is no evidence that the use of chromates as wood preservatives offers any hazard of cancer.

Dosage Response   Judging from urinary excretion, absorption of chromium at a rate of not less than 0.02 mg/kg/day led to serious illness; twice that rate of absorption also produced liver injury in other workers, although no symptoms appeared. A ceiling concentration in the working atmosphere of 100 μg

Cr(VI) per cubic meter has been recommended [Occupational Safety and Health Administration (OSHA), 1998].

Laboratory Findings   Chromium can be detected in almost every sample of normal tissue. For most organs, the median value for concentration is close to the limits of detection. For example, the median concentration in the liver ash is 0.7 ppm or about 0.009 ppm, wet weight. The concentration in plasma does not exceed 0.04 ppm (Gofman *et al.*, 1964). The lung and skin, however, have median concentrations in the order of 0.17 and 0.22 ppm, wet weight, presumably because of their direct exposure to contamination. Most investigators have found similar results in the United States (Tipton and Cook, 1963).

Investigations by Guthrie *et al.* (1978), Kayne *et al.* (1978), and Andersen (1981) indicate that measurements of chromium by atomic absorption in normal blood and urine before 1978 were probably too high due to inadequate background correction. Mean or median normal levels in the general population with ranges in parentheses are as follows (ATSDR, 2000): serum 0.006 μg/l (0.1–0.17 μg/l); urine 0.4 μg/l (0.24–1.8); hair 0.234 mg/g (not available); and breast milk 0.30 μg/l (0.06–1.56).

Treatment of Poisoning   Chromium is chelated by dimercaprol and by calcium disodium edetate, of which the latter is preferred (Hayes, 1975). Otherwise treatment is symptomatic (Hayes, 1975). Chelating agents are also valuable for treating chrome ulcers of the skin. A 10% calcium disodium edetate ointment was effective in treating all of 54 chrome skin ulcers. In about 90% of cases, the complex chrome salts adherent to the base of the ulcer could be removed painlessly after the ointment had been applied for 24 hr. In the remaining cases, removal of the adherent chrome could be carried out after 48 or at most 72 hr. Once its base had been cleared of chrome salts, the ulcer healed promptly (Maloof, 1955).

61.3 COPPER

Copper compounds are not an important source of poisoning [for a general review, see U.S. Environmental Protection Agency (U.S. EPA, 1987)]. With few exceptions, those used as pesticides owe their mammalian toxicity to a massive overdose of copper ions, especially the cupric ion. Because many of the compounds do not dissolve readily, their toxicity is low. However, copper sulfate is a soluble, ionizable compound. It has been the cause of the majority of cases of poisoning involving copper compounds, and its effects are typical of those involving an excess of copper ions.

The toxicities of copper acetoarsenite and copper arsenate are related to their arsenic content (see Section 61.12).

Copper is an essential element. It is closely associated with the absorption and metabolism of iron. Zinc and molybdenum also interact with copper. Copper is necessary for the formation of hemoglobin, although it is not part of the molecule. When copper is deficient, hemoglobin is not formed at the normal rate even though there is a reserve of iron in the liver. Copper is also required for bone formation. The element is also essential for carbohydrate metabolism, catecholamine biosynthesis, and the cross-linking of collagen, elastin, and hair keratin. Copper is an integral part of more than 12 specific proteins, including cytochrome oxidase, tyrosinase, ascorbic acid oxidase, uricase, catalase, and peroxidase.

Deficiency of copper occurs occasionally in domestic animals and is easily produced experimentally. Signs of copper deficiency include anemia, gastrointestinal disturbances, depressed growth, dystrophy of bone, depigmentation of hair or wool, impaired reproduction, and heart failure (Underwood, 1977). Copper deficiency has not been described in humans, probably because adequate copper occurs in such a wide variety of human food.

Many vegetables, cereals, and meats contain between 1 and 10 ppm of copper, but liver contains about 24 ppm and oysters about 36 ppm. The normal dietary intake of copper usually does not exceed 5 mg/day but usually does exceed 2 mg/day (Davies and Bennett, 1983). Kehoe *et al.* (1940) reported an average intake of 2.32 mg/day. Additional intake such as that from occupational exposure leads to little increase in the retention of copper. Drinking water is not an important source of copper except in rare cases where soft water has been contained in copper piping for long periods (Piscator, 1979). The existence of a hereditary disease (hepatolenticular degeneration or Wilson's disease) characterized by abnormal absorption and retention of copper from a normal diet calls attention to the precision with which copper metabolism is regulated in healthy persons. Some information on the concentration of copper in different normal tissues is given in Section 61.3.1.3.

61.3.1 COPPER SULFATE

61.3.1.1 Identity, Properties, and Uses

Chemical Name   Cupric sulfate.

Structure $CuSO_4$.

Synonyms   Copper sulfate also is known as blue copperas, bluestone, blue vitrol, Roman vitrol, and Salzburg vitrol. It occurs in nature as the mineral hydrocyanite. The CAS registry no. is 7758-98-7.

Physical and Chemical Properties   Copper sulfate occurs as the anhydride, a monohydrate, and, the pentahydrate, which is the form used as a fungicide or algicide. The molecular weight for the anhydride is 159.61, and that for the pentahydrate is 267.6. The pentahydrate forms a blue, crystalline, odorless solid with a metallic taste. It occurs in nature as the mineral chalcanthite. Its density at 15.6°C is 2.286. Most formulations of copper sulfate contain 98–99% pure salt. The compound is soluble in water (316 g/l at 0°C) but insoluble in ethanol and most organic solvents. Copper sulfate solutions are strongly corrosive

to iron and galvanized iron. The crystals are slightly efflorescent in air.

History, Formulations, and Uses   The fungicidal activity of soluble copper salts was discovered in 1807 by B. Prévost. The algicidal properties of the salts came into practical use about 1895. Copper sulfate is used as a fungicide for control of downy mildew, blights, leaf spots, apple scab, bitter rot, and peachleaf curl. It also is used as an herbicide for the control of algae in water. Copper compounds are also used as algicides and insecticides. Products containing copper compounds are frequently used with other chemicals. Bordeaux mixture, formed from $CuSO_4$ and $Ca(OH)_2$, is used as a fungicide and seed treatment.

61.3.1.2 Toxicity to Laboratory Animals

Basic Findings   The oral LD 50 of copper sulfate for the rat is 960 mg/kg (Stokinger, 1981) and in mice is 87 mg/kg (Jones *et al.*, 1980). The reason for large species differences is not known. Poisoned animals show violent retching, muscular spasms, and collapse. The onset is within a few minutes of dosing, and many rats die within an hour. However, some survive the gastrointestinal irritation only to die several days later of systemic effects (Lehman, 1951, 1952).

Rats fed copper sulfate for 4 weeks at a dietary level of 500 ppm as copper (about 25 mg/kg/day) showed slightly decreased food intake and a slight decrease in growth rate but appeared entirely normal. Higher dietary levels of copper led to progressively greater food refusal. Rats fed 4000 ppm ate less than one-fifth the normal amount of food, lost weight, and died within a week. Part of their trouble was starvation, for they ingested less copper (7.6 mg/rat/day) than rats that survived 4 weeks when fed 2000 ppm (9.8–11.8 mg/rat/day) (Boyden *et al.*, 1938). Pigs maintained on diets supplemented with copper sulfate (250–425 ppm) for 48–79 days exhibited a gradual development of anemia, jaundice, hepatic necrosis, gastrointestinal hemorrhage, and decreased weight gain (Suttle and Mills, 1966a, b). Pigs exposed to 100–500 ppm of copper ulfate in the diet for 54–88 days experienced reductions in hemoglobin and hematocrit and reduced weight gain (Kline *et al.*, 1971). Lifetime exposure of mice to copper gluconate in drinking water (42.4 mg Cu/kg/day) resulted in a 13% decrease in maximal life span from 986 to 874 days (Massie and Aiella, 1984).

Two inhalation studies (Johansson *et al.*, 1984; Lundborg and Camner, 1984) found no toxic effects in the lungs of rabbits exposed to 0.6 mg/m^3 of copper chloride 6 hr/day, 5 days/week for up to 6 weeks. Pimentel and Marques (1969) exposed 12 guinea pigs to a saturated atmosphere of Bordeaux mixture for 6.5 months, three times daily (the duration of each exposure was not reported), and found micronodular lesions and hystiocytic granulomas. In a brief report, Eckert and Jerochin (1982) claim that copper sulfate is the principal toxic agent in Bordeaux mixtures.

Absorption, Distribution, Metabolism, and Excretion   Copper absorption after an oral dose occurs in the upper gastrointestinal tract in mammals (Evans, 1973). Two mechanisms are involved. One is an energy-dependent process involving copper–amino acid complexes (Kirchgessner *et al.*, 1967) and the other involves an inducible carrier protein (Evans and Johnson, 1978). The gastrointestinal absorption of copper is affected by several factors: (1) competition with other metals; (2) the amount of copper ingested; (3) certain dietary components such as phytates and fiber; and (4) the chemical form of copper (for details, see ATSDR, 1990).

Absorbed copper is predominantly bound to albumin and is transported to the liver, which is the main storage organ. Copper is incorporated into a number of enzymes. It is secreted in bile and also incorporated into ceruloplasm, an alpha globulin that accounts for about 90% of all copper in plasma. Ceruloplasmin is a major regulator of copper retention and storage. The major route of excretion is the feces via secretion in bile. Urinary excretion is a minor route (Underwood, 1977).

Mode of Action   The corrosive effect of large doses of copper sulfate in the gastrointestinal tract leads to shock, which may be the cause of death. Damage to the erythrocytes, liver, and kidney may combine to kill patients who survive the initial effects. The biochemical mechanism of excessive doses of copper is not well understood.

61.3.1.3 Toxicity to Humans

Therapeutic Use   Copper sulfate (300 mg in 100 ml of water) has been used as an emetic in cases of known or suspected poisoning by other compounds. If vomiting did not occur, intestinal colic, diarrhea, and systemic symptoms often appeared (Sollmann, 1957).

Accidental and Intentional Poisoning   At least until recently, practically all systemic illness attributed to copper sulfate was the result of accidental or suicidal ingestion. Although such acute poisoning is uncommon in the United States, it is common in some countries (Chawla and Mehta, 1973).

The corrosive action of the copper may produce a characteristic stain of the mucous membranes of the mouth and pharynx and will certainly produce severe painful gastrointestinal irritation, nausea, and diarrhea. The repeated vomiting of blue-green masses is common. The stools are profuse and watery at first and later contain blood. Patients often die in shock 2 or 3 hours after ingestion of the poison. If they survive, the absorption of copper produces severe hemolysis so that hemoglobinuria and anemia are present in 5–6 hours, and icterus appears soon after. If the patient survives a few days, signs of liver damage and renal tubular damage may appear. A fatal case was described in detail by Chugh *et al.* (1975). In one series of cases, 11 of 29 patients developed acute renal failure. Intravascular hemolysis appeared to be the chief factor responsible for the renal lesions. Although uremia was controlled adequately by dialysis, only 6 of the 11 patients recovered. Septicemia was responsible for

death in 3, hepatic failure in 1, and methemoglobinemia in another (Chugh *et al.*, 1977). Katoh *et al.* (1977) reported a case that was typical in showing the usual initial signs followed by severe anemia, icterus, and kidney failure but very unusual in that the patient died after surviving 40 days.

A disease known as Indian childhood cirrhosis has been associated with high intakes of copper (Sharda, 1984). The disease is characterized by hepatic necrosis, Mallory's hyaline inclusions in many hepatocytes, intralobular fibrosis, and very high copper content in liver (Pundit and Bhave, 1983). It is generally believed that water and milk stored in copper or brass vessels lead to high intakes in children.

Use Experience   Ordinary occupational exposure may lead to an itching, papulovesicular eczema. Contact with the eye by copper sulfate dust or even strong solutions may produce conjunctivitis or ulceration of the cornea.

Two cases of pneumoconiosis were described in sprayers who had applied Bordeaux mixture to vineyards for several years. Symptoms included shortness of breath, weakness, loss of weight, and cough productive of a thick, yellow sputum. Although no tubercle bacilli were found, tuberculosis was diagnosed on the basis of diffusely abnormal chest X-rays. In hospital, both patients improved slowly, both clinically and radiologically. However, recovery was incomplete, and symptoms recurred as soon as the men were reexposed to Bordeaux mixture spray (Pimentel and Marques, 1969). The account indicated that the condition responded to cessation of exposure and may have been improved by rest, but there was no evidence that drugs intended for tuberculosis are beneficial against copper pneumoconiosis. Later study showed that some patients presented not with characteristic respiratory symptoms but with chills, fever, joint and muscular pain, weakness, and/or anorexia that became severe enough to cause hospitalization only 2 or 3 weeks after onset. Although no pathological organism was identified, it was assumed that persons suffering from vineyard sprayer's lung were unusually susceptible to infection. Regardless of the exact mechanism, the condition certainly was the cause of death in many in whom it was recognized (Pimentel and Menezes, 1975, 1976). Apparently no evaluation of the hazard of using Bordeaux mixture sprays has been made. One paper (Pimentel and Menezes, 1976) was based on 30 autopsies, but there was no indication of the size of the population of workers with similar exposure from whom this sample was drawn. Be that as it may, it is astonishing that so serious a disease was recognized so recently in connection with a kind of occupational exposure that began in 1882. In fact the recent recognition of the condition and the restricted geographical distribution of cases recognized so far forces one to consider the possibility that some unrecognized factor may be critical to development of the condition. Epidemiological study certainly is needed.

Dosage Response   The fatal dose tor humans is difficult to estimate because of vomiting, but it is about 10 g for adults or

140 mg/kg. This estimate of the fatal ingested dosage is not inconsistent with the observed fatal retained dosage mentioned earlier. An 18-month-old boy narrowly survived a dosage estimated at 262 mg/kg that was reduced to an unknown degree by vomiting and gastric lavage (Walsh *et al.*, 1977). The usual emetic dose of copper sulfate is 4.3 mg/kg or slightly more. However, an accidental dosage probably no more than half as large as regards copper ion may cause vomiting, diarrhea, and abdominal cramps (Pennypacker *et al.*, 1975). The average normal intake of copper ion is about 0.03 mg/kg/day. The occupational health saftey limit (threshold limit value) is 0.2 mg/m^3 for copper fumes and 1.0 mg/m^3 for copper dusts and mists [American Conference of Governmental Industrial Hygienists (ACGIH), 1988].

Laboratory Findings The peak blood copper level in a fatal case was 82.67 ppm (Chugh *et al.*, 1975). A child who narrawly survived had an initial serum level of 16.5 ppm (Walsh *et al.*, 1977).

The milk of female vineyard workers, who were exposed to copper sulfate and a variety of other pesticides, contained 6.2 times as much copper as the milk of milkmaids who did equally hard work but were not exposed to pesticides. Placentas from the vineyard workers contained 4.7 times more copper than those from milkmaids (Nikitina, 1974).

Copper is essential to life and occurs in all tissues. Kehoe *et al.* (1940) reported that the concentrations in blood, muscle, and most of the viscera range from 0.85 to 1.90 ppm. Values for plasma lie in the narrow range 1.16–1.42 ppm (Gofman *et al.*, 1964). The concentrations in the brain (2.2–6.8 ppm), liver (7.1 ppm in adults and 24 ppm in infants), and bone (3.7–4.7 ppm in rib and 6.8 ppm in long bones) are higher. The concentration in erythrocytes is slightly greater than that in the plasma. The values reported by Tipton and Cook (1963) and by Liebscher and Smith (1968) are basically similar but expressed on a different basis. The organs of Orientals frequently contain more copper than those of Americans (Tipton *et al.*, 1965). The concentration of copper in the urine varies from 0.01 to 0.08 and averages about 0.034 ppm (Kehoe *et al.*, 1940). Fecal excretion is greater than urinary excretion and averages 1.96 ing/day according to Kehoe *et al.* (1940).

Pathology Persons who die soon after ingestion of copper sulfate show on autopsy a characteristic staining of the lining of the digestive tract and fatty degeneration of the liver, kidney, and to some degree other organs. Persons who develop acute renal failure as part of acute poisoning by copper sulfate may or may not show well established acute tubular necrosis. In those who survive long enough, granulomatous lesions of the kidney may develop (Chugh *et al.*, 1977).

Biopsy revealed nodules containing copper in the lungs of men who developed pneumoconiosis following years of exposure to Bordeaux mixture (Pimentel and Marques, 1969). Later study of biopsy and autopsy material from workers exposed to Bordeaux mixture sprays for 3 to 35 years revealed that many rural workers who developed pulmonary granulomas

developed liver granulomas also, and in some the liver was enlarged. The liver granulomas varied, with all transitional forms, from those consisting entirely of histiocytic cells to those consisting of clusters of epithelioid cells perfectly organized in sarcoid-type follicles. No giant cells or lymphocytic borders were observed. A finely granular material in the granuloma cells and in prominent Kupffer cells did not stain for ferric iron but was positive for copper when stained with rubeanic acid. No copper was demonstrable in the hepatocytes. Thus the distribution of copper in the liver was entirely different from that in any previously described granulomatosis of whatever origin. Some of the patients also had micronodular cirrhosis or fatty change of the liver, but it was thought that this might be due to alcoholism. Angiosarcoma and idiopathic portal hypertension also were seen (Pimentel and Menezes, 1975, 1976).

Treatment of Poisoning Treatment should include a prompt effort to prevent absorption and later the use of a chelating agent. The protein of milk or egg white combines with copper to form an insoluble copper proteinate. However, the product must be removed by vomiting or lavage before it is digested and the copper released. Copper may also be precipitated by potassium ferrocyanide given in a dose of 600 mg in a glass of water.

British anti-lewisite (BAL), dicalcium EDTA, and penicillamine are all effective in binding copper. Penicillamine is definitely the drug of choice in Wilson's disease. There is less experience on which to base a choice in the treatment of acute poisoning.

61.4 ZINC

Zinc follows copper in the periodic table, and, like copper, it is an essential element. More than 20 metalloenzymes containing zinc have been identified. These include alcohol dehydrogenase, alkaline phosphatase, carbonic anhydrase, and DNA polymerase [National Research Council (NRC), 1979]. Zinc forms a necessary part of carbonic anhydrase, carboxypeptidase, alcohol dehydrogenase, lactic acid dehydrogenase, glutamic dehydrogenase, and alkaline dehydrogenase molecules (Vallee, 1959, 1962). Zinc also plays an essential role in maintaining the structure of nucleic acids in genes, such as the zinc finger structures (ATSDR, 1994).

It has been known for some time that a deficiency of zinc leads to testicular atrophy and failure of body growth in animals. Zinc deficiency, complicated only by iron deficiency, has been found in patients from villages in the Middle East who exhibited severe growth retardation and sexual hypofunction. In adolescent patients, zinc supplementation alone resulted in body growth, gonadal development, and the appearance of secondary sexual characteristics. Some of the dwarfs who received reagent grade iron but no zinc failed to develop sexually, and their growth rate was less than that following zinc (Prasad, 1966). Dermatitis also is seen in zinc deficiency. Animal experiments indicate that simultaneous administration of cadmium will exacerbate the effects of zinc deficiency (Petering *et al.*, 1971). Poor intestinal absorption of zinc is believed to be a factor in the familial disease acrodermatitis enterohepatica (Moynahan, 1974).

Zinc is a normal constituent of food, and only rarely is it possible to avoid an adequate intake. The average daily intake of zinc in different areas of the world ranges from 5 to 22 mg in adults (Halsted *et al.*, 1974). Protein-rich foods, especially marine organisms sach as oysters, have the highest levels (10–50 mg/kg wet weight), whereas concentrations in grains, vegetables, and fruits are relatively low, usually less than 5 mg/kg fresh weight (Great Britain Ministry of Agriculture, Fisheries, and Food, 1981). The concentration in drinking water is usually the same as in freshwater and seawater (1–10 µg/l) but may be much higher if the water is passed through zinc-coated pipes (Sharrett *et al.*, 1982). Information on the concentration of zinc in normal human tissue is given in Section 61.4.1.3.

Pesticides containing zinc may be divided into four classes: (*a*) Most inorganic and certain organic compounds of zinc that are toxic because sufficient doses supply an excess of zinc ions. Examples include zinc chloride and zinc acetate. These compounds are discussed in the following section. (*b*) Complexes of zinc with other elements, the greater toxicity of which predominates in the effect of the complex regardless of the exact chemical combination. An example is zinc arsenate. (*c*) Zinc phosphide, which owes its toxicity to the phosphine (PH_3) it produces (see Section 61.4.2 and see Section 14.6.2 of the first edition of this Handbook). (*d*) Certain organic compounds of zinc, the toxicity of which is not essentially different from those of similar compounds that are salts of other metals. An example is zineb (see Section 21.12.5 of the first edition of this Handbook).

61.4.1 ZINC CHLORIDE

61.4.1.1 Identity, Properties, and Uses

Chemical Name   Zinc chloride.

Structure $ZnCl_2$.

Synonyms   Other names include butter of zinc and zinc dichloride. The CAS registry no. is 7646-85-7.

Physical and Chemical Properties   Zinc chloride has the empirical formula Cl_2Zn and a molecular weight of 136.29. It forms white, odorless, very deliquescent granules with a density of 2.907. It has a melting point of approximately 290°C and a boiling point of 732°C. One gram of zinc chloride dissolves in 0.5 ml water, 1.3 ml ethanol, or 2 ml glycerol. The compound is freely soluble in acetone. Zinc oxychloride is formed in the presence of water.

Formulations and Uses   Technical grade is at least 95% pure, the remainder being mostly water and oxychloride. Zinc chloride may be used with copper and chromium compounds as a

wood preservative. Zinc chloride is also used as an herbicide [Hazardous Substances Data Bank (HSDB), 1993].

61.4.1.2 Toxicity to Laboratory Animals

Basic Findings   Zinc chloride may be taken as typical of those compounds that owe their toxicity to the zinc ion. However, to gain a reasonably complete picture of the toxicity of the ion it is necessary to refer to other compounds also. The small differences in toxicity between most zinc compounds are explained by differences in their solubility and degree of ionization.

The acute (less than 14 days oral intake) and the intermediate (14 days to 1 year) LD 50s are in the range 100–1000 mg Zn/kg/day in rats and mice (ATSDR, 1994) for zinc chloride and similar compounds of zinc. Oral administration of zinc compounds can depress hemoglobin levels. The lowest reported observed effects level in rats was 12 mg Zn/kg/day as zinc chloride given over 4 weeks in the drinking water (Zaporowska and Wasilewski, 1992). However, most studies report lowest observed effects levels above 100 mg/kg/day (ATSDR, 1994).

Absorption, Distribution, Metabolism, and Excretion
Early studies (Drinker *et al.*, 1927a, b) indicate that animals can regulate zinc absorption such that large oral doses produce minimal change in tissue levels. Thus intestinal absorption is highly variable (10–90%), depending on zinc status and the magnitude of the oral dose. Also, calcium and phytates in food interfere with zinc absorption (Becker and Hoekstra, 1971). Metallothionein may play a role in regulation of zinc absorption (Richards and Cousins, 1976). Another protein, also rich in cysteine residues, also plays a role (Hempe and Cousins, 1991).

In the plasma, albumin is the primary carrier of zinc, which represents the metabolically active pool (ATSDR, 1994). Zinc is initially concentrated in the liver after ingestion, and is subsequently delivered throughout the body. The liver, pancreas, bone, kidneys, and muscle are the major tissue storage sites.

Zinc is secreted in bile (Barrowman *et al.*, 1973) and fecal excretion is considerably greater than urinary excretion in both animals (Schryver *et al.*, 1980) and humans (Aamodt *et al.*, 1979). Biliary secretion may be a glutation-dependent process (Alexander *et al.*, 1981).

Mode of Action   The mechanism of toxicity of zinc in general is not well understood. The lowered hemoglobin levels are believed to be due to competition of zinc with copper to produce a relative copper deficiency (ATSDR, 1994).

Treatment of Poisoning in Animals   By using ^{65}Zn injected intravenously as the chloride, it was shown that the intramuscular injection of BAL doubled the concentration of zinc in the red cells, increased urinary excretion as much as 20 times (from a level of 4% or less of the administered dose), and decreased fecal excretion (from a level of 31% to 42% of the administered dose in rats that received no BAL). Total excretion of zinc was increased. Under the conditions used, the injection of BAL completely eliminated acute toxicity but did not prevent death

72–96 hours after injection. In fact, BAL seemed to accentuate the renal damage caused by sufficient zinc (Bruner, 1950). The study throws no light on the question of whether BAL would divert a harmful amount of zinc through the kidneys under practical conditions of accidental poisoning.

61.4.1.3 Toxicity to Humans

Therapeutic Use Zinc oxide and zinc carbonate, which are highly insoluble, are applied liberally to inflamed skin in the form of powder, calamine lotion, and the like. Zinc chloride, sulfate, and acetate have been used for their antiseptic, astringent, or caustic properties. Their use is limited by difficulty of local control, not by systemic effects. Zinc sulfate has been used as an emetic at an oral dose of 1000 or 2000 mg in a glass of water (Sollmann, 1957). This dose intentionally produces a concentration in the water well above the threshold (675-2280 ppm) that may lead to vomiting if taken on an empty stomach, as sometimes happens accidentally when fruit juice or other acid drinks are stored in galvanized vessels.

Accidents and Use Experience Zinc chloride is caustic. Stokinger (1963) recorded without detail or reference that it has caused dermatitis in men working with railroad crossties treated with the compound as a fungicide. More direct contact with zinc chloride, as in its use as a soldering flux, may cause ulceration of the fingers, hands, and forearms. Respiratory exposure to a sufficient concentration of zinc chloride smoke is highly irritating to the mucous membranes of the nasopharynx, trachea, and bronchi and may be fatal (Evans, 1945). Schaidt *et al.* (1979) have proposed that the high toxicity of $ZnCl_2$ in the lung is due to the formation of hydrochloric acid.

Zinc chloride intended for use as a pesticide apparently has not led to injury other than dermatitis. Ingestion undoubtedly would produce illness similar to that caused by copper sulfate. In several instances, the preparation or storage of an acid food in a galvanized or zinc-plated vessel has led to severe vomiting and to headache and discomfort in the chest (Hegsted *et al.*, 1945).

Dosage Response The lethal dose in humans is unknown but has been estimated at 3000–5000 mg (43–71 mg/kg). The emetic dosage is 14–28 mg/kg. Zinc intake from food and water is usually at the rate of about 0.14–0.21 mg/kg/day but in some communities it may reach 0.75 mg/kg/day without injury. To prevent respiratory irritation and other effects of fumes from $ZnCl_2$, the American Conference of Governmental Industrial Hygienists (ACGIH, 1981) have set a threshold limit value of $1 \, mg/m^3$ and a short-term exposure limit of $2 \, mg/m^3$.

Laboratory Findings There is only moderate variation between the normal concentrations of zinc in different tissues; in most organs it is about 20–30 ppm; in liver, bone, and voluntary muscle it is from 60 to 180 ppm. Higher concentrations are found in the prostate (860 ppm) and the retina (500–1000 ppm), whereas blood contains 6.6–8.8 ppm, of which the greater part

is in the red cells. The plasma contains only 0.93–1.03 ppm (Gofman *et al.*, 1964), but whole blood contains 0.60–19.87 ppm with a mean of 5.30 ppm (Kubota *et al.*, 1968). Excretion of zinc is chiefly via the feces (Vallee, 1959). The daily urinary output is about 0.5 mg (Elinder *et al.*, 1978; Halsted *et al.*, 1974).

In studies of normal unexposed humans, the biological half-life of zinc is in the range 160–500 days (Aamodt *et al.*, 1975). Bone and muscle, which contain the major amount of the body's zinc, have longer biological half-lives than other tissues, for example, liver (NRC, 1979).

61.4.2 ZINC PHOSPHIDE

61.4.2.1 Identity, Properties, and Uses

Chemical Name Zinc phosphide.

Structure Zn_3P_2.

Synonyms As a rodenticide, zinc phosphide has been manufactured under tradenames Fasco Field rat powder®, Kilrat®, Mouse-Con®, and Rumetan®. The CAS registry no. is 1314-84-7.

Physical and Chemical Properties Zinc phosphide has the empirical formula P_2Zn_3 and a molecular weight of 258.09. It forms a gray-black crystalline powder with a faint garlic odor and taste. It has a density of 4.55, a melting point above 420°C, and a boiling point of 1100°C. It is insoluble in water and alcohol. Zinc phosphide is stable when dry but spontaneously flammable on contact with acids. It is decomposed by acids into phosphine and is slightly corrosive to metals.

Formulations and Uses Technical zinc phosphide is 80–90% pure. Rodenticidal baits contain 0.5 or 1.0% of the compound; pastes contain 5–10%. As reviewed by von Oettingen (1947), zinc phosphide has been used not only as a rodenticide but also as an insecticide for control of mole crickets.

61.4.2.2 Toxicity to Laboratory Animals

Basic Findings The oral LD 50 of zinc phosphide for rats is 40.5 mg/kg (Dieke and Richter, 1946). Because the complete reaction of 40.5 mg of zinc phosphide produces 10.6 mg of phosphine and because the fatal dosage of phosphine for rats exposed to vapor concentrations ranging from 564 to $7.5 \, mg/m^3$ varies from only 13.5 to 8.9 mg/kg (see Section 14.6.2.2 in the first edition of this Handbook), the toxicity of zinc phosphide is fully accounted for by the toxicity of the phosphine it produces when hydrolyzed by the acid of the stomach. The symptoms produced by the two compounds are similar except that respiratory exposure to the gas may have a slightly greater tendency to produce pulmonary edema and associated symptoms. However, the emetic action of its zinc moiety reduces the toxicity of zinc phosphide to humans and other animals that can vomit. The usual emetic doses of hydrated zinc sulfate in humans (1000–2000 mg) are equivalent to zinc intakes of 3.2–6.4 mg/kg, whereas the oral LD 50 of zinc phosphide for rats is equivalent to a zinc uptake of 30.8 mg/kg. Thus, a dangerous dose has a powerful emetic action in humans. At the same time, little injury from a dangerous dose of zinc phosphide can be attributed to the zinc moiety.

Absorption, Distribution, Metabolism, and Excretion   According to Curry *et al.* (1959), both phosphide and phosphine were demonstrated in the liver of rats poisoned by zinc phosphide, but were only demonstrable in those that had survived long enough to excrete most of the poison. Although this conclusion probably is correct, the data do not support the authors' assumption that phosphide is absorbed in paniculate form.

It is reported that the main urinary excretion product of zinc phosphide in rats and guinea pigs is hypophosphite (Curry *et al.*, 1959).

61.4.2.3 Toxicity to Humans

Accidental and Intentional Poisoning   One of the best-described cases of poisoning by zinc phosphide involved a 37-year-old woman who, with suicidal intent, drank a mixture of 180 g of the rodenticide with water. Vomiting began 1 hr after ingestion and was frequent and violent. She was discovered in a state of shock after about 5 hr. On admission to hospital, her skin was cold and blue; the heart was inaudible, no limb pulses were palpable, and blood pressure was unobtainable. The carotid pulse was 80 per minute. The breath smelled of phosphine. Rectal temperature was 33°C. Treatment was entirely appropriate and almost certainly prolonged the patient's life. Besides very thorough gastric lavage and the use of detoxifying antidotes, the important features of treatment included rehydration and efforts to combat severe metabolic acidosis. Within 8 hr, 1200 mEq of sodium bicarbonate was administered. An attempt to induce diuresis was promptly but only briefly successful. Peripheral limb pulses returned, blood pressure reached 90/60 mm Hg, and by 21 hr after ingestion the patient was conscious, rational, and oriented, and she gave a lucid account of the events leading to her condition. However, complications had developed already and others appeared later. By 16 hr after ingestion, serum bilirubin had risen to 2.2 mg/100 ml. Hepatic tenderness appeared, and other tests of liver function became abnormal. Blood pressure and urine output decreased, and blood urea reached 30 mg/100 ml. A thrombotest showed 28% of normal coagulation activity. Variable tetany appeared; although blood calcium was low (3.3 mEq/l), the condition did not respond to injection of calcium gluconate. Abdominal pain became severe. The extremities again became pulseless and icy cold. Fever and rapid breathing preceded a rapidly developing cortfusional state. For a brief period, the patient seemed to suffer terrifying hallucinations, and toward the end she screeched repeatedly. Unexpected cardiac arrest occurred 41 hr after ingestion (Stephenson, 1967).

In a drunken state, a 19-year-old woman in her 30th or 31st week of pregnancy ingested an unknown amount of zinc phosphide intended as a rodent bait. She soon lost consciousness and was cyanotic when brought to hospital. However, her pulse was detectable and her blood pressure normal. Treatment included gastric lavage and supportive measures. Recovery was complete by the third day. A baby girl later was born at term by normal labor; she was normal at birth and in subsequent development (Kuptsov and Aslanov, 1970).

Symptoms are basically the same regardless of route of administration whether oral, vaginal (Santini, 1955), respiratory (Elbel and Holsten, 1936), or directly into the subcutaneous and muscular tissues (Blisnakov and Iskrov, 1961).

In a review of cases where there was enough information to reach a conclusion, it was found that there was no mortality following three industrial accidents with zinc phosphide. However, mortality was 66% in 3 domestic accidents, 69% in 26 suicides, and 38% in 8 attempted murders. Ten patients who died did so within 7–58 hr after ingestion, with an average of 24.6 hr. Patients who survived for 3 days were out of danger, although some suffered liver and/or kidney injury for days before full recovery (Stephenson, 1967). Apparently no exception to this rule regarding survival has been observed even though Rimalis and Bochkarnikov (1978) reported a case in which hepatorenal insufficiency was noted 5 days after ingestion, and the patient was not discharged until 36 days after ingestion.

Use Experience   Zinc phosphide has given rise only rarely to occupational poisoning, although accidental poisoning of children by the baits is a real possibility. In one case, inhalation of dust from grain coated with the compound was followed several hours later by vomiting, diarrhea, cyanosis, rales, tachycardia, meteorism, restlessness, fever, albuminuria, and eventual recovery (Elbel and Holsten, 1936). In another instance reviewed by von Oettingen (1947) it apparently was not the applicator but workers in a fish-processing plant who were affected by phosphine generated from zinc phosphide after the rodenticide had come in contact with acid brine used for curing fish.

Dosage Response   Adults have been killed by doses of 4000 or 5000 mg (Frketić *et al.*, 1957; Gili, 1948). However, others have survived as much as 25,000 mg (Paszko, 1961), 50,000 mg (Simonović, 1954), or even 100,000 mg (Rimalis and Bochkarnikov, 1978). Early vomiting improves the prognosis. In fact, one of two young women who had ingested similar amounts of zinc phosphide in a suicide pact survived with only transient symptoms because she had been induced to vomit; the other, who would not vomit, died in spite of gastric lavage 1 hr after ingestion (Mannaioni, 1960).

Laboratory Findings   Phosphine may be detected most readily by odor. The concentration of zinc in the tissues is increased; in one case the serum level was between 5.9 and 6.1 ppm (Stephenson, 1967). For zinc in normal tissues, see Section 61.4.1.3. Other findings may include metabolic acidosis, reducing agents in the urine, increased serum bilirubin and other abnormal tests of liver function, thrombocytopenia, methemoglobin, and electrocardiogram (ECG) abnormalities.

The reducing substances in the urine include glucose but may induce hypophosphite and dissolved phosphine (Stephenson, 1967).

Pathology   When death is rapid, abnormal findings may be restricted to pulmonary edema (Frketić *et al.*, 1957; Mannaioni, 1960; Paszko, 1961; Puccini, 1961; Stephenson, 1967) or to this and cerebral edema (Mannaioni, 1960; Puccini, 1961). Other findings that may be present especially in persons who survive longer include centrilobular necrosis of the liver, tubular necrosis of the kidneys, mucosal hemorrhage of the stomach, and bloody pleural, peritoneal, or pericardial fluid (Stephenson, 1967).

Treatment of Poisoning   Treatment is entirely symptomatic (Hayes, 1975).

61.5 CADMIUM

Cadmium is a metal in the same periodic group as zinc and mercury. The toxicity of cadmium is especially evident when there is a deficiency of zinc, and within limits cadmium toxicity may be counteracted by supplementing the diet with zinc.

A wide range of cadmium concentrations are in human food—0.005–0.1 mg/kg wet weight. Kidney and oysters may have concentrations exceeding 1 mg/kg. Drinking water usually has concentrations below 5 µg/l, but higher levels may be found due to cadmium impurities in the zinc of galvanized pipes and cadmium-containing solders in pipe fittings. More details are available in reviews of cadmium toxicity (Foulkes, 1974; Friberg *et al.*, 1986).

Several cadmium salts showed some promise as insecticides, but their use never became extensive. A number of cadmium salts have been used as fungicides on turf.

61.5.1 CADMIUM CHLORIDE

61.5.1.1 Identity, Properties, and Uses

Chemical Name   Cadmium chloride.

Structure $CdCl_2$.

Synonyms   The CAS registry no. for cadmium chloride is 10108-64-2.

Physical and Chemical Properties   The empirical formula for cadmium chloride is $CdCl_2$ and the molecular weight is 183.32. The compound forms colorless, odorless crystals with a density of 4.05, a melting point of 568°C, and a boiling point of 960°C. It is freely soluble in water and acetone, slightly soluble in methanol and ethanol, and practically insoluble in ether.

Use   Cadmium chloride is a fungicide for turf.

61.5.1.2 Toxicity to Laboratory Animals

Basic Findings   Acute exposures (less than 14 days) to aerosols of cadmium chloride or similar soluble compounds result in a lethal outcome in mice, rats, and other small mammals at air concentrations generally above 10 mg Cd/m^3; intermediate exposures (2 weeks to 1 year), at levels above 0.1 mg Cd/m^3; and longer exposures, at levels above 0.05 mg Cd/m^3 (ATSDR, 1997).

Acute exposures (less than 14 days) to orally administered cadmium chloride and chemically similar cadmium compounds are lethal to rats at intakes above 10 mg Cd/kg/day, and intermediate (2 weeks to 1 year) exposures at intakes above 1 mg Cd/kg/day (ATSDR, 1997).

Cadmium compounds can produce a number of serious systemic effects, including anemia, kidney damage (the main target organ after long-term exposures), and skeletal disturbances such as osteoporosis. The latter may be due, at least in part, to alterations in renal metabolism of vitamin D.

In rats and mice, acute oral exposure at near lethal doses can produce testicular atrophy and necrosis (Andersen *et al.*, 1988; Bomhard *et al.*, 1987). Cadmium inhalation can cause lung cancer but only in rats (Oldiges *et al.*, 1989; Takenaka *et al.*, 1983).

Absorption, Distribution, Metabolism, and Excretion   Absorption from the gastrointestinal tract usually is limited by rapid and violent vomiting. Absorption may occur from the respiratory tract following exposure to dusts and aerosols. Dermal absorption is not significant.

Once absorbed, cadmium is tenaciously stored and only slowly excreted. Cadmium is believed to be carried to the liver attached to serum albumin. In the liver, it induces metallothionein, a protein of molecular weight 6000 that avidly binds cadmium. It is lost from the liver as a cadmium–metallothionein complex, filtered as the glomerulus, and take up by the proximal tubular cells of the kidney. Once inside the kidney cell, the metallothionein–cadmium complex is broken down by lysosomes to release free cadmium. The latter can induce metallothionein synthesis in the kidney cells. However, if the rate of release of cadmium exceeds the ability of the cell to produce metallothionein, the cadmium will attach to other "sensitive sites" and damage the cell. The ability of cadmium to induce metallothionein and to bind avidly to this protein is believed to account for its long-term storage in the body (Friberg *et al.*, 1986). Storage is mainly in the pancreas, liver, and kidney (Friberg, 1956) and, following respiratory exposure, in the lung.

Biochemical Effects   Nonfatal doses of cadmium induce the synthesis of metallothionein, as just discussed, and may cause an increased tolerance for the ion. When groups of mice were given four-tenths of the LD 50 dosage of cadmium chloride previously determined for the strain and then challenged 48 hr later, the intraperitoneal LD 50 was increased from 5.2 mg/kg in controls to 6.7 mg/kg. The difference was statistically significant. A significant increase was obtained with cadmium acetate also (Jones *et al.*, 1979).

61.5.1.3 Toxicity to Humans

Accidental and Intentional Poisoning   Apparently, the limited use of cadmium chloride as a pesticide has not led to poisoning of anyone. However, the evidence that has accumulated about the high toxicity of cadmium and its very tenacious storage leave no doubt that cadmium in any form should not be used as a pesticide.

Dramatic but not fatal poisoning used to occur fairly frequently when fruit juices or other acid foods were held for a time in cadmium-plated vessels. The citric or other organic salts formed on standing were fully ionized in the presence of hydrochloric acid in the stomach. Signs and symptoms included salivation, nausea, persistent vomiting, mild diarrhea, abdominal pain, and tenesmus. Illness often began suddenly 0.25–5 hr after ingestion; the interval was usually less than 2 hr unless food was eaten at the same time. Recovery usually was well advanced in 1–2 hr (Cangelosi, 1941; Frant and Kleeman, 1941). The amount of cadmium necessary to produce these effects was not great. Schwartze and Alsberg (1923) cited a case of voluntary ingestion of cadmium sulfate, equivalent to about 18 mg of metallic cadmium, which produced vomiting. Mild illness is produced by concentrations as low as 15 ppm.

Use Experience and Environmental Exposure   The few episodes of acute occupational poisoning by cadmium have all been associated with inhalation of dust or fumes. The cases were characterized by severe pulmonary irritation, and persons who died showed marked hyperplasia of the lung epithelium and thickening and edema of the alveolar septa. Signs of severe gastrointestinal irritation were present in a high proportion of cases.

Less severe but more prolonged occupational exposure to cadmium may produce a distinctive form of emphysema leading to dyspnea and often accompanied by a low-grade anemia. The most typical feature of chronic cadmium poisoning is kidney damage. The first sign is the excretion of low-molecular-weight proteins. This condition is known as tubular proteinuria because these proteins are normally reabsorbed by the tubular cells in the kidney (Friberg, 1950; Piscator, 1966). At high exposure, more severe effects in kidney function occur, such as aminoaciduria (Clarkson and Kench, 1956), glucosuria, and phosphaturia (Piscator, 1966).

By far the largest number of cases of cadmium poisoning have occurred in Japan as a result of environmental exposure. These cases differed greatly from those caused by cadmium under other circumstances, being characterized by osteomalacia, skeletal deformity, and very severe pain. In fact, the condition took its name "itai-itai disease" from the predominance of pain. The entire matter has been reviewed critically by Friberg *et al.* (1974), who concluded that there was no doubt that cadmium was the cause but that there was reason to believe that high intake of cadmium and deficient consumption of certain essential food items, especially calcium and vitamin D, had been contributing factors. In spite of the very different clinical manifestations seen in itai-itai disease, it is thought that the basic injury is to the kidney as in other forms of chronic poisoning by cadmium and that the osteomalacia is secondary.

The World Health Organization (WHO) has proposed a guideline for drinking water of 5 μg Cd/l (WHO, 1984a) and a provisional tolerable weekly intake of 0.4–0.5 mg (WHO, 1984b). The U.S. Occupational Safety and Health Administration recommends a permissible exposure limit for all cadmium compounds of 5 μg Cd/m^3 in the occupational setting (OSHA, 1992).

Dosage Response   Apparently, no information is available on the minimal dosage of a cadmium salt that has been fatal in humans. According to reports cited by Schwartze and Alsberg (1923) doses of 250–1000 mg of cadmium bromide produced illness, and a 3-mg dose of cadmium sulfate produced vomiting.

The World Health Organization (WHO) has proposed a guideline for drinking water of 5 μg Cd/l (WHO, 1984a) and a provisional tolerable weekly intake of 0.4–0.5 mg (WHO, 1984b). The U.S. Occupational Safety and Health Administration recommends a permissible exposure limit for all cadmium compounds of 5 μg Cd/m^3 in the occupational setting (OSHA, 1992).

Laboratory Findings   Friberg *et al.* (1974) have given reasons for thinking that some of the early reports of concentrations of cadmium in environmental samples and human tissues were incorrectly high because the chemical methods used formerly were not entirely specific. This is an unusual situation because improvement in chemical methods often leads to more complete recovery and recognition of the material analyzed and thus to higher values. Considering only results based on dependable chemical methods, it now seems likely that blood levels in normal adults usually are <0.01 ppm. The renal cortex usually contains cadmium at concentrations of 20–50 ppm, higher than the concentrations in any other tissue. The highest concentration is reached at about 50 years of age, and levels then decline gradually. The kidneys contain about one-third of the total body burden, and the kidneys and liver together contain about half the body burden. Normal urinary excretion is about 0.002 mg/person/day or less, but levels increase with age.

Intake is about 0.05 mg/person/day from food, with much less from water, air, and even cigarette smoking. The amount of cadmium in ordinary food is one-seventh to one-fifth of the intake thought to be required to produce the storage of 200 ppm in the kidney and consequent kidney damage. Absorption of cadmium ingested in food and water ranges from 4.7 to 7.0% but may be higher if calcium and protein are deficient. Retention of cadmium from smoke or fumes may be 25–50%.

The placenta is an efficient barrier to small concentrations of cadmium; the newborn contains less than 0.001 mg. The biological half-life for cadmium in the whole body lies between 20 and 30 years. Thus cadmium has an unusually great tendency to accumulate in the body (Friberg *et al.*, 1974). In workers, cadmium in the blood is mainly in the cells; the concentration in whole blood usually is between 0.01 and 0.1 ppm. Concentrations in the kidney cortex may be around 300 ppm. The liver may contain proportionately more than would be expected in persons without special exposure. Cadmium is transported in the circulation at least in part bound to metallothionein. When workers begin to excrete protein in their urine, their excretion of cadmium increases, sometimes dramatically, and their blood levels fall correspondingly. Based on results in animals and on autopsy findings in workers, a concentration of 200 ppm in the kidney is the threshold for kidney injury as reflected by kidney function tests and the urinary excretion of protein. More recent data are available based on direct *in vivo* measurement of the kidney content of cadmium in occupationally exposed workers using a neutron activation technique (Ellis *et al.*, 1984). This has allowed the development of more sophisticated dosage–response models (Kjellström, 1985) that estimate, for example, that a daily intake of about 200 μg Cd via food for 45 years will give a 10% chance of mild kidney effects. The equivalent occupational exposure would be 10 years at about 50 μg Cd/m^3.

Besides the proteinuria, other laboratory findings may include mild hypochronic anemia, mild jaundice, and the presence of microscopic blood in the urine.

Persons mildly poisoned by cadmium may show blood levels as high as 6.2 ppm and urinary levels as high as 2.2 ppm (Cotter, 1958).

Treatment of Poisoning   Cotter (1958) treated three patients whose major exposure was to cadmium, including at least one without any other exposure. The patients suffered one or more of the following: mental disturbance, cough and other respiratory disturbance, mild jaundice, mild anemia, and abnormal urinary findings. Treatment consisted of 500 mg of calcium disodium EDTA by mouth every 2 hr while the patient was awake and for a period of 1 week. All the patients showed marked clinical improvement. There was no evidence of kidney damage from the treatment, and in fact the proteinuria present before treatment gradually cleared completely. Icterus disappeared, and the red cell count and hemoglobin level improved. Before treatment, blood cadmium levels in the three patients were 0.022–6.2 ppm, and urinary cadmium was 0.036–2.2 ppm. The concentrations fell to undetectable levels following treatment.

A patient who had marked irregularity of the heartbeat and other ECG abnormalities 3 hr after ingesting cadmium showed marked improvement following intravenous injection of calcium gluconate and magnesium sulfate, and she was almost normal within 48 hr after ingestion (Lydtin *et al.*, 1965). However, evidence from animals indicates that some chelating agents such as EDTA can cause renal accumulation by redistribution from other tissues, and therefore application of chelating agents to cases of human poisoning should be viewed with great caution.

61.6 MERCURY

There is no evidence that any quantity of mercury is beneficial to any form of life. However, the element is widely distributed in the environment, and traces of it occur in food, water, and tissues even in the absence of occupational exposure.

Mercury is toxic no matter what its chemical combination. However, different forms of mercury have different absorption, distribution, and excretion characteristics; at the same rate of intake, they reach and maintain different concentrations in different tissues. For this and perhaps other reasons they have distinguishable toxic effects.

In the late twentieth century the only mercury pesticides used in significant amounts were organic compounds; some of them constitute a real hazard. It is said that mercury vapor formerly was used in India for the disinfection of stored grain. Several inorganic mercury salts are still listed as fungicides. There is no evidence that the use of mercury vapor or inorganic mercury compounds as pesticides constitutes a significant hazard at this time, largely because such use is limited. Even so, some information on the toxicity of these forms of mercury is necessary for understanding the toxicology of the organic mercury fungicides. Finally, among the organic mercurials, the short-chain alkyl compounds are far more toxic than the phenyl or alkoxyalkyl compounds as discussed in Section 61.6.3.

Valuable reviews (Berlin, 1986; Berlin *et al.*, 1969c; Bidstrup, 1964; Clarkson, 1972; WHO, 1976) of the toxicology of mercury and its compounds are available.

61.6.1 ELEMENTAL MERCURY

61.6.1.1 Identity, Properties, and Uses

Synonyms   Synonyms for elemental mercury (Hg) include mercure (French), mercurio (Italian), kwik (Dutch), Quecksilber (German), quicksilver, and RTEC (Polish). The CAS registry no. is 7439-97-6.

Physical and Chemical Properties   Elemental mercury is a heavy, silver-white metal which is liquid at room temperature. Its atomic number is 80, and its atomic weight is 200.59. Mercury has a melting point of $-38.9°C$, a boiling point of $356.9°C$, and a density at $0°C$ of 13.5955. The vapor pressure is 2×10^{-3} mm at $25°C$; air saturated at this temperature contains 19.5 mg of mercury (Giese, 1940). Mercury is insoluble in water, alkalies, and most common solvents. Mercury is not attacked by dilute hydrochloride and sulfuric acids but will dissolve in dilute nitric acid and hot, concentrated sulfuric acid. It oxidizes slowly.

Use   See Section 61.6.

61.6.1.2 Toxicity to Laboratory Animals

Basic Findings   The toxicity of elemental mercury is essentially limited to the vapor, and, therefore, it is not convenient to determine dosage on a milligram-per-kilogram basis.

Exposure of rats or rabbits to concentrations of elemental mercury vapor at air concentrations of about 30 mg/m^3 for periods of a few hours produced death or severe tissue damage.

Exposures at air concentrations of 3–6 mg Hg/m^3 produced pathological changes in kidney and brain as well as behavioral abnormalities (ATSDR, 1999). Both rabbits and dogs tolerated an exposure of 7 hr/day, 5 days/week for over 70 weeks at 0.1 mg Hg/m^3 without functional or microscopic injury (Ashe et al., 1953).

Rats apparently are less susceptible. When they were exposed for only 2 hr each day for 30 days at a concentration of 17 mg/m^3, they developed only a delay in escape response plus an increase in the duration and severity of reflexive fighting behavior and of actual fighting (Beliles et al., 1968).

Absorption, Distribution, Metabolism, and Excretion   Inhaled mercury vapor diffuses across the alveolar regions of the lung into the bloodstream (Berlin et al., 1969a). Mercury vapor is a monatomic gas which is highly diffusible and lipid soluble (Hursh, 1985). Once in the bloodstream, mercury vapor enters the red blood cells, where it is oxidized to divalent inorganic mercury under the influence of catalase (Halbach and Clarkson, 1978; Magos et al., 1978). The oxidation can be inhibited by alcohol, thereby decreasing the retention of inhaled vapor (Nielsen-Kudsk, 1965, 1969). Despite oxidation in the red blood cells, dissolved mercury vapor persists in the plasma for sufficient time for it to be transported to other tissues. This explains why 10 times more mercury is retained in the brain after exposure to mercury vapor than after an equivalent intravenous dose of mercuric mercury in both mice (Berlin and Johansson, 1964) and primates (Berlin et al., 1969b). Placental transport of mercury is also greater after exposure to the vapor (Clarkson et al., 1972). Oxidation by catalase also takes place in fetal tissues (Dencker et al., 1983).

Except for these differences, the pattern of organ distribution of mercury after exposure to vapor or mercuric salts is generally similar, with the highest concentrations always found in the kidney cortex. Excretion is mainly by urine and feces at roughly similar rates but there is a small loss of mercury in expired breath (Clarkson and Rothstein, 1964; Rothstein and Hayes, 1960, 1964).

61.6.1.3 Toxicity to Humans

Experimental Exposure   Using a group of four volunteers in each experiment, the concentrations of radioactive mercury vapor in the inspired and expired air were compared. The inspired air contained from 0.050 to 0.350 mg/m^3. The dead space for the vapor corresponded to the physiological dead space, indicating that all mercury vapor that reached the alveoli was absorbed (Nielsen-Kudsk, 1965, 1969; Teisinger and Fiserova-Bergerova, 1965). A later study in five volunteers confirmed that retention occurs almost entirely in the alveoli. Overall retention was 74%. Examination of the subjects in a whole-body counter yielded average half-lives for mercury as follows: lung, 1.7 days; head, 21 days; kidney region, 64 days; and standard chair position, 58 days (Hursh et al., 1976).

Use Experience   Acute poisoning by metallic mercury is rare. Inhalation of vapor by laboratory workers in a closed space led to bronchial irritation, violent coughing, and severe headache, followed in a few hours by fever, dyspnea, and nausea. Stomatitis appeared in 3 days. Dyspnea and fatigue lasted several months (Christensen et al., 1937). Both renal and nervous involvement are unusual in acute poisoning (Browning, 1969).

Neal et al. (1937, 1941a) gave a very thorough account of chronic mercurialism in the fur-cutting and felt-hat industries. Although mercuric nitrate was the material used to treat fur from which felt was made, the mercury was gradually released from the fur and felt in the form of metallic mercury vapor. Thus the workers had a mixed exposure to dust of mercury compounds (especially the nitrate) and to vapor of the element. The clinical picture of poisoning was similar to that observed among smaller groups whose occupational exposure involved metallic mercury only (Browning, 1969; West and Lim, 1968).

The incidence of chronic mercurialism is roughly proportional to the concentration of mercury in the air at concentrations of 0.1 mg/m^3 and upward, and within each range of concentration the incidence increases with duration of employment (Neal et al., 1941a). Patients often gave a history of gastrointestinal disturbances and sore mouth. Salivation, gingivitis, and the loss of teeth were common. However, the major signs included fine tremors and psychic disturbances often called erethism. The tremor usually was noticed first in the hands and later ia the tongue, eyelids, face, and legs. It became worse during intentional movement or after the slightest emotional strain. The psychic disturbance took the form of irritability, excitability, timidity, irascibility, and difficulty in getting along with people. These signs were noted more frequently by an examiner than they were reported by the patient. They tended to be replaced by depression or despondency. Headache, drowsiness, insomnia, weakness, slurred speech, excessive sweating, dermographia, and vasomotor disorders all pointed to disorder of some part of the nervous system. Ataxia was seen occasionally and hemiplegia more rarely. In advanced cases there might be hallucinations, loss of memory, and intellectual deterioration. Death might follow symptoms resembling cerebral pachymeningitis (Neal et al., 1941a).

More recent studies have indicated that a number of nonspecific symptoms, such as insomnia, introversion, and anxiety, may be produced at concentrations somewhat below 0.1 mg/m^3 (for review, see ATSDR, 1999).

Laboratory Findings   Effects on renal function may be severe (the nephrotic syndrome) at high exposure (Friberg et al., 1953; Kazantzis et al., 1962). Air concentrations in the occupational setting in the range of 0.05–0.1 mg Hg/m^3 have been associated with increased urinary excretion of biochemical biomarkers of kidney cellular changes such as renal enzymes and antigens without compromised kidney function (ATSDR, 1999).

Treatment of Poisoning   Conflicting reports have been published about the value of both BAL and calcium disodium EDTA for treating chronic poisoning by mercury vapor (Browning, 1969). Sunderman (1978) found that BAL (2,3-dimercapto-

l-propanol) was more effective in alleviating the signs and symptoms of mercury vapor poisoning than D-penicillamine or sodium diethyldithiocarbamate. However, treatment with complexing agents may not be necessary as the prognosis is good with virtually complete regression if exposure ceases (Berlin, 1986).

61.6.2 MERCURIC CHLORIDE

61.6.2.1 Identity, Properties, and Uses

Chemical Name   Mercuric chloride.

Structure $HgCl_2$.

Synonyms   Mercuric chloride also is known as corrosive sublimate, mercury bichloride, and mercury perchloride. The CAS registry no. is 7487-94-7.

Physical and Chemical Properties   Mercuric chloride has the empirical formula Cl_2Hg and a molecular weight of 271.52. It is an odorless, white, crystalline powder with a metallic taste. At 25°C, it has a density of 5.4. It melts at 277°C, and sublimes unchanged at about 300°C. Its vapor pressure is 1.4×10^{-4} torr at 35°C. Mercuric chloride is soluble in ethanol, methanol, acetone, ethyl acetate, and diethyl ester. It is slightly soluble in acetic acid, pyridine, and carbon disulfide. Its solubility in water at 20°C is 69 g/l. Mercuric chloride is unstable in the presence of alkalies and is decomposed to metallic mercury by sunlight in the presence of organic matter. It is readily reduced to mercurous chloride and elemental mercury.

History, Formulations, and Uses   Mercuric chloride first was used for crop protection in 1891. It formerly was used as a fungicide in soil application to control potato scab and clubroot of brassicas and as an insecticide against root maggots of crucifers. It now is used in seed treatment of potatoes and as a wood preservative. Formulations include wettable powders, dusts, and solutions for injection into tree trunks.

61.6.2.2 Toxicity to Laboratory Animals

Basic Findings   Oral doses of mercuric chloride in the range 15–60 mg Hg/kg/day given daily for 2 weeks or less to rats or mice produce death through kidney failure. Daily oral exposure from 2 to 26 weeks at 1–28 mg Hg/kg produces mainly kidney damage and weight loss (for a review, see ATSDR, 1999). Exposure of rats for 2 years, 5 days/week at 1.9 mg Hg/kg produced pathological changes in kidney morphology (NTP, 1993).

Absorption, Distribution, Metabolism, and Excretion
Gastrointestinal absorption of oral doses of mercury chloride in rats or mice ranges from 1 to 40% of the dose. Several factors influence the degree of absorption including diet and age of the animal. Suckling animals have higher absorption rates. The

kidneys are the main site of deposition with considerably less mercury crossing the blood–brain barrier or placenta compared to inhaled mercury vapor or methyl mercury compounds.

Inorganic mercury is excreted in both urine and feces. Studies on dogs revealed the inorganic mercury in urine originates from inorganic mercury in renal tissues (Hursh *et al.*, 1985). Inorganic mercury is readily eliminated in milk according to experiments in guinea pigs (Yoshida *et al.*, 1992).

Effect on Organs and Tissues   Mercuric ion in sufficient concentration causes a reversible precipitation of protein. Concentrations of the ion high enough to cause this effect may be reached as a result of direct contact with the skin, the mucous membranes of the eye, or the mucosa of the gastrointestinal tract. However, the mercuric ion produces systemic toxicity at much lower concentrations through inhibition of many enzymes, especially those containing the SH group. After a large dose, death is due to shock and circulatory collapse; arrhythmias may be present, and ventricular fibrillation may be the terminal event. After a somewhat smaller dose, death is due to renal damage leading to anuria.

The necrosis of the kidney tubule cells of rats following subcutaneous injection of mercuric chloride at dosage of 0.1–4.0 mg/kg/day for several days was reflected not only by characteristic histology but by the shedding of cells in the urine and by an increase of urinary glutamic-oxaloacetic transaminase activity in the intact animal. The urinary output of cells reached a peak in a few days and then declined in spite of continued administration of the compound. The peak came earlier at higher dosage levels. A transient increase in transaminase corresponded with the peak of renal cell exfoliation, but the enzyme activity was a less sensitive test. Histological examination showed that the decline in cellular exfoliation was associated with tubular regeneration. The new cells were relatively immune to the effects of mercuric ion, but the basis of the tolerance is unknown (Prescott and Ansari, 1969).

Mercuric chloride at a concentration of 3.5×10^{-5} M acted as a mitogen in cultures of lymphoid cells from rats, guinea pigs, and rabbits (Pauly *et al.*, 1969).

61.6.2.3 Toxicity to Humans

Accidental and Intentional Poisoning   Ingestion of mercuric chloride leads immediately to a burning metallic taste, thirst, and soreness of the throat followed soon by salivation, severe gastric pain, bloody diarrhea, and often vomiting.

If the patient does not die promptly in shock following a dose of about 1 g, the onset is delayed for a few hours. Damage to the capillaries leads to stomatitis, loosening of the teeth, progressive renal damage, and continuing diarrhea. If the blood pressure is maintained, there may be an initial diuresis resulting from suppression of the renal tubular resorption. Progressive injury leads to a diminished flow of urine and eventually to anuria.

Inorganic mercury is excreted so efficiently that persons who survive one or a few doses usually recover completely.

Laboratory Findings   See Section 61.6.3.4.

Pathology Local corrosive effects may be the only indication of injury of persons who die rapidly of shock following a large dose of mercuric chloride. In case of longer survival, renal tubular necrosis is the major finding.

Treatment of Poisoning Both BAL and penicillamine are effective in treating poisoning by inorganic mercury compounds (Hayes, 1975).

61.6.3 ORGANIC MERCURY COMPOUNDS: SIMILARITIES AND DISTINCTIONS

61.6.3.1 Uses

The organic mercury compounds are used as seed dressings for the prevention of seed-borne disease of grains, vegetables, cotton, peanuts, soybeans, sugar beets, and ornamentals. They may be used for the control of fungus diseases of turf, fruits, cereals, and vegetables but not under conditions that will leave any measurable residue in the food of humans or animals. At least in other countries, organic mercury compounds have been used for the preservation of wood (Ahlmark, 1948) and in the paper, plastics, and fabric industries (Lundgren and Swensson, 1960).

About 1915, phenylmercury fungicides began to replace mercuric chloride, which had been in use for seed treatment before the turn of the century. Alkyloxyalkyl mercury compounds were introduced next, and ethyl mercury was tested as early as 1929. Alkyl mercury fungicides were used extensively in the 1940s and thereafter.

The following discussion is necessarily incomplete. Additional information may be found in a book by Bidstrup (1964) and in a health criteria document issued by the WHO (1976) The first of these references is notable for a tabulated description of cases caused by different forms of mercury.

61.6.3.2 Compounds and Their Characteristics

Mercury is bivalent in the organic compounds used as fungicides. Most of these compounds fall into three major classes depending on whether the organomercury cation involves an (*a*) alkyl (e.g., methyl or ethyl), (*b*) phenyl, or (*c*) alkoxyalkyl (e.g., methoxyethyl) group. Compounds of each group may involve a wide range of inorganic or organic anions, including chloride, bromide, iodide, nitrate, hydroxide, acetate, dicyandiamide, toluene-sulfonate, benzoate, methanedinaphthyldisulfonate, and others. There are other bivalent organomercury compounds not used as fungicides, for example, dialkyl mercury compounds, certain local antiseptics, and the mercurial difuretics, but they are not discussed further here.

Vapor pressure is an important factor determining the availability of organic mercury compounds for absorption. Table 61.1, derived in part from a detailed review by Swensson and Ulfvarson (1963), shows the concentrations of mercury and some of its compounds in saturated atmospheres. This helps to explain the observed extreme hazard of methyl mercury compounds in workplaces. Only a lack of use limits the hazards of

Table 61.1

Saturated Vapor Concentration of Mercury and Certain Groups of Its Compounds at 20°C

Group	Concentrations (mg/m^3)
Metallic mercury	14
Dialkyl compounds	10,000
Methyl compounds	0.3–94
Ethyl compounds	0.05–9.0
Phenyl compounds	0.001–0.017
Methoxyethyl compounds	0.002–2.6

the very highly volatile dialkyl compounds. The high reported range of volatility of some alkoxyalkyl compounds depends at least in part on the fact that they often contain metallic mercury as a contaminant (Lindström, 1961). In fact, commercial formulations of all organic mercury compounds are likely to contain related compounds and metallic mercury resulting from the manufacturing process or from slow decompensation catalyzed by light.

61.6.3.3 Absorption, Distribution, Metabolism, and Excretion

Absorption These compounds are absorbed slowly by the skin and more efficiently by the respiratory and gastrointestinal tracts. Some of the alkyl compounds are highly volatile thus increasing the hazard of their inhalation. There is no indication of any significant difference in the rate of absorption of different compounds at the same rate of dosage.

Distribution and Storage Alkyl and aryl mercury compounds, like metallic mercury vapor, are transported mainly in association with the erythrocytes. This is in contrast to the inorganic mercury ion, which is bound mainly to plasma protein. Methoxyethyl compounds are evenly distributed between red cells and plasma.

There are striking differences in the distribution and storage of different classes of organic mercury compounds, and this appears to be the basis for the differences in their toxic effects when given in repeated doses. The mercury content of different organs of rats following repeated doses of typical compounds is shown in Table 61.2. It may be seen that mercury from methoxyethyl mercuric hydroxide reaches about the same concentrations in the blood and vital organs as those from mercuric nitrate. However, the distribution of mercury derived from methylmercuric hydroxide is entirely different, being about 15 times as high in the brain, 100 times as high in the blood, but only one-tenth as high in the kidney. The behavior of mercury derived from phenylmercuric hydroxide is intermediate between that of alkyl mercury and inorganic mercury but much more nearly like the latter (Ulfvarson, 1962). Similar results were obtained in chickens (Swensson and Ulfvarson, 1968a).

Table 61.2
Average Mercury Content of Fresh Tissue of Rats[a,b]

Compound	Blood (ppm)	Liver (ppm)	Kidney (ppm)	Brain (ppm)
Hg(NO$_3$)$_2$	0.028	0.372	20.1	0.024
Methyl Hg OH	3.04	0.676	2.9	0.155
Phenyl Hg OH	0.313	0.566	26.2	0.008
Methoxyethyl Hg OH	0.033	0.248	26.9	0.009

[a] From data of Ulfvarson (1962).
[b] Treatment of rats is 0.1 mg Hg/day every other day for 2 weeks.

Metabolism Differences in distribution and storage of organic mercury pesticides are generally assumed to be due to differences in mobility across cell membranes, affinities for tissue ligands, and rates of metabolism to inorganic mercury. The latter is illustrated by the greater stability of alkyl compounds as compared to the more rapid degradation of methoxyethyl and phenol compounds (Daniel *et al.*, 1971; Gage, 1964; Norseth and Clarkson, 1970).

Methyl mercury is readily transported across the placenta in rodents (Childs, 1973). In humans, cord blood levels closely parallel and are about 20% higher than the corresponding levels in maternal blood (Bakir *et al.*, 1973; Skerfving, 1974).

Species vary considerably in the relative distribution of alkyl mercury between brain and blood (Berlin *et al.*, 1969b).

Table 61.2 shows that somewhat more mercury was stored in the liver and kidney when a phenyl compound was injected for 2 weeks than when inorganic mercury was injected at an equivalent rate. The same thing was seen in much exaggerated form when phenylmercuric acetate and mercuric acetate were fed at equivalent doses for a year or more; there was 10 to 20 or more times greater storage of the phenyl compound depending on dosage. The difference was attributed at least in part to greater absorption of the phenyl compound (Fitzhugh *et al.*, 1950).

Excretion Following injection of equivalent amounts of mercury, urinary excretion of phenyl compounds is almost twice that of inorganic mercury and more than 10 times greater than that of methyl mercury (Friberg, 1959; Swensson and Ulfvarson, 1959). That is, the same level of excretion is achieved only at high blood and tissue levels of alkyl compounds.

In rats, following a single dose, the excretion of various forms of mercury was more rapid at first and then slower. For both mercuric nitrate and phenylmercuric hydroxide the "half-lives" were 5 days during the first 9 days and 10 days during the subsequent 30 days. The half-lives were 16 and 26 days for methylmercuric hydroxide during the same intervals (Swensson and Ulfvarson, 1968b).

Half-lives may be different in different species. The half-life of methyl mercury in the mouse is about 7 days compared to an average 70 days in humans and may be as high as 700 days in certain marine mammals (for review, see Clarkson, 1972).

The half-life of methyl mercury in blood in humans averages about 50 days, whereas that of inorganic mercury is about 30 days (for review, see Clarkson *et al.*, 1988). Information on phenyl mercury compounds is not available.

Although dimethyl mercury apparently has not been used as a pesticide, it is of interest because of its formation in aquatic environments. Most of the dimethyl mercury injected into mice was rapidly exhaled. The remaining part was metabolized to methyl mercury, on which the entire toxic effect depended (Oestlund, 1969).

61.6.3.4 Laboratory Findings in Humans

The record of mercury levels in human tissues and excreta is complicated by the fact that early analytical methods lacked the necessary sensitivity and made no distinction between inorganic and organic mercury. In fact, this distinction has not yet been made for many different occupational situations or for a reasonably complete spectrum of dietary patterns. As a result, the mercury concentrations in human tissues discussed next are expressed in terms of total mercury.

Blood Goldwater and Hoover (1967) have reported blood levels of mercury in 812 people from 15 countries with no known special exposure to mercury. Approximately 75% of the samples were less than 0.5 µg/l and about 90% were less than 20 µg/l. Mercury in blood is greatly influenced by dietary fish consumption in otherwise nonexposed people. Methyl mercury in fish can make a substantial and dominant contribution to blood levels. Certain populations that depend on fish for their main source of protein can develop levels in excess of 299 µg/l (for review, see WHO, 1976).

In groups occupationally exposed to mercury vapor, blood levels are proportional to time-weighted average air concentrations for long-term exposures (1 year or more) and on a group basis (Smith *et al.*, 1970). In general, time-weighted air concentrations in the range 50–100 µg Hg/m^3—values corresponding to maximum allowable limits—correspond to blood levels in the range 35–70 µg/l. Values of 500 to 1000 or 1300 µg/l have been reported in patients (Berlin *et al.*, 1969c; Birke *et al.*, 1967).

Urine A study of urine samples from 1107 people in 15 different countries (Goldwater and Hoover, 1967) revealed that approximately 80% of the samples had mercury concentrations below 0.5 µg/l (the detection limit of the analytical method), 90% were below 10 µg/l, and 95% were below 20 µg. Studies in other populations are consistent with these figures (Buchet *et al.*, 1980; Gotelli *et al.*, 1985).

Smith *et al.* (1970) have reported that urine concentrations of mercury are proportional to the time-weighted average air concentrations of mercury vapor in groups of exposed workers. In general, average air concentrations in the range 50–100 µg Hg/m^3 (the maximum values expected in industrial atmosphere) would correspond to urine concentrations in the range 100–200 µg/l (WHO, 1980).

Exposure to alkyl mercury compounds results in elevated urinary concentrations of mercury (Bakir *et al.*, 1973) but the icrease is small and urinary concentrations are not a viable biological indicator (for discussion, see Clarkson *et al.*, 1988). Urinary concentrations may be markedly increased after occupational (Goldwater, 1973) or accidental (Gotelli *et al.*, 1985) exposure to aryl mercury compounds. However, the quantitative relations between exposure and urinary excretion have not been described.

Hair In a study of 559 samples in 13 countries, Airey (1983) noted a correlation between hair concentrations and average fish consumption. Thus he found the mean hair concentration to be 1.4 ppm in individuals consuming fish once or less per month, 1.9 ppm for consumption once every 2 weeks, 2.5 ppm for consumption once a week, and 11.6 ppm for consumption once or more per day.

This correlation is probably due to intake of methyl mercury in fish. A close correlation has been noted in both population (Amin-Zaki *et al.*, 1976; Birke *et al.*, 1972; Phelps *et al.*, 1980) and experimental (Hislop *et al.*, 1963; Kershaw *et al.*, 1980) studies between mercury concentration in hair next to the scalp and the simultaneous blood concentration after exposure to methyl mercury. The average ratio of hair to blood concentrations is about 250:1. Studies in volunteers who received measured amounts of methyl mercury in fish indicate that there is a 20-day delay between the blood concentration and the appearance of mercury in hair next to the scalp (Hislop *et al.*, 1963). Methyl mercury appears to be incorporated into the hair during its formation and remains stable. Because there is little variation in the rate of growth of head hair (1.15 cm/month) it is possible to determine the sequence of past exposures of persons to methyl mercury (Al-Shahristani and Shihab, 1976; Amin-Zaki *et al.*, 1976).

Hair concentrations after exposure to other forms of mercury (mercury vapor, inorganic and aryl compounds) have not been reported in any detail. In the case of occupational exposure, the probability of external contamination should be considered. Factors affecting hair concentration and the use of washing procedures have been reviewed by Airey (1983).

Tissues Information on tissue levels of mercury are generally restricted to the chief target tissues such as brain, kidney, and liver. Measurements have also been reported on placental tissues from the viewpoint of biological monitoring. Determinations on tissue in the early part of the twentieth century are not included because of the possibility of contamination with mercury added to tissue fixatives.

Studies of the outbreak of methyl mercury poisoning in Minamata, Japan, in the 1950s provided data on control (nonexposed) groups. Brain levels were reported to be less than 0.1 ppm (for review, see Takeuchi and Eto, 1977). Five autopsy cases in Yugoslavia (Kosta *et al.*, 1975) revealed values in the brain in the range 0.001–0.007 ppm. Mottet and Brody (1974) reported levels in 60 hospital autopsy cases in the United States with no known exposure to mercury in the range 0.006–0.965 for the cerebellum and 0.008–0.470 for the cerebrum. A more recent report (Nylander *et al.*, 1987) suggests that brain levels

in otherwise nonexposed individuals increased according to the number of mercury amalgam tooth fillings. Measurements in the occipital lobe cortex in 34 individuals yielded an average value of 0.011 ppm with a range of 0.002 to 0.029 ppm. Linear regression analysis indicated that the mercury concentrations increased with the number of amalgam surfaces in the teeth.

Kidney values for nonexposed people are reported to be in the range 0.18–2.6 ppm in Japan (Takeuchi and Eto, 1977), 0.01–0.37 ppm in Yugoslavia (Kosta *et al.*, 1975), 0.006–0.4 ppm in the United States (Mottet and Brody, 1974), and average values of 0.433 ppm in seven people with mercury amalgams and 0.049 ppm in five people with no mercury amalgams in Sweden (Nylander *et al.*, 1987).

Liver levels in nonexposed people are reported to be 0.16–1.3 ppm in Japan (Tsubaki and Irukayama, 1977), 0.01–0.05 ppm in Yugoslavia (Kosta *et al.*, 1975), and 0.008–1.43 ppm in the United States (Mottet and Brody, 1974).

Fatal cases of methyl mercury poisoning in Minamata had brain levels in the range 2.6–25 ppm, liver levels in the range 22–70 ppm, and kidney levels in the range 21–144 ppm. These individuals had died about 3 months after the end of exposure. Liver levels in the autopsy cases after an outbreak of methyl mercury in Iraq (Magos *et al.*, 1976) were reported to be in the range 1.4–76 ppm (Takeuchi and Eto, 1977).

Little information is available on human tissue levels after exposure to other forms of mercury. Kosta *et al.* (1975) noted elevated levels (sometimes a thousandfold higher than in controls) in thyroid, pituitary, kidney, and liver in mercury miners who had died many years after retirement.

The average level of mercury in 38 placentas from residents in Iowa (United States) was 2.3 ppm. In another study, in Ohio, 29 placentas yielded an average of 6.7 ppm, of which 5.3 ppm was in the inorganic form.

Other Findings A close correlation between selenium and mercury concentrations in a variety of autopsy tissues from retired miners and other residents of the mining village of Idria, Yugoslavia, was reported by Kosta *et al.* (1975). The atomic ratio of selenium to mercury was almost exactly 1:1 over a wide range of concentrations. These observations, along with experimental data on animals (for a more recent report, see Magos *et al.*, 1984), suggest that inorganic mercury forms a complex with selenium that may persist for long periods in human tissues.

61.6.3.5 Treatment of Poisoning in Animals and Humans

Treatment in Animals The literature on the treatment of poisoning by mercury in animals and people was already very extensive in 1967 when Swensson and Ulfvarson reviewed it and added their own thorough studies in animals. On the basis of information on both animals and humans, they emphasized that therapeutic effect depends on the form of mercury causing poisoning and also on whether treatment begins early in the course of acute poisoning or after chronic poisoning already is established. Of compounds that they tested and that have ever been put to clinical use, BAL and D-penicillamine had a therapeutic effect in acute poisoning by inorganic mercury salts. BAL was also useful in acute poisoning by phenyl mercury. No useful treatment was found for acute poisoning by methyl mercury. Whereas penicillamine may have conferred some benefit in acute poisoning by methoxyethyl mercury, BAL did great harm: all animals died in convulsions following the second dose. AH of the chelating agents had some influence on the distribution of mercury in different organs and on its excretion. However, there was no definite connection between the lifesaving effect of an antidote and its effect on distribution or excretion of mercury. An increase in excretion of mercury was not a precondition for lifesaving effect. On the other hand, each chelating agent not only has its own toxicity but also may increase the toxicity of one or more forms of mercury, whether by increasing its concentration in the brain or kidney or in some other way.

Zimmer and Carter (1979) confirmed that BAL is useless in methyl mercury poisoning but, contrary to some earlier results, found that D-penicillamine enhanced weight gain and prevented further development of neurotoxic signs in rats poisoned by methyl mercury chloride.

In some instances, studies concerned directly with therapy have been confirmed by studies on distribution. For example Berlin and Ullberg (1963) showed that BAL greatly increased the uptake of phenyl mercury or methyl mercury by the brain. Zimmer and Carter (1979) reported a similar result with methyl mercury.

More recent work has served to confirm most of the findings, but further progress has been limited. To be sure, an almost endless array of new chelating agents have been synthesized and tested for ability to increase the excretion of mercury, to cause a redistribution of it, and/or to increase the survival of experimental animals. There has been progress in understanding the complications of using systemically acting chelating agents. Following intravenous injection of mercuric chloride, Gabard (1976) tabulated not only the urinary and fecal excretion of ^{203}Hg but also its distribution in red cells, plasma, liver, kidneys, brain, femur, muscle, spleen, and intestine of different groups of rats following treatment with one of 15 chelating agents. It was concluded that the only agent that had a truly favorable effect was sodium 2,3-dimercaptopropane-l-sulfonate (DMPS). Whether this would be true in humans as well as the rat is, of course, unproved. It seems certain, however, that the general problem of complex effects on distribution of metals following systemic chelation applies to all species.

The possible danger that a systemic chelating agent will increase the toxicity of mercury may be avoided completely by using a nonabsorbable chelating agent that serves to reduce the absorption or reabsorption of mercury from the intestine and thus to promote fecal excretion. One of these mercury-binding polymers (MBP) decreased the half-life of intraperitoneally administered methyl mercury in mice from 10.0 to 4.5 days and increased the LD 50 from 10.0 to 12.7 or 13.4 mg/kg, depending on the exact method of administration of the antidote (Harbison *et al.*, 1977).

A possible new approach to the treatment of poisoning by mercury, especially methyl mercury, was suggested by Kostyniak *et al.* (1975). In an *in vitro* study, they used a soluble and dialyzable chelating agent to free methyl mercury from protein binding and then removed the complex by passing the blood through a semipermeable dialysis tube. Using cysteine at a concentration of 10 mM in whole blood, up to 44% of methyl mercury and up to 94% of the cysteine were removed by one pass through die dialyzer.

Treatment in Humans Although BAL has been widely and successfully used in the treatment of inorganic mercury poisoning, the treatment of methyl mercury poisoning with chelating agents has not been successful (Nierenberg *et al.*, 1998). The reason is that, by the time symptoms and signs of poisoning appear, irreversible damage has been inflicted on the target tissue, the brain.

There have not been enough cases of poisoning by alkoxy or phenyl mercury compounds to reach any conclusions regarding the effectiveness of chelation therapy. Animal experiments suggest that BAL may be dangerous to use in the case of alkoxyalkyl mercury poisoning (for a review, see Swensson and Ulfvarson, 1967).

A neuromuscular disorder similar to myasthenia gravis and responsive to neostigmine was uncovered in the course of electrophysiological testing of Iraqi patients poisoned by methyl mercury. Subsequently, neostigmine therapy (gradually increased to 15–22.5 mg plus 2–3 mg of atropine sulfate intramuscularly daily in split doses) produced a remarkable clinical improvement. Substitution of a placebo resulted in substantial loss of strength that was restored when therapy was resumed (Rustam *et al.*, 1975).

61.6.4 ALKYL MERCURY COMPOUNDS

61.6.4.1 Identity, Properties, and Uses

Compounds and Synonyms Of the entire range of alkyl mercury compounds, ethyl and methyl compounds have been used as pesticides. Methyl mercury was available in the form of several salt—each sold under one or more proprietary names, including the bis-methylmercuric sulfate (Cerewet®), the cyanoguanidine or dicyandiamide (Agrosol®, Morsodren®, Panogen®, Panospray®), the nitrile (Chipcote®), and the propionate (Metasol MP®). Ethyl mercury also was available in the form of several salts, including the chloride (Ceresan®, Granosan®), the phosphate (Lignasan®, New Improved Ceresan®, New Improved Granosan®), the *p*-toluenesulfonanilide (Ceresan M®, Granosan M®), the 1,2,3,6-tetrahydro-3,6-endomethano-3,4,5,6,7,7-hexachlorophthalimide (50-CS46, Emmi®, PX-332), and the thiosalicylate (Elcide®, Merfamin®, Mertorgan®, Merzonin®). Ethylmercuricthiosalicylate also was known by the nonproprietary names mercurothiolate, thimerosal, and thiomersalate.

Properties See Section 61.6.3.2.

Uses Most of the individual compounds are used as fungicides in treating seeds, especially those of cereals, sorghum, sugar beets, cotton, and flax. Used in this way, they control diseases caused by seed-borne infection and protect germinating seedlings from soil-borne pathogens (WHO, 1974).

61.6.4.2 Toxicity to Laboratory Animals

Basic Findings The acute oral LD 50 value for representative compounds in rats is approximately 30 mg/kg (Lehman, 1951, 1952). The total dose of an alkyl mercury compound necessary to produce chronic poisoning in cats is about the same, that is, 6–24 mg/kg expressed as mercury (Kurland *et al.*, 1960).

Rats tolerated 0.5 mg (about 2.8 mg/kg/day) of ethyl mercury chloride daily for 150 days without sign of poisoning, but twice that dosage produced typical signs in 34 to 84 days (Akitake, 1968).

Methyl mercury affects mainly the central nervous system. However, the effects differ markedly for adult versus prenatal exposures, so the two situations will be discussed separately.

Effects on the Mature Nervous System Methyl mercury produces focal damage to specific areas of the brain—the neuronal cells of the visual cortex, particularly neurons situated in the deep sulci, appear to be most susceptible to damage (for a review, see Berlin, 1986). Effects most similar to those observed in humans are seen in nonhuman primates and rats.

Inhibition of protein synthesis is one of the earliest biochemical effects that precede the appearance of overt signs of intoxication in animals.

Effects on the Developing Nervous System Spyker *et al.* (1972) treated mice on day 7 and day 9 of pregnancy with a single (8 mg/kg) dose of methyl mercury. The young did not differ from the controls in size, weight, and appearance. However, when tested at 30 days of age, their behavior was abnormal in an open field test and in swimming. The brain showed abnormalities in the Purkinje and granule cells of the cerebellum (Chang *et al.*, 1977). More recently, Sager *et al.* (1984) reported that after a single (8 or 4 mg/kg) dose of methyl mercury to neonatal mice, the cell division of cerebellar granule cells was drastically reduced. The lower dose produced effects in male mice but not in females. It is thought that methyl mercury produces these effects by damaging microtubules, essential for cell division. For further discussion, see Sager and Matheson (1988).

61.6.4.3 Toxicity to Humans

Alkyl mercury fungicides commonly have been the cause of occupational poisoning even in developed countries, especially when anything but the best equipment was used for applying them to seed. Furthermore, their application to seed created the possibility that they would be eaten in quantity, especially by peasants who were hungry and did not know about either the delayed onset of symptoms or the impossibility of adequately decontaminating the seed (see Section 7.1.2.4 of Hayes, 1975). Finally, outbreaks of poisoning clinically similar to that caused by eating treated seed resulted from eating animals that had consumed contaminated feed or from eating fish that had absorbed alkyl mercury from industrial wastes.

Symptomatology Acute poisoning by organic mercury has been reported infrequently in humans, although cases of such poisoning by methyl (Swensson, 1952) and other alkyl compounds (Lundgren and Swensson, 1949; Veichenblau, 1932) have occurred. There have been many cases of chronic poisoning involving organic mercury.

The classical description of poisoning by an alkyl mercury compound is that of Edwards (1865). The patient may complain of headache; paresthesia of the tongue, lips, fingers, and toes; and other nonspecific dysfunction. In mild cases, the symptoms do not develop beyond this point, and in such instances they usually disappear gradually.

Some but not all workers equally exposed to alkyl mercury compounds complain of a metallic taste in the mouth and slight gastrointestinal disturbances, such as excessive flatus and diarrhea (Bloom *et al.*, 1955; Ritter and Nussbaum, 1945). However, the acute symptoms associated with irritation of the gastrointestinal system and renal failure caused by inorganic mercury compounds are seldom observed in poisoning by alkyl mercury compounds and then almost exclusively in acute poisoning. Even the mild digestive disturbances and sore mouth seen in moderate, chronic, occupational poisoning by inorganic mercury are relatively rare. Instead, the nervous symptoms appear first, sometimes after relatively slight exposure and after weeks or months of latency. Diagnosis is complicated not only by the latency but also by the insidiousness of the onset. The patient may be unable to state with any certainty when he or she first noticed important symptoms.

Early signs of more severe poisoning include fine tremors of the extended hands, loss of side vision, and slight loss of coordination, especially with the eyes closed as in the finger-to-nose test. Incoordination is especially noticeable in speech, writing, and gait. Incoordination may progress to the point of inability to stand or to carry out other voluntary movements. Occasionally there is muscle atrophy and flexure contractures. In other cases, there are generalized myoclonic movements. There may be difficulty in understanding ordinary speech, although hearing and the understanding of slow deliberate speech often remain unaffected. Irritability and bad temper are frequently present and may progress to mania. Occasionally the mental picture deteriorates to stupor or coma (Ahlborg and Ahlmark, 1949; Ahlmark, 1948; Herner, 1945; Hunter *et al.*, 1940). Especially in children, mental retardation may be added to the symptoms of poisoning already mentioned (Engleson and Herner, 1952; Kurland *et al.*, 1960).

Patients frequently become gradually much worse after their illness is recognized and exposure is stopped.

The alkyl mercury compounds are strong irritants of the skin and may cause blisters or other dermatitis with or without associated systemic illness (Hunter *et al.*, 1940; Vintinner, 1940).

Study of 43 cases in the 1972 outbreak in Iraq showed that a few entered hospital with complaints that suggested psychiatric disturbances, and over half of them were consistently depressed. Blood mercury levels were consistently higher in depressed than in nondepressed patients (Maghazaji, 1974).

Signs and symptoms of poisoning in children are similar to those in adults (Nagi and Yassin, 1974).

Duration of Illness The duration of illness in fatal cases ranged from about a month to 15 years (Hunter *et al.*, 1940). Intercurrent infection, aspiration pneumonia, and inanition are the immediate causes of death in protracted cases (Kurland *et al.*, 1960). Ten years after poisoning, neurological disorders persisted with little or no improvement among 26 victims of Minamata disease (Tokutomi *et al.*, 1961). Symptoms often persist for years even in mild poisoning (Tsubaki, 1968).

Recovery from poisoning by alkyl mercury is so slow and the effects of chelation therapy are so unimpressive that it was thought some years ago that no recovery is possible. Observations repeated at long intervals have indicated that some improvement does occur except perhaps in very severe cases.

Twelve patients who were poisoned by ethyl mercury during the 1960 outbreak in Iraq were reexamined in 1973 and showed considerable improvement (Al-Damluji, 1976a). The most severely poisoned patients who survived the 1971–1972 outbreak caused by methyl mercury improved slowly, although ataxia, diminution of visual fields and visual acuity, and paresthesias were still present 2 years later. During the same period, most patients originally graded mild or moderate lost their symptoms completely (Al-Damluji, 1976b). Some children who had suffered mild or moderate poisoning by methyl mercury recovered completely in the course of 2 years. Over half of the children who had suffered severe poisoning remained physically and mentally incapacitated. The degree of clinical progress shown by the children in Iraq was better than that of some other groups, but the difference may have depended on the prompt termination of exposure rather than on the age of the patients (Amin-Zaki *et al.*, 1978).

Perinatal Poisoning Infants exposed to methyl mercury *in utero* may be severely and permanently injured even though their mothers remain asymptomatic. On the other hand, infants who received no mercury *in utero* but received it in their mother's milk may escape without clinical signs. Such cases were observed in association with the outbreak of methyl mercury poisoning in Iraq during the winter and spring of 1971 to 1972. Four infants had blood levels above 1.0 ppm, and one had levels above 1.5 ppm without sign of injury, even though 0.2 ppm is the minimal toxic level for adults (Amin-Zaki *et al.*, 1974a).

In the Minamata area during the period 1955–1959, 22 infants of a total of about 400 were born defective. Most of the mothers of these defective children did not have typical Minamata disease, but most of them experienced numbness during pregnancy. All ate fish frequently (Kutsuna, 1966). Experience in Iraq was quite different: in only one of 15 infant–mother pairs exposed to methyl mercury was the infant affected and the mother free of clinical signs (Amin-Zaki *et al.*, 1974b).

The cause of the difference is uncertain, but it might be associated with the stages of gestation at which exposure occurred. Whether teratogenesis occurs, as distinct from fetal intoxication, has been discussed (Berlin *et al.*, 1969b) but is not yet clear.

Follow-up studies of prenatally exposed infants in Iraq have revealed a milder form of affliction characterized by delayed achievement of developmental milestones, abnormal reflexes, and a history of seizures (Marsh *et al.*, 1980, 1981).

Possible Distinctions between Poisoning by Methyl Mercury and Ethyl Mercury There is some indication that, compared to methyl compounds, the illness produced by ethylmercuric compounds involves relatively greater injury to the gastrointestinal system (aphthous stomatitis, catarrhal gingivitis, nausea, liquid stool, pain, and laboratory evidence of liver disorder) and the cardiovascular and hematopoietic systems and less disorder of sensation and coordination (deafness, ataxia) (Alekseyeva and Mishin, 1971; Bogomaz, 1969; D'yachuk, 1972; Shustov and Tsyganova, 1970; WHO, 1962). The contrast between the two has been pointed out on the basis of outbreaks in Iraq, the one in 1960 caused by ethyl mercury and the one in 1972 caused by methyl mercury (Al-Damluji, 1976b). However, poisoning by ethyl mercury may be fatal (Gis' and Pozner, 1970; Ljubetskii *et al.*, 1961; Mal'tsev, 1972), and those who survive may have residual nervous symptoms (Gis' and Pozner, 1970; Mal'tsev, 1972). A description of poisoning by ethyl mercury in children (Mal'tsev, 1972) makes it appear impossible to distinguish poisoning by ethyl and methyl mercury. At present it is unclear whether an important, clinical distinction is justified between poisoning by ethyl and methyl mercury either in adults or in children.

Outbreaks from Eating Treated Grain Several outbreaks caused by eating seeds dressed with methyl or ethyl mercury are listed in Table 7.14 in the first edition of this Handbook and are discussed briefly in the associated text. Findings reached in study of these and some other outbreaks have been used as appropriate throughout this section and Section 61.6.3. However, no attempt is made here to describe the epidemics themselves. The largest one, in which 6148 patients were admitted to hospital and 452 died there, was described at length in the proceedings of a Conference on Intoxication Due to Alkylmercury-Treated Seed (WHO, 1976) and was summarized by Skerfving and Copplestone (1976).

Outbreaks from Eating Poisoned Animals and Fish In December 1969, an 8-year-old girl developed ataxia, decreased vision, and depression of consciousness progressing to coma over a period of 3 weeks. Two weeks after she became sick, her 13-year-old brother developed a similar illness, which also progressed to coma in 2–3 weeks. At the end of December, their 20-year-old sister developed similar symptoms and became semicomatose. All were hospitalized and given supportive therapy. The use of chelating drugs was of very doubtful value. In May, two patients remained comatose, the other semi-comatose (Likosky *et al.*, 1970; Storrs *et al.*, 1970a, b). The 40-year-old mother in the family was pregnant at the time. She did not become ill, and she ate no more pork after the sixth month of gestation. However, her urinary mercury levels were elevated during the 7th and 8th months. A 3062-g male infant was delivered at term. He became dusky at 1 minute of life, and intermittent gross tremulous movements of the extremities persisted for several days. The cry was weak and high pitched, but otherwise the child seemed clinically normal. Urinary mercury values were markedly elevated. The electroencephalogram (EEG) and electromyogram (EMG) were normal 3 days after birth and remained so at 6 weeks. However, at 3 months of age the EEG was abnormal, and remained so. Clinical abnormality progressed even more rapidly with increased tone of the extremities at 6 weeks, generalized myoclonic jerks by 6 months, and hypertonicity, irritability, and nystagmoid eye movements without fixation of the eyes at 8 months. These effects were the result of mercury via the placenta, for the child was never breast-fed (Snyder, 1971, 1972).

During the investigation it was learned that in October 1969, 14 of 17 hogs owned by the family became ill with blindness and a gait disturbance; 12 of these 14 died, and 2 became blind. In September, one hog had been butchered for family food and the meat was eaten by seven of nine family members from September through December. Further investigation revealed that, in August 1969, the father had obtained floor sweepings from a plant for treating seed grain with methyl mercury dicyandiamide and had included this grain in food for the hogs.

High levels of mercury were found in the urine of the patients (0.16–0.21 ppm) and of other members of the family who remained well (0.06–0.20 ppm). The seed grain and pork contained almost equal concentrations of mercury (32.8 and 27.5 ppm, respectively) (Curley *et al.*, 1971; Storrs *et al.*, 1970a, b). Mass spectral analysis demonstrated the presence of methyl, ethyl, and probably methoxyethyl mercury in what was left of the waste grain that had been fed to the hogs (Curley *et al.*, 1971). Thus, poisoning had been caused by a mixture of alkyl compounds.

At least two epidemics were associated with the ingestion of seafood contaminated by industrial waste (Kurland *et al.*, 1960; Tsubaki and Irukayama, 1977).

The first of these outbreaks, which occurred at Minamata, Japan, alerted the medical community to the great danger, and Minamata disease became a synonym for chronic poisoning by organic mercury compounds. There is now considerable evidence that the compound in seafood responsible for poisoning is dimethyl mercuric sulfide ($CH_3-Hg-S-CH_3$) (Tokutomi *et al.*, 1961).

Dosage Response Apparently no useful information on dosage response to alkyl mercury compounds has come from accidents resulting from occupational exposure. Epidemiological studies of populations exposed to unusually high concentrations of methyl mercury in food have defined three categories differing in intensity and duration of exposure. People were poisoned

in Iraq when they consumed contaminated grain for an average of 1–2 months at an average mercury intake of 0.08 mg/kg/day and a maximum of about 0.2 mg/kg/day. People were poisoned in Japan when they ate contaminated fish for months or a few years at average and maximal mercury intakes of about 0.03 and 0.10 mg/kg/day. People in Sweden and various other parts of the world where fish have relatively high levels of methyl mercury were not affected by a maximal mercury intake of 0.005 mg/kg/day lasting many years or for life (WHO, 1976). A dosage–response analysis of both adult and prenatal exposures in Iraq revealed that the developing nervous system is more susceptible than the mature nervous system, probably by a factor of 3 (Clarkson *et al.*, 1981).

Laboratory Findings Three men each swallowed 0.01 mg of ^{203}Hg in the form of methylmercuric nitrate. Whole-body counting indicated that mercury accumulated mainly in the liver (50% of dose) and the head (10%). The main excretion route was the feces but urinary excretion (as a fraction of total excretion) increased with time up to 30 days after intake. The whole-body retention curves followed a single exponential curve with half-lives between 70 and 74 days (Aberg *et al.*, 1969). Similar data were obtained by Miettinen (1973). See also Section 61.6.3.4.

Treatment See Section 61.6.3.6 and see Section 8.2 in the first edition of this Handbook.

Pathology Extensive and relatively characteristic pathology has been reported in humans and experimental animals killed by alkyl mercury compounds. The most common findings are (*a*) bilateral cortical atrophy around the anterior end of the calcarine fissure with disappearances of the striation of Gennari (associated with constriction of the visual fields) and (*b*) gross atrophy of the folia in the depths of the sulci of the lateral lobes and the declive of the cerebellum involving the granule cell layer (associated with ataxia). The hypothalamus, midbrain, and basal ganglia may be involved. The changes in the brain involve gliosis as well as abnormality and loss of specific neurons. The bodies of the Purkinje cells are spared, although the axons are affected. The classical description of the pathology is that of Hunter and Russell (1954) based on a patient who had had industrial exposure to methyl mercury for only 4 months and who had been followed medically from the time of onset until his death from pneumonia and complications a little over 15 years later. The disease had progressed slowly at first, but by the end of the first year the patient was quite helpless although still alert and intelligent, and he remained so until his death. Reference to poisoning by alkyl mercury as the "Hunter–Russel syndrome" may be traced to this paper, which pointed out, among other things, the marked difference of pathology associated with alkyl mercury in humans and in experimental animals. Changes in peripheral nerves and the posterior columns have been reported in animals (Hunter *et al.*, 1940; Swensson, 1952), but Hunter was unable to find such changes in humans.

61.6.5 ALKOXYALKYL MERCURY COMPOUNDS

61.6.5.1 Identity, Properties, and Uses

Methoxyethyl mercury silicate frequently was formulated with other fungicides or insecticides for protection of cereal grain against both fungi and insects. Examples of proprietary names, which designate each total formulation and must not be confused with formulations of ethyl mercury involving the word "Ceresan®" include Ceresan-Aldrin® (with aldrin and HCB), Ceresan Gamma M® (with anthraquinone, hexachlorobenzene, and lindane), Ceresan-Morkit® (with anthraquinone and hexachlorobenzene), and Ceresan Universal Trockenbeize® (methoxyethyl mercuric silicate with hexachlorobenzene). Methoxyethylmercuric chloride was known by several proprietary names, including Agallol®, Aretan®, and Ceresan Universal Nassbeize®. For a comparison of the vapor pressures of alkoxyalkyl compounds with those of other organic mercury compounds, see Section 61.6.3.2.

61.6.5.2 Toxicity to Laboratory Animals

No information on the toxicity of alkoxyalkyl mercury compounds has been found.

61.6.5.3 Toxicity to Humans

Poisoning by alkoxyalkyl mercury compounds usually begins with loss of appetite, flatulence, and diarrhea. The patient may complain of loss of weight, exhaustion, and headache. Albuminuria is a common finding and may be accompanied by generalized edema. Signs of injury of the central nervous system are less prominent than in poisoning by alkyl mercury compounds, but numbness of the fingers and toes and some degree of ataxia and weakness may occur (Bonnin, 1951; Dérobert and Marcus, 1956; Wilkening and Litzner, 1952; Zeyer, 1952).

Acrodynia was recognized in a 5-year-old boy exposed on a farm to a methyloxyethyl mercury seed disinfectant. The symptoms, which were typical, included an exanthem with scaling of the skin of the hands and feet, extreme apathy, anorexia, photophobia, sleeping during the day and inability to sleep at night, muscular weakness with tremor of the extremities, heavy sweating, hypertension, and tachycardia. The concentrations of mercury in the blood and urine were 0.04 and 0.055 ppm, respectively. The clinical picture improved within 4 weeks; the skin cleared in 2 months, and the patient gained weight; hypertension and tachycardia disappeared slowly (Prediger, 1976). It is unclear whether treatment with cortisone was helpful.

A disease of children eventually named acrodynia because of the severe pain it caused in the extremities or "pink disease" because of the dusky pink color of these parts was described at least as early as 1828. There was no constructive clue to its cause until Warkany and Hubbard (1948) reported that mercury was present in the urine in 18 of 20 suspected cases, and the concentration exceeded 0.05 ppm in 15 of them. The two cases without mercury already had been recognized as atypical, but they indicated that an acrodynia-like condition may occur without demonstrable mercury. The paper also pointed out that the concentration of mercury in the urine of children treated with calomel often exceeds 0.05 ppm, and, therefore, some special susceptibility must be involved in the relatively few instances in which exposure to mercury is followed by acrodynia. A great many more cases confirmed the relationship (Warkany and Hubbard, 1951, 1953). When measures were taken by physicians, pharmaceutical companies, and regulatory agencies to stop the mercurial medication of infants and children, acrodynia became extremely rare (Warkany, 1966).

Following communications with Warkany, Bivings and Lewis (1948) first used BAL to treat acrodynia. The value of such treatment remains unclear.

The alkoxyalkyl mercury compounds, like the alkyl ones, can cause toxic dermatitis ranging from mild irritation to the production of slowly healing ulcers.

Treatment is symptomatic. See Section 61.6.3.6 and see Section 8.2 of the first edition of this Handbook.

61.6.6 ARYL MERCURY COMPOUNDS

61.6.6.1 Identity, Properties, and Uses

Compounds and Synonyms Phenyl mercury was available in the form of several salts each sold under one or more proprietary names, including the acetate (Gallotox®, Liquiphene®, Mersolite®, Nylmerate®, Phix®, Riogen®, Scutl®, Tag Fungicide®, Tag HL-331®, also known by the acronyms PMA, PMAC, PMAS), the nitrate (Merphenyl®, Phenmerzyl nitrate®, Phermerite®), the cyanamide (also known as barbak), the methylenebis(2-naphthyl-3-sulfonic) acid (Conotrane®, phenyl mercuric Fixtan®, Fibrotan®, Hydraphen®, Penotrane®, Septotan®, Versotrane®, also known as P.M.F. and as hydrargaphen), the borate (Famosept®, Imerfen®, Merfen®), the dimethyldithiocarbamate (Merbam®), the monoethanolammonium lactate (Puratized Agricultural Spray®, Puratized N5E®), the N-urea (Puratized Apple Spray®), the propionate (Metasol P-6®), the quinolinate (Metasol DPO®), the triethanolamine lactate (Dowicide la®, Dowicide 1®, Leytosan®, Natriphene®), and the hyrdoxychlorophenol (Semesan®, Uspulun®).

Properties For a comparison of the vapor pressure of phenyl mercury with that of other organic mercury compounds see Section 61.6.3.2.

Uses The individual compounds are used as fungicides for apples, pears, and other fruits, potatoes, tree wounds, bulbs, textiles, timber, leather, and wood pulp. A few are used as topical antiseptics and bactericides. The acetate is used as an herbicide for crabgrass as well as a fungicide.

61.6.6.2 Toxicity to Laboratory Animals

Basic Findings The oral LD 50 of phenyl mercury acetate in rats was found to be 60 mg/kg (Piechocka, 1968). The same parameter for another phenyl mercury compound was 30 mg/kg (Lehman, 1951, 1952). In mice, oral LD 50 values for phenylmercuric acetate and another phenylmercuric salt were both 70 mg/kg (Goldberg *et al.*, 1950).

Dietary mercury levels of 40 ppm (about 2 mg/kg/day) or lower in the form of either mercuric acetate or phenylmercuric acetate were tolerated by rats for 2 years without any change in rate of growth, mortality, or organ weights. A dietary level of 160 ppm (about 8 mg/kg/day) of mercuric acetate produced slight reduction in growth of male rats only, whereas the same rate of ingestion of phenylmercuric acetate interfered to a marked degree with the growth of both sexes and shortened their survival. The action of both compounds in the rat appeared to be on the kidney. A dietary level of 0.5 ppm of the phenyl compound produced detectable histological change in the kidney, but 10–20 times as much mercuric acetate was required to produce the same effect (Fitzhugh *et al.*, 1950). Solecki *et al.* (1991) observed that rats exposed to phenylmercuric acetate at 5 mg per liter of drinking water for 2 years showed an acceleration in the development of age-associated chronic nephrosis compared to controls.

61.6.6.3 Toxicity to Humans

Accidental and Intentional Poisoning Poisoning by aryl mercury compounds usually involves the blood, with symptoms of weakness secondary to anemia and infection secondary to leukopenia (Cotter, 1947). In some instances, a nonspecific neurasthenia occurs even though anemia is mild (Massmann, 1957) or absent (Swensson and Ulfvarson, 1963). In reporting an unsuccessful suicide with phenyl mercury, Ishida (1970) noted that the patient displayed no significant neurological manifestations.

Use Experience In many instances phenyl mercury fungicides have been used extensively without untoward effect even though workers may have increased levels of mercury in their hair (Kinoshita and Ogima, 1968; Tokutomi, 1968).

Three cases of acrodynia were reported in several thousand infants exposed to a phenyl mercury acetate added to a diaper wash as a fungicide (Gotelli *et al.*, 1985). A follow-up investigation of several hundred of these infants revealed urinary levels of mercury up to 500 μg/l. No clinical effects were found. Some infants had a mild enzymuria that subsequently disappeared.

Laboratory Findings See Section 61.6.3.4.

Pathology Decrease in anterior horn cells with demyelination of the lateral columns of the spinal cord (associated with a case said to resemble amyotrophic sclerosis) has been reported; the difference may be related to the fact that a phenyl mercury compound was involved (Brown, 1954).

Treatment of Poisoning See Section 61.6.3.6 and see Section 8.2 in the first edition of this Handbook.

61.7 THALLIUM

Thallium stands between mercury and lead in the periodic table. It has no known essential function in the body.

Most cases of poisoning by compounds of thallium, including even the small number that are truly occupational, involve compounds intended for use as pesticides. Most of the cases involve accidental ingestion, suicide, or murder. Moeschlin (1965) stated that in Europe thallium had replaced arsenic as a homicidal poison.

Thallium sulfate has been more widely used as a pesticide than any other compound of thallium. It has produced many cases of poisoning and serves as a good example of the toxicity of thallium generally.

A very thorough review of the toxicology of thallium is that of Heyroth (1947).

61.7.1 THALLIUM SULFATE

61.7.1.1 Identity, Properties, and Uses

Chemical Name   Thallous sulfate.

Structure Tl_2SO_4.

Synonyms   Proprietary names for thallium sulfate include Bonide Antzix ant killer®, GTA ant bane®, GTA bait®, Magikil Jelly ant bait®, Martin's Rat-Stop®, Liquid Mission Brank ant–roach killer®, and Rex ant bait®. The CAS registry no. is 7446-18-6.

Physical and Chemical Properties   Thallium sulfate has the empirical formula O_4STl_2 and a molecular weight of 504.85. It forms a colorless, odorless, dense powder of rhomboid prisms, with a density of 6.77 and a melting point of 632°C. Its vapor pressure is inappreciable. Its solubility in water at 20°C is 4.87%; at 100°C, 18.45%.

History, Formulations, and Uses   Thallium sulfate was introduced as a rodenticide in the United States during the 1930s. Syrups and jeilies for sweet-eating ants and grain baits for ground squirrels and prairie dogs formerly were available with concentrations as high as 3%. The use of thallium compounds as pesticides was banned by the USEPA in 1972 (U.S. EPA, 1985) but its use probably continues in some other countries.

61.7.1.2 Toxicity to Laboratory Animals

Basic Findings   Work in the first half of these twentieth century indicated that the oral LD 50 was in the range 7–24 mg Tl/kg (Dieke and Richter, 1946; Gettler and Weiss, 1943; Lehman, 1951, 1952; Munch and Silver, 1931). An extensive toxicological study on a number of thallium compounds by Down *et al.* (1960) indicated that the LD 50 for the acetate and oxide of thallium was in the range 12–30 mg Tl/kg in rats, guinea pigs, rabbits, and dogs. Diets fed to rats for 15 weeks showed increased mortality at levels of 4.5 mg Tl/kg as thallic oxide and 2.3 mg Tl/kg as thallium acetate. Rats given 1.4 mg Tl/kg/day in the drinking water as thallium sulfate exhibited 21% mortality after 240 days (Manzo *et al.*, 1983).

Absorption, Distribution, Metabolism, and Excretion
Thallium compounds are well absorbed in the gastrointestinal tract (Lie *et al.*, 1960). In industry, absorption is mainly respiratory, whereas nearly all accidental and intentional poisoning involves ingestion.

Thallium rapidly distributes from the bloodstream to all tissues in the body. The kidneys tend to have the highest concentrations. Thallium also accumulates in active hair follicles, much less so in follicles in the resting state. There is indirect evidence of enterohepatic circulation as the portal vein contains higher levels than in peripheral blood (Frey and Schlechter, 1939).

In rats, the fecal route is the predominant pathway of excretion. In studies using a radioactive tracer, Lie *et al.* (1960) observed a half-life of 3.3 days in rats.

Thallium crosses the placental barrier in rats and mice (Gibson *et al.*, 1967), in rabbits (Frey and Schlechter, 1939), and in humans. Characteristic hair loss and nail bands were seen in a baby born 60 days after the mother ingested 750 mg of thallium sulfate (von Martius, 1953).

Pathology   By far the most thorough study of tissue changes in rats poisoned by thallium is that of Herman and Bensch (1967), which must be consulted for details. Briefly, renal eosinophilic casts, enteritis, and severe colitis were present consistently in acute poisoning. In subacute poisoning, the brain contained frequent foci of perivascular cuffing and rare foci of recent necrosis. In chronic poisoning, no abnormality was visible by light microscopy, but degenerative changes frequently were present in the mitochondria of the kidney, liver, and intestines, and sometimes in those of the brain, seminal vesicles, and pancreas. Other changes included autophagic vacuoles and lipid droplets. The changes were not specific for thallium. These findings were similar to but more detailed than those of Cortella (1928).

Treatment of Poisoning in Animals   A number of antidotes have been used in the treatment of thallium poisoning in animals. These include BAL (Braun *et al.*, 1946; Lund, 1956; Moeschlin, 1965; Thyresson, 1951), cysteamine (Moeschlin, 1965), dithizone (Lund, 1956), cystine (Thyresson, 1951), and potassium chloride (Lund, 1956). The outcomes with these antidotes were equivocal.

The agent of choice is Prussian blue [potassium ferrohexacyanoferrate(II), having the empirical formula $KFe^{III}Fe^{II}(CN)_6 \cdot nH_2O$]. Given orally at 200 mg/kg daily for nine days, Prussian blue was found to be effective in rats (Heydlauf, 1969). Other investigators also found that Prussian blue was effective in experimental animals (for a review, see Stevens *et al.*, 1974).

61.7.1.3 Toxicity to Humans

The most complete review of human thallotoxicosis is that of Munch (1934). For more recent reviews, see ATSDR (1992b) and Goyer (1991).

Therapeutic Use   Apparently thallium sulfate has not been used as a drug. Thallium acetate was used as a dipilatory agent in treating fungal infections of the hair. Single oral doses at the rate of 4–10 mg/kg were employed. An interval of 2–6 months (usually 3 months) was recommended before readministration. Use of thallium was discontinued because it was found impossible to adjust the dosage so that the toxic effects were restricted to the loss of hair. However, children who survived treatment were reported to grow normally.

A review (Munch, 1934) showed there was serious poisoning in 5.5% of 8006 cases treated with a single oral dose of thallium acetate at different recommended dosage rates, mostly 8 mg/kg. There were 8 deaths in the series. No deaths were reported at dosages lower than 8 mg/kg, but such dosages were unreliable in causing hair loss, and one case of poisoning occurred at a dosage of 4 mg/kg.

Adults were more susceptible to poisoning than children, so the drug was given orally only to children under 10 or 12 years of age (Felden, 1928). However, thallium acetate ointments were used for treating hypertrichosis in adults. Munch (1934) tabulated 59 intoxications, some involving severe polyneuropathy, muscular atrophy, marked cerebral involvement, and blindness following use of 3–8% ointments for 1 week to several months. There were no deaths in this series.

Accidental and Intentional Poisoning   Signs and symptoms are referable mainly to the gastrointestinal tract, nervous system, and the hair and nails; the heart and kidneys may also be involved. After large doses, gastroenteritis is evident in about 12–14 hours, whereas neurological symptoms may be delayed 2–5 days. Following smaller doses, onset may be delayed as much as 3 weeks (Reed *et al.*, 1963).

Gastrointestinal manifestations include severe paroxysmal abdominal pain, vomiting, diarrhea, anorexia, stomatitis, salivation, and weight loss. Neurological manifestations during the first days of illness may include paresthesias, headache, cranial nerve damage (ptosis, strabismus, optic atrophy), myoclonic or choreiform movements, convulsions, delirium, and coma. The occurrence of high fever is probably the result of brain injury; it indicates a bad prognosis. Vascular collapse and death may occur in 24–48 hours, but the course is usually more prolonged. Death may be caused by respiratory paralysis, pneumonia, or circulatory disturbances. Peripheral neuropathy, particularly in the legs, is common with severe pain, paresthesias, muscle weakness, tremor, ataxia, and atrophy (Sollmann, 1957). Obstinate constipation may interfere with treatment. Loss of hair begins after 1 to 2 weeks have elapsed. Several days before spontaneous shedding, impending alopecia is indicated by the ease with which the hair may be pulled out. In the more protracted cases, ataxia, choreiform movements, dementia, depression, and psychosis may be prominent. The neurological changes must be characterized as diverse (Steinberg, 1961) and sometimes as bizarre. Neurologic damage may be permanent. In fact, chronic neurological defects were found in 54% of 48 patients who survived and were followed up. A blue gingival line and dermatological abnormalities, including white bands in the nails, may appear. Liver damage occurs but is not prominent clinically. Kidney damage may occur (Chamberlain et al., 1958; Munch et al., 1933; Reed et al., 1963).

Death may occur promptly from shock, or it may be delayed as much as 19 days after onset (Cavanagh et al., 1974). In a series of 72 children who ingested thallium, 9 died and 26 (36%) were left with persistent neurological damage. Prognostically unfavorable signs were gastrointestinal disturbances, cardiovascular abnormalities, coma, convulsions, and mental ion (Reed et al., 1963).

An outbreak of poisoning resulting from the use of thallium-treated grain as food is listed in Table 7.14 of the first edition of this Handbook.

In chronic poisoning, symptoms can be nonspecific, and thallium intoxication may not be suspected unless depilation occurs. Although characteristic of thallium toxicity, hair loss also can result from poisoning with other metals and certain drugs. The same is true of the white bands on the nails.

The findings already summarized are confirmed in many other reports of accidents, murders, and especially suicides (Bank et al., 1972; Bental et al., 1961; Chinen et al., 1977; Curry et al., 1969; Freund et al., 1971; Gastel et al., 1978; Gefel et al., 1970; Gerdts, 1964; Gharib, 1970; Goulon, 1963; Grulee and Clark, 1951; Hausman and Wilson, 1964; Koblenzer and Weiner, 1969; Marten, 1969; Ossa et al., 1975; Potes-Gutierrez and Del Real, 1966; Reibscheid et al., 1966; Sørensen, 1965; Taber, 1964; Vasil'eva et al., 1978).

Dosage Response   Even in children, who are less susceptible than adults, serious poisoning has followed a single dose of thallium acetate at a rate of 4 mg/kg. Twice that dosage poif soned 5.5% of treated patients. Moeschlin (1965) reported that death of an adult had followed a dosage of only 8 mg/kg, but that most fatalities involved dosages in the range 10–15 mg/kg or higher.

Laboratory Findings   Diagnosis of poisoning often can be confirmed by analysis for thallium in urine, blood, or hair. The concentration of thallium in normal tissue is low. The concentration in serum does not exceed 0.03 ppm (Gofman et al., 1964). The values for urine of unexposed individuals are below 1 μg Tl/g creatinine (Schaller et al., 1980). Urinary levels as high as 10–15 ppm have been found in a patient who survived (Mathews and Anzarut, 1968). In a group of poisoned children 1–6 years of age, the excretion of thallium soon after hospitalization was usually 1–3 mg/24 hr, but in one patient it reached a level of 15.4 mg/24 hr (Chamberlain et al., 1958). Similar concentrations (2–4 ppm) were found in a poisoned adult (Gettler and Weiss, 1943). In a case of subacute, nonfatal poisoning, the concentration of thallium in the urine varied from 0.2 to 0.3

ppm when first measured a month after ingestion and then declined more and more slowly to values of 0.05 to 0.06 ppm 20 days later (Rodermund et al., 1968).

Proteinuria, cylindruria, and sometimes hematuria and oliguria may be present as indications of renal damage. Liver function tests may be abnormal. The blood picture and bone marrow are usually normal. However, there may be increased coproporphyrin and/or, more rarely, uroporphyrin in the urine. The serum iron may be slightly increased, suggesting a disturbance in the uptake of iron by the reticuloendothelial system. According to Moeschlin (1965), the spinal fluid shows a marked increase in protein, sometimes involving the globulin, but no increase in cells; a slight gold-sol and mastix reaction of the parenchymatous type may be present also. In other cases, the spinal fluid may be entirely normal (Chamberlain et al., 1958). Examination of the spinal fluid is not useful in prognosis (Reed et al., 1963).

One or more bands of dark pigment may be demonstrated in hair near the root in as little as 4 days after ingestion. The bands do not contain increased thallium (Moeschlin, 1965).

In many patients there is flattening or inversion of the T-waves in some leads of the electrocardiogram.

In the few patients who have epileptic seizures, the electroencephalogram shows long stretches of low-voltage theta waves and low-voltage fast activity interrupted at intervals by slow high-amplitude waves that may be single or in groups, including regular runs of waves at the rate of 6 or 7 per second (Moeschlin, 1965). Other investigators have emphasized the slow, high-amplitude waves. Patients with abnormal electroencephalographic findings frequently die or fail to recover completely, while those with normal records usually survive without sequelae (Reed et al., 1963).

Pathology   Only visceral congestion and hyperemia and punctate hemorrhages of the gastrointestinal tract may be found if death occurs soon after exposure. In cases with longer survival, alopecia may be present. The skin is dry, and microscopic examination reveals marked lesions of the epithelium, follicles, and glands. Damage to the intestinal mucosa is common. There may be fatty degeneration of the heart and liver, degeneration of kidney tubules and the adrenal medulla, and edema and congestion of the lungs. At least a part of the varied tissue damage is explained by histological damage in the capillaries. Degeneration and demyelination occur in peripheral nerves. Similar changes have been found in one or more cases in the paravertebral sympathetic chain, the fasciculus gracilis, and in various other tracts or nerves, including the optic nerve. There may be retrograde injury to neurons in ganglia and nerve nuclei (Bank et al., 1972; Gettler and Weiss, 1943; Heyroth, 1947; Karkos, 1971; Moeschlin, 1965). The dying back may affect both motor and sensory nerves (Cavanagh et al., 1974). Finally, severe damage to a wide range of brain nuclei may be found (Kennedy and Cavanagh, 1976).

Treatment of Poisoning   The treatment of choice (following efforts to remove as much ingested poison as possible) would appear to include ferric ferrocyanide (Prussian blue) or activated charcoal, forced diuresis (with a moderate supplementation of total potassium chloride), and supportive measures as required. Among the latter, trihexyphenidyl (Artane) may be of value in selected cases. This compound, which is ordinarily used to treat Parkinsonism, caused a striking reduction in tremors in one series of cases of thallium poisoning (Stein and Perlstein, 1959).

Ferric ferrocyanide in divided oral doses at a total rate of 250 mg/kg/day or even greater should be administered to minimize absorption of thallium from the intestine. Daily doses should be given to reduce reabsorption of the poison from the intestine. Although fecal excretion of thallium is ordinarily small in humans, the material is excreted into the gastrointestinal tract as in animals. Frey and Schlechter (1939) reported a case in which moderate quantities of thallium were found in the vomitus as late as the 35th day after onset.

Rauws and van Heyst (1979) found that different preparations of Prussian blue differed in their ability to adsorb thallium. In general, colloidally soluble preparations are effective, but ideally every batch intended for antidotal use should be tested for thallium-binding capacity.

No side effects were seen from ferric ferrocyanide even at a dosage of 416 mg/kg/day. Duodenal intubation is not required for administering this material. Its effects are dramatic when administered soon after ingestion and rewarding even when given in long-standing intoxication. It may promote substantial fecal excretion, even though the concentration of thallium in the urine has decreased to less than 0.5 mg/24 hr (Barbier, 1974). On the contrary, when hemodialysis, forced diuresis, and Prussian blue were used in combined treatment, slightly more thallium was recovered in the urine than in the dialysate and only very little was found in the feces (Drasch and Hauck, 1977). It is not yet clear how the different forms of removal of thallium compete with one another, just which method is best, or whether combined treatment is necessarily better than the best single treatment.

If ferric ferrocyanide is not available at once, the patient should be treated with repeated doses of activated charcoal (500 mg/kg twice daily) until Prussian blue can be obtained.

Prussian blue, taken orally, is nonabsorbable. It is believed to trap thallium ions in the intestinal tract via exchange with potassium ions in the Prussian blue mineral matrix (Stevens *et al.*, 1974).

Many other antidotes have been tested but with equivocal results (Bass, 1963; Foreman, 1961; Reed *et al.*, 1963).

61.8 LEAD

The present minor importance of lead compounds as pesticide would justify very little attention to them in this book. However, the great importance of other lead compounds as causes of accidental poisoning and the long persistence of lead arsenate following its earlier heavy use as a pesticide require some discussion of lead here. Those requiring additional information

may find it in several reviews (Aub *et al.*, 1926; Browning, 1969; Cantarow and Trumpeter, 1944; Goldwater, 1972; Goyer, 1974; Kehoe, 1964; U.S. Public Health Service, 1966; WHO, 1977).

61.8.1 LEAD ARSENATE

61.8.1.1 Identity, Properties, and Uses

Chemical Name Lead arsenate.

Structure $PbHAsO_4$.

Synonyms Other names for lead arsenate include acid lead arsenate, dibasic lead arsenate, dilead arsenate, dilead orthoarsenate, diplumbic hydrogen arsenate, lead hydrogen arsenate, and standard lead arsenate. Trade names include Arsinette®, Gypsine®, Ortho L10 Dust®, and Ortho L40 Dust®. The GAS registry no. is 10102-48-4.

Physical and Chemical Properties Lead arsenate has the empirical formula $AsHO_4Pb$ and a molecular weight of 347.13. It is a white, odorless powder with a density of 5.79. It decomposes above 280°C. It is soluble in dilute nitric acid and alkali but insoluble in water. It is stable to light, air, and water. It is not stable in acid, alkali, or sulfides.

History, Formulations, and Uses Lead arsenate first was used as an insecticide in 1894. It is used for the control of moths, leaf rollers, and other chewing insects and in soil treatments for Japanese and Asiatic beetles in lawns. It is formulated as pastes or powders. Pastes contain at least 28.4% PbO, 14% As_2O_5; powder contains at least 62% PbO, 32% As_2O_5; neither contains more than 0.25% As_2O_5 in water-soluble form. Lead arsenate may be used with summer oil emulsions, spray lime, wettable sulfur, and certain hydrocarbons and nicotine sulfate. An indefinite lead arsenate mixture called basic lead arsenate (see Table 61.4 in Section 61.12, also is used in the form of dusts, with sulfur or clay, and in water suspensions. Production of lead arsenate and of calcium arsenate is illustrated in Fig. 1.8) in the first edition of this Handbook.

61.8.1.2 Toxicity to Laboratory Animals

Symptomatology The signs of acute poisoning by lead arsenate in rats are similar to those of other arsenic compounds (see Section 61.12.1). The animals show violent gastroenteritis and diarrhea and die from exhaustion and dehydration. Convulsions and general paralysis may occur before the onset of gastroenteritis. Death may occur within a few hours to several days.

Following repeated doses, dogs may develop convulsions and paralysis not unlike the signs of encephalopathy seen in subacute poisoning in humans. Rats show nephropathy at least histologically and thus reproduce another injury seen in humans. Anemia is commonly present. Many of the subtle effects of chronic lead poisoning observed in humans are poorly reproduced in animals, although Aub *et al.* (1926) produced a convincing "wristdrop" in cats by weighting the paw.

Dosage Response Voight *et al.* (1948) reported a marked difference between the oral LD 50 values of lead arsenate in the rabbit (125 mg/kg) and rat (825 mg/kg). However, Lehman (1951, 1952) reported a value for the rat (100 mg/kg) not very different from that reported earlier for the rabbit.

Dogs fed lead at rates of 0.33–1.10 mg/kg developed signs of poisoning in 120–215 days, and only some of them survived 229 days until the end of the experiment. Young animals were more susceptible than old ones. Dogs fed lead at rates of 1.8–2.6 mg/kg/day developed the first signs of poisoning in 14–44 days, and most of them died following convulsions and paralysis in 51–84 days after the beginning of feeding. Within the dosage range used, there was an approximately straight-line inverse relationship between rate of intake and the time at which signs of poisoning began. Dogs fed arsenic trioxide at arsenic rates corresponding to those obtained from lead arsenate remained well (Calvery *et al.*, 1938). A no-effect level for lead was not demonstrated.

Male rats, but not females, were said to show decreased growth rate when fed lead arsenate at an average lead rate of about 0.21 mg/ kg/day (Laug and Morris, 1938), but the difference was of questionable statistical significance. There was a slight increase in the dry weight of the kidney relative to body weight, but this may have been the result of a nutritional disturb bance caused by pair feedings. It is possible that 0.21 mg/kg/day is a threshold level for toxicity in the rat. This result is very similar to that reported earlier by Smyth and Smyth (1932), who found a dosage of 0.265 mg/kg/day for 16 weeks harmless, 1.03 mg/kg/day questionably harmful, and a dosage of 3.93 mg/kg/day definitely harmful.

Fairhall and Miller (1941) found that a dosage of 24 mg/kg/day caused some failure of growth in the course of a 2-year experiment. Horwitt and Cowgil (hor7) found that an intake of about 5 mg/kg/day produced no effect on growth, but an intake of about 10 mg/kg/day did produce anemia and growth retardation. Slight but reproducible growth retardation was reported by Laug and Morris (1938) in an experiment in which rats on a special low-lead diet received a supplement that added only 0.213 mg/kg/day to their lead intake.

Absorption, Distribution, Metabolism, and Excretion Absorption of lead arsenate is generally gastrointestinal. This is likely to be true following respiratory exposure to coarse dusts as well as after ingestion. Dermal absorption is extremely small.

Lead and arsenic derived from lead arsenate are distributed separately in the body. Lead is stored in highest concentration in the bone with much lower concentrations in soft tissues. Arsenic, although constituting a smaller proportion of the molecule, is stored in the liver and in some instances in the kidney at higher concentrations than those for lead (Fairhall and Miller, 1941).

Lead is transferred to the fetus of animals and humans (Calvery, 1938; Horiuchi *et al.*, 1959; Legge and Goadby, 1912; Morris *et al.*, 1938).

Dogs and rats fed lead at a constant rate store less lead when fed a normal or high-calcium diet than when fed a low-calcium diet (Calvery *et al.*, 1938; Grant *et al.*, 1938). In fact, the metabolism of lead is very similar to that of calcium. The same factors act on both, and each tends to displace the other.

Rats store lead at the lowest measurable dietary intake, and storage is proportional to intake (Laug and Morris, 1938).

When rats ingest lead at ordinary dietary levels, it is stored in highest concentration in bone, but when feeding is at a high level for a few weeks, the highest concentration is in the kidney (Laug and Morris, 1938).

Mode of Action Because lead arsenate contains two toxic elements, it might be predicted that its toxicity would show an influence of both kinds of poisoning. Fairhall and Miller (1941) reported evidence that this is true; for example, it was clear that increased hemosiderin of the spleen was an effect of arsenic, whereas certain inclusion bodies in the kidney were an effect of lead. Furthermore, as described later, this study suggests that rats are more susceptible to mortality caused by prolonged exposure to the arsenic moiety of lead arsenate, whereas the work of Calvery *et al.* (1938) suggests that dogs are more susceptible to the lead moiety.

One group of rats was fed lead arsenate at an approximate rate of 10 mg/rat/day, which would be about 40 mg/kg/day when they reached adulthood. Other groups were fed lead carbonate and calcium arsenate at such a rate that they received an equivalent dosage of lead and arsenic, respectively. A control group received the same diet but none of the chemicals. During the 2-year course of the experiment, lead carbonate did not increase the mortality significantly over that of the controls (42%). However, both arsenic compounds caused an approximately equal increase in mortality (56% or more after 2 years). At the end of 1 year, half of the living animals were killed and their tissues analyzed. Similar analyses were made on the rats that survived for 2 years. Animals fed lead arsenate stored more arsenic than lead in their soft tissues, even though the rate of arsenic intake was less (21.6% of molecule as compared to 60.7%). The storage of lead in bone was very great, as expected. More interesting was the fact that (with the possible exception of arsenic in the liver) all organs stored less arsenic and less lead when they were fed simultaneously as lead arsenate than when fed separately at the same rates. The difference (at least for lead) was attributed to decreased absorption or increased excretion, but the possibility that solubility might be involved could not be excluded (Fairhall and Miller, 1941).

Treatment of Poisoning in Animals CaNa₂-EDTA was more effective than unithiol in promoting excretion of lead (Soroka and Sorokina, 1969).

61.8.1.3 Toxicity to Humans

Experimental Exposure One man was given lead arsenate at the rate of 40 mg/day or about 0.57 mg/kg/day for 50 days without ill effect (Cardiff, 1940). In a separate study, two men ingested lead arsenate at a rate of 100 mg/man/day for 10 days without injury (Fairhall and Neal, 1938). These levels are far above the level of lead in soluble form found to produce mild poisoning in a somewhat longer period. The difference in effect presumably is due to the insolubility of lead arsenate, although duration of exposure may play a part also.

Accidental and Intentional Poisoning There have been astonishingly few reports of poisoning by lead arsenate. Tobaldin *et al.* (1966) did report cases of nonfatal poisoning in two girls, ages 8 and 10 years. The initial symptoms of gastrointestinal irritation were what one would expect in acute poisoning by a metal salt. The authors concluded that the effects were the result of both elements.

Use Experience In an apple-raising area, many people, including children, ate apples sprayed with lead arsenate so that the average intake of the compound was about 5 mg/person/day. They suffered no ill effect, and the only change was a marginal increase in the levels of lead in the blood and of lead and arsenic in the urine as compared with samples from an urban community (Neal *et al.*, 1941b).

In a 14-month study of 542 formulators and applicators of lead arsenate sprays for apple orchards, Neal *et al.* (1941b) found only 7 who had a combination of clinical and laboratory findings directly referable to the absorption of the compound. Whether the very mild observed conditions represented poisoning was left moot, but it was noted that not a single case met the criteria established by the Committee on Lead Poisoning of the American Public Health Association. Dermatitis was infrequent and not related to exposure to lead arsenate. The fertility of married orchardists was normal. The degree exposure of these orchardists was indicated by average lead concentrations of 5.74 mg/m^3 during mixing and 0.45 mg/m^3 during spraying. Arsenic values were proportionally smaller.

These orchardists, who had had many years of heavy exposure to lead arsenate as applicators and the arsenic content of whose urine in 1938 averaged 0.141 ppm (men) and 0.098 ppm (women), were studied again in 1968 and 1969. The standard total mortality ratio (SMR) for the orchardists compared to the general population of the same state was only 0.65. The corresponding SMRs for heart disease, cancer, and stroke were 0.60, 0.66, and 0.76, respectively, indicating that this cohort experienced less total mortality and less mortality from heart disease, cancer, and stroke (Nelson *et al.*, 1973).

61.9 TIN

Tin is in the same periodic group as lead. Under conditions of use, inorganic tin compounds have proved essentially harmless, although inhalation of stannic oxide commonly leads to

a benign pneumoconiosis. Organic tin compounds have produced gastrointestinal disturbances, tremor, convulsions, paralysis, and death in animals. Triethyltin compounds, which readily cross the blood–brain barrier, produce severe neurological disturbances in both animals and humans (see Section 61.9.2). Thus lead and tin may injure the same organs, and some alkyl compounds of both are especially dangerous. However, the situation is far from simple. Alkyl derivatives of lead, like those of antimony, bismuth, and mercury, damage nerve cells, whereas triethyltin produces an interstitial edema of the white matter without damage to the cells. Some tin compounds that are closely related chemically have very different toxic effects. Triethyltin causes edema of the central nervous system; diethyltin causes hypertrophy of the bile ducts in some species. The same compound may be highly toxic to one species and essentially harmless to another. An example is dibutyltin, which is highly toxic to rats but not to guinea pigs. In addition to these differences observed in the same laboratory, there are unusually large quantitative differences in the toxicity of certain compounds (e.g., triphenyltin) as observed in different laboratories. Unexplored possibilities to explain the quantitative differences include the strain of rat and the supply of essential trace elements such as zinc.

Traces of inorganic tin are widely distributed in nature. In addition to the amount naturally present in food, tin may be added from foil and plated cans used as containers. Organic tin does not occur naturally. No conclusion about its safety can be drawn from experience with inorganic compounds. Organic tin compounds have some importance as fungicides and they have been proposed as insecticides or antifeeding compounds for insects. So far, these uses have led to no serious difficulty. However, the fact that related compounds have produced serious injury and death in humans serves as a warning that any tin compound proposed for use as a pesticide should be studied with particular care.

The following sections are confined to recognized pesticides and to an extremely brief summary of ethyltin compounds. Although the latter compounds have only been proposed as pesticides, it is necessary to keep them in mind in any consideration of pest control based on tin. Comprehensive reviews of the toxicology of tin are those of Barnes and Stoner (1959), LeBreton (1962), and ATSDR (1992c).

61.9.1 FENTIN ACETATE

61.9.1.1 Identity, Properties, and Uses

Chemical Name Triphenyltin acetate.

Structure (C$_6$H$_5$)$_3$Sn—OC(O)—CH$_3$.

Synonyms Fentin acetate (BSI, ISO) is the common name in use. A trade name for the compound is Brestan, Code designations include ENT-25,208, GC-6,936, Hoe-2,824, and VP-1,940. The CAS registry no. is 900-95-8.

Physical and Chemical Properties Fentin acetate has the empirical formula $C_{20}H_{18}O_2Sn$ and a molecular weight of 409.06. It forms white odorless crystals that melt at 122–124°C. The vapor pressure at 30°C is 1.33×10^{-6} torr. Its solubility in water at 20°C is 28 mg/l. It is poorly soluble in organic solvents. Fentin acetate is stable when dry but rapidly hydrolyzed by water to the hydroxide, a white solid that melts at 118–120°C. The hydroxide practically is insoluble in water but is soluble in most organic solvents.

History, Formulations, and Uses Fentin acetate was introduced in 1954. It is used as a fungicide on turnips, potatoes, celery, beans, and other crops. The technical product is 90–95% pure. It is formulated as wettable powders of 20 and 60% concentration and applied at a rate of approximately 160–260 g of active ingredient per hectare. Fentin acetate also is used as an antifeeding compound for insect control.

61.9.1.2 Toxicity to Laboratory Animals

Basic Findings Rats poisoned by a single dose of fentin acetate show sluggishness, unsteadiness, moderate diarrhea, anorexia, bloody stain around the nose and eyes, and wheezing.

The acute toxicity of fentin acetate is shown in Table 61.3. It is clear that absorption from the gastrointestinal tract is poor compared with that from the peritoneum.

Klimmer (1964) found that 70% of rats dosed by stomach tube at a daily rate considered equivalent to 50 ppm in the diet died of secondary infection in an average of 26.6 days. Stoner (1966) found that rats survived a dietary level of 200 ppm for 10 weeks, but most died when the concentration was raised to 300 ppm. The difference in response almost certainly depended

Table 61.3
Acute Toxicity of Fentin Acetate

Species	Route	LD 50 (mg/kg)	Reference
Rat	Oral	136[a]	Klimmer (1964)
Rat, F	Oral	491[b]	Stoner (1966)
Rat	Dermal	450	Klimmer (1964)
Rat	Intraperitoneal	13.2	Klimmer (1964)
Rat, M	Intraperitoneal	8.5	Stoner (1966)
Rat, F	Intraperitoneal	11.9	Stoner (1966)
Mouse, M	Oral	81.3	Stoner (1966)
Mouse, M	Intraperitoneal	7.9	Stoner (1966)
Guinea pig	Oral	21	Klimmer (1964)
Guinea pig, M	Oral	10	Stoner et al. (1955)
Guinea pig	Intraperitoneal	5.3	Klimmer (1964)
Guinea pig, M	Intraperitoneal	3.74	Stoner (1966)
Rabbit	Oral	30–50	Klimmer (1964)
Rabbit	Intraperitoneal	10	Klimmer (1964)

[a] In methylcellulose.
[b] In arachis oil.

on the dosage schedule. Even a level of 25 ppm may reduce food intake, growth, and the number of leukocytes in the blood (Verschuuren et al., 1966).

Guinea pigs are more susceptible than rats to triphenyltin acetate, on both an acute and a long-term basis. Dietary levels of 50 ppm are fatal in a few weeks. Levels as low as 5 ppm cause growth inhibition and reduction in hemoglobin and white cells in the blood (Stoner, 1966; Verschuuren et al., 1966). Even at 1 ppm, food intake was reduced (Stoner, 1966). The injury is not merely one of starvation; treated guinea pigs grow more slowly than pair-fed controls (Stoner and Heath, 1967).

The effect of fentin acetate is highly cumulative in the guinea pig. The logarithmic mean survival time on 25 ppm was twice that on 50 ppm (Stoner, 1966). However, the log mean survival time (>190 days) on 12 ppm was greater than would be predicted on the basis of a completely cumulative effect (Stoner and Heath, 1967).

Histologically, only a few animals fed triphenyltin acetate displayed interstitial edema of the brain. Dietary levels of 20 ppm and higher significantly increased the water content of the brain and spinal cord in guinea pigs. A dietary level of 500 ppm significantly increased the water content of the spinal cord of rats, but only in the females (Verschuuren et al., 1966). In spite of these morphological and chemical changes in the brain and spinal cord at high levels of intake, the symptomatology does not suggest that injury to the central nervous system is critical in poisoning by triphenyltin acetate.

Triphenyltin acetate (and chloride) produced marked testicular atrophy in rats when fed for 20 days at a concentration giving an intake of 20 mg/kg/day (Pate and Hays, 1968). The effect was more striking than that reported for triphenyltin hydroxide but the difference probably was explained by the higher dosage involved.

The second segment of the log(time)–log(dosage) curve for fatal dosages of triphenyltin acetate in guinea pigs was presented by Scholz (1965). As expected (see Section 1.2.3,2), it closely fits a straight line.

Fentin acetate was not tumorigenic when administered to mice for about 18 months at the maximal tolerated level (Innes et al., 1969).

Sachsse et al. (1987) found no adverse effects in dogs given 0.6 mg/kg/day in the feed for 1 year. Tennekes et al. (1989), in studies of rats given triphenyltin in the diet for 2 years, found evidence of tubular atrophy of the testes and atrophy of the sciatic nerve at dosage rates down to 0.3 mg/kg/day. Lowest effect levels in mice for chronic oral exposures appear to be higher than those for the rat. For example, a National Cancer Institute study (NCI, 1978) did not find adverse effects at 3.75 mg/kg/day over a 78-week oral exposure.

The Agency for Toxic Substances and Disease Registry (ATSDR, 1992c) have reviewed evidence for the tumorigenicity of triphenyltin compounds in animal studies. Most tumors are found in the endocrine glands. Tumors have also been found in testicular Leydig cells and in hepatic cells.

Absorption, Distribution, Metabolism, and Excretion Absorption from the skin is poor (Stoner, 1966). During oral dosing of sheep for 20 days with fentin acetate at the rate of 10 mg/day, [113]Sn was found in the milk at an average concentration of 0.0017 ppm. Tin was present as fentin acetate and in two unidentified forms. Seventeen days after dosing was stopped, the concentration had fallen to the limits of detectability. During treatment, the concentration 0.0029 ppm in the blood and 0.0075 ppm in the urine. Eight days after dosing was stopped, the liver, kidney, lung, pancreas, gallbladder, and brain contained higher concentrations of [113]Sn than did other organs, and the level was still increased in the liver after 218 days (Herok and Götte, 1964). In cows and sheep, triphenyltin is excreted chiefly in the feces (Brügemann *et al.*, 1964; Herok and Götte, 1964).

Triphenyltin is rapidly distributed to all tissues, including the brain of rats. It can still be detected in the brains of rats and guinea pigs more than 30 days after a single dose (Heath, 1966).

Mode of Action A single dose in the fatal range produces irritation of mucous membranes and death due to respiratory failure. Repeated doses produce no injury unless they are large enough to interfere with food intake. However, the cause of death following repeated doses is not clear. Starvation undoubtedly contributes. In some but not all laboratories, secondary infection has been an important cause of death of animals receiving this compound (Klimmer, 1964; Verschuuren *et al.*, 1966). A basis for susceptibility to infection was found in guinea pigs, which showed reduced lymphopoiesis, including atrophy of the white pulp of the spleen (Verschuuren *et al.*, 1966). It may be that increased susceptibility to infection explains the morbidity and mortality caused by fentin acetate to a far greater extent than has been proved. Infection is difficult to recognize in the absence of inflammation.

61.9.1.3 Toxicity to Humans

Poisoning of two pilots and three mechanics followed the aerial application to field crops of a mixture of fentin acetate and manganese ethylenedithiocarbamate without stringent observation of safety regulations. The pilots were severely ill. Gastrointestinal irritation was the main problem, but the liver was affected in one. Illness in the mechanics was mainly subjective (Horacek and Demcik, 1970).

Laboratory Findings Apparently there is no report of tissue levels of tin following poisoning by fentin acetate. The occurrence of tin in normal people is discussed in Section 61.9.2.3.

61.9.2 ETHYLTIN AND RELATED COMPOUNDS

61.9.2.1 Identity, Properties, and Uses

Compounds and Their Characteristics Alkyltin compounds occur in the following forms: $RSnX_3$, R_2SnX_2, R_3SnX, and R_4Sn, where R is an alkyl group linked directly to tin and X is a simple or complex ion. It has been found that the toxicity of these compounds and of certain phenyltin compounds to mammals and fungi depends mostly on the R constituent and to only a minor degree on the nature of X. Tributylin salts have the greatest fungicidal activity, and the effectiveness decreases with changes in the R component in the following order: tributyl > tri-*n*-propyl = tri-*iso* propyl > triethyl = diethylphenyl > triphenyl > trihexyl > trimethyl > trioctyl = diethyl. The monoethyl- and tetraethyl-tin compounds were ineffective as fungicides (Van der Kerk and Luijten, 1954). Triethyltin salts have the greatest toxicity for mammals.

61.9.2.2 Toxicity to Laboratory Animals

Basic Findings The toxicity of ethyltin trichloride is low. An intravenous dose at the rate of 70–150 mg/kg quickly produced hyperpnea, vasodilatation, prostration, and muscular tremors in rabbits, but they recovered in about an hour. Rats showed no distinctive signs after an intraperitoneal dose of 200 mg/kg (Stoner *et al.*, 1955).

Diethyltin compounds do not produce clearly neurological effects. They produce a more generalized illness similar to that caused by the triphenyltin. They also produce in the rat and mouse but not the rabbit, guinea pig, cat, or hen a characteristic injury of the bile ducts (Barnes and Stoner, 1959). The lesion was first described in great detail in connection with dibutyltin dichloride (Barnes and Magee, 1958). The injury starts within 60 min of an intravenous dose or 4 hr of an oral dose as a localized lesion of the lower part of the bile duct. The initial lesion, accompanied by an apparently minor extravasation of bile into the surrounding pancreatic tissue, sets up a chain of events leading to: (*a*) partial blockage of the bile duct and its great dilatation, (*b*) inflammation of the walls of the main vessels of the portal tracts, (*c*) thrombosis in some of these vessels, and (*d*) sharply localized areas of necrosis resembling infarcts within the liver parenchyma. The bile duct may rupture, leading to peritonitis and fat necrosis. It is of interest that this unusual injury apparently occurs only in species in which the pancreatic ducts enter the lower part of the common bile duct rather than entering the duodenum directly. It is also of interest that the general toxic effects of dibutyltin are prevented by BAL, but the local action on the biliary tract is not prevented

Triethyltin produces significant swelling of the brain and spinal cord and a striking noninflammatory interstitial edema of their white matter without detectable damage to the nerve cells. Chemical study indicates that the fluid between the fibers is an ultrafiltrate of plasma. Even among compounds that produce brain edema, triethyltin was considered unique in not affecting the gray matter (Magee *et al.*, 1957). Later it was found that hexachloraphene produces a similar lesion (Kimbrough and Gaines, 1971). Poisoning by triethyltin is manifested by progressive weakness, paralysis, and convulsions. In rats, the sulfate is about equally toxic orally, intravenously, or intraperitoneally. The intraperitoneal LD 50 is 5.7 mg/kg (Stoner *et al.*, 1955). Rats fed triethyltin hydroxide at a dietary level of 20 ppm lost weight, but only a little more rapidly than pair-fed controls. Unlike the controls, they showed ataxia of the hind legs in 7–9 days when they had consumed a total of about 10 mg/kg. Weakness progressed until the hind legs lay motionless while the rats dragged themselves about using their front legs. The hind legs were not completely paralyzed and could be withdrawn if pinched. If feeding were continued, the front legs, too, became weak, and the rats lay helplessly on their sides, although they would still attempt to eat. About two-thirds of them died during the third week, but the remainder appeared to become resistant. Their food intake increased and they showed partial recovery. Recovery was more certain if they were transferred to a dietary level of 10 ppm when they first reached a state of prostration. Such rats appeared almost normal after 6 weeks on the lower concentration, although there was some wasting of the muscles of the hind legs and some difficulty in balancing on the edge of a cage. No further improvement occurred even if the rats were returned to a normal diet, but the histological lesion cleared. If, on the other hand, the rats were continued on diets containing triethyltin hydroxide, they gradually became irritable, tremorous, and unwell. The tremor was made worse by intentional movement. Some of these rats suffered intermittent or almost continuous convulsions (Magee *et al.*, 1957; Stoner *et al.*, 1955).

Tetraethyltin has the same effect as triethyltin but acts more slowly because its toxic action really depends on its metabolism to triethyltin (Cremer, 1958).

In general, methyltin compounds are less toxic than corresponding ethyltin compounds. For trialkyl compounds, the toxicity decreases gradually as the length of the side chains is increased beyond 2. In the dialkyl series, the propyl and butyl compounds are more toxic than either ethyl or methyl, and toxicity remains high through octyl (Barnes and Magee, 1958).

Single oral doses in the hamster, monkey, and gerbil produce neurological damage at 3 mg Sn/kg (Brown *et al.*, 1979). One study in rats claims to find marked proximal tubular necrosis in rats after a single oral dose of 10 mg Sn/kg (Opacka and Sparrow, 1985). It is difficult to find long-term studies on ethyltin and related compounds. Brown *et al.* (1979) conducted a 4-week study of rats given daily oral doses of triethyltin chloride. Neuronal alterations were seen at a dosage rate of 4 mg Sn/kg/day.

Absorption, Distribution, Metabolism, and Excretion There is considerable variation in the absorption of alkyltin compounds. For example, in the rat triethyltin is equally toxic by mouth and by intraperitoneal injection, but in the hen it is not toxic orally. In the rat, diethyltin is toxic when given by stomach tube, but it apparently reacts with some constituent in the food so that even high dietary concentrations are without effect.

Ethyltin trichloride injected intraperitoneally is almost all excreted unmetabolized in the urine, with only trace amounts in the bile; when the compound is given by mouth it is excreted in the feces, indicating very limited absorption from the gastrointestinal tract (Bridges *et al.*, 1967).

Diethyltin dichloride injected intraperitoneally is partially metabolized to ethyltin, much of which is excreted in the urine; a portion of the unmetabolized compound is excreted in the bile and eventually appears in the feces. The conversion of diethyltin to ethyltin apparently occurs in the tissues and in the gut, although the conversion has been demonstrated *in vitro* only in cecal contents and not in liver homogenate (Bridges *et al.*, 1967).

When the triethyltin chloride is injected intravenously into rats, guinea pigs, or hamsters, it reaches a higher concentration in the liver than in other tissues, including the brain. In the rat, this relative distribution is maintained from 10 min to 5 days after injection. In 4 days, rats excrete about 50% of an intravenous dose, mostly in the feces. The compound is probably excreted in the bile of rats, and it certainly reaches high concentrations in the bile of guinea pigs and hamsters (Rose and Aldridge, 1968).

Mode of Action Dialkyltin compounds inhibit α-keto oxidase activity leading to the accumulation of pyruvate. This is considered important in the toxic action. BAL blocks this inhibition and the acute toxicity (Aldridge and Cremer, 1955; Barnes and Stoner, 1959).

Triethyltin is the most effective known inhibitor of oxidative phosphorylation, being active at 1×10^{-7} M *in vitro*. This inhibition is not blocked by BAL (Aldridge and Cremer, 1955).

Inhibition of phosphorylation must interfere with energy exchange everywhere in the body. It does not explain why the visible lesion is confined to the white matter of the central nervous system (Barnes and Stoner, 1959).

61.9.2.3 Toxicity to Humans

Therapeutic Use Tin and various inorganic compounds of it were promoted during the early part of the twentieth century for treating staphylococcal infection or helminthic infestation. These treatments were usually harmless to patients and pathogens alike, although Bar (1956) reported a case of poisoning by stannous oxide. However, in 1953, a large outbreak of poisoning followed the introduction in France of an organic tin preparation called "Stalinon" for treating staphylococcal infection of the skin, osteomyelitis, anthrax, and acne. The preparation was supposed to be diethyltin diiodide, but it contained about 10% of triethyltin iodide and a little less ethyltin triiodide. One report tabulated 224 cases, including 103 deaths (LeBreton, 1962). There were a few additional cases and deaths reported by others. It was estimated that about 1000 people took the medicine.

Symptoms began in 1–30 days after dosage was started. The total dose varied from 81 to 1094 mg or about 1–16 mg/kg in fatal cases. Signs and symptoms included headache, vomiting, photophobia, dizziness, abdominal pain, marked weight loss, hypothermia, bradycardia, retention of urine, alteration of consciousness, psychic changes, convulsions, coma, and paralysis. In spite of this array of abnormalities and the high mortality rate, many patients presented without any diagnostic signs. Some patients had abnormalities of the fundus of the eye, the spinal fluid, or the electroencephalogram, but these changes were often absent in patients who went on to die. The level of consciousness was the best prognostic sign; only one patient who became comatose survived. A few patients recovered rapidly, but most who lived required several months to recover, and one required 18 months. Still others were left with permanent sequelae, including blindness and severe, flaccid paraplegia. Death occurred as early as the day of onset; in most instances it came 1–13 weeks after onset but was delayed 36 days in one case.

The symptomatology and the autopsy findings indicated edema of the white matter of the brain as the cause of death. Consistent with this view was the finding that surgical decompression of the brain constituted the only useful treatment; six of eight patients treated in this way survived (Alajouanine et al., 1959; LeBreton, 1962). Thus, the action was characteristic of triethyltin, not of diethyltin, which constituted a little more than 80% of the preparation. It appears that humans react the same as other animals to triethyltin but are far more sensitive.

Laboratory Findings In the victims of "Stalinon," the concentration of tin was similar in the heart, lung, liver, and kidney, although it tended to be slightly lower in the heart and higher in the liver. The range for pooled viscera was 1.5–16 ppm with a mean of 5.6 ppm. The concentration in die brain was consistently higher, with a range of 5.1-39 ppm and a mean of 17.3 ppm (LeBreton, 1962).

In the United States and France, tin may be found in most samples of all organs except the brain, which rarely contains a detectabte quantity in normal people. The median concentration in most organs is no more than 1 ppm (Kehoe et al., 1940; LeBreton, 1962; Tipton and Cook, 1963).

The concentration of tin in the blood of normal Americans averages 0.14 ppm and that in urine 0.018 ppm (Kehoe et al., 1940). The concentration in normal plasma does not exceed 0.47 ppm (Gofman et al., 1964).

The distribution of tin in the organs of the French patients was entirely different from that found in experimental animals injected intravenously with triethyltin chloride, where more tin is retained by the liver than by the brain. Whether the difference depends on species or on the fact that "Stalinon" was a mixture is not clear.

61.10 BISMUTH

Bismuth is a heavy metal immediately following lead in the periodic table. It is in the same group as arsenic and antimony.

Bismuth compounds used as pesticides are highly insoluble. They have proved safe when used as drugs in doses far larger than any likely to arise from their use as pesticides.

In persons without special exposure, the concentration of bismuth in the plasma does not exceed 0.20 ppm (Gofman et al., 1964).

61.10.1 BISMUTH SUBCARBONATE

61.10.1.1 Identity, Properties, and Uses

Chemical Name Bismuth subcarbonate.

Structure $(BiO)_2CO_3$.

Synonyms Synonyms include bismuth oxycarbonate and basic bismuth carbonate. The CAS registry no. is 5892-10-4.

Physical and Chemical Properties Bismuth subcarbonate has the empirical formula CBi_2O_5 and a molecular weight of 510.01. It is an odorless, tasteless powder that is practically insoluble in water or alcohol but soluble in mineral acids and concentrated acetic acid.

Use When added to arsenical and fluoride formulations, bismuth subcarbonate tended to increase the feeding of insects on poisoned foliage.

61.10.1.2 Toxicity to Laboratory Animals

Basic Findings Apparently the toxicology of the specific bismuth compounds used or proposed as pesticides has not been studied in animals. It seems reasonable to suppose, however, that sufficient dosages of relatively insoluble pesticides would produce changes similar to all but the most acute injuries produced by soluble bismuth compounds.

Sollmann and Seifter (1942) found that intravenous doses of sodium bismuth citrate and bismuth glycolate were lethal to rabbits in a dosage range of 2.5–5 mg Bi/kg. Death appeared to be due to renal failure. The oral LD 50 is 22 g/kg for rats and is 0.5 g/kg for rabbits according to Kruger et al. (1985). The acute toxicity of bismuth depends greatly on the solubility of the compound under study.

Pathology The tissue changes in rabbits caused by several bismuth compounds used in the treatment of syphilis were found to be characteristic of bismuth and not dependent on specific compounds or any particular route of administration. The major lesion involved the epithelium of the convoluted tubules of the kidney. These cells showed all types of degeneration from cloudy swelling to calcification. The glomeruli did not appear primarily damaged, but the glomerular capillaries frequently contained coagulated masses of erythrocytes. The lesions of the liver were much less conspicuous than those of the kidney, but cloudy swelling and small areas of necrosis flooded by erythrocytes did occur. Other organs showed no dependable or characteristic pathology.

61.10.1.3 Toxicity to Humans

Therapeutic Use Bismuth subcarbonate is used to furnish mechanical protection and to exclude irritants from external ulcers, fistulas, or inflamed mucous membranes or from gastrointestinal inflammations or ulcers. It helps to allay diarrhea.

Formerly it was used as an adjuvant to more active amoe-bacides against intestinal amoebae and as an opaque medium in roentgenoscopy. The usual oral dose in treating peptic ulcer is 1000–2000 mg suspended in fluid before each meal. The material is harmless unless applied to extensive burns or ulcers or left in fistulas for long periods. Formerly the compound was given as an X-ray contrast medium al a dose of about 50,000 mg. The disadvantage compared to barium sulfate was not toxicity but a delay in emptying of the stomach (Sollmann, 1957).

Treatment of Poisoning BAL has been used for treating poisoning by any bismuth compound. Other treatment is symptomatic.

61.10.2 BISMUTH SUBSALICYLATE

61.10.2.1 Identity, Properties, and Uses

Chemical Name Bismuth subsalicylate.

Structure See Fig. 61.1.

Synonyms Other names for bismuth subsalicylate include basic bismuth salicylate and salicylic acid basic bismuth salt. The CAS registry no. is 14882-18-9.

Physical and Chemical Properties Bismuth subsalicylate has the empirical formula $C_7H_5BiO_4$ and a molecular weight of 362.11. It forms microscopic prisms mat are decomposed by boiling water and by alkalies into a more basic salt. It is almost insoluble in water or alcohol.

Use Bismuth subsalicylate is a fungicide, especially for the control of bluemold disease of tobacco seedlings.

61.10.2.2 Toxicity to Laboratory Animals

See Section 61.10.1.2.

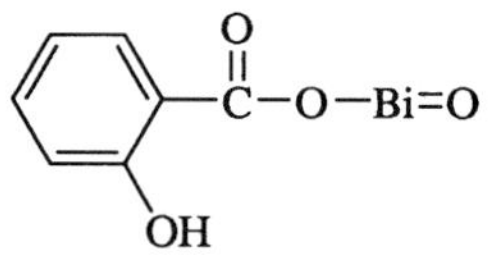

Bismuth subsalicylate

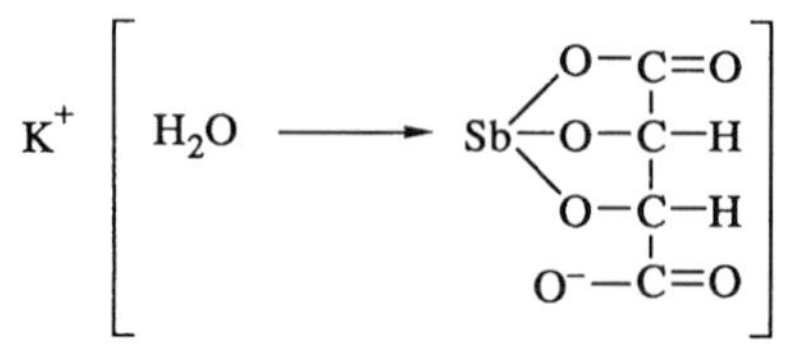

Antimony potassium tartrate

Figure 61.1 Two organometallic pesticides.

61.10.2.3 Toxicity to Humans

Therapeutic Use The compound is sometimes used orally to allay diarrhea or to soothe gastritis or peptic ulcer. The dose varies from 500 to 2000 mg and may be given three times a day. Before the advent of penicillin, bismuth subsalicylate was much used in the treatment of syphilis, and it may still be used in patients who are intolerant to penicillin. It is given by intramuscular injection as a 10% suspension in oil at the rate of 130 mg/week, usually for 8–10 weeks. This treatment results within about 3 weeks in a urinary excretion of about 1 mg/day. By using a dose of 260 mg, a urinary level of 2 mg/day can be achieved in 1 week.

Even when its use was extensive, the gradual intramuscular injection used against syphilis rarely led to serious poisoning. It was customary to stop treatment if gingivitis, albuminuria, cutaneous eruptions, or marked diarrhea appeared. If one of these signs was ignored and dosing continued, serious ulcerative stomatitis with salivation was likely to appear and soon be followed by one or more of the following: malaise, headache, insomnia, depression, asthenia, joint pains, nausea, loss of appetite, diarrhea, loss of weight, albuminuria, and skin reactions (such as puritis, herpes zoster, purpura, and sometimes serious exfoliative dermatitis). Jaundice and conjunctival hemorrhage were rare complications of treatment. A line of bismuth sulfide often appeared at the gingival margin along with similar blotches on the mucosae of the mouth, tongue, throat, colon, rectum, cecum, and appendix. The bismuth line was not a contraindication to treatment. Even when illness occurred, it was usually less severe than that associated with other heavy metals. Specifically, the stomatitis and albuminuria were less severe than those caused by mercury and the cutaneous eruptions less severe than those caused by arsphenamine (Sollmann, 1957).

After treatment, the highest concentration of bismuth was found in the kidneys ami the lowest in the brain and blood. Bismuth freely crosses the placental barrier (Sollmann, 1957).

Pathology Two patients who died following bismuth therapy but not as a result of it both showed refractile globules in the nuclei and cytoplasm of the epithelium of the convoluted tubules. Similar globules were found in the renal epithelial cells of rats following injection with one of the same compounds (Pappenheimer and Maechling, 1934).

Treatment of Poisoning BAL has been used for treatment of poisoning by any bismuth compound. Other treatment is symptomatic.

61.11 ANTIMONY

Antimony is a metal. It follows tin in the periodic table, and it belongs to the same group as arsenic. The trivalent compounds of antimony, like those of arsenic, are more toxic than the pentavalent ones. The toxic effects of antimony compounds closely resemble those of arsenic compounds, but antimony causes greater vomiting and is excreted more rapidly.

Traces of antimony are widely distributed in the environment.

Eight or more compounds of antimony had some use as insecticides before DDT became available. However, antimony potassium tartrate was the only one of much commercial importance. The toxicity of this compound is typical of the group.

Two useful reviews of the toxicology of antimony, which emphasize the industrial aspects, are those of Fairhall and Hyslop (1947) and ATSDR (1992d).

61.11.1 ANTIMONY POTASSIUM TARTRATE

61.11.1.1 Identity, Properties, and Uses

Chemical Name Antimony potassium tartrate.

Structure See Fig. 61.1.

Synonyms Other names include antimony tartrate, potassium antimonyl tartrate, tartar emetic, tartarized antimony, and tartrated antimony. A code designation is ENT-50,434. The CAS registry no. is 28300-74-5.

Physical and Chemical Properties Antimony potassium tartrate has the empirical formula $C_4H_4KO_7Sb$ and a molecular weight of 324.92. It forms transparent crystals or powder with a sweetish, metallic taste. The density is 2.6. It is soluble in water and glycerol, insoluble in alcohol. Crystals effloresce upon exposure to air.

Formulations and Uses The compound serves as a poison in baits to control insects, especially thrips, and as an emetic (for people or pets) in baits to control rodents. The insect baits usually are applied as sprays containing 0.36–0.48% of the compound in the liquid formulation. The rodent baits are pastes or solids containing 0.3–3% of the compound, specifically 0.30% with thallium sulfate and zinc phosphide, 1.12% with arsenic trioxide, and 3.00% with ANTU.

61.11.1.2 Toxicity to Laboratory Animals

Basic Findings The intraperitoneal LD 50 for mice is 46–50 mg/kg for the different isomers of antimony potassium tartrate (Haskins and Luttermoser, 1950). The subcutaneous and intravenous LD 50 values in mice are 55 and 65 mg/kg, respectively (Ercoli, 1968). The oral LD 50 for the same species is 600 mg/kg. The marked difference between these values is an indication of poor gastrointestinal absorption even in an animal that does not vomit. Other species are somewhat more susceptible, with an intraperitoneal LD 50 of 30 mg/kg (11 mg/kg as antimony) in rats and 25 mg/kg in guinea pigs (Bradley and Fredrick, 1941). Lifetime exposure of rats (Schroeder et al., 1970) and mice (Kanisawa and Schroeder, 1969; Schroeder et al., 1968) to antimony potassium tartrate produced a significant decrease in life span at a daily dosage of about 0.3 mg Sb/kg.

Animals poisoned by antimony compounds showed dyspnea, loss of weight, weakness, loss of hair, and evidence of cardiac insufficiency. Those that survived began to regain weight within 5–10 days (Bradley and Fredrick, 1941).

Absorption, Distribution, Metabolism, and Storage Ingestion of the compound usually leads to repeated vomiting, Thus, removal of the material from the gastrointestinal tract and inherently poor absorption combine to limit the amount of the compound reaching the tissues. Excretion is mainly urinary. It is much faster than that of arsenic and is almost complete in 72 hr (Osol et al., 1967). The rate of excretion varies considerably in different species, being slower in rnice and monkeys and more rapid in rats. The synergistic action of salts of tris(p-aminophenyl)carbonium on the toxicity of tartar emetic to Schistosoma mansoni was not accompanied by any significant effect on the distribution or rate of excretion of tartar emetic and must, therefore, have involved the parasite only (Waitz et al., 1965).

Although the acute toxicity of soluble antimony is greater than that of soluble lead, the excretion of antimony is sufficientiy rapid that no significant storage occurs (Bradley and Fredrick, 1941).

Following single or repeated doses of tartar emetic, there was no really marked accumulation of antimony in any organ, but the concentration was always greatest in the liver, and it reached an average of 65 ppm in hamsters kilted by repeated intraperitoneal injection (Gellhorn et al., 1946). A similar relationship was found in dogs, where the concentration of antimony decreased in the following order: liver > thyroid > parasites > kidney cortex > other organs (Brady et al., 1945).

Mode of Action Antimony combines with sulfydryl groups including those in several enzymes important for tissue respiration. The antidotal action of BAL depends on its ability to prevent or break the union between antimony and vital enzymes (Sollmann, 1957).

The most characteristic toxic effect is vomiting, which is largely reflex in origin. Although vomiting may occur after intravenous injection, a larger dose is required and the action is nore delayed than when the drug is given by mouth (Sollmann, 1957). Furthermore, the action is largely reflex even after injection, for the compound is excreted through the walls of the stomach (Osol et al., 1967).

The cause of death is essentially the same as that in acute arsenic poisoning. Serious injury almost always involves the gastrointestinal system and may involve the cardiovascular system, the kidneys, or other organs leading in any event to a condition of shock. The rapid excretion of antimony makes important sequelae or delayed death unusual.

Pathology Rats killed by an intraperitoneal injection of tartar emetic showed degenerative changes of the myocardium, congestion of the glomeruli and degeneration of the tubules of the kidney, and extensive centrolobular hepatic necrosis. Injury to the heart was detected histologically in rats receiving daily doses of antimony too small to reduce the rate of growth. On the contrary, antimony produced no serious blood changes following either single or repeated doses (Bradley and Fredrick, 1941).

61.11.1.3 Toxicity to Humans

Therapeutic Use When antimony potassium tartrate is rubbed on the skin in the form of an ointment, it produces little irritation at first but produces a pustular eruption if applied for long periods. This is due to decomposition of the double salt by the acid secretions of the follicles, leading to formation of the more irritant antimonous oxide and other compounds (Sollmann, 1957).

Antimony potassium tartrate was once used as an emetic for treating patients poisoned by a wide variety of compounds. The drug still has some use as a diaphoretic or expectorant in certain cough syrups. It has been used for treating a number of tropical diseases, and it still is the drug of choice for treating infection by *Schistosoma japonicum*. It is not used to treat *S. mansoni* or *S. haematobium* infections because less toxic agents are effective [American Medical Association (AMA) 1977].

The dose of tartar emetic varies greatly according to these different uses. As an emetic, the dose was usually 30–60 mg. The small safety factor is indicated by the fact that in one case a dose of 130 mg proved fatal (Osol *et al.*, 1967). The dose in cough remedies or expectorants varies from 1 to 8 mg repeated two or three times daily. As an intravenous injection for treating *S. japonicum* infection in adults, a freshly prepared 0.5% solution should be injected extremely slowly on alternate days according to the following schedule: 8 ml initially increased by 4 ml with each subsequent dose until the 11th day (when 28 ml is given) and then 28 ml on alternate days until a total of 500 ml (2500 mg) has been given or until side effects become severe. Each dose should be given 2 hr after a light meal and the patient should remain recumbent for 1 hr after treatment (AMA, 1977). These therapeutic doses may be compared with 5 mg/person/day, the rate of respiratory intake of antimony considered safe for workers exposed to various antimony compounds.

Use of antimony potassium tartrate has been abandoned as an emetic to give patients, but it is still used as an emetic to combine with certain rodenticides to make them less harmful if they are accidentally consumed by people or pets. Presumably the compound is more stable in rodenticide formulations than ipecac, which now is considered a faster and safer emetic for patients.

The doses of antimony potassium tartrate received from cough medicines generally cause no side effects. Excessive doses either by mouth or intravenously produce symptoms resembling those of acute or subacute arsenic poisoning. In fact, the resemblance is so close that a distinction may be impossible unless the cause is known as the result of history or chemical analysis. There is, however, a tendency for antimony to produce earlier more profuse vomiting, less systemic absorption, more rapid excretion, and thus a shorter course without severe neurological sequelae. Symptoms include a metallic taste, extreme nausea, copious vomiting, frequent hiccough, burning pain in the stomach, colic, frequent stools and tenesmus, fainting, bradycardia often with EGG irregularities, hypotension, difficult and irregular breathing, cutaneous anesthesia, convulsive movements, painful cramps in the legs or joints, jaundice, anuria, prostration, and death (Osol *et al.*, 1967; AMA, 1977).

Laboratory Findings Antimony is found in all tissues and organs of "unexposed" people. Autopsy data on Japanese (Sumino *et al.*, 1975) indicate a uniform distribution throughout the body with concentrations generally between 0.01 and 0.05 µg Sb per gram wet weight. The average hair level was 0.12 µg/g but others have reported a range of 0.08–6.6 µg/g (Liebscher and Smith, 1968). The average blood level in the Japanese study was 0.016 µg/g.

Following intravenous injection of tartar emetic, only about 2.5% of the dose was recovered from the urine during the first 24 hr. The rate of recovery fell only very slowly in subsequent days (Boyd and Roy, 1929).

Analysis of 315 electrocardiograms taken on 100 patients during various stages of treatment with tartar emetic and Fuadin for schistosomiasis revealed one or another abnormality in 11–99% of the patients. Abnormalities in one or more leads included increased amplitude of P waves, a fusion of ST segment and T wave, decreased amplitude of T wave, and prolongation of the Q–T interval. The duration of these changes was variable but was noted up to 2 months after treatment stopped (Schroeder *et al.*, 1946).

Pathology At autopsy of persons who have died following ingestion of a large dose, ulcerations usually are found in the esophagus and stomach but not in the intestine. In subacute cases, fatty degeneration of the liver, kidney, and heart may be present; degenerative changes in the nervous system are less common. Persons who died, perhaps as a result of individual susceptibility, following the usual, intravenous, therapeutic dose of tartar emetic showed marked degeneration of the liver, some necrosis of the renal tubular epithelium, and varying degrees of hemorrhage (McKenzie, 1932).

Treatment of Poisoning BAL is effective in treating poisoning by antimony potassium tartrate, but this is not true of all organic antimony compounds.

61.12 ARSENIC

Arsenic is a metalloid. It belongs to the same group as phosphorus. Each of these elements combines with hydrogen to form a highly toxic gas, arsine and phosphine, respectively. Arsenic is followed in the periodic table by selenium, an essential element which also finds applications as a pesticide.

Arsenic compounds occur in many rocks and thus find their way into soil, water, and food, being especially high (3–170 ppm) in some seafood (Monier-Williams, 1949). Arsenic is a normal constituent of the human body, a fact recognized since the work of Gautier (1899). Two laboratories have independently reported that arsenic, at least in the inorganic form, is an essential nutrient in minipigs and goats (Anke *et al.*, 1976, 1978) and in rats and chicks (Nielsen *et al.*, 1975; Uthus and Nielsen, 1985). If an element is found to be essential in animals, it is highly probable it is essential in humans. However, we lack knowledge of a biochemical mechanism and physiologic role of arsenic.

For reviews of arsenic, see WHO (1981), U.S. EPA (1983), Ishinishi *et al.* (1986), and ATSDR (1998).

61.12.1 ARSENICAL PESTICIDES

61.12.1.1 Identity, Properties, and Uses

Compounds and Their Characteristics Elementary arsenic forms two oxides: the trioxide, As_2O_3, and the pentoxide, AS_2O_5. Arsenic trioxide (trivalent) reacts with water to form arsenous acid, H_3AsO_3, which is known only in solution and forms three series of salts: orthoarsenites (e.g., Na_3AsO_3), metaarsenites (e.g., $NaAsO_2$), and pyroarsenites (e.g., $Na_4As_2O_5$). Arsenic pentoxide (pentavalent) reacts with water to form three acids that may be isolated: orthoarsenic acid, H_3AsO_4; metaarsenic acid, $HAsO_3$; and pyroarsenic acid, $H_4As_2O_7$. These acids form the corresponding salts: orthoarsenates, metaarsenates, and pyroarsenates. A few organic arsenic compounds also are used as pesticides. Although a great many arsenicals have had some use as pesticides, the ones shown in Table 61.4 are of the greatest importance.

It is beyond the scope of this book to discuss the highly toxic compounds of arsenic (arsine and certain war gases) or those of

Table 61.4
Some Arsenical Pesticides

Name	Synonym	Formula
Arsenic trioxide	White arsenic	As_2O_3
Sodium arsenite		Na_3AsO_3, $NaAsO_2$
		$Na_4As_2O_5$
Paris green	Cooper aceto-meta-arsenite	$Cu(CH_3COO)_2\ 3Cu(AsO_2)_2$
Lead arsenate	Acid lead arsenate	$PbHAsO_4$
	Standard lead arsenate	
	Dilead arsenate	
Basic lead arsenate	Lead hydroxy-arsenate	$Pb_4(PbOH)(AsO_4)_3 \cdot H_2O$
Calcium arsenate		A complex mixture
Dimethylarsinic acid	Arsan®	$(CH_3)_2AsO(OH)$
	Cacodylic acid	
	Phytar®	
	Silvisar®	
Disodium methyl arsenate		$Na_2CH_3AsO_3 \cdot 6H_2O$

low toxicity employed therapeutically in medicine and agriculture (drugs and feed additives).

Formulations, Uses, and Production Arsenites are more soluble and more rapidly toxic than corresponding arsenates; therefore, arsenites are used as rodenticides and herbicides and in insecticidal baits. Paris green, although an arsenite, may be applied to foliage, but inorganic arsenates are less phytotoxic and, therefore, preferred for application to crops as insecticides. Some organic arsenates (dimethylarsinic acid and disodium methyl arsenate) are herbicides. The use of arsenical insecticides in agriculture decreased greatly following the introduction of DDT and later poisons, but the use of arsenical herbicides has increased. Starting about 1975, the uses of arsenic compounds as wood preservatives began to grow. By 1980, 70% of the arsenic consumed in the United States was used by the wood preservative industry (Loebenstein, 1994).

61.12.1.2 Toxicity to Laboratory Animals

Symptomatology The acute effects of arsenic in animals are similar to those observed in humans (see Section 61.12.1.3). The degree of irritation of the gastrointestinal tract involved in poisoning by arsenic trioxide depends on its purity. A commercial preparation that was 97.8% pure was much more irritant yet slightly less toxic than a sample of greater man 99.999% purity (Harrisson *et al.*, 1958).

Dogs fed sodium arsenite at a rate of about 2.7 mg/kg/day showed anorexia, listlessness, and weight loss leading to cachexia and eventually death (Kiyono *et al.*, 1974). Mild to moderate anemia was present prior to death. Neither skin lesions nor polyneuropathy apparently has been observed in experimental animals. Thus, except for weight loss and anemia in some species, arsenic poisoning as it occurs in humans is poorly reproduced in animals.

Dosage Response The literature indicates a tremendous variation in the oral toxicity of arsenic compounds. Table 61.5, prepared from a careful study of arsenic trioxide by Harrisson *et al.* (1958), shows that the variation is real but can be accounted for largely by whether the compound is administered dry or in solution and to a lesser extent by the purity of the sample and by the species, strain, and weight of the experimental animals. Harrisson and his colleagues found no significant difference in the response of males and females. They acknowledged that arsenic of coarse grind might less easily dissolved and hence less toxic than fine powder. However, in the particular samples they studied, the coarser preparation was actually more toxic because of its greater purity. Thus a combination of variables must be taken into account.

The LD 50 values of suspensions of calcium arsenate (298 mg/kg) and of Paris green (100 mg/kg) in rats are similar to that of powdered arsenic trioxide. The LD 50 value of lead arsenate is distinctly higher (1050 mg/kg) (Gaines, 1969).

Long-term feeding of dogs (Byron *et al.*, 1967) or monkeys (Heywood and Sortwell, 1979) causes death at a dosage rate

Table 61.5
Effect of Purity and Dosage Form of Arsenic Trioxide on Its Oral Toxicity in Male Animals of Different Species, Strains, and Weights[a]

Experimental animal	Weight (g)	Dosage form	LD 50 value (mg As/kg) 97.8% As_2O_3	99.999% As_2O_3
Swiss mouse	20–25	Solution	42.9 ± 2.1	39.4 ± 4.7
Swiss mouse	35–40	Solution		47.6 ± 3.3
C57HI6 mouse		Solution		25.8 ± 1.8
Dba2 mouse		Solution		32.4 ± 2.3
C3H mouse		Solution		25.8 ± 1.8
Sprague–Dawley rat	125–200	Solution	23.6 ± 1.4	15.1 ± 1.8
Sprague–Dawley rat	125–200	Dry	214.0 ± 8.4	145.2 ± 8.7

[a]From data of Harrisson *et al.* (1958).

of about 3 mg/kg/day as arsenate or arsenite. A marked enlargement of the common bile duct is a characteristic feature. A no-adverse-effect level in rats is about 1.6 mg As/kg/day as arsenite and about twice as high for sodium arsenate. Dogs appear to be somewhat more susceptible than rats. Neither skin lesions nor polyneuropathy has been observed in experimental animals.

Absorption, Distribution, Metabolism, and Excretion   Arsenic is absorbed chiefly by the gastrointestinal and respiratory tracts. However, some is absorbed by the intact skin, and systemic illness may follow application of arsenical ointment to eczematous skin.

Gastrointestinal absorption of the soluble trivalent compounds of arsenic appears to be high (Buchet *et al.*, 1981a, b; Charbonneau *et al.*, 1978; Coulson *et al.*, 1935; Crecelius, 1977; Freeman *et al.*, 1993; Mappes, 1977; Marafante and Vahter, 1987; Marafante *et al.*, 1987; Vahter, 1981; Vahter and Norin, 1980; Yamauchi and Yamamura, 1985) in both animals and humans. The organic form of arsenic present in shellfish and other marine foods is also well absorbed from the gastrointestinal tract. Soluble arsenates are also well absorbed.

Arsenic is rapidly cleared from the bloodstream except in the case of rats, where its methylated derivatives bind to hemoglobin. In fact, both trivalent and pentavalent forms of arsenic are rapidly methylated, so their distributions are somewhat similar. Initial accumulation is in liver, kidneys, and lung, from which arsenic is cleared rapidly; long-term accumulation is in skin, squamous epithelium of the upper gastrointestinal tract, thyroid, the lens of the eye, and the skeleton. It is also accumulated in hair. Human autopsies have also confirmed accumulation in keratinized tissues and the skeleton.

Both trivalent and pentavalent forms of arsenic readily cross the placenta (for review, see Clarkson *et al.*, 1983). The pentavalent form accumulated in the skeleton of the fetus in late gestation. Little arsenic crossed the blood–brain barrier.

Most arsenic in tissues is found to be protein bound. Trivalent arsenic is well known to bind to tissue −SH groups (Webb, 1966).

Both trivalent and pentavalent arsenic can be interconverted by oxidations–reduction reactions in mammalian tissues. The biochemical mechanisms are not known. Monomethyl and dimethyl derivatives are produced in experimental animals and humans presumably by methylation of the trivalent form. Substantial species differences exist in methylation rates and in the relative proportions of the monomethyl and dimethyl forms. Arsenobetaine, the organic form of arsenic in marine organisms, is not further metabolized in the body.

Methylation of arsenic may be regarded as a detoxication process, as the methylated derivative is less toxic than the inorganic form. Factors affecting the methylation rate are therefore important. There is evidence that the efficiency of methylation decreases at higher doses. Populations having certain dietary deficiencies (e.g., in methionine) may be more susceptible to arsenic poisoning.

After absorption of either the trivalent or pentavalent form, urinary excretion is the dominant pathway. In chronic exposure, this route accounts for 60–70% of total excretion. Methylation rate is important, as the methylated species is more rapidly excreted than the inorganic form. For example, urinary excreition is lowest in the marmoset monkey, which is unable to methylate arsenic (Vahter *et al.*, 1982). Excretion also takes place by feces, skin, hair, and milk. Fecal excretion may be preceded by extensive enterohepatic recirculation according to data for experimental animals (Klaassen, 1974).

Tolerance   It was reported during the nineteenth century that the mountaineers of Styria and certain other regions ate arsenic once or twice a week as a tonic and thus accustomed themselves to doses of 400 mg or more per day. Their blood and urinary arsenic levels and even the absorbability of the material they ate are apparently unknown. However, the reality of tolerance to inorganic arsenic has been demonstrated by tests in dogs (Cloetta, 1906), rabbits (Cloetta, 1906), and rats (Joschimoglu, 1916; Norris and Elliott, 1945). Tolerance does not depend on decreased absorption from the gastrointestinal tract, for it may be induced by intraperitoneal injection (Norris and Elliott, 1945).

Biochemical Effects   Arsenic inhibits pyruvate oxidase and the phosphatases. The blood level of pyruvate increases in poisoned animals or people. There is a reduction of tissue respiration leading to a wide range of functional and some morphological changes. Many other sulfhydryl-containing enzymes are involved also, and it is impossible to assign relative importance to them. However, studies on antidotes have made it clear that chemical reaction of trivalent arsenic with sulfhydryl groups, including those in susceptible enzymes, is the biochemical lesion (Peters, 1952). Further studies by Peters' group (for review, see Clarkson, 1983) revealed that the inhibition of pyruvate oxidase was due to the binding of trivalent arsenic, as the oxyanion, to neighboring −SH groups of α-lipoic acid. Pentavalent arsenic, also as the oxyanion, is able to substitute for phosphate anions in the cell's transport and enzymic processes. The result is replacement of phosphates by arsenate in high-energy phosphorylated substrates, leading to uncoupling of oxidative phosphorylation reactions (for a review, see Jennette, 1981).

Altered biochemical functions in the liver mitochondria of rats fed arsenic are associated with considerable physical distortion of the mitochondrial membrane components. The same degree of biochemical change is associated with less electron microscopic change in the mouse (Fowler and Woods, 1979).

Although arsenic inhibits many enzymes, it increases the activity of liver microsomal enzymes. Arsenic trioxide at a dietary level of 1000 ppm for 15 days induced several enzymes, and even at 100 ppm hexobarbital sleeping time was decreased. Rats develop some tolerance to arsenic, and its toxicity is decreased by phenobarbital (Kourounakis *et al.*, 1973; Wagstaff, 1972).

Effects on Organs and Tissues   The chief pharmacodynarnic action is dilatation and increased permeability of the capillaries. This action is strongest in the intestines, regardless of route of absorption. Local action on capillaries causes congestion, stasis, thrombosis, ischemia, and necrosis. Such necrosis extends into the bone in some instances. Injury to the kidneys is due primarily to capillary injury, but there is always some injury to the epithelium. Initial injury to the nervous system is also based on circulatory disturbance, but later there is direct injury to the nerve cells. Injury to the liver by arsenic is usually minor. A few single cases or clusters of cases involving cirrhosis have been described. In many of these cases, alcohol was a complicating and perhaps critical factor in the etiology.

The cause of death depends on the size of the dose and, therefore, on the speed of action. If death occurs within a day or two, it is caused by shock characterized by a severe fall in blood pressure. Vasodilatation is most marked in the splanchnic area, but death occurs in experimental animals even if the intestines are tied off early. The action on capillaries is direct, for it follows perfusion of excised organs with solutions of arsenic. The dilatation is not due to a loss of contractility; the vessels continue to react to splanchnic stimulation until very late, and they react to epinephrine even later (Loeb, 1912).

If death is delayed 3–14 days, it is caused by dehydration, electrolyte imbalance, and a more gradual fall in blood pressure.

Most animal studies testing for carcinogenicity of arsenic have been negative (for review, see U.S. EPA, 1983). Studies on rats should be viewed with caution in view of the unusual metabolism of arsenic in this species.

Effects on Reproduction and Development   Few studies have been made on the effect of arsenic on reproduction and development. Treatment of pregnant animals with high doses of inorganic arsenic results in fetal resorptions and, in surviving offspring, defects in the genitourinary tract. Studies to date indicate that effects on the fetus are not produced at dosages below those causing maternal toxicity (for reviews, see ATSDR, 1998; Clarkson *et al.*, 1983).

Pathology   The injury produced by arsenic compounds in most species is not characteristic although the enlargement of the rat's common bile duct by sodium arsenite and sodium arsenate is indeed striking. Using a strain of rat that occasionally showed spontaneous enlargement of the duct, Byron *et al.* (1967) found that the duct enlarged in 45 of 49 rats fed sodium arsenite at a dietary As level of 250 pptn and in 42 of 48 rats fed sodium arsenate at a dietary As level of 400 ppm. Lower dietary levels produced a lower incidence of enlargement. Some of the ducts measured more than 7 mm in diameter, and their walls were as much as 10 times thicker than normal. The condition was reminiscent of that produced in rats by dibutyltin dichloride and a few nonmetal compounds. No parallel condition in humans has been recognized.

Treatment of Poisoning in Animals   Dimercaptosuccinic acid increased the rate of excretion of radioactive arsenic by poisoned rats and increased their survival compared with controls (Okonishnikova, 1965).

61.12.1.3 Toxicity to Humans

Experimental Exposure   See Laboratory Findings.

Therapeutic Use   Arsenic in the form of arsenic trioxide, potassium arsenite solution (Fowler's solution), or arsenious acid solution formerly was used extensively as a tonic in treating nutritional disturbances, neuralgia, rheumatism, arthritis, asthma, chorea, malaria, syphilis, tuberculosis, diabetes, skin disease, and every kind of blood disturbance. Some skin conditions were treated locally, and arsenic was used to destroy some superficial epitheliomas. In fact, both Hippocrates and Galen recommended a naturally occurring arsenic disulfide for treating ulcers, and cautery of tumors by arsenic salts was practiced by Avicenna in the tenth century and by Guy de Chauliac in the fourteenth. Fowler's solution was used in some treatment of leukemia until rather recently (Sollmann, 1957).

Experience in the systemic use of inorganic arsenicals showed that their prolonged administration at the usual rate of 0.04–0.09 mg/kg/day frequently produced mild poisoning. The various systemic and cutaneous effects described under Use Experience have been produced by arsenical therapy also.

Accidental and Intentional Poisoning   For many years, arsenic has been the most important single cause of accidental deaths associated with pesticides in the United States. It caused 36, 26, 29, 31, and 17% of such cases in 1956, 1961, 1969, 1973, and 1974, respectively (Hayes and Vaughn, 1977). Accidental poisoning by arsenic pesticides is almost always and often involves children. Experience in many other countries, for example, Poland (Brodniewicz and Szuber, 1960), Australia (Southby, 1965), and New Zealand (Bailey, 1964; Kennedy, 1961), has indicated the disproportionate importance of arsenical pesticides as a cause of pesticide poisoning.

Contamination of well-water by arsenical pesticides has been a cause of outbreaks of poisoning in Russia (Khasanov,

1971; Planques *et al.*, 1960) and possibly in Hungary (Nagy *et al.*, 1975a, b).

The first symptom is often a feeling of constriction of the throat, followed by difficulty in swallowing and epigastric discomfort. Abdominal pain and vomiting often start within an hour of ingestion, although the onset may be delayed until the next day, particularly if foul play is involved and the dosage is controlled. Death may result from a severe fall in blood pressure and collapse as in "dry" cholera. Generally, death is delayed for 1.5–3 days after onset and sometimes as much as 14 days. In this event, death follows vomiting and profuse, watery, painful diarrhea; the clinical picture is similar to cholera because of the "rice water" character of the stools and the great dehydration of the patient. Although arsenic is not truly corrosive, the extreme distention of the capillaries may lead to their rupture and thus to ecchymoses or even bleeding into the stomach or intestine and eventually, but infrequently, bloody vomiting and diarrhea. The patient has great thirst and difficulty in swallowing and articulation. Although the abdomen is painful, it is not tender. Descriptions of cases of this kind can be found in great profusion in the older literature, for example, Orfila (1814–1815) and Christison (1845).

If the patient survives the acute phase, skin eruptions, a moderate depression of blood cells, and polyneuropathy may appear.

The pseudoinflammatory reaction may extend to the conjunctiva, gums, mouth, pharynx, and bronchi, and it may persist in the gastrointestinal tract. Thus, conjunctivitis, rhinitis, cough, or bronchopneumonia may be present. Dermatitis is especially prominent in the palms and soles and other areas subject to pressure. White transverse bands in the nails frequently appear in about 6 weeks and may accompany polyneuropathy, which often appears 1–3 weeks after ingestion. The bands migrate to the free edge of the nails at approximately the normal rate of about 5 months from matrix to edge. Although these lines, first described by Mees (1919), may have other causes, their occurrence in conjunction with polyneuropathy is almost pathognomonic of arsenic poisoning. Skin eruptions may progress to exfoliative dermatitis, especially following exposure to organic arsenicals. Peripheral circulatory difficulty characterized by blanching or flushing of the skin may be present, especially in the fingers.

Some authors (Leng-Levy *et al.*, 1969) have emphasized the importance of cardiac involvement in the total syndrome, and the frequency of ECG changes would support this view. Among various forms of cardiac involvement, Wang and Mazzia (1969) emphasized the unusual susceptibility of persons severely poisoned by arsenic to ventricular fibrillation and cardiac arrest during anesthesia.

Arsenical polyneuropathy involves paresthesia, pain, burning, and tenderness of the affected limbs (Heyman *et al.*, 1956). Trouble in walking or in grasping objects may at first be secondary to pain. Later the pain may disappear with astonishing suddenness, but the patient may be left with loss of (*a*) proprioception, (*b*) other sensory functions, and (*c*) motor function. The relative importance of different changes varies from case to case. The legs and arms are affected about equally, although difficulty usually is first noticed in the feet. Muscle atrophy may be pronounced (McCutchen and Utterback, 1966). Tendon reflexes are, of course, weak or absent. Mental confusion may be present and may be evident as an apparent inability of the patient to grasp the seriousness of the condition or the possible implications of foul play.

Tsuchiya (1977) reviewed an outbreak of arsenic poisoning that differed from others in two ways: most of the victims were less man 12 months of age, and the compound involved was found to be pentavalent. The arsenic was a contaminant of sodium phosphate intentionally added to milk as a stabilizer. Different lots of the powdered milk product contained 0–34 ppm of arsenic. Symptoms began early in the summer of 1955; following investigation, sale of this milk powder was banned on August 24, 1955, Many of the signs and symptoms (diarrhea, vomiting, anorexia, and others) were typical of acute poisoning by trivalent arsenic but the prominence of many other difficulties (dermatitis, loss of hair, melanosis, leukoderma, and irritation of the eyes and upper respiratory system) was typical of subchronic or chronic poisoning, as one might expect with exposure lasting several months. However, neuritis was not observed, and electrical measurements indicated no dysfunction of the peripheral nervous system. In view of the fact that there were a total of 12,131 cases and 130 deaths, one would have expected hundreds if not thousands of cases of polyneuropathy if trivalent arsenic had been involved. Other differences from ordinary arsenic poisoning were the presence of fever and of liver swelling in the majority of cases. The contrast is especially remarkable in view of the demonstrated interconversion of the two valence forms. The poisoned infants were treated with BAL; rapid weight gain was considered the most striking benefit. Survivors were examined in June 1956, and it was concluded that most were normal—another contrast in view of the severity of the initial illness.

It seems clear that the majority of cases of arsenic poisoning have been associated with trivalent compounds, but in some instances the identity—and thus the valence—of the offending compound has not been reported. The large outbreak just mentioned suggests that there are two distinctly different forms of arsenic poisoning, depending on valence.

Arsine (AsH_3) is not used as a pesticide and ordinarily plays no part in the danger of arsenical pesticides. However, arsine was the cause of the illness of eight children and one adult who 48 hr earlier had helped to clean a dip vat that had been charged with chlordimeform and monobasic calcium phosphate. All of the patients showed albuminuria, and some showed hematuria, abdominal pain, dysuria, and headache. A diagnosis of arsine poisoning was made in the absence of any known source of arsenic. However, the next day, the farmer recalled that an arsenical dip had been used in the vat 2 years earlier, and arsenic later was measured in the acid mud (pH 6.5) of the vat and in the urine of the patients. Fortunately (and consistently with the delayed onset), all the cases were mild and the recoveries complete (Rathus *et al.*, 1979).

Use Experience Poisoning has not been a significant problem in pesticide applicators; cases reported in vineyard workers in Germany may have involved the drinking of contaminated wine. Poisoning is well known from other occupational sources, including the manufacture of pesticides. However, according to Buchanan (1962), who reviewed the industrial toxicology of arsenic in detail, even the use of arsenic compounds in industry has not proved an important cause of occupational morbidity and mortality.

Poisoning that is caused by repeated occupational exposure usually involves the frequently insidious onset of loss of appetite, weight loss, weakness, nausea, alternating diarrhea and constipation, colic, peripheral neuropathy, dermatitis, some loss of hair, giddiness, and headache. In general, gastrointestinal involvement is less and dermal involvement is greater than in poisoning caused by one or a few doses. Prolonged exposure may lead to gradual mental and physical deterioration and a state of cachexia suggestive of a malignant or endocrine disorder. Cyanosis of the face may be present as a result of statis in the injured capillaries rather than systemic anoxia. The dermatitis may be erythrematous, pustular, or even ulcerative. Burning and itching may be present and there may be serous discharge. With most arsenic compounds, the skin lesions tend to be most marked in the area of greatest contact. They are considered mainly the result of direct toxic action. The eruption may involve the face, eyelids, conjunctivae, or even cornea. There may be irritation of the nose, pharynx, and trachea leading to hoarseness and chronic cough. Perforation of the nasal septum has occurred.

A highly characteristic dermatitis confined to the scrotum, inguinal area, and nasolabial folds may follow moderate occupational exposure to Paris green. The lesions begin with erythema, frequently become eczematous and weeping, and may start to heal with the formation of a black scab. A sensitization reaction may be involved because the distribution does not correspond to the distribution of insecticide on the skin, and the dermatitis generally occurs in the absence of typical systemic poisoning.

In less acute cases, hyperkeratosis, hyperhidrosis, or melanosis may occur. These changes are considered evidence of chronic systemic action. The hyperpigmentation is most marked on surfaces exposed to light; it does not extend to mucous membranes. There may be a speckled depigmentation of pigmented areas giving the so-called raindrop appearance.

In persons exposed to sufficient arsenical dust, the onset of illness is characterized by dyspnea and oppression and pain in the chest. These symptoms may be followed by nausea, diarrhea, and other usual signs of poisoning but generally of a mild degree.

The polyneuropathy that may follow repeated exposure to arsenic resembles that seen in persons who survive one or a few doses. Disturbance of sight, taste, and smell may occur. There may be disturbance of bladder function. It is said that arsenical polyneuropathy is particularly severe and unremitting in chronic alcoholics.

There is no doubt that compounds similar or identical to those used as pesticides have caused skin cancer in humans. The earliest evidence comes from patients treated with potassium arsenite (Fowler's solution) (Fierz, 1966; Hutchinson, 1887; Minkowitz, 1964; Neubauer, 1947; Sanderson, 1963; Sommers and McManus, 1953) and from people who consumed water with a naturally high arsenic content (Hsueh et al., 1995; Neubauer, 1947; Tseng et al., 1968). In these instances, intake of arsenic was oral. The situation was somewhat less clear in connection with certain winegrowers in Germany and France (Denk et al., 1969; Galy et al., 1963a, b; Latarjet et al., 1964; L'Epee et al., 1973; Liebegott, 1952; Roth, 1957a). Whereas the initial impression was that exposure to lead arsenate was dermal and respiratory—as, indeed, it was—the critical intake of arsenic may have been oral and associated with contamination of wine by arsenic, making the exposure of the winegrowers entirely similar to that of people who drank arsenic in Fowler's solution or in water.

Two histopathological types of skin cancer have been associated with arsenic—squamous carcinomas in the keratin areas and basal cell carcinomas. Skin cancers caused by arsenic differ from those resulting from ultraviolet light by occurring in areas of the body not exposed to sunlight, e.g., soles of the feet. The appearance of skin cancer is preceded by a characteristic sequence of changes in skin epithelium.

Hyperpigmentation is followed by hyperkeratosis, which, histologically, has been described as keratin proliferation of a verrucose nature with derangement of the squamous portions of the epithelium. The latent period for initiation of exposure to appearance of skin cancer ranges from 6 to 50 years when arsenic was used medicinally, e.g., Fowler's solution. When exposure was from contaminated drinking water, the shortest latency was about 24 hours.

There is now mounting evidence that ingestion of arsenic may increase the risk of internal cancers as well. In large-scale epidemiological studies in Taiwan, where exposure is mainly from drinking water, clear associations are reported with tumors of the bladder, kidney, liver, and lung (Chen and Wang, 1990; Chen et al., 1985, 1986, 1988a, b, c; 1992; Chiang et al., 1988; Chou et al., 1995; Wu et al., 1989).

Increased risk of bladder cancer has been reported for populations in Argentina (Hopenhayn-Rich et al., 1996) and in Chile (Moore et al., 1997) from arsenic in drinking water. Cuzick et al. (1992) reported on follow-up findings of a cohort in Lancashire who had been tested with Fowler's solution (potassium arsenite) during 1945–1969. A significant excess bladder cancer mortality was found.

A considerable body of evidence now associates lung cancer with occupational exposure to arsenic. Perry et al. (1948) in the United Kingdom and Ott et al. (1974), Baetjer et al. (1975), and Mabuchi et al. (1979) in the United States found an excess risk of lung cancer associated with exposure to arsenic in industries manufacturing arsenic pesticides. A number of studies of copper smelters in the United States, Sweden, and Japan (for review, see U.S. EPA, 1984) have also implicated arsenic as a cause of lung cancer.

Arsenic has been mentioned in connection with the carcinogenicity of cigarettes (Satterlee, 1956), and it is true that residues of arsenic in tobacco increased from an average of 16.2 ppm in 1932–1934 to an average of 42 ppm in 1950–1951 (Satterlee, 1956). However, the concentration of arsenic in tobacco decreased later, so that in 1958 the average concentration in 17 brands was only 6.2 ppm (Guthrie *et al.*, 1959).

In a few instances, people with arsenical keratoses or other late effects of arsenic ingestion have presented with a wide variety of internal cancers, and the possibility that the internal cancers were caused by arsenic has been raised (Atkinson, 1969; Brady *et al.*, 1977; Roth, 1957b). However, more recent reviews (e.g., U.S. EPA, 1984) regard the evidence as equivocal.

Dosage Response A dose of 5–50 mg of arsenic trioxide is toxic. A dose of 128 mg (about 1.8 mg/kg) is said to have proved fatal to an unhabituated adult, but recovery has occurred after much larger doses. In fact, recovery occurred in one case after what was thought to be 20,000 mg (Cosic and Kusic, 1966). Very young children may be more susceptible. Study of 291 exposure incidents involving a single kind of ant bait in the form of a bottle containing one-half ounce (15 ml) of sweetened 0.61% sodium arsenite solution permitted a poison control center to conclude that a dosage of less than 1 mg/kg can cause serious illness in a child and 2 mg/kg can cause death (Peoples *et al.*, 1977).

The effectiveness of arsenical rat poisons varies greatly with the grind of the powder; very fine powders approach the toxicity of solutions containing an equivalent amount of arsenic. Thus, the ease of absorption influences the toxicity to a marked degree.

The repeated dose necessary to produce poisoning is less well known. The "therapeutic" dose of arsenic trioxide (1–2 mg three times daily) that used to be employed as a tonic frequently led to mild poisoning. Two milligrams three times a day for an adult is a rate of only about 0.06 mg/kg/day expressed as As. The Agency for Toxic Substances and Disease Registry (ATSDR, 1998) has estimated an upper no-adverse-effect level for skin lesions (blackfoot disease, hyperkeratosis, hyperpigmentation) to be 0.8 µg As/kg/day.

Cancer associated with arsenic has not been reported in persons exposed to air concentrations of 0.1 mg/m^3 or less even for long periods. It has been estimated that exposure to air concentrations of 50 µg As/m^3 occupationally for 24 years would result in a 200% excess risk of lung cancer (WHO, 1981). Data from a population in Taiwan (Tseng, 1977) led a WHO Task Group on Environmental Health Criteria for Arsenic (WHO, 1981) to conclude that the lifetime risk for skin cancer due to arsenic in drinking water is about 5% for a total dose of 10 g in an assumed life span of 70 years.

Absorption, Distribution, Metabolism, and Excretion Arsenic has been measured in human tissue and body fluids in both "nonexposed" and exposed individuals. In people exposed to normal environmental levels, hair and nails have the highest concentration with skin and lung next in order (Liebscher and Smith, 1968). Unfortunately, only total arsenic is reported, and we do not know the levels of specific forms of arsenic.

Tissue levels change rapidly after a single dose of arsenic. In six human subjects who ingested a tracer dose of arsenate labeled with the ^{74}As isotope, more than 5% of the dose was excreted in urine within 5 days (Tam *et al.*, 1979). In three people who ingested 500 µg of arsenic as arsenate in drinking water, 45% of the dose was excreted in urine within 45 days. Ingestion of the same amount of arsenic as the mono- or dimethyl derivative resulted in about 75% of the dose being excreted in urine within 4 days (Buchet *et al.*, 1981a).

Arsenic is rapidly cleared from blood in humans (for review, see U.S. EPA, 1984). If exposure is continuous, blood levels should quickly attain a steady state and should be proportional to average daily intake. However, it was not possible to detect any increase in blood levels in individuals exposed to arsenic in drinking water until the level in drinking water rose to 100–300 µg As/l (Valentine *et al.*, 1979). Most drinking water samples are below 10 µg As/l (WHO, 1981).

Normal concentrations in blood of nonexposed adults are in the range 1–4 µg As/l. Individuals exposed to elevated arsenic in drinking water may have blood levels up to 50–60 µg As/l (for review, see Vahter, 1988). When considering blood levels in nonexposed people, the possibility of intake of organic arsenic in seafood should be taken into account. Ingestion of shrimp with a high natural arsenic content causes blood levels to rise to 50 µg As/l within 2 hr (Vahter, 1988).

Levels of total arsenic in urine in nonexposed people are in the range 5–50 µg As/l. However, ingestion of seafood can increase urinary levels up to 1000 µg As/l. Urinary arsenic in occupational exposure is usually in the range of hundreds of micrograms per liter—values that can easily be confounded by ingestion of seafood. Vahter (1988) has reviewed published studies indicating that long-term daily ingestion of drinking water at 100 µg As/l results in an average urinary concentration of 60 µg As/l. Vahter (1988) goes on to suggest that a better index of exposure to inorganic arsenic may be obtained by measuring the urinary concentrations of inorganic arsenic and the two metabolites mono- and di-methyl arsenic.

Hair concentrations of total arsenic in nonexposed individuals are usually less than 2 µg As/g. In subjects occupationally exposed or ingesting arsenic in contaminated drinking water, hair concentrations can rise to 50 µg As/g.

The methylated derivatives of arsenic and the organic arsenic in seafood are not accumulated in the hair (Vahter, 1988), so total arsenic in hair should reflect the body levels of inorganic arsenic. Inorganic arsenic is accumulated into hair at the time of formation of the hair strand. Once incorporated into the strand, its concentration remains unchanged. Thus the "segmental" analysis of hair section by section measured from the scalp should quantitatively reveal the sequence of part absorption (Smith, 1964).

The use of hair as a monitor of absorbed inorganic arsenic is limited by the possibilities of external contamination from water, soaps, and shampoos. No satisfactory washing procedure has been developed for removing external arsenic from the hair sample (Atalla *et al.*, 1965). Because trivalent arsenic is known to bind selectively to the −SH groups of keratin in hair, it is likely that accumulation in hair may depend not only on inorganic versus organic forms of arsenic but also on the oxidation state of inorganic arsenic.

Concentrations of arsenic in nails in nonexposed persons are in the range of 0.01–3 μg As/g with an average of about 0.3 μg As/g. Values over 100 μg As/g have been reported in cases of chronic arsenic poisoning (see Vahter, 1988). Arsenic is probably incorporated into the growing tissue of nails, so its concentration may vary along the growth direction of the nail.

The concentrations of arsenic in the organs of people in the general population and in persons killed by arsenic are shown in Table 61.6. There should be no difficulty in confirming a diagnosis of poisoning by analysis of organs if the deceased person had no occupational exposure to arsenic and if arsenical embalming fluid does not complicate the picture. Apparently no information is available on the concentration of arsenic in the organs of occupationally exposed persons who died of unrelated causes. Thus, it is not certain whether the analysis of organs always offers clear evidence about whether the death of a person with occupational or other special exposure to arsenic was or was not caused by the material. In any event, levels less than 0.2 ppm (dry weight) should be ignored; levels higher than 0.2 ppm should be evaluated carefully, although they occasionally occur in normal persons.

Pathology In acute poisoning, erosion and inflammation of the stomach and upper intestinal tract may be marked. The liver may show degenerative lesions. Unless death is very rapid, the severe dehydration produced by acute poisoning gives the body an emaciated appearance, even though a normal amount of fat may remain. The alimentary canal shows a large amount of fluid, shreds of mucus, and false membrane in the absence of marked corrosion—a picture similar to that in cholera. Central necrosis may be found in the follicles of the spleen and the tonsils. The body may decay more slowly than would be expected in the same amount of time at the same temperature.

When death follows long repeated exposure, there is usually fatty degeneration of the myocardium, kidney, and liver, and the liver is often enlarged. Cachexia may be marked, and severe edema may be present. The nerves may show demyelinization and disintegration of axons.

Treatment of Poisoning If ingestion is suspected, the stomach should be emptied by vomiting or lavage with warm water and activated charcoal followed by a saline cathartic. BAL (dimercaprol) is a specific antidote. Dehydration should be combated with saline infusions, guided, where possible, by laboratory studies. If available, an artificial kidney may be used. According to Lasch (1961), much arsenic can be removed by hemodialysis. The diet should be liquid and supplemented with vitamins. D-Penicillamine has been found at least as effective as BAL fof treating human cases, and it has been recommended in all situations in which oral administration is appropriate (Peterson and Rumack, 1977). Soviet authors generally prefer unithiol to BAL for treating poisoning by arsenic compounds other than arsine (Mizyukova and Petrun'kin, 1974), and they are almost certainly correct on the basis of both effectiveness and safety. The relative value of unithiol and D-penicillamine is uncertain.

61.13 PHOSPHORUS

Compounds of phosphorus are a major constituent of protoplasm and essential to life. However, the element itself in its reactive white or yellow form is highly toxic. Red phosphorus and the less common black phosphorus are much less reactive and, therefore, relatively harmless.

61.13.1 PHOSPHORUS

61.13.1.1 Identity, Properties, and Uses

Chemical Name White phosphorus.

Synonyms Because of discoloring impurities, white phosphorus is sometimes known as yellow phosphorus. Trade names for the rodenticide include Bonide Blue Death rat killer®, Common Sense cockroach and rat preparations®, and RatNip®. The CAS registry no. is 7723-14-0.

Physical and Chemical Properties Phosphorus has an atomic weight of 30.97376. It has three main allotropic forms: white, black, and red, all of which melt to form the same liquid. White phosphorus is the most highly reactive solid form, and it is the only one used as a pesticide. Red phosphorus is used for the manufacture of some fertilizers and pesticides. Under ordinary

Table 61.6
Concentration of Arsenic in Human Organs

Sample	General population (ppm)	Persons killed by arsenic (ppm)
Brain	0.001–0.036[a,b]	0.5–20[c]
Kidney	0.002–0.363[a,b]	5–150[c]
Liver	0.005–0.246[a,b]	10–500[c]
		7–127[d]
		110–132[a,e]
		1.2–73[g]
Spleen	0.001–0.132[a,b]	5–250[c]
Lung		1.6[f]

[a] Concentration in dry tissue.
[b] Liebscher and Smith (1968).
[c] Sollmann (1957).
[d] Gonzales *et al.* (1954).
[e] Boylen and Hardy (1967).
[f] Buchanan (1962).
[g] Hayes and Vaughn (1977).

conditions, phosphorus is present as the molecule P_4. White phosphorus is a colorless or pale yellow crystalline solid with a waxy appearance and garlic-like odor. When stored in water, it increases the water's acidity and corrodes the container at the liquids–air interface. The density of white phosphorus at 20°C is 1.83. It has a melting point of 44.1°C and a boiling point of 280°C. It is practically insoluble in water but soluble in absolute alcohol (1 g/400 ml); in benzene (1 g/31.5 ml); in chloroform (1 g/40 ml); in oil of turpentine (1 g/60 ml); and in almond oil (1 g/100 ml). White phosphorus ignites spontaneously in moist air at about 30°C and in dry air at a higher temperature.

Formulations and Uses Pastes in collapsible tubes and jars containing 1.5–2% or even as much as 5% phosphorus were formerly used for rat, mouse, and cockroach control.

61.13.1.2 Toxicity to Experimental Animals

Oral and subcutaneous lethal doses of 2–12 mg/kg for rabbits and dogs are quoted from the literature around 1900 (Spector, 1955). It appears that no measurement of the acute or chronic toxicity of phosphorus has been made in a way that would permit proper quantitation. Rabbits and guinea pigs were not killed by a dosage of 0.66 mg/kg/day but they developed a cirrhosis-like condition (Mallory, 1933).

To assess risks to wildlife arising from use and environmental dispersal of white phosphorus pellets, mallard ducks were subjected to acute toxicity tests (Sparling et al., 1997). The 24-hour median oral lethal dose (LD 50) for white phosphorus dissolved in oil was similar in both sexes: 6.55 mg/kg in adult males and 7 mg/kg in adult females. The LD 50 for the ecologically more relevant pelletized form of white phosphorus was 4 mg/kg in adult males.

Absorption, Distribution, Metabolism, and Excretion
Phosphorus is absorbed from the respiratory and gastrointestinal tracts. It can cause severe burns to the skin, but it is said that not enough is absorbed from the burned areas to cause systemic poisoning. The dead tissue may be protective by permitting time for complete oxidation to phosphoric acid. Whether dilute formulations such as may occur in the gastrointestinal tract would be absorbed from the skin in harmful amounts has not been tested.

Unreacted elemental phosphorus may be demonstrated in the tissues of people who die several days after ingesting phosphorus but not in those who die after longer periods.

No quantitative study of the excretion of phosphorus seems to have been made.

Mode of Action The mode of action is unknown. It has not been possible to associate the main clinical or pathological features of intoxication with inhibition of any particular enzyme or class of enzymes, although some are inhibited. It is common to speak of phosphorus as a protoplasmic poison, but it is difficult to distinguish its possible direct effects on the liver, kidney, brain, and heart from the effects of anoxia on those organs. The peripheral vascular dilatation, which is the first and

most pervasive systemic effect of phosphorus, contributes to all the disorders that may be seen in various organs. However, the mechanism of this dilatation is not clear.

Phosphorus not only leads to structural damage of vital organs but also produces serious disruption of their metabolic function, as evidenced by hypoglycemia, azotemia, inhibition of glycogen formation in the liver, and many other disorders. Apparently there has been no recent review of the metabolic effects of phosphorus. Early reviews (Rubitsky and Myerson, 1949; Sollmann, 1957) list a great variety of biochemical effects, but nothing that could be termed a biochemical lesion.

It is interesting that the signs and symptoms of poisoning by phosphorus are similar to those of poisoning by phosphine. This is especially true if one considers poisoning by zinc phosphide or aluminum phosphide, in which phosphine is released in the stomach and symptoms involving direct irritation of the lungs are minimal. Poisoning by phosphorus apparently has not been studied quantitatively in rats. Therefore, it is not possible to compare in this species the toxicity of preformed phosphine and of phosphine equivalent from phosphorus. It can be stated that in the rat the LD 50 for phosphine gas is 8.9 mg/kg (Section 14.6.2 of the first edition of this Handbook) and that for phosphine derived from zinc phosphide is 10.6 mg/kg (Section 61.4.2.2), whereas that for white phosphorus (expressed as phorphine equivalent) in humans may be estimated at roughly 16 mg/kg. The values are certainly of the same order of magnitude. The difference is in the direction one would expect if the conversion of phosphorus to phosphine is incomplete. Such differences as exist in the kind of injury caused by ingested phosphorus and ingested phosphine (in the form of a phosphide) might be due to differences in distribution of phosphine in the tissue related to the place of its formation.

These qualitative and quantitative relationships could be explained if phosphorus were converted to phosphine in the intestine before absorption or in the liver after absorption. Such conversion probably has not been looked for and certainly has not been demonstrated, although it commonly is stated that small quantities of phosphine are formed in the putrefaction of organic matter containing phosphorus.

Treatment of Poisoning in Animals Mineral oil (50 to 100 ml) prolonged the life of some 10- to 12-kg dogs and saved others from a 500-mg dose of phosphorus, which was uniformly fatal to controls that received saline cathartics or no treatment (Atkinson, 1921).

61.13.1.3 Toxicity to Humans

Therapeutic Use It was observed about 100 years ago that continued small doses of phosphorus to growing animals result in a layer of dense bone under the proliferating epiphyseal cartilage. In adults, the haversian and narrow canals are gradually filled with dense bone. These observations led to the illadvised use of phosphorus in treating rickets, osteoporosis, and fractures (Sollmann, 1957). It was claimed that children up to 8 years old suffered no dangerous effects from 0.5 rag/day, although some vomited at first. The smallest dosage that exceptionally produced dangerous effects was 1 mg/day. The effects included gastrointestinal disturbance, necrosis of the jaw, and rarely typical phosphorus poisoning.

Accidental and Intentional Poisoning Apparently the most thorough clinical study of poisoning by phosphorus is that of Díaz-Rivera *et al.* (1950, 1961) based on a series of 56 cases involving suicide. Practically all poisoning by phosphorus has been caused by accidental or suicidal ingestion or occasionally by murder. The mortality was high.

It has been conventional to describe phosphorus poisoning in three stages: initial, latent, and systemic. This convention was recognized by the turn of the last century (Hann and Veale, 1910) and was followed in a review by Rubitsky and Myerson (1949). It is universally agreed that persons who ingest large doses die quickly in profound shock. Thus, the three stages are possibly applicable only in cases in which the dose is small enough to permit survival for a week or more. Even in regard to such cases, there is apparent disagreement concerning the distinctness of the three stages.

The initial symptoms include nausea, severe epigastric pain, headache, dizziness, and weakness. Diarrhea is uncommon. Vomoting is frequent but does not occur in all cases. Hematomesis may be present. The patient may be very nervous. These symptoms are commonly attributed directly or indirectly to irritation of the gastric mucosa (Díaz-Rivera *et al.*, 1950). However, absorption of phosphorus must begin at once, for the very first symptoms are similar regardless of the severity of poisoning, and in severe cases the absorption of a fatal dose requires only a few bours.

The initial symptoms are usually very distressing so that victims of accidental poisoning and many suicides seek medical attention promptly. However, LaDue *et al.* (1944) reported the death of a 15-month-old girl on the fifth by of illness, although the symptoms (abdominal pain and interminent vomiting) during the first 4 days were so mild they did not interfere with the child's play; diagnosis was on the basis of autopsy findings and not confirmed by chemical analysis or a history of ingestion.

The onset of poisonmg may be delayed as much as 5 hr but is often within half an hour or less.

The latent stage is characterized by a temporary and misleading improvement in the patient's condition and sense of well being. However, according to Díaz-Rivera *et al.* (1950), the so-called asymptomatic period is seldom as pleasant as may appear in the literature. In spite of some apparent improvement, their patients were seldom free of nausea, anorexia, a dissagreable taste in the mouth, eructations, or epigastric or generalized abdominal pain; some had constipation, and a few vomited. This period of relative relief starts within the first 48 hr, and the severe symptoms observed in those not destined to survive begin within the first 4–5 days. In some cases the latent stage may last until 10 days after ingestion (Rubitsky and Myerson, 1949).

In some cases, the improvement leading to what might otherwise constitute a latent phase is retained, and the patient goes on to complete recovery (LaDue *et al.*, 1944).

The third stage is ushered in by the reappearance of severe vomiting, abdominal pain, and sometimes hermitemesis. Severe damage to several organs becomes apparent. The liver is usually enlarged and very tender; jaundice, hypoprothrombinemia, and a bleeding tendency appear. Hypoglycemia is severe in some cases. Bleeding may be from the gums, stomach, intestine, or kidney, or in rare cases there may be extensive superficial ecchymoses (Hann and Veale, 1910). Injury to the kidney is evident by oligoria and azotemia. Injury to the brain rezults in severe restlessness, toxic delirium, and toxic insanity. These have been attributed to cerebral anoxia, but it seems impossible to exclude the possibility of direct toxic effects. The early appearance and rapid progression of hepatic, renal, or cerebral signs portend a best prognosis, and death frequently occurs by the eighth day or earlier. Severe agitation, coma, shock, earty azotemia, and severe hypoglycemia are the most certain signs of impending death. However, the actual occurrence of death is often sudden. Occasionally death is due to massive hemsternesis but more often has been attributed to cardiac arrest.

In cases destined to survive, the third or systemic stage of poisoning begins relatively late, and the signs and symptoms are relatively mild compared to those in fatal cases. Recovery is usually established by the 14th day, although asymptomatic hepatomegaly may persist as long as 30 days after intoxication, and abnormalities of the electrocardiogram have been found as much as 27 days after ingestion.

Although cirrhosis of the liver may be a sequela of poisoning (LaDue *et al.*, 1944; Moeschlin, 1965), recovery in other cases is complete.

A 30-year-old man who had swallowed a substantial dose of phosphorus presumably with suicidal intent developed in addition to the usual symptoms and signs of poisoning also symptoms, signs, and ECG changes indicating myocardial infarction. The patient recovered. On the ninth day, the acute S–T segment changes began to resolve, and 2 days later the Q wave changes diagnostic of infarct were no longer visible. Following more specialized ECG studies, it was concluded that ischemic myocardial necrosis had not occurred, and the ECG changes had been the result of metabolic derangement secondary to poisoning (Pietras *et al.*, 1968).

A positive Chvostek sign and increased neuromuscular irritability were observed on the 15th day of acute, typical phosphorus poisoning from which the patient had already recovered to a considerable degree. Blood levels of calcium and phosphate were low, and urinary excretion of calcium exceeded intake. Both the clinical and laboratory findings spontaneously reverted to normal in 3 days. The lesion was considered to have been in the proximal renal tubules. Three other cases of hypocalcemia in phosphorus poisoning were reviewed and it was concluded that this complication may be more frequent than formerly supposed (Cushman and Alexander, 1966).

Phosphorus may be effective as an abortifacient, although it may kill the mother also (Piribauer and Wallenko, 1961).

Use Experience Formerly, chronic poisoning, characterized by necrosis of the mandible and maxillary bone, was caused by prolonged inhalation of phosphorus in industry. This kind of phosphorus poisoning might be accompanied by signs of mild liver and kidney damage, but in some cases necrosis of die jaw was the only evidence of injury (Heimann, 1946). The history of the condition commonly called "phossy jaw" has been reviewed in detail by Hughes *et al.* (1962), who also described the much milder condition that still occasionally occurs in industry. In spite of continuing clinical observation and modern biochemical studies, the cause of the condition remains obscure. However, it appears to be an osteomyelitis that progresses because of a local, probiotic effect of elemental phorus. Although the condition is an osteomyelitis, it differs clinically and radiologically from other osteomyelitis. The organisms involved vary from case to case and may not even be recognized pathogens.

Under present conditions, phosphorus is not an important problem in industry. In a similar way, phosphorus used as a rodenticide is rarely a source of occupational poisoning, but it is highly dangerous to children who find and ingest it.

Dosage Response A daily dose of 1 mg given with therapeutic intent sometimes produced gastrointestinal disturbance, necrosis of the jaw, and rarely typical phosphorus poisoning.

A dose of 15 mg may be severely toxic, and as little as 50 mg (about 0.7 mg/kg) has proved fatal to an adult (Sollmann, 1957). As little as 2 mg is reported to have killed an infant (Rabinowitch, 1943). On the contrary, patients have recovered after doses thought to range from 350 to 715 mg (Caley and Kellock, 1955; Fletcher and Galambos, 1963).

Phosphorus is better absorbed and more toxic if ingested in a finely divided state rather than in lumps. Díaz-Rivera *et al.* (1950) gave evidence that even a uniform, finely ground paste of phosphorus was more quickly and completely absorbed when suspended in water, or especially when dissolved in an alcoholic beverage. Study of a series of 56 cases, in which a single formulation of phosphorus was ingested with suicidal intent, revealed a clear relationship between the amount ingested and the severity and outcome of intoxication. In this particular series, the smallest fatal dose was estimated as 190 mg (about 3 mg/kg). In 33 cases in which the dose ingested was 780 mg or less (up to about 13 mg/kg), the mortality was 18% and the time from ingestion to death was 4 days or more. In 21 individuals who ingested 1570 mg (about 26 mg/kg), the mortality was 90% and death occurred in a few hours to 3 days. Higher doses were uniformly, rapidly fatal.

Laboratory Findings Urinalysis may show albuminuria, cylindruria, hematuria, and grossly abnormal concentrations of several amino acids. Liver function tests, including prothrombin time, become abnormal but usually not before hepatomegaly and jaundice are evident. Hypoglycemia may be severe; blood urea nitrogen, creatinine, and ammonia may be elevated. Any changes in the peripheral blood are small in degree and in no way characteristic. The phosphorus content of the blood is usually normal. Electrogardiogram changes have been described in detail by Díaz-Rivera *et al.* (1961).

In the absence of a history of exposure, the garlic-like odor of the patient's breath often gives the first indication that phosphorus is involved. In addition, phosphorus may be detected in vomitus and feces—and, according to Rubitsky and Myerson (1949), in the breath—by the light it emits in a dark room. Elementary phosphorus may be detected in excreta, gastric contents, and tissues in smaller concentration but with no greater certainty by chemical analysis. It is claimed that phosphorus and phosphine in tissue can be separately demonstrated (Curry *et al.*, 1958).

Pathology If death is sufficiently prompt, there is no pathology except irritation of the esophagus and stomach. Perforation may occur. Following survival for several days, fatty degeneration is striking in the liver, heart, and kidney but may be found in all organs, including the brain. Hepatic necrosis may be extensive, with changes occurring first in the periphery of lobules. The earliest signs of definite morphological change of the liver were found in a patient who died 6 hr after ingesting phosphorus.

Periportal necrosis with degenerative changes extending toward the center of the lobules have been observed in biopsies from patients who survived. Later biopsies showed that fibrosis occurred in some but not all cases. When present, the fibrosis was periportal, sometimes forming septa between portal areas. The degree of fibrosis could not be explained by dosage or by the degree of injury evident during the acute phase and must have depended in part on one or more unidentified factors (Fletcher and Galambos, 1963; Greenberger *et al.*, 1964; LaDue *et al.*, 1944).

Differential Diagnosis If history of phosphorus exposure is unavailable, the initial symptoms may be confused with the gastroenteritis caused by agents such as arsenic. There is a characteristic odor of garlic to the breath and vomitus in phosphorus poisoning. Luminescence of the gastric contents or feces in a darkened room is pathognomonic. Diagnosis in the absence of a history of exposure is much easier if the patient survives long enough to develop signs of hepatic, renal, and central nervous system dysfunction.

Treatment of Poisoning Because there is no specific therapy, the removal of phosphorus by vomiting or gastric lavage with large volumes of fluid is of utmost importance. According to Díaz-Rivera *et al.* (1950), early vomiting or gastric lavage may be of benefit, and at times lifesaving among patients ingesting doses of 780 mg or less, but for larger doses the outcome is almost always death, regardless of treatment. Potassium permanganate, 0.1% solution, or 2% hydrogen peroxide is used in preference to water because they may oxidize phosphorus to harmless phosphates. Mineral oil (200–250 ml), which helps to prevent phosphorus absorption, should be administered by gastric tube. Additional doses of 30–40 ml should be given by mouth every 3 hr for the first 24 hr. Absorption can be increased by digestible fats and oils, and for that reason they are contraindicated. The treatment of shock and acute hepatic or renal failure is instituted when necessary. According to some authors, shock caused by phosphorus responds to vasopressor agents, but in connection with poisoning associated with suicide Díaz-Rivera *et al.* (1950) found these agents generally ineffective.

A high carbohydrate, high protein, low fat diet supplemented with heavy doses of vitamin B and crude liver extract is generally advised. It has been reported but not confirmed that a combination of methionine and cystine can prevent necrosis of the liver (Rubitsky and Myerson, 1949).

The use of cortisone acetate resulted in dramatic improvement in one case of severe poisoning after the ingestion of 825 mg of phosphorus, which is ordinarily a fatal dose. The drug was given in an initial intramuscular dose of 200 mg followed by 50 mg ever 6 hr. Oral administration was used after 48 hr. Doses were decreased on the 8th day and again later, and eventually stopped on the 65th day. The drug was given in the hope that it would improve both glycogen deposition and detoxification in the liver (Bayne *et al.*, 1952).

It should be mentioned that although BAL has been tried in the treatment of phosphorus poisoning, there is neither clinical nor theoretical justification for it. If signs of calcium deficiency appear, calcium gluconate should be given.

If phosphorus contacts the skin, it should be removed with water and later with a 1% solution of copper sulfate. Additional details about the treatment of phosphorus burns were given by Rabinowitch (1943).

61.14 SULFUR

Sulfur follows phosphorus in the periodic table. It is in the same group as oxygen and selenium. Sulfur is an important constituent of protoplasm.

61.14.1 ELEMENTAL SULFUR

61.14.1.1 Identity, Properties, and Uses

Chemical Name Sulfur.

Synonyms Synonyms for sulfur include brimstone, colsul, flour sulfur, and flowers of sulfur. Trade names include Corosul D and S®, Kolofog®, Kolospray®, Magnetic 70, 90, and 95®, Spersul®, Sulforon®, and Thiovit®. The CAS registry no. is 7704-34-9.

Physical and Chemical Properties The atomic weight of sulfur is 32.064. The element exists in several allotropic forms of which the orthorhombic, cyclooctasulfur (also called α-sulfur) is stable at ordinary temperatures and pressures. The stable form consists of amber-colored crystals with a density of 2.06. When this is heated to 94.5°C, it forms monoclinic, cyclooctasulfur (β-sulfur), which melts at 115°C and boils at about 444.6°C. The vapor pressure of sulfur is 3.96×10^{-6} torr at 30.4°C. Sulfur is soluble in carbon disulfide, slightly soluble in petroleum ether and alcohols, and insoluble in water.

Formulations and Uses Sulfur is used as an acaricide and fungicide in the form of dusts, wettable powders, and pastes.

61.14.1.2 Toxicity to Laboratory Animals

In the intestine, sulfur is converted to hydrogen sulfide; the reaction is more rapid and complete if the sulfur is in colloidal rather than crystalline or powdered form. With the colloid, an oral dosage of 175 mg/kg was rapidly fatal to some rabbits; prior to death they showed convulsions, unconsciousness, a hydrogen sulfide odor of the breath, a fall in blood pressure, bradycardia, and stimulation of respiration followed by respiratory arrest (Greengard and Woolley, 1940a). Part of the absorbed sulfur is excreted and part enters into the general metabolic pool. When radioactive sulfur was fed to sheep, activity appeared in their wool within 2 weeks, and continued feeding of sulfur changed the physical properties of the fibers by changing the number of disulfide linages (Clark and Buhrke, 1954).

61.14.1.3 Toxicity to Humans

Experimental Exposure Volunteers who ingested daily doses of 500 or 750 mg of colloidal sulfur absorbed it completely and excreted most of it, mainly as the sulfate, within 24 hr. Fecal excretion of sulfur was not measurably increased. After ingestion of a single dose, excretion rose to a peak within the first 2–4 hr and then declined gradually to normal in 14–20 hr. Absorption of powdered (100 mesh) sulfur was far less complete and was delayed until 8–16 hr after ingestion (Greengard and Woolley, 1940b).

Therapeutic Use Binz (1897) cited an earlier reference on the medicinal use of sulfur by the followers of Hippocrates. In relatively recent times elemental sulfur has been used as a laxative and as an ointment for treatment of scabies and fungal infections. These uses were effective. In addition, sulfur ointments were used for various other skin diseases, and colloidal sulfur was injected either intravenously or intramuscularly for treatment of tuberculosis, syphilis, and especially arthritis (Sollmann, 1957). The injections especially for arthritis were probably an extension of the traditional treatment of rheumatisni and various other conditions by baths in water from sulfur springs.

The oral, purgative dose of noncolloidal sulfur was 2000–4000 mg. Sulfur in combination with molasses constituted a favorite "spring tonic" of earlier times. Its purgative action was due to hydrogen sulfide, which was formed by gradual reduction of a part of the sulfur. If the dose were retained, a dangerous amount of hydrogen sulfide might be formed, but this was rare and is unlikely in the absence of mechanical obstruction. It has long been recognized that hydrogen sulfide was formed and was exhaled in the breath and apparently secreted by the skin. Silver ornaments worn by patients treated with sulfur were turned black (Binz, 1897).

Accidental and Intentional Poisoning Poisoning by lime sulfur (calcium polysulfides) probably should be attributed to sulfur because it decomposes to form sulfur in the presence of acid, including that in the stomach. Wakasugi and Fukui (1974) reported the suicide of a 22-year-old student who was found dead beside a 400-ml bottle labeled calcium polysulfide. The yellowish material with a sulfide odor was found on the face and hands as well in the stomach. Findings at autopsy were numerous but nonspecific.

61.15 SELENIUM

Selenium is a metalloid. It follows arsenic in the periodic table and falls in the same group as sulfur, which it resembles in many of its chemical reactions.

The toxic properties of plants grown on certain soils and eventually shown to depend on selenium have been known for a long time. In fact, the loss of hooves by horses and cows that eat these poisonous plants is so characteristic, one can be confident this was the disease observed by Marco Polo (1254–1327) in western China and described by him. The disease has been carefully studied and its quantitative relationship to selenium established.

It is only recently that selenium has been shown to be an essential trace element. Thus, selenium is one of those elements known first as a poison but later found necessary for life. The difference is one of dosage. Deficient diets contain less than 0.1 ppm of selenium; normal diets contain 0.1 ppm or somewhat more; toxic diets may contain as little as 5 ppm, but toxicity is more likely at concentrations of about 25 ppm.

Selenium is widely, but unevenly, distributed in nature. Traces of it ranging from 0.0000 to 0.01 ppm are found in community drinking water (Taylor, 1962). Food also contains selenium. For example, commercial wheat contains from 0.1 to 1.9 ppm. Selenium often is found in relatively high concentrations in acid soils of semiarid areas. Soils containing more than 0.5 ppm may lead to concentrations greater than 5 ppm in plants sometimes eaten by livestock and thus constitute a potential hazard. Much higher concentrations may occur in plants either because the soil in which they grow contains up to 30 ppm or because certain ones, namely some species of *Astragalus* and all species of *Stanleya, Oonopsis,* and *Xylorrhizia* (Kingsbury, 1964), are especially adapted to high concentrations of selenium and, in fact, are dependent on the element. The highest concentration of selenium repotted in field-grown wheat is 63 ppm (Moxon, 1958). Most vegetables contain far less but onions may contain up to 17.8 ppm (Underwood, 1956). (Indicator plants of the genera just mentioned may contain concentrations approaching 15,000 ppm (Trelease and Beath, 1949).) Livestock do not eat these plants unless driven by starvation, but their presence indicates the possibility of a problem in the soil, and if they are eaten, only a small amount of such plants may cause poisoning.

At least a portion of the selenium in plant tissues is in the form of analogs of ordinary sulfur compounds. Thus Se-methyl-selenocysteine has been identified in plant tissue but

is difficult to separate from its sulfur analog (Trelease *et al.,* 1960).

If a high proportion of their diet contains high residues of selenium, livestock, especially cattle, at first become depressed and unaware of their surroundings. Gastrointestinal stasis leads to pain indicated by grunting, grinding of the teeth, and excessive salivation. A period of excitement may follow in which the animals wander aimlessly. There may be partial blindness and usually is some degree of paralysis. The aimless, stumbling wandering is recalled by the term "blind staggers," which is the common name for this form of poisoning.

Autopsy usually reveals multiple small hemorrhages in the heart, kidney, and spleen. Gastroenteritis may be present and the kidney may be soft and friable (Radeleff, 1964).

If the intake of selenium is smaller but more prolonged, livestock develop a more chronic condition called alkali disease. It may even be intermittent if the animals receive excessive residues only part of the time. The disease is characterized by emaciation, lack of vitality, loss of long hair from the tails of horses and cattle and from the manes of horses, and deformity of the hooves leading to pain and lameness. In severe cases, the hooves may be lost. The animals are often anemic. Congestive heart failure is common, and on autopsy atrophy and fibrosis of the heart are prominent. Cirrhosis of the liver and scarring of the kidney and erosion of the joints of the long bones may also be found at death (Radeleff, 1964).

Rats fed grain grown in affected areas show many of the signs seen in poisoned livestock, including reduced food intake, weight loss, paralysis of the hind legs, hemorrhage into the gastrointestinal tract and the subcutaneous tissues and muscle fascia near the joints, and atrophy of the thymus and reproductive organs. Pathology is not marked in rats that die early because it requires some time to develop. Animals receiving smaller doses develop anemia and characteristic liver changes involving necrosis and atrophy accompanied by regeneration and leading to a grossly nodular appearance and to edema and other secondary changes (Franke, 1934).

Adult sheep are not very susceptible to selenium poisoning. However, lambs born to ewes fed high levels of this element may have abnormal eyes and deformed feet.

Dietary levels above 5 ppm are teratogenic to poultry (Franke and Tully, 1935).

It was shown by Schwarz *et al.* (1957) and by Schwarz and Foltz (1958) that rats maintained on a diet containing an undetectable amount of selenium (less than 0.1 ppm) develop liver necrosis, and chicks onthe same diet develop an exudative diathesis. The selenium normally present in the diet of animals is in organic form. However, the rats and chicks remained healthy and developed normally when their deficient diet was supplemented by selenium at a dietary level of 0.04 ppm (rats) or 0.1 ppm (chicks). Selenium was equally effective whether in the form of sodium selenite or some organic selenium compounds. However, selenium is an integral part of Factor 3, a normally occurring dietary agent mat prevents liver necrosis in the rat (Schwarz and Foltz, 1957), and, on a molar basis, the selenium in Factor 3 is some three to four times more effective than the other forms of selenium studied (Schwarz and Foltz, 1958). Even elementary selenium was effective if fed at a substantially higher level. This result was confirmed and extended by many authors. Although the actions of selenium and vitamin E are similar in many respects, it has been shown that selenium is an essential nutrient in both rats (McCoy and Weswig, 1969) and chicks (Thompson and Scott, 1970) even when their diet is fully supplemented by the vitamin.

More recent progress in showing that selenium is a necessary constituent of certain enzymes and other critical molecules was reviewed by Stadtman (1974) and by Underwood (1977). Although most details cannot be given here, the essentiality of selenium is emphasized by the finding that, at least in *Escherichia coli,* selenium in the form of 4-selenouridine is an integral part of RNA (Hoffman and McConnell, 1974). Selenium is known to be an essential part of the enzymes glutathione peroxidase and type I iodothyronine 5′-deiodinase (Lockitch, 1989).

It was later found that muscular dystrophy (white muscle disease), a spontaneous myopathy of lambs raised in certain areas, could be prevented to a large extent by supplementing the deficient diet of their mothers with selenium at the rate of 0.1 ppm using sodium selenite (Muth *et al.,* 1958). The disease can be prevented (or, if not too advanced, it can be cured) by subcutaneous injection of 1 mg of sodium selenate per lamb (Lagacé, 1961). Radeleff (1964) mentions that traces of selenium will prevent certain myodystrophic conditions of horses as well as those of cattle and sheep. In addition to muscular dystrophy in several species and exudative diathesis in chickens, other diseases of domestic animals that occur spontaneously in selenium-deficient areas and may be corrected by selenium supplements include pancreatic fibrosis in chickens, hepatosis dietetica in pigs, unthriftiness in sheep and cattle, and reproductive disorders in various species (Underwood, 1977).

The beneficial effects of selenium may be due in part to interaction with other metals. For example, micromolar concentrations of selenium partially prevented the *in vitro* inhibition of colony formation by mouse bone marrow cells and by certain tumor cells caused by low concentrations of organic and inorganic mercury (Strom *et al.,* 1979).

Even dietary levels that permit reproduction and lead to no recognizable disease may be inadequate for maximal growth. On the other hand, the optimal level of dietary selenium is astonishly close to the toxic level, as was discussed in connection with the logprobit model and quantitative study of the effects of small dosages (Section 1.2.7.4).

Although illness of people has been attributed to excessive industrial environmental exposure to selenium (Dudley, 1938; Lemley, 1940; Lemley and Merryman, 1941), there is no agreement about the nature of the disease, and its existence has been questioned (Smith, 1941). The fact that people remain healthy in areas where livestock are subject to alkali disease has been explained by the facts that human diet is more varied and that much human food is brought in from other areas so that the dosage received by people is less than that received by livestock. This argument was less applicable in pioneer times, when both food and feed were raised locally. It remains true, of course, that people eat only plants that are relatively inefficient in accumulating selenium. Animals may be driven by starvation to eat plants of high selenium content. Thus people tend to receive a lower dosage than livestock living in the same areas and the people probably have a higher protein intake. However, the urinary excretion of selenium by healthy people living on seleniferous soil varies from 0.02 to 1.33 ppm (Smith and Westfall, 1936), and the daily output of some workers may reach 5 mg (Vesce, 1947). There is, therefore, some evidence that humans are less susceptible than livestock to poisoning by selenium.

Nearly all injury caused by a wide variety of selenium compounds in industry arises not from their systemic toxicity but from their irritation of the skin, eyes, and respiratory tract (Browning, 1969).

Apparently no form of uncomplicated selenium deficiency has been reported in people. However, increased growth in children suffering from kwashiorkor (Schwarz, 1961) and other malnutrition (Majaj and Hopkins, 1966) has been reported following administration of selenium.

Additional information on the toxic and nutritional effects of selenium may be found in reviews by Frost and Lish (1975), Underwood (1977), and Lockitch (1989).

61.15.1 SODIUM SELENATE

61.15.1.1 Identity, Properties, and Uses

Chemical Name   Sodium selenate.

Structure $Na_2SeO_4 \cdot 10H_2O$.

Synonyms   Trade names include Sel-Kaps®, Sel-Tox®, SS02®, and SS-20®. Code designations for the compound include P-40. The CAS registry no. is 10112-94-4.

Physical and Chemical Properties   Sodium selenate has the empirical formula Na_2O_4Se. The anhydrous salt and the hydrate have molecular weights of 188.94 and 369.11, respectively. The compound forms white, nonflammable crystals which have a density of 3.098 and are very water-soluble.

Use   Sodium selenate is an insecticide used in horticulture for the control of mites, aphids, and mealybugs. It is also used as a fungicide (ATSDR, 1996).

61.15.1.2 Toxicity to Laboratory Animals

Basic Findings   Animals given enough of a selenium compound to produce poisoning in 15 min show spasmotic contractions of the flanks, dyspnea, tetanic spasms, and death from respiratory failure (Franke and Moxon, 1936). Pathological changes include congestion of the liver with areas of focal necrosis; congestion of the kidney; endocarditis; myocarditis; and atony of smooth muscle of the gastrointestinal tract, gallbladder, and bladder.

The intraperitoneal dosage of selenium (as sodium selenate) that kills 75% of rats in 48 hr is 5.25–5.75 mg/kg. The lowest dosage causing death is 3.75 mg/kg. Sodium selenate is only slightly less toxic than sodium selenite (Franke and Moxon, 1936). Lehman (1951, 1952) reported the oral LD 50 values of both compounds as 2.5 mg/kg. The intravenous dosage of selenium (as sodium selenate) fatal to 50% of rats lies between 3 and 4 mg/kg. Rabbits are more susceptible; an intravenous dosage of 2.5 mg/kg killed all those tested, as was true of an oral dosage of 4.0 mg/kg (Smith *et al.*, 1937).

Animals showing signs of poisoning have urinary concentrations of selenium ranging from 0.6 to 3.0 ppm (Smith, 1941).

The National Toxicology Program (NTP, 1994) conducted a 13-week study of rats and mice given sodium selenate in their feed. 100% mortality was seen in rats at a dosage rate of 2.5 mg Se/kg/day, cholestasis at 1.6 mg Se/kg/day, minimal degeneration of renal papilla at 0.5 mg Se/kg/day, and an 11% decrease in epididymal sperm count at about 0.2 mg Se/kg/day, the latter probably being the lowest adverse effect dosage. In mice, increased kidney weight associated with decreased water intake was seen at about 2 mg Se/kg/day and changes in estrus timing were seen at about 1 mg/kg/day, which appears to be the lowest adverse effect dosage level.

Rats maintained on a diet deficient in protein (10%) were severely poisoned by a wheat selenium at a dietary level of 10 ppm, but the same concentration of selenium had virtually no effect on rats maintained on an isocaloric diet containing adequate protein, whether obtained from casein, wheat protein, lactalbumin, ovalbumin, yeast protein, liver protein, or even gelatin. Several individual amino acids were not protective (Gortner, 1940; Lewis *et al.*, 1940; Smith, 1939, 1941; Smith and Stohlman, 1940).

Oral intake of selenium compounds leads to restricted food intake and marked loss of weight. Weight loss also occurred in an experiment involving subcutaneous administration, even though food intake was increased above the control level (Cameron, 1947). In spite of this difference, the rats showed many changes found in the other studies, including both atrophy and hypertrophy of liver lobes. Curiously enough, there was no cirrhosis (the injured liver was smooth), and the lobular distribution of hypertrophy and atrophy were reported to be opposite to that described and clearly illustrated by Franke (1934).

Absorption, Distribution, Metabolism, and Excretion
Most selenium compounds including sodium selenate are well absorbed (80–100% of intake) in laboratory animals, including rats, mice, dogs, and monkeys (Furchner *et al.*, 1975; Thomson and Stewart, 1973). Absorption takes place mainly in the duodenum (Whanger *et al.*, 1976).

In rats and dogs, selenium arising from intake of sodium selenite in the diet or in drinking water distributes widely throughout the body although concentrated in liver and kidneys (Furchner *et al.*, 1975; Sohn *et al.*, 1991; Thomson and Stewart, 1973). Selenomethionine is accumulated in tissues to a greater extent than the inorganic compounds (Behne *et al.*, 1991; Butler *et al.*, 1990; Ip and Hayes, 1989; Salbe and Levander, 1990).

Selenium, being an essential trace element, undergoes extensive metabolism. It is incorporated into numerous selenoproteins (Sunde, 1990). Selenomethionine, which cannot be synthesized in the body, competes with methionine at methionine codons as does selenocysteine with cysteine at cysteine codons. Selenium can be methylated. Dimethylselenide is exhaled and trimethylselenium ion is a major metabolite in urine. Methylation is believed to be a detoxication pathway (ATSDR, 1996).

Selenium is excreted chiefly in the urine but about 3–10% is metabolized and excreted by the lungs, and there is some fecal excretion even when sodium selenate is administered subcutaneously (McConnell, 1942). When sodium selenite is administered in the same way, 17–52% is exhaled within 8 hr (Schultz and Lewis, 1940).

Selenium crosses the placental barrier in both animals and humans (Hadjimarkos *et al.*, 1959; Westfall *et al.*, 1938) and is found in human milk (Archimbaud *et al.*, 1992; Chhabra and Rao, 1994; Choy *et al.*, 1993; Hawkes *et al.*, 1994; Jandial *et al.*, 1976; Parizek *et al.*, 1971; Willhite *et al.*, 1990). The concentration varied from 0.13 to 0.24 ppm in the placenta and from 0.07 to 0.18 ppm in cord blood.

Carcinogenicity   When the possible carcinogenicity of selenium and its compounds was reviewed by an IARC Working Group, it was concluded that the available data were insufficient to allow an evaluation of the carcinogenicity of large dosages of selenium compounds in animals. The group concluded that the data provided no suggestion that selenium is carcinogenic in humans. They found evidence for a negative correlation between regional cancer death rates and selenium not convincing, even though they cited considerable evidence along this line as well as evidence that small dosages of selenium tend to protect animals from naturally occurring cancer or cancer induced by classical carcinogens (WHO, 1975). The Agency for Toxic Substances and Disease Registry (ATSDR, 1996) also concluded that "the majority of subsequent studies of humans and animals have revealed either no association between selenium intake and the incidence of cancer or a chemopreventive association."

61.15.1.3 Toxicity to Humans

Accidental and Intentional Poisoning   Apparently there is no record of human poisoning by sodium selenate. Ingestion of about 1000 mg of sodium selenite caused a condition similar to arsenic poisoning with death in 5 hr (Moeschlin, 1965).

Laboratory Findings   The levels of selenium in human tissues and body fluids is affected by geographic differences in dietary intakes (for a review, see ATSDR, 1996). For example, average plasma or serum level in the United States is 0.13 µg Se/ml; in Scandinavia, 0.052 µg Se/ml; and in New Zealand, 0.03 µg Se/ml. Most human tissue levels in the United States are below 1 µg/g with the thyroid showing some of the highest levels.

Treatment of Poisoning   The treatment of selenium poisoning is essentially unknown. A high-protein diet may be helpful.

Arsenical feed supplements are beneficial in animals. BAL is not indicated. Some evidence from animal studies suggests that BAL decreases injury to the liver, increases injury to the kidneys, and has no effect on survival.

61.16 FLUORINE

Fluorine is the halogen of lightest atomic weight. Its salts are widely distributed in soil and water and occur in all tissues. The toxic effects of excessive doses of various fluorides have been known for many years. Since about 1940 it has been known that children develop a high level of dental caries if they live where the drinking water contains much less than 1 ppm of the fluoride ion. Children who live where there is naturally a good supply of fluoride in the local water or children whose supply of fluoride is supplemented develop teeth that are more resistant to rotting. Thus fluoride is essential to human health if not to human life.

Conflicting results have been obtained in animal experiments addressing the question of whether fluorine is an essential trace element. The difficulty is in preparing animal feed free of fluorine without changing other key nutrients in the diet. The National Research Council concluded that the data do not yet justify classifying fluorine as essential (NRC, 1989). On the other hand, the World Health Organization lists fluorine as essential for animal life without giving the supporting data (WHO, 1973).

Sodium fluoride is the prototype of inorganic fluorides used as pesticides. It has received some study in this connection and a great deal more in connection with industrial air pollution on the one hand and the prevention of dental caries on the other. The remaining inorganic fluoride pesticides, cryolite, sodium fluorosilicate, and even zinc hexafluorosilicate, owe their toxicity to fluoride ion, which they release slowly on contact with water. Through their often careless use, the inorganic fluoride pesticides have been an important cause of accidental acute poisoning. There is no indication that they have been a source of any chronic condition. The fluorine compounds that have given rise to chronic effects (mainly fluorosis of teeth and bone) in both humans and animals are in all instances not pesticides.

For those several reasons, it seems best to confine the sections on fluoride pesticides to information on the compounds themselves, emphasizing acute effects, and to outline what is known of the long-term environmental and occupational effects of fluorine compounds in this section. These long-term effects offer the best available indication of what continuing rate of intake of fluoride pesticides would be required to produce chronic injury.

The only moderately common effect of continued excessive intake of fluoride in humans is mottling of the enamel of the teeth. This effect involves chalky patches alternating with areas of staining. No mottling has been reported where the concentration of fluoride in drinking water is less than 0.3 ppm and practically none at levels below 0.6 ppm. Mottling is exceptional and slight when the concentration in drinking water is 1 ppm. The incidence and degree of mottling increase in proportion to the fluoride concentration in water within the range 2–10 ppm.

Chronic fluorosis was first described as occurring among animals that obtained excessive fluorides from their pastures. The residues deposited on vegetation consist of dust from indigenous soil (certain phosphate deposits or volcanic ash) or from the stack of gases of factories making phosphate fertilizer, some other phosphorus chemicals, steel, and aluminum. The compounds include native minerals, silicon tetrafluoride, and hydrofluorosilicic acid. Affected animals have stiff-legged gait, swollen hock joints, palpable lumps on their bones, and severely and irregularly worn teeth (Heyroth, 1963).

The pain the animals show is a direct result of the deformity of their bones and the erosion of their articular surfaces. Lameness may lead to inability to feed; this contributes to weight loss, rough coat, reduced milk production, and infertility often seen in poisoned animals (Radeleff, 1964).

Under field conditions, cattle are most susceptible, and other species are less so in the following order: cattle > sheep > swine > horses > turkeys > chickens (Radeleff, 1964). An extensive review of die literature (Schmidt and Rand, 1952) revealed that the highest dosages that did not produce fluorosis were 1–3 mg/kg/day in cattle, 5–12 mg/kg/day in swine, 10–20 mg/kg/day in rats and guinea pigs, and 35–70 mg/kg/day in chickens.

Mottling of the enamel in humans does not occur if excessive exposure to fluorides begins after the permanent teeth are formed. Although the bones may be affected at any time of life, even mild effects of this kind generally occur only after prolonged, poorly regulated, generally industrial exposure and, therefore, only in adults. It is probably because of this age distribution that essentially all reports of fluorosis in people involve osteosclerotic changes in bone marked by greater opacity to X-ray, thickening of the lamina, exostoses, and calcification or the ligamentous attachments.

Table 61.7 shows various indices of excessive repeated fluoride intake that have been associated with detectable effects in humans. In most instances, even workers who exhibit radiological evidence of skeletal fluorosis suffer no disabling symptoms. However, about half of a group with an average urinary concentration of 16.1 ppm and with urinary levels up to 43.4 ppm complained of lack of appetite, nausea, and shortness of breath and showed some degree of anemia. A smaller proportion of the men had other complaints (Brun *et al.*, 1941, or Roholm, 1937).

The beneficial effect of fluoride in reducing the prevalence of dental caries was discovered much more recently than the toxic effects of higher doses. The beginning of this discovery, which has permitted our children's teeth to be so much better than our own, has been traced back to (*a*) the observation of Eager (1901) connecting "Chiaie teeth" (now called mottled teeth) with drinking water and air charged with volcanic vapors now known to be fluorides and (*b*) the subsequent demonstration by Dean (1942a, b) of a quantitative relationship between caries in 7257 children and the concentrations of fluoride in their drinking waters. The decrease in caries is a linear func-

Table 61.7
Effect of Prolonged Intake of Fluoride in Humans

Concentration		Approximate intake (mg/kg/day)	Urinary output	Effect	Reference
Water (ppm)	Air (mg/m³)				
<0.6		<0.01	<0.6 ppm	Rotting of teeth	
1		0.03	~1 ppm	Optimal tooth development; no injury	
6		0.17	7.8 ppm	Mottled dental enamel	
		0.2–0.35		Fluorosis in many	Møller and Gudjonsson (1932)
	12–26[a]	0.2–1.0	16.1	Fluorosis[b]	Roholm (1937)
			2.4–43.4 ppm	Fluorosis progressive with duration of employment	Brun et al. (1941)
	0.14–3.43		<9.03 mg/24 hr	Fluorosis by X-ray in some	Agate et al. (1949)
			≥10	Fluorosis by X-ray	Largent et al. (1951)
			6 ppm	Slight fluorosis in a few	Heyroth (1952)

[a] Fluoride content calculated from gravimetric measurement of cryolite dust, slightly over half of which was of respirable size.
[b] First detectable by X-ray after an avenge of 8.0 years of exposure, the shortest time observed being 2.8 years.

tion of the logarithm of fluoride concentration (Hodge, 1950). The use of fluoridation has been reviewed in detail (Campbell, 1963; Shaw, 1954). Briefly, when the concentration of fluoride is optimum, no ill effects will result and caries rates will be only 35–40% of those in communities using water supplies with little or no fluoride. The optimal concentration is about 1 ppm. However, the dosage obtained from drinking water depends on the average amount of water consumed, and this depends on temperature. Therefore, the official recommendation for a particular community depends on its annual average maximal daily air temperatures as shown in Table 61.8. The recommendations take into account the usual range of fluoride intake from food.

Of 165 community water supplies analyzed for fluorine in 1961, 81 fell below the lowest optimal average of 0.7 ppm, whereas only 21 were above the highest optimal average of 1.2 ppm, and only 6 supplies had an average concentration above 1.29 ppm. The highest observed value was 10 ppm (Taylor, 1962).

Table 61.8
Recommended Limits for Fluoride in Drinking Water[a]

Annual average of maximum daily air temperatures[b]		Lower level (ppm)	Optimum level (ppm)	Upper level (ppm)
(°F)	(°C)			
50.0–53.7	10.0–12.0	0.9	1.2	1.7
53.8–58.3	12.1–14.6	0.8	1.1	1.5
58.4–63.8	14.7–17.6	0.8	1.0	1.3
63.9–70.6	17.7–21.4	0.7	0.9	1.2
70.7–79.2	21.5–26.2	0.7	0.8	1.0
79.3–90.5	26.3–32.5	0.6	0.7	0.8

[a] Modified from U.S. Public Health Service (1962).
[b] Based on temperature data obtained for a minimum of 5 years.

More information on the value of fluoride and on the injuries produced by both deficient and excessive intake of it may be found in a WHO monograph entitled *Fluorides and Human Health* (WHO, 1970). Another valuable source of information that emphasizes effects on domestic animals is a chapter by Underwood (1977). More general works on the pharmacology and toxicology of fluorides are those by Roholm (1937), Largent (1961), Hodge and Smith (1965), Smith (1966, 1970), and ATSDR (1991).

61.16.1 SODIUM FLUORIDE

61.16.1.1 Identity, Properties, and Uses

Chemical Name Sodium fluoride.

Structure NaF.

Synonyms Trade names for sodium fluoride include Floridine®, Florocid®, Flura-Drops®, Karidium®, Pergantine®, T-Fluoride®, and Villiaumite®. Code designations include FDA-101. The CAS registry no. is 7681-49-4.

Physical and Chemical Properties Sodium fluoride has the empirical formula FNa and a molecular weight of 41.99. It forms an odorless, noninflammable, white crystalline powder with a salty taste. It has a density of 2.78, a melting point of 993°C, and a boiling point of 1704°C. It is soluble in water and slightly soluble in alcohol.

Formulations and Uses Sodium fluoride is toxic to all forms of life. It has been used as an insecticide, rodenticide, and herbicide and as a fungicide for preservation of timber. Its toxicity to plants generally has restricted its use as an insecticide to bait formulations. The commercial product varies in purity from 93 to 99%. It should be colored to help distinguish it from table salt or flour.

61.16.1.2 Toxicity to Laboratory Animals

Oral LD 50 values ranging from 31 to 200 mg/kg have been reported in rats (DeLopez *et al.*, 1976; Lehman, 1951, 1952; Lim *et al.*, 1978; Skare *et al.*, 1986; Smyth *et al.*, 1969). Strain and gender differences contribute to this wide range in values. An LD 50 of 44 mg of fluoride per kilogram was reported for mice (Lim *et al.*, 1978).

Animal studies on reproductive toxicity of sodium fluoride have been equivocal. Some have reported no effects on sperm and no accumulation of fluoride in the testes (Dunipace *et al.*, 1989; Li *et al.*, 1987; Skare *et al.*, 1986) whereas others have reported decreased male fertility (Araibi *et al.*, 1989). Decreased female fertility has been observed at levels producing other signs of toxicity (Messer *et al.*, 1973). However, others have claimed that fluoride can actually enhance fertility by increasing the absorption of iron (Messer *et al.*, 1973; Tao and Suttie, 1976).

The National Toxicology Testing program conducted two studies of chronic oral toxicity on rats (F334/N) and mice (B6C3F1) of sodium fluoride added to drinking water (Bucher *et al.*, 1991; NTP, 1990). The first study was compromised due to suspected dietary deficiencies. Based on the findings of the second study, the NTP concluded that there was "equivocal evidence of carcinogenic activity of sodium fluoride in male rats." No evidence of carcinogenicity was found in female rats or in mice of either sex.

Absorption, Distribution, Metabolism, and Excretion Dietary fluoride is well absorbed from the gastrointestinal tract as the undissociated hydrogen fluoride molecule by passive absorption (Whitford and Pashley, 1984). The absorption of soluble fluoride is therefore rapid and complete in all species, including humans (Carlson *et al.*, 1960a; Ekstrand *et al.*, 1977, 1983), with maximum plasma fluoride concentrations attained as early as 30 min following exposure (Ekstrand *et al.*, 1977). Long-term retention of fluoride is mainly in calcified tissues (Wagner *et al.*, 1958) but soft-tissue levels do rise transiently following ingestion (Carlson *et al.*, 1960b). Excretion is mainly via the urine (Spencer *et al.*, 1970).

Biochemical Effects In fluorosis uncomplicated by systemic illness, fluoride ion appears to be deposited in place of hydroxyl ion in the hydroxyapatite of bone (McCann, 1953; Neuman *et al.*, 1950). There is little or no change in the calcium (Lantz and Smith, 1934; McClure and Mitchell, 1931) or phosphate (Phillips, 1932; Smith and Lantz, 1935) content of the bone. A part of the fluorine deposited in bone is readily excreted after fluoride feeding is stopped, but another part is more firmly held (Miller and Phillips, 1953; Savchuck and Armstrong, 1951).

61.16.1.3 Toxicity to Humans

Therapeutic Use In areas where there is a deficiency of fluoride in the drinking water, the incidence of dental caries can be reduced by administering sodium fluoride at a rate of 2.2 mg/day (Arnold *et al.*, 1960). However, to be of value the drug must be taken consistently during the years when the permanent teeth are being formed. Because few children or their parents can remember to carry out this preventive procedure, it is much more efficient to treat municipal water supplies so that the concentration of fluoride ion is in the range 0.7–1.2 ppm. This may be done by adding sodium fluoride at a rate of 1.5–3.0 ppm.

Larger doses given therapeutically are discussed under Dosage Response.

Accidental and Intentional Poisoning Acute, nonfatal poisoning is characterized by gastroenteritis (sudden nausea and vomiting, abdominal cramps, burning pain, and diarrhea) lasting for 3–6 hr and followed by collapse involving stupor and weakness lasting for about 36 hr (Sharkey and Simpson, 1933; Vallee, 1920). Tetany may occur as a result of calcium depletion. In fatal poisoning, muscular weakness appears early and is accompanied by a marked fall in blood pressure; tremor may be followed by clonic convulsions; dyspnea may be accompanied by a grayish-blue cyanosis. Death from respiratory and cardiac arrest may occur a few minutes to 10 hr or more after ingestion but usually in 3 or 4 hr.

Table 7.14 in the first edition of this Handbook lists a large outbreak of poisoning caused by the eating of sodium fluoride. In a much smaller outbreak, two people were killed by the compound when it was sold and used as flour (Fazekas, 1968).

Dosage Response Hodge and Smith (1965) estimated the certainly lethal dose for a 70-kg adult to be in the range 5–10 g of sodium fluoride (32–64 mg of fluoride per kilogram) based on reports of fatal poisonings. Children may be more sensitive. Whitford (1990) reported that a dose of only 8 mg of fluoride per kilogram was responsible for the death of a 27-month-old child.

Two adults were able to withstand a dose of 250 mg with minimal illness. One volunteer experienced slight nausea and epigastric distress lasting about 5 hr and salivation, which was intense for 15–30 min and stopped in half an hour; an itching sensation on his hands and feet lasted for about a week (Rabuteau, 1867). Another volunteer, who took 250 mg of sodium fluoride on an empty stomach, experienced nausea, which appeared in 2 min and in 20 min increased to a maximum accompanied by greatly increased salivation and some retching but no vomiting. Two hours after the dose, lunch was eaten but was immediately vomited. Slight nausea continued throughout the following day but disappeared on the second day (Baldwin, 1899). Therapeutic usages of sodium fluoride in the early part of the twentieth century suggested that adults might tolerate doses of 80 mg four times daily and children 20–50 mg four times daily for periods of several months (Black *et al.*, 1949).

Table 61.9
Concentration of Fluoride in Drinking Water and in the Urine of Persons Who Drink This Water[a]

Fluoride in water (ppm)	Mean urinary output (ppm)
2	2.09
5.5	5.46
6	7.80
8	8.71

[a] Modified from Heyroth (1963), by permission of John Wiley and Sons, Inc.

Laboratory Findings   In the general population, levels of fluorine in tissues and body fluids depend, inter alia, on consumption of fluoridated water. In fact the concentration of fluoride in urine corresponds numerically with the concentration in drinking water as shown in Table 61.9. When the concentration of fluoride in water was reduced from 8 ppm to 1 ppm, the corresponding concentrations in urine decreased from 6–8 ppm to about 2 ppm in the course of 27 months (Likins *et al.*, 1956).

The mean fluoride concentration in plasma is in the range 0.14–0.19 ppm even when the fluoride concentration in drinking water varies from 0.15 to 2.5 ppm (WHO, 1970). Sequestration in bone and urinary excretion may act to control plasma levels (Hodge, 1961).

The normal concentration of fluoride in soft tissues is in the range 0.5–1.0 ppm. Bones and teeth contain much higher concentrations, usually in the range 100–300 ppm (Hodge and Smith, 1965).

In cases of poisoning, plasma calcium may be decreased and there is generally a disruption of fluid balance as a result of vomiting. Albuminuria is common.

Pathology   In acute fatal poisoning there is corrosion of the stomach and sometimes other parts of the gastrointestinal tract. Frequently there is edema of the brain and lungs and petechial hemorrhages of the lungs and heart.

Treatment of Poisoning   Vomiting should be promoted or gastric lavage carried out if the poison itself has not already produced copious vomiting. Liquid given between bouts of vomiting or used for gastric lavage should contain calcium (lime water, 1% calcium chloride solution, calcium gluconate, or even milk) to form the highly insoluble calcium fluoride. After the stomach has been cleared, a cathartic should be given. Milk of magnesia is best because it precipitates fluoride as well as clearing the intestine. Vomitus and excreta should be washed away quickly to prevent burns (Peters, 1948).

Calcium gluconate (20 ml of a 10 or 20% solution) should be given intravenously at once. It should be repeated as required by the blood calcium level. It not only may alleviate carpopedal spasm but may raise the blood pressure to normal from a shock level (Rao *et al.*, 1969).

Additional treatment should be symptomatic depending on the progress of the case but should emphasize restoration of fluid balance. In one very severe case, an intravenous atrial pacemaker was necessary to control ventricular fibrillation; feeding through a gastrostomy was necessary for 30 days (Abukurah *et al.*, 1973).

61.16.2 SULFURYL FLUORIDE

61.16.2.1 Identity, Properties, and Uses

Chemical Name   Sulfuryl fluoride.

Structure SO_2F_2.

Synonyms   Sulfuryl fluoride is manufactured under the trade name Vikane®. The CAS registry no. is 2699-79-8.

Physical and Chemical Properties   Sulfuryl fluoride has the empirical formula F_2O_2S and a molecular weight of 102.07. It is an odorless, colorless gas with a melting point of $-135.82°C$ and a boiling point of $-55.38°C$. The vapor pressure is 13×10^3 torr at 25°C. The solubility in water at 25°C is 0.75 g/kg. Sulfuryl fluoride is of low solubility in most organic solvents but is miscible with methyl bromide. It is stable and noncorrosive. It is not hydrolyzed by water, but by NaOH solution.

History, Formulations, and Uses   Sulfuryl fluoride was first introduced in 1957. It is used for the fumigation of structures against drywood termites. Technical sulfuryl fluoride is 95% pure.

61.16.2.2 Toxicity to Laboratory Animals

Both sexes of rats, guinea pigs, and rabbits and female rhesus monkeys tolerated air concentrations of 100 ppm (417 mg/m³) without apparent adverse effect when exposed 7 hr a day, 5 days a week, for 6 months. Observations included survival, general appearance, behavior, and the appearance of internal organs of animals killed at the end of the experiment (Stewart, 1957). Later it was reported that a concentration of 20 ppm produced detectable effects in rats, mice, and guinea pigs exposed 7 hr a day for 6 months, but the injury present after 12 months was reversible when exposure was discontinued. Some evidence of fluorosis was observed in the incisors of mice but not in those of rats or guinea pigs (ACGIH, 1971).

Although the long-term effects of sulfuryl fluoride are those of excess fluoride, it seems possible that some or all of the acute effects are those of the intact molecule.

Biochemical Effects   In the absence of studies on mammals, it is necessary to refer to an excellent study on termites. First it was shown that termites fumigated with a nonlethal concentration of [³⁵S]sulfuryl fluoride excreted inorganic sulfate, indicating that fluoride had been released. Then, using the labeled metabolic pool technique (see Section 3.3.3 in Hayes,

1975), separate studies of termites prefed sodium [^{14}C]acetate or on [^{32}P]phosphate showed that fumigated termites exhibited a spectrum of metabolic changes characteristic of fluoride toxicity (Meikle *et al.*, 1963).

61.16.2.3 Toxicity to Humans

Accidental and Intentional Poisoning   A case attributed to sulfuryl fluoride involved a 30-year-old man who was exposed for about 4 hr to unknown concentrations of a 99:1 mixture of it with chloropicrin. While still at work, he experienced nausea, vomiting, crampy abdominal pain, and itching. When admitted to hospital soon afterward, vital signs were normal; the only abnormalities observed were reddening of the conjunctival, pharyngeal, and nasal mucosae; diffuse rhonchi; and paresthesia of the lateral surface of the right leg. The serum was positive for fluoride. The signs and symptoms resolved quickly; the patient was discharged on the fourth hospital day. He returned three times as an outpatient, complaining of persistent scratching of the throat, flatulence, and difficulty in reading. Ophthalmological examination revealed no abnormality, and the patient was discharged with a strong suspicion that emotional factors played a significant role in his disorder (Taxay, 1966). In his discussion of the case, Taxay reviewed unpublished reports of animal experiments apparently indicating that dosages sufficient to produce illness from a single exposure produce respiratory irritation, central nervous system depression, and possible liver and kidney injury. Certainly the patient's major objective findings involved irritation of the eyes and respiratory tract. Only a series of cases would reveal whether the patient's signs and symptoms were typical or even whether they were due primarily to sulfuryl fluoride.

Dosage Response   The threshold limit value (20 mg/m^3) would permit occupational exposure at the rate of 2.86 mg/kg/day, equivalent to a fluoride exposure of 0.42 mg/kg/day.

Treatment of Poisoning   Treatment is symptomatic (see Section 61.16.1.3 and see Section 8.2 of the first edition of this Handbook).

61.16.3 ZINC HEXAFLUOROSILICATE

61.16.3.1 Identity, Properties, and Uses

Chemical Name   Zinc hexafluorosilicate.

Structure $ZnSiF_6 \cdot 6H_2O$.

Synonyms   Other names for zinc hexafluorosilicate include zinc fluosilicate, zinc fluorosilicate, and zinc silicofluoride. The CAS registry no. is 16871-71-9.

Physical and Chemical Properties   The anhydride of zinc hexafluorosilicate has the empirical formula F_6SiZn and a molecular weight of 207.46. The hexahydrate forms white crystals which are soluble in water.

Use   Mothproofing agent.

61.16.3.2 Toxicity to Laboratory Animals

The oral lethal dose for the guinea pig was reported as 100 mg/kg (Simonin and Pierron, 1937).

61.16.3.3 Toxity to Humans

Accidental and Intentional Poisoning   A suicide served to show that poisoning by zinc hexafluorosilicate is typical of poisoning by the fluoride ion. A 35-year-old man drank half a glassful of a 5–10% solution of a commercial formulation. Following ingestion, emesis and tetanic convulsions occurred in 3.4 hr and death in 4.5 hr. Pathology was typical of fluoride poisoning (von Kraemer and Giebelmann, 1975).

Laboratory Findings   In two cases, including the suicide just mentioned, analysis showed that the concentration of zinc was increased over normal values more dependably in the blood than in the liver or kidneys. In fact, in the suicide, the concentration of zinc in these organs was within the range of normal (Giebelmann and Peplow, 1974). Even in cases in which analysis of stomach contents for zinc hexafluorosilicate is definitive, it would seem best to analyze the tissues for fluoride.

Treatment of Poisoning   See Section 61.16.1.3 and see Section 1.8 of the first edition of this Handbook.

61.17 CHLORINE

Chlorine is a halogen that can occur as the highly toxic gas Cl_2. However, the chloride ion is essential to life. Its concentration as NaCl in normal human blood is 4500–5000 ppm.

Unlike compounds of lead or mercury, which have toxic properties common to the element, compounds of chlorine, whether inorganic or organic, have little in common, although certain groups of them may exhibit similarities. Thus there seems to be no characteristic chlorine toxicity as there is a mercury toxicity. This does not deny that the toxicity of many organic compounds can be modified and often substantially increased by chlorine substitution in the molecule. Such substitutions have been developed by living organisms and much more recently by chemists. Examples of naturally occurring organic chlorine compounds include ochratoxin A (Van der Merwe *et al.*, 1965), the compound now called penitrem A (Wilson *et al.*, 1968), and cyclochlorotine (Ishikawa *et al.*, 1970).

61.17.1 SODIUM CHLORATE

61.17.1.1 Identity, Properties, and Uses

Chemical Name   Sodium chlorate.

Structure $NaClO_3$.

Synonyms Trade names for sodium chlorate include Altacide®, Chlorax®, De-Fol-Ate®, Drop Leaf®, Klorex®, Ortho-C-1-Defoliant®, Rasikal®, Shed-A-Leaf®, Val-Drop®, and Weed Killer®. The CAS registry no. is 775-09-9.

Physical and Chemical Properties Sodium chlorate has the empirical formula $ClNaO_3$ and a molecular weight of 106.45. It forms an odorless white powder with a density of 2.5 and a melting point of 248°C. It liberates oxygen at about 300°C and decomposes upon heating. The solubility of sodium chlorate in water at 0°C is 790 g/l. It is soluble in ethanol and glycerol. A strong oxidizing agent, sodium chlorate reacts with organic materials in the presence of sunlight.

History, Formulations, and Uses Sodium chlorate has been in use as a weed killer since 1910. The commercial product is about 99% pure and is applied at rates of about 100 to 200 kg/ha. In some formulations, sodium chloride or other salts are included as fire retardants. Sodium borate may be formulated with sodium chlorate for both its fire retardant and herbicidal action.

61.17.1.2 Toxicity to Laboratory Animals

The oral LD 50 of sodium chlorate in the rat is 1200 mg/kg (Edson, 1960). The intraperitoneal LD 50 in the mouse is 596 mg/kg (Nofre *et al.*, 1963).

Sodium chlorate is a strong oxidizing agent. In the body it produces methemoglobin, a process involving the conversion of iron from the normal ferrous state to the ferric state. In addition, chlorate destroys red blood corpuscles, liberating hemoglobin and other proteins. The intact red cell has considerable power to reduce methemoglobin, but the mechanism apparently cannot operate after hemolysis. Thus, a high percentage of hemoglobin in the plasma may be in the form of methemoglobin whereas the percentage of metaglobin in the intact cells is low (Knight *et al.*, 1967).

Repeated doses of chlorate, large enough to produce illness and weight loss but too small to be harmful if given only once, injure the kidney tubules severely without producing detectable methemoglobinemia (Richardson, 1937). This situation apparently has no parallel in human clinical experience but could be involved with livestock.

61.17.1.3 Toxicity to Humans

Accidental and Intentional Poisoning The majority of deaths caused by sodium chlorate have been the result of suicide (Mengele *et al.*, 1969; Motin *et al.*, 1970; Oliver *et al.*, 1972; Timperman and Maes, 1966). The chance of ingesting a fatal dose accidentally is small unless the compound is mistaken for a drug and taken purposely, as occurred when the potassium salt mistakenly was substituted for potassium chloride (Cochrane and Smith, 1940). However, completely typical, near-fatal poisoning occurred when a 13-year-old boy "tasted" crystals of this weed killer which he found in his father's shed. In spite of

intensive treatment, recovery did not begin until about the 15th day and required a little over 40 days (Starvou *et al.*, 1978).

Poisoning is characterized by gastritis (nausea, vomiting, and pain), anoxia (cyanosis, collapse, and terminal convulsions) secondary to methemoglobinemia, possible liver injury, and nephritis (lumbar pain and oliguria). Nephritis presumably is the direct result of chlorate ion as well as secondary to the destruction of corpuscles. The blood pressure tends to fall and the heartbeat becomes irregular. The liver and spleen may be enlarged and tender. The urine, if any, is brown or black in color and contains casts, red cells, free hemoglobin, and methemoglobin. The blood is brownish in color, and the plasma contains free hemoglobin and free methemoglobin. The red cell count is very low and the white cell count high (Knight *et al.*, 1967; Sollmann, 1957).

Onset may be delayed as much as 12 hr (Mengele *et al.*, 1969).

Death from sodium chlorate poisoning has occurred from 4 hr to 34 days after ingestion with an average of just over 4 days (Knight *et al.*, 1967; Mengele *et al.*, 1969; Motin *et al.*, 1970).

An entirely different kind of danger also arises from the strong oxidizing action of sodium chlorate. Its storage constitutes a special fire hazard.

Sodium chlorate can explode if subjected to intense heat with or without sudden pressure. If mixed with sulfur, sugar, or some other oxidizable materials, it forms an explosive mixture that may be more powerful than gunpowder (in which the oxidant is KNO_3). McGregor and Jackson (1969) described the pattern of hand injuries resulting from the accidental explosion of homemade sodium chlorate mixture bombs in 11 teenage patients and discussed the management of the injury.

Use Experience When used as a pesticide, sodium chlorate may cause irritation of the skin, eyes, or upper respiratory tract.

Dosage Response Dermal absorption associated with agricultural use of sodium chlorate is not sufficient to cause systemic poisoning. Even by mouth, a large dose is required to produce illness. A 6.35% solution of potassium chlorate was long used as a gargle, or a 300-mg tablet was allowed to dissolve slowly in the mouth to treat pharyngitis before modern antibiotics became available. The toxicities of the sodium and potassium salts are similar. It was considered that a dose of 10,000 mg was toxic and 15,000–20,000 mg was fatal (Cochrane and Smith, 1940; Sollmann, 1957). The smallest recorded fatal dose was 7500 mg (Bernstein, 1930). However, vigorous treatment saved one person who had ingested about 40,000 mg (Knight *et al.*, 1967).

Laboratory Findings In a fatal case in which chlorate could not be demonstrated in the blood or organs, it was found at a concentration of 6000 ppm in the urine (Oliver *et al.*, 1972).

Methemoglobin levels of workers exposed to sodium chlorate were greater than those of a control group but always less than 10% (Maki, 1972).

In acute poisoning, blood potassium and urea may be increased. Even in a patient who eventually survives, the plasma may have a dark, opaque, muddy brown appearance, and spectroscopy may show hemoglobin, oxyhemoglobin, methemoglobin, and methemalbumin. The red cells may appear black and shiny like coal dust. During recovery, kidney function may return to normal very slowly and not always completely (Knight et al., 1967).

Treatment of Poisoning   In case of irritation of the skin or mucous membranes, the area should be thoroughly flushed with water. Every effort should be made to remove the material if ingestion has occurred. There is no specific antidote, but oxygen, peritoneal dialysis, and exchange transfusions may be lifesaving even after a dose as high as 40 g. Dialysis is important because 95% of small doses of chlorate are excreted by the kidney, but larger doses so injure that organ that the body is almost powerless to remove the poison unaided (Knight et al., 1967).

61.18 BORON

Boron has atomic number 5 and an atomic weight of 10.81. It precedes carbon in the periodic table and is in the same group as aluminum.

Although boron has long been recognized as essential to the growth of higher plants, there is no evidence so far that it is essential for animals. The lowest dietary level yet attained was 0.15 ppm (Underwood, 1977). On the other hand, the addition of 5 ppm boron (as sodium metaborate) to the drinking water of mice during their entire lifetime was without effect on their body weight, tumor incidence, or longevity (Schroeder and Mitchener, 1975).

As might be expected of an element essential to plants, boron is found in all animal tissues. As reviewed by Underwood (1977) measurements of daily intake of boron have varied from 0.4 to 20 mg/person/day, depending largely if not entirely on the quantity of fruits and vegetables in the diet. The concentrations in normal human soft tissues, including brain, range from 0.06 to 0.6 ppm; concentrations in bone and teeth are somewhat higher, especially in hard-water areas.

Boron has been used as an insecticide in the form of boric acid and borax, both mainly for the control of cockroaches. The acid is slightly more toxic, but the kind of illness produced by the two compounds is the same.

61.18.1 BORIC ACID

61.18.1.1 Identity, Properties, and Uses

Chemical Name   Boric acid.

Structure H_3BO_3.

Synonyms   Boric acid also is known as boracic acid and as orthoboric acid. The CAS registry no. is 10043-35-3.

Physical and Chemical Properties   Boric acid has the empirical formula BH_3O_3 and a molecular weight of 61.84. It forms odorless, white crystals with a pearly lustre and faintly bitter taste. It is slightly corrosive at room temperature. The density of boric acid is 1.435 at 15°C. It has a melting point of about 171°C but also may decompose upon heating. Its solubility in water at 20°C is 4.88 g/100 ml; in cold alcohol, 1 g/18 ml; in boiling alcohol, 1 g/6 ml; and in glycerine, 1 g/4 ml. It is stable up to 100°C.

Formulations and Uses   Boric acid has slight fungicidal properties. Its main use as a pesticide is in the form of tablets for the control of roaches.

61.18.1.2 Toxicity to Laboratory Animals

Basic Findings   The oral LD 50 values of boric acid are 2660 and 3450 mg/kg in rats and mice, respectively. The corresponding intravenous values are 1330 and 1780 mg/kg (Pfeiffer et al., 1945), indicating relatively rapid and complete absorption from the gastrointestinal tract. Animals poisoned by boric acid showed depression, ataxia (occasionally convulsions), a fall in body temperature, a violet-red color of the skin and mucous membranes, and, in dogs, persistent vomiting and meningismus (Pfeiffer et al., 1945).

Growth of rats was inhibited when their drinking water contained boric acid at a concentration of 2500 ppm, resulting in a dosage of about 325 mg/kg/day; growth was unaffected at a concentration of 1000 ppm (about 130 mg/kg/day).

The mechanism of the toxic action of boron is not known. However, it is clear that no injury is done unless one or a few doses overpower the body's rather considerable ability to excrete the ion so that its concentration in the tissues and especially in the brain increases to >10 ppm from the normal level of <1 ppm.

Absorption, Distribution, Metabolism, and Excretion   The similarity of the oral and intravenous LD 50 values indicates that absorption from the gastrointestinal tract is rapid and virtually complete.

Following intraperitoneal injection, a peak concentration was reached in about 1.0–1.5 hr in the brain and in about 0.5 hr in other tissues. The concentrations of borate in the tissues were directly proportional to dosage over the range 18–700 mg/kg (Locksley and Sweet, 1954).

In acute poisoning, the concentration of boric acid reaches high levels in all tissues, the high concentration in the brain being especially noteworthy. In a typical experiment, the concentrations were about 1110, 910, and 260 ppm in brain, liver, and body fat, respectively (Pfeiffer et al., 1945).

Boric acid is excreted unchanged in the urine. Following intravenous injection in dogs, this excretion became maximal in 1–2 hr and then declined gradually; at the same time, there was an initial, brief depression of phosphorus excretion followed by a gradual rise, which at 6 hr exceeded the control value for phosphorus by five times (Pfeiffer et al., 1945). The significance of this increase in excretion of phosphorus is unknown.

The half-life of boric acid in the blood of mice is about 65 min (Locksley and Sweet, 1954).

61.18.1.3 Toxicity to Humans

Experimental Exposure Pfeiffer *et al.* (1945) demonstrated by animal studies and by a review of human case histories that boric acid is absorbed easily from injured skin. By studies in adult volunteers who were heavily exposed to 5% solution or to 10% boric acid ointment, they showed by analysis of the urine that no detectable boron was absorbed from the intact skin. Goldbloom and Goldbloom (1953) confirmed this negative result in 10 volunteers.

Accidental and Intentional Exposure Most poisoning by boric acid has occurred in connection with its former use as a local antiseptic applied to irritated skin, bums, or wounds or from its mistaken inclusion in the feeding formula for babies. However, children also have ingested the compressed tablets made to combat roaches.

Illness usually begins about 8 hr after ingestion. Signs include vomiting, diarrhea, rapidly progressing prostration, tremors, meningismus, and convulsions. An erythematous eruption of the skin that may progress to exfoliative dermatitis is characteristic. The eruption tends to be prominent on the palms, soles, and buttocks. Death may occur in less than a day or after as much as a week (Goldbloom and Goldbloom, 1953; Pfeiffer *et al.*, 1945; Wong *et al.*, 1964; Young *et al.*, 1949). In very severe cases, onset may be within an hour and death within 4 hr (McNally and Rukstinat, 1947).

Goldbloom and Goldbloom (1953) raised the possibility that Ritter's disease was, in fact, acute boric acid poisoning.

Dosage Response The fatal dose is thought to be 2000-3000 mg for infants, 5000–6000 mg for children, and 15,000–20,000 mg for adults (Young *et al.*, 1949).

When through error a 42-year-old patient received an intravenous infusion of about 15,000 mg of boric acid as a 2.5% solution with 10% dextrose, she showed slight flushing, slight nausea, one episode of vomiting, and no further trouble. A total of 14,650 mg of boric acid was recovered from the urine (McIntyre and Burke, 1937). It is not clear whether this case is to be viewed as an example of individual variation—and good luck—or whether it reflects the relative protective effect of very gradual administration.

In newborns, who may be more susceptible than older infants, active treatment was successful in saving all those thought to have ingested 4000 mg and one thought to have ingested 4500 mg, but was not successful against higher doses (Wong *et al.*, 1964).

Laboratory Findings Fisher and Freimuth (1958) reported the cases of two children who failed to show any illness after drinking a solution of boric acid; their blood boron levels when first examined were 13.0 and 13.8 ppm, respectively. The authors questioned an earlier report that 8.7 ppm is a fatal level

and stated that, in their experience, levels of 87–175 ppm or higher (500–1000 ppm or more expressed as boric acid) are found in cases of fatal poisoning. These results are consistent with those of Boggs and Anrode (1955), who reported the recovery of a mildly ill infant whose initial blood boron level of 48 ppm was soon reduced to 31 ppm by an exchange transfusion. The report by others of low blood boron values associated with serious or fatal poisoning may have been the result of faulty analytical techniques. One baby whose initial blood boron level was 94 ppm died in spite of vigorous treatment, but two with initial levels of 49 and 34 ppm survived (Segar, 1960).

In fatal cases the concentration of boric acid in the brain has ranged from 250 to 2555 ppm (Fellows *et al.*, 1948; McNally and Rust, 1928; Young *et al.*, 1949), that is, boron levels of 44–447 ppm. In many cases, the highest concentration was found in the brain, but in some instances the highest concentration was in the lung or liver.

Metabolic acidosis, jaundice, and increased blood urea may be present (Wong *et al.*, 1964).

Pathology In fatal cases, pathological changes may be minimal but may include degeneration of the kidney tubules; slight degeneration of liver cells; engorgement, focal hemorrhage, and leukocytic infiltration of the skin; and edema and congestion of the brain and spinal cord (Goldbloom and Goldbloom, 1953; Wong *et al.*, 1964).

Treatment of Poisoning Treatment of poisoning by boron is symptomatic. There is no pharmacological or specific antidote. Therefore removal of the poison is of particular importance.

Boggs and Anrode (1955) demonstrated the effectiveness of exchange transfusion in removing boric acid from the body. Later, Segar (1960) showed that 4 hr of peritoneal dialysis removed about the same amount of bone acid as one exchange transfusion and concluded that continuous dialysis for 24–28 hr is, therefore, much more efficient than exchange transfusion for this purpose. Peritoneal dialysis was also used and recommended by Wong *et al.* (1964).

Animal experiments showing that the compound is excreted readily in the urine (Pfeiffer *et al.*, 1945) would justify the use of forced diuresis.

REFERENCES

Aamodt, R. L., Ramble, W. F., O'Reilly, S., Johnston, E., and Henkin, R. I. (1975). Studies on he metabolism of Zn-65 in man. *Fed. Proc., Fed. Am. Soc. Exp. Biol.* **34**, 922 (Abstr. 3981).

Aamodt, R. L., Ramble, W. F., Johnston, G. S., Foster, D., and Henkin, R. I. (1979). Zinc metabolism in humans after oral and intervenous administration of Zn-69m. *Am. J. Clin. Nutr.* **32**, 559–569.

Aberg, B., Ekman, L., Falk, R., Greitz, U., Presson, G., and Snihs, J.-O. (1969). Metabolism of methyl mercury (203-Hg) compounds in man. *Arch. Environ. Health* **19**, 478–484.

Abukurah, A. R., Moser, A. M., Baird, C. L., Randall, R. E., Jr., Setter, J. G., and Blanke, R. V. (1973). Acute sodium fluoride poisoning. *Fluoride* **6**, 68–69.

Agate, J. N., Bell, G. H., Boddie, C. F., Bowler, R. G., Bucknell, M., Cheeseman, E. A., Douglas, T. H. J., Druett, H. A., Garrad, J., Hunter, D., Perry, K. M. A., Richardson, J. D., and Weir, J. B. V. (1949). "Industrial Fluorosis." Memo. No. 22, Med. Res. Counc. Br., London.

Agency for Toxic Substances and Disease Registry (ATSDR) (1990). "Toxicological Profile for Copper." ATSDR, Atlanta.

Agency for Toxic Substances and Disease Registry (ATSDR) (1991). "Toxicological Profile for Fluorides, Hydrogen Fluoride and Fluorine." ATSDR, Atlanta.

Agency for Toxic Substances and Disease Registry (ATSDR) (1992a). "Toxicological Profile for Barium." ATSDR, Atlanta.

Agency for Toxic Substances and Disease Registry (ATSDR) (1992b). "Toxicological Profile for Thallium." ATSDR, Atlanta

Agency for Toxic Substances and Disease Registry (ATSDR) (1992c). "Toxicological Profile for Tin." ATSDR, Atlanta.

Agency for Toxic Substances and Disease Registry (ATSDR) (1992d). "Toxicological Profile for Antimony." ATSDR, Atlanta.

Agency for Toxic Substances and Disease Registry (ATSDR) (1994). "Toxicological Profile for Zinc (Update)." ATSDR, Atlanta.

Agency for Toxic Substances and Disease Registry (ATSDR) (1996). "Toxicological Profile for Selenium (Update)." ATSDR, Atlanta.

Agency for Toxic Substances and Disease Registry (ATSDR) (1997). "Toxicological Profile for Cadmium (Update)." ATSDR, Atlanta.

Agency for Toxic Substances and Disease Registry (ATSDR) (1998). "Toxicological Profile for Arsenic (Update)." ATSDR, Atlanta.

Agency for Toxic Substances and Disease Registry (ATSDR) (1999). "Toxicological Profile for Mercury (Update)." ATSDR, Atlanta.

Agency for Toxic Substances and Disease Registry (ATSDR) (2000). "Toxicological Profile for Chromium." ATSDR, Atlanta.

Ahlborg, G., and Ahlmark, A. (1949). Alkyl mercury compound poisoning: Clinical aspect and risks of exposure. Nord. Med. **41**, 503–504.

Ahlmark, A. (1948). Poisoning by methyl mercury compounds. Br. J. Ind. Med. **5**, 117–119.

Airey, D. (1983). Total mercury concentrations in human hair from 13 countries in relation to fish consumption and location. Sci. Total Environ. **31**, 157–180.

Akitake, T. (1968). Experimental study on poisoning by organic mercury, compounds. Igaku Kentyu **38**, 357–378 (in Japanese).

Alajouanine, T., Derobert, L., and Thieffry, S. (1958). Clinical study of a group of 210 cases of intoxication by organic salts of tin. Rev. Neurol. **98**, 85–96 (in French).

Al-Damluji, S. F. (1976a). Organomercury poisoning in Iraq: History prior to the 1971–72 outbreak. Bull. W.H.O. **53**(Suppl.), 11–13.

Al-Damluji, S. F. (1976b). Intoxication due to alkylmercury-treated seed—1971–72 outbreak in Iraq: Clinical aspects. Bull. W.H.O. **53**(Suppl.), 65–81.

Aldridge, W. N., and Cremer, J. E. (1955). The biochemistry of organotin compounds diethyltin dichloride and triethyltin sulphate. Biochem. J. **61**, 406–418.

Alekseyeva, T. I., and Mishin, G. P. (1971). Treatment of cases of Granosan poisoning. Sov. Med. **5**, 137–138 (in Russian).

Alexander, J., Aaseth, J., and Refsvik, T. (1981). Excretion of zinc in rat bile—a role of glutathione. Acta Pharmacol. Toxicol. **49**, 190–194.

Al-Shahristani, H., and Shihab, K. (1976). Mercury in hair as an indicator of total body burden. Bull. W.H.O. **53**(Suppl.), 105–112.

American Conference of Governmental Industrial Hygienists (ACGIH) (1971). "Documentation of the Threshold Limit Value for Substances in Workroom Air." Am. Conf. Govt. Ind. Hyg., Cincinnati, OH.

American Conference of Governmental Industrial Hygienists (ACGIH) (1981). "Documentation of the Threshold Limit Values," pp. 283–285. Am. Conf. Govt. Ind. Hyg., Cincinnati, OH.

American Conference of Governmental Industrial Hygienists (ACGIH) (1988). "Threshold Limit Values and Biological Exposure Indices for 1988–1989." Am. Conf. Govt. Ind. Hyg., Cincinnati, OH.

American Medical Association (AMA) (1977). "AMA Drug Evaluations." Publishing Sciences Group, Littleton, MA.

Amin-Zaki, L., Elhassani, S., Majeed, M. A., Clarkson, T. W., Doherty, R. A., and Greenwood, M. R. (1974a). Studies of infants postnatally exposed to methylmercury. J. Pediatr. **85**, 81–84.

Amin-Zaki, L., Elhassani, S., Majeed, M. A., Clarkson, T. W., Doherty, R. A., and Greenwood, M. (1974b). Intra-uterine methylmercury poisoning in Iraq. Pediatrics **54**, 587–595.

Amin-Zaki, L., Elhassani, S., Majeed, M. A., Clarkson, T. W., Doherty, R. A., Greenwood, M. R., and Giovanoli-Jakubczak, T. (1976). Perinatal methylmercury poisoning in Iraq. Am. J. Dis. Child. **130**, 1070–1076.

Amin-Zaki, L., Majeed, M. A., Clarkson, T. W., and Greenwood, M. R. (1978). Methylmercury poisoning in Iraqi children: Clinical observations over two years. Br. Med. J. **1**, 613–616.

Andersen, R. A. (1981). Nutritional role of chromium. Sci. Total Environ. **17**, 13–19.

Andersen, O., Nielsen, J. B., and Svendsen, P. (1988). Oral cadmium chloride intoxication in mice: Effects of dose on tissue damage, intestinal absorption and relative organ distribution. Toxicology **48**, 225–236.

Anke, M., Gran, M., and Parschefeld, M. (1976). The essentiality of arsenic for animals. Trace Subst. Environ. Health **10**, 403–409.

Anke, M., Gran, M., Parschefeld, M., Groppel, B., and Hennig, A. (1978). Essentiality and function of arsenic. In Trace Elem. Metab. Man Anim., Proc. Int. Symp., 3rd, 1977," pp. 248–252.

Araibi, A. A., Yousif, W. H., and Al-Dewachi, O. S. (1989). Effect of high fluoride on the reproductive performance of the male rat. J. Biol. Sci. Res. **20**, 19–30.

Archimbaud, Y., Grillon, G., Poncy, J. S., et al. (1992). Selenium-75 transfer via placenta and milk—distribution and retention in fetal, young, and adult rat. Radiat. Protection Dosimetry **41**(2–4), 147–151.

Arnold, F. A., Jr., McClure, F. J., and White, C. L. (1960). Sodium fluocide tablets for children. Dent. Prog. **1**, 8–12.

Ashe, W. F., Largent, E. J., Dutra, F. R., Hubbard, D. M., and Blackstone, M. (1953). Behavior of mercury in the animal organism following inhalation. Arch. Ind. Hyg. Occup. Med. **7**, 19–43.

Atalla, L. T., Silva, C. M., and Lima, F. W. (1965). Activation analysis of arsenic in human hair—some observations on the problem of external contamination. An. Acad. Bras. Cienc. **37**, 433–441.

Atkinson, H. V. (1921). The treatment of acute phosphorus poisoning. J. Lab. Clin. Med. **7**, 148–150.

Atkinson, S. C. (1969). Arsenical teratotes and internal cancer (urinary bladder and nasopharynx). Arch. Dermatol. **99**, 237–238.

Aub, J. C., Fairhall, L. T., Minot, A. S., Reznikoff, P., and Hamilton, A. (1926). Lead poisoning. In "Medicine Monograph," Vol. 7, pp. i–x and 1–265. Williams & Wilkins, Baltimore.

Baetjer, A. M., Damron, C., and Budacz, V. (1959). The distribution and retention of chromium in men and animals. Arch. Ind. Health **20**, 136–150.

Baetjer, A. M., Lilienfeld, A. M., and Levin, M. L. (1975). Cancer and occupational exposure to inorganic arsenic. In "Proc. Int. Congr. Occup. Health, 18th, 1975." Abstr., p. 393.

Bailey, R. R. (1964). The farmer and his poisons. N. Z. Med. J. **63**, 655–659.

Bakir, F., Damluji, S. F., Amin-Zaki, L., Murtadha, M., Khalidi, A., Al-Rawi, N. Y., Tikriti, S., Dhahir, H. I., Clarkson, T. W., Smith, J. C., and Doherty, R. A. (1973). Methylmercury poisoning in Iraq. Science **181**, 230–241.

Bakir, F., Al-Khalidi, A., Clarkson, T. W., and Greenwood, R. (1976). Clinical observations on treatment of alkylmercury poisoning in hospital patients. Bull. W.H.O. **53**(Suppl.), 87–92.

Baldwin, H. (1899). The toxic action of sodium fluoride. J. Am. Chem. Soc. **21**, 517–521.

Bank, W. J., Pleasure, D. E., Suzuki, K., Nigro, M., and Katz, R. (1972). Thallium poisoning. Arch. Neurol. (Chicago) **26**, 456–464.

Bar, M. J. (1956). Concerning an accident due to tin. Arch. Mat. Prof., Med. Trav. Secur. Soc. **17**, 506–508 (in French).

Barbier, F. (1974). Treatment of thallium poisoning. Lancet **2**, 1528.

Barnes, J. M., and Magee, P. N. (1958). The biliary and hepatic lesion produced experimentally by dibutyltin salts. J. Pathol. **75**, 267–279.

Barnes, J. M., and Stoner, H. B. (1958). Toxic properties of some dialkyl and trialkyl tin salts. Br. J. Ind. Med. **15**, 15–22.

Barnes, J. M., and Stoner, H. B. (1959). The toxicology of tin compounds. *Pharmacot. Rev.* **11**, 211–231.

Barrowman, J. A., Bonnett, R., and Bray, P. J. (1973). Biliary excretion of zinc in rats. *Biochem. Soc. Trans.* **1**, 985–989.

Bass, M. (1963). Thallium poisoning: A preliminary report. *J. Am. Osteopath. Assoc.* **63**, 229–235.

Bauer, G. C. H., Carlsson, A., and Lindquist, B. (1956). A comparative study of metabolism of ^{140}Ba and ^{45}Ca in rats. *Biochem. J.* **63**, 535–542.

Bauer, G. C. H., Carlsson, A., and Lindquist, B. (1957). Metabolism of Ba^{140} in man. *Acta Orthop. Scand.* **26**, 241–254.

Bayne, J. R. D., Beck, J. C., Lowenstein, L., and Browne, J. S. L. (1952). Cortisone acetate in file treatment of acute phosphorus poisoning. *Can. Med. Assoc. J.* **67**, 465–467.

Becker, W. M., and Hoekstra, W. G. (1971). Ion transport in plant cells. *In* "Intestinal Absorption of Metal Ions, Trace Elements and Radionuclides" (S. C. Skovya and D. Waldron-Edward, eds.), pp. 229–256. Pergamon, New York.

Behne, D., Kyriakopoulos, A., Scheid, S., *et al.* (1991). Effects of chemical form and dosage on the incorporation of selenium into tissue proteins in rats. *J. Nutr.* **121**(6), 806–814.

Behrbohm, P. (1957). Allergic contact eczema from chromate wood preservatives. *Berfus-dermatosen* **5**, 271–282 (in German).

Beliles, R. P., Clark, R. S., and Yuile, C. L. (1968). The effects of exposure to mercury vapor on behavior of rats. *Toxicol. Appl. Pharmacol.* **12**, 15–21.

Bental, E., Lavy, S., and Amir, N. (1961). Electroencephalographic changes due to arsenic, thallium and strychnine poisoning. *Confin. Neurol.* **21**, 233–240.

Berlin, M. H. (1986). Mercury. *In* "Handbook on the Toxicology of Metals" (L. Friberg, G. F. Nordberg, and V. B. Vouk, eds.), 2nd ed., Vol. 2, pp. 387–445. Elsevier, Amsterdam.

Berlin, M. H., and Johansson, L. G. (1964). Mercury in mouse brain after inhalation of mercury vapor and after intravenous injection of mercury salt. *Nature (London)* **204**, 85–86.

Berlin, M. H., and Ullberg, S. (1963). Increased uptake of mercury in mouse brain caused by 2,3-dimercaptopropanol. *Nature (London)* **197**, 84–85.

Berlin, M. H., Nordberg, G. F., and Serenius, F. (1969a). On the site and mechanism of mercury vapor resorption in the lung. A study in the guinea pig using mercuric nitrate Hg-203. *Arch. Environ. Health* **18**, 42–50.

Berlin, M. H., Fazackerley, J., and Nordberg, G. (1969b). The uptake of mercury in the brain of mammals exposed to mercury vapor and to mercuric salts. *Arch. Environ. Health* **18**, 719–729.

Berlin, M. H., Clarkson, T. W., Friberg, L. T, Gage, J. C., Goldwater, L. J., Jernelov, A., Kazantzis, G., Magos, L., Nordberg, G. F., Radford, E. P., Ramel, C., Skerfving, S., Smith, R., Suzuki, T., Swensson, A., Tejning, S., Truhart, R., and Vostal, J. (1969c). Maximal allowable concentrations of mercury compounds. *Arch. Environ. Health* **19**, 891–905.

Bernstein, R. (1930). Potassium chlorate poisoning (suicide by means of Pebeco toothpaste). *Sommerkersamml. Vergiftungsfallen* **1**(A7), 15–16.

Berry, J. P., Hourdig, J., Galle, P., and Laquie, G. (1978). Chromium concentration by proximal renal tubule cells: An ultrastructural microanalytical and cytochemical study. *J. Histochem. Cytochem.* **26**, 651–657.

Bidstrup, P. L. (1964), "Toxicity of Mercury and Its Compounds." Elsevier, Amsterdam.

Binz, C. (1897). "Lectures on Pharmacology for Practitioners and Students" (P. W. Latham, ed.), Vol. II. New Sydenham Society, London.

Birke, G., Johnels, A. G., Plantin, L. O., Sjöstrand, B., and Westermark, T. (1967). Mercury poisoning through eating fish? *Sven. Laekaritidn.* **64**, 3628–3637.

Birke, G., Johnels, A. G., Plantin, L. O., Sjöstrand, B., Skerfving, S., and Westermark, T. (1972). Studies on humans exposed to methyl mercury through fish consumption. *Arch. Environ. Health* **25**, 77–91.

Bivings, L., and Lewis, G. (1948). Acrodynia: A new treatment with BAL. *J. Pediatr.* **32**, 63–65.

Black, M. M., Kleiner, I. S., and Btoker, H. (1949). The toxicity of sodium fluoride in man. *N.Y. State J. Med.* **49**, 1187–1188.

Bligh, P. H., and Taylor, D. M. (1963). Comparative studies of the metabolism of strontium and barium in the rat. *Biochem. J.* **87**, 612–618.

Blisnakov, C., and Iskrov, G. (1961). Fatal poisoning by parenteral injection of zinc phosphide. *Folia Med.* **3**, 73–76 (in German).

Bloom, G., Lundgren, K.-D., and Swensson, A. (1955). Exposure and hazards from organic mercury compounds in connection with seed dressing on small farms. *Nord. Hyg. Tidskr.* **36**, 110–117.

Boggs, T. R., and Anrode, H. G. (1955). Boric acid poisoning treated by exchange transfusion. *Pediatrics* **16**, 109–114.

Bogomaz, M. S. (1969). Food poisoning with Granosan. *Vrach. Delo* **1**, 142–143.

Bomhard, E., Vogel, O., and Loser, E. (1987). Chronic effects on single and multiple oral and subcutaneous cadmium administration on the testes of Wistar rats. *Cancer Lett.* **36**, 307–315.

Bonnin, M. (1951). Organic mercury dust poisoning. *Rep. Adelaide Hosp.* **31**, 11–13.

Borneff, I., Engelhardt, K., Griem, W., *et al.* (1968). Carcinogenic substances in water and soil. XXII. Mouse drinking study with 3,4-benzpyrene and potassium chromate. *Arch. Hyg.* **152**, 45–53 (in German).

Boyd, T. C., and Roy, A. C. (1929). Observations on the excretion of Sb in urine. *Indian J. Med. Res.* **17**, 94–108.

Boyden, R., Potter, V. R., and Elvehjen, C. A. (1938). Effect of feeding high levels of copper to albino rats. *J. Nutr.* **15**, 397–402.

Boylen, G. W., Jr., and Hardy, H. L. (1967). Distribution of arsenic in nonexposed persons (hair, liver, and urine). *Am. Ind. Hyg. Assoc. J.* **28**, 148–150.

Bradley, W. R., and Fredrick, W. G. (1941). Toxicity of antimony—animal studies. *Ind. Med. (Ind. Hyg. Sect.)* **2**, 15–22.

Brady, F. J., Lawton, A. H., Cowie, D. B., Andrews, H. L., Ness, A. T., and Ogden, G. E. (1945). Localization of trivalent radio-active Sb following intravenous administration to dogs infected with *Diofilaria immitis*. *Am. J. Trop. Med.* **25**, 103–107.

Brady, J., Liberatore, F., Harper, P., Greenwald, P., Burnett, W., Davies, J. N. P., Polan, A., Vianna, N., and Bishop, M. (1977). Angiosarcoma of the liver: An epidemiologic survey. *J. Natl. Cancer Inst. (U.S.)* **59**, 1383–1385.

Braun, H. A., Lusky, L. M., and Calvery, H. O. (1946). The efficacy of 2,3-dimercaptopropanol (BAL) in the therapy of poisoning by compounds of antimony, bismuth, chromium, mercury and nickel. *J. Pharmacol. Exp. Ther.* **87**(Suppl.), 119–125.

Brenniman, G. R., and Levy, P. S. (1985). Epidemiological study of barium in Illinois drinking water supplies. *In* "Inorganics in water and cardiovascular disease" (E. J. Calabrese, R. W. Tuthill, and L. Codie, eds.), pp. 231–240. Princeton Sci. Pub., Princeton, NJ.

Brenniman, G. R., Hamekata, T., Kojola, W. H., Carnow, B. W., and Levy, P. S. (1979). Cardiovascular disease death rates in communities with elevated levels of barium in drinking water. *Environ. Res.* **20**, 318–324.

Bridges, J. W., Davis, D. S., and Williams, R. T. (1967). The fate of ethyltin and diethyltin derivatives in the rat. *Biochem. J.* **105**, 1261–1267.

Brodniewicz, A., and Szuber, T. (1960). Poisoning of the population with rodenticides in Poland. *Zdrowie* **75**, 159–167 (in Polish).

Brown, A. W., Aldridge, W. N., and Verschoyle, R. D. (1979). The behavioral and neuropathologic sequelae of intoxication by trimethyltin compounds in the rat. *Am. J. Pathol.* **97**, 59–76.

Brown, I. A. (1954). Chronic mercurialism. *Arch. Neurol. Psychiatry* **72**, 674–681.

Browning, E. (1969). "Toxicity of Industrial Metals," 2nd ed. Appleton–Century–Crofts, New York.

Brügemann, J., Barth, K., and Niesar, K. H. (1964). Part II. Experimental studies on the occurrence of triphenylacetate residues in beet leaves and silage, in animals fed them, and in their excretions. *Zentralbl. Veterinaermed., Reihe A* **11**, 4–19 (in German).

Brun, G. C., Buchwald, H., and Roholm, K. (1941). Excretion of fluoride in urine in chronic fluoride poisoning of cryolite workers. *Acta Med. Scand.* **106**, 261–273 (in German).

Bruner, H. D. (1950). Effect of BAL on distribution of intravenously administered zinc using Zn^{65}. *Fed. Proc., Fed. Am. Soc. Exp. Biol.* **9**, 260.

Buchanan, W. D. (1962). "Toxicity of Arsenic Compounds." Am. Elsevier, New York.

Bucher, J. R., Hejtmancik, M. R., Toft, J. D., II *et al.* (1991). Results and conclusions of the national toxicology program's rodent carcinogenicity studies with sodium fluoride. *Int. J. Cancer* **48**, 733–737.

Buchet, J. P., Roels, H., Bernard, A., and Lauwerys, R. (1980). Assessment of renal function of workers exposed to inorganic lead, cadmium and mercury vapor. *Occup. Med.* **22**, 741–750.

Buchet, J. P., Lauwerys, R., and Roels, H. (1981a). Comparison of the urinary excretion of arsenic metabolites after a single oral dose of sodium arsenite, monomethyl arsonate and dimethyl arsinate in man. *Int. Arch. Occup. Environ. Health* **48**, 71–79.

Buchet, J. P., Lauwerys, R., and Roels, H. (1981b). Urinary excretion of inorganic arsenic and its metabolites after repeated ingestion of sodium meta arsenite by volunteers. *Int. Arch. Occup. Environ. Health* **48**, 111–118.

Butler, J. A., Whanger, P. D., Kaneps, A. J., *et al.* (1990). Metabolism of selenite and selenomethionine in the rhesus monkey. *J. Nutr.* **120**(7), 751–759.

Byron, W. R., Bierbower, G. W., Brouwer, J. B., and Hansen, W. H. (1967). Pathologic changes in rats and dogs from two-year feeding of sodium arsenite or sodium arsenate. *Toxicol. Appl. Pharmacol.* **10**, 132–147.

Caley, J. P., and Kellock, I. A. (1955). Acute yellow phosphorus poisoning with recovery. *Lancet* **1**, 539–541.

Calvery, H. O. (1938). Chronic effects of ingested lead and arsenic. A review and correlation. *JAMA, J. Am. Med. Assoc.* **111**, 1723–1729.

Calvery, H. O., Laug, E. P., and Morris, H. J. (1938). The chronic effects on dogs of feeding diets containing lead acetate, lead arsenate, and arsenic trioxide in varying concentrations. *J. Pharmacol. Exp. Ther.* **64**, 364–387.

Cameron, G. R. (1947). Liver atrophy produced by chronic selenium intoxication. *J. Pathol. Bacteriol.* **59**, 539–545.

Campbell, I. R. (1963). "The Role of Fluoride in Public Health—The Soundness of Fluoridation of Communal Water Supplies." Kettering Laboratory, University of Cincinnati, Cincinnati, OH.

Cangelosi, J. T. (1941). Acute cadmium metal poisoning. *U.S. Nav. Med. Bull.* **39**, 408–410.

Cantarow, A., and Trumpeter, M. (1944). "Lead Poisoning." Williams & Wilkins, Baltimore.

Cardiff, I. D. (1940). How toxic is arsenate of lead? *J. Ind. Hyg.* **22**, 333–346.

Carlson, C. H., Armstrong, W. D., and Singer, L. (1960a). Distribution and excretion of radiofluoride in the human. *Proc. Soc. Exp. Biol. Med.* **104**, 235–239.

Carlson, C. H., Singer, L., and Armstrong, W. D. (1960b). Radiofluoride distribution in tissues of normal and nephrectomized rats. *Proc. Soc. Exp. Biol. Med.* **103**, 418–420.

Cavanagh, J. B., Fuller, N. H., Johnson, H. R. M., and Rudge, P. (1974). The effects of thallium salts, with particular reference to the nervous system changes. *Q. J. Med.* **43**, 293–319.

Chamberlain, P. H., Stavinoh, W. B., Davies, H., Kniker, W. T., and Panos, T. C. (1958). Thallium poisoning. *Pediatrics* **22**, 1170–1182.

Chang, L. W., Reuhl, K. R., and Spyker, J. M. (1977). Ultrastructural study of the latent effects of methyl mercury on the nervous system after prenatal exposure. *Environ. Res.* **13**, 171–185.

Charbonneau, S. M., Spencer, K., Bryce, F., *et al.* (1978). Arsenic excretion by monkeys dosed with arsenic-containing fish or with inorganic arsenic. *Bull. Environ. Contam. Toxicol.* **20**, 470–477.

Chawla, S. C., and Mehta, S. P. (1973). A study of host and environmental factors in cases of accidental poisoning admitted in Irwin Hospital. *Indian J. Med. Res.* **61**, 724–731.

Chen, C. J., and Wang, C. J. (1990). Ecological correlation between arsenic level in well water and age-adjusted mortality from malignant neoplasms. *Cancer Res.* **50**, 5470–5474.

Chen, C. J., Chen, C. W., Wu, M. M., *et al.* (1992). Dose–response relationship between ischemic heart disease mortality and long-term arsenic exposure. *Arterioscler. Thromb. Vasc. Biol.* **16**(4), 504–510.

Chen, C. J., Chuang, Y. C., Lin, T. M., *et al.* (1985). Malignant neoplasms among residents of a blackfoot disease–endemic area in Taiwan: High-arsenic artesian well water and cancers. *Cancer Res.* **45**, 5895–5899.

Chen, C. J., Chuang, Y. C., You, S. L., *et al.* (1986). A retrospective study on malignant neoplasms of bladder, lung, and liver in blackfoot disease endemic area in Taiwan. *Br. J. Cancer* **53**, 399–405.

Chen, C. J., Kuo, T. W., and Wu, M. M. (1988a). Arsenic and cancers [Letter]. *Lancet* (February 20), 414–415.

Chen, C. J., Wu, M.-M., Leer, S.-S., *et al.* (1988b). Atherogenicity and carcinogenicity of high-arsenic artesian well water. Multiple risk factors and related malignant neoplasms of blackfoot disease. *Arteriosclerosis* **8**, 452–460.

Chen, K. S., Huang, C. C., Liaw, C. C., *et al.* (1988c). Multiple primary cancers in blackfoot endemic area: Report of a case. *J. Formosan Med. Assoc.* **87**, 1125–1128 (in Chinese).

Chhabra, S. K., and Rao, A. R. (1994). Translactational exposure of F' mouse pups to selenium. *Food Chem. Toxicol.* **32**(6), 527–531.

Chiang, H.-S., Hong, C.-L., Guo, H.-R., *et al.* (1988). Comparative study on the high prevalence of bladder cancer in the blackfoot disease endemic area in Taiwan. *J. Formosan Med. Assoc.* **87**, 1074–1080.

Childs, E. A. (1973). Kinetics of transplacental movement of mercury fed in a tuna matrix to mice. *Arch. Environ. Health* **27**, 50–52.

Chinen, M., Mori, T., Anjirei, K., Nakamura, Y., Tamanaha, E., Kiyamu, M., and Nakamoto, F. (1977). Six cases of intoxication due to thallium in a single district. *Acta Paediatr. Jpn., Overseas Ed.* **81**, 1125–1126 (in Japanese).

Chou, H. Y., Hsueh, Y. M., Liaw, K. F., *et al.* (1995). Incidence of internal cancers and ingested inorganic arsenic. A seven-year follow-up study in Taiwan. *Cancer Res.* **55**(6), 1296–1300.

Choy, W. N., Henika, P. R., Willhite, C. C., *et al.* (1993). Incorporation of a micronucleus study into a developmental toxicology and pharmacokinetic study of L-selenomethionine in nonhuman primates. *Environ. Mol. Mutagen.* **21**(1), 73–80.

Christensen, H., Krogh, M., and Nielsen, M. (1937). Acute mercury poisoning in a respiration chamber. *Nature (London)* **139**, 626–627.

Christison, R. (1845). "A Treatise on Poisons in Relation to Medical Jurisprudence, Physiology, and the Practice of Physic." E. Barrington and G. D. Haswell. Philadelphia.

Chugh, K. S., Singhal, P. C., and Sharma, B. K. (1975). Methemoglobinemia in acute copper sulfate poisoning. *Ann. Intern. Med.* **82**, 226–227.

Chugh, K. S., Singhal, P. C., Sharma, B. K., Das, K. C., and Datta, B. N. (1977). Acute renal failure following copper sulphate intoxication. *Postgrad. Med. J.* **53**, 18–23.

Clark, G. L., and Buhrke, V. E. (1954). Effect of elemental sulfur in the diet on load–extension hysteresis in single wood fibers. *Science* **120**, 40.

Clarkson, T. W. (1972). Recent advances in the toxicology of mercury with emphasis on the alkylmercurials. *CRC Crit. Rev. Toxicol.* **1**, 203–234.

Clarkson, T. W. (1983). Molecular targets of metal toxicity. *In* "Chemical Toxicity and Clinical Chemistry of Metals" (S. S. Brown and J. Savory, eds.), pp. 211–226. Academic Press, New York.

Clarkson, T. W., and Kench, J. E. (1956). Urinary excretion of amino acids by men absorbing heavy metals. *Biochem. J.* **62**, 361–372.

Clarkson, T. W., and Rothstein, A. (1964). Excretion of volatile mercury in rats injected with mercuric salts. *Health Phys.* **10**, 1115–1121.

Clarkson, T. W., Magos, L., and Greenwood, M. R. (1972). The transport of elemental mercury into fetal tissue. *Biol. Neonate* **21**, 239–244.

Clarkson, T. W., Cox, C., Marsh, D. O., Myers, G. J., Al-Tikriti, S., Amin-Zaki, L., and Dabbagh, A. R. (1981). Dose–response relationships for adult and prenatal exposures to methylmercury. *In* "Measurement of Risk" (G. G. Berg and H. D. Maillie, eds.), pp. 111–130. Plenum, New York.

Clarkson, T. W., Nordberg, G. F., Sager, P. *et al.* (1983). An overview of the reproductive and developmental toxicity of metals. *In* "Reproductive and Developmental Toxicity of Metals" (T. W. Clarkson, G. F. Nordberg, and P. R. Sager, eds.), pp. 1–26. Plenum, New York.

Clarkson, T. W., Hursh, J. B., Sager, P. R., and Syversen, T. L. M. (1988). Mercury. *In* "Biological Monitoring of Toxic Metals" (T. W. Clarkson, L. Friberg, G. F. Nordberg, and P. R. Sager, eds.), pp. 199–246. Plenum, New York.

Cloetta, M. (1906). On the cause of tolerance to arsenic. *Arch. Exp. Pathol. Pharmakol.* **54**, 196–205 (in German).

Cochrane, W. J., and Smith, R. P. (1940). A fatal case of accidental poisoning by chlorate of potassium: With a review of the literature. *Can. Med. Assoc. J.* **42**, 23–26.

Cortella, E. (1928). Research on changes in the central nervous system in intoxication by thallium acetate. *G. Ital. Dermatol. Sifilol.* **69**, 1167–1176.

Cosic, V., and Kusic, R. (1966). Acute poisoning with arsenic trioxide. *Vojnosanit. Pregl.* **23**, 601–603 (in Serbo-Croatian).

Cotter, L. H. (1947). Hazard of phenylmercuric salts. *Occup. Med.* **4**, 305–309.

Cotter, L. H. (1958). Treatment of cadmium poisoning with EDTA. *JAMA, J. Am. Med. Assoc.* **166**, 735–736.

Coulson, E. J., Remington, R. E., and Lynch, K. M. (1935). Metabolism in the rat of the naturally occurring arsenic of shrimp as compared with arsenic trioxide. *J. Nutr.* **10**, 255–270.

Cox, C. J. (1954). Acute fluoride poisoning and crippling chronic fluorosis. In "Fluorides as a Public Health Measure" (J. H. Shaw, ed.). Am. Assoc. Adv. Sci., Washington, DC.

Crecelius, E. A. (1977). Changes in the chemical speciation of arsenic following ingestion by man. *Environ. Health Perspect.* **19**, 147–150.

Cremer, J. E. (1958). The biochemistry of organotin compounds. The conversion of tetraethyltin into triemyltin in mammals. *Biochem. J.* **68**, 685–692.

Cuddihy, R. G., and Griffith, W. C. (1972). A biological model describing tissue distribution and whole-body retention of barium and lantanum in beagle dogs after inhalation and gavage. *Health Phys.* **23**, 621–633.

Curley, A., Sedlak, V. A., Girling, E. F., Hawk, R. E., Barthel, W. F., Pierce, P. E., and Likosky, W. H. (1971). Organic mercury identified as the cause of poisoning in humans and hogs. *Science* **172**, 65–67.

Curry, A. S., Rutter, E. R., and Lim, C. H. (1958). The detection of yellow phosphorus and phosphides in biological material. *J. Pharm. Pharmacol.* **10**, 635–637.

Curry, A. S., Price, D. E., and Tryhorn, F. G. (1959). Absorption of zinc phosphide particles. *Nature (London)* **184**, 642–643.

Curry, A. S., Green, J. L., Spiteri, L., and Vassallo, L. (1969). Death from thallium poisoning: A case report. *Eur. J. Toxicol.* **2**, 260–269.

Cushman, P., Jr., and Alexander, B. H. (1966). Renal phosphate and calcium excretory defects in a case of acute phosphorus poisoning. *Nephron* **3**, 123–128.

Cuzick, J., Sasieni, P., and Evans, S. (1992). Ingested arsenic, keratoses, and bladder cancer. *Am. J. Epidemiol.* **136**(4), 417–421.

Daniel, J. W., Gage, J. C., and Lefevre, P. A. (1971). Metabolism of methoxyethylmercury salts. *Biochem. J.* **121**, 411–415.

Davies, D. J. A., and Bennett, B. G. (1983). Summary exposure assessment—copper. In "Exposure Commitment Assessments of Environmental Pollutants," Vol. 3, p. 15. MARC, Global Environ. Monk. Syst., University of London, London.

Dean, G. (1950). Seven cases of barium carbonate poisoning. *Br. Med. J.* **2**, 817–818.

Dean, H. T. (1942a). Geographical distribution of endemic dental fluorosis (mottled enamel). In "Fluorine and Dental Health" (F. R. Mouton, ed.), pp. 6–11. Am. Assoc. Adv. Sci., Washington, DC.

Dean, H. T. (1942b). The investigation of physiological effects by the epidemiological method. In "Fluorine and Dental Health" (F. R. Moulton, ed.), pp. 23–31. Am. Assoc. Adv. Sci., Washington, DC.

DeLopez, O. H., Smith, F. A., and Hodge, H. C. (1976). Plasma fluoride concentrations in rats acutely poisoned with sodium fluoride. *Toxicol. Appl. Pharmacol.* **37**, 75–83.

Dencker, L., Nillson, A., Ronnback, C., and Walinder, G. (1976). Uptake and retention of ^{133}Ba and ^{140}Ba$-^{140}$La in mouse tissue. *Acta Radiol: Ther., Phys., Biol. [N.S.]* **15**, 273–287.

Dencker, L., Danielsson, B., Knayat, A., and Lindren, A. (1983). Deposition of metals in the embryo and fetus. In "Reproductive and Developmental Toxicity of Metals" (T. W. Clarkson, G. F. Nordberg, and P. R. Sager, eds.), pp. 607–631. Plenum, New York.

Denk, R., Holzmann, H., Lange, H. J., and Greve, D. (1969). Chronic arsenic injuries in autopsied Moselle winegrowers. *Med. Welt* **20**, 557–567 (in German).

Dérobert, L., and Marcus, O. (1956). Occupational poisoning by inhalation of organic mercury compounds. *Ann. Méd. Lég.* **36**, 294–296 (in French).

Díaz-Rivera, R. S., Collazo, P. J., Pons, E. R., and Torregrosa, M. V. (1950). Acute phosphorus poisoning in man: A study of 56 cases. *Medicine (Baltimore)* **29**, 269–298.

Díaz-Rivera, R. S., Ramos-Morales, F., Garcia-Palmieri, M. R., and Ramirez, E. A. (1961). The electrocardiographic changes in acute phosphorus poisoning in man. *Am. J. Med. Sci.* **241**, 758–765.

Dieke, S. H., and Richter, C. P. (1946). Comparative assays of rodenticides on wild Norway rats. *Public Health Rep.* **61**, 672–679.

Diengott, D., Rozsa, O., Levy, N., and Muammar, S. (1964). Hypokalaemia in barium poisoning. *Lancet* **2**, 343–344.

Donaldson, R. B., and Barreras, R. F. (1966). Intestinal absorption of trace quantities of chromium. *J. Lab. Clin. Med.* **68**, 484–493.

Down, W. L., Scott, J. K., Steadman, L. T., et al. (1960). Acute and sub-acute toxicity studies of thallium compounds. *Am. Ind. Hyg. Assoc. J.* **21**, 399–406.

Drasch G., and Hauck, G. (1977). Monitoring the progress of intensive treatment of thallium poisoning. *Arch. Toxicol.* **38**, 209–215 (in German).

Drinker, K. R., Thompson, P. K., and Marsh, M. (1927a). An investigation of the effect of long-continued ingestion of zinc in the form of zinc oxide, by cats and dogs, together with observations upon the excretion and storage of zinc. *Am. J. Physiol.* **80**, 31–64.

Drinker, K. R., Thompson, P. K., and Marsh, M. (1927b). An investigation of the effect upon rats of long-continued ingestion of zinc compounds, with special reference to the relation of zinc excretion to zinc intake. *Am. J. Physiol.* **81**, 284–306.

Dudley, H. C. (1938). Toxicology of selenium. Toxic and vesicant properties of Se oxychloride. *Public Health Rep.* **53**, 94.

Dunipace, A. J., Zhang, W., Noblitt, T. W., et al. (1989). Genotoxic evaluation of chronic fluoride exposure: Micronucleus and sperm morphology studies. *J. Dent. Res.* **68**, 1525–1528.

D'yachuk, I. A. (1972). Hygienic assessment of the working conditions in seed treatment facilities. *Gig. Tr. Prof. Zabol.* **16**, 45–47 (in Russian).

Eager, J. M. (1901). Denti di Chiaie (Chiaie teeth). *Public Health Rep.* **16**, 2576–2577.

Eckert, H., and Jerochin, S. (1982). Copper sulfate mediated changes of the lung: An experimental contribution to pathogenesis of vineyard sprayer's lung. *Z. Erkr. Atmungsorgane* **148**, 270–276.

Edson, E. F. (1960). Applied toxicology of pesticides. *Pharm. J.* **185**, 361–367.

Edwards, G. N. (1865). Two cases of poisoning by mercuric methide. *St. Bart's Hosp. Rep.* **1**, 141.

Ekstrand, J., Alván, G., Boréus, L. O., et al. (1977). Pharmacokinetics of fluoride in man after single and multiple oral doses. *Eur. J. Clin. Pharmacol.* **12**, 311–317.

Ekstrand, J., Koch, G., and Petersson, L. G. (1983). Plasma fluoride concentrations in pre-school children after ingestion of fluoride tablets and toothpaste. *Caries Res.* **17**, 379–384.

Elbel, H., and Holsten, K. (1936). On the hazard of the mouse poison "Delicia." *Dtsch. Z. Gesamte Gerichtl. Med.* **26**, 178–180 (in German).

Elinder, C.-F., Kjellström, T., Linnman, L., and Pershagen, G. (1978). Urinary excretion of cadmium and zinc among persons from Sweden. *Environ. Res.* **15**, 473–484.

Ellis, K. J., Yuen, K., Yasumura, S., and Cohen, S. H. (1984). Dose–response analysis of cadmium in man: Body burden vs kidney dysfunction. *Environ. Res.* **33**, 216–226.

Elwood, P. C., Abernethy, M., and Morton, M. (1974). Mortality in adults and trace elements in water. *Lancet* 1470–1472.

Engleson, G., and Herner, T. (1952). Alkyl mercury poisoning. *Acta Paediatr.* **41**, 289–294.

Ercoli, N. (1968). Chemotherapeutic and toxicological properties of antimonyl tartrate–dimethylcysteine chelates. *Proc. Soc. Exp. Biol. Med.* **129**, 284–290.

Evan, A. P., and Dail, W. G. (1974). The effects of sodium chromate on the proximal tubules of the kidney. *Lab. Invest.* **30**, 704–715.

Evans, E. H. (1945). Casualties following exposure to zinc chloride smoke. *Lancet* **249**, 368–370.

Evans, G. W. (1973). Copper homeostasis in the mammalian system. *Physiol. Rev.* **53**, 535–570.

Evans, G. W., and Johnson, P. E. (1978). Copper and zinc binding ligands in the intestinal mucosa. In "Trace Elem. Metab. Man Anim., Proc. Int. Symp. 3rd, 1977," pp. 98–105.

Fairhall, L. T., and Hyslop, F. (1947). The toxicology of antimony. *Public Health Rep., Suppl.* **195**.

Fairhall, L. T., and Miller, J. W. (1941). A study of the relative toxicity of the molecular components of lead arsenate. *Public Health Rep.* **56**, 1610–1625.

Fairhall, L. T., and Neal, P. A. (1938). The absorption and excretion of lead arsenate in man. *Public Health Rep.* **53**, 1231–1245.

Fazekas, I. G. (1968). Two fatal cases on sodium fluoride poisoning. *Orv. Hetil.* **100**, 2493–2496 (in Hungarian).

Felden, B. F. (1928). Epilation with thallium acetate in the treatment of ringworm of the scalp in children. *Arch. Dermatol.* **17**, 182–193.

Fellows, A. W., Campbell, J. S., and Wadsworth, R. C. (1948). Boric acid—poison. *J. Maine Med. Assoc.* **39**, 339–350.

Fierz, U. (1966). Studies on the side-effects of therapy of skin diseases with arsenic based on patients' histories. *Arch. Klin. Exp. Dermatol.* **227**, 286–290 (in German).

Fisher, R. S., and Freimuth, H. C. (1958). Blood boron levels in human infants. *J. Invest. Dermatol.* **30**, 85–86.

Fitzhugh, O. G., Nelson, A. A., Laug, E. P., and Kunze, F. M. (1950). Chronic oral toxicities of mercuriphenyl- and mercuric salts. *Arch. Ind. Hyg.* **2**, 433–442.

Fletcher, G. F., and Galambos, J. T. (1963). Phosphorus poisoning in humans. *Arch. Intern. Med.* **112**, 846–852.

Foreman, H. (1961). Use of chelating agents in treatment of metal poisoning (with special emphasis on lead). *Fed. Proc., Fed. Am. Soc. Exp. Biol.* **20**, 191–196.

Foulkes, E. C. (1974). Excretion and retention of cadmium, zinc, and mercury by rabbit kidney. *Am. J. Physiol.* **227**, 1356–1360.

Fowler, B. A., and Woods, J. S. (1979). The effects of prolonged oral arsenate exposure on liver mitochondria of mice: Morphometric and biochemical studies. *Toxicol. Appl. Pharmacol.* **50**, 177–187.

Franke, K. W. (1934). A new toxicant occurring naturally in certain samples of plant foodstuffs. I. Results obtained in preliminary feeding trials. *J. Nutr.* **8**, 597–608,

Franke, K. W., and Moxon, A. L. (1936). A comparison of the minimum fatal doses of selenium, tellurium, arsenic, and vanadium. *J. Pharmacol. Exp. Ther.* **58**, 454–459.

Franke, K. W., and Tully, W. C. (1935). Low hatchability due to deformities in chicks. *Poult. Sci.* **14**, 273–277.

Frant, S., and Kleeman, I. (1941). Cadmium food poisoning. *JAMA, J. Am. Med. Assoc.* **117**, 86–89.

Freeman, G. B., Johnason, J. D., Killinger, J. M., *et al.* (1993). Bioavailability of arsenic in soil impacted by smelter activities following oral administration in rabbits. *Fundam. Appl. Toxicol.* **21**(1), 83–88.

Freund, M., Leffkowitz, M., and Elian, M. (1971). Clinical manifestations of thallium poisoning. *Harefuah* **81**, 140–141 (in Hebrew).

Frey, J., and Schlechter, M. (1939). Experimental investigation of the quantitative excretion of thallium in various body fluids. *Naunyn-Schmiedebergs Arch. Exp. Pathol. Pharmakol.* **193**, 530–538 (in German).

Friberg, L. (1950). Health hazards in the manufacture of alkaline accumulators with special reference to chronic cadmium poisoning. *Acid Med. Scand., Suppl.* **240**, 1–124.

Friberg, L. (1956). Edathamil calcium disodium in cadmium poisoning. *Arch. Ind. Health* **13**, 18–23.

Friberg, L. (1959). Studies on the metabolism of mercuric chloride and methyl mercuric dicyandiamide. *Arch. Ind. Health* **20**, 42–49.

Friberg, L., Hammarström, S., and Nyström, A. (1953). Kidney injury after chronic exposure to inorganic mercury. *Arch. Ind. Hyg. Occup. Health* **8**, 149–153.

Friberg, L., Kjellström, T., and Nordberg, G. F. (1986). Cadmium. *In* "Handbook on the Toxicology of Metals" (L. Friberg, G. F. Nordberg, and V. B. Vouk, eds.), 2nd ed., Vol. 2, pp. 130–184. Elsevier, Amsterdam.

Friberg, L., Piscator, M., Nordberg, G. F., and Kjellström, T. (1974). "Cadmium in the Environment." CRC Press, Cleveland.

Frketić, J., Magdić, A., and Stajdaker-Djević, Z. (1957). Zn phosphide poisoning. *Arh. Hig. Rada Toksikol.* **8**, 15–24.

Frost, D. V., and Lish, P. M. (1975). Selenium in biology. *Annu. Rev. Pharmacol.* **15**, 259–284.

Furchner, J. E., London, J. E., and Wilson, J. S. (1975). Comparative metabolism of radionuclides in mammals. IX. Retention of 75Se in the mouse, rat, monkey and dog. *Health Phys.* **29**, 641–648.

Gabard, B. (1976). The excretion and distribution of inorganic mercury in the rat as influenced by several chalating agents. *Arch. Toxicol.* **35**, 15–24.

Gage, J. C. (1964). Distribution and excretion of methyl and phenyl mercury salts. *Br. J. Ind. Med.* **21**, 197–201.

Gaines, T. B. (1969). Acute toxicity of pesticides. *Toxicol. Appl. Pharmacol.* **14**, 515–534.

Galy, P., Touraine, R., Bruno, J., Gallos, P., Roudier, R., Lotre, R., l'Heureux, P., and Wissendenger, T. (1963a). Bronchopulmonary cancers in chronic arsenic poisoning of winegrowers of Bonjolsis. *Lyon Med.* **210**, 735–744 (in French).

Galy, P., Touraine, R., Bruno, J., Roudier, P., and Gallois, P. (1963b). Pulmonary cancer from arsenic in winegrowers of Besujolais. *J. Fr. Med. Chir. Thorac.* **17**, 303–311 (in French).

Gastel, B., Innis, R., and Moses, H., III (1978). Thallium poisoning. *Johns Hopkins Med. J.* **142**, 27–31.

Gautier, A. (1899). On the normal occurrence of arsenic in animals and its localization in certain organs. *C. R. Hebd. Scéances Acad. Sci. Sér. D* **12**, 929–936 (in French).

Gefel, A., Liron, M., and Hirach, W. (1970). Chronic thallium poisoning. *Isr. J. Med. Sci.* **6**, 380–382.

Gellhorn, A., Tupikova, N. A., and van Dyke, H. B. (1946). Tissue distribution and excretion of 4 organic anti???? after single or repeated administration to normal hamsters. *J. Pharmacol. Exp. Ther.* **87**, 169–180.

Gerdts, E. (1964). Thallium poisoning. *Tidsskr. Nor. Lasgeforen.* **84**, 1556–1558.

Gettler, A. O., and Weiss, L. (1943). Thallium poisoning. III. Clinical toxicology of thallium. *Am. J. Clin. Pathol.* **13**, 422–429.

Gharib, M. (1970). Esigmetic alopecia. *Clin. Pediatr.* **9**, 622.

Gibson, J. E., Sigdestad, C. P., and Becker, B. A. (1967). Placental transport and distribution of thallium-204 sulfate in newborn rats and mice. *Toxicol. Appl. Pharmacol.* **10**, 408.

Giebelmann, V. R., and Peplow, E. (1974). Concentration of zinc in man following poisoning by zinc hexafluorosilicate. *Dtsch. Gesund???.* **29**, 1378–1379 (in German).

Giese, A. C. (1940). Mercury poisoning. *Science* **91**, 476–477.

Gili, R. (1948). On a case of acute fatal poisoning by zinc phosphide. *Zacchia* **23**, 144–152.

Gis', Yu. F., and Pozner, A. Z. (1970). The clinical picture of Grancean intoxication in children. *Pediatrija (Moscow)* **49**, 80–81 (in Russian).

Gofman, J. W., deLalla, O. F., Kovich, E. L., Lows, O., Martin, W., Piloso, D. L., Tandy, R. K., and Upham, F. (1964). Chemical elements of the blood of man. *Arch. Environ. Health* **8**, 105–109.

Goldberg, A. A., Shapiro, M., and Wilder, E. (1950). Antibacterial colloidal electrolyte: The potentistion of the activitica of mercuric-, phenylmercuric-, and silver ions by colloidal sulphonic anion. *J. Pharm. Pharmacol.* **2**, 20–26.

Goldbloom, R. B., and Goldbloom, A. (1953). Boric acid poisoning. Report of four cases and a review of 109 cases from the world literature. *J. Pediatr.* **43**, 631–643.

Goldwater, L. J. (1972). An assessment of the scientific justification for establishing 2 μg/m^3 as the maximum safe level for airborne lead. *Ind. Med. Surg.* **41**(7), 13–18.

Goldwater, L. J. (1973). Acryl and alkoxyalkylmercurinic. *In* "Mercury, Mercurisis and Mercuphaus" (M. W. Miller and T. W. Clarkson, eds.), pp. 56–67. Thomas, Springfield, IL.

Goldwater, L. J., and Hoover, A. W. (1967). An international study of "normal" levels of lead in blood and urine. *Arch. Environ. Health* **15**, 60–63.

Goldwater, L. J., Ladd, A. C., Berkhorst, P. G., and Jacobs, M. B. (1964). Acute exposure to phenylmercuric acetate. *J. Occup. Med.* **6**, 227–228.

Gonzales, T. A., Vance, M., Helpern, M., and Umberger, C. (1954). "Legal Medicine Pathology and Toxicology," 2nd ed. Appletorr–Century–Crofta, New York.

Gortner, R. A., Jr. (1940). Chronic ???? poisoning of rats as influenced by dietary protein. *J. Nutr.* **19**, 105.

Gotelli, C. A., Astroid, E., Con, C., Carniari, E., and Clarkson, T. W. (1985). Early biochemical effects of an organic mercury fungicide on infants: "Dose makes the poison." *Science* **227**, 638–640.

Goulon, M. (1963). Intoxication by thallium. *Rev. Prat.* **13**, 1321–1324.

Goyer, R. A., ed. (1974). Perspective on low level lead toxicity. *Environ. Health Perspect.* **7**, 1–252.

Goyer, R.A. (1991). Toxic effects of metals. *In* "Toxicology—The Basic Science of Poisons" (M. O. Amdur, J. Doull, and C. D. Klaassen, eds.), 4th ed., p. 670. McGraw–Hill, New York.

Grant, R. L., Calvery, H. O., Laug, E. P., and Morris, H. J. (1938). The influence of calcium and phosphorus on the storage and toxicity of lead and arsenic. *J. Pharmacol. Exp. Ther.* **64**, 446–457.

Great Britain Ministry of Agriculture, Fisheries, and Food. (1981). "Survey of Copper and Zinc in Food." Food Serveilance Paper No. 5, H. M. Stationary Office, London.

Greenberger, N. J., Robinson, W. L., and Izzelbacher, K. I. (1964). Toxic ?????? after ingestion of phosphorus with subsequent recovery. *Gastroenterology* **47**, 179–183.

Greengard, H., and Woolley, J. R. (1940a). Studies on colloidal sulfur–polysulphide mixture. I. Toxicity. *J. Am. Pharm. Assoc., Sci. Ed.* **29**, 289–292.

Greengard, H., and Woolley, J. R. (1940b). Studies on colloidal sulfur–polysulphide mixture. Absorption and oxidation after oral administration. *J. Biol. Chem.* **132**, 83–89.

Gross, W. G., and Heller, V. G. (1946). Chromates in animal nutrition. *J. Ind. Hyg.* **78**, 52–56.

Grulee, C. G., Jr., and Clark, E. H. (1951). Thallotoxiconics in a preschool mercury. *Am. J. Dis. Child.* **81**, 47–51.

Guthrie, F. E., Wolf, W. R., and Willson, C. (1978). Background correction and method problems in the determination of chromium in urine by graphite forces atomic absorption spectrophotometry. *Anal. Chem.* **50**, 1900–1902.

Guthrie, F. E., McCants, C. B., and Small, H. G., Jr. (1959). Arsenic content of commercial tobacco, 1917–1958. *Tob. Sci.* **3**, 62–64.

Hadjimarkos, D. M., Bonborat, C. W., and Matrice, J. J. (1959). The selesium concentration in placental tissue and foetal cord blood. *J. Pediatr.* **54**, 296–298.

Halbach, S., and Clarkson, T. W. (1978). Enzymic oxidation of mercury vapor by erythrocytes. *Biochim. Biophys. Acta* **523**, 522–531.

Halsted, J. A., Smith, J. C., and Irwin, M. I. (1974). A conspectus of research on zinc requirements of man. *J. Nutr.* **104**, 345–378.

Hann, R. G., and Veale, R. A. (1910). A fatal case of poisoning by phosphorus with unusual subcutaneous haemorrhages. *Lancet* **1**, 163–164.

Harbison, R. D., Jones, M. M., MacDonald, J. S., Pratt, T. H., and Coates, R. L. (1977). Synthesis and pharmacological study of a polymer which selectively binds mercury. *Toxicol. Appl. Pharmacol.* **42**, 445–454.

Harrisson, J. W. E., Packman, E. W., and Abbott, D. D. (1958). Acute oral toxicity and chemical and physical properties of arsenic trioxides. *Arch. Ind. Health* **17**, 118–123.

Haskins, W. T., and Luttermoser, G. W. (1950). The comparative toxicities of the antimonyl derivatives of the four isomeric potassium acid tartrates. *Am. J. Trop. Med.* **30**, 591–592.

Hausman, R., and Wilson, W. J., Jr. (1964). Thallotoxicosis: A social menace. *J. Forensic Sci.* **9**, 71–88.

Hawkes, W. C., Whillhite, C. C., Omaye, S. T., *et al.* (1994). Selenium kinetics, placenta transfer, and neonatal exposure in cynomolgus macaques (*Macaca fascicularis*). *Teratology* **50**, 148–159.

Hayes, W. J., Jr. (1975). "Toxicology of Pesticides." Williams & Wilkins, Baltimore.

Hayes, W. J., Jr., and Vaughn, W. K. (1977). Mortality from pesticides in the United States in 1973 and 1974. *Toxicol. Appl. Pharmacol.* **42**, 235–252.

Hazardous Substances Data Bank (HSDB) (1993). National Library of Medicine, National Toxicology Information Program, Bethesda, MD.

Heath, D. F. (1966). The retention of triphenyltin and dieldrin and its relevance to the toxic effects of multiple dosing. *In* "Radioisotopes in the Detection of Pesticide Residues." Int. At. Energy Agency, Vienna.

Hegsted, D. M., McKirbbin, J. M., and Drinker, C. K. (1945). The biological, hygienic, and medical properties of zinc and zinc compounds. *Public Health Rep., Suppl.* **179**.

Heimann, H. (1946). Chronic phosphorus poisoning. *J. Ind. Hyg. Toxicol.* **28**, 142–150.

Hempe, J. M., and Cousins, R. J. (1991). Cysteine-rich intestinal protein binds zinc during transmucosal zinc transport. *Proc. Natl. Acad. Sci.* **88**(121), 9671–9674.

Henderson, R. F., Rebar, A. H., Pickrell, J. A., *et al.* (1979). Early damage indicators in the lung. III. Biochemical and cytological response of the lung to inhaled metal salts. *Toxicol. Appl. Pharmacol.* **50**, 123–136.

Herman, M. M., and Bensch, K. G. (1967). Light and electron microscopic studies of acute and chronic thallium intoxication in rats. *Toxicol. Appl. Pharmacol.* **10**, 199–222.

Herner, T. (1945). Intoxication with organic compounds of mercury. *Nord. Med., NM* **26**, 833–836.

Herok, J., and Götte, H. (1964). Part III. Radioactive metabolic balance studies with tin triphenylacetate in the lactating sheep. *Zentralbl. Veterinaermed., Reihe A* **11**, 20–28 (in German).

Heydlauf, H. (1969). Ferric-cyanoferrate (II): An effective antidote in thallium poisoning. *Eur. J. Pharmacol.* **6**, 340–344.

Heyman, A., Pfeiffer, J. B., Willett, R. W., and Taylor, H. M. (1956). Peripheral neuropathy caused by arsenical intoxication. *N. Engl. J. Med.* **254**, 401–409.

Heyroth, F. F. (1947). Thallium—a review and summary of medical literature. *Public Health Rep., Suppl.* **197**, 1–23.

Heyroth, F. F. (1952). Toxicological evidence for the safety of the fluoridation of public water supplies. Am. *J. Public Health* **42**, 1568–1575.

Heyroth, F. F. (1963). Halogens. *In* "Industrial Hygiene and Toxicology" (F. A. Patty, ed.), 2nd rev. ed., pp. 831–856. Wiley (Interscience), New York.

Heywood, R., and Sortwell, R. J. (1979). Arsenic intoxication in the rhesus monkey. *Toxicol. Lett.* **3**, 137–144.

Hislop, J. S., Collier, T. R., White, G. F., Khathing, D. T., and French, E. (1963). The use of keratinised tissues to monitor the detailed exposure of man to methylmercury from fish. *In* "Chemical Toxicology and Clinical Chemistry of Metals" (S. S. Brown and J. Savory, eds.), pp. 145–148. Academic Press, New York.

Hodge, H. C. (1950). The concentration of fluorides in drinking water to give the point of minimum caries with maximum safety. *J. Am. Dent. Assoc.* **40**, 436–439.

Hodge, H. C. (1961). Metabolism of fluorides. *JAMA, J. Am. Med. Assoc.* **177**, 313–316.

Hodge, H. C., and Smith, F. A. (1965). Biological properties of inorganic fluorides. *In* "Fluorine Chemistry" (J. H. Simmons, ed.), Vol. 4, pp. 2–16. Academic Press, New York.

Hoffman, J., and McConnell, K. (1974). The presence of 4-selenouridine in *Escherichia coli* tRNA. *Biochim. Biophys. Acta* **366**, 109–113.

Hopenhayn-Rich, C., Biggs, M. L., Fuchs, A., *et al.* (1996). Bladder cancer mortality associated with arsenic in drinking water in Argentina [see comments]. *Epidemiology* **7**(2), 117–124. [published erratum appears in *Epidemiology* (1997) **8**(3), 334.]

Horacek, V., and Demcik, K. (1970). Group poisoning in the spraying of field crops with Brestan-60 (triphenyltin acetate). *Prac. Lek.* **22**, 61–66 (in Czech).

Horiuchi, K., Horiguchi, S., and Suekane, M. (1959). Studies on the industrial lead poisoning. I. Absorption, transportation, deposition and excretion of lead. 6. The lead contents in organ tissues of the normal Japanese. *Osaka City Med. J.* **5**, 41–70.

Horwitt, M. K., and Cowgil, G. R. (1937). The effects of ingested lead on the organism. I. Studies on the rat. *J. Pharmacol. Exp. Ther.* **61**, 300–310.

Hsueh, Y. M., Cheng, G. S., Wu, M. M., *et al.* (1995). Multiple risk factors associated with arsenic-induced skin cancer: Effects of chronic liver disease and malnutritional status. *Br. J. Cancer* **71**(1), 109–114.

Hughes, J. P. W., Baron, R., Buckland, D. H., Cooke, M. A., Craig, J. D., Duffield, D. P., Grosart, A. W., Parkes, P. W. J., and Porter, A. (1962). Phosphorus necrosis of the jaw: A present-day study. *Br. J. Ind. Med.* **19**, 83–99.

Hunter, D., and Russell, D. S. (1954). Focal cerebral and cerebellar atrophy in a human subject due to organic mercury compounds. *J. Neurol., Neurosurg. Psychiatry* **17**, 235–241.

Hunter, D., Bomford, R. R., and Russels, D. S. (1940). Poisoning by methyl mercury compounds. *Q. J. Med.* **33**, 192–213.

Hursh, J. B. (1985). Partition coefficients of mercury (^{203}Hg) vapor between air and biological fluids. *J. Appl. Toxicol.* **5**, 327–332.

Hursh, J. B., Clarkson, T. W., Cherian, M. G., Vostad, J. J., and Vander Mallie, R. (1976). Clearance of mercury (mercury-197, mercury-203) vapor inhaled by human subjects. *Arch. Environ. Health* **31**, 302–309.

Hursh, J. B., Clarkson, T. W., Nowak, T. V., Pabico, R. C., McKenna, B. A., Miles, E. F., and Gibb, R. F. (1985). Prediction of kidney mercury content by isotope techniques. *Kidney Int.* **27**, 898–907.

Hutchinson, J. (1887). Arsenic cancer. *Br. Med. J.* **2**, 1280–1281.

Innes, J. R. M., Ulland, B. M., Valerio, M. G., Petrucelli, L., Fishbein, L., Hart, E. R., Pallotta, A. J., Bates, R. R., Falk, H. L., Gart, J. J., Klein, M., Mitchell, I., and Peters, J. (1969). Bioassay of pesticides and industrial chemicals for tumorigenicity in mice: A preliminary note. *J. Natl. Cancer Inst. (U.S.)* **42**, 1101–1114.

International Agency for Research on Cancer (IARC) (1980). IARC monographs on the evaluation of the carcinogenic risk of chemicals to humans: Some metals and metallic compounds. *IARC Sci. Publ.* **23**, 205–323.

Ip, C., and Hayes, C. (1989). Tissue selenium levels in selenium-supplemented rats and their relevance in mammary cancer protection. *Carcinogenesis* **10**(5), 921–925.

Ishida, F. (1970). Studies on organic mercury poisoning. *Kumamoto Med. J.* **44**, 638–652 (in Japanese).

Ishikawa, I., Ueno, Y., and Tsunoda, H. (1970). Chemical determinations of the chlorine-containing peptide, a hepatotoxic mycotoxin of *Penicillium islandicum* Sopp. *J. Biochem. (Tokyo)* **67**, 753.

Ishinishi, N., Tsuchiya, K., Vahter, M., and Fowler, B. A. (1986). Arsenic. *In* "Handbook on the Toxicology of Metals" (L. Friberg, G. F. Nordberg, and V. B. Vouk, eds.), 2nd ed., Vol. 2, pp. 43–83. Am. Elsevier, New York.

Jandial, V., Handerson, P., and MacGillivray, I. (1976). Placental transfer of radioactive selenomethionine in late pregnancy. *Eur. J. Obstet. Gynocol. Reprod. Biol.* **6**, 295–300.

Jennette, K. W. (1981). The role of metals in carcinogenesis: Biochemistry and metabolism. *Environ. Health Perspect.* **40**, 233–252.

Joschimoglu, G. (1916). On the question of tolerance to arsenic. *Arch. Exp. Pathol. Pharmakol.* **79**, 419–442 (in German).

Johansson, A. T., Curstedt, T., Robertson, B., and Camner, P. (1984). Lung morphology and phospholipids after experimental inhalation of soluble cadmium, copper and cobalt. *Environ. Res.* **34**, 295–309.

Jones, M. J., Schoenheit, J. E., and Weaver, A. D. (1979). Pretreatment and heavy metal LD50 values. *Toxicol. Appl. Pharmacol.* **49**, 41–44.

Jones, M. M., Basinger, M. A., and Tarka, M. P. (1980). The relative effectiveness of some chelating agents in acute copper intoxication in the mouse. *Res. Commun. Chem. Pathol. Pharmacol.* **27**, 571–577.

Kanisawa, M., and Schroeder, H. A. (1969). Life terms studies on the effects of trace elements on spontaneous tumors in mice and rats. *Cancer Res.* **29**, 892–895.

Karkos, J. (1971). Neuropathological findings in thallium encephalopathy. *Neurol. Neurochir. Pol.* **21**, 911–915 (in Polish).

Katoh, Y., Torikai, S., Ohkubo, Y., and Kigawada, R. (1977). A case of acute renal insufficiency due to copper sulfate. *J. Kanagawa Med. Assoc.* **4**, 39 (in Japanese).

Kayne, K. J., Komar, G., Laboda, H., and Vanderlinde, R. E. (1978). Atomic absorption spectrophotometry of chromium in serum and urine with a modified Perkin-Elmer 603 atomic absorption spectrophotometer. *Clin. Chem. (Winston-Salem, N.C.)* **24**, 2151–2154.

Kazantzis, G., Schiller, K. F. R., Asscher, A. W., and Drew, R. G. (1962). Albuminuria and the nephrolic syndrome following exposure to mercury and its compounds. *Q. J. Exp. Med.* **31**, 403–418.

Kehoe, R. A., Cholak, J., and Storey, R. V. (1940). A spectrochemical study of the normal ranges of concentration of certain trace metals in biological materials. *J. Nutr.* **19**, 579–592.

Kehoe, R. A. (1964). Normal metabolism of lead. *Arch. Environ. Health* **8**, 232–235.

Kennedy, D. (1961). Notes on the casualties with poisons in New Zealand. *In* "WHO Inf. Circ. Toxic. Pestic. Man," No. 7, p. 5. WHO, Geneva.

Kennedy, P., and Cavanagh, J. B. (1976). Spinal changes in the neuropathy of thallium poisoning. *J. Neurol. Sci.* **29**, 295–301.

Kershaw, T. G., Dhahir, P. J., and Clarkson, T. W. (1980). The relationship between blood levels and dose of methylmercury in man. *Arch. Environ. Health* **35**, 8–35.

Khasanov, Y. Kh. (1971). A rare case of poisoning with pesticide-contaminated water. *Gig. Sanit.* **36**, 96 (in Russian).

Kimbrough, R. D., and Gaines, T. B. (1971). Hexachlorophene effects on the rat brain: Study of high doses by light and electron microscopy. *Arch. Environ. Health* **23**, 114–118.

Kingsbury, J. M. (1964). "Poisonous Plants of the United States and Canada." Prentice-Hall, Englewood Cliffs, NJ.

Kinoshita, Y., and Ogima, I. (1968). Symposium on clinical observations on public nuisances and agricultural pesticide poisonings. 4. Pesticide pneumonitis. *Nippon Naika Gakkai Zasshi* **57**, 1219–1221 (in Japanese).

Kirchgessner, M., Weser, U., and Muller, H. L. (1967). Dynamics of copper absorption. 7. Copper absorption with supplements of gluconic, citric, salicylic, and oxalic acids. *Z. Tierphysiol. Tierenaehr. Futtermittelkd.* **23**, 28–30 (in German).

Kirschbaum, B. B., Sprinkel, F. M., and Oken, D. E. (1981). Proximal tubule brush border alterations during the course of chromate nephropathy. *Toxicol. Appl. Pharmacol.* **58**, 19–30.

Kiyono, S., Hasui, K., Takasu, K., and Seo, M. (1974). Toxic effect of arsenic trioxide in infant rats. *J. Physiol. Soc. Jpn.* **36**, 253–254.

Kjellström, T. (1985). Critical organs, critical concentrations and whole-body dose–response relationships. *In* "Cadmium and Health: A Toxicological and Epidemiological Appraisal" (L. Friberg, C.-G. Elinder, T. Kjellström, and G. F. Nordberg, eds.), pp. 231–246. CRC Press, Boca Raton, FL.

Klaassen, C. D. (1974). Biliary excretion of arsenic in rats, rabbits, and dogs. *Toxicol. Appl. Pharmacol.* **29**, 447–457.

Klimmer, O. R. (1964). Part IV. Toxicological studies on triphenylacetate of tin (TPZA). *Zentralbl. Veterinaermed., Reihe A* **11**, 29–39.

Kline, R. D., Hayes, V. W., and Cromwell, G. L. (1971). Effects of copper, molybdenum and sulfate on performance, hematology and copper stores of pigs and lambs. *J. Anim. Sci.* **33**, 771.

Knight, R. K., Trounce, J. R., and Cameron, J. S. (1967). Suicidal chlorate poisoning treated with peritoneal dialysis. *Br. Med. J.* **3**, 601–602.

Koblenzer, P. J., and Weiner, L. B. (1969). Alopecia secondary to thallium intoxication. *Arch. Dermatol.* **99**, 777.

Kosta, L., Byrne, A. R., and Zelenko, V. (1975). Correlation between selenium and mercury in man following exposure to inorganic mercury. *Nature (London)* **254**, 238–239.

Kostyniak, P. J., Clarkson, T. W., Cestero, R. V., Freeman, R. B., and Abbasi, A. H. (1975). An extracorporeal complexing hemodialysis system for the treatment of methylmercury poisoning. I. In vitro studies of the effects of four complexing agents on the distribution and dialyzability of methylmercury in human blood. *J. Pharmacol. Exp. Ther.* **192**, 260–269.

Kourounakis, P., Szabo, S., Villeneuve, C., and Gagnon, M. (1973). Effect of pharmacologic or surgical conditioning upon intoxication with arsenicals. *J. Eur. Toxicol.* **6**, 232–236.

Kruger, J., Winkler, P., Lüderitz, E., Lück, M., and Wolf, H. U. (1985). Bismuth, bismuth alloys and bismuth compounds. *In* "Ullman's Encyclopedia of Industrial Chemistry," 5th ed., Vol. A4, pp. 171–189. VCH Verlagsgesellschaft, Deerfield Beach, FL.

Kubota, J., Lazar, V. A., and Losee, F. (1968). Copper, zinc, cadmium, and lead in human blood from 19 locations in the United Slates. *Arch. Environ. Health* **16**, 788–793.

Kuptsov, V. V., and Aslanov, M. O. (1970). A case of a favorable course of pregnancy and birth after severe poisoning with zinc phosphide. *Pediatr., Akush. Ginekol.* **32**, 61 (in Ukrainian).

Kurland, L. T., Faro, S. N., and Siedler, H. (1960). Minamata disease. *World Neurol.* **1**, 370–394.

Kutsuna, M., ed. (1966). "Minamata Disease: An Investigation of Intoxication by Organic Mercury." Kumamoto University Medical School, Kumamoto, Japan (see Berlin *et al.*, 1969c).

LaDue, J. S., Schenken, J. R., and Kuker, L. H. (1944). Phosphorus poisoning: A report of sixteen cases with repeated liver biopsies in a recovered case. *Am. J. Med. Sci.* **208**, 223–234.

Lagacé, A. (1961). White muscle disease in lambs. *J. Am. Vet. Med. Assoc.* **138**, 188.

Lantz, E. M., and Smith, M. C. (1934). The effect of fluorine on calcium and phosphorus metabolism in albino rats. *Am. J. Physiol.* **109**, 645–654.

Largent, E. J. (1961). "Fluorosis, the Health Aspects of Fluorine Compounds." Ohio State Univ. Press, Columbus, OH.

Largent, E. J., Bovard, P. G., and Heyroth, F. F. (1951). Roentgenographic changes and urinary fluoride excretion among workmen engaged in the manufacture of inorganic fluorides. *Am. J. Roentgenol. Radium Ther.* **65**, 42–48.

Lasch, F. (1961). Successful treatment of an acute severe arsenic poisoning. *Med. Klin. (Munich)* **56**, 62–63 (in German).

Latarjet, R., Galy, P., Maret, G., and Gallois, P. (1964). Bronchopulmonary cancers and arsenic poisoning in winegrowers of Beaujolais. *Mem. Acad. Chir.* **90**, 384–390 (in French).

Laug, E. P., and Morris, H. P. (1938). The effect of lead on rats fed diets containing lead arsenate and lead acetate. *J. Pharmacol. Exp. Ther.* **64**, 388–410.

LeBreton, R. (1962). "Toxicological Study of Tin and Its Derivatives." Tours Imp. Mame., France (in French).

Legge, T. M., and Goadby, K. W. (1912). "Lead Poisoning and Lead Absorption." Longmans, Green, New York.

Lehman, A. J. (1951). Chemicals in foods: A report to the Association of Food and Drug Officials on current developments. II. Pesticides. Section I. Introduction. *Q. Bull.—Assoc. Food Drug Off.* **15**(I), 122–133.

Lehman, A. J. (1952). Chemicals in foods: A report to the Association of Food and Drug Officials on current developments. II. Pesticides. Section II. Dermal toxicity. Section III. Subacute and chronic toxicity. Section IV. Biochemistry. Section V. Pathology. *Q. Bull.—Assoc. Food Drug Off.* **16** (II), 3–9; (III), 47–53; (IV), 85–91; (V), 126–132.

Lemley, R. E. (1940). Selenium poisoning in the human. *Lancet* **60**, 528–536.

Lemley, R. E., and Merryman, M. P. (1941). Selenium poisoning in the human subject. *Lancet* **61**, 435–438.

Leng-Levy, J., Aubertin, J., Leng, B., Magendie, P., Marion, J., and Mauriac, M. (1969). Myocardiac attacks in the course of occupational arsenic poisoning. *Arch. Mat. Prof. Med. Trav. Secur. Soc.* **30**, 434–436 (in French).

L'Epee, P., Texier, L., Lazarini, H. J., Ducombs, G., Doignon, J., Larcebau, S., and Miegeville, M. J. (1973). Late-developing cutaneous arsenicalism. Arsenical cancers. *Arch. Mat. Prof. Med. Trav. Secur. Soc.* **34**, 457–461 (in French).

Lewi, Z., and Bar-Khayim, Y. (1964). Food poisoning from barium carbonate. *Lancet* **2**, 342–343.

Lewis, H. B., Schulz, J., and Gortner, R. A., Jr. (1940). Dietary protein and the toxicity of sodium selenite in the white rat. *J. Pharmacol. Exp. Ther.* **68**, 292–299.

Li, Y. M., Dunipace, A. J., and Stookey, G. K. (1987). Effects of fluoride on the mouse sperm morphology test. *J. Dent. Res.* **66**, 1509–1511.

Lie, R., Thomas, R., and Scott, J. (1960). The distribution and excretion of thallium-204 in the rat, with suggested MPC's and a bio-assay procedure. *Health Phys.* **2**, 334–340.

Liebegott, G. (1952). On the relations between chronic arsenic poisoning and malignant neoplasms. *Zentralbl. Arbeitsmed. Arbeitsschutz* **2**, 15 (in German).

Liebscher, K., and Smith, H. (1968). Essential and nonessential trace elements. A method of determining whether an element is essential or nonessential in human tissue. *Arch. Environ. Health* **17**, 881–890.

Likins, R. C., McClure, F. J., and Steere, A. C. (1956). Urinary excretion of fluoride following defluoridation of a water supply. *Public Health Rep.* **71**, 217–220.

Likosky, W. H., Hinman, A. R., and Barthel, W. F. (1970). Organic mercury poisoning, New Mexico. *Neurology* **20**, 401.

Lim, J. K., Renaldo, G. J., and Chapman, P. (1978). LD50 of stannous fluoride, sodium fluoride and sodium mono-fluoro phosphate in the mouse compared to the rat. *Caries Res.* **12**, 17–179.

Lindström, O. (1961). Liquid seed treatment studies. *Trans. R. Inst. Technol., Stockholm* **185**.

Ljubetskii, K. Z., Krazil'shchikov, D. G., and Reshetova, T. E. (1961). On the problem of food poisoning with Granosan. *Gig. Sanit.* **26**, 68–71.

Lockitch, G. (1989). Selenium: Clinical significance and analytical concepts. *Crit. Rev. Clin. Lab. Sci.* **27**(6), 483–541.

Locksley, H. B., and Sweet, W. H. (1954). Tissue distribution of boron compounds in relation to neutron-capture therapy of cancer. *Proc. Soc. Exp. Biol. Med.* **86**, 56–63.

Loeb, A. (1912). On the vascular action of arsenic. *Verh. Ges. Disch. Naturforsch. Aerzie* **2**, 489–491 (in German).

Loebenstein, J. R. (1994) "The Materials Flow of Arsenic in the United States <note> Information Circular/1994 (Final)." BUMINESIC-9382, Bureau of Mines, Division of Mineral Commodities, United States Department of the Interior, Washington, DC.

Lund, A. (1956). The effect of various substances on the excretion and the toxicity of thallium in the rat. *Acta Pharmacol. Toxicol.* **12**, 260–268.

Lundborg, M., and Camner, P. (1984). Lysozyme levels in rabbit lung after inhalation of nickel, cadmium, cobalt and copper chlorides. *Environ. Res.* **34**, 335–342.

Lundgren, K.-D., and Swensson, A. (1949). Occupational poisoning by alkyl mercury compounds. *J. Ind. Hyg. Toxicol.* **31**, 190–200.

Lundgren, K.-D., and Swensson, A. (1960). A survey of results of investigations on some organic mercury compounds used as fungicides. *Am. Ind. Hyg. Assoc. J.* **21**, 308–311.

Lydtin, H., Korfmacher, I., Frank, U., and Zollner, N. (1965). Barium poisoning. *Muench. Med. Wochenschr.* **107**, 1045–1048 (in German).

Mabuchi, K. A., Lilienfeld, A. M., and Snell, L. (1979). Lung cancer among pesticide workers exposed to inorganic arsenicals. *Arch. Environ. Health* **34**, 312–319.

MacKenzie, R. D., Brerrum, R. U., Decker, G. F, Hoppert, C. A., and Laugham, R. F. (1958). Chronic toxicity studies. II. Hexavalent and trivalent chromium administered in drinking water to rats. *AMA Arch. Ind. Health* **18**, 232–234.

MacKenzie, R. D., Anwar, R. A., Byerrum, R. U., and Hoppert, C. A. (1959). Absorption and distribution of ^{51}Cr in the albino rat. *Arch. Biochem. Biophys.* **79**, 200–205.

Magee, P. N., Stoner, H. B., and Bames, J. M. (1957). The experimental production of oedema in the central nervous system of the rat by triethyltin compounds. *J. Pathol. Bacteriol.* **73**, 107–124.

Maghazaji, H. I. (1974). Psychiatric aspects of methylmercury poisoning. *J. Neurol., Neurosurg. Psychiatry* **37**, 954–958.

Magos, L., Bakir, F., Clarkson, T. W., Al-Jawad, A. M., and Al-Soffi, M. H. (1976). Tissue levels of mercury in autopsy specimens of liver and kidney. *Bull. W.H.O.* **53**(Suppl.), 93–97.

Magos, L., Clarkson, T. W., and Hudson, A. R. (1984). Differences in the effects of selenite and biological selenium on the chemical form and distribution of mercury after the simultaneous administration of $HgCl_2$ and selenium to rats. *J. Pharmacol. Exp. Ther.* **228**, 478–483.

Magos, L., Halbach, S., and Clarkson, T. W. (1978). Role of catalase in the oxidation of mercury vapor. *Biochem. Pharmacol.* **27**, 1373–1377.

Majaj, A. S., and Hopkins, L. L., Jr. (1966). Selenium and kwashiorkor. *Lancet* **2**, 592–593.

Maki, S. (1972). Agricultural chemicals and their toxicity. *Ringyo to Yakuzai* **39**, 15–20 (in Japanese).

Mallory, F. B. (1933). Phosphorus and alcoholic cirrhosis. *Am. J. Pathol.* **9**, 557–567.

Maloof, C. C. (1955). Use of edathamil calcium in treatment of chrome ulcers of the skin. *AMA Arch. Ind. Health* **11**, 123–125.

Mal'tsev, P. V. (1972). Granosan poisoning in children. *Fel'dsher Akush.* **37**, 14–16 (in Russian).

Mannaioni, P. F. (1960). Clinical–toxicological considerations in some cases of acute poisoning by zinc phosphide. *Minerva Med.* **51**, 3721–3724.

Manzo, L., Scelsi, R., Moglia, A., *et al.* (1983). Long-term toxicity of thallium in the rat. *In* "Chemical Toxicology and Clinical Chemistry of Metals," pp. 401–405. Academic Press, London.

Mappes, R. (1977). Experiments on the excretion of arsenic in urine. *Int. Arch. Occup. Environ. Health* **40**, 267–272.

Marafante, E., and Vahter, M. (1987). Solubility, retention and metabolism of intratracheally and orally administered inorganic arsenic compounds in the hamster. *Environ. Res.* **42**, 72–82.

Marafante, E., Lundborg, M., Vahter, M., *et al.* (1987). Dissolution of two arsenic compounds by rabbit alveolar macrophages *in vitro. Fundam. Appl. Toxicol.* **8**, 382–388.

Marsh, D. O., Myers, G. J., Clarkson, T. W., Amin-Zaki, L., Tikriti, S., and Majeed, M. A. (1980). Fetal mefhylmercury poisoning: Clinical and toxicological data in 29 cases. *Ann. Neurol.* **7**, 348–355.

Marsh, D. O., Myers, G. J., Clarkson, T. W., Amin-Zaki, L., Tikriti, S., and Majeed, M. A. (1981). Dose–response relationship for human fetal exposure to methylmercury. *Clin. Toxicol.* **18**, 1311–1318.

Marten, J. (1969). Acute thallium poisoning in an eleven-year-old boy. *Cesk. Pediatr.* **24**, 233–237.

Massie, H. R., and Aiella, V. R. (1984). Excessive intake of copper: Influence on longevity and cadmium accumulation in mice. *Mech. Ageing Dev.* **26**, 195–203.

Massmann, W. (1957). Observations on the circulation with phenylmercury pyrocatechol. *Zentralbl. Arbeitsmed. Arbeitsschutz* **7**, 9–13 (in German).

Mathews, J., and Anzarut, A. (1968). Thallium poisoning. *Can. Med. Assoc. J.* **99**, 72–75.

Mathur, A. K., Chandra, S. V., and Tandon, S. K. (1977). Comparative toxicity of trivalent and hexavalent chromium in rabbits. III. Morphological changes in some organs. *Toxicology* **8**, 53–61.

McCann, H. G. (1953). Reactions of fluoride ion with hydroxapatite. *J. Biol. Chem.* **201**, 247–259.

McClure, F. J., and Mitchell, H. H. (1931). The effect of fluorine on the calcium metabolism of albino rats and the composition of the bones. *J. Biol. Chem.* **90**, 297–320.

McConnell, K. P. (1942). Respiratory excretion of selenium studied with the radioactive isotope. *J. Biol. Chem.* **145**, 55–60.

McCoy, K. E. M., and Weswig, P. H. (1969). Some selenium responses in the rat not related to vitamin E. *J. Nutr.* **98**, 383–389.

McCutchen, J. J., and Utterback, R. A. (1966). Chronic arsenic poisoning resembling muscular dystrophy. *South. Med. J.* **59**, 1139–1145.

McGregor, I. A., and Jackson, I. T. (1969). Sodium chlorate bomb injuries of the hand. *Br. J. Plast. Surg.* **22**, 16–29.

McIntyre, A. R., and Burke, J. C. (1937). Intravenous boric acid poisoning in man. *J. Pharmacol. Exp. Ther.* **60**, 112–113.

McKenzie, A. (1932). Fatalities following administration of intravenous tartar emetic. *Trans. R. Soc. Trop. Med. Hyg.* **25**, 407–410.

McNally, W. D., and Rukstinat, G. (1947). Two deaths due to boric acid. *Med. Rec.* **160**, 284–288.

McNally, W. D., and Rust, C. A. (1928). The distribution of boric acid in human organs in six deaths due to boric acid poisoning. *JAMA, J. Am. Med. Assoc.* **90**, 382–383.

Mees, R. A. (1919). Nails with arsenical polyneuritis. *JAMA, J. Am. Med. Assoc.* **72**, 1337.

Meikle, R. W., Stewart, D., and Globus, O. A. (1963). Drywood termite metabolism of Vikane fumigant as shown by labeled pool technique. *J. Agric. Food Chem.* **11**, 226–230.

Mengele, K., Schwarzmeier, J., Schmidt, P., and Moser, K. (1969). Clinical aspects and studies of eiythrocyte metabolism in poisoning by sodium chlorate. *Int. Z. Klin. Pharmakol., Ther. Toxikol.* **2**, 120–125 (in German).

Mertz, W. (1967). Biological role of chromium. *Fed. Proc., Fed. Am. Soc. Exp. Biol.* **26**, 186–193.

Messer, H. H., Armstrong, W. D., and Singer, L. (1973). Influence of fluoride intake on reproduction in mice. *J. Nutr.* **103**, 1319–1326.

Miettinen, J. K. (1973). Absorption and elimination of dietary (Hg^{2+}) and methyl mercury in man. *In* "Mercury, Mercurials and Mercaptans" (M. W. Miller and T. W. Clarkson, eds.), pp. 233–246. Thomas, Springfield, IL.

Miller, R. F., and Phillips, P. H. (1953). The metabolism of fluorine in the bones of the fluorine-poisoned rat. *J. Nutr.* **51**, 273–281.

Minkowitz, S. (1964). Multiple carcinomata following ingestion of medicinal arsenic. *Ann. Intern. Med.* **61**, 296–299.

Mizyukova, I. G., and Petrun'kin, V. Y. (1974). Unithiol and mercaptide as antidotes in poisonings with arsenic-containing substances. *Vrach. Delo* **2**, 126–129 (in German).

Moeschlin, S. (1965). "Poisoning Diagnosis and Treatment," 1st Am. ed. Grune & Stratton, New York.

Møller, F., and Gudjonsson, S. V. (1932). Cases of massive fluorosis of the bones and tendons (fluorosis in workmen handling cryolite). *Acta Radiol.* **13**, 269–294.

Monier-Williams, G . W. (1949). "Trace Elements in Food." Chapman & Hall, London.

Moore, L. E., Smith, A. H., Hopenhayn-Rich, C., *et al.* (1997). Micronuclei in exfoliated bladder cells among individuals chronically exposed to arsenic in drinking water. *Cancer Epidemiol. Biomarkers Prev.* **6**(1), 31–36.

Morris, H. P., Laug, E. P., Morris, H. J., and Grant, R. L. (1938). The growth and reproduction of rats fed diets containing lead acetate and arsenic trioxide and the lead and arsenic content of newborn and suckling rats. *J. Pharmacol. Exp. Ther.* **64**, 420–445.

Morton, W. (1945). Poisoning by barium carbonate. *Lancet* **2**, 738–739.

Motin, J., Maret, G., Traeger, J., Fries, D., and Guibaud, P. (1970). Attempted suicide with sodium chlorate. *Bull. Med. Leg. Toxicol. Med.* **13**, 177–179 (in French).

Mottet, N. K., and Brody, R. L. (1974). Mercury burden in human autopsy organs and tissues. *Arch. Environ. Health* **29**, 18–24.

Moxon, A. L. (1958). Selenium. *In* "Trace Elements" (C. A. Lamb, O. G. Bentley, and J. M. Beattie, eds.). Academic Press, New York.

Moynahan, E. J. (1974). Acrodermatitis enteropathica: A lethal inherited human zinc-deficiency disorder. *Lancet* **2**, 399–400.

Munch, J. C. (1934). Human thallotoxicosis. *JAMA, J. Am. Med. Assoc.* **102**, 1929–1934.

Munch, J. C., and Silver, J. (1931). "The Pharmacology of Thallium and Its Use in Rodent Control." Tech. Bull. No. 238, pp. 1–28. U.S. Dept. Agric., Washington, DC.

Munch, J. C., Ginsburg, H. M., and Nixon, C. E. (1933). The 1932 thallotoxicosis outbreak in California. *JAMA, J. Am. Med. Assoc.* **100**, 1315–1319.

Muth, O. H., Oldfield, J. E., Remmert, L. F., and Schubert, J. R. (1958). Effects of selenium and vitamin E on white muscle disease. *Science* **128**, 1090.

Nagi, N. A., and Yassin, A. K. (1974). Organic mercury poisoning in children. *J. Trop. Med. Hyg.* **77**, 128–132.

Nagy, G., Varga, G., Thurzo, A., and Szilagyi, M. (1975a). Endemic chronic arsenic poisoning caused by water. *Borgyogy. Venerol. Sz.* **51**, 19–26 (in Hungarian).

Nagy, G., Varga, G., and Thurzo, T. (1975b). Clinical and hygienic aspects of chronic endemic poisonings due to contaminated drinking-water. *Orv. Hetil.* **116**, 497–500 (in Hungarian).

National Cancer Institute (NCI) (1978). "Bioassay of triphenyltin hydroxide for possible carcinogenicity." NCI-CG-TR 139, NTIS No. PB 287399, Division of Cancer Cause and Prevention, National Cancer Institute, Bethesda, MD.

National Research Council (NRC) (1979). "Zinc." University Park Press, Baltimore.

National Research Council (NRC) (1989). "Recommended Dietary Allowance," 10th ed., pp. 235–239. Subcommittee on the Tenth Edition of the RDAs Food and Nutrition Board, Commission on Life Sciences, National Academy of Science. Nat. Acad. Press, Washington, DC.

National Toxicology Program (NTP) (1990). "NTP Technical Report on the Toxicology and Carcinogenesis Studies of Sodium Fluoride in F344/N Rats and B6C3F$_1$ Mice (Drinking Water Studies)." NTTP TR 393, NIH Publication No. 90-2848, National Toxicology Program, Department of Health, Education, and Welfare, Washington, DC.

National Toxicology Program (NTP) (1993). "Toxicology and Carcinogenesis Studies of Mercuric Chloride (CAS No. 7487-94-7) in F344/N Rats and B6C3F$_1$ Mice (Gavage Studies)." NTP TR 408, NIH Publication No. 91-3139, National Institutes of Health, Research Triangle Park, NC.

National Toxicology Program (NTP) (1994).

National Toxicology Program (NTP) (1996a). "Final Report on the Reproductive Toxicity of Potassium Dichromate (Hexavalent) (CAS No. 7778-50-9) Administered in Diet to SD Rats." NTIS No. PB97-125355, National Institute of Environmental Health Sciences.

National Toxicology Program (NTP) (1996b). "Final Report on the Reproductive Toxicity of Potassium Dichromate (Hexavalent) (CAS No. 7778-50-9) Administered in Diet to BALB/c Mice." NTIS No. PB97-125363, National Institute of Environmental Health Sciences.

Neal, P. A., Jones, R. R., Bloomfield, J. J., Dalla Valle, J. M., and Edwards, T. I. (1937). A study of chronic mercurialism in the hatters' fur-cutting industry. *Public Health Bull.* **234**, 1–70.

Neal, P. A., Flinn, R. H., Edwards, T. I., Reinhart, W. H., Hough, J. W., Dalla Valle, J. M., Goldman, F. H., Armstrong, D. W., Gray, A. S., Coleman, A. L., and Postman, B. F. (1941a). Mercurialism and its control in the felt hat industry. *Public Health Bull.* **263**, 1–34.

Neal, P. A., Dreessen, W. C., Edwards, T. I., Reinhart, W. H., Webster, S. H., Castberg, H. T., and Firhall, L. T. (1941b). A study of the effect of lead arsenate exposure on orchardists and consumers of sprayed fruit. *Public Health Bull.* **267**, 1–181.

Nelson, W. C., Lykins, M. H., Mackey, J., Newill, V. A., Finklea, J. F., and Hammer, D. I. (1973). Mortality among orchard workers exposed to lead arsenate spray: A cohort study. *J. Chronic Dis.* **26**, 105–118.

Neubauer, O. (1947). Arsenical cancer. A review. *Br. J. Cancer* **1**, 192–251.

Neuman, W. F., Neuman, M. W., Main, E. R., O'Leary, J., and Smith, F. A. (1950). The surface chemistry of bone. II. Fluoride deposition. *J. Biol. Chem.* **187**, 655–661.

Nielsen, F. H., Givand, S. H., and Myron, D. R. (1975). Evidence of a possible requirement for arsenic in ihe rat. *Fed. Proc., Fed. Am. Soc. Exp. Biol.* **34**, 923.

Nielsen-Kudsk, F. N. (1965). Absorption of mercury vapor from the respiratory tract in man. *Acta Pharmacol. Toxicol.* **23**, 250–262 (in Danish).

Nielsen-Kudsk, F. N. (1969). Uptake of mercury vapor in blood *in vivo* and *in vitro* from Hg-container air. *Acta Pharmacol. Toxicol.* **27**, 149–160.

Nierenberg, D. W., Nordgren, R. E., Chang, M. B., *et al.* (1998). Delayed cerebellar disease and death after accidental exposure to dimethylmercury. *N. Engl. J. Med.* **338**(23), 1672–1676.

Nikitina, Y. I. (1974). Course of labor and puerperium in me vineyard workers and milkmaids in Crimea. *Gig. Tr. Prof. Zabol.* **18**, 17–20.

Nofre, C., Dufour, H., and Cier, A. (1963). Comparative general toxicity of mineral anions in the mouse. *C. R. Hebd, Séances Acad. Sci., Sér. D* **257**, 791–794 (in French).

Norris, E. R., and Elliott, N. W. (1945). Tolerance to arsenic trioxide in the albino rat. *Am. J. Physiol.* **143**, 635–638.

Norseth, T., and Clarkson, T. W. (1970). Studies on the biotransformation of 203-Hg-labeled methyl mercury chloride in rats. *Arch. Environ. Health* **21**, 717–727.

Nylander, M., Friberg, L., and Lind, B. (1987). Mercury concentration in the human brain and kidneys in relation to exposure from dental amalgam fillings, *Swed. Dent. J.* **11**, 179–187.

Occupational Safety and Health Administration (OSHA) (1992). 29 CFR 1910.1027 (c).

Occupational Safety and Health Administration (OSHA) (1998). Air contaminants; final rule. U.S. Department of Labor. *Federal Register* **54**, 2930.

Oestlund, K. (1969). Studies on me metabolism of methyl mercury and dimethyl mercury in mice. *Acta Pharmacol. Toxicol.* **27**(Suppl. 1), 1–132.

Ogawa, E. (1976). Experimental study on absorption, distribution and excretion of trivalent and hexavalent chromes. *Jpn. J. Pharmacol.* **26**, 92.

Okonishnikova, I. E. (1965). Experimental therapy and prophylaxis of acute poisoning with arsenic compounds. *Gig. Tr. Prof. Zabol.* **9**, 38–43.

Oldiges, H., Hochrainer, D., and Glaser, U. (1989). Long-term inhalation study with Wistar rats and four cadmium compounds. *Toxicol. Environ. Chem.* **19**, 217–222.

Oliver, J. S., Smith, H., and Watson, A. A. (1972). Sodium chlorate poisoning. *J. Forensic Sci. Soc.* **12**, 445–448.

Opacka, J., and Sparrow, S. (1985). Nephrotoxic effect of trimethyltin in rats. *Toxicol. Lett.* **27**, 97–102.

Orfila, M. J. B. (1814–1815). "Traité des Poisons Tirés des Règnes Minéral, Végétal et Animal ou Toxicologie Genérale Considérée sous les Rapports de la Pathologie et de la Médecine Légale." Crochard, Paris.

Osol, A., Pratt, R., and Altschule, M. D. (1967). "The United States Dispensatory and Physicians' Pharmacology," 26th ed. Lippincott, Philadelphia.

Ossa, A. P., Soto, H. R., Wolff, F. C., and Armas, M. R. (1975). Acute thallium poisoning. *Rev. Med. Chile* **103**, 256–259.

Ott, G. O., Holder, B. B., and Gordon, H. L. (1974). Respiratory cancer and occupational exposure to arsenicals. *Arch. Environ. Health* **29**, 250–255.

Pappenheimer, A. M., and Maechling, E. H. (1934). Inclusions in renal epithelial cells following the use of certain bismuth preparations. *Am. J. Pathol.* **10**, 577–588.

Parizek, J., Ostadalova, I., Kalouskova, J., *et al.* (1971). Effect of mercuric compounds on the maternal transmission of selenium in the pregnant and lactating rat. *J. Prod. Fertil.* **25**, 157–170.

Paszko, W. (1961). A case of zinc phosphide poisoning. *Pol. Tyg. Lek.* **16**, 1618–1619 (in Polish).

Pate, B. D., and Hays, R. L. (1968). Histological studies of testes in rats treated with certain insect chemosterilants. *J. Econ. Entomol.* **61**, 32–34.

Pauly, J. L., Caron, G. A., and Suskind, R. R. (1969). Blast transformation of lymphocytes from guinea pigs, rats and rabbits induced by mercuric chloride in *vitro. J. Cell Biol.* **41**, 847–850.

Pennypacker, E., Shrair, H. R., Lane, W. T., and Schrack, W. D., Jr. (1975). Acute copper poisoning—Pennsylvania. *Morbid. Mortal. Wkly. Rep.* **24**, 99.

Peoples, S. A., Maddy, K. T., Johnston, L., Ray, C., and Weindler, F. (1977). Poison exposures of children in California due to ingestion of liquid-formation pesticides containing sodium arsenite. *Clin. Toxicol.* **10**, 477.

Perry, K., Bowler, R. G., Buckell, H. M., Druett, H. A., and Schilling, R. S. F. (1948). Studies in the incidence of cancer in a factory handling inorganic compounds of arsenic. II. Clinical and environmental investigations. *Br. J. Ind. Med.* **5**, 6.

Petering, H. O., Johnsson, M. A., and Temmer, K. L. (1971). Studies of zinc metabolism in the rat. 1. Dose–response effects of cadmium. *Arch. Environ. Health* **23**, 93–101.

Peters, J. H. (1948). Therapy of acute fluoride poisoning. *Am. J. Med. Sci.* **216**, 278–285.

Peters, R. A. (1952). British anti-Lewisite. I. The biochemistry of arsenic. *R. Inst. Public Health Hyg. J.* **15**, 89–103.

Peterson, R. G., and Rumack, B. H. (1977). D-Penicillamine therapy of acute arsenic poisoning. *J. Pediatr.* **91**, 661–666.

Pfeiffer, C. C., Hallman, L. F., and Gersh, I. (1945). Boric acid ointment. A study of possible intoxication in the treatment of burns. *JAMA, J. Am. Med. Assoc.* **128**, 266–274.

Phelps, R. W., Clarkson, T. W., Kershaw, T. G., and Wheatley, B. (1980). Interrelationships of blood and hair mercury concentrations in a North American population exposed to methylmercury. *Arch. Environ. Health* **35**, 161–168.

Phillips, P. H. (1932). Plasma phosphatase in dairy cows suffering from fluorosis. *Science* **76**, 239–240.

Piechocka, J. (1968). Chemical and toxicological studies of the fungicide phenylmercury acetate. 2. Studies of mercury absorption by some organs in the rat and mercury excretion following poisoning with phenylmercury acetate as compared to mercury chloride. *Rocz. Panstw. Zakl. Hig.* **19**, 389–393.

Pietras, R. J., Stavrakos, C., Gunnar, R. M., and Tobin, J. R., Jr. (1968). Phosphorus poisoning simulating acute myocardial infarction. *Arch. Intern. Med.* **22**, 430–434.

Pimentel, J. C., and Marques, F. (1969). Vineyard sprayer's lung: A new occupational disease. *Thorax* **24**, 678–688.

Pimentel, J. C., and Menezes, A. P. (1975). Liver granulomas containing copper in vineyard sprayer's lung. A new etiology of hepatic granulomatosis. *Am. Rev. Respir. Dis.* **111**, 189–195.

Pimentel, J. C., and Menezes, A. P. (1976). Liver damage in vineyard fungicide applicators. *J. Med. (Lisbon)* **90**, 409–415.

Piribauer, J., and Wallenko, H. (1961). Fatal phosphorus poisoning. *Med. Klin. (Munich)* **56**, 1043–1046 (in German).

Piscator, M. (1966). "Proteinuria in Chronic Cadmium Poisoning." Beckman's, Stockholm.

Piscator, M. (1979). Copper. *In* "Handbook on the Toxicology of Metals" (L. Friberg, G. Nordberg, and V. Vouk, eds.), pp. 411–420. Elsevier/North-Holland Biomedical Press, Amsterdam.

Planques, J., Brustier, V., Bourbon, P., Pitet, G., and Broussy, G. (1960). Distribution of arsenic in the human organism in an outbreak of chronic poisoning. *Ann. Med. Leg.* **40**, 509–515.

Potes-Gutierrez, J., and Del Real, E. (1966). Acute thallium intoxication. *Ind. Med. Surg.* **35**, 618–619.

Prasad, A. S. (1966). Metabolism of zinc and its deficiency in human subjects. *In* "Zinc Metabolism" (A. S. Prasad, ed.), pp. 250–303. Thomas, Springfield, IL.

Prediger, V. (1976). Seed disinfectants as a cause of acrodynia. *Monatsschr. Kinderheilkd.* **124**, 36–37 (in German).

Prescott, L. F., and Ansari, S. (1969). The effects of repeated administration of mercuric chloride on exfoliation of renal tubular cells and urinary glutamicoxaloacetic transaminase activity in the rat. *Toxicol. Appl. Pharmacol.* **14**, 97–107.

Puccini, C. (1961). On poisoning by zinc phosphide. *Minerva Med.* **81**, 216–223.

Pundit, A. N., and Bhave, S. A. (1983). Copper and Indian childhood cirrhosis. *Indian Pediatr.* **20**, 893–899.

Rabinowitch, I. M. (1943). Treatment of phosphorus burns. *Can. Med. Assoc. J.* **48**, 291–296.

Rabinowitz, M. B., Wetherill, G. W., and Kopple, J. D. (1974). Studies of human lead metabolism by use of stable isotope tracers. *Environ. Health Perspect.* **7**, 145–153.

Rabuteau, A. P. A. (1867). Experimental study of the physiological effects of fluorides and of metal compounds in general (in French). Thesis, Paris (cited by Cox, 1954).

Radeleff, R. D. (1964). "Veterinary Toxicology." Lea & Febiger, Philadelphia.

Rahill, W. J., and Walser, M. (1965). Renal tubular resorption of trace alkaline earths compared with calcium. *Am. J. Physiol.* **208**, 1165–1170.

Rao, S. H., Gopal, E. R., and Raj, R. (1969). A case of acute sodium fluoride intoxication. *J. Assoc. Physicians India* **17**, 373–374.

Rathus, E., Stinton, R. G., and Putnam, J. L. (1979). Arsine poisoning, country style. *Med. J. Aust.* **1**, 163–166.

Rauws, A. G., and van Heyst, A. N. (1979). Check of Prussian blue for antidotal efficacy in thallium intoxication. *Arch. Toxicol.* **43**, 153–154.

Reed, D., Crawley, J., Faro, S. N., Pieper, S. J., and Kurland, L. T. (1963). Thallotoxicosis. *JAMA, J. Am. Med. Assoc.* **183**, 516–522.

Reibscheid, S., Stella, S., and de Padua Vilela, M. (1966). Poisoning with thallium. Report of two cases. *Hospital (Rio de Janeiro)* **70**, 715–724 (in Portuguese).

Richards, M. P., and Cousins, R. J. (1976). Metallothionein and its relationship to the metabolism of dietary zinc in rats. *J. Nutr.* **106**, 1591–1599.

Richardson, A. P. (1937). Toxic potentialities of continued administration of chlorate for blood and tissues. *J. Pharmacol. Exp. Ther.* **59**, 101–113.

Rimalis, B. T., and Bochkarnikov, V. V. (1978). Acute hepatorenal insufficiency in some rare acute exogenous poisoning. *Klin. Med. (Moscow)* **56**, 125–128 (in Russian).

Ritter, W. L., and Nussbaum, M. A. (1945). Occupational illnesses in cotton industries. III. The mercury hazard in seed treating. *Miss. Doct.* **22**, 262–264.

Rodermund, O. E., Goenechea, S., and Sellier, K. (1968). Poisoning with thallium. Report of two cases. *Hospital (Rio de Janeiro)* **70**, 715–724.

Roholm, K. (1937). "Fluorine Intoxication." H. K. Lewis and Co., London.

Rose, M. S., and Aldridge, W. N. (1968). The interaction of triethyltin with components of animal tissues, *Biochem. J.* **106**, 821–828.

Roth, F. (1957a). On the late effects of chronic arsenicism of Mosel winegrowers. *Dtsch. Med. Wochenschr.* **82**, 468 (in German).

Roth, F. (1957b). Arsenic liver tumors (hemangioendotheliomas). *Z. Krebsforsch.* **61**, 468–503.

Rothstein, A., and Hayes, A. L. (1960). Metabolism of mercury in the rat studied by isotope techniques. *J. Pharmacol. Exp. Ther.* **130**, 166–176.

Rothstein, A., and Hayes, A. L. (1964). The turnover of mercury in rats exposed repeatedly to mercury vapor. *Health Phys.* **10**, 1099–1113.

Rubitsky, H. J., and Myerson, R. M. (1949). Acute phosphorus poisoning. *Arch. Intern. Med.* **83**, 164–178.

Rustam, H., von Burg, R., Amin-Zaki, L., and El Hassani, S. (1975). Evidence for a neuromuscular disorder in methylmercury poisoning. *Arch. Environ. Health* **30**, 190–195.

Sachsse, K., Frei, T., Luethemeier, H., *et al.* (1987). TPTH-substance technical (HOE029664 of 2097004) chronic oral toxicity 52-week feeding study in beagle dogs. American Hoecht Corporation, Somerville, NJ.

Sager, P. R., and Matheson, D. W. (1988). Mechanisms of neurotoxicily related to selective disruption of microtubules and intermediate filaments. *Toxicology* **49**, 479–492.

Sager, P. R., Aschner, M., and Rodier, P. M. (1984). Persistent, differential alterations in developing cerebellar cortex of male and female mice after methylmercury exposure. *Dev. Brain Res.* **12**, 1–11.

Salbe, A. D., and Levander, O. A. (1990). Effect of various dietary factors in the deposition of selenium in the hair and nails of rats. *J. Nutr.* **120**(2), 200–206.

Sanderson, K. V. (1963). Arsenic and skin cancer. *Trans. St. Johns Hosp. Dermatol. Soc.* **49**, 115–122.

Santini, M. (1955). Poisoning by zinc phosphide introduced per vagina. *G. Med. Leg. Infortunistica Tossicol.* **1**, 104–110.

Satterlee, H. S. (1956). The problem of arsenic in American cigarette tobacco. *N. Engl. J. Med.* **254**, 1150–1154.

Savchuck, W. B., and Armstrong, W. D. (1951). Metabolic turnover of fluoride by the skeleton of the rat. *J. Biol. Chem.* **193**, 575–585.

Sayato, Y., Nakamuro, K., Matsui, S., *et al.* (1980). Metabolic fate of chromium compounds. I. Comparative behavior of chromium in rat administered with Na_2 $^{51}CrO_4$ and $^{51}CrCl_3$. *J. Pharm. Dyn.* **3**, 17–23.

Schaidt, G., Geldmacher-von Mallinckrodt, M., and Opitz, O. (1979). On the distribution of zinc in the body fluids and organs following fatal zinc poisoning. *Beitr. Gerich. Med.* **37**, 351–355.

Schaller, K. H., Manke, G., Raithel, H. J., *et al.* (1980). Investigations of thallium-exposed workers in cement factories. *Int. Arch. Occup. Environ. Health* **47**, 223–231.

Schmidt, H. J., and Rand, W. E. (1952). A critical study of the literature on fluoride toxicology with respect to cattle damage. *Am. J. Vet. Res.* **13**, 38–49.

Scholz, J. (1965). Chronic toxicity testing. *Nature (London)* **207**, 870–871.

Schroeder, E. G., Rose, F. A., and Most, H. (1946). Effect of antimony on the electrocardiogram. *Am. J. Med. Sci.* **212**, 697–706.

Schroeder, H. A. (1973). Recondite toxicity of trace elements. *Essays Toxicol.* **4**, 108–199.

Schroeder, H. A., and Kraemer, L. A. (1974). Cardiovascular mortality, municipal water, and corrosion. *Arch. Environ. Health* **28**, 303–311.

Schroeder H. A., and Mitchener, M. (1975). Life-term effects of mercury, methyl mercury, and nine other trace metals on mice. *J. Nutr.* **105**, 452–458.

Schroeder, H. A., Mitchener, M., Balassa, J. J., *et al.* (1968). Zirconium, niobium, antimony, and fluorine in mice: Effects on growth, survival and tissue levels. *J. Nutr.* **95**, 95–101.

Schroeder, H. A., Mitchener, M., and Nason, A. P. (1970). Zirconium, niobium, antimony, vanadium and lead in rats: Life term studies. *J. Nutr.* **100**, 59–68.

Schryver, H. F., Hintz, H. F., and Lowe, J. W. (1980). Absorption, excretion and tissue distribution of stable zinc and ^{65}zinc in ponies. *J. Anim. Sci.* **51**, 896–902.

Schultz, J., and Lewis, H. B. (1940). The excretion of volatile selenium compounds after the administration of sodium selenite to white rats. *J. Biol. Chem.* **133**, 199–207.

Schwartze, E. W., and Alsberg, C. L. (1923). Studies on the pharmacology of cadmium and zinc with particular reference to emesis. *J. Pharmacol. Exp. Ther.* **21**, 1–22.

Schwarz, K. (1961). Development and status of experimental work on Factor 3–selenium. *Fed. Proc., Fed. Am. Soc. Exp. Biol.* **20**(Pt. I), 666–673.

Schwarz, K., and Foltz, C. M. (1957). Selenium as an integral part of Factor 3 against dietary necrotic liver degeneration. *J. Am. Chem. Soc.* **79**, 3292–3293.

Schwarz, K., and Foltz, C. M. (1958). Factor 3 activity of selenium compounds. *J. Biol. Chem.* **233**, 245–251.

Schwarz, K., Bieri, J. G., Briggs, G. M., and Scott, M. L. (1957). Prevention of exudative diathesis in chicks by Factor 3 and Se. *Proc. Soc. Exp. Biol. Med.* **95**, 621–625.

Segar, W. E. (1960). Peritoneal dialysis in the treatment of boric acid poisoning. *N. Engl. J. Med.* **262**, 798–800.

Sharda, B. (1984). Indian childhood cirrhosis: Dietary copper. *Indian Pediatr.* **21**, 182.

Sharkey, T. P., and Simpson, W. M. (1933). Accidental sodium fluoride poisoning. *JAMA, J. Am. Med. Assoc.* **100**, 97–100.

Sharrett, A. R., Carter, A. P., Orheim, R. M., and Feinleib, M. (1982). Daily intake of lead, cadmium, copper and zinc from drinking water: The Seattle study of trace metal exposure. *Environ. Res.* **28**, 456–475.

Shaw, J. J., ed. (1954). "Fluoridation as a Public Health Measure." Am. Assoc. Adv. Sci. Washington, DC.

Shustov, V. I. A., and Tsyganova, S. I. (1970). Clinical aspects of subacute intoxication with Granosan. *Kazan. Med. Zh.* **2**, 78–79.

Simonin, P., and Pierron, A. (1937). Acute toxicity of fluorine compounds. *C. R. Seance Soc. Biol. Ses. Fil.* **124**, 133–134 (in German).

Simonović, I. (1954). Zinc phosphide poisoning. *Arh. Hig. Rada* **5**, 355–358.

Skare, J. A., Schrotel, K. R., and Nixon, G. A. (1986). Lack of DNA-strand breaks in rat testicular cells after *in vivo* treatment with sodium fluoride. *Mutat. Res.* **170**, 85–92.

Skerfving, S. (1974). Methylmercury exposure, mercury levels in blood and hair, and health status in Swedes consuming contaminated fish. *Toxicology* **2**, 3–23.

Skerfving, S. B., and Copplestone, J. F. (1976). Poisoning caused by the consumption of organomercury-dressed seed in Iraq. *Bull. W.H.O.* **54**, 111–112.

Smith, F. A., ed. (1966). "Handbuch der Experimentellen Pharmakologie," Vol. 20, Part 1. Springer-Verlag, Berlin.

Smith, F. A., ed. (1970). "Handbuch der Experimentellen Pharmakologie," Vol. 20, Part 2. Springer-Verlag, Berlin.

Smith, H. (1964). The interpretation of the arsenic content of hair. *J. Forensic Sci. Soc.* **4**, 192–199.

Smith, M. C., and Lantz, E. M. (1935). The effect of fluorine upon the phosphatase content of plasma, bones, and teeth of albino rats. *J. Biol. Chem.* **112**, 303–311.

Smith, M. I. (1939). The influence of diet on the chronic toxicily of selenium. *Public Health Rep.* **54**, 1441–1453.

Smith, M. I. (1941). Chronic endemic selenium poisoning. A review of the more recent field and laboratory studies. *JAMA, J. Am. Med. Assoc.* **116**, 562–567.

Smith, M. I., and Stohlman, E. F. (1940). Further observations on the influence of dietary protein on the toxicity of selenium. *J. Pharmacol. Exp. Ther.* **70**, 270–278.

Smith, M. I., and Westfall, B. B. (1936). The selenium problem in relation to public health. *Public Health Rep.* **51**, 1496.

Smith, M. I., Westfall, B. B., and Stohlman, E. F. (1937). Elimination of Se and its distribution in tissues. *Public Health Rep.* **52**, 1171.

Smith, R. G., Vorwald, A. J., Patil, L. S., and Mooney, T. F. (1970). Effects of exposure to mercury in the manufacture of chlorine. *Am. Ind. Hyg. Assoc. J.* **31**, 687–700.

Smyth, H. F., and Smyth, H. F., Jr. (1932). Relative toxicity of some fluoride and arsenical insecticides. *Ind. Eng. Chem.* **24**, 229–232.

Smyth, H. F., Jr., Carpenter, C. P., Weil, C. S., Pozzani, U. C., Striegel, J. A., and Nycum, J. S. (1969). Range-finding toxicity data: List VII. *Am. Ind. Hyg. Assoc. J.* **30**, 470–476.

Snowden, E. M. (1958). Trace elements in human tissue. 3. Strontium and barium in non-skeletal tissue. *Biochem. J.* **70**, 712–715.

Snowden, E. M., and Stitch, S. R. (1957). Trace elements in human tissue. 2. Estimation of the concentrations of stable strontium and barium in human bone. *Biochem. J.* **67**, 104–109.

Snyder, R. D. (1971). Congenital mercury poisoning. *N. Engl. J. Med.* **284**, 1014–1016.

Snyder, R. D. (1972). The involuntary movements of chronic mercury poisoning. *Arch. Neurol. (Chicago)* **26**, 379–381.

Sohn, O. S., Blackwell, L., Mathis, J., *et al.* (1991). Excretion and tissue distribution of selenium following treatment of male F344 rats with benzylselenocyanate or sodium selenite. *Drug Metab. Dispos. Biol. Fate Chem.* **19**(5), 865–870.

Solecki, R., Hothorn, L., Holzweissig, M., *et al.* (1991). Computerised analysis of pathological findings in longterm trials with phenylmercuric acetate in rats. *Arch. Toxicol.*, Suppl. 14, 100–103.

Sollmann, T. (1957). "A Manual of Pharmacology and Its Applications to Toxicology and Therapeutics," 8th ed. Saunders, Philadelphia.

Sollmann, T., and Seifter, J. (1942). Intravenous injection of soluble bismuth compounds. *J. Pharmacol. Exp. Ther.* **74**, 134–154.

Sommers, S. C., and McManus, R. G. (1953). Multiple arsenical cancers of skin and internal organs. *Cancer (Philadelphia)* **6**, 347.

Sørensen, O. H. (1965). Thallium poisoning. *Ugeskr. Laeg.* **127**, 804–807.

Soroka, V. P., and Sorokina, A. A. (1969). The effect of unithiol and $CaNa_2$–EDTA on urinary trace element excretion in dogs. *Gig. Tr. Prof. Zabol.* **13**, 40–41.

Southby, R. (1965). Fatal poisoning in children under five years of age: A survey in Victoria for the years 1955 to 1963. *Med. J. Aust.* **1**, 533–538.

Sparling, D. W., Gustafson, M., Klein, P., and Karouna-Renier, N. (1997). Toxicity of white phosphorus to waterfowl: Acute exposure in mallards. *J. Wildlif. Dis.* **33**(2), 187–197.

Spector, W. S. (1955). "Handbook of Toxicology." Carpenter Litho and Printing Co., Springfield, IL.

Spencer, H., Lewin, I., Wistrowski, E., *et al.* (1970). Fluoride metabolism in man. *Am. J. Med.* **49**, 807–813.

Spyker, J. M., Sparber, S. B., and Goldberg, A. M. (1972). Subtle consequences of methylmercury exposure: Behavioral deviations in offspring of treated mothers. *Science* **177**, 621–623.

Stadtman, T. C. (1974). Selenium biochemistry. *Science* **183**, 915–922.

Starvou, A., Butcher, R., and Sakula, A. (1978). Accidental self-poisoning by sodium chlorate weedkiller. *Practitioner* **221**, 397–399.

Stein, M. D., and Perlstein, M. A. (1959). Thallium poisoning: Report of two cases. *Am. J. Dis. Child.* **98**, 80–85.

Steinberg, H. J. (1961). Accidental thallium poisoning in adults. *South. Med. J.* **54**, 6–9.

Stephenson, J. B. P. (1967). Zinc phosphide poisoning. *Arch. Environ. Health* **15**, 83–88.

Stevens, W., Van Peteghem, C., Heyndrickx, A., and Barbier, F. (1974). Eleven cases of thallium intoxication treated with Prussian blue. *Int. J. Clin. Pharmacol., Ther. Toxicol.* **10**, 1–22

Stewart, D. (1957). Sulfuryl fluoride: A new fumigant for control of the drywood termite *Kalotermes minor* Hagen. *J. Econ. Entomol.* **50**, 7–11.

Stokinger, H. H. (1963). The metals (excluding lead). *In* "Industrial Hygiene and Toxicology" (F. A. Patty, ed.), Vol. 2, pp. 987–1194. Wiley (Interscience), New York.

Stokinger, H. E. (1981). Copper. *In* "Patty's Industrial Hygiene and Toxicology" (G. D. Clayton and F. E. Clayton, eds.), 3rd rev. ed., Vol. 2A, pp. 1620–1630. Wiley, New York.

Stoner, H. B. (1966). Toxicity of triphenyltin. *Br. J. Ind. Med.* **23**, 222–229.

Stoner, H. B., and Heath, D. F. (1967). The cumulative action of triphenyltin. *Food Cosmet. Toxicol.* **5**, 285–286.

Stoner, H. B., Banes, J. M., and Duff, J. I. (1955). Studies on the toxicity of alkyl tin compounds. *Br. J. Pharmacol. Chemother.* **10**, 16–25.

Storrs, B., Thomson, J., Fair, G., Dickerson, M. S., Nickey, L., Barthel, W., and Spaulding, J. E. (1970a). Organic mercury poisoning. Alamogordo, New Mexico. *Morbid. Mortal. Wkly. Rep.* **19**, 25–26.

Storrs, B., Thompson, J., Nickey, L., Barthel, W., and Spaulding, J. E. (1970b). Follow-up organic mercury poisoning—New Mexico. *Morbid. Mortal. Wkly. Rep.* **19**, 169–170.

Strom, S., Johnson, R. L., and Uyeki, E. M. (1979). Mercury toxicity to hemopoietic and tumor colony-forming cells and its reversal by selenium *in vitro. Toxicol. Appl. Pharmacol.* **49**, 431–436.

Sumino, K., Hayakawa, K., Shibata, T., *et al.* (1975). Heavy metals in normal Japanese tissues. *Arch. Environ. Health* **30**, 487–494.

Sunde, R. A. (1990). Molecular biology of selenoproteins. *Annu. Rev. Nutr.* **10**, 451–474.

Sunderman, F. W., Sr. (1978). Clinical response to therapeutic agents in poisoning from mercury vapor. *Ann. Chem. Lab. Sci.* **8**, 259–269.

Suttle, N. F., and Mills, C. F. (1966a). Studies on the toxicity of copper to pigs. 1. Effects of oral supplements of zinc and iron salts on the development of copper toxicosis. *Br. J. Nutr.* **20**, 135–145.

Suttle, N. F., and Mills, C. F. (1966b). Studies on the toxicity of copper to pigs. 2. Effects of protein source and other dietary components on the response to high and moderate intakes of copper. *Br. J. Nutr.* **20**, 149.

Swensson, A. (1952). Investigations on the toxicity of some organic mercury compounds which are used as seed disinfectants. *Acta Med. Scand.* **143**, 365–384.

Swensson, A., and Ulfvarson, U. (1963). Toxicology of organic mercury compounds used as fungicides. *Occup. Health Rev.* **15**, 5–11.

Swensson, A., and Ulfvarson, U. (1967). Experiments with different antidotes in acute poisoning by different mercury compounds: Effects on survival and on distribution and excretion of mercury. *Int. Arch. Gewerbepathol. Gewerbehyg.* **24**, 12–50.

Swensson, A., and Ulfvarson, U. (1968a). Distribution and excretion of various mercury compounds after single injections in poultry. *Acta Pharmacol. Toxicol.* **26**, 259–272.

Swensson, A., and Ulfvarson, U. (1968b). Distribution and excretion of mercury compounds in rats over a long period after a single injection. *Acta Pharmacol. Toxicol.* **26**, 273–283.

Swensson, A., Lundgren, K. D., and Lindström, O. (1959). Distribution and excretion of mercury compounds after single injection. *A.M.A., Arch. Ind. Health* **20**, 432–443.

Syed, I. B., and Hosain, F. (1972). Determination of LD50 of barium chloride and allied agents. *Toxicol. Appl. Pharmacol.* **22**, 150–152.

Taber, P. (1964). Chronic thallium poisoning: Rapid diagnosis and treatment. *J. Pediatr.* **65**, 461–463.

Takenaka, S., Oldiges, H., Konnig, H., *et al.* (1983). Carcinogenicity of cadmium chloride aerosols in Wistar rats. *J. Natl. Cancer Inst.* **70**, 367–373.

Takeuchi, T., and Eto, K. (1977). Pathology and pathogenesis of Minamata disease. *In* "Minamata Disease" (T. Tsubaki and K. Irukayama, eds.), pp. 103–142. Am. Elsevier, New York.

Tam, G. K. H., Charbonneau, S. M., Bryce, F., Pomroy, C., and Sandi, E. (1979). Metabolism of inorganic arsenic (^{74}As) in humans following oral ingestion. *Toxicol. Appl. Pharmacol.* **50**, 319–322.

Tao, S., and Suttie, J. W. (1976). Evidence for a lack of an effect of dietary fluoride level on reproduction in mice. *J. Nutr.* **106**, 1115–1122.

Taxay, E. (1966). Vikane inhalation. *J. Occup. Med.* **8**, 425–426.

Taylor, D. M., Bligh, P. H., and Duggan, M. H. (1962). The absorption of calcium, strontium, barium and radium from the gastrointestinal tract of the rat. *Biochem. J.* **83**, 25–29.

Taylor, F. B. (1962). Effectiveness of water utility quality control practices. *J. Am. Water Works Assoc.* **54**, 1257–1264.

Teisinger, J., and Fiserova-Bergerova, V. (1965). Pulmonary retention and excretion of mercury vapors in man. *Ind. Med. Surg.* **34**, 580–584.

Tennekes, H., Horst, K., Leuthemeier H., *et al.* (1989). "TPTH Technical (Code: HOE029664 of ZD97004) Oncogenicity Study in Mice." Hoechst Celanese Corporation, Somerville, NJ.

Thompson, J. N., and Scott, M. L. (1970). Impaired lipid and vitamin E absorption related to atrophy of the pancreas in selenium-deficient chicks. *J. Nutr.* **100**, 797–809.

Thomson, C. D., and Stewart, R. D. H. (1973). Metabolic studies of [75Se] selenomethionine and [75Se] selenite in the rat. *Br. J. Nutr.* **30**, 139–147.

Thyresson, N. (1951). Experimental investigation on thallium poisoning in the rat. *Acta Derm.-Venereol.* **31**, 3–27.

Timperman, J., and Maes, R. (1966). Suicidal poisoning by sodium chlorate. A report of three cases. *J. Forensic Med.* **13**, 123–129.

Tipton, I. H., and Cook, M. J. (1963). Trace elements in human tissue. Part II. Adult subjects from the United States. *Health Phys.* **9**, 103–145.

Tipton, I. H., Schroeder, H. A., Peny, H. M., Jr., and Cook, M. J. (1965). Trace elements in human tissue. Part III. Subjects from Africa, the Near and Far East and Europe. *Health Phys.* **11**, 403–451.

Tobaldin, G., Castellani, E., Ferrari, B., and Montanari, M. G. (1966). Acute intoxication by lead arsenate. *Arcisp. S. Anna Ferrara* **19**, 177–1006.

Tokutomi, H. (1968). Symposium on clinical observations on public nuisances and agricultural pesticide poisonings. 3. Organic mercury poisoning. *Nippon Naika Gakkai Zasshi* **57**, 1212–1216.

Tokutomi, H., Okajima, T., Kanai, J., Tsunoda, M., Ichiyasu, Y., Misumi, H., Shimomura, K., and Takaba, M. (1961). Minamata disease: An unusual neurological disorder occuring in Minamata, Japan. *Kumamoto Med. J.* **14**, 47–64.

Trelease, S. F., and Beath, O. A. (1949). "Selenium." Published by the authors, New York.

Trelease, S. F., DiSomma, A. A., and Jacobs, A, L. (1960). Seleno-amino acid found in *Astragalus bisulcatus. Science* **132**, 618.

Tseng, W. P. (1977). Effects and dose–response relationships of skin cancer and blackfoot disease with arsenic. *Environ. Health Perspect.* **19**, 109–119.

Tseng, W. P., Chu, H. M., How, S. W., Fong, J. M., Lin, C. S., and Yeh, S. (1968). Prevalence of skin cancer in an endemic area of chronic arsenicism in Taiwan. *J. Natl. Cancer Inst. (U.S.)* **40**, 453.

Tsubaki, T. (1968). Symposium on clinical observations on public nuisances and agricultural pesticide poisonings. 3. Organic mercury poisoning. 3a. Clinical features of organic mercury intoxication. *J. Jpn. Soc. Intern. Med.* **57**, 1217–1218 (in Japanese).

Tsubaki, T., and Irukayama, K., eds. (1977). "Minamata Disease: Methylmercury Poisoning in Minamata and Nigata, Japan." Am. Elsevier, New York.

Tsuchiya, K. (1977). Various effects of arsenic in Japan depending on type of exposure. *Environ. Health Perspect.* **19**, 35–42.

Ulfvarson, U. (1962). Distribution and excretion of some mercury compounds after long term exposure. *Int. Arch. Gewerbepathol. Gewerbehyg.* **19**, 412–422.

Underwood, E. J. (1956). "Trace Elements in Human and Animal Nutrition." Academic Press, New York.

Underwood, E. J. (1977). "Trace Elements in Human and Animal Nutrition," 4th ed. Academic Press, New York.

U.S. Environmental Protection Agency (U.S. EPA) (1983). "Health Assessment Document for Inorganic Arsenic." Rep. No. EPA-600/8-83-021F, U.S. Environ. Prot. Agency, Washington, DC.

U.S. Environmental Protection Agency (U.S. EPA) (1984). "Mercury Health Effects Update. Health Issue Assessment." Rep. No. EPA-600/8-84-019F, U.S. Environ. Prot. Agency, Washington, DC.

U.S. Environmental Protection Agency (U.S. EPA) (1985). "Suspended, Cancelled and Restricted Pesticides." Office of Pesticides and Toxic Substances Compliance, U.S. Environ. Prot. Agency, Washington, DC.

U.S. Environmental Protection Agency (U.S. EPA) (1987). "Summary Review of the Health Effects Associated with Copper." Rep. No. EPA 600/8-87-001, U.S. Environ. Prot. Agency, Washington, DC.

U.S. Public Health Service (1962). "Public Health Service Drinking Water Standards." Publ. No. 956, U.S. Public Health Serv., Washington, DC.

U.S. Public Health Service (1966). "Symposium on Environmental Lead Contamination." Publ. No. 1440, U.S. Public Health Serv., Washington, DC.

Uthus, E. O., and Nielsen, F. H. (1985). Consequence of arsenic deprivation in laboratory animals. *In* "Arsenic, Industrial, Biomedical and Environmental Perspectives" (W. H. Lederer, ed.), pp. 173–189. Van Nostrand–Reinhold, New York.

Vahter, M. (1981). Biotransformation of trivalent and pentavalent inorganic arsenic in mice and rats. *Environ. Res.* **25**, 286–293.

Vahter, M. E. (1988). Arsenic. *In* "Biological Monitoring of Toxic Metals" (T. W. Clarkson, L. Friberg, G. F. Nordberg, and P. R. Sager, eds.), pp. 303–321. Plenum, New York.

Vahter, M., and Norin, H. (1980). Metabolism of ^{74}As-labeled trivalent and pentavalent inorganic arsenic in mice. *Environ. Res.* **21**, 446–457.

Vahter, M. E., Marafante, E., Lindgren, A., and Dencker, L. (1982). Tissue distribution and subcellular binding of arsenic to marmoset monkeys after injection of ^{74}As-arsenite. *Arch. Toxicol.* **51**, 65–77.

Valentine, J. L., Kang, H. K., and Spivey, G. (1979). Arsenic levels in human blood, urine and hair in response to exposure via drinking water. *Environ. Res.* **20**, 24–32.

Vallee, B. L. (1959). Biochemistry, physiology, and pathology of zinc. *Physiol. Rev.* **39**, 443–490.

Vallee, B. L. (1962). Zinc. *In* "Mineral Metabolism: An Advanced Treatise" (C. L. Comar and F. Bronner, eds.), Vol. 2B, pp. 443–482. Academic Press, New York.

Vallee, C. (1920). Nonfatal poisoning by sodium fluoride. *J. Pharm. Chim.* **21**, 5–8.

Van der Kerk, G. J. M., and Luijten, J. G. A. (1954). Investigations on organotin compounds. III. The biocidal properties of organo-tin compounds. *J. Appl. Chem.* **4**, 314–319.

Van der Merwe, K. J., Steyn, P. S., and Fourie, L. (1965). Mycotoxins. Part II. The constitution of ochratoxins A, B, and C. Metabolites of *Aspergillus ochraceus* Wilh. *J. Chem. Soc., London*, 7083–7088.

Vasil'eva, S. N., Aleksandrova, T. G., Rybakova, M. G., Bryukhanov, V. A., Bulavintseva, O. A., and Bulavintsev, A. G. (1978). Domestic poisoning with thallium. *Klin. Med. (Moscow)* **56**, 130–132 (in Russian).

Veichenblau, L. (1932). New occupational illnesses in agriculture. *Muench. Med. Wochenschr.* **79**, 432–433 (in German).

Verschuuren, H. G., Kroes, R., Vink, H. H., and Van Esch, G. J. (1966). Short-term toxicity studies with triphenyltin compounds in rats and guinea pig. *Food Cosmet. Toxicol.* **4**, 35–45.

Vesce, C. A. (1947). Experimental intoxication by selenium: Morphological changes of the endocrine glands. *Folia Med. (Naples)* **30**, 209–217.

Vintinner, F. J. (1940). Dermatitis venenata resulting from contact with an aqueous solution of elhyl mercury phosphate. *J. Ind. Hyg.* **22**, 297–299.

Voight, J. L., Edwards, L. D., and Johnson, C. H. (1948). Acute toxicity of arsenate of lead to animals. *J. Am. Pharm. Assoc., Sci. Ed.* **37**, 122–123.

von Kraemer, M., and Giebelmann, R. (1975). Fatal poisoning by zinc hexafluorosilicate. *Dtsch. Gesundheitswes.* **29**, 1378–1379 (in German).

von Martius, C. O. (1953). Clinical and spectroanalytic observations on acute poisoning by thallium sulphate. *Dtsch. Arch. Klin. Med.* **200**, 596–602 (in German).

von Oettingen, E. W. (1947). The toxicity and potential dangers of zinc phosphide and of hydrogen phosphide (phosphine). *Public Health Rep., Suppl.* **203**, 1–17.

Wagner, M. J., Stookey, C. K., and Muhler, K. (1958). Deposition of fluoride in soft tissue following skeletal saturation. *Proc. Soc. Exp. Biol. Med.* **99**, 102–105.

Wagstaff, D. J. (1972). Arsenic trioxide: Stimulation of liver enzyme detoxication activity. *Toxicol. Appl. Pharmacol.* **22**, 310.

Wahlberg, J. E. (1965). Percutaneous absorption of trivalent and hexavalent chromium. *Arch. Dermatol.* **92**, 315–318.

Waitz, A., Ober, R. E., Meisenhelder, J. E., and Thompson, P. E. (1965). Physiological distribution of Sb after administration of [124]Sb-labeled tartar emetic to rats, mice, and monkeys, and the effects of tris (*p*-aminophenyl)carbonium pamoate on this distribution. *Bull. W.H.O.* **33**, 537–546.

Wakasugi, C., and Fukui, M. (1974). A case report of fatal intoxication by ingestion of calcium polysulfide. *Nippon Hoigaku Zasshi* **28**, 102–103 (in Japanese).

Walsh, F. M., Crosson, F. J., Bayley, M., McReynolds, J., and Pearson, B. J. (1977). Acute copper intoxication. Pathophysiology and therapy with a case report. *Am. J. Dis. Child.* **131**, 149–151.

Wang, B. C., and Mazzia, V. D. B. (1969). Arsenic poisoning as anesthetic risk. *N.Y. State J. Med.* **69**, 2911–2912.

Warkany, J. (1966). Postmortem of a disease. *Am. J. Dis. Child.* **112**, 147–156.

Warkany, J., and Hubbard, D. M. (1948). Mercury in the urine of children with acrodynia. *Lancet* **204**, 829–830.

Warkany, J., and Hubbard, D. M. (1951). Adverse mercurial reactions in the form of acrodynia and related conditions. *Am. J. Dis. Child.* **81**, 335–373.

Warkany, J., and Hubbard, D. M. (1953). Acrodynia and mercury. *J. Pediatr.* **42**, 365–386.

Webb, J. L. (1966). Arsenicals. *In* "Enzyme and Metabolic Inhibitors" (J. L. Webb, ed.), Vol. 3, pp. 595–793. Academic Press, New York.

West, I., and Lim, J. (1968). Mercury poisoning among workers in California's mercury mills. *J. Occup. Med.* **10**, 697–701.

Westfall, B. B., Stohlman, E. F., and Smith, M. I. (1938). The placental transmission of selenium. *J. Pharmacol. Exp. Ther.* **64**, 55–57.

Whanger, P. D., Pedersen, N. D., Hatfield, J., *et al.* (1976). Absorption of selenite and selenomethionine from ligated digestive tract segments in rats (39531). *Proc. Soc. Exp. Biol. Med.* **153**, 295–297.

Whitford, G. M. (1990). The physiological and toxicological characteristics of fluoride. *J. Dent. Res.* **69**, 539–549 (special issue).

Whitford, G. M., and Pashley, D. H. (1984). Fluoride absorption: The influence of gastric acidity. *Calcif. Tissue Int.* **36**, 302–307.

Wilkening, H., and Litzner, St. (1952). Injuries especially to the kidney from alkylmercury compounds. *Dtsch. Med. Wochenschr.* **77**, 432–434 (in German).

Willhite, C. C., Ferm, V. H., and Zeise, L. (1990). Route-dependent pharmacokinetics, distribution, and placental permeability of organic and inorganic selenium in hamsters. *Teratology* **42**(4), 359–371.

Wilson, B. J., Wilson, C. H., and Hayes, A. W. (1968). Tremorgenic toxin from *Penicillium cyclopium* grown on food materials. *Nature (London)* **220**, 77–78.

Wong, L. C., Heimbach, M. D., Truscott, D. R., and Duncan, B. D. (1964). Boric acid poisoning. Report of 11 cases. *Can. Med. Assoc. J.* **90**, 1018–1023.

World Health Organization (WHO) (1962). Accidental food poisoning with Agrosan. Communication to World Health Organization from S. A. Raza Ali. *In* "WHO Inf. Circ. Toxic. Pestic. Man," No. 9, p. 23. WHO, Geneva.

World Health Organization (WHO) (1970). "Fluorides and Human Health." WHO, Geneva.

World Health Organization (WHO) (1973). "Trace Elements in Nutrition: A Report of a WHO Expert Committee." Technical Report Series No. 532, WHO, Geneva.

World Health Organization (WHO) (1974). The use of mercury and alternative compounds as seed dressings. Report of a Joint FAO/WHO Meeting. *W.H.O. Tech. Rep. Ser.* **555**.

World Health Organization (WHO) (1975). Some aziridines, N-, S-, and O-mustards and selenium. *IARC Monogr. Eval. Carcinog. Risk Chem. Man* **9**, 1–268.

World Health Organization (WHO) (1976). "Environmental Health Criteria. I. Mercury." WHO, Geneva.

World Health Organization (WHO) (1977). "Environmental Health Criteria. 3 Lead." WHO, Geneva.

World Health Organization (WHO) (1980). Recommended health-based limits in occupational exposure to heavy metals. *W.H.O. Tech. Rep. Ser.* **647**.

World Health Organization (WHO) (1981). "Environmental Health Criteria 18. Arsenic." WHO, Geneva.

World Health Organization (WHO) (1984a). "Recommendations," Guidelines for Drinking-Water Quality, Vol. 1. WHO, Geneva.

World Health Organization (WHO) (1984b). "Health Criteria and Other Supporting Information," Guidelines for Drinking Water Quality, Vol. 2. WHO, Geneva.

Wu, M. M., Kuo, T. L., Hwang, Y. H., *et al.* (1989). Dose–response relation between arsenic concentration in well water and mortality from cancers and vascular diseases. *Am. J. Epidemiol.* **130**, 1123–1132.

Yamauchi, H., and Yamamura, Y. (1985). Metabolism and excretion of orally administered arsenic trioxide in the hamster. *Toxicology* **34**, 113–121.

Yoshida, M., Satoh, H., and Kishimoto, T. (1992). Exposure to mercury via breast milk in suckling offspring of maternal guinea pigs exposed to mercury vapor after parturition. *J. Toxicol. Environ. Health* **35**(2), 135–139.

Young, E. G., Smith, R. P., and MacIntosh, O. C. (1949). Boric acid as a poison. *Can. Med. Assoc. J.* **61**, 447–450.

Zaporowska, H., and Wasilewski, W. (1992). Combined effect of vanadium and zinc on certain selected hematological indices in rats. *Comp. Biochem. Physiol.* **103C**(1), 143–147.

Zeyer, H. G. (1952). Melhoxyethylmercury oxalate poisoning. *Zentralbl. Arbeitsmed. Arbeitsschutz* **2**, 68–72 (in German).

Zimmer, L., and Carter, D. E. (1979). Effects of complexing treatment administered with the onset of methyl mercury neurotoxic signs. *Toxicol. Appl. Pharmacol.* **51**, 29–38.

Boric Acid and Inorganic Borate Pesticides

Philip L. Strong
U.S. Borax Inc.

62.1 INTRODUCTION

Boric acid and inorganic borates are water-soluble, low-acute-toxicity, low-volatility white powders, which have been used in registered pesticide applications since 1948. They are non-mutagenic and noncarcinogenic. Animal studies at higher doses show reproductive toxicity, primarily male effects (decreased spermiation and testicular atrophy). Exposures during pregnancy to mice, rats, and rabbits resulted in developmental effects (i.e., low birth weight and skeletal defects). The reported NOAEL (No-Observed-Adverse-Effect Level) is 10 mg B/kg/day based on the most sensitive effect, low fetal body weight in rats.

Recent reports involving adult accidental poisonings report minimal or no toxicity and recommend that aggressive treatment is not necessary for most patients. Earlier reported infant poisonings are based on outdated applications and misuse. The chronic "No Effect" level for humans was reported to be about 2.5 mg B/kg/day and the chronic "Adverse Effect" level was 5 mg B/kg/day. Cattle have been reported to eat sufficient quantities of borate fertilizer from open bags left in the field to result in death.

Oral absorption is nearly 100%. Dermal absorption from intact skin is very low. Borates are distributed throughout the total body water. Bone is the only tissue that accumulates boron significantly above blood levels. Boric acid and inorganic borates are not metabolized below the $B(OH)_3$ structure. Excretion is primarily in urine with the reported excretion half-life between 13 and 24 hours. Recent studies are demonstrating that low levels of boron are important nutritionally for both animals and humans.

62.2 BACKGROUND

This chapter focuses on boric acid and inorganic borates, primarily borax and disodium octaborate tetrahydrate and their derivatives, since the major pesticide uses involve these three materials. Dilute aqueous solutions of boric acid and borax yield identical species, most frequently boric acid, at physiological pH; therefore, toxicological data for systemic and chronic toxicity are used interchangeably for boric acid and the borate chemicals considered here. In order to allow comparisons from one chemical to another, the data are often reported in terms of the boron content, expressed as boron equivalents. The element boron does not exist in nature; it is always combined with oxygen in the form of borates. To convert boric acid data to boron equivalents, the multiplication factor is 0.1750, for borax it is 0.1134, and for disodium octaborate tetrahydrate the factor is 0.2096. Acute data, such as for dermal and respiratory toxicity, are considered separately based upon studies of the individual chemicals (i.e., boric acid and borax).

62.2.1 CHEMICAL NAMES (SYNONYMS) AND FORMULAS

1. Boric acid (boracic acid, orthoboric acid) $B(OH)_3$
2. Disodium tetraborate decahydrate (sodium tetraborate decahydrate, borax, borax decahydrate, borax 10-mole) $Na_2B_4O_7 \cdot 10H_2O$
3. Disodium octaborate tetrahydrate (none) $Na_2B_8O_{13} \cdot 4H_2O$ (The chemical composition formula given above is an approximate composition of the solid material. The solid is amorphous and the exact structure is not known. It is the composition that gives the maximum water solubility of all the sodium borate species.)

62.2.2 PHYSICAL AND CHEMICAL PROPERTIES

1. Boric acid (CAS No. 10043-35-3)—white crystalline powder; molecular weight, 61.88; melting point, $170.9°C \pm 0.2°C$; vapor pressure, less than 10^{-4} torr at 20°C; water solubility, 4.72% at 20°C; octanol/water partition coefficient: 0.175; pH: 5.1 (1% solution) at 20°C; specific gravity, 1.51.

2. Disodium tetraborate decahydrate (borax) (CAS No. 1303-96-4)—white crystalline powder; molecular weight, 381.87; melting point, 62°C (begins to dissolve in water of hydration); vapor pressure, less than 10^{-6} torr at 20°C; water solubility, 4.71% at 20°C; pH, 9.24 (1% solution) at 20°C; specific gravity, 1.71.

3. Disodium octaborate tetrahydrate (CAS No. 12280-03-4)— white amorphous powder; molecular weight, 412.52; melting point, 815°C; vapor pressure, negligible at 20°C; water solubility, 9.5% at 20°C; pH, 8.5 (1% at 23°C); bulk density, 320 to 480 kg/m^3.

62.2.3 HISTORY, FORMULATIONS, AND USES

Boric acid was first registered in the United States for pesticide use in 1948. As of September 1993, there were 189 registered products containing boric acid and its salts. Many formulations are marketed, including liquids, soluble and emulsifiable concentrates, granulars, powders, dusts, pellets, tablets, solids, paste, baits, and crystalline rods (U.S. Environmental Protection Agency, 1993). Uses include insecticides, fungicides, and algaecides, with very little herbicide usage remaining. The major borate pesticide usage includes control of cockroaches, wood-destroying insects (including termites) and fungi, and ants. Borates are used for stump treatment (sapstain) and algae control in swimming pools. They are also used for flea control in carpets, although this use has been controversial due to some high application rates reported and to concern for exposures to children and pets.

62.3 TOXICITY TO ANIMALS

A number of excellent reviews have been published on the toxicology of boric acid and inorganic borates (ATSDR, 1992; Culver *et al.*, 1994b; ECETOC, 1995; Fail *et al.*, 1998; Hubbard, 1998; Hubbard and Sullivan, 1996; IPCS, 1998; Moore, 1997; Murray, 1995).

62.3.1 EXPERIMENTAL LABORATORY STUDIES

62.3.1.1 Acute Studies

In general, acute toxicity of boric acid and inorganic borates is considered to be low. Acute oral LD_{50}-values in rats range from 2500 to almost 5000 mg/kg body weight (Smyth *et al.*, 1969; Weir and Fisher, 1972). Dermal LD_{50} values in rabbits are greater than 2000 mg/kg body weight. Symptoms of acute toxicity include central nervous system (CNS) depression, ataxia, convulsions, and death. They are not skin irritants or sensitizers. Boric acid and disodium octaborate tetrahydrate produced mild eye irritation in the Draize test in rabbits. Borax yielded severe eye irritation in the same test. The U.S. EPA reports a Category 3 for eye irritation for boric acid and disodium octaborate

tetrahydrate and a Category 1 for borax (U.S. Environmental Protection Agency, 1993).

62.3.1.2 Chronic Studies

Mutagenicity No evidence for mutagenic activity has been reported from a number of *in vivo* and *in vitro* studies (Bakke, 1991, 1992; Benson *et al.*, 1984; Hayworth *et al.*, 1983; Landolf, 1985; McGregor *et al.*, 1988; National Toxicology Program, 1987; O'Loughlin, 1991; Stewart, 1991).

Carcinogenicity The U.S. EPA Office of Pesticide Programs Carcinogenicity Peer Review Committee has classified boric acid as a "Group E" carcinogen, "evidence of noncarcinogenicity for humans" (U.S. Environmental Protection Agency, 1993). This classification is based on the results of two 2-year chronic feeding studies: one in rats (Weir and Fisher, 1972) and one in B6C3F1 mice (National Toxicology Program, 1987).

Reproductive Toxicity Most of the toxicological studies on boric acid and inorganic borates have involved either reproductive or developmental end points. The reviews, mentioned at the beginning of Section 62.3 do a good job of discussing these effects. The first reports of reproductive effects from borate exposure came from France (Caujolle *et al.*, 1962; Truhaut *et al.*, 1964) in which sterility was reported in rats after ingestion of repeated high doses in the range of 1 to 24 g/kg body weight. These reports were followed up by a series of studies known as the Weir and Fisher studies (Weir and Fisher, 1972) utilizing rats and dogs in parallel studies with both boric acid and borax. This series of studies, published as final reports to U.S. Borax by Hazelton Laboratories in eight separate volumes, was summarized in one publication (Weir and Fisher, 1972). These reports were far ahead of their time for the details reported and included 2-year dietary rat and dog studies, 38-week dog studies, and three-generation reproduction studies in rats. Each study was carried out separately for boric acid and borax and confirmed that effects observed are equivalent for both materials based on boron content. Testicular degeneration, including atrophy and sterility in both rats and dogs, was reported at 1170 ppm boron levels in the feed (equivalent to 6880 ppm boric acid and 10,300 ppm borax in the feed). The NOAEL dose was 350 ppm B (2000 ppm boric acid and 3090 ppm borax). The dog study NOAEL results are equivalent to a dose of 8.8 mg B/kg body weight, which is the lowest reported NOAEL. This Weir–Fisher dog study NOAEL has been used as the key study for risk assessment in the past, and still is the study upon which the current EPA reference dose of 0.09 mg B/kg/day is based (U.S. EPA, 1998). However, the U.S. EPA is currently reevaluating the RfD for boron. Reasons for not selecting the older Weir and Fisher dog study as the pivotal study for risk assessment of boric acid and inorganic borates were recently elucidated and include use of only one dog per group for some observations and problems with the control group (Murray, 1996). Recent risk assessments use a more current rat developmental study as the key study for risk assessment purposes (ECETOC, 1995; IPCS, 1998; Moore, 1997; Murray, 1995). This new rat developmental study is discussed in Section Developmental Toxicity.

Following the Weir and Fisher studies, there have been numerous animal studies reporting reproductive effects from boric acid and inorganic borates. Species included are mice, rats, and dogs (Chapin and Ku, 1994; Dixon *et al.*, 1976, 1979; Fail *et al.*, 1989, 1991; Krasovskii *et al.*, 1976; Ku and Chapin, 1994; Ku *et al.*, 1991, 1993a, b; Lee *et al.*, 1976; National Toxicology Program, 1987; Silaev *et al.*, 1977; Treinen and Chapin, 1991). Rats were fed 9000 ppm boric acid in their chow for up to four weeks; the first testicular effect observed by light microscopy was inhibited spermiation (Treinen and Chapin, 1991). At similar dose levels over a one-week-period, rats were killed at 1, 2, 3, 4, and 7 days after exposure was begun, and several soft-tissue boron levels were measured and compared to bone and serum levels. Steady-state levels (12–40 μg B/g) were reached in 3 to 4 days; no accumulation of boron above plasma levels was observed in any tissue except for bone. Bone boron levels increased throughout the 7 days, reaching 40–50 μg B/g (Ku *et al.*, 1991). In a third study, rats were fed boric acid in their feed at 3000, 4500, 6000, and 9000 ppm for up to 9 weeks. Rats were sacrificed weekly and examined for multiple end points including serum and tissue boron levels, testis histology, weight, and sperm count. Inhibited spermiation was separated from atrophy based on dose, with inhibited spermiation observed at 3000- to 4500-ppm levels and atrophy at 6000 to 9000 ppm. Inhibited spermiation was reversible and atrophy was not (Ku *et al.*, 1993a). An *in vitro* study using several testicular cell culture systems was carried out to investigate possible mechanisms for boric acid reproductive toxicity. No effects on steroidogenic function were observed in the isolated Leydig cells. The most sensitive *in vitro* effect involved a reduction in DNA synthesis of mitotic/meiotic germ cells, and next was an effect on energy metabolism in Sertoli or germ cells (Ku *et al.*, 1993b). In addition to the three-generation rat study (Weir and Fisher, 1972), a mouse reproductive study utilizing the continuous breeding protocol has been reported (Fail *et al.*, 1991). Doses of 0, 1000, 4500, and 9000 ppm boric acid in the feed were utilized. No litters were obtained at 9000 ppm. All measured parameters, including fertility and litter size, were reduced at 4500 ppm. There were no differences from the controls noted for the 1000-ppm group during the 14-week continuous breeding period. The final litters from the 1000-ppm and control groups were allowed to mature and breed an F_2 litter. A decrease in the adjusted body weight of the F_2 was reported. In addition, a crossover mating trial was carried out which established the male as the affected sex (Fail *et al.*, 1991).

Developmental Toxicity   Developmental effects related to exposure to boric acid and inorganic borates have been reported in mice, rats, and rabbits (Heindel *et al.*, 1992; Price *et al.*, 1996a, b). Boric acid was dosed in the feed of Swiss mice at average doses of 248, 452, and 1003 mg boric acid/kg/day throughout gestation. Some maternal toxicity was reported at

all dose groups (mild renal lesions in the low-dose mice). A reduction in fetal body weight was observed in the mid-dose group, and increased incidence of resorptions and malformed fetuses was observed at the highest dose. Short rib XIII (a malformation) and an increased incidence of rudimentary or missing ribs at lumbar I (a variation) were also reported. The developmental NOAEL was 248 mg boric acid/kg/day (Heindel *et al.*, 1992). In Sprague Dawley rats, the average dose of boric acid in the feed was 78, 163, and 330 mg boric acid/kg/day (also throughout gestation). However, a higher dose, 539 mg boric acid/kg/day, was tested on gestational days 6 to 15 only. Maternal rats showed some toxicity at all doses except the lowest dose. A reduction in fetal body weight was observed at all doses. Prenatal mortality was increased at the 539 mg/kg dose. Fetal malformations were increased over controls at all doses except the lowest, with enlarged lateral ventricles of the brain and shortening of rib XIII the most frequent. The NOAEL for maternal toxicity was 78 mg boric acid/kg/day. The NOAEL for developmental toxicity in rats was not reached in this study (Heindel *et al.*, 1992). Two rat studies were conducted to elucidate the Heindel observation of enlarged lateral ventricles of the brain at the two highest doses, 330 and 539 mg boric acid/kg/day (Price *et al.*, 1994a, b). The first study was carried out at 0.8, 1.6, and 2.4% boric acid in the diet during gestation days 14–17, and showed that this was not a sensitive period for boric acid-induced ventricular enlargement (Price *et al.*, 1994a). The second study incorporated boric acid in the feed at 0.4, 0.5, 0.6, and 0.8% during gestation days 6–15, attempting to reproduce the effects reported by Heindel *et al.* and to demonstrate dose dependence. After adjusting for body weight effects, there were no significant dose-related enlarged lateral ventricles, either incidence or severity. Hydrocephaly was reported to be significant in the 0.8% group (2% in controls and 15% at the highest dose) (Price *et al.*, 1994b). In New Zealand White rabbits, the boric acid dose was delivered by gavage on gestation days 6–19 (Price *et al.*, 1994a). In this study, boric acid was provided at 62.5, 125, and 250 mg boric acid/kg/day. Maternal toxicity was observed only at the highest dose. At this high dose, significant prenatal mortality was reported (90% versus 6% in controls). Malformed fetuses were also increased at the highest dose, with defects being primarily cardiovascular (intraventricular septal defect). No significant maternal or developmental toxicity was reported at the lowest two doses. The NOAEL, for both maternal and fetal developmental effects, was 125 mg boric acid/kg/day. There has been significant interest in the increase in reduction of extra lumbar ribs and in whether a reduction of a "variation" is adverse or not (Moore, 1997). A recent study in rats (Narotsky *et al.*, 1998) has investigated this effect, utilizing two daily gavage doses of 500 mg boric acid/kg. This very high twice-daily gavage dose level was utilized in order to increase the incidence of rib skeletal changes for meaningful observation and to provide a methodology for studying the mechanism of these changes. In this study, Narotsky noted that the types of rib changes observed depend on the days of exposure during gestation and that the changes are specific for specific exposure days. Shortening or absence of rib XIII was observed in the gestation day (GD) 5–9 and the GD 6–10 exposure groups. About 90% of the fetuses had only six cervical vertebrae in the GD-9 exposure group, while the GD-10 exposure group showed missing thoracic and lumbar vertebrae in 60% of the fetuses. The findings of Narotsky *et al.* show the critical periods for axial development in the rat (at least at these high dose levels), and provide an experimental model for the study of rib and vertebral changes (Narotsky *et al.*, 1998).

Since a developmental NOAEL was not obtained in the original rat study (Heindel *et al.*, 1992), and the rat was found to be the most sensitive mammal (based on reduced fetal body weight), a second study was carried out (Price *et al.*, 1996b). This second study was carried out in the same laboratory as the first study and was designed to repeat the first study as closely as possible; but additional, lower-dose exposures were included in order to tightly bracket the NOAEL dose. The average oral doses reported in the feed were 19, 36, 55, 75, and 144 mg boric acid/kg/day. The upper two doses were identical to those from the previous study (Heindel *et al.*, 1992). This new study (Price *et al.*, 1996b) consisted of two phases, allowing for one group to survive for postnatal observations. The study was successful in reproducing the earlier skeletal effects at the overlapping doses and reported a developmental NOAEL for rats of 55 mg boric acid/kg/day on gestation day 20 and of 74 mg boric acid/kg/day on postnatal day 21. Some reversibility of skeletal abnormalities was also reported; the incidence of short rib XIII was increased at 76 mg/kg on gestation day 20. On postnatal day 21, short rib XIII was only increased at 144 mg/kg/day. Wavy ribs, however, were completely reversed by postnatal day 21 (Price *et al.*, 1996b). The data from this last study were utilized in the determination of a Benchmark Dose for boric acid in rats, which was reported to be 59 mg boric acid/kg/day, in good agreement with the reported NOAEL (Allen *et al.*, 1996). Blood boron concentrations from the animals used in the NOAEL study have been reported (Price *et al.*, 1997). Increasing dietary doses of boric acid were positively correlated with blood boron concentrations in pregnant rats. Blood boron concentrations of 1.27 ± 0.298 and 1.53 ± 0.546 µg boron/g blood were associated with the NOAEL of 55 mg boric acid/kg/day and the LOAEL of 75 mg boric acid/kg/day reported above, respectively.

62.3.2 ACCIDENTAL POISONINGS IN ANIMALS

62.3.2.1 Cattle

One should not become complacent in handling borates just because these materials are considered to be of low toxicity. A herd of 85 mixed-breed, 350- to 400-kg beef cows were allowed to forage in a recently harvested peanut field along the edge of which a bag of borate fertilizer had been inadvertently left. The fertilizer bag was completely torn apart and 26 cows subsequently died (Sisk *et al.*, 1988). Clinical signs were weakness, mild ataxia, general depression, and mild shivering in the neck, shoulder, and hindquarter muscles. Two cows

suffered seizures. Greenish diarrhea and dehydration were observed in most affected cattle before death. A group of Herford heifers was investigated for tolerance to elevated boron levels in drinking water (Green and Weeth, 1977). When given a choice, the heifers discriminated against concentrations greater than 29 ppm boron (added as borax) and rejected concentrations above 95 ppm. None chose boron water over tap water. The safe tolerance was not determined in this study, but was proposed to be between 40 and 150 ppm boron. In a study in yearling heifers, the boron status of cattle was found to correlate with plasma and urine concentrations (Weeth *et al.*, 1981).

62.3.2.2 Sheep

A study was designed to produce toxicosis in goats and to study blood and cerebrospinal fluid parameters at selected dose periods (Sisk *et al.*, 1990). Numerous blood factors were affected. There was evidence of CNS activity, including seizures.

62.4 TOXICITY TO HUMANS

A review of the health effects in humans from exposure to inorganic borates is available in which the purpose was to provide information to assist in risk assessment and in to provide helpful guidance for clinical judgment (Culver and Hubbard, 1996). The chronic "No Effect" levels for humans was reported to be about 1 g/day of boric acid (2.5 mg B/kg/day), and the chronic adverse effect level (based on anorexia, indigestion, and exfoliative dermatitis) was 5 mg B/kg/day.

62.4.1 ACUTE EXPOSURES IN INFANTS AND CHILDREN

Numerous instances of infant deaths from accidental poisonings and medical misuse have been reported in the early literature (Goldbloom and Goldbloom, 1953; Valdes-Dapena and Arey, 1962; Wong *et al.*, 1964). Dose–response data from these reports are difficult to obtain due to lack of information on the initial dose, as well as on the actual quantity absorbed and on complications from vomiting, plus the rapid excretion over time. Reported blood and urine boron levels must be evaluated carefully, considering the time lapse between intake and sampling.

Analytical values reported in the earlier literature tend to be significantly higher (by an order of magnitude) than values reported by current inductively coupled plasma analytical techniques. Most of the infant poisonings were due to accidental ingestion of boric acid solutions in hospitals (usually from mistaking saturated boric acid solutions intended for disinfectant use and using them in infant formulations instead of water). Also, 100% boric acid powders were used to treat diaper rash. Both of these use patterns have been discontinued, and the serious poisoning incidents have essentially disappeared. Reported symptoms included diarrhea, vomiting, erythema, exfoliation, desquamation of the skin, and central nervous system irritation.

A more recent incident in Malasia may or may not involve boric acid poisoning (Chao *et al.*, 1991a, b). An outbreak of food poisoning resulting in the deaths of 13 children in Malasia was attributed to aflatoxin or boric acid. In some countries in the Far East, boric acid is sometimes illegally used as a food preservative in noodles. All of the victims had consumed the same type of noodles. Boric acid (boron—current analytical methods do not report the boron chemical species) was found in the blood, urine, and liver of some patients, but the level was not reported. Boron would be found normally in all tissues at low levels. Aflatoxin, the likely cause, was found at toxic levels in the tissues of victims.

62.4.2 ACUTE EXPOSURES IN ADULTS

Recent reports indicate that acute boric acid accidental ingestions are not as serious as is indicated by some of the earlier literature. Two publications, summarizing borate poisoning experience from three national poison control centers, report that acute boric acid ingestions produce minimal or no toxicity, and that aggressive treatment is not necessary for most patients (Linden *et al.*, 1986; Litovitz *et al.*, 1988). At the Rocky Mountain Poison Control Center in 1983–1984, of 364 cases of boric acid exposure, there was only one fatality, and that was a suspected chronic exposure. No systemic effects were reported from the acute exposures, including four patients who had ingested 10 to 297 grams (Linden *et al.*, 1986). Of a total of 782 acute ingestions studied during 1981 to 1985 at two Poison Centers, no patients developed severe manifestations of toxicity. The most common symptoms were vomiting, abdominal pain, and diarrhea, with less frequent symptoms of lethargy, headache, lightheadedness, and pain. A half-life for boric acid was reported as 13.4 hours. Hemodialysis shortened the half-life (three patients). These authors suggest that aggressive treatment is not necessary in most patients (Litovitz *et al.*, 1988). A Japanese clinical report on one incident of ingestion of 21 g of boric acid concluded that hemodialysis was helpful and reported a serum half-life decrease from 13.46 hr to 3.76 hr. The total body clearance was 0.99 liter/hr and increased to 3.53 liter/hr by hemodialysis (Teshima *et al.*, 1992).

62.4.3 CHRONIC EXPOSURES IN INFANTS

Two reports of chronic borate toxicity in infants (Gordon *et al.*, 1973; O'Sullivan and Taylor, 1983) both involve borax and honey used on infant pacifiers as a soothing agent. These reports are reviewed by Culver and Hubbard (1996). The symptoms of chronic exposure are different than those described for acute exposures. Nine infants had suffered various seizure episodes; each had been exposed to the borax and honey pacifiers for more than four weeks. The seizures stopped when the honey and borax treatments were removed. The mean intake was calculated to be 98 mg boric acid/kg/day (Culver and Hubbard, 1996). Some vomiting and diarrhea were also involved.

62.4.4 CHRONIC EXPOSURES IN ADULTS

Some very high chronic borax and boric acid exposures over many years were reported as a result of an epilepsy treatment (Kliegel, 1980). Exposures were on the order of one to two grams per day. Symptoms included skin rash, indigestion, anorexia, exfoliative dermatitis, and alopecia. When the patients were removed from the borate treatments, the symptoms stopped and no remaining effects were noted. In one study involving adult males receiving 500 mg boric acid per day for 50 days, no adverse symptoms were reported (Wiley, 1904).

Occupation-related chronic exposures at considerably lower levels have also been reported. An extensive study of respiratory effects from sodium borate exposures over a 7-year period in a California mining operation has been described (Wegman *et al.*, 1994). No significant adverse effects from these exposures were reported. This study also evaluated acute sensory irritant effects (eye, nose, and throat). Most of the incidences reported were nasal irritation, but all three types of irritation were reported. Severity was rated on a 13-point scale, with zero equal to "not at all," 1 as "very little," 2 as "fairly little," 3 as "moderate," 4 as "pretty much," 5 as "a lot"-... 7 as "very much,"..., and 10 as "very, very much." Among all symptoms, 91% were reported as ≤3 and 96% were ≤4. Irritation was described as "moderate" for borate respiratory exposures (Wegman *et al.*, 1994). Because of the numerous reports of reproductive effects in animal studies, an epidemiology study was initiated at the same mining facility as the Wegman study above, utilizing the same exposure data (Whorton *et al.*, 1994a, b). The methodology involved both questionnaires and interviews and utilized the "Standard Birth Ratio" for statistical comparisons. The measured end point was "live births." No adverse reproductive effects were found. There was a nonstatistically significant excess of female offspring, which was subsequently reported to be *not* dose-related. A third study on the same workforce investigated the relationship of blood and urine boron content to dust exposure levels at the mine packaging and shipping facilities, where the exposures were the highest (Culver *et al.*, 1994a). Dust concentrations in the air ranged from 3.3 mg borax/m^3 to 18 mg borax/m^3. Mean blood boron concentrations varied from 0.11 to 0.26 µg/g, and mean urine concentrations ranged from 3.16 to 10.72 µg/mg creatinine. No increase in boron accumulation was observed during the course of the workweek. The highest worker exposure, which included both dietary boron and inhaled borate dust, was 0.38 mg boron/kg/day. The mean boron level measured for these workers was 0.26 µg boron/g blood. This value was reported to be a factor of 10 lower than corresponding boron blood values found in the rat and dog at NAOEL exposure levels (Culver *et al.*, 1994a).

There have been some epidemiology studies in Turkey comparing family birth rates in boron rich areas with those in lower-boron areas (Sayli *et al.*, 1998; Sayli, 1998; Tuccar *et al.*, 1998). Some village drinking waters are reported with boron levels as high as 29 ppm B. No evidence of reproductive toxicity was found in this population. Two Russian studies report adverse reproductive effects in humans, one from drinking-water exposures to 0.3 mg B/kg (Krasovskii *et al.*, 1976) and the other from occupational exposures to high boric acid dust concentrations (Tarasenko *et al.*, 1972). Both studies utilize a similar epidemiology study questionnaire that is not fully described, and insufficient details are reported to adequately evaluate the studies. Krasovskii reports a limited study on the sexual function of some men with no actual numbers reported. Tarasenko's study involves 28 men between the ages of 30 and 40 years who had worked at a boric acid plant for more than 10 years, and a control group of 10 men. They report a reduction in "sexual activity" (undescribed) and gave results of semen analysis on six men. The semen analysis (details not reported) showed reduced volume, fewer spermatozoa, and a lower percentage of motile sperm.

62.5 PHARMACOKINETICS

The pharmacokinetics of boric acid and inorganic borates have been reviewed previously in the literature (ECETOC, 1995; IPCS, 1998; Moore, 1997; Murray, 1998).

62.5.1 ABSORPTION

62.5.1.1 Oral Absorption

Boric acid and borates are reported to be 100% absorbed by the oral route in both animals and humans. Six adult men given 750 mg of boric acid in water solution excreted 94% of the dose in 96 hours (Schou *et al.*, 1984). Eight young adult males infused with 600 mg of boric acid excreted 98.7% of the dose in 120 hours; total clearance was 54.6 ml/min/1.73 m^2; and $t_{1/2}$ = 21 hr (Jansen *et al.*, 1984). In another experiment, 10 students who drank spa water containing 102 mg boron excreted 92% of the boron, in the urine within a 4-day period (Job, 1973). A 1-ml oral dose of borax solution was given orally to male Wistar rats (n = 20 per group) at eleven concentrations (0, 100, 200, 300, 400, 500, 600, 700, 800, 900, and 1000 mg boron/liter). Twenty-four-hour urine samples were analyzed and the reported recovery was 99.6±7.9% (Usada *et al.*, 1998). There was a linear correlation between dose and excretion (r-0.999) suggesting complete oral absorption. In the same study, a group of rats (n = 10) was dosed intravenously with borax at 0.4 mg boron/100 g of body weight. The following kinetic parameters were reported: absorption $t_{1/2}$ = 0.608 hr; elimination $t_{1/2}$ = 4.64 hr; total clearance = 0.359 ml/min per 100 g body weight. Serum boron concentrations also indicate that borate was rapidly and completely absorbed. This study suggests that borates are not strongly bound by body proteins or tissues, and that these materials are eliminated by glomerular filtration. A study with Sprague-Dawley rats reports a positive correlation between dietary boron concentrations and whole blood concentrations (Price *et al.*, 1997).

62.5.1.2 Dermal Absorption

Because of conflicting reports in the literature regarding the degree of absorption of borates through intact human skin, partially due to difficulties in analytical sensitivity in earlier studies, a recent study was conducted, utilizing both *in vivo* and *in vitro* methods. In addition, a sensitive inductively coupled plasma mass spectrometry analytical technique involving enriched boron-10 isotope was included (Wester *et al.*, 1998a, b, c). Results from the *in vivo* clinical study suggest that dermal absorption of boric acid, borax, and disodium octaborate tetrahydrate, in intact human skin, is low and is significantly less than the normal dietary intake. The *in vitro* results agreed best with the *in vivo* study when the available dose levels were equivalent. Another human study that also reports minimal dermal absorption involved 18 females and 4 males performing a Jazzercise™ routine on nylon carpet to which disodium octaborate tetrahydrate had been applied (Krieger *et al.*, 1996). Studies are needed to access dermal absorption in damaged skin. It is known from early reports of toxicity (including death) that significant absorption occurs from exposures through damaged skin, that is, burns, injuries, and extensive diaper rash (Goldbloom and Goldbloom, 1953; Pfeiffer *et al.*, 1945; Valdes-Dapena and Arey, 1962).

62.5.2 DISTRIBUTION

Boric acid is rapidly distributed throughout the body water in both animals and humans. The only tissue that appears to accumulate boron significantly above blood levels is bone. In humans, elevated levels in bone have been reported (Alexander *et al.*, 1951; Ward, 1987). In rats fed boric acid in the chow, boron was reported in bone at levels four times those in blood; all other tissues were not significantly different than blood (Ku *et al.*, 1991). Adipose tissue contained 20% of the level found in rat blood. In another rat study, steady-state tissue levels were obtained three to four days after dosing (Treinen and Chapin, 1991).

62.5.3 METABOLISM

Boric acid and borates are not metabolized beyond the boric acid structure B(OH$_3$). Metabolism in biological systems is not feasible due to the high-energy requirements of breaking the boron–oxygen bond (Emsley, 1989). However, boric acid (the primary chemical structure in dilute solution at physiological pH, whether boric acid or borax is ingested) does form reversible coordination bonds with many biological chemicals, particularly those with adjacent hydroxyl groups. Much of its biological activity is thought to arise from these types of complexes (Woods, 1994).

62.5.4 EXCRETION

Boric acid is excreted primarily in the urine in both animals and humans. In humans, the reported excretion half-life is between 13 and 21 hr (Jansen *et al.*, 1984; Litovitz *et al.*, 1988; Schou *et al.*, 1984; Teshima *et al.*, 1992). The elimination half-life reported for rats is 4.6 hr (Usada *et al.*, 1998).

62.6 BENEFICIAL EFFECTS OF BORIC ACID AND INORGANIC BORATES

It has been known since the 1920s that boron is a required nutrient for healthy plants. Its use in fertilizers is well known. More recently, numerous publications from the USDA Human Nutrition Research Center in Grand Forks, North Dakota have reported beneficial effects from dietary boron in both animals and humans (Hunt, 1994, 1998; Hunt and Neilsen, 1981; Nielsen, 1991, 1994, 1998). Reports on the nutritional essentiality for boron in animals have been published for frogs (Fort *et al.*, 1998, 1999) and for fish (Eckhert, 1998; Eckhert and Rowe, 1999; Rowe *et al.*, 1998). In both frogs and fish, low boron environments have led to death of the embryo at very early developmental stages. Typical of other nutritionally essential elements, the dose–response curves are U-shaped. Similar studies are underway in rats and mice (Lanoue *et al.*, 1998, 1999). Adverse effects on blastocyst development were observed in mice.

REFERENCES

Agency for Toxic Substances and Disease Registry (ATSDR) (1992). "Toxicological Profile for Boron." U.S. Department of Health and Human Services, Washington, DC.

Alexander, G. V., Nusbaum, R. E., and MacDonald, N. S. (1951). The boron and lithium content of humen bones, *J. Biol. Chem.* **192**, 489–496.

Allen, B. C., Strong, P. L., Price, C. J., Hubbard, S. A., and Daston, G. P. (1996). Benchmark dose analysis of developmental toxicity in rats exposed to boric acid. *Fund. Appl. Toxicol.* **32**, 194–204.

Bakke, J. P. (1991, 1992). "Evaluation of the Potential of Boric Acid to Induce Unscheduled DNA Repair Assay using the Male F-344 Rat," Study No. 2389-V500-91 and Amendment 1 to the original report. SRI International, Menlo Park, CA. (Unpublished report to U.S. Borax Inc.)

Benson, W. H., Birge, W. J., and Dorough, H. W. (1984). Absence of mutagenic activity of sodium borate (borax) and boric acid in the Salmonella preincubation test. *Environ. Toxicol. Chem.* **3**, 209–214.

Caujolle, F., Familiades, C., Souard, J., and Gout, R. (1962). Limite de tolerance du rat a l'acide borique. *Compt. Rend. Acad. Sci.* **254**, 3449–3451.

Chao, T. C., Maxwell, S. M., Lyen, K., Wang, D., and Chia, H. K. (1991a). Mass poisoning in Perak, Malaysia or the tale of the nine emperor gods and rat tail noodles. *J. Forensic Sci. Soc.* **31**, 283–288.

Chao, T. C., Maxwell, S. M., and Wong, S. Y. (1991b). An outbreak of aflatoxicosis and boric acid poisoning in Malaysia: A clinicopathological study. *J. Pathology* **164**, 225–233.

Chapin, R. E., and Ku, W. W. (1994). The reproductive toxicity of boric acid. *Environ. Health Perspect.* **102**(Suppl. 7), 87–91.

Culver, B. D., and Hubbard, S. A. (1996). Inorganic boron health effects in humans: An aid to risk assessment and clinical judgment. *J. Trace Elem. Exp. Med.* **9**, 175–184.

Culver, B. D., Shen, P. T., Taylor, T. H., Lee-Feldstein, A., Anton-Culver, H., and Strong, P. L. (1994a). The relationship of blood- and urine-boron to boron exposure in borax workers and the usefulness of urine-boron as an exposure marker. *Env. Health Perspect.* **102**(Suppl. 7), 133–137.

Culver, B. D., Smith, R. G., Brotherton, R. J., Strong, P. L., and Gray, T. M. (1994b). Boron. *In* "Patty's Industrial Hygiene and Toxicology" (G. Clayton and F. Clayton, eds.), Vol. 2, Part F, pp. 4411–4448. John Wiley & Sons, Inc., New York.

Dixon, R. L., Lee, I. P., and Sherins, R. J. (1976). Methods to assess reproductive effects of environmental chemicals: Studies of cadmium and boron administered orally. *Env. Health Perspect.* **13**, 59–67.

Dixon, R. L., Sherins, R. J., and Lee, I. P. (1979). Assessment of environmental factors affecting male fertility. *Env. Health Perspect.* **30**, 53–68.

Eckhert, C. D. (1998). Boron stimulates embryonic trout growth. *J. Nutr.* **128**, 2488–2493.

Eckhert, C. D., and Rowe, R. I. (1999). Embryonic dysplasia and adult retinal dystrophy in boron deficient zebrafish. *J. Trace Elem. Exp. Med.* **12**(3), 213–220.

Emsley, J. (1989). "The Elements," p. 32. Oxford University Press (Clarendon Press), New York.

European Center for Ecotoxicology and Toxicology of Chemicals (ECETOC) (1995). "Reproductive and General Toxicology of Some Inorganic Borates and Risk Assessment for Human Beings." Tech. Rep. No 63, ECETOC, Brussels.

Fail, P. A., Chapin, R. E., Price, C. J., and Heindel, J. J. (1998). General, reproductive, developmental, and endocrine toxicity of boronated compounds. *Repro. Toxicol.* **12**(1), 1–18.

Fail, P. A., George, J. D., Sauls, H. R., Dennis, S. W., and Seely, J. C. (1989). Effect of boric acid on reproduction and fertility of rodents. *Adv. Contracept. Delivery Syst.* **5**(3–4), 324–333.

Fail, P. A., George, J. D., Seely, J. C., Grizzle, T. B., and Heindel, J. J. (1991). Reproductive toxicity of boric acid in swiss (CD-1) mice: Assessment using the continuous breeding protocol. *Fund. Appl. Toxicol.* **17**, 225–239.

Fort, D. J., Propst, T. L., Stover, E. L., Murray, F. J., and Strong, P. L. (1999). Adverse effects from low dietary and environmental boron exposure on reproduction, development, and maturation in *Xenopus laevis*. *J. Trace Elements in Exp. Med.* **12**(3), 75–185.

Fort, D. J., Propst, T. L., Stover, E. L., Strong, P. L., and Murray, F. J. (1998). Adverse reproductive and developmental effects in *Xenopus* from insufficient boron. *Biological Trace Element Research* **66**(1–3), 237–260.

Goldbloom, R. B., and Goldbloom, A. (1953). Boric acid poisoning: Report of four cases and a review of 109 cases from the world literature. *J. Pediatrics* **43**, 631–643.

Gordon, A. S., Prichard, J. S., and Freedman, M. H. (1973). Seizure disorders and anemia associated with chronic borax intoxication. *Can. Med. Assoc. J.* **108**, 719–721; **108**, 724.

Green, G. H., and Weeth, H. J. (1977). Responses of heifers ingesting boron in water. *J. Animal Sci.* **45**(4), 812–818.

Hayworth, S., Lawlor, T., Mortelmans, K., Speck, W., and Zeiger, E. (1983). Salmonella mutagenicity test results for 250 chemicals. *Environ. Mutagen* **1**(suppl.), 3–142.

Heindel, J. J., Price, C. J., Field, E. A., Marr, M. C., Myers, C. B., Morrissey, R. E., and Schwetz, B. A. (1992). Developmental toxicity of boric acid in mice and rats. *Fund. Appl. Toxicol.* **34**, 266–277.

Hubbard, S. A. (1998). Comparative toxicology of borates. *Biological Trace Element Research* **66**(1–3), 343–357.

Hubbard, S. A., and Sullivan, F. M. (1996). Toxicological effects of inorganic boron compounds in animals: A review of the literature. *J. Trace Elements in Exp. Med.* **9**, 165–173.

Hunt, C. D. (1994). The biochemical effects of physiologic amounts of dietary boron in animal nutrition models. *Env. Health Perspect.* **102**(Suppl. 7), 35–43.

Hunt, C. D. (1998). Regulation of enzymatic activity; one possible role of dietary boron in higher animals and humans. *Biological Trace Element Research* **66**(1–3), 205–225.

Hunt, C. D., and Nielsen, F. H. (1981). Interaction between boron and cholecalciferol in the chick. *Trace Element Metabolism in Man and Animals* **4**, 597–600.

International Program on Chemical Safety (IPCS) (1998). "Boron." Environmental Health Criteria 204. World Health Organization, Geneva.

Jansen, J. A., Anderson, J., and Schou, J. S. (1984). Boric acid single dose pharmacokinetics after intravenous administration to man. *Arch. Toxicol.* **55**, 64–67.

Job, C. (1973). Resorption und ausscheidung von peroral zugefuhrtem Bor. *Zeitschrift fur augewandte Bader und Kleinaheilkunde* **20**, 137–142.

Kliegel, W. (1980). "BOR in Biologie, Medizin und Pharmazie." Springer-Verlag, Berlin, Heidelberg, New York.

Krasovskii, G. N., Varshavskaya, S. P., and Borisov, A. I. (1976). Toxic and gonadotropic effects of cadmium and boron relative to standards for these substances in drinking water. *Env. Health Perspect.* **13**, 69–75.

Krieger, R. I., Dinoff, T. M., and Peterson, J. (1996). Human disodium octaborate tetrahydrate exposure following carpet flea treatment is not associated with significant dermal absorption. *J. Exposure Anal. Env. Epidemiology* **6**(3), 279–288.

Ku, W. W., and Chapin, R. E. (1994). Mechanism of the testicular toxicity of boric acid in rats: In Vivo and In Vitro studies. *Environ. Health Perspect.* **102**(Suppl. 7), 99–105.

Ku, W. W., Chapin, R. E., Moseman, R. F., Brink, R. E., Pierce, K. D., and Adams, K. Y. (1991). Tissue disposition of boron in male Fischer rats. *Toxicol. Appl. Pharmacol.* **111**, 145–151.

Ku, W. W., Chapin, R. E., Wine, R. N., and Gladen, B. C. (1993a). Testicular toxicity of boric acid (BA): Relationship of dose to lesion development and recovery in the F344 rat. *Repro. Toxicol.* **7**, 305–319.

Ku, W. W., Shih, L. M., and Chapin, R. E. (1993b). The effects of boric acid (BA) on testicular cells in culture. *Repro. Toxicol.* **7**, 321–331.

Landolf, J. R. (1985). Cytotoxicity and negligible genotoxicity of borax and borax ores to cultured mammalian cells. *Am. J. Ind. Med.* **7**, 31–43.

Lanoue, L., Strong, P. L., and Keen, C. L. (1999). Adverse effects of a low boron environment on the preimplantation development of mouse embryos in vitro. *J. Trace Elem. Exp. Med.* **12**(3), 235–250.

Lanoue, L., Taubeneck, M. W., Muniz, J., Hanna, L. A., Strong, P. L., Murray, F. J., Nielsen, F. H., Hunt, C. D., and Keen, C. L. (1998). Assessing the effects of low boron diets on embryonic and fetal development in rodents using in vitro and in vivo model systems. *Biological Trace Element Research* **66**(1–3), 271–298.

Lee, I. P., Sherins, R. J., and Dixon, R. L. (1976). Evidence for induction of germinal aplasia in male rats by environmental exposure to boron. *Toxicol. Appl. Pharmacol.* **13**, 59–67.

Linden, C. H., Hall, A. H., Kulig, K. W., and Rumack, B. H. (1986). Acute ingestions of boric acid. *Clin. Toxicol.* **24**(4), 269–279.

Litovitz, T. L., Klein-Schwartz, W., Oderda, G. M., and Schmitz, B. F. (1988). Clinical manifestations of toxicity in a series of 784 boric acid ingestions. *Am. J. Emerg. Med.* **6**(3), 209–213.

Magour, S., Schramel, P., Ovcar, J., and Maser, H. (1982). Uptake and distribution of boron in rats: Interaction with ethanol and hexobarbital in the brain. *Arch. Environ. Contam. Toxicol.* **11**, 521–525.

McGregor, D. B., Brown, A., Cattanach, P., Edwards, I., McBride, D., Riach, C., and Caspari, W. J. (1988). Responses of the L5178Y tk-/tk- mouse lymphoma cell forward mutation assay: III. 72 coded chemicals. *Environ. Mol. Mutagen* **12**, 85–154.

Moore, J. A. (1997). An assessment of boric acid and borax using the IEHR evaluative process for assessing human developmental and reproductive toxicity of agents. *Repro. Toxicol.* **11**(1), 123–160.

Murray, F. J. (1995). A human health risk assessment of boron (boric acid and borax) in drinking water. *Regul. Toxicol. and Pharmacol.* **22**, 221–230.

Murray, F. J. (1996). Issues in boron risk assessment: Pivotal study, uncertainty factors, and ADI's. *J. Trace Elem. Exp. Med.* **9**, 231–243.

Murray, F. J. (1998). A comparative review of the pharmacokinetics of boric acic in rodents and humans. *Biological Trace Element Research* **66**(1–3), 331–342.

Narotsky, M. G., Schmid, J. E., Andrews, J. E., and Kavlock, R. J. (1998). Effects of boric acid on axial skeletal development in rats. *Biological Trace Element Research* **66**(1–3), 373–394.

National Toxicology Program (1987). Toxicology and Carcinogenesis Studies of Boric Acid (CAS No. 10043-35-3) in B6C3F Mice (Feed Studies). Technical Report No. 324, National Institute of Health. U.S. Department of Health and Human Services, Washington, DC.

Nielsen, F. H. (1991). The saga of boron in food: From a banished food preservative to a beneficial nutrient for humans. *Curr. Top. Plant Biochem. Physiol.* **10**, 274–286.

Nielsen, F. H. (1994). Biochemical and physiologic consequences of boron deprivation in humans. *Env. Health Perspect.* **102**(Suppl. 7), 59–63.

Nielsen, F. H. (1998). The justification for providing dietary guidance for the nutritional intake of boron. *Biological Trace Element Research* **66**(1–3), 319–330.

O'Loughlin, K. G. (1991). "Bone Marrow Erythrocyte Micronucleus Assay of Boric Acid in Swiss-Webster Mice," Study No. 2389-C400-91. SRI International, Menlo Park, CA. (Unpublished report to U.S. Borax Inc.)

O'Sullivan, K., and Taylor, M. (1983). Chronic boric acid poisoning in infants. *Arch. Disease in Childhood* **58**, 737–739.

Pfeiffer, C. C., Hallman, L. F., and Gersh, I. (1945). Boric acid ointment: A study of possible intoxication in the treatment of burns. *J. Am. Med. Assoc.* **128**(4), 266–274.

Price, C. J., Bates, H. K., Kebede, G. A., Marr, M. C., Myers, C. B., Heindel, J. J., and Schwetz, B. A. (1994a). "Final Report on the CNS Developmental Toxicity of Boric Acid (CAS #10042-35-3) in Sprague-Dawley CD Rats Exposed on Gestation Days 14–17," National Toxicology Program Report No. TER90123.

Price, C. J., Hunter, E. S., Shelby, M. D., and Schwetz, B. A. (1994b). "Final Report on the CNS Developmental Toxicity of Boric Acid (CAS #10043-35-3) in Sprague-Dawley CD Rats Exposed on Gestation Days 6–15," National Toxicology Program Report No. TER93138.

Price, C. J., Marr, M. C., Myers, C. B., Seely, J. C., Heindel, J. J., and Schwetz, B. A. (1996a). The developmental toxicity of boric acid in rabbits. *Fund. Appl. Toxicol.* **34**, 176–187.

Price, C. J., Strong, P. L., Marr, M. C., Myers, C. B., and Murray, F. J. (1996b). Developmental toxicity NOAEL and postnatal recovery in rats fed boric acid during gestation. *Fund. Appl. Toxicol.* **32**, 179–193.

Price, C. J., Strong, P. L., Murray, F. J., and Goldberg, M. M. (1997). Blood boron concentrations in pregnant rats fed boric acid throughout gestation. *Repro. Toxicol.* **11**(6), 833–842.

Rowe, R. I., Bouzan, C., Nabili, S., and Eckhert, C. D. (1998). The response of trout and zebrafish embryos to low and high boron concentrations is U-shaped. *Biological Trace Element Research* **66**(1–3), 261–270.

Sayli, B. S. (1998). An assessment of fertility in boron-exposed Turkish subpopulations: 2: Evidence that boron has no effect on human reproduction. *Biological Trace Element Research* **66**(1–3), 409–422.

Sayli, B. S., Tuccar, E., and Elhan, A. H. (1998). An assessment of fertility in boron-exposed Turkish subpopulations. *Repro. Toxicol.* **12**(3), 297–304.

Schou, J. S., Jansen, J. A., and Aggerbeck, B. (1984). Human pharmacokinetics and safety of boric acid. *Arch. Toxicol. Suppl.* **7**, 232–235.

Silaev, A. A., Kasparov, A. A., and Korolev, V. V. (1977). Ultrastructure of the spermatogenic epithelium following boric acid poisoning. *Gigiena Truda i Professionalnye Zabolevaniya* **2**, 34–37.

Sisk, D. B., Colvin, B. M., and Bridges, C. R. (1988). Acute, fatal illness in cattle exposed to boron fertilizer. *J. Am. Vet. Med. Assoc.* **193**(8), 943–945.

Sisk, D. B., Colvin, B. M., Merrill, A., Bondar, K., and Bowen, J. M. (1990). Experimental acute inorganic boron toxicosis in the goat: Effects on serum chemistry and CSF biogenic amines. *Vet. Hum. Toxicol.* **32**(3), 205–211.

Smyth, H. F., Jr., Carpenter, J. P., Weil, C. S., Pozzanni, U. C., Streigel, J. A., and Nycum, J. S. (1969). Range finding toxicity data: List VII. *Am. Ind. Hyg. Assoc. J.* **30**, 470–476.

Stewart, K. R. (1991). "Salmonella/Microsome Plate Incorporation Assay of Boric Acid," Study No. 2389-A200-91. SRI International, Menlo Park, CA. (Unpublished report to U.S. Borax Inc.)

Tarasenko, N. Y., Kasparova, A. A., and Strongina, O. M. (1972). Effect of boric acid on the generative function in males. *Gigiena Truda i Professionalnye Zabolevaniya* **11**, 13–16.

Teshima, D., Morishita, K., Ueda, Y., Futagami, K., Higuchi, S., Komoda, T., Nanishi, F., Taniyama, T., Yoshitake, J., and Aoyama, T. (1992). Clinical management of boric acid ingestion: Pharmacokinetic assessment of efficacy of hemodialysis for treatment of acute boric acid poisoning.

Treinen, K. A., and Chapin, R. E. (1991). Development of testicular lesions in F344 rats after treatment with boric acid. *Toxicol. Appl. Pharmacol.* **107**, 325–335.

Truhaut, R., Phu-Lich, N., and Lousillier, F. (1964). Sur les effets de l'ingestion repetee de petites doses de derives du bore sur les fonctions de reproduction du rat. *Compt. Rend. Acad. Sci.* **258**, 5099–5102.

Tuccar, E., Elhan, A. H., Yavuz, Y., and Sayli, B. S. (1998). Comparison of infertility rates in communities from boron-rich and -poor territories. *Biological Trace Element Research* **66**(1–3), 401–408.

United States Environmental Protection Agency (U.S. EPA) (1993). "Reregistration Eligibility Decision (RED) Boric Acid and its Sodium Salts," EPA 738-R-93-017, Washington, DC.

United States Environmental Protection Agency (U.S. EPA) (1998). "Boron. Integrated Risk Information System (IRIS)," Washington, DC.

Usada, K., Kono, K., Orita, Y., Dote, T., Iguchi, K., Nishiura, H., Tominaga, M., Tagawa, T., Goto, E., and Shirai, Y. (1998). Serum and urinary boron levels in rats after single administration of sodium tetraborate. *Arch. Toxicol.* **72**, 468–474.

Valdes-Dapena, M. A., and Arey, J. B. (1962). Boric acid poisoning; Three fatal cases with pancreatic inclusions and a review of the literature. *J. Pediatrics* **61**(4), 531–546.

Ward, N. L. (1987). The determination of boron in biological materials by neutron irradiation and prompt gamma-ray spectrometry. *J. Radioanalytical and Nuclear Chemistry* **110**(2), 633–639.

Weeth, H. J., Speth, C. F., and Hanks, D. R. (1981). Boron content of plasma and urine as indicators of boron intake in cattle. *Am. J. Vet. Res.* **42**(3), 474–477.

Wegman, D. H., Eisen, E. A., Xiaohank, H., Woskie, S. R., Smith, R. G., and Garabrant, D. H. (1994). Acute and chronic respiratory effects of sodium borate particulate exposures. *Env. Health Perspect.* **102**(Suppl. 7), 119–128.

Weir, R. J., and Fisher, R. S. (1972). Toxicologic studies on borax and boric acid. *Toxicol. Appl. Pharmacol.* **23**, 351–364.

Wester, R. C., Hartway, T., Maibach, H. I., Schell, M. J., Northington, D. J., Strong, P. L., and Culver, B. D. (1998c). Summary: In vitro percutaneous absorption of boron as boric acid, borax and disodium octaborate tetrahydrate in human skin. *Biological Trace Element Research* **66**(1–3), 111–120.

Wester, R. C., Hui, X., Hartway, T., Maibach, H. I., Bell, K., Schell, M. J., Northington, D. J., Strong, P. L., and Culver, B. D. (1998a). In vivo percutaneous absorption of boric acid, borax, and disodium octaborate tetrahydrate in humans compared to in vitro absorption in human skin from infinite and finite doses. *Toxicol. Sci.* **45**, 42–51.

Wester, R. C., Hui, X., Maibach, H. I., Bell, K., Schell, M. J., Northington, D. J., Strong, P., and Culver, B. D. (1998b). Summary: In vivo percutaneous absorption of boron as boric acid, borax and disodium octaborate tetrahydrate in humans. *Biological Trace Element Research* **66**(1–3), 101–110.

Whorton, D., Haas, J., and Trent, L. (1994a). Reproductive effects of inorganic borates on male employees: Birth rate assessment. *Env. Health Perspect.* **102**(Suppl. 7), 129–131.

Whorton, M. D., Haas, J. L., Trent, L., and Wong, W. (1994b). Reproductive effects of sodium borates on male employees: Birth rate assessment. *Occup. Env. Med.* **51**, 761–767.

Wiley, W. W. (1904). "Influence of Food Preservatives and Artificial Colors on Digestion and Health. 1. Boric Acid and Borax," Bulletin No. 84, Part 1, Bureau of Chemistry, U.S. Department of Agriculture, Washington, DC.

Wong, L. C., Heimbach, M. D., Truscott, D. R., and Duncan, B. D. (1964). Boric acid poisoning: Report of 11 cases. *Canad. Med. Assoc. J.* **90**, 1018–1023.

Woods, W. G. (1994). An introduction to boron: History, sources, uses, and chemistry. *Env. Health Perspect.* **102**(Suppl. 7), 5–11.

DEET

Gerald P. Schoenig

Toxicology/Regulatory Services, Inc.

Thomas G. Osimitz

S.C. Johnson and Son, Inc.

63.1 INTRODUCTION

DEET is a personal insect repellent that has been shown to repel biting flies, biting midges, black flies, chiggers, deer flies, fleas, gnats, horse flies, mosquitoes, no-see-ums, sand flies, small flying insects, stable flies, and ticks (U.S. EPA, 1998). In addition to its nuisance prevention value, DEET has public health benefits because of its efficacy against mosquitoes that can transmit malaria, yellow fever, denque fever, and encepholitis and ticks that carry Rocky Mountain Spotted Fever and Lyme Disease. DEET was first developed in 1946 for use by the military and was registered with the U.S. Environmental Protection Agency for use by the general public in 1957 (U.S. EPA, 1980). Unlike most pesticides, it has no food uses. DEET is applied directly to the human body and to clothing. It also is used to repel insect pests on cats, dogs, and horses and in pet living quarters.

DEET is sold in a variety of product forms including liquids (including pump sprays), pressurized and nonpressurized aerosols, formulated lotions, and impregnated materials (such as towelettes and wrist bands). Recently, products combining DEET with sunscreens have become available. The concentration of DEET in these products ranges from 4 to 100%. The most commonly used solvents in formulated products are ethanol and isopropanol.

DEET is used in approximately 21% of households in the United States, or by about 30% of the U.S. population annually (U.S. EPA, 1998). This corresponds to about 27% of adult males, 31% of adult females, and 34% of children.

63.2 CHEMISTRY

DEET (CAS Registry No. 134-62-3) is a member of the N,N-dialkylamide family of chemicals. Its chemical name is N,N-diethyl-m-toluamide. Its chemical structure is presented in Fig. 63.1. The empirical formula and molecular weight of DEET are $C_{12}H_{17}NO$ and 191.26 grams/mole, respectively.

Technical-grade DEET is a liquid with color ranging from water-white to amber and a faint characteristic odor. Its boiling point is 160°C at 19 mm Hg. The specific gravity at 20°C is 0.996 and its viscosity is 13.3 mPa/s at 30°C. The vapor pressure is 0.0017 and 0.0056 mm Hg at 20 and 25°C, respectively. The octanol/water partition coefficient (log K_{ow}) is 2.00 to 2.02. DEET is practically insoluble in water and glycerin, very soluble in alcohol, ether and benzene, and sparingly soluble in petroleum ether. DEET is miscible in most petroleum hydrocarbons, alcohols, chlorinated solvents, and cottonseed oil.

63.3 TOXICOLOGY

Toxicology data have been generated on DEET for the past 50 years. However, because the state of the art in toxicology testing has changed over these 50 years, most of the early studies do not meet current standards. As a result, during the reregistration process initiated by U.S. EPA (U.S. EPA, 1980), a new state-of-the-art safety database was developed by the major manufacturers and formulators of DEET. This work was conducted under the auspices of the DEET Joint Venture (DJV) and the Chemical Specialties Manufacturers Association (Washington, DC). The discussions presented below focus on the studies that were conducted as part of this comprehensive data development program. Other studies from the open literature are discussed briefly and referenced at the end of each section. All of the studies conducted by the DJV followed applicable U.S. EPA Testing Guidelines (U.S. EPA, 1984), where applicable, and were conducted in accordance with U.S. EPA Good Laboratory Practice Standards (40 CFR Part 160).

Even though the principal route of exposure in humans is dermal, most of the studies conducted by the DJV were conducted by the oral route of exposure. The reason the oral route of exposure was selected for many of these studies is because little or no toxicity can be demonstrated in laboratory animals at the maximum dose level that can be applied by the dermal route of exposure, i.e., 1000 mg/kg/day. Therefore, in order to

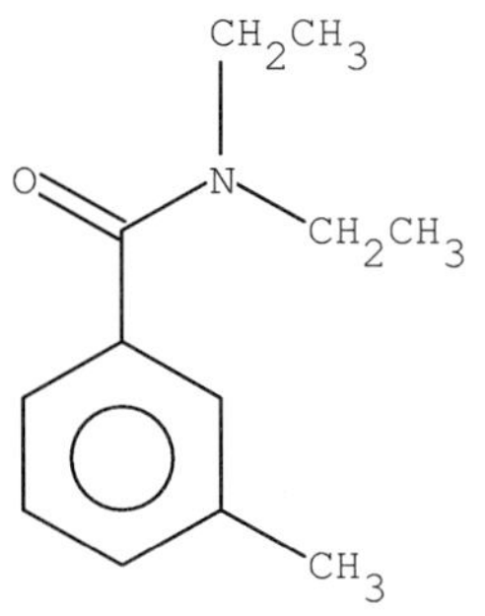

Figure 63.1 Molecular structure of DEET.

satisfy the criteria for evaluating a maximum tolerated dose, the oral route of exposure was selected in order to evaluate the critical endpoints of developmental effects, reproductive effects, neurotoxicity, chronic toxicity, and oncogenicity. The exposure pattern that most closely simulates human exposure, i.e., subchronic exposure, was evaluated by both the oral and dermal routes of exposure. The absorption, distribution, metabolism, and excretion of DEET also was examined by both of these routes of administration.

63.3.1 ACUTE TOXICITY STUDIES

Technical grade DEET has a low order of acute toxicity by the oral, dermal, and inhalation routes of exposure. In a recent set of full guideline GLP studies conducted on typical production grade DEET by one of the major DEET manufacturers (Moore, 2000), the rat oral LD_{50} was found to be 1892 mg/kg, the rat dermal LD_{50} was > 5000 mg/kg, and the rat 4-hr LC_{50} was > 2.0 mg/liter. In this same set of studies, technical grade DEET was shown to produce moderate erythema and edema to the skin of albino rabbits following a 4-hr occluded exposure. All skin irritation subsided within seven days. When instilled into the rabbit's eye, slight corneal opacity and slight to moderate conjunctive irritation in the form of redness, swelling, and discharge were observed. All ocular irritation cleared within seven days. In a skin sensitization study conducted using the Buehler method, no evidence of skin sensitization was observed.

The acute toxicity of DEET also is discussed in a number of publications in the open literature (Ambrose *et al.*, 1959; Macko and Weeks, 1980; Weil, 1973). The findings reported in these publications are consistent with those described above. In an acute oral toxicity study conducted in rats of different ages, it was shown that the acute oral LD_{50} of DEET increased four- to fivefold between the ages of 11 days and 47–56 days of age (Verschoyle *et al.*, 1992). Two publications describe findings in cats and dogs that were simultaneously administered DEET and fenvalerate, a combination of ingredients used in a commercial tick and flea spray (Dorman *et al.*, 1990; Mount *et al.*, 1991). Three other publications describe studies in which potential interactions between DEET, permethrin, and/or pyridostigmine were evaluated (Abou-Donia and Wilmarth, 1996; Chaney *et al.*, 1999; McCain *et al.*, 1995). The interest in this combination of chemicals arose from the fact that servicemen

in the Persian Gulf War potentially could have been exposed simultaneously to these chemicals. While the findings presented in these publications provide suggestive evidence for some sort of interaction between DEET and these other chemicals, the evidence for actual chemical synergy is far from conclusive. Also, because DEET was administered orally, subcutaneously or intraperitoneally at lethal or near lethal dose levels in the laboratory studies, the relevance of these findings to normal human exposure is limited.

63.3.2 SUBCHRONIC TOXICITY STUDIES

A number of subchronic studies were conducted as part of the DJV Data Development Program. These studies were conducted to develop data that could be used to select dose levels for longer term studies, to satisfy regulatory requirements for 90-day oral and dermal toxicity studies, to determine the palatability of DEET in the diet, to explore other ways of administering DEET orally when palatability in the diet was a problem, and to further address findings in other subchronic studies.

63.3.2.1 Rat 90-Day Dietary Toxicity (Johnson, 1987a)

This study was conducted in order to assess the potential for DEET to produce subchronic oral toxicity and to develop data that could be used to select dose levels for a rat two-generation reproduction study and a rat chronic toxicity/oncogenicity study. DEET was incorporated into the diet and administered to Charles River CD® rats at concentrations such that dose levels of 0, 100, 500, 1000, 2000, and 4000 mg/kg/day could be evaluated. Fifteen male and 15 female rats were evaluated at each level. Due to rejection of the treated diets and subsequent body weight depression and mortality, the 4000 mg/kg/day group was discontinued after 7 days. Animals in the remaining groups continued through to the end of the 90-day test period. At the dose levels that were evaluated for 90 days, no treatment-related clinical signs or effects on hematology, clinical chemistry, or gross pathology were observed. Decreased body weight and food consumption were observed at dose levels ≥500 mg/kg/day and signs of inanition were evident at 2000 mg/kg/day. Nonspecific liver weight increases without correlative microscopic findings occurred in all treatment groups except the 100 mg/kg/day females. Renal lesions were observed microscopically in males at all concentrations and included granular cast formation, multifocal chronic inflammation, regenerative tubular epithelium, and hyaline droplets. These renal lesions were considered to be reflective of α_{2u}-globulin induced nephropathy, a condition which is unique to certain strains of male rats (Goldenthal, 1992).

63.3.2.2 Mouse 90-Day Dietary Toxicity (Johnson, 1987b)

The purpose of this study was to develop data that could be used to select dose levels for an 18-month mouse oncogenicity study. DEET was incorporated into the diet and administered to Charles River CD®-1 mice at concentrations such that dose levels of 0, 300, 1000, 3000, 6000, and, 10,000 mg/kg/day could be evaluated. Fifteen male and 15 female mice were evaluated at each level. Due to rejection of the treated diets, the 6000 and 10,000 mg/kg/day dose groups were discontinued after two weeks. Animals in the remaining groups continued through to the end of the 90-day test period. At the dose levels that were evaluated for 90 days, no treatment-related clinical signs or effects on food consumption or gross pathological observations were noted in any dose group. Decreased defecation early in the study and decreased body weight gain were observed in animals in the 3000 mg/kg/day dose group. Absolute and relative liver weights were increased in both males and females at dose levels ≥1000 mg/kg/day and in females at 300 mg/kg/day. Multifocal hepatocellular hypertrophy was observed at a high incidence in males and females at 3000 mg/kg/day and at a lower incidence in females at 1000 mg/kg/day. The increased liver weights and the corresponding hypertrophy were considered to be adaptive changes rather than an indication of systemic toxicity. No other gross or microscopic changes were observed. Hematology and clinical chemistry evaluations were not included in this dose range-finding study.

63.3.2.3 Hamster 90-Day Dietary Toxicity (Goldenthal, 1989a)

This study was conducted to evaluate further the renal lesions observed in the rat 90-day dietary toxicity study and to develop data that could be used to set dose levels for a chronic toxicity/oncogenicity study in hamsters in the event that it was determined that the rat was not the most suitable animal model for evaluating chronic effects. DEET was incorporated into the diet and administered to Golden Syrian VAF/Plus® hamsters at 0, 1000, 5000, 10,000, and 15,000 ppm. Fifteen male and 15 female hamsters were evaluated at each dietary concentration. Clinical signs including labored breathing, decreased defecation, decreased activity, pale skin, and mortality were observed at 15,000 ppm. Decreased body weights and food consumption were observed in males at 5000 ppm and in males and females at ≥10,000 ppm. The testes and epididymides appeared smaller and decreased testis weights were observed at ≥10,000 ppm. These observations were accompanied by an increased incidence of tubular degeneration in the testes and an associated accumulation of cellular lumenal debris in the epididymides. Blood potassium levels were elevated at 15,000 ppm. No other effects on the hematological or clinical chemistry parameters were observed. The renal lesions observed in the rat 90-day dietary toxicity study were not observed in this study.

63.3.2.4 Dog Dietary Palatability Studies (Goldenthal, 1994a, 1994b, 1995a)

Three dog dietary palatability studies were conducted in order to determine the maximum concentration of DEET that dogs would consume as part of the diet and to develop data that potentially could be used to set dose levels for a chronic toxicity

study. The first study was two weeks in duration in which DEET dietary concentrations corresponding to 0, 300, 1000, 3000, and 10,000 ppm were evaluated. One male and one female dog were evaluated at each concentration. Clear evidence of diet rejection was observed at a dietary concentration of 10,000 ppm. The findings with regard to palatability at dietary concentrations ≤3000 ppm were inconclusive.

The second palatability study was eight weeks in duration and dietary concentrations of 0, 300, 1000, 3000, and 6000 ppm were evaluated. Two male and two female dogs were evaluated at each dietary concentration. Due to rejection of the treated diet, the dogs in the 6000 ppm dose group were administered diet containing DEET at a concentration of 4500 ppm during study weeks 4 and 5 and 3000 ppm during study weeks 7 and 8. Control diet was offered to dogs in this group during study weeks 3 and 6. No treatment-related clinical signs or effects on body weight, food consumption, hematology, clinical chemistry, organ weights, or gross or microscopic pathology were observed at dietary concentrations ≤3000 ppm. Clinical signs including thinness throughout the study and decreased activity during study weeks 3 and 5 were observed in all dogs in the 6000/4500/3000 ppm dose group. Decreased body weights and food consumption also were observed in this group throughout the study except during study weeks 3 and 6 when the control diet was administered. Food consumption by the dogs in this group was much lower when offered diet at 3000 ppm during study week 8 compared to that of the dogs offered diet at 3000 ppm throughout the study, indicating that these dogs had developed an aversion to the taste of the test substance by exposure to diets containing 6000 and 4500 ppm DEET. On the basis of the results of this study, it was determined that DEET does not produce toxicity in dogs when administered in the diet at concentrations up to 3000 ppm (approximately 75 mg/kg/day), while diets containing greater than 3000 ppm are not palatable to the beagle dog.

The third palatability study was three weeks in duration and evaluated dietary concentrations of 0 and 4000 ppm. Two male and two female dogs were evaluated at each level. Depressed food consumption, decreased body weight, decreased defecation, thin and/or dehydrated appearance, and emesis were observed in the 4000 ppm treatment group. The results of this study confirmed that the highest concentration of DEET in the diet that is palatable to dogs is 3000 ppm (approximately 75 mg/kg/day).

63.3.2.5 Dog Oral Toxicity Studies Using Gelatin Capsule Administration (Goldenthal, 1994c, 1995b, 1997)

Because palatability limited the dose level of DEET that could be administered in the diet to approximately 75 mg/kg/day (3000 ppm), three studies were conducted in order to determine if higher dose levels could be administered to dogs as bolus doses using gelatin capsules. In the first of these studies, DEET was administered daily as a single bolus dose, at levels of 0, 62.5, 125, 250, and 500 mg/kg/day for a period of two weeks.

One male and one female dog were evaluated at each dose level. Food was allowed *ad libitum*. No treatment-related effects on body weight or food consumption were observed. At 250 and 500 mg/kg/day emesis, ptyalism and nodding or twitching of the head and neck were observed occasionally. The male dog at 500 mg/kg also exhibited ptosis, ataxia, and convulsions. Clinical signs were observed shortly after dosing and the affected animals fully recovered shortly after their occurrence. No treatment-related clinical signs were observed at the two lower dose levels.

In the second gelatin capsule study, DEET was scheduled to be administered daily as a single bolus dose at levels of 0, 75, 125, 175, and 225 mg/kg/day for a period of eight weeks. Two male and two female dogs were evaluated at each dose level. Food was allowed *ad libitum*. At dose levels ≥125 mg/kg/day, emesis, ptyalism, abnormal biting and scratching, and abnormal head movements were observed in one or more animals in each group during the first five days of the study. Ataxia and ptosis also were observed in some dogs at 175 and 225 mg/kg/day. In addition, convulsions were observed following the first dose in a female dog in the 225 mg/kg/day dose group and following the third dose in a male dog in the 125 mg/kg/day dose group. Clinical signs occurred shortly after dosing, after which recovery was observed. Because of the unexpected nature and severity of the clinical signs, this study was terminated after five days.

The results of the first two gelatin capsule studies demonstrated that oral administration of DEET as a single bolus dose is not a suitable method of dose administration for a chronic toxicity study. Therefore, in a third study this procedure was modified by allowing the dogs access to food only for a 1-hr period prior to dose administration (thereby assuring that the dogs would not be receiving the bolus dose of DEET on an empty stomach) and dividing equally the daily dose into one morning and one afternoon dose. In addition to allowing a higher daily dose of DEET to be administered, this dosing procedure was considered to have the added advantage of more closely simulating the time frame of exposure humans receive under normal conditions of use. In this study, DEET was administered orally to beagle dogs via gelatin capsules at dosage levels of 0, 50, 100, 200, and 400 mg/kg/day for a period of eight weeks. Two male and two female dogs were evaluated at each dose level. No treatment-related clinical signs or effects on body weight, food consumption, hematology, clinical chemistry, organ weights, or gross and microscopic pathology were observed at dose levels of 50 and 100 mg/kg/day. Clinical observations including abnormal head movements and ptyalism were observed at 400 mg/kg/day. Ptyalism also was observed occasionally at 200 mg/kg/day. These effects generally were observed within 1 hr of dosing and were considered to be related to the administration of DEET. Additional treatment-related effects observed at 400 mg/kg/day included decreased body weight gain in dogs of both sexes, decreased food consumption for females, and a slight decrease in cholesterol levels for males. The results of this study demonstrated that the oral administration of DEET in divided daily doses via gelatin capsules in nonfasted dogs

offered advantages over dietary administration and represented an appropriate means of orally administering DEET in a dog chronic toxicity study. Oral dose levels of 0, 30, 100, and 400 mg/kg/day were selected for the 1-year chronic dog toxicity study.

63.3.2.6 Rat 90-Day Dermal Toxicity (Johnson, 1987c)

The purpose of this study was to evaluate the potential for DEET to produce toxicity by the dermal route of exposure in a definitive 90-day study. DEET was applied dermally to the shaven backs of Charles River CD® rats five days per week for 13 weeks at dosage levels of 0, 100, 300, and 1000 mg/kg/day. The 1000 mg/kg/day dose level represented the maximum dose of DEET that could be applied dermally without significant runoff. Fifteen male and 15 female rats were evaluated at each dosage level. Treatment-related effects included dermal irritation, body weight depression in males at the 1000 mg/kg/day dose level, and renal lesions that were observed in males at all dose levels. Microscopically, these lesions were described as granular cast formation, multifocal inflammation, regenerative tubular epithelium, and hyaline droplets. The dermal irritation was confirmed microscopically in the form of acanthosis and/or hyperkeratosis. The renal lesions were accompanied by elevated kidney weights and slightly increased urea nitrogen levels at 13 weeks at the 300 and 1000 mg/kg/day dose levels. Increased liver weights also were observed in male and female rats in the 1000 mg/kg/day dose level. No treatment-related clinical signs or effects on food consumption, hematology, or ophthalmology were observed in any of the treatment groups. As was the case in the 90-day oral toxicity study, the renal lesions observed in the male rats were attributed to $alpha_{2u}$-globulin nephropathy.

63.3.2.7 Micropig® 90-Day Dermal Toxicity (Goldenthal, 1991)

The purpose of this study was to evaluate the potential for DEET to produce toxicity by the dermal route of exposure in a nonrodent species and to develop data to demonstrate that the renal lesions observed in the rat 90-day oral and dermal toxicity studies do not occur in a nonrodent species. DEET was applied dermally to the shaven backs of Charles River micropigs® five days per week for 13 weeks at dosage levels of 0, 100, 300, and 1000 mg/kg/day. Four male and four female micropigs® were evaluated at each level. Parameters evaluated included observations for clinical signs, dermal irritation, body weight, food consumption (approximated), hematology, clinical chemistry, organ weights, and gross and microscopic pathology. With the exception of slight skin irritation at the application site in all treatment groups, no treatment-related effects were noted in this study. The grossly observed skin irritation was confirmed microscopically in the form of acanthosis and/or hyperkeratosis.

63.3.2.8 Subchronic Studies to Evaluate Further Male Rat Kidney Lesions

The findings from the rat 90-day oral and dermal toxicity studies discussed above indicated that DEET produces kidney lesions in male Charles River CD® rats that are characteristic of the renal lesions produced by a wide range of chemicals that induce $alpha_{2u}$-globulin accumulation in the epithelial cells of renal proximal tubules. These lesions were not observed in female CD® rats nor in animals of any other species in which 90-day toxicity studies were conducted. In order to investigate further the correlation between the renal findings observed in the rat subchronic toxicity studies and $alpha_{2u}$-globulin, two additional 90-day studies were undertaken by the DJV. The first study investigated renal effects of DEET in three different strains of male rats, two strains that produce $alpha_{2u}$-globulin and one that does not produce $alpha_{2u}$-globulin. The second study investigated the effect of castration on the renal toxicity of DEET to male rats. This study was of interest because the synthesis of $alpha_{2u}$-globulin is influenced by the level of circulating androgens.

Rat 90-Day Oral Toxicity: Multistrain Study (Goldenthal, 1992) DEET was incorporated into the diet and administered to three different strains of male rats such that dose levels of 0 and 400 mg/kg/day could be evaluated. The three rat strains utilized were CD®, Fischer 344, and NCI Black-Reiter (NBR). CD® and Fischer rats produce high levels of $alpha_{2u}$-globulin, while NBR rats do not produce $alpha_{2u}$-globulin. Ten male rats of each strain were evaluated at the 0 and 400 mg/kg/day dose levels. A limited set of parameters was evaluated, including clinical observations, body weight and food consumption measurements, kidney weight measurements, and gross and microscopic examination of the kidneys. Hematoxylin and eosin and Mallory–Heidenhain stained slides of the kidney of each rat were examined microscopically.

Treatment-related clinical findings in this study included slightly decreased body weights for CD® and NBR treated rats as compared with their respective control groups. In addition, slightly decreased food consumption was observed for treated CD® rats as compared with the CD® rat control group. An increase in microscopic kidney lesions, including granular cast formation (CD® only), chronic inflammation, regenerative tubular epithelium and hyaline droplets, was observed in the CD® and Fischer 344 rats but not in the NBR rats. The distribution of microscopic kidney lesions in the three strains of rats supports the correlation of DEET kidney toxicity in male rats with $alpha_{2u}$-globulin nephrotoxicity.

Castrated Rat 90-Day Dermal Toxicity (Goldenthal, 1989b) DEET was applied to the shaven backs of castrated Charles River CD® rats at dose levels of 0 or 1000 mg/kg/day. In addition, noncastrated CD® rats were administered DEET dermally at a dose level of 1000 mg/kg/day. Fifteen rats were evaluated in each dose group for parameters including clinical observations, dermal irritation, body weight and food consumption measurements, kidney weight measurements, and microscopic examination of the kidney. One kidney from each rat was processed for $alpha_{2u}$-globulin analysis by immunocytochemistry using the method described in Olson *et al.* (1987).

Microscopic examination of the kidney revealed renal lesions in both the castrated and noncastrated DEET-treated rats. These lesions included hyaline and granular cast formation, chronic inflammation, regenerative tubular epithelium, and hyaline droplets. The incidence and severity of these lesions was greater in the noncastrated treated group. No treatment-related lesions were noted in the castrated control group. Immunocytochemical techniques confirmed the presence of hyaline droplets containing $alpha_{2u}$-globulin in the kidneys of the noncastrated and castrated treated animals. No $alpha_{2u}$-globulin was observed in kidneys of the castrated control group. The results of this study showed that while castration reduced the renal effects of DEET, it did not completely eliminate them. The most likely explanation for the incomplete modulation of the renal effects by castration is that $alpha_{2u}$-globulin synthesis is regulated by other hormones besides androgens (Roy, 1973; Sippel *et al.*, 1975).

Conclusions Regarding Male Rat Kidney Lesions Considerable evidence currently is available to support the position that the renal lesions observed in male rats following DEET administration are associated with accumulation of $alpha_{2u}$-globulin. First, the microscopic changes that were observed are characteristic of the lesions produced by other chemicals that produce these effects via this mechanism. Second, the lesions were not observed in DEET treated female rats or in mice, hamsters, dogs, or micropigs of either sex. Third, it has been shown that castration modifies the response and that similar lesions are not observed in a strain of male rat that does not produce $alpha_{2u}$-globulin. It also was shown that $alpha_{2u}$-globulin was present in the hyaline droplets that occur in the renal tubule cells of DEET treated rats. Since $alpha_{2u}$-globulin induced nephropathy is not observed in humans, the renal lesions observed in male rats in several DEET studies are not considered to be relevant to human risk assessment. This position was supported by the U.S. EPA Risk Assessment Forum in 1991.

63.3.2.9 Subchronic Studies Referenced in the Open Literature

Three other studies in which the subchronic toxicity of DEET was evaluated by dietary incorporation in the rat (Ambrose *et al.*, 1959), by inhalation exposure in the rat (Macko and Bergman, 1980), and by oral gavage in the rabbit (Haight *et al.*, 1980) are described in the open literature. None of these studies comes close to meeting current testing standards and the findings, for the most part, are similar to those observed in the DJV studies.

63.3.3 TERATOLOGY STUDIES

63.3.3.1 Rat Teratology (Schoenig *et al.*, 1994)

Dose range-finding and definitive teratology studies were conducted with Charles River CD® rats. In both studies, DEET was administered undiluted by oral gavage on gestation days 6–15. Control animals received corn oil at the volume used in the highest dose group in each study. In the dose range-finding study, five mated female rats per group were evaluated at levels of 0, 62.5, 125, 250, 500, and 1000 mg/kg/day. In the definitive study, 25 mated female rats per group were evaluated at levels of 0, 125, 250, and 750 mg/kg/day. Parameters evaluated in both studies included observations for clinical signs, body weights, food consumption, maternal liver and gravid uterine weights, maternal ovarian and uterine exams, and fetal external examinations. In the definitive study, the fetuses also were given detailed internal soft-tissue and skeletal examinations.

In the dose range-finding study, maternal toxicity in the form of mortality, decreased body weights, decreased food consumption, hypoactivity, ataxia, prostration, unkempt appearance, urine stains, and perioral wetness was observed at 1000 mg/kg/day. No maternal effects were observed at levels below 1000 mg/kg/day and no evidence of developmental toxicity was observed at any dose. On the basis of these results, dose levels of 0, 125, 250, and 750 mg/kg/day were selected for the definitive study. In the definitive study, maternal toxicity, including mortality, decreased body weight gain, decreased body weights, decreased food consumption, hypoactivity, ataxia, decreased muscle tone, urine stains, foot splay, perinasal encrustation, perioral wetness, and increased liver weights, was observed at 750 mg/kg/day. Remarkably, the only fetotoxic effect at this clearly toxic maternal dose level was a reduction in fetal body weights per litter. The incidence of external, visceral, and skeletal variations and/or malformations were comparable in the control and treatment groups.

63.3.3.2 Rabbit Teratology (Schoenig *et al.*, 1994)

Dose range-finding and definitive teratology studies were conducted in female New Zealand White rabbits. In both studies, DEET was administered undiluted by oral gavage on gestation days 6–18. Control animals received corn oil at the volume used in the highest dose group in each study. In the dose range-finding study, five mated female rabbits per group were evaluated at levels of 0, 62.5, 125, 250, 500, and 1000 mg/kg/day. In the definitive study, 16 mated female rabbits per group were evaluated at levels of 0, 30, 100, and 325 mg/kg/day. Parameters evaluated in both studies included observations for clinical signs, body weights, food consumption, maternal liver and gravid uterine weights, maternal ovarian and uterine exams, and fetal external examinations. In the definitive study, the fetuses also were given detailed internal soft-tissue and skeletal examinations.

In the dose range-finding study, clinical signs of maternal toxicity in the form of mortality, hypoactivity, ataxia, slow or rapid respiration, and gasping were observed at 1000 mg/kg/day. Mortality and rapid respiration also were noted at 500 mg/kg/day and rapid respiration was observed at 250 mg/kg/day. Decreased body weight gain and food consumption were observed at ≥500 mg/kg/day. There were no signs of maternal toxicity at 125 mg/kg/day and below and no signs of fetotoxicity or developmental toxicity at any dose level. On the basis of these results, dose levels of 0, 30, 100, and 325 mg/kg/day were selected for the definitive study. Maternal toxicity in the form of decreased body weight gain and food consumption was observed in the 325 mg/kg/day group. No evidence of fetotoxicity was observed and the incidence of external, visceral, and skeletal variations and/or malformations were comparable in the control and treatment groups.

63.3.3.3 Teratology Studies Referenced in the Open Literature

Four other developmental toxicity studies are described in the open literature. Three of these studies were conducted in rats by the oral (Sterner, 1977), dermal (Gleiberman *et al.*, 1975), and subcutaneous (Wright *et al.*, 1992) routes of administration, respectively. The fourth study was conducted in rabbits by the dermal route of administration (Angerhofer and Weeks, 1980). None of these studies came close to meeting today's standards for developmental toxicity studies. While no increases in malformations or variations were described, evidence of fetotoxicity at maternally toxic doses was noted in three studies (Angerhofer and Weeks, 1980; Gleiberman *et al.*, 1975; Sterner, 1977).

63.3.4 REPRODUCTIVE TOXICITY STUDIES

63.3.4.1 Rat Two-Generation Reproduction Study (Schardein, 1989)

A two-generation reproduction study was conducted in Charles River CD® rats. DEET was incorporated into the diet and administered to the rats at concentrations of 0, 500, 2000, and 5000 ppm. The F_0 parental generation consisted of 28 males and 28 females per group which were administered treated or control diet for at least 80 days prior to mating. Twenty-eight male and 28 female offspring per group from the F_1 generation were selected randomly to become the parents of the F_2 generation. These animals were treated for at least 93 days prior to mating. For both parental groups, treatment was continued through gestation and lactation. Parameters evaluated in the parental rats included observations for clinical signs, body weight and food consumption measurements, gross necropsy, and microscopic examination of gross lesions and reproductive tract organs. Reproductive and litter parameters that were evaluated included male and female fertility indices, events at parturition, gestation duration, litter size, numbers of viable and stillborn pups, and pup survival and growth during lactation.

Parental toxicity in the form of decreased body weight and food consumption was noted for males and females in the F_0 and F_1 generations at 5000 ppm, and decreased body weight was noted for males in the F_0 generation at 2000 ppm. A slight increase in hair loss was observed in the F_0 and F_1 females at 5000 ppm. In the F_1 adult males, kidney lesions including mottled kidneys, hyaline droplets, chronic inflammation, regenerative tubules, and renal granular cast formation were observed. These kidney effects occurred in a dose-related manner in all treatment groups and were characteristic of $alpha_{2u}$-globulin nephropathy. No other treatment-related effects were observed in the parental generations at 500 ppm. Neonatal toxicity as evidenced by reduced pup sizes and weights in both generations was noted for males and females in the 5000 ppm group. No treatment-related effects were observed in pups at ≤2000 ppm. No treatment-related effects on reproduction or fertility were observed at any of the dose levels evaluated in this study.

63.3.4.2 Reproductive Toxicity Studies Referenced in the Open Literature

Three other nonguideline, non-GLP studies that address reproductive toxicity are described in the open literature. One study was a subchronic study conducted in rats by the subcutaneous route of exposure that was designed to evaluate dominant lethal effects and male fertility (Wright *et al.*, 1992). A second was a rat subchronic inhalation study in which testicular weights and sperm morphology were evaluated (Macko and Bergman, 1980). The third was a rat subchronic dermal toxicity study in which sperm morphology was evaluated (Brusick, 1980). An increase in the incidence of abnormal sperm was reported in the latter two studies; however, the evidence for this finding is very weak.

63.3.5 CHRONIC TOXICITY AND ONCOGENICITY STUDIES

63.3.5.1 Dog Chronic Toxicity (Schoenig *et al.*, 1999)

DEET was administered orally for one year to purebred beagle dogs via gelatin capsules at 0, 30, 100, and 400 mg/kg/day. The daily dose of DEET was divided equally into two doses administered in the morning and afternoon following a 1-hr period of food availability. Four male and four female dogs were evaluated at each dose level. Parameters evaluated in this study included observations for clinical signs, body weight and food consumption measurements, hematology, clinical chemistry, urinalysis, ophthalmology, organ weights, and gross and microscopic pathology. Treatment-related effects were observed only in the 400 mg/kg/day group and included emesis, ptyalism, decreased body weights, and decreased food consumption for both males and females. One male in the 400 mg/kg/day group also exhibited occasional ataxia, tremors, abnormal head movements, and convulsions. These clinical signs generally occurred shortly after dosing and were followed by complete recovery before the succeeding dose. Other treatment-related effects observed in the 400 mg/kg/day group included transient reduction

in hemoglobin and hematocrit levels, increased alkaline phosphatase levels (males only), decreased cholesterol levels, and increased potassium levels (males only).

63.3.5.2 Mouse Oncogenicity Study (Schoenig *et al.*, 1999)

DEET was incorporated into the diet and administered for 78 weeks to Charles River CD®-1 mice at concentrations such that dose levels of 250, 500, and 1000 mg/kg/day could be evaluated. Sixty male and 60 female mice were evaluated at each dose level. In addition, two independent untreated control groups, each consisting of 60 male and 60 female mice, were included in the study. Parameters evaluated included observations for clinical signs and palpable masses, measurements, of body weight and food consumption, hematology, organ weight measurements, and gross and microscopic pathology. A slight decrease in body weight and food consumption was noted at the 1000 mg/kg/day dose level and an increase in liver weights was noted in male and female mice at 500 and 1000 mg/kg/day. The liver weight increases were considered to be adaptive in nature, since no corroborative microscopic findings were observed. No other treatment-related effects were observed and DEET administration had no effect on survival or tumor incidence.

63.3.5.3 Rat Chronic Toxicity/Oncogenicity (Schoenig *et al.*, 1999)

DEET was incorporated into the diet and administered for two years to Charles River CD® rats at dietary concentrations such that dosage levels of 10, 30, and 100 mg/kg/day for males and 30, 100, and 400 mg/kg/day for females could be evaluated. Lower dosage levels were selected for the males because it was felt that $alpha_{2u}$-globulin induced renal lesions that were observed in male rats in the subchronic toxicity studies would jeopardize survival of the male rats at dose levels above 100 mg/kg/day. Sixty male and 60 female rats were evaluated at each dose level. In addition, two independent untreated control groups were included, each consisting of 60 male and 60 female rats. Parameters evaluated included observations for clinical signs and palpable masses, body weight and food consumption measurements, hematology, clinical chemistry, urinalysis, ophthalmology, organ weight measurements, and gross and microscopic pathology.

Decreased body weight and food consumption and slightly increased cholesterol levels were observed in the female rats at 400 mg/kg/day. No other treatment-related effects were noted and DEET administration did not have any effect on survival or tumor incidence.

63.3.5.4 Chronic Toxicity/Oncogenicity Studies Referenced in the Open Literature

Two other chronic toxicity/oncogenicity studies are reported in the open literature. In one of these studies, DEET was applied dermally to mice for 120 weeks (Stenbäck, 1976). In the other,

DEET was applied dermally to the ears of rabbits for 95 weeks (Stenbäck, 1976). No treatment-related increase in tumors was observed in either study. Both studies had many major deficiencies relative to today's standards for conducting chronic toxicity/oncogenicity studies.

63.3.6 NEUROTOXICITY STUDIES

63.3.6.1 Acute Neurotoxicity Study (Schoenig *et al.*, 1993)

The neurotoxicity potential of DEET was evaluated in Charles River Crl:CD® VAF/Plus® rats. A single dose of undiluted DEET was administered by oral gavage at dose levels of 0, 50, 200, or 500 mg/kg and the rats were observed for 14 days following dose administration. These dose levels were selected on the basis of findings in a dose range-finding study in which mortality was observed at a dose level of 1000 mg/kg and pharmacotoxic signs were evident at dose levels of 500 and 1000 mg/kg. Ten male and 10 female rats were evaluated at each dose level. Parameters evaluated included observations for clinical signs and measurements of body weight and food consumption. In addition, functional observational battery (FOB), thermal response test, and motor activity measurements were made at 1 hr, 24 hr, and 14 days following dose administration. No clinical signs of toxicity were observed in any animals and there were no treatment-related effects on body weight or food consumption. No effects related to DEET exposure were observed in the FOB. Animals in the 500 mg/kg dose group exhibited an increased response time to heat in the thermal response test and slightly decreased rearing activity in the motor activity test. These effects occurred in animals of both sexes at the 1-hr post-treatment observation interval but were not observed at 24 hr or 14 days post-treatment. No other treatment-related effects were observed during this study.

63.3.6.2 Chronic Neurotoxicity Study (Schoenig *et al.*, 1993)

The neurotoxicity potential of DEET was evaluated following multigeneration plus chronic administration. The animals used in this study were second generation (F_2) offspring from the rat multigeneration reproductive toxicity study in which DEET was administered continuously over two generations at dietary concentrations of 0, 500, 2000, and 5000 ppm. The dietary concentration of 5000 ppm meets the criteria for a maximum tolerated dose (MTD) based upon traditional chronic toxicology assessments. Following weaning, all control offspring and two male and two female F_2 generation pups from 21 to 25 litters per treatment group were selected and maintained on the treated diets for an additional 9 months. During the 9-month dietary administration period, the rats were observed for clinical signs, and body weight and food consumption measurements were made. At the end of this 9-month period, one male and one female from each of 20 litters were selected for the neurotoxicity evaluations. An additional control group of the 10 males and 10

females was selected from the rats maintained on basal diet for use as a sham group in the passive avoidance test. Neurotoxicity evaluations included a functional observational battery, motor activity testing, M-water maze, acoustic startle habituation, and passive avoidance. In addition, comprehensive neuropathological examinations were performed on 1 male and 1 female from each of 10 litters per group. The following tissues were included in this neuropathological examination: forebrain, center of cerebrum, midbrain, cerebellum, pons, medulla oblongata, proximal sciatic nerve, sural nerve, tibial nerve, spinal cord at cervical swelling (C_3–C_6) and lumbar swelling (L_1–L_4), gasserian ganglia, dorsal root ganglia (C_3–C_6, L_1–L_4), and dorsal and ventral root fibers (C_3–C_6, L_1–L_4). At the time that these neurotoxicity evaluations were performed, all animals were approximately 40 weeks of age.

No clinical signs of toxicity were noted throughout the 9-month dietary administration period; however, decreased body weights relative to the control animals were observed for all treatment groups. These findings were somewhat unexpected at 500 and 2000 ppm, since decreased body weights in the original multigeneration study were observed only at 5000 ppm. The decreased body weights at 500 and 2000 ppm may have been due to random selection of the animals at study start, since the treatment groups were not balanced with respect to animal weight at the time of selection. In the in-life neurotoxicity evaluation, the only treatment-related finding was a transient increase in exploratory locomotor activity at 5000 ppm. Equivocal findings were noted in the M-water maze, in which a decrease in initial choice accuracy on reversal was observed in all of the treated groups as compared with the controls. However, the effect was not dose-dependent, and no confirmatory evidence was found for a DEET-related reversal learning effect on response times and total errors, which are the primary measures of performance recorded for this task. Therefore, this finding was not considered to be adequate evidence of an effect of DEET on learning. No treatment-related effects were observed in the comprehensive neuropathological examinations performed on the central and peripheral nervous tissues. Since the only potential neurotoxic effect that was observed in this study was observed at 5000 ppm, a dose level at which other toxic effects have been observed, the results of this study demonstrate that the nervous system does not appear to be a selective target when DEET is administered chronically at dose levels up to and including the MTD. In addition, the results of this study demonstrate that the chronic administration of DEET at a MTD dose does not result in any morphologic changes in the tissues of the nervous system.

63.3.6.3 Studies Referenced in the Open Literature that Describe Neurotoxic Effects in Laboratory Animals

Six other studies that describe neurotoxic effects associated with DEET administration are described in the open literature. One study is an acute inhalation study conducted in rats (Sherman, 1980). A second is an acute oral toxicity study in rats

(Verschoyle *et al.*, 1992). A third is a subchronic inhalation study in rats (Macko and Bergman, 1980). The fourth is a sub-chronic oral toxicity study conducted in rats (Campbell, 1986). The fifth is a developmental toxicity study conducted in rats by the subcutaneous route of administration (Wright *et al.*, 1992). The sixth is a study designed to evaluate dominant lethal effects and male fertility in which DEET was administered subcutaneously to male rats (Wright *et al.*, 1992). None of these studies came close to meeting current standards for neurotoxicity testing and most reported effects were observed at lethal or near lethal dose levels.

63.3.7 GENOTOXICITY STUDIES

63.3.7.1 *Salmonella*/Mammalian-Microsome Plate Incorporation Assay (Ames Test) (San and Schadly, 1989)

Five strains of *Salmonella typhimurium*, TA98, TA100, TA1535, TA1537, and TA1538, were used. Each strain was tested in the presence and absence of metabolic activation by a rat liver S-9 system induced with Aroclor 1254. The concentrations of DEET evaluated in these studies (with and without metabolic activation) ranged from 278 to 8333 µg/plate. Mutagenic frequency did not increase in any of the tester strains. Results from the initial assay were confirmed in an independent repeat assay.

63.3.7.2 Chromosomal Aberrations in Chinese Hamster Ovary Cells (Putman and Morris, 1989)

This assay was conducted in Chinese Hamster Ovary cells in the presence and absence of metabolic activation with a rat liver S-9 fraction after induction by Aroclor 1254. In the absence of metabolic activation, the concentrations of DEET evaluated were 0.063, 0.125, 0.25, 0.5, and 1 µl/ml while, with activation, the concentrations of DEET evaluated were 0.032, 0.063, 0.125, 0.25, and 0.5 µl/ml. No increase in chromosomal aberrations was observed with or without metabolic activation.

63.3.7.3 Unscheduled DNA Synthesis in Rat Primary Hepatocytes (Curren, 1989)

This assay was conducted in rat primary hepatocytes. DEET concentrations of 0.003, 0.01, 0.03, 0.1, and 0.2 µl/ml were evaluated in an initial assay and DEET concentrations of 0.01, 0.03, 0.1, 0.2, and 0.3 µl/ml were evaluated in a confirmatory assay. No increase in DNA synthesis was observed in either assay.

63.3.7.4 Genotoxicity Studies Referenced in the Open Literature

One study evaluated reverse gene mutation in *Salmonella typhimurium* (Zeiger *et al.*, 1992) and two studies evaluated both reverse gene mutation in *Salmonella typhimurium* and *Saccharomyces cerevisiae* (Brusick, 1976; Macko and Weeks, 1980).

A dominant lethal assay in Swiss white mice is reported by Swentzel (1978). No significant activity was observed in any of these studies

63.3.8 PHARMACOKINETIC STUDIES

63.3.8.1 Absorption, Distribution, Metabolism, and Excretion in Rats (Schoenig *et al.*, 1996)

Absorption, distribution, metabolism, and excretion (ADME) was evaluated in Charles River CD® rats following oral or dermal administration of [^{14}C]DEET. Six experiments were conducted using separate treatment groups, each consisting of five male and five female rats. Four experiments involved the evaluation of ADME patterns following administration of [^{14}C]DEET orally as a single low dose of 100 mg/kg, orally as a single high dose of 500 mg/kg, orally as a single low dose following 13 days of oral dosing at 100 mg/kg/day with nonradiolabeled DEET, and dermally as a single low dose of 100 mg/kg. Urine and feces were collected over a 7-day post-treatment period, after which the animals were humanely sacrificed and selected tissues and organs were harvested. Urine, feces, and tissues were analyzed for ^{14}C content and the major urinary metabolites were identified. The remaining two experiments examined the distribution of radioactivity in tissues of animals humanely sacrificed at peak ^{14}C blood levels after receiving a single dose of 100 mg/kg [^{14}C]DEET by the oral or dermal route of administration.

In the three experiments designed to determine the ADME patterns of DEET after oral administration, 85 to 91% of administered radioactivity was found in the urine and 3 to 5% was found in the feces. Quantitatively, the overall amount of radioactivity excreted into the urine and feces was similar for males and females in the three groups, but the rate at which radioactivity appeared in the urine differed significantly between the three dosing regimens. The fastest rate of excretion of radioactivity into the urine was observed in the rats that received the repeated oral low dose, followed by the single oral low dose and the single oral high dose groups. This pattern of excretion suggests that the rate of excretion is closely related to the rate of metabolism and that repeated dose administration induces the enzymes responsible for the metabolism of DEET.

In the group of rats that received the dermal low dose, 74 to 78% of administered radioactivity was found in the urine and 4 to 7% was found in the feces, with an additional 6.5% found on the skin surface at the application site or associated with the occlusive enclosure. Slightly less radioactivity was recovered in the urine and slightly more was recovered in the feces for females than for males in this dosing regimen. Overall, the rate of excretion of radioactivity into the urine and feces was much slower after dermal administration than after any of the oral dosing regimens.

Total tissue residues of ^{14}C activity at 7 days post-treatment ranged from 0.15 to 0.67% of administered radioactivity for all four dosage regimens. At peak ^{14}C blood levels (0.5 hr for males and 2 hr for females), the percent of administered radioactivity reaching systemic circulation and the tissues was much higher for animals administered [^{14}C]DEET orally than for animals administered [^{14}C]DEET dermally. In both cases, the only tissues with ^{14}C residues consistently higher than plasma ^{14}C residues were the liver, kidney, and fat.

DEET was metabolized completely in all treatment groups, with little or no parent compound excreted in the urine. Two major urinary metabolites were identified in the urine by mass spectroscopy as *m*-[(*N*,*N*-diethylamino)carbonyl]benzoic acid and *m*-[(ethylamino)carbonyl]benzoic acid. Both metabolites involved oxidation of the aromatic methyl substituent in the DEET molecule to a carboxylic acid moiety. In addition, one of the metabolites also had undergone *N*-dealkylation of an ethyl substituent on the amide moiety. Based upon the metabolites observed, a metabolic pathway was proposed for DEET as shown in Fig. 63.2.

63.3.8.2 Absorption, Metabolism, and Excretion in Humans (Selim *et al.*, 1995)

The absorption, metabolism, and excretion of DEET following dermal application of [^{14}C]DEET to male human volunteers was evaluated. DEET was applied to the forearm of two groups of six volunteers either as the undiluted technical grade material or as a 15% (w/w) solution in ethanol. The material was left in contact with the skin for 8 hr and then rinsed off the skin. Serial blood samples and all urine and feces were collected for 5 days after application. The application sites also were stripped with

tape at 1, 23, and 45 hr following rinsing. All samples collected were analyzed for total radioactivity. Urine samples also were analyzed by HPLC for metabolite characterization.

Absorption of DEET as evidenced by the appearance of radioactivity in the plasma occurred within 2 hr after dermal dose administration. Elimination of radioactivity from the plasma was rapid, with measurable levels of radioactivity remaining in the plasma only up to 4 hr after the application period. Most of the excreted radioactivity was found in the urine, with an average recovery of 5.61 and 8.33% of the applied dose in the undiluted DEET and 15% DEET in ethanol groups, respectively. Less than 0.08% of the applied dose was recovered in the feces in both groups. Total excretion in the urine and feces of applied radioactivity ranged from 3 to 8% with a mean of 5.6% in the volunteers that applied undiluted DEET and from 4 to 14% with a mean of 8.4% in the volunteers that applied 15% DEET in ethanol. The recovery of radioactivity in the tape strips was very low, indicating that DEET did not accumulate in the superficial layers of the skin. Most of the applied radioactivity was recovered in the skin rinses. Absorbed DEET was metabolized completely and six major metabolites were observed in the urine. Based upon a comparison of their HPLC retention times with the two major rat urinary metabolites, the two human urinary metabolites tentatively were identified as *m*-[(*N*,*N*-diethylamino)carbonyl]benzoic acid and *m*-[(ethylamino)carbonyl]benzoic acid. The results of this study showed that DEET is absorbed slowly and excreted rapidly when applied to human skin. It also shows that DEET is metabolized completely prior to urinary excretion and that the

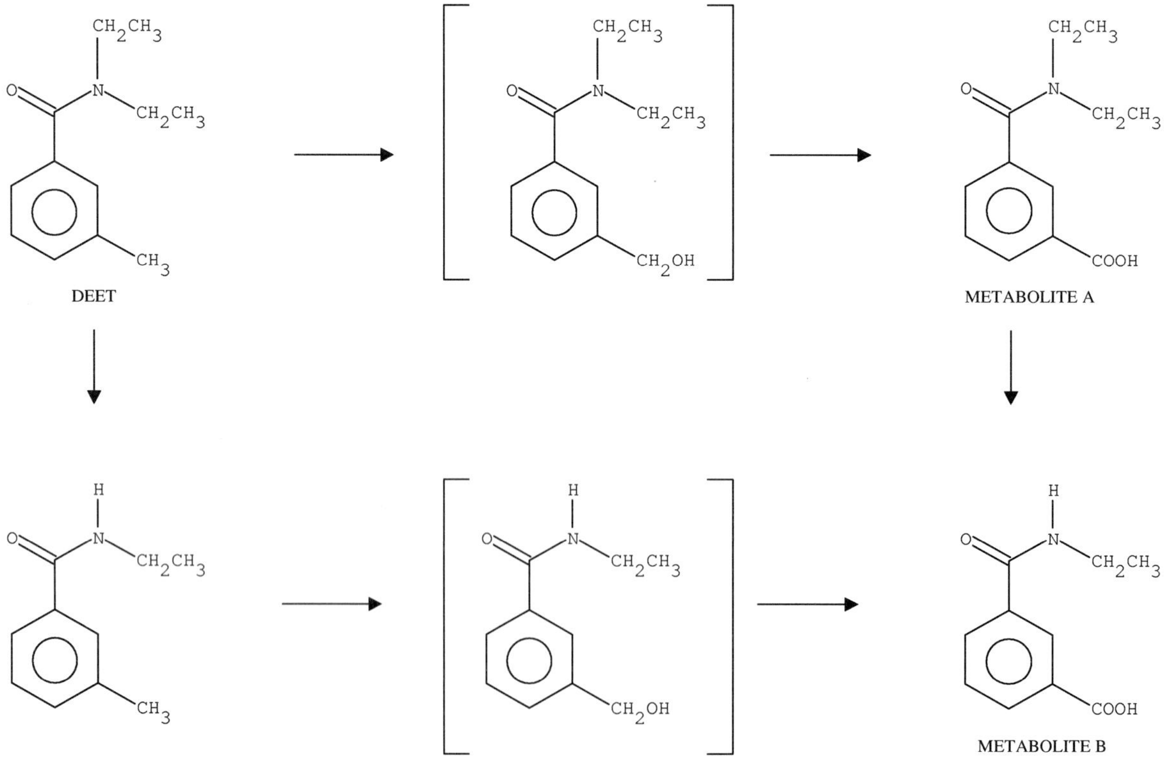

Figure 63.2 Proposed metabolic pathway for DEET in rats (Selim *et al.*, 1995).

metabolic pattern in humans is similar to that observed in rats. The latter finding is important since it supports the relevance of the findings observed in the toxicology studies conducted in this animal model.

63.3.8.3 Studies in the Open Literature that Address the Pharmacokinetics of DEET

A large number of other nonguideline, non-GLP studies that were designed to evaluate one or more of the pharmacokinetic properties of DEET are available in the open literature. These studies were conducted by the dermal route of administration in mice (Blomquist and Thorsell, 1977), rats (Moody and Nadeau, 1993; Moody *et al.*, 1989; Snodgrass *et al.*, 1982), guinea pigs (Moody and Nadeau, 1993; Schmidt *et al.*, 1959), rabbits (Hannibal, 1992; Snodgrass *et al.*, 1982), dogs (Reifenrath *et al.*, 1980, 1981; Snodgrass *et al.*, 1982), cattle (Taylor *et al.*, 1994), monkeys (Moody *et al.*, 1989), and humans (Blomquist and Thorsell, 1977; Feldman and Maibach, 1970; Wu *et al.*, 1979), by intravenous injection in mice (Blomquist *et al.*, 1975), and using *in vitro* methods (Baynes *et al.*, 1997; Taylor, 1986; Windheuser *et al.*, 1982; Yeung and Taylor, 1988).

Overall, these studies, along with those conducted by the DJV, show that DEET is well absorbed by the oral route of administration in all animal species. By the dermal route of exposure, absorption ranged from 7.9 to 92.5% in the vari-ous laboratory animal species. In humans, dermal absorption ranged from 4.6 to 16.7%. The site of application, the method of application (occluded or unoccluded) and vehicle were shown to influence dermal absorption. There is little evidence for tissue accumulation and, for the most part, DEET was found to be quantitatively metabolized and excreted in the urine.

63.4 HUMAN ASPECTS

63.4.1 CLINICAL CASE REPORTS

63.4.1.1 Dermal Exposure

The analysis of the available case reports on DEET is difficult because of limited clinical details provided. Nonetheless, these reports often are cited in discussions of DEET safety. Over the past 40 years, 14 reports have appeared in the medical literature associating clinical illness with dermal DEET exposure in 20 individuals (Osimitz and Murphy, 1997). Fourteen individuals had neurologic symptoms (Table 63.1), one had an acute manic psychosis (Snyder *et al.*, 1986), one had anaphylaxis (Miller, 1982), and one had a cardiovascular event (Clem *et al.*, 1993). Three were newborns who were reported to have alleged teratogenic effects from DEET (Hall *et al.*, 1975).

Thirteen of the reported 14 patients with neurologic symptoms were less than 8 years old (Table 63.1). The DEET con-

Table 63.1
Case Studies in which Neurological Symptoms Were Reported Following the Topical Application of DEET

Patient	Sex/Age (y)	% DEET used	Pattern of use	Symptoms	Laboratory	Outcome	Possible alternative diagnosis
1 (Gryboski *et al.*, 1961)	F/3.5	15	Daily × 2 wks	Seizures	Normal CSF	Full recovery	Idiopathic seizure
2 (Hall *et al.*, 1975)	F/5	10	Nightly × 3 mos	Headaches, ataxia, seizures, agitation	185 WBC in CSF	Death	Encephalitis, parainfectious encephalopathy
3 (Hall *et al.*, 1975)	F/7.5	10	Application & ingestion	Opisthotonos	?? cells	Full recovery	Encephalitis, parainfectious encephalopathy
4 (Zadikoff, 1979)	F/8	15	10 occasions	Headaches, ataxia, disoriented	Hyperammonemia	Death	OCT heterozygote
5 (de Garbino and Laborde, 1983)	F/1.5	NA	Frequent	"acute encephalopathy"	Normal	Death	?
6 (Roland *et al.*, 1985)	F/8	15 and 100	Copius X4 d	Rash, restlessness, seizures	Abnormal EEG	Recovery	Idiopathic seizure nonspecific rash
7 (Edwards and Johnson, 1987)	F/1.5	20	3 mos	Ataxia, movement disorder, drooling, opisthotonos, opsoclonus, myoclonus	14 WBC in CSF	Recovery	Encephalitis, parainfectious encephalopathy, myclonic encephalopathy
8–11 (Oransky *et al.*, 1989)	M/3-7	NA	NA	Seizures	Normal	Recovery	Idiopathic seizure
12 (Oransky *et al.*, 1989)	M/28	NA	NA	Seizures	Normal	Recovery	Idiopathic seizure
13 (Oransky, 1991)	?/8	NA	Hours	Seizure	Unknown	Unknown	Idiopathic seizure
14 (Lipscomb *et al.*, 1992)	M/5	100 and 15	Brief	Seizures	Normal CSF, normal CT	Recovery	Idiopathic seizure

Key: NA, not available; WBC, white blood cells; OCT, ornithine carbamoyl transferase; EEG, electroencephalogram; CSF, cerebrospinal fluid; CT, cranial computed tomography.

centration of the products used is known for 7 of the 14 patients. Of these 7, 5 developed symptoms following use of products with less than 20% DEET. The other two had applications of both 15% and 100% DEET. The most commonly reported neurologic symptom was convulsions. This was the only symptom in eight patients (patients 1 and 8 through 14), leaving the impression that a single seizure was the only symptom. All eight of these patients recovered. One 8-year-old girl had seizures and a rash on her extremities, with spontaneous resolution of symptoms (patient 6). She is the only patient in this series with a rash. Since exanthematous illnesses in children are not infrequently associated with convulsions, an infectious disease is not excluded (Modlin, 1995).

In pediatric patients, single seizures in otherwise normal children may be idiopathic events. In fact, about 2% of U.S. children have had isolated, idiopathic, nonfebrile seizures by the time they reach age 10 (Annegers, 1993). Considering that, if 2% of the 37,459,000 children in the United States that are less than 10 years old (or 750,000 children) have had single seizures by the age of 10 and, if 25% of these events (or 187,500) occur during the three summer months when DEET is most used (hence, approximately 18,750 seizures among this cohort each summer), on many occasions the use of DEET and appearance of a seizure may be temporally associated only by chance. It is interesting to note that there are no reports of DEET seizures in children with epilepsy (close to 1% of children; Annegers, 1993). These children may be exposed to DEET as frequently as children without epilepsy, and the risk in this population merits evaluation.

Three patients, one of whom died, had more complex neurologic symptoms (patients 2, 3, and 7). All had cerebrospinal fluid pleocytosis, suggesting either an inflammatory response to DEET or the possibility of infectious (Whitley, 1994) or parainfectious disease (Marks et al., 1988) processes involving the central nervous system.

Patient 4 was a heterozygote for ornithine carbamoyl transferase (OCT) deficiency and suffered neurologic symptoms, coma, and death following DEET exposure. She had suffered prior hyperammonemic episodes not associated with the use of DEET. Heterozygosity for OCT deficiency is known as a potentially lethal hyperammonemic condition (Rowe et al., 1986). The specific effect of DEET on ammonia metabolism is unknown, but DEET does not inhibit human OCT in vitro (Rej et al., 1990).

In summary, 9 of the 14 patients with neurological symptoms (patients 1, 6, and 8–14) may have had idiopathic seizures, one may have had an exanthematous illness and a convulsion, three may have had an inflammatory process affecting the central nervous system, and one was heterozygous for OCT deficiency but synergism with DEET is not excluded. Insufficient information is available on patient 5 to determine if there are alternate explanations for the patient's encephalopathy. The authors of 7 of the 10 reports of neurologic adversity after DEET exposure were contacted in 1997 and no additional information on this cohort of patients was available (Osimitz and Murphy, 1997).

Of the six clinical cases not involving neurologic symptoms, one describes a woman with anaphylactic symptoms following brief exposure to DEET who also had very similar symptoms following re-exposure to DEET in an emergency room setting (Miller, 1982). She is thought to represent an allergic hypersensitivity to DEET. Given the unique nature of the events in the other five patients, i.e., acute manic psychosis (Miller, 1982), a cardiovascular event (Clem et al., 1993), and fetal malformations (Hall et al., 1975; Schaefer and Peters, 1992), as well as the possibility of alternative etiologies (e.g., gestational urinary tract infection; Schaefer and Peters, 1992) and familial predisposition (Hall et al., 1975), it is difficult to establish a cause and effect relationship.

63.4.1.2 Oral Ingestion

In addition to the above case reports that involved dermal application, two investigators have reported adverse reactions to intentional oral ingestion of DEET by six patients (Fraser et al., 1995; Tenenbein, 1987). Of the five patients described by Tenenbein, two died and three resolved with no sequelae. The common symptoms included coma, seizures, and hypotension observed within 1 hr of ingestion. Alcohol and/or other drugs were present in three of the five patients. The two patients who died had serum DEET levels of 1.68 mg/ml and 2.4 mg/ml. This compares with a recent report showing peak serum levels of 0.52 µg/ml in humans following a single dermal application of 100% DEET at the 95th percentile of human use (Osimitz et al., 1997). One of the fatalities reported by Tenenbein had a blood ethanol level of 13.0 mg/ml and was also positive for cannabinoids. The other individual who died was found with empty bottles of chlorpromazine-HCl and hydralazine-HCl.

Fraser et al. (1995) reported the intentional ingestion of 15 to 25 ml 95% DEET by a 19-year-old woman with a history of psychiatric disorders. An EKG shortly after admission to the hospital (1 to 2 hr after ingestion) showed left and right atrial enlargement, diffuse ST-T abnormalities and a normal QT interval. The EKG was normal within 12 hr and the patient recovered completely. Analysis of the serum indicated a DEET level of 63 mg/liter about 2 hr after ingestion. Because of the intentional nature of the ingestions reported above and the fact that peak plasma levels were in excess of 1000 times higher than that seen during normal use of DEET, such cases are not relevant for the assessment of adverse effects following typical consumer use of DEET.

63.4.1.3 Occupational Exposure

The Hazards Evaluation and Technical Assistance Branch of The National Institute for Occupational Safety and Health used a survey interview to evaluate occupational exposure to DEET and self-reported health effects among adults employed at Everglades National Park in Florida (McConnell et al., 1986). Higher exposure to DEET was associated with a higher prevalence of insomnia, muscle cramps, mood disturbances, rashes, or difficulty in micturition. The subjects with higher exposure also were more likely to work at sites distant from the park headquarters, to use pesticides on a regular basis, to consume more alcohol, and to have had a job with prior chemical exposure. Whether any of the factors, alone or in combination with DEET, could account for the symptoms, was not explored.

A follow-up comparison of the workers pre-exposure (March) and post-exposure (August) did not support the findings of the initial survey. Any relationship, if it existed at all, between DEET exposure and reported neurologic symptoms was confounded by other factors.

63.4.1.4 Poison Control Center Data

Further information of the human experience with DEET comes from a review of adverse effect reports following DEET exposure from the 71 Poison Control Centers (PCCs) participating in the American Association of Poison Control Centers' National Data Collection System between 1985 and 1989 (Veltri *et al.*, 1994). The participating centers covered a wide area of the United States with a population of over 180 million people. Trained poison control specialists assessed the cases as minor, moderate, or major at the conclusion of patient contact.

There were 9086 human exposures involving DEET-containing insect repellents reported to PCCs from 1985–1989. Of these, 98.9% experienced either no effect or had short-lived symptoms. These involved mild irritation to the skin or mucous membranes. Sixty-six patients had symptoms classified as moderate, i.e., more pronounced or more prolonged than the minor effects, but all symptoms resolved without sequelae.

Five patients had symptoms classified as major. All five patients experiencing a major effect were exposed to products containing 11–50% DEET. Two of the five patients experienced eye irritation which was treated at home. One patient, a 17-year-old male who had saturated his clothing with 17.9% DEET, was ataxic and may have had a seizure. A 33-year-old male reported diminished sensation and hypotension one week after using a DEET product. Both were discharged after emergency room evaluation and recovered fully. The fifth patient had a dystonic reaction responding to diphenhydramine. Earlier in the day, he had ingested prochlorperazine, a known cause of dystonia, but synergism with DEET is not excluded. One patient ingested 8 oz. of DEET in a successful suicide attempt. Symptoms included cardiorespiratory arrest and status epilepticus.

Beginning in 1995, the DJV contracted Pegus Research, Inc. (Salt Lake City, UT) to establish the National Registry of Human Exposures to DEET. The purpose is to collect detailed information from individuals who use DEET-containing insect repellents and report serious adverse effects that are either neurologic or systemic. The Registry has been designed to overcome some of the limitations inherent in retrospective analysis of PCC data. Because of its prospective nature, the Registry allows for the quick and thorough follow-up on individual cases to determine the circumstances surrounding the case, the medical features, and to attempt to determine the relationship between the exposure and the symptoms (causality). The results of this ongoing effort, which will be published shortly in the literature, will provide important insight into the human safety of DEET.

63.5 RISK ASSESSMENT CONSIDERATIONS

63.5.1 INTRODUCTION

The risk assessment for DEET can be approached in a number of different ways. One is the traditional method of defining toxicity endpoints of concern from the existing toxicology database and comparing the no-effect levels for these endpoints to some estimate of human exposure. In the case of DEET, there are at least two problems associated with this approach. One is that little or no toxicity can be produced in laboratory animals by the principal (dermal) route of exposure, to which humans are exposed. The second is that, while toxic effects can be produced by the oral, inhalation, and subcutaneous routes of exposure, because of the large differences in how DEET would be expected to be handled in the body by these other routes of administration, it is questionable as to whether toxicity endpoints identified by these other routes of administration are applicable to human risk assessment. For example, it has been demonstrated that neurotoxic effects can be produced in laboratory animals when DEET is administered orally as a bolus dose. However, as data that are presented below show, if these effects are related to the peak levels of DEET in the blood, then they probably have little or no applicability to human risk by the dermal route of exposure. On the other hand, since it has been shown that DEET is not a teratogen, a reproductive toxin, or an oncogen at maximum tolerated doses by the more rigorous oral route of administration, a risk assessor can feel quite confident that developmental, reproductive, or oncogenic effects are not toxicity endpoints of concern for DEET. This is the type of reasoning that went into U.S. EPA's recent decision, as stated in the DEET Reregistration Eligibility Document, that there are no significant endpoints of toxicity concern for DEET and that a comprehensive, quantitative risk assessment is not warranted (U.S. EPA, 1998).

While the DJV agreed with the approach taken by the U.S. EPA, it felt that additional data were needed to aid in the risk assessment process. Therefore, five blood level studies designed to define the profile of systemic exposure that occurs under four different exposure scenarios were undertaken. The exposure scenarios that were evaluated were: (1) in humans following single and repeated dermal applications of DEET at the 95th percentile of human exposure; (2) in dogs under the conditions in which neurotoxic signs were observed following single and repeated oral dose administration via gelatin capsules; (3) in rats under the conditions in which potential neurotoxic effects were observed following acute oral administration by gastric gavage; and (4) in rats under the conditions of the 90-day dermal toxicity study.

These studies, in which systemic exposure was measured in terms of DEET plasma levels, were intended to demonstrate two points. One is that the systemic exposure laboratory animals receive following oral dose administration (especially oral bolus dosing) is very different than that which humans receive by the dermal route of exposure. This is an important consideration for the risk assessment process since treatment-related effects have been observed in a number of oral toxicity studies. A second point that these blood level data were intended to demonstrate is that the subchronic dermal toxicity studies conducted in rats and micropigs provide the most meaningful data for human risk assessment. The design and results of these blood level studies are discussed below.

63.5.2 BLOOD LEVEL STUDIES

63.5.2.1 Blood Level Study to Define DEET Plasma Profile in Humans Following Single and Repeated Dermal Applications of DEET at the 95th Percentile of Human Exposure (Ohayon *et al.*, 1997)

In this study, three male and three female human volunteers were administered undiluted DEET by the dermal route of administration at the 95th percentile of human use (3 g/day for females and 4 g/day for males). Both single and repeated (8 hr per day for four consecutive days) applications were evaluated. DEET plasma levels were profiled on the first and fourth days of the study. The DEET plasma profiles for humans under this scenario are presented in Fig. 63.3 and are summarized in Table 63.2.

The findings from this study show that DEET does not appear in the blood of humans until 1 to 2 hr after dermal application, after which time the DEET plasma levels gradually increase until the material is washed off 8 hr after application. The DEET plasma profiles and peak plasma levels were similar in males and females and did not increase after repeated dosing. The overall mean peak plasma level was 0.45 μg/ml. The overall mean area under the DEET plasma concentration versus time curve (AUC) was 3.51 μg hr/ml.

63.5.2.2 Blood Level Study to Define DEET Plasma Profile in Dogs under Conditions in which Neurotoxic Signs Were Observed Following Single and Repeated Oral Dose Administration (Badalone, 1997)

As discussed previously in Section 63.3.2.5 clinical signs indicative of neurotoxicity were observed in two studies in which undiluted DEET was administered to dogs as a single oral bolus dose via gelatin capsules. In order to compare the systemic exposure that the dogs received under the dosage regimen employed in these studies to that of humans under normal conditions of use, a blood level study was conducted in dogs ad-

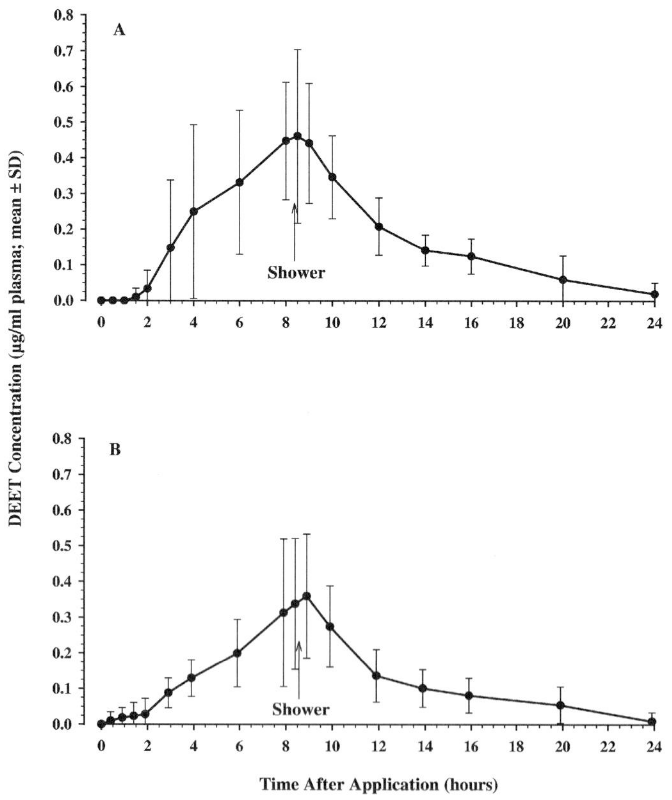

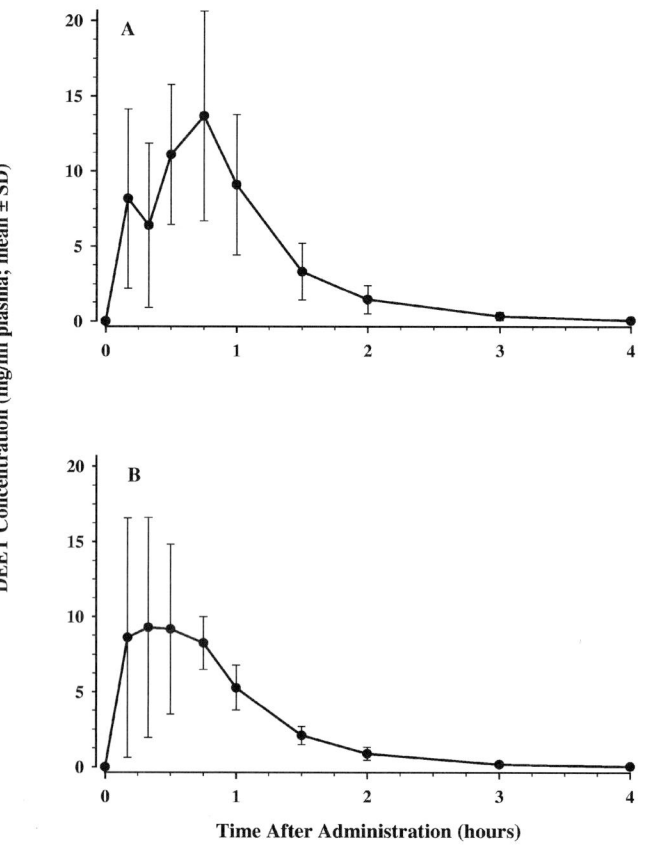

Figure 63.3 DEET plasma profile in human volunteers administered DEET dermally at the 95th percentile of human use during and following the first of four (A) and fourth of four (B) daily 8-hr dermal applications. Each value represents the mean of six individual values (three males and three females).

Figure 63.4 DEET plasma profile in dogs during and following the first of four (A) and fourth of four (B) daily oral bolus doses of DEET at a level of 75 mg/kg/day. Each value represents the mean of eight individual values (four males and four females).

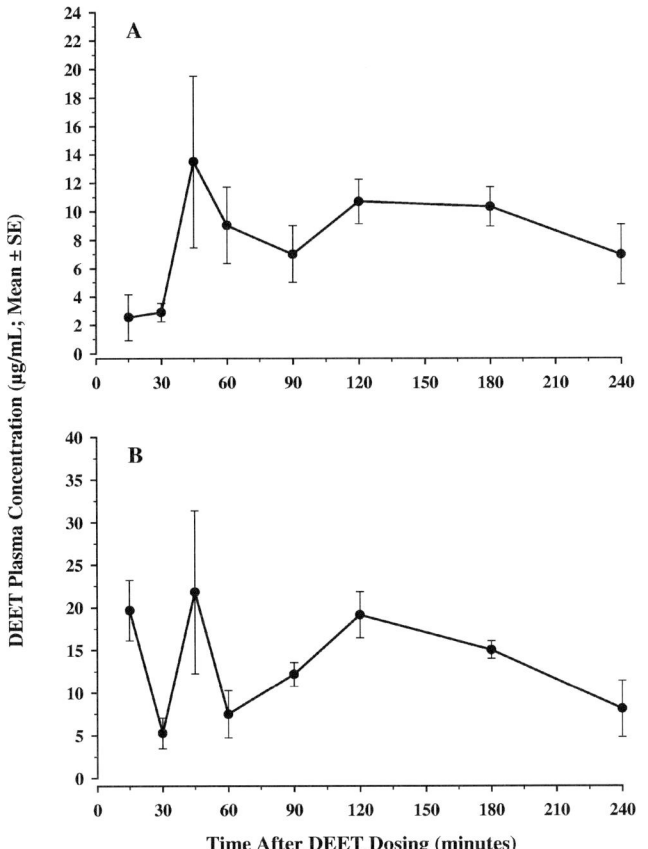

Figure 63.5 DEET plasma profile over a 4-hr period in male (A) and female (B) rats following a single oral bolus dose of DEET at a dose level of 200 mg/kg. Each value represents the mean of three individual values.

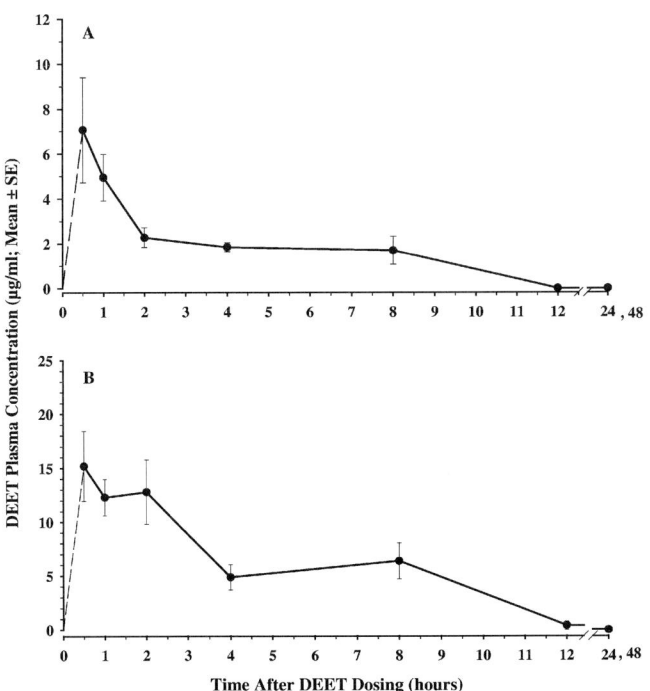

Figure 63.6 DEET plasma profile over a 48-hr period in male (A) and female (B) rats following a single oral bolus dose of DEET at a dose level of 200 mg/kg. Each value represents the mean of five individual values.

ministered DEET as a daily oral bolus dose via gelatin capsules at the NOAEL for effects in the dog studies, i.e., 75 mg/kg/day. Four male and four female dogs were utilized in this four day study. DEET plasma levels were profiled on the first and last days of this study. The DEET plasma profile for dogs under this dosing regimen is presented in Fig. 63.4 and is summarized in Table 63.3.

In this study, both the blood profiles and peak blood levels observed in these dogs were much different than those observed in humans. For example, peak plasma levels were observed within 30 minutes after dosing and plasma levels were back below the limit of quantitation within 3 to 4 hr after dose administration. Consistent with humans, no differences were observed between male and female dogs and there was no evidence of accumulation of DEET in the blood following repeated doses. The overall mean peak plasma level was 14.7 µg/ml. The overall mean AUC was 12.59 µg hr/ml.

Since the effects that were observed in the dogs occurred shortly after dosing, they appear to be closely associated with the time frame in which peak plasma levels would have occurred. A comparison of the overall mean peak plasma levels between dogs and humans showed a 33-fold difference, i.e., 14.7 versus 0.45 µg/ml. Since these plasma level data provide a direct comparison of the true systemic exposure, all of the un-

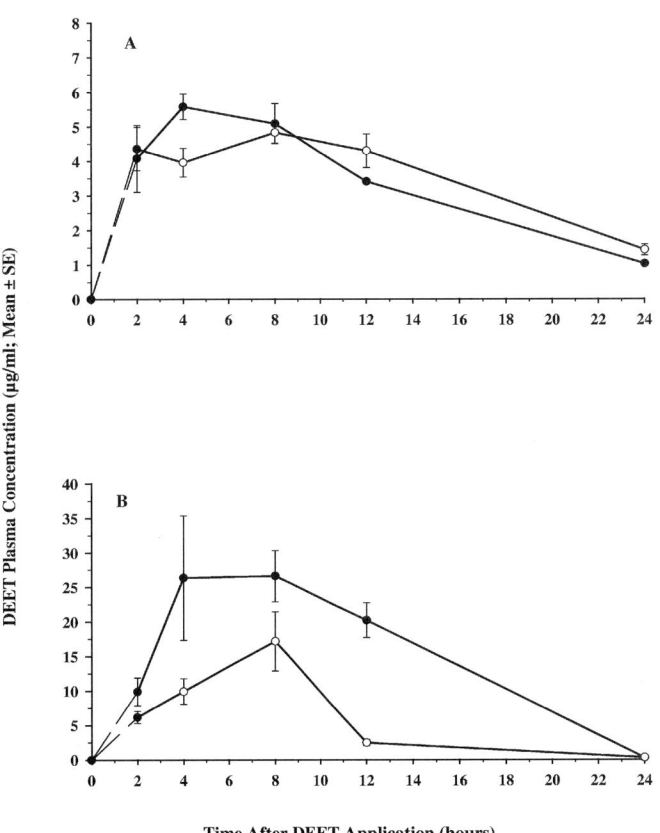

Figure 63.7 DEET plasma profile in male (A) and female (B) rats during and following the first and fifth of five consecutive dermal applications of DEET at a dose level of 1000 mg/kg/day. Each value represents the mean of four individual values. (●) First application. (○) Fifth application.

Table 63.2
DEET Plasma Levels in Human Volunteers Administered DEET Dermally at the 95th Percentile of Human Use

DEET exposure metric	Single exposure[a]			Repeated exposure[b]		
	Male	Female	Mean	Male	Female	Mean
Mean maximum						
Plasma level (μg/ml)	0.62	0.43	0.52	0.49	0.25	0.37
AUC[c] (μg hr/ml)	5.11	3.07	4.09	3.76	2.10	2.93

[a] From data collected during and following the first of four daily dermal applications of technical grade DEET at dose levels of 4 g/day for males and 3 g/day for females.
[b] From data collected during and following the fourth of four daily dermal applications of technical grade DEET at dose levels of 4 g/day for males and 3 g/day for females.
[c] AUC = area under the DEET plasma concentration versus time curve.

Table 63.3
DEET Plasma Levels in Dogs Administered DEET in Gelatin Capsules at a Dose Level of 75 mg/kg/day

DEET exposure metric	Single exposure[a]			Repeated exposure[b]		
	Male	Female	Mean	Male	Female	Mean
Mean maximum						
Plasma level (μg/ml)	18.26	13.97	16.11	14.25	12.48	13.36
AUC (μg hr/ml)[c]	15.87	13.45	14.66	11.21	10.17	10.69

[a] From data collected during and following the first of four daily oral doses of technical grade DEET.
[b] From data collected during and following the fourth of four daily oral doses of technical grade DEET.
[c] AUC = area under the DEET plasma concentration versus time curve.

certainties associated with making similar comparisons based on whole body exposure on a mg/kg basis have been eliminated. Because of this reduction in uncertainty, a 10-fold difference in plasma levels generally is considered to be at least equivalent to a 100-fold safety factor or margin of exposure (MOE) based on whole body exposure on a mg/kg basis.[1] Therefore, the observed 33-fold difference in overall mean peak plasma levels is at least equivalent to a 300-fold safety factor or MOE developed on the basis of whole body exposure.

The data obtained in this dog blood level study also are applicable to the eight-week and chronic dog studies since peak blood levels were observed within 30 minutes after dosing and blood levels returned to baseline within 3 to 4 hr in the blood level study. Because the dogs were fed just prior to dose administration in the subchronic and chronic studies, the peak blood levels after the a.m. dose may have been slightly lower due to the influence food may have had on absorption. However, if this were the case, the peak blood levels following the p.m. dose probably would have been as high or higher because the blood levels probably would not have returned to baseline prior to the p.m. dose.

63.5.2.3 Blood Level Study to Define Plasma Profile in Rats Administered DEET under the Conditions in which Potential Neurotoxic Effects Were Observed Following Acute Oral Administration by Gastric Gavage (Goldenthal, 1999; Laveglia, 1998a)

As discussed in Section 63.3.6.1 an increase in time to respond in a thermal response test and decreased rearing activity detected by two measures of vertical movement (vertical activity

and vertical time) in a motor activity test were observed in a rat acute neurotoxicity study. These findings were observed in animals of both sexes but only at the 1-hr post-treatment time point and only at the 500 mg/kg dose level. Other time points at which these parameters were evaluated were 24 hr and 14 days post-treatment. The NOEL in this study was 200 mg/kg.

In order to compare the systemic exposure to DEET that rats received under this dosage regimen to that of humans under simulated conditions of human use, a blood level study was conducted at the highest level at which no effects were observed in the rat study, i.e., 200 mg/kg. Eight groups, each consisting of three male and three female rats, were employed in this study. One group of rats was humanely sacrificed for blood collection and subsequent DEET plasma analysis at each of eight different time intervals over a 4-hr time period following oral dose administration.

The DEET plasma profiles for male and female rats under the scenario described above are presented in Fig. 63.5 and are summarized in Table 63.4.

As was the case with dogs, the blood profiles and peak blood levels observed in these rats were much different than those observed in humans under normal use conditions. For example, peak plasma levels were observed within 15 to 45 minutes after dosing, after which time a plateau level or gradual decrease in plasma levels was observed during the 4-hr time period in which the plasma levels were measured. Average peak plasma levels were 9.58 μg/ml in male rats and 13.61 μg/ml in female rats. AUC values could not be determined because DEET plasma levels did not return to baseline over the 4-hr period in which they were measured in this study. However, since the effects that were observed in the rats occurred shortly after dosing, they appear to be closely associated with the time frame during which peak plasma levels would have been expected to occur in the rat acute neurotoxicity study rather than AUC. A comparison of peak plasma levels between the rats and humans shows 21- to 30-fold differences.

In order to characterize more fully the time course of elimination of DEET from the plasma following an oral bolus dose, a second oral blood level study was conducted in rats. In the second study, the same dose level (200 mg/kg) was adminis-

---

[1] While these types of blood level data are not usually available for pesticides and insect repellenys, they are routinely developed and used for risk assessment for pharmaceutical products by U.S. FDA. A 10-fold difference in plasma levels is used as the benchmark for safety for pharmaceutical products in much the same manner as other regulatory agencies use an MOE of 100 for nondrug products such as pesticides.

Table 63.4
DEET Plasma Levels in Rats Administered DEET by Gastric Gavage at a Dose Level of 200 mg/kg

DEET exposure metric	Male	Female
Mean maximum Plasma level (μg/ml)[a]	9.58	13.61

[a]Peak plasma level during a 4-hr period following dose administration.

Table 63.5
DEET Plasma Levels in Rats Administered DEET by Gastric Gavage at a Dose Level of 200 mg/kg

DEET exposure metric	Male	Female
Mean maximum Plasma level (μg/ml)[a]	7.06	15.18
AUC (μg hr/ml)[b]	22.91	79.18

[a]Peak plasma level during a 48-hr period following dose administration.
[b]AUC = area under the DEET plasma concentration versus time curve (48-hr time period).

Table 63.6
DEET Plasma Levels in Rats Administered DEET Dermally at 1000 mg/kg/day

DEET exposure metric	Single exposure[a]		Repeated exposure[b]	
	Male	Female	Male	Female
Mean maximum plasma level (μg/ml)	4.56	24.37	4.37	17.14
AUC (μg hr/ml)[c]	89.5	368.2	100.8	134.8

[a]From data collected during and following the first of four daily dermal applications.
[b]From data collected during and following the fourth of four daily dermal applications.
[c]AUC = area under the DEET plasma concentration versus time curve.

tered; however, the DEET plasma profile was evaluated over a 48-hr rather than a 4-hr period of time, and groups consisting of five male and five female rats were humanely sacrificed at each time interval. The DEET plasma profiles for rats in this study are presented in Fig. 63.6 and are summarized in Table 63.5.

The data from this study showed that peak plasma levels occurred 30 minutes after dosing and that there was a distinct difference between both male and female rats in both maximum plasma levels and AUC. In this study, the elimination of DEET from plasma after reaching peak levels was biphasic, indicating that DEET was rapidly absorbed from the stomach, distributed in the body within 2 to 4 hr of administration, and subsequently eliminated from plasma within 12 hr. A comparison of peak plasma levels between rats and humans shows that the levels in male and female rats under these experimental conditions were 16 to 34 times higher than in humans, respectively.

The data developed in these rat acute oral blood level studies also can be used to support the position that the clinical signs observed in the rat teratology study are not relevant to human health. Since the exposure was more severe (due to repeated daily dosing) and the NOAEL was higher in the teratology study than it was in the acute neurotoxicity study (250 versus 200 mg/kg), systemic exposure at the NOAEL in the teratology study would be expected to be greater than the acute neurotoxicity study in which DEET peak plasma levels were 16 to 34 times higher than humans at the 95th percentile of human use.

63.5.2.4 Blood Level Studies to Define the Plasma Profile in Rats Administered DEET under the Conditions of the Rat 90-Day Dermal Toxicity Study (Laveglia, 1998b)

Because human exposure to DEET is by the dermal route of exposure and is, for the most part, seasonal, the rat and mi-

cropig 90-day dermal toxicity studies appear to be the most appropriate studies for human risk assessment. There also is considerable evidence that rat skin is more permeable than human skin to xenobiotics like DEET, and that the permeability of the skin of the pig is considered to be similar to that of man. Therefore, systemic exposure to DEET in these two animal models would be expected to exceed or mimic systemic human exposure by the dermal route. In these studies, undiluted DEET was administered to rats and micropigs at dose levels of 100, 300, and 1000 mg/kg/day five days per week for a period of 13 weeks. The 1000 mg/kg/day dose level represents the highest dose level that can be applied without runoff and the NOAEL for biologically meaningful effects.

In order to compare the systemic exposure to DEET that rats received under this dosage regimen to that of humans under normal use conditions, a blood level study was conducted at a dose level of 1000 mg/kg/day under conditions that simulated the exposure the rats received in the 90-day dermal toxicity study. Ten groups, each consisting of four male and four female rats, were employed in this study. One group of rats was humanely sacrificed for blood collection and subsequent DEET plasma analysis at each of 10 different time intervals over a 24-hr period following a single or following the fifth daily dermal dose. The data from this study are presented in Fig. 63.7 and are summarized in Table 63.6.

Unlike the data obtained in the dog and rat blood level studies in which DEET was administered orally as a bolus dose, the DEET plasma profile in the rat dermal blood level study was qualitatively similar to that obtained in the human dermal blood level study. DEET did not accumulate in the plasma and the DEET plasma levels in rats decreased to about baseline levels within 24 hr in a manner similar to that of the human volunteers, even though no attempt was made to remove the material after 8 hr of exposure.

The data from the rat dermal blood level study can be compared to the data from the human blood level study in two ways. One is on the basis of peak plasma levels and the other is on the basis of the area under the DEET plasma versus time curve. In this case, the AUC data are considered to be more appropriate because no clinical signs were observed in the laboratory animal studies and because plasma profiles were qualitatively similar over the entire 24-hr period. A comparison of the mean AUC data shows 27- and 72-fold differences between humans and male and female rats, respectively.[2]

63.5.3 RISK ASSESSMENT CONCLUSIONS

Because of the large differences in actual systemic exposure, the studies conducted with DEET by the oral route of administration are not amenable for defining endpoints for toxicity concern or quantitative risk assessment. However, the teratology, reproductive toxicity, neurotoxicity, and oncogenicity studies that were conducted at MTD doses by the more rigorous oral route of administration are useful from the perspective that they demonstrate that DEET is not a teratogen, reproductive toxin, selective neurotoxin, or oncogen. In the studies that are most appropriate for use in human risk assessment, i.e., 90-day dermal toxicity studies in rats and micropigs, no significant endpoints for toxicity concern were observed at the highest dose that could be applied in these animal model systems, i.e., 1000 mg/kg/day. The blood level studies that examined actual systemic exposure to DEET under key exposure scenarios support these conclusions and provide useful data for quantitative risk assessment.

63.6 CONCLUSIONS

Over the past 50 years, DEET has been proven to be a safe and effective personal insect repellent that provides public health benefits. In addition to its safe history of human use, it is one of the most thoroughly studied chemicals known to man and a state-of-the-art toxicology database recently has been developed. These studies show that, by the most relevant route of human exposure, DEET is practically nontoxic in laboratory animals. Because systemic toxicity cannot be produced in laboratory animals by the dermal route of exposure, most of the key studies that are traditionally used to define endpoints of toxicity concern were conducted by the more rigorous oral route of exposure in order to satisfy the maximum tolerated dose criteria. Under these conditions, it has been shown that DEET is not a teratogen, reproductive toxin, selective neurotoxin, or oncogen. In addition, while clinical signs of toxicity can be produced by administering DEET as an oral bolus dose, blood level studies have demonstrated that the DEET plasma profile following oral bolus dosing is much different than that observed following dermal administration. Therefore, it is unlikely that the findings observed under these conditions have any relevance to human health under the conditions that DEET is intended to be used. Relative to the millions of people who use DEET each year, there have been relatively few reported cases of serious illness

associated with its use. However, there are approximately 14 case reports involving 20 individuals in the open literature in which a purported relationship between DEET exposure and serious effects have been reported. A review of these cases provided alternative etiologies for the symptoms reported in most patients (Osimitz and Murphy, 1997). Therefore, consistent with the recent opinion of the U.S. EPA (U.S. EPA, 1998), there are no endpoints for toxicity concern for DEET and its use as an insect repellent does not pose a significant health risk to the general population.

REFERENCES

Abou-Donia, M. B., and Wilmarth, K. R. (1996). Neurotoxicity resulting from coexposure to pyridostigmine bromide, DEET, and permethrin: Implications of Gulf War Chemical Exposures. *J. Toxicol. Environ. Health* **48**, 35–56.

Ambrose, A. M., Huffman, D. K., and Salamone, R. T. (1959). Pharmacologic and toxicologic studies on N,N-diethyltoluamide 1. N,N-diethyl-m-toluamide. *Toxicology* **1**, 97–115.

Angerhofer, R. A., and Weeks, M. H. (1980). Phase 7—Effect of dermal applications of N,N-diethyl-m-toluamide (m-Det) on the embryonic development of rabbits. Unpublished study conducted at U.S. Army Environmental Hygiene Agency.

Annegers, J. F. (1993). Epidemiology of childhood seizures. *In* "Pediatric Epilepsy: Diagnosis and Therapy" (W. E. Dodson and J. M. Pellock, eds.), pp. 57–62. Demos, New York.

Badalone, V. (1997). Blood level study in dogs following oral administration, via gelatin capsules, of N,N-diethyl-m-toluamide (DEET). Unpublished study conducted at Bio-Research Laboratories Ltd. under the sponsorship of the DEET Joint Venture/Chemical Specialties Manufacturers Association.

Baynes, R. E., Halling, K. B., and Riviere, J. E. (1997). The influence of diethyl-m-toluamide (DEET) on the percutaneous absorption of permethrin and carbaryl. *Toxicol. Appl. Pharmacol.* **144**, 332–339.

Blomquist, L., Ström, L., and Thorsell, W. (1975). Distribution and fate of the insect repellent ^{14}C-N,N-diethyl-m-toluamide in the animal body. I. Distribution and excretion after injection into mice. *Acta Pharmacol. Toxicol.* **37**, 121–133.

Blomquist, L., and Thorsell, W. (1977). Distribution and fate of the insect repellent ^{14}C-N,N-diethyl-m-toluamide in the animal body. II. Distribution and excretion after cutaneous application. *Acta Pharmacol. Toxicol.* **41**, 235–243.

Brusick, D. J. (1976). Mutagenicity evaluation of m-DEET. Unpublished study conducted at Litton Bionetics, Inc. under the sponsorship of McLaughlin Gormley King Co.

Brusick, D. J. (1980). The effect of DEET (N,N-diethyltoluamide) on the morphology, viability, and count of sperm in rats exposed by dermal administration. Unpublished study conducted at Litton Bionetics, Inc. under the sponsorship of McLaughlin Gormley King Co.

Campbell, K. R. (1986). "An *In Vitro* Study of N,N-Diethyl-m-Toluamide (DEET) as a Neurotoxin." Thesis, Air Force Institute of Technology, Air University, Department of the Air Force, Wright–Patterson Force Base, Ohio.

Chaney, L. A., Rockhold, R. W., Wineman, R. W., and Hume, A. S. (1999). Anticonvulsant-resistant seizures following pyridostigmine bromide (PB) and N,N-diethyl-m-toluamide (DEET). *Toxicol. Sci.* **49**, 301–311.

Clem, J. R., Havemann, D. F., and Raebel, M. A. (1993). Insect repellent (N-N-diethyl-m-toluamide) cardiovascular toxicity in an adult. *Ann. Pharmacother.* **27**, 289–293.

Curren, R. D. (1989). Unscheduled DNA synthesis assay in rat primary hepatocytes with a confirmatory assay. Unpublished study conducted at Microbiological Associates, Inc. under the sponsorship of the DEET Joint Venture/Chemical Specialties Manufacturers Association.

---

[2]In the human blood level study, no differences were noted between male and female volunteers or between single and repeated exposure scenarios, and the overall mean AUC value was 3.51 µg hr/ml. For male rats, the corresponding value is 95.25 µg hr/ml. For female rats, the corresponding value is 251.5 µg hr/ml.

de Garbino, J. P., and Laborde, A. (1983). Toxicity of an insect repellent: *N*,*N*-diethyltoluamide. *Vet. Hum. Toxicol.* **24**, 422–423.

Dorman, D. C., Buck, W. B., Trammel, H. L., Jones, R. D., and Beasley, V. R. (1990). Fenvalerate/*N*,*N*-diethyl-*m*-toluamide (DEET) toxicosis in two cats. *J. Amer. Vet. Med. Association* **196**(1), 100–102.

Edwards, D. L., and Johnson, J. E. (1987). Insect-repellent-induced toxic encephalopathy in a child. *Clin. Pharmacol.* **6**, 496–498.

Feldman, R. J., and Maibach, H. I. (1970). Absorption of some organic compounds through the skin in man. *J. Invest. Dermatol.* **54**(5), 399–404.

Fraser, D., MacNeil, A., Theriault, M., and Morzycki, W. (1995). Analysis of DEET following intentional oral ingestion of Muscol®. *Analyt. Toxicol.* **19**, 197–199.

Gleiberman, S. E., Volkova, A. P., Nikolaev, G. M., and Zhukova, E. V. (1975). An investigation of the embryotoxic properties of the repellent diethyltoluamide. *Farmakol. Toksikol.* **38**(2), 202–205.

Goldenthal, E. I. (1989a). Evaluation of DEET in a 90-day dose range findings study in hamsters. Unpublished study conducted at International Research and Development Corporation under the sponsorship of the DEET Joint Venture/Chemical Specialties Manufacturers Association.

Goldenthal, E. I. (1989b). Evaluation of DEET in a 90-day dermal toxicity study in castrated male rats. Unpublished study conducted at International Research and Development Corporation under the sponsorship of the DEET Joint Venture/Chemical Specialties Manufacturers Association.

Goldenthal, E. I. (1991). Evaluation of DEET in a 90-day subchronic dermal toxicity study in micropigs®. Unpublished study conducted at International Research and Development Corporation under the sponsorship of the DEET Joint Venture/Chemical Specialties Manufacturers Association.

Goldenthal, E. I. (1992). Evaluation of DEET in a multistrain 90-day dietary renal toxicity study in rats. Unpublished study conducted at International Research and Development Corporation under the sponsorship of the DEET Joint Venture/Chemical Specialties Manufacturers Association.

Goldenthal, E. I. (1994a). Evaluation of DEET in a two-week palatability study in dogs. Unpublished study conducted at International Research and Development Corporation under the sponsorship of the DEET Joint Venture/Chemical Specialties Manufacturers Association.

Goldenthal, E. I. (1994b). Evaluation of DEET in a three week toxicity study in dogs. Unpublished study conducted at International Research and Development Corporation under the sponsorship of the DEET Joint Venture/Chemical Specialties Manufacturers Association.

Goldenthal, E. I. (1994c). Evaluation of DEET in a two-week oral gelatin capsule toxicity study in dogs. Unpublished study conducted at International Research and Development Corporation under the sponsorship of the DEET Joint Venture/Chemical Specialties Manufacturers Association.

Goldenthal, E. I. (1995a). Evaluation of DEEt in an eight-week dietary toxicity study in dogs. Unpublished study conducted at International Research and Development Corporation under the sponsorship of the DEET Joint Venture/Chemical Specialties Manufacturers Association.

Goldenthal, E. I. (1995b). Evaluation of DEET in an eight-week oral gelatin capsule toxicity study in dogs. Unpublished study conducted at International Research and Development Corporation under the sponsorship of the DEET Joint Venture/Chemical Specialties Manufacturers Association.

Goldenthal, E. I. (1997). Evaluation of DEET in a eight-week oral toxicity study in dogs. Unpublished study conducted at MPI Research (formerly International Research and Development Corporation) under the sponsorship of the DEET Joint Venture/Chemical Specialties Manufacturers Association.

Goldenthal, E. I. (1999). 48-hour blood level study in rats following a single oral bolus administration of *N*,*N*-diethyl-*m*-toluamide (DEET) in the rat. Unpublished study conducted at MPI Research (formerly International Research and Development Corporation) under the sponsorship of the DEET Joint Venture/Chemical Specialties Manufacturers Association.

Gryboski, J., Weinstein, D., and Ordway, K. (1961). Toxic encephalopathy apparently related to the use of an insect repellent. *N. Engl. J. Med.* **264**, 289–291.

Haight, E. A., Harvey, J. G., Jr., and Singer, A. W. (1980). Phase 5, Subchronic oral toxicity of the insect repellent *N*,*N*-diethyl-*m*-toluamide (m-DET)

study. Unpublished study conducted at U.S. Army Environmental and Hygiene Agency.

Hall, J. G., McLaughlin, J. F., and Stamm, S. (1975). Coarctation of the aorta in male cousins with similar maternal environmental exposure to insect repellent and insecticides. *Pediatrics* **55**, 425–427.

Hannibal, D. (1992). A comparison of the absolute bioavailability of C-14 radiolabelled diethyltoluamide from a 10% alcoholic solution and from Skedaddle® after a single exposure in rabbits. Unpublished study conducted at Nova Pharmaceutical Corporation under the sponsorship of LittlePoint Corporation.

Johnson, D. E. (1987a). Evaluation of DEET in a 90-day oral dose range finding study in rats. Unpublished study conducted at International Research and Development Corporation under the sponsorship of the DEET Joint Venture/Chemical Specialties Manufacturers Association.

Johnson, D. E. (1987b). Evaluation of DEET in a 90-day oral dose range finding study in mice. Unpublished study conducted at International Research and Development Corporation under the sponsorship of the DEET Joint Venture/Chemical Specialties Manufacturers Association.

Johnson, D. E. (1987c). Evaluation of DEET in a 90-day subchronic dermal toxicity study in rats. Unpublished study conducted at International Research and Development Corporation under the sponsorship of the DEET Joint Venture/Chemical Specialties Manufacturers Association.

Laveglia, J. (1998a). Blood level study in rats following a single oral bolus administration of *N*,*N*-diethyl-*m*-toluamide (DEET). Unpublished study conducted at MPI Research, Inc. (formerly International Research and Development Corporation) under the sponsorship of the DEET Joint Venture/Chemical Specialties Manufacturers Association.

Laveglia, J. (1998b). Blood level study in rats following single and repeated dermal applications of *N*,*N*-diethyl-*m*-toluamide (DEET). Unpublished study conducted at MPI Research, Inc. (formerly International Research and Development Corporation) under the sponsorship of the DEET Joint Venture/Chemical Specialties Manufacturers Association.

Lipscomb, J. W., Kramer, J. E., and Leikin, J. B. (1992). Seizure following brief exposure to the insect repellent *N*-*N*-diethyl-*m*-toluamide. *Ann. Emerg. Med.* **21**, 315–317.

Macko, J. A., and Bergman, J. D. (1980). Phase 4—Inhalation toxicities of *N*,*N*-diethyl-*meta*-toluamide (M-Det). Unpublished study conducted at U.S. Army Environmental Hygiene Agency.

Macko, J. A., and Weeks, M. H. (1980). Phase 6, Acute toxicity evaluation of *N*,*N*-diethyl-*meta*-toluamide (M-Det). Unpublished study conducted at U.S. Army Environmental Hygiene Agency under the sponsorship of S.C. Johnson & Son, Inc.

Marks, W. A., Bodensteiner, J. B., Bobele, G. B., Hamza, M., and Wilson, D. A. (1988). Parainflammatory leukoencephalomyelitis: Clinical and magnetic resonance imaging findings. *J. Child Neurol.* **3**, 205–213.

McCain, W. C. *et al.* (1995).

McCain, W. C., Lee, R., Johnson, M. S., Whaley, J. E., Ferguson, J. W., Beall, P., and Leach, G. (1997). Acute oral toxicity study of pyridostigmine bromide, permethrin, and DEET in the laboratory rat. *J. Toxicol. Environ. Health* **50**, 113–124.

McConnell, R., Fidler, A. T., and Chrislip, D. (1986). Health Hazard Evaluation Report No. 85-05, National Institute for Occupational Safety and Health, Public Health Service Centers for Disease Control, U.S. Department of Health and Human Services, HETA 83-085-1757.

Miller, J. D. (1982). Anaphylaxis associated with insect repellent. *N. Eng. J. Med.* **307**, 1341–1342.

Modlin, J. F. (1995). Coxsackieviruses, echoviruses, and new enteroviruses. *In* "Principles and Practice of Infectious Diseases" (G. L. Mandell, J. E. Bennett, and R. Dolin, eds.), pp. 620–636. Churchill Livingstone, New York.

Moody, R. P., Benoit, F. M., Riedel, D., and Ritter, L. (1989). Dermal absorption of the insect repellent DEET (*N*,*N*-diethyl-*m*-toluamide) in rats and monkeys: Effect of anatomical site and multiple exposure. *J. Toxicol. Environ. Health* **26**(2), 137–147.

Moody, R. P., and Nadeau, B. (1993). An automated *in vitro* dermal absorption procedure: III *In vivo* and *in vitro* comparison with the insect repellent *N*,*N*-diethyl-toluamide in mouse, rat, guinea pig, human, and tissue-cultured skin. *Toxic. in Vitro* **7**(2), 167–176.

Moore, G. E. (2000). Acute oral, dermal and inhalation toxicity, primary skin and eye irritation and dermal sensitization studies with DEET insect repellent. Unpublished studies conducted at Product Safety Labs under the sponsorship of Morflex, Inc.

Mount, M. E., Moller, G., Cook, J., Holstege, D. H., Richardson, E. R., and Ardans, A. (1991). Clinical illness associated with a commercial tick and flea product in dogs and cats. *Vet. Hum. Toxicol.* **33**(1), 19–27.

Ohayon, A., Ehler, L., and Denver, K. (1997). A blood level study in humans following topical application of *N,N*-diethyl-*m*-toluamide (DEET). Unpublished study conducted at L.A.B. Pharmacological Research International, Inc. under the sponsorship of the DEET Joint Venture/Chemical Specialties Manufacturers Association.

Olson, M. J., Garg, B. D., Murty, C. V. R., and Roy, A. K. (1987). Accumulation of α_{2u}-globulin in the renal proximal tubules of male rats exposed to unleaded gasoline. *Toxicol. Appl. Pharmacol.* **90**, 43–51.

Oransky, S., Roseman, B., Fish, D., Gentile, M. S., Melius, J., and Cartter, M. L. (1989). Seizures temporally associated with use of DEET insect repellent. *M.M.W.R. (New York and Connecticut)* **38**, 378–680.

Oransky, S. (1991). Letter on file with the Department of Environment, Bureau of Pesticides Management, Albany, NY.

Osimitz, T. G., Gill, M. W., Gabriel, K. L., Ouellette, R. E., and Schoenig, G. P. (1997). DEET blood level studies in humans following dermal application and in dogs following oral administration. *Toxicologist* **36**, 343.

Osimitz, T. G., and Murphy, J. V. (1997). Neurological effects associated with use of the insect repellent *N,N*-diethyl-*m*-toluamide (DEET). *Clin. Toxicol.* **35**(5), 435–441.

Putman, D. L., and Morris, M. J. (1989). Chromosome aberrations in Chinese hamster ovary (CHO) cells. Unpublished study conducted at Microbiological Associates, Inc. under the sponsorship of the DEET Joint Venture/Chemical Specialties Manufacturers Association.

Reifenrath, W. G., Hill, J. A., Robinson, P. B., McVey, D. L., and Akers, W. A. (1980). Percutaneous absorption of carbon 14 labeled insect repellents in hairless dogs. *J. Environ. Pathol. Toxicol.* **4**, 249–256.

Reifenrath, W. G., Robinson, P. B., Bolton, V. D., and Aliff, R. E. (1981). Percutaneous penetration of mosquito repellents in the hairless dog: Effect of dose on percentage penetration. *Food Cosmet. Toxicol.* **19**, 195–199.

Rej, R., Loux, M., and Copeland, W. (1990). Effect of diethyl-toluamide on human ornithine carbamoyltransferase. *Clin. Chem.* **36**, 1143.

Roland, E. H., Jan, C. E., and Rigg, M. J. (1985). Toxic encephalopathy in a child after brief exposure to insect repellents. *Can. Med. Assoc. J.* **132**, 155–156.

Rowe, P. C., Newman, S. L., and Brusilow, S. W. (1986). Natural history of symptomatic partial ornithine transcarbamylase deficiency. *N. Engl. J. Med.* **314**, 541–547.

Roy, A. K. (1973). Androgen-dependent synthesis of α_{2u}-globulin in the rat: Role of the pituitary gland. *J. Endocrinol.* **56**, 295–301.

San, R. H. C., and Schadly, M. B. (1989). *Salmonella*/mammalian-microsome plate incorporation mutagenicity assay (Ames test) with a confirmatory assay. Unpublished study conducted at Microbiological Associates, Inc. under the sponsorship of the DEET Joint Venture/Chemical Specialties Manufacturers Association.

Schaefer, C., and Peters, P. W. (1992). Intrauterine diethyltoluamide exposure and fetal outcome. *Reprod. Toxicol.* **6**, 175–176.

Schardein, J. L. (1989). Evaluation of DEET in a two generation reproduction/fertility study in rats. Unpublished study conducted at International Research and Development Corporation under the sponsorship of the DEET Joint Venture/Chemical Manufacturers Association.

Schmidt, C. H., Acree, F., Jr., and Bowman, M. C. (1959). Fate of C[14]-diethyltoluamide applied to guinea pigs. *J. Econ. Entomol.* **52**(5), 928–930.

Schoenig, G. P., Hartnagel, R. E., Jr., Schardein, J. L., and Vorhees, C. V. (1993). Neurotoxicity evaluation of *N,N*-diethyl-*m*-toluamide (DEET) in rats. *Fund. Appl. Toxicol.* **21**, 355–365.

Schoenig, G. P., Neeper-Bradley, T. L., Fisher, L. C., and Hartnagel, R. E., Jr. (1994). Teratologic evaluations of *N,N*-diethyl-*m*-toluamide (DEET) in rats and rabbits. *Fund. Appl. Toxicol.* **23**, 63–69.

Schoenig, G. P., Hartnagel, R. E., Jr., Osimitz, T. G., and Llanso, S. (1996). Absorption, distribution, metabolism, and excretion of *N,N*-diethyl-*m*-toluamide in the rat. *Drug Metab. Disposition* **24**(2), 156–163.

Schoenig, G. P., Osimitz, T. G., Gabriel, K. L., Hartnagel, R., Gill, M. W., and Goldenthal, E. I. (1999). Evaluation of the chronic toxicity and oncogenicity of *N,N*-diethyl-*m*-toluamide (DEEt). *Toxicol. Sci.* **47**, 99–109.

Selim, S., Hartnagel, R. E., Jr., Osimitz, T. G., Gabriel, K. L., and Schoenig, G. P. (1995). Absorption, metabolism, and excretion of *N,N*-diethyl-*m*-toluamide following dermal application to human volunteers. *Fund. Appl. Toxicol.* **25**, 95–100.

Sherman, R. A. (1980). Phase 2—Behavioral effects of acute aerosol exposure to *N,N*-diethyl-*meta*-toluamide (M-Det). Unpublished study conducted at U.S. Army Environmental Hygiene Agency.

Sippel, A. E., Feigelson, P., and Roy, A. K. (1975). Hormonal regulation of the hepatic messenger RNA levels for α_{2u}-globulin. *Biochemistry* **14**, 825–829.

Snodgrass, H. L., Nelson, D. C., and Weeks, M. H. (1982). Dermal penetration and potential for placental transfer of the insect repellent *N,N*-diethyl-*m*-toluamide. *Am. Ind. Hyg. Assoc. J.* **43**(10), 747–754.

Snyder, J. W., Poe, R. O., Stubbins, J. F., and Garrettson, L. K. (1986). Acute manic psychosis following the dermal application of *N-N*-diethyl-*m*-toluamide. *J. Toxicol. Clin. Toxicol.* **24**, 429–439.

Stenbäck, F. (1976). Testing of cosmetics, ingredients of sunscreen ointments, insect repellents, and detergents on skin of mice and rabbits: Lifespan studies. Unpublished study conducted at the Eppley Institute for Research in Cancer and Allied Diseases under the sponsorship of Morflex Chemical Co., Inc.

Sterner, W. (1977). Effect of "MGK Diethyltoluamide" on the embryonic development of rats after oral application. Unpublished study conducted at International Bio-Research, Inc. under the sponsorship of McLaughlin Gormley King Co.

Swentzel, K. C. (1978). Investigation of *N,N*-diethyl-*m*-toluamide (M-Det) for dominant lethal effects in the mouse study. Unpublished study conducted at U.S. Army Environmental Hygiene Agency.

Taylor, W. G. (1986). Metabolism of *N,N*-diethyl-*meta*-toluamide by rat liver microsomes. *Drug Metab. Disp.* **14**(5), 532–539.

Taylor, W. G., Danielson, T. J., Spooner, R. W., and Golsteyn, L. R. (1994). Pharmacokinetic assessment of the dermal absorption of *N,N*-diethyl-*m*-toluamide (DEET). *Drug Metab. Disp.* **22**(1), 106–112.

Tenenbein, M. (1987). Severe toxic reactions and death following the ingestion of diethyltoluamide-containing insect repellents. *J. Am. Med. Assoc.* **258**(11), 1509–1511.

U.S. EPA (1980). Pesticide Registration Standard—DEET. Registration Division and Special Pesticide Review Division. U.S. Environmental Protection Agency, Washington, DC.

U.S. EPA (1984). Pesticide Assessment Guidelines, Subdivision F, Hazard Evaluation: Human and Domestic Animals (Revised). Hazard Evaluation Division, Office of Pesticide Programs, U.S. Environmental Protection Agency, Washington, DC.

U.S. EPA (1998). Reregistration Eligibility Document on DEET. Office of Pesticide Programs, U.S. Environmental Protection Agency, Washington, DC.

Veltri, J. C., Osimitz, T. G., Bradford, D. C., and Page, B. C. (1994). Retrospective analysis of calls to poison control centers resulting from exposure to the insect repellent *N,N*-diethyl-*m*-toluamide (DEET) from 1985–1989. *J. Toxicol. Clin. Toxicol.* **32**, 1–16.

Verschoyle, R. D., Brown, A. W., Nolan, C., Ray, D. E., and Lister, T. (1992). A comparison of the acute toxicity, neuropathology, and electrophysiology of *N,N*-diethyl-*m*-toluamide and *N,N*-dimethyl-2,2-diphenylacetamide in rats. *Fund. Appl. Toxicol.* **18**, 79–88.

Weil, C. S. (1973). *N,N*-diethyl-*m*-toluamide range finding toxicity studies. Unpublished studies conducted at Carnegie-Mellon University under the sponsorship of Union Carbide Corporation.

Whitley, R. J. (1994). Viral encephalitis. Diagnosis and treatment. *C.N.S. Drugs* **2**, 355–366.

Windheuser, J. J., Haslam, J. L., Cadwell, L., and Shaffer, R. D. (1982). The use of *N,N*-diethyl-*m*-toluamide to enhance dermal and transdermal delivery of drugs. *J. Pharmaceut. Sci.* **71**(11), 1211–1213.

Wright, D. M., Hardin, B. D., Goad, P. W., and Chrislip, D. W. (1992). Reproductive and developmental toxicity of N,N-diethyl-m-toluamide in rats. *Fund. Appl. Toxicol.* **19**, 33–42.

Wu, A., Pearson, M. L., Shekoski, D. L., Soto, R. J., and Stewart, R. D. (1979). High resolution gas chromatography/mass spectrometric characterization of urinary metabolites of N,N-diethyl-m-toluamide (DEET) in man. *J. High Resolut. Chromatogr. Commun.* **2**, 558–562.

Yeung, J. M., and Taylor, W. G. (1988). Metabolism of N,N-diethyl-m-toluamide (DEET) by liver microsomes from male and female rats: Simultaneous quantitation of DEET and its metabolites by high performance liquid chromatography. *Drug Metab. Disp.* **16**(4), 600–604.

Zadikoff, C. M. (1979). Toxic encephalopathy associated with use of insect repellent. *J. Pediatr.* **95**, 140–142.

Zeiger, E., Anderson, B., Haworth, S., Lawlor, T., and Mortelmans, K. (1992). *Salmonella* mutagenicity tests: V. Results from the testing of 311 chemicals. *Environ. Mol. Mutagen.* **19**(Suppl. 21), 2–141.

The Safety Assessment
of Piperonyl Butoxide

Thomas G. Osimitz
S.C. Johnson and Sons, Inc.

Ruaidhri Breathnach
University College Dublin

64.1 CHEMISTRY AND FORMULATIONS

Piperonyl butoxide (PBO), 2-(2-butoxyethoxy)ethyl 6-propyl-piperonyl ether (IUPAC), is an insecticide synergist produced from the condensation of the sodium salt of 2-(2-butoxyethoxy) ethanol and the chloromethyl derivative of hydrogenated safrole (Fig. 64.1). The methylenedioxyphenyl moiety constitutes over half of the PBO molecule by weight and is derived from sassafras oil. Sassafras oil is an essential oil distilled from several species of trees found in Brazil, China, and Viet Nam.

Current world production of PBO averages 92% pure. In the early days, PBO contained small but detectable amounts of safrole and dihydrosafrole (DHS). However, refinements in distillation have resulted in safrole and DHS levels usually below the 40 ppm detection limit by high resolution gas chromatography (Di Blashi, 1998).

The development of PBO grew out of a need in the late 1930s and early 1940s to extend the usefulness of the naturally derived insecticide pyrethrum, which was considered a strategic insecticide against mosquitoes and other disease-carrying insects. The chemicals that were developed had little intrinsic pesticidal activity of their own; however, they did increase the effectiveness of a given dose of pyrethrins and were thus called synergists. PBO was one of a series of molecules synthesized (Wachs, 1947).

PBO is usually formulated with natural pyrethrins or synthetic pyrethroids in ratios (PBO : pyrethrins) ranging from 5:1 to 20:1. Formulations of PBO and carbamates are also available, although their use is minor relative to that of PBO and pyrethrins/pyrethroids.

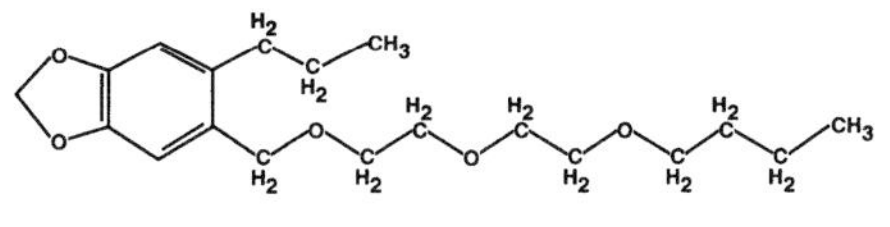

64.2 USES

As a synergist, PBO inhibits the mixed function oxidase (MFO) system of insects, thereby reducing the oxidative breakdown of other pesticides like pyrethrum and the synthetic pyrethroids (Casida, 1970). The precise mechanism of inhibition is unknown, but speculation is that a carbene derivative forms and binds to the heme moiety of the cytochrome P-450 enzyme, thereby rendering it inactive (Dahl and Brenzinski, 1985; Delaforge et al., 1985; Franklin, 1976; Hodgson et al., 1973; Murray and Reidy, 1989; Philpot and Hodgson, 1971, 1972a, 1972b). The result is that higher levels of the insecticide remain in the insect and are thereby available to exercise their lethal effect on the insect. PBO enhances the pesticidal activity of a given level of active ingredient, thus promoting reduced use of the pesticide.

Appearing in several thousand U.S. Environmental Protection Agency (U.S. EPA)-registered products, PBO is one of the most commonly registered pesticides in terms of the number of formulas in which it is present. It is approved for preharvest application to a wide variety of crops including fruits and vegetables. The application rates are low; the highest single rate is 0.386 lbs PBO/acre. It is also used extensively in combination with pyrethrins and some synthetic pyrethroids to control insect pests in and around the home and in food handling establishments. A wide variety of water-based PBO-containing products such as crack and crevice sprays, total release foggers, and flying insect sprays are made for use by consumers in the home.

Annual use of PBO in the United States is approximately 1.3–1.5 million pounds (PBOTF, 1997). About 47% of this total

Figure 64.1 Chemical structure of piperonyl butoxide (PBO).

is used for indoor residential purposes, 17% for indoor food uses in warehouses and food handling establishments, and only 13% goes for agricultural crop applications.

Piperonyl butoxide has also been allowed as a food additive in Japan since 1955, its maximum approved level being 0.024 g/kg (24 ppm) in raw cereals.

64.3 HAZARD IDENTIFICATION

64.3.1 ACUTE TOXICITY

Numerous acute studies have been conducted over the years with PBO in a variety of species and by various exposure routes. This body of data, including the most recent studies, indicates that PBO is generally of low acute toxicity to animals. It is mildly irritating to the eye and skin. It is not a dermal sensitizer. Table 64.1 summarizes this acute toxicity data as well as European Economic Commission (EEC) labeling classifications and U.S. EPA toxicity categories.

64.3.2 SUBCHRONIC TOXICITY

PBO has been tested in dogs, mice, rats, rabbits, and African green monkeys for subchronic toxicity. A summary of the subchronic toxicity studies discussed below is presented in Table 64.2.

64.3.2.1 Dogs

Lorber (1972) reported unexpected alterations in blood counts of intact and splenectomized dogs after use of a fogger (containing PBO among other chemicals). The fogger bathed the animals inadvertently in a "dense pesticide mist." The dogs were part of a research project investigating the relationship of spleen, bone marrow, and blood cells. Further work was undertaken in which 17 intact, 12 splenectomized, and 7 partially

splenectomized dogs were purposefully exposed to deodorized kerosene containing only PBO (1.5%). Exposure periods consisted of four intervals of 5 minutes duration, with an 8-minute interval between each exposure. The splenectomized dogs showed a reduction in serum platelet count and an occasional increase in reticulocytes. The authors concluded that the demonstrated greater resistance of intact dogs to the hematotoxic potential of the tested chemicals may have been in part due to the larger spleens in these animals which could perhaps sequester the chemical(s) more effectively. Moreover, they felt that the normal hepatic blood flow in these animals could also enhance the removal of the chemical(s) from the systemic circulation.

Goldenthal (1993a) conducted a range-finding study as a prelude to a 1-year chronic study. PBO was administered in the diet to dogs (4 animals/sex/dose level) for 8 weeks. The dosage levels were 500, 1000, 2000, and 3000 ppm (approximately equivalent to 12.5, 25, 50, and 75 mg/kg body weight/day, respectively). All dogs survived to study termination. All animals in the 3000 ppm dose group had decreased appetites and reduced defecation during the first week. No other abnormal clinical signs were present. Three out of four dogs lost weight in the highest dose group. Even at 1000 ppm PBO in the diet, weight gains were lower than the control group. Food intake was similar between treated and control groups, except for a slight reduction in some animals at the 3000 ppm dosage level. There were no treatment-related effects on hematological parameters at any dose level, but slight increases in alkaline phosphatase values and slight decreases in cholesterol were noted at doses ≥2000 ppm. No treatment-related microscopic changes were noted at necropsy in any group, but a compound-related increase in absolute and relative liver and gall bladder weights was recorded in males. Upon histopathologic examination, hypertrophy of hepatocytes was noted in males of all dose levels and in females at dosages 2000 ppm and above. This finding was consistent with the increases in liver weights and serum alkaline phosphatase levels described above. No other

Table 64.1
Summary of Acute Toxicity Data and Classifications

Route	Species	Result	EEC labeling classification	U.S. EPA toxicity category	Reference
Oral LD$_{50}$	Rat	>4 g/kg (male) >7 g/kg (female)	Unclassified	Category IV	Gabriel (1991a)
Dermal LD$_{50}$	Rabbit	>2 g/kg	Unclassified	Category IV	Gabriel (1991b)
Inhalation LC$_{50}$	Rat	>5.9 mg/L air	Harmful	Category III	Hoffman (1991)
Eye irritation	Rabbit	Minimally irritating	Labeling not indicated	Category III	Romanelli (1991a)
Skin irritation	Rabbit	Minimally irritating	Labeling not indicated	Category IV	Romanelli (1991b)
Skin sensitization (Buehler)	Guinea pig	Negative	Labeling not indicated	Category IV	Romanelli (1991c)

treatment-related microscopic changes were evident. There was a decrease in the absolute and relative weights of the testes and epididymis in the groups treated with 2000 and 3000 ppm. The dose level of 500 ppm was set as a NOAEL for this study because the changes recorded in the liver were considered adaptive in nature rather than adverse and were not accompanied by any systemic signs of toxicity.

64.3.2.2 Mice

Fujitani *et al.* (1993) reported the results of dosing CD-1 mice (10 animals/sex/dose level) with 1000, 3000, or 9000 ppm (approximately equivalent to 150, 450, and 1350 mg/kg body weight/day, respectively) PBO in the diet for 20 days. Body weights were depressed in the high-dose animals (about 15%) and in the mid-dose females (about 8%). Kidney and spleen weights were also reduced in the high-dose group. A treatment-related elevation in liver weights was noted with a 79% increase in the high-dose males. Females in the high-dose group showed higher levels of γ-glutamyl transpeptidase (GGT) activity. The high-dose males and females featured higher levels of cholesterol, phospholipids, and total serum proteins. Hepatocyte hypertrophy, single cell necrosis, and inflammation, most

Table 64.2
Summary of Results of Subchronic Toxicity Studies with PBO

Species	Route	Dose	Duration	NOAEL	Comments	Reference
Dog	Inhalation	15,000 ppm	Four 5 min intervals	Not applicable	Reduction in serum platelet count, increase in reticulocytes (splenectomized animals)	Lorber (1972)
	Diet	500–3000 ppm (~12.5–75 mg/kg body weight/day)	8 wks	500 ppm (~12.5 mg/kg body weight/day)	Decreased body weight, increased liver weight, hepatocyte hypertrophy	Goldenthal (1993a)
Mouse	Diet	1000–9000 ppm (~150–1350 mg/kg body weight/day)	20 days	1000 ppm (~150 mg/kg body weight/day)	Increased liver weight, hepatocyte hypertrophy, necrosis, inflammatory cell infiltration	Fujitani *et al.* (1993)
	Oral	10–1000 mg/kg body weight/day	90 days	30 mg/kg body weight/day	Increased liver weight, liver necrosis, centrilobular hypertrophy	Chun and Wagner (1993)
	Oral	1500–6000 ppm (236–880 mg/kg body weight/day)	7 wks	Not established	Alterations in motor activity	Tanaka (1993)
Rat	Gavage	2.5–5 ml/kg body weight/day	31 days	Not established	Anorexia, loss of weight, death	Sarles and Vandergrift (1952)
	Oral	1857 mg/kg body weight/day	90 days	Not applicable	40% mortality, increased liver weight	Bond *et al.* (1973)
	Diet	62.5–2000 mg/kg body weight/day	28 days	125 mg/kg body weight/day	Increased liver weight, microscopic changes in liver	Modeweg-Hausen *et al.* (1984)
	Oral	6000–24,000 ppm (~300–1200 mg/kg body weight/day)	13 wks	Not established	Decreased body weight, increased liver and kidney weights, hepatocyte hypertrophy	Fujitani *et al.* (1992)
	Gavage	250–4000 mg/kg body weight/day	10 days	250 mg/kg body weight/day	Ataxia, twitching, dyspnoea, gastric ulceration	Chun and Neeper-Bradley (1992)
	Inhalation	15–512 mg/m^3	90 days	155 mg/m^3	Alterations in clinical chemistry parameters, increased liver and kidney weights	Newton (1992)
Rabbit	Oral	1 or 4 ml/kg body weight/wk (5% emulsion)	3 wks	Not applicable	No signs of toxicity	Sarles *et al.* (1949)
	Dermal	100–1000 mg/kg body weight/day	3 wks	1000 mg/kg body weight/day (systemic toxicity) 100 mg/kg body weight/day (local effects)	Slight erythema/edema, fissuring/inflammation of skin	Goldenthal (1992)
Monkey	Oral	0.03 or 0.1 ml/kg body weight/day	4 wks	Not applicable	Minor changes in liver	Sarles and Vandergrift (1952)

prominently in the centrilobular region, were also seen in the livers of the mid- and high-dose groups. The NOAEL for this study, based on liver toxicity, was 1000 ppm.

As a prelude to a 2-year bioassay, Chun and Wagner (1993) report the conduct of a 90-day oral toxicity study in CD-1 mice (15 animals/sex/dose level) using dose levels of 10, 30, 100, 300, and 1000 mg PBO/kg body weight/day in the diet. A significant decrease in body weight was noted in the high-dose males (−34% versus controls). The target organ for toxicity was the liver as indicated by increased liver weights, hepatocyte necrosis, and centrilobular hypertrophy (NOAEL = 30 mg/kg body weight/day).

Tanaka (1993) reported the results of a study in male CD-1 mice designed to probe neurobehavioral endpoints. Male mice were fed PBO daily from 5–12 weeks of age at concentrations of 1500, 3000, or 6000 ppm (equivalent to 236, 448, and 880 mg/kg body weight/day, respectively as averaged over the 5–11 week period). Twenty animals were used per dose level. No significant adverse effects were observed in water T-maze performance. Significant changes were noted, however, in exploratory behavior at 8 and 11 weeks of age. The incidence of defecation was increased at all dose levels at 8 weeks. Numerous parameters were affected at 11 weeks [i.e., number of movements, movement time, number of horizontal activities, total distance (all dose levels), number of turnings, average distance (all dose levels) and average speed]. The authors concluded that piperonyl butoxide has an influence on the motor activity of exploratory behavior in mice at 11 weeks of age.

64.3.2.3 Rats

Sarles and Vandergrift (1952) gavaged six male and six female rats with PBO daily, 6 days/week for 31 days. The first seven doses were at 2.5 ml/kg body weight. Two animals died on the third and fourth days. The remaining animals improved after some initial clinical signs of toxicity. They were dosed with a second seven doses of 3.5 mL/kg body weight each. Little toxicity was noted at this dose level. Hence, the animals thereafter received doses of 5 ml/kg body weight. Clinical signs of toxicity included anorexia and loss of weight. Additional animal deaths occurred from the 17th to 24th days of testing; the next and last death was at 31 days.

Bond *et al.* (1973) administered 1857 mg PBO/kg body weight/day orally to a single group of 20 rats for 90 days. Forty percent of the rats died prior to conclusion of the study. The most significant finding was a dramatic increase in liver weight (i.e., 2.4 times that of untreated controls). The authors also allude to another study they performed, which is unpublished, in which rats were fed 500 mg PBO/kg body weight/day. These animals were reported to have liver and kidney damage.

A 4-week range-finding study was conducted by Modeweg-Hausen *et al.* (1984). Rats (10 animals/sex/dose level) were fed 62.5, 125, 250, 500, 1000, or 2000 mg PBO/kg body weight/day. Hepatic eosinophilic infiltration and the increased vacuolization of hepatocytes were seen with increasing severity among the mid- and high-dose groups. These effects were

viewed as being degenerative changes representing chronic toxicity. Liver weights were elevated at 250 mg/kg body weight/day and above in the males and at 500 mg/kg body weight/day and above in the females. Except for an increase in alkaline phosphatase at the highest dose level, no treatment-related changes were reported in hematologic and clinical chemical parameters. Based on the observed liver toxicity, the NOAEL for this study is 125 mg/kg body weight/day.

A 13-week subacute oral toxicity study was performed in Fischer F344 rats (10 animals/sex/dose level) at levels of 6000, 12,000, or 24,000 ppm (approximately equivalent to 300, 600, or 1200 mg/kg body weight/day, respectively) PBO in the diet (Fujitani *et al.*, 1992). No mortality occurred. Nasal bleeding and dose-related abdominal distension were reported. A significant decrease in body weight was evident in the high-dose groups (36% decrease in males, 24% decrease in females). Blood hemoglobin levels were reduced in both sexes in the high-dose group and in mid-dose females. Biochemical changes in the high-dose group consisted of increases in albumin, cholesterol, urea, and GGT activity. Liver and kidney weights were increased in a dose-dependent manner. Histopathologic examination revealed hypertrophic hepatocytes (containing a basophilic granular substance) and vacuolation of hepatocytes in periportal areas. Coagulative necrosis and oval cell proliferation were occasionally seen. Atrophy of the epithelial lining of the proximal convoluted tubules in the renal cortex was present in some male rats. A NOAEL for PBO could not be established in this study owing to the presence of liver and kidney effects even at the "low" dose of 6000 ppm.

Marked clinical signs of subacute toxicity were seen in the dams of a range-finding study conducted to select doses for a developmental toxicology study (Chun and Neeper-Bradley, 1992). Pregnant female rats (15 animals/dose level) were gavaged on gestational days 6–15 with PBO at levels of 250, 500, 1000, 2000, or 4000 mg/kg body weight/day. Signs of general stress, such as urogenital wetness and periocular encrustation, were evident in many animals during the first three days of the study at dose levels of at least 500 mg/kg body weight/day. At levels of 2000 mg/kg body weight/day, more severe clinical signs such as ataxia, twitching, prostration, dyspnea, gasping, and lacrimation were noted. Ulceration of the lining of the glandular region of the stomach as well as hemorrhage and sloughing of the lining of the nonglandular region were noted at necropsy.

In the only subchronic study conducted by the inhalation route, Newton (1992) exposed CD rats (15 animals/sex/dose level) for 6 hr/day, 5 days/week, for 90 days in whole body exposure chambers. PBO was aerosolized to achieve exposure concentrations of 15, 74, 155, and 512 mg PBO/m^3 (MMAD of the aerosol was 1.7 μm). Neither body weight gain nor food intake was affected by exposure. In the high-dose group, serum alanine transaminase, aspartate transaminase, and glucose levels were decreased, whereas BUN, total protein, and albumin levels were increased. However, not all of these effects were statistically significant, and there was no clear dose–response relationship. Both absolute and relative liver and kidney weights were elevated in the high-dose group.

Minimal to slight irritation of the larynx was observed upon necropsy in all treatment groups. Inflammation, congestion, edema, and debris in the lumen were noted as well. Squamous metaplasia of the laryngeal epithelium was noted in all groups but was most marked in both sexes at the highest dose level. These changes are considered to represent an adaptive response to mild irritation and do not represent systemic toxicity. Moreover, there is no evidence that such metaplasia in the absence of atypia is preneoplastic (Brown, 1990; Monticello *et al.*, 1990).

64.3.2.4 Rabbits

Sarles *et al.* (1949) performed a subacute oral toxicity experiment in rabbits. A 5% PBO emulsion was fed once weekly in the diet to three rabbits over a 3-week period. The dosage used varied between 1.0 and 4.0 ml/kg body weight/week. There was neither mortality nor clinical signs of toxicity. The rabbit that received the highest dosage was sacrificed 1 week after the last treatment, but no lesions were detected at postmortem examination.

A 21-day subchronic dermal toxicity study was conducted in rabbits (5 animals/sex/dose level) in which 100, 300, or 1000 mg PBO/kg body weight was applied topically once a day, 5 days a week, for 3 consecutive weeks (Goldenthal, 1992). Treatment-related effects were limited to minor skin changes at the application site. Dermal irritation was present in all treatment groups (although to a lesser extent and incidence at the 100 mg/kg body weight/day dose level). Dermal lesions consisted of very slight erythema and edema. This irritation usually appeared by day 5 and persisted for the remainder of the study. Desquamation and fissuring of the skin appeared in the 300 and 1000 mg/kg body weight/day groups. Moderate acanthosis, hyperkeratosis, and chronic inflammation of the epidermis were present. The severity of these lesions increased with increasing dosage. Body weights were comparable with those in the control group, and food intake was only slightly lower in treated animals. No treatment-related changes were seen in hematology and clinical chemistry, and no signs of systemic toxicity were present at any dosage level. The NOAEL is 100 mg/kg body weight/day for local effects whereas the NOAEL for systemic toxicity is 1000 mg/kg body weight/day.

64.3.2.5 Other Species

A 4-week oral toxicity study was performed by Sarles and Vandergrift (1952) in which two African Green monkeys were fed PBO by capsule, 6 days a week (for 4 weeks), at a dosage level of 0.03 or 0.1 ml/kg body weight/day (one monkey at each dosage level). No gross pathological lesions were evident in the treated monkeys' livers. Upon histopathologic examination of the liver, the monkey on the higher dose level showed evidence of minimal dystrophy and dysplasia, occasional acidophilic and hyaline-necrosis cells, as well as hydropic swelling.

64.3.3 REPRODUCTIVE AND DEVELOPMENTAL TOXICITY

A summary of the results of the reproductive and developmental toxicity studies discussed below is presented in Tables 64.3 and 64.4.

64.3.3.1 Reproductive Toxicity

Mice A three-generation, one litter per generation, reproductive toxicity study was performed in CD-1 mice by Tanaka *et al.* (1992). Ten animals of either sex were incorporated at each dosage level and PBO dosage rates were set at 1000, 2000, 4000, and 8000 ppm (purity not specified) in the diet. These dose levels are equivalent to 268, 506, 936, and 1583 mg PBO/kg body weight/day as averaged over F_0 and F_1 generations from preconception through lactation. Food intake was reduced in the F_0 generation at the 8000 ppm dose, except during the mating period, and was also reduced during the lactation period in the F_1 generation, also at 8000 ppm. The 4000 ppm treatment groups of both the F_0 and the F_1 generations also had a reduction in food intake during the lactation period. Mean F_1 litter weight was significantly decreased (38%) at 8000 ppm and reduced by 18% at the 4000 ppm treatment level. However, litter size remained unchanged at all levels. Pups born in the 8000 ppm treated group of the F_1 generation had a lower survival index at postpartum day 21 (63% versus 91% for males of control group; 79% versus 89% for females of control group). Pup weights in the F_1 generation were decreased for all dosage groups, but there was no dose-related response at lower or mid-dose levels. No treatment-related effects were noted in neurobehavioral tests conducted in the F_1 animals.

The mean F_2 litter size was significantly decreased at the 4000 and 8000 ppm treatment levels. Mean F_2 litter weights were decreased in all treated groups. Pups in the 8000 ppm treated group of the F_2 generation had a lower survival index than controls at day 21 postpartum (59% in males and 79% in females versus 100% in male and female control groups). Pup weights in the F_2 generation were decreased at dosage levels of 2000 ppm and above on postnatal days 4, 7, 14, and 21. Pup weights were reduced on postnatal days 4 and 7 at the 1000 ppm dosage level. No clear dose–response relationship was evident in the neurobehavioral tests conducted with F_2 animals. Because pup weights were reduced at all doses tested, a NOAEL could not be set for this study.

Tanaka (1992) further probed the developmental neurotoxicity of PBO in CD-1 mice in a subsequent study. Ten mice of either sex per group received diets containing 1500, 3000, or 6000 ppm (approximately equivalent to 400, 700, and 1250 mg/kg body weight/day, respectively, based on food consumption values in Tanaka *et al.*, 1992) PBO during a 4-week period prior to mating (F_0), during gestation and through the time that the F_1 generation was 8 weeks old. The open field test demonstrated a dose-dependent decrease in ambulating and rearing in F_0 male mice. However, because of the excessive dosage levels incorporated in this study, pup body weights were

Table 64.3
Summary of Results from Reproductive Studies with PBO

Species	Route	Dose	Study type	NOAEL	Comments	Reference
Mice	Diet	1000–8000 ppm (268–1583 mg/kg body weight/day)	Three-generation	Not established	Pup weights reduced at all dose levels.	Tanaka et al. (1992)
	Diet	1500–6000 ppm (~400–1250 mg/kg body weight/day)	Two-generation	Not established	Excessive dose levels resulted in decreased pup weights in all treated animals.	Tanaka (1992)
Rat	Diet	100–25,000 ppm (~8–2000 mg/kg body weight/day)	Three-generation	1000 ppm (~8 mg/kg body weight/day)	Very high maternal toxicity at two highest dose levels resulting in marked reductions in the incidence of pregnancies, numbers of litters per dam, general health of the offspring, and average weanling weights of pups.	Sarles and Vandergrift (1952)
	Diet	300–5000 ppm (~24–400 mg/kg body weight/day)	Two-generation	Parental toxicity/ pup development: 1000 ppm (~80 mg/kg body weight/day) Reproductive toxicity: 5000 ppm (~400 mg/kg body weight/day)	Body weights of pups born to dams treated at the highest dose level were reduced in the early postpartum period.	Robinson et al. (1986)
	Diet	30–500 mg/kg body weight/day	2-yr chronic	Not applicable	Increases in ovarian weight observed in some females at highest dose level.	Butler et al. (1998)
Dog	Diet	500—3000 ppm (~12.5–75 mg/kg body weight/day)	Range-finding	Not applicable	Increased absolute and relative weights of testis and epididymis noted. No microscopic abnormalities observed in the testis.	Goldenthal (1993a)

reduced at birth in all treated animals. By postpartum day 21, the mean pup body weight in the mid-dose group was 7% lower than controls. The mean body weight of high-dose pups was decreased 41%. The survival index for pups at postpartum day 21 was 79.2% (controls), 92.9% (low-dose group), 80.0% (mid-dose group), and 51.7% (high-dose group). There were no significant differences in the behavioral test during the lactation period, except for a reduction in olfactory orientation in mid- and high-dose group animals. Other than sporadic non-dose-dependent changes, the open field test and multiple water T-maze tests were not significantly altered by PBO.

Rats   In a reproductive toxicity study reported by Sarles and Vandergrift (1952), groups of 12 male and 12 female rats per dose level were fed diets containing 100, 1000, 10,000, or 25,000 ppm (approximately equivalent to 8, 80, 800, or 2000 mg/kg body weight/day, respectively) of PBO (technical grade, 80% purity), for three generations. None of the female rats at the highest dose level were fertile and there were marked reductions in the incidence of pregnancies, numbers of litters per dam, general health of the offspring, and average weanling

weights of pups born to dams treated at 10,000 ppm. These findings are clearly a result of the high maternal toxicity, especially at 10,000 and 25,000 ppm. No adverse effect on reproduction was observed in three generations of progeny in the 100 and 1000 ppm groups (NOAEL = 1000 ppm).

A two-generation reproduction study was performed in rats with PBO by Robinson et al. (1986). Groups of 26 male and 26 female Sprague–Dawley rats were utilized and adults of the F_0 and F_1 generations were treated at dose levels of 300, 1000, or 5000 ppm (approximately equivalent to 24, 80, or 400 mg/kg body weight/day, respectively) in the diet. Animals were treated for 83 to 85 days prior to placement for mating, and treatment continued throughout mating, pregnancy, and lactation. The only consistent finding throughout the study period was a lower body weight gain at the highest dosage level. This tendency was partially reversed during the lactation period, when females at this dose level showed higher weight gains when compared with control rats. For both F_1 and F_2 generation pups, the viability, survival, and lactation indices were unaffected by treatment. There were no treatment-related abnormal findings for the pups, and weanlings did not reveal any treatment-related

Table 64.4
Summary of Results from Developmental Studies with PBO

Species	Route	Dose	NOAEL	Comments	Reference
Mice	Gavage	1065–1800 mg/kg body weight/day	Not established	Total resorption rates significantly increased in mid- and high-dose groups. Significant decrease in body weights of male and female fetuses, appearing to be dose-dependent.	Tanaka *et al.* (1994)
Rat	Gavage	300 or 1000 mg/kg body weight/day	*Maternal toxicity*: Not established *Developmental toxicity*: 1000 mg/kg body weight/day	Maternal body weights were reduced at both dose levels tested.	Kennedy *et al.* (1977)
	Gavage	62.5–500 mg/kg body weight/day	*Maternal and developmental toxicity*: 500 mg/kg body weight/day	No signs of either maternal or embryo-fetotoxicity.	Khera *et al.* (1979)
	Gavage	200–1000 mg/kg body weight/day	*Maternal toxicity*: 200 mg/kg body weight/day *Developmental toxicity*: 1000 mg/kg body weight/day	Gestational body weights and body weight gains were reduced in the 500 and 1000 mg/kg body weight/day groups.	Chun and Neeper-Bradley (1991)
Rabbit	Gavage	50–200 mg/kg body weight/day	*Maternal toxicity*: 50 mg/kg body weight/day *Developmental toxicity*: 200 mg/kg body weight/day	Maternal toxicity was evident at 100 and 200 mg/kg body weight/day manifested by decreased defecation and a dose-dependent weight loss during the treatment period.	Leng *et al.* (1986)

adverse effects. Body weights of pups born to dams treated at the highest dose level were reduced in the early postpartum period. The NOAEL for parental toxicity and pup development was thus 1000 ppm PBO in the diet. The NOAEL for reproductive toxicity was set at 5000 ppm PBO in the diet.

Other Studies In an 8-week dietary range-finding toxicity study in dogs, PBO was fed daily in the diet to beagles at dose rates of 500, 1000, 2000, or 3000 ppm (approximately equivalent to 12.5, 25, 50, or 75 mg/kg body weight/day, respectively) (Goldenthal, 1993a). There was an increase in the absolute and relative weights of the testes and epididymides. No microscopic abnormalities were noted in the testes. Spermatozoa were being produced. Other details of the study are presented in Section 64.3.2.1.

In a 2-year chronic oral toxicity study in Sprague–Dawley rats, animals received dietary administration of 15, 30, 100, or 500 mg PBO/kg body weight/day (89% purity) (Butler *et al.*, 1998). Only changes in the reproductive system are discussed here. Full details of the study are presented in Section 64.3.4.3. Increases in ovarian weights were observed among some females receiving 500 mg/kg body weight/day, although no histopathologic changes were noted. Atrophy of the testes was seen histologically in all male groups and when bilateral atrophy was considered alone, there was an increased incidence in the intermediate and high-dose groups with a corresponding reduction in the incidence of unilateral atrophy. However,

the finding is unlikely to be related to treatment because the dose–response relationship was unclear and the atrophy was not accompanied by changes in the seminiferous tubules or sperm production. Moreover, there were no statistically significant increases or decreases in testes weight when expressed as either absolute weight or relative-to-brain weight.

64.3.3.2 Developmental Toxicity

Mice Tanaka *et al.* (1994) reported a study conducted in CD-1 mice in which PBO was administered by gavage on day 9 of gestation to groups of 20 animals at doses of 1065, 1385, or 1800 mg/kg body weight (>95% purity; PBO dissolved in olive oil). No abnormal behavior or mortality patterns were observed in dams. Three abortions occurred in the mid- and high-dose groups. Four litters were resorbed in the two higher dosage groups, but maternal body weights were comparable between all groups. Total resorption rates were significantly increased in the mid-dose (26%) and the high-dose groups (32%) when compared with the control value (6%). The number of viable fetuses per dam was comparable between all dosage groups. There was a significant decrease in body weights of male and female fetuses derived from treated dams, which did appear to be dose-dependent. Certain external malformations such as exencephaly, craniochisis, open eyelids, omphalocele, kinky tail, and *talipes varus* were observed in all groups (including controls) and oligodactyly was recorded in the forelimbs of some fetuses derived from treated dams. The incidence of this latter defect was 6% in those fetuses derived from the highest dosage group. The authors concluded that a single high dose of PBO (1065 mg/kg body weight or above), when given orally to pregnant mice on day 9 of gestation, could cause embryo-fetal toxicity with associated oligodactyly of the forelimbs. The high dose levels of this study make it difficult to interpret the significance of this finding.

Rats Kennedy *et al.* (1977) performed a teratogenicity study with PBO in pregnant rats. Twenty female animals per dose level were gavaged with PBO in corn oil at 300 or 1000 mg PBO/kg body weight/day. Other than a decline in body weight gain in both treated groups (especially in the later stages of gestation), no other treatment-related signs of toxicity occurred. The reproductive parameters of the dams were not significantly affected by treatment. One female from each treatment group resorbed most or all of her litter. The fetuses derived from each treatment group exhibited no internal or external skeletal malformations that could be related to treatment. Because maternal body weights were reduced at both doses tested, a NOAEL was not established for maternal toxicity. Because no developmental effects were seen, the NOAEL for embryo-fetal toxicity for this study was 1000 mg/kg body weight/day.

Pregnant female Wistar rats (17–20 per dosage group) were dosed with PBO levels of 62.5, 125, 250, or 500 mg/kg body weight/day from day 6 to day 15 of gestation in a study performed by Khera *et al.* (1979). The types and incidences of anomalies in fetuses derived from treated dams were comparable with those of the control group and it was concluded that doses as high as 500 mg/kg body weight/day produced no signs of either maternal or embryo-fetal toxicity.

A developmental toxicity study with PBO was performed in Sprague–Dawley rats by Chun and Neeper-Bradley (1991). Timed pregnant rats were administered PBO (90.78% purity) by gavage on gestation days 6 to 15. The dosage levels were 200, 500, and 1000 mg/kg body weight/day and 25 animals were included in each group. The pregnancy rate was equivalent among groups and ranged from 88% to 96%. No females aborted, delivered early, or were removed from the study. Gestational body weights and body weight gains were reduced in the 500 and 1000 mg/kg body weight/day groups, as was food intake for the first 7 days, indicating that a sufficiently high dose was achieved. Treatment had no effect on gestational parameters including resorption, pre- and postimplantation losses, percentage of live fetuses, and sex ratios nor did it affect the fetal body weights or the incidence of fetal malformations. However, two common skeletal variations (i.e., nonossification of centrum of vertebrae 5 or 6) had a higher incidence in the two highest dosage groups. These findings were not considered treatment-related, as adjacent vertebrae did not have delayed ossification. The NOAEL for maternal toxicity in the rat was 200 mg/kg body weight/day and the NOAEL for developmental toxicity was at least 1000 mg/kg body weight/day.

Rabbits New Zealand White female rabbits were gavaged with PBO (purity 100%) in corn oil at levels of 50, 100, or 200 mg/kg body weight between day 7 and day 19 of pregnancy (Leng *et al.*, 1986). Caesarian sections were performed on day 29 of gestation. Maternal toxicity was evident at 100 and 200 mg/kg body weight/day manifested by decreased defecation and a dose-dependent weight loss during the treatment period (these weight losses were recovered post-treatment). Common developmental defects, including an increase in the number of full ribs and the presence of more than 27 presacral vertebrae, were recorded in all dose groups. However, no dose–response relationship was apparent. The number of litters in the treated groups with these observations was not increased when compared with control values. The NOAEL for maternal toxicity was 50 mg/kg body weight/day, whereas the NOAEL for developmental toxicity was 200 mg/kg body weight/day.

64.3.4 CHRONIC TOXICITY/ONCOGENICITY

Numerous long-term toxicity and oncogenicity studies have been undertaken on piperonyl butoxide over the past 50 years in various species. As evidenced in these studies, the primary target organ is the liver. The results of the studies discussed below are summarized in Table 64.5.

64.3.4.1 Dogs

PBO was administered to dogs in capsule form for a 1-year chronic dietary toxicity study (Sarles and Vandergrift, 1952). Groups of four dogs each were treated at dose levels corresponding to 3, 32, 160, or 320 mg/kg body weight/day. The dosage was adjusted in accordance with any alteration in body weight to maintain the same dose in mg/kg body weight, except for one individual animal per dosage group, which received a constant absolute dose throughout the trial. All dogs belonging to the two highest dosage groups lost weight; however, meaningful comparisons between the lower dose groups and control animals were not possible owing to large variations in body weight gains and the small number of animals involved. All dogs at the highest dosage level died. However, no toxic reaction was seen at 3 mg/kg body weight/day. Red blood cell (RBC) and white blood cell (WBC) counts were unchanged at all dose levels. There was a dose-dependent increase in liver, kidney, and adrenal weights. Microscopic changes were quite similar to those in long-term toxicity studies performed in rats, with the liver again being the major target organ for toxicity. Hydropic swelling was evident in hepatocytes in the mid-dose group, with hepatic dystrophy and dysplasia becoming more obvious at the two highest dosage levels. The NOAEL for this study was 32 mg/kg body weight/day.

A more recent 1-year chronic dietary toxicity study was conducted with PBO in the beagle dog (Goldenthal, 1993b). Groups of four males and four females were fed PBO for 1 year at doses of 100, 600, or 2000 ppm (approximately equivalent to 2.5, 15, or 50 mg/kg body weight/day, respectively) in the diet. All animals survived to study termination. A reduction in

Table 64.5
Summary of Results of Chronic Toxicity/Oncogenicity Studies with PBO

Species	Route	Dose	Duration	NOAEL	Comments	Reference
Dog	Oral	3–320 mg/kg body weight/day	1 yr	32 mg/kg body weight/day	Increased liver and kidney weights, hepatic dystrophy and dysplasia	Sarles and Vandergrift (1952)
	Diet	100–2000 ppm (~2.5–50 mg/kg body weight/day)	1 yr	600 ppm (~15 mg/kg body weight/day)	Increased liver and gall bladder weights, hypertrophy of hepatocytes	Goldenthal (1993b)
Mouse	Diet	300 or 1112 ppm (~45 or 167 mg/kg body weight/day)	69 wks	Not applicable	No significant increase in tumor incidence	Innes *et al.* (1969)
	Diet	45 or 133 mg/kg body weight/day	18 months	45 mg/kg body weight/day	No signs of toxicity	Bond *et al.* (1973)
	Diet	1036–2804 ppm (~148–298 mg/kg body weight/day)	112 wks	Not established	Decreased body weight in both sexes, hepatic nodular hyperplasia in males	U.S. National Cancer Institute (1979)
	Diet	6000–12,000 ppm (960–1920 mg/kg body weight/day)	1 yr	Not established	Hepatic adenomas and hepatocarcinomas	Takahashi *et al.* (1994b)
	Diet	30–300 mg/kg body weight/day	78 wks	30 mg/kg body weight/day	Increased liver weight, benign hepatic adenomas	Butler *et al.* (1998)
Rat	Diet	100–25,000 ppm (~5–1250 mg/kg body weight/day)	2 yr	100 ppm (~5 mg/kg body weight/day)	No significant increase in tumor incidence; severe liver damage, increased incidence of liver "hyperdysplastic" nodules	Sarles and Vandergrift (1952)
	Diet	~90 mg/kg body weight/day	2 yr	Not applicable	Decreased body weight	Hunter *et al.* (1977)
	Diet	5000–10,000 ppm (~250–500 mg/kg body weight/day)	107 wks	Not established	Dose-related increase in hepatocytomegaly, dose-related increase in lymphomas in female rats, but incidence in controls was also high	Cardy *et al.* (1979)
	Diet	5000–10,000 ppm (~250–500 mg/kg body weight/day)	2 yr	Not established	No significant increase in tumor incidence; dose-related increase in ileocaecal ulcers	Maekawa *et al.* (1985)
	Diet	6000–24,000 ppm (526–2187 mg/kg body weight/day)	95–96 wks	Not established	Hepatic adenomas and hepatocarcinoma at mid- and high-dose levels, caecal hemorrhaging, severe general and hepatic toxicity	Takahashi *et al.* (1994a)
	Diet	15–500 mg/kg body weight/day	2 yr	30 mg/kg body weight/day	Increased liver and kidney weights, centrilobular hepatocyte hypertrophy, focal hyperplasia	Butler *et al.* (1998)
Goat	Diet	2.0 mL/day (~1000 ppm)	1 yr	Not applicable	Slight hepatic dystrophy and dysplasia	Sarles and Vandergrift (1952)

body weight gain and food intake was evident in the 2000 ppm group. Physical examinations were otherwise normal throughout the test period. Biochemical analysis showed increases in serum alkaline phosphatase levels at 6 and 12 months in the highest dosage group. Female beagles showed a decrease in serum cholesterol at the 2000 ppm dosage level. Increased liver and gall bladder weights, with mild hypertrophy of hepatocytes, were also recorded at this highest dosage level. A small increase in thyroid gland and parathyroid gland weights was also noted. However, no microscopic abnormalities were detected in the thyroid gland. No treatment-related histopathologic changes

were seen on the study. Based on the changes seen in the liver, the NOAEL for this study was 600 ppm.

64.3.4.2 Mice

Innes and co-workers (1969) studied the effect of PBO on tumorigenicity in mice by administering the maximal tolerated dose. Animals (18/sex/strain) from two hybrid stocks (C57BL/6 × C3H/Anf or C57BL/6 × AKR) were gavaged with 100 mg undiluted PBO/kg body weight or 464 mg PBO/kg body weight in solvent vehicle from 7 to 28 days of age. Thereafter, they received 300 ppm undiluted PBO or 1112 ppm PBO in solvent vehicle (approximately equivalent to 45 and 167 mg/kg body weight/day, respectively) in the diet for 69 weeks. These researchers found no significant increase in tumor incidence as a result of PBO treatment.

Bond *et al.* (1973) reported no adverse effects following dosing of mice with 45 or 133 mg/kg body weight/day PBO in the diet for 18 months. Few details are available for this early study, however.

The U.S. National Cancer Institute (1979) conducted a mouse carcinogenicity study in which male and female B6C3F1 animals (50/sex/dose level) were initially dosed with 2500 or 5000 ppm of PBO in the diet. Toxicity appearing in both these groups resulted in a reduction in the doses to 500 and 2000 ppm, respectively after 30 weeks of dosing. The time-weighted average doses in the diets were approximately 1036 and 2804 ppm (approximately equivalent to 148 and 298 mg/kg body weight/day, respectively). Dose-dependent decreases in body weight and body weight gains were observed in both dose groups and both sexes. Nodular hyperplasia of the liver was slightly elevated in males. Although tumors were observed in the liver and lacrimal gland, the incidence was not statistically significant. Thus, the authors concluded that PBO was not oncogenic.

The Tokyo Metropolitan Research Laboratory reported the results of a 1-year chronic toxicity study conducted in CD-1 mice using dietary doses of 6000 and 12,000 ppm PBO (equivalent to 960 and 1920 mg/kg body weight/day, respectively) (Takahashi *et al.*, 1994b). Animals were allocated to three groups consisting of 52, 53, and 100 animals for dose levels of 0, 6000, and 12,000 ppm, respectively. Significant depressions in body weight and body weight gain were noted for low and high doses of PBO. Only 81% of the high-dose animals survived the 12-month study period compared to 98% and 94% of the animals in the low-dose and control groups, respectively. Hepatic adenomas and hepatocarcinomas were observed in both treatment groups as were hemangiosarcomas and hemangio-endothelial sarcomas. However, the doses used in this study are clearly in excess of internationally accepted maximum tolerated dose (MTD) criteria and thus they are of questionable relevance in determining the hazard and risk for humans of PBO exposure.

Butler *et al.* (1998) report a study in which groups of 60 male and 60 female CD-1 mice were administered PBO in the diet at doses of 0 (two separate control groups), 30, 100, or 300 mg/kg body weight/day for at least 78 weeks. No treatment-related clinical signs of toxicity or changes in food consumption or clinical chemistry were observed. The mean absolute body weight and mean body weight gains were generally slightly decreased throughout the study at the high dose in both males and females, indicating that the MTD was reached.

A dose-related increase in the mean absolute and relative liver weights was seen in the mid- and high-dose groups of both sexes. The mean absolute and relative liver weights of the low-dose group of male mice were also slightly increased. Both males and females clearly showed an increased incidence of be-

nign hepatic nodules diagnosed as adenomas. The further characterization of the adenomas showed that the increased burden of lesions was due to the increased incidence of eosinophilic adenomas, similar to the lesions induced by a range of enzyme inducers in the mouse (Butler, 1996). There was no increase of either basophilic adenomas or hepatocarcinomas. The NOAEL in this study was 30 mg/kg body weight/day.

64.3.4.3 Rats

In an early study, Sarles and Vandergrift (1952) fed Wistar rats with diets containing from 100 to 25,000 ppm (approximately equivalent to 5 to 1250 mg/kg body weight/day) PBO for 2 years. Twelve males and 12 females were used at each dose level. The entire high-dose group died by week 68 and showed severe liver damage upon necropsy. An increased incidence of "hyperdysplastic" hepatic nodules, characterized by the authors as the appearance of larger cells and increased polyploidy, was seen in the treated groups. Dystrophy and dysplasias were also observed in the livers from animals fed 1000 ppm or greater PBO. The authors concluded that there was no evidence of carcinogenicity; the 100 ppm dose level was considered "nontoxic."

Because PBO is most often used as a synergist with pyrethrins, a 2-year dietary study was conducted in Sprague–Dawley rats using a mixture of pyrethrins (53.1% purity) and piperonyl butoxide (95% purity) (Hunter *et al.*, 1977). Forty-five males and 45 females were fed diets containing 400 ppm pyrethrins plus 2000 ppm piperonyl butoxide. The average daily doses received by the animals over the study period were 16 + 79 mg/kg body weight/day (pyrethrins + PBO) for males and 20 + 101 mg/kg body weight/day (pyrethrins + PBO) for females. Body weights were depressed in the females during the first 78 weeks of treatment and among males during the first 26 weeks of treatment. No other treatment-related effects were noted and no treatment-related change in tumor incidence was seen.

The U.S. National Cancer Institute conducted a two-year cancer bioassay in Fisher 344 rats (Cardy *et al.*, 1979). Fifty male and 50 female animals per dose level were allocated to low- and high-dose groups which received PBO (88.4% purity) in the diet at 5000 or 10,000 ppm (approximately equivalent to 250 or 500 mg/kg body weight/day, respectively) for 107 weeks. A dose-dependent decrease in the mean body weights of treated groups was noted. Other than increased hepatocytomegaly, no dose-related increases in the incidence of tumors or other microscopic findings were observed in the liver. The hepatocytomegaly consisted of foci of enlarged hepatocytes, often associated with large, vesicular nuclei and numerous cytoplasmic vacuoles, giving the cytoplasm a "ground glass" appearance. Distortion of lobular architecture in these foci was minimal, and trabeculae were continuous with adjacent normal hepatocytes. These lesions appear similar to those described by Squire and Levitt (1975) as "eosinophilic foci," "ground glass foci," or "clear cell foci."

Although a dose-dependent increase in lymphomas was noted in females, the incidence of lymphomas, leukemias, and reticuloses observed was not significantly different from the historical rates from the laboratory. Thus, this study showed that, under the conditions of the bioassay, PBO was not carcinogenic in Fischer 344 rats.

The carcinogenicity of piperonyl butoxide was also studied in F344/DuCrj rats by Maekawa *et al.* (1985). Animals (50 sex/dose level) were fed a dietary level of 5000 or 10,000 ppm (approximately equivalent to 250 and 500 mg/kg body weight/day, respectively) for 2 years but no significant dose-related increase in the incidence of any tumor was found. A dose-related incidence of ileocaecal ulcers, however, was found in animals of both sexes.

The Tokyo Metropolitan Research Laboratory conducted a 2-year chronic toxicity study in the rat at dose levels up 24,000 ppm (1000 times the maximum level approved in raw cereals in Japan) (Takahashi *et al.*, 1994a). Fischer F344/DuCrj rats (30–33 per group) received a diet containing PBO at 6,000, 12,000 or 24,000 ppm (equivalent to 526, 1052, or 2187 mg/kg body weight/day, respectively) for 95–96 weeks. Beginning at about 40 weeks, 10 rats in the 12,000 ppm male group died due to caecal hemorrhages. By the end of the study, gastrointestinal hemorrhage occurred at all dose levels. Organ weights (with the exception of the liver) were reduced in all animals in the high-dose group. "Probable essential thrombocytopenia" was present in all treated male groups. Body weight gains relative to controls were reduced in all treated groups of both sexes and reached approximately 50% in the high-dose group. A dose-dependent increase in hepatocellular hyperplasia (seen as liver nodules) was reported. Although the nomenclature is different, these lesions are much like those described by Sarles and Vandergrift (1952) at toxic doses of PBO. Takahashi also reported hepatocellular adenomas and carcinomas in the mid- and high-dose groups.

It is important to note that the study was not intended to be a carcinogenicity study and the procedures for collecting and examining tissues were not performed according to current USEPA/OECD standards. Thus, not all tissues were taken or prepared for histological examination. Because of the high-dose levels used and resulting toxicity, it is difficult to interpret the carcinogenicity findings and their relevance for hazard assessment. Moreover, several investigators have reported that hepatotoxicity, and the resulting regenerative hyperplasia, can contribute to the formation of liver tumors by nongenotoxic mechanisms (Kociba *et al.*, 1978; McClean *et al.*, 1990; Mutai *et al.*, 1990; Tatematsu *et al.*, 1990; Van Miller *et al.*, 1977). This and other mechanistic aspects of this oncogenicity response are discussed in Section 64.3.5.

The most recent report is from another dietary study in which the Sprague–Dawley rat was utilized (Butler *et al.*, 1998). Animals were divided into groups of 60 animals of each sex and were administered 15, 30, 100, or 500 mg PBO/kg body weight/day. Three control groups were included. Because a 4-week range-finding study did not provide clear evidence of a NOAEL with respect to minor alterations in liver cell morphology, additional animals were used during the early stages of this study. Thus, after completion of 4 weeks of treatment, 10 males

and 10 females from each low-dose group and a special control group consisting of 10 males and 10 females were sacrificed for both gross pathological and histopathologic examinations of the liver. Since the results of the histopathologic examination showed no abnormal findings in the livers of these rats, the low dose level of 30 mg/kg body weight/day was continued on the 2-year study. The 15 mg/kg body weight/day group was discontinued.

No adverse treatment-related effects on survival and no treatment-related clinical signs were seen. A reduced growth rate and a minimal reduction in food intake were noted for males and females receiving 500 mg/kg body weight/day. These females were shown to have increased serum cholesterol levels and slightly higher total serum protein levels. The blood urea nitrogen levels were also slightly higher in this group on one occasion. Dose-related increases in liver and kidney weights were noted in both sexes at 100 and 500 mg/kg body weight/day.

Histologically, the most common effect in the liver was centrilobular hepatocyte hypertrophy and the presence of eosinophilic and mixed (basophilic and eosinophilic) cell foci. The severity of focal hyperplasia in the liver was also greater in the intermediate- and high-dose groups. The hyperplastic foci contained either basophilic, normal, or enlarged eosinophilic cells that were variable in size. Normal lobular architecture was retained. Portal triads and central veins were present in the lesions. Neither the incidence of adenomas nor incidence of carcinomas was increased. Pituitary adenomas were common in both males and females but showed no treatment-related effect upon incidence of the adenomas.

Thyroid changes, including increased pigment in colloid, and follicular hyperplasia (particularly at 500 mg/kg body weight/day) were seen in both sexes at the end of the study as well as in the high-dose group males dying or sacrificed during the study.

In the kidney, glomerulonephritis was more common in the male than the female. No significant increase in the incidence of glomerulonephritis was observed, but the severity of the lesions was increased slightly in the intermediate- and high-dose groups.

The non-neoplastic changes observed in this rat study are consistent with induction of the hepatic mixed function oxidase system. The liver observations such as increased liver weight, centrilobular hypertrophy, eosinophilic foci, and eosinophilic focal hyperplasia are probably due to enzyme induction. Likewise, the thyroid follicular hyperplasia is a likely secondary response of the thyroid gland to prolonged TSH stimulation resulting from decreased circulating levels of T_3 and T_4. Reduced T_3 and T_4 levels are due to increased conjugation and excretion of the thyroid hormones resulting from liver enzyme induction. This pattern has been observed with other liver enzyme inducers such as phenobarbital (McClain, 1989). Given these considerations, the authors concluded that there was no evidence of carcinogenic activity and that the NOAEL based on liver changes was 30 mg/kg body weight/day.

64.3.4.4 Other Species

Sarles and Vandergrift (1952) also reported a chronic oral toxicity experiment where a mature female goat was fed a daily dose of 2.0 mL PBO by capsule, 6 days a week, for 1 year. This dose equated to approximately 1000 ppm PBO in the diet. The dose started 4 days after the goat gave birth to a female kid, with both dam and offspring being observed for 1 year to ascertain any signs of direct or indirect (i.e., PBO in dam's milk) toxic effects. The general health of both dam and kid was unaffected by treatment. The kid was nursed by the treated dam for approximately 6 months and continued to grow and thrive as expected. RBC and WBC counts were unremarkable. At postmortem examination, the dam's liver revealed slight dystrophy and dysplasia, with central hydrophic swelling and slight fatty accumulation. No abnormalities were detected in the organs of the kid goat.

64.3.5 MECHANISTIC CONSIDERATIONS FOR ONCOGENICITY

The chronic toxicity/oncogenicity studies discussed in Section 64.3.4 indicate that liver is a target for both oncogenic and nononcogenic changes in both the mouse and the rat. In addition, one study showed an apparent hyperplastic response in the thyroid (Butler *et al.*, 1998).

Many nongenotoxic compounds have been shown to induce tumors in rodents (Ames *et al.*, 1993; Butler, 1996; Cohen and Ellwein, 1990; Grasso and Hinton, 1991; Grasso *et al.*, 1991; Loury *et al.*, 1987; Wilson *et al.*, 1992). Although the mechanism(s) of liver tumor production by nongenotoxic inducers of hepatic xenobiotic metabolism, such as sodium phenobarbital (NaPB), remains to be fully elucidated (Grasso and Hinton, 1991; Grasso *et al.*, 1991), it is clear that the mitogenic and promotional effects of such agents are important. Tumor formation may involve the promotion of particular populations of hepatocytes through differential effects on cell replication, growth factors, intercellular communication, etc. (Anderson *et al.*, 1995; Grasso and Hinton, 1991; Grasso *et al.*, 1991; Jirtle, 1994; Law, 1991; Lubet *et al.*, 1989; Neveu *et al.*, 1994; Whysner *et al.*, 1996).

It is important to note that threshold doses have been reported for both liver enlargement/enzyme induction and, at higher dose levels, for tumor formation (Grasso and Hinton, 1991; Grasso *et al.*, 1991). There is evidence that such lesions may regress upon withdrawal of the inducing compound (Evans *et al.*, 1992; Ito *et al.*, 1976; Malarkey *et al.*, 1995). Other studies have shown that the lesions found in MFO-induced mice are fundamentally different from both spontaneous lesions and those induced by genotoxic carcinogens in that they do not express oncogenes (Fox *et al.*, 1990; Rumsby *et al.*, 1991) and fail to grow in semisolid agar (Pedrick *et al.*, 1994). Thus, although these lesions are usually diagnosed as adenomas, the evidence suggests that the lesions are compound-dependent, rather than autonomous, and do not progress to hepatic carcinoma.

Besides the additive hyperplasia that may occur from mitogenic and promotional agents, tumors may also result from regenerative hyperplasia produced in response to cell necrosis (as with chloroform and furan). Such a mechanism would also be expected to demonstrate a threshold for effects, including tumorigenesis. Substantial evidence suggests that both additive and regenerative hyperplasia may result from sufficiently high doses of PBO.

Several studies have shown that PBO is an inducer of hepatic xenobiotic metabolism in the mouse and rat (Fennell *et al.*, 1980; Goldstein *et al.*, 1973; Lake *et al.*, 1973; Phillips *et al.*, 1997; Wagstaff and Short, 1971). Phillips *et al.* (1997) characterized the induction of enzyme activities in both the mouse and rat and compared it to the classic inducer, phenobarbital. Four groups of 16 male F-344 rats were fed PBO in the diet at 100, 550, 1050, or 1850 mg/kg body weight/day. Animals were treated for either 7 or 42 days and were sacrificed, and liver studies were performed. Even the low-dose group (100 mg/kg body weight/day PBO) showed increased relative liver weights and microsomal protein content (42 days treatment), increased cytochrome P-450 levels (7 days treatment), increased GGT levels (42 days treatment), and increases in certain MFO enzyme activities. PBO appeared to be a mixed-type enzyme inducer in the rat in that it induced hepatic cytochrome P450 isoenzymes in the CYP1A, CYP2B, and CYP3A subfamilies.

Recent work by Watanabe *et al.* (1998) in the rat is in agreement with these findings of Phillips. These workers also noted weak induction of the CYP4A isozyme. The induction pattern was similar to that they observed for NaPB, with the exception that NaPB did not induce CYP1A. A NOEL of 0.05% PBO in the diet (approximately 50 mg/kg body weight) over 4 weeks was reported for this enzyme induction.

PBO treatment of the mouse by Phillips and co-workers also resulted in a dose-related induction of cytochrome P450 content and ethylmorphine demethylase activity (CYP3A). Taken with other studies that have shown induction of CYP1A and CYP2B isoenzymes in mouse liver (Adams *et al.*, 1993; Fennell *et al.*, 1980), PBO appears to be able to induce CYP1A, CYP2B, and CYP3A isoenzymes in CD-1 mouse liver as well.

Aside from the enzyme induction discussed above, certain nongenotoxic rodent liver carcinogens produce either a transient or a sustained stimulation of cell replication (Goldsworthy *et al.*, 1991). Both PBO and NaPB produced a stimulation of cell replication after 7 but not 42 days of treatment in the mouse (Phillips *et al.*, 1997). Like NaPB, PBO also increased relative liver weight in CD-1 mice and produced liver hypertrophy, although a difference in the lobular distribution of this effect was noted. Generally, the effects of PBO on relative liver weight, liver morphology, replicative DNA synthesis, and xenobiotic metabolism occurred at the 100 and 300 mg/kg body weight/day dose levels, the same doses where eosinophilic nodules were observed in a 2-year study by Butler *et al.* (1998). In addition, the eosinophilic nodules produced by PBO in mouse liver (Butler, 1996) appear similar to those formed by NaPB (Evans *et al.*, 1992).

Thus, the data show that PBO is an inducer of the MFO enzymes and hepatocyte proliferation in the mouse and such induction results in enlarged livers, centrilobular hypertrophy and hyperplasia, and an increase of benign eosinophilic adenomas by a mechanism similar to that of NaPB (Butler, 1996; Evans *et al.*, 1986; Jones and Butler, 1975; Phillips *et al.*, 1997).

With respect to the rat, Watanabe *et al.* (1998), demonstrated the production of centrilobular hypertrophy in the rat liver following 4 weeks of dosing with 2% PBO in the diet. The degree of response was similar to that observed after 4 weeks dosing with 0.1% NaPB.

Further evidence of the similarity between the action of PBO and NaPB comes from a report by Okamiya *et al.* (1998) showing an increase in proliferating cell nuclear antigen in rats fed 0.2% PBO in the diet for 4 weeks. They also demonstrated a decrease in the gap junction protein connexin 32 (Cx32) at the highest dose tested (2.0%) after dosing for 1, 2, but not 4 weeks.

Phillips *et al.* (1997) reported that high doses of PBO (1850 mg/kg body weight/day) given to rats caused a significant reduction of body weight gain and of food consumption throughout the 42 days of dosing. Morphological examination of liver showed individual cell necrosis in rats dosed with 1050 and 1850 mg PBO/kg body weight/day. While the severity of the individual cell necrosis was similar in rats given 1050 and 1850 mg PBO/kg body weight/day, the incidence was greater (seven of eight animals examined) in rats given 1850 mg/kg body weight/day. Like NaPB, the increase in relative liver weight in PBO-treated animals was associated with hypertrophy, although a difference in the lobular distribution of this effect was noted. Replicative DNA synthesis was stimulated by 550 and 1050 mg PBO/kg body weight/day and 0.05% NaPB after 7 days of administration, most likely due to transient mitogenesis typical of enzyme inducers. In contrast, the stimulation of cell replication observed after 42 days treatment by 1050 mg/kg body weight/day is more likely to be associated with the onset of a regenerative hyperplasia. The mitogenic and hypertrophic effects of PBO were observed at doses (e.g., 550 mg/kg body weight/day) lower than those required to produce individual cell necrosis, where a high incidence of necrosis was only observed in rats given 1850 mg/kg body weight/day for 42 days. Chronic treatment (i.e., >42 days) with PBO at high-dose levels such as that in an oncogenesis study could result in a sustained stimulation of replicative DNA synthesis and an increased likelihood of oncogenesis. It is important to note that Takahashi *et al.* (1994b) reported no increase in liver tumors following 2 years of dosing at the lowest study dose of 547 mg/kg body weight/day, a dose calculated by the authors to be about 18,000 times the allowable daily intake (ADI) for humans. In contrast, higher doses of PBO were both toxic to the rat liver and produced tumors.

Thus, the data suggest that eosinophilic nodules in mouse liver may result from a mechanism similar to that of NaPB and other enzyme inducers, whereas tumor formation in rats at greater than MTD doses is most likely related both to significant induction of hepatic metabolism in conjunction with a regenerative hyperplasia resulting from PBO-induced hepatotoxicity. Both of these mechanisms are threshold phenomenon

and suggest that at doses likely to be encountered by humans, PBO poses essentially no oncogenic risk.

64.3.6 GENOTOXICITY

Piperonyl butoxide has shown no evidence of mutagenic activity in a number of bacterial assays involving *Salmonella typhimurium*, *Bacillus subtilis*, and *Escherichia coli* both in the presence or absence of rat liver microsomes (S-9) (Ashwood-Smith *et al.*, 1972; Butler *et al.*, 1996; Ishidate *et al.*, 1984; Kawachi *et al.*, 1980; Moriye *et al.*, 1983; White *et al.*, 1977).

Most of the studies in systems using mammalian cells in culture show no evidence of mutation or a chromosome damaging effect. Galloway *et al.* (1987) investigated a wide range of compounds including piperonyl butoxide in Chinese hamster ovary cells and failed to find chromosome aberrations and sister chromatid exchange in the presence or absence of rat liver S-9. PBO had no effect on Chinese hamster ovary cells in the report of Butler *et al.* (1996), and produced a small increase in sister chromatid exchanges only in the absence of S-9 in the recent study by Tayama (1996). Tayama also concluded that the metabolites of PBO are unlikely to be genotoxic. In addition, piperonyl butoxide did not produce chromosomal aberrations in Chinese hamster lung cells (Ishidate *et al.*, 1984, 1988; Kawachi *et al.*, 1980) or induce mutations in the CHO/HGPT assay (Butler *et al.*, 1996).

However, in L5178Y mouse lymphoma cells, piperonyl butoxide showed evidence of mutagenic activity only in the absence of additional metabolic activation. In this study, the mutagenic activity was observed only where cytotoxicity was evident. The relative total cell growth at the lowest mutagenic concentration of 30 μg/mL was around 60% (McGregor *et al.*, 1988). Piperonyl butoxide also induced cell transformation in Syrian hamster embryo cells (Amacher and Zelljadt, 1983). In this study, three dose levels (0.5, 1.0, and 3.0 μg/ml), were used and only 2 transformed colonies out of 2761 were observed. No indication is given of the dose level that caused the 2 transformed colonies. Suzuki and Suzuki (1995) investigated the mutagenicity of piperonyl butoxide in human RSA cells, a cell line of double transformed human embryonal fibroblasts considered to be hypermutable, by determining ouabain resistance. The results show an unusual dose response in that despite having little effect upon survival at dose levels above 0.2 μg/ml piperonyl butoxide, the incidence of mutation declined. The authors also report mutation of K-*ras* codon 12 with an apparent similar dose response. While K-*ras* mutation has been reported in human tumors at various sites (Almoguera *et al.*, 1988; Bos *et al.*, 1987) no such association has been observed in rodent liver tumors the apparent target site of piperonyl butoxide (Maronpot *et al.*, 1995).

Butler *et al.* (1996) reported that PBO did not induce unscheduled DNA synthesis in rat hepatocytes. Moreover, Beamand *et al.* (1996) showed a similar negative response to PBO in cultured human hepatocytes.

In vivo studies have also failed to demonstrate convincing genotoxic effects of piperonyl butoxide. A dominant lethal assay in ICR/Ha Swiss mice using both single and multiple doses of piperonyl butoxide given either by intraperitoneal injection or by gavage resulted in toxicity and death of the male mice. Although there was some evidence of reduced reproductive efficiency and an increase in early fetal death, the results were not consistent and the authors concluded the study was equivocal (Epstein *et al.*, 1972). Other studies have been reported only briefly as abstracts and have stated that no chromosomal aberrations or sister chromatid exchanges were produced in either rat or mouse bone marrow (Ivett and Tice, 1983; Kawachi *et al.*, 1980).

64.3.7 HUMAN STUDIES

Wintersteiger and Juan (1991) investigated the absorption of combination pyrethrin and PBO sprays across the skin of six healthy subjects in Austria. The spray was applied over a wide area of the back with a total dose of approximately 3.3 mg pyrethrum extract and 13.2 mg PBO being applied. No untoward clinical signs were noted. Cutaneous absorption of PBO was shown to be extremely low, with plasma samples containing no more than 10 ng PBO/mL. Wester *et al.* (1994) investigated the percutaneous absorption of both PBO and pyrethrin compounds across the skin of the ventral forearm in six volunteers. Based on the recovery of radioactivity in the urine, it was calculated that 2.1% ± 0.6% of the dose of PBO was absorbed through the skin. Not surprisingly, higher levels of absorption of PBO were achieved when the compound was applied to the skin of the scalp (8.3%). There was no evidence of any local or systemic toxicity of PBO when used as a topical agent in humans.

Selim (1995) investigated the absorption, excretion, and mass balance of ^{14}C PBO from two different formulations following dermal application to healthy volunteers. The first preparation applied was a 4% (w/w) solution of PBO in an aqueous formulation. This product was applied to four healthy human volunteers. The second preparation tested was a 3% (w/w) solution of PBO in isopropyl alcohol. In the former case, the mean amount of PBO applied was 3.8 mg per volunteer (approximately 39.9 μCi of radioactivity per volunteer), while the average exposure was 3.0 mg PBO per volunteer (approximately 40 μCi of radioactivity per volunteer) in the case of the isopropyl alcohol solution. Results from this study show that there was a similar dermal absorption pattern for both formulations. The principal route of excretion of absorbed radioactivity was via urine. Fecal samples from volunteers contained negligible levels of radioactivity. Dermally applied PBO was rapidly excreted from the volunteers. The majority of the applied radioactivity remained at the application site, with less than 3% of the applied dose being absorbed during the 8-hour test period. Radioactivity did not accumulate in the skin.

The only study to examine the ability of PBO to inhibit xenobiotic metabolism in humans was that by Conney *et al.* (1972). Using the rate of antipyrine metabolism as a gauge of P-450 activity, two healthy men (weighing 87.4 kg and 82.6 kg, respectively) were given capsules containing increasing amounts

(5, 10, 20, and 50 mg) of PBO at consecutive intervals of approximately 1 week. No signs of toxicity were seen. Clinical chemical analysis of blood and urine samples taken at 4, 8, and 24 hours after ingestion of the capsules did not reveal any adverse effects. In a subsequent study, eight men were given PBO as a single dose of 0.71 mg/kg body weight. A control group received a placebo. Two hours later, both the treated and control groups received a 250 mg oral dose of antipyrine. Antipyrine was analyzed in blood samples taken at intervals over the next 31 hours. PBO had no effect on the rate of clearance of antipyrine.

Although no systematic epidemiology studies have been conducted on PBO-exposed individuals, no evidence suggests that PBO has resulted in any significant adverse effects to human health.

Occupational health data collected at a PBO manufacturing site in Italy, consisting of routine health checks, have been made on potentially exposed workers from 1974 to 1994. Sixty workers were examined, 11 of which were employed in the manufacture of PBO for periods of 15–26 years. Workers received x-rays and spirometric evaluations every three years and annual clinical chemistry analysis. No adverse clinical signs or symptoms related to PBO were found (Endura, 1996).

Similarly, at a manufacturing site in Scotland, where PBO was made from 1962 to 1990, "no cases of toxic symptoms or adverse effects attributable to PBO manufacture" were noted in production workers at the plant. Moreover, no adverse effects were reported in operations involved in the handling and use of PBO at a site in England (JMPR, 1993; Pitman Moore, 1990; Wellcome, 1991). The only clinical report referring to PBO exposure is the case of two sisters who gave birth, within 2 weeks of each other, to children who each had coarction of the aorta (Hall *et al.*, 1975). Both mothers had been on a camping trip at 2 months gestation where they used "large amounts" of insect repellents and insecticides containing, among other chemicals, PBO, pyrethrins, DEET, and DDVP. No cause-and-effect relationship was established.

There have been no reported suicide attempts by humans with PBO. Based on its acute toxicity to experimental animals, a probable oral lethal dose for humans is estimated to be 5–15 g/kg body weight (i.e., approximately 300 to 900 g PBO for a 60 kg human).

64.4 PHARMACODYNAMICS

Yamamoto (1973) suggests that the primary function of synergists such as PBO when formulated with pyrethrins or pyrethroids is to provide an alternative substrate for the MFO enzyme system, which would normally metabolize such insecticides. Inhibition of MFO-mediated oxidation of the transmethyl groups and the alcohol moiety on the pyrethrin molecule appear to be the most important functions of PBO. Inhibition of ester hydrolysis may also contribute to the effectiveness of PBO as a synergist.

As a known alternative substrate for the liver microsomal enzyme system, PBO will inhibit the metabolism of many xenobiotics including drugs and pesticides. Brown (1970) reported that the detoxification of certain drugs such as pentobarbital, zoxazolamine, antipyrine, and benzopyrene were inhibited by PBO, presumably due to the inhibition of their microsomal oxidation. Conney *et al.* (1972) investigated the inhibition of antipyrine metabolism in rats and mice. Both species were treated intraperitoneally (i.p.) with a single dose of PBO, followed by a further i.p. injection of antipyrine (200 mg/kg body weight) 1 hour later. A marked species difference was noted in the response; the NOEL for inhibition of antipyrine metabolism in the mouse was 0.5–1.0 mg PBO/kg body weight, whereas the NOEL for the rat was 100 mg PBO/kg body weight.

The effects of PBO on the metabolism of benzopyrene in Sprague–Dawley rats were studied by Falk *et al.* (1965). PBO was administered by the oral, intraperitoneal (i.p.), or intravenous (i.v.) routes at various times before the i.v. injection of labeled benzopyrene. The level of radioactivity was then measured in bile at frequent intervals up to 4 hours. This author demonstrated marked inhibition of benzopyrene metabolism when PBO was administered i.v. at 262 mg/kg body weight, some 5 minutes to 16 hours before the administration of benzopyrene. However, this effect is much reduced at 121 mg/kg body weight. Virtually no effect is seen at 25 hours postdosing. This implies that single large doses of PBO are quickly metabolized by rats. Administration of PBO by the oral and i.p. routes resulted in a greatly reduced effect when compared with the i.v. route. A second similar study performed by Conney *et al.* (1972), where the effects of i.p. administration of PBO on the metabolism of benzopyrene were investigated, showed less sensitive results when rats of lighter weight were used (approximately 180 g versus 400 g in Falk's study). It was postulated by Brown (1970) that the extra fat in the animals in Falk's study could possibly act as a reservoir of PBO and lead to a longer duration of action. It would appear from these studies in rats that 250 mg of PBO per kg body weight is the minimum oral dose required to give any significant effect on benzopyrene metabolism.

Whereas a single dose of PBO will generally inhibit the metabolism of pentobarbital, repeated PBO doses will generally induce the metabolism of phenobarbital and other xenobiotics. Brown (1970) reports an experiment in rats where a single i.p. dose of PBO (333–1000 mg/kg body weight) increased the sleeping time of the animals following administration of pentobarbital. However, the i.p. administration of eight injections of 50 mg PBO/kg body weight, each at 12-hour intervals, followed by the injection of pentobarbital some 18 hours later, caused a reduction in sleeping time in rats. The administration of 50 mg PBO per kg body weight i.p. to rats (Anders, 1968) and mice (Graham *et al.*, 1970) prior to treatment with hexobarbital approximately doubled the sleeping time of both species.

CD-1 mice given a single i.p. dose of 600 mg PBO per kg body weight were found to have suffered less hepatotoxicity when treated with acetaminophen (600 mg/kg body weight, p.o.) at either 2 hours prior to or 1 hour following PBO administration. This reduced hepatotoxicity was measured via GSH and sorbitol dehydrogenase levels, as well as subsequent histopathology of the liver. Since the hepatic MFO system metabolizes acetaminophen to a toxic metabolite, the decreased toxicity seen in this experiment is likely due to inhibition of such oxidase enzymes by PBO (Brady *et al.*, 1988).

Many other studies have been undertaken relevant to the pharmacodynamics of PBO and are reported elsewhere (Skrinijaric-Spoljar *et al.*, 1971; Conney *et al.*, 1972; Goldstein *et al.*, 1973). More recent work is discussed in Section 64.3.5 of this chapter.

64.5 RISK CHARACTERIZATION

The U.S. EPA evaluated the weight of evidence relating to the potential oncogenicity of PBO and classified it as a Group C-Possible Human Carcinogen (U.S. EPA, 1995a). This was based on the increases in hepatocellular tumors in both male and female mice (adenomas, carcinomas, and combined adenomas and carcinomas in the males and adenomas only in the females). However, because of the generally low concern for mutagenicity, and the minor significance of other tumors observed in the rat studies, rather than recommend the Q_1^* linearized multistage model for risk characterization based on oncogenicity, the U.S. EPA endorsed the use of a Reference Dose (RfD) and Margin of Exposure (MOE) approaches using non-oncogenic endpoints, such as body weight changes.

The Joint FAO/WHO Meeting on Pesticide Residues (JMPR) evaluated the toxicology of PBO in 1965, 1966, 1972, 1992, and, most recently in 1995. They recognized that, at doses up to internationally accepted standards for a Maximum Tolerated Dose, PBO is not oncogenic in the mouse or rat. Thus, based on the NOAEL of 600 ppm (16 mg/kg body weight/day) in the most sensitive toxicology study (1 year feeding study in dogs), they established an ADI for humans of 0.2 mg/kg body weight.

64.6 EXPOSURE AND RISK ASSESSMENT

The first formal discussion of human exposure to PBO took place at a joint FAO/WHO Codex Alimentarius in 1987. FAO/WHO estimated that the average daily human diet (1.4 kg) might contain as much as 1 ppm of PBO, corresponding to a daily dose of 1.4 mg. This is likely an overestimation as cooking may destroy up to 90% of PBO present. FAO/WHO estimated the exposure from aerosol consumer products (from ingestion and inhalation) to be approximately 0.63 mg/day. Thus, the total intake from dietary and nondietary sources was estimated to be approximately 2.03 mg/day. This corresponds to a daily dose of 0.029 mg/kg body weight for a 70 kg adult and 0.14 mg/kg body weight for a 15 kg child, well below the ADI for humans of 0.2 mg/kg body weight for PBO set by the JMPR (1995). In a refinement of this exposure estimate, Crampton (1994) calculated that the daily exposure of adults to PBO residues in food was 0.0037 mg/kg body weight/day, less than 1/50th the ADI set by JMPR.

From the 1990s and through the present, the PBO Task Force (PBTF) and a subsequent entity, the Non-Dietary Exposure Task Force (NDETF), both consortia of PBO producers and marketers, have been developing exposure data for PBO. Their goal has been to estimate the aggregate human exposure to PBO from both dietary and nondietary routes. The PBTF conducted a series of crop residue studies on various crops representing 12 crop groups. In addition, studies were conducted where residue levels and transfer factors were obtained following application of PBO to livestock, and estimation of potential dietary intake of PBO was done using DietRisk™, a software tool that incorporates the USEPA's Dietary Risk Evaluation System (Burin, 2000). Determination of chronic dietary exposure requires the use of the anticipated PBO levels in a given food commodity (obtained from field studies) and the quantity of the commodity ingested. In addition, because PBO is not used widely on any given commodity, the anticipated value is adjusted by an estimate of the percentage of the crop that it is treated.

Given the above information, the estimated dietary intake of PBO was 2.34 ug/kg body weight/day, about 1.2% of the JMPR ADI, and 7.8% of the U.S. EPA RfD. Because many conservative assumptions were built into this assessment (e.g., no account for losses during washing and cooking of foods), it is likely that the actual human exposure is much lower.

The NDETF is also currently conducting studies to define the various dermal and hand-to-mouth "transferability" parameters to support the development of a predictive stochastic model estimating potential distributions of postapplication exposure and absorbed doses following different residential exposure scenarios (e.g., indoor foggers, carpet and room aerosol sprays). This work is ongoing and will be published when available. As a precursor to the exposure monitoring program, the NDETF performed conservative screening-level assessments, based on existing information and default assumptions, to deterministically estimate potential exposures following the use of a PBO-containing total release indoor fogger (Dragula *et al.*, 1996). Such products are typically used to combat flea and roach infestations. Given the intermittent nature of this exposure scenario and most nondietary exposures to PBO-based consumer products, subchronic toxicity endpoints were used as the basis for calculation of margins of exposure (MOEs). Thus, MOEs were derived using the most sensitive subchronic study, the 90-day rat inhalation study. The NOAEL for systemic toxicity in this study was 155 mg/m^3 that converts to 15 mg/kg body weight using a conversion factor relating lung ventilation to body weight (0.365 ml/min/g; U.S. EPA, 1988). For purposes of the screening-level assessment for indoor foggers containing PBO, potential adult applicator exposures were estimated using relevant surrogate data from the EPA's Pesticide Handlers Exposure Database (U.S. EPA, 1995a, b). Potential postapplication exposures were estimated using the conservative assumption that consumers reenter treated areas immediately postapplication (when surface residues dry) and remain

Table 64.6
PBO Route-Specific and Total Absorbed Doses (Day of Application), and Corresponding MOE, associated with Exposures to Adults Involved in Application of an Indoor Fogger Product and Post-Application Activities in a Treated Residence

Exposure period	Daily dose (mg/kg body weight/day)	
	Inhalation	Dermal
Application	1.8×10^{-5}	3.5×10^{-5}
Postapplication	7.2×10^{-4}	3.5×10^{-5} + 1.0×10^{-6}
Route-specific total	7.4×10^{-4}	7.1×10^{-5}
Total daily absorbed dose (mg/kg body weight/day)	8.1×10^{-4}	
MOE (based on total daily absorbed dose)	19,000	

in these areas throughout the day. Inhalation exposures via indoor air, dermal exposures via contact with surface residue levels, and, in the case of toddlers, incidental ingestion exposures resulting from hand-to-mouth activities were estimated on the day of application. Inhalation exposures were conservatively based on surrogate data from an indoor chamber study and assumptions regarding exposure duration (i.e., 8 hours in the treated room). The assessment also assumed no decline in surface residues during this time. In the case of the postapplication dermal (for adults and children) and incidental ingestion (children) routes, conservative estimates were based on surrogate postapplication dermal (including hand measurements used in children's hand-to-mouth exposure estimation) exposure monitoring studies involving high contact activities (i.e., Jazzercizing®) (Ross *et al.*, 1990).

The resulting absorbed doses for adults, including application and postapplication exposures, are shown in Table 64.6. The associated MOE (using the systemic NOAEL of 15 mg/kg body weight/day) for the estimated total absorbed dose across both routes is also shown in Table 64.6. The screening-level MOE exceed 100, indicating this particular adult, nondietary exposure scenario presents an insignificant health risk. The postapplication daily absorbed dose of PBO from inhalation, dermal contact, and incidental ingestion for a 10.2 kg toddler (child) are estimated to be 1.5×10^{-3}, 1.3×10^{-7}, and 3.9×10^{-6} mg/kg body weight/day, respectively. For these calculations, dermal absorption was estimated to be 0.58% for aqueous/water-based formulations and 2.4% for isopropanol/solvent-based formulations based on Selim (1995). The total absorbed dose (sum across the three routes) is estimated to be approximately 1.5×10^{-3} mg/kg body weight/day. The MOE based on this simplistic point estimate of total absorbed dose is approximately 10,000 (using the systemic NOAEL of 15 mg/kg body weight/day), indicating no significant health risk for this particular age group.

REFERENCES

Adams, N. H., Levi, P. E., and Hodgson, E. (1993). Regulation of cytochrome *P*-450 isozymes by methylenedioxyphenyl compounds. *Chem.–Biol. Interact.* **86**, 255–274.

Almoguera, C., Shibatan, D., Forrester, K., Martin, J., Arnheim, N., and Peruduo, M. (1988). Most human carcinogenesis of the exocrine pancreas contain mutant c-K-*ras* genes. *Cell* **53**, 549–554.

Amacher, D. E., and Zelljadt, I. (1983). The morphological transformation of Syrian hamster embryo cells by chemicals repeatedly non-mutagenic to Salmonella typhimurium. *Carcinogenesis* **4**, 291–295.

Ames, B. N., Shigenaga, M. K., and Gold, L. S. (1993). DNA lesions, inducible DNA repair, and cell division: Three key factors in mutagenesis and carcinogenesis. *Environ. Health Perspect.* **101**(Suppl. 5), 35–44.

Anders, M. W. (1968). Inhibition of microsomal drug metabolism by methylenedioxybenzenes. *Biochem. Pharmacol.* **17**, 2367–2370.

Anderson, M. E., Mills, J. J., Jirtle, R. L., and Greenlee, W. F. (1995). Negative selection in hepatic tumor promotion in relation to cancer risk assessment. *Toxicology* **102**, 223–237.

Ashwood-Smith, M. J., Trevino, J., and Ring, R. (1972). Mutagenicity of dichlorvos. *Nature (London)* **240**, 418.

Beamand, J. A., Price, R. J., Phillips, J. C., Butler, W. H., Glynne Jones, G. D., Osimitz, T. G., Gabriel, K. L., Preiss, F. J., and Lake, B. G. (1996). Lack of effect of piperonyl butoxide on unscheduled DNA synthesis in precision-cut human liver slices. *Mutation Res.* **371**, 273–282.

Bond, H., Mauger, K., and DeFeo, J. J. (1973). The oral toxicity of pyrethrum, alone and combined with synergists. *Pyreth. Post* **12**, 59.

Bos, J. L., Fearson, E. R., Hamilton, S. R., Verlaan-de Uries, M., Van Boom, J. H., van der Eb, A. J., and Vogelstein, B. (1987). Prevalence of *ras* gene mutations in human colorectal cancers. *Nature* **327**, 293–297.

Brady, J. T., Montelius, D. A., Beierschmitt, W. P., Wyand, D. S., Khairalla, E. A., and Cohen, S. D. (1988). Effect of piperonyl butoxide post-treatment on acetaminophen hepatotoxicity. *Biochem. Pharmacol.* **37**, 2097–2099.

Brown, H. R. (1990). Neoplastic and potentially preneoplastic changes in the upper respiratory tract of rats and mice. *Environ. Health Perspec.* **85**, 281–304.

Brown, N. C. (1970). Report A28/52, Research and Development, The Wellcome Foundation, UK.

Burin, G. J. (2000). "Chronic Dietary Exposure and Risk Assessment for the Agricultural Uses of PBO Based upon Anticipated Residues." Prepared by Technology Sciences Group Inc. for the Non-Dietary Task Force.

Burke, M. D., Thompson, S., Elcombe, C. R., Halpert, J., Haaparanta, T., and Mayer, R. T. (1985). Ethoxy-, pentoxy- and benzyloxyphenoxazones and homologues: A series of substrates to distinguish between different induced cytochromes P-450. *Biochem. Pharmacol.* **34**, 3337–3345.

Butler, W. H. (1996). A review of the hepatic tumours related to mixed-function oxidase induction in the mouse. *Toxicol. Pathol.* **24**, 484–492.

Butler, W. H., Gabriel, K. L., Preiss, F. J., and Osimitz, T. G. (1996). Lack of genotoxicity of PBO. *Mutation Res.* **371**, 249–258.

Butler, W. H., Gabriel, K. L., Osimitz, T. G., and Preiss, F. J. (1998). Oncogenicity studies of PBO in rats and mice. *Hum. Exper. Toxicol.* **17**, 323–330.

Cardy, R. H., Renne, R. A., Warner, J. W., and Cypher, R. L. (1979). Carcinogenesis bioassay of technical-grade piperonyl butoxide in F344 rats. *J. Nat. Canc. Inst.* **62**, 569–578.

Casida, J. E. (1970). MFO involvement in the biochemistry of insecticide synergists. *J. Agric. Food. Chem.* **18**, 753–772.

Chun, J. S., and Neeper-Bradley, T. L. (1991). "Developmental Toxicity Evaluation of Piperonyl Butoxide Administered by Gavage to CD® (Sprague–Dawley) Rats." Unpublished Rep. 54-586 from Bushy Run Research Center, undertaken for the PBO Task Force, Washington, DC.

Chun, J. S., and Neeper-Bradley, T. L. (1992). "Developmental Toxicity Dose Range-Finding Study of Piperonyl Butoxide Administered by Gavage to CD® (Sprague–Dawley) Rats." Unpublished Rep. 54-578 from Bushy Run Research Center, undertaken for the PBO Task Force, Washington, DC.

Chun, J. S., and Wagner, C. L. (1993). "90 Day Dose Range-Finding Study with PBO in Mice." Study No. 91 N0052, Bushy Run Research Centre, Union Carbide Chemicals and Plastics Company Inc., Export, PA, undertaken for the PBO Task Force, Washington, DC.

Cohen, S. M., and Ellwein, L. B. (1990). Cell proliferation in carcinogenesis. *Science* **249**, 1007–1011.

Conney, A. H., Chang, R., Levin, W. M., Garbut, A., Munro-Faure, A. D., Peck, A. W., and Bye, A. (1972). Effects of piperonyl butoxide on drug metabolism in rodents and man. *Arch. Environ. Health* **24**, 97–106.

Crampton, P. L. (1994). Piperonyl butoxide human intake estimates. (Europe) G. R. 94-0009.

Dahl, A. R. and Brenzinski, D. A. (1985). Inhibition of rabbit nasal and hepatic cytochrome P-450-dependent hexamethylphosphoramide (HMPA)-*N*-demethylase by methylenedioxyphenyl compounds. *Biochem. Pharmacol.* **34**, 631–636.

Delaforge, M., Ioannides, C. and Parke, D. V. (1985). Ligand-complex formation between cytochrome P-450 and P-448 and methylenedioxyphenyl compounds. *Xenobiotica* **15**, 333–342.

Di Blashi, G. (1998). A review of the chemistry of PBO. *In* "PBO—The Insecticide Synergist" (D. Glynne Jones, ed.). Academic Press, San Diego.

Dragula, C., Driver, J. H., Whitmyre, G. K., and Burin, G. J. (1996). "Evaluation of the Potential Health Risks Associated with Indoor, Non-food, Consumer Uses of Piperonyl Butoxide—Volume II: Indoor Total Release Fogger." Prepared by Technology Sciences Group Inc. for Piperonyl Butoxide Task Force.

Driver *et al.* (1996).

Endura. (1996). Personal correspondence. Endura, SpA, Bologna, Italy.

Epstein, S. S., Arnold, E., Andrea, J., Bass, W., and Bishop, Y. (1972). Detection of chemical mutagens by the dominant lethal assay in the mouse. *Toxicol. Appl. Pharmacol.* **233**, 288–325.

Evans, J. G., Collins, M. A., Savage, S. A., Lake, B. G., and Butler, W. H. (1986). The histology and development of hepatic nodules in C3H/He mice following chronic administration of phenobarbitone. *Carcinogenesis* **7**, 627–631.

Evans, J. G., Collins, M. A., Lake, B. G., and Butler, W. H. (1992). The histology and development of hepatic nodules and carcinoma in C3H/He and C57BL/6 mice following chronic phenobarbitone administration. *Toxicol. Pathol.* **20**, 585–594.

Falk, H. L., Thompson, S. J., and Kotin, P. (1965). Carcinogenic potential of pesticides. *Arch. Environ. Health* **10**, 847–858.

Fennell, T. R., Sweatman, B. C., and Bridges, J. W. (1980). The induction of hepatic cytochrome *P*-450 in C57BL/10 and DBA/2 mice by isosafrole and piperonyl butoxide. A comparative study with other inducing agents. *Chem.–Biol. Interact.* **31**, 189–201.

Fox, T. R., Schumann, A. M., Watanabe, P. G., Yano, B. L., Maher, V. M., and McCormick, J. J. (1990). Mutational analysis of the H-ras oncogene in spontaneous C57BL/6X C3H/He mouse liver tumors and tumors induced with genotoxic and non-genotoxic hepatocarcinogens. *Cancer Res.* **50**, 4014–4018.

Franklin, M. R. (1976). Methylenedioxyphenyl insecticide synergists as potential human health hazards. *Environ. Health Perspec.* **14**, 29–37.

Fujitani, T., Ando, H., Fujitani, K., Ikeda, T., Kojima, A., Kubo, Y., Ogata, A., Oishi, S., Takahashi, H., Takahashi, O., and Yoneyama, M. (1992). Subacute toxicity of piperonyl butoxide in F344 rats. *Toxicology* **72**(3), 291–293.

Fujitani, T., Tanaka, T., Hashimoto, Y. and Yoneyama, M. . (1993). Subacute toxicity of piperonyl butoxide in ICR mice. *Toxicology* **83**, 93–100.

Gabriel, D. (1991a). "Acute Oral Toxicity, LD50—Rats." Unpublished Rep. 91-7317A from Biosearch Inc., Philadelphia, PA, undertaken for the PBO Task Force, Washington, DC.

Gabriel, D. (1991b). "Acute Dermal Toxicity, Single Level—Rabbits." Unpublished Rep. 91-7317A from Biosearch Inc., Philadelphia, PA, undertaken for the PBO Task Force, Washington, DC.

Galloway, S. M., Armstrong, M. J., Reubec, C., Coleman, S., Brown, B., Cannen, C., Bloom, A. D., Nakamura, F., Alimed, F. M., Duk, S., Rimpo, J., Margolin, B. H., Resnick, M. A., Anderson, B., and Zeiger, E. (1987). Chromosome aberrations and sister chromatid exchanges in Chinese hamster ovary cells. *Environ. Mol. Mutagen.* **10**(Suppl. 10), 1–175.

Goldenthal, E. I. (1992). "21-day Repeated Dose Dermal Toxicity Study with Piperonyl Butoxide in Rabbits." Unpublished Rep. 542-007 from International Research and Development Corp., Mattawan, Michigan, undertaken of the PBO Task Force, Washington, DC.

Goldenthal, E. I. (1993a). "Evaluation of Piperonyl Butoxide in an Eight-Week Toxicity Study in Dogs." Unpublished Rep. 542-004 from International Research and Development Corp., Mattawan, Michigan, undertaken for the PBO Task Force, Washington, DC.

Goldenthal, E. I. (1993b). "Evaluation of Piperonyl Butoxide in a One Year Chronic Dietary Toxicity Study in Dogs." Unpublished Rep. 542-005 from International Research and Development Corp., Mattawan, Michigan, undertaken for the PBO Task Force, Washington, DC.

Goldstein, J. A., Hickman, P., and Kimbrough, R. D. (1973). Effects of purified and technical piperonyl butoxide on drug-metabolizing enzymes and ultrastructure of rat liver. *Toxicol. Appl. Pharmacol.* **26**, 444–458.

Goldsworthy, T. L., Morgan, K. T., Popp, J. A., and Butterworth, B. E. (1991). Guidelines for measuring chemically-induced cell proliferation in specific rodent target organs. *In* "Chemically Induced Cell Proliferation: Implications for Risk Assessment" (B. E. Butterworth, T. D. Slaga, W. Farland, and M. McClain, eds.), pp. 253–284. Wiley-Liss, New York.

Graham, D. (1987). "24-Month Dietary Toxicity and Carcinogenicity Study of Piperonyl Butoxide in the Albino Rat." Unpublished Rep. 81690 from Bio-Research Ltd. Laboratory, Senneville, Quebec, Canada, undertaken for the PBO Task Force, Washington, DC.

Graham, P. W., Hellyer, R. O., and Ryan, A. J. (1970). The kinetics of inhibition of drug metabolism in vitro by some naturally occurring compounds. *Biochem. Pharmacol.* **19**, 769–775.

Grasso, P., and Hinton, R. H. (1991). Evidence for and possible mechanisms of nongenotoxic carcinogenesis in rodent liver. *Chem.–Biol. Interact.* **248**, 271–290.

Grasso, P., Sharratt, M., and Cohen, A. J. (1991). Role of persistent, nongenotoxic tissue damage in rodent cancer and relevance to humans. *Annu. Rev. Pharmacol. Toxicol.* **31**, 253–287.

Hall, J. G., McLaughlin, J. F., and Stamm, S. (1975). Coarctation of the aorta in male cousins with similar maternal environmental exposure to insect repellent and insecticides. *Pediatrics* **55**, 425–427.

Hodgson, E., Philpot, R. M., Backer, R. C., and Mailman, R. B. (1973). Effect of synergists on drug metabolism. *Drug Metab. Dispos.* **1**, 391–401.

Hoffman, G. M. (1991). "An Acute Inhalation Toxicity Study of Piperonyl Butoxide in the Rat." Unpublished Rep. 91-8330 from Bio/dynamics, East Millstone, NJ, undertaken for the PBO Task Force, Washington, DC.

Hunter, B., Bridges, J. L., and Prentice, D. G. (1977). "Long Term Feeding of Pyrethrins and PBO to Rats." Conducted by Huntingdon Research Center for the Pyrethrum Board of Kenya.

Innes, J., Ulland, B., Valerio, M., Petrucelli, L., Fishbein, L., Hart, E. and Pallotta, A. (1969). Bioassay of pesticides and industrial chemicals for tumorigenicity in mice: A preliminary note. *J. Nat. Canc. Inst.* **42**, 1101–1114.

Ishidate, M., Sofuri, T., Yoshikawa, K., Hayashi, M., Nohmi, T., Sawada, M., and Matsnoka, A. (1984). Primary mutagenicity screening of food additives currently used in Japan. *Food. Chem. Toxicol.* **22**, 623–636.

Ishidate, M., Harnois, M. C., and Sofuni, T. (1988). A comparative analysis of data on the clastogenicity of 951 substances tested in mammalian cell cultures. *Mutation Res.* **195**, 151–213.

Ito, N., Hananouchi, M., Sugihara, S., Shirai, T., and Tsuda, H. (1976). Reversibility and irreversibility of liver tumors in mice induced by the isomer of 1,2,3,4,5,6-hexachlorocyclohexane. *Cancer Res.* **36**, 2227–2234.

Ivett, J. L., and Tice, R. R. (1983). Response of C57BL/6 and DBA/2 mouse strains to benzene-induced genotoxicity after inhibition of cytochrome P-450. *Environ. Mutagen.* **5**, 450–451.

Jirtle, R. L. (1994). Liver tumor promotion and breast cancer chemoprevention: Common mechanisms. *In* "Nongenotoxic Carcinogenesis: Ernst Schering Research Foundation Workshop 10" (A. Cockburn and L. Smith, eds.), pp. 157–171. Springer-Verlag, Berlin.

Jones, G., and Butler, W. H. (1975). Morphology of spontaneous and induced neoplasia. *In* "Mouse Hepatic Neoplasia" (W. H. Butler and P. M. Newberne, eds.), pp. 21–59. Elsevier, Amsterdam.

JMPR (1993). Piperonyl butoxide. *In* "Pesticide Residues in Food—1992," Toxicology Evaluations, pp. 317–334. World Health Organization, Geneva.

JMPR (1995). "Piperonyl Butoxide." A monograph prepared by the Joint FAO/WHO Meeting on Pesticide Residues, Geneva.

Kawachi, T., Komatsu, T., Kada, T., Ishidate, M., Sasaki, M., Sugiyama, T., and Tazima, Y. (1980). Results of recent studies on the relevance of various short-term screening tests in Japan. *Appl. Methods Oncol.* **3**, 253–276.

Kennedy, G. L., Smith, S. H., Kinoshita, F. K., Keplinger, M. L., and Calandra, J. C. (1977). Teratogenic evaluation of piperonyl butoxide in the rat. *Food Cosmet. Toxicol.* **15**, 337–339.

Khera, K. S., Whalen, C., Angers, G., and Trivett, G. (1979). Assessment of the teratogenic potential of piperonyl butoxide, biphenyl and phosalone in the rat. *Toxicol. Appl. Pharmacol.* **47**, 353–358.

Kociba, R. J., Keyes, D. G., Beyer, J. E., Carreon, R. M., Wade, C. E., Dittenber, D. A., Kalnins, R. P., Frauson, L. E., Park, C. N., Barnard, S. D., Hummel, R. A., and Humiston, C. G. (1978). Results of a two-year chronic toxicity and oncogenicity study of 2,3,7,8-tetrachlorodibenzo-*p*-dioxin in rats. *Toxicol. Appl. Pharmacol.* **46**(2), 279–303.

Lake, B. G., Hopkins, R., Chakraborty, J., Bridges, J. W., and Parke, D. V. (1973). The influence of some hepatic enzyme inducers and inhibitors on extrahepatic drug metabolism. *Drug Metab. Dispos.* **1**, 342–349.

Law, M. G. (1991). Susceptibility to phenobarbital promotion of hepatotumorigenesis: correlation with differential expression and induction of hepatic drug-metabolizing enzymes in heavy and light male (C3H x VY) F1 hybrid mice. *Carcinogenesis* **12**, 911–915.

Leng, J. M., Schwartz, C. A., and Schardein, J. L. (1986). "Teratology Study in Rabbits." Unpublished Rep. 542-002 from International Research and Development Corp., Mattawan, Michigan, submitted to WHO by Endura SA, Bologna, Italy, for the Piperonyl Butoxide Task Force, Washington, DC.

Lorber, M. (1972). Hematotoxicity of synergized pyrethrum insecticides and related chemicals in intact and totally and subtotally splenectomized dogs. *Acta Hepato-Gastroenterol.* **19**, 66–78.

Loury, D. J., Goldsworthy, T. L., and Butterworth, B. E. (1987). The value of measuring cell replication as a predictive index of tissue-specific tumorigenic potential. *In* "Nongenotoxic Mechanisms in Carcinogenesis" (B. E. Butterworth and T. J. Slaga, eds.), pp. 119–136. Cold Spring Harbor Laboratories, Cold Spring Harbor, NY (Banbury Report 25).

Lubet, R. A., Nims, R. W., Ward, J. M., Rice, J. M., and Diwan, B. A. (1989). Induction of cytochrome P450b and its relationship to liver tumor promotion. *J. Am. Coll. Toxicol.* **8**, 259–268.

Maekawa, A., Onodera, H., Furuta, K., Tanigawa, H., Ogiu, T., and Hayashi, T. (1985). Lack of evidence of carcinogenicity of technical-grade piperonyl butoxide in F344 rats: Selective induction of ileocaecal ulcers. *Fd. Chem. Toxic.* **23**(7), 675–682.

Malarkey, D. E., Devereus, T. R., Dime, G. E., and Maronpot, R. R. (1995). Hepatocarcinogenicity of chlordane in B6C3F1 and B6C2F1 male mice. Evidence for regression in B6C3F1 mice and carcinogenesis independent of *ras* proto-oncogene activation. *Carcinogenesis* **16**, 2617–2625.

Maronpot, R. R., Fox, T., Malarkey, D. E., and Goldsworthy, T. L. (1995). Mutations in the *ras* proto-oncogene: clues to etiology and molecular pathogenesis of mouse liver tumors. *Toxicology* **101**, 125–156.

McClain, R. M. (1989). The significance of hepatic microsomal enzyme induction and altered thyroid function in rats: Implications for thyroid gland neoplasia. *Toxicol. Path.* **17**, 294–303.

McClean, E. M., Driver, H., and McDanell, R. (1990). Nutrition and enzyme inducers in liver tumor promotion in human and rat. *Bull. Cancer* **77**(5), 505–508.

McGregor, D. B., Brown, A., Cattanach, P., Edwards, I., McBride, D., Riach, C., and Caspary, W. J. (1988). Response of the L5178Y TK+/TK- mouse lymphoma cell forward mutation assay III, 72 coded chemicals. *Environ. Mol. Mutagenesis* **12**, 85–154.

Modeweg-Hausen, L., Lalande, M., Bier, C., Lossos, G., and Osborne, B. E. (1984). "A Dietary Dose Range-Finding Study of Piperonyl Butoxide in the Albino Rat." Unpublished Rep. 81820B from Bio-Research Laboratories, Edgewater, MD, undertaken for the PBO Task Force, Washington, DC.

Monticello, T. M., Morgan, K. T., and Uraih, L. (1990). Nonneoplastic nasal lesions in rats and mice. *Environ. Hleath Perspec.* **85**, 249–274.

Moriye, M., Ohta, T., Watanabe, K., Miyazawa, T., Kato, K., and Sturaso, Y. (1983). Further mutagenicity studies on pesticides in bacterial reversion assay systems. *Mutation Res.* **116**, 185–216.

Murray, M., and Reidy, G. F. (1989). *In vitro* formation of an inhibitory complex between an isosafrole metabolite and rat hepatic cytochrome P-450. *Drug Metab. Dispos.* **17**, 449–454.

Mutai, M., Tatematsu, M., Aoki, T., Wada, S., and Ito, N. (1990). Modulatory interaction between initial clofibrate treatment and subsequent administration of 2-acetylaminofluorene or sodium phenobarbital on glutathione S-transferase positive lesion development. *Cancer Lett.* **49**(2), 127–132.

Neveu, M. J., Babcock, K. L., Hertzberg, E. L., Paul, E. L., Nicholson, B. J., and Pitot, H. C. (1994). Colocalized alterations in connexin 32 and cytochrome P450IIB1/2 by phenobarbital and related liver tumor promoters. *Cancer Res.* **54**, 3145–3152.

Newton, P. E. (1992). A subchronic (3-month) inhalation toxicity study of piperonyl butoxide in the rat via whole-body exposures. Unpublished Rep. 91-8333 from Bio/Dynamics, East Millstone, NJ, undertaken for the PBO Task Force, Washington, DC.

Okamiya, H., Onodera, H., Ito, S., Imazawa, T., Yasuhara, K., and Takahashi, M. (1998). Mechanistic study on liver tumor promoting effects of PBO in rats. *Arch. Toxicol.* **72**(11), 744–750.

Okey, A. B. (1990). Enzyme induction in the cytochrome P-450 system. *Pharmacol. Ther.* **45**, 241–298.

Pedrick, M. S., Rumsby, P. C., Wright, V., Phillimore, H. E., Butler, W. H., and Evans, J. G. (1994). Growth characteristics and Ha-*ras* mutations of all cultures isolated from chemically induced mouse liver tumors. *Carcinogenesis* **15**, 1847–1852.

Phillips, J. C., Cunningham, M. E., Price, R. J., Osimitz, T. G., Gabriel, K. L., Preiss, F. J., Butler, W. H., and Lake, B. G. (1997). Effect of piperonyl butoxide on cell replication and xenobiotic metabolism in rat liver. *Fund. Appl. Toxicol.* **38**, 64–74.

Philpot, R. M., and Hodgson, E. (1971). A cytochrome P-450-piperonyl butoxide spectrum similar to that produced by ethyl isocyanide. *Life Sci. II* **10**, 503–512.

Philpot, R. M., and Hodgson, E. (1972a). The production and modification of cytochrome P-450 difference spectra by *in vivo* administration of methylenedioxyphenyl compounds. *Chem. Biol. Interactions* **4**, 185–194.

Philpot, R. M., and Hodgson, E. (1972b). The effect of piperonyl butoxide concentration on the formation of cytochrome P-450 difference spectra in hepatic microsomes for mice. *Mol. Pharmacol.* **8**, 204–214.

Pitman Moore (1990). Manufacturers of PBO in Scotland, 1962–1990.

Robinson, K., Pinsonneault, L., and Procter, B. G. (1986). "A Two-Generation (Two-Litter) Reproduction Study of Piperonyl Butoxide Administered in the Diet to the Rat." Unpublished Rep. 81689 from Bio-Research Laboratories Ltd., Montreal, Canada, undertaken for the PBO Task Force, Washington, DC.

Romanelli, P. (1991a). "Primary Eye Irritation—Rabbits." Unpublished Rep. 91-7317A from Biosearch Inc., Philadelphia, undertaken for the PBO Task Force, Washington, DC.

Romanelli, P. (1991b). "Primary Skin Irritation—Rabbits." Unpublished Rep. 91-7317A from Biosearch Inc., Philadelphia, undertaken for the PBO Task Force, Washington, DC.

Romanelli, P. (1991c). "Guinea Pig Dermal Sensitization—Modified Buehler Method." Unpublished Rep. 91-7317A from Biosearch Inc., Philadelphia, undertaken for the PBO Task Force, Washington, DC.

Ross, J., Thongsinthusak, T., Fong, H. R., Margetich, S., and Krieger, R. (1990). Measuring potential dermal transfer of surface pesticide residue generated from indoor fogger use: An interim report. *Chemosphere* **20**, 349–360.

Rumsby, P. C., Barrass, N. C., Phillimore, H. E., and Evans, J. G. (1991). Analysis of the Ha-ras oncogene in C3H/H3 mouse liver tumours derived spontaneously or induced with diethylnitrosamine or phenobarbitone. *Carcinogenesis* **12**, 2331–2336.

Sarles, M. P., Dove, W. E., and Moore, D. H. (1949). Acute toxicity and irritation tests on animals with the new insecticide, piperonyl butoxide. *Am. J. Trop. Med.* **29**, 151–166.

Sarles, M. P., and Vandergrift, W. B. (1952). Chronic toxicity and related studies on animals with the insecticide and pyrethrum synergist piperonyl butoxide. *Am. J. Trop. Med.* **1**, 862–883.

Selim, S. (1995). "Absorption, Excretion, and Mass Balance of ^{14}C Piperonyl Butoxide from Two Different Formulations after Dermal Application to Healthy Volunteers." Unpublished Rep. PO594006 from Biological Test Center, Irvine, CA, undertaken for the PBO Task Force, Washington, DC.

Skrinijaric-Spoljar, M., Matthew, H. B., Engel, J. L., and Casida, J. E. (1971). Response of hepatic microsomal mixed-function oxidases to various types of insecticide chemical synergists administered to mice. *Biochem. Pharmacol.* **20**, 1607–1618.

Squire, R. A., and Levitt, M. H. (1975). Report of a workshop on classification of specific hepatocellular lesions in rats. *Cancer Res.* **35**, 3214–3223.

Suzuki, H., and Suzuki, N. (1995). Piperonyl butoxide mutagenicity in human RSa cells. *Mutation Res.* **344**, 27–30.

Takahashi, O., Oishi, T., Fujitani, T., Tanaka, T., and Yoneyama, M. (1994a). Chronic toxicity studies of piperonyl butoxide in F344 rats: Induction of hepatocellular carcinoma. *Fundam. Appl. Toxicol.* **22**, 293–303.

Takahashi, O., Oishi, T., Fujitani, T., Tanaka, T., and Yoneyama, M. (1994b). PBO induces hepatocellular carcinoma in CD1 mice. *Arch. Toxicol.* **68**, 467–469.

Tanaka, T. (1992). Effects of piperonyl butoxide on F1 generation mice. *Toxicol. Lett.* **60**, 83–90.

Tanaka, T. (1993). Behavioral effects of piperonyl butoxide in male mice. *Toxicol. Lett.* **69**, 155–161.

Tanaka, T., Takahashi, O., and Oishi, S. (1992). Reproductive and neurobehavioral effects in three-generation toxicity study of piperonyl butoxide administered to mice. *Food Chem. Toxicol.* **30**, 1015–1019.

Tanaka, T., Fujitani, T., Takahashi, O., and Oishi, S. (1994). Developmental toxicity evaluation of piperonyl butoxide in CD-1 mice. *Toxicol. Lett.* **71**, 123–129.

Tatematsu, M., Ozaki, K., Mutai, M., Shichino, Y., Furihata, C., and Ito, N. (1990). Enhancing effects of various gastric carcinogens on development of pepsinogen-altered pyloric glands in rats. *Carcinogenesis* **11**(11), 1975–1978.

Tayama, S. (1996). Cytogenic effects of PBO and safrole in CHO-K1 cells. *Mutation Res.* **368**, 249–260.

U.S. Environmental Protection Agency (U.S. EPA) (1988). "Standard Evaluation Procedure for Inhalation Studies." USEPA, Washington, DC.

U.S. Environmental Protection Agency (U.S. EPA) (1995a). "List of Chemicals Evaluated for Carcinogenic Potential." Office of Pesticide Programs, Washington, DC.

U.S. Environmental Protection Agency (U.S. EPA) (1995b). "Pesticide Handlers Exposure Database (PHED) Evaluation Guidance," PHED V1. 1. Occupational and Residential Exposure Branch, Office of Pesticide Programs, Washington, DC.

U.S. National Cancer Institute (1979). "Bioassay of Piperonyl Butoxide for Possible Carcinogenicity." DHEW Publ. 79-1375, Bethesda, MD, U.S. Department of Health, Education and Welfare.

Van Miller, J. P., Lalich, J. J., and Allen, J. R. (1977). Increased incidence of neoplasms in rats exposed to low levels of 2,3,7,8-tetrachlorodibenzo-rhodioxin. *Chemosphere* **6**(9), 537–544.

Wachs, H. (1947). Synergistic insecticides. *Science* **105**, 397–401.

Waf, D. J., and Short, C. R. (1971). Induction of hepatic microsomal hydroxylating enzymes by technical piperonyl butoxide and some of its analogues. *Toxicol. Appl. Pharmacol.* **19**, 54–61.

Wagstaff, D. J., and Short, C. R. (1971). Induction of hepatic microsomal hydroxylating enzymes by technical piperonyl butoxide and some of its analogues. *Toxicol. Appl. Pharmacol.* **19**, 54–61.

Watanabe, T., Manabe, S., Ohashi, Y., Okamiya, H., Onodera, H., and Mitsumori, K. (1998). Comparison of the induction profile of hepatic drug-metabolizing enzymes between piperonyl butoxide and phenobarbital in rats. *J. Toxicol. Pathol.* **11**, 1–10.

Wellcome Environmental Health Unit (1991). Users of PBO.

Wester, R. C., Bucks, D. A. W., and Maibach, H. I. (1994). Human *in vivo* percutaneous absorption of pyrethrin and piperonyl butoxide. *Food Chem. Toxicol.* **32**, 51–53.

White, T. J., Goodman, D., Shulgin, A. T., Castagnoli, N., Jr., Lee, R., and Petrakis, N. L. (1977). Mutagenic activity of some centrally active aromatic amines in Salmonella typhimurium. *Mutat. Res.* **56**, 199–202.

Whysner, J., Ross, P. M., and Williams, G. M. (1996). Phenobarbital mechanistic data and risk assessment: Enzyme induction, enhanced cell proliferation, and tumor promotion. *Pharmacol. Ther.* **71**, 153–191.

Wilson, D. M., Goldsworthy, T. L., Popp, J. A., and Butterworth, B. E. (1992). Evaluation of genotoxicity, pathological lesions, and cell proliferation in livers of rats and mice treated with furan. *Environ. Mol. Mutagen.* **19**, 209–222.

Wintersteiger, R., and Juan, H. (1991). "Resorption Study of Tyrason after Dermal Application (Study Performed on Healthy Subjects)." J.S.W.—Experimental Research, Studie Analytik. 01/91, p. 1.

Yamamoto, I. (1973). Mode of action of synergists in enhancing the insecticidal activity of pyrethrum and pyrethroids. *In* "Pyrethrum—Natural Insecticide," pp. 195–210. Academic Press, London/New York.

Pentachlorophenol

Gay Goodman
Human Health Risk Resources, Inc.

65.1 IDENTITY, PROPERTIES, AND USES

65.1.1 CHEMICAL NAME

Pentachlorophenol is the chemical name.

65.1.2 STRUCTURE

See Figure 65.1 for molecular structure.

65.1.3 SYNONYMS

Pentachlorophenol, commonly abbreviated as PCP, is also known as penta, chlorophen, penchlorol, pentachlorofenol, and pentachlorofenolo. Current and former trade names include Dowicide 7, Dowicide EC-7, Dow Pentachlorophenol DP-2 Antimicrobial, Fungifen, Fungol, Glazd Penta, Permacide, Permagard, Permasa, Permatox, Permite, Santophen, Term-i-Trol, Thompson's Wood Fix, Weedone, and Witophen P.

65.1.4 PHYSICAL AND CHEMICAL PROPERTIES

Pentachlorophenol (PCP) is a chlorinated derivative of phenol with empirical formula C_6Cl_5OH and molecular weight 266.34.

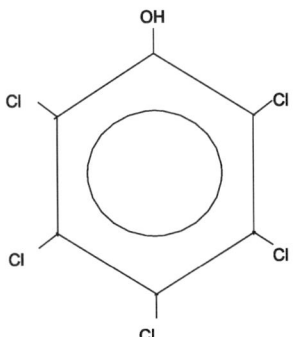

Figure 65.1 Molecular structure of pentachlorophenol.

The compound consists of needlelike crystals. PCP of 98% purity has been described as cream-colored, while technical-grade PCP is pale brown in color (NTP, 1989). PCP is almost insoluble in water (8 mg in 100 ml), freely soluble in alcohol or ether, soluble in benzene, and slightly soluble in cold petroleum ether (Budavari, 1996). Sodium pentachlorophenate (NaPCP), the sodium salt of the anion, has empirical formula $C_6Cl_5O^-Na^+$ and molecular weight 288.32. NaPCP is freely soluble in water. PCP has a pungent odor when heated. The odor threshold in humans is approximately 1.6 mg/l (WHO, 1987).

65.1.5 HISTORY, FORMULATIONS, AND USES

PCP, in common with other chlorophenols, has a broad range of biocidal activity. In particular, PCP has been found to be effective as an algicide, bactericide, fungicide, herbicide, insecticide, and molluscicide (WHO, 1987).

Collectively, PCP and its sodium salt previously constituted one of the most heavily used pesticides in the United States. Net production of the three U.S. manufacturers active in 1980 was 30,600 tons (Jones, 1981). Usage patterns tabulated around that time indicate that 95–98% of North American PCP production (of which 94% originated in the United States) was employed directly or indirectly in wood treatment (Economist Intelligence Unit, 1981). Wood preservation uses of PCP and NaPCP included commercial wood treatment, fence-post treatment, paint treatment, and sapstain control in pressboard and other wood-derived materials (WHO, 1987).

65.1.5.1 U.S. Federal Regulation of Pesticidal Use

Pesticidal use of PCP is regulated at the federal level under the Federal Insecticide, Fungicide, and Rodenticide Act (FIFRA). PCP was designated a Restricted Use pesticide on July 13, 1984 by the Office of Pesticide Programs (U.S. EPA, 1984a). Most uses as an herbicide, antimicrobial agent (e.g., in cooling towers), defoliant, disinfectant, and molluscicide (e.g., in marine paint) were discontinued at that time. It is permitted to use PCP as a biocidal agent on wood, but not on wood to be used for log homes or the interiors of buildings. It is also permitted to use PCP as a biocide in oil field flood waters and in pulp and paper mill solutions. The label is required to state that PCP can only be sold to and used by certified pesticide applicators who must wear specific items of protective clothing and take specific handling precautions. The label also must state that application to logs for use in the construction of log homes is explicitly prohibited (U.S. EPA, 1986).

65.1.5.2 U.S. Federal Regulation of Toxic Contaminants

Levels of the most toxic contaminants of PCP and PCP salts are regulated by U.S. federal statute. Both hexachlorodibenzo-*p*-dioxin (HxCDD) and hexachlorobenzene (HCB) are considered by the U.S. EPA to pose potential carcinogenic, teratogenic, and fetotoxic risks. As of February 2, 1989, the maximum allowable level of HxCDD is 4 ppm in any batch and the maximum allowable monthly average is 2 ppm (U.S. EPA, 1987). Registrants are instructed that the method used to lower HxCDD is not to increase concentrations of HCB and polychlorodibenzofurans (pCDFs) "above the levels in products marketed at the time of publication of this Notice" (U.S. EPA, 1984a); for HCB the maximum level was later specified as 75 ppm (U.S. EPA, 1987). The other contaminant specifically regulated in the earlier ruling was the potent rodent carcinogen 2,3,7,8-tetrachlorodibenzo-*p*-dioxin (TCDD), which was required to be below detection by an acceptable method (U.S. EPA, 1984a, b). The later ruling established that the detection limit for TCDD shall be no higher than 1 ppb (U.S. EPA, 1987).

65.1.5.3 U.S. Federal Drinking Water Standards and Guidelines

Pursuant to the requirements of the Safe Drinking Water Act, the U.S. EPA established the level of PCP permissible in drinking water: the maximum contaminant level (MCL) was set at 0.001 mg/l (U.S. EPA, 1991a). Based upon potential carcinogenicity, the maximum contaminant level goal (MCLG) was set at zero mg/l (U.S. EPA, 1991b).

65.2 PHARMACOKINETICS

65.2.1 ABSORPTION

PCP is readily absorbed by oral, inhalation, and dermal routes of exposure.

65.2.1.1 Oral

Absorption of PCP or NaPCP by the oral route has been studied in the mouse (Reigner *et al.*, 1992a), rat (Braun *et al.*, 1977; Reigner *et al.*, 1991; Yuan *et al.*, 1994), rhesus monkey (Braun and Sauerhoff, 1976), and human (Braun *et al.*, 1979). The time for peak plasma levels to be attained following an oral dose of PCP has been found to be comparable in rodents (1.5–6 hr) and humans (4 hr) but longer in monkeys (12–24 hr). The oral absorption efficiency was found to be greater than 90% in rats,

monkeys, and humans for doses in the range 0.1–15 mg/kg. Approximately 4–20% (dependent on dose and species) of a single ingested dose of PCP is excreted in the feces, while essentially all of the remainder appears in the urine. The slow time course of excretion along with the completeness of absorption into the bloodstream are evidence that enterohepatic recirculation plays an important role in the disposition of PCP in all species examined.

65.2.1.2 Inhalation

Absorption of an aerosol of NaPCP was studied in rats by Hoben *et al.* (1976a); approximately 80% of the inhaled dose (6 mg/kg over 20 minutes) was excreted unmetabolized in urine during the 72-hr period following exposure. However, actual absorption must have been greater than 80% because urinary excretion of the major metabolite in rodents was not quantified (see Section 65.2.3). An estimate of the amount of inhaled PCP absorbed by humans under conditions in which dermal exposure was expected to be insignificant was obtained in two volunteers with no previous occupational exposure to PCP (Casarett *et al.*, 1969). The two subjects were exposed to mean ambient PCP concentrations of 230 and 432 mg/m^3 PCP, respectively, for 45 minutes in a wood-treatment plant during brush application of PCP. Calculated exposure doses were 91 and 147 µg. Based upon chemical analysis of PCP in the 7-day urine, respiratory tract absorption was calculated as 88% for the volunteer exposed to the lower concentration. A less complete accounting of absorption (76%) was available for the other volunteer, as urinary PCP levels were still well above baseline at the end of the 5-day collection period.

65.2.1.3 Dermal

Wester *et al.* (1993) measured dermal absorption of PCP in four female rhesus monkeys. ^{14}C-labeled PCP (98.6% pure) was prepared in either acetone or premoistened soil and applied topically to an area of shaved abdominal skin. The PCP doses applied were 0.8 µg/cm^2 for the acetone sample and 0.7 µg/cm^2 for the soil sample. Urine was collected for 14 days. The percentage of the applied dose absorbed percutaneously was determined to be 29 ± 6% of the acetone sample and 24 ± 6% of the soil sample.

65.2.2 DISTRIBUTION AND ELIMINATION

The kinetics of removal from plasma are summarized in Table 65.1, while Table 65.2 summarizes the kinetics of excretion via the urine and feces. There is good agreement in the published literature on plasma half-lives of PCP in various experimental animals. Following oral or intravenous (i.v.) administration, mean half-lives of 5–6 hr in mice, 2–11 hr in rats, and 72–84 hr in monkeys have been calculated based on a first-order model representing the major portion of plasma PCP. Urinary excretion rates are similar to the corresponding plasma distribution rates, with estimated mean half-lives of 13 hr in rats

Table 65.1
Kinetics of PCP Removal from Plasma in Mice, Rats, Monkeys, and Humans Following Single-Dose Exposure[a]

Study	Route	Species	Sex	No.	Dose (mg/kg)	Collection period	Analytical method	Mean half-life in plasma (hr)
Reigner et al., 1992a	oral	mouse	M	6	15	36 hr	Chem.	5.8[b]
Reigner et al., 1992a	i.v.	mouse	M	6	15	36 hr	Chem.	5.2[b]
Braun et al., 1977	oral	rat	M	2[d]	10	6 days	[14]C	6.9, (24)[c,e]
Braun et al., 1977	oral	rat	F	2[d]	10	6 days	[14]C	11, (30)[c,e]
Reigner et al., 1991	oral	rat	M	5	2.5	48 hr	Chem.	7.5[b]
Reigner et al., 1991	i.v.	rat	M	5	2.5	48 hr	Chem.	(0.7), 7.1[e]
Reigner et al., 1991	i.v.	rat	M	1	20	96 hr	Chem.	4.1, (36)
Reigner et al., 1991	i.v.	rat	M	1	20	96 hr	[14]C	4.5, (45)
Yuan et al., 1994	oral	rat	M	3[d]	9.5	40 hr	Chem.	8.6[b]
Yuan et al., 1994	oral	rat	M	3[d]	38	60 hr	Chem.	6.3[b]
Yuan et al., 1994	i.v.	rat	M	3[d]	5	20 hr	Chem.	<3[f], 5.6[e]
Yuan et al., 1994	i.v.	rat	F	3[d]	5	20 hr	Chem.	<4[f], 9.5[e]
Meerman et al., 1983	i.v.	rat	M	2[d]	10.7	36 hr	Chem.	2.2, 7.2[e]
Braun and Sauerhoff, 1976	n.g.	monkey	M	3	10	7 days	[14]C/Chem.	72[b]
Braun and Sauerhoff, 1976	n.g.	monkey	F	3	10	7 days	[14]C/Chem.	84[b]
Braun et al., 1979	oral	human	M	4	0.1	6 days	Chem.	30[b]

[a]Abbreviations: [14]C, radioactive counts; Chem., chemical analysis; i.v., intravenous; n.g., nasogastric.
[b]Monophasic model.
[c]Value estimated using linear extrapolation from data in Fig. 2 of the citation.
[d]Number of animals sacrificed or sampled per time point.
[e]Biphasic model. Half-lives accounting for only a minor portion of PCP are in parenthesis.
[f]Upper limit of initial-phase half-life estimated from inspection of data in Fig. 1 of the citation.

Table 65.2
Kinetics of PCP Excretion in Rats, Monkeys, and Humans Following Single-Dose Exposure[a]

Study	Route	Species	Sex	No.	Dose (mg/kg)	Collection period	Analytical method	Mean elimination half-life[b] (hr)	Mean urinary elimination half-life (hr)
Braun et al., 1977	oral	rat	M	3	10	9 days	[14]C	17.4, (40.2)[c]	—
Braun et al., 1977	oral	rat	F	3	10	9 days	[14]C	13.4, (32.5)[c]	—
Braun et al., 1977	oral	rat	M	3	100	8 days	[14]C	12.8, (121)[c]	—
Braun et al., 1977	oral	rat	F	3	100	8 days	[14]C	27.2[d]	—
Braun et al., 1977	oral	rat	n.s.	3	100	8 days	[14]C	—	13, (31)[c,e]
Braun and Sauerhoff, 1976	n.g.	monkey	M	3	10	7 days	[14]C/Chem.	—	41[d]
Braun and Sauerhoff, 1976	n.g.	monkey	F	3	10	7 days	[14]C/Chem.	—	92[d]
Braun et al., 1979	oral	human	M	4	0.1	6 days	Chem.	—	33[d]
Uhl et al., 1986	oral	human	M	1	0.016	53 days	[13]C	—	432[d]
Uhl et al., 1986	oral	human	M	1	0.31	70 days	Chem.	—	480[d]
Uhl et al., 1986	oral	human	M	3	0.055–0.15	6–14 days	Chem.	—	≤144[d,f]
Young and Haley, 1978	oral	human	M	1	≥2400[g]	7 days	Chem.	116[d]	128[d]

[a]Abbreviations: [13]C, isotopic substitution; ^{14}C, radioactive counts; Chem., chemical analysis; i.v., intravenous; n.g., nasogastric; n.s., not specified.
[b]Combined urinary and fecal excretion.
[c]Biphasic model. Half-lives accounting for only a minor portion of PCP are in parenthesis.
[d]Monophasic model.
[e]Values estimated using linear extrapolation from data in Fig. 4 of the citation.
[f]Estimated from Fig. 1 of the citation.
[g]Accidental poisoning case study.

and 41–92 hr in monkeys. In rats, excretion by combined urinary and fecal routes has also been measured; the major portion of dose is excreted with an estimated mean half-life of 13–27 hr. The single human study to examine the rate of PCP elimination from plasma reported a mean half-life of 30 hr, nearly identical to the mean half-life for urinary excretion found in the same study (33 hr). Other human studies of urinary excretion reported much longer half-lives (128–480 hr). The disparity in reported values is unexplained.

65.2.3 METABOLISM

An across-study comparison of urinary excretion profiles indicates that the disposition of PCP in rodents is qualitatively and quantitatively dissimilar to its disposition in monkeys and humans. In mice and rats, a substantial, dose-dependent fraction (16–48%) of ingested PCP is excreted in the urine as tetrachloro-1,4-hydroquinone (TCHQ). By contrast, every experimental study entailing administration of PCP to humans or monkeys has failed to find any evidence for the metabolism of PCP to TCHQ. In two male and two female rhesus monkeys given [^{14}C]PCP by nasogastric intubation at a single dose of 10 mg/kg, all recovered urinary radioactivity occurred as PCP (Braun and Sauerhoff, 1976). Using gas chromatography/mass spectrometry (GC/MS), Braun et al. (1979) found no trace of TCHQ in the urine of four human male volunteers exposed orally to non-radiolabeled PCP at a single dose of 0.1 mg/kg. Using a more sensitive method, GC/MS detection of ^{13}C-labelled compounds, Uhl et al. (1986) failed to find detectable levels of [^{13}C]-labeled TCHQ, 2,3,4,5-tetrachlorophenol, or 2,3,4,6-tetrachlorophenol in the urine of two human volunteers exposed orally to [^{13}C]PCP at a single dose of 0.98 or 2.4 mg/kg.

Nevertheless, the absence of PCP metabolism in humans remains controversial. Using GC/MS, Ahlborg et al. (1974) identified (without quantification) both TCHQ and PCP in the urine of two occupationally exposed male pesticide applicators. Because complete exposure profiles for the applicators were not obtained, one cannot rule out the possibility of concurrent exposure to the pesticide lindane (γ-hexachlorocyclohexane). It is known that lindane undergoes hydroxylation followed by aromatization (Gopalaswamy and Aiyar, 1986) to form 2,3,4,6- and 2,3,5,6-tetrachlorophenol as major metabolites in the rat (Engst et al., 1976), while TCHQ is the primary metabolite of 2,3,5,6-tetrachlorophenol administered to rats (Ahlborg and Larsson, 1978). This pathway does not entail formation of PCP. Furthermore, tetrachlorophenol is a contaminant of the commercial product (i.e., technical-grade PCP). The percentage tetrachlorophenol in technical-grade PCP varies over time and from product to product, but as examples, the two PCP formulations tested in a mouse carcinogenicity bioassay by the National Toxicology Program contained tetrachlorophenol at levels of 3.8% and 9.4%, respectively (NTP, 1989).

Another finding in apparent conflict with the in vivo observations of no PCP metabolism to TCHQ is the in vitro result of Juhl et al. (1985), who found evidence of PCP metabolism to TCHQ in a microsomal extract (S-9 fraction) of human liver (from a 61-year-old woman) and compared the time course of metabolite formation in the human liver S-9 to that in rat liver S-9. The rate of formation of TCHQ in the rat and human S-9 fractions during the first half-hour of incubation with the same (unspecified) PCP concentration can be estimated from Fig. 1 of Juhl et al. (1985): approximately 0.93 pmol/mg protein/min in human liver S-9 and 1.7 pmol/mg protein/min in rat liver S-9. Without information as to the concentration of PCP in the incubation mixtures, it is impossible to judge the relevance of this in vitro result to human exposures in vivo.

The inducible cytochrome P450 family of enzymes (the mixed-function oxygenase system) plays an important role in the Phase I biotransformation of a broad spectrum of endogenous compounds and xenobiotics (Sipes and Gandolfi, 1991). Rats and humans differ substantially with respect to cytochrome P450 subtypes (Paine, 1995). The human P450 3A isozymes function as mediators of the hydroxylation of steroids and various drugs. Human P450 3A3/4 and 3A7 variants are found in both adult and fetal liver (Hakkola et al., 1994). The gene for the human P450 3A4 variant has been expressed in a strain of the yeast Saccharomyces cerevisiae, in which it was able to catalyze the oxidative transformation of an extremely diverse group of molecules (Brian et al., 1990). Mehmood et al. (1996) used this yeast system to express human P450 3A4 and found that in both intact yeast cultures and microsomal extracts, PCP is transformed to TCHQ in a process dependent upon the presence of the cytochrome, oxygen, and NADPH. The affinity constant (K_a) for PCP was reported to be 85 μM, although data used in the derivation of this value were not given. In microsomal extracts, incubation for 30 min in the presence of 113 μM PCP produced 8 pmol TCHQ/nmol P450/min.

Taken together, these data suggest that humans, like rodents, possess the enzymatic capability to metabolize PCP to TCHQ, but in both the human and the rhesus monkey (the only nonhuman primate species tested) this enzymatic pathway is unimportant, at least when PCP is given in a single dose as large as 2.4 mg/kg (human) or 10 mg/kg (monkey). Reigner et al. (1992b) suggested that the failure of some investigators to find TCHQ in the urine of humans exposed to PCP may reflect the instability of this compound in urine. However, it is difficult to imagine why the breakdown product(s) would not then be detected, especially in the [^{13}C]PCP experiment of Uhl et al. (1986).

The question of whether humans metabolize PCP to TCHQ to any significant extent is more than academic: TCHQ has been demonstrated to be genotoxic in numerous short-term tests (including those for mutagenicity), whereas the data base on the genotoxicity of PCP consists of essentially negative or equivocal results (see Section 65.6). If, at a given PCP dose level, TCHQ is formed to a significant extent in mice but not humans, then very likely the carcinogenic potency of PCP in mice is not relevant to humans. Given the importance of this question, it is surprising how little attention has been focused on resolving

Table 65.3
Relative Amounts of Conjugated and Nonconjugated PCP and TCHQ in Urine Following Single-Dose Exposure to PCP[a]

Study	Species	Sex	Route	Collection period	Dose (mg/kg)	Percent of total urinary recovery[b]			
						PCP	PCP-c	TCHQ	TCHQ-c
Jakobson and Yllner, 1971	mouse	F	i.p.	24 hr	7.4–8.2	54%[c]		44%[c]	
Jakobson and Yllner, 1971	mouse	F	i.p.	24 hr	15–19	54%	12%	33%[c,d]	
Jakobson and Yllner, 1971	mouse	F	i.p.	24 hr	36–37	50%	20%	48%[c,d]	
Ahlborg et al., 1974	mouse	n.s.	i.p.	24 hr	10–25	41%	13%	24%	22%
Reigner et al., 1992a	mouse	M	gav.	48 hr	15	8%	51%	5%	47%
Ahlborg et al., 1978	rat	n.s.	i.p.	24 hr	10	60%	9–16%	7%	22%
Braun et al., 1977	rat	M/F	gav.	8 days	100	75%	9%	16%[c]	
Braun and Sauerhoff, 1976	monkey	M/F	n.g.	7–15 days	10	100%[c]		n.d.[c]	
Braun et al., 1979	human	M	oral	7 days	0.1	86%	14%	n.d.	n.d.
Uhl et al., 1986	human	M	oral	24 hr[e]	0.31	71%	29%	n.d.	n.d.

[a]*Abbreviations:* gav., gavage; i.p., intraperitoneal; n.d., none detected; n.g., nasogastric; n.s., not specified; PCP-c, PCP conjugate; TCHQ-c, TCHQ conjugate.
[b]Mean values except as indicated.
[c]The conjugated and nonconjugated forms were not differentiated.
[d]Value for the single animal tested.
[e]Single sample collected 24 hr after dosing.

the discrepancy between the *in vivo* and *in vitro* findings. An attempt should be made to replicate the *in vitro* results of Juhl *et al.* (1985), at the same time improving upon the study design. It would be useful to learn how the rate of TCHQ formation in intact rodent and human liver cells as well as microsomes depends on PCP, particularly at concentrations expected to occur in blood following administration of PCP at doses tested in the pharmacokinetic studies. It would also be helpful to know whether [^{13}C]TCHQ or its metabolites are excreted by humans or nonhuman primates during multiday exposure to [^{13}C]PCP.

The discovery that horseradish peroxidase can catalyze the hydroperoxide-dependent oxidation of PCP to TCHQ *in vitro* has led to speculation that mammalian peroxidases might catalyze this transformation *in vivo* as well (Samokyszyn *et al.*, 1995). Whether this possible pathway is relevant to interspecies differences in PCP metabolism remains to be discovered.

The potential influence of exposure route on the metabolism of PCP has not been studied methodically. However, there is no evidence to suggest route dependence of either rates or pathways.

Glucuronide and sulfide conjugates of PCP and TCHQ contribute to the total urinary excretion, as revealed by complete hydrolysis (Ahlborg *et al.*, 1978; Edgerton and Moseman, 1979). Experimentally observed urinary excretion profiles of free and conjugated PCP and TCHQ following single-dose administration of PCP are given in Table 65.3.

65.2.4 PLASMA PROTEIN BINDING

In plasma isolated from Sprague-Dawley (SD) rats, PCP was found to have high- and low-affinity binding constants of approximately 10^6 and 10^4 M^{-1}, respectively, suggesting that binding is strong enough to influence distribution and

metabolism (Braun *et al.*, 1977). In an *in vivo* study in the same rat strain, 81% of plasma PCP was found to be bound to protein (Gómez-Catalán *et al.*, 1991) Hoben *et al.* (1976b) reported that the ratio of bound PCP to albumin (mol/mol) was 1.3 for human plasma and 0.86 for plasma from an unspecified rat strain; the investigators suggested that this difference, which reflects differential binding to nonalbumin sites, may contribute to the longer retention time of PCP in human plasma.

65.2.5 PROTEIN ADDUCTS OF REACTIVE METABOLITES

Waidyanatha *et al.* (1996) found that PCP-derived adducts of hemoglobin and albumin occurred in a dose-dependent manner in SD rats given a single gavage dose of PCP at 5 to 40 mg/kg. The investigators demonstrated that the adducts resulted from reaction of protein binding sites with the quinones tetrachloro-1,4-benzoquinone (TC-1,4-BQ) and tetrachloro-1,2-benzoquinone (TC-1,2-BQ) and the semiquinones tetrachloro-1,4-benzosemiquinone (TC-1,4-BSQ) and tetrachloro-1,2-benzosemiquinone (TC-1,2-BSQ), all of which are formed by metabolism of PCP via TCHQ or tetrachlorocatechol (TCC):

$$PCP \rightarrow TCHQ \rightarrow TC\text{-}1,4\text{-}BSQ \rightarrow TC\text{-}1,4\text{-}BQ$$
$$PCP \rightarrow TCC \rightarrow TC\text{-}1,2\text{-}BSQ \rightarrow TC\text{-}1,2\text{-}BQ$$

In lifetime carcinogenicity bioassays, PCP produces liver tumors in mice but not rats (see Section 65.5). Lin *et al.* (1999) measured the *in vivo* formation of PCP-derived benzoquinone and benzosemiquinone adducts of liver cytosolic and nuclear proteins in B6C3F$_1$ mice and SD rats and attempted to interpret the results in light of the known interspecies difference in liver tumorigenicity. Rats and mice were given a single gavage dose of PCP at 5 to 40 mg/kg and sacrificed 24 hr later. The extent and type of adduct formation apparently differed between mice and rats. The primary differences appear to have been: (a) rats formed adducts of TC-1,2-BSQ and TC-1,4-BSQ in both cytosolic and nuclear protein whereas mice formed the cytosolic adducts (at an order of magnitude lower rate) but not the nuclear adducts, and (b) mice formed mono-S-substituted adducts of TC-1,2-BQ in both cytosolic and nuclear protein whereas rats formed neither. The authors argued that adduct formation in mice was linear in dose whereas that in rats was sublinear, but in fact, one or more minor (benzosemiquinone) adducts in both species demonstrated sublinearity while the major (benzoquinone) adducts were about equally linear in dose in both species. Based on the results described, one might tentatively hypothesize that PCP is able to produce liver tumors in B6C3F$_1$ mice but not SD rats (Section 65.5) because the mice form mono-S-substituted TC-1,2-BQ protein adducts while the rats do not. However, in the absence of plausible data showing that the ability to form this particular adduct above all others determines PCP tumorigenicity in mice, it is tempting to argue that the results of Lin et al. (1999) provide evidence against the hypothesis that protein adduct formation is related to the liver tumorigenicity of PCP.

44-min exposures to an aerosol of NaPCP containing PCP at approximately 1 ppm resulted in 33 to 83% mortality. Based on the assumption that the inhalation volume was 80 ml/min, the corresponding range of PCP doses was calculated as 10 to 14.5 mg/kg and the LD$_{50}$ as 12 mg/kg (Hoben et al., 1976c). Oral LD$_{50}$ values in rats for an unspecified grade of PCP were reported to be 146 mg/kg for males and 175 mg/kg for females (Gaines, 1969). Renner et al. (1986) tested purified PCP in mice and found oral and intraperitoneal (i.p.) LD$_{50}$ values of approximately 130 and 60 mg/kg, respectively, in both sexes. Similar oral LD$_{50}$ values for purified PCP in mice (177 mg/kg for males and 117 mg/kg for females) were reported by Borzelleca et al. (1985). In an earlier study in female mice, Ahlborg and Larsson (1978) tested an unspecified grade of PCP delivered in 40% ethanol and found oral and i.p. LD$_{50}$ values of 74 and 32 mg/kg, respectively. See Gasiewicz (1991) for a summary of dermal, subcutaneous, and earlier oral and i.p. studies and Goodman et al. (1998) for descriptions of several unpublished studies.

65.3 ACUTE TOXICITY

The acute toxicity of PCP appears to be greatest when the route of exposure is inhalation. In a study in male rats, 28- to

65.4 SUBCHRONIC TOXICITY

The results of subchronic toxicity studies of PCP in mice and rats are summarized in Table 65.4.

Table 65.4
Subchronic Toxicity of PCP in Dietary Exposure Studies in Mice and Rats[a]

Study	Strain/species/ sex	Duration	PCP grade	Effects at LOEL[b]	LOEL (mg/kg-day)	NOEL (mg/kg-day)
NTP, 1989[c]	B6C3F$_1$ Mouse, M/F	30 days	TGC	↑ serum cholesterol (F); ↑ liver porphyrins (M); ↑ liver lesions[d] (M/F); ↑ platelets (M/F)	102	2.8
NTP, 1989[c]	B6C3F$_1$ Mouse, M/F	30 days	EC-7	↑ serum cholesterol (F); ↑ liver porphyrins (M); ↓ reticulocytes (F); ↑ γ-globulin (F)	24	4.3
NTP, 1989[c]	B6C3F$_1$ Mouse, M/F	30 days	AG	↑ liver porphyrins (M); ↑ liver lesions[d] (F)	27	4.1
NTP, 1989[c]	B6C3F$_1$ Mouse, M/F	6 months	TGC, DP-2	Liver lesions[d] (M/F); urinary bladder changes (M/F); immune suppression (M/F)	43	None
NTP, 1989[c]	B6C3F$_1$ Mouse, M/F	6 months	EC-7, AG	Liver lesions[d] (M/F); urinary bladder changes (M/F)	54	None
Renner et al., 1987	Sprague-Dawley Rat, F	28 days	AG	Liver lesions[d]; ↑ relative liver and kidney weights; mild anemia	53	None
NTP, 1999	F344 Rat, M/F	28 days	AG	↑ absolute and relative liver weights (F)	20	None
Kurtz and Hejtmancik, 1993[e]	F344 Rat, M/F	27 weeks	AG	Liver cell hypertrophy, necrosis (minimal), and enzyme changes (M/F); ↓ body weight gain (M/F)	71	None

[a]Abbreviations: AG, analytical-grade PCP; LOEL, lowest-observed-effect level; NOEL, no-observed-effect level; TGC, technical-grade composite.
[b]Sex affected at the LOEL is in parenthesis.
[c]With additional data provided by the NTP.
[d]Liver lesions included cytomegaly, karyomegaly, nuclear atypia, hepatocellular degeneration, and necrosis.
[e]Interim sacrifice of the 2-year bioassay described in NTP (1999).

65.4.1 MOUSE

The NTP (1989) conducted 30-day and 6-month dietary exposure studies of PCP in B6C3F$_1$ mice. Three PCP formulations were tested in the 30-day study: analytical-grade (AG-PCP), a partially purified product (EC-7), and a technical-grade composite (TGC-PCP). Two formulations were tested in the 6-month study: AG-PCP and a technical-grade product (DP-2). All formulations produced liver lesions in both sexes (NTP, 1989). Hematologic changes (altered platelet or reticulocyte counts) developed upon exposure to TGC-PCP and EC-7 but not AG-PCP, suggesting that one or more contaminants were intrinsic to these responses. In the 30-day study, no-observed-effect levels (NOELs) in male and female mice were 2.8, 4.3, and 4.1 mg/kg-day for TGC-PCP, EC-7, and AG-PCP, respectively. In the 6-month study, lowest-observed-effect levels (LOELs) in male and female mice were 43 mg/kg-d for TGC-PCP and DP-2 and 54 mg/kg-d for EC-7 and AG-PCP, the lowest doses tested.

The major contaminants of the test substances EC-7, DP-2, and TGC-PCP were other chlorophenols. For example, tetrachlorophenol comprised 9.4% of EC-7 and 3.8% of TGC-PCP. Hexachlorobenzene was also a contaminant of these three formulations, present in EC-7 and TGC-PCP at 65 and 50 ppm, respectively (NTP, 1989). The extent of contamination of the test substances with polychlorinated dibenzodioxin (pCDD) and pCDF compounds is shown in Table 65.5.

65.4.2 RAT

In an NTP study in rats, dietary exposure to purified PCP for 27 weeks at 71 mg/kg-day, the only dose tested, produced liver le-

Table 65.5
Chlorinated Dibenzodioxin and Dibenzofuran Contaminants of PCP Formulations Tested by the NTP in Toxicity Studies in Mice[a]

| Contaminant | PCP formulation | | | |
	EC-7 (91% PCP)[b]	TGC (90% PCP)[b]	DP-2 (91.6% PCP)[c]	AG (98.6% PCP)[b,c]
TCDD	<0.04 ppm	n.d.	n.d.	n.d.
HxCDD	0.19 ppm	10.1 ppm	0.59	<1
HpCDD	0.53 ppm	296 ppm	0.28	n.d.
OCDD	0.69 ppm	1386 ppm	173	<1
PCDF	n.d.	1.4 ppm	n.d.	n.d.
HxCDF	0.13 ppm	9.9 ppm	13.0	n.d.
HpCDF	0.15 ppm	88 ppm	172	n.d.
OCDF	n.d.	43 ppm	320	n.d.

[a]Information drawn from Table 3 of NTP (1989). *Abbreviations:* AG, analytical grade; HpCDD, heptachlorodibenzo-*p*-dioxin; HpCDF, heptachlorodibenzofuran; HxCDD, hexachlorodibenzo-*p*-dioxin; HxCDF, hexachlorodibenzofuran; OCDD, octachlorodibenzo-*p*-dioxin; OCDF, octachlorodibenzofuran; PCDF, pentachlorodibenzofuran; TGC, technical-grade composite; n.d., nondetectable (detection limit not given).
[b]Used in the 30-day study. TCDD was nondetectable at the detection limit of 40 ppb.
[c]Used in the 6-month study.

sions in both sexes (Kurtz and Hejtmancik, 1993). Minimal to mild degeneration of hepatocytes was observed in both male and female rats given purified PCP for 28 days at doses of 40 mg/kg-day and above (NTP, 1999). Mild anemia and elevated kidney weights were also found in female rats in response to 28-day dietary exposure to purified PCP at the only dose tested, 53 mg/kg-day (Renner *et al.*, 1987).

A subchronic exposure study of PCP, limited to histologic examination of the sciatic nerve, liver, and kidney, was conducted in Chile by Villena *et al.* (1992). The investigators reported that young male Wistar rats were exposed to analytical-grade PCP in drinking water at 0.3 mM (80 mg/l) for 60 days, 1.0 mM (270 mg/l) for 60 or 90 days, or 3.0 mM (800 mg/l) for 120 days. Assuming default values for drinking-water consumption and body weight of 0.032 l/day and 0.217 kg, respectively (U.S. EPA, 1988), the PCP doses can be estimated as 12, 39, and 120 mg/kg-day. Presumably, animals in each exposure group were sacrificed at the end of their exposure period. The four exposure groups were compared to a single control group; it is not clear at what stage the control animals were sacrificed.

In rats exposed to 1.0 mM (39 mg/kg-day) for 90 days or 3.0 mM (120 mg/kg-day) for 120 days, the investigators reported myelin degeneration of the sciatic nerve, hepatocellular degeneration, hepatic vascular congestion, glomerular congestion of the renal cortex, and turbid tumefaction of the renal proximal tubules. However, the reliability of this study is questionable in light of several flaws and insufficient provision of experimental details. One major problem with this study is that the solubility of PCP in water is only 20 mg/l at 30°C (IPCS, 1987), a factor of 4–40 less than the target doses. The investigators apparently did not measure the actual concentrations attained. It is conceivable that PCP precipitated out of solution and sank to the bottom of the water bottles, resulting in higher doses than intended. Measurement of food intake, body weight, and organ weight constitutes minimal insurance against exceeding the maximum tolerated dose; none of these parameters was reported. An additional concern is that standard laboratory practices do not appear to have been followed concerning quantification of the observed histologic effects. Still another problem is that control animals were not sacrificed at the same times as exposure groups, i.e., at 60, 90, and 120 days. Thus, age-related effects, unintentional cross-contamination with other toxic agents, or other laboratory error cannot be excluded. Because of these concerns, and principally because the doses must be considered unspecified, the study is not included in Table 65.4.

65.4.3 COW

A 5-month ingestion experiment in yearling Holstein cows was performed by McConnell *et al.* (1980). The data are useful for discriminating the effects of PCP from those of its technical-grade contaminants. Three heifers per group were given a diet containing one of the following four mixtures of AG and TG

PCP: 100% AG, 90% AG/10% TG, 65% AG/35% TG, and 100% TG. A control group of three heifers received an untreated diet. The dose in all treatment groups was originally set at 20 mg/kg-day but after 42 days was reduced to 15 mg/kg-day because of concerns about decreased body-weight gain compared to the controls. The overall time-weighted average dose was 16.3 mg/kg-day in all treatment groups. The distribution of chlorinated nonphenolic contaminants in the TG-PCP was similar to that in the TGC-PCP used in the NTP mouse study (Table 65.5). The purity of the AG-PCP was 99%.

Statistically significant decreases in serum thyroxine (29–40%) and serum triiodothyronine (35–44%) occurred in all four PCP-treatment groups. These changes echo those seen by van Raaij *et al.* (1991b) and Jekat *et al.* (1994) in rats exposed to PCP acutely and subchronically, respectively (see Section 65.7.1).

The proliferative response of peripheral blood lymphocytes (PBLs) to *in vitro* stimulation by T-cell mitogens was increased with increasing percentage TG-PCP and exposure duration. By contrast, in PBLs from cows treated with 100% AG-PCP there was a nonsignificant decrease in the proliferative response. This result is consistent with the report by Kerkvliet *et al.* (1982a) that *in vivo* T-cell activation in mice is unaffected by treatment with analytical-grade PCP. Dose-dependent, statistically significant perturbations in serum immunoglobulins were observed in the TG-PCP groups. In the 100% AG-PCP group the changes in immunoglobulin levels were in the same direction as in the TG-PCP groups, but smaller and not statistically significant.

In all treatment groups there was a marked, highly significant depression of thymus weight, both absolute and relative to body weight. Macroscopic changes were observed in the spleens of some cows in the 35% and 100% TG-PCP groups; microscopic examination revealed hyper- or hypoplastic foci in these animals.

Relative liver weights were significantly elevated in all treatment groups, but absolute liver weights were significantly increased only in TG-PCP groups. Increased serum γ-glutamyl transpeptidase was seen only in the TG-PCP groups. This is indicative of cholestasis, a condition generally associated with lesions of the liver or bile secretory system; histopathologic examination revealed damage to the liver, bile duct, and gall bladder in animals receiving 100% TG-PCP. Although increased amounts of smooth endoplasmic reticulum were found in the 100% AG-PCP group, no other microscopic signs of liver toxicity occurred in these animals. In the absence of other signs of toxicity, an increase in SER might reflect an adaptive response to the xenobiotic load.

65.5 CARCINOGENICITY AND CHRONIC TOXICITY

Two rodent bioassays conducted by the NTP provide the most useful information on the carcinogenicity of PCP in these species. The NTP rat bioassay tested analytical-grade (99% pure) PCP, whereas the NTP mouse bioassay tested technical-grade and partially purified PCP formulations. Given the fact that several of the impurities are known or suspected carcinogens, the absence of interstudy consistency in the materials tested makes it difficult to compare the underlying carcinogenicity of PCP in mice and rats. Tables 65.6 (mice) and 65.7 (rats) give the incidence rates of exposure-related neoplastic and non-neoplastic lesions observed in these two studies.

Table 65.6
Summary of the Carcinogenicity and Chronic Toxicity of PCP Formulations Tested in Dietary Exposure Studies in Mice[a]

B6C3F$_1$ Mice (NTP, 1989; McConnell *et al.*, 1991)	Males		Females	
	TGC	EC-7	TGC	EC-7
Doses in feed	0, 100, 200 ppm (0, 18, 35 mg/kg-day)	0, 100, 200, 600 ppm (0, 18, 37, 118 mg/kg-day)	0, 100, 200 ppm (0, 17, 35 mg/kg-day)	0, 100, 200, 600 ppm (0, 17, 34, 114 mg/kg-day)
Nonneoplastic lesions				
Adrenal gland medulla:				
Hyperplasia	3%, **22%**, **22%**	3%, **40%**, **27%**, 2%	0%, 8%, 4%	6%, 2%, 11%, **35%**
Neoplastic lesions				
Adrenal gland medulla:				
Benign pheochromocytoma	0%, **22%**, **51%**	3%, 8%, **44%**, **90%**	0%, 4%, 2%	0%, 2%, 4%, **78%**
Liver:				
Adenoma	16%, **43%**, **69%**	14%, 27%, **35%**, **65%**	9%, 16%, 16%	3%, 6%, 12%, **63%**
Carcinoma	6%, 21%, **25%**	3%, 15%, 15%, **18%**	0%, 2%, 2%	0%, 2%, 0%, 4%
Adenoma or Carcinoma	22%, **55%**, **77%**	17%, **40%**, **44%**, **69%**	9%, 18%, 18%	3%, 8%, 12%, **65%**
Liver or spleen:				
Hemangiosarcoma	0%, 4%, 2%	0%, 8%, 4%, 6%	0%, 6%, **12%**	0%, 2%, 6%, **16%**

[a]Incidence rates in **bold** were significantly elevated ($p < 0.05$) relative to the control group. *Abbreviation*: TGC, technical-grade composite.

Table 65.7
Summary of the Carcinogenicity and Chronic Toxicity of 99% Pure PCP in Dietary Exposure Studies in Rats[a]

F344/N Rats (NTP, 1999; Chhabra *et al.*, 1999)	Males		Females	
	2-Year Exposure	1-Year On/1-Year Off Stop-Exposure	2-Year Exposure	1-Year On/1-Year Off Stop-Exposure
Doses in feed	0, 200, 400, 600 ppm (0, 10, 20, 30 mg/kg-day)	1000 ppm (60 mg/kg-day)	0, 100, 200 ppm (0, 17, 35 mg/kg-day)	0, 100, 200, 600 ppm (0, 17, 34, 114 mg/kg-day)
Nonneoplastic lesions	No exposure-related increase at any site	Increased hepatocyte centrilobular hypertrophy and cytoplasmic vacuolization at 7-month sacrifice but not at terminal sacrifice	No exposure-related increase at any site	Increased hepatocyte centrilobular hypertrophy at 7-month sacrifice but not at terminal sacrifice
Neoplastic lesions				
Malignant mesothelioma	2%, 0%, 4%, 0%	**18%**	0%, 0%, 0%	0%, 0%, 0%, 0%
Nasal squamous cell carcinoma	2%, 6%, 2%, 0%	10%	0%, 0%, 0%	0%, 0%, 0%, 0%

[a]Incidence rates in **bold** were significantly elevated ($p < 0.05$) relative to the control group.

65.5.1 TWO-YEAR EXPOSURE IN MICE

The NTP conducted a 2-year feed study of PCP in B6C3F₁ mice (McConnell *et al.*, 1991; NTP, 1989). The technical-grade composite (TGC) and partially purified (EC-7) PCP formulations tested are described in Section 65.4.1. Fifty animals per sex per group received TGC-PCP at 100 or 200 ppm diet (18 or 35 mg/kg-day) or EC-7 at 100, 200, or 600 ppm diet (18, 36, or 116 mg/kg-day). Separate control groups for the two formulations each consisted of 35 animals of each sex.

65.5.1.1 Neoplastic Lesions of the Liver

In male mice, both EC-7 and TGC-PCP produced dose-related increases in benign and malignant liver tumors (hepatocellular adenoma and carcinoma). There was a significantly ($p < 0.05$) elevated incidence of adenoma in males exposed to TGC-PCP at either dose or to EC-7 at 200 ppm or higher, while a significantly elevated incidence of carcinoma occurred in males treated with 200 ppm TGC-PCP or 600 ppm EC-7. In female mice, a significant elevation of adenoma occurred only in the 600 ppm EC-7 group.

65.5.1.2 Non-neoplastic Lesions of the Liver

A large proportion of male and female mice treated with either EC-7 or TGC-PCP developed dose-related, non-neoplastic liver and bile-duct lesions (including cytomegaly, multifocal proliferation of hematopoietic cells, diffuse chronic inflammation, and acute diffuse necrosis). In low-dose TGC-PCP males and females the incidence rates for acute diffuse necrosis were 87% and 90%, respectively, while in low-dose EC-7 males and females the incidence rates were 98% and 42%, respectively.

65.5.1.3 Neoplastic Lesions of the Adrenal Medulla

In male mice, TGC-PCP and EC-7 produced similar, dose-related increases in benign pheochromocytoma, with significant elevation in animals receiving 100 ppm TGC-PCP or 200 ppm EC-7. In female mice, significant elevation of pheochromocytoma occurred only in the 600 ppm EC-7 group.

65.5.1.4 Non-neoplastic Lesions of the Adrenal Medulla

In male mice, statistically significant increases in hyperplasia of the adrenal medulla were produced at both doses of TGC-PCP and at the two lower doses (but not the high dose) of EC-7. Incidence rates were 0%, 40%, 27%, and 2% in the 0, 100, 200, and 600 ppm EC-7 groups, respectively. The U-shaped dose–response observed in EC-7 males reflects the existence of a morphologic continuum leading to benign pheochromocytoma, which increased sharply between 200 and 600 ppm in parallel with the decline in hyperplasia. In female mice, hyperplasia of the adrenal medulla was significantly elevated only in the group receiving 600 ppm EC-7.

65.5.1.5 Neoplastic Lesions of the Vascular System

The incidence of a malignant tumor of the blood vessels (hemangiosarcoma) was significantly elevated in female mice treated with 200 ppm TGC-PCP or 600 ppm EC-7. The investigators indicated that these tumors occurred mostly in the spleen while a few were found in the liver.

65.5.1.6 Non-neoplastic Lesions of the Vascular System

Diffuse hematopoietic cell proliferation in the red pulp of the spleen (extramedullary hematopoiesis) was increased in male and female mice at both doses of TGC-PCP. Incidence rates in the control, 100 ppm, and 200 ppm groups were 17%, 65%, and 39% in males and 6%, 31%, and 23% in females, respectively. The U-shaped dose–response observed in both males and females may be partially explained by the existence of a morphologic continuum leading to splenic hemangiosarcoma, but there were too few males with this tumor at the 200 ppm dose (6%) to account for the magnitude of the downturn.

With respect to the argument that the liver toxicity attributable to pCDD or pCDF contaminants was responsible for the observed hepatocarcinogenicity, the investigators noted that while non-neoplastic lesions of identical morphology and approximately equal severity occurred in females treated with EC-7 at 200 and 600 ppm, liver neoplasms were significantly elevated only in the 600 ppm group. The investigators performed separate analyses for benign adenoma, malignant carcinoma, and the presence of adenoma *or* carcinoma. It is the combined adenoma/carcinoma category which provides the strongest statistical association with PCP exposure. The use of such a category is not unusual and rests upon histologic evidence that hepatocellular adenoma and carcinoma are part of a physiological continuum (Bannasch *et al.*, 1986). It is noteworthy that the incidence of adenoma/carcinoma in males on the 200 ppm EC-7 regime (44%) was lower than the rate in males receiving TGC-PCP at 200 ppm (77%). Similarly, the incidence rates for hemangiosarcoma in females in the 100 and 200 ppm EC-7 dose groups were lower (2% and 6%) than in females given TGC-PCP at the same levels (6% and 12%). If PCP alone were responsible for the neoplastic response in liver and blood vessels, one expects that the incidence rates at a given dose level of TGC-PCP and EC-7 would have been roughly the same because both formulations contain approximately 90% PCP. The fact that TGC-PCP was more potent suggests that the contaminants in TGC-PCP acted as co-carcinogens.

Concerning the argument (noted above) that the liver tumorigenicity of the PCP formulations may have been secondary to toxicity, the Environmental Health Committee of U.S. EPA's Science Advisory Board was asked to examine the results of the study and consider this question, among other issues. The Committee recommended that "the observed dose-dependent increase in the incidence of hepatocellular carcinomas and adenomas be considered a valid indicator" of the carcinogenic potential of PCP. The Committee also pointed out that the mouse strain tested in the study, B6C3F$_1$, is extremely sensitive to hepatocarcinogenesis and therefore recommended that exposure-related liver tumors be considered less relevant to human risk than the production of hemangiosarcomas (U.S. EPA SAB, 1991).

The incidence rates for benign pheochromocytoma in male mice were approximately the same in the 200 ppm TGC-PCP and EC-7 groups (51% and 44%, respectively), while the rate in the 100 ppm TGC-PCP group was notably higher than in the 100 ppm EC-7 group (22% vs. 8%). These results suggest that the technical-grade impurities were key to the response at the 100 ppm dose but less important at the 200 ppm dose, when PCP played a partial role in the formation of pheochromocy-

tomas. In female mice, the only elevated pheochromocytoma incidence occurred in groups treated with 600 ppm EC-7 (78%), with a sharp increase over rates in the 100 and 200 ppm groups (4% in both). This was similar to the dose–response relationship observed for hepatocellular adenoma/carcinoma in the female EC-7 groups.

The NTP concluded that there was *clear evidence of carcinogenic activity* in male B6C3F$_1$ mice exposed to TGC-PCP or EC-7, *clear evidence of carcinogenic activity* in female B6C3F$_1$ mice exposed to EC-7, and *some evidence of carcinogenic activity* in female B6C3F$_1$ mice exposed to TGC-PCP (NTP, 1989).

65.5.2 INITIATION/PROMOTION IN MICE

Umemura *et al.* (1999) conducted an initiation/promotion study of 99% pure PCP in male B6C3F$_1$ mice to investigate the mechanism by which PCP produces liver cancer. In the portion of the study devoted to evaluating the ability of PCP to act as a promoter, groups of 20 mice received PCP at 0, 300, or 600 ppm diet for 25 weeks following preinitiation with diethylnitrosamine (DEN). The incidence of animals bearing liver adenoma or carcinoma was significantly elevated in both the 300 ppm (10/15, $p < 0.05$) and 600 ppm (13/18, $p < 0.01$) PCP groups relative to DEN treatment alone (4/15). The liver tumor incidence was 0/19 in mice receiving PCP for 25 weeks without prior DEN treatment. In the portion of the study devoted to evaluating the ability of PCP to act as an initiator, groups of 20 mice were given PCP at 600 or 1200 ppm diet for 13 weeks followed by phenobarbital in drinking water at 500 ppm for 29 weeks. No liver tumors were observed.

The study by Umemura *et al.* (1999) demonstrated that 99% pure PCP at 300 ppm diet has the ability to promote liver carcinogenesis in preinitiated male B6C3F$_1$ mice. The study also revealed that purified PCP at 1200 ppm diet for 13 weeks does not appear to initiate liver tumors.

65.5.3 TWO-YEAR EXPOSURE AND STOP-EXPOSURE IN RATS

The NTP conducted a 2-year, dietary-exposure study of 99% pure PCP in F344/N rats (Chhabra *et al.*, 1999; NTP, 1999). Rats on the standard regime were given PCP at 200, 400, or 600 ppm diet (10, 20, or 30 mg/kg-day) for two years, while rats on the stop-exposure regime were given a diet containing PCP at 1000 ppm the first year and no PCP the second year (time-averaged dose = 60 mg/kg-day). A total of 50 rats per sex per dose were on the standard regime while 60 rats per sex were on the stop-exposure regime. Ten rats of each sex in the stop-exposure group were necropsied after 7 months of exposure.

65.5.3.1 Neoplastic Lesions

There was no evidence of exposure-related neoplasia in male or female rats at any dose on the standard regime or in stop-exposure female rats. By the end of the two-year study, stop-exposure male rats had an increased incidence of malignant mesothelioma relative to the controls (18% vs. 2%). The incidence of nasal squamous cell carcinoma was likewise elevated relative to the controls in stop-exposure male rats (10% vs. 2%), but this difference was not statistically significant ($p > 0.05$). However, the incidence of nasal cell carcinoma in this group was significantly elevated relative to that in NTP historical controls (0.4% ± 1.0%).

65.5.3.2 Non-neoplastic Lesions

At the 7-month interim evaluation of the stop-exposure groups, an increased incidence of centrilobular hepatocyte hypertrophy was observed in both males and females, while hepatocyte cytoplasmic vacuolization was elevated in males only. At the 2-year sacrifice there was no hepatocyte hypertrophy and no elevation of hepatocyte cytoplasmic vacuolization, nor was there any exposure-related increase in non-neoplastic lesions at any site.

The NTP concluded that there was *no evidence of carcinogenic activity* in male or female F344/N rats fed diets containing 99% pure PCP at 200, 400, or 600 ppm for 2 years, *some evidence of carcinogenicity* in male F344/N rats fed a diet containing 99% pure PCP at 1000 ppm for 1 year followed by a control diet for 1 year, and *no evidence of carcinogenic activity* in female F344/N rats fed a diet containing 99% pure PCP at 1000 ppm for 1 year followed by a control diet for 1 year (NTP, 1999).

65.6 GENOTOXICITY OF PCP AND TCHQ

PCP is almost a textbook example of a nonmutagenic, non-DNA-reactive compound. Because PCP has been tested numerous times for genotoxicity, it is expected that false positives will have occurred at a rate consistent with the overall false-positive rate of the tests applied. All positive genotoxicity tests performed in the presence of microsomal extracts are likely to reflect the genotoxicity of TCHQ or other DNA-reactive metabolites rather than the parent compound. Van Ommen *et al.* (1986) demonstrated that the rate of PCP binding to calf thymus DNA in the presence of rat liver microsomes is correlated with the formation of TCHQ and the 1,2-isomer of TCHQ. Keeping in mind that yeast are rich in cytochrome P450, it is reasonable to wonder whether observations that PCP is mutagenic or recombinogenic in these lower eukaryotes might be explained by conversion to TCHQ or other metabolites. It would clarify matters if metabolite concentrations were routinely measured whenever genotoxicity testing of PCP is performed.

65.6.1 SHORT-TERM TESTS OF PCP

65.6.1.1 Isolated DNA

PCP at concentrations up to 100 mM (27 mg/ml) did not bind covalently to calf-thymus DNA and produced no single-strand DNA breaks in bacteriophage DNA (Witte *et al.*, 1985).

65.6.1.2 Bacteria

A comprehensive review of the literature by Seiler (1991) and a more concise review by an anonymous author (NTP, 1989) both indicated that PCP was almost uniformly negative for induction of gene mutation in bacteria. The one exception was a study by Nishimura *et al.* (1982), performed in the presence of activated rat liver microsomes (S9). More recently, Gopalaswamy and Nair (1992) reported that PCP was mutagenic in *Salmonella typhimurium* in the presence of activated S9. Note, however, that Haworth *et al.* (1983) found that technical-grade PCP was negative for mutagenicity in four *S. typhimurium* strains in both the presence and absence of activated S9.

65.6.1.3 Lower Eukaryotes

PCP generally has been found to be positive for genotoxicity in yeast and mold, although most studies were inadequate or inadequately reported (reviewed by Seiler, 1991). Fahrig *et al.* (1978) found evidence for mutation and intragenic (but not intergenic) recombination in yeast incubated with PCP at 400 µg/ml. A separate group of investigators reported both positive (Simmon *et al.*, 1979) and negative (Simmon and Kauhanen, 1978) results for mitotic recombination in yeast.

65.6.1.4 Mammalian Cells *In Vitro*

Ehrlich (1990) found no evidence of DNA single-strand breaks or alkali-labile sites in Chinese hamster ovary (CHO) cells cultured in the presence of PCP at concentrations up to 10 µg/ml. Wang and Lin (1995) found no evidence of increased DNA breakage in mouse embryonic fibroblasts cultured with PCP at concentrations up to 240 µM (64 µg/ml). Jansson and Jansson (1986) found no induction of point mutations in Chinese hamster lung fibroblasts (V79 cells) with PCP concentrations in the range 6–50 µg/ml. Galloway *et al.* (1987) looked for cytogenetic changes in CHO cells treated with the same technical-grade PCP formulation used in the NTP mouse chronic carcinogenicity study (NTP, 1989). In the absence of S9 the assay was clearly negative for chromosomal aberrations (CAbs); in the presence of S9 the results were positive in one trial and equivocal in another. In the presence of S9 the sister chromatid exchange (SCE) response was clearly negative. The SCE response was said to be "weakly positive" in the absence of S9, but this conclusion does not appear to be supported by the data. In the absence of exogenous metabolic activation, Ishidate (1988) found no induction of CAbs in cultured Chinese hamster lung fibroblasts at PCP concentrations up to 60 µg/ml; when the toxic threshold was raised by changing to an intermittent treatment regimen, CAbs were induced at a PCP concentration of 300 µg/ml. Ziemsen *et al.* (1987) found no elevation of SCEs or CAbs in lymphocytes from healthy donors following incubation with technical-grade NaPCP at concentrations up to 90 µg/ml. It should be noted that the *in vitro* SCE assay appears to be of little value to cancer risk assessment owing to its low specificity (Ashby, 1993; Tennant *et al.*, 1987).

65.6.1.5 Mice Exposed *In Vivo*

A mammalian spot test (designed to reveal mutation, deletion, and recombination events) of purified PCP in hybrid mice yielded equivocal results. Single transplacental injection of 152, 86, or 40 females, respectively, with maternal PCP doses of 0, 50, or 100 mg/kg produced color spots said to be of "definite" genetic relevance in 1/967 (0.10%), 2/316 (0.63%), and 2/157 (1.3%) offspring (Fahrig *et al.*, 1978). The response was dose-related, but the small numbers easily could have arisen by chance. A negative interpretation is supported by the finding, in the same test system, that treatment with purified PCP at 50 mg/kg had no effect on the incidence of genetically relevant color spots produced by ethylnitrosourea (Fahrig and Steinkamp-Zucht, 1996). Male mice injected i.p. with technical- or reagent-grade PCP at doses up to 50 mg/kg-day for 5 days did not exhibit dose-related increases in the frequency of abnormal sperm morphology 35 days after the initial injection (Osterloh *et al.*, 1983).

65.6.2 OCCUPATIONAL EXPOSURE TO PCP

An investigation of CAbs and SCEs was performed on the peripheral blood lymphocytes of 22 male workers engaged in the production of PCP or NaPCP (Bauchinger *et al.*, 1982). At the time of the measurements the mean length of employment was 11.4 years. All 22 of the PCP/NaPCP-exposed men were smokers while the sex- and age-matched control group included 9 smokers and 13 nonsmokers. The percentage of cells containing CAbs was significantly elevated in the exposed workers vs. the controls ($p < 0.004$), primarily due to elevation of dicentrics ($p = 0.020$) and acentrics ($p = 0.037$). Comparison of the exposed workers to the smoking controls also revealed elevation of dicentrics ($p = 0.021$) and acentrics ($p = 0.043$). A slight elevation of SCEs in the exposed workers vs. the controls was no longer significant when the comparison was limited to smoking controls.

Several factors complicate interpretation of the results of Bauchinger *et al.* (1982). For one, the investigators did not indicate whether chromosome analyses were conducted in a blind fashion with respect to exposure status. In addition, the degree to which smoking may have confounded the CAb results is not clear because the authors did not report individual CAb data or summary statistics for the 9 controls who smoked. Without such data it is not possible to compare the exposed workers and smoking controls with respect to the percentage of cells containing CAbs or to discern the influence of individual controls on the overall comparison. It is also worrisome that there was no mention of a relationship between exposure level and CAb incidence even though the workers were divided into low- and high-exposure groups. The failure to note the existence of such a relationship can only be interpreted as signifying that no dose dependence was found. Given the apparent absence of a dose-response and the relatively low CAb frequency in the exposed workers (i.e., within the range considered normal), the overall response must be considered equivocal.

Ziemsen *et al.* (1987) examined CAb and SCE frequencies in the lymphocytes of 20 workers occupationally exposed to PCP. Mean blood PCP levels in the low- and high-exposure groups were 58 and 330 μg/ml, respectively. There was no control group. The average number of CAbs per cell was slightly greater in the high-exposure group (0.040 vs. 0.026), but the difference was not statistically significant. The frequency of SCEs was similar in the two groups. Consideration of the smokers separately yielded negative results as well.

65.6.3 GENOTOXICITY OF TCHQ

Unlike PCP, TCHQ binds isolated DNA covalently and produces single-strand breaks (Witte *et al.*, 1985). TCHQ is clearly mutagenic and damaging to DNA in cultured mammalian cells in the absence of metabolic activation. TCHQ at concentrations as low as 20–25 μM (5–6 μg/ml) produced single-strand breaks and formed DNA adducts in CHO and V79 cells (Dahlhaus *et al.*, 1995, 1996; Ehrlich, 1990) and increased the frequency of mutations at a distinct genetic locus in V79 cells (Jansson and Jansson, 1991). TCHQ concentrations as low as 10 μM (2.5 μg/ml) induced micronuclei in V79 cells (Jansson and Jansson, 1992). One or more reactive oxygen species (including hydrogen peroxide) produced through reaction of an autooxidation product, the semiquinone radical, are implicated in the DNA-damaging actions of TCHQ (Carstens *et al.*, 1990; Naito *et al.*, 1994).

65.7 REPRODUCTIVE AND ENDOCRINE TOXICITY

Several acute, subchronic, and reproductive studies in rats, mink, and sheep have examined the effects of PCP on reproductive and endocrine function. The results of these studies are summarized in Table 65.8. The most consistent outcome was a decrease in serum thyroxine (T_4), a potentially adverse effect. A LOEL between 0.6 and 1 mg/kg-day for the effect of PCP on serum T_4 has been observed in rats, mink, and sheep. No NOEL for this endpoint has been identified.

The effects of PCP on serum T_4 are similar to those produced by much lower concentrations of TCDD. Sewall *et al.* (1995) found that serum total thyroxine (TT_4) levels were significantly depressed following 30-week administration of TCDD to rats at doses as low as 11 ng/kg-day, while a TCDD dose of 125 ng/kg-day produced a degree of depression comparable to that observed at a PCP dose of 3 mg/kg-day. TCDD at 125 ng/kg-day also produced a 2.5-fold increase in serum thyrotropin (TSH). By contrast, PCP-induced depression of T_4 has been found to be associated with *decreased* serum TSH and thyroid mass. The latter relationship between T_4 and TSH is found in a limited set of physiological conditions, including caloric restriction (Scanlon and Toft, 1996). The disparity in the direction of the TSH change produced by TCDD and PCP suggests that these substances act via dissimilar mechanisms to depress T_4 levels.

Table 65.8
Summary of the Reproductive and Endocrine Toxicity of PCP[a]

Study	Route	PCP/NaPCP grade	Doses	Effects at the LOEL	LOEL	NOEL
Thyroid-hormone related effects in rats						
van Raaij *et al.*, 1991b, 1993 (acute exposure study in males)	i.p.	AG-PCP	0, 0.6, 1.1, 1.8, 28 mg/kg	↓ serum TT_4 and FT_4	1.8 mg/kg	1.1 mg/kg
van Raaij *et al.*, 1994 (acute exposure study in males)	i.p.	AG-PCP	0, 7, 14, 28 mg/kg	↓ uptake of T_4 into cerebrospinal fluid and brain	7 mg/kg	n.d.
Jekat *et al.*, 1994 (28-day exposure study in females)	gav.	TG-NaPCP; AG-PCP	vehicle, 3 mg/kg-day TG-PCP, 3 and 30 mg/kg-day AG-PCP	TG-NaPCP: ↓ serum TT_4, TT_3, TT_4:TT_3, and TSH AG-PCP: ↓ serum TT_4 and TSH	TG-NaPCP, AG-PCP: 3 mg/kg-day	TG-NaPCP, AG-PCP: n.d.
Reproductive effects in rats						
Schwetz *et al.*, 1978 (one-generation study)	diet	TG-PCP	0, 3, 30 mg/kg-day	↓ maternal and neonatal body weight; ↓ pup survival	30 mg/kg-day	3 mg/kg-day
Reproductive effects in mink						
Beard *et al.*, 1997 (one-generation study; maternal exposure only)	diet	AG-PCP	0, 1 mg/kg-day (target)	↓ whelping rate; ↑ severity of maternal uterine cysts	1 mg/kg-day	n.d.
Beard and Rawlings, 1998 (three-generation study: in F_1, maternal exposure only)	diet	AG-PCP	1 mg/kg-day (target)	↓ serum T_4 in F_2 and F_3 males and F_3 females; ↓ thyroid mass in F_3 females; ↑ severity of testicular hyperplasia in F_3 males; ↑ incidence of mild, multifocal, cystic hyperplasia of the prostate in F_2 and F_3	1 mg/kg-day	n.d.
Endocrine-related effects in ewes						
Rawlings *et al.*, 1998 (43-day study, twice weekly dosing)	i.g.	AG-PCP	vehicle, 2 mg/kg (time-averaged: 0.6 mg/kg-day)	↓ serum T_4; ↑ serum insulin; ↑ severity of oviductal intraepithelial cysts	0.6 mg/kg-day	n.d.
Reproductive effects in sheep						
Beard *et al.*, 1999a (one-generation study: maternal exposure only)	diet	AG-PCP	0, 1 mg/kg-day (target)	↓ maternal serum TT_4; ↑ maternal thyroid follicle size and lymphocytic infiltration into the uterine endometrium; ↓ weaning weight of female lambs	1 mg/kg-day	n.d.
Beard *et al.*, 1999b (two-generation study: in F_1, maternal exposure only; in F_2, exposure of rams only)	diet	AG-PCP	0, 1 mg/kg-day (target)	In F_2: ↓ serum TT_4; ↑ scrotal size; ↑ severity of semiferous tubule atrophy; ↓ sperm density	1 mg/kg-day	n.d.

[a]*Abbreviations*: AG, analytical or purified grade; FT_3, free triiodothyronine; FT_4, free thyroxine; gav., gavage; i.g., intragastric; i.p., intraperitoneal; n.d., none determined; TG, technical grade; TSH, thyrotropin; TT_4, total thyroxine.

The effect of PCP on T_4 levels suggests a role for this molecule, the principal metabolite of hexachlorobenzene (HCB), in the altered thyroid function accompanying HCB-induced porphyria (Kleiman de Pisarev *et al.*, 1990; Rozman *et al.*, 1986). In *ex vivo* experiments, PCP, but not TCHQ, was a competitive inhibitor of T_4 binding to rat sera, indicating that PCP depression of T_4 levels does not involve metabolism to TCHQ (van Raaij *et al.*, 1991a).

65.7.1 THYROID HORMONE EFFECTS IN RATS

Two studies in male, 12-week-old Wistar rats examined the effects of a single i.p. dose of purified PCP on serum levels of thyroid hormones. Maximum depression of TT_4 was observed at 4–6 hr postexposure with recovery within 48 hr. Serum TT_4 was depressed at a dose of 1.8 mg/kg ($p < 0.001$) but not at 0.6 mg/kg (van Raaij *et al.*, 1991b) or 1.1 mg/kg (van Raaij *et al.*, 1993). Depression of serum free thyroxine (FT_4) demonstrated a similar dose–response (van Raaij *et al.*, 1993). The results of these studies indicate an acute, i.p. NOEL in rats of 1.1 mg/kg for decreased serum TT_4 and FT_4.

The same group of investigators found that single i.p. doses of purified PCP at 7, 14, or 28 mg/kg decreased the uptake of T_4 into the cerebrospinal fluid of male Wistar rats by 34, 60, or 75%, respectively, while uptake of T_4 into total brain tissue and specific brain structures was also decreased (van Raaij *et al.*, 1994).

Jekat *et al.* (1994) studied the effects of subchronic exposure to PCP on serum TSH, TT_4, and total triiodothyronine (TT_3) in female Wistar rats. Eight animals per group were treated twice daily by gavage for 28 days with purified PCP at 3 or 30 mg/kg-day or with technical-grade NaPCP (TG-NaPCP) at 3 mg PCP/kg-day. The control group received the gavage vehicle. Mean serum TT_4 was approximately 50% of the control value in both the TG-NaPCP and low-dose PCP groups and approximately 30% of the control value in the high-dose PCP group ($p < 0.0025$). Lesser reductions were seen for serum TT_3 with TG-NaPCP ($p < 0.05$) and with the high dose of purified PCP ($p < 0.01$). The serum $TT_4 : TT_3$ ratio was substantially reduced in all treatment groups ($p < 0.0025$). Serum TSH was approximately 70% of the control level in all treatment groups ($p < 0.05$).

65.7.2 REPRODUCTIVE EFFECTS IN RATS

In a single-generation, dietary exposure study of reproductive toxicity, technical-grade PCP at 0, 3, or 30 mg/kg-day was fed to groups of 10 male and 20 female SD rats for 62 days before mating, throughout gestation, and for 21 days postpartum (Schwetz *et al.*, 1978). The maternal NOEL was 3 mg/kg-day based on reduced body weight at 30 mg/kg-day. The NOEL for the offspring was 3 mg/kg-day based on reproductive effects at 30 mg/kg-day (reduced pup survival across litters and reduced neonatal body weight). The study design was limited: only one generation, only two treatment groups, and too few males under test. The reproductive effects observed were likely to have been secondary to maternal toxicity.

65.7.3 REPRODUCTIVE AND ENDOCRINE EFFECTS IN MINK

The effects of analytical-grade PCP on fertility, hormone levels, and histopathology were examined in a single-generation study in mink (Beard *et al.*, 1997). PCP at a target dose of 1 mg/kg-day was fed to 10 female mink; a control group of 10 females received no treatment. PCP was "sprayed evenly onto a weekly supply of the pelleted ration" which was mixed with other dietary components before feeding. The investigators apparently did not verify the PCP content of the feed or the uniformity of distribution. The PCP-containing diet was fed to adult females for 3 weeks before mating, throughout gestation, and until 8 weeks postpartum, when weaning occurred and the maternal mink were sacrificed.

Where treatment-related effects on fertility were noted the absolute differences were small; the low number of animals tested rendered the results ambiguous. The fraction of mated females that subsequently accepted the second mating was significantly decreased in the PCP group (5/9 vs. 7/8, $p < 0.01$). The toxicological relevance of such a measure is obscure. A better measure of fertility, the fraction of mated females that subsequently whelped (whelping rate), was also significantly reduced in PCP-treated animals (5/9 vs. 7/8, $p < 0.01$). Nonsignificant reductions were observed in the proportion of mated females with implantation sites visible at necropsy (7/9 vs. 8/8), the mean number of implantation sites per animal (4.6 vs. 6.8), and the mean litter size of mink that whelped (3.4 vs. 4.5). PCP exposure had no effect on maternal serum levels of the measured hormones (progesterone, estradiol, cortisol, and T_4). The maternal tissues subject to histopathologic examination were not specified. The only treatment-related histologic change reported was an increased severity score for uterine cysts ($p < 0.05$).

The same laboratory conducted a three-generation reproductive toxicity study of analytical-grade PCP in mink, continuing to apply their method of spraying PCP onto a weekly supply of pelleted ration to deliver a target dose of 1 mg/kg-day (Beard and Rawlings, 1998). The F_2 mink in this study were the offspring from the one-generation study discussed above. Thus, the F_2 mink (8 males, 8 females) were born to mothers exposed from 3 weeks prior to mating, while the F_3 mink (8 males, 10 females) were born to mothers exposed from the point of conception.

Implantation sites were not counted, but otherwise the tests of fertility was the same as those applied in the one-generation study. No evidence of treatment-related effects on fertility was observed. Measurement of serum progesterone, estradiol, cortisol, T_4, and testosterone at sacrifice revealed depression of T_4 in all treatment groups, achieving statistical significance in F_2 males, F_3 males, and F_3 females ($p < 0.05$).

The animals were necropsied and all major organs subjected to histopathologic examination. Mass or size changes in the thyroid gland, adrenal glands, and testis were reported; only the effect on the thyroid appears to have been of potential toxicological relevance. Thyroid mass was lower in all PCP treatment groups, achieving statistical significance only in F_3 females ($p < 0.05$). Adrenal mass was higher in F_2 females, but this difference probably reflected unusually low values in the control group. Mean adrenal mass values in F_2 and F_3 control females were 0.105 and 0.150 mg/kg, while mean values in F_2

and F_3 treated females were 0.149 and 0.146 mg/kg. During development, testis length in the F_2 was smaller ($p < 0.05$), but body-weight adjusted testis length was not. Testis mass and length at autopsy were unaltered by treatment in either the F_2 or F_3. Testicular hyperplasia was more severe in PCP-treated than untreated F_2 males ($p < 0.05$). Fifty percent of PCP-treated males had mild, multifocal, cystic hyperplasia of the prostate; the control incidence was not given. Treated males displaying multifocal cystic hyperplasia had twofold higher mean serum testosterone levels than treated males without the lesion. In treated F_2 females and F_3 males, the severity of adrenal cortex vacuolization was *less severe* than in their respective control groups.

65.7.4 REPRODUCTIVE, ENDOCRINE, AND HISTOLOGIC EFFECTS IN SHEEP

Rawlings *et al.* (1998) conducted a study of the effects of analytical-grade PCP on hormone levels and histopathology in adult ewes. Six ewes were given PCP intragastrically (i.g.) in gelatin capsules twice weekly for 43 days at a dose of 2 mg/kg. A designated control group of six age- and weight-matched ewes received empty capsules. Two other control groups for experiments not entailing PCP were started 22 and 11 days earlier. Ewes were estrus-synchronized during treatment. On treatment day 36, ewes were bled at regular intervals to detect any changes in the pulsatile patterns of luteinizing hormone (LH) and follicle-stimulating hormone (FSH) secretion. In addition, serum levels of progesterone, estradiol, cortisol, T_4 (presumably TT_4), insulin, LH, and FSH were measured in blood pooled over each hour of collection. At the end of the treatment period, animals were necropsied and histopathologic examination performed on all major tissues.

The only treatment-related effects on hormones were significant T_4 depression ($p < 0.05$) and insulin elevation ($p < 0.05$) on the day of the intensive bleed. The only treatment-related histopathologic change noted was increased severity of oviductal intraepithelial cysts; data supporting this observation were not provided. It was generally not clear whether a given analysis reflected comparison to the designated or combined controls.

The same laboratory conducted a single-generation study of the effects of PCP on reproductive and general endocrine function in ewes (Beard *et al.*, 1999a). Two groups of 13 ewes were given a control diet or feed treated with PCP to deliver a target dose of 1 mg/kg-day. Treated feed, prepared weekly, consisted of alfalfa pellets sprayed with PCP. The PCP-containing diet was fed to adult females for 5 weeks before mating, throughout gestation, and until 2 weeks after weaning, when the ewes were sacrificed. The investigators argued that it was not necessary to adjust the dose based on feed intake because each ewe consumed all alfalfa pellets offered. Ewes were estrus-synchronized prior to mating. Blood samples were taken frequently from the ewes during pregnancy and lactation. On postweaning day 5, six ewes per group were bled at regular intervals during the day and night for determination of pulsatile

LH and FSH secretion. Two days later the same ewes were bled at regular intervals for 1 hr before and 5 hr after injection of a mixture of gonadotropin-releasing hormone (GnRH), bovine TSH, and adrenocorticotropin (ACTH). The same serum hormones measured by Rawlings *et al.* (1998) were obtained in hourly pooled blood drawn during the periods of intensive bleeding. Fertility parameters (size and number of ovarian follicles and corpora lutea) and fetal growth rate (head diameter) were obtained *in vivo* using ultrasonography. At the end of the treatment period, ewes were necropsied and histopathologic examination performed on all major tissues.

The weaning weight of female lambs was depressed compared to the female controls, consistent with there being slightly more lambs per ewe (fewer singletons) in the PCP groups. Cortisol levels in both control and PCP-treated ewes were highly variable. PCP-treated ewes exhibited significant depression of T_4 throughout pregnancy and lactation and on postweaning day 5 ($p < 0.05$). PCP had no effect on the response to stimulation with the trophic hormones. Histopathologic examination revealed increased thyroid follicle size ($p < 0.01$) and increased lymphocytic infiltration into the uterine endometrium ($p < 0.05$).

The same laboratory also conducted a study of reproductive and endocrine function in rams exposed to PCP, using the same method of treating the feed to deliver a target PCP dose of 1 mg/kg-day (Beard *et al.*, 1999b). Beginning 5 weeks prior to conception, maternal ewes were fed either a control diet or a PCP-containing diet. Ewes received the treated diet through weaning; the 5 male offspring in the PCP group were maintained on the same treated diet until sacrifice at age 28 weeks. Tests of testicular growth (using ultrasound), sperm quality, and sexual behavior were performed at appropriate time points during development. When the rams were 27 weeks of age, levels of the same serum hormones as those measured by Rawlings *et al.* (1998) plus testosterone were evaluated before and after stimulation with a mixture of GnRH, TSH, and ACTH. Hormones were also monitored in blood samples taken every 2 weeks beginning at age 6 weeks. At sacrifice, animals were necropsied and the pituitary, adrenal, thyroid, pancreas, and reproductive tissues were subjected to histopathologic examination.

Rams in the PCP group had increased testicular development; scrotal circumference was approximately 10 to 15% greater than that of the controls throughout the measurement period ($p < 0.05$). The only effect of PCP on hormones was decreased T_4 in rams prior to 18 weeks of age. From age 18 to 26 weeks, T_4 levels in the treatment group were indistinguishable from control values. At age 28 weeks a significant decrease was again observed. At necropsy, the only possibly treatment-related effect noted was a nonsignificant increase in mean testes weight in the PCP group (586 g) compared to the controls (496 g), a finding in support of the larger scrotal circumference observed in the PCP-treated animals during life. Histologic examination revealed that PCP-treated rams had higher severity scores for seminiferous tubule atrophy ($p < 0.05$) and reduced sperm density in the body of the epididymides ($p < 0.05$). Because sperm quality in the living rams was unaffected by PCP treatment, the reported histopathologic findings must be considered tentative in the absence of independent replication.

65.8 DEVELOPMENTAL TOXICITY

Four teratology studies of oral PCP were identified, three in rats and one in rabbits. The rabbit study and the most recent rat study were performed by the same laboratory. These two studies tested recent (*c.* 1992) lots of a commercially available, technical-grade PCP. Results of the teratology studies in rats and rabbits are summarized in Table 65.9.

65.8.1 RAT

Hoberman (1994a) performed a teratology study of technical-grade PCP (89% pure) in a strain of CD rats under contract to the Pentachlorophenol Task Force, an industry group. Twenty-five female rats per group were mated and then administered PCP by gavage at dose levels of 0, 10, 30, or 80 mg/kg-day on gestation days 6–15.

The litter and/or fetal incidences of various malformations or variations were increased (significantly or otherwise) at 80 mg/kg-day. The incidence of "slight to moderate" dilatation of the kidney pelvis was significantly elevated at the high dose ($p \leq 0.01$), occurring in 4/22 litters (4 fetuses) at this dose, 1/23 litters (1 fetus) at 30 mg/kg-day, and in none of the low-dose or

Table 65.9
Summary of the Developmental Toxicity of PCP in Rats and Rabbits

Species/strain: study	Route	PCP grade	Effects at LOEL	LOEL	NOEL
				(mg/kg-day)	
CD rat: Hoberman (1994a)	gavage	technical	Maternal: ↓ weight gain.	80	30
			Developmental: ↑ gross malformations (external, soft tissue); ↑ skeletal anomalies (delayed or residual ossification at multiple sites, extra vertebra and rib pair)	80	30
Sprague-Dawley rat: Schwetz *et al.* (1974)	gavage	technical and purified	Maternal: ↓ weight gain	technical: 30 purified: 34.7	technical: 15 purified: 15
			Developmental: ↑ percentage males; ↓ fetal body weight; ↑ subcutaneous edema; ↑ skeletal anomalies (lumbar spurs, delayed skull ossification)	technical: 15 purified: 5.0	technical: 5.8 purified: n.d.
Sprague-Dawley rat: Welsh *et al.* (1987)	diet	purified	Maternal: ↓ weight gain; ↑ "ringed eye"; ↑ vaginal hemorrhaging	43	13
			Developmental: ↓ fetal body weight; ↑ skeletal anomalies (misshapen centra)	13	4
New Zealand rabbit: Hoberman (1994b)	gavage	technical	Maternal: ↓ weight gain	15	7.5
			Developmental: No effects	None	30 (highest dose tested)

control litters. The only other gross external or tissue lesion in the 30 mg/kg-day group was a ventricular septal defect. Minor ossification changes observed at 30 mg/kg-day are judged to be of no developmental significance. Based on malformations and other effects observed at the high dose, the developmental NOEL for this study was 30 mg/kg-day. Aside from the difference in rat strains, there is no obvious explanation for why the NOEL observed in this study was so much higher than the NOELs found in the two other rat studies discussed below.

Schwetz et al. (1974) evaluated the teratogenic potential of sample lots of commercial (TG) and purified PCP in SD rats. The test substances were given by gavage on gestation days 6–15 at dose levels of 5.8, 15, 34.7, or 50 mg/kg-day for TG-PCP and 5.0, 15, 30, or 50 mg/kg-day for purified PCP, with one control group for both PCP formulations. The TG-PCP doses of 5.8 and 34.7 mg/kg-day were chosen to correspond to PCP doses of 5.0 and 30 mg/kg-day, respectively. Both the TG-PCP and purified PCP contained nondetectable levels of TCDD, but the detection limit at that time was quite high (50 ppb). The TG-PCP contained levels of the nonphenolic contaminants Hx-CDD, HxCDF, HpCDF, OCDF, HpCDD, and OCDD at 4, 30, 80, and 80, 125, and 2500 ppm, respectively.

Between days 6 and 21, average maternal weight gains in the 30 mg/kg-day purified PCP and 34.7 mg/kg-day TG-PCP groups were, respectively, 26% and 74% of the control value. The maternal NOEL was 15 mg/kg-day for both PCP grades.

The percentages of resorbed fetuses per animal and per litter were significantly increased in groups receiving TG-PCP at doses $\geq$15 mg/kg-day or purified PCP at doses $\geq$30 mg/kg-day. Even though the LOEL for fetal resorption was lower for animals given TG-PCP, at the two highest dose levels (30/34.7 and 50 mg/kg-day) the percentage of resorbed fetuses was greater for purified PCP (98 and 100%) than for TG-PCP (27 and 58%). There were no data on fetal sex, weight, and length for the 50 mg/kg-day purified PCP group because all fetuses were resorbed. The sex ratio of surviving pups was markedly altered at the higher doses, with male to female ratios of 3.8 to 1 in the 50 mg/kg-day TG-PCP group and 4.9 to 1 in the 30 mg/kg-day purified PCP group. Fetal body weights were significantly decreased at the 30 mg/kg-day dose of purified PCP and at TG-PCP doses $\geq$34.7 mg/kg-day. Crown-rump length was significantly decreased in the 30 mg/kg-day purified PCP group. At 5.0 mg/kg-day purified PCP, the percentage of litters with delayed skull ossification was significantly elevated (9/15 vs. 6/31 in controls). Based on the dose-related effects on fetal development observed at all doses, this study produced no NOEL for the developmental toxicity of purified PCP. In the 15 mg/kg-day TG-PCP group, the percentage of litters with subcutaneous edema or lumbar spurs was significantly elevated. In the absence of other signs of teratogenicity at the lowest dose, the developmental NOEL for the technical-grade PCP tested was 5.8 mg/kg-day based on skeletal and soft tissue anomalies detected at higher dose levels.

The results of Schwetz et al. (1974) seem to suggest that impurities present in technical-grade PCP are responsible for diminishing some of the maternal and developmental toxicity of PCP by unknown mechanisms. The differential toxicity of the TG-PCP and purified PCP formulations cannot be explained by small differences in their relative PCP content; for example, the incidence of delayed ossification for the 15 mg/kg-day purified PCP group was approximately twice that of the TG-PCP group receiving nominally double the dose (30 mg/kg-day). Whatever the explanation for the differential toxicity of the two formulations, this study showed that the developmental toxicity of PCP does not result from impurities present in the TG product.

A study performed by the U.S. Food and Drug Administration examined the teratogenic potential of purified PCP in SD rats (Welsh et al., 1987). Weanling animals of both sexes received PCP at 0, 60, 200, or 600 ppm diet (corresponding to average daily intakes of 0, 4.0, 13, or 43 mg/kg-day for females). After 181 days on this dietary regimen, males and females were permitted to mate with animals from the same dose group. For the teratology phase, females in each group were continued on the same daily dose until Caesarian section on gestation day 20. The test compound was a highly purified product recrystallized from >99% pure PCP. The only pCDD detected was 1.3 ppb OCDD; no pCDF impurities were found.

Signs of maternal toxicity observed at the highest dose were reduced body weight gain, "ringed eye" (50% incidence), and vaginal hemorrhaging (25% incidence). The maternal NOEL was 13 mg/kg-day. At a maternal dose of 43 mg/kg-day, essentially complete resorption of fetuses (99.5%) was observed, indicating a profound effect on reproductive competence. In the 13 mg/kg-day group, the percentage of dams with two or more resorbed fetuses was twice as great as in the control group. At this dose, the major fetal effects were a highly significant ($p < 0.01$) increase in misshapen centra by litter and by fetus and an approximately 10% weight reduction in fetuses of both sexes. Fetal body weight was depressed to a lesser extent (3–4%) in male and female pups in the 4.0 mg/kg-day group, approaching statistical significance for males ($p = 0.06$). There were no fetal abnormalities at the low dose. The developmental NOEL for highly purified PCP was 4.0 mg/kg-day based on fetal weight reduction and skeletal abnormalities at 13 and 43 mg/kg-day.

Unlike the study performed by Schwetz et al. (1974) in the same rat strain, Welsh et al. (1987) found no evidence for delayed skull ossification. Potential explanations for this discrepancy may lie in differences in exposure route and onset (dietary exposure from weaning vs. gavage exposure on gestation days 6–15). It is conceivable that adaptive tolerance played a role in limiting the toxic effects of PCP in the FDA study.

65.8.2 RABBIT

Hoberman (1994b) performed a developmental toxicity study of technical-grade PCP (88–89% pure) in New Zealand white rabbits under contract to the Pentachlorophenol Task Force. Twenty does per group were artificially inseminated, presumed pregnant, and then administered PCP by gavage at dose levels of 0, 7.5, 15, or 30 mg/kg-day on gestation days 6–18. At Caesarian section on gestation day 29, the number of litters was 17 in the control group and 17, 13, and 18 in the low-, middle-, and high-dose PCP groups, respectively.

Mean maternal body weight gain in the 15 mg/kg-day group was marginally ($\leq 2.5\%$) but significantly depressed during the dosing period but recovered by gestation day 19. Mean maternal body weight gain in the 30 mg/kg-day group was likewise marginally ($\leq 3.5\%$) but significantly depressed during the dosing period and remained depressed ($\leq 3.8\%$) throughout the entire 29 days of gestation. The maternal NOEL was 7.5 mg/kg-day based on transient decreased weight gain in animals receiving 15 mg/kg-day and lasting decreased weight gain in animals receiving 30 mg/kg-day.

No deaths, abortions, or preliminary deliveries occurred. No treatment-related developmental toxicity was observed at any dose. The developmental NOEL was 30 mg/kg-day based on the observation of no developmental effects at the highest dose tested.

65.9 IMMUNOTOXICITY

In several studies, TG-PCP was found to suppress humoral immunity in mice treated subchronically at oral doses as low as 9 or 10 mg/kg-day; no NOEL was identified. There is suggestive evidence for a developmental immunotoxic effect of PCP; partially purified PCP suppressed delayed-type hypersensitivity and humoral immunity in rats exposed prenatally and then subchronically to oral doses as low as an estimated 0.74 mg/kg-day, the lowest dose tested. However, confidence in that finding is weak because of the absence of dose dependence.

The only clearly dose-related immunotoxic response to AG-PCP was the unexpected occurrence of splenic tumors in mice surviving primary challenge with tumor virus and secondary challenge with virus-transformed sarcoma cells; the LOEL was 9 mg/kg-day (the lowest dose tested). This finding suggests that PCP possesses a partial complement of the immunosuppressive activity associated with the technical-grade formulation. Apparently there has not yet been any attempt to replicate the result. Nevertheless, the observation of increased susceptibility to invasive tumorigenesis must be considered as evidence of a potentially important immunotoxic effect of PCP.

Studies are presented chronologically within Sections 65.9.1–65.9.3.

65.9.1 RAT

65.9.1.1 Two-Generation Dietary Exposure

Female SD rats were fed partially purified (97%) PCP at 0, 5, 50, or 500 ppm diet from weaning, throughout mating, gestation, and lactation (Exon and Koller, 1983). Progeny were weaned at 3 weeks and maintained on the maternal exposure regime until commencement of immunotoxicity testing at 13 weeks. Based on recommended values for body weight and food consumption for female and weanling SD rats in subchronic studies (U.S. EPA, 1988), the average PCP dose

levels can be estimated as 0.49, 4.9, and 49 mg/kg-day for the dams and 0.74, 7.4, and 74 mg/kg-day for the weanlings. Delayed-type hypersensitivity (DTH), humoral immunity, and macrophage activation were assayed following *in vivo* antigen challenge.

The investigators found evidence for suppression of DTH and humoral immunity in PCP-treated progeny, but dose dependence was lacking. The DTH response was significantly depressed in all PCP treatment groups ($p \leq 0.03$); mean values were 82%, 72%, and 74% of controls in the 5, 50, and 500 ppm groups. Humoral immunity (serum antibody response to bovine serum albumin) was likewise reported to be significantly depressed in all treatment groups ($p \leq 0.0001$); mean values were 44%, 58%, and 45% of controls in the 5, 50, and 500 ppm groups. Without further information it is not possible to distinguish between a saturated response (spanning two orders of magnitude in dose) and a spurious result. Clear evidence of dose-related immunoactivation (increased phagocytosis by macrophages) was observed, with statistical significance achieved at the two highest doses ($p \leq 0.01$).

65.9.1.2 Twenty-Eight-Day Dietary Exposure

Blakley *et al.* (1998) administered 99% pure PCP via oral gavage to 10 male F344 rats twice weekly for 28 days at a dose of 2.0 mg/kg (time-averaged dose, 0.57 mg/kg-day). A control group of 10 rats received the olive oil vehicle. At the end of the exposure period animals were sacrificed and organ weights recorded. Immune parameters assayed were IgM antibody plaque formation (following immunization with sheep red blood cells) and lymphocyte blastogenesis in spleen cell suspensions, phagocytic function of peritoneal macrophages, and lymphocyte surface marker expression in whole blood.

Mean body-weight gain, kidney/body-weight ratio, and liver/body-weight ratio were moderately increased in PCP-treated animals. PCP inhibited background lymphocyte blastogenesis but not mitogen-stimulated blastogenesis, an effect that cannot by itself be considered a sign of reduced humoral immunity. PCP exposure did not affect the number of plaque-forming colonies (PFCs) per spleen, despite the fact that the number of PFCs per unit viable cells was reduced to 61% of the control value ($p = 0.006$). These results are difficult to interpret. As discussed by the investigators, increased spleen cellularity (in compensation for diminished lymphocyte function) is an unlikely explanation because the spleen/body-weight ratio was not at all increased by PCP treatment. Based on the absence of effects in the other tests applied, PCP treatment did not appear to affect humoral immunity overall.

65.9.2 MOUSE

65.9.2.1 Subchronic Dietary Exposure

Kerkvliet *et al.* (1982a) fed male B6 mice a diet containing 50 or 500 ppm AG-PCP (>99% pure), 50 or 500 ppm TG-PCP (86% pure), or a control diet for 10–12 weeks prior to immunotoxicity testing. Measured concentrations of both PCP grades were within 15% of target levels. B6 mice (along with C3 mice) are progenitors of the B6C3F$_1$ mice routinely used by the NTP in toxicity and carcinogenicity studies. Recommended body weight and food consumption values for B6C3F$_1$ mice in subchronic studies are available (U.S. EPA, 1988); based on those recommended values, PCP dose levels in the study by Kerkvliet *et al.* (1982a) can be estimated as 9.0 and 90 mg/kg-day for AG-PCP and 7.7 and 77 mg/kg-day for TG-PCP. Immunocompetence was measured with tests of host susceptibility to virus infection and tumor growth. Components of the immune response presumed to underlie an organism's net infectibility and tumor susceptibility (i.e., macrophage phagocytic activity and T-cell cytotoxicity) were tested separately following *in vivo* antigen challenge.

Mice given TG-PCP exhibited a dose-related increase in tumor incidence following challenge with syngeneic sarcoma cells, with statistically significant elevation at the high dose. In mice given a primary challenge with Moloney sarcoma virus (MSV), TG-PCP at 500 ppm diet produced progressive (i.e., fatal) primary tumors in 6/11 mice compared to 0/11 in the 50 ppm group and 0/16 in the controls. Fifteen weeks later, survivors were given a secondary challenge with MSV-transformed sarcoma cells (MSB). The incidence of progressive secondary tumors in PCP-treated mice was elevated, but the elevation was not significant and not dose-dependent. Necropsy of animals resistant to both the MSV and MSB challenges revealed splenic tumor formation in 0/13, 3/6, and 0/3 of the mice given 0, 50, and 500 ppm TG-PCP, respectively. An *in vitro* test of T-cell activity following *in vivo* sensitization revealed a dose-related decrease in cytotoxicity that could be explained by a diminished number of lysing units per spleen. In contrast to its immunosuppressive actions, TG-PCP improved resistance to a lethal virus, but not significantly. Resistance to EMCV-induced mortality is considered to be macrophage-dependent; a direct test of macrophage activation *in vitro* (following *in vivo* sensitization) revealed a dose-related enhancement of phagocytosis.

Contrary to the results with TG-PCP, animals exposed to AG-PCP showed no alteration in host susceptibility to syngeneic tumor cells, primary challenge with MSV, or secondary challenge with MSB. T-cell activation and macrophage phagocytic activity were similarly unaffected by AG-PCP. However, necropsy of animals resistant to both primary MSV and secondary MSB challenges revealed splenic tumor formation in 0/13, 2/9, and 4/9 of mice given 0, 50, and 500 ppm AG-PCP, respectively. These findings suggest that the PCP molecule, apart from contaminants present in technical-grade formulations, possesses immunosuppressive activity.

Kerkvliet *et al.* (1982b) further assessed the differential immunotoxicity of TG-PCP (86% PCP) and AG-PCP (>99% PCP) in female mice. Groups of 7–10 Swiss-Webster (SW) or B6 mice were exposed to TG-PCP at 0, 50, 100, 250, or 500 ppm diet for 8 weeks prior to primary immunization. Groups of 15–16 SW or B6 mice were exposed to AG-PCP at 0 or 1000 ppm diet. Based on recommended default values for body weight and food consumption in B6C3F$_1$ mice in subchronic studies (U.S. EPA, 1988), the five PCP dose levels can

be calculated as 9, 18, 45, 90, and 180 mg/kg-day for AG-PCP and 7.7, 15, 39, 77, and 155 mg/kg-day for TG-PCP. Humoral immune responses to *in vivo* antigen challenge were assessed with assays for hemolytic antibody isotope release, hemolytic plaque formation, and serum hemagglutination. Several measures of humoral immunity were significantly depressed at all TG-PCP levels tested (50–500 ppm), while no depression of humoral immunity was observed at the only AG-PCP level tested (1000 ppm).

65.9.2.2 Fourteen-Day Gavage Exposure

A study in female B6C3F$_1$ mice conducted by Holsapple *et al.* (1987) also differentiated the immunosuppressive properties of two grades of PCP: partially purified (EC-7) and TG-PCP. Eight mice per dose group were given TG-PCP at 0, 10, 30, or 100 mg/kg-day or EC-7 at 100 mg/kg-day by corn oil gavage for 14 days. The effect of PCP administration on humoral immunity was measured as the spleen-cell antibody response to antigenic activation *in vivo* and *in vitro*. The results of *in vivo* antigen challenge in this study were in agreement with the results of Kerkvliet *et al.* (1982a); i.e., TG-PCP but not EC-7 was found to suppress the spleen-cell antibody response. However, the *in vitro* antigen challenge assay revealed no evidence for suppression of the spleen-cell antibody response by TG-PCP. The negative result in the *in vitro* assay suggests that TG-PCP produces an immunosuppressive action on spleen cells *in vivo* though a mechanism external to the spleen. By contrast, the *in vivo* immunosuppressive action of HCDD (a major contaminant of TG-PCP) can be reproduced in the *in vitro* spleen cell assay (Holsapple *et al.*, 1984).

65.9.2.3 Acute Gavage Exposure

Various contaminant TG-PCP fractions and purified isomers isolated from TG-PCP were examined for their effect on humoral immunity (splenic plasma-cell antibody response to *in vivo* antibody challenge) in an acute gavage exposure study in B6 mice of both sexes (Kerkvliet *et al.*, 1985). Outcomes were compared to those for acute exposure to the TG-PCP and AG-PCP formulations tested by Kerkvliet *et al.* (1982a, b).

The investigators found that a pCDD/pCDF fraction was significantly immunosuppressive. The oral dose at which 50% immunosuppression occurred (ID$_{50}$) was calculated as 7.1, 85, and 208 µg/kg for HxCDD, HpCDD, and HpCDF, respectively. OCDD was not immunosuppressive at doses up to 500 µg/kg, the highest dose tested. For comparison, the investigators calculated an ID$_{50}$ of 83 mg/kg for TG-PCP containing < 5 ppm HxCDD and 88 ppm HpCDD. AG-PCP was not immunosuppressive at doses up to 120 mg/kg, the highest dose tested. Co-administration of HxCDD and HpCDD produced an additive immunosuppressive effect, suggesting that toxic pCDD isomers present in TG-PCP act in concert. Co-administration of 60 mg/kg AG-PCP and 100 µg/kg HpCDD resulted in no increase over the degree of immunosuppression produced by HpCDD alone. For the TG-PCP tested, the full extent of immunosuppression observed in the splenic plasma-cell antibody response assay could be explained by a combination of the pCDDs present as impurities.

65.9.3 *IN VITRO* EXPOSURE

Holsapple *et al.* (1987) compared the effect of two grades of PCP on the spleen cell antigen-specific IgM response in spleen cells isolated from untreated female B6C3F$_1$ mice. Spleen cells were cultured with one of three antigens in the presence of TG-PCP or EC-7. The PCP concentration range is given in the text of the citation as 0.05–50 mg/culture and in Table 3 of the citation as 0.05–50 μg/culture. Both TG-PCP and EC-7 suppressed the immune response to one or more antigens at concentrations above 5 mg (or 5 μg) per culture. However, the investigators stated that immunosuppression was associated with markedly decreased viability in all cases, indicating that cytotoxicity interfered with the test. Thus, the results of this study cannot be interpreted as having demonstrated a specific immunotoxic effect of TG-PCP or EC-7.

Lang and Mueller-Ruchholtz (1991) investigated the effect of *in vitro* exposure to TG or partially purified (Dowicide 7) PCP on the immunocompetence of peripheral blood lymphocytes (PBLs) isolated from 7–12 healthy human donors. The TG-PCP contained 2040 ppm pCDDs and pCDFs. The Dowicide 7 was >99% pure and contained 6 ppm pCDDs and pCDFs. Final concentrations of PCP in the lymphocyte culture media were in the range 2.7 to 54 mg/l (approximately 10 to 200 μM). Immunocompetence was measured with assays of mitogen responsiveness, interleukin-2 (IL-2) production, and stimulated (T-cell-dependent or independent) synthesis of IgM and IgG. Viability was found to be unaffected at PCP concentrations ≤40 μM. *In vitro* exposure of lymphocytes to TG-PCP resulted in stimulated synthesis of both IgM and IgG at concentrations ≥10 or 20 μM. Dose-related suppression of IL-2 occurred only at concentrations ≥80 μM, above the threshold for cytotoxicity. Similar results were obtained in experiments with Dowicide 7.

The concordant *in vitro* results for Dowicide 7 and TG-PCP obtained by Lang and Mueller-Ruchholtz (1991) are in stark contrast with the results of animal studies showing that TG-PCP but not AG-PCP suppresses antibody release and T-cell activation in response to *in vivo* antigen challenge (Exon and Koller, 1983; Kerkvliet *et al.*, 1982a, b, 1985; Holsapple *et al.*, 1987). However, Kerkvliet *et al.* (1982a) also found that exposure of mice to AG-PCP resulted in increased susceptibility of the spleen to viral tumorigenesis, indicating that isolated tests of humoral and T-cell-mediated immunity may have been inadequate to detect a more complex immunosuppressive response.

65.10 BIOCHEMICAL MECHANISMS

TCHQ is clearly DNA-reactive and mutagenic whereas the weight of evidence suggests little or no genotoxicity for PCP. Because TCHQ is the major metabolite of PCP in rodents, it seems plausible that the DNA reactivity attributed to PCP in rodent experiments (or in mammalian cells incubated with a microsomal extract of rat liver) is actually a consequence of TCHQ formation.

The ability to promote oxidative DNA damage is typically regarded as being indicative of a potential to initiate carcinogenesis. PCP at 60 mg/kg given to male B6C3F$_1$ mice as a single gavage dose resulted in significant elevation of 8-hydroxydeoxyguanosine (8-OH-dG) adducts in liver nuclear DNA at 6 hr but not at 24 hr (Sai-Kato *et al.*, 1995). Curiously, TCHQ given to male B6C3F$_1$ mice as a single i.p. dose of 50 mg/kg produced no elevation of 8-OH-dG adducts in liver nuclear DNA at 6 hr (Dahlhaus *et al.*, 1994). One possible explanation of these findings is that when TCHQ was administered i.p., adducts were formed rapidly and DNA repair was complete by the 6-hr mark, whereas when PCP was administered by gavage, the rate of absorption or metabolism to TCHQ slowed the rate of adduct formation, which was therefore incomplete at 6 hr postexposure.

PCP is an uncoupler of oxidative phosphorylation in intact mitochondria, an effect observable at micromolar PCP concentrations (Weinbach, 1957). The ratio of phosphate to oxygen consumed (P : O ratio) was approximately halved when rat liver mitochondria were incubated in the presence of 5 μM PCP (Weinbach and Garbus, 1965), while a concentration of 0.5 μM produced a substantial increase in oxygen consumption consistent with the action of an uncoupler (Arrhenius *et al.*, 1977). It is perhaps conceivable that mitochondrial uncoupling could play a role in the hepatotoxicity or immunotoxicity of PCP; this hypothesis has not been tested.

PCP inhibits the binding of T$_4$ to thyroid hormone receptors. An IC$_{50}$ of approximately 0.05 μM was found by van Raaij *et al.* (1991a) for PCP displacement of T$_4$ from rat serum binding sites *in vitro*. Depression of serum T$_4$ levels in PCP-exposed animals is likely to be a consequence of negative feedback originating from PCP occupation of the receptors.

In a yeast strain engineered to express the human progesterone receptor (hPR), PCP antagonized the action of 10 nM progesterone with an IC$_{50}$ of approximately 0.7 μM. Binding of 1 nM synthetic progesterone to hPR was inhibited by PCP with an IC$_{50}$ of approximately 0.4 μM (Tran *et al.*, 1996).

PCP inhibits hepatic phenol sulfotransferase with high specificity and inhibits several other metabolizing enzymes and cytochrome P450 activities with lower efficiency. The IC$_{50}$ for PCP inhibition of 4′-hydroxypropranolol sulfation by canine hepatic cytosol was approximately 0.2 μM; in a partially purified phenol sulfotransferase fraction, the IC$_{50}$ was approximately 0.1 μM (Christ and Walle, 1989). An IC$_{50}$ value two orders of magnitude larger (approximately 20 μM) was found for PCP inhibition of 1-chloro-2,4-dinitrobenzene sulfation by purified equine liver glutathione S-transferase (Moorthy and Randerath, 1996). IC$_{50}$ values of 12 to 25 μM were observed for PCP inhibition of O-acetylation of N-hydroxyarylamines in liver cytosol from hamster and rat (Shinohara *et al.*, 1986). Higher IC$_{50}$ values have been observed for inhibition of N-acetyltransferase, N,O-acetyltransferase, and epoxide hydrolase activities in liver extracts from one or more rodent species (Moorthy and Randerath, 1996; Shinohara *et al.*, 1986).

Each of the hepatic enzyme activities inhibited by PCP is implicated in both activating and deactivating pathways in the metabolism of one or more class of xenobiotics. Studies in rats designed to elucidate potentially carcinogenic products of xenobiotic metabolism have found an inhibitory effect of PCP pretreatment or cotreatment on hepatic DNA adduct formation produced by *N*-hydroxy-2-acetylaminofluorene or dinitrotoluene (Kedderis *et al.*, 1984; Meerman *et al.*, 1981), hepatic unscheduled DNA synthesis produced by 2-acetylaminofluorene (Monteith, 1992), hepatic cytogenetic changes produced by safrole (Daimon *et al.*, 1997–98), initiation and promotion of hepatic foci and tumors produced by 1′-hydroxysafrole (Boberg *et al.*, 1987), and growth of hepatic foci promoted by *N*-hydroxy-2-acetylaminofluorene (Kroese *et al.*, 1988). In mice, pretreatment with PCP inhibited DNA adduct and hepatoma formation produced by 1′-hydroxy-2′,3′-dehydroestragole (Fennell *et al.*, 1985). All of the anti-DNA-reactive and antitumorigenic actions of PCP described in this paragraph are likely to be explained, at least in part, by inhibition of sulfotransferase activity.

The above evidence suggests that PCP at subcarcinogenic doses inhibits the metabolism of many xenobiotics to DNA-reactive compounds and therefore would have a mitigating effect overall on the initiation of carcinogenesis by those compounds. On the other hand, i.p. administration of PCP (>99% pure) to mice at 20 mg/kg daily on each of the four days on which tamoxifen was administered increased the sulfotransferase-dependent DNA adduct formation produced by tamoxifen (Randerath *et al.*, 1994). Also, there is some evidence for a promotional effect of PCP that could, at sufficiently high doses, counteract the anti-initiating effect. Umemura *et al.* (1999) found that in male B6C3F$_1$ mice fed 99% pure PCP at 300 ppm diet for 25 weeks following pre-initiation with diethylnitrosamine, promotion of liver tumors occurred (discussed in Section 65.5.2). When co-administered to rats chronically with 2-hydroxyethylnitrosourea, technical-grade (86% pure) PCP at 500 ppm diet (dose estimated as 22 mg/kg-day based on NTP, 1999) increased the incidence of acute myelocytic leukemia in males from 20% to 60% (Mirvish *et al.*, 1991). However, the technical-grade contaminants, including TCDD (25 ppb diet) and 2,3,7,8-tetrachlorodibenzofuran (TCDF, 670 ppb diet), might have been relevant to the observed promoting action. Promotional potential may also be indicated by the ability of PCP (>99% pure) to interfere with gap junctional communication in cultured rat liver epithelial cells (Sai *et al.*, 1998). In that study, the IC$_{50}$ for PCP was >40 μM (the highest concentration tested) for 4-hr incubation and 30–40 μM for 24-hr incubation. Although no statistical analysis was presented, the data shown indicated a threshold above 10 μM for 4-hr incubation and <10 μM (the lowest concentration tested) for 24-hr incubation. The fact that the extent of inhibition increased between 4 and 24 hr suggests that the mechanism is indirect, perhaps a buildup of damage arising as a consequence of PCP inhibition of oxidative phosphorylation, buildup that might not occur in vascularized tissue *in vivo*. Therefore, in the event that PCP treatment *in vivo* is able to interfere with gap junctional communication, it is likely that much higher concentrations would be required to produce a given level of inhibition.

65.11 HUMAN HEALTH EFFECTS

65.11.1 SHORT-TERM EXPOSURE

65.11.1.1 Occupational Case Reports

The occupational case report literature on PCP includes evidence that short-term inhalation of vapors in an unventilated area or prolonged dermal contact can result in hemotoxicity, including aplastic anemia and thrombocytopenic purpura (Hay and Singer, 1991; Rugman and Cosstick, 1990), toxicity to the nervous system, including excessive sweating, tachycardia, tachypnea, anorexia, fever, and death (Bergner *et al.*, 1965; Gordon, 1956; Menon, 1958), and hepatic and pulmonary damage combined with pancreatitis (Cooper and Macauley, 1982).

65.11.1.2 Nonoccupational Case Reports

In a hospital nursery, poisoning of neonates occurred when diapers and bed linens were laundered with PCP. Twenty exposed infants manifested symptoms potentially associated with neurotoxicity (excessive sweating, tachycardia, tachypnea, respiratory distress, and metabolic acidosis); autopsy of the two fatal cases revealed hepatic and renal pathology (Armstrong *et al.*, 1969; Robson *et al.*, 1969). Three cases of dermal toxicity (*pemphigus vulgaris* and urticaria) were reported to be associated with short-term residential exposure to PCP-treated wood; serum PCP levels in the cases at presentation were 47–114 μg/l.

65.11.2 SUBCHRONIC AND CHRONIC EXPOSURE

65.11.2.1 Case Reports

The case report literature on the toxicity of subchronic exposures to PCP is primarily indicative of hemotoxicity (Roberts, 1990). Roberts (1983) described six cases of aplastic anemia or red cell aplasia associated with exposure to PCP. In one of the cases of aplastic anemia, the patient, a 21-year-old male, had handled wet lumber processed with a commercial product containing 3% PCP and 1.5% tetrachlorophenol during the year prior to onset of clinical symptoms. Handling resulted in dermal and oral (hand-to-mouth) exposure to the wood preservative. The patient died of related causes 5 months after clinical onset. In another case, a 27-year-old male worked at building a log cabin one day per month. Using cloth gloves, he applied a 5% PCP solution with a brush after diluting a 40% solution with fuel oil. Symptoms were established within 9 months of the initial PCP exposure. Multiple medical measures were taken, but death occurred 6 months later. The other cases summarized by Roberts (1983) include a 24-year-old male exposed to PCP while working in construction who developed aplastic anemia and Hodgkin's disease 2 years after initial exposure, resulting in death; a 21-year-old male who applied PCP to furniture for 2 days, allowed the furniture to remain in his room, and developed aplastic anemia 1 month later; a 73-year-old male who repeatedly applied undiluted PCP to wood in a poorly ventilated barn, wearing no protective clothing, and developed pure red cell aplasia 4 years after initial exposure, resulting in death; and a 47-year-old male who dipped window frames into PCP at work and developed pure red cell aplasia 2 years after initial exposure, with death due to acute leukemia 2 years later. Rugman and Cosstick (1990) reported one case of fatal aplastic anemia in a 28-year-old male who applied PCP to timber over a period of months while renovating an old building.

De Maeyer *et al.* (1995) described the cases of two women who suffered multiple miscarriages following introduction of PCP-treated wood products into their homes. Serum PCP levels recorded around the time of the miscarriages were ≤ 62 μg/l in one woman and ≤ 31 μg/l in the other.

Roberts (1997) reported symptoms and laboratory findings for a family of five who had burned PCP-treated logs in their fireplace and whose home had been sided with PCP-treated lumber. The family reported intense irritation of the eyes and respiratory tract, recurrent infections, and neuropsychiatric symptoms. Laboratory findings included antinuclear antibody positivity, high serum rheumatoid factor titer, low serum complement 4, and elevated urinary porphyrins.

65.11.2.2 Case-Control Studies: Cancer

In a case-control study, Pearce *et al.* (1986a) investigated whether the incidence of non-Hodgkin's lymphoma (NHL) in New Zealand was associated with the performance of occupational tasks entailing likely exposure to pentachlorophenol or other chlorophenols. The case population consisted of male patients with a confirmed diagnosis of NHL other than lymphosarcoma or reticulosarcoma during the years 1977–1981; the number of cases in the final sample was 83. Two sets of controls were chosen, one from the general population and one from patients with other types of cancer. A telephone questionnaire was used to elicit information concerning occupation and potential occupational exposures. The criterion selected for statistical significance was $p < 0.1$. The relative risk for fencing contractors was nonsignificantly elevated against the cancer controls and significantly elevated against the population controls; for the latter, the odds ratio (OR) was 6.1 and the 90% lower confidence limit (LCL) was 1.5. The relative risk for fencing as a farmer was significantly elevated against the cancer controls (OR = 1.9, 90% LCL = 1.1) and nonsignificantly elevated against the population controls. For employment in the pelt department of a meat works (a source of potential exposure to 2,4,6,-trichlorophenol), the relative risk was significantly elevated against the population controls (OR = 4.1, 90% LCL = 1.1) and nonsignificantly elevated against the cancer controls. There was no increased relative risk of NHL for sawmill/timber

merchants or for persons in the category "potential chlorophenol exposure at sawmill or timber merchant." The investigators suggested that some nonchlorophenol exposure (such as a tumor virus) may have been responsible for the elevated NHL risk observed in meat workers.

Pearce *et al.* (1987) expanded the case-control study of Pearce *et al.* (1986a) to include lymphosarcoma and reticulosarcoma diagnoses among the NHL cases; a total of 183 male NHL cases were included in the final sample. Controls were drawn from patients diagnosed with other types of cancer. The criterion selected for statistical significance was $p < 0.1$. The relative risk for fencing work was nonsignificantly elevated (OR = 1.4, 90% LCL = 1.0), as was the relative risk for employment in the pelt department of a meat works (OR = 1.9, 90% LCL = 0.9). For employment in any meat works job, the elevation was statistically significant (OR = 1.8, 90% LCL = 1.2). Once again there was no increased risk of NHL for sawmill/timber merchants or for persons in the category "potential chlorophenol exposure at sawmill or timber merchant."

In both studies by Pearce and co-workers (1986a, 1987), sawmill workers were expected to have had the most PCP exposure but did not exhibit an elevated relative risk for NHL. Although NHL was found to be associated with fencing work, the investigators concluded that this finding was not relevant to any potential association between PCP and NHL. This can be understood from the investigators' observation that the principal method for preserving fencing timber in New Zealand is by vacuum-pressure impregnation with chromated copper arsenate and that since 1955, less than 1% of posts have been preserved with PCP. Although NaPCP was probably applied to some percentage of fencing-post timber as an antisapstain agent, any resultant exposure to fencing workers was still expected to be less than that for exposure at a sawmill or timber merchant (Pearce *et al.*, 1986a). Nevertheless, it is difficult to assess the relevance of the fencing-work associations because neither absolute nor relative PCP exposure estimates were provided. It would be helpful also to have more information about the plausibility of a link between NHL and chromated copper arsenate.

Hardell *et al.* (1981, 1994) reported results for 105 confirmed cases of NHL in males diagnosed in Umea, Sweden during the years 1974–1978. Living and deceased controls were drawn from national registries of population and death. A self-administered questionnaire was used to elicit information concerning chemical exposures and occupation. The criterion selected for statistical significance was $p < 0.05$. A nonsignificantly elevated relative risk was found for sawmill workers (OR = 1.5, 95% LCL = 0.7). A significantly elevated relative risk was found for high-grade PCP exposure, i.e., more than 1 week continuously or one month total (OR = 8.8; 95% LCL = 3.4).

Pearce *et al.* (1986b) interviewed 76 male cancer patients in New Zealand who had been diagnosed with multiple myeloma (MM) during the years 1977–1981 and looked for associations with occupational exposures to chlorophenols. Controls were drawn from patients diagnosed with other types of cancer. A telephone questionnaire was used to elicit information concerning occupation and potential occupational exposures. The criterion selected for statistical significance was $p < 0.05$. Relative risk for MM was nonsignificantly elevated for fencing work (OR = 1.6, 95% LCL = 0.9), fencing work with self-treated posts (OR = 1.1, 95% LCL = 0.2), work at a saw mill or timber merchant (OR = 1.1, 95% LCL = 0.5), potential occupational exposure to chlorophenols at a sawmill or timber merchant (OR = 1.4, 95% LCL = 0.5), and meat works employment (OR = 1.3, 95% LCL = 0.7).

Smith *et al.* (1984) interviewed 82 male cancer patients in New Zealand diagnosed with soft-tissue sarcoma (STS) during the years 1976–1980 and looked for associations with occupational exposures to chlorophenols. Controls were drawn from patients diagnosed with other types of cancer. A telephone questionnaire was used to elicit information concerning occupation and potential occupational exposures. The criterion selected for statistical significance was $p < 0.1$. Nonsignificantly elevated relative risks for STS were found for fencing contractors (OR = 1.9, 90% LCL = 0.5), saw mill or timber merchants (OR = 1.3, 90% LCL = 0.6), employment in the pelt department of a meat works (OR = 4.7, 90% LCL = 0.6), and tannery or meat-works pelt department work (OR = 7.2, 90% LCL = 1.0). The only significantly elevated relative risk was for meat works employment (OR = 2.8, 90% LCL = 1.3). There was no elevation of relative risk linked to the job classification with the highest potential exposure to PCP, "potential chlorophenol exposure at saw mill or timber merchant."

Eriksson *et al.* (1990) performed a case-control study based on confirmed cases of STS in males diagnosed in Uppsala, Sweden during the years 1978–1986. Assessment of exposure to PCP and other chlorophenols was determined by questionnaire and follow-up interview. The final case group size was 78 alive and 140 deceased. Controls were drawn from the national population registry. The criterion selected for statistical significance was $p < 0.05$. Relative risk was significantly elevated for high-grade exposure to PCP (i.e., at least 1 week continuously or at least 1 month total) in the absence of exposure to phenoxyacetic acid herbicides (OR = 3.9, 95% LCL = 1.2).

Potential Confounding by TCDD/pCDD Contamination In laboratory tests conducted in the late 1970s, TCDD levels in the range 0.25 to 1.1 ppb were measured in commercial PCP (IPCS, 1987). Thus, it is expected that this range approximates the TCDD contamination associated with PCP exposures discussed in case reports and epidemiological studies of that time period and earlier. Exposure to TCDD has been linked to STS in several epidemiologic studies. Fingerhut *et al.* (1991) examined a cohort consisting of essentially all U.S. chemical workers occupationally exposed to TCDD; a significantly increased risk of cancer mortality, mostly due to STS, was found in the sub-cohort with at least 1 year of exposure and at least 20 years latency. STS was found to be associated with self-reported exposures to TCDD and more highly chlorinated pCDDs in a Swedish case-control study (Eriksson *et al.*, 1990). Although that study found larger odds ratios associated with exposures to

PCP than to TCDD and higher pCDDs, the design did not allow assessment of exposure to TCDD and pCDDS among those with self-reported exposures to those agents relative to those with self-reported exposures to PCP.

65.11.2.3 Cohort Studies

Mortality Ramlow *et al.* (1996) conducted a mortality study of PCP manufacturing workers, part of a larger cohort of Dow Chemical Company workers in Michigan with potential exposure to pCDDs. The final PCP cohort consisted of 770 workers employed between 1940 and 1989, followed through 1989. Relative risks were based on comparison with age- and period-specific death rates for white males in the U.S. population. In cohort members with at least 15 years latency, a nonsignificant elevation was observed for mortality from lymphopoietic cancer other than Hodgkin's disease, leukemia, or aleukemia (SMR = 2.0, 95% LCL = 0.54). The only statistically significant finding for the group with 15 years latency was for mortality from gastric or duodenal ulcer (SMR = 5.6, 95% LCL = 1.8). Dividing the entire cohort into low and high-exposure categories revealed significantly elevated mortality in the high-exposure group for cancer of the kidney (SMR = 4.2, LCL = 1.4) and nonmalignant digestive system disease (including gastric or duodenal ulcer and liver cirrhosis). Also in the high-exposure group, mortality from lymphopoietic cancer other than leukemia was nonsignificantly elevated (SMR = 2.6, 95% LCL = 0.98).

Immunotoxicity and Clinical Pathology Klemmer *et al.* (1980) performed a clinical study of wood-treatment workers, pest-control operators (PCOs), farmers, and nonoccupationally exposed controls in Hawaii. A single, cross-sectional measurement of blood PCP concentration was used as a surrogate measure of long-term exposure. The mean blood PCP concentration in the wood-treatment workers ("PCP-exposed") was 2.7 mg/l. The mean blood PCP concentration in the PCOs, farmers, and controls ("non-PCP-exposed") was 0.26 mg/l. Routine clinical testing of blood was performed; results were reported for only 45% (189/422) of the available study population, those for whom a complete set was available. Of these, 17 were wood-treatment workers, 155 were PCOs or farmers, and 17 were controls. In the PCP-exposed group there was significant elevation of the number of immature leukocytes ($p < 0.005$), plasma cholinesterase levels ($p < 0.05$), and alkaline phosphatase levels ($p < 0.05$); the observed values were within ranges considered normal. The study's ability to detect an effect of PCP exposure was limited by the fact that the "non-PCP-exposed" population had serum PCP levels far higher than what can be considered background exposure.

McConnachie and Zahalsky (1991) performed a cross-sectional study on peripheral blood lymphocytes (PBLs) from 38 individuals in 10 families living in PCP-treated log homes in Indiana and Kentucky. The cohort consisted of 21 males and 17 females, 8–60 years of age (mean, 30 years). Exposure duration was 1–13 years (mean, 7.4 years). The elapsed time between the last exposure and performance of PBL testing was 0–9 years (mean, 4 years). There were 39 male and 81 female controls, 11–67 years of age. Controls had no known hematologic disorders or illness. No exclusions or data corrections were made for other potentially confounding factors such as smoking. The results of measuring antibody expression, T-cell activation, functional immunity, B-cell regulation, autoantibody expression, and natural killer cell function provided a reasonably coherent body of evidence suggesting that production of autoimmunity and depression of the T-cell proliferative response are associated with residence in log cabins treated with PCP. For the most part, the results were consistent with observations that T-cell response and general immunocompetence were suppressed in experimental animals treated with technical-grade PCP manufactured in the same decade (1980s) that the cabins were constructed. The findings suggest an immunotoxic effect of subchronic exposure to technical-grade PCP that is not reversed upon removal of exposure. Information on the postexposure time course of the observed outcomes would aid in the interpretation of this study.

Colosio *et al.* (1993) evaluated clinical and immunologic parameters in a cross-sectional study of 32 workers with prolonged exposure to PCP in a northern Italian wood factory. Of these, 14 subjects (the high-exposure group) had been engaged in brush application of PCP for at least 10 years. The remaining 18 subjects (the low-exposure group) had only indirect exposure to PCP in the work place. The control group consisted of 37 subjects who worked in a marble factory in the same valley. Mean plasma PCP concentrations in the high-exposure, low-exposure, and control groups were 289, 145, and 9 µg/l, respectively. Routine clinical chemistry testing of blood and urine was performed. Fasting levels of serum bile acids (SBAs) and urinary excretion of D-glucaric acid (a degradation product of SBAs), porphyrins, and 6-β-hydroxycortisol were determined as additional measures of liver function. Tests of humoral and cellular immunity were also performed. In the high-exposure group, plasma levels of some SBAs were found to be significantly elevated relative to the controls, while the T-cell response to mitogen was significantly reduced relative to the low-exposure group as well as the controls. The results demonstrated a potentially adverse effect on the liver associated with long-term occupational exposure to technical-grade PCP. The observation of depressed T-cell response to mitogen was consistent with the results of treating animals with technical-grade PCP. However, suppression of humoral immunity was invariably produced in the animal studies of technical-grade PCP while none was observed in this study. The finding in this study of depressed T-cell activation in occupationally exposed workers is consistent with a similar finding in residents of PCP-treated log homes, reported by McConnachie and Zahalsky (1991).

Daniel *et al.* (1995) identified 188 patients with >6 months exposure to PCP-containing pesticides. The investigators, who were based in a hospital immunology department, did not indicate the circumstances under which the patients had originally presented themselves. Presumably the patients had symptoms of suspected immune dysfunction, although those with chronic infections, rheumatic diseases, or other chronic diseases were excluded from the study population. *In vitro* responses to mitogenic and allogenic stimulation were determined in 163 patients, lymphocyte subpopulations in 157 patients, plasma neopterin levels in 118 patients, and plasma cytokine and cytokine receptor levels in 100 patients. By the criteria for impaired lymphocyte stimulation established within the study, a significantly greater fraction of patients with blood PCP > 10 µg/l exhibited impairment than those with blood PCP $\leq$ 10 µg/l (91/133 vs. 15/30, $p < 0.05$). In addition, IL-8 levels were reported to correlate with blood PCP levels. Finally, all 11 patients with both impaired lymphocyte stimulation and an abnormally low CD4/CD8 ratio had blood PCP levels > 10 µg/l. Although the results of this study are intriguing, the presentation of data was far too incomplete to engender confidence in the results. Also, in the absence of a comparison group consisting of persons chosen from the general population, it is not possible to assess the clinical relevance of the study findings. These and other problems with the study were discussed by Triebig (1997).

Neurotoxicity A longitudinal study of nerve conduction velocity (NCV) in the peripheral nervous system was performed by Triebig *et al.* (1987) in 10 chemical-company workers in Germany. The 7 men and 3 women had been in contact with PCP for a duration of 4–24 years (mean, 16 years). NCV values measured in 1980 and 1984 and were in the low-normal range; mean serum PCP levels were 368 µg/l in 1980 and 346 µg/l in 1984. The only conclusion that can be drawn from the results is that four additional years of PCP exposure apparently did not diminish NCV in subjects with ongoing occupational exposure to PCP. The study did not address the question of whether PCP exposure was at all related to the clinically unremarkable finding of low-normal NCV values.

Peper *et al.* (1999) identified 15 women who met the following criteria: residential exposure to wood-preserving chemicals for > 5 years, serum PCP > 25 µg/l, and serum lindane > 0.1 µg/l. This cohort of PCP-exposed women was drawn from a population of 2000 women presenting with infertility or gynecological problems. The exposure group was matched pairwise (for age, education, demographics, and education) with a control group of 15 women drawn from the same population. Subjective complaints were ascertained by questionnaire. Although a variety of the self-reported complaints surveyed were significantly higher in the exposure group, the investigators found that none was meaningfully correlated with serum PCP level. Standardized tests of cognitive function, psychomotor speed, attention, learning, and memory were administered. The PCP exposure group did significantly less well than the controls on several subtests. A rank correlation analysis of subtest score vs. serum PCP level revealed significant negative correlations for four subtests: reading speed, naming speed, paired associations, and visual retention. Unfortunately, the raw data were not supplied and the investigators apparently did not examine to data to discover whether an effect threshold could be discerned (i.e., a serum PCP level below which the correlations would be absent). Given the potential importance of the finding that neurobehavioral test scores were correlated with serum PCP, the study warrants repeating with a larger sample size, a higher ratio of controls to exposed, and a more detailed analysis of the relationship between serum PCP and the outcome variables.

Endocrine Toxicity   Gerhard *et al.* (1999) conducted a study of endocrine parameters in a cohort of 171 women presenting with infertility, a gynecological problem, or an endocrine problem with gynecologic ramifications. Serum PCP levels > 20 µg/l were measured for 65 of the women; these were considered to be the exposed population. The control group consisted of 105 women with serum PCP < 20 µg/l, matched for age, underlying condition, and geographical region. It is difficult to understand what was meant by matching on the basis of "underlying condition" because in the exposure group relative to the controls, primary infertility was under-represented (26% vs. 58%) while habitual abortions (22% vs. 8%) and alopecia (22% vs. 0.9%) were over-represented. The investigators reported that the exposed and control populations had significantly different levels of various hormones. However, all differences in mean values were small and almost certainly clinically unimportant. For example, mean ($\pm$SD) values of FSH were 7.8 $\pm$ 12.2 mE/ml in the exposure group and 8.1 $\pm$ 7.5 mE/ml in the controls, while the normal range was given as 1–10 mE/ml. Despite the low p value reported for the comparison (0.005), it is doubtful that the observed difference was meaningful. At a minimum, the investigators should have investigated the reproducibility of intergroup differences in measurements made at different times.

Reproductive Toxicity   Dimich-Ward *et al.* (1996) identified 19,675 births in British Columbia between 1952 and 1988 as the children of a cohort of 9512 fathers with potential exposure to PCP prior to the births. The fathers were part of a larger cohort of men who had worked at least one year in a sawmill where chlorophenate wood preservatives had been used. A nested case-referent (i.e., case-control) strategy was adopted. Five referents were matched for birth year; gender was either matched or treated as a covariate. The investigators indicated that the referents "were selected from all the offspring at risk when the case occurred." Presumably this meant all births recorded in British Columbia during the appropriate year. Chlorophenate exposure for three cumulative exposure periods (two preconception, one postconception) and maximal annual preconception exposure were estimated for each father for each birth. The investigators calculated odds ratios for five major indicators of reproductive health and 18 categories of congenital anomalies. The criterion for statistical significance was $p < 0.05$ (two-tailed test). None of the reproductive health indicators (prematurity, small size, low birthweight, stillbirth, or neonatal death) was significantly associated with any measure of chlorophenate exposure. Two of the congenital-anomaly categories were positively associated ($p < 0.05$) with one

exposure measure: increased incidence of anenceephaly/spina bifida was associated with maximal preconception exposure (OR = 1.11) and increased incidence of genital-organ anomalies was associated with cumulative exposure during pregnancy (OR = 1.05). One of the congenital-anomaly categories was *negatively* associated ($p < 0.05$) with one exposure measure: decreased incidence of other limb was associated with maximal preconception exposure. Considering the number of comparisons made (18 $\times$ 4 = 72), 1 or 2 positive and 1 or 2 negative associations with two-tailed p values <0.05 would be expected to arise by chance (2.5% of 72 = 1.8). Thus, the above results are consistent with no effect of chlorophenates. However, congenital anomalies of the eye exhibited positive associations with three exposure measures, and two of these were highly significant ($p < 0.005$): increased incidence of eye anomalies with cumulative exposure 3 months prior to conception (OR = 2.01) and during pregnancy (OR = 1.21). Analysis by subcategories revealed that the associations pertained primarily to cataracts and the relative risk for cataracts was significantly greater in those with the most exposure (75th percentile) than those with the least (25th percentile).

The results of Dimich-Ward *et al.* (1996) suggest that congenital cataracts may be related to paternal chlorophenate exposure occurring prior to conception and during pregnancy. If this relationship turns out to be real, it will be important to discover whether the causative agent is PCP, its technical-grade impurities, or some other chlorophenate. Despite the slant of the investigators, the study results do not necessarily indicate an effect on the male reproductive system. Alternative explanations exist, including the possibility that the causative agent contaminated the residential environment and was absorbed by the mother, impacting her reproductive function or affecting the fetus directly.

ACKNOWLEDGMENT

The author evaluated many of the studies discussed in this chapter while a Staff Toxicologist in the Medical Toxicology Branch of the California Environmental Protection Agency's Department of Pesticide Regulation (DPR) during the years 1993 to 1996. She wishes to thank two former colleagues in the Medical Toxicology Branch, Charles N. Aldous, Ph.D. and Earl Meierhenry, D.V.M., Ph.D. for the valuable gift of their counsel. Dr. Aldous performed initial data review on the major PCP toxicology studies, identifying any deficiencies in methodology or in the reporting of results. At numerous times during the course of evaluating PCP toxicology studies, the author called upon Dr. Meierhenry to contribute his insight and expertise as a veterinary pathologist.

REFERENCES

Ahlborg, U. G., Lindgren, J.-E., and Mercier, M. (1974). Metabolism of pentachlorophenol. *Arch. Toxicol.* **32**, 271–281.

Ahlborg, U. G., and Larsson, K. (1978). Metabolism of tetrachlorophenols in the rat. *Arch. Toxicol.* **40**, 63–74.

Ahlborg, U. G., Larsson, K., and Thunberg, T. (1978). Metabolism of pentachlorophenol *in vivo* and *in vitro*. *Arch. Toxicol.* **40**, 45–53.

Armstrong, R. W., Eichner, E. R., Klein, D. E., Barthel, W. F., *et al.* (1969). Pentachlorophenol poisoning in a nursery for newborn infants. II. Epidemiologic and toxicologic studies. *J. Pediatr.* **75**, 317–325.

Arrhenius, E., Renberg, L., Johansson, L., and Zetterqvist, M.-A. (1977). Disturbance of microsomal detoxication mechanisms in liver by chlorophenol pesticides. *Chem.–Biol. Interactions* **18**, 35–46.

Ashby, J. (1993). Gambling and the conduct of genetic toxicology tests. *Mutation Res.* **319**, 151–153.

Bannasch, P., Griesemer, R. A., Anders, F., Becker, R., Cabral, J. R., et al. (1986). Early preneoplastic lesions. *In* "Long-Term and Short-Term Assays for Carcinogens: A Critical Appraisal," IARC Scientific Publications No. 83, pp. 85–101. International Agency for Research on Cancer, Lyon.

Bauchinger, M., Dresp, J., Schmid, E., and Hauf, R. (1982). Chromosome changes in lymphocytes after occupational exposure to pentachlorophenol (PCP). *Mutation Res.* **102**, 83–88.

Beard, A. P., and Rawlings, N. C. (1998). Reproductive effects in mink (Mustela vison) exposed to the pesticides lindane, carbofuran and pentachlorophenol in a multigeneration study. *J. Reprod. Fertility* **113**, 95–104.

Beard, A. P., McRae, A. C., and Rawlings, N. C. (1997). Reproductive efficiency in mink (Mustela vison) treated with the pesticides lindane, carbofuran and pentachlorophenol. *J. Reprod. Fertility* **111**, 21–28.

Beard, A. P., Bartlewski, P. M., and Rawlings, N. C. (1999a). Endocrine and reproductive function in ewes exposed to the organochlorine pesticides lindane or pentachlorophenol. *J. Toxicol. Environ. Health* **56**, 23–46.

Beard, A. P., Bartlewski, P. M., Chandolia, A., Honaramooz, A., and Rawlings, N. C. (1999b). Endocrine and reproductive function in ewes exposed to the organochlorine pesticides lindane or pentachlorophenol. *J. Reprod. Fertil.* **115**, 303–414.

Bergner, H., Constantinidis, P., and Martin, J. H. (1965). Industrial pentachlorophenol poisoning in Winnipeg. *Can. Med. Assoc. J.* **92**, 448–451. As cited in U.S. EPA, 1991 (op. cit.).

Blakley, B. R., Yole, M. J., Brousseau, P., Boermans, H., and Fournier, M. (1998). Effect of pentachlorophenol on immune function. *Toxicology* **125**, 141–148.

Boberg, E. W., Liem, A., Miller, E. C., and Miller, J. A. (1987). Inhibition by pentachlorophenol of the initiating and promoting activities of 1'-hydroxysafrole for the formation of enzyme-altered foci and tumors in rat liver. *Carcinogenesis* **8**, 531–539.

Borzelleca, J. F., Hayes, J. R., Condie, L. W., and Egle, J. L., Jr. (1985). Acute toxicity of monochlorophenols, dichlorophenols and pentachlorophenol in the mouse. *Toxicol. Lett.* **29**, 39–42.

Braun, W. H., and Sauerhoff, M. W. (1976). The pharmacokinetic profile of pentachlorophenol in monkeys. *Toxicol. Appl. Pharmacol.* **38**, 525–533.

Braun, W. H., Young, J. D., Blau, G. E., and Gehring, P. J. (1977). The pharmacokinetics and metabolism of pentachlorophenol in rats. *Toxicol. Appl. Pharmacol.* **41**, 395–406.

Braun, W. H., Blau, G. E., and Chenoweth, M. B. (1979). The metabolism/pharmacokinetics of pentachlorophenol in man, and a comparison with the rat and monkey. *In* "Toxicology and Occupational Medicine" (W. B. Deichmann, ed.), pp. 289–296. Elsevier/North Holland, New York.

Brian, W. R., Sari, M. A. Iwasaki, M., Shimada, T., Kaminsky, L. S., and Guengerich, F. P. (1990). Catalytic activities of human liver cytochrome P-450 IIA4 expressed in *Saccharomyces cerevisiae*. *Biochemistry* **29**, 11280–11292.

Budavari, S. (ed.) (1996). "The Merck Index," 12th ed., p. 1222. Merck & Co., Whitehouse Station, NJ.

Carstens, C.-P., Blum, J. K., and Witte, I. (1990). The role of hydroxyl radicals in tetrachlorohydroquinone induced DNA strand break formation in PM2 DNA and human fibroblasts. *Chem.–Biol. Interactions* **74**, 305–314.

Casarett, L. J., Bevenue, A., Yauger, W. L., Jr., and Whalen, S. A. (1969). Observations on pentachlorophenol in human blood and urine. *Am. Indust. Hyg. Assoc. J.* **30**, 360–366.

Chhabra, R. S., Maronpot, R. M., Bucher, J. R., Haseman, J. K., Toft, J. D., and Hejtmancik, M. R. (1999). Toxicology and carcinogenesis studies of pentachlorophenol in rats. *Toxicol. Sci.* **48**, 14–20.

Christ, D. D., and Walle, T. (1989). Stereoselective sulfation of R,S-4'-hydroxypropranolol by canine hepatic cytosol and partially purified phenolsulfotransferases. *J. Pharmacol. Exp. Ther.* **251**, 949–955.

Colosio, C., Maroni, M., Barcellini, W., Meroni, P., et al. (1993). Toxicological and immune findings in workers exposed to pentachlorophenol (PCP). *Arch. Environ. Health* **48**, 81–88.

Cooper, R. G., and Macauley, M. B. (1982). Pentachlorophenol pancreatitis. *Lancet* **1**, 517.

Dahlhaus, M., Almstadt, E., and Appel, K. E. (1994). The pentachlorophenol metabolite tetrachloro-p-hydroquinone induces the formation of 8-hydroxy-2-deoxyguanosine in liver DNA of male B6C3F1 mice. *Toxicol. Lett.* **74**, 265–274.

Dahlhaus, M., Almstadt, E., Henschke, P., Lüttgert, S., and Appel, K. E. (1995). Induction of 8-hydroxy-2-deoxyguanosine and single-strand breaks in DNA of V79 cells by tetrachloro-p-hydroquinone. *Mutation Res.* **329**, 29–36.

Dahlhaus, M., Almstadt, E., Henschke, P., Lüttgert, S., and Appel, K. E. (1996). Oxidative DNA lesions in V79 cells mediated by pentachlorophenol metabolites. *Arch. Toxicol.* **70**, 457–460.

Daimon, H., Sawada, S., Asakura, S., and Sagami, F. (1997–98). Inhibition of sulfotransferase affecting *in vivo* genotoxicity and DNA adducts induced by safrole in rat liver. *Teratog. Carcinog. Mutagen.* **17**, 327–337.

Daniel, V., Huber, W., Bauer, K., and Opelz, G. (1995). Impaired *in-vitro* lymphocyte responses in patients with elevated pentachlorophenol (PCP) levels. *Arch. Environ. Health* **50**, 287–292.

De Maeyer, J., Schepens, P. J. C., Jorens, P. G., and Verstraete, R. (1995). Exposure to pentachlorophenol as a possible cause of miscarriages. *Brit. J. Obs. Gyn.* **102**, 1010–1011.

Dimich-Ward, H., Hertzman, C., Teschke, K., Hershler, R., Marion, S. A., Ostry, A., Kelly, S. (1996). Reproductive effects of paternal exposure to chlorophenate wood preservatives in the sawmill industry. *Scand. J. Work Environ. Health* **22**, 267–273.

Economist Intelligence Unit (1981). "Economic Implications of Abatement Measures of Water Pollution Due to Hexachlorobutadiene, Endosulfan, Trichlorophenol, and Pentachlorophenol." Report prepared for Environment and Consumer Protection Service, Commission of the European Communities, Brussels. As cited in WHO, 1987 (op. cit.).

Edgerton, T. R., and Moseman, R. F. (1979). Determination of pentachlorophenol in urine: the importance of hydrolysis. *J. Agric. Food Chem.* **27**, 197–199.

Ehrlich, W. (1990). The effect of pentachlorophenol and its metabolite tetrachlorohydroquinone on cell growth and the induction of DNA damage in Chinese hamster ovary cells. *Mutation Res.* **244**, 299–302.

Engst, R., Macholz, R. M., Kujaws, M., Lewerenz, H.-J., and Plass, R. (1976). The metabolism of lindane and its metabolites gamma-2,3,4,5,6-pentachlorocyclohexane, pentachlorobenzene, and pentachlorophenol in rats and the pathways of lindane metabolism. *J. Environ. Sci. Health* **11**, 95–117.

Eriksson, M., Hardell, L., and Adami, H. O. (1990). Exposure to dioxins as a risk factor for soft tissue sarcoma: A population-based case-control study. *J. Natl. Cancer Inst.* **82**, 486–490.

Exon, J. H., and Koller, L. D. (1983). Effects of chlorinated phenols on immunity in rats. *Int. J. Immunopharmacol.* **5**, 131–136.

Fahrig, R., Nilsson, C.-A., and Rappe, C. (1978). Genetic activity of chlorophenols and chlorophenol impurities. *In* "Pentachlorophenol: Chemistry, Pharmacology, and Environmental Toxicology" (K. R. Rao, ed.), pp. 325–338. Plenum, New York.

Fahrig, R., and Steinkamp-Zucht, A. (1996). Co-recombinogenic and antimutagenic effects of diethylhexylphthalate, inactiveness of pentachlorophenol in the spot test with mice. *Mutation Res.* **354**, 59–67.

Fennell, T. R., Wiseman, R. W., Miller, J. A., and Miller, E. C. (1985). Major role of hepatic sulfotransferase activity in the metabolic activation, DNA adduct formation, and carcinogenicity of 1'-hydroxy-2',3'-dehydroestragole in infant male C57BL/6J x C3H/HeJ F1 mice. *Cancer Res.* **45**, 5310–5320.

Fingerhut, M. A., Halperin, W. E., Marlow, D. A., Piacitelli, L. A., et al. (1991). Cancer mortality in workers exposed to 2,3,7,8-tetrachlorodibenzo-p-dioxin. *N. Engl. J. Med.* **324**, 212–218.

Gaines, T. (1969). Acute toxicity of pesticides. *Toxicol. Appl. Pharmacol.* **14**, 515–534.

Galloway, S. M., Armstrong, M. J., Reuben, C., Colman, S., Brown, B., Cannon, C., Bloom, A. D., Nakamura, F., Ahmed, M., Duk, S., Rimpo, J., Margolin, B. H., Resnick, M. A., Anderson, B., and Zeiger, E. (1987). Chromosome aberrations and sister chromatid exchanges in Chinese hamster ovary cells: Evaluations of 108 chemicals. *Environ. Molec. Mutagen.* **10**(Suppl. 10), 1–175.

Gasiewicz, T. A. (1991). Pentachlorophenol. In "Handbook of Pesticide Toxicology, Volume 3" (W. J. Hayes and E. R. Laws, eds.), pp. 1206–1216. Academic Press, San Diego.

Gerhard, I., Frick, A., Monga, B., and Runnebaum, B. (1999). Pentachlorophenol exposure in women with gynecological and endocrine dysfunction. *Environ. Res.* **30**, 383–388.

Gómez-Catalán, J., To-Figueras, J., Rodamilans, M., and Corbella, J. (1991). Transport of organochlorine residues in the rat and human blood. *Arch. Environ. Contam. Toxicol.* **20**, 61–66.

Goodman, G., Aldous, C. N., and Rech, C. J. (1998). "Pentachlorophenol (PCP): Risk Characterization Document." Medical Toxicology and Worker Health & Safety Branches, Department of Pesticide Regulation, California Environmental Protection Agency.

Gopalaswamy, U. V., and Aiyar, A. S. (1986). Biotransformation and toxicity of lindane and its metabolite hexachlorobenzene in mammals. In "Hexachlorobenzene: Proceedings of an International Symposium," IARC Scientific Publications No. 77 (C. R. Morris and J. R. P. Cabral, eds.), pp. 267–276. International Agency for Research on Cancer, Lyon.

Gopalaswamy, U. V., and Nair, C. K. K. (1992). DNA binding and mutagenicity of lindane and its metabolites. *Bull. Environ. Contam. Toxicol.* **49**, 300–305.

Gordon, D. (1956). How dangerous is pentachlorophenol? *Med. J. Austral.* **43**, 485–488. As cited in U.S. EPA, 1991 (*op. cit.*).

Hakkola, J., Pasanen, M., Purkunen, R. Saarikoski, S., Pelkonen, O., Maenpaa, J., Rane, A., and Raunio, H. (1994). Expression of xenobiotic-metabolizing cytochrome P450 forms in human adult and fetal liver. *Biochem. Pharmacol.* **48**, 59–64.

Hardell, L., Eriksson, M., Lenner, P., and Lundgren, E. (1981). Malignant lymphoma and exposure to chemicals, especially organic solvents, chlorophenols and phenoxy acids: A case-control study. *Brit. J. Cancer* **43**, 169–176.

Hardell, L., Eriksson, M., and Degerman, A. (1994). Exposure to phenoxyacetic acids, chlorophenols, or organic solvents in relation to histopathology, stage, and anatomical localization of non-Hodgkin's Lymphoma. *Cancer Res.* **54**, 2386–2389.

Haworth, S., Lawlor, T., Mortelmans, K., Speck, W., and Zeiger, E. (1983). *Salmonella* mutagenicity test results for 250 chemicals. *Environ. Mutagen.* **5**(Suppl. 1), 3–142. As cited in NTP, 1989 (*op. cit.*).

Hay, A., and Singer, C. R. J. (1991). Wood preservatives, solvents, and thrombocytopenic purpura (Letter). *Lancet* **338**, 766.

Hoben, H. J., Ching, S. A., and Casarett, L. J. (1976a). A study of inhalation of pentachlorophenol by rats IV. Distribution and excretion of inhaled pentachlorophenol. *Bull. Environ. Contam. Toxicol.* **15**, 466–474.

Hoben, H. J., Ching, S. A., Young, R. A., and Casarett, L. J. (1976b). A study of the inhalation of pentachlorophenol by rats, part V. A protein binding study of pentachlorophenol. *Bull. Environ. Contam. Toxicol.* **16**, 225–232.

Hoben, H. J., Ching, S. A., and Casarett, L. J. (1976c). A study of inhalation of pentachlorophenol by rats III. Inhalation toxicity study. *Bull. Environ. Contam. Toxicol.* **15**, 463–465.

Hoberman, A. M. (1994a). "Developmental Toxicity (Embryo-Fetal Toxicity and Teratogenic Potential) Study of Pentachlorophenol Administered Orally via Gavage to Crl:CD® BR VAF/Plus® Presumed Pregnant Rats." Argus Research Laboratories, Horsham, PA.

Hoberman, A. M. (1994b). "Developmental Toxicity (Embryo-Fetal Toxicity and Teratogenic Potential) Study of Pentachlorophenol Administered Orally via Stomach Tube to New Zealand White Rabbits." Argus Research Laboratories, Horsham, PA.

Holsapple, M. P., McNerney, P. J., and McCay, J. A. (1984). Suppression of humoral antibody production by exposure to 1,2,3,6,7,8-hexachlordibenzo-*p*-dioxin. *J. Pharmacol. Exp. Therap.* **231**, 518–526.

Holsapple, M. P., McNerney, P. J., and McCay, J. A. (1987). Effects of pentachlorophenol on the *in vitro* and *in vivo* antibody response. *J. Toxicol. Environ. Health* **20**, 229–239.

IPCS (International Programme on Chemical Safety) (1987). "Environmental Health Criteria," Vol. 71, *Pentachlorophenol.* World Health Organization, Geneva.

Ishidate, M., Jr. (1988). "Data Book of Chromosomal Aberration Test *in Vitro*," revised edition (English translation), pp. 312–313. Elsevier, New York. As cited in Seiler, 1991 (*op. cit.*).

Jakobson, I., and Yllner, S. (1971). Metabolism of ^{14}C-pentachlorophenol in the mouse. *Acta Pharmacol. Toxicol.* **29**, 513–524.

Jansson, K., and Jansson, V. (1986). Inability of chlorophenols to induce 6-thioguanine-resistant mutants in V79 Chinese hamster cells. *Mutation Res.* **171**, 165–168.

Jansson, K., and Jansson, V. (1991). Induction of mutation in V79 Chinese hamster cells by tetrachlorohydroquinone, a metabolite of pentachlorophenol. *Mutation Res.* **260**, 83–87.

Jansson, K., and Jansson, V. (1992). Induction of micronuclei in V79 Chinese hamster cells by tetrachlorohydroquinone, a metabolite of pentachlorophenol. *Mutation Res.* **279**, 205–208.

Jekat, F. W., Meisel, M. L., Eckard, R., and Winterhoff, H. (1994). Effects of pentachlorophenol (PCP) on the pituitary and thyroidal hormone regulation in the rat. *Toxicol. Lett.* **71**, 9–25.

Jones, P. A. (1981). "Chlorophenols and Their Impurities in the Canadian Environment." Rep. EPS 3-EC-81-2, Environment Canada, Ottawa. As cited in WHO, 1987 (*op. cit.*).

Juhl, U., Witte, I., and Butte, W. (1985). Metabolism of pentachlorophenol to tetrachlorohydroquinone by human liver homogenate. *Bull. Environ. Contam. Toxicol.* **35**, 596–601.

Kedderis, G. L., Dyroff, M. C., and Rickert, D. E. (1984). Hepatic macromolecular covalent binding of the hepatocarcinogen 2,6,-dinitrotoluene and its 2,4-isomer *in vivo*: Modulation by the sulfotransferase inhibitors pentachlorophenol and 2,6-dichloro-4-nitrophenol. *Carcinogenesis* **5**, 1199–1204.

Kerkvliet, N. I., Baecher-Steppan, L., and Schmitz, J. A. (1982a). Immunotoxicity of pentachlorophenol (PCP): Increased susceptibility to tumor growth in adult mice fed technical PCP-contaminated diets. *Toxicol. Appl. Pharmacol.* **62**, 55–64.

Kerkvliet, N. I., Baecher-Steppan, L., Claycomb, A. T., Craig, A. M., and Sheggeby, G. G. (1982b). Immunotoxicity of technical pentachlorophenol (PCP-T): Depressed humoral immune responses to T-dependent and T-independent antigen stimulation in PCP-T exposed mice. *Fundam. Appl. Toxicol.* **2**, 90–99.

Kerkvliet, N. I., Brauner, J. A., and Matlock, J. P. (1985). Humoral immunotoxicity of polychlorinated diphenyl ethers, phenoxyphenols, dioxins and furans present as contaminants of technical grade pentachlorophenol. *Toxicology* **36**, 307–324.

Kleiman de Pisarev, D. L., del Carmen Rios de Molina, M., and San Martin de Viale, L. C. (1990). Thyroid function and thyroxine metabolism in hexachlorobenzene-induced porphyria. *Biochem. Pharmacol.* **39**, 817–825.

Klemmer, H. W., Wong, L., Sato, M. M., Reichert, E. L., Korsak, R. J., and Rashad, M. N. (1980). Clinical findings in workers exposed to pentachlorophenol. *Arch. Environ. Contam. Toxicol.* **9**, 715–725.

Kroese, E. D., van de Poll, M. L., Mulder, G. J., and Meerman, J. H. (1988). The role of *N*-sulfation in the *N*-hydroxy-2-acetylaminofluorene-mediated outgrowth of diethylnitrosamine-initiated hepatocytes to gamma-glutamyltranspeptidase-positive foci in male rat liver. *Carcinogenesis* **9**, 1953–1958.

Kurtz, P. J., and Hejtmancik, M. R., Jr. (1993). "Current In-Life Data and the 27-Week Interim Sacrifice Data Summary (Abbreviated) For the Chronic Dosed-Feed Study of Pentachlorophenol in F344 Rats." Battelle, Columbus, under contract to the National Toxicology Program.

Lang, D., and Mueller-Ruchholtz, W. (1991). Human lymphocyte reactivity after *in vitro* exposure to technical and analytical grade pentachlorophenol. *Toxicology* **70**, 271–282.

Lin, P.-H., Waidyanatha, S., Pollack, G. M., Swenberg, J. A., and Rappaport, S. M. (1999). Dose-specific production of chlorinated quinone and semiquinone adducts in rodent livers following administration of pentachlorophenol. *Toxicol. Sci.* **47**, 126–133.

McConnachie, P. R., and Zahalsky, A. C. (1991). Immunological consequences of exposure to pentachlorophenol. *Arch. Environ. Health* **46**, 249–253.

McConnell, E. E., Moore, J. A., Gupta, B. N., Rakes, A. H., Luster, M. I., Goldstein, J. A., Haseman, J. K., and Parker C. E. (1980). The chronic toxicity of technical and analytical pentachlorophenol in cattle. I. Clinicopathology. *Toxicol. Appl. Pharmacol.* **52**, 468–490.

McConnell, E. E., Huff, J. E., Hejtmancik, M., Peters, A. C., and Persing, R. (1991). Toxicology and carcinogenesis studies of two grades of pentachlorophenol in B6C3F$_1$ mice. *Fund. Appl. Toxicol.* **17**, 519–532.

Meerman, J. H., Beland, F. A., and Mulder, G. J. (1981). Role of sulfation in the formation of DNA adducts from *N*-hydroxy-2-acetylaminofluorene in rat liver *in vivo*. Inhibition of *N*-acetylated aminofluorene adduct formation by pentachlorophenol. *Carcinogenesis* **2**, 413–416.

Meerman, J. H. N., Sterenborg, H. M. J., and Mulder, G. J. (1983). Use of pentachlorophenol as long-term inhibitor of sulfation of phenols and hydroxamic acids in the rat *in vivo*. *Biochem. Pharmacol.* **32**, 1587–1593.

Mehmood, Z., Williamson, M. P., Kelly, D. E., and Kelly, S. L. (1996). Metabolism of organochlorine pesticides: The role of human cytochrome P450 3A4. *Chemosphere* **33**, 759–769.

Menon, J. A. (1958). Tropical hazards associated with the use of pentachlorophenol. *Brit. Med. J.* **1**, 1156–1158. As cited in U.S. EPA, 1991 (*op. cit.*).

Mirvish, S. S., Nickols, J., Weisenburger, D. D., Johnson, D., Joshi, S. S., Kaplan, P., Gross, M., and Tong, H. Y. (1991). Effects of 2,4,5-trichlorophenoxyacetic acid, pentachlorophenol, methylprednisolone, and Freund's adjuvant on 2-hydroxyethylnitrosourea carcinogenesis in MRC-Wistar rats. *J. Toxicol. Environ. Health* **32**, 59–74.

Monteith, D. K. (1992). Inhibition of sulfotransferase affecting unscheduled DNA synthesis induced by 2-acetylaminofluorene: An *in vivo* and *in vitro* comparison. *Mutation Res.* **282**, 253–258.

Moorthy, B., and Randerath, K. (1996). Pentachlorophenol enhances 9-hydroxybenzo[a]pyrene-induced hepatic DNA adduct formation *in vivo* and inhibits microsomal epoxide hydrolase and glutathione S-transferase activities *in vitro*: likely inhibition of epoxide detoxification by pentachlorophenol. *Arch. Toxicol.* **70**, 696–703.

Naito, S., Ono, Y., Somiya, I., Inoue, S., Ito, K., Yamamoto, K., and Kawanishi, S. (1994). Role of active oxygen species in DNA damage by pentachlorophenol metabolites. *Mutation Res.* **310**, 79–88.

National Toxicology Program (NTP) (1989). "Toxicology and Carcinogenesis Studies of Two Pentachlorophenol Technical-Grade Mixtures (CAS No. 87-86-5) in B6C3F$_1$ Mice (Feed Studies)." Technical Rep. TR-349.

National Toxicology Program (NTP) (1999). "Toxicology and Carcinogenesis Studies of Pentachlorophenol (CAS No. 87-86-5) in F344/N Rats (Feed Studies)." Technical Rep. TR-483.

Nishimura, N., Nishimura, H., and Oshima, H. (1982). Survey on mutagenicity of pesticides by the *Salmonella*-microsome test. *Aichi Ika Daigaku Igakukai Zasshi (J. Aichi Med. Univ. Ass.)* **10**, 305–312. As cited in NTP, 1989 (*op. cit.*).

Osterloh, J., Letz, G., Pond, S., and Becker, C. (1983). An assessment of the potential testicular toxicity of 10 pesticides using the mouse-sperm morphology assay. *Mutation Res.* **116**, 407–415.

Paine, A. J. (1995). Heterogeneity of cytochrome P450 and its toxicological significance. *Human Exper. Toxicol.* **14**, 1–7.

Pearce, N. E., Smith, A. H., Howard, J. K., Sheppard, R. A., Giles, H. J., and Teague, C. A. (1986a). Non-Hodgkin's lymphoma and exposure to phenoxyherbicides, chlorophenols, fencing work, and meat works employment: A case-control study. *Brit. J. Indust. Med.* **43**, 75–83.

Pearce, N. E., Smith, A. H., Howard, J. K., Sheppard, R. A., Giles, H. J., and Teague, C. A. (1986b). Case-control study of multiple myeloma and farming. *Brit. J. Cancer* **54**, 493–500.

Pearce, N. E., Sheppard, R. A., Smith, A. H., and Teague, C. A. (1987). Non-Hodgkin's lymphoma and farming: An expanded case-control study. *Int. J. Cancer* **39**, 155–161.

Peper, M., Ertl, M., and Gerhard, I. (1999). Long-term exposure to wood-preserving chemicals containing pentachlorophenol and lindane is related to neurobehavioral performance in women. *Amer. J. Indust. Med.* **35**, 632–641.

Ramlow, J. M., Spadacene, N. W., Hoag, S. R., Stafford, B. A., Cartmill, J. B., and Lerner, P. J. (1996). Mortality in a cohort of pentachlorophenol manufacturing workers, 1940–1989. *Amer. J. Indust. Med.* **30**, 180–194.

Randerath, K., Bi, J., Mabon, N., Sriram, P., and Moorthy, B. (1994). Strong intensification of mouse hepatic tamoxifen DNA adduct formation by pretreatment with the sulfotransferase inhibitor and ubiquitous environmental pollutant pentachlorophenol. *Carcinogenesis* **15**, 797–800.

Rawlings, N. C., Cook, S. J., and Waldbillig, D. (1998). Effects of the pesticides carbofuran, chlorpyrifos, dimethoate, lindane, triallate, trifuralin, 2,4-D, and pentachlorophenol on the metabolic endocrine and reproductive endocrine system in ewes. *J. Toxicol. Environ. Health* **54**, 21–36.

Reigner, B. G., Gungon, R. S., Hoag, M. K., and Tozer, T. N. (1991). Pentachlorophenol toxicokinetics after intravenous and oral administration to rat. *Xenobiotica* **21**, 1547–1558.

Reigner, B. G., Rigod, J. F., and Tozer, T. N. (1992a). Disposition, bioavailability, and serum protein binding of pentachlorophenol in the B6C3F$_1$ mouse. *Pharmaceut. Res.* **9**, 1053–1057.

Reigner, B. G., Bois, F. Y., and Tozer, T. N. (1992b). Assessment of pentachlorophenol exposure in humans using the clearance concept. *Human Exp. Toxicol.* **11**, 17–26.

Renner, G., Hopfer, C., and Gokel, J. M. (1986). Acute toxicities of pentachlorophenol, pentachloroanisole, tetrachlorohydroquinone, tetrachlorocatechol, tetrachlororesorcinol, tetrachlorodimethoxybenzenes and tetrachlorobenzenediol diacetates administered to mice. *Toxicol. Environ. Chem.* **11**, 37–50.

Renner, G., Hopfer, C., Gokel, J. M., Braun, S., and Mücke, W. (1987). Subacute toxicity studies on pentachlorophenol (PCP), and the isomeric tetrachlorobenzenediols tetrachlorohydroquinone (TCH), tetrachlorocatechol (TCC), and tetrachlororesorcinol (TCR). *Toxicol. Environ. Chem.* **15**, 301–312.

Roberts, H. J. (1983). Aplastic anemia and red cell aplasia due to pentachlorophenol. *Southern Med. J.* **76**, 45–48.

Roberts, H. J. (1990). Pentachlorophenol-associated aplastic anemia, red cell aplasia, leukemia and other blood disorders. *J. Florida M. A.* **77**, 86–90.

Roberts, H. J. (1997). Effects of pentachlorophenol exposure. *Lancet* **340**, 1917.

Robson, A. M., Kissane, J. M., Elvick, N. H., and Pundavela, L. (1969). Pentachlorophenol poisoning in a nursery for newborn infants. I. Clinical features and treatment. *J. Pediatr.* **75**, 309–316.

Rozman, K., Gorski, J. R., Rozman, P., and Parkinson, A. (1986). Reduced serum thyroid hormone levels in hexachlorobenzene-induced porphyria. *Toxicol. Lett.* **30**, 71–78.

Rugman, F. P., and Cosstick, R. (1990). Aplastic anaemia associated with organochlorine pesticides: Case reports and review of evidence. *J. Clin. Pathol.* **43**, 98–101.

Sai, K., Upham, B. L., Kang, K.-S., Hasegawa, R., Inoue, T., and Trosko, J. E. (1998). Inhibitory effect of pentachlorophenol on gap junctional intercellular communication in rat liver epithelial cells *in vitro*. *Cancer Lett.* **130**, 9–17.

Sai-Kato, K., Umemura, T., Takagi, A., Hasegawa, R., Tanimura, A., and Kurokawa, Y. (1995). Pentachlorophenol-induced oxidative DNA damage in mouse liver and protective effect of antioxidants. *Fd. Chem. Toxicol.* **33**, 877–882.

Samokyszyn, V. M., Freeman, J. P., Maddipati, K. R., and Lloyd, R. V. (1995). Peroxidase-catalyzed oxidation of pentachlorophenol. *Chem. Res. Toxicol.* **8**, 349–355.

Scanlon, M. F., and Toft, A. D. (1996). Regulation of thyrotropin secretion. *In* "Werner and Ingbar's The Thyroid," 7th ed. (L. E. Braverman and R. D. Utiger, eds.), pp. 220–240. Lippincott-Raven, Philadelphia.

Schwetz, B. A., Keeler, P. A., and Gehring, P. J. (1974). The effect of purified and commercial grade pentachlorophenol on rat embryonal and fetal development. *Toxicol. Appl. Pharmacol.* **28**, 151–161.

Schwetz, B. A., Quast, J. F., Keeler, P. A., Humiston, C. G., and Kociba, R. J. (1978). Results of two-year toxicity and reproduction studies on pentachlorophenol in rats. *In* "Pentachlorophenol: Chemistry, Pharmacology, and Environmental Toxicology" (K. R. Rao, ed.), pp. 301–309. Plenum, New York.

Seiler, J. P. (1991). Pentachlorophenol. *Mutation Res.* **257**, 27–47.

Sewall, C. H., Flagler, N., Vanden Heuvel, J. P., Clark, G. C., Tritscher, A. M., Maronpot, R. M., and Lucier, G. W. (1995). Alterations in thyroid function in female Sprague–Dawley rats following chronic treatment with 2,3,7,8-tetrachlorodibenzo-*p*-dioxin. *Toxicol. Appl. Pharmacol.* **132**, 237–244.

Shinohara, A. Saito, K., Yamazoe, Y., Kamataki, T., and Kato, R. (1986). Inhibition of acetyl-coenzyme A dependent activation of *N*-hydroxyarylamines by phenolic compounds, pentachlorophenol and 1-nitro-2-naphthol. *Chem. Biol. Interact.* **60**, 275–285.

Simmon, V. F., and Kauhanen, K. (1978). "*In Vitro* Microbiological Mutagenicity Assays of Pentachlorophenol." Final report, Stanford Research Institute (SRI) Project LSU-5612, U.S. Environmental Protection Agency, National Environmental Research Center, Cincinnati, OH. 13 pp. As cited in NTP, 1989 (*op. cit.*).

Simmon, V. F., Riccio, E. S., and Peirce, M. V. (1979). "*In Vitro* Microbiological Genotoxicity Assays of Pentachlorophenol and 2,4,5-T Acid." Final report, Stanford Research Institute (SRI) Project LSU-7558.

Sipes, G. I., and Gandolfi, J. A. (1991). Biotransformation of toxicants. *In* "Casarett and Doull's Toxicology: The Basic Science of Poisons," (M. A. Amdur, J. Doull, and C. D. Klaassen, eds.), 4th ed., pp. 88–126. Pergamon, New York.

Smith, A. H., Pearce, N. E., Fisher, D. O., Giles, H. J., Teague, C. A., and Howard, J. K. (1984). Soft tissue sarcoma and exposure to phenoxy-herbicides and chlorophenols in New Zealand. *J. Natl. Cancer Inst.* **73**, 1111–1117.

Tennant, R. W., Margolin, B. H., Shelby, M. D., Zeiger, E., Haseman, J. K, Spalding J., Caspary, W., Resnick, M., Stasiewicz, S., Anderson, B., and Minor, R. (1987). Prediction of chemical carcinogenicity in rodents from in vitro genetic toxicity assays. *Science* **236**, 933–941.

Tran, D. Q., Klotz, D. M., Ladlie, B. L., Ide, C. F., McLachlan, J. A., and Arnold, S. F. (1996). *Biochem. Biophys. Res. Commun.* **229**, 518–523.

Triebig, G., Csuzda, I., Krekeler, H. J., and Schaller, K. H. (1987). Pentachlorophenol and the peripheral nervous system: A longitudinal study in exposed workers. *Brit. J. Indust. Med.* **44**, 638–641.

Triebig, G. (1997). Untitled letter. *Arch. Environ. Health* **52**, 148.

Uhl, S., Schmid, P., and Schlatter, C. (1986). Pharmacokinetics of pentachlorophenol in man. *Arch. Toxicol.* **58**, 182–186.

Umemura, T., Kai, S., Hasegawa, R., Sai, K., Kurokawa, Y., and Williams, G. M. (1999). Pentachlorophenol (PCP) produces liver oxidative stress and promotes but does not initiate hepatocarcinogenesis in B6C3F$_1$ mice. *Carcinogenesis* **20**, 1115–1120.

United States Environmental Protection Agency (U.S. EPA) (1984a). Creosote, pentachlorophenol, and inorganic arsenicals; notice of intent to cancel; notice of determination; notice of availability of position document. *Federal Reg.* **49**(136), 28666–28689; OPP-30000/28F; PH-FRL-2630-4.

United States Environmental Protection Agency (U.S. EPA) (1984b). "Wood Preservative Pesticides: Creosote, Pentachlorophenol, and Inorganic Arsenicals," Position Document 4, Office of Pesticides and Toxic Substances, Washington.

United States Environmental Protection Agency (U.S. EPA) (1986). "Creosote, Pentachlorophenol, and Inorganic Arsenicals; Amendment of Notice of Intent to Cancel Registrations; Notice." *Federal Reg.* **51**(7), 1334–1348; OPP-30000/28H; FRL-2952-6.

United States Environmental Protection Agency (U.S. EPA) (1987). Pentachlorophenol; Amendment of notice of intent to cancel registrations. *Federal Reg.* **52**(1), 140–148; OPP-30000/28M; FRL-3137-3.

United States Environmental Protection Agency (U.S. EPA) (1988). "Recommendations for and Documentation of Biological Values for Use in Risk Assessment." EPA/600/6-87/008, PB88-179874, Environmental Criteria and Assessment Office, Office of Health and Environmental Assessment, Cincinnati.

United States Environmental Protection Agency (U.S. EPA) (1991a). *Federal Reg.* 56 FR 3600 (1/30/91); 56 FR 3526 (1/30/91); 56 FR 30266 (7/1/91).

United States Environmental Protection Agency (U.S. EPA) (1991b). *Federal Reg.* 56 FR 3600 (1/30/91); 56 FR 30266 (7/1/91).

United States Environmental Protection Agency, Science Advisory Board (U.S. EPA SAB) (1991). "Report of Science Advisory Board's Review of Issues Concerning the Health Effects of Ingested Pentachlorophenol," Environmental Health Committee, EPA-SAB-EHC-91-002.

van Ommen, B., Adang, A. Müller, F., and van Bladeren, P. J. (1986). The microsomal metabolism of pentachlorophenol and its covalent binding to protein and DNA. *Chem.–Biol. Interactions* **60**, 1–11.

van Raaij., J. A. G. M., van den Berg, K. J., and Notten, W. R. F. (1991a). Hexachlorobenzene and its metabolites pentachlorophenol and tetrachlorohydroquinone: Interaction with thyroxine binding sites of rat thyroid hormone carriers *ex vivo* and *in vitro*. *Toxicol. Lett.* **59**, 101–107.

van Raaij., J. A. G. M., van den Berg, K. J., Engel, R., Bragt, P. C., and Notten, W. R. F. (1991b). Effects of hexachlorobenzene and its metabolites pentachlorophenol and tetrachlorohydroquinone on serum thyroid hormone levels in rats. *Toxicology* **67**, 107–116.

van Raaij., J. A. G. M., Frijters, C. M. G., and van den Berg, K. J. (1993). Hexachlorobenzene-induced hypothyroidism: Involvement of different mechanisms by parent compound and metabolite. *Biochem. Pharmacol.* **46**, 1385–1391.

van Raaij., J. A. G. M., Frijters, C. M. G., Wong Yen Kong, L., van den Berg, K. J., and Notten, W. R. F. (1994). Reduction of thyroxine uptake into cerebrospinal fluid and rat brain by hexachlorobenzene and pentachlorophenol. *Toxicology* **94**, 197–208.

Villena, F., Montoya, G., Klaasen, R., Fleckenstein, R., and Suwalsky, M. (1992). Morphological changes on nerves and histopathological effects on liver and kidney of rats by pentachlorophenol (PCP). *Comp. Biochem. Physiol.* **101**, 353–363.

Waidyanatha, S., Lin, P.-H., and Rappaport, S. M. (1996). Characterization of chlorinated adducts of hemoglobin and albumin following administration of pentachlorophenol to rats. *Chem. Res. Toxicol.* **9**, 647–653.

Wang, Y. J., and Lin, J. K. (1995). Estimation of selected phenols in drinking water with *in situ* acetylation and study on the DNA damaging properties of polychlorinated phenols. *Arch. Environ. Contam. Toxicol.* **28**, 537–542.

Weinbach, E. C. (1957). Biochemical basis for the toxicity of pentachlorophenol. *Proc. Natl. Acad. Sci. USA* **43**, 393–397.

Weinbach, E. C., and Garbus, J. (1965). The interaction of uncoupling phenols with mitochondria and with mitochondrial protein. *J. Biol. Chem.* **240**, 1811–1819.

Welsh, J. J., Collins, T. F. X., Black, T. N., Graham, S. L., and O'Donnell, M. W., Jr. (1987). Teratogenic potential of purified pentachlorophenol and pentachloroanisole in subchronically exposed Sprague–Dawley rats. *Fd. Chem. Toxic.* **25**, 163–172.

Wester, R. C., Maibach, H. I., Sedik, L., Melendres, J., Wade, M., and DiZio, S. (1993). Percutaneous absorption of pentachlorophenol from soil. *Fundam. Appl. Toxicol.* **20**, 68–71.

Witte, I., Juhl, U., and Butte, W. (1985). DNA-damaging properties and cytotoxicity in human fibroblasts of tetrachlorohydroquinone, a pentachlorophenol metabolite. *Mutation Res.* **145**, 71–75.

WHO (World Health Organization). (1987). "Pentachlorophenol. Environmental Health Criteria 71," IPCS, International Programme on Chemical Safety, World Health Organization, Geneva.

Young, J. F., and Haley, T. J. (1978). A pharmacokinetic study of pentachlorophenol poisoning and the effect of forced diuresis. *Clin. Toxicol.* **12**, 41–48.

Yuan, J. H., Goehl, T. J., Murrill, E., Moore, R., Clark, J., Hong, H. L., and Irwin, R. D. (1994). Toxicokinetics of pentachlorophenol in the F344 rat: Gavage and dosed feed studies. *Xenobiotica* **24**, 553–560.

Ziemsen, B., Angerer, J., and Lehnert, G. (1987). Sister chromatid exchange and chromosomal breakage in pentachlorophenol (PCP) exposed workers. *Int. Arch. Occup. Environ. Health* **59**, 413–417.

CHAPTER

66

Symmetrical and Asymmetrical Triazine Herbicides

James T. Stevens, Charles B. Breckenridge
Novartis Crop Protection

James Simpkins
University of North Texas

J. Charles Eldridge
Wake Forest University

66.1 INTRODUCTION

Triazines have been used extensively as selective herbicides in agriculture in the United States and other parts of the world for more than 35 years (Stevens and Sumner, 1991). The triazines inhibit photosynthesis (Gysin and Knuesli, 1960). Even after more than three decades of use, certain of these triazine herbicides remain agronomically and commercially important, especially for the pre-emergent control of broadleaf weeds. They have become important "mixing partners" for many of the newer herbicides since they offer a broad spectrum of weed control (Gressel *et al.*, 1982). Because of their continued widespread use, the safety of this class of chemistry has been continually reassessed.

66.1.1 CHEMISTRY AND FORMULATIONS

These inhibitors of photosynthesis include the asymmetrical triazines or triazinones, such as metribuzin, and the symmetrical triazine herbicides. The major commercial symmetrical triazines are further divided into chloro-*s*-triazines: simazine, atrazine, propazine, cyanazine; the thiomethyl-*s*-triazines: ametryn, prometryn, terbutryn; and the methoxy-*s*-triazine prometon. The symmetrical triazines (*s*-triazines) have a chlorine, sulfur, or oxygen atom at the 2-position of the ring and are usually substituted in the 4- and 6-positions with alkylamino-group (Fig. 66.1).

Cyanazine contains a 2-cyano-isopropylamino-substituent at the 4-position on the ring. The asymmetrical triazine, metribuzin, retains the triazine ring, but since the nitrogen atoms are unevenly spaced, aromaticity is maintained by the presence of the carbonyl group. Metribuzin adheres to the class by containing a thiomethyl-substituent on the ring.

These herbicides are formulated into various water and lipid soluble products for commercial sales. Most of these formulations are identified with trade names and major manufacturers in Table 66.1.

66.1.2 USES

Mode of action of the triazine and triazinone herbicides is inhibition of photosynthetic electron transport in most plants and generally have low toxicity to animals. The mode of action and uses of these chemicals are shown in Table 66.2.

66.1.3 HAZARD IDENTIFICATION

Hazards were identified for all the triazine and triazinone herbicides based upon protocols established under the Federal Insecticide, Fungicide, and Rodenticide Act (U.S. EPA, 1982) and the studies were conducted according to Good Laboratory Practices (U.S. EPA, 1979).

66.1.4 ACUTE STUDIES

Triazine herbicides are acutely relatively nontoxic, they are not remarkably irritating to the skin or eye, nor are they generally skin sensitizers (Table 66.3). The exceptions are atrazine, which is a skin sensitizer, and cyanazine, which is acute by the oral route.

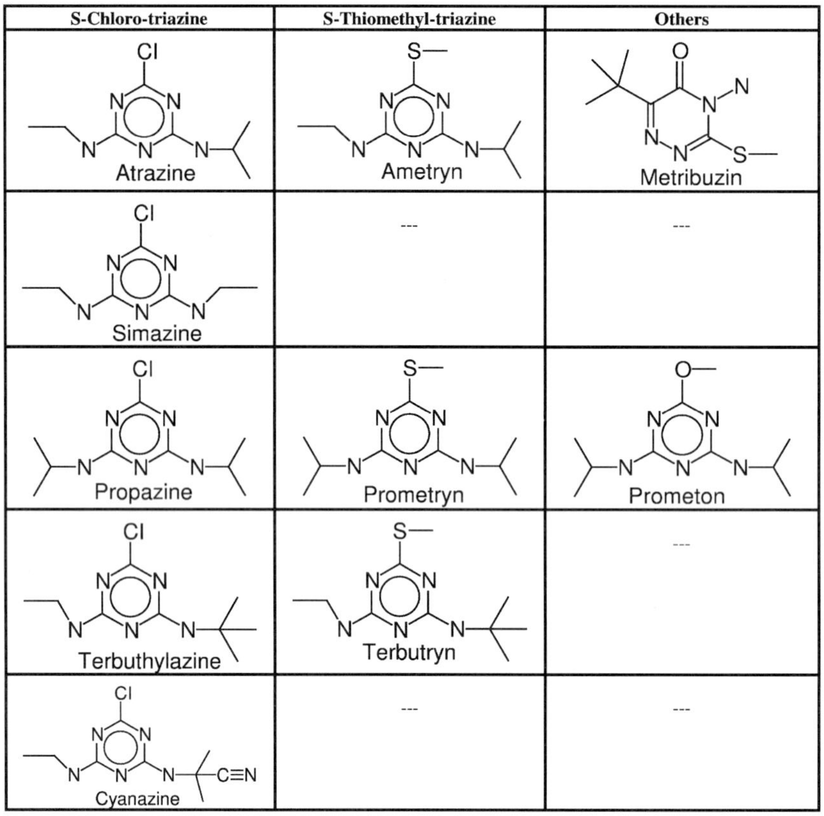

Figure 66.1   Structures of symmetrical and asymmetrical triazine herbicides.

66.1.5 SUBCHRONIC/CHRONIC TOXICITY

The United States Environmental Protection Agency guidelines (U.S. EPA, 1982, 1998a) for subchronic studies for pesticides specify treatment of rats, mice, or dogs with the chemical for various lengths of time. Rat and mouse studies are 90 days in duration, and lifetime studies are typically 24 and 18 months,

respectively. In dogs, the studies are usually conducted for 90 days, 1 year, or 2 years. In all cases, animals are divided into test groups, 10 to 50 rats or mice and 4 to 6 dogs. At least four test groups are used in each study, one group receiving no chemical (controls) and three groups receiving low, medium, or high concentrations of the chemical in their diets. In these studies, urinalysis, hematology, and clinical chemistry

Table 66.1
Chemical Key Trade Name, Major Manufacturer, and Formulations for the Selected Triazines and Triazinone

Chemical	Trade name	Major manufacturer	Water soluble granule/powder	Emulifiable concentrate	Other
Ametryn	EVIK®	Novartis	80W	NA[a]	NA
Atrazine	AATREX®	Novartis	Nine-0	4l (90%)	NA
Cyanazine	BLADEX®	DuPont	NA	4L (90%)	NA
Metribuzin	SENCOR®	Miles	DF (75%)	4 (75%)	NA
Prometon	PRAMITOL®	Novartis	NA	25E (25%)	5PS (5%)
Prometryn	CAPAROL®	Novartis	WG (80%)	4L (90%)	NA
Propazine	Milo-Pro*	Griffin	80 WP (80%)	NA	NA
Simazine	PRINCEP®	Novartis	80 WG (80%)	4L (90%)	NA
Terbuthylazine	Gardoprim®	Novartis	WG	NA	NA
Terbutryn	Terbutrex*	Makhteshim Agan	50 WP	L	NA

[a]NA = not available.

Table 66.2
Mode of Action and Uses for the Selected Triazines and Triazinone

Chemical	Reference	Mode of herbicide action	Uses
Ametryn	Tomlin (1997a)	Selective systemic	Control of annual grasses and broad-leaved weeds in pineapples
Atrazine	Tomlin (1997b)	Selective systemic	Control of annual grasses and broad-leafs in corn, sorghum and sugar cane
Cyanazine	Tomlin (1997c)	Selective systemic	General weed control in beans, maize and peas
Metribuzin	Tomlin (1997d)	Selective systemic	Control of many grasses and broad-leaved weeds in soya beans, maize and corn
Prometon	Tomlin (1997e)	Non-selective systemic	Controls most grasses, many broad-leaved weeds and brush
Prometryn	Tomlin (1997f)	Selective systemic	Pre-emergent use in cotton, sun flowers, peanuts and vegetables
Propazine	Tomlin (1997g)	Selective systemic	Preplant and pre-emergent use for weeds in sorghum
Simazine	Tomlin (1997h)	Selective systemic	Control of annual grasses and broad-leaved weeds in pome fruit, stone fruit, cane fruit, citrus, vines, strawberries, nuts, olives, pineapples, beans, peas, corn, aparagus, hops, alfalfa, coffee, rubber, oil palms, tea, and turef
Terbuthylazine	Tomlin (1997i)	Systemic	Broad-spectrum pre- or postemergence weed control in corn, sorghum, vines, fruit trees, citrus, coffee, oil palm , cocoa, olives, potatoes, peas, beans, sugar cane, rubber, and tree nurseries
Terbutryn	Tomlin (1997j)	Selective systemic	Pre-emergence weed control in cereals, sugar cane, and sunflowers; postemergence uses in cereals, sugar cane, and corn

parameters are evaluated, and gross and microscopic pathological examinations are performed on up to 50 tissues. Maximally tolerated doses are tested in order to demonstrate toxicity (up to 1000 mg/kg/day in the diets). In this fashion, it is possible to determine whether a chemical damages or alters any organ or tissue, and to establish levels of the chemical which produce no observable effects (the NOEL), and the lowest level at which effects are noted (the LOEL). The responses of repeated exposure of rats and dogs to the selected triazine herbicides are presented in Table 66.4.

With the exception of rats and dogs fed terbuthylazine and cyanazine, the NOEL values were generally 2.5 mg/kg/day or higher, and LOEL values were 15 mg/kg/day or higher. The most common observation was not a specific organ or tissue,

but a reduction in body weight gain. Microscopically, the liver was the most common target organ.

66.1.6 DEVELOPMENTAL AND REPRODUCTIVE TOXICITY

Developmental toxicity studies, formerly called teratology studies, are required to be performed both in rats and rabbits; a two-generation reproduction study is conducted in rats (U.S. EPA, 1998a). The results of such studies conducted with the selected triazine herbicides are presented in Table 66.5.

The triazine herbicides, with the exception of cyanazine, did not produce developmental or reproductive effects. Cyanazine produced developmental effects in the rat and rabbit at the high-

Table 66.3
EPA Acute Hazard Classification of the Technical Grade For Selected Triazine Herbicides[a]

Triazine technical[a] Group	Chemical	Eye Irritation	Skin Irritation	Oral LD$_{50}$ (mg/kg)	Dermal LD$_{50}$ (mg/kg)	Inhalation LC$_{50}$ (mg/L)	Sensitization potential	Signal word
s-Cl	Atrazine	Nonirritating		3090	>3100	>5	Sensitizer	Caution
	Simazine	Nonirritating	Mild	>5000	>3100	>5.5	Nonsensitizer	Caution
	Propazine	Mild	Nonirritating	>7000	>3100	>2.0	Nonsensitizer	Caution
	Terbuthylazine	Nonirritating	Mild	1590–2000	>2000	>5.3	Nonsensitizer	Caution
	Cyanazine	Nonirritating	Nonirritating	182–334	>2000	0.81	Nonsensitizer	Warning
s-SCH3	Ametryn	Nonirritating	Nonirritating	1160	>2020	>5.1	Sensitizer	Caution
	Prometryn	Slight irritation	Nonirritating	4550	>2020	>5.1	Nonsensitizer	Caution
	Terbutryn	Nonirritating	Nonirritating	2500	>2000	>2.2	Nonsensitizer	Caution
s-OCH3	Prometon	Irritating	Mild	1518–4345	>2020	>3.2	Nonsensitizer	Caution
Asym.	Metribuzin	Nonirritating	Nonirritating	1090–1206	>20,000	>0.65	Nonsensitizer	Caution

[a]This table lists only technical products; formulated products used for agriculture may have more restrictive labeling due to the formulants used. Commercial formulations of prometon (Danger, Corrosive) and the 4L formulation of prometryn (Warning) carry more restrictive signal words due to formulants.

Table 66.4
Hazard Assessment for Repeat Exposure to the Selected Triazine Herbicides

Triazine Group	Chemical	Species/study	mg/kg/day NOEL[a]	mg/kg/day LOEL[b]	Target organ Tissue or system
s-Cl	Atrazine	Rat/90-day oral	3.4	33	Body weight
		Dog/52-week oral	7.5	25	Heart/myocardium
	Simazine	Rat/90-day oral	12.6	126	Body weight
		Dog/90-day oral	7.5	134	Body weight
	Propazine	Rat/90-day oral	13	50	Body weight
		Dog/90-day oral	7	25	Body weight
	Terbutylazine	Rat/90-day oral	2.1	7.1	Body weight
		Dog/52-week oral	0.4	1.6	Body weight
	Cyanazine	Rat/90-day oral	1.5	15.0	Body weight
		Dog/52-week oral	0.8	7.5	Hematology effects
s-SCH$_3$	Ametryn	Rat/90-day oral	8.6	86	Liver
		Dog/52-week oral	5.0	50	Liver
	Prometryn	Rat/90-day oral	50	>500	75% mortality
		Dog/104-week oral	3.7	37.5	Liver, kidney, bone marrow
	Terbutryn	Rat/90-day oral	50	140	Body weight
		Dog/26-week oral	10	25	Stomach
s-OCH$_3$	Prometon	Rat/90-day oral	5	15	Body weight
		Dog/52-week oral	5	20	Body weight
Asymmetric	Metribuzin	Rat/104-week oral	5	15.0	Body weight, liver, kidney
		Dog/104-week oral	2.5	37.5	Body weight, liver, kidney

[a] No observable effect level.
[b] Lowest observable effect level.

est doses tested. Effects noted at doses that were toxic to the mothers were cyclopia and diaphragmatic hernia in rabbits, and an apparent increase in the incidence of skeletal variations (i.e., anomalies) in rats (U.S. EPA, 1994).

66.2 MUTAGENICITY

Weisburger (1975) noted that certain chemical carcinogens are capable of interacting directly with genetic material such as DNA. Based upon this association, several short-term tests to identify the alteration of genetic material or mutation were introduced into hazard testing for crop protection chemicals. These include tests to examine the possible (1) interaction with genes (gene mutation tests), (2) interaction with the chromosome (clastogenic tests), and (3) direct interaction with DNA (classified as other tests). The results for the selected triazine herbicides are presented in Table 66.6.

All of the triazines were negative in the specific tests listed in Table 66.6. The overall mutagenic potentials of atrazine, simazine, and cyanazine have been reviewed by Brusick (1994), Hauswirth and Wetzel (1998), and Bogdanffy et al. (1999), respectively. The weight of the evidence indicates that these s-chloro-triazines are not mutagenic. Metribuzin is also negative in the standard battery of mutagenicity studies.

66.2.1 ONCOGENICITY ASSESSMENT

The triazine and triazinone herbicides have been evaluated in lifetime animal bioassays. In these studies, groups of mice and rats are fed selected concentrations of the test chemical in their diet for 18 and 24 months, respectively. The levels of the test chemical administered in the diet are generally selected from repeat dose feeding studies at least 90-day in duration, and normally used to establish the NOEL, LOEL, and the maximum tolerated dose (MTD) (Farber, 1987). The MTD is defined as the highest concentration of test chemical that can be administrated without causing the death of the animal; often a 10% reduction in body weight gain has been used as criteria for establishing the MTD (Foran et al., 1997).

Following lifetime feeding of the chemical at the prescribed levels, veterinary pathologists microscopically examine approximately 50 tissues from each animal for the presence of tumors or other evidence of tissue damage. The results of such oncogenicity studies conducted in the mice are presented in Table 66.7.

None of the selected triazines showed any evidence of the induction of tumors in either male or female mice despite high feeding levels, ranging from 76 to 1400 mg/kg/day doses, that were equal to or exceeding the MTD. The chloro-s-triazines, atrazine, cyanazine, propazine, and simazine, all resulted in either an increased incidence or an earlier onset of mammary tumors when administered to female S-D rats at high feeding

Table 66.5
Summary of the Results of Rat and Rabbit Developmental and a Two-Generation Rat Reproduction Study with Triazine Herbicides

Triazine Group	Chemical	Study/Species	Developmental/ reproduction	Toxicity observed	mg/kg/day HDT[a]	LOEL[b]	NOEL[c]
s-Cl	Atrazine	Developmental/rat	None	↓ Body wt. gain	700	70	10
		Developmental/rabbit	None	↓ Body wt. gain	75	75	5
		Reproductive/rat	None	↓ Body wt. gain	35	35	3.5
	Simazine	Developmental/rat	None	↓ Body wt. gain	600	300	30
		Developmental/rabbit	None	↓ Body wt. gain	200	75	5
		Reproductive/rat	None	↓ Body wt. gain	30	6	0.6
	Propazine	Developmental/rat	None	↓ Body wt. gain	600	100	10
		Developmental/rabbit	None	↓ Body wt. gain	—	—	—
		Reproductive/rat	None	↓ Body wt. gain	50	50	5
	Terbuthylazine	Developmental/rat	None	↓ Body wt. gain	30	30	5
		Developmental/rabbit	None	↓ Body wt. gain	5	5	0.4
		Reproductive/rat	None	↓ Body wt. gain	15	3	0.3
	Cyanazine	Developmental/rat	Positive	↑ Malformations	75	5	>5
		Developmental/rabbit	Positive	↑ Malformations	4	2	1
		Reproductive/rat	None	↓ Body wt. gain	15	5	1.5
s-S–CH₃	Ametryn	Developmental/rat	None	↓ Body wt. gain	250	50	5
		Developmental/rabbit	None	↓ Body wt. gain	60	60	10
		Reproductive/rat	None	↓ Body wt. gain	100	10	1
	Prometryn	Developmental/rat	None	↓ Body wt. gain	250	250	>250
		Developmental/rabbit	None	↓ Body wt. gain	72	72	12
		Reproductive/rat	None	↓ Body wt. gain	5	5	>5
	Terbutryn	Developmental/rat	None	↓ Body wt. gain	500	500	50
		Developmental/rabbit	None	↓ Ossified sternabra	75	75	10
		Reproductive/rat	None	↓ Body wt. gain	150	150	15
s-OCH₃	Prometon	Developmental/rat	None	↓ Body wt. gain	360	120	36
		Developmental/rabbit	None	↓ Body wt. gain	25	25	3.5
		Reproductive/rat	None	↓ Body wt. gain	75	25	1
Assymet.	Metribuzin	Developmental/rat	None	↓ Body wt. gain	100	100	>100
		Developmental/rabbit	None	↓ Body wt. gain	135	45	>45
		Reproductive/rat	None	↓ Body wt. gain	15	7.5	1.5

[a]Highest dose tested.
[b]Lowest observable effect level.
[c]No observable effect level.

Table 66.6
Results of Mutagenicity Studies with the Selected Triazine Herbicides

Triazine Group	Chemical	Gene mutation Ames	E. Coli REC	Mouse lymphoma	Clastogenic Micronucleus	Other DNA repair	Dominant lethal
s-Cl	Atrazine	Negative	Negative	Negative	Negative	Negative	Negative
	Simazine	Negative	—	Negative	Negative	Negative	—
	Propazine	Negative	Negative	Negative	Negative	Negative	—
	Terbuthylazine	Negative	Negative	Negative	Negative	Negative	—
	Cyanazine	Negative	—	Negative	Negative	Negative	—
s-SCH3	Ametryn	Negative	—	Negative	Negative	Negative	Negative
	Prometryn	Negative	Negative	Negative	Negative	Negative	—
	Terbutryn	Negative	—	—	Negative	Negative	Negative
s-OCH3	Prometon	Negative	—	—	Negative	Negative	—
Asymmetric	Metribuzin	Negative	Negative	—	Negative	Negative	Negative

Table 66.7
Results of Carcinogenicity Studies in the Mouse

Group	Triazine Chemical[a]	Cancer potential	Feeding level (mg/kg/day) HDT[b]	NOEL[c]	LOEL[d]	Other effects	Reference
s-Cl	Atrazine	Negative	386[e]	38	38	↓ Body weight gain and thrombi in both sexes	Hauswirth and Wetzel (1998)
	Simazine	Negative	544[e]	5.7	132	↓ Body weight gain in both sexes	Hauswirth and Wetzel (1998)
	Propazine	Negative	450[e]	15	450	Cardiac fibrosis and focal degeneration	IRIS (1997a)
	Terbuthylazine	Negative	76[e]	15	76	↓ Body weight gain in both sexes; hematologic changes in males	Stevens et al. (1994)
	Cyanazine	Negative	143	1.4	3.6	↓ Body weight gain in both sexes	U.S. EPA (1994)
s-SCH3	Ametryn	Negative	100[e]	0.5	50	↓ Body weight gain in both sexes	Ahrens (1994a)
	Prometryn	Negative	429	1.4	143	↓ Body weight gain in both sexes	Ahrens (1994b)
	Terbutryn	Negative	429[e]	429	>429	No effects observed	Jessup (1980)
s-OCH3	Prometon	Negative	1400[e]	70	700	↓ Body weight gain and ↑ mortality in both sexes	Ahrens (1994c)
Asymmet.	Metribuzin	Negative	480	120	120	↓ Hematocrit, ↑ Liver, kidney and spleen weight	IRIS (1997b)

[a] CD1 mice were tested for all chemical except terbuthylazine where Tif : MAGf was used.
[b] Highest dose tested.
[c] Lowest observable effect level.
[d] No observable effect.
[e] Maximum tolerated dose exceeded.

Table 66.8
Results of Carcinogenicity Studies in the Rat

Group	Triazine Chemical[a]	Tumor response	Feeding level (mg/kg/day) HDT[b]	NOEL[c]	LOEL[d]	Other effects	Reference
s-Cl	Atrazine	Mammary (S-D)[a]	50[e]	3.5	20	↓ Body weight gain in both sexes	Stevens et al. (1999)
	Simazine	Mammary (S-D)	50[e]	0.5	5.3	↓ Body weight gain in both sexes; hematologic effects and ↑ mortality in females	Stevens et al. (1994)
	Propazine	Mammary (S-D)	50[e]	5.8	50	↓ Body weight gain in both sexes	Stevens et al. (1994)
	Terbuthylazine	Negative (Tif : RAI)	33[e]	0.2	1.1	↓ Body weight gain in both sexes	Stevens et al. (1994)
	Cyanazine	Mammary (S-D)	2.5[e]	0.2	1.0	↓ Body weight gain in females; ↑ hyperactivity in the males	U.S. EPA (1994)
s-SCH3	Ametryn	Negative (S-D)	100[e]	2.5	25	↓ Body weight gain in both sexes; hematological effects in females	Stevens et al. (1994)
	Prometryn	Negative (S-D)	75[e]	5.0	37	↓ Body weight gain in both sexes	Stevens et al. (1994)
	Terbutryn	Mammary, Thyroid, Liver (S-D)	150[e]	0.1	15	↓ Body weight gain in both sexes	Stevens et al. (1994)
s-OCH3	Prometon	Negative (S-D)	75	1	25	↓ Body weight gain in both sexes	Stevens et al. (1994)
Assymet	Metribuzin	Negative (Wistar)	15	5.0	15	↓ Body weight gain; ↑ liver and kidney weight; uterine and mammary gland pathology	IRIS (1997b); Ahrens (1994d)

[a] Strain of rat tested (S-D = Sprague–Dawley).
[b] Highest dose tested.
[c] Lowest observable effect level.
[d] No observable effect level.
[e] Maximum tolerated dose exceeded.

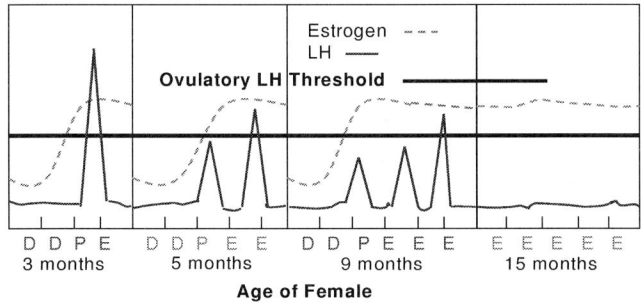

Figure 66.2 Representation of effect of normal reproductive aging on the ovulatory LH surge in S-D female rat.

levels, whereas male rats did not respond (Hauswirth and Wetzel, 1998). These finding are presented in Table 66.8.

The thiomethyl- and methoxy-*s*-triazines, as well as asymmetrical triazine, metribuzin, were not carcinogenic, even at feeding levels exceeding the MTD; the exception was terbutryn where an increased incidence of mammary, thyroid, and liver tumors were observed in female S-D rats at feeding levels that exceeded the MTD.

The female S-D rat has limitations in evaluating the effects of chemicals on the endocrine system because of the high degree of spontaneous tumor formation seen in the pituitary and mammary gland. At about 9 to 12 months of age the S-D rat begins to experience prolonged periods of estrus (Eldridge *et al.*, 1996; Simpkins *et al.*, 1998). Most laboratory rats, and S-D rats prior to 9–12 months, spend about 20 to 25% of their time in estrus. In the S-D rat, after this period, the animals spend increasing amounts of time in estrus. By 12 months of age, they often reach 40% of the time in estrus and eventually display persistent estrus (Eldridge *et al.*, 1998). This normal process of reproductive aging in the female S-D rat is depicted in Fig. 66.2.

The failure of reproduction in the female S-D rat is most probably related to a deficient neuroendocrine control of gonadotropin releasing hormone (GnRH) secretion from the hypothalmus. With decreasing release of GnRH, the pituitary secretion of lutenizing hormone (LH) gradually decreases until it is inadequate to stimulate ovulation. As a result of the failed ovulation and the resulting prolonged periods of estrus, the rats experience prolonged exposure to estrogen and prolactin produced by the ovary and pituitary, respectively (Simpkins *et al.*, 1998). Both of these hormones are known to enhance the growth rate of mammary tumors in rats (Cutts and Noble, 1964).

The reproductive aging process observed in the female S-D rat appears to be species specific. Other strains of rats, like the Fischer 344 rat, do not demonstrate this deficiency and do not have a high spontaneous incidence of mammary or pituitary tumors (Eldridge *et al.*, 1998).

Detailed studies on atrazine have shown that Fischer 344 rats administered high doses of atrazine do not develop either an increased incidence or an early onset of mammary tumors (Thakur *et al.*, 1998; Wetzel *et al.*, 1994), unlike the findings noted in similarly treated female S-D rats (Hauswirth and Wetzel, 1998; Stevens *et al.*, 1994; Wetzel *et al.*, 1994). Furthermore, when the major internal source of estrogen was removed from the female S-D rats by surgical removal of the ovaries at the beginning of the study, no mammary tumors were found after 2 years of atrazine treatment (Stevens *et al.*, 1999).

Examination of the reproductive cycles of intact female S-D rats fed high doses of atrazine over their lifetimes showed that prolonged periods of estrus occurred earlier in the treated group than in control group (Hauswirth and Wetzel, 1998). Subsequent studies showed that high doses of atrazine administered to female S-D rats reduced the magnitude of the LH, resulting in a failure of ovulation to occur (Simpkins *et al.*, 1998). However, low doses of atrazine had no effect on the LH surge, the estrous cycle, or the rate of appearance of mammary tumors (Simpkins *et al.*, 1998), indicating that even in female S-D rats there is a threshold dose below which there are no adverse effects on reproductive processes. Finally, when high-dose atrazine-treated animals were given GnRH, the hormone that is responsible for triggering the LH surge, the LH surge was restored. This finding suggests that the pituitary LH releasing mechanisms function normally in atrazine-treated animals (Cooper *et al.*, 1995). Presumably then the effect of atrazine treatment at high doses is at the level of the hypothalamus.

High doses of chloro-*s*-triazines appear to accelerate the development of mammary tumors in the S-D rat; This phenomenon occurs in a strain of rat that is already prone to spontaneously developing mammary tumors because of an inherent age-dependent deficiency in the regulation of the estrous cycle. The earlier appearance of mammary tumors in female S-D rats treated with high doses of atrazine is attributed to an increased exposure to endogenous estrogen and prolactin, secondary to the lengthening of the estrous cycle. Removal of endogenous estrogen in female S-D rats by ovariectomy prevents the appearance of mammary tumors, even in animals that have received high doses of atrazine for 2 years. In the S-D female there is a dose of atrazine (approximately 2.5 mg/kg) that has no effect on the estrous cycle or mammary tumor incidence and/or onset. The mammary tumor response to high doses of atrazine is unique to the female S-D rat; the response was not observed in male or female CD-1 mice, Fischer 344 rats, or male S-D rats.

66.2.2 TOXICOLOGY IN HUMANS

The reproductive aging process observed in female S-D rats is not relevant to human female since reproductive senescence in women is characterized principally as a ovarian failure. Human menopause commences with a decrease in endogenous estrogen, instead of an increase that is characteristic of the female S-D rat in a state of persistent estrus. The lack of relevance of these data to humans is supported by about 40 years of manufacturing and use history for atrazine and other triazine herbicides; To date there is no evidence linking atrazine exposure to any human health effects (Loosli, 1995; Neuberger, 1996; Sathiakumur *et al.*, 1992).

66.2.3 SUMMARY RISK CHARACTERIZATION

Evaluation of hazard profiles of the triazine herbicides revealed that these products are relatively nontoxic acutely, are well tolerated when administered to animals over a long duration of time, are not developmental or reproductive toxins, and are not mutagenic nor carcinogenic in mice or male rats. The exception is cyanazine, which is more acutely toxic, is weakly mutagenic, and results in developmental toxicity, presumably because of the presence of the cyanomoiety. The chloro-*s*-triazines appear to produce an earlier onset or an excess of mammary tumors in female S-D rats at high doses. Because of the unique nature of reproductive aging in female S-D rats, the carcinogenic response in this strain of rat is not considered relevant for human risk assessment.

REFERENCES

Ahrens, W. H. (1994a). Ametryn. *In* "Herbicide Handbook," 7th ed., pp. 12–14. Weed Science Society of America, Champaign, IL.

Ahrens, W. H. (1994b). Prometryn. *In* "Herbicide Handbook," 7th ed., pp. 245–247. Weed Science Society of America, Champaign, IL.

Ahrens, W. H. (1994c). Prometryn. *In* "Herbicide Handbook," 7th ed., pp. 243–245. Weed Science Society of America, Champaign, IL.

Ahrens, W. H. (1994d). Metribuzin. *In* "Herbicide Handbook," 7th ed., pp. 200–203. Weed Science Society of America, Champaign, IL.

Bakke, J. E., Larson, J. R., and Price, C. E. (1972). Metabolism of atrazine and 2-hydroxyatrazine by the rat. *J. Agric. Food Chem.* **20**, 603–607.

Bogdanffy, M. S., O'Connor, J. C., Hansen, J. F., Gaddamidi, V., Van Pelt, C. S., and Cook, J. C. (1999). Chronic toxicity and oncogenicity bioassay in rats with the chloro-S-triazine herbicide cyanazine. *J. Toxicol. Environ. Health*, Accepted for publication.

Brusick, D. J. (1994). An assessment of the genetic toxicity of atrazine: Relevance to health and effects. *Mutation Res.* **317**, 133–144.

Cooper, R. L., Parrish, M. B., McElroy, W. K., Rehnberg, G. L., Hein, J. F., Goldmann, J. M., Stoker, T., and Tyrey, L. (1995). Effect of atrazine on the hormonal control of the ovary. *The Toxicologist* **15**, 294.

Cutts, J. H., and Noble, R. L. (1964). Estrone-induced mammary tumors in the rat—II. Effect of alteration in hormonal environment on tumor induction, behavior, and growth. *Cancer Res.* **24**, 1124–1130.

Eldridge, J. C., Stevens, J. T., Wetzel, L. T., Tisdel, M. O., Breckenridge, C. B., McConnell, R. F., and Simpkins, J. W. (1996). Atrazine: Mechanisms of hormonal imbalance in female SD rats. *Fund. Appl. Toxicol.* **24**(12), 2–5.

Eldridge, J. C., McConnell, R. F., Wetzel, L. T., and Tisdel, M. O. (1998). Appearance of mammary tumors in atrazine-treated female rats: Probable mode of action involving strain-related control of ovulation and estrous cycling. *In* "Triazine Herbicides: Risk Assessment" (L. G. Ballantine, J. E. McFarland, and D. S. Hackett, eds.), Chap. 32, pp. 414–423. American Chemical Society, Washington, DC.

Farber, T. M. (1987). "Pesticide Assessment Guidelines, Subdivision F, Position Document: Selection of a Maximum Tolerated Dose (MTD) in Oncogenicity Studies." Toxicology Branch, Hazard Evaluation Division, Office of Pesticides Programs, U.S. Environmental Protection Agency, NTIS PB88-116736.

Foran, J., and the ILSI Risk Science Working Group on Dose Selection. (1997). Principles for the selection of doses in chronic rodent bioassays. *Environ. Health Perspect.* **105**(1), 18–20.

Gressel, J., Ammon, H. U., Fogelfors, H., Gasquez, J., Kay, Q. O. N., and Kees, H. (1982). Discovery and distribution of herbicide-resistant weeds outside of North America. *In* "Herbicide Resistance in Plants" (H. M. LeBaron and J. Gressel, eds.), pp. 31–46. Wiley, New York.

Gysin, H., and Knuesli, E. (1960). Chemistry and herbicidal properties of triazine derivatives. *In* "Advances in Pest Control Research" (R. Metcalf, ed.), Vol. III, pp. 289–358. Wiley Interscience, New York.

Hauswirth, J. W., and Wetzel, L. T. (1998). Toxicity characteristics of the 2-chlorotriazines, atrazine and simazine. *In* "Triazine Herbicides: Risk Assessment" (L. G. Ballantine, J. E. McFarland, and D. S, Hackett, eds.), pp. 370–383. American Chemical Society, Washington, DC.

Jessup, D. C. (1980). "Terbutryn Technical Two-Year Carcinogenicity Study in Mice." Project Rep. 382-005, International Research and Development Corporation. Mattawan, MI (unpublished).

IRIS (1997a). Propazino. CASRN 139-40-2. EPA. http://Narero.epa.gov/ngispgrn3/iris/subst/0187.htm

IRIS (1997b). Metribuzin. CASRN 21087-64.9. EPA. http://Narero.epa.gov/ngispgrn3/iris/subst/. 0075htm

Loosli, R. (1995). Epidemiology of atrazine. *Rev. Environ. Contam. Toxicol.* **143**, 47–57.

Neuberger, J. S. (1996). Atrazine and/or triazine herbicides exposure and cancer: An epidemiologic review. *J. Agromed.* **3**(2), 9–30.

Sathiakumur, N., Delzell, E., Austin, H., and Cole, P. (1992). A follow-up study of agricultural chemical production workers. *Am. J. Ind. Med.* **21**, 321–330.

Simpkins, J. W., Eldridge, J. C., and Wetzel, L. T. (1998). Role of strain-specific reproductive patterns in the appearance of mammary tumors in atrazine-treated rats. *In* "Triazine Herbicides: Risk Assessment" (L. G. Ballantine, J. E. McFarland, and D. S. Hackett, eds.), Chap. 31, pp. 399–413. American Chemical Society, Washington, DC.

Stevens, J. T., and Sumner, D. D. (1991). Herbicides. *In* "Handbook of Pesticide Toxicology" (W. J. Hayes and E. R. Laws, eds.), Vol. 3, pp. 1317–1408. Academic Press, San Diego.

Stevens, J. T., Breckenridge, C. B., Wetzel, L. T., Gillis, J., and Luempert, III, L. C. (1994). Hypothesis for mammary tumorigenesis in Sprague–Dawley rats exposed to certain triazine herbicides. *J. Toxicol. Environ. Health* **43**, 139–153.

Stevens, J. T., Breckenridge, C. B., Wetzel, L. T., Thakur, A. J., Liu, C., Werner, C., Luempert, III, L. C., and Eldridge, J. C. (1999). A risk characterization for atrazine: Oncogenicity profile. *J. Toxicol. Environ. Health* **56**, 69–109.

Sumner, D. D., Luempert, III, L. C., and Stevens, J. T. (1995). Agricultural chemicals: The impact of regulation under FIFRA on science and economics. *In* "Primer on Regulatory Toxicology" (C. Chenzelis, J. Holson, and S. Gad, eds.), pp. 133–163. Raven Press, New York.

Thakur, A. J., Wetzel, L. T., Voelker, R. W., and Wakefield, A. E. (1998). Results of a two-year oncogenicity study in Fischer 344 rats with atrazine. *In* "Triazine Herbicides: Risk Assessment" (L. G. Ballantine, J. E. McFarland, and D. S. Hackett, eds.), pp. 384–398. American Chemical Society, Washington, DC.

Tomlin, C. D. S. (1997a). Ametryn. *In* "A World Compendium: The Pesticide Manual," 11th ed., pp. 35–36. British Crop Protection Council, Farnham, Surrey.

Tomlin, C. D. S. (1997b). Atrazine. *In* "A World Compendium: The Pesticide Manual," 11th ed., pp. 55–57. British Crop Protection Council, Farnham, Surrey.

Tomlin, C. D. S. (1997c). Cyanazine. *In* "A World Compendium: The Pesticide Manual," 11th ed., pp. 280–282. British Crop Protection Council, Farnham, Surrey.

Tomlin, C. D. S. (1997d). Metribuzin. *In* "A World Compendium: The Pesticide Manual," 11th ed., pp. 840–841. British Crop Protection Council, Farnham, Surrey.

Tomlin, C. D. S. (1997e). Prometon. *In* "A World Compendium: The Pesticide Manual," 11th ed., pp. 1010–1011. British Crop Protection Council, Farnham, Surrey.

Tomlin, C. D. S. (1997f). Prometryn. *In* "A World Compendium: The Pesticide Manual," 11th ed., pp. 1011–1012. British Crop Protection Council, Farnham, Surrey.

Tomlin, C. D. S. (1997g). Propazine. *In* "A World Compendium: The Pesticide Manual," 11th ed., pp. 1024–1026. British Crop Protection Council, Farnham, Surrey.

Tomlin, C. D. S. (1997h). Simazine. *In* "A World Compendium: The Pesticide Manual," 11th ed., pp. 1106–1108. British Crop Protection Council, Farnham, Surrey.

Tomlin, C. D. S. (1997i). Terbuthylazine. *In* "A World Compendium: The Pesticide Manual," 11th ed., pp. 1168–1170. British Crop Protection Council, Farnham, Surrey.

Tomlin, C. D. S. (1997j). Terbutryn. *In* "A World Compendium: The Pesticide Manual," 11th ed., pp. 1170–1172. British Crop Protection Council, Farnham, Surrey.

U.S. Environmental Protection Agency (EPA) (1979). "Federal Insecticide, Fungicide, and Rodenticide Act (FIFRA); Good Laboratory Practice Standards—Final Rules. 40 CFR Part 160." *Fed. Reg.* **44**(91), 27362–27407.

U.S. Environmental Protection Agency (EPA) (1982). "Pesticide Assessment Guidelines, Subdivision F. Hazard Evaluation: Human and Domestic An-imals." Environmental Protection Agency—540/9-82-025. Available from NTIS, Springfield, VA.

U.S. Environmental Protection Agency (EPA) (1994). Atrazine, simazine, and cyanazine; Notice of initiation of special review. *Fed. Reg.* **59**(225), 60412–60443.

U.S. Environmental Protection Agency (EPA) (1997). Propazine. Pesticide tolerance petition filing. *Fed. Reg.* **63**(193), 53657–53660.

U.S. Environmental Protection Agency (EPA) (1998a). "Pesticide Assessment Guidelines," http://www. epa. gov/opptsfrs/OPPTS Harmonized/870 Health Effects Test Guidelines /Series (accessed 3/99).

U.S. Environmental Protection Agency (EPA). (1998b). Prometryn: Pesticide tolerances. *Fed. Reg.* **63**(37), 9494–9499.

Weisburger, J. H. (1975). *In* "Toxicology, The Basic Science of Poisons" (L. J. Casarett and J. Duoll, eds.), p. 333. MacMillan, New York.

Wetzel *et al.* (1994).

Phenylurea Herbicides

Jing Liu
Oklahoma State University

67.1 INTRODUCTION

Substituted phenylurea herbicides are a group of pesticides used for general weed control in agricultural and nonagricultural practices, for example, along railroads, utilities' rights-of-way, and in industrial areas. The first phenylurea herbicide, *N,N*-dimethyl-*N'*-(4-chlorophenyl)-urea, was introduced in 1952 by Du Pont under the common name of monuron. In subsequent years, many more derivatives of this class of compounds have been marketed. The phenylurea herbicides are now manufactured and distributed under the names of anisuron, buturon, chlorbromuron, chlortoluron, chloroxuron, difenoxuron, diuron, fenuron, fluometuron, isoproturon, linuron, methiuron, metobromuron, metoxuron, monuron, neburon, parafluron, siduron, tebuthiuron, tetrafluron, and thidiazuron. Of these, diuron and fluometuron are the most commonly used in the United States. Isoproturon has been reported to be the most widely used phenylurea herbicide in other countries, for example, India.

The herbicidal action of these compounds is based on their ability to inhibit photosynthesis. Typical phenylurea herbicides, such as diuron, fluometuron, and isoproturon, are photosystem II inhibitors. Photosystem II is a multisubunit enzyme complex which uses light energy to catalyze the photooxidation of water to reducing equivalents and oxygen. The reaction center in photosystem II is composed of the proteins D1, D2, CP43, CP47, and the light-harvesting complex II (Rhee *et al.*, 1998). Substituted phenylurea herbicides inhibit photodependent electron transfer by binding to the D1 protein (Arnaud *et al.*, 1994).

Degradation of phenylurea herbicides in nature can be a relatively slow process. These pesticides can be decomposed by ultraviolet (UV) irradiation or by acidic or alkaline conditions. There are four basic types of reactions in the photochemistry of the substituted phenylurea herbicides; they are photolysis of the $-C-X$ bond on aromatics (X = Cl, Br), photoeliminations (Norrish-Type II reactions), photooxidations, and photorearrangements (Kotzias and Korte, 1981).

Biological degradation of the compounds in plants and soil is carried out by microflora and microfauna. Vroumsia and co-workers (1996) reported that *Rhizoctonia solani* (agonomycetes) was the most efficient microorganism tested at degrading diuron, chlortoluron, and isoproturon. The basic reactions of the biological metabolism of phenylurea herbicides are N-demethylation followed by oxidation of the aromatic ring. The compounds are gradually transformed by microorganisms to 3-arylureas, which are then metabolized to arylamines, carbon dioxide, and ammonia (Cernakova, 1995; Engelhard *et al.*, 1972).

Human cytochrome P_{450} 3A4 (CYP3A4) expressed in yeast has been reported to catalyze the metabolism of chlortoluron (Mehmood *et al.*, 1995). The metabolism was absolutely dependent on NADPH. Chlortoluron was degraded by CYP3A4 into four major metabolites, hydroxylated-N-monodemethylated, hydroxylated ring methylated, N-didemethylated, and N-monodemethylated products. Other cytochrome P_{450}-mediated reactions have not been reported.

While over 20 different phenylureas have been marketed for use as herbicides, little information is available on the toxicity of most of these compounds. More specific information on three of the most common phenylureas, diuron, fluometuron, and isoproturon, is provided.

67.2 DIURON

Synonyms: *N'*-(3,4-Dichlorophenyl)-*N,N*-dimethylurea; 3-(3,4-Dichlorophenyl)-1,1-dimethylurea; DCMU; DMU

Chemical abstract number (CAS#): 330541

Molecular formula: $C_9H_{10}Cl_2N_2O$ (233.1)

Chemical structure:

Trade names and available formulations: Karmex, Karmex DL, Diuron 80WP, Diuron 4L, Direx 4L, Di-on, Diurex, Duirol, Dailon, Rout, Diater, Unidron, Crisuron, and Cekiuron.

67.2.1 PHYSICAL AND CHEMICAL PROPERTIES

Diuron is a white, odorless, crystalline solid with a melting point of 158–159°C, and a boiling point of 180–190°C. Diuron has a water solubility of about 42 ppm (mg/l) at 25°C. Under room temperature and neutral pH, hydrolysis of diuron is negligible. Diuron is stable to oxygen and moisture (Worthing, 1983).

67.2.2 USAGE

Diuron was introduced in 1954 by E. I. Du Pont de Nemours & Co. (Inc.) under the trademark "Karmex" and is mainly used as a pre-emergence herbicide for general weed control on noncrop lands. It is also used as a soil sterilant. The industrial use of diuron, for example, along railroad rights-of-way, represents 57% of the total usage. As of 1995, the estimated usage of diuron in the United States was about 2–4 million pounds (Aspelin, 1997). Diuron is also used selectively before emergence on crops such as asparagus, citrus, pineapple, sugarcane, and cotton. Tolerance for diuron residues was established at 1 ppm on fruits and vegetables in Canada (Chapman, 1967). The occupational exposure limit (TWA, i.e., 8-hour time-weighted average) for diuron in workplace air was established at 10 mg/m³ by ACGIH in the United States (International Labor Office, 1980), which indicates that occupational intake at a rate of 1.4 mg/kg/day is considered safe (Stevens and Sumner, 1991).

67.2.3 ABSORPTION, METABOLISM, AND EXCRETION

Diuron is readily absorbed through the gastrointestinal tract in rats and dogs. Tissue levels of diuron were positively correlated with dosage. No apparent storage of diuron in tissues was noted (Hodge *et al.*, 1967). In mammals, diuron is mainly metabolized by dealkylation of the urea methyl groups. Hydrolysis of diuron to 3,4-dichloroaniline and oxidation to 3,4-dichlorophenol as well as hydroxylation at carbon 2 and/or 6 of the benzene ring, have also been reported. The predominant metabolite of diuron in urine was N-(3,4-dichlorophenyl)-urea. Diuron is also partially excreted unchanged in feces and urine (Boehme and Ernst, 1965; Hodge *et al.*, 1967). Metabolites found in mammals were qualitatively similar to those found in soil and plants wherein dealkylation was also the major metabolic pathway (Dalton *et al.*, 1966; Geissbuhler *et al.*, 1963).

67.2.4 TOXICITY TO LABORATORY ANIMALS

67.2.4.1 Acute Toxicity

The oral LD_{50} (14 days) for diuron in male rats was 3.4 g/kg with 95% confidence limits of 2.9–4.0 g/kg (Hodge *et al.*,

1967). It has been reported (Boyd and Krupa, 1970) that protein content in the diet can influence the acute toxicity of diuron. For example, the LD_{50} of diuron in weanling rats fed a protein-deficient diet (i.e., about 14% of the normal protein intake) was 0.4 ± 0.1 g/kg, whereas the LD_{50} was 2.4 ± 1.4 g/kg in weanling rats fed a protein-enriched diet. Weanling rats fed normal laboratory chow exhibited intermediate sensitivity ($LD_{50} = 1.0 \pm 0.2$ g/kg).

Signs of acute toxicity following near-lethal dosages of diuron in rats included drowsiness, ataxia, decrease and subsequent increase in reflexes, irritability, and bradypnea. Diarrhea, diuresis, shedding of bloody tears, and nosebleed were also noted. Animals treated with diuron exhibited significant loss of body weight, along with a decrease in food and water intake. Hypothermia, glucosuria, proteinuria, and aciduria were detected at 24 hours after exposure. Respiratory failure was the immediate cause of death. The intensity of the signs of toxicity was dose-dependent. Recovery in surviving animals began at 24 hours, and most of the signs disappeared by 72 hours after exposure (Boyd and Krupa, 1970). No signs of skin irritation or sensitization were noted in dermally exposed guinea pigs (Hodge *et al.*, 1967).

Pathological examination revealed local gastroenteritis, gastric ulcers, and capillary-venous congestion of the gastrointestinal mucosa. Stress reactions were also seen in the adrenal and thymus glands and in the spleen. Young animals may exhibit signs of kwashiorkor, such as developmental retardation of the adrenal and thymus glands, gastrointestinal tracts, and especially the testes (Boyd and Krupa, 1970). Other pathological changes included an enlarged, congested spleen (Hodge *et al.*, 1967).

67.2.4.2 Subacute Toxicity

Rats treated with 1 g/kg of diuron daily for 10 days did not show any lethality but exhibited weight gain retardation. Pathologic changes in the spleen and bone marrow were noted at autopsy 3 and 11 days after the final dose (Hodge *et al.*, 1967).

67.2.4.3 Subchronic and Chronic Toxicity

Rats fed a diuron-containing diet (200, 400, 2000, 4000, or 8000 ppm) for 30 days showed growth retardation and anemia at dosages of 4000 and 8000 ppm. Red blood cell counts and hemoglobin levels were also reduced. Lethality occurred only at 8000 ppm. Congestion and an increase in spleen weight were also observed with the highest dose (Hodge *et al.*, 1967).

In 90-day feeding studies (Hodge *et al.*, 1967), 50 and 250 ppm diuron did not cause any toxic effects in rats of either sex: Female rats treated with 500 ppm diuron showed cyanotic discoloration and less weight gain, while the males exhibited literally no signs of toxicity. Reductions in red blood cell counts and hemoglobin levels accompanied by a compensatory bone marrow hyperplasia were observed in rats fed 2500 or 5000 ppm diuron. Growth retardation and decreased food consumption were also noted. All these effects of diuron were greater in females than in males.

Two-year feeding studies in rats and dogs revealed no significant adverse effects at the dietary levels of 25, 125, or 250 ppm diuron except for an inconsistent and sporadic slight anemia. Growth depression was seen with 250 ppm diuron (Hodge *et al.*, 1967).

67.2.4.4 Hematotoxicity

Female Sprague-Dawley rats fed 250, 500, or 1000 mg/kg diuron in the diet for 14 months exhibited biochemical and morphological changes in the circulatory system (Wang *et al.*, 1993). Relative spleen weight was significantly increased in a dose-dependent manner. Hemoglobin levels and erythrocyte counts were significantly reduced, while methemoglobin concentration and white blood cell counts were increased. Hemoglobin adduct of the released parent aromatic amine, 3,4-DCA, was detected at dose-related levels in animals fed 500 or 1000 mg/kg diuron. Increased pigmentation (hemosiderin) in the spleen was seen histologically, reflecting a response to the hemolytic anemia and methemoglobinemia induced by the herbicide. Morphological examination of the red blood cells revealed changes such as erythrocytes with the shape of a spindle or with a centrally stained area associated with abnormal hemoglobin, polychromatic erythrocytes, and hypochromic erythrocytes with a large area of central pallor presumably due to the decreased hemoglobin content.

67.2.4.5 Genotoxicity and Carcinogenesis

It has been reported that a single dose of 170 or 340 mg/kg diuron given intraperitoneally induced the formation of micronuclei in bone marrow cells in mice at 30 and 48 hours after the treatment (Agrawal *et al.*, 1996). Seiler (1978), however, reported that diuron was incapable of inducing micronuclei in erythrocytes when given as a single dose by gavage at 1 or 2 g/kg in mice. In other mutagenicity tests, such as the testicular DNA synthesis inhibition test and the Ames test, diuron exhibited mutagenic activity (Seiler, 1978). Diuron was a suspect genotoxicant, directly or after S-9 activation, at the lowest detected concentrations (LCD) of 900 or 112.5 μg/l, respectively, in the *Vibrio fischeri*/Mutatox™ test (Canna-Michaelidou and Nicolaou, 1996).

Antony and co-workers (1989) reported that topical application of diuron at the rate of 250 mg/kg, three times a week for 3 weeks followed by multiple application of a known skin tumor promotor (12-*O*-tetradecanoyl phorbol 13-acetate, TPA) initiated neoplastic transformation and development of skin tumors in mice. Multiple skin applications of diuron alone for up to 52 weeks, however, did not show any tumor-inducing activity.

There was no evidence in two-year bioassays that diuron was carcinogenic in rats or dogs (Hodge *et al.*, 1967). Mice given 464 mg/kg diuron daily from 7 to 28 days of age followed by 1000 ppm diuron daily in the diet for 18 months showed no signs of increased tumor formation (Reinhold, 1987).

67.2.4.6 Teratogenicity

In a study in which the formulation Karmex® (containing 80% diuron) was given by gastric intubation to pregnant rats from gestation days 6–15 at levels of 125, 250, or 500 mg/kg/day, only the highest dosage reduced both maternal and fetal body weights. Wavy ribs were seen at the dosages of 250 and 500 mg/kg, and delayed ossification of the calvarium was noted in fetuses whose dams received 125 mg/kg diuron (Khera *et al.*, 1979). Diuron showed no teratogenic activity in mice, however (Reinhold, 1987).

A multigeneration reproductive toxicity study in rats given 125 ppm diuron in the diet revealed no significant changes in reproductive performance endpoints. Post-weaning growth of the F_{2b} and F_{3a} generations was moderately affected, however (Hodge *et al.*, 1967).

67.2.4.7 Biochemical Effects

Diuron, a dihalogenated substituted urea herbicide, has been reported to be a more potent inducer of hepatic metabolizing enzymes [e.g., benzo(*a*)pyrene mono-oxygenase (BP-MOO), 7-ethoxycoumarin *O*-deethylase (ECOD), and 7-ethoxyresorufin *O*-deethylase (EROD)] compared to those phenylurea herbicides with one or no halogen substitutions, for example, chlortoluron and isoproturon (Schoket and Vincze, 1985, 1986, 1990). Schoket and co-workers (1987) found that repeated diuron exposures (1/6 LD_{50} for 3 days) decreased the plasma half-life of antipyrine significantly, indicating hepatic cytochrome P_{450} isozymes were induced. Close correlations ($r = 0.98$–0.99) were found between the induction of BP-MOO, ECOD, and EROD and the increase of antipyrine metabolism after diuron treatment. Moreover, hepatic enzymes such as cytochrome P_{450}, BP-MOO, microsomal epoxide hydrolase, glutathione S-transferase, and UDP-glucuronyltransferase were all induced by diuron in a dose-related manner (oral dosing 1/20 to 1/4 LD_{50}) in rats (Schoket and Vincze, 1990). Dose-related induction of hepatic microsomal enzymes was also seen in rats fed a diuron-containing diet (100, 250, 500, 1000, and 2000 ppm) for 13 weeks (Kinoshita and DuBois, 1970). Maximum induction occurred within the first 3 weeks of feeding and then decreased afterwards. Moreover, a sex difference was noted in the response of the animals, that is, male rats were more sensitive than females to the enzyme-inducing activity of diuron.

67.2.4.8 Aquatic Toxicity

Diuron used for weed control in water may interfere with the growth of fish and food-chain microfauna, such as *Daphnia* (Crosby and Tucker, 1966). The LC_{50} of diuron in *Daphnia magna* or *Daphnia pulex* at 24 or 48 hours is 1.4 mg/l. The LC_{50}s of diuron in the warm-water fish *Lepomis macrochirus* and the cold-water fish *Oncorhynchus kisutch* are 7.4 and 16.0 mg/l at 48 hours, respectively (Ramamoorthy and Baddaloo, 1995).

67.3 FLUOMETURON

Synonym: 1,1-dimethyl-3-[3-(trifluoromethyl)phenyl]urea

Chemical abstract number (CAS#): 2164-17-2

Molecular formula: $C_{10}H_{11}F_3N_2O$ (232.2)

Chemical structure:

Trade names and available formulations: Cotoran, Cotoran 4L, Cotoran 85DF, Meturon 4L, Ciba 2059, Cottonex, Lanex, Herbicide C-2059, Pakhtaran

67.3.1 PHYSICAL AND CHEMICAL PROPERTIES

Fluometuron is a colorless, crystalline, sandlike material with a melting point of 163–164.5°C and a vapor pressure of 5×10^{-7} mm Hg at 20°C. Its solubility in water and acetone at 20°C is about 105 mg/l (ppm) and 105 g/l (ppt), respectively. Fluometuron is soluble in most organic solvents (IARC Monographs, 1983; Worthing, 1983).

67.3.2 USAGE

Fluometuron has been used as a herbicide in the United States for more than three decades. Since being introduced as a commercial chemical in 1960 by Ciba-Geigy AG under the trademark "Cotoran" (Worthing, 1983), fluometuron has been widely used to control broadleaf weeds and grasses on agricultural crops, for example, cotton and sugarcane. The amount of fluometuron used in the United States in 1976 and 1978 was estimated to be 5.3 and 2.9 million pounds, respectively (IARC Monographs, 1983). As of 1995, the approximate quantity of fluometuron used annually in U.S. agricultural practices was about 5–9 million pounds (Aspelin, 1997).

The tolerance for fluometuron in or on raw agricultural commodities, cottonseed, and sugarcane was set at 0.1 ppm in the United States (U.S. Environmental Protection Agency, 1980a). In or on sugarcane bagasse, a tolerance of 0.2 ppm was established (U.S. Environmental Protection Agency, 1980b). Maximum occupational exposure to fluometuron was established at the level of 5 mg/m³ in workplace air in the USSR (International Labor Office, 1980).

67.3.3 TOXICITY TO LABORATORY ANIMALS

67.3.3.1 Acute Toxicity

The oral LD_{50} of fluometuron was about 8.9 g/kg in rats of both sexes (Ben-Dyke et al., 1970), 0.9 and 2.4 g/kg in male and female mice, and greater than 10 g/kg in rabbits and dogs (Spencer, 1968). The dermal LD_{50} in rats and rabbits was > 2 and 10 g/kg, respectively (Ben-Dyke et al., 1970; Worthing, 1983). LC_{50}s (96 hours) for rainbow trout, crucian carp, and bluegill were 47, 17, and 96 mg/l, respectively (Worthing, 1983). Animals treated with lethal dosages of fluometuron exhibited signs of depression, gasping, hyperpnea, lacrimation, and peripheral vasoconstriction (National Cancer Institute, 1980).

Toxicity of fluometuron in 6- to 9-month-old desert sheep has been seen with a single oral dose of 0.8 or 4 g/kg (Mohamed et al., 1995). Signs of toxicity appeared within 15 minutes after exposure and included depression, salivation, grinding of the teeth, chewing movement of the jaws, mydriasis, dyspnea, incoordination of movements, and drowsiness. Similar signs of toxicity were also seen in animals treated with repeated daily dosages of 25 or 200 mg/kg fluometuron. Laboratory testing revealed increased activities of serum alanine aminotransferase (ALT), aspartate transaminase (AST), and lactate dehydrogenase. Blood urea nitrogen was also elevated. Total serum protein and calcium were significantly decreased.

67.3.3.2 Subchronic Toxicity

In 90-day feeding studies where rats or mice of both sexes were treated with 250, 500, 1000, 2000, 4000, 8000, or 16,000 ppm fluometuron, less weight gain was seen with the three highest doses in both male and female rats (National Cancer Institute, 1980). Deaths occurred in male rats fed 8000 and 16,000 ppm fluometuron and in females receiving 16,000 ppm. Various degrees of spleen enlargement were observed in rats of both sexes treated with 2000 ppm or more of fluometuron. Dose-related pathological changes in rats included mild to severe congestion of the red pulp with corresponding atrophy of the white pulp and depletion of the lymphocytic elements. There were essentially no signs of toxicity observed in mice in these subchronic studies except for a moderate decrease (about 10%) in body weight gain in both sexes at levels of 4000 ppm and greater.

67.3.3.3 Mutagenicity

Fluometuron given as a single dose by gavage in mice exhibited mutagenic activity in both the testicular DNA synthesis inhibition test and the erythrocyte micronucleus test at levels of 1 and 2 g/kg. In the in vitro Ames test, fluometuron also showed mutagenic activity (Seiler, 1978).

67.3.3.4 Carcinogenicity

Mice of both sexes (7 weeks old) fed a diet containing 500 or 1000 mg/kg fluometuron for 103 weeks showed similar incidences of both neoplastic and non-neoplastic lesions compared to the control animals. A nonsignificant increase in the incidences of hepatocellular adenomas or carcinomas and tumors in the hematopoietic system (e.g., lymphoma and leukemia) was seen in male mice. Carcinogenicity studies in rats fed 125 or 250 mg/kg fluometuron-containing diet for 103 weeks were negative (IARC Monographs, 1983; National Cancer Institute, 1980).

67.4 ISOPROTURON

Synonyms: (*N,N*-dimethyl-*N'*-[4-(1-methylethyl)phenyl]urea; 3-(4-isopropylphenyl)-1,1-dimethylurea

Chemical abstract number (CAS#): 34123-59-6

Molecular formula: $C_{12}H_{18}N_2O$ (206.3)

Chemical structure:

Trade names and available formulations: Arelon, Graminon

67.4.1 PHYSICAL AND CHEMICAL PROPERTIES

Isoproturon is a colorless powder with a melting point of 155–156°C and a vapor pressure of 2.5×10^{-8} mm Hg at 20°C. Its water solubility is about 55 ppm at 20°C. Isoproturon is soluble in most organic solvents and is stable to light, acids, and alkalis (Worthing, 1983).

67.4.2 USAGE

Isoproturon was introduced as a herbicide by Hoechst AG under the tradename of "Arelon," by Ciba-Geigy AG under the tradename of "Graminon", and by Rhone-Poulenc as Phytosanitaire. Isoproturon is used to control selectively germinating broadleaf and grass weeds in sugarcane, citrus, cotton, and asparagus. It is widely used abroad. About 3 million pounds of isoproturon are used annually in India.

67.4.3 TOXICITY TO LABORATORY ANIMALS

67.4.3.1 Basic Findings

The acute oral LD_{50} of isoproturon in rats was estimated at 1.8–2.4 g/kg, while the acute dermal LD_{50} was >3.2 g/kg (Worthing, 1983). An acute oral LD_{50} of 1 g/kg in rats has also been reported (Behera and Bhunya, 1990).

In 90-day feeding studies, the no observed adverse effect level was reported to be 400 mg/kg/day in rats and 50 mg/kg/day in dogs (Worthing, 1983).

The 96-hour LC_{50}s of isoproturon for carp and rainbow trout were 193 and 240 mg/l, respectively (Worthing, 1983).

67.4.3.2 Subacute and Subchronic Toxicity

Repeated dermal exposure of isoproturon technical (IPT; 250, 500, or 1000 mg/kg/day) and its wettable powder formulation (IPF; 750, 1500, or 2250 mg/kg/day) in rats of both sexes for 21 days produced no clear overt signs of toxicity (Dikshith *et al.*, 1990). Increased organ:body weight ratios (e.g., liver, kidney, adrenal, and spleen) were seen more in the females with both IPT and IPF, especially with the highest dosages. Hematological studies showed that all three dosages of IPT decreased red blood cell counts in males, while only the highest dosage caused a slight reduction in erythrocyte counts in females. Hemoglobin levels in both sexes were reduced by all three dosages of isoproturon (IPT). Neutrophils were decreased and lymphocytes were increased by all IPT exposures. IPF, on the other hand, did not produce any hematological changes. Activities of ALT and AST and protein content in the liver and serum were also altered by IPT or IPF in one or both sexes of the rats. For example, females had an increase in serum AST activity, a decrease in liver ALT, and a significant reduction in serum protein after repeated IPT. Repeated IPF exposure reduced serum ALT activity in male rats and lowered total serum proteins in female rats.

No overt signs of toxicity were observed in rats treated orally with 200, 400, or 800 mg/kg/day of isoproturon for 42 and 60 days (Sarkar *et al.*, 1995). The highest dosage of the chemical, however, did significantly decrease body weight. Moreover, a dose-dependent increase in the liver weight was noted. Isoproturon also increased the weights of the kidney and the heart. Histopathological changes included hepatocellular degeneration and focal necrosis in the liver, glomerular and tubular degeneration in the kidney, and hemosiderosis in the spleen.

67.4.3.3 Genotoxicity

Isoproturon and its structural analogs fluometuron and monuron have all been reported to be genotoxic (Behera and Bhunya, 1990; Garrett *et al.*, 1986; Seiler, 1978). Behera and Bhunya (1990) found that 100, 150, and 200 mg/kg of isoproturon given intraperitoneally to adult Swiss albino mice induced various types of chromosomal aberrations in bone marrow cells, for example, chromatid gaps, chromatid breaks, acentric fragments, chromatid exchanges, ring chromosomes, and metacentric chromosomes. The highest dosage of isoproturon also induced the formation of micronuclei in bone marrow cells. Pregnant rats treated orally with 180 mg/kg of isoproturon daily from gestation day 6 to gestation day 20 also exhibited chromatid breaks in bone marrow cells (Srivastava and Raizada, 1995).

67.4.3.4 Reproductive Toxicity

Isoproturon has been found to induce abnormalities in sperm shape in a dose-dependent manner in mice (Behera and Bhunya, 1990). The sperm would either have hammer, mushroom, or amorphous shaped heads, or hook and beak shaped acrosomal ends. Sarkar and co-workers (1997) also reported the potential toxic effects of isoproturon on the male reproductive system in rats. When isoproturon was given orally to rats 6 days/week at the rate of 200, 400, or 800 mg/kg/day for 10 weeks, the highest dosage decreased epididymal sperm counts and the percentage of motile sperm and increased the percentage of abnormal sperm (e.g., distorted heads, atypical tails, bent necks or midpieces). Degeneration and desquamation of germinal layer cells were observed in the testis. Tubular lumens of the testis and the epididymis exhibited reduced numbers of spermatids and spermatozoa, respectively (Sarkar *et al.*, 1995). The activities of androgen biosynthesis-related enzymes, for example, glucose-6-phosphate dehydrogenase and Δ5-3β-hydroxy steroid dehydrogenase, were reduced in a dose-related manner (Sarkar *et al.*, 1997). Overall, isoproturon has been suggested to have the potential to cause maturational malformation of sperm cells and retarded spermatogenesis in rats.

67.4.3.5 Fetotoxicity and Teratogenicity

Isoproturon (45, 90, or 180 mg/kg/day) given orally to pregnant rats from gestation days 6–20 caused no observable fetotoxic and/or teratogenic effects. The numbers of implantations and resorptions, fetal body weights, and external, visceral, and skeletal structures were all comparable to those in the controls (Srivastava and Raizada, 1995). With higher dosages of isoproturon (225, 450, and 900 mg/kg/day) given orally from gestation days 6–15 (Sarkar and Gupta, 1993a), however, dose-related depression and drowsiness of the dams were observed. Though there was no lethality associated with isoproturon exposures, decreased maternal body weight was noted during later pregnancy (gestation days 15–20) with the dosages of 450 and 900 mg/kg. Litter size, fetal weights, and crown-rump and transumbilical lengths were all decreased by 450 mg/kg or more of isoproturon. Moreover, there was a significant increase in the frequency of fetal resorptions and the number of fetuses with retarded growth. Again, no major visceral and/or skeletal malformations were observed.

67.4.3.6 Neurological Effects

Neurotoxic effects of isoproturon in mice have been reported by Sarkar and Gupta (1993b). They found a single oral dose of isoproturon (0.5, 1.0, or 2.0 g/kg) potentiated both pentobarbital- and barbital-induced sleeping time. Spontaneous and forced locomotor activity were reduced by 1.0 and 2.0 mg/kg isoproturon. In addition, isoproturon exhibited anticonvulsant activity against electroshock and pentylenetetrazol-induced convulsions. The mechanisms of these inhibitory effects of isoproturon on the central nervous system are unclear.

67.4.3.7 Biochemical Effects

Isoproturon given by gavage to rats at the dose of 1/6 LD_{50} for 3 consecutive days induced significantly the activities of hepatic enzymes, for example, NADPH-cytochrome c reductase, microsomal epoxide hydrolase, 7-ethoxycoumarin O-deethylase, aldrin epoxidase, UDP-glucuronyl-transferase, and glutathion-S-transferase (Schoket and Vincze, 1985, 1986). Antipyrine plasma half-life, however, was not affected by the isoproturon treatment, suggesting that hepatic cytochrome P-450 isozymes, for example, benzo(a)pyrene monooxygenase and 7-ethoxyresorufin O-deethylase, were not induced by isoproturon (Schoket *et al.*, 1987).

REFERENCES

Agrawal, R. C., Kumar, S., and Mehrotra, N. K. (1996). Micronucleus induction by diuron in mouse bone marrow. *Toxicol. Lett.* **89**, 1–4.

Antony, M., Shukla, Y., and Mehrotra, N. K. (1989). Tumor initiatory activity of a herbicide diuron on mouse skin. *Cancer Lett.* **48**, 125–128.

Arnaud, L., Taillandier, G., Kaouadji, M., Ravanel, P., and Tissut, M. (1994). Photosynthesis inhibition by phenylureas: A QSAR approach. *Ecotoxicol. Environ. Safety* **28**, 121–133.

Aspelin, A. L. (1997). "Pesticides Industry Sales and Usage: 1994 and 1995 Market Estimates," EPA 733-R-97-002, Office of Prevention, Pesticides and Toxic Substances (7503W), United States Environmental Protection Agency, Washington, DC.

Behera, B. C., and Bhunya, S. P. (1990). Genotoxic effect of isoproturon (herbicide) as revealed by three mammalian *in vivo* mutagenic bioassays. *Indian J. Exper. Biol.* **28**, 862–867.

Ben-Dyke, R., Sanderson, D. M., and Noakes, D. N. (1970). Acute toxicity data for pesticides. *World Rev. Pest. Contr.* **9**(3), 119–127.

Boehme, C., and Ernst, W. (1965). The metabolism of urea-herbicides in the rat. 2. Diuron and linuron. *Food Cosmet. Toxicol.* **3**, 797–802. [In German].

Boyd, E. M., and Krupa, V. (1970). Protein-deficient diet and diuron toxicity. *J. Agr. Food Chem.* **18**(6), 1104–1107.

Canna-Michaelidou, S., and Nicolaou, A.-S. (1996). Evaluation of the genotoxicity potential (by Mutatox™) test of ten pesticides found as water pollutants in Cyprus. *Sci. Total Environ.* **193**, 27–35.

Cernakova, M. (1995). Biological degradation of isoproturon, chlortoluron and fenitrothion. *Folia Microbiol.* **40**(2), 201–206.

Chapman, R. A. (1967). "Tolerances for Residues of Pesticide Chemicals," T.I.L. No. 290. Food and Drug Directorate, Department of National Health and Welfare, Ottawa.

Crosby, D. G., and Tucker, R. K. (1966). Toxicity of aquatic herbicides to Daphnia magna. *Science* **154**, 289–290.

Dalton, R. L., Evans, A. W., and Rhodes, R. C. (1966). Disappearance of diuron in cotton field soils. *Weeds* **14**, 31–33.

Dikshith, T. S. S., Raizada, R. B., and Srivastava, M. K. (1990). Dermal toxicity to rats of isoproturon technical and formulation. *Vet. Hum. Toxicol.* **32**(5), 432–434.

Engelhard, G., Wallnofer, P. R., and Plapp, K. (1972). Identification of N,O-dimethylhydroxylamine as microbial degradation product of the herbicide linuron. *Appl. Microbiol.* **23**, 664–666.

Garrett, N. E., Stack, H. F., and Waters, M. D. (1986). Evaluation of the genetic activity profiles of 65 pesticides. *Mut. Res.* **168**, 301–325.

Geissbuhler, H. C., Haselback, C., Aebi, H., and Ebner, L. (1963). The fate of N'-(4-chlorophenoxy)-phenyl-N,N-dimethylurea (C-1983) in soils and plants. III. Breakdown in soils. *Weed Res.* **3**, 277–297.

Hodge, H. C., Downs, W. L., Panner, B. S., Smith, D. W., and Maynard, E. A. (1967). Oral toxicity and metabolism of diuron (N-(3,4-dichlorophenyl)-N',N'-dimethylurea) in rats and dogs. *Food Cosmet. Toxicol.* **5**, 513–531.

IARC Monographs (1983). Fluometuron. *IRAC Monographs on the Evaluation of the Carcinogenic Risk of Chemicals to Man* **30**, 245–253.

International Labor Office (1980). "Occupational Exposure Limits for Airborn Toxic Substances," 2nd (revised) ed., Occupational Safety and Health Series, No. 37, pp. 106; 118–119. Geneva.

Khera, K. S., Whalen, C., Trivett, G., and Angers, G. (1979). Teratogenicity studies on pesticidal formulations of dimethoate, diuron and lindane in rats. *Bull. Environ. Contam. Toxicol.* **22**, 522–529.

Kinoshita, F. K., and DuBois, K. P. (1970). Induction of hepatic microsomal enzymes by Herban, diuron and other substituted urea hericides. *Toxicol. Appl. Pharmacol.* **17**, 406–417.

Kotzias, D., and Korte, F. (1981). Photochemistry of phenylurea herbicides and their reactions in the environment. *Ecotoxicol. Environ. Safety* **5**, 503–512.

Mehmood, Z., Kelly, D. E., and Kelly, S. L. (1995). Metabolism of the herbicide chlortoluron by human cytochrome P450 3A4. *Chemosphere* **31**(11/12), 4515–4529.

Mohamed, O. S. A., Ahmed, K. E., Adam, S. E. I., and Idris, O. F. (1995). Toxicity of cotoran (fluometuron) in desert sheep. *Vet. Hum. Toxicol.* **37**(3), 214–216.

National Cancer Institute (1980). "Bioassay of Fluometuron for Possible Carcinogenicity." Carcinogenesis Technical Report Series. CAS No. 2164-17-2, NCI-CG-TR-195, NTP-80-11.

Ramamoorthy, S., and Baddaloo, E. G. (1995). Aquatic toxicity data. *In* "Handbook of Chemical Toxicity Profiles of Biological Species. Volume I: Aquatic Species," pp. 165, 172, 251, 284. CRC Press, Boca Raton, FL.

Reinhold, V. N. (1987). Diuron, a review. *Dangerous Properties of Industrial Material Report* **7**(5), 49–55.

Rhee, K. H., Morris, E. P., Barber, J., and Kuhlbrandt, W. (1998). Three-dimensional structure of the plant photosystem II reaction centre at 8 A resolution. *Nature* **398**(19), 283–286.

Sarkar, S. N., Chattopadhyay, S. K., and Majumdar, A. C. (1995). Subacute toxicity of urea herbicide, isoproturon, in rats. *Indian J. Exper. Biol.* **33**, 851–856.

Sarkar, S. N., and Gupta, P. K. (1993a). Fetotoxic and teratogenic potential of substituted phenylurea herbicide, isoproturon, in rats. *Indian J. Exper. Biol.* **31**, 280–282.

Sarkar, S. N., and Gupta, P. K. (1993b). Neurotoxicity of isoproturon, a substituted phenylurea herbicide, in mice. *Indian J. Exper. Biol.* **31**, 977–981.

Sarkar, S. N., Majumdar, A. C., and Chattopadhyay, S. K. (1997). Effect of isoproturon on male reproductive system: Clinical, histological and histoenzymological studies in rats. *Indian J. Exper. Biol.* **35**, 133–138.

Schoket, B., and Vincze, I. (1985). Induction of rat hepatic drug metabolizing enzymes by substituted urea herbicides. *Acta Pharmacol. Toxicol.* **56**, 283–288.

Schoket, B., and Vincze, I. (1986). Induction of rat hepatic microsomal epoxide hydrolase by substituted urea herbicides. *Acta Pharmacol. Toxicol.* **58**, 156–158.

Schoket, B., and Vincze, I. (1990). Dose-related induction of rat hepatic drug-metabolizing enzymes by diuron and chlorotoluron, two substituted phenylurea herbicides. *Toxicol. Lett.* **50**, 1–7.

Schoket, B., Zilahy, Z., Molnar, J., and Vincze, I. (1987). Comparative investigation of antipyrine half-life and induction of cytochrome P-450 dependent monooxygenases in rats treated with phenylurea herbicides. *In Vivo* **1**, 185–188.

Seiler, J. P. (1978). Herbicidal phenylalkylureas as possible mutagens I. Mutagenicity tests with some urea herbicides. *Mut. Res.* **58**, 353–359.

Spencer, E. Y. (1968). "Guide to the Chemicals Used in Crop Protection," 5th ed. Research Branch Agriculture Canada Publication 1093, University of Western Ontario, London, Ontario.

Srivastava, M. K., and Raizada, R. B. (1995). Developmental toxicity of the substituted phenylurea herbicide isoproturon in rats. *Vet. Hum. Toxicol.* **37**(3), 220–223.

Stevens, J. T., and Sumner, D. D. (1991). Herbicides. *In* "Handbook of Pesticide Toxicology. Vol. 3. Classes of Pesticides" (W. J. Hayes, Jr. and E. R. Laws, Jr., eds.), pp. 1349–1350. Academic Press, San Diego, CA.

U.S. Environmental Protection Agency (1980a). "Protection of Environment." US Code of Federal Regulations, Title 40, part 180.229.

U.S. Environmental Protection Agency (1980b). "Food and Drugs." US Code of Federal Regulations, Title 21, part 561.240.

Vroumsia, T., Steiman, R., Seigle-Murandi, F., Benoit-Guyod, J. L., and Khadrani, A. (1996). Biodegradation of three substituted phenylurea herbicides (chlortoluron, diuron, and isoproturon) by soil fungi. A comparative study. *Chemosphere* **33**(10), 2045–2056.

Wang, S. W., Chu, C. Y., Hsu, J. D., and Wang, C. J. (1993). Haemotoxic effect of phenylurea herbicides in rats: Role of haemoglobin-adduct formation in splenic toxicity. *Food Chem. Toxic.* **31**(4), 285–295.

Worthing, C. R. (1983). "The Pesticide Manual: A World Compendium," 7th ed., pp. 226, 281, 329. BCPC.

CHAPTER

68

Protoporphyrinogen Oxidase Inhibitors

Franck E. Dayan, Joanne G. Romagni, and Stephen O. Duke
United States Department of Agriculture

68.1 INTRODUCTION

Protoporphyrinogen oxidase (Protox)–inhibiting herbicides have been used since the 1960s and now represent a relatively large (ca. 10%) and growing segment of the herbicide market. Before their molecular target, Protox, was discovered (Matringe et al., 1989a, b), this category of herbicides was often termed "diphenyl ether–type herbicides." At that time, almost all of the Protox inhibitors were diphenyl ethers. This nomenclature led to some confusion in herbicide classification, because other "diphenyl ether" herbicides have an entirely different molecular site of action (i.e., inhibition of acetyl CoA carboxylase). Now, many other structural classes of Protox inhibitors are commercialized. In general, the newer products are more potent Protox inhibitors, resulting in lower application rates than the older herbicides of this class. Some of them appear to be analogs of the substrate or a substrate/product transition state of the enzyme (Reddy et al., 1998).

There are several previous reviews of the Protox inhibitors, both before (Böger, 1984; Gilham and Dodge, 1987; Kunert et al., 1987; Matsunaka, 1976) and after (Dayan and Duke, 1996, 1997; Duke et al., 1991; Nandihalli and Duke, 1993; Reddy et al., 1998; Scalla and Matringe, 1994) their target site was known. The emphasis in most of these previous reviews was on the mode of action. An entire book dealing mainly with Protox inhibitors is available (Duke and Rebeiz, 1994). This review updates and supplements these previous publications.

68.2 COMMERCIALLY AVAILABLE PROTOX INHIBITORS

68.2.1 DIPHENYL ETHER PROTOPORPHYRINOGEN OXIDASE INHIBITORS

Nitrofen was the first Protox-inhibiting herbicide to be introduced for commercial use in 1964. This diphenyl ether (DPE) herbicide was eventually recognized as a relatively weak inhibitor of Protox (Nandihalli et al., 1992), but was a lead compound of an entire class of structurally related herbicides that were much more active. Several DPE herbicides (see Table 68.1) have been successfully commercialized (Anderson et al., 1994). Although many of these older commercialized DPEs have a p-nitrophenyl substitution, newer DPE-like herbicides more commonly contain p-trifluoromethyl phenyl substitutions. These new herbicides are heterocyclic phenyl ethers (structurally related to DPEs), where one of the phenyl rings of ether is replaced by an aromatic heterocycle. Recently reported examples include 6-aryloxy-1H-benzotriazoles (Condon et al., 1995), aryloxyindolin-2(3H)-ones (Karp et al., 1995), 5-aryloxybenzisoxazoles (Wepplo et al., 1995), 6-aryloxyquinoxalin-2,3-diones (Anderson et al., 1994), benzheterocycles (Lee et al., 1995), and benzoxazines (Sumida et al., 1995). Pyrazolyl, pyridyl, and furyl rings have also been investigated as the heterocyclic component (Anderson et al., 1994; Armbruster et al., 1993; Clark, 1994; 1996; Sherman et al., 1991).

68.2.2 NON–DIPHENYL ETHER PROTOPORPHYRINOGEN OXIDASE INHIBITORS

Whereas the first generation of Protox inhibitors (with the exception of oxadiazon) was primarily based on the DPE backbone, numerous non-oxygen-bridged compounds with this same site of action have been discovered (Table 68.2). These compounds invariably consist of heterobicyclic structures with one phenyl ring attached to a heterocyclic ring. The linkage can consist of a carbon–carbon bridge, as with the isoxazole carboxamides (Dayan et al., 1997a; Hamper et al., 1995), but more often consists of a carbon–nitrogen bridge, as with the phenyl imides (Lyga et al., 1991; Mito et al., 1991; Sato et al., 1987), triazolinones (Amuti et al., 1997; Dayan et al., 1997b, c; Theodoridis, 1997; Theodoridis et al., 1992, 1995), oxadia-

Table 68.1
Commercially Available DPE and DPE-like Protox-Inhibiting Herbicides[a]

Common name	U.S. trade name	Primary source	Chemical structure
Acifluorfen	Blazer[®]	BASF	
Bifenox	Foxpro[®]	Rhône-Poulenc	
Fluoroglycofen	Complete[®]	Rohm and Haas	
Fomesafen	Reflex[®]	Zeneca	
Lactofen	Cobra[®]	Valent	
Oxyfluorfen	Goal[®]	Rohm and Haas	

[a] Information from Ahrens (1994).

zolones (Dickmann *et al.*, 1997), and pyrazoles (Prosch *et al.*, 1997).

There are several reasons for the high level of interest among agrochemical companies in the discovery and development of new Protox inhibitors. For one thing, weeds have not shown a propensity to develop resistance to these herbicides. It is likely that Protox inhibitors may soon supplant acetolactate synthase inhibitors as the preferred herbicides for broad-spectrum weed control in soybean fields. Additionally, the market niche for Protox inhibitor is beginning to expand to weed control in monocot crops, with the marketing of newer compounds such as carfentrazone, JV 485, and oxadiargyl (Table 68.3). Finally, Protox seems to be a particularly good target that can be inhibited by structurally diverse classes of herbicides, allowing for the development of a new chemistry not yet patented by other companies.

68.3 AGRICULTURAL USE

68.3.1 CROPS AND WEEDS

Protox inhibitors have historically been used for broad-spectrum weed control in soybean fields (Table 68.3). Dayan and Duke (1996) proposed that the market share of Protox in-

hibitors could be increased by developing compounds for use in monocot crops. Several non-DPE herbicides based on the triazolinone and the oxadiazole structures have been, or will soon be, registered for weed control in cereal crops. At the moment, most of the compounds, with selectivity for cereals and small grains (bifenox, carfentrazone, and fluoroglycofen), are currently not available in the U.S. market. Finally, compounds with the highest biological activity, such as oxyfluorfen and azafenidin, have also been developed for use as nonselective herbicides in noncrop areas and nurseries.

As a group, Protox-inhibiting herbicides control both monocotyledonous and dicotyledonous weeds. The market for weed control in soybean fields is intense because a similar spectrum of weed control can be obtained with herbicides with other sites of action. In particular, acetolactate synthase (ALS) inhibitors, such as the imidazolinones and sulfonyl ureas, have become important tools for soybean growers. The situation may be changing, though, as many weeds have become resistant to the ALS-inhibiting herbicides by evolving herbicide-insensitive forms of the enzyme. In contrast, no cases of evolved resistance to Protox inhibitors have been reported. Possible reasons for this will be discussed in Section 68.4.3. As a result, agrochemical companies are actively pursuing the development of new Protox inhibitors in order to replace ALS-inhibiting herbicides as resistant weeds become more widespread in soybean fields.

Table 68.2
Non-Oxygen-Bridged Protox-Inhibiting Herbicides

Common name	Trade name	Primary source	Chemical structure
Azafenidin[a]	—	Dupont	
Carfentrazone[b]	Affinity®	FMC	
Flumiclorac[c]	Resource®	Valent	
JV-485[d]	—	Monsanto	
Oxadiargyl[e]	—	Rhône-Poulenc	
Oxadiazon[c]	Ronstar®	Rhône-Poulenc	
Sulfentrazone[f]	Authority®	FMC Corporation	

[a] Amuti *et al.* (1997).
[b] Anonymous (1995b).
[c] Ahrens (1994).
[d] Prosch *et al.* (1997).
[e] Dickmann *et al.* (1997).
[f] Anonymous (1995a).

68.3.2 MODE OF APPLICATION

For the most part, Protox-inhibiting herbicides are applied postemergence during the early stages of weed development. The rate of application ranges widely among Protox inhibitors. Most of the DPE herbicides (such as acifluorfen and lactofen) are applied at rates of 100 to 500 g active ingredient per hectare. Fluoroglycofen is more active and can be applied at rates 10-fold lower. The most active of these herbicides can be applied at rates as low as 1 g active ingredient per hectare.

With a few exceptions, these compounds do not have preemergence activity and have little residual activity in soils. However, more recently discovered structures such as sulfentrazone have excellent preemergence activity (Table 68.3) (Theodoridis *et al.*, 1992). The preemergence-applied Protox inhibitors are active at concentrations ranging from 2 to 4 kg active ingredient per hectare for oxadiazon to 100 g active ingredient per hectare for sulfentrazone.

68.4 BEHAVIOR IN PLANTS

Protox inhibitors cause rapid photobleaching and light-dependent desiccation of foliage. The symptoms observed on the

Table 68.3
Targeted Crops and Mode of Application of Commercially Available Protox-Inhibiting Herbicides

Common name	Main crop	Application[a]
Acifluorfen[a]	Soybean, peanut, rice	Postemergence
Azafenidin[b]	Perennial crops/forestry	Preemergence
Bifenox[a]	Small grain	Preemergence/postemergence
Carfentrazone[c]	Cereal crops	Postemergence
Flumiclorac[a]	Soybean and maize	Preemergence/postemergence
Fluoroglycofen[a]	Cereal crops	Postemergence
Fomesafen[a]	Soybean	Postemergence
JV-485[d]	Winter wheat	Preemergence
Lactofen[a]	Soybean	Postemergence
Oxadiargyl[e]	Rice/sugarcane	Preemergence
Oxadiazon[a]	Grasses and ornamentals	Postemergence
Oxyfluorfen[a]	Vegetable crops	Preemergence/postemergence
Sulfentrazone[f]	Soybean, sugarcane, tobacco	Preemergence

[a] Ahrens (1994).
[b] Amuti *et al.* (1997).
[c] Anonymous (1995b).
[d] Prosch *et al.* (1997).
[e] Dickmann *et al.* (1997).
[f] Anonymous (1995a).

foliage of DPE-treated plants include leaf cupping, crinkling, bronzing, and necrosis (Johnson *et al.*, 1978). The lesions on the foliage are due to loss of membrane integrity that leads to cellular leakage (Fig. 68.1) (Dayan *et al.*, 1997c, 1998; Kenyon *et al.*, 1985; Lee *et al.*, 1995). Other physiological responses include inhibition of photosynthesis; evolution of ethylene, ethane, and malondialdehyde; and, finally, bleaching of chloroplast pigments (Kenyon *et al.*, 1985). Protox inhibitors are known to cause temporary injury to the foliage of treated

crops (particularly soybean). However, crops generally recover rapidly, and yields are not affected (Vidrine *et al.*, 1993, 1994, 1996; Walker *et al.*, 1992). Though not desirable, crop injury on soybean is not unusual and farmers have become accustomed to this phenomenon as the use of ALS-inhibiting herbicides has become more widespread.

68.4.1 ABSORPTION, TRANSLOCATION, AND METABOLISM

Most postemergence-applied Protox inhibitors are readily absorbed through the leaves (Dayan *et al.*, 1996, 1997b; Ritter and Coble, 1981a). Root uptake of foliar active compounds is generally poor (Ritter and Coble, 1981b). Once absorbed into the foliage, little translocation is observed. Most of the DPE herbicides (such as acifluorfen, lactofen, and fluoroglycofen) are not translocated beyond the point of absorption. However, some of them, such as fomesafen, can be readily translocated by the xylem. Some studies demonstrate that absorption and translocation of DPE herbicides may be affected by temperature and humidity (Ritter and Coble, 1981a; Wills and McWhorter, 1981).

Soil active compounds, such as sulfentrazone, are readily taken up by the roots and translocated through the xylem along the transpiration flow (Wehtje *et al.*, 1997). Radiolabeled pulse–chase studies show that nearly all of the herbicide taken up by the roots is translocated to the foliage within 24 h (Fig. 68.2) (Dayan *et al.*, 1996, 1997c). Interestingly, the related sensitive (coffee senna) and resistant (sicklepod) weeds absorbed and translocated sulfentrazone in the same manner (Fig. 68.2).

The selectivity of Protox inhibitors lies primarily in the differential rate of metabolism. In the case of DPE herbicides, such as acifluorfen and fluorodifen, the resistance of soybean is achieved by metabolic cleavage of the ether bridge, followed

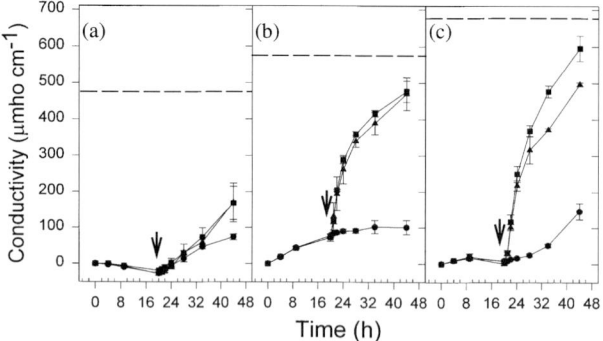

Figure 68.1 Herbicidal activity of carfentrazone-ethyl and deethylated carfentrazone metabolite as measured by electrolyte leakage from leaf discs of (a) soybean (*Glycine max*), (b) velvetleaf (*Abutilon theophrasti*), and (c) ivyleaf morninglory (*Ipomoea hederacea*). Leaf discs were incubated in the presence of no inhibitor (●), 10 μM carfentrazone-ethyl (■), or the free-acid metabolite (▲) for 20 h in darkness and then exposed to continuous light. The arrows indicate the beginning of light exposure and the dotted lines indicate maximum conductivity from boiled samples. Data are the average of three replications ± SD (from Dayan *et al.*, 1997b).

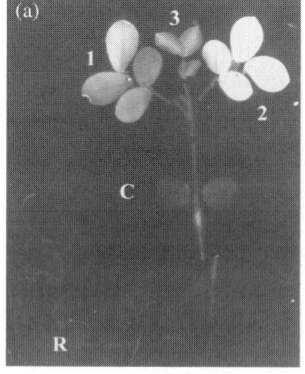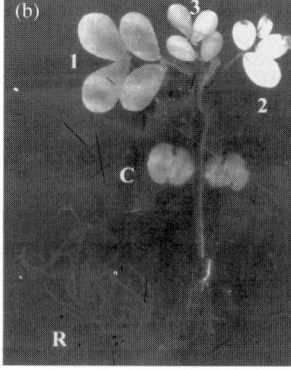

Figure 68.2 Uptake and translocation of ^{14}C-sulfentrazone in (a) coffee senna (*Senna occidentalis*) and (b) sicklepod (*Cassia obtusifolia*). Autoradiograms were obtained by incubating the roots of both plants in a solution containing ^{14}C-sulfentrazone for 3 h and transferring the plants to nonlabeled solutions for another 21 h. R, root; C, cotyledons; 1, 2, and 3 refer to the first, second, and third true leaves. Notice that no radioactivity remained in the roots and that most of the radioactivity accumulated in the fully expanded leaves (1 and 2).

by rapid conjugation of the phenyl rings to cysteine, homoglutathione, and glucose (Fig. 68.3) (Frear and Swanson, 1973; Frear *et al.*, 1983). In the case of non-DPE structures, such as sulfentrazone, resistance is achieved via rapid oxidative degradation followed by conjugation (Dayan *et al.*, 1996, 1997c). The nature of the conjugated metabolites was not determined in this study, but 90% of the herbicide was transformed into extremely water-soluble metabolites within 24 h from the time of application (Dayan *et al.*, 1996, 1997c). Sensitive weeds are apparently unable to oxidize sulfentrazone (Dayan *et al.*, 1996). Further studies on the biological activity of the primary metabolites of sulfentrazone showed that the initial oxidative step leading the hydroxylation of the methyl group on the triazolinone ring did not reduce the biological activity of sulfentrazone. Further oxidation of the moiety led to the formation of less active compounds (Dayan *et al.*, 1998).

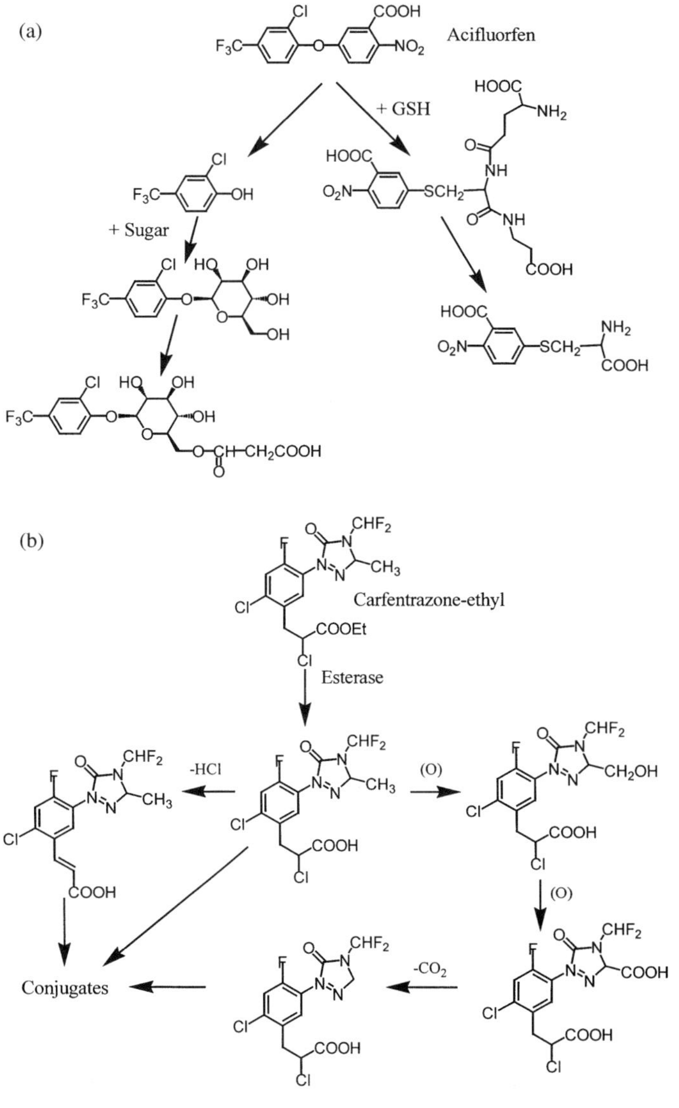

68.4.2 MODE OF ACTION

Early investigations on the mode of action of Protox inhibitors determined that light was needed for herbicidal activity (Matsunaka, 1969); yet, photosynthesis was not involved in the mechanism (Duke and Kenyon, 1986). There was good evidence that the observed peroxidative damage was due to a process involving a photodynamic pigment [reviewed by Scalla and Matringe (1994)]. Matringe and Scalla (1988) demonstrated that the chlorophyll precursor protoporphyrin IX (Proto) accumulated in acifluorfen-treated plant tissues. Proto is a photodynamic pigment (Cox *et al.*, 1982), and its content in Protox inhibitor-treated plant tissues correlated well with peroxidative damage (e.g., Becerril and Duke, 1989). Matringe *et al.* (1989a, b) discovered that Proto accumulated in response to the inhibition of the enzyme responsible for its synthesis (Fig. 68.4). This apparently contradictory situation is mirrored by the accumulation of Proto in humans with the genetic disease variegate porphyria that results from a deficiency of Protox activity (Deybach *et al.*, 1981). The paradox of inhibition of an enzyme leading to the accumulation of its catalytic product is explained by altered compartmentalization of porphyrin intermediates (Jacobs *et al.*, 1991; Lee *et al.*, 1993). Inhibition of Protox induces an uncontrolled accumulation of protoporphyrinogen IX (Protogen), which leaks out of the chloroplast outer membrane into the cytoplasm where it is converted into the highly photodynamic Proto (Fig. 68.5). In the presence of light, this

Figure 68.3 Examples of hydrolytic and oxidative metabolic degradation of various Protox inhibitors in plants. (a) Metabolism of the diphenyl ether acifluorfen in soybean plants (Frear *et al.*, 1983) and (b) metabolism of the triazolinone carfentrazone (Anonymous, 1995b).

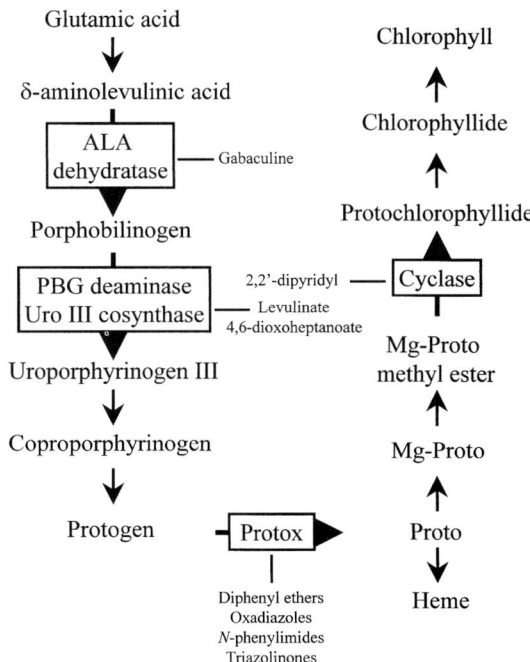

Figure 68.4 Simplified pathway of chlorophyll and heme biosynthesis in plants showing the enzymes known to be sensitive to chemical inhibition (boxes). ALA dehydratase, aminolevulinic acid dehydratase; PBG deaminase/Uro III cosynthase, porphobilinogen deaminase/uroporphyrinogen III cosynthase; Protox, protoporphyrinogen oxidase (redrawn from Reddy *et al.*, 1998).

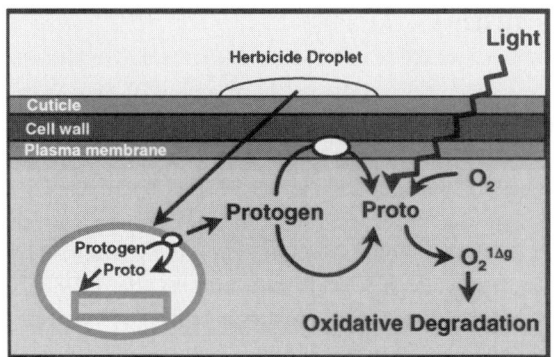

Figure 68.5 Mode of action of Protox-inhibiting herbicides. The initial step consists of the foliar absorption and translocation of the herbicide. Inhibition of Protox (localized in the outer membrane of chloroplasts) causes an unregulated accumulation of Protogen, which is oxidized (either enzymatically or chemically) to Proto. Proto is energized by light and causes formation of reactive singlet oxygen species that can lead to oxidative membrane degradation (redrawn from Dayan and Duke, 1997).

photosensitized Proto generates a highly reactive singlet oxygen that induces lipid peroxidation of the relatively unprotected plasma membrane (Fig. 68.5) (Devine *et al.*, 1993; Lee *et al.*, 1993). This phenomenon explains the light-dependent nature of the mode of action of Protox inhibitors.

A large number of Protox inhibitors exists, and in spite of their structural differences, they apparently all compete for the same site on the enzyme, suggesting that the binding pocket is very promiscuous. Figure 68.6 demonstrates the competitive binding between the natural substrate and various synthetic herbicides belonging to structurally different chemical classes. The regression of the lines intersecting with each other at the level of the *y* axis on a double reciprocal plot is typical of competitive binding. These graphs also enable the calculation of binding constants for each inhibitor. As would be expected, the inhibition of Protox is proportional to the ability of each compound to bind to that particular site on Protox. Early studies on DPE

herbicides indicated that these molecules compete for the binding site by mimicking half of the natural substrate Protogen (Nandihalli *et al.*, 1992). However, no such clear resemblance to Protogen can be easily established with non-oxygen-bridged Protox inhibitors (Dayan *et al.*, 1997a–c; Reddy *et al.*, 1998).

Two-dimensional quantitative structure–activity relationship (QSAR) analyses have been somewhat successful in predicting the herbicidal activities of these compounds (Nandihalli *et al.*, 1992; Reddy *et al.*, 1995, 1998). However, equations derived from three-dimensional (3-D) QSAR have been more reliable at predicting the activity of various structurally related groups of Protox-inhibiting herbicides, as well as differentiating active from inactive stereoisomers (Dayan *et al.*, 1999).

68.4.3 MODES OF RESISTANCE

Plants can be resistant to herbicides via physical, physiological, and/or biochemical mechanisms. Most often, resistance is achieved via slow uptake and translocation, rapid metabolic degradation, and/or resistance at the molecular site. The complex mode of action of Protox inhibitors provides several more unusual sites for possible herbicide resistance (Fig. 68.7) (Duke *et al.*, 1997).

Reduced uptake and translocation of Protox-inhibiting herbicides through the shoots may account for the resistance of some species (Matsumoto *et al.*, 1994) but does not play a major role in resistance to those that are soil applied (Dayan *et al.*, 1996, 1997b, c). On the other hand, metabolic degradation of Protox inhibitors seems to plays a key role in crop resistance to these herbicides. Resistance of soybean to acifluorfen and two phenyl triazolinones is due primarily to rapid metabolic degradation of the herbicides (Dayan *et al.*, 1996, 1997b, c; Frear *et al.*, 1983). However, these herbicides act so rapidly that metabolic degradation does not provide a large safety margin, and some crop damage, often referred to as "bronzing," is com-

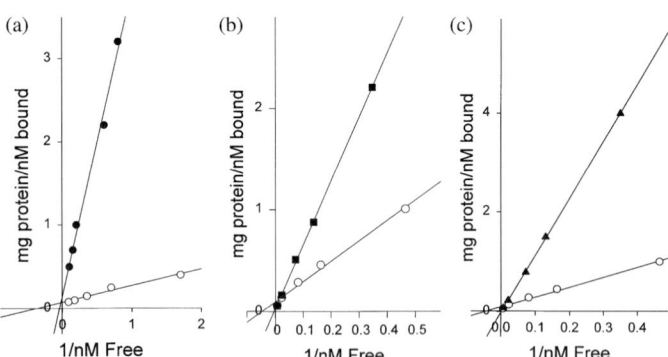

Figure 68.6 Competitive binding between the radiolabeled acifluorfen (DPE herbicide), Protogen (the natural substrate of Protox), and various Protox inhibitors on isolated etioplasts. The graphs illustrate the competitive nature of the binding between acifluorfen (○) and (a) Protogen (●), (b) a triazolinone-type Protox inhibitor (■), and (c) an isoxazole carboxamide-type Protox inhibitor (▲) (redrawn, respectively, from Matringe *et al.*, 1992; Dayan *et al.*, 1997b; Dayan *et al.*, 1997a).

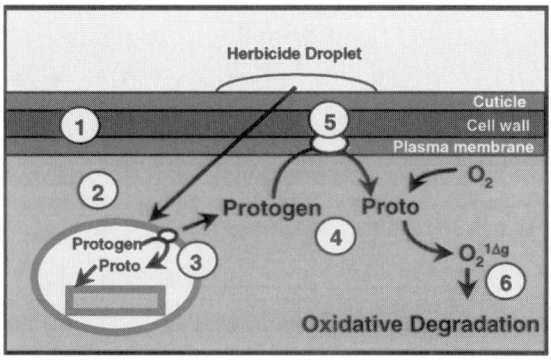

Figure 68.7 Schematic of possible mechanisms of resistance to Protox-inhibiting herbicides. Potential sites of resistance are in boldface numbers: 1, inhibition of uptake or sequestration of the herbicide; 2, rapid metabolic degradation of the herbicide; 3, herbicide-resistant Protox; 4, degradation of extraplastidic Protogen and/or Proto; 5, inactivated herbicide-resistant, extraplastidic Protox; 6, quenching of singlet oxygen and other toxic oxygen species (redrawn from Dayan and Duke, 1996).

mon. The extent of injury might be greater with those herbicides that have longer soil persistence.

There are no cases of natural resistance in whole plants associated with herbicide-insensitive chloroplastic Protox. Nevertheless, herbicide-resistant Protox has been isolated from tobacco (Ichinose *et al.*, 1995) and soybean cell cultures selected with Protox inhibitors (Pornprom *et al.*, 1994). Overexpression of mitochondrial Protox in photomixotrophic tobacco cells lines can result in resistance to Protox inhibitors (Watanabe *et al.*, 1998). This result suggests that if sufficient uninhibited mitochondrial Protox is available, Protogen leaking from inhibited plastids can be rapidly converted to heme by the mitochondria before it can accumulate as damaging extraorganellar Proto. Whole plants have not been regenerated from any of these cell lines.

Rice appears to be more naturally resistant to the oxidative stress induced by Protox inhibitors relative to the targeted weeds (Matsumoto *et al.*, 1994). That is, the plant generates Proto in response to the herbicides, but appears to have the ability to cope with the resulting singlet oxygen and the toxic compounds (hydroxyl radical, lipid peroxides, etc.) resulting from it. We have reported that a similar mechanism may be involved in the differential sensitivity of soybean cultivars to sulfentrazone (Dayan *et al.*, 1997c). Other species (e.g., mustards) and older tissues of some species that are sensitive in the seedling stage are apparently resistant due to enzymatic degradation of Protogen to nontoxic compounds (Jacobs *et al.*, 1996).

The complex mechanism of action of Protox inhibitors provides several potential mechanisms for evolved resistance in weeds (Fig. 68.7). Yet, no cases of evolved resistance in the field have been verified. This could be due, in part, to the relatively short-lived selection pressure of these fast-acting, foliar-applied herbicides. However, the recent development of more persistent soil-active Protox inhibitors will increase the selection pressure, increasing the probability of the evolution of resistance. No resistant mutants were obtained when hundreds of thousands of mutagenized *Arabidopsis thialiana* seeds were tested with a Protox inhibitor (M. Yamamoto and S. O. Duke, unpublished).

Recent patents (e.g., Ward and Volrath, 1995) propose to produce Protox inhibitor–resistant crops through a variety of molecular genetics approaches. To date, the only published successful genetically engineered crop resistant to Protox inhibitors was obtained by transforming tobacco with a herbicide-resistant form of Protox from bacteria (Choi *et al.*, 1998).

68.5 ENVIRONMENTAL IMPACT

68.5.1 INTERACTION WITH SOIL

As mentioned previously, the crop selectivity of Protox inhibitors is, for the most part, limited to soybean. Although no significant limitation on crop rotations has been associated with foliar-applied Protox inhibitors, there are some limitations with the more persistent Protox inhibitors (e.g., fomesafen

and sulfentrazone). Nevertheless, the excellent broad-spectrum preemergence activity associated with greater soil persistence of sulfentrazone, relative to other Protox-inhibiting herbicides, makes this herbicide unique in its class for the moment.

The combination of relatively high soil adsorption and rapid microbial degradation strongly limits soil leaching of most Protox-inhibiting herbicides. None of the Protox inhibitors has volatilization problems (vapor pressure lower than 10^{-7} mm Hg at 25°C), and none has caused drift-related injury to nontarget crops when properly applied.

It is important to note that soil quality may affect leaching of fluoroglycofen, and metabolites of lactofen may be highly mobile in soil (Ahrens, 1994). In the case of soil active Protox inhibitors, mobility may be of some concern. The herbicide bifenox is quite mobile in spite of its relatively high soil sorption (Table 68.4); fortunately, its half-life is fairly short. Sulfentrazone is not as mobile, but its sorption appears to be affected by pH and soil mobility may be a problem at pH greater than its pK_a (6.6) (Anonymous, 1995a; Grey *et al.*, 1997). Typical soils of soybean fields can be as high as pH 7.5. Such pH might lead to significant levels of leaching. This problem may be compounded by the relatively long half-life of sulfentrazone (Table 68.4).

68.5.2 DEGRADATION IN THE ENVIRONMENT

Protox inhibitors are not known to be a threat to the environment. The principal form of degradation is associated with microbial activity, though some of these herbicides (e.g., DPEs) are also susceptible to photodegradation (Table 68.4). The half-lives of this class of herbicides vary greatly and are affected by soil quality. Half-life can be very short (i.e., less than a week for lactofen) but can be as long as 280 days (e.g., sulfentrazone) (Table 68.4) (Anonymous, 1995a).

In an aquatic environment, photodegradation of most Protox inhibitors is very rapid ($<$5 days). Some Protox inhibitors, such as JV-485 (Prosch *et al.*, 1997) and fomesafen (Ahrens, 1994), have low water solubility and are, therefore, considered a low risk to groundwater or surface water runoff and, consequently, to aquatic wildlife. Others, such as oxadiargyl (Dickmann *et al.*, 1997), dissipate rapidly from water and do not persist in the aquatic environment. Oxadiazon, oxyfluorfen, and lactofen (Ahrens, 1994) are strongly adsorbed by the soil and, therefore, do not leach into groundwater, presenting a diminished toxicological risk to aquatic wildlife.

68.5.3 ECOTOXICOLOGY

With the exception of acifluorfen, the majority of Protox inhibitors are not harmful to avian wildlife (Table 68.5). In general, they present a low risk to the environment (Table 68.4) and terrestrial animals (Table 68.6). Of the herbicides tested against insects, flumiclorac, fluoroglycofen, lactofen, oxyfluorfen, and JV-485 presented extremely low risk of toxicity.

Table 68.4
Fate of Protox-Inhibiting Herbicides in the Environment

Common name	Sorption (K_{oc}, ml/g)	Degradation	Mobility	Volatilization	Half-life (days)
Acifluorfen[a]	113	Photo/microbiol.	Negligible	Negligible	14–60
Azafenidin[b]	n/a	Photo/microbiol.	Negligible	Negligible	25–40
Bifenox[a]	10,000	Microbiol.	Significant	Negligible	7–14
Carfentrazone[c]	n/a	Photo/microbiol.	Low	Negligible	60
Flumiclorac[a]	Strong	Photo/hydrol.	Negligible	Negligible	1–6
Fluoroglycofen[a]	1,364	Photo/microbiol.	Moderate	Negligible	7–21
Fomesafen[a]	60	Photo	Moderate	Negligible	100
JV-485[d]	250	Microbiol.	Negligible	Negligible	40–70
Lactofen[a]	10,000	Microbiol.	Negligible	Negligible	3–7
Oxadiargyl[e]	n/a	Microbiol.	Negligible	Not available	40
Oxadiazon[a]	3,200	Not available	Low	Negligible	60
Oxyfluorfen[a]	100,000	Photo/microbiol.	Negligible/low	Low	30–40
Sulfentrazone[f]	160–192[g]	Microbiol.	Moderate	Negligible	110–280

[a] Ahrens (1994).
[b] Amuti *et al.* (1997).
[c] Anonymous (1995b).
[d] Prosch *et al.* (1997).
[e] Dickmann *et al.* (1997).
[f] Anonymous (1995a).
[g] K. N. Reddy, M. A. Locke, and L. A. Gaston (1997), personal communication.

Fomesafen was the only inhibitor tested that exhibited moderate toxicity to bees.

Aquatic wildlife is generally more susceptible to Protox inhibitors than avian wildlife. Photodegradation times in water for most of these is very short (<5 days). Some Protox inhibitors, such as JV-485 (Prosch *et al.*, 1997) and fomesafen (Ahrens, 1994), have low water solubility and are, therefore, considered a low risk to groundwater or surface water runoff and, consequently, to aquatic wildlife following soil application. Others, such as oxadiargyl (Dickmann *et al.*, 1997), dissipate rapidly from water and do not persist in the aquatic environment. When applied directly in water, oxadiazon, oxyfluorfen, and lactofen are strongly adsorbed by the soil and, therefore do not leach into the groundwater, presenting a diminished toxicological risk to aquatic wildlife (Ahrens, 1994). Many Protox-inhibiting herbicides, such as carfentrazone and flumiclorac, are highly toxic to algae, but are only moderately toxic to fish. Others, such as sulfentrazone and fomesafen, are essentially nontoxic to fish (Ahrens, 1994; Anonymous, 1995a). Finally, bifenox and oxyfluorfen are highly toxic to aquatic wildlife (Ahrens, 1994).

68.6 MAMMALIAN TOXICOLOGY

68.6.1 SKIN AND ORAL

All Protox-inhibiting herbicides have passed toxicological evaluations prior to registration. Table 68.6 provides toxicological information on most commercial Protox inhibitors. Although most of these approvals were granted before the molecular target site of these herbicides was identified, Protox inhibitors have been shown to have little acute toxicity. It is now known that the target site is Protox, the last common enzyme in the biosynthesis of heme and chlorophylls. Protox-inhibiting herbicides appear to be as inhibitory to mammalian mitochondrial Protox as to that of chloroplast (e.g., Matringe *et al.*, 1989b). These compounds cause an increase in porphyrin levels in animals when administered by oral doses (see Section 68.6.3). However, the herbicides appear to be effectively metabolized and/or excreted (Adler *et al.*, 1977; Hunt *et al.*, 1977; Leung *et al.*, 1991), and thus porphyrin levels return to normal within a few days. Interestingly, many of the primary mammalian metabolites formed are the same as photochemical degradation products (Hunt *et al.*, 1977). Even under exaggerated dietary doses (>100× recommended field rates), there appears to be little bioaccumulation risk in animals (e.g., Leung *et al.*, 1991). In general, for healthy individuals, these compounds are not considered to pose any significant toxicological risk.

68.6.2 TERATOGENICITY AND MUTAGENICITY

All compounds have been tested under a series of mutagenicity studies, and the overwhelming weight of evidence supports the conclusion that, with the exception of oxyfluorofen and sulfentrazone, Protox inhibitors are not genotoxic (Table 68.6). Teratology studies conducted on rat and rabbit, have demonstrated that the majority of the compounds are not teratogenic. Chronic toxicity/oncogenicity studies of carfentrazone (Anonymous, 1995b) are still in progress at the time of this writing.

Table 68.5
Ecotoxicity of Protoporphyrin Oxidase-Inhibiting Herbicides

| Common name | Avian | | Fish | | Others | |
	Test species	Oral LD$_{50}$ (mg/kg)	Test species	LC$_{50}$ (mg/l) (96 h)	Test species	Oral LD$_{50}$
Acifluorfen[a]	Bobwhite quail	325	Bluegill sunfish	62	n/a	
	Mallard duck	4,187	Rainbow trout	17		
Azafenidin[b]	Bobwhite quail	>2,500	Bluegill sunfish	48	n/a	
	Mallard duck	>2,500	Rainbow trout	33		
Bifenox[a]	Mallard duck	>5,000	Bluegill sunfish	0.64	n/a	
	Pheasant	>5,000	Rainbow trout	0.87		
Carfentrazone[c]	Bobwhite quail	>2,250	Bluegill sunfish	2.0	n/a	
	Mallard duck	>5,620	Rainbow trout	1.6		
Flumiclorac[a]	Bobwhite quail	>2,250	Bluegill sunfish	17.4	Honey bee	>106 μg/bee
	Mallard duck	>5,620	Rainbow trout	1.1		
Fluoroglycofen[a]	Bobwhite quail	>1,075	Bluegill sunfish	1.5	Honey bee	>100 μg/bee
	Mallard duck	>5,000	Rainbow trout	23		
Fomesafen[a]	Bobwhite quail	>2,000	Bluegill sunfish	6,000	Honey bee	>50 μg/bee
	Mallard duck	>5,000	Rainbow trout	680		
JV-485[d]	Bobwhite quail	>2,130	Bluegill sunfish	>0.045 mg a.i./l	Earthworm	>1,170 mg/kg soil
	Mallard duck	>2,130	Rainbow trout	>0.045 mg a.i./l		
Lactofen[a]	Bobwhite quail	>2,510	Bluegill sunfish	>560	Honey bee	>160 μg/bee
	Mallard duck	>5,620	Rainbow trout	>0.1		
Oxadiargyl[e]	Bobwhite quail	>2,000	Bluegill sunfish	Below detection	n/a	
			Rainbow trout	Below detection		
Oxadiazon[a]	Bobwhite quail	6,000	Catfish	≥15.4	n/a	
	Mallard duck	>1,000	Rainbow trout	>9		
Oxyfluorfen[a]	Bobwhite quail	>2,200	Bluegill sunfish	0.2	Honey bee	>10,000 ppm
	Mallard duck	>4,000	Rainbow trout	0.4	Fiddler crab	>1,000 mg/l
Sulfentrazone[f]	Bobwhite quail	>5,620	Bluegill sunfish	93.8	n/a	
	Mallard duck	>5,620	Rainbow trout	>130		

[a] Ahrens (1994).
[b] Amuti *et al.* (1997).
[c] Anonymous (1995b).
[d] Prosch *et al.* (1997).
[e] Dickmann *et al.* (1997).
[f] Anonymous (1995a).

68.6.3 EFFECTS ON MAMMALIAN PORPHYRIN METABOLISM

In healthy individuals, approved Protox-inhibiting herbicides are not considered to be of significant toxicological risk due to their effects on porphyrin metabolism. To date, no health problems have been associated with human consumption of crops treated with these compounds (Duke and Rebeiz, 1994). Mammalian Protox is as sensitive to Protox-inhibiting herbicides as chloroplastic Protox (Birchfield and Casida, 1997; Krijt *et al.*, 1994; Scalla and Matringe, 1994), and these compounds can cause greatly elevated levels of porphyrins in animals administered with oral doses of these compounds (Krijt *et al.*, 1994). However, these herbicides are either not readily absorbed by the body during digestion and/or are rapidly degraded

by metabolism (Adler *et al.*, 1977; Hunt *et al.*, 1977; Leung *et al.*, 1991).

In mammals, there are remarkable species differences in the levels of porphyrin accumulation resulting from exposure to Protox inhibitors, and developmental toxicity correlates with Proto accumulation (Kawamura *et al.*, 1996). Rats and mice seem to be particularly sensitive to Protox inhibitors. Variegate porphyria, a human disease characterized by accumulation of Proto and other porphyrins, is caused by a deficiency of Protox. Variegate porphyria–like symptoms can be generated in mice with high doses of herbicidal Protox inhibitors (Krijt *et al.*, 1997). However, neither of two structurally divergent Protox inhibitors (oxadiazon and oxyfluorfen) affected Protox activity of the brain and liver. How this relates to human risk assessment is unknown. In general, however, relatively high doses

Table 68.6
Mammalian Toxicity of Protoporphyrin Oxidase-Inhibiting Herbicides

Common name	Test	Test species	LD_{50} (mg/kg)	Mutagenicity	Teratogenicity (mg/kg/day)
Acifluorfen[a]	Acute oral	Rat	1,540	Negative	n/a
	Acute dermal	Rabbit	—	>2000 mg/kg	
Azafenidin[b]	Acute oral	Rat	>5,000	Negative	n/a
	Acute dermal	Rabbit	>2,000		
Bifenox[a]	Acute oral	Rat	>5,000	n/a	None at 200
		Mouse	>4,556		
	Acute dermal	Rabbit	>2,000		
Carfentrazone[c]	Acute oral	Rat	>5,000	Negative	Negative
	Acute dermal	Rat	>4,000		
Flumiclorac[a]	Acute oral	Rat/mouse	>5,000	Negative	>1500 (rat)
	Acute dermal	Rat	>2,000		
Fluoroglycofen[a]	Acute oral	Rat	1,500	Negative	Negative (rat/rabbit)
	Acute dermal	Rabbit	>5,000		
Fomesafen[a]	Acute oral	Rat	24,000	Negative	Negative
	Acute dermal	Rabbit	>1,683		
JV-485[d]	Acute oral	Rat	>5,000	Negative	Negative
	Acute dermal	Rat	>5,000		
Lactofen[a]	Acute oral	Rat	>5,000	Negative	Negative
	Acute dermal	Rabbit	>2,000		
Oxadiargyl[e]	Acute oral	Rat	>5,000	Negative	n/a
	Acute dermal	Rat	>2,000		
Oxadiazon[a]	Acute oral	Rat	>5,000	n/a	n/a
	Acute dermal	Rat	>8,000		
Oxyfluorfen[a]	Acute oral	Rat/dog	>5,000	Positive	Toxic at 150
	Acute dermal	Rabbit/rat	>5,000		
Sulfentrazone[f]	Acute oral	Rat	>2,000	Negative	Toxic at 25
	Acute dermal	Rabbit/rat	>2,000		

[a] Ahrens (1994).
[b] Amuti *et al.* (1997).
[c] Anonymous (1995b).
[d] Prosch *et al.* (1997).
[e] Dickmann *et al.* (1997).
[f] Anonymous (1995a).

of herbicides are required to elicit an effect, and porphyrin levels return to normal within days after withdrawal of the herbicide.

Finally, Protox inhibitors have been proposed as pharmaceuticals for use in tumor phototherapy (Halling *et al.*, 1994). Some Protox inhibitors may preferentially accumulate in tumors, resulting in sufficient differences between tumor Proto accumulation and that in adjacent tissues for exploitation in phototherapy.

68.6.4 METABOLIC DEGRADATION IN ANIMALS

There are few studies that document metabolism of DPE herbicides and other Protox inhibitors in animals and wildlife. In general, the primary form of metabolite excretion is through urine and feces (Hunt *et al.*, 1977; Leung *et al.*, 1991). A variety of animals, including rats, rabbits, goats, sheep, cattle, and chickens, have been tested. General classes of metabolic degradation of these compounds by animals include nitro reduction, deesterification, and conjugation to glutathione, cysteine, and carbohydrates.

All commercial diphenyl ether herbicides contain a *p*-nitrophenyl substituent. In animals, this moiety is readily reduced to an amine group. Some DPE herbicides contain a carboxyester group at the *meta* position on the nitrophenyl ring. This ester is readily hydrolyzed to produce a very polar carboxylic acid derivative. DPEs are also easily inactivated by cleavage of the ether bridge, followed by conjugation to glutathione (Aizawa and Brown, 1999). Other conjugated metabolites have been identified with glucuronic acid. Most of the primary metabolites are the same as those formed in plants (see Fig. 68.3a).

The DPE herbicides fluoroglycofen ethyl and bifenox are readily deesterified in animals. In fact, the initial steps of fluoroglycofen ethyl metabolism lead to the formation of acifluorofen (Aizawa and Brown, 1999). In animals, bifenox, following deesterification, forms 5-(2,4-dichlorophenoxy)-2-nitrobenzoic acid.

The 4-hydroxyphenyl ether metabolite of nitrofen was identified as a major derivative in rabbits (Bray *et al.*, 1953). This metabolite was excreted primarily as a glucuronide conjugate, with small amounts of free 4,4'-dihydroxydiphenyl ether also present. Another study demonstrated that rabbits further degraded these metabolites to yield their corresponding hydroxy derivatives (Matsunaka, 1976).

Studies of the metabolic degradation of oxyflurofen in animals showed that most of the metabolic products were excreted in the feces, with small amounts remaining in the urine (2% in males; 4% in females) (Adler *et al.*, 1977). A common metabolite consisted of an amino derivative of nitro-substituted primary metabolite 4-[2-chloro-4-(trifluoromethyl)phenoxy]-2-ethoxybenzenamine. This amino derivative was further degraded with the consecutive conversion of the amino group to an acetamido group to yield another common metabolite (*N*-[4-[2-chloro-4-(trifluoromethyl)phenoxy]-2-hydroxy-phenyl]acetamide).

All non-oxygen-bridged Protox inhibitors (i.e., those structurally different from DPEs) appear to follow a similar metabolic degradation pattern. In rats and goats, most of the herbicide metabolites are found in urine, with small amounts excreted in feces and milk. In chickens, approximately 95% of the metabolites are eliminated in excreta, with small amounts (0.09%) eliminated in the eggs (Leung *et al.*, 1991).

The carboxyester group of the triazolinone herbicide carfentrazone ethyl is initially metabolized to a carboxylic acid group. Further metabolites identified in rats and lactating goats included hydroxymethylpropionic acid and cinnamic acid derivatives (Aizawa and Brown, 1999). In mammals, the propionic acid metabolites undergo further oxidation of the methyl group by the cytochrome P-450. Finally, the cinnamic acid conjugate may be further metabolized to yield a benzoic acid derivative (Aizawa and Brown, 1999).

Metabolism of the triazolinone herbicide sulfentrazone has been tested in rats, goats, and hens. The primary metabolite (88–95%) is 3-hydroxymethyl sulfentrazone. Other metabolites include 3-desmethyl sulfentrazone and 2,3-dihydroxymethyl sulfentrazone. Overall, triazolinone herbicides such as sulfentrazone are rapidly metabolized, with most of the compound being excreted within 3–5 days (Leung *et al.*, 1991).

68.7 CONCLUDING COMMENTS

Protox-inhibiting herbicides may play a more important role in the future agrochemical market for several reasons. These compounds are effective at very low application rates and have generally good ecotoxicology and human toxicology profiles at recommended application rates. Many are highly compatible with the trend toward no-tillage agriculture. Furthermore, unlike with some of the other herbicide classes, weeds have not been able to evolve resistance at this particular site of action. As a result, these herbicides might replace comparable products currently available for broad-spectrum weed control in soybean fields to which weeds are rapidly becoming resistant. The success of Protox inhibitors is dependent on broadening their use to include other major crops such as maize and in enhancing the resistance of crops for which these herbicides are currently being marketed. Following the promise shown by the commercialization of genetically engineered glyphosate-resistant soybean (Cole, 1994), intensive research to generate crops resistant to Protox inhibitors is in progress (e.g., Choi *et al.*, 1998). Although we are aware of no evidence of any significant environmental or toxicological risks of approved Protox inhibitor herbicides, the fact that all mitochondrial Protox forms tested so far are highly sensitive might provide a clue for toxicologists (mammalian and environmental) to find overlooked effects. However, the relatively low dose rates required for herbicidal activity may be far below the dose needed to adversely affect porphyrin metabolism in animals in field situations or humans as a result of exposures in food, water, air, or during application. This appears to the case with at least one other herbicide (glufosinate) that is equally effective on the plant and animal forms of the enzyme glutamine synthetase (Lydon and Duke, 1998).

REFERENCES

Ahrens, W. H. (ed.) (1994). "Herbicide Handbook," 7th ed. Weed Science Society of America, Champaign, IL.

Aizawa, K., and Brown, H. M. (1999). Metabolism and degradation of porphyrin biosynthesis inhibitor herbicides. *In* "Peroxidizing Herbicides" (P. Böger and K. Wakabayashi, eds.), pp. 371–383. Springer-Verlag, Berlin.

Adler, I. L., Jones, B. M., and Wargo, J. P., Jr. (1977). Fate of 2-chloro-1-(3-ethoxy-4-nitrophenoxy)-4-(trifluoromethyl)benzene (oxyfluorfen) in rats. *J. Agric. Food Chem.* **25**, 1339–1341.

Amuti, K., Trombinin, A., Giammarrusti, L., Sbriscia, C., Harder, H., and Gabard, J. (1997). Azafenidin, a new low use rate herbicide for weed control in perennial crops, industrial weed control and forestry. *In* "Brighton Crop Protection Conference," pp. 59–66.

Anderson, R. J., Norris, A. E., and Hess, F. D. (1994). Synthetic organic chemicals that act through the porphyrin pathway. *Am. Chem. Soc. Symp. Ser.* **559**, 18–33.

Anonymous (1995a). "Authority Herbicide." Technical Information Bulletin, FMC Corporation.

Anonymous (1995b). "Carfentrazone-Ethyl Herbicide." Technical Information Bulletin, FMC Corporation.

Armbruster, B. L., Clark, R. D., Sharp, C. R., and Dill, G. M. (1993). Herbicidal action of nitrophenyl pyrazole ether MON 12800: Immunolocalization, ultrastructural, and physiological studies. *Pestic. Sci.* **47**, 21–35.

Becerril, J. M., and Duke, S. O. (1989). Protoporphyrin IX content correlates with activity of photobleaching herbicides. *Plant Physiol.* **90**, 1175–1181.

Birchfield, N. B., and Casida, J. E. (1997). Protoporphyrinogen oxidase of mouse and maize: Target site selectivity and thiol effects on peroxidizing herbicide action. *Pestic. Biochem. Physiol.* **57**, 36–43.

Böger, P. (1984). Multiple modes of action of diphenyl ethers. *Z. Naturforsch, C: Biosci.* **39**, 468–475.

Bray, H. G., James, S. P., Thorpe, W. V., and Wasdell, M. R. (1953). The metabolism of ethers in the rabbit. *Biochem. J.* **54**, 547–551.

Choi, K. W., Han, O., Lee, H. J., Yun, Y. C., Moon, Y. H., Kim, M., Kuk, Y. I., Han, S. U., and Guh, J. O. (1998). Generation of resistance to the diphenyl ether herbicide, oxyfluorfen via expression of the *Bacillus subtilis* protoporphyrinogen oxidase gene in transgenic: on tobacco plants. *Biosci. Biotechnol. Biochem.* **62**, 558–560.

Clark, R. D. (1994). Synthesis of protoporphyrinogen oxidase inhibitors. *Am. Chem. Soc. Symp. Ser.* **559**, 34–47.

Clark, R. D. (1996). Synthesis and QSAR of herbicidal 3-pyrazoyl α, α, α-trifluorotolyl ethers. *J. Agric. Food Chem.* **44**, 3643–3652.

Cole, D. J. (1994). Introduction of herbicide resistant crops. *Pestic. Outlook* **5**, 32–36.

Condon, M. E., Alvarado, S. I., Arthen, F. J., Birk, J. H., Brady, T. E., Crews, A. D., Marc, J. H., Karp, G. M., Lavanish, J. M., Nielsen, D. R., and Lies, T. A. (1995). 6-aryloxy-1*H*-benzotriazoles. *Am. Chem. Soc. Symp. Ser.* **584**, 123–135.

Cox, G. S., Krieg, M., and Whitten, D. G. (1982). Self-sensitized photooxidation of protoporphyrin IX derivatives in aqueous surfactant solutions: Product and mechanistic studies. *J. Am. Chem. Soc.* **104**, 6930–6937.

Dayan, F. E., and Duke, S. O. (1996). Porphyrin-generating herbicides. *Pestic. Outlook* **7**, 22–27.

Dayan, F. E., and Duke, S. O. (1997). Phytotoxicity of protoporphyrinogen oxidase inhibitors: Phenomenology, mode of action and mechanisms of resistance. *In* "Herbicide Activity: Toxicology, Biochemistry and Molecular Biology" (R. M. Roe, J. D. Burton, and R. J. Kuhr, eds.), pp. 11–35. IOS Press, The Netherlands.

Dayan, F. E., Armstrong, B. M., and Weete, J. D. (1998). Inhibitory activity of sulfentrazone and its metabolic derivatives on soybean (*Glycine max*) protoporphyrinogen oxidase. *J. Agric. Food Chem.* **46**, 2024–2029.

Dayan, F. E., Duke, S. O., Reddy, K. N., Hamper, B. C., and Leschinsky, K. L. (1997a). Effect of isoxazole herbicides on protoporphyrinogen oxidase and porphyrin physiology. *J. Agric. Food Chem.* **45**, 967–975.

Dayan, F. E., Duke, S. O., Weete, J. D., and Hancock, H. G. (1997b). Selectivity and mode of action of carfentrazone-ethyl, a novel phenyl triazolinone herbicide. *Pestic. Sci.* **51**, 65–73.

Dayan, F. E., Reddy, K. N., and Duke, S. O. (1999). Structure–activity relationships of diphenyl ethers and other oxygen-bridged protoporphyrinogen oxidase inhibitors. *In* "Peroxidizing Herbicides" (P. Böger and K. Wakabayashi, eds.), pp. 144–162. Springer-Verlag, Berlin.

Dayan, F. E., Weete, J. D., Duke, S. O., and Hancock, H. G. (1997c). Soybean (*Glycine max*) cultivar differences in response to sulfentrazone. *Weed Sci.* **45**, 634–641.

Dayan, F. E., Weete, J. D., and Hancock, H. G. (1996). Physiological basis for differential sensitivity to sulfentrazone by sicklepod (*Senna obtusifolia*) and coffee senna (*Cassia occidentalis*). *Weed Sci.* **44**, 12–17.

Devine, M. D., Duke, S. O., and Fedtke, C. (1993). Oxygen toxicity and herbicidal action. *In* "Physiology of Herbicide Action," pp. 177–189. Prentice Hall, Englewood Cliffs, NJ.

Deybach, J. C., de Verneuil, H., and Nordmann, Y. (1981). The inherited enzymatic defect in porphyria variegata. *Hum. Genet.* **58**, 425–428.

Dickmann, R., Melgarejo, J., Loubiere, P., and Montagnon, M. (1997). Oxadiargyl, a novel herbicide for rice and sugarcane. *In* "Brighton Crop Protection Conference," pp. 51–57.

Duke, S. O., and Kenyon, W. H. (1986). Photosynthesis is not involved in the mechanism of action of acifluorfen in cucumber (*Cucumis sativus* L.). *Plant Physiol.* **81**, 882–888.

Duke, S. O., and Rebeiz, C. A. (1994). Porphyric pesticides: Chemistry, toxicology, and pharmaceutical applications. *Am. Chem. Soc. Symp. Series* **559**.

Duke, S. O., Lee, H. J., Duke, M. V., Reddy, K. N., Sherman, T. D., Becerril, J. M., Nandihalli, U. B., Matsumoto, H., Jacobs N. J., and Jacobs, J. M. (1997). Mechanisms of resistance to protoporphyrinogen oxidase–inhibiting herbicides. *In* "Herbicide Resistance in Crops and Weeds" (R. DePrado, L. García-Torres, and J. Jorrin, eds.), pp. 155–160. Kluwer Academic, Amsterdam.

Duke, S. O., Lydon, J., Becerril, J., Sherman, T. D., Lehnen, L. P., and Matsumoto, M. (1991). Protoporphyrinogen oxidase-inhibiting herbicides. *Weed Sci.* **39**, 465–473.

Frear, D. S., and Swanson, H. R. (1973). Metabolism of substituted diphenyl ether herbicides in plants. I. Enzymic cleavage of fluorodifen in peas (*Pisum sativum*). *Pestic. Biochem. Physiol.* **3**, 473–482.

Frear, D. S., Swanson, H. R., and Mansager, E. R. (1983). Acifluorfen metabolism in soybean: Diphenyl ether bond cleavage and the formation of homoglutathione, cysteine and glucose conjugates. *Pestic. Biochem. Physiol.* **20**, 299–310.

Gilham, D. J., and Dodge, A. D. (1987). The mode of action of nitro-diphenyl ether herbicides. *In* "Progress in Pesticide Biochemistry and Physiology" (D. H. Hutson and T. R. Roberts, eds.), Vol. 7, pp. 147–167. Wiley, New York.

Grey, T. L., Walker, R. H., Wehtje, G. R., and Hancock, H. G. (1997). Sulfentrazone adsorption and mobility as affected by soil and pH. *Weed Sci.* **45**, 733–738.

Halling, B. P., Yuhas, D. A., Fingar, V. F., and Winkelmann, J. W. (1994). Protoporphyrinogen oxidase inhibitors for tumor therapy. *Am. Chem. Soc. Symp. Ser.* **559**, 280–290.

Hamper, B. C., Leschinsky, K. L., Massey, S. S., Bell, C. L., Brannigan, L. H., and Prosch, S. D. (1995). Synthesis and herbicidal activity of 3-aryl-5-(haloalkyl)-4-isoxazolecarboxamides and their derivatives. *J. Agric. Food Chem.* **43**, 219–228.

Hunt, L. M., Chamberlain, W. F., Gilbert, B. N., Hopkins, D. E., and Gingrich, A. R. (1977). Absorption, excretion, and metabolism of nitrofen by a sheep. *J. Agric. Food Chem.* **25**, 1062–1065.

Ichinose, K., Che, F.-S., Kimura, Y., Matsunobu, A., Sato, F., and Yoshida, S. (1995). Selection and characterization of protoporphyrinogen oxidase inhibiting herbicide (S23142) resistant photomixotrophic cultured cells of *Nicotiana tabacum*. *J. Plant Physiol.* **146**, 693–698.

Jacobs, J. M., Jacobs, N. J., and Duke, S. O. (1996). Protoporphyrinogen destruction by plant extracts and correlation with tolerance to protoporphyrinogen oxidase inhibiting herbicides. *Pestic. Biochem. Physiol.* **55**, 77–83.

Jacobs, J. M., Jacobs, N. J., Sherman, T. D., and Duke, S. O. (1991). Effect of diphenyl ether herbicides on oxidation of protoporphyrinogen to protoporphyrin in organellar and plasma membrane-enriched fractions of barley. *Plant Physiol.* **97**, 197–203.

Johnson, W. O., Kollman, G. E., Swithenbank, C., and Yih, R. Y. (1978). RH-6201 (Blazer): A new broad spectrum herbicide for postemergence use in soybean. *J. Agric. Food Chem.* **26**, 285–286.

Karp, G. M., Condon, M. E., Arthen, F. J., Birk, J. H., Marc, P. A., Hunt, D. A., Lavanish, J. M., and Schwindeman, J. A. (1995). Aryloxyindolin-2(3*H*)-ones. *Am. Chem. Soc. Symp. Ser.* **584**, 136–148.

Kawamura, S., Kato, T., Matsuo, M., Katsuda, Y., and Yasuda, M. (1996). Species difference in protoporphyrin IX accumulation produced by an *N*-phenylimide herbicide in embryos between rats and rabbits. *Toxicol. Appl. Pharmacol.* **141**, 520–525.

Kenyon, W. H., Duke, S. O., and Vaughn, K. C. (1985). Sequences of effects of acifluorfen on physiological and ultrastructural parameters in cucumber cotyledon discs. *Pestic. Biochem. Physiol.* **24**, 240–250.

Krijt, J., Stranska, P., Maruna, P., Vokurka, M., and Sanitrák, J. (1997). Herbicide-induced experimental variegate porphyria in mice: Tissue porphyrinogen accumulation and response to porphyrogenic drugs. *Can. J. Physiol. Pharmacol.* **75**, 1181–1187.

Krijt, J., Vokurda, M., Sanitrák, J., and Janousek, V. (1994). Effect of protoporphyrinogen oxidase inhibition on mammalian porphyrin metabolism. *Am. Chem. Soc. Symp. Series.* **559**, 247–254.

Kunert, K. J., Sandmann, G., and Böger, P. (1987). Modes of action of diphenyl ethers. *Rev. Weed Sci.* **3**, 35–55.

Lee, H. J., Duke, M. V., Birk, J. H., Yamamoto, M., and Duke, S. O. (1995). Biochemical and physiological effects of benzheterocycles and related compounds. *J. Agric. Food Chem.* **43**, 2722–2727.

Lee, H. J., Duke, M. V., and Duke, S. O. (1993). Cellular localization of protoporphyrinogen-oxidizing activities of etiolated barley (*Hordeum vulgare* L.) leaves. *Plant Physiol.* **102**, 881–889.

Leung, L. Y., Lyga, J. W., and Robinson, R. A. (1991). Metabolism and distribution of the experimental triazolinone herbicide sulfentrazone in the rat, goat and hen. *J. Agric. Food Chem.* **39**, 1509–1514.

Lydon, J., and Duke, S. O. (1998). Inhibitors of glutamine biosynthesis. *In* "Plant Amino Acids: Biochemistry and Biotechnology" (B. K. Singh, ed.), pp. 445–463. Dekker, New York.

Lyga, J. W., Patera, R. M., Theodoridis, G., Halling, B. P., Hotzman, F. W., and Plummer, M. J. (1991). Synthesis and quantitative structure–activity relationships of herbicidal *N*-(2-fluoro-5-methoxyphenyl)-3,4,5,6-tetrahydrophthalimides. *J. Agric. Food Chem.* **39**, 1667–1673.

Matringe, M., and Scalla, R. (1988). Effects of acifluorfen-methyl on cucumber cotyledons: Protoporphyrin accumulation. *Pestic. Biochem. Physiol.* **32**, 164–168.

Matringe, M., Camadro, J.-M., Labbe, P., and Scalla, R. (1989a). Protoporphyrinogen oxidase as a molecular target for diphenyl ether herbicides. *Biochem. J.* **260**, 231–235.

Matringe, M., Camadro, J.-M., Labbe, P., and Scalla, R. (1989b). Protoporphyrinogen oxidase inhibition by three peroxidizing herbicides: Oxadiazon, LS 82-556 and M&B 39279. *FEBS Lett.* **245**, 35–38.

Matringe, M., Mornet, R., and Scalla, R. (1992). Characterization of [3H]acifluorfen binding to purified pea etioplasts, and evidence that protoporphyrinogen oxidase specifically binds acifluorfen. *Eur. J. Biochem.* **209**, 861–868.

Matsumoto, H., Lee, J. J., and Ishizuka, K. (1994). Variation in crop response to protoporphyrinogen oxidase inhibitors. *Am. Chem. Soc. Symp. Ser.* **559**, 120–132.

Matsunaka, S. (1969). Acceptor of light energy in photoactivation of diphenyl ether herbicides. *J. Agric. Food Chem.* **17**, 171–175.

Matsunaka, S. (1976). Diphenyl ether herbicides. *In* "Herbicides: Chemistry, Degradation and Mode of Action" (P. C. Kearney and D. D. Kaufman, eds.), Vol. 2, pp. 709–739. Dekker, New York.

Mito, N., Sato, R., Miyakado, M., Oshio, H., and Tanaka, S. (1991). *In vitro* mode of action of *N*-phenylimide photobleaching herbicides. *Pestic. Biochem. Physiol.* **40**, 128–135.

Nandihalli, U. B., and Duke, S. O. (1993). The porphyrin pathway as a herbicide target site. *Am. Chem. Soc. Symp. Ser.* **524**, 62–78.

Nandihalli, U. B., Duke, M. V., and Duke, S. O. (1992). Quantitative structure–activity relationships of protoporphyrinogen oxidase–inhibiting diphenyl ether herbicides. *Pestic. Biochem. Physiol.* **43**, 193–211.

Pornprom, T., Matsumoto, H., Usui, K., and Ishizuka, K. (1994). Characterization of oxyfluorfen tolerance in selected soybean line. *Pestic. Biochem. Physiol.* **50**, 107–114.

Prosch, S. D., Ciha, A. J., Grogna, R., Hamper, B. C., Feucht, D., and Dreist, M. (1997). JV 485: A new herbicide for pre-emergence broad spectrum weed control in winter wheat. *In* "Brighton Crop Protection Conference," pp. 45–50.

Reddy, K. N., Dayan, F. E., and Duke, S. O. (1998). QSAR analysis of protoporphyrinogen oxidase inhibitors. *In* "Comparative QSAR" (J. Devillers, ed.), pp. 197–234. Taylor & Francis, London.

Reddy, K. N., Nandihalli, U. B., Lee, H. J., Duke, M. V., and Duke, S. O. (1995). Predicting activity of protoporphyrinogen oxidase inhibitors by computer-aided molecular modeling. *Am. Chem. Soc. Symp. Series.* **589**, 221–224.

Ritter, R. L., and Coble, H. D. (1981a). Influence of temperature and relative humidity on the activity of acifluorfen. *Weed Sci.* **29**, 480–485.

Ritter, R. L., and Coble H. D. (1981b). Penetration, translocation, and metabolism of acifluorfen in soybean (*Glycine max*), common ragweed

(*Ambrosia artemissifolia*), and cocklebur (*Xanthium pensylvanicum*). *Weed Sci.* **29**, 474–480.

Sato, R., Nagano, E., Oshio, H., and Kamoshita, K. (1987). Diphenylether-like physiological and biochemical actions of S-23142, a novel *N*-phenylimide herbicide. *Pestic. Biochem. Physiol.* **28**, 194–200.

Scalla, R., and Matringe, M. (1994). Inhibitors of protoporphyrinogen oxidase as herbicides: Diphenyl ethers and related photobleaching molecules. *Rev. Weed Sci.* **6**, 103–132.

Sherman, T. D., Duke, M. V., Clark, R. D., Sanders, E. F., Matsumoto, H., and Duke, S. O. (1991). Pyrazole phenyl ether herbicides inhibit protoporphyrinogen oxidase. *Pestic. Biochem. Physiol.* **40**, 236–245.

Sumida, M., Niwata, S., Fukami, H., Tanaka, T., Wakabayashi, K., and Böger, P. (1995). Synthesis of novel diphenyl ether herbicides. *J. Agric. Food Chem.* **43**, 1929–1934.

Theodoridis, G. (1997). Structure–activity relationships of herbicidal aryltriazolinones. *Pestic. Sci.* **50**, 283–290.

Theodoridis, G., Bahr, J. T., Davidson, B. L., Hart, S. E., Hotzman, F. W., Baum, J. S., Hotzman, F. W., Poss, K. M., and Tutt, S. F. (1995). Alkyl 3-[2,4-disubstituted-4,5-dihydro-3-methyl-5-oxo-1*H*-1,2,4-triazol-1-yl)phenyl]propenoate derivatives: Synthesis and structure–activity relationships. *Am. Chem. Soc. Symp. Ser.* **584**, 90–99.

Theodoridis, G., Baum, J. S., Hotzman, F. W., Manfredi, M. C., Maravetz, L. L., Lyga, J. W., Tymonko, J. M., Wilson, K. R., Poss, K. M., and Wyle, M. J. (1992). Synthesis and herbicidal properties of aryltriazolinones. A new class of pre- and postemergence herbicides. *Am. Chem. Soc. Symp. Ser.* **504**, 135–146.

Vidrine, P. R., Griffin, J. L., Jordan, D. L., and Reynolds, D. B. (1996). Broadleaf weed control in soybean (*Glycine max*) with sulfentrazone. *Weed Technol.* **10**, 762–765.

Vidrine, P. R., Jordan, D. L., and Girlinghouse, J. M. (1994). Efficacy of F-6285 in soybeans. *Proc. South. Weed Sci. Soc.* **47**, 62.

Vidrine, P. R., Reynolds, D. B., and Griffin, J. L. (1993). Weed control in soybean (*Glycine max*) with lactofen plus chlorimuron. *Weed Technol.* **7**, 311–316.

Walker, R. H., Richburg, J. S., and Jones, R. E. (1992). F6285 efficacy as affected by rate and method of application. *Proc. South. Weed Sci. Soc.* **45**, 51.

Ward, E. R., and Volrath, S. (1995). "Manipulation of Protoporphyrinogen Oxidase Enzyme Activity in Eukaryotic Organisms." International Patent Application WO 95/34659.

Watanabe, N., Che, F. S., Iwano, M., Nakano, T., Takayama, S., Yoshida, S., and Isogai, A. (1998). Molecular characterization of photomixotrophic tobacco cells resistant to photoporphyrinogen oxidase-inhibiting herbicides. *Plant Physiol.* **118**, 451–458.

Wehtje, G. R., Walker, R. H., Grey, T. L., and Hancock, H. G. (1997). Response of purple (*Cyperus rotundus*) and yellow nutsedge (*Cyperus esculentus*) to selective placement of sulfentrazone. *Weed Sci.* **45**, 382–387.

Wepplo, P., Birk, J. H., Lavanish, J. M., Mandredi, M., and Nielsen, D. R. (1995). 5-Aryloxybenzisoxazole esters. *Am. Chem. Soc. Symp. Ser.* **584**, 149–160.

Wills, G. D., and McWhorter, C. G. (1981). Effect of environment on the translocation and toxicity of acifluorfen to showy crotalaria (*Crotalaria spectabilis*). *Weed Sci.* **29**, 397–401.

Chloracetanilides

William F. Heydens
Monsanto Company

Ian C. Lamb
Pioneer Hi-Bred International, Inc.

Alan G. E. Wilson
Pharmacia Corporation

69.1 INTRODUCTION

This chapter describes the toxicology of several chloracetanilide herbicides, a subclass of the acetamides [general structure $R_1-C(O)-N(R_2R_3)$] that have as a common structural feature a ClH_2C group as the R_1 substitution. Information is provided for alachlor, acetochlor, butachlor, metolachlor, and propachlor (see Fig. 69.1 for chemical structures); all of these herbicides, with the exception of butachlor, are sold in the United States, used primarily on corn, and collectively have the largest share in this market.

The herbicidal mode of action for chloracetaniiides is not totally understood. It is known that this class of herbicides inhibits the biosynthesis of lipids, alcohols, fatty acids, proteins, isoprenoids, and flavonoids. By inhibiting synthesis of various terpenoid precursors (e.g., kaurene), these herbicides appear to interfere with the production of gibberellin. Terpenes and waxes are formed via different biosynthetic pathways both using coenzyme A intermediates and substrates; interference with the synthesis of both substances may indicate a common mechanism of inhibition through actions on coenzyme A. Furthermore, it has been shown that chloracetaniiides are detoxified in plants by conjugation with glutathione. This has also led to the suggestion that these compounds cause their herbicidal effect via conjugation of acctyl coenzyme A and other sulfhydryl-containing enzymes, with consequent inhibition of some critical function needed for the germination or survival of seedlings.

69.2 ALACHLOR

69.2.1 IDENTITY, PROPERTIES, AND USES

69.2.1.1 Chemical Name

Alachlor is N-methoxymethyl-2′,6′-diethyl-2-chloroacetanilide.

69.2.1.2 Structures

See Fig. 69.1.

69.2.1.3 Synonyms

The common name alachlor is in general use. The major trade name for alachlor products in the United States is Lasso®. The CAS registry number for alachlor is 15972-60-8.

69.2.1.4 Physical and Chemical Properties

Alachlor has the empirical formula of $C_{14}H_{20}NO_2Cl$ and a molecular weight of 269.8. It is an odorless solid at room temperature with a melting point of approximately 38°C and has a vapor pressure of 1.6×10^{-5} mm Hg at 25°C. The solubility of alachlor in water is 242 ppm at 25°C. Alachlor is also soluble in ether, acetone, benzene, chloroform, ethanol, and ethyl acetate; it is slightly soluble in heptane.

69.2.1.5 History, Formulations, and Uses

Alachlor was registered and introduced in 1967 for the preplant or preemergence control of a broad spectrum of grass, sedge, and broadleaf weeds. It is used in corn, soybeans, dry beans, cotton, sorghum, sunflowers, peanuts, and other crops.

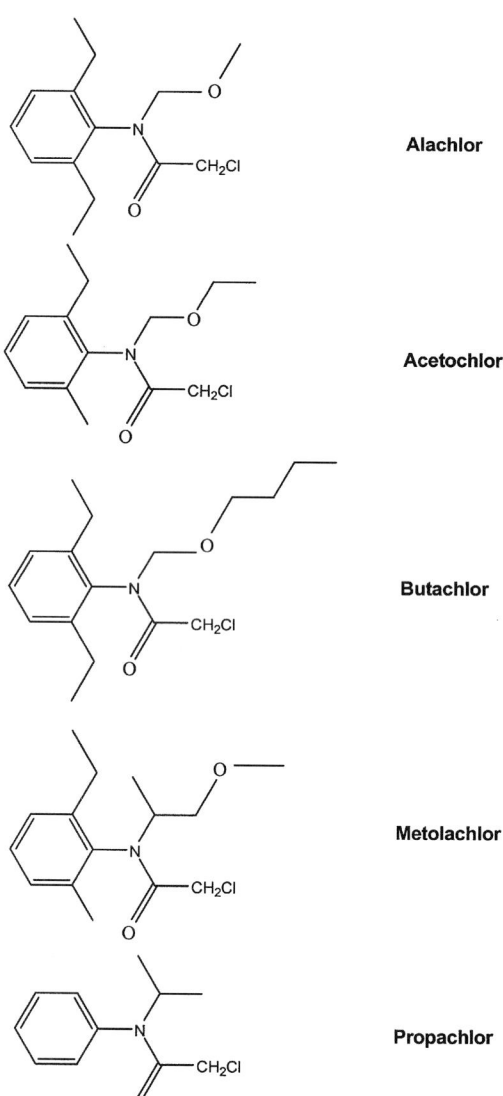

Figure 69.1 Structures of Acetanilides.

69.2.2 TOXICITY TO LABORATORY ANIMALS

69.2.2.1 Irritation and Sensitization

Eye and skin irritation studies conducted in rabbits showed alachlor to be nonirritating to the eye and slightly irritating to the skin. Alachlor produced skin sensitization in guinea pigs (Ahrens, 1994).

69.2.2.2 Acute Studies

Acute toxicity data have been reported by Ahrens (1994). The oral LD_{50} in rats ranges from 930 to 1350 mg/kg, while the dermal LD_{50} is reported to be 13,300 mg/kg. The 4-h inhalation LC_{50} in rats was shown to be greater than 5.1 mg/l, the highest concentration tested (Monsanto, 1997a).

69.2.2.3 Repeated Dose Studies

Several subchronic and chronic toxicology studies of alachlor have been conducted, the results of which have recently been reported by the U.S. Environmental Protection Agency EPA (1998a) and Heydens (1998). The major studies are summarized next.

Administration of alachlor to beagle dogs for 6 months at dose levels of 5, 25, 50, and 75 mg/kg/day produced changes indicative of liver toxicity; the effect at the lowest dose was limited to a slight elevation in the liver weights of male dogs only. In a subsequent 1-year dog study, a no observable effect level (NOEL) was established at 1 mg/kg/day based on evidence of slight anemia at 3 mg/kg/day in two animals.

In the first of two chronic studies conducted in Long–Evans rats, alachlor was administered in the diet at doses of 14, 42, and 126 mg/kg/day for approximately 2 years. Hepatotoxicity was evident at all dose levels. Eye examinations revealed the presence of an ocular lesion, progressive uveal degeneration syndrome (UDS). This syndrome was noted at the two highest doses tested, and may also have occurred in two rats at 14 mg/kg/day. This ocular lesion was considered to be unique to the Long–Evans rat because the response has not been observed in other strains of rats, mice, or dogs. Furthermore, the effect has not been observed in humans involved in the manufacture of alachlor (see Section 69.2.3). The second long-term feeding study in rats was conducted at dose levels of 0.5, 2.5, and 15 mg/kg/day for approximately 25 months. Liver and ocular effects were not observed at any dose level; the NOEL was 2.5 mg/kg/day based on nasal hyperplasia and submucosal gland hyperplasia at the highest dose tested. In conclusion, the lowest NOEL for all subchronic and chronic effects was determined to be 1 mg/kg/day in the 1-year dog study.

69.2.2.4 Pharmacokinetic Studies

The absorption, metabolism, and excretion of alachlor has been extensively studied in rats, mice, and monkeys (EPA, 1998a; Heydens et al., 1998).

Alachlor is well absorbed in rats following oral administration. The metabolism of alachlor in rats is complex due to extensive biliary excretion, intestinal microbial metabolism, and enterohepatic circulation of metabolites. In excess of 30 metabolites of alachlor have been identified in rat excreta, with approximately equal quantities appearing in urine and feces. Nearly 90% of the administered dose was eliminated in 10 days. Qualitatively, alachlor metabolism in the mouse is similar to the rat; however, there are significant quantitative differences between the two species. In contrast, alachlor is metabolized in monkeys to a limited number of glutathione and glucuronide conjugates, which are excreted primarily via the kidney. Excretion in monkeys is more rapid than in rodents, with ≥90% or more of an administered dose being excreted in the urine within 48 h.

The large differences in metabolic profile patterns and urinary excretion rates between rats and monkeys is thought to be due to a physiological phenomenon commonly referred to as the molecular weight threshold for biliary excretion. Being of intermediate molecular weight (i.e., 300–500 g/mol), alachlor metabolites have been shown to undergo biliary excretion and enterohepatic recirculation in rodents, but are not good candidates for biliary excretion in primates (Millburn, 1975; Williams, 1971).

The dermal penetration of alachlor has been investigated in monkeys and shown to be relatively low. One study showed that penetration rates (i.e., percentage of applied dose that is absorbed) for the emulsifiable concentrate (EC) formulation over a 12-h period were 7.7 and 9.1% for the undiluted formulation and diluted spray solution, respectively; values of 2.7 and 5.0% were reported for the microencapsulated product (Kronenberg et al., 1988). Another study done with a spray dilution of the EC formulation reported that the penetration rate ranged from 15 to 21% after a continuous 24-h exposure (Wester et al., 1992).

69.2.2.5 Genotoxicity Studies

Numerous genetic toxicology studies have been conducted that assessed a variety of in vitro and in vivo endpoints. These include studies generated for regulatory purposes using established testing guidelines conducted under good laboratory practices (GLPs) and studies published in the scientific literature, some of which have a limited amount of validation data and/or employ questionable assay conditions. The results of all these studies provide no evidence that neoplastic responses observed in the rat (discussed later) arise through a genotoxic mode of action, and the weight of evidence indicates that alachlor does not have general genotoxic potential in mammals.

The most relevant studies for evaluating genotoxic potential are well-validated, standard assays required/recommended by regulatory authorities worldwide. Alachlor has been tested in several of these test systems (Kier et al., 1996). Ames/Salmonella assays conducted on alachlor as well as urine and bile samples from alachlor-treated rats showed no mutagenic activity. Alachlor was negative in a CHO/HGPRT mammalian cell gene mutation assay when tested up to cytotoxic levels. In an in vivo cytogenetics assay, alachlor was not clastogenic to rat bone marrow cells when given orally at dose levels up to 1000 mg/kg. Alachlor was negative in rat and mouse micronucleus assays conducted at doses of 600 mg/kg (ip) and 1000 mg/kg (po), respectively. In two in vivo/in vitro UDS assays, variable responses were seen at 1000 mg/kg, but alachlor was clearly negative at all other doses below that level. The 1000 mg/kg dose is near the oral LD_{50} and has been shown to produce severe hepatotoxicity under the conditions employed in the UDS assay. Therefore, the biological relevance of the results at this high dose is doubtful.

Two specialized studies have also been conducted to assess possible interactions with nasal tissue DNA in vivo (Heydens et al., 1998). The first study was conducted to determine if alachlor bound to DNA in rat nasal tissue. Following administration of ^{14}C-labeled alachlor at a dose of 125 mg/kg, DNA and protein were purified and harvested from nasal turbinate tissue. There was an extremely low level of net radioactivity

(<5 dpm/mg DNA) associated with nasal tissue DNA, the nature of the bound radioactivity was not determined, and it was difficult to eliminate the possibility that the apparent binding represented protein contamination. Nevertheless, the results do represent an upper bound on the possible level of DNA binding. The possible biological significance of this DNA-associated radioactivity was evaluated by comparing the covalent binding index (CBI) to alachlor's oncogenic potential expressed as the TD_{50} (Gold et al., 1984). Using a relationship developed for hepatocarcinogens (Lutz, 1986), it was concluded that the radioactivity was much too low to be consistent with a genotoxic mode of action for the induction of nasal tumors in rats. The second study investigated the ability of alachlor to produce DNA damage following administration in the diet at a dose of 126 mg/kg/day for 7 days. No evidence of DNA strand breakage was observed in the nasal cells. These studies support the conclusion that alachlor produces nasal tumors in rats via a mechanism that does not involve the initial induction of DNA damage.

A number of studies evaluating the genotoxic potential of alachlor have been reported in the literature. General conclusions from the major studies can be summarized as follows: Alachlor has been tested for mutagenicity in 14 bacterial test systems. While one spot test and one plate incorporation test were reported positive, the other 12 tests showed a uniform and consistent pattern of negative results. Both positive and negative results have been reported for a number of in vitro studies conducted to assess chromosome effects. Some of the studies reporting positive effects were conducted using alachlor samples that were produced by inexpensive, alternative manufacturing processes that are not used by Monsanto. One of these processes was known to involve the use of the alkylating agent, chloromethyl methyl ether, which is a known mutagen and carcinogen. The test materials used in these studies (Georgian et al., 1983; Lin et al., 1987) were substantially more toxic (10- to >100-fold) to the mammalian cells tested than alachlor produced by a high-quality manufacturing process. Therefore, results from these studies are not applicable to quality-produced, name brand alachlor products and should not be included in an assessment of alachlor's genotoxic potential. Conflicting results have been reported for two other in vitro mammalian chromosome effect studies using alachlor of high purity (Erexson et al., 1993; Meisner et al., 1992). Use of nonstandard procedures (e.g., extended treatment period) and an unusual frequency of aberrant human lymphocytes in the control group of the study reporting positive effects were undoubtedly important factors. DNA strand breakage has also been reported in vitro at concentrations eliciting cytotoxicity and which, using pharmacokinetic analyses, would be associated with lethality in vivo (Bonfanti et al., 1992). In vivo DNA strand breakage studies in rats and mice showed no evidence of DNA damage (Taningher et al., 1993). These studies, along with the other negative in vivo work described previously, clearly demonstrate that the in vitro DNA damage findings reported by some investigators are not reflective of the universally negative in vivo mammalian effects.

69.2.2.6 Carcinogenicity Studies

The oncogenic potential of alachlor has been assessed in two bioassays conducted with the Long–Evans strain of rat and in two studies done with CD-1 mice (EPA, 1998a; Heydens, 1998). Alachlor produced significant increases in glandular stomach and thyroid follicular tumors in rats at the highest dose tested, a level exceeding the maximum tolerated dose (MTD); nasal epithelial (olfactory) tumors were also observed at lower doses. Based on these findings, the EPA had previously classified alachlor as a Group B2 carcinogen. However, the EPA's Cancer Peer Review Committee (CPRC) reconsidered the weight of evidence for alachlor, taking into account new mechanistic information (Section 69.7) in accordance with its Proposed Guidelines for Carcinogen Risk Assessment (EPA, 1996). Alachlor was reclassified as "likely" at high doses but "not likely" at low doses to be a human carcinogen. The term "low doses" denotes anticipated human exposures resulting from pesticide use. The EPA, in the Reregistration Eligibility Decision (RED) document for alachlor, agreed that a nonlinear approach (margin of exposure, or MOE) should be used for the purpose of risk assessment (EPA, 1998a).

In the first rat bioassay, alachlor was administered in the diet at dose levels of 14, 42, and 126 mg/kg/day. Surviving male rats were sacrificed after 27 months while females were sacrificed after 25 months on study. In the second study, which was conducted to follow-up on non-neoplastic effects observed in the first bioassay, rats received alachlor in their diets at dose levels equivalent to 0.5, 2.5, 15, and 126 mg/kg/day. The highest dose level of 126 mg/kg/day exceeded the maximum tolerated dose (MTD) as evidenced by excessive body weight loss (>30% below controls), hepatocellular necrosis, and decreased survival. Neoplastic responses attributable to alachlor administration were observed in the nasal turbinate mucosa and glandular stomach mucosa of both sexes and in the thyroid follicular epithelium of male rats. Significant increases in stomach and thyroid tumors were restricted to the highest dose tested. One benign nasal tumor was noted at 2.5 mg/kg/day. Although single nasal tumors of this type are occasionally observed in control animals, the tumor at 2.5 mg/kg/day was considered to be treatment related by the EPA and the definitive NOEL for oncogenicity is, therefore, 0.5 mg/kg/day. Subsequent mode-of-action investigations have shown that the nasal, stomach, and thyroid tumors are produced via non-genotoxic, threshold-sensitive mechanisms. The studies supporting this conclusion are described in Section 69.7.

The first oncogenicity study in mice was conducted at dose levels of 26, 78, and 260 mg/kg/day for approximately 19 months. The only notable finding was the occurrence of benign lung (bronchoalveolar) tumors in high-dose females. Although the incidence was statistically different from concurrent controls, it was within the range expected for untreated animals. Due to this equivocal finding and the overall poor survival of animals in this study, a second mouse bioassay was conducted at dose levels of 20, 78, and 331 mg/kg/day for 18 months. There was no dose–response relationship for the incidence of lung tumors and no other indication that the tumors were related to administration of the test material. Based on all the available information, it was concluded that alachlor was not oncogenic in the mouse.

69.2.2.7 Development and Reproduction Studies

The reproductive and developmental toxicity database has been reported by Heydens (1998) and recently evaluated by the EPA (1998a). The EPA's assessment included special consideration of possible effects on infants and children as required by the Food Quality Protection Act (FQPA) of 1996. This provision of the FQPA requires the use of an additional safety factor for the protection of infants and children when warranted by the severity of effects observed in toxicology studies. The EPA considered the alachlor database to be complete, and the NOELs for developmental effects were equal to or greater than those for maternal effects in both developmental toxicity studies. Therefore, the EPA concluded there is no unique sensitivity from prenatal exposure. Likewise, in the reproduction study, the reproductive NOEL is greater than the systemic NOEL. Thus, no special sensitivity for infants or children was indicated. Brief details of the studies supporting these conclusions are given next.

Alachlor was fed to male and female rats at doses of 3, 10, and 30 mg/kg/day throughout premating, mating, gestation, and lactation periods for three successive generations. Nephritis and an apparent decrease in ovarian weights were noted in high-dose adults. The significance of the latter finding is doubtful because there was no microscopic change in the tissue and no effects on reproductive parameters. The systemic and reproductive toxicity NOELs were 10 and 30 (or more) mg/kg/day, respectively. In a developmental toxicity study with rats, alachlor was administered by gavage at doses of 50, 150, and 400 mg/kg/day on gestation days 6–19. Maternal and fetal toxicity were noted at the highest dose tested as evidenced by maternal deaths and decreased body weight gains, a slight decrease in fetal body weight, and a slight increase in postimplantation loss. The NOEL for developmental toxicity in the rat was 150 mg/kg/day. Oral administration of alachlor to rabbits at doses of 50, 100, and 150 mg/kg/day on gestation days 7–19 produced maternal toxicity at the highest dose tested but no effects on the fetus. Therefore, the NOEL for developmental toxicity in the rabbit was greater than or equal to 150 mg/kg/day.

69.2.3 HUMAN EXPERIENCE

A large number of workers have had long-term occupational exposure to alachlor at the Monsanto manufacturing facility for this herbicide, which has been in continuous operation since 1968. An exposure analysis indicated that exposure of these workers exceeded that of farmers and herbicide applicators (Acquavella et al., 1994). These manufacturing workers therefore presented an opportunity to assess alachlor's potential to produce adverse health affects in humans. Three epidemiological studies were conducted on these individuals, the focus of which was the ocular and oncogenic effects observed in the chronic rat studies.

In an evaluation of ocular health, the eyes of 135 workers judged to have the highest alachlor exposure were examined for the presence of a specific eye abnormality termed pigmentary dispersion syndrome (PDS) (Ireland *et al.*, 1994). This lesion is analogous to the initiating lesion that occurred in one specific strain of rat from the chronic alachlor studies. Eye examinations were also given to an unexposed control group. PDS was not found in any of the exposed workers, and other eye abnormalities occurred at similar rates in exposed and unexposed individuals. These results indicate that humans exposed to alachlor are not at an increased risk of developing ocular disease.

Mortality and cancer incidence studies for the period 1970–1990 were originally reported in 1994 (Leet *et al.*, 1996) and have been updated with additional data through 1993 (Acquavella *et al.*, 1996). The mortality cohort comprised 1199 workers employed for at least 1 year between 1961 and 1993. The cancer incidence cohort was a subset of 1169 of the mortality cohort whose members lived in Iowa for some time during the period 1969–1993. Using an in-depth knowledge of the plant and process, all job titles and descriptions used in personnel records were allocated into occupational exposure categories. Each such category was assigned a qualitative exposure rank (high, medium, low, or negligible) for alachlor.

A total of 1036 workers who had potential alachlor exposure met the criteria for inclusion in the mortality analysis. Mortality from all causes among workers judged to have high alachlor exposure was lower than expected (standardized mortality ratio, SMR = 0.7), and mortality from cancer was similar to that for the state of Iowa (SMR = 0.9). Likewise, there was no increased cancer mortality among those workers with 5 or more years of exposure and 15 or more years since first exposure, the group in which occupationally related cancers would be mostly to occur. There were no deaths from nasal, stomach, or thyroid cancers.

There were 1025 workers who met the criteria for cancer incidence analysis, and 701 (68%) of them belonged to the high-exposure category. The cancer incidence for workers with high-exposure potential was similar to that of the Iowa population (standardized incidence ratio, SIR = 1.2), especially for those exposed for 5 or more years and with at least 15 years since exposure began (SIR = 1.0). There were no cases of thyroid, stomach, or nasal cancers. These results indicate that alachlor exposure had no effect on cancer incidence rates in the workers.

Thus, there was no indication of increased mortality rates from cancer or any other causes among alachlor manufacturing workers with up to 25 years of follow-up. It is especially noteworthy that cancer rates were not elevated in the highest exposed alachlor workers and that there were no cases of thyroid, stomach, or nasal cancers, which were the oncogenic responses observed in the rat bioassays.

The production workers were exposed to alachlor during the year at a level that exceeded that of agricultural exposure; in fact, exposure to manufacturing personnel was estimated to exceed that of pesticide applicators by a factor of 10,000 or more (Acquavella *et al.*, 1994). Dietary exposure is even lower than that of applicators. Therefore, the absence of ocular effects, elevated mortality, and increased cancer incidence in production workers serves as an important indicator of the low potential for adverse effects among the general population, which is exposed to extremely low levels of alachlor.

69.3 ACETOCHLOR

69.3.1 IDENTITY, PROPERTIES, AND USES

69.3.1.1 Chemical Name

Acetochlor is 2-chloro-*N*-ethoxymethyl-*N*-(2′-ethyl-6′-methylphenyl)acetamide.

69.3.1.2 Structure

See Fig. 69.1.

69.3.1.3 Synonyms

The common name acetochlor is in general use. The CAS registry number for acetochlor is 34256-82-1.

69.3.1.4 Physical and Chemical Properties

Acetochlor has the empirical formula of $C_{14}H_{20}NO_2Cl$ and a molecular weight of 269.77. It is a light amber to violet-colored oily liquid at room temperature with a specific gravity of 1.110 g/ml at 30°C. Acetochlor has a boiling point of 162°C at 7 mm Hg and a vapor pressure of 3.4×10^{-8} at 25°C. Solubility in water is 233 ppm at 25°C. Acetochlor is also soluble in organic solvents including alcohol, acetone, toluene, and carbon tetrachloride.

69.3.1.5 History, Formulations, and Uses

This herbicide was registered in the United States in 1994 by the Acetochlor Registration Partnership (ARP), which is now a partnership between Monsanto Company and Dow Agro Sciences. The registration of acetochlor is owned by the ARP, but both companies compete in the marketplace with different formulations. Acetochlor is a selective herbicide that controls a broad spectrum of annual grasses, sedge, and broadleaf weeds primarily in corn. Monsanto manufactures a number of formulations under the trade name Harness®. Formulations produced by Zeneca are sold under the trade name Surpass®.

Prior to formation of the ARP, two companies had separately pursued registration with independently generated toxicology databases. Therefore, there are two or more studies for each type of toxicology test performed for regulatory purposes.

69.3.2 TOXICITY TO LABORATORY ANIMALS

69.3.2.1 Irritation and Sensitization

Acetochlor has been shown to be practically nonirritating to the eyes and skin of rabbits. A dermal sensitization study in guinea pigs was positive (Monsanto, 1997b).

69.3.2.2 Acute Studies

The acute oral and dermal toxicity of acetochlor is low. The oral LD_{50} value is 2148 mg/kg in the rat (Monsanto, 1997b). Dermal LD_{50} values were shown to be greater than 2000 mg/kg in both rats and rabbits.

69.3.2.3 Repeat Dose Studies

Several subchronic and chronic toxicology studies have been conducted with acetochlor. The results have been reported by the EPA (1994) and are summarized next.

A 21-day dermal study in rats at dose levels ranging from 0.1 to 100 mg/kg/day resulted in mild to minimal skin irritation but no systemic effects. In a second study conducted with rabbits at doses of 100 to 1200 mg/kg/day, the NOEL for systemic toxicity was 400 mg/kg/day. The main effects in two 90-day feeding studies with rats were reductions in body weight and food consumption. The lowest observed effect levels (LOELs) in both studies were 100 mg/kg/day; the NOELs were 10 and 40 mg/kg/day.

Oral administration to dogs for 12 months at 4, 12, and 40 mg/kg/day resulted in decreased food consumption, body weight loss, testicular atrophy, and an increase in relative liver weights at the highest dose tested. The NOEL was 12 mg/kg/day. In a second 12-month dog study, the NOEL was 2 mg/kg/day based on changes in serum chemistry values as well as renal and testicular effects in males at 10 mg/kg/day.

Dietary administration of acetochlor to CD-1 mice for 23 months produced excessive mortality, body weight loss, anemia, interstitial nephritis, and changes indicative of liver damage at the highest dose tested (5000 ppm); this level clearly exceeded the MTD. Increased liver, kidney, and adrenal weights were observed at lower dose levels (500 and 1500 ppm). In a second mouse study conducted at dietary levels of 10, 100, and 1000 ppm for 18 months, the NOEL for systemic toxicity was 10 ppm (1.1 mg/kg/day) in males based on renal changes and 100 ppm (~13 mg/kg/day) in females. The administration of acetochlor to rats at doses of 500–5000 ppm (26–297 mg/kg/day) for 27 months exceeded the MTD at the highest dose tested. This was evidenced by increased mortality, excessive body weight loss, hepatocellular necrosis, and other effects. A NOEL for chronic effects was not established. In two subsequent 24-month studies conducted at lower dose levels, the lowest NOEL was determined to be 7.4 mg/kg/day based on decreased body weight gain and indications of liver toxicity.

69.3.2.4 Pharmacokinetic Studies

Rats were found to rapidly metabolize acetochlor to numerous polar metabolites, which were then quickly excreted in the urine and feces; more than 95% of the recovered dose was excreted within 72 h. Blood was the only tissue in which significant retention of radioactivity was observed (2–3% of the dose), and the activity was shown to be associated with hemoglobin. The major metabolite, as well as some minor degradates, were identified and shown to be a result of the mercapturic acid pathway formed by initial glutathione conjugation. The glucuronide conjugate is the major metabolite in bile, and enterohepatic recirculation is known to occur as discussed previously for alachlor. In the mouse, little or no enterohepatic recirculation occurs and the glucuronide is the major urinary metabolite.

The dermal penetration of acetochlor was measured in rhesus monkeys following a 24-h exposure. The penetration of the concentrated material was 4.9%, while that of a 1:70 spray dilution was 17.3% (Wester et al., 1996).

69.3.2.5 Genotoxicity Studies

Acetochlor gave uniformly negative results in a wide range of in vivo rodent genetic toxicity studies conducted in rats and mice at and below toxic levels. This inactivity is consistent with its lack of in vitro gene mutation and DNA-damaging activity. Several negative in vivo clastogenicity assays indicate that acetochlor's in vitro clastogenicity is not relevant to its activity in vivo or to its ability to produce tumors in rodents (discussed later). This conclusion is further supported by the fact that acetochlor is not genotoxic to the olfactory nasal epithelium of rats, the primary site of its rodent carcinogenicity. Detailed discussions of the genetic toxicity data for acetochlor have been published (Ashby et al., 1996, 1997); a summary of those studies is provided next.

An extensive set of studies have led to the conclusion that acetochlor is not mutagenic to Salmonella typhimurium. The experiments included observations made with strains TA98, TA100, TA1535, TA1537, and TA1538 using S9 mixes derived from rats pretreated with either aroclor or a combination of phenobarbitone/beta naphthoflavone.

Acetochlor was inactive in an in vitro assay for unscheduled DNA synthesis (UDS) using isolated primary rat hepatocytes. In two CHO/HGPRT gene mutation assays conducted at the same concentrations, acetochlor marginally increased the mutation frequency at toxic dose levels and in the presence of S9 mix in one investigation, and produced a clearly negative response in the second assay. Acetochlor is clastogenic to human lymphocytes in vitro at cytotoxic dose levels. The nonclastogenicity of the deschloro analog of acetochlor and the clastogenicity of the desoxy (N-butyl) analog indicate that the chloroacetyl substituent on acetochlor is the clastogenic moiety. Although relatively inert, this substituent can react with sulfhydryl (−SH) groups such as that present on reduced glutathione (Ashby et al., 1996). This reactivity most likely accounts for the clastogenicity of acetochlor in isolated lymphocytes that have extremely low levels of protective glutathione. Acetochlor gave a weak positive response in the mouse lymphoma TK$^\pm$ mutation assay when tested in the presence of S9 mix at excessively toxic levels ($\leq$10% relative survival of cells). It is concluded that acetochlor is not directly mutagenic to DNA, but that it is clastogenic *in vitro* by virtue of the sulfur reactivity of its chloroacetyl substituent. *In vivo*, normal levels of glutathione protect against this activity.

Several *in vivo* assays have been conducted and provide important information regarding the relevance of the *in vitro* assay results. Negative results have been obtained in six separate *in vivo* assays assessing chromosome aberration activity in somatic and germ cells. Acetochlor was negative in an *in vivo* rat bone marrow cytogenetic assay, in two mouse bone marrow micronucleus assays, and in two rat and a mouse dominant lethal assays. In the first rat dominant lethal assay (single oral dose), a reversible toxic effect, which was observed only at supra-MTD dose levels, led to a reduction in litter sizes at the 3-week sampling period (2000 mg/kg). This effect was not observed in either the mouse or the second rat dominant lethal assay or in multigeneration studies conducted using the dietary route up to the MTD of acetochlor. Clearly, the clastogenic activity observed *in vitro* was not expressed *in vivo* in the primary rodent cytogenetic assays.

Acetochlor gave a negative response in the rat liver unscheduled DNA synthesis (UDS) assay when tested at dose levels up to, and including, the MTD. At a supra-MTD dose level (2000 mg/kg), a weak positive UDS response was observed. However, this dose depressed hepatic glutathione levels by up to 80% and was associated with severe liver necrosis, substantial release of hepatic enzymes, and lethality among the treated animals (up to 30%). Acetochlor gave negative results in assays for DNA damage (comet assays) conducted using nasal tissue (respiratory and olfactory) derived from rats treated with the supra-MTD dose of 1750 ppm of acetochlor in the diet for either 7 days or 18 weeks. These negative data are particularly relevant, given that the primary target for acetochlor carcinogenesis in the rat is the olfactory nasal epithelium.

69.3.2.6 Carcinogenicity Studies

Acetochlor has been assessed for oncogenic potential in a total of five dietary studies (three rat and two mouse). These studies have been discussed by Ashby *et al.* (1996) and are summarized next. Although tumors were reported at various sites, the only potentially toxicologically significant effects are nasal and thyroid tumors in the rat. In 1986, acetochlor was classified as a Group B2 carcinogen by the EPA. However, this evaluation was conducted prior to the availability of recent negative *in vivo* genotoxicity studies and mechanistic information. The negative *in vivo* genotoxicity results, along with the absence of tumors below the MTD, provide evidence that the oncogenic responses arise through non-genotoxic, threshold-sensitive mechanisms. This conclusion is further supported by the results of the mechanistic investigations (see Section 69.7). The European Union's

DGXI Labelling Committee did consider all relevant information in 1997, and concluded that acetochlor should not be classified as a carcinogen.

The oncogenic potential of acetochlor in rats was assessed in one study at dietary levels of 500, 1500, and 5000 ppm (equivalent to 26, 81, and 297 mg/kg/day) and in a follow-up study at doses of 40, 200, and 1000 ppm (equivalent to 2, 10.5, and 54 mg/kg/day). The third rat bioassay was conducted at dietary levels of 8, 175, and 1750 ppm (equivalent to 0.8, 7.9, and 80 mg/kg/day). The dose of 54 mg/kg/day represented an MTD based on a 10% depression in body weight gain. A marginal increase in liver tumors was seen but only at a dose (297 mg/kg/day) that greatly exceeded the MTD. Nasal epithelial (olfactory) adenomas and small increases in thyroid follicular tumors occurred at and above the MTD. The NOEL for oncogenic effects was 26 mg/kg/day.

Acetochlor's oncogenic potential in mice was evaluated in one study conducted at dietary doses of 500, 1500, and 5000 ppm (equivalent to 85, 254, and 973 mg/kg/day) for 23 months, and in a second study at dietary doses of 10, 100, and 1000 ppm (equivalent to 1.2, 12, and 126 mg/kg/day) for 18 months. In the first study, the dose of 973 mg/kg/day greatly exceeded the MTD as evidenced by decreased body weight gain (males, 70%; females, 24%), increased mortality, and organ toxicity. Under these excessively toxic conditions, the incidence of liver tumors was increased. The only consistent finding in the mouse across the two studies was a marginal increase in the incidence of lung tumors, predominantly adenomas in female mice. These tumors are common in the mouse strain (CD-1) employed in these studies and occur spontaneously at variable incidences. The incidences observed in treated animals from the acetochlor studies were within the historical control range. An apparent increase in the incidence of uterine histiocytic sarcomas was noted in all treatment groups in the first mouse study. However, there was clearly no dose–response relationship across the 10-fold range of doses tested, and there was no increase in the second study. Based on these and other factors, the higher incidence of histiocytic sarcomas was not clearly related to acetochlor administration and is most likely the result of normal variation.

69.3.2.7 Development and Reproduction Studies

Developmental toxicity has been assessed in two rat and two rabbit studies in which acetochlor was administered by gavage (EPA, 1994). Acetochlor did not produce a teratogenic response in any of these studies. In each of the two rat studies, maternal and fetal toxicity were noted at the highest dose tested (400 and 600 mg/kg/day). The NOEL for both maternal and developmental toxicity was shown to be 150 mg/kg/day in one study and 200 mg/kg/day in the other. In a study with rabbits, acetochlor did not produce developmental toxicity at doses up to 190 mg/kg/day, the highest dose tested; the NOEL for maternal toxicity in this study was 50 mg/kg/day. The second rabbit study was conducted at levels up to 300 mg/kg/day without producing any developmental toxicity. Because the

NOELs for developmental effects were equal to or greater than the NOELs for maternal effects in all three studies, it was concluded that there is no unique sensitivity from prenatal exposure.

The reproductive toxicity of acetochlor has been evaluated in two 2-generation rat reproduction studies (EPA, 1994). The first study resulted in decreased body weight gain and reduced viable litter size at dietary concentrations of 1500 and 5000 ppm. The highest dose of 5000 ppm ($\sim$400 mg/kg/day) exceeded the MTD. The NOEL for reproductive toxicity was 500 ppm (30.4 and 44.9 mg/kg/day for males and females, respectively). In the second study, systemic toxicity was observed in parental animals at 160 mg/kg/day, which was the highest dose tested. Acetochlor had no effects on reproductive performance, but probably because of a slightly reduced body weight gain in offspring late in lactation at 160 mg/kg/day, the reproductive NOEL was considered to be 21 mg/kg/day.

69.4 BUTACHLOR

69.4.1 IDENTITY, PROPERTIES, AND USES

69.4.1.1 Chemical Name

Butachlor is *N*-(butoxymethyl)-2-chloro-2′,6′-diethylacetanilide.

69.4.1.2 Structure

See Fig. 69.1.

69.4.1.3 Synonyms

The common name butachlor is in general use. The CAS registry number for butachlor is 23184-66-9.

69.4.1.4 Physical and Chemical Properties

Butachlor has the chemical formula $C_{17}H_{26}NO_2Cl$ and a molecular weight of 311.89. It is a liquid at room temperature with a vapor pressure of 1.8×10^{-6} mm Hg at 25°C. The solubility of butachlor in water is 20 ppm at 25°C. Butachlor is miscible with alcohol, ether, acetone, and benzene.

69.4.1.5 History, Formulations, and Uses

Butachlor was developed for the preemergent control of grass and broadleaf weeds in rice and barley. Butachlor is available as emulsifiable concentrate and granular formulations sold under the trade name Machete®.

69.4.2 TOXICITY TO LABORATORY ANIMALS

69.4.2.1 Irritation and Sensitization

In studies with rabbits, butachlor was practically nonirritating to the skin and moderately irritating to the eye; dermal sensitization was observed in a study with guinea pigs (Monsanto, 1991).

69.4.2.2 Acute Studies

Butachlor is slightly to practically nontoxic in standard animal tests. The oral LD_{50} in rats is 2000 mg/kg, and the dermal LD_{50} is 13,300 mg/kg (Monsanto, 1991).

69.4.2.3 Repeat Dose Studies

New Zealand white rabbits were exposed to butachlor dermally for 21 days at dose levels up to 2500 mg/kg/day; the only sign of toxicity was dermal irritation, and the systemic NOEL was the highest dose tested. Feeding studies of 90 days' duration have been performed with the Fischer 344, Sprague–Dawley, and Wistar strains of rats at dietary concentrations ranging from 300 to 40,000 ppm. Toxicity was manifest in one or more strains as decreased survival, body weight depression, anemia, and effects in the liver, kidney, and bladder. The lowest NOEL was observed in the Fischer rat at 300 ppm ($\sim$18 mg/kg/day). A 90-day feeding study in CD-1 mice at dietary concentrations ranging from 1000 to 6000 ppm resulted in liver and kidney toxicity; the NOEL was determined to be less than 1000 ppm due to increased liver weights in male mice at the lowest dose tested. An 8-week oral capsule study was performed in beagle dogs at dose levels ranging from 10 to 100 mg/kg/day. The subchronic NOEL in dogs was 10 mg/kg/day based on indications of liver toxicity (Wilson and Takei, 1999).

The chronic toxicity of butachlor has also been evaluated in dogs, mice, and rats. As in the subchronic studies, the liver, kidney, and bladder were the primary target organs in one or more species. The chronic NOELs in dogs and mice were 5 and 8 mg/kg/day, respectively. Chronic NOELs of 4 and 5 mg/kg/day were established in Fischer 344 and Sprague–Dawley rats, respectively (Wilson and Takei, 1999).

69.4.2.4 Pharmacokinetic Studies

Similar to alachlor and acetochlor, investigations into the metabolism and pharmacokinetics of butachlor have revealed species differences in the way that this molecule is biotransformed and eliminated from the body. Butachlor metabolism in rats is complex due to extensive biliary excretion, intestinal microbial metabolism, and enterohepatic circulation of metabolites. Metabolism in rats follows three major pathways: (1) initial conjugation with glutathione followed by mercapturic acid pathway metabolism; (2) cytochrome P-450-mediated hydroxylation of the aromatic ring, its ethyl groups, and the *N*-butoxymethylene group; and (3) cleavage of the amide bonds via aryl amidase to form 2,6-diethylaniline, which is further oxidized to 4-amino-3,5-diethylphenol. Approximately 85% of an orally administered dose is eliminated in 48 h; 60% of the excreted material is found in feces and 40% in urine.

The results of dermal penetration studies with rhesus monkeys indicate that butachlor is poorly absorbed through the skin. In studies employing a 6-h topical exposure period, only 0.02%

of the dose was systemically absorbed during exposure to a granular formulation, and 5% of the dose was absorbed when an EC formulation was applied (Wilson and Takei, 1999).

69.4.2.5 Genotoxicity Studies

The genotoxic potential of butachlor has been evaluated in numerous assay systems, using a variety of species, metabolic activation conditions, and endpoints. Results from an extensive battery of well-validated tests conducted under GLPs have shown that butachlor is not genotoxic. Butachlor produced no response in the *Escherichia coli* wp2 reverse mutation assay. A weak positive response was observed in the TA100 strain of *Salmonella* in one Ames assay; however, this finding was not reproduced in subsequent assays. When tested in cultured Chinese hamster ovary (CHO) cells, there was no mutagenic response in the HGPRT forward gene mutation assay. A CHO *in vitro* cytogenetics assay was also negative for clastogenicity. A bone marrow cytogenetics assay and a mouse micronucleus assay conducted at ip dose levels up to 750 and 1000 mg/kg, respectively, were both negative. Exposure of CD-1 male mice to butachlor for 7 weeks at dietary concentrations up to 5000 ppm produced significant body weight depression but no evidence of dominant lethal effects. An *in vivo/in vitro* DNA assay in F-344 rats at oral dose levels ranging from 50 to 1000 mg/kg produced no increase in unscheduled DNA synthesis (Wilson and Takei, 1999).

69.4.2.6 Carcinogenicity Studies

Butachlor has been evaluated for oncogenic potential in two strains of rats (Sprague–Dawley and Fischer 344) and in CD-1 mice. Butachlor administration induced nasal, stomach, and thyroid tumors only in the Sprague–Dawley rat, but not in the Fischer 344 rat or the CD-1 mouse. In the Sprague–Dawley rat, the tumors were similar to those seen with alachlor and occurred only above toxic dose levels (i.e., $\geq$MTD). Mechanistic studies have been conducted that support the conclusion that these tumors are not relevant in assessing the oncogenic risk to humans. The results of these investigations are presented in Section 69.7.

Butachlor was administered to Sprague–Dawley rats in the diet at concentrations of 100, 1000, and 3000 ppm for 26 months. Increases in neoplastic lesions were observed in the olfactory epithelium of the nasal turbinate, glandular stomach mucosa, and thyroid follicular epithelium. The stomach tumors were observed only at the 3000-ppm level. This dose level exceeded the MTD as evidenced by reduced survival and severe body weight depression ($>20\%$). Increased incidences of nasal and thyroid tumors occurred only at levels of 1000 ppm and above. No treatment-related tumors were noted in Fischer 344 rats fed butachlor at concentrations of 10, 100, and 1000 ppm for 24 months. Butachlor was administered in the diet to mice at concentrations of 50, 500, and 2000 ppm. This study provided no convincing evidence of oncogenic potential (Wilson and Takei, 1999).

69.4.2.7 Development and Reproduction Studies

The potential of butachlor to produce developmental toxicity has been evaluated in both rats and rabbits. The ability of butachlor to impair normal reproduction following continuous oral exposure over two generations was evaluated in rats. The results of these studies showed that butachlor was not a teratogen or reproductive toxin.

The rat and rabbit developmental toxicity studies were conducted at dose levels ranging from 49 to 490 mg/kg/day and 50 to 250 mg/kg/day, respectively. In rats, maternal toxicity was observed at the highest dose tested, but there was no effect on the developing fetus. In the rabbit study, a slight increase in postimplantation loss and decreased fetal weights were observed at maternally toxic dose levels (150 and 250 mg/kg/day). The NOEL for maternal and fetal effects was 50 mg/kg/day. Butachlor administration at dietary concentrations of 100–3000 ppm over two successive generations did not adversely affect reproductive performance or pup survival (Wilson and Takei, 1999).

69.5 METOLACHLOR

69.5.1 IDENTITY, PROPERTIES, AND USES

69.5.1.1 Chemical Name

Metolachlor is 2-chloro-2′-ethyl-6′-methyl-*N*-(2-methoxy-1-methylethyl)acetanilide.

69.5.1.2 Structure

See Fig. 69.1.

69.5.1.3 Synonyms

The common name metolachlor is in general use. A code designation is CGA-24,705. The CAS registry number for metolachlor is 51218-45-2.

69.5.1.4 Physical and Chemical Properties

Metolachlor has the chemical formula $C_{15}H_{22}NO_2Cl$ and a molecular weight of 283.8. It is a liquid that is white to tan in color. Metolachlor has a vapor pressure of 1.3×10^{-6} and a boiling point of 100°C at 0.001 mm Hg. The solubility of metolachlor in water is 530 ppm at 20°C. Metolachlor is miscible with most organic solvents.

69.5.1.5 History, Formulations, and Uses

Metolachlor was registered with the EPA in 1976. It is a selective herbicide for the control of annual grass weeds, yellow nutsedge, and some broadleaf species. Metolachlor is used in corn, peanuts, and soybeans. S-metolachlor, which contains a higher percentage of the more active of two isomers, was registered in 1997. Its formulations are sold under trade names such as Dual® Magnum®.

69.5.2 TOXICITY TO LABORATORY ANIMALS

69.5.2.1 Irritation and Sensitization

Metolachlor did not produce eye or skin irritation in rabbits; the material was positive in a dermal sensitization study with guinea pigs (EPA, 1995).

69.5.2.2 Acute Studies

Oral (rats) and dermal (rabbits) LD_{50} values for metolachlor are 2780 and more than 10,000 mg/kg, respectively (EPA, 1995). Inhalation LC_{50} values (rats) of more than 1.75 mg/l (EPA, 1995) and more than 4.3 mg/l (Ahrens, 1994) have been published.

69.5.2.3 Repeat Dose Studies

The results of subchronic and chronic studies have been summarized in the Reregistration Eligibility Decision (RED) document issued by the EPA (1995), and are briefly described next.

A 21-day dermal study was conducted with New Zealand white rabbits at dose levels of 10, 100, and 1000 mg/kg/day. Effects observed in high-dose animals were increased bilirubin, liver weights (males), and kidney weights (females); the systemic NOEL was 100 mg/kg/day. A 3-month feeding study conducted in beagle dogs produced no effects at dose levels of 500 and 1000 ppm. In a 6-month feeding study with dogs, the NOEL was 300 ppm (approximately 7.5 mg/kg/day) based on decreased food consumption and body weight gain at 1000 ppm (25 mg/kg/day), the highest dose tested.

Beagle dogs were fed metolachlor at dose levels of 100, 300, and 1000 ppm for 1 year. The NOEL for female dogs was 300 ppm (9.7 mg/kg/day) based on decreased body weight gain. In another chronic toxicity study, metolachlor was fed to Sprague–Dawley rats at dietary levels of 30, 300, and 3000 ppm (approximately 1.5, 15, and 150 mg/kg/day) for 2 years. At the high dose level, decreased body weight gain and increased liver weights (males) were observed. The NOEL for systemic toxicity was 300 ppm.

69.5.2.4 Pharmacokinetic Studies

Data reviewed by the EPA (1995) indicate that metolachlor is readily absorbed following oral exposure and excreted in the urine and feces (approximately 50% in each component) over 3 days. Dermal absorption was assumed to be 62.8% in the human based on the results from an *in vitro* study with rat skin.

69.5.2.5 Genotoxicity Studies

Metolachlor produced negative results in the genotoxicity assays conducted with the material (EPA, 1995). No gene mutations were detected in the Ames/*Salmonella* assay or the L5178/TK$^\pm$ mouse lymphoma test. No chromosome aberrations were observed in a hamster micronucleus assay and a dominant lethal assay in mice. Metolachlor was negative in

DNA damage/repair assays in rat liver cells and human fibroblasts. An *in vivo/in vitro* unscheduled DNA synthesis assay also produced no adverse effects.

69.5.2.6 Carcinogenicity Studies

The oncogenic potential of metolachlor has been assessed in two bioassays with CD-1 mice and in two studies using Sprague–Dawley rats (EPA, 1995). The EPA's CPRC classified metolachlor as a Group C (possible human) carcinogen. This classification was based on an increased incidence of liver tumors observed in female rats, an effect that was reproduced in the second rat study. The CPRC also recommended that a margin of exposure (MOE) methodology be used for the estimation of human risk (EPA, 1995) rather than a cancer potency factor calculation.

Dose levels in the 2-year mouse studies ranged from 30 to 3000 ppm in the diet. No treatment-related carcinogenic effects were noted in these studies. In a feeding study with rats, metolachlor was administered at dietary concentrations of 30, 300, and 3000 ppm. The incidence of benign liver tumors was significantly increased in high-dose females (150 mg/kg/day). This effect was reproduced in a second rat bioassay. Nasal tumors (one adenocarcinoma, one fibrosarcoma) were observed in high-dose males (vs. zero in controls); however, the EPA stated it was not clear that an obvious toxic effect was exerted on the nasal tissue (EPA, 1997).

69.5.2.7 Development and Reproduction Studies

Two developmental toxicity studies have been conducted in Sprague–Dawley rats and another was performed using New Zealand white rabbits (EPA, 1995). The dose levels in the two rat studies ranged from 60 to 1000 mg/kg/day. The NOELs for maternal and developmental toxicity were 300 mg/kg/day based on effects at 1000 mg/kg/day. Maternal toxicity was manifested by mortality, convulsions, and reduced body weight gain and food consumption. The effects observed in offspring were reduced mean body weight and an increase in resorptions. Rabbits were evaluated for developmental effects at doses of 36, 120, and 360 mg/kg/day. Maternal toxicity was observed at the highest dose tested, but there was no evidence of developmental toxicity at any dose level.

A two-generation rat reproduction study was conducted at doses of 30, 300, and 1000 ppm in the diet (EPA, 1995). The reproductive NOEL was 300 ppm (23.5 and 26.0 mg/kg/day for males and females, respectively) based on reduced pup weights in the F1a and F2a litters. No toxicity was observed in parental animals.

69.6 PROPACHLOR

69.6.1 IDENTITY, PROPERTIES, AND USES

69.6.1.1 Chemical Name

Propachlor is 2-chloro-*N*-isopropylacetanilide.

69.6.1.2 Structure

See Fig. 69.1.

69.6.1.3 Synonyms

The common name propachlor is in general use. The major trade name for propachlor products in the United States is Ramrod®. The CAS registry number for propachlor is 1918-16-7.

69.6.1.4 Physical and Chemical Properties

Propachlor has the empirical formula of $C_{11}H_{14}ClNO$ and a molecular weight of 211.7. It is a tan solid with a melting point of 77°C and has a vapor pressure of 7.9×10^{-5} mm Hg at 25°C. The solubility of propachlor in water is 613 ppm at 25°C. Propachlor is soluble in most organic solvents except aliphatic hydrocarbons (Monsanto, 1995; WHO, 1993).

69.6.1.5 History, Formulations, and Uses

Propachlor was introduced by Monsanto in 1965. It is a pre-emergence herbicide for annual grass and broadleaf weed control in corn and sorghum. Propachlor is available as a granular and flowable formulation; it is also available as a prepack formulation with atrazine.

69.6.2 TOXICITY TO LABORATORY ANIMALS

69.6.2.1 Irritation and Sensitization

Eye and skin irritation studies conducted in rabbits showed propachlor to be severely irritating to the eye and slightly irritating to the skin. Propachlor produced skin sensitization in guinea pigs (EPA, 1998b).

69.6.2.2 Acute Studies

Acute toxicity data have been reported by the WHO (1993). The oral LD_{50} in rats ranges from 550 to 1700 mg/kg, while the dermal LD_{50} is reported to be greater than 20,000 mg/kg in the rabbit. The inhalation (4-h) LC_{50} in rats is greater than 1.2 mg/l, the maximum attainable concentration achieved in the study (EPA, 1998b).

69.6.2.3 Repeat Dose Studies

Two chronic toxicity studies of propachlor have been conducted in both the rat and the mouse. No treatment-related effects were observed in the first study for either species (WHO, 1993), in which the highest dietary level was 500 ppm, and it was concluded that the dose level selection for these studies was inadequate. In the second study conducted in the rat (EPA, 1998b) at dietary levels up to 2500 (males)/5000 (females) ppm, the NOEL was 300 ppm (~6 mg/kg/day) based on changes observed in the pyloric region of the stomach (erosion, ulceration, and hyperplasia of the mucosa and herniated mucosal

glands) and centrilobular/midzonal region of the liver (hepatocellular hypertrophy and eosinophilic foci). In the second study conducted in the mouse (EPA, 1998b) at dietary levels up to 6000 ppm, the NOEL was 14.6 and 19.3 mg/kg/day in male and female mice, respectively, based on changes observed in the glandular region of the stomach (erosion and ulceration of the mucosa and herniated mucosal glands) and centrilobular/midzonal region of the liver (hepatocellular hypertrophy and necrosis and eosinophilic foci). Administration of propachlor to beagle dogs for 1 year at dietary levels of 0, 25, 250, and 1000 ppm resulted in reductions in body weight gain and food consumption at the highest concentration (~33 mg/kg/day). These effects may have resulted from poor diet palatability. The NOEL was approximately 6 mg/kg/day (EPA, 1998b). No adverse effects were observed in a 3-week dermal toxicity study of propachlor conducted in rats; the no observed adverse effect level (NOAEL) was 500 mg/kg/day (Rush, 1998).

69.6.2.4 Pharmacokinetic Studies

The absorption, distribution, metabolism, and excretion of propachlor has been studied extensively in the rat (WHO, 1993). Propachlor is well absorbed following oral administration; following a single oral dose, approximately 70% is recovered in urine 48–56 hours after administration. The biotransformation of propachlor is complex due to extensive biliary excretion, intestinal microbial metabolism, and enterohepatic recirculation of metabolites. Propachlor is initially metabolized via the mercapturic acid pathway; the molecule is conjugated to glutathione and excreted in the bile along with the catabolites cysteinyl-glycine, cysteine, and N-acetylcysteine-mercapturic acid. The biliary mercapturic acid metabolites undergo deconjugation via intestinal/microbial carbon-sulfur (C-S) lyase activity and can be reabsorbed. The reabsorbed metabolites are subsequently glucuronidated and eliminated in the urine or bile. Glucuronides eliminated in the bile can subsequently undergo further enterohepatic recirculation. Elimination of propachlor is rapid; more than 90% of a single dose is excreted within 48 h, primarily in the urine. Dermal penetration studies of propachlor have not been conducted. However, such data are available for one liquid formulated product; the dermal penetration rates were 20% and 51% for undiluted and diluted spray formulations, respectively (van de Sandt, 2000).

69.6.2.5 Genotoxicity Studies

Negative results were observed in in vitro prokaryote (Ames/Salmonella) and mammalian gene mutation (CHO/HGPRT) assays of propachlor (WHO, 1993). Propachlor had no effect on DNA repair in rat hepatocytes following the conduct of in vitro and in vivo/in vitro UDS assays (EPA, 1998b). A possible weak clastogenic response was observed in an in vitro mammalian (CHO) assay in the presence of metabolic activation; no evidence of clastogenic activity was observed in the absence of a metabolic activation system (EPA, 1998b). In vivo, there was no evidence of a clastogenic response in a rat bone marrow cytogenetics assay (EPA, 1998b). Propachlor had no effects on germ cells in a dominant lethal study (EPA, 1998b) conducted in rats at dietary concentrations up to 2500 ppm (111.8 mg/kg/day). Overall, the weight of evidence indicates that propachlor is not genotoxic or clastogenic in mammals.

69.6.2.6 Carcinogenicity Studies

Two carcinogenicity studies of propachlor have been conducted in both the rat and the mouse (WHO, 1993). No treatment-related carcinogenic effects were observed in the first study for either species in which the highest dietary level was 500 ppm. In the second study conducted in the rat (EPA, 1998b) at dietary levels up to 2500 (males)/5000 (females) ppm, the only evidence of a possible oncogenic effect was a single carcinoma observed in the pyloric (nonglandular) region of the stomach in one male only, at the highest dietary level (2500 ppm). No carcinogenic effects were seen in the female stomach at twice this dietary concentration (5000 ppm). Erosion and proliferation of the pyloric mucosa were observed microscopically at this dietary concentration (2500/5000 ppm); these findings were dose dependent, showed a clear threshold, and are consistent with a non-genotoxic mode of action. In the second study conducted in the mouse (EPA, 1998b) at dietary concentrations up to 6000 ppm, a statistically significant increase in hepatic adenomas was observed in males at the highest dietary level only. Administration of propachlor to male CD-1 mice in their diet for a period of 3 months produced a statistically significant increase in hepatic cell proliferation at 6000 ppm (Hotz and Wilson, 1998); the increased cell proliferation was shown to be dose dependent with a clear threshold at 1000 ppm (NOEL). The increase in hepatic cell proliferation is believed to represent a regenerative response to the underlying severe non-neoplastic changes observed in this organ (see Section 69.6.2.3). These data provide support for a non-genotoxic, threshold-sensitive mechanism (cell proliferation) being responsible for the increase in the predominantly benign hepatic tumors observed in male mice at a dietary concentration of 6000 ppm.

69.6.2.7 Development and Reproduction Studies

Two reproduction studies have been conducted in the rat with propachlor; in the first study (EPA, 1998b), parental toxicity was observed at the high dose level only (30 mg/kg/day), by reductions in food consumption and body weight and microscopic changes to the liver (eosinophilia and hypertrophy). No treatment-related reproductive effects were observed in the study and the NOELs for systemic and reproductive toxicity were 3 and 30 (or more) mg/kg/day, respectively. In the second reproduction study (EPA, 1998b), the parental MTD was clearly exceeded at the highest dietary concentration of 2500 (males)/5000 ppm (females); offspring survival and weights were also adversely affected and this dietary level was discontinued after the first litter was weaned. Parental toxicity was observed at a dietary level of 1000 ppm by reductions in weight gain and a microscopic change in the liver (hepatocyte hypertrophy). Slight effects on offspring weight were observed late in the lactation period at a dietary concentration of 1000 ppm. The NOEL for systemic toxicity to parents and offspring was 100 ppm (~7 mg/kg/day), and the NOEL for reproductive effects was 1000 ppm (~75 mg/kg/day). In a developmental toxicity study in the rabbit (EPA, 1998b), propachlor was administered by gavage at doses of 5.8, 58.3, and 116.7 mg/kg/day on gestation days 7–19. The maternal MTD was exceeded at the highest dose, as indicated by mortality, clinical signs, body weight loss, and reduced food consumption. Slight effects on postimplantation loss, the number of viable fetuses, and fetal weight were observed at the highest dose. None of the effects was statistically significant, and all values were within the relevant laboratory historical control ranges; however, they were considered to be possible effects of treatment. The NOEL for maternal and developmental toxicity was 58.3 mg/kg/day. In a developmental toxicity study in the rat (EPA, 1998b), propachlor was administered by gavage at doses of 20, 60, and 200 mg/kg/day on gestation days 6–19. The NOEL was 200 mg/kg/day. Propachlor had no effect on germ cells in male rats at a dietary concentration up to 2500 ppm (111.8 mg/kg/day). Overall, the weight of evidence indicates that propachlor does not produce developmental or reproductive effects.

69.6.3 HUMAN EXPERIENCE

Effects reported in humans occupationally exposed to propachlor have been limited to local skin changes (Von Schubert, 1979). Positive responses have been observed following controlled skin patch testing (Iden and Schroeter, 1977). This is consistent with observations made in experimental animals.

69.7 MODE-OF-ACTION EVALUATIONS: ONCOGENICITY

As discussed previously, chronic administration of chloracetanide herbicides has resulted in the production of nasal, stomach, liver, and thyroid tumors in rats. Most tumors occurred at excessively toxic dose levels, at or above the MTD. Such oncogenic responses are of questionable significance because of the extreme doses required to produce them. A weight-of-evidence analysis of mutagenicity results indicates that chloracetanides have no significant genotoxic potential in mammalian systems. This suggests that the oncogenic responses in rats arise through non-genotoxic, threshold-sensitive mechanisms.

To better understand the relevance of the rat nasal, thyroid, and stomach tumors to humans, extensive mechanistic investigations were undertaken with alachlor, acetochlor, and butachlor.

69.7.1 RAT NASAL TUMORS

69.7.1.1 Alachlor

Two metabolic pathways have been proposed to explain the development of chloracetanilide-induced nasal tumors in rats. The first scheme involves the generation of formaldehyde, while the second pathway leads to quinone mine metabolite formation. The formaldehyde theory has not been supported by the available data and is only briefly mentioned here. This is followed by a discussion of the quinone mine pathway, which is widely accepted as being involved in nasal tumor induction.

Alachlor and other chloracetanllfde herbicides undergo O-demethylation with the release of formaldehyde (Brown *et al.*, 1988; Jacobsen *et al.*, 1991). This led to the suggestion that formaldehyde may be involved in the nasal carcinogenicity of alachlor and other chtoracetanilide herbicides. However, although formaldehyde is known to produce rat nasal tumors upon inhalation exposure, the nature and distribution of these tumors are quite different from those seen with the chloracetanilide herbicides. For example, formaldehyde-induced nasal lesions are essentially confined to the anterior nose, in regions lined by transitional or respiratory epithelium (Morgan *et al.*, 1986), whereas chloracetanilide-induced lesions are essentially confined to the posterior region, lined by olfactory epithelium (Morgan *et al.*, 1997). In addition, formaldehyde nasal tumors are characterized by marked irritancy and involve carcinomas of the squamous epithelium, the squamous cell metaplasia being a consequence of the severe damage produced in the nasal epithelium due to the irritant properties of the molecule. In contrast, there is no evidence of irritancy with the chloracetanilides, and the tumors are predominately benign adenomas of the olfactory epithelium. In addition, as mentioned previously, primary O-deatkylation of alachlor occurs in the liver and there is little evidence of unchanged alachlor reaching the nasal turbinate area. Thus, any formaldehyde released during the metabolism of alachlor in the rat liver would be expected to rapidly undergo further metabolism and not be available in the systemic circulation to reach the olfactory area. Therefore, the available evidence does not support formaldehyde as the metabolite responsible for the nasal carcinogenicity observed with chloracetanilide herbicides.

Investigations to understand the mechanism by which chloracetanilides produce nasal tumors in rats were initially undertaken with alachlor. Early whole-body autoradiography (WBA) work showed that alachlor-derived radioactivity specifically localized in the nasal mucosa of rats but not mice or monkeys. In another WBA study, the tertiary amide methylsulfide metabolite of alachlor, a metabolite arising only through enterohepatic circulation, was orally administered to rats. Specific localization in nasal mucosa was again observed. The intensity of the labeling was greater than that observed when parent alachlor was administered. These findings showed the importance of metabolic processes in the localization of alachlor metabolites in rat nasal tissue and provided evidence implicating metabolism in the production of nasal tumors.

Significant species differences in metabolism were demonstrated that provided a mechanistic basis for the rat-specific production of nasal tumors. In rats, alachlor is initially metabolized primarily in the liver via the P-450 pathway and by glutathione conjugation (Feng and Patanella, 1988, 1989). The glutathione conjugates and their metabolites undergo enterohepatic circulation with further metabolism in liver and nasal tissue to form the putative carcinogenic metabolite, a diethyl quinoneimine (DEIQ). Higher rates of intestinal microbial metabolism, enterohepatic circulation, and target tissue metabolism result in a greater conversion of alachlor to DEIQ in rat nasal mucosa as compared to other species (Feng *et al.*, 1990).

Quinone imines such as DEIQ are electrophilic, deplete glutathione (GSH), and can exert toxicity by binding to cellular proteins. It has been shown that a DEIQ protein adduct is the major alachlor-derived protein adduct in rat nasal mucosa (Wilson *et al.*, 1995a); however, no evidence of this adduct was observed in the nasal tissue of mice or monkeys (Heydens *et al.*, 1998). The binding of DEIQ to nasal protein is thought to disturb cell structure and function, which leads to cytotoxicity, prolonged regenerative cell proliferation, and the eventual development of nasal tumors. Increased cell proliferation was shown in rats but not mice, and a clear threshold was demonstrated; the proliferation was sustained during treatment and reversible after dosing was terminated (Heydens *et al.*, 1998). These findings indicate that increased cell turnover is a prerequisite for tumor development and that its induction is threshold sensitive.

Critical differences in metabolic capability result in much higher formation of DEIQ in the nasal mucosa of rats than other species. For example, the ability of rat nasal tissue to convert the secondary sulfide metabolite of alachlor to 2,6-DEA-phenol, the proximate metabolite of DEIQ, is more than 30 times greater than that of monkeys (Li *et al.*, 1992) and 751 times higher than that of human nasal tissue (Wilson *et al.*, 1995b). Further, species differences are even greater when the relative enzymatic rate of alachlor conjugation to GSH (the initial metabolic step) is included in the overall rate of DEA-phenol formation from alachlor; the overall ability of rats to convert alachlor to DEA-phenol is 3000- and 22,000-fold greater than that of humans when the initial GSH conjugation occurs in the liver or nose, respectively (Wilson *et al.*, 1995b). These data indicate that the potential for the formation of the reactive DEIQ metabolite in human nasal tissue is negligible. The results further indicate that the rat is not an appropriate model for assessing alachlor's oncogenic risk to humans.

69.7.1.2 Butachlor

The metabolism of butachlor closely parallels that of alachlor. The only difference between these two molecules is the length of the *N*-alkoxymethyl side chain. An important, common step in the metabolism of alachlor and butachlor is P-450-mediated *N*-dealkylation of this side chain. Once this occurs, the product of the two parent molecules is identical, and the subsequent metabolism to DEIQ and toxicologic response would be the same. Indeed, it has been shown that oral administration of butachlor results in the same rat-specific nasal localization and induction of cell proliferation observed with alachlor. Similar differences in nasal metabolism across species as observed with alachlor are also apparent for butachlor; with the potential for DEIQ formation substantially higher in the rat.

69.7.1.3 Acetochlor

The metabolism of acetochlor has also been extensively studied. These studies have confirmed that the overall metabolism of acetochlor shares critical commonality with alachlor and butachlor. In rats, metabolism in the liver and gastrointestinal tract produces sulfur-containing metabolites that are delivered to the nose and undergo further metabolism. WBA studies corresponding to those described previously for alachlor have been conducted for acetochlor. Acetochlor-derived radioactivity localized in the nasal turbinates of rats but not in mice. Analysis of protein adducts found in nasal tissue from rats treated with acetochlor or its methylsulfide metabolite confirmed that the major adducts involved EMIQ, the acetochlor quinone imine metabolite analogous to DEIQ from alachlor. As with alachlor, these adducts were not found in the nasal tissues of mice or monkeys.

Similarly, when acetochlor was fed to rats at doses that produced nasal tumors in the chronic studies, prolonged cell proliferation was observed. Acetochlor administration did not induce cell proliferation at the same dose level in mice. Acetochlor administration to rats at 200 ppm, a nononcogenic dose level, did not cause increased cell proliferation.

In vitro metabolism studies similar to those done with alachlor have measured the enzymatic activities involved in the conversion of acetochlor and key metabolites to EMIQ. The data showed that the potential for EMIQ formation is significantly lower in the mouse and monkey than the rat. Overall, the relative rates for conversion of acetochlor to quinone imines in rat, mouse, and monkey were very similar to those seen with alachlor, suggesting that the differences between rat and human nasal tissue for acetochlor would also be comparable to that seen with alachlor.

69.7.2 RAT STOMACH TUMORS

Butachlor and alachlor are close structural analogs that produce the same stomach tumors in rats. An extensive mechanistic research program was undertaken to understand the mechanism by which these tumors are induced. A stomach tumor initiation–promotion study demonstrated that butachlor was not active as an initiator, but it did promote the formation of tumors after treatment with *N*-methyl-*N'*-nitro-*N*-nitrosoguanidine (MNNG), a known initiator (Branch *et al.*, 1995). A subsequent tumor promotion study with alachlor showed that it, too, produced stomach tumors by the same promotional activity. The results of these studies provided direct

experimental evidence indicating that the stomach tumors are produced by a non-genotoxic mode of action.

Mechanistic studies with butachlor have shown that chloracetanilide-induced gastric neoplasia involves toxicity (atrophy) to the fundic mucosa as an initial event following high dose exposure (Hard *et al.*, 1995; Thake *et al.*, 1995). This atrophy then results in compensatory cell proliferation in the fundic mucosa. The accompanying profound loss of parietal cells leads to an extensive gastric hypochlorhydria and a subsequent increase in pH of the gastric contents. This increase causes excessive gastrin production, resulting in a substantial elevation of serum gastrin levels. The tropic effect of long-term stimulation of enterochromaffin-like (ECL) cells and fundic stem cells by gastrin further drives a sustained regenerative cell proliferation response that ultimately results in the induction of the gastric neoplasms observed in the chronic studies. Additional work demonstrated that high-dose alachlor exposure also induces the same mucosal atrophy, hypochlorhydria, and hypergastrinemia that characterize the unique oncogenic mechanism demonstrated with butachlor. Mucosal atrophy did not occur at a lower, nononcogenic dose of alachlor.

Prolonged exposure to toxic doses of alachlor and butachlor were required to produce stomach tumors in rats. Such exposure would not occur in humans; results from a study with rhesus monkeys showed that mucosal atrophy, the initial preneoplastic event, did not occur at doses ranging from 100 to 400 mg/kg/day. These doses are comparable to, and higher than, the oncogenic dose (150 mg/kg/day) in rats. Based on all the data, it was concluded that these chloracetanilide-induced stomach tumors are not relevant to humans (Heydens *et al.*, 1998).

69.7.3 RAT THYROID TUMORS

Various studies have shown that the prolonged alteration of thyroid homeostasis can lead to the development of thyroid follicular tumors in rats (Hill *et al.*, 1989; Thomas and Williams, 1991; Zbinden, 1989). The oncogenic response is mediated via increased levels of circulating thyroid stimulating hormone (TSH), which result in hyperplasia and, ultimately, neoplasia. One mechanism causing such a thyroid imbalance involves the induction of liver enzymes (McClain, 1989). This induction increases the rate of thyroid hormone excretion and is responsible for the compensatory elevation in TSH observed.

Separate studies were conducted to determine if alachlor, acetochlor, and butachlor produce thyroid tumors by this mechanism (Ashby *et al.*, 1996; Wilson and Takei, 1999; Wilson *et al.*, 1996). The results of these studies showed that the administration of each chloracetanilide at the dose level producing thyroid neoplasia in the chronic studies caused significant increases in liver weight and T4-UDPGT (thyroxine–uridine diphosphate glucuronosyl transferase) activity, serum TSH levels, and thyroid weight at several time points. These changes were observed as early as 7–14 days after dosing began and continued throughout 2 or more months of dosing. Reversibility studies with alachlor and butachlor showed that serum TSH and hepatic UDPGT activity returned to normal after dosing was discontinued.

Rats are especially sensitive to altered thyroid function by this mechanism because of their susceptibility to liver enzyme induction and lack of thyroid binding globulin in plasma, making thyroid hormone more susceptible to metabolic activity. Furthermore, because this mechanism is believed to be a threshold-sensitive phenomenon, it is not expected to be relevant for humans under actual exposure scenarios with chloracetanilide herbicides.

69.8 COMMON MECHANISM OF TOXICITY

The Food Quality Protection Act of 1996 requires the EPA to perform a combined risk assessment for chemicals that produce adverse effects by a common mechanism of toxicity. The extensive database of mechanistic information, developed (see Section 69.7) to support (1) a nongenotoxic threshold mechanism of action and (2) lack of relevance to humans for the nasal turbinate, stomach, and/or thyroid oncogenic effects produced in rats for alachlor, acetochlor, and butachlor, provides the basis for considering whether these chemicals can be grouped based on a common mechanism of toxicity. The data support grouping alachlor, acetochlor, and butachlor with respect to a common mechanism of toxicity for nasal turbinate and thyroid tumors, and alachlor and butachlor for stomach tumors.

REFERENCES

Acquavella, J. F., Ireland, B., Leet, T., Anne, M., Farrell, T., and Martens, M. (1994). Epidemiological studies of morbidity and mortality among alachlor manufacturing workers. *In* "Proceedings of the XII Joint CIGR, IAAMRH, IUFRO International Symposium: Health, Safety and Ergonomic Aspects in Use of Chemicals in Agriculture and Forestry," pp. 184–194.

Acquavella, J. F., Riordan, S. G., Anne, M., Lynch, C. F., Collins, J. J., Ireland, B. K., and Heydens, W. F. (1996). Evaluation of mortality and cancer incidence among alachlor manufacturing workers. *Environ. Health Perspect.* **104**, 728–733.

Ahrens, W. H. (1994). "Herbicide Handbook of the Weed Science Society of America," 7th ed. Weed Sci. Soc. Am., Champaign, IL.

Ashby, J., Kier, L., Wilson, A. G. E., Green, T., Lefevre, P. A., Tinwell, H., Willis, G. A., Heydens, W. F., and Clapp, M. J. L. (1996). Evaluation of the potential carcinogenicity and genetic toxicity to humans of the herbicide acetochlor. *Hum. Exp. Toxicol.* **15**, 702–735.

Ashby, J., Tinwell, H., Lefevre, P. A., Williams, J., Kier, L., Adler, I.-D., and Clapp, M. J. L. (1997). Evaluation of the mutagenicity of acetochlor to male rat germ cells. *Mutat. Res.* **393**, 263–281.

Bonfanti, M., Taverna, P., Chiappetta, L., Villa, P., D'Incalci, M., Bagnati, R., and Fanelli, R. (1992). DNA damage induced by alachlor after *in vitro* activation by rat hepatocytes. *Toxicology* **72**, 207–219.

Branch, D. K., Shibata, M., Thake, D. C., and Wilson, A. G. E. (1995). "Gastric Tumor Initiation/Promotion Study of Butachlor in Sprague–Dawley Rats." Presented at Annual Conference of International Federation of Societies of Toxicologic Pathologists, Tours, France.

Brown, M. A., Kimmel, E. C., and Casida, J. E. (1988). DNA adduct formation by alachlor metabolites. *Life Sci.* **43**, 2087–2094.

Erexson, G. L., Bryant, M. F., Doer, C. L., Kwanyuen, P., and Kligerman, A. D. (1993). Cytogenetic analyses of human peripheral blood lymphocytes exposed to alachlor *in vitro*. *Environ. Mol. Mutagen.* **21**, 19.

Feng, P. C. C., and Patanella, J. E. (1988). Identification of mercapturic acid pathway metabolites of alachlor formed by liver and kidney homogenates of rats, mice, and monkeys. *Pestic. Biochem. Physiol.* **31**, 84–90.

Feng, P. C. C., and Patanella, J. E. (1989). *In vitro* oxidation of alachlor by liver microsomal enzymes from rats, mice, and monkeys. *Pestic. Biochem. Physiol.* **33**, 16–25.

Feng, P., Wilson, A., McClanahan, R., Patanella, J., and Wratten, S. (1990). Metabolism of alachlor by rat and mouse liver and nasal turbinate tissues. *Drug Metab. Dispos.* **18**, 373–377.

Georgian, L., Moraru, I., Draghicescu, T., Dinu, I., and Ghizelea, G. (1983). Cytogenetic effects of alachlor and mancozeb. *Mutat. Res.* **116**, 341–348.

Gold, L. S., Sawyer, C. B., Magaw, R., Backman, G. M., deVediana, M., Levinson, R., Hooper, N. K., Havender, W. R., Bernstein, L., Peto, R., Pike, M. C., and Ames, B. N. (1984). A carcinogenic potency data base of the standardized results from animal bioassays. *Environ. Health Perspect.* **58**, 9–319.

Hard, G. C., Iatropoulos, M. J., Thake, D. C., Wheeler, D., Tatematsu, M., Hagiwara, A., Williams, G. M., and Wilson, A. G. E. (1995). Identity and pathogenesis of stomach tumors in Sprague–Dawley rats associated with the dietary administration of butachlor. *Exp. Toxicol. Pathol.* **47**, 95–105.

Heydens, W. F. (1998). Summary of toxicology studies with alachlor. *J. Pestic. Sci.* **24**, 75–82.

Heydens, W. F., Wilson, A. G. E., Kier, L. D., Lau, H., Thake, D. C., and Martens, M. A. (1998). An evaluation of the carcinogenic potential of the herbicide alachlor to humans. *Hum. Exp. Toxicol.* **18**, 363–391.

Hill, R. N., Erdreich, L. S., Paynter, O. E., Roberts, P. A., Rosenthal, S. L., and Wilkinson, C. F. (1989). Thyroid follicular cell carcinogenesis. *Fundam. Appl. Toxicol.* **12**, 629–698.

Hotz, K. J., and Wilson, A. G. E. (1998). "Effect of Propachlor on Cell Proliferation in the Liver of Male Mice." Monsanto Unpublished Report.

Iden, D. L., and Schroeter, A. L. (1977). Allergic contact dermatitis to herbicides. *Arch. Dermatol.* **113**, 983.

Ireland, B., Acquavella, J., Farrell, T., Anne, M., and Fuhremann, T. (1994). Evaluation of ocular health among alachlor manufacturing workers. *J. Occup. Med.* **36**, 738–742.

Jacobsen, N. E., Sanders, M., Toia, R. F., and Casida, J. E. (1991). Alachlor and its analogues as metabolic progenitors of formaldehyde: Fate of N-methoxymethyl and other N-alkoxylalkyl substituents. *J. Agric. Food Chem.* **39**, 1342–1350.

Kier, L. D., Heydens, W. F., Lau, H., Thake, D. C., and Wilson, A. G. E. (1996). Genotoxicity studies of alachlor. *Toxicologist* **30**, 231.

Kronenberg, J. M., Fuhremann, T. W., and Johnson, D. E. (1988). Percutaneous absorption and excretion of alachlor in rhesus monkeys. *Fundam. Appl. Toxicol.* **10**, 664–671.

Leet, T., Acquavella, J., Lynch, C., Anne, M., Weiss, N., Vaughan, T., and Checkoway, H. (1996). Cancer incidence among alachlor manufacturing workers. *Am. J. Ind. Med.* **30**, 300–306.

Li, A. A., Asbury, K. J., Hopkins, W. E., Feng, P. C., and Wilson, A. G. E. (1992). Metabolism of alachlor by rat and monkey liver and nasal turbinate tissue. *Drug Metab. Dispos.* **20**, 616–618.

Lin, M. F., Wu, C. L., and Wang, T. C. (1987). Pesticide clastogenicity in Chinese hamster ovary cells. *Mutat. Res.* **88**, 241–250.

Lutz, W. K. (1986). Quantitative evaluation of DNA binding data for risk estimation and for classification of direct and indirect carcinogens. *J. Cancer Res. Clin. Oncol.* **112**, 85–91.

McClain, R. (1989). The significance of hepatic microsomal enzyme induction and altered thyroid function in rats: Implications for thyroid gland neoplasia. *Toxicol. Pathol.* **17**, 294–306.

Meisner, L. F., Belluck, D. A., and Roloff, B. D. (1992). Cytogenetic effects of alachlor and/or atrazine *in vivo* and *in vitro*. *Environ. Mol. Mutagen.* **19**, 77–82.

Millburn, P. (1975). Excretion of xenobiotic compounds in bile. *In* "The Hepatobiology System: Fundamental and Pathological Mechanisms" (W. Taylor, ed.), p. 109. Plenum, New York.

Monsanto Company (1991). "Material Safety Data Sheet: Butachlor Technical." Monsanto Company, St. Louis, MO.

Monsanto Company (1995). "Material Safety Data Sheet: Propachlor Technical." Monsanto Company, St. Louis, MO.

Monsanto Company (1997a). "Material Safety Data Sheet: Alachlor Technical." Monsanto Company, St. Louis, MO.

Monsanto Company (1997b). "Material Safety Data Sheet: Acetochlor Technical." Monsanto Company, St. Louis, MO.

Morgan, K. T., Gross, E. A., Joyner, D. R., Ishmael, J., and Thake, D. (1997). Proliferative nasal lesions induced in rats by alachlor, acetochlor, and butachlor originate in specific regions of the olfactory mucosa. *Toxicologist* **36**, 12.

Morgan, K. T., Jiang, X. Z., Starr, T. B., and Kerns. W. D. (1986). More precise localization of nasal tumors associated with chronic exposure of F-344 rats to formaldehyde gas. *Toxicol. Appl. Pharmacol.* **82**, 264–271.

Rush, R. E. (1998). "Propachlor: A 21-Day Dermal Toxicity Study in Rats." Monsanto Unpublished Report.

Taningher, M., Terranove, M. P., Airoldi, L., Chiappetta, L., and Parodi, S. (1993). Lack of alachlor induced DNA damage as assayed in rodent liver by the alkaline elution test. *Toxicology* **85**, 117–122.

Thake, D. C., Iatropoulos, M. J., Hard, G. C., Hotz, K. J., Wang, C.-X., Williams, G. M., and Wilson, A. G. E. (1995). A study of the mechanism of butachlor-associated gastric neoplasms in Sprague–Dawley rats. *Exp. Toxicol. Pathol.* **47**, 107–116.

Thomas, G., and Williams, E. (1991). Evidence for and possible mechanisms of non-genotoxic carcinogenesis in the rodent thyroid. *Mutat. Res.* **248**, 357–370.

U.S. Environmental Protection Agency (EPA) (1994). Decision Document, Conditional Registration of the New Chemical Acetochlor. Office of Pesticide Programs, Washington, DC.

U.S. Environmental Protection Agency (EPA) (1995). Metolachlor Reregistration Eligibility Decision Document, Office of Pesticide Programs, Washington, DC.

U.S. Environmental Protection Agency (EPA) (1996). Proposed guidelines for carcinogen risk assessment: Notice. *Fed. Reg.* 17960–18011.

U.S. Environmental Protection Agency (EPA) (1997). "Common Mechanism of Toxicity." Presentation to the Scientific Advisory Panel, Washington, DC.

U.S. Environmental Protection Agency (EPA) (1998a). Alachlor Reregistration Eligibility Decision Document, Office of Pesticide Programs, Washington, DC.

U.S. Environmental Protection Agency (EPA) (1998b). Propachlor Reregistration Eligibility Decision Document, Office of Pesticide Programs, Washington, DC.

U.S. Environmental Protection Agency (EPA) (2001). The Grouping of a Series of Chloroacetanilide Pesticides Based on a Common Mechanism of Toxicity, Office of Pesticide Programs, Washington, DC.

van de Sandt, J. J. M. (2000). "In Vitro Percutaneous Absorption Study with Propachlor in Ramrod® SC through Viable Human Skin Membranes." Monsanto Unpublished Report.

Von Schubert, H. (1979). Allergic contact dermatitis caused by propachlor. *Dermatol. Monatsschr.* **165**, 495–498 (In German).

Wester, R. C., Melendres, J., and Maibach, H. I. (1992). *In vivo* percutaneous absorption and skin decontamination of alachlor in rhesus monkey. *J. Toxicol. Environ. Health* **36**, 1–12.

Wester, R. C., Melendres, J. L., and Maibach, H. I. (1996). *In vivo* percutaneous absorption of acetochlor in the rhesus monkey: Dose–response and exposure risk assessment. *Food Chem. Toxicol.* **34**, 979–983.

Williams, R. (1971). Species variations in drug biotransformations. *In* "Fundamentals of Drug Metabolism and Drug Disposition" (B. Lau, H. Mandel, and E. Way, eds.), p. 187. Williams & Wilkins, Baltimore.

Wilson, A. G. E., and Takei, A. S. (1999). Summary of toxicology studies with butachlor. *J. Pestic. Sci.* **25**, 75–83.

Wilson, A. G. E., Lau, H., Asbury, K. J., Thake, D. C., and Heydens, W. F. (1995a). "Mechanistic Basis for the Rat Specific Nasal Tumors Observed with Alachlor." Abstract, International Congress of Toxicology—VII, Seattle.

Wilson, A. G. E., Lau, H., Asbury, K. J., and Heydens, W. F. (1995b). Metabolism of alachlor by human nasal tissue. *Fundam. Appl. Toxicol.* **15**, 1398.

Wilson, A. G. E., Thake, D. C., Heydens, W. F., Brewster, D. W., and Hotz, K. J. (1996). Mode of action of thyroid tumor formation in the male Long–Evans rat administered high doses of alachlor. *Fundam. Appl. Toxicol.* **33**, 16–23.

World Health Organization (WHO) (1993). "Propachlor." Environmental Health Criteria Document 147 (prepared by L. Ivanova-Chemishanka).

Zbinden, G. (1989). Hyperplastic and neoplastic responses of the thyroid gland in toxicological studies. *Arch. Toxicol.* **12**, 98–106.

Paraquat

Edward A. Lock
Syngenta Central Toxicology Laboratory
Martin F. Wilks
Syngenta Crop Protection AG

70.1 IDENTITY, PROPERTIES, AND USE

70.1.1 CHEMICAL NAME

Paraquat is 1,1′-dimethyl-4,4′-bipyridinium ion (IUPAC, CAS RN *[4685-14-7]*), also known as the 1,1′-dimethyl-4,4′-bipyridyldiylium ion.

70.1.2 STRUCTURE

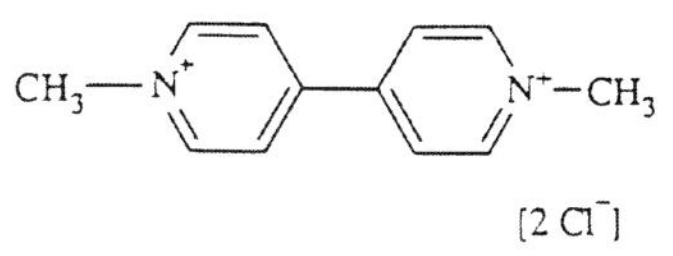

Paraquat dichloride

Figure 70.1

70.1.3 SYNONYMS

The common name paraquat is in general use (BSI, E-ISO, ANSI, WSSA, JMAF), except in Germany. Paraquat is usually formulated as the dichloride salt (also known as methyl viologen) (CAS MR *[1910-42-5]*). The bis(methyl sulphate) salt (CAS NR *[2074-50-2]*) is no longer commercialized. Code designations for the material are PP148 (for the dichloride salt) and PP910 (for the bis(methyl sulphate) salt). Trade names for paraquat dichloride formulations include Crisquat®, Cyclone®, Dextrone X®, Esgram®, Efoxon®, Goldquat® 276, Gramoxone®, Herbaxon®, Katalon®, Osaquat Super®, Pilarxone®, R-Bix®, Speeder®, Starfire®, Sweep®, Total®, and Weedless®. Mixtures of paraquat with diquat are sold under trade names including Actor®, Dukatalon®, Opal®, Pathclear® (also includes simazine and aminotriazole), Preeglox®, Preglone®, Seccatuto®, Spray Seed®, and Weedol®. Trade names of mixtures with urea herbicides include Dexuron®, Gramocil®, Gramonol®, Gramuron®, and Tota-Col®.

70.1.4 PHYSICAL AND CHEMICAL PROPERTIES

The molecular formula of the cation is $C_{12}H_{14}N_2$ with a molecular weight of 186.3. The dichloride salt has the formula $C_{12}H_{14}Cl_2N_2$ and a molecular weight of 257.2. Paraquat dichloride forms colorless, hygroscopic crystals which decompose at 300°C. It is practically nonvolatile with a vapor pressure of <0.1 mPa. It is very soluble in water (700 g/l at 20°C) and practically insoluble in most other organic solvents. It is stable in neutral and acidic media but readily hydrolyzed in alkaline media. Paraquat is photochemically decomposed by ultraviolet radiation in aqueous solution.

70.1.5 HISTORY, FORMULATIONS, AND USES

Paraquat was first described in 1882 by Weidel and Russo. In 1933, Michaelis and Hill discovered its redox properties and called the compound methyl viologen. The herbicidal properties of paraquat were first described by Brian *et al.* (1958) and it became commercially available in 1962. Paraquat is mainly formulated as an aqueous solution with surface-active agents. In some countries, a low-strength granular formulation (also containing diquat) is available. Paraquat is a fast-acting, nonselective contact herbicide, absorbed by the foliage with some translocation in the xylem. It is used for broadspectrum control of broad-leaved weeds and grasses in fruit orchards and plantations, and for inter-row weed control in many crops. It is also used for general weed control on noncrop land, as a defoliant on cotton and hops, for destruction of potato haulms, as a desiccant, and for control of aquatic weeds. Paraquat is rapidly deactivated upon contact with the soil and does not leach.

1559

70.2 TOXICITY TO LABORATORY ANIMALS

70.2.1 SIGNS OF TOXICITY

Following a lethal dose of paraquat to rats mortality is first seen on days 2–5 after dosing but deaths can also occur around days 10–12 (Clark *et al.*, 1966; Sharp *et al.*, 1972; Smith and Rose, 1977), indicating there is considerable interindividual animal response to the chemical. The major cause of death after a median lethal dose is due to lung damage. The animals develop acute pulmonary edema with signs of labored respiration and ultimately die of respiratory failure (Clark *et al.*, 1966; Kimbrough and Gaines, 1970; Murray and Gibson, 1972; Sharp *et al.*, 1972). Rabbits, however, do not show signs of respiratory distress. They stop eating and drinking and tend to die without overt toxicity, following oral dosing (Butler and Kleinerman, 1971; Clark *et al.*, 1966). Rats and mice given doses above the maximum lethal dose (MLD), by intraperitoneal (ip) or subcutaneous (sc) administration show signs of hyperexcitability, ataxia, and convulsions and usually die within a few hours of dosing, indicative of an effect on the central nervous system (Bagetta *et al.*, 1992; Clark *et al.*, 1966). Following chronic exposure signs of toxicity are few but may include respiratory effects.

70.2.2 ACUTE TOXICITY

The acute oral toxicity of paraquat to the rat is shown in Table 70.1. The ask for of pure paraquat dichloride expressed as the cation was about 150 mg/kg to female rats and ranged from 100 to 143 mg/kg in a number of different strains from a number of different laboratories. No sex difference in toxicity was seen and the toxicity was similar for the two different salts of paraquat (Table 70.1). Fasting rats prior to oral administration of paraquat made little difference to the toxicity. The 7 day MLD with 95% confidence limits were 143 (123–166), 130 (106–159), and 126 (102–156) mg paraquat ion/kg, respectively, for rats fasted for 0, 4, and 8 hr (Murray and Gibson, 1971). Mice are less sensitive than the rats to orally administered paraquat, while guinea pigs, cats, monkeys, and rabbits are more susceptible (Table 70.2).

Paraquat was more toxic when given by the ip or intravenous (iv) routes with a MLD of approximately 20 mg paraquat ion/kg (Table 70.3), indicating that following oral dosing the compound is poorly absorbed from the gastrointestinal tract (see

Table 70.1
Acute Toxicity of Paraquat to the Rat (Data Expressed as mg Paraquat ion/kg)

Paraquat dichloride	Sex	Strain	Route of administration	Median lethal dose (time studied)	Reference
Pure salts	F	NS[a]	po	112 (104–122), 150 (139–162), 141[b] (140–142) (14 days)	Clark *et al.*, 1966
Pure salt	F	NS	po	150 (110–173) (21 days)	Mehani, 1972
Formulation	M	Sprague–Dawley	po	143 (123–166) (7 days)	Murray and Gibson, 1971
Formulation	M	Sherman	po	100 (87–117) (15 days)	Kimbrough and Gaines, 1970
Formulation	F	Sherman	po	110 (90–134) (15 days)	Kimbrough and Gaines, 1970
Formulation	M	Sprague–Dawley	po	115 (90–150) (30 days)	Sharp *et al.*, 1972
Formulation	M	Wistar	po	95 (79–114) (30 days)	Sharp *et al.*, 1972
Pure salt	F	NS	ip	19 (16–21) 16[b] (14–19)	Clark *et al.*, 1966
Pure salt	F	NS	ip	16 (10–26) (21 days)	Mehani, 1972
Formulation	M	Sprague–Dawley	iv	21 (19–25)	Sharp *et al.*, 1972

[a] Not stated.
[b] Dimethosulphate salt.

Table 70.2
Acute Toxicity of Paraquat to Laboratory Animals (Data Expressed as mg Paraquat Ion/kg)

Species	Sex	Route of administration	Median lethal dose	Reference
Mouse	F[a]	ip	30[c]	Ecker et al., 1975b;
	F		30[c] (26.5–35.1)	Bus et al., 1976a
Mouse	F	po	196[c]	Bus et al., 1976b
Guinea pig	F	ip	3	Clark et al., 1966
Guinea pig	M[b]	po	30 (22–41)	Clark et al., 1966
Guinea pig	M & F	po	22[c] (15–33)	Murray and Gibson, 1972
Cat	F	po	35 (27–46)	Clark et al., 1966
Monkey (Macaca fascicularis)	M & F	po	50[c]	Murray and Gibson, 1972
Rabbit	M	po	100[c]	Kuo and Nanikawa, 1990
Rabbit	M	po	50 (45–58)	Mehani, 1972
Rabbit	M	ip	25 (15–30)	Mehani, 1972
Rabbit	M	ip	18 (11–31)	McElligott, 1972
Dog	M	sc	1.8[c] (1–6.1)	Nagata et al., 1992a
Dog	F	sc	3.5[c] (2.4–10.1)	Nagata et al., 1992a

[a]Female.
[b]Male.
[c]Reference refers to paraquat, not clear if salt or ion.

later). The guinea pig and dog (Nagata et al., 1992a) are also more sensitive to systemic administration with a MLD of 2–3 mg/kg (Table 70.2), reflecting poor or incomplete absorption of paraquat from the gastrointestinal tract after oral administration. Rabbits given a single iv dose of paraquat at 40 or 80 mg/kg died within 24 h; while they survived a single dose of 10 mg/kg iv, no lung lesions were seen at these doses (Ilett et al., 1974). The vehicle used to administer paraquat can influence lethality in mice. For example, paraquat was more toxic when given by the ip or sc route in water than in isotonic saline, suggesting that the solvent may influence the absorption from the site of injection and hence the amount delivered to the lung (Drew and Gram, 1979).

The dermal toxicity of paraquat has been studied in rabbits (Table 70.3). The precise technique of application of paraquat to the skin, whether the site of application is open to the air or covered and whether the rabbits are prevented from grooming, affects the findings (Clark et al., 1966; McElligott, 1972). Rabbits fitted with restraining collars to reduce grooming the site of ap-

plication, followed by decontamination of the skin and removal of the collars, showed glossitis, anorexia, weakness, and loss of weight with some skin erythema followed by hyperkeratosis and desquamation at the higher doses, indicating that some oral ingestion had still occurred. This technique resulted in a MLD following a single application of 236 mg paraquat ion/kg. If, however, the restraining collars were not removed, then the erythema and desquamation was mild and the extent of glossitis and hence body weight loss was less. Under these conditions the MLD was found to be >480 mg ion/kg, the maximum dose possible to apply in a satisfactory manner (McElligott, 1972). Thus, when compared to the systemic MLD of 18 mg ion/kg (Table 70.2). It indicates that little of the applied dose has been absorbed through intact skin. Dermal exposure of rats to paraquat gave an MLD of 80–90 mg paraquat ion/kg (Table 70.3). However these authors (Kimbrough and Gaines, 1970) gave no information on the state of the skin after application, whether the site was occluded or free for the rats to groom. The absorption of paraquat across the skin has been reviewed by Smith (1988),

Table 70.3
Acute Toxicity of Paraquat to Laboratory Animals Following Dermal Application or Inhalation Exposure (Data Expressed as mg Paraquat Ion/kg)

Species	Sex	Route of administration	Median lethal dose	Reference
Rat	M	Dermal	80 (60–96)	Kimbrough and Gaines, 1970
Rat	F	Dermal	90 (74–110)	Kimbrough and Gaines, 1970
Rabbit	M	Dermal	236 (collars removed)	Clark et al., 1966;
			>480 (with collars)	McElligott, 1972
Rat	M & F	Inhalation	6 μg/l/h	Gage, 1968a

who concluded that paraquat is poorly absorbed by intact skin and raised technical concerns about the validity of the earlier dermal studies reported by Kimbrough and Gaines (1970).

Paraquat is not volatile, but following inhalation exposure to an aerosol is irritant to the respiratory tract. At lethal concentrations under these conditions, death is usually delayed for several days and is due to respiratory failure. Following single exposures the MLD is a function of both the amount and duration of exposure, which in the rat is approximately 6 µg/l/hr (Table 70.3). Guinea pigs and male mice are of similar sensitivity to the rat, while female rats and rabbits are less sensitive. Dogs can tolerate a concentration–time product of 25 µg/l/hr without ill effects (Gage, 1968a). The toxicity is also a function of particle size, and 3 µm was the most lethal to the rat. Large particles do not reach the alveolar region and are less toxic. Under normal conditions of manufacture, handling, and use, inhalation exposure is not considered to be a hazard.

Studies with rabbits have shown that the lung is susceptible to paraquat injury following intrabronchial deposition (Zavala and Rhodes, 1978) and inhalation exposure (Seidenfeld et al., 1978), although as mentioned above it is refractory following oral or intraperitoneal administration. Local instillation of paraquat in the lungs of rats will also produce local injury and fibrosis (Kimbrough and Gaines, 1970; Wyatt et al., 1981).

70.2.3 IRRITATION AND SENSITIZATION

Paraquat is a skin and eye irritant but is not a skin sensitizer (Bainova, 1969). As discussed earlier skin irritation has been reported in rabbits when the area of application is occluded (Clark et al., 1966; McElligott, 1972), resulting in local erythema followed by hyperkeratosis and desquamation.

Instillation of a 0.29% aqueous solution of paraquat into the rabbit eye produced no effect. However, more concentrated solutions produced inflammation of the conjunctiva and nictitating membrane. This response developed gradually over 12 h and lasted for 48–96 h (Clark et al., 1966). Instillation of higher concentrations of paraquat (3–48 mg contained in 0.2 ml of water) into the rabbit eye produced a dose-related increase in ocular injury with doses of 48 mg (about 16 mg/kg) and above producing fatalities (Sinow and Wei, 1973). These findings indicate that absorption of paraquat from the eye is similar to that following systemic administration.

70.2.4 SUBCHRONIC TOXICITY

Daily administration of paraquat in the diet of rats at an inclusion rate of 100 ppm (about 5 mg ion/kg/day) was tolerated for several months. However, if increased to 250 ppm (about 12.5 mg ion/kg/day) the rats became ill and died within 27 to 57 days. Females appeared to be more susceptible than males, the primary target organ for toxicity being the lungs (Clark et al., 1966). A number of other studies have shown that moderate daily doses of paraquat can be tolerated. Rats fed 125 ppm (about 6.25 mg/kg/day) for 2 years showed no toxic effects

and dogs tolerated 50 ppm (about 0.9 mg/kg/day) for 2 years (Howe and Wright, 1965). Rats given paraquat in their drinking water at 1.3 or 2.6 mg/l for 2 years showed some mortality and histological changes in the lung at the highest dose, while only minimal changes to the lung were seen at the lower dose (Bainova and Vulcheva, 1977). The MLD for paraquat fed in the diet for 90 days has been determined. Groups of female rats were fed 300, 400, 500, 600, and 700 ppm paraquat and their food consumption was recorded at intervals to enable the dose in mg/kg/day to be calculated. After 90 days the surviving rats were held for 2 weeks to allow time for any delayed deaths. The MLD was 21 mg/kg/day, giving a subchronic toxicity factor of 5.2 (ratio of acute to subchronic MLD's), indicating that paraquat has a moderate cumulative toxicity in this species (Kimbrough and Gaines, 1970).

Rabbits given paraquat ip at 10 or 20 mg/kg at 48 h intervals showed marked signs of toxicity with a high mortality following three to five doses. There was little evidence of lung damage and it is likely that the animals died from multiorgan failure (Butler and Kleinerman, 1971). Rabbits can, however, tolerate 3 mg/kg day ip for up to 14 days, but when increased to 6 mg/kg/day significant mortality was seen (Hassan et al., 1989). Daily oral dosing at 11 mg/kg/day to male rabbits for 30 days produced few signs of toxicity, with only one animal showing lung damage (Dikshith et al., 1979).

Subchronic exposure following dermal application has been examined in rabbits. The mortality observed with repeated daily applications beneath an occlusive dressing gave a MLD of 6.24 (4.6–8.5) mg ion/kg/day of paraquat over 20 days (McElligott, 1972). At the higher doses the skin was reddened and sloughing with local edema, while at the lowest dose some scab formation was seen after about 7 days of application. Systemic effects at postmortem included renal tubular necrosis, focal hepatocellular necrosis, and pulmonary congestion. Studies were also conducted where the skin was not occluded; rabbits were fitted with collars and these were either removed after decontamination of the skin or at the end of the observation period. The MLD for 20 days exposure was between 7.25 and 14.5 mg paraquat ion/kg/day for the animals where the collars were removed after decontamination and at least 24 mg ion/kg/day for those where the collars were left on all the time. The rabbits showed marked signs of salivation, which was associated with glossitis and ulceration of the tongue. The animals refused to eat and death occurred in a state of cachexia; this effect was less marked at the lower doses when the collars were kept in place all the time (McElligott, 1972). When the "Gramoxone" formulation of paraquat was diluted to spray strength and applied to the skin of rabbits for 20 days (2.4 mg ion/kg/day) no clinical signs of toxicity or pathological changes were seen (McElligott, 1972).

Daily subcutaneous dosing of paraquat to dogs for 4 weeks resulted in some animals being terminated at the top dose of 0.495 mg/kg/day, while at the other doses of 0.165 and 0.055 mg/kg/day all animals appeared well (Nagata et al., 1992b). Histopathology of the lungs showed proliferation of alveolar lining cells and some fibrosis at the top dose and pulmonary changes (thickening of the alveolar wall and pleura) at all doses. The 28 day MLD from this study was about 0.5 mg/kg/day.

Repeated exposure of rats to a respirable aerosol of paraquat (approx. 90% < 2.5 μm) by inhalation at 0.4 μg/l for 6 hr per day for 15 days, over 3 weeks, led to intermittent respiratory problems after about four exposures. At postmortem after 15 exposures the animals showed marginal paraquat-related pathology to the lungs. Exposure to 0.1 μg/l for 15 daily, 6 hr periods showed no signs of toxicity or pathology in the lungs (Gage, 1968a). Rats exposed to 0.003 μg/l for 6 hr a day for 5 days per week for 2 months put on body weight, remained in good condition, and showed no histopathological evidence of lung damage. Bainova *et al.* (1972) exposed rats to a respirable paraquat aerosol at 1.1 or 0.05 mg/L for 6 hr/day for 4.5 months and found evidence of lung damage at the higher dose, with little effect at the lower dose. Seidenfeld *et al.* (1978) exposed rabbits by inhalation to paraquat by an ultrasonic nebulizer (mean particle size 4 μm) at a concentration of 0.1 mg/ml of aqueous solution for 2 hr/day for 5 days per week for 3 months and found no lung damage. However rabbits exposed to 2 mg/ml of aqueous solution for 2 hr/day could only tolerate three exposures and developed a reduced arterial oxygen tension and specific compliance which was associated with marked lung injury.

Overall these studies show that following acute and chronic exposure the primary target organ for toxicity is the lung, with deaths from lung damage frequently taking many days to occur following a single dose. The rabbit is unusual in that it does not readily develop a lung lesion following oral or parenteral exposure, but if instilled into the lung or exposed via inhalation, lung injury ensues. Renal functional impairment with some renal tubular necrosis is the other major organ affected. Dose levels of paraquat that do not cause lung damage in laboratory animals following acute and chronic exposure have been clearly established.

70.2.5 MUTAGENIC AND CARCINOGENIC POTENTIAL

Paraquat is not carcinogenic in either rats or mice. The activity seen in some short-term assays for mutagenesis is associated with cytotoxicity and is believed to arise as a consequence of the redox cycling ability of paraquat, leading to superoxide anion formation.

Paraquat has minimal to no genotoxic activity when evaluated in a wide range of *in vitro* and *in vivo* test systems. Many groups have reported the absence of an effect while others have reported weakly positive effects (Dabney, 1995; IPCS, 1984; Ribas *et al.*, 1995 and references therein). These later effects were usually associated with high cytotoxicity or mortality and are believed to arise as a consequence of the redox cycling ability of paraquat. It is known that DNA damage frequently occurs when cells are exposed to oxidative stress (Brawn and Fridovich, 1981; Repine *et al.*, 1981).

Paraquat-mediated effects on DNA have been reported in bacteria (Moody and Hassan, 1982; Yonei *et al.*, 1986), Chinese hamster cells (Nicotera *et al.*, 1985; Sofuni *et al.*, 1985; Tanaka and Amano, 1989), isolated alveolar macrophages and epithelial type II cells (Dusinska *et al.*, 1998), and in a few cases cells from treated mice (He and Yasumoto, 1994; Rios *et al.*, 1995). These responses are all considered to be secondary to superoxide anion generation.

Studies with cultured mammalian cells have shown that paraquat inhibits DNA synthesis leading to the arrest of the cells in S-phase (Tomita, 1996; Yamagami *et al.*, 1994). This effect occurs prior to the onset of cytotoxicity and is thought to be part of a cascade of events initiated by the production of oxygen free radicals by the redox cycling of paraquat. These findings have been extended to rat lung cells exposed to paraquat *in vivo* which also showed S-phase arrest at early times after dosing. Prior treatment of the rats with a diet enriched in sodium tungstate, an inhibitor of xanthine oxidase to reduce the production of free radicals, prevented the S-phase arrest produced by paraquat (Matsubara *et al.*, 1996) and reduced mortality (Kitazawa *et al.*, 1991). Once inside a cell, paraquat can redox cycle, producing oxygen free radicals that can cause cell cycle arrest and inhibit DNA synthesis. These findings are consistent with early studies showing that paraquat reduces DNA synthesis at early times after dosing (Smith and Rose, 1977; Van Osten and Gibson, 1975).

Paraquat has been evaluated for its carcinogenic potential in both rats and mice and it was concluded that at all doses up to the maximum tolerated dose, paraquat did not result in a compound related increase in tumour incidence (Bainova and Vulcheva, 1977; FAO/WHO, 1986).

70.2.6 EFFECTS ON REPRODUCTION, EMBRYOTOXICITY AND TERATOGENICITY

Paraquat has no effect on fertility, is not teratogenic, and only produces fetotoxicity at doses that are maternally toxic. The main finding in multigeneration studies was lung damage.

Paraquat does not readily cross the placenta and enter the embryo of mice when given either orally or by ip administration (Bus *et al.*, 1975). In contrast, paraquat appears to readily cross the placenta of rats, being detected in fetuses within 30 min of an iv injection to 20 day pregnant rats (Ingebrigtsen *et al.*, 1984). A three-generation reproduction study in rats maintained on dietary levels of paraquat of 30 or 100 ppm showed no effect on food intake, fertility, fecundity, neonatal morbidity, mortality. No teratogenesis or other changes in gross or histological morphology were seen, except for a slight increase in the incidence of renal hydropic degeneration in the 3–4 week old young receiving 100 ppm (about 10 mg/kg/day). Pregnant and young animals did not appear to be more susceptible than adults (FAO/WHO, 1973). A two-generation reproduction study in mice maintained on dietary levels of 45, 90, or 125 ppm showed no effects on age to parturition, number born, or abnormalities in the pups in the first generation following 45 or 90 ppm. However, at 125 ppm an increase in mortality was seen in the dams and pups during the first few weeks of life (Dial and Dial, 1987). The second generation mice were more resistant to the effects of paraquat, the only effect being an increase in the age of the mothers at second parturition on the highest dose of paraquat (Dial and Dial, 1987). Subsequent studies to explore the basis for the high mortality in the first generation dams, and pups exposed to 125 ppm paraquat in the diet showed that they almost certainly died from lung damage. This only occurred in pups exposed prenatally via the placenta, not in pups exposed postnatally (Dial and Dial, 1989). Bus and Gibson (1975) also reported that paraquat given to mice in their drinking water at either 50 or 100 ppm from day 8 of gestation and to the young until 42 days of age increased pup mortality at 100 ppm but not 50 ppm. The lungs of mice killed 42 days after 100 ppm snowed extensive alveolar consolidation and collapse, supporting the view that the deaths at this dose were probably due to lung damage. No dominant lethal effects were seen in mice exposed to paraquat at oral doses up to 4 mg/kg/day for 5 days (Anderson et al., 1976).

High doses of paraquat injected ip into pregnant rats or mice on various days of gestation can produce significant maternal toxicity (Bus et al., 1975; Khera et al., 1970). Examination of the fetuses of mice exposed to 1.67 or 3.35 mg/kg ip or 20 mg/kg per os po daily on days 8–16 of gestation induced no teratogenic effects, although a slight increase in nonossification of the sternbrae was seen (Bus et al., 1975).

70.2.7 PATHOLOGY OF THE LUNG

The toxic effects of paraquat were first described by Clark et al. (1966) who reported that the histological effects of paraquat in rats, mice, and dogs are similar. The lung, liver, kidney, and thymus were affected, the lung being the major target. The effect of paraquat in the cynomologus monkey is similar to that in rats (Murray and Gibson, 1972). In contrast, as mentioned previously, rabbits do not develop lung lesions following acute oral or ip administration (Butler and Kleinerman, 1971; Ilett et al., 1974; Mehani, 1972; Zavala and Rhodes, 1978). There is one report of daily administration of paraquat in the drinking water to rabbits over several days leading to lung damage that resembles that seen in rats (Restuccia et al., 1974). Inhalation exposure to paraquat produces lung damage in the rabbit (Seidenfeld et al., 1978). The hamster responds in a similar way, being refractory to a single sc dose of paraquat, but lung fibrosis is produced by repeated sc injections (Butler, 1975).

The most extensive studies on the pathogenesis of lung damage produced by paraquat have been conducted in rats. The time course of development of the injury in rats given a single MLD ip was reported by Vijeyaratnam and Corrin (1971) and Smith and Heath (1974a). Damage to the type I and II alveolar epithelial cells was seen within a day of dosing. This damage was more marked by days 2–4 with large areas of the alveolar epithelium being completely lost. Alveolar edema developed and in some areas hemorrhage into the air spaces occurred. At this time there was extensive infiltration of inflammatory cells into the alveolar interstitium, air spaces, and perivascular areas, although the alveolar endothelial capillaries were mainly spared. The animals died as a consequence of severe anoxia usually within the first few days after dosing and this has been confirmed by others (Clark et al., 1966; Sharp et al., 1972; Smith and Rose, 1977). This phase has been called the destructive phase (Smith and Heath, 1976). Similar early pathological changes have been reported by Kimbrough and Gaines (1970), Brooks (1971), Modee et al. (1972), Wasan and McElligott (1972), Smith et al. (1974), Sykes et al. (1977), and Smith and Heath (1976). Some rats that survive for up to 10–12 days after dosing develop an extensive hypercellular lesion in the lung which is dominated by proliferation of fibroblasts. This phase of the lesion is called the proliferative phase and is characterized by attempts by the epithelium to regenerate and restore normal architecture of the alveolar epithelium (Kimbrough and Gaines, 1970; Smith and Heath, 1974a; Vijeyaratnam and Corrin, 1971). The findings in these animals are typically extensive intraalveolar and interalveolar fibrosis, which in association with residual edema reduces gaseous exchange results in death from anoxia. It appears that the initial damage to the alveolar epithelium, produced by paraquat, is the primary event in the development of the lung injury, with the proliferative fibrosis being a consequence of the extensive damage produced. For a more detailed review on pulmonary injury see Smith and Heath (1976).

70.2.8 ABSORPTION

The first studies on the absorption and excretion of paraquat from the gastrointestinal tract were conducted by Daniel and Gage (1966) in rats. Following a single oral dose of 4, 6, or 50 mg/kg [^{14}C-methyl] paraquat dichloride, most of the radioactivity was excreted within 48 h. Occasionally some appeared in the feces 3 and 4 days after dosing at the higher doses, with small amounts also in the urine. Between 6 and 14% of the dose was excreted in the urine over 48 h when given as the dichloride salt, and 16–23% when given as the dimethylthiosulphate salt, the remainder being in the feces. In contrast, when paraquat as either salt was given sc, the bulk of the radioactivity appeared in the urine within 24 h of dosing, showing that paraquat is poorly absorbed across the gastrointestinal tract of the rat. Subsequent studies have extended and essentially confirmed these findings (Chui et al., 1988; Lock and Ishmael, 1979; Molnar and Hayes, 1971; Murray and Gibson, 1974).

The concentration of paraquat in the plasma following an oral dose to the rat is determined largely by the amount of paraquat present in the small intestine (Smith et al., 1974). Studies in the dog using tracer doses (129 μg/kg) of [^{14}C-methyl]paraquat support this. Peak plasma concentrations following oral dosing were observed at 75–90 min (Fig. 70.2), with about 46–66% of the dose absorbed, as judged by the amount excreted in the urine at 6 h (Davies et al., 1977). Thus,

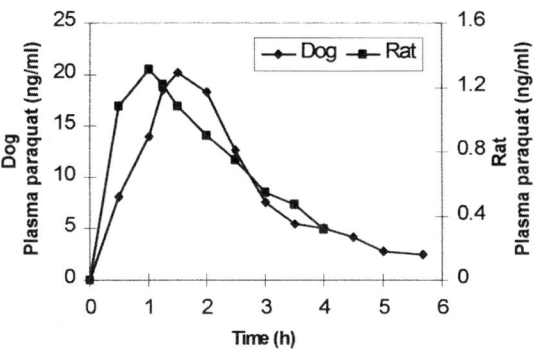

Figure 70.2 Plasma levels of paraquat in the rat and dog following a single nontoxic oral dose. The dog was given a total dose of 1.03 mg of paraquat, while the rats were dosed at 0.038 mg/kg. Data adapted from (Davies *et al.*, 1977; Chui *et al.*, 1988).

the dog absorbs a greater percentage of an orally administered dose of paraquat than the rat, which is consistent with the greater susceptibility of the dog to paraquat by this route of administration. Pretreatment of dogs with a drug that will block gastric emptying delayed the peak plasma concentration by 3 to 6 h, indicating that the stomach is not the major site of absorption (Bennett *et al.*, 1976).

These data in both rats and dogs indicate that the absorption of paraquat from the gastrointestinal tract occurs somewhere beyond the stomach. It is assumed this is similar for humans but there is limited evidence to support this. Based on the cationic nature of paraquat, it would not be expected to readily cross cellular membranes, and it seems unlikely that simple diffusion would explain the rapid but incomplete absorption seen in the rat and dog. Studies *in vitro* with isolated mucosa from a number of different regions of the rat gastrointestinal tract (Steffen and Konder, 1979) have confirmed that the jejunum and ileum have the greatest capacity to transport paraquat from the lumen into the bloodstream and also showed that a component of the transport is facilitated (Heylings, 1991).

Following oral administration of paraquat to rats, the peak plasma concentration is seen between 30 and 60 min (Figs. 70.2 and 70.3) following either a tracer dose (Chui *et al.*, 1988) or a toxic dose (Murray and Gibson, 1974). This profile is similar to that seen in the dog (Fig. 70.2) (Davies *et al.*, 1977). The peak plasma concentration in the monkey and guinea pig occurs within the first hour (Fig. 70.2) and 30 min respectively following a toxic oral dose (Murray and Gibson, 1974). Overall, these studies indicate that paraquat is rapidly but incompletely absorbed from the gastrointestinal tract of laboratory animals and humans (see later), with peak plasma concentrations occurring within 30–90 min.

Paraquat is poorly absorbed across human skin *in vitro*, human skin being less permeable to paraquat than the skin of rats, rabbits, or guinea pigs (Walker *et al.*, 1983). Application of a low dose of [^{14}C] paraquat (150 nmol/kg) in acetone to rat skin resulted in a peak blood level about 1 hr after dosing and a total of 3.5% of the dose absorbed (Chui *et al.*, 1988). It should be pointed out that an occlusive dressing was applied in these studies which has previously been shown to greatly enhance the percutaneous absorption of paraquat in animals (McElligott, 1972). Overall, these studies, plus those of Hoffer *et al.* (1989) on rabbits, indicate that paraquat is poorly absorbed across the intact skin of laboratory animals.

70.2.9 DISTRIBUTION

In the rat, after a lethal oral dose, the plasma paraquat concentration remained relatively constant after the initial peak for up to 32 h (Murray and Gibson, 1974; Rose *et al.*, 1976a). During this time the concentration in the lung rose progressively to several times that found in the plasma. In no other organ, apart from the kidney, the major organ for the excretion of paraquat, was a time-dependent accumulation of paraquat detected (Murray and Gibson, 1974; Rose *et al.*, 1976a). These findings, plus the earlier observation of Sharp *et al.* (1972) who

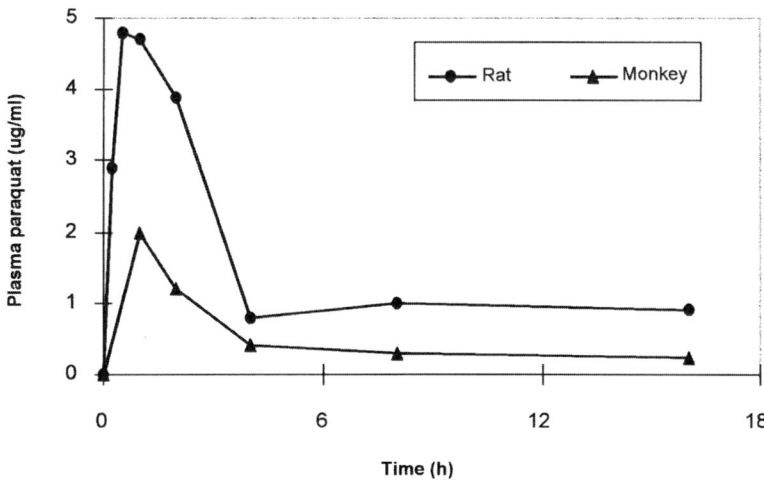

Figure 70.3 Plasma levels of paraquat in the rat and monkey following a single toxic oral dose. The rats were given 126 mg/kg paraquat while the monkeys received 50 mg/kg. Data adapted from (Murray and Gibson, 1974).

administered paraquat iv and showed that paraquat was retained in the lung with a half-life of 50 h, provided the key evidence showing that those organs that had the highest concentration of paraquat were those that were susceptible to injury, namely the lung and kidney. Many other groups have subsequently examined the pharmacokinetics and elimination of paraquat in the rat (Chui *et al.*, 1988; Dey *et al.*, 1990; Maling *et al.*, 1978), dog (Giri *et al.*, 1982; Hawksworth *et al.*, 1981; Pond *et al.*, 1993), rabbit (Ilett *et al.*, 1974; Yonemitsu, 1986; Yu *et al.*, 1994), and mouse (Drew and Gram, 1979). The distribution of paraquat in the body is best described by a three-compartment model, with input to and removal from the central plasma compartment. Simulations of plasma concentrations in the peripheral compartments show there is a compartment with rapid uptake and removal of paraquat, which was assumed to be the highly vascular tissues such as the kidney, and a slow uptake compartment reaching a maximum about 4–5 h after iv dosing, which may be the lung (Hawksworth *et al.*, 1981).

Using lung slices, Rose *et al.* (1974a) first described the time-dependent accumulation of paraquat into lung tissue. This process was shown to be energy-dependent in that it could be inhibited by the addition of the metabolic inhibitors cyanide plus iodoacetate to the incubation medium. The accumulation of paraquat into rat lung was shown to obey saturation kinetics with an apparent K_m of 70 μM and a V_{max} of 300 nmol/h/g wet weight of lung slice (Table 70.4) (Rose *et al.*, 1974a). Other aspects of the accumulation of paraquat into the lung will be discussed in more detail later. Hawksworth *et al.* (1981) also showed that early onset of renal failure markedly affected the concentration of paraquat in the peripheral compartments, suggesting that any reduction in renal excretion of paraquat may allow more of the chemical to be transported into the lung. The distribution in the rabbit, which is refractory to lung damage following a single systemic dose, showed the organs with the highest concentration of paraquat were the lung and kidney at 6 and 24 h after dosing, but the concentration in rabbit lung appeared to decline more rapidly than from rat lung (Ilett *et al.*, 1974).

Whole body autoradiography studies have provided valuable information on the tissue distribution of paraquat; early studies by Litchfield *et al.* (1973) in mice given iv [^{14}C methyl]-paraquat showed retention in the lung. A more detailed study using [^{3}H-methyl]-paraquat and thin tissue sections revealed localization of radioactivity at all time intervals after dosing in the

Table 70.4

Kinetic Constants for the Accumulation of Paraquat and Putrescine by Rat and Human Lung Slices or Isolated Alveolar Type II Cells

Species/ tissue	Paraquat accumulation		Putrescine accumulation		Reference
	K_m (μM)	V_{max}[a]	K_m (μM)	V_{max}[b]	
Rat-lung slice	70	300			Rose *et al.*, 1974a
	210	710			Ross and Krieger, 1981
	119	636	8	480	Karl and Friedman, 1983
			7	330	Smith and Wyatt, 1981
			31	870	Nemery *et al.*, 1987
			12–18		O'Sullivan *et al.*, 1991
			13.5	720	Hardwick *et al.*, 1990
			13.1	723	Smith *et al.*, 1982
Human-lung slice	40	300			Rose *et al.*, 1974a
	244	370	7	376	Hoet *et al.*, 1994
			2–11	99–249	Brooke-Taylor *et al.*, 1983
			7	414	Hoffer *et al.*, 1993
Cultured rat-type II cells			5	18	Lewis, 1989
			8–14	58	Richards *et al.*, 1987
	29				Van der Wal *et al.*, 1990
	64		15	128	Oreffo *et al.*, 1991
Suspensions of rat-type II cells	88	29	2.5	34	Chen *et al.*, 1992
Cultured human-type II cells			6–8	12–14	Hoet *et al.*, 1994

[a] V_{max} in lung slices expressed as nmol/h/g wet weight of slice.

[b] V_{max} Alveolar type II cells expressed as pmol/h/μM DNA.

lung, choroid plexus, muscle, and melanin in addition to excretory pathways such as the proximal tubules of the kidney, urine, liver, gall bladder, and intestinal contents of the mouse (Waddell and Marlowe, 1980). Radioactivity in the lungs appeared to be higher in certain areas and higher cellular resolution autoradiography revealed that the radioactivity was confined to alveolar type II cells, which are one of the major target cells for paraquat toxicity. In these studies it was essential to keep the tissue frozen at all times to prevent diffusion of paraquat which is highly polar. An association of paraquat with melanin has been demonstrated and this is probably due to an ionic interaction (Larsson et al., 1977, 1978; Lindquist et al., 1988). Immunohistochemical approaches utilizing specific antibodies to paraquat have shown immunoreactive material localized primarily in bronchiolar epithelial cells and walls of blood vessels in the lungs of rats, 3 h to 10 days after an iv dose. Other studies have localized immunoreactive material in the intestine, liver, kidneys, and brain to capillary walls and glial cells but not neurones, after paraquat administration (Nagao et al., 1990, 1991, 1993).

70.2.10 METABOLISM

Paraquat is very poorly metabolized with the bulk of the administered dose being excreted unchanged in the urine and faeces. Daniel and Gage (1966) compared the colorimetric assay for paraquat with that found by radiochemical detection on the urine and feces of rats dosed with paraquat and demonstrated that there was very close agreement. Chromatography of the urine and lung tissue from rats treated with paraquat also showed no evidence of biotransformation (Hughes et al., 1973; Murray and Gibson, 1974; Rose et al., 1974a). No radioactivity was excreted in expired air following paraquat administration to rats, indicating that it did not undergo metabolism to CO_2 (Murray and Gibson, 1974). Incubation of paraquat with rat caecal contents for up to 24 h showed up to a 50% loss, indicating microbial metabolism. The loss was not seen when the contents of the caecum were heat treated (Daniel and Gage, 1966). However, in vivo studies in rats, guinea pigs, and dogs showed little

evidence of biotransformation, indicating that the in vitro studies had overpredicted the likely metabolism (Summers, 1980). The overriding weight of evidence is that metabolism does not contribute to the toxicity of paraquat.

70.2.11 EXCRETION

Elimination of paraquat from the body is almost exclusively via the kidneys. The renal clearance of paraquat is greater than that of creatinine in the rat (Chan et al., 1997; Lock, 1979), dog (Hawksworth et al., 1981), sheep (Webb, 1983), monkey (Purser and Rose, 1979), and humans (Bismuth et al., 1982); see later for a more detailed discussion on humans. Thus paraquat is actively secreted by the kidney. Renal tubular secretion was completely inhibited by N'-methylnicotinamide, suggesting that paraquat is secreted via a cationic transport system (Hawksworth et al., 1981).

The transport mechanisms for organic cations in renal proximal tubular cells is not fully understood. Recently two membrane proteins, organic cation transporter 1 (Grundemann et al., 1994) and organic cation transporter 2 (Okuda et al., 1996), have been isolated from rat kidney. The organic cation transporter 1 located on the basolateral membrane will transport tetraethylammonium, and this can be inhibited by other organic cations such as quinine. The organic cation transporter 2, which is predominantly expressed in the kidney, stimulates the uptake of tetraethylammonium and this can be markedly inhibited by cimetidine. Studies using freshly isolated renal proximal tubules and renal cell lines have shown that paraquat is transported across the basolateral membrane (from the bloodstream into the renal tubular epithelial cell) using an organic cation transport system (Chan et al., 1996a, b, 1997, 1998; Groves et al., 1995). The transport of paraquat can be blocked by the addition of the divalent cation quinine, cimetidine, and to a lesser extent tetraethylammonium (Chan et al., 1996b), suggesting that paraquat may be transported by both transport systems (Fig. 70.4).

Exit across the apical membrane into the tubular lumen is also an active process; current evidence suggests that there are

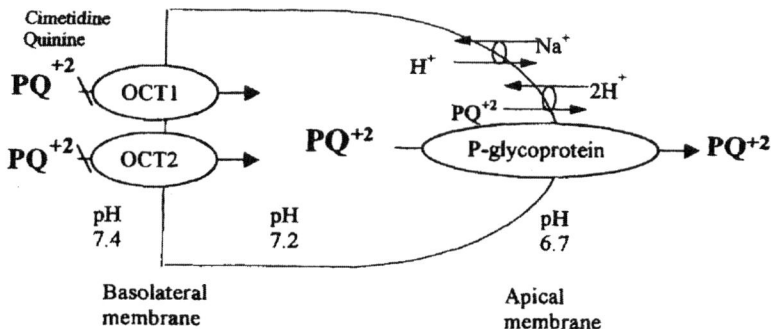

Figure 70.4 Mechanism of paraquat transport across renal tubular cells. A schematic representation of the proposed transport systems for paraquat across renal tubular cells. The transporters are OCT 1 at the basolateral membrane and P-glycoprotein and the cation/H^+ exchange system at the brush border membrane. Adapted from (Chan et al., 1998). Reproduced with permission from © 1998.

two cation transport systems, an electroneutral organic cation /H^+ exchange (Sokol *et al.*, 1988) and P-glycoprotein (Dutt *et al.*, 1992). Studies with rabbit brush-border membrane vesicles have shown that paraquat is a substrate for the cation/H^+ exchange transporter and further that it can inhibit the transport of other monovalent cations such as tetraethylammonium (Wright and Wunz, 1995).

In the rat *in vivo*, the fractional excretion of paraquat decreased from 2.1 at a plasma concentration of about 0.4 nmol/ml to 1.2 at a plasma concentration of 21 nmol/ml, demonstrating that the excretion of paraquat is greater than the glomerular filtration rate and that the process is saturable (Chan *et al.*, 1997). Thus, at low plasma concentrations paraquat will be readily cleared from the body; however, at higher plasma concentrations the system will become saturated and less paraquat will be cleared. At toxic doses it is well established that paraquat can cause renal functional impairment. In rats, given 126 mg ion/kg po (Lock, 1979), and mice given 50 mg ion/kg iv (Ecker *et al.*, 1975b) renal impairment was observed 17–24 h after dosing. In the cynomologus monkey given 85 mg ion/kg po the decline in renal clearance was seen 12 h after dosing, the first time examined (Purser and Rose, 1979). In dogs given 20 mg ion/kg iv (Hawksworth *et al.*, 1981) renal impairment was observed as early as 2.5 h after dosing. An early report on the renal handling of paraquat by the dog suggested that paraquat was reabsorbed by the proximal tubules. This study was conducted at high plasma concentrations (54–810 nmol/ml) where the transport system will have been saturated and function impairment almost certainly will have occurred (Ferguson, 1973). The weight of evidence strongly supports the view that paraquat is actively secreted by the kidney of laboratory animals and humans (see later). The implication of impairment of renal excretion is that more paraquat is available in the plasma to accumulate into the lung.

Whole body autoradiography has shown that paraquat was present in the gall bladder of mice, indicating some biliary excretion (Waddell and Marlowe, 1980). The extent of biliary excretion of paraquat was <5% when dosed to bile cannulated rats, rabbits, or guinea pigs and measured over a 3 h period (Hughes *et al.*, 1973). The bulk of the dose appeared unchanged in the urine. These authors suggest that the molecular weight of paraquat at 186 was below the minimal molecular weight of about 500 for chemicals that are excreted in bile. Radioactivity from paraquat was also detected in the bile of dogs given a single iv dose, indicating some biliary excretion in this species (Giri *et al.*, 1982).

70.2.12 ACCUMULATION OF PARAQUAT INTO THE LUNG

The original discovery of an energy-dependent accumulation of paraquat into rat lung tissue (Rose *et al.*, 1974a) lead to studies to look for this transport system in the lung of other species, including human. The accumulation of paraquat by slices of lung from a number of species was reported by Rose *et al.* (1976a). The apparent kinetic constants for the uptake process were very similar for all species examined except the rabbit. Slices of rabbit had a very high affinity, but low capacity, to accumulate paraquat which is consistent with the *in vivo* findings that show that following oral or parenteral administration of paraquat the rabbit does not develop a lung lesion. For the rat the derived K_m was 70 μM with a V_{max} of 300 nmol/h/g wet weight of lung (Table 70.4). The kinetic constants for rat and human lung were very similar, suggesting that the rat lung was a good surrogate for studying paraquat uptake into human lung (Rose *et al.*, 1976a). The kinetics of accumulation of paraquat into human lung slices has been confirmed by others, the V_{max} being similar at 370 nmol/h/g wet weight while the K_m was lower at 244 μM (Hoet *et al.*, 1994). Considerable interindividual variation is seen in paraquat accumulation into human lung slices (Brooke-Taylor *et al.*, 1983) which may either reflect individual variability or more likely the state of the tissue and delay between removal of the tissue and analysis of paraquat transport. Table 70.4 summarizes the available data on the transport kinetics for paraquat in rat and human lung tissue. These observations, coupled with the finding that paraquat is not metabolized by the lung nor covalently bound to any degree (Forman *et al.*, 1982; Ilett *et al.*, 1974; Sullivan and Montgomery, 1983), suggests that this accumulation is mediated through binding to and subsequent translocation into lung cells by a carrier-mediated system.

The finding that paraquat was actively transported into lung slices lead to a search for chemicals that might inhibit this process (Dunbar *et al.*, 1988; Lock *et al.*, 1976; Maling *et al.*, 1978; Ross and Krieger, 1981; Smith *et al.*, 1981) and hence provide protection against paraquat-induced lung toxicity. A number of chemicals were identified that could block paraquat uptake into lung slices but none of these were effective in the whole animal (see later under treatment of poisoning).

Studies were also undertaken to try and identify the endogenous chemicals for this transport system. A wide range of chemicals was examined and a number of naturally occurring amines were identified as the most effective inhibitors of paraquat accumulation into slices of rat lung, and which themselves act as substrates. These amines include the diamine putrescine, the oligoamines spermidine and spermine (Gordonsmith *et al.*, 1983; Smith and Wyatt, 1981; Smith *et al.*, 1982), and the disulphide cystamine (Lewis *et al.*, 1989). The physiological role for this transport system is not known, but it has been suggested that polyamines, which are known to regulate cell growth, may play a role in the differentiation of alveolar type II cells to type I cells (Smith, 1982). It has also been proposed that cystamine represents a source of taurine, which may have an antioxidant role in the lung (Lewis *et al.*, 1989; Wright *et al.*, 1986). Cystamine has also been implicated in playing a role in regulating cellular NADPH levels in response to oxidative stress (Brigelius, 1985). The structural requirements of substrates for this system have been examined and at least two charged nitrogen atoms separated by a distance of at least four methylene groups (about 6.6°A) is essential for uptake (Gordonsmith *et al.*, 1983; O'Sullivan *et al.*, 1991; Ross and Krieger,

1981). It is probable that paraquat, which meets these criteria, is recognized as a substrate and thereby accumulated (Smith, 1987).

Paraquat accumulation into rat lung slices is reduced in the presence of putrescine in a dose-related manner (Karl and Friedman, 1983; Smith and Wyatt, 1981). Subsequent studies showed that putrescine was accumulated into slices of rat lung by saturable energy-dependent process with an apparent K_m of 7 µM and a V_{max} of 330 nmol/h/g wet weight of lung. The K_m is about 10-fold lower than that for paraquat, indicating that the endogenous substrate has a higher affinity for the uptake process than paraquat (Table 70.4). These studies stimulated work to try and identify the specific cell types into which both paraquat and putrescine are accumulated. Slices of rat lung from rats treated with paraquat, which had been shown to cause selective damage to alveolar type I and type II cells, had a decreased ability to accumulate both paraquat and putrescine, suggesting that the transport system resides at least in part in these cell types (Smith *et al.*, 1976; Smith and Wyatt, 1981). This finding is consistent with the autoradiographic studies reported by Waddell and Marlowe (1980), who showed the distribution of paraquat in mouse lung following iv administration to be consistent with localization in alveolar type II cells. Studies with rat lung slices *in vitro* have shown localization of [^{3}H]-paraquat to alveolar type II cells (Wyatt *et al.*, 1988). Similar studies with rat lung slices using [^{3}H]-putrescine, [^{3}H]-spermine have also shown localization to alveolar type II cells and in addition provided evidence for accumulation of radiolabel in bronchiolar Clara cells and possibly alveolar type I cells (Wyatt *et al.*, 1988). Similar localization of [^{3}H]-putrescine was reported by Nemery *et al.* (1987) and the localization confirmed by electron microscopy to the type I and type II alveolar epithelial cells and Clara cells (Dinsdale *et al.*, 1991). In contrast, in rabbit lung slices [^{3}H]-putrescine was localized to alveolar type II cells and macrophages but not in Clara cells (Saunders *et al.*, 1988). More recent studies with slices of human lung have established that [^{3}H]-putrescine also accumulates into type I and type II alveolar epithelial cells (Hoet *et al.*, 1993).

Paraquat accumulation has also been demonstrated in isolated alveolar type II cells from rat and rabbit lung (Chen *et al.*, 1992; Forman *et al.*, 1982; Horton *et al.*, 1986) and in isolated Clara cells from rabbit lung (Horton *et al.*, 1986), suggesting that paraquat transport resides in both cell types. Paraquat is toxic to isolated mouse Clara cells and the addition of putrescine affords some protection (Masek and Richard, 1990). No accumulation of paraquat was, however, detected in isolated rabbit lung macrophages, although Saunders *et al.* (1988) have reported putrescine accumulation by rabbit lung macrophages. The basis for this difference is currently not clear but it is now well established that polyamine transport systems are present in a number of transformed and nontransformed blood cells (see Smith *et al.*, 1990).

The kinetics of transport of paraquat into isolated type II alveolar epithelial cells has been reported by Chen *et al.* (1992). Using freshly isolated cell suspensions, they found a K_m of 88 µM with a V_{max} of 20 pmol/h/µM DNA. They also examined putrescine transport in these alveolar type II suspensions and found a K_m of 2.5 µM with a V_{max} of 33 pmol/h/µM DNA. This finding is in broad agreement with that for rat lung slices where the V_{max} is very similar for both substrates while the K_m for putrescine is higher than that for paraquat (Table 70.4). The accumulation of both spermidine and putrescine has been characterized in rat alveolar type II cells in culture (Kameji *et al.*, 1989; Oreffo *et al.*, 1991; Richards *et al.*, 1987). The uptake of spermidine into isolated cells was inhibited by putrescine, spermine, and paraquat as described for slices of rat lung. The accumulation of putrescine has also been studied in human alveolar type II cells in culture. The uptake of putrescine and the competitive inhibition by paraquat was essentially the same as that seen in human lung slices (Hoet *et al.*, 1994). Some difficulties have been experienced by several groups in determining the kinetics of transport of paraquat into isolated alveolar type II cells in culture. This may reflect changes to the cell membrane during the isolation procedure, such that the findings in these cells may not accurately reflect that occurring *in vivo*.

A summary of the kinetic constants for the accumulation of both paraquat and putrescine by lung slices and isolated alveolar type II cells for rats and humans is shown in Table 70.4. These data show that paraquat and putrescine are accumulated by lung slices and alveolar type II cells from both rats and humans and that putrescine has a higher affinity for this system than paraquat.

70.2.13 EFFLUX OF PARAQUAT FROM THE LUNG

The amount of paraquat that accumulates into the lung is determined by both the rate of accumulation and the rate of efflux from the cells in which it concentrates. The loss of paraquat from rat lung following *in vivo* administration is slow. There appears to be a rapid phase of elimination over the first 20–30 min following iv administration of paraquat which is then followed by slower loss that obeys first-order kinetics with a half-life of about 50 h (Sharp *et al.*, 1972). Similar studies by Smith *et al.* (1978) and Dey *et al.* (1990) showed a rapid phase of elimination that was similar to that reported by Sharp *et al.* (1972) while the second phase showed a half-life for paraquat loss from the lung of approximately 20 h, which was independent of the plasma concentration. Studies *in vitro* using lung slices from rats dosed *in vivo* with paraquat also showed a biphasic elimination, with a rapid loss within 30 min presumably reflecting loss from the extracellular space followed by a slower phase with a half-life of 17 h similar to that seen *in vivo* (Smith *et al.*, 1981).

Thus, the basis for the selective toxicity of paraquat to the lung resides in paraquat's ability to become concentrated in alveolar type I and II cells and Clara cells. The concentration of paraquat retained in the lung is a combination of that retained during the time of the peak plasma concentration, plus that accumulated via the carrier-mediated process. Paraquat, once accumulated into lung cells, is not then readily lost.

70.2.14 BIOCHEMICAL MECHANISMS OF PARAQUAT TOXICITY

Paraquat can be reduced to form a free radical which is stable in aqueous solution in the absence of oxygen (Michaelis and Hill, 1933):

$$PQ^{2+} + e^- \rightarrow PQ^{+\cdot}$$

In the presence of oxygen, in biological systems, the radical will rapidly reoxidize to the cation with the concomitant production of superoxide anion $O_2^{-\cdot}$ (Farrington *et al.*, 1973):

$$PQ^{+\cdot} + O_2 \rightarrow PQ^{2+} + O_2^{-\cdot}$$

Thus, once paraquat enters a cell it will undergo alternate reduction followed by reoxidation, a process known as redox cycling. Gage (1968b) first reported that the paraquat cation could be reduced by rat liver NADPH-dependent microsomal flavoprotein reductase to form the radical, with the concomitant oxidation of NADPH. Redox cycling of paraquat has also been reported in microsomal preparations of lung, liver, and kidney (Baldwin *et al.*, 1975) and in lung microsomal and slice systems (Adam *et al.*, 1990). Studies using antibodies against NADPH-cytochrome *c* reductase have shown that paraquat radical formation can be blocked, demonstrating a role for this enzyme in the reduction process (Bus *et al.*, 1974; Horton *et al.*, 1986). Further support for a key role for NADPH-cytochrome *c* reductase comes from the studies of Kelner and Bagnell (1989) using a lymphoblastoid cell line with a specific deficiency in this enzyme which they reported was very resistant to paraquat toxicity. Thus, provided there is sufficient NADPH as an electron donor and O_2 as an electron acceptor, paraquat will redox cycle inside a cell, generating superoxide anion and consuming NADPH. This reaction is believed to be a key step in the mechanism of paraquat toxicity. However, the biochemical consequences of this reaction which leads to lung cell death are complex and still not fully understood. Recent studies with endothelial cells in culture have indicated that xanthine oxidase can also mediate redox cycling of paraquat to produce superoxide anion (Sakai *et al.*, 1995), indicating that two intracellular enzyme systems are probably involved.

Mammalian cells have many enzyme systems which provide them with protection against free radical attack and it is assumed that once these defenses have been overwhelmed that cell death occurs. Superoxide dismutase (SOD) is a family of metalloenzymes that can dismutate superoxide anion to hydrogen peroxide and oxygen:

$$O_2^{-\cdot} + O_2^{-\cdot} \rightarrow H_2O_2 + O_2$$

The importance of this enzyme in cellular toxicity comes from studies where cellular SOD activity has been genetically modified either by spontaneous mutation or by the transfection of SOD genes. Bilinski and Litwinska (1987) isolated a mutant yeast deficient in SOD activity, which had a greater sensitivity to paraquat than its isogenic wild type. In contrast, Hela cells which possess a higher content of both manganese and copper/zinc SOD had an increased resistance to paraquat (Krall *et al.*, 1988). Transfection of human copper/zinc SOD into various cell lines also lead to resistance to paraquat toxicity (Elroy-Stein *et al.*, 1986; Krall *et al.*, 1988). Recent studies have shown that mice lacking copper/zinc SOD show a marked increase in sensitivity to paraquat (Fig. 70.5) $Sod^{-/-}$ mice showed a median survival time of about 1.5 days after 10 mg/kg ip, while the $Sod^{+/-}$ and $Sod^{+/+}$ mice appeared normal at the end of 7 days of observation (Ho *et al.*, 1998). These studies provide strong evidence for a role for superoxide anion radical in the mechanism of cellular toxicity and for the role of copper/zinc SOD in protecting the lungs against paraquat toxicity.

However, superoxide anion itself is unlikely to be the ultimate toxic species as it has limited reactivity in biological systems (Halliwell and Gutteridge, 1984). Dismutation of superoxide anion leads to hydrogen peroxide formation which can undergo detoxification by catalase and glutathione peroxidase. Studies with genetically engineered cells have shown that the balance between these two enzymes plays an important role in cellular toxicity of paraquat. Increasing intracellular concentra-

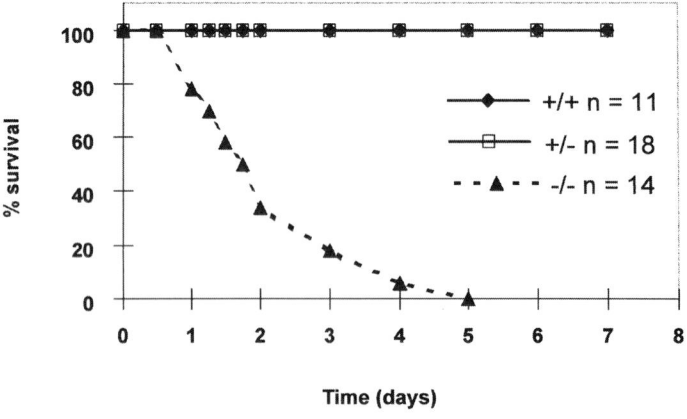

Figure 70.5 Increased susceptibility of mice lacking Cu/Zn superoxide dismutase to paraquat. The survival times of age-matched, male $Sod1^{+/+}$, $Sod1^{+/-}$, and $Sod1^{-/-}$ mice was determined following ip administration of paraquat at 10 mg/kg. From (Ho *et al.*, 1998). Reproduced with permission from © 1998.

tions of SOD to high levels can alter the balance of metabolism of hydrogen peroxide from two electron addition via catalase and glutathione peroxidase to produce water to allow an increase in one electron metabolism to form hydroxyl radical:

$$H_2O_2 \to^{e^-} \to OH^{\cdot} \to^{e^-} \to H_2O$$
$$\downarrow$$
$$2e^-$$
$$\downarrow \text{ catalase/GSH peroxidase}$$
$$H_2O$$

Increasing intracellular SOD content to a very high level ultimately leads to an increase in toxicity to paraquat in a number of transfected cells or *Escherichia coli* (Bloch and Ausubel, 1986; Elroy-Stein *et al.*, 1986; Scott and Eaton, 1996; Scott *et al.*, 1987). In contrast, cells having an increase in both SOD and catalase exhibited a greater resistance to paraquat than with just SOD alone (Krall *et al.*, 1988).

Generation of hydroxyl radical has been proposed as the critical event in the toxicology of paraquat. This reaction requires the presence of iron and is generated by the Fenton reaction. In this reaction ferrous ions react with hydrogen peroxide to generate hydroxyl radicals:

$$Fe^{2+} + H_2O_2 \to Fe^{3+} + OH^- + OH^{\cdot}$$

Under physiological conditions free iron predominately exists in the ferric form (Fe^{3+}) as a chelate with ADP, ATP, and citrate. The reduction of ferric iron may be achieved directly by the paraquat radical (Sutton *et al.*, 1987; Winterbourn and Sutton, 1984) or indirectly by superoxide anion generated from the redox cycling of paraquat (McCord and Da, 1987).

A role for transition metals such as iron in the toxicity is supported by studies showing that paraquat toxicity is reduced by removal of iron and enhanced by its addition (Kohen and Chevion, 1985; Sion *et al.*, 1989; Van der Wal *et al.*, 1990). The role of the iron chelator desferrioxamine in affording some protection against paraquat toxicity will be discussed in the section on antidotes.

Many other studies too numerous to mention have been conducted both *in vitro* and *in vivo* to explore the effect of altered antioxidant status on the toxicology of paraquat. Examples include the role of GSH and GSH reductase (Bus *et al.*, 1976a; Hardwick *et al.*, 1990; Keeling *et al.*, 1982), the role of selenium deficiency, vitamin E, and glutathione peroxidase (Block, 1979; Bus *et al.*, 1976b; Cagen and Gibson, 1977; Kelner *et al.*, 1995; Omaye *et al.*, 1978), and the role of metallothionein (Lazo *et al.*, 1995; Satoh *et al.*, 1992). Metallothionein appears to have play a role as a free radical scavenger in addition to its well established role as a heavy metal chelator. Metallothionein has been reported to quench both superoxide anion and hydroxyl radicals, with a significantly higher reactivity toward hydroxyl radicals (Thornalley and Vasak, 1985). Genetically engineered animals have been used as tools to elucidate the function of the various antioxidant defense mechanisms against paraquat-induced oxidant injury. In addition to the discussion above regarding mice deficient in copper/zinc SOD, Sato *et al.*

(1996) found mice deficient in metallothionein I and II genes to be more susceptible to paraquat toxicity. Glutathione peroxidase deficient mice show an increased susceptibility to paraquat toxicity with a mean survival time of 5 h compared to the wild type of 69 h following an ip dose of 50 mg/kg (Cheng *et al.*, 1998). Mice overexpressing glutathione peroxidase are more tolerant to paraquat toxicity; wild type mice given a large 125 mg/kg ip dose of paraquat died within 5 h while the mice overexpressing the enzyme lived for about 54 h (Cheng *et al.*, 1998).

Figure 70.6 shows a schematic representation of the key requirements to enable paraquat to enter a cell and the subsequent redox cycling steps believed to lead to cytotoxicity. Three hypotheses have been proposed to account for the ensuing cytotoxicity, one involving lipid peroxidation, another the oxidation of NADPH, and the third mitochondrial toxicity; none of these hypotheses are mutually exclusive.

70.2.15 LIPID PEROXIDATION HYPOTHESIS

Bus and co-workers (1974, 1976a) proposed the sequential generation of superoxide anion and hydroxyl radical and the initiation of lipid peroxidation as the mechanism of cellular toxicity of paraquat. However, there is little direct evidence which demonstrates lipid peroxidation occurs in the lung of animals dosed with paraquat before there is morphological evidence of cell damage. Paraquat-induced lipid peroxidation has been demonstrated *in vitro* in broken cell systems and isolated cells from the lung and liver (Aldrich *et al.*, 1983; Bus *et al.*, 1976a; Kornbrust and Mavis, 1980; Saito *et al.*, 1985; Sandy *et al.*, 1986; Sata *et al.*, 1983; Trush *et al.*, 1981) and *in vivo* (Burk *et al.*, 1980; Bus *et al.*, 1976b; Reddy *et al.*, 1977). However, others have questioned its significance in the toxicity. For example Steffen *et al.* (1980) only found a small increase in the exhalation of ethane (a marker of lipid peroxidation) in rats suffering from respiratory distress following exposure to paraquat and oxygen. Similarly, others have been unable to find evidence of lipid peroxidation in the lungs of mice given large doses of paraquat (Shu *et al.*, 1979; Younes *et al.*, 1985) or it is only detected as a late event in the toxicity (Ogata and Manabe, 1990). So the question remains as to whether lipid peroxidation is a cause, or a consequence, of the toxicity. These contrasting findings *in vivo* may also reflect the difficulty in detecting a small but critical increase in lipid peroxidation in the alveolar type I and II cells and Clara cells that are only a small population of the total cells in the lung.

70.2.16 OXIDATION OF NADPH HYPOTHESIS

Intracellular redox cycling of paraquat results in the oxidation of NADPH leading to cellular depletion such that those cells that selectively accumulate paraquat can longer function normally. Fisher *et al.* (1975) first suggested that the redox potential of lung cells may be altered by the redox cycling of paraquat. A marked stimulation of the activity of the pentose

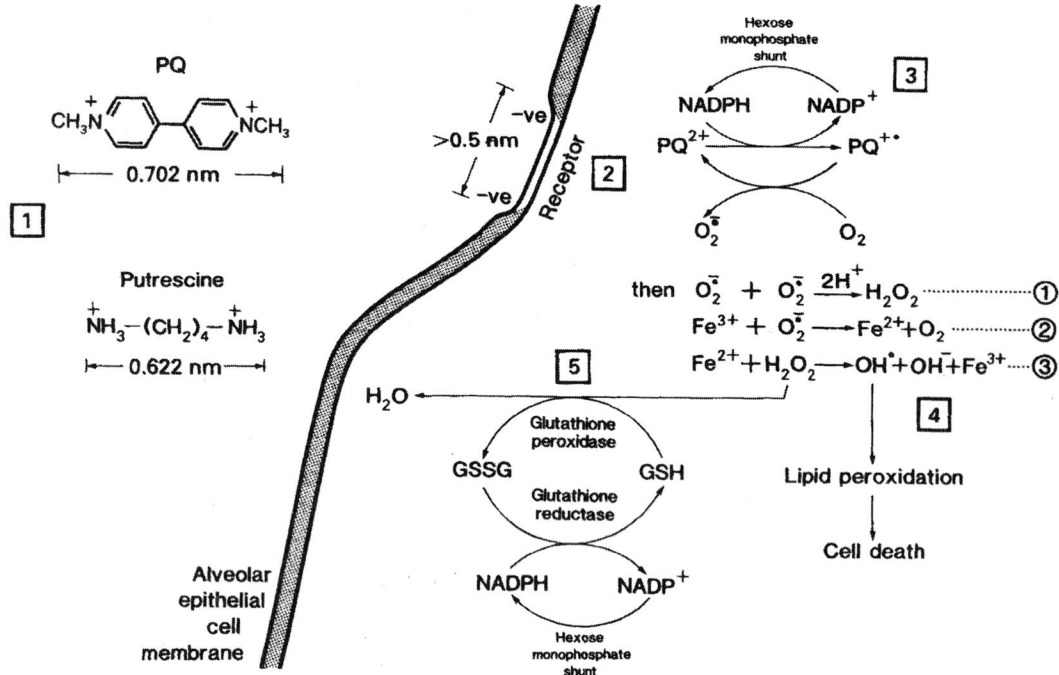

Figure 70.6   Mechanism of toxicity of paraquat. A schematic representation of the mechanism of toxicity of paraquat. 1 = structure of paraquat and putrescine showing the geometric standards of the distance between the nitrogen atoms; 2 = transport system which recognizes paraquat, minimum separation of charge of approximately 0.5 nm; 3 = redox cycling or paraquat utilizing NADPH; 4 = formation of hydroxyl radical leading to lipid peroxidation; 5 = detoxification of H_2O_2 via glutathione reductase/peroxidase couple, utilizing NADPH. From (Smith, 1987). Reproduced with permission from © 1987.

phosphate pathway in the lung has been observed following exposure to paraquat (Bassett and Fisher, 1978; Fisher *et al.*, 1975; Fisher and Reicherter, 1984; Keeling *et al.*, 1982; Rose *et al.*, 1976b). Since this pathway represents the major cellular source of NADPH, it is inferred that this response represents an attempt by lung cells to maintain their levels of reducing equivalents under conditions of oxidative stress. In those cells in which paraquat is accumulated, the concentration may be very high and result in very fast rates of NADPH oxidation. If the rate of consumption exceeds the rate of formation via the pentose phosphate pathway, the concentration of NADPH will fall below that required to maintain cell viability. Witschi *et al.* (1977) first demonstrated that the NADPH/NADP$^+$ ratio in the lungs of rats dosed iv with paraquat was decreased, suggesting that oxidation of the reduced nucleotide had occurred. Later studies by Keeling and Smith (1982) demonstrated that the shift in NADPH/NADP$^+$ ratio in the lung following sc administration of paraquat was the result of NADPH loss from the lung. A consequence of depletion of cellular NADPH is that the cell shuts down it synthetic pathways which are dependent on this nucleotide, such as the synthesis of fatty acids (Keeling *et al.*, 1982). A loss of NADPH may also have particular importance for alveolar type II cells which produce pulmonary surfactant (Brigelius *et al.*, 1986).

NADPH is also consumed in an attempt by the lung to detoxify hydrogen peroxide that is formed via the glutathione peroxidase/reductase enzyme system (Fig. 70.6) to regenerate

reduced glutathione (GSH) from its oxidized form (GSSG). In general large changes in lung GSH and GSSG are not seen after paraquat administration (Bus *et al.*, 1976a; Keeling and Smith, 1982; Shu *et al.*, 1979; Reddy *et al.*, 1977). This may explain why lipid peroxidation has not been conclusively demonstrated *in vivo* as this would not become apparent until both NADPH and GSH were markedly reduced. However, formation of protein mixed disulphides is increased in the lung *in vivo* (Keeling *et al.*, 1982; Keeling and Smith, 1982) and in perfused liver (Brigelius *et al.*, 1982). These changes in protein mixed disulphides in the lung are presumably a response to oxidative stress and may not be critical to the cellular toxicity. This notion is supported by studies with the bipyridyl diquat which can undergo redox cycling in the lung (Rose *et al.*, 1976b; Witschi *et al.*, 1977). Diquat also produced increases in protein mixed disulphide content in the lung without affecting NADPH content at a dose that did not cause lung injury (Keeling and Smith, 1982). This indicates that NADPH depletion subsequent to redox cycling is a critical step in the mechanism of paraquat toxicity.

70.2.17   THE ROLE OF MITOCHONDRIA IN THE TOXICITY

Another hypothesis that has been proposed is that paraquat toxicity is due to mitochondrial damage, based on morphological findings of early mitochondrial changes in alveolar type II cells

(Hirai *et al.*, 1985). Ultrastructural studies of the time course of development of paraquat-induced lung injury have also reported early changes to mitochondria such as swelling and altered staining density (Keeling *et al.*, 1981; Smith and Heath, 1974a; Sykes *et al.*, 1977). These mitochondrial changes were also observed in the lungs of rats exposed to paraquat and 85% oxygen, which enhances paraquat toxicity to the lung (Keeling *et al.*, 1981). However, as discussed with regard to the lipid peroxidation hypothesis, the question is: are the effects on mitochondria a cause, or a consequence, of paraquat toxicity? Early studies with isolated liver mitochondria reported only minor changes in mitochondria respiration by paraquat (Gage, 1968b). More recent studies have reported that paraquat cation can be reduced by NADH-ubiquinone oxidoreductase (Complex I) located on the inner mitochondrial membrane (Fukushima *et al.*, 1993; Shimada *et al.*, 1998). These authors also showed that paraquat was able to stimulate lipid peroxidation in submitochondrial particles (Yamada and Fukushima, 1993). These findings show that mitochondria have the potential to generate superoxide anion from paraquat provided it can gain access. In general, studies with intact mitochondria support the orginal findings of Gage (1968b) showing that little or no effects are seen (Costantini *et al.*, 1995; Lambert and Bondy, 1989) unless very high concentrations of paraquat are present (Kopazyk-Locke, 1977; Yamamoto *et al.*, 1987; Thakar and Hassan, 1988; Palmeira *et al.*, 1995). Paraquat has been shown to induce a Ca^{2+}-dependent permeability transition of the inner mitochondrial membrane leading to membrane depolarization, uncoupling, and matrix swelling in isolate rat liver mitochondria (Costantini *et al.*, 1995). This opening of the membrane permeability pore does not occur in the absence of added Ca^{2+} and requires the presence of rotenone, leading one to question the relevance of this observation to the *in vivo* situation. It seems likely that any intracellular increases in Ca^{2+} would only occur once paraquat had entered the lung cell, undergone redox cycling, and altered mixed disulphide status. In summary, mitochondrial damage has been observed in the lung prior to cell death; it seems likely that this response is secondary to changes taking place in the cytosol.

70.2.18 THE INVOLVEMENT OF OXYGEN

As discussed earlier, the redox cycling of paraquat to form superoxide anion requires oxygen and hence oxygen plays a critical role in the toxic process. It has been known for many years that hyperoxia is toxic to the lung, causing damage to endothelial cells through a mechanism that involves the formation of reactive oxygen species (Frank and Massaro, 1979; Jenkinson, 1982). One of the therapeutic measures for anoxia in human cases of paraquat poisoning was the addition of air supplemented with oxygen (see treatment of human poisoning). However, it has been shown that increasing the oxygen concentration potentiates the lethality of paraquat to rats (Douze and van Heijst, 1977; Fisher *et al.*, 1973; Keeling *et al.*, 1981; Kehrer *et al.*, 1979) by increasing the injury to the lung. The

converse is also true; rats exposed to paraquat in a hypoxic environment are protected relative to those exposed to paraquat in air (Rhodes *et al.*, 1976). Detailed histopathology on the lungs of rats exposed to paraquat alone or paraquat in an atmosphere of 85% oxygen showed that the damage was primarily localized to the alveolar type I and II cells with little evidence of endothelial cell damage, showing that oxygen potentiated paraquat toxicity (Keeling *et al.*, 1981). These findings have recently been reproduced using isolated rat and human alveolar type II cells exposed to either paraquat in air or paraquat and increasing concentrations of oxygen. Increasing the oxygen concentration in the atmosphere potentiated the toxicity of paraquat, while lowering the oxygen concentration to 10% afforded some protection (Hoet *et al.*, 1997). The mechanism underlying this synergistic effect of oxygen on paraquat toxicity is not entirely clear. It seems unlikely that oxygen would normally be rate limiting for paraquat to redox cycle. A more likely explanation is that the cellular defense mechanisms that protect against oxygen and paraquat toxicity are more rapidly overwhelmed.

In summary, the key events leading to cellular toxicity are (1) accumulation of paraquat into the cell and (2) its ability to redox cycle and produce oxidative stress. It seems likely that a combination of depletion of NADPH plus the generation of hydroxyl radical leading to lipid peroxidation and mitochondrial dysfunction is involved but the precise temporal relationships have not as yet been established.

70.2.19 EFFECTS ON THE KIDNEY

The major route of elimination for paraquat once it has entered the bloodstream is via the kidneys where it is actively secreted by organic cation transport systems (see review by Chan *et al.*, 1998). This process becomes saturated at fairly low plasma concentrations (3–4 nmol/ml; 0.5–0.7 µg/ml) in the rat (Chan *et al.*, 1997). At higher plasma concentrations paraquat is nephrotoxic. Large oral or systemic doses administered to rats or mice produce morphological changes to the proximal renal tubules, including hydropic degeneration with occasional evidence of necrotic epithelial cells and of renal tubular regeneration (Clark *et al.*, 1966; Lock and Ishmael, 1979). Chronic exposure to mice via their drinking water showed ultrastructural evidence for proliferation of smooth endoplasmic reticulum and the presence of lipid containing bodies in proximal tubule cells (Fowler and Brooks, 1971). Renal tubular necrosis is more marked in the dog and rabbit following large toxic doses with clear evidence of degeneration of proximal tubular cells with the presence of casts in the tubular lumen (Clark *et al.*, 1966; Giri *et al.*, 1982; McElligott, 1972; Nagata *et al.*, 1992a; Yonemitsu, 1986). Prior to the onset of renal tubular necrosis, paraquat-induced renal functional changes occur including diuresis, albuminuria, glucosuria, and elevations in plasma urea and creatinine in the rat (Lock and Ishmael, 1979), dog (Giri *et al.*, 1982; Nagata *et al.*, 1992a), and cynomologus monkey (Purser and Rose, 1979). The precise mechanism of renal functional impairment is not known; it probably involves altered renal hemodynamics as well as accumulation of paraquat into proximal renal tubules leading to cellular necrosis. There is some evidence that paraquat may reduce renal blood flow based on the finding of elevated renal plasma renin activity in the dog after dosing (Giri *et al.*, 1982) and hypovolaemia in the rat (Lock, 1979). Paraquat is thought to enter renal tubular cells by an organic cation transport system, thereby enabling it to concentrate to many times that present in the plasma (Chan *et al.*, 1996a, 1996b, 1997; Ecker *et al.*, 1975a; Groves *et al.*, 1995; Hawksworth *et al.*, 1981; Lock and Ishmael, 1979; Wright and Wunz, 1995). The accumulation can be blocked by other organic cations such as tetraethylammonium and quinine but is not affected by the polyamines, putrescine, or spermine (Chan *et al.*, 1996a; Groves *et al.*, 1995). Thus the accumulation of paraquat into renal tubular cells occurs via a different transport system to that which leads to its accumulation in the lung. Once inside a renal tubular cell paraquat can redox cycle (Baldwin *et al.*, 1975; Tomita, 1991), producing superoxide anion and hence trigger the cascade of biochemical events leading to cytotoxicity similar to that discussed for the lung (Lock and Ishmael, 1979; Molck and Friis, 1997).

Regardless of the mechanism, the consequence of a reduced renal excretion is that more paraquat is available in the plasma to accumulate into the lung. Thus, maintenance of renal function to facilitate paraquat excretion from the body is critically important for cases of human poisoning (see later).

70.2.20 EFFECTS ON THE CENTRAL NERVOUS SYSTEM

No signs of neurotoxicity or neuropathological changes have been reported following oral gavage or dietary administration of paraquat to rodents or dogs (IPCS, 1984). Paraquat as a di-cation does not readily cross the blood–brain barrier and enter the rat brain after either oral or systemic administration (Corasaniti *et al.*, 1991; Corasaniti and Nistico, 1993; Dey *et al.*, 1990; Naylor *et al.*, 1995; Rose *et al.*, 1976a; Widdowson *et al.*, 1996a, b). The concentration associated with the rat brain is always lower than that in the plasma and decreases with time. The initial concentration detected in the brain may be largely associated with blood (Dey *et al.*, 1990; Naylor *et al.*, 1995; Rose *et al.*, 1976a). Paraquat was, however, detected in brain regions such as the olfactory bulb, area postrema, and hypothalamus, which do not possess an effective blood–brain barrier. Autoradiographic studies have detected paraquat in these regions and in the cerebrospinal fluid (ventricles and choroid plexus) but the concentrations were low and only represent a very small percentage of the administered dose, about 0.05% at the time of maximal blood concentration 1 h after dosing (Naylor *et al.*, 1995; Waddell and Marlowe, 1980). Immunohistochemical localization of paraquat in rat brain has shown it is present in capillary walls and glial cells but was not detected in neurones (Nagao *et al.*, 1991).

Recent studies in the rat, using parenteral doses of paraquat at or above the MLD (20–100 mg/kg, ip), produced signs of neurotoxicity with muscle fasciculation, some tremors and "wet-dog" shakes, and at the higher doses myoclonus, typically within 30 min of dosing (Bagetta *et al.*, 1992; Corasaniti *et al.*, 1992; Hara *et al.*, 1993), which is the time of peak blood and brain concentrations. These authors also reported neuronal cell necrosis in the pyriform cortex of these animals 24 h after dosing (Bagetta *et al.*, 1992; Corasaniti *et al.*, 1992). The neuronal cell necrosis could be reduced by administration of atropine but not methylatropine (Bagetta *et al.*, 1992), suggesting some involvement of central muscarinic receptors. No effects were seen after 5 mg/kg ip paraquat. The basis for the selective injury to the pyriform cortex is currently not known, but it does not reflect the brain region with the highest concentration of paraquat (Corasaniti and Nistico, 1993; Naylor *et al.*, 1995). Others have reported that paraquat (20 mg/kg, sc) does not produce neuronal cell necrosis in the pyriform cortex of perfused-fixed material from rats 24 and 48 h after dosing (Naylor *et al.*, 1995; Widdowson *et al.*, 1996a) and have suggested the effect reported by the Italian group may be a fixation artifact. The precise basis for this variance is currently not understood. Similarly, daily oral dosing of paraquat at 5 mg/kg/day for 14 days to rats produced no evidence of neuronal cell necrosis, despite particular emphasis on the pathology of the pyriform cortex, nigro-stratial region, and hypothalamus or behavioral changes indicative of neurotoxicity (Widdowson *et al.*, 1996b).

Direct administration of paraquat into the ventricles or infusion into certain brain regions produced signs of neurotoxicity in rats which were associated with neuronal cell damage (Bagetta *et al.*, 1992, 1994; Calo *et al.*, 1990; Corasaniti *et al.*, 1992; De Gori *et al.*, 1988; Liou *et al.*, 1996; Liu *et al.*, 1995; Yoshimura *et al.*, 1993). These effects were seen at low doses of paraquat 2–20 μg injections. These observations lend support to the view that little paraquat enters the brain following systemic administration (20 mg/kg, sc or 4000 μg/200 g rat) or oral administration (126 mg/kg or 25,200 μg/200 g rat) as no neuronal cell toxicity was seen at these doses.

Comparisons have been drawn to the structural similarity between paraquat and 1-methyl-4-phenylpyridinium ion (MPP^+), the active metabolite of 1-methyl-4-phenyl-1,2,3,6-tetrahydropyridine (MPTP) which can induce a Parkinson-like syndrome in monkeys and humans. Administration of MPTP to susceptible animal species produces selective damage to dopaminergic neurons in the substantia nigra leading to a marked loss of dopamine and clear signs of neurotoxicity.

The mechanism for MPTP toxicity (see Markey *et al.*, 1986; Tipton and Singer, 1993) is due to its ability to cross the blood–brain barrier and enter glial cells where it can undergo oxidative metabolism by the enzyme monoamine oxidase B to form MPP^+. This metabolite then accumulates selectively into dopaminergic neurons via the dopamine transport system, leading to inhibition of mitochondrial respiration which ultimately leads to the demise of the neurone. Structure-activity relationships suggest that, despite their apparent similarity, paraquat and MPTP are two very different chemicals (Koller, 1986). MPTP is uncharged and lipophilic and thereby able to cross the blood–brain barrier, whereas paraquat is charged and hydrophilic and does not readily enter the brain. Also, MPTP is a monoamine whose metabolite MPP$^+$, the proximate toxin, is able to use a specific uptake system, particularly in the substantia nigra, whereas paraquat is a diamine. It is also very relevant that administration of MPP$^+$ to experimental animals did not produce neurotoxicity, due to its poor entry across the blood–brain barrier (Tipton and Singer, 1993). Thus like paraquat, MPP$^+$ does not readily enter the brain. Consistent with this, systemic administration of paraquat to C57 black mice or rats did not lead to dopamine depletion or neuronal cell death in the striatum, like that seen with MPTP (Perry *et al.*, 1986; Widdowson *et al.*, 1996b). Others have reported changes in brain dopamine content following paraquat administration to mice (Endo *et al.*, 1988; Fredriksson *et al.*, 1993). In the latter case, paraquat was administered to pups on days 10 and 11 after birth at a time when the brain is undergoing rapid growth and hence might be a more vulnerable to chemical insult. The authors reported a small loss of dopamine and its metabolites and a decreased behavioral activity when measured at about 4 months of age (Fredriksson *et al.*, 1993). This suggests that the developing brain is potentially more sensitive to insult. However, adverse effects have not been detected in developmental toxicity or multigeneration studies, where paraquat was given to pregnant rats and their offspring (see earlier section). Attempts to reproduce the findings of Fredriksson *et al.* (1993) in C57 black mice, in another laboratory, have not proved possible (David Ray, personal communication). Thus, paraquat as a charged di-cation does not readily enter the brain. The behavioral effects observed in rats only occur at lethal systemic doses.

70.2.21 EFFECTS ON OTHER ORGANS

Following oral ingestion of paraquat by humans, ulceration of the pharyngeal, oesophageal, and gastric mucosa has been reported (see Section 70.3). In animal studies there is often no direct contact with these tissues when gavage dosing is employed. However, focal necrosis of the gastrointestinal tract has been observed in primates, demonstrating the topical irritant nature of high oral doses of paraquat (Murray and Gibson, 1972).

Paraquat administration to the rat produced an increased synthesis of liver glycogen and an increase in blood glucose that appeared to be mediated by the adrenal, since adrenalectomy prevented these changes (Rose *et al.*, 1974b). These effects seen following paraquat and the related bipyridyl diquat are thought to be due to catecholamine release and high circulating concentrations of corticosteroids (Rose *et al.*, 1974b). This response is thought to be unrelated to the pulmonary damage produced by paraquat but may account for some of the effects seen with paraquat on the adrenal and lymphoid tissues such as the spleen and thymus (Butler and Kleinerman, 1971; Clark *et al.*, 1966; Fisher *et al.*, 1973). The increase in circulating corticosterone seen with paraquat can also be prevented by lesioning the area postrema (Edmonds and Edwards, 1996). This area of the brain also controls the taste aversion to paraquat seen in rats (Dey *et al.*, 1987; Edmonds and Edwards, 1996).

Liver damage is not a major finding after paraquat administration: after large doses some central lobular necrosis has been reported in most species examined (Cagen *et al.*, 1976; Clark *et al.*, 1966; Giri *et al.*, 1982; Murray and Gibson, 1972; Nagata *et al.*, 1992a). Since paraquat is delivered to the liver following dosing and hepatocytes possess the relevant enzymes to facilitate redox cycling, presumably paraquat does not normally accumulate in hepatocytes to a sufficient concentration to overwhelm the protective antioxidant defence enzymes and produce necrosis. However, both mice and rats made selenium deficient show marked liver injury following paraquat administration (Burk *et al.*, 1980; Cagen and Gibson, 1977) supporting the view that selenium dependent enzymes such as glutathione peroxidase play an important protective role. These findings are consistent with recent studies using transgenic mice where glutathione peroxidase has either been deleted or overexpressed, showing that this selenium-dependent enzyme plays a key role in paraquat-induced tissue injury (Cheng *et al.*, 1998; de Haan *et al.*, 1998).

70.2.22 TREATMENT OF POISONING IN ANIMALS

Over the past 30 years a variety of attempts to modify the toxicity of paraquat in experimental animals have been examined. To date the only approach that has been shown to clearly reduce mortality in rats is purgation of the gastrointestinal tract with a diatomaceous clay (bentonite or Fuller's earth) along with a cathartic (e.g., magnesium sulphate) (Clark, 1971; Smith *et al.*, 1974). Attempts to modify paraquat toxicity have been based on its known mechanism of toxicity and will be briefly discussed under the following headings: (*a*) prevention of absorption from the gastrointestinal tract, (*b*) removal from the bloodstream, (*c*) prevention of accumulation into the lung, (*d*) attempts to scavenge oxygen free radicals, and (*e*) attempts to prevent lung fibrosis. This aspect of paraquat toxicity has been reviewed by others. See Bateman (1987), Meredith and Vale (1995), Jaeger *et al.* (1995), and Section 70.3 on human poisoning in this review.

70.2.23 ADSORPTION FROM THE GASTROINTESTINAL TRACT

As discussed earlier, paraquat is poorly absorbed from the gastrointestinal tract and therefore attempts to reduce its entry into the bloodstream could be beneficial. Peak blood levels are detected within 60–90 min in rats, dogs, and monkeys (Figs. 70.2 and 70.3). Therefore any interventions must be taken quickly after poisoning if they are to be effective. The bipyridilium herbicides have been shown to bind very strongly to soil and clay minerals (Knight and Tomlinson, 1967). Clark (1971) demonstrated that bentonite and Fuller's earth where able to reduce mortality in rats given a lethal dose of paraquat when delayed for 2 or 3 h after paraquat administration. Smith *et al.* (1974) subsequently showed that repeated doses of a bentonite, castor oil, and magnesium sulphate mixture protected rats against the lethal effects of paraquat when given 4 h after exposure and this regimen also reduced mortality when delayed for as long as 10 h after exposure. The basis for the protection was shown to be due to a reduction in the concentration of paraquat in the bloodstream and a concomitant reduction in the amount accumulated into the lung (Smith et al., 1974). Several other absorbent or binding agents have been examined. Activated charcoal was shown to be very effective in rats (Okonek et al., 1982) and in mice in combination with magnesium citrate, the magnesium salt affording some protection on its own (Gaudreault et al., 1985). Kayexalate (sodium polystyrene sulphate), Kalimate (calcium polystyrene sulphate), sodium dextrin sulphate, sodium glucose sulphate, and a variety of alkylsulphates and alkylsulphonates have been shown to afford some protection in rats and mice (Nokata et al., 1984; Tsuchiya et al., 1995; Ukai et al., 1987). The use of this approach in clinical practice will be discussed in more detail later.

70.2.24 REMOVAL FROM THE BLOODSTREAM

Both peritoneal dialysis and hemodialysis have been suggested for removing paraquat from the bloodstream and thereby reducing availability to the lungs. Charcoal hemoperfusion was initially demonstrated to remove paraquat from the blood of beagle dogs (Maini and Winchester, 1975). Hemoperfusion appeared to reduce mortality in dogs when given within 12 h of administration of paraquat (Widdop et al., 1975), although more recent studies in the dog have indicated that unless started within 2 h of exposure it is unlikely to reduce the paraquat content in the lungs (Pond et al., 1993).

70.2.25 PREVENTION OF ACCUMULATION INTO THE LUNG

Paraquat is actively transported into alveolar type I and II cells where it accumulates. Studies in vitro using polyamines, diaminoalkanes, and a number of other chemicals have identified chemicals that can reduce paraquat accumulation (Gordonsmith et al., 1983; Lock et al., 1976; Maling et al., 1978; Ross and Krieger, 1981; Smith and Wyatt, 1981). However, attempts to reduce paraquat mortality in rats with these agents have failed to demonstrate significant protection (Dunbar et al., 1988; Maling et al., 1978).

Another approach has been to use antibodies to paraquat (polyclonal, monoclonal, or specific Fab fragments) to try and reduce toxicity to the lung. This approach has been shown to reduce paraquat uptake and cytotoxicity in rat lung slices and isolated alveolar type II cells (Chen et al., 1994; Wright et al., 1987a). However, treatment of paraquat-intoxicated mice (Cadot et al., 1985; Wright et al., 1987b) or rats (Nagao et al., 1989) by immunotherapy did not reduce the concentration of paraquat in the lung or affect the mortality.

70.2.26 FREE RADICAL SCAVENGING

As discussed earlier, once inside a cell paraquat can redox cycle and produce superoxide anion, singlet oxygen, and hydroxyl radicals. Many studies have been aimed at attempting to scavenge the radicals formed to reduce or protect the lung injury. In many of these cases significant protection can be demonstrated using isolated cell systems, but in whole animals the protection is limited or equivocal.

Superoxide dismutase has been reported to increase survival in rats exposed to paraquat (Autor, 1974; Wasserman and Block, 1978), while other studies have failed to confirm these observations (Frank, 1983; Patterson and Rhodes, 1982). The short plasma half-life of exogenous superoxide dismutase and the fact that it does not enter cells accounts for the lack of protection. A more recent report indicated that a low molecular weight metalloporphyrin superoxide dismutase mimetic afforded some protection against paraquat-induced injury to the lung, but its effect on mortality was not examined and its effect is likely to have been marginal (Day and Crapo, 1996).

Desferrioxamine (DF) is an iron chelating agent which has been used to scavenge free iron and thereby reduce hydroxyl radical production. Studies in mice suggested that DF given 24 h before and regularly after an acute dose of paraquat reduced mortality (Kohen and Chevion, 1985). In this same model these workers showed that iron increased paraquat toxicity. In rats, however, DF appeared to afford no protection (Hoffer et al., 1992; Osheroff et al., 1985). Van Asbeck et al. (1989) gave DF by continuous infusion to vitamin E deficient rats and showed it prevented the lung injury and hence reduced mortality. This group also examined the effect of DF and CP51 an hydroxypyridin-4-one iron chelator in rats with a normal vitamin E status and found no protection with DF while CP51 increased survival (Van der Wal et al., 1992).

Xanthine oxidase inhibitors may also reduce superoxide anion formation and rats fed a diet rich in tungstenate showed a better survival following paraquat exposure than rats fed the diet alone (Kitazawa et al., 1991).

Clofibrate induces hepatic peroxisomes in rodents and thereby increases hepatic catalase activity, and it was postulated that a similar effect in the lung might afford protection against paraquat toxicity. Prior administration of clofibrate to rats for 6 days followed by paraquat afforded significant protection. However, when clofibrate was administered after paraquat it gave no protection (Frank et al., 1982).

Vitamin E is a lipid soluble antioxidant and radical scavenger. Some early studies showed that vitamin E deficient animals were more susceptible to paraquat than those with a normal vitamin E status (Block, 1979; Bus et al., 1975). Acute administration of vitamin E to normal mice or rats did not, however, significantly protect against the toxicity (Bus et al., 1976a; Redetzki et al., 1980) even when instilled into the trachea in a liposome either alone or in combination with reduced glutathione (Suntres and Shek, 1995, 1996).

The protective effect of selenium has been reported, animals fed selenium deficient diets being more sensitive to paraquat toxicity (Cagen and Gibson, 1977; Omaye *et al.*, 1978). This is probably related to the selenium-dependant enzyme glutathione peroxidase which plays an important role in protecting cells against oxidative stress. Evidence that glutathione peroxidase plays a key role in protecting animals against paraquat toxicity comes from recent studies in transgenic mice where deletion of this enzyme enhances toxicity while addition affords some protection (Cheng *et al.*, 1998; de Haan *et al.*, 1998).

Vitamin C, water soluble antioxidant, has provided equivocal data with one study suggesting it might protect while others showed it either had no effect or enhanced paraquat toxicity (Matkovics *et al.*, 1980; McArn *et al.*, 1980; Minakata *et al.*, 1996; Montgomery *et al.*, 1982; Sullivan and Montgomery, 1984). A combination of vitamin C and riboflavin in rats produced a significant improvement in paraquat mortality (Schvartsman *et al.*, 1984), while vitamin C or riboflavin alone was not protective. These authors suggested that perhaps the combination of antioxidant plus an effect of riboflavin on glutathione reductase activity may have contributed to the protection.

Niacin has been reported to modestly reduce paraquat mortality in rats. This may be due to an effect of niacin on NAD synthesis which is reduced by paraquat (Brown *et al.*, 1981); however, subsequent studies were unable to confirm any protection with niacin (Hooper *et al.*, 1983).

A number of sulphydryl compounds have been examined based on their antioxidant ability, and on an early observation by Bus *et al.* (1976b) showing that diethylmaleate, which depletes glutathione, enhanced paraquat toxicity. In general precursors of glutathione synthesis which increase intracellular cysteine content have been shown by some workers to provide some increased survival in mice or rats, while others have found these reagents to produce equivocal effects. The protection may be due to alteration of the pharmacokinetics of paraquat or induction of some of the enzymes involved in providing protection against free radical damage. The following have been examined *N*-acetylcysteine (Cramp, 1985; Hoffer *et al.*, 1993; Hybertson *et al.*, 1995; Shum *et al.*, 1982; Wegener *et al.*, 1988), glutathione (Matkovics *et al.*, 1980; Szabo *et al.*, 1986), cysteine and cystine (Kojima *et al.*, 1992; Szabo *et al.*, 1986), L-2-oxothiazolidine-4-carboxylate (Ali *et al.*, 1996); D-penicillamine (Szabo *et al.*, 1986), and sulphite or thiosulphate (Yamamoto, 1993).

The effect of the lung-surfactant stimulating drug ambroxol has been examined in rats and was shown to increase the rate of survival after paraquat (Salmona *et al.*, 1992) while Nemery *et al.* (1992) found no protective effect.

70.2.27 PREVENTION OF LUNG FIBROSIS

Since delayed deaths with pulmonary fibrosis are a characteristic of paraquat poisoning in experimental animals and humans (see later) a number of agents have been examined to ameliorate the fibrotic response. Immunosuppressants such as methylprednisolone, dexamethasone, and cyclophosphamide have been examined in experimental animals and in general they were either without effect (Seidenfeld, 1985) or only afforded some protection when give prior to paraquat, but not when given simultaneously (Kitazawa *et al.*, 1988; Reddy *et al.*, 1976; Smith and Watson, 1987). Lung irradiation (Saenghirunvattana *et al.*, 1992) and collagen synthesis inhibitors such as D,L-3,4-dehydroproline (Akahori and Oehme, 1983) were not effective in reducing paraquat lung damage.

A recent suggestion has been mechanical ventilation with additional inhalation of nitric oxide, based on nitric oxide's vasodilatory effect on the lungs (Berisha *et al.*, 1994). This approach has not been examined in experimental animals but some clinical experience in combination with other antidotes has been examined (see later).

In summary, removal of the ingested material by emesis and purgation of the gastrointestinal tract is currently the most effective method after paraquat exposure in experimental animals. As discussed later, a cocktail of many of these approaches is often used in cases of human poisonings.

70.3 TOXICITY TO HUMANS

70.3.1 EXPERIMENTAL EXPOSURE

The percutaneous absorption of radiolabelled paraquat has been determined in humans (Wester *et al.*, 1984). Following application of 9 $\mu g/cm^2$ the amount absorbed was 0.29% for the leg, 0.23% for the hand, and 0.29% for the forearm. This gave a calculated *in vivo* absorption rate of 0.03 $\mu g/cm^2$ for the 24 h exposure period. Paraquat was thus only minimally absorbed, especially in comparison with other commonly available pesticides (Wester and Maibach, 1985).

70.3.2 ACCIDENTAL AND INTENTIONAL POISONING

The first case fatalities described involved accidental ingestion of the 20% paraquat concentrate (Bullivant, 1966; Campbell, 1968; Oreopoulos *et al.*, 1968; Swan, 1967). A major source of poisoning was the decanting into unlabelled drinks bottles and other containers (Malone *et al.*, 1971). Throughout the 1970s the number of reported cases continued to rise; however, there was a noticeable shift in the circumstances. For example, in the Republic of Ireland the number of accidents due to decanting decreased between 1967 and 1977 from 45% to 4% of total cases (Fitzgerald *et al.*, 1978b). Further analysis of the circumstances of poisoning showed that before 1975 there was an approximately equal proportion of accidental and suicidal cases, whereas after that date suicides accounted for over 90% of cases and all fatalities. A similar pattern was described in Northern Ireland (Carson and Carson, 1976) and the United Kingdom (Bramley and Hart, 1983; Howard, 1979a). A review of deaths from pesticide poisoning in the United Kingdom between 1945 and 1989 showed that the number of paraquat-associated deaths rose continuously from 1973 onward and peaked in 1981. Since then, the number has steadily declined to pre-1973 levels (Casey and Vale, 1994).

With the increasing use of paraquat throughout the world during the 1970s and 1980s it became apparent that the problem of accidental and intentional poisoning had shifted away from the British Isles and Europe (Onyon and Volans, 1987). A high incidence was reported in particular from Asian countries such as Japan (Naito and Yamashita, 1987), Malaysia (Amarasingham and Lee, unpublished report), Sri Lanka (Hettiarachi and Kodithuwakku, 1989), and Fiji (Goundar, 1984). Paraquat was also the most widely used chemical suicidal agent in Trinidad (Hutchinson *et al.*, 1991) and Surinam (Perriens *et al.*, 1989).

In Costa Rica, Wesseling *et al.* (1993) examined records of the Forensic Medical Department which showed that over the 7 year period from 1980 to 1986 a total of 169 fatalities had occurred from paraquat poisoning. The pathologists had classified the overwhelming majority as suicide-related, although the authors suggested that misclassification occurred in some cases. However, a detailed examination of case records of the Forensic Medical Department between 1990 and 1992 showed that 74 out of 76 paraquat related fatalities were due to suicide from oral ingestion, with 2 fatalities occurring from accidental ingestion (Vargas and Sabapathy, 1995). Government statistics for 1995 and 1996 showed that 62 out of a total of 72 pesticide related fatalities (no compound mentioned) were due to suicide and 2 due to homicide, 8 fatalities were classified as nonoccupational, and there were no occupationally related fatalities (Ministerio de Salud, 1997).

Paraquat poisoning is uncommon in the United States the world's largest market for paraquat-containing products. A 10 year survey of calls to U.S. poison centers showed that paraquat (and diquat)-related enquiries accounted for only around 0.01% of the total (Hall, 1995). Most cases showed either no or minor symptoms, with less than two fatalities occurring annually, almost all of them related to suicides.

Data on mortality from paraquat poisoning are difficult to compare because of differences in circumstances, treatment, and reporting systems. In a collection of data from 14 publications compiled by the International Programme on Chemical Safety (IPCS, 1984), mortality ranged from 36% to 100%, with an overall mortality of 48% (446 of 925 cases). A difference in mortality between ingestion of the liquid concentrate (20% paraquat ion) and a granular product (2.5% paraquat, 2.5% diquat) has been described by some authors. Park *et al.* (1975) found that the fatality rate was 15 of 23 (65%) in patients who had ingested liquid concentrate and 3 of 8 (38%) in patients ingesting the granular product. Fitzgerald and Barniville (1978) reported no deaths in 14 patients ingesting the granular product compared to a mortality of 74% in 118 cases of ingestion of the liquid concentrate. In the series published by Howard (1979a) there were 36 deaths from 41 cases (88%) where liquid concentrate was ingested, and 5 deaths from 27 cases (19%) involving the granular product. These differences are largely a reflection of the size of dose ingested.

While suicidal ingestion of paraquat concentrate accounts for most of the recorded fatalities, the problem of accidental

ingestion prompted the principal manufacturer of paraquat to introduce formulation changes to the liquid concentrate in the late 1970s and early 1980s (Sabapathy, 1995). A blue color was added to prevent confusion with drinks, a stenching agent was introduced to alert users, and an emetic was included. In addition, packaging and labelling was improved to prevent decanting of the product, and education and training efforts were directed in particular toward smallholder farmers in developing countries, where the majority of incidents occurred. The effect of these efforts is believed to have made a significant contribution to the decrease of accidental paraquat ingestion in many countries (Sabapathy, 1995; Wesseling *et al.*, 1997).

Although ingestion is the route of entry into the body for the overwhelming majority of poisoning cases, there are a few reports of systemic effects from inhalation and dermal exposure (localized skin, eye, and upper respiratory effects will be discussed in Section 70.3.4). Inhalation exposure is not a prominent feature in paraquat poisoning cases because of the extremely low (not measurable) vapor pressure of paraquat. Respiratory exposure to paraquat during spray applications is very low because the large droplet size will prevent the material from going beyond the nasal cavity. Concerns about oral exposure to spray droplets as a result of drainage into the oral cavity and swallowing appear unwarranted because the typical spray concentration of paraquat for hand-held spray applications is 0.1–0.2% and would thus require a dose of 1–2 liters of spray solution directly into the nose and into the oral cavity to achieve a lethal dose (Howard, 1980). It is therefore not surprising that there are no reports in the published literature of deaths arising from inhalation exposure. A review of 30 cases of presumed inhalation exposure found no evidence for systemic poisoning (Vlachos and Kontoes, 1987). Where paraquat was measured it was undetectable or at the limit of detection. Patients were either asymptomatic or had nonspecific symptoms such as headache, nausea, or feeling unwell. Two patients described nosebleeds. In two patients who presented with cough and fever, pneumonia was established as clinical diagnosis. A recent review (Garnier, 1995) concluded that there was only one convincing reported case of possible systemic poisoning following inhalational exposure to paraquat and signs of toxicity were very mild and the patient made a full recovery (Fitzgerald *et al.*, 1978a). In this case, a 43 year old market gardener sprayed a "stronger than usual" solution (no details of spray concentration available) in a greenhouse and complained of a burning sensation in throat and mouth and weakness. There was biochemical evidence of mild renal failure, but liver function tests and chest x-ray were normal. Paraquat tested positive in urine. Renal function parameters returned to normal within 10 days after exposure.

It has already been mentioned that paraquat absorption across intact human skin is extremely low both *in vitro* (Walker *et al.*, 1983) and *in vivo* (Wester *et al.*, 1984). In 15 cases of single exposures of the skin and eyes during work with paraquat solutions only localized lesions (dermatitis, vesicles, bums, conjunctivitis) were found (Hoffer and Taitelmann, 1989). Paraquat was undetectable in plasma except for three cases where it was at the limit of detection. There were no manifestations of systemic toxicity. A small number of case reports describe systemic paraquat poisoning and fatalities from dermal exposure. In six cases there was deliberate or accidental application of paraquat concentrate to the skin, usually in the unfortunate mistaken belief that it could act against parasitic disease (Binns, 1976; Garnier *et al.*, 1994; Ongom *et al.*, 1974; Tungsanga *et al.*, 1983; Wohlfahrt, 1982 (2 cases)). Three cases (Okonek *et al.*, 1983; Waight, 1979; Wesseling *et al.*, 1997) involved widespread accidental contamination of the lower abdomen and legs with the 20% concentrate.

In two cases (Jaros *et al.*, 1978; Levin *et al.*, 1979) it was evident that a far too concentrated paraquat dilution (28 g/l; 2.8% and 40 g/l; 4%, respectively) was applied combined with faulty leaking spray equipment and lack of skin decontamination. In a further case (Athanaselis *et al.*, 1983) it is explicitly claimed that a correct dilution of 0.5% paraquat was used (the maximum recommended rate for knapsack). However, subsequent investigation (Hart, 1984) led to the conclusion that, in fact, a more concentrated paraquat solution, probably in excess of 1.5%, was used.

In one case (Fitzgerald *et al.*, 1978a) the combination of paraquat exposure and pre-existing skin disease caused the death of the person involved, although very few details are given. Another case (Garnier *et al.*, 1994) involved the application of multiple herbicidal mixtures, including paraquat, over several days by a man with a history of psoriasis. This man suffered a febrile lung disease but made a complete recovery.

Four cases involving prolonged skin contact with "diluted" paraquat without pre-existing skin lesions should be mentioned. The two cases described by Wohlfahrt (1982) give very few date which would be useful in this context. In the third case (Papiris *et al.*, 1995), a farmer was exposed for 5–6 h to diluted paraquat from a leaking sprayer which caused burning, blisters, and erosions in his scrotal area. This patient survived after hospital treatment. In the fourth case (Wesseling *et al.*, 1997), a plantation worker experienced chemical burns on his back, scrotum, and inner parts of both thighs after spraying paraquat with a leaking knapsack sprayer for three consecutive days. He subsequently died from interstitial fibrosis of the lung.

Thus, there is no indication that paraquat has caused fatal poisoning through skin contact in normal occupational use. The few cases described in the literature occurred as a result of a combination of factors such as misuse (wrong dilution), pre-existing extensive skin disease, faulty equipment, prolonged extensive skin contact, and disregard of safety procedures (no decontamination following significant exposure).

70.3.3 USE EXPERIENCE

Exposure to paraquat under actual field conditions has been assessed in studies with hand-held (knapsack), vehicle mounted, and aerial applications. Dermal exposure was measured either in patches placed on different body regions or, more recently, using whole body exposure assessments. Inhalation exposure (including oral exposure) was determined using personal air sampling and the air concentration of different particle sizes was measured. Internal dose was assessed using biological monitoring, for which paraquat is an ideal candidate: it is not metabolized, it is rapidly and completely excreted via the kidneys, it is stable in urine, and there are sensitive analytical techniques available. The data from these studies are summarized in Table 70.5.

There is an enormous variation in dermal exposure evident in the studies found in the literature. This is not surprising given the differences in spray strength, volume applied, application technique, environmental conditions, use of personal protective equipment, and differences in study design. Nevertheless, some patterns emerge across the variety of study conditions encountered. It is evident that skin exposure represents by far the most significant route of exposure for paraquat. For hand-held applications, total dermal exposure was more than an order of magnitude higher than exposure to uncovered body parts (Chester and Woollen, 1981; Van Wendel de Joode *et al.*, 1996). A similar difference was seen for vehicle-mounted spray applications (Staiff *et al.*, 1975; Wojeck *et al.*, 1983). The lowest dermal exposure was seen for pilots applying paraquat (Chester and Ward, 1984), whereas the total dermal exposure of flaggers is comparable to exposure of uncovered body parts in other spray applications.

Inhalation exposure was approximately three orders of magnitude lower than skin exposure (Chester and Ward, 1984; Chester and Woollen, 1981; Singmaster and Liu, 1998; Staiff *et al.*, 1975; Van Wendel de Joode *et al.*, 1996; Wojeck *et al.*, 1983). Paraquat proved to be below the limit of detection in most samples. Furthermore, the inhalation potential of respirable droplets was found to be negligible since no respirable paraquat could be measured in the breathing zone of exposed workers (Chester and Ward, 1984). The most recent study (Singmaster and Liu, 1998) showed that even under difficult spraying conditions (heavy exertion while spraying on hillsides) paraquat was below the limit of detection.

Paraquat is an ideal candidate for biological monitoring because it is excreted unchanged in urine, where it is comparatively stable. Most of the worker exposure studies mentioned above included measurement of paraquat in urine. Overall, the paraquat concentration in urine was low, with the majority of samples being below the limit of detection. None of the samples contained paraquat at levels which would be indicative of a risk of poisoning (see below).

Topical effects from contact with paraquat during spray operations can occur due to a delayed caustic action of paraquat as a result of poor working practice and hygiene (Howard, 1980). Discoloration (white bands), paronychia, and partial or complete loss of nails has been described following contact with concentrated (Samman and Johnston, 1969) and prolonged exposure to diluted paraquat solutions (Hearn and Keir, 1971). Upon cessation of exposure, normal nail growth resumes. Irritant dermatitis, burns, and blistering can occur from skin exposure to paraquat concentrate or as a result of prolonged skin contact with contaminated clothing or from leaking spray

Table 70.5
Worker Exposure and Absorption of Paraquat

Reference	Country	Application method	Spray dilution (%w/v)	Dermal exposure (mg/h)	Inhalation exposure (mg/h)	Urine level (mg/l)
Swan, 1969	Malaysia	Hand held	0.05	–	–	<0.01 −0.32
Hogarty, 1976	Ireland	Hand held	–	–	<0.003	ND
Staiff et al., 1975	USA	Vehicle mounted	0.1	0.01–3.4[a]	0–0.002	<0.02
		Hand held	0.2	0.01–0.57[a]	<0.001	<0.02
Chester and Woollen, 1981	Malaysia	Hand held	0.1–0.2	<0.01–12[a] 12–170[b]	0–0.005	<0.05 −0.76
Wojeck et al., 1983	USA	Vehicle mounted	0.05–0.1	7.0–42[a] 12–169[b]	0–0.07	<0.02 −0.03
Chester and Ward, 1984	USA	Aerial	0.3	0.1–2.4[b,c] 0.05–0.26[b,d]	0–0.047[c] 0–0.06[d]	–
Chester et al., 1993	Sri Lanka	Hand held	0.03–0.04	0.94–2.71[b,e]	–	<0.03
Van Wendel de Joode et al., 1996	Costa Rica	Hand held	0.1–0.2	0.2–5.7[a]	0–0.043	<0.03 −0.24
Singmaster and Liu, 1998	Puerto Rico	Hand held	0.1	–	<0.007	–

ND = not detected.
[a] Exposure to uncovered skin.
[b] Total dermal exposure.
[c] Aerial—flagger.
[d] Aerial—pilot.
[e] Mg/g paraquat sprayed.
[f] Extrapolation from indirect measurement using copper as marker.

equipment (Swan, 1969; Van Wendel de Joode et al., 1996). Epistaxis has been described (Swan, 1969; Van Wendel de Joode et al., 1996), most likely from breathing in spray mist or contact with contaminated fingers. No serious or long-term effects have been described. There are a number of case reports of eye damage resulting from splashes with paraquat concentrate (Cant and Lewis, 1968; Deveckova and Mydlik, 1980; Joyce, 1969; Peyresblanques, 1969; Watanabe et al., 1979). Apart from eye irritation and blepharitis, more serious, delayed ocular damage may occur such as destruction of the bulbar and tarsal conjunctiva and erosion of the corneal epithelium. Anterior uveitis has also been noted. Progressive keratitis and decreased visual acuity may occur and persist for several weeks. However, complete restoration of vision is normal.

Attempts have been made to establish the frequency of topical effects from paraquat exposure, particularly for hand-held applications in developing countries. Surveys have been carried out interviewing 400 smallholder farmers using paraquat in Malaysia (Whitaker, 1989a), 365 smallholders in Central America (Whitaker, 1989b), and 732 smallholders in Thailand (Whitaker et al., 1993). These surveys showed that, in general, farmers were aware of the potentially fatal consequences of swallowing small quantities of the concentrate. Spray practices and standards of personal hygiene were generally adequate, although the wider use of gloves and eye protection when handling the concentrate needed to be encouraged. In all three surveys, approximately 10% of respondents had experienced health effects attributed to the use of paraquat. These were predominantly skin irritation (mainly on hands and feet), nausea and headaches associated with the smell of the product (due to the added stenching agent), and, to a lesser extent, eye irritation, nail damage, and epistaxis. Ramasamy and Nursiah (1988) interviewed 1219 Malaysian estate workers, rice farmers, vegetable growers, and smallholders about health effects from pesticide use. They found that exposure to organophosphorous insecticides was associated with giddiness and nausea, whereas the main effects associated with paraquat exposure were eye irritation, nail damage, and nasal bleeding. However, their survey did not establish cause effect relationships with exposure to specific products. Only three cases of hospitalization were described among their study population.

The State of California has probably the most comprehensive surveillance system of pesticide-related illness in the world. Between 1971 and 1985 a total of 231 cases of ill health attributed to paraquat were notified to the Worker Health and Safety Branch, California Department of Food and Agriculture (Weinbaum *et al.*, 1995). Of these, 38.5% were listed as systemic effects (mainly dizziness, nausea, lightheadedness, headache, chest pain, vomiting, and tiredness), 32% were eye effects (burning, itching, redness), 26% were skin effects (rash and irritation, itching) and 3.5% were local respiratory irritant effects (epistaxis, sore throat). There were no cases of pulmonary fibrosis. Analysis of data from 1981 to 1985 showed that the overall incidence of illness was low at 0.6 per 1000 paraquat applications.

Detailed medical surveys have been carried out to determine whether the long term exposure to paraquat leads to chronic health effects in workers and spray applicators. Swan (1969) found no abnormalities in chest radiographs of groups of Malaysian rubber plantation workers during paraquat applications over several weeks. Howard (1979b) studied two groups of paraquat formulation workers in the United Kingdom and Malaysia. Mean exposure duration for the UK workers was 5 years, and 2.3 years for the Malaysian workers. A history of skin rashes was found in half of the Malaysian workers, but not in the UK workers where the most common finding was epistaxis and nail damage. Eye irritation was more common in the Malaysian than in the UK workers. There was no evidence of any longterm or permanent skin or eye damage.

The most comprehensive medical surveys in paraquat-exposed spray operators were carried out in Malaysia (Howard *et al.*, 1981) and Sri Lanka (Senawayake *et al.*, 1993). In both studies there were detailed clinical examinations, lung function measurements (including CO diffusion capacity), hematological and biochemical investigations, and, in the Sri Lankan study, a chest radiograph was taken. In the Malaysian survey, 27 paraquat spraymen (mean spraying time 5.3 years; mean individual annual quantity of paraquat handled 67.2 kg as paraquat ion) were compared with two control groups comprising 24 general plantation workers and 23 latex factory workers, respectively. In the Sri Lankan survey, 85 paraquat spraymen (mean spraying time 12 years) were compared with two groups of 76 factory workers and 79 general workers, respectively. In both studies there were no clinically significant differences in any of the parameters studies; in particular, the results of the lung function tests showed similar results for exposed and control groups. It was concluded that the long term spraying of paraquat was not associated with any measurable adverse health effects.

A recently published study was carried out in Nicaragua (Castro-Gutierrez *et al.*, 1997), although the investigation dates back to 1987/88. A population of 134 spray workers with at least 2 years spraying experience with paraquat from 15 banana plantations was interviewed, 63 out of which had not experienced skin irritation, and 71 who had a history of skin rash or burn (used as a surrogate measure of intensity of exposure). A questionnaire was used to check for symptoms of respiratory illness and Forced Vital Capacity (FVC) and Forced Expiratory Volume in 1 second (FEV_1) were measured. The results were compared with a control population of 152 unexposed workers. There was a difference in male : female ratio between the exposed and unexposed groups (100:34 and 88:64, respectively). Paraquat-exposed workers gave a significantly more frequent

history of Grade 3 dyspnea, but not Grade 1 or 2 dyspnea. There was no difference in the occurrence of chronic bronchitis, and episodic dyspnea with wheezing was more frequent in the group with topical effects only. However, there were no differences between exposed and control workers with regard to restrictive (FVC < 80% of predicted value) or obstructive (FEV1:FVC < 70% of predicted value) spirometry parameters. In fact, the lowest incidence of restrictive changes was found in the "intensive exposure" group.

70.3.4 ATYPICAL CASES OF VARIOUS ORIGINS

In a case described by Newhouse *et al.* (1978), a farner's wife had been spraying paraquat in an orchard for many days. This case is unique in that her complaints started with scratches on arms and legs which proved nonhealing over four weeks. She was then hospitalized for two weeks and discharged without diagnosis. Two and a half weeks later she was readmitted to the hospital because of increased dyspnoea and wheeziness. She was diagnosed as suffering from systemic arteritis and died 12 days after final admission, some 8 weeks after initial exposure. Although the paper links her disease to paraquat exposure, it is doubtful if paraquat was the cause. First, at no time was paraquat measured in blood or urine. Second, the time from exposure to her death was more than 8 weeks, which is highly unusual for paraquat poisoning. Third, she had a clinical diagnosis (systemic arteritis) which did not include any reference to paraquat poisoning.

George and Hedworth-Whitty (1980) attributed a case of nonfatal lung disease to the inhalation of nebulised paraquat. A 64 year old woman noticed spray mist drifting into her garden from a spraying operation in an adjacent field. After some 10 minutes she noticed a chest tightening, and over the next week she became gradually more breathless. She was initially treated with a short course of steroids without much effect. Pulmonary function evaluation some two months later showed severe restriction, but there were no abnormalities in the chest radiograph. She was kept on systemic steroids and her lung function had markedly improved some 7 months after the original incident. Hart (1980) commented that the diagnosis of paraquat-induced lung injury was doubtful. The woman had a history of allergic rhinitis and chronic sinusitis. No previous lung function recording was available and no transfer factor was measured at the time of assessment. The chest radiograph was clear and the description of exposure did not provide convincing arguments for a significant inhalation exposure.

In the case described by Katopodis *et al.* (1993), a 31 year old woman was admitted 4 days after ingestion of 2 g paraquat. The urine test for paraquat was still positive, but her plasma concentration was only 10 μg/l. Charcoal hemoperfusion was carried out over the next 5 days. Paraquat levels became undetectable in plasma on day 6 and in urine on day 8. The patient survived without evidence of pulmonary involvement. The authors attributed the favorable outcome to the hemoperfusion therapy even at such a late stage after ingestion. However, the low paraquat plasma concentration at the time of admission would have suggested a good chance of survival anyway (see below and Table 70.5).

Ragoucy-Sengler and Pileire (1996b) reported a case of paraquat poisoning in an HIV positive patient. Indices of severity of the poisoning suggested a survival probability of 30% on admission, and 3% after 72 h. The clinical course included acute renal failure and severe hypoxia; however, pulmonary fibrosis did not develop. The patient was discharged with normal pulmonary function 18 days after admission. The authors suggested that the immune deficiency on the basis of the patient's HIV infection may have prevented the development of pulmonary fibrosis.

In a case described by Ernouf et al. (1998) a 47 year old man, while under the influence of alcohol, ingested paraquat which had been decanted into an unmarked a red wine bottle. The patient was a chronic alcoholic. He was admitted to hospital within 3 h and treated with gastric elimination and antioxidant therapy. Evolution of plasma paraquat concentrations pointed toward a prognosis of delayed death from pulmonary fibrosis. However, the patient died on the fourth day after admission from persistent hemodynamic shock and hypoxaemia. The authors speculated that co-ingestion of ethanol may have enhanced the toxicity of paraquat through increased absorption from the gastrointestinal tract and/or decreased renal clearance. However, it has also been suggested that alcoholism may have a protective effect against paraquat toxicity on the basis of increased synthesis of superoxide dismutase (Ragoucy-Sengler et al., 1991).

Methemoglobinemia was described in a patient who ingested "Gramonol," formulation containing 100 g/l paraquat and 140 g/l monolinuron (Ng et al., 1982). The authors speculated that the superoxide anion and hydrogen peroxide generated by paraquat could oxidize hemoglobin to methemoglobin. However, in response, Proudfoot (1982) pointed out that monolinuron, along with other substituted urea herbicides, is metabolized to aniline derivatives which are well known methemoglinemia and hemolysis causing agents. Furthermore, administration of monolinuron alone had produced methemoglobinemia in experimental animals. Instead of a new feature of paraquat poisoning, it appeared therefore that Ng et al. had reported the first human case of monolinuron toxicity. Since then, a further case of paraquat-monolinuron poisoning has been described (Casey et al., 1994) in which the severe methenoglobinemia (52%) was successfully treated with methylene blue. However, the patient died after 10 days from the consequences of paraquat poisoning.

In 1975 the Government of Mexico began an aerial spraying program, financed by the United States, to destroy marijuana fields with paraquat. In 1978 analyses showed that 21% of 61 marijuana samples confiscated in California, Arizona, and Texas contained paraquat residues between 3 and >2000 ppm (Turner et al., 1978). Further work demonstrated that, nationally, 0.63% of over 100,000 kg marijuana seized contained detectable paraquat levels with a median of 52 ppm (Liddle et

al., 1980). Over 70% of the contaminated samples were found in the Southwest region of the United States, originating almost exclusively from Mexico. Combustion testing suggested that around 0.2% of the paraquat residue would pass unchanged into marijuana smoke (Brine et al., 1981). On the basis of a worst case epidemiological risk assessment it was suggested that some marijuana smokers in the Southwest region might have been at risk of health effects from paraquat inhalation (Landrigan et al., 1983). However, no clinical cases were identified during these studies.

A possible association between paraquat exposure and the development of Parkinson's disease has been the subject of much speculation. The reason for this is, as previously discussed, the apparent structural similarity between paraquat and the synthetic pyridine MPTP which produced severe neuropathies in several dozen drug users in southern California (Langston et al., 1983; Lewin, 1984). The first epidemiological work to draw attention to a possible role of pesticides in Parkinson's disease was published by Barbeau et al. (1986), who showed that the regional incidence of the illness in Canada was nonuniform and correlated with a genetically determined enzyme deficiency. While there was certainly a strong correlation between disease incidence and pesticide use, such a correlation was also found for industrial areas and wood processing regions. Since then a number of case-control studies have been published, with varying methodologies and conflicting results. Some studies suggested that the use of herbicides was significantly associated with the development of Parkinson's disease (Golbe et al., 1990; Ho et al., 1989; Semchuk et al., 1991); in two studies this was specifically linked to paraquat exposure (Hertzman et al., 1990; Liou et al., 1997). Others have found no such association (Koller et al., 1990; Ohlson and Hogstedt, 1981; Tanner et al., 1989; Tanner et al., 1990; Zayed et al., 1990).

Structure-activity relationships suggest that, despite their apparent similarity, paraquat and MPTP are two very different chemicals (Koller, 1986; see above). Barbeau's hypothesis that Parkinson patients may be more likely to have a specific hydroxylation defect in the P450 enzyme system which might inhibit their ability to metabolize toxins (Barbeau et al., 1985) does not apply to paraquat because it is not metabolized in mammals. Furthermore, none of the health surveys of paraquat-exposed workers (see above) has revealed any neurological deficits, let alone Parkinson's disease. The strongest evidence against paraquat as a causative factor in Parkinson's disease, however, comes from the many published case reports of paraquat poisoning. There is no evidence of a specific effect of paraquat on the nervous system, nor have neurological sequelae been noticed in survivors of paraquat poisoning (Vieregge et al., 1988). Zilker et al. (1988) carried out detailed neurological follow-up examinations in four survivors of paraquat poisoning (latency period between ingestion and follow-up 5–10 years) and three patients who had had skin contact with paraquat. It was possible to exclude Parkinsonism in all patients. One patient exhibited tardive dyskinesia most likely due to long term therapy with neuroleptic drugs. The authors concluded that acute paraquat exposure does not lead to Parkinson's disease.

70.3.5 CLINICAL FINDINGS AND DOSAGE RESPONSE

Information on the clinical course of paraquat poisoning is mainly based on case reports of patients who swallowed paraquat concentrate with suicidal intent. However, the systemic toxic effects are similar regardless of the route of absorption. Paraquat causes nausea which may be prolonged especially following ingestion of emeticized formulations (Meredith and Vale, 1987), as well as vomiting and diarrhea as a result of its local irritant effect on the gastrointestinal tract. Patients may develop a burning sensation, soreness, and pain in the mouth, throat, chest, and abdomen (Vale *et al.*, 1987). Ulceration in the mourn and throat, an inability to swallow saliva, dysphagia, and aphonia are common. The presence of buccopharyngeal lesions has no prognostic value (Bismuth *et al.*, 1995), in contrast to oesophageal and, in particular, gastric ulcerations which indicate a poor prognosis (Bismuth *et al.*, 1982). Prominent pharyngeal membranes ("pseudodiphtheria") have been reported (Stephens *et al.*, 1981) and perforation of the oesophagus may result in mediastinitis, surgical emphysema, and pneumothorax (Ackrill *et al.*, 1978).

The further clinical course is dependent on the amount of paraquat absorbed into the body (usually following ingestion). Attempts have been made to quantify the toxic dose from estimates based on the information given by patients. Although such estimates are often unreliable, a consensus has emerged which is based on experience with many patients. This has allowed the identification of three degrees of intoxication which are summarized below (for further details see Vale *et al.*, 1987, and Bismuth *et al.*, 1995).

70.3.5.1 Mild or Subacute Poisoning

The smallest fatal dose has been quoted as 16.7 mg/kg (Stevens and Sumner, 1991). However, the original reference (FAO/WHO, 1973) makes clear that this value is erroneously low, since the formulation ("Weedol") also contained an equal amount of diquat, so that the total bipyridyl ingestion was approximately 35 mg/kg. This is in line with clinical experience which shows that ingestion of less than 20–30 mg paraquat ion/kg has rarely serious consequences. Patients are either asymptomatic or develop nausea and vomiting. Renal and hepatic lesions are minimal or absent. An initial decrease of the diffusing capacity may be apparent in lung function measurements, but full recovery is normal.

70.3.5.2 Moderate to Severe Acute Poisoning

This occurs following ingestion of more than 20–30, but less than 40 to 50 mg/kg. Apart from the localized lesions described above, patients in this group develop renal failure, usually between the second and fifth day after ingestion. Hepatocellular

necrosis may occur. Both these lesions are fully reversible. Delayed development of pulmonary fibrosis is responsible for the generally poor prognosis in this group. Clinically and radiologically this appears around 7 days after ingestion, but subtle abnormalities are present much earlier, such as a decreased diffusing capacity. The x-ray often shows patchy infiltration which may progress to opacification in one or both lungs. In thin section computerized tomography, the most common pattern on initial scans is ground-glass attenuation, followed by consolidation with bronchiectasis (Lee *et al.*, 1995). In most cases, pulmonary fibrosis leads to development of refractory hypoxaemia, resulting in death over a period of 5 days to several weeks.

70.3.5.3 Fulminant or Hyperacute Poisoning

In cases of massive ingestion (usually well above 40–55 mg/kg paraquat ion) patients survive less than 4 days and die in cardiogenic shock and multiorgan failure. Apart from renal and hepatic failure, alveolitis and noncardiogenic pulmonary oedema are observed. Other organ systems (adrenal glands, pancreas, heart) are affected and mortality in this group has been suggested to approach 100%.

While this categorization reflects experience with a large number of cases, it has to be emphasized that there are a significant number of cases reported in the literature where there was survival following the ingestion of alleged doses well above of what is usually considered to be fatal. Table 70.6 shows that there are 52 case reports where a dose apparently in excess of 55 mg/kg has been survived. While inaccuracies in estimating the dose may have led to exaggeration of the dose in some cases, this appears unlikely in many others.

Talbot *et al.* (1988b) reported a series of nine cases of suicidal paraquat poisoning in pregnant women. In the cases where the outcome was known, one fetus died probably unrelated to paraquat, three died in utero or after delivery but associated with respiratory distress in the mothers, two died in utero (one mother survived and subsequently had a normal pregnancy with no evidence of teratogenicity from the previous paraquat intoxication), one and fetus was aborted. Previously, Fennelly *et al.* (1968) had reported the case of a woman who was 28 weeks pregnant and died 20 days after paraquat ingestion. Upon autopsy the fetus showed no abnormalities. A 20 week pregnant patient survived the ingestion of a small dose of paraquat and subsequently delivered a normal child (Musson and Porter, 1982).

There are now sufficient case reports in the literature to demonstrate that the development of pulmonary lesions is not inevitably fatal. Fitzgerald *et al.* (1979b) examined 13 survivors of acute paraquat poisoning after a minimum of 1 year. In two children, no clinical, functional, or radiological abnormalities were seen. Of the 11 adults, 5 nonsmokers also showed no evidence of pulmonary disease. Four smokers were considered normal on clinical and radiological criteria, but had a mild deficit in pulmonary function which could reasonably be attributed to smoking. Two patients had pronounced arterial hypoxemia, both having had pre-existing pulmonary disease. In

Table 70.6
Summary of Case Reports with Doses above 55 mg/kg Taken by Survivors of Paraquat Poisoning by Ingestion

Calculated ingested dose (mg/kg)[a]	Dose stated[b]	Number of cases	Body weight (kg)[c]	Age Range (years)	References
55–75	15–20 ml (9 cases) 1–2 mouthful one sachet (2 cases)	13	25–70	3–75	Addo *et al.*, 1984 Iff *et al.*, 1971 Lloyd 1969 (cited in Cavalli, 1977) Mahieu *et al.*, 1977 Ming *et al.*, 1980 Mirchev, 1977 Taki *et al.*, 1996 Talbot *et al.*, 1988a
76–100	10–40 ml (14 cases) 1–2 mouthful (4 cases)	18	25–70	3–65	Addo *et al.*, 1984 Douze *et al.*, 1977 Malone *et al.*, 1971 McKean, 1968 Ragoucy-Sengler *et al.*, 1991 Shahar *et al.*, 1980 Tabei *et al.*, 1982 Taki *et al.*, 1996 Thomas *et al.*, 1977 Tsatsakis *et al.*, 1996
101–200	40–>50 ml (7 cases) 3–4 mouthful (2 cases)	9	70	17–59	Addo *et al.*, 1984 Douze *et al.*, 1974, 1977 Florkowski *et al.*, 1992 Grundies *et al.*, 1971 Lheureux *et al.*, 1995 Okonek *et al.*, 1980
>201	50–150 ml (8 cases) 3–4 mouthful (2 cases) one glass or cup (2 cases)	12	40–70	10–50	Addo *et al.*, 1984 Douze *et al.*, 1974, 1977 Malone *et al.*, 1971 Okonek *et al.*, 1979 1980 Tabei *et al.*, 1982 Tsatsakis *et al.*, 1996

[a] All doses expressed as paraquat ion.
[b] Volumes (ml) refer to the 20% liquid concentrate. A volume of 17.5 ml has been used for "a mouthful." "Sachet" refers to a granular formulation containing 2.5% paraquat and 2.5 g diquat.
[c] Where the body weight was not explicitly stated, the following assumption were used: 3–6 years, 25 kg; 7–11 years, 40 kg; 12–16 years, 50 kg; 17 years and above, 70 kg.

one of these two patients new and persistent infiltrates were seen in radiography which could be ascribed to paraquat lung damage. Hudson *et al.* (1991) described persistent radiological changes in three survivors of paraquat poisoning. In one case the patient died a year after her first intoxication from a second massive dose of paraquat. Upon autopsy pulmonary changes from the first as well as the second intoxication were present. Lin *et al.* (1995) studied 16 survivors of moderate to severe paraquat poisoning after 3 months. Detailed lung function showed significant improvements over time. This was confirmed by improvements in chest radiographs which showed some residual interstitial fibrosis, especially in the lower lobes. Bismuth *et al.* (1995) reported five cases, all of which had developed a restrictive pulmonary lesion, but who survived. Two patients were followed up for 4 and 10 years, respectively. In the first patient there was an obstructive component to his pulmonary insufficiency (from smoking) which persisted over time. However, the restrictive component gradually improved

Table 70.7

Predictive Plasma Paraquat Concentrations beyond 24 Hours Separating Surviving and Nonsurviving Patients (from Scherrmann, 1995)

Time (h)	Plasma paraquat concentration (ng/ml)
24	100
48	86
72	74
96	63
120	54
144	48
168	42
192	37
216	32
240	27
264	23.5
288	20
312	18

over several years, with eventual return to near baseline state. In the second patient (a 13 year old adolescent at the time of intoxication) pulmonary function tests were completely normal 10 years after the poisoning. He had also been able to actively participate in sports.

The measurement of paraquat plasma concentration has proved to be a reliable indicator of the prognosis of the intoxication. Levitt (1979) was the first to demonstrate a relationship between plasma concentration of paraquat, the estimated time after ingestion, and the eventual outcome. Based on results from 79 patients with a reasonably well established time of ingestion, Proudfoot *et al.* (1979) found that those patients whose plasma paraquat concentration did not exceed 2.0, 0.6, 0.3, 0.16, and 0.1 mg/l at 4, 6, 10, 16, and 24 h after ingestion survived. This semilogarithmic plot has become known as the predictive line, or "Proudfoot's curve." Because of the rapidly decreasing plasma concentration in the first few hours following ingestion no accurate prognosis could be given prior to 4 h. The authors emphasized that the line to separate survivors and nonsurvivors was meant to be an approximate guide, and the main use should be to help clinicians in deciding which patients needed urgent aggressive treatment. Subsequently, several other methods have been described to establish the prognosis from plasma paraquat concentrations. None of those methods have been found to invalidate the original estimate by Proudfoot *et al.*, but they have added other dimensions which may be of help to clinicians. Scherrmann *et al.* (1987) used data from 30 patients to extrapolate the predictive line beyond 24 h up to 15 days after intoxication; this was later modified (Scherrmann, 1995) with data from a total of 52 patients (Table 70.7). The same authors evaluated the relationship between early urine concentrations and clinical prognosis. They also attempted to correlate urine results obtained by radioimmunoassay with those given by the simple colorimetric dithionite test. Data from 75 patients showed a wide variation in urine concentrations within

24 h of ingestion. All 17 patients with concentrations of less than 1 μg/ml survived, whereas 51 out of 58 patients with urine paraquat concentrations of more than 1 μg/ml died. No color was observed in the dithionite test at paraquat concentrations below 0.5 μg/ml (Scherrmann *et al.*, 1987; Scherrmann, 1995).

Using a sample size of 219 patients, Hart *et al.* (1984) were able to calculate the probability of survival of the patient from the initial paraquat plasma concentration (Fig. 70.7). It was noted that the line denoting a 50% probability of survival correlated well with Proudfoot's curve. Sawada *et al.* (1988) categorized their patients into three groups: survivors ($n = 10$), nonsurvivors who died from respiratory failure ($n = 9$), and nonsurvivors who died from circulatory failure ($n = 11$). They calculated a severity index of paraquat poisoning (SIPP) from time to treatment since ingestion of paraquat multiplied by the serum level at admission (μg/ml). A boundary SIPP of 10 separated survival from death by either cause, whereas a SIPP of 50 separated deaths from respiratory failure and deaths from circulatory failure. Using data from 128 patients, Ikebuchi *et al.* (1993) separated survivors and fatal cases by multivariate analysis and established a discriminate function D. Their toxicological index of paraquat (TIP) could then be divided into three types. TIP 1 is characterized by $D > 0.1$ (100% survival probability). TIP 2 has the characteristic $-0.1 < D < 0.1$ and here urgent treatment may influence the outcome. In TIP 3 the discriminate function $D < -0.1$, and the probability of a fatal outcome is 100%.

All these methods depend on the availability of paraquat analysis, and this is often not the case, or at least not in a timely fashion. Investigators have therefore attempted to predict the outcome of the intoxication using biological indices rather than plasma paraquat concentrations. Suzuki *et al.* (1989) measured the respiratory index (RI) from blood gas analysis and used it as an index of lung oxygenation in 51 patients. Progressive deterioration of the RI above 1.5 was found in 43 nonsurvivors, whereas the RI remained below 1.5 in the 8 survivors. Furthermore, the time taken from ingestion for the RI to exceed 1.5 was found to be a good indicator for predicting the survival period in fatal cases. The major weakness of this method is that it cannot predict the outcome at the point of first contact with the patient, unlike the methods relying on plasma paraquat analysis. Also, conditions which may influence the RI such as pneumothorax, cardio-pulmonary rescuscitation, septic shock, pulmonary edema, and pneumonia limit the usefulness of this method. On the other hand, it can be used at any time after the intoxication, and it is independent from an estimate of time of ingestion. Yamaguchi *et al.* (1990) reviewed the medical records of 160 patients who had ingested paraquat and calculated an equation derived from serum creatinine and potassium concentrations and arterial blood bicarbonate level. When plotted against time of ingestion they were able to estimate the probability of survival in three categories (90%, 38%, and 3%). Most recently, a different biological index using creatinine measurement from 18 patients has been proposed by Ragoucy-Sengler and Pileire (1996a). They found that the time evolution of blood creatinine in intoxicated patients was linear during the first 24 h

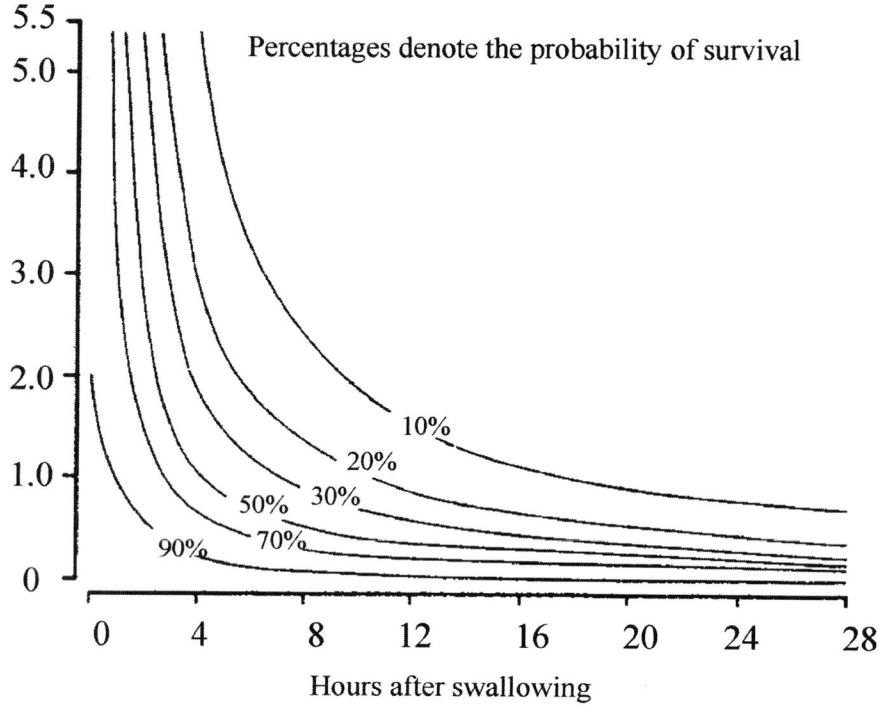

Figure 70.7 Relationship between the concentration of paraquat in the plasma and the survival of the patient. From (Hart *et al.*, 1984), reproduced with permission © 1984.

after admission. The rate of increase of creatinine in the patients with fatal outcome was equal to a constant (zero order kinetics). A rate of creatinine increase over 5 h (dCreat/dt) of >3 μmol/l/h was found in the 12 fatal cases whereas this value remained <1.26 for the survivors. As with the method of Suzuki *et al.* (1989) this biological index is independent of an estimate of time elapsed since ingestion. It has the advantage that a prognosis can be established within a few hours after admission of the patient using a standard biochemical analysis. However, it is currently based on data from a relatively small number of patients and will thus require further confirmation from a larger dataset.

70.3.6 LABORATORY FINDINGS

If performed early and serially, pulmonary function tests may be of diagnostic value. However, it has been pointed out that any changes seen are not specific for paraquat poisoning, since they may also occur in other clinical conditions such as pneumonia, pulmonary edema, pulmonary thromboembolism, and advanced degrees of the alveolar capillary block syndrome (Cooke *et al.*, 1973). The abnormalities must be interpreted in conjunction with the clinical picture. As mentioned above, pulmonary function tests in patients with moderate to severe paraquat poisoning are likely to be abnormal much earlier than clinical or radiological findings. A decrease in the carbon monoxide diffusing capacity or transfer factor (DL_{CO} or TL_{CO}) can be noted as early as the first day after intoxication (Baguley *et al.*, 1983). Beginning between the fifth and sixth

day there may be a restriction of the FEV_1 and the FVC. These changes are followed by a drop in the arterial oxygen tension and an increase in the gradient of alveolar to arterial tension. Finally, there is the development of a functional shunt by which a decreasing fraction of the blood passing through the lungs is oxygenated (Cooke *et al.*, 1973).

In patients who died within 11–14 days, the extent of lipid peroxidation, expressed as malondialdehyde, was higher than in controls or in patients who survived. Massive doses (death in 1–3 days) did not result in increased levels of malondialdehyde (Yasaka *et al.*, 1981, 1986). Serum superoxide dismutase (SOD) levels were significantly decreased in cases of lethal paraquat poisoning (Nemeth *et al.*, 1985). Better clinical courses were detected if SOD levels were normal or slightly elevated. Extremely increased levels were measured several times in the terminal state and were interpreted as the consequence of liver cell necrosis and intravascular haemolysis.

Other laboratory findings, including those reflecting renal and hepatic failure, are nonspecific. Detailed renal function studies were performed in three cases of paraquat poisoning who developed acute renal failure (Vaziri *et al.*, 1979). The glomerular filtration rate (estimated by using creatinine clearance) improved for two patients who survived two weeks, illustrating the reversible nature of the renal failure. A mild to moderate transient proteinuria but little albuminuria was observed during the first two weeks after intoxication. Other findings consistent with proximal tubular dysfunction included glucosuria, amino aciduria, and increased fractional excretion of phosphorus, sodium, and uric acid.

Many case reports have shown a transient rise in liver enzymes such as ALT and AST, reflecting the centrilobular necrosis and cholestasis often seen at autopsy (Vale *et al.*, 1987). Serum protein was decreased in one case (Bullivant, 1966) but increased in another with a large increase in the globulin fractions (Matthew *et al.*, 1968). Peak total serum bilirubin concentration correlated significantly with the alveolar–arterial oxygen difference in a series of 21 patients (Lin *et al.*, 1995).

Normochromic anemia developed rapidly in five cases reported by Lautenschläger *et al.* (1974). This was accompanied by suppression of erythropoietin in the bone marrow but had little effect on other aspects of hematopoesis. The bone marrow had returned to normal in one patient who survived and was re-examined 6 months after the intoxication. In the above mentioned study by Lin *et al.* (1995), the alveolar–arterial oxygen difference also showed a negative correlation with the initial platelet count.

Paraquat analysis in plasma and urine has already been mentioned as the key to diagnosis and prognosis of paraquat poisoning. A simple spot test can be performed with urine or gastric aspirate and is based on the reduction of paraquat cation to a blue radical in the presence of alkali and sodium dithionite (Berry and Grove, 1971; Widdop, 1976). These methods can detect concentrations of paraquat in urine down to 1–2 μg/ml and may be made semiquantitative if a range of standards are prepared in control samples. Quantitative methods based on the dithionite reaction with a spectrophotometric endpoint have also been described to determine paraquat in plasma (Jarvie and Stewart, 1979; Knepil, 1977). An improved spot test using extraction with a silica cartridge has allowed lower detection limits between 0.1 and 0.5 μg/ml (Woollen and Mahler, 1987). The lower limit of detection for paraquat using spectrophotometry following solid phase extraction was 45 ng/ml (Smith *et al.*, 1993).

Other methods which have been described include a radioimmunoassay with a sensitivity of 6 ng/ml (Levitt, 1979). Gas chromatography and mass spectroscopy have been used (Draffan *et al.*, 1977), giving a sensitivity of 25 ng/ml. A fluoroimmunoassay achieved a sensitivity of 20 ng/ml (Coxon *et al.*, 1988). Gill *et al.* (1983) described a high performance liquid chromatography method involving ion-pair extraction on disposable cartridges of octadecyl silica. Most of these methods can be applied to the analysis of plasma, urine, and tissue samples.

70.3.7 ABSORPTION

No adequate data exist on absorption of paraquat in humans. However, Davies (1987) has pointed out that early estimates of an absorption of less than 5% of an ingested dose (Conning *et al.*, 1969) may be an underestimate. He suggested that absorption kinetics in man may be more similar to those seen in the dog, where a rapid but incomplete paraquat absorption occurs, with peak plasma levels occurring at 75–90 minutes, and almost 40% of the dose absorbed in 6 h, as judged by the amount

excreted in urine (Bennett *et al.*, 1976; Davies *et al.*, 1977). Limited clinical data suggest that having a full stomach may effectively decrease the bioavailability of paraquat (Bismuth *et al.*, 1982, 1995).

In humans, the precise time at which the plasma paraquat concentration peaks is unknown. However, paraquat may be detected in urine as early as 1 h after ingestion (Meredith and Vale, 1987). To judge by the plasma concentration data published by Proudfoot *et al.* (1979), peak plasma concentrations in humans are certainly attained within 4 h. This is in line with the toxicokinetic analysis of data from 18 patients by Houze *et al.* (1990), who estimated peak plasma concentrations to occur between 2 and 4 h. However, most patients were admitted to hospital comparatively late, and they could measure peak plasma concentrations in only two case; in both they were seen around 3.5 h after ingestion.

70.3.8 DISTRIBUTION

The distribution of paraquat appears to be similar in humans and dogs (Davies *et al.*, 1977; Van den Bogaerde *et al.*, 1984), suggesting that the three compartment model described by Hawksworth *et al.* (1981) (see above) in the dog is also applicable to humans. Smith (1987) pointed out that the concentration of paraquat in plasma in human poisoning cases falls rapidly to much lower levels than described in the rat. In their series, Houze *et al.* (1990) found that the concentration–time curve in 15 adult patients (not hemodialyzed) was best described by a biexponential curve, with the elimination half-lives of the early and late phase being 5 and 84 h, respectively. These patients could be divided into three groups:

1. Patients admitted early and having a rapidly fatal course from cardiovascular collapse showed only monoexponential decreases with a mean half-life of 7 h. However, because of the early death of the patients, evaluation of the late phase was precluded.

2. The second group included patients who were admitted early and survived long enough for an evaluation of the late phase. They showed a biexponential decrease with mean half-lives of 7 and 103 h, respectively.

3. In the third group hospital admission was delayed and only late paraquat plasma concentrations could be measured. Accordingly, a monoexponential decrease in plasma paraquat concentrations was observed with a mean half-life of 101 h.

Acute renal failure occurred in all but one of the patients. The terminal half-life, however, was very long even in the patient with normal renal function, suggesting that the prolonged elimination phase depends not only on renal function but also on the gradual release of paraquat by extravascular tissue into the blood circulation.

In six of their cases with fatal outcome, Houze *et al.* (1990) also determined tissue paraquat concentrations. High concentrations were found in the lungs, kidneys, heart, and liver and much lower concentrations in lipophilic organs such as brain and adipose tissue. The apparent volume of distribution ranged from 1.2 to 1.5 l/kg, compared to 2.75 l/kg in the study by Davies *et al.* (1977). The mean value of the distribution half-life in humans is greater than that reported from animal studies (see above). Assuming a first-order distribution rate constant and an early half-life of 5 h, paraquat distribution would be achieved within approximately 30 to 40 h (Houze *et al.*, 1990).

The active transport of paraquat into lung tissue in different species, including humans, has been described in detail above. Paraquat accumulation in tissue could be considered as a slow process from a pharmacological point of view, but it is rapid in clinical terms (Bismuth *et al.*, 1987). In a study of the kinetics of paraquat through the heart–lung block, Baud *et al.* (1988) showed that concentrations in the radial artery were usually higher than or equal to the corresponding value in the pulmonary artery. Only one patient who was examined approximately 4 h after ingestion showed a pulmonary artery concentration clearly higher than that in the radial artery, providing evidence of pulmonary uptake of paraquat. The arteriovenous difference disappeared approximately 8 h after ingestion followed by inversion of this ratio. This suggests that lethal concentrations of paraquat in the lung may be reached less than 10 h after ingestion.

Paraquat crosses the placenta and a case reported by Talbot *et al.* (1988b) suggests that it is concentrated in the fetus. Following suicidal ingestion of paraquat a premature infant (32 weeks) was delivered by Caesarean section. Both mother and infant died shortly thereafter. Paraquat was measured in maternal blood at 5.6 µg/ml and in the infant's blood at 20.6 µg/ml.

70.3.9 METABOLISM

As in experimental animals, paraquat is not metabolized in humans but is reduced to an unstable free radical which is then reoxidized to produce a superoxide radical (see above). Paraquat is excreted unchanged in urine.

70.3.10 EXCRETION

As in experimental animals, paraquat elimination is essentially renal via glomerular filtration with an element of tubular secretion (Bismuth *et al.*, 1988). With normal renal function, clearance of paraquat is greater than creatinine clearance, which enables excretion of high concentrations and large amounts of paraquat within the first hours after ingestion (Davies *et al.*, 1977; Scherrmann *et al.*, 1983). However, ingestion of large doses of paraquat causes tubular necrosis with a rapid decrease of glomerular filtration and tubular secretion.

In four cases described by Houze *et al.* (1990), renal paraquat clearance was lower than creatinine clearance, even in a patient with apparently normal creatinine clearance. Urinary and plasma elimination half-lives correlated well. Paraquat may be detectable in urine for a long period of time. Beebeejaun *et*

al. (1971) found paraquat excreted in urine until 26 days after ingestion. In the case of a 14 month old boy, Houze *et al.* (1990) could detect paraquat in urine for up to 3 months after ingestion, suggesting ongoing release of paraquat from a deep body compartment.

Small amounts of paraquat have been recovered in bile samples at postmortem examination, suggesting that a minor enterohepatic cycle may exist in humans (Van Dijck *et al.*, 1975). As in experimental animals, the amount of paraquat excreted in feces corresponds to 60–70% of the ingested dose in humans. This excretion may be prolonged (Van Dijck *et al.*, 1975).

70.3.11 PATHOLOGY

Pathological findings upon autopsy in humans fatalities from paraquat poisoning are similar to those seen in experimental animals, in particular the rat (for a detailed review see Smith and Heath, 1976). The lung is the organ showing the most severe changes in paraquat poisoning. Pulmonary pathology has been divided into two phases which correspond with the early and late stages of the clinical signs and symptoms (Smith and Heath, 1975).

70.3.11.1 The Destructive Phase

This occurs during the first few days after paraquat poisoning and is rarely seen in human autopsy cases, but it has been described in a case where an early biopsy was performed (Toner *et al.*, 1970). It is characterized by swelling of the alveolar epithelium which sloughs off and is thought to be related to early development of pulmonary edema with congestion and fibrin exudate (Smith and Heath, 1974a). Death due to this pulmonary pathology is rare.

70.3.11.2 The Proliferative Phase

This phase is usually seen in patients who survive for longer than 1 week. Pulmonary congestion with interstitial and alveolar edema continues, sometimes associated with hemorrhage. There is lymphocytic and other inflammatory cell infiltration and occasional proliferation of cells lining the alveolar wall (Bullivant, 1966). The most specific feature is the presence of large quantities of fibroblastic tissue which is perivascular and peribronchial early on, but later more diffuse (Smith and Heath, 1974b). The pulmonary fibrosis is sometimes associated with an early honeycomb appearance of the lung parenchyma. However, in contrast to a true honeycomb lung the cystic air spaces are dilated respiratory bronchioles and their, walls consist of fibrosed, collapsed alveoli.

Renal pathology is common, but it is rarely responsible for the death of the patient. Macroscopically, the kidneys are swollen and soft. There is degeneration or necrosis of proximal tubular cells (Bullivant, 1966; Campbell, 1968) with nuclear loss and cast formation (Parkinson, 1980). Depending on the time after poisoning, there may be signs of regeneration.

While early studies made little mention of liver damage, Mullick *et al.* (1981) found evidence of cholestasis, usually localized to the centrilobular region in the majority of their 13 autopsy cases. There was cholangiocellular injury involving the small- and medium-sized bile ducts in portal areas. The authors hypothesized that paraquat injury to the liver is biphasic with an initial hepatocellular injury followed after 2 days by a cholangiocellular phase.

Toxic myocarditis is frequently seen in cases with ingestion of larger amounts of paraquat. Parkinson (1980) described a patchy but widespread polymorphonuclear leucocyte infiltration in the presence of normal myocardial fibers.

In some cases adrenal cortical necrosis has been described (Nagi, 1969; Reif and Lewinsohn, 1983) in patients who died early after ingestion of paraquat. This lesion was diffuse and involved mainly the zona fasciculata and zona reticularis. Fitzgerald *et al.* (1977) found adrenal cortical necrosis upon autopsy in 12 of 23 patients. The severity of the lesion appeared dose-related with patients showing complete cortical necrosis after ingestion of higher doses.

Brain pathology has been studied in a series of eight patients (Grant *et al.*, 1980). Changes included generalized edema, hemorrhages (these two findings being the most consistent changes), glial reactions, and meningeal inflammation. The authors suggested that paraquat may damage the cerebral blood vessels. These changes were also seen in a case reported by Hughes (1988) who suggested that, apart from a direct toxicity of paraquat on cerebral blood vessels, the neuronal depletion, myelin breakdown, and astrocytic fibrous gliosis seen were a secondary effect due to prolonged anoxia.

70.3.12 TREATMENT OF POISONING

The therapy of paraquat intoxication has focused on three main areas: prevention of absorption from the gastrointestinal tract, enhancement of elimination of paraquat from the body, and therapy directed against the mechanisms of toxicity. In addition, there have been attempts to use lung transplantation as a means to overcome the consequences of paraquat lung toxicity.

70.3.12.1 Prevention of Absorption

Following the first reports of paraquat poisoning it was suggested that the immediate therapy of paraquat poisoning should be directed toward prevention of absorption from the gastrointestinal tract (Malone *et al.*, 1971). There is little information available on the use of gastric lavage in paraquat poisoned patients. Bismuth *et al.* (1982) were not able to establish a beneficial effect from gastric lavage in their series of 28 patients. Bramley and Hart (1983) did not find an improved prognosis resulting from the use of gastric lavage in a series of 262 patients. McDonah and Martin (1970) proposed urgent gastric lavage with a 1% bentonite solution to inactivate paraquat. Following the studies by Clark (1971) who found that bentonite (sodium montmorillonite) and Fuller's Earth (calcium montmorillonite) had a high adsorption capacity for paraquat, Douglas

et al. (1973) reported three cases of survival after paraquat poisoning, two of which had been treated with 7% bentonite as adsorbent. Smith *et al.* (1974) suggested a treatment regime of repeated administration of cathartics together with large volumes of Fuller's Earth or bentonite which had been shown to effectively protect rats against an otherwise lethal dose of paraquat. Vale *et al.* (1977) used this approach together with charcoal hemoperfusion in 10 patients with paraquat poisoning. Only 1 patient who had the initially lowest plasma paraquat concentration survived, prompting the authors to conclude that the treatment was likely to be of benefit only in less severely poisoned patients. This was also the conclusion of Fitzgerald *et al.* (1979a) who analyzed 62 cases of paraquat poisoning with respect to treatment with Fuller's Earth and survival. They found that the majority of patients who survived had not taken what was regarded as a lethal dose. Also, death occurred in all patients who had ingested more than 30 ml of the concentrate, irrespective of therapy. In the group of patients who ingested between 5 and 30 ml and who received therapy within 6 h after ingestion 4 out of 7 survivors and 2 out of 5 nonsurvivors had received Fuller's Earth. The authors suggested that Fuller's Earth may have been of benefit in a few cases who had taken slightly in excess of the lethal dosage, but it was unlikely to affect the outcome in the majority of patients with paraquat poisoning.

While Fuller's Earth is still widely used in the first-line treatment of paraquat poisoning, the original claim by Clark (1971) that activated charcoal did not bind paraquat has been disputed. On the basis of *in vitro* binding studies and *in vivo* experiments, Okonek *et al.* (1982) suggested that the use of activated charcoal instead of Fuller's Earth was equally effective. This has prompted a revision of the advice given to medical practitioners in the United Kingdom (Department of Health, 1996) since activated charcoal is more likely to be immediately available in most hospitals and treatment centers. Other adsorbents such as the cation exchange resin kayexalate have been used (Yamashita *et al.*, 1987) but it is doubtful whether these have any benefit over the use of Fuller's Earth and activated charcoal.

From 1979 onward a potent emetic, the phosphodiesterase inhibitor PP796, was gradually introduced in all paraquat formulations made by the major manufacturer (Denduyts-Whitehead *et al.*, 1985). It has been shown that following ingestion of emeticized formulations vomiting occurs earlier and is more profuse and prolonged than following ingestion of nonemeticized product (Meredith and Vale, 1987). However, a comparison of data from patients who had ingested paraquat concentrate with or without added emetic failed to show an overall benefit of the emetic on survival rate (Bismuth *et al.*, 1982; Bramley and Hart, 1983; Onyon and Volans, 1987). Nevertheless, the emetic has been retained with the rationale that in particular accidental paraquat ingestions usually involve small quantities of the product, where early gastric emptying could have an effect on the outcome.

It can be concluded that there is no clear evidence that gastric emptying and the use of adsorbents have improved the survival of patients with paraquat poisoning. The main reasons for this are the high dose of paraquat ingested by the majority of patients with deliberate ingestion and the frequent delay in hospital admission. Most authors concede that, on theoretical grounds, therapy designed to prevent absorption of paraquat should be able to help those patients who have a realistic chance of survival. However, clear evidence for this from clinical studies has so far not been obtained.

70.3.12.2 Elimination of Paraquat from the Body

Since the kidney is the primary excretory organ for absorbed paraquat, enhancement of urinary elimination was one of the first therapeutic options considered. Kerr *et al.* (1968) published the first case report where forced diuresis had been used to treat paraquat poisoning. The exact fluid volume was not given, but their patient's urine excretion was more than 11 liters over 24 h. The total urine excretion of paraquat was 46 mg and the patient survived. Another patient was treated with a total of 27 liters of fluid over 48 h (Fennelly *et al.*, 1971). During the course of the forced diuresis he developed seizures, a metabolic alkalosis, and electrolyte disturbances, but the therapy was successfully completed. He developed transient mild hepatic and renal failure, but the only sign of pulmonary involvement was a slight temporary reduction in transfer factor. The authors suggested that this was a case of severe poisoning but were unable to attribute his survival to the forced diuresis therapy because the patient had also received immunosuppressive therapy with azathioprin and prednisolone. Bismuth *et al.* (1982) suggested that forced diuresis per se does not enhance the urinary elimination of paraquat. Nevertheless, they believed the therapy might be of value in the prevention of paraquat-induced renal damage because of a reduction in the tubular concentration of paraquat. However, of the 18 patients with developing renal failure who were treated with frusemide, only 1 survived despite the fact that diuresis was maintained in nine patients.

Removal of paraquat by means of peritoneal dialysis, hemodialysis, and hemoperfusion has been advocated to reduce paraquat plasma concentrations and enhance elimination. Of these, dialysis procedures were found to be ineffective (Bismuth *et al.*, 1982; Vale *et al.*, 1977) and the value of charcoal hemoperfusion remains controversial. Experimental hemoperfusion in dogs was able to improve survival (Widdop *et al.*, 1977), but early results in paraquat poisoned patients were disappointing (Vale *et al.*, 1977). In 1979, Okonek and co-workers published a report on the successful treatment of two patients with what they described as "continuous hemoperfusion." Plasma paraquat analysis prior to hemoperfusion indicated a very poor prognosis, but under an aggressive hemoperfusion therapy over several weeks both survived. Subsequently, a further 6 patients were treated with this regime and had a positive outcome (Okonek *et al.*, 1982/83). However, these apparent successes proved to be rare. Hampson and Pond (1988) carried out a meta-analysis of data from 35 cases published in the literature and 7 cases from their own hospital which had sufficient comparative data, as well as details of the haemoperfusion procedure. They showed that none of the patients whose initial

plasma paraquat concentration was higher than 3 mg/l survived, regardless of time after ingestion and treatment. Overall, the outcome was in line with predictions and did not appear to be affected by hemoperfusion, single or repeated. The authors concluded that hemoperfusion should only be considered for patients whose initial plasma concentration was below 3 mg/l, those in whom the probability of survival was between 20 and 70%, and those who present within a few hours of ingestion. Subsequently, Böhler *et al.* (1992) reported a case where the use of continuous arterio-venous hemoperfusion was effective in lowering the plasma paraquat concentration below the limit of detection. However, the patient died on the second day after ingestion from gastrointestinal complications. Suzuki *et al.* (1993) compared the effect of "aggressive" (>10 hours in the first 24 h after ingestion) vs "conventional" (<10 h) hemoperfusion on the outcome of the intoxication in 40 patients. Aggressive hemoperfusion did not improve the overall outcome but significantly increased survival time. Finally, Lee and Lee (1995) found that 8 out of 18 patients treated with hemoperfusion survived, whereas none of 20 who did not receive hemoperfusion died. No plasma paraquat concentrations were measured, but the authors stated that the estimated volume ingested was not significantly different between the two groups.

In conclusion, no clear benefit has been demonstrated from therapies aimed at enhancing elimination of paraquat from the body. The best chances appear to lie in the maintenance of renal function through adequate diuresis. As for extracorporeal elimination, hemoperfusion appears to be the only technique which may be of benefit in some patients, and the early and aggressive use of this technique may have contributed to survival in a few cases.

70.3.12.3 Pathophysiological Treatment

A wide range of therapeutic substances have been studied experimentally in an attempt to prevent the specific lung toxicity of paraquat from occurring. Some have been used in humans, but most of the published work is based on single or a small number of cases. Usually, more than one therapy was employed, and information on the severity of poisoning and the initial probability of survival is often limited. For these reasons a critical evaluation of the benefit of any one therapy is difficult and, in many cases, impossible.

Since oxygen is required to set off the biochemical cascade of paraquat toxicity the use of supplementary oxygen should be avoided as long as possible. Bismuth *et al.* (1982) used a hypoxic breathing mixture and hypothermia in six patients. The arterial oxygen tension was maintained below 6.6 kPa. Only one patient survived who had clinical evidence of only mild poisoning. In the other patients, the FiO_2 had to be increased on a daily basis, all of them requiring >0.5 (50%) prior to their death.

Since redox cycling and the generation of free radicals are considered to be the principal a steps in the development of alveolar epithelial cell damage, a number of agents which, at least theoretically, interfere with this process have been tried therapeutically. One of the first steps in the biochemical cascade of injury is the generation of the superoxide anion which is detoxified by the enzyme superoxide dismutase. This has been given either intravenously (Davies and Connolly, 1975), intramuscularly (Harley *et al.*, 1977), intrapulmonary during fiberoptic bronchoscopy (Bateman, 1987), or as a nebulized aerosol (Davies and Connolly, 1975; Hong *et al.*, 1996). In some cases there was co-administration with the antioxidants vitamin C (Hong *et al.*, 1996) or vitamin E (Harley *et al.*, 1977) which has also been given on its own (Shahar *et al.*, 1980). The doses given appeared to have been determined empirically, and no conclusive evidence of a beneficial effect has so far been shown. *N*-acetyl cysteine (NAC) is a glutathione precursor which readily crosses the cell membrane, and glutathione depletion is one of the features of paraquat-induced cellular damage, Lheureux *et al.* (1995) treated a patient with high doses of NAC (300 mg/kg/day) over 3 weeks. However, the patient who survived also received early hemodialysis and desferrioxamine. The latter, an iron chelating agent, has been proposed because iron has a catalytic effect in the production of hydroxyl radicals. However, no other data exist on its clinical use.

70.3.12.4 Prevention of Lung Fibrosis

The development of the paraquat lung lesion is characterized by early infiltration of inflammatory cells, followed by fibroblast proliferation. Attempts have therefore been made to halt this process by giving immunosuppressive therapy. A few case reports involved the use of azathioprine, in one case with successful outcome (Laithwaitte, 1975); in two other cases the patients died (Malcolmson and Beesley, 1975). In one patient who survived, bleomycin was used over 3 days (Mahieu *et al.*, 1977). Most experience exists with a combination treatment of cyclophosphamide and corticosteroids which was first advocated by Malone *et al.* (1971). Addo *et al.* (1984) claimed a 75% survival rate in 20 patients treated with, cyclophosphamide (5 mg/kg/day to a maximum total of 4 g) and dexamethasone (8 mg t.i.d. over 2 weeks). Two years later they published a case series using the same regime with 72 patients, 52 (72%) of which survived (Addo and Poon-King, 1986). However, the plasma paraquat data of 25 patients showed that 7 survivors had no measurable paraquat levels, and of the other 18 only the 6 patients with the lowest plasma concentration survived. Following a preliminary report (Lin *et al.*, 1996) on the use of pulse therapy with cyclophosphamide (1 g/day over 2 days) and methylprednisolone (1 g/day over 3 days), Lin *et al.* (1999) reported results of a prospective study in 142 patients. Seventy-one patients died from fulminant poisoning within 1 week, and cyclophosphamide did not make any difference. In the group of moderately to severely poisoned patients, only 4/22 patients treated with cyclophosphamide died, compared to 16/28 in the control group. Plasma paraquat concentrations were not available, but the authors stated that there was no difference in severity of poisoning between the two groups based on the urine dithionite test. However, the beneficial effects of the cyclophosphamide–dexamethasone regime have been disputed

(Nogue *et al.*, 1989), and in a prospective study Perriens *et al.* (1992) did not find any difference in mortality between 14 patients who had received standard treatment and the 33 patients who had received high-dose cyclophosphamide and dexamethasone. A final answer regarding the usefulness of this therapy can therefore not been given at this stage.

Because of the radiosensitivity of fibroblasts *in vitro*, Webb *et al.* (1984) treated a patient who had developed diffuse alveolar damage following paraquat ingestion initially with cyclophosphamide and, after further deterioration, with fractionated radiotherapy over 11 days. The patient survived. It was noted that the severity of poisoning in this patient was mild (Proudfoot *et al.*, 1984) and the majority of patients in subsequent reports died (Bloodworth *et al.*, 1986; Williams and Webb, 1987). This may have been due to differences in the severity of intoxication, as well as the therapy employed. Following the successful treatment of a patient with poor prognosis (Talbot *et al.*, 1988a), Talbot and Barnes (1988) treated a further eight patients with radiotherapy. Only two survived and the authors suggested that a definite benefit of radiotherapy could not be demonstrated in their study.

70.3.12.5 Other Treatments

Beta-blocking agents such as propranolol have been shown to block the uptake of paraquat into the lung (Maling *et al.*, 1978). However, their limited therapeutic use has not been successful (Davies and Connolly, 1975; Fairshter *et al.*, 1976, 1979).

Recently, there have been two case reports on the use of nitrogen oxide inhalation (NO) in paraquat poisoning. On the basis that NO is a potent endogenous vasodilator and that NO inhalation exerts a beneficial effect on pulmonary gas exchange, Köppel *et al.* (1994) treated a 52 year old patient with severe paraquat poisoning (plasma concentration 4 days after ingestion 1 mg/l). She received 25 ppm in the inhalation mixture, her respiratory parameters improved immediately, and she was stabilized for 3 days. However, the patient died with massive pleural effusions and ventilatory failure on day 11 after ingestion. In the second case, Eisenman *et al.* (1998) treated a 52 year old male whose plasma paraquat concentration predicted only a 30% chance of survival, with NO because of developing respiratory distress. In addition, the patient had received Fuller's Earth, forced diuresis, hemofiltration, *N*-acetyl cysteine, methyl prednisolone, cyclophosphamide, vitamin E, and colchicine. Because of the multiple therapy it was impossible to be sure which of the therapeutic measures had contributed to this patient's survival. Nevertheless, it was felt that the use of NO deserved further evaluation (Hall, 1998).

There are five reports in the literature where lung transplantation has been performed after paraquat poisoning. Matthew *et al.* (1968) described a single lung transplantation 6 days after accidental paraquat ingestion in a 15 year old boy whose plasma paraquat levels at the time of the operation were still at toxic levels (0.4 μg/ml). The patient died 13 days after the operation in respiratory failure and the autopsy showed changes typical for paraquat poisoning, although no paraquat was measurable in the transplanted lung. A contribution of rejection to the disease process could not be excluded. The same group subsequently reported a further unsuccessful lung transplantation in an 18 year old farm worker (Cooke *et al.*, 1973). A further single lung transplantation with fatal outcome in a 25 year old man was reported in 1984 by Kamholz *et al.* This patient died after 45 days from the consequences of a bronchopleural fistula. A sequential bilateral lung transplantation was described by the Toronto Lung Transplant Group (Saunders *et al.*, 1985). This 31 year old patient had received a lung transplant at a time when his plasma paraquat levels were below what was considered to be a toxic level (0.03 μg/ml). In the postoperative period there was a sevenfold increase in paraquat plasma levels, possibly due to the release of paraquat from muscle stores. The transplanted lung failed and following several days of intensive therapy including hemoperfusion a second transplant was undertaken. The transplant worked well over 2 months; however, the patient developed a progressive toxic myopathy and ultimately died from a cerebrovascular accident. Nevertheless, this case showed the feasibility of lung transplantation in paraquat poisoning. The most recent case (Licker *et al.*, 1998) is the only one with a successful outcome. A 17 year old farmer developed respiratory failure of unknown origin. Repeated plasma paraquat measurements were negative. Following mechanical ventilation for 5 weeks a single lung transplantation was carried out. Recovery was complicated by myopathy, and paraquat was confirmed in the excised lung and a muscle biopsy. The patient subsequently admitted to having taken paraquat. The patient was discharged after 88 days and was able to lead an independent life at the last follow-up 13 months after transplantation.

These cases demonstrate that, over the years, lung transplantation has become feasible in cases of paraquat poisoning. While the early attempts were hampered by problems with immune suppression as well as a lack of understanding of the pathophysiological events following paraquat poisoning, these problems appear now to have been satisfactorily resolved. However, the authors of the latest paper make the point that the use of such a scarce and expensive resource is questionable in cases of deliberate self-harm.

Disclaimer The positions on certain aspects of the toxicology of paraquat in this chapter may not be aligned with the Syngenta positions; the latter are derived mainly from internal Syngenta reports many of which have not been published in the open literature.

REFERENCES

Ackrill, P., Hasleton, P. S., and Ralston, A. J. (1978). Oesphagal perforation due to paraquat. *Br. Med. J.* **1**, 1252–1253.

Adam, A., Smith, L. L., and Cohen, G. M. (1990). An evaluation of the redox cycling potencies of paraquat and nitrofurantoin in microsomal and lung slice systems. *Biochem. Pharmacol.* **40**, 1533–1539.

Addo, E., and Poon-King, T. (1986). Leucocyte suppression in treatment of 72 patients with paraquat poisoning. *The Lancet* **I**, 1117–1120.

Addo, E., Ramdial, S., and Poon-King, T. (1984). High dosage cyclophosphamide and dexamethasone treatment of paraquat poisoning with 75% survival. *West. Indian Med. J.* **33**, 220.

Akahori, F., and Oehme, F. W. (1983). Inhibition of collagen synthesis as a treatment for paraquat poisoning. *Vet. Human Toxicol.* **25**, 321–327.

Aldrich, T. K., Fisher, A. B., Cadenas, E., and Cnance, B. (1983). Evidence for lipid peroxidation by paraquat in the perfused rat lung. *J. Lab. Clin. Med.* **101**, 66–73.

Ali, S., Abdulla, M., and Athar, M. (1996). L-2-oxothiazolidine-4-carboxylate, an *in situ* inducer of glutathione, protects against paraquat-mediated pulmonary damage in rat. *Med. Sci. Res.* **24**, 699–701.

Amarasingham, R. D., and Lee, S. E. (1977–1981). A review of human poisoning cases examined by the Toxicology Division of the Department of Chemistry, Petaling Jaya, Malaysia, unpublished report.

Anderson, D., McGregor, D. B., and Purchase, I. F. H. (1976). Dominant lethal studies with paraquat and diquat in male CD-1 mice. *Mutat. Res.* **40**, 349–358.

Athanaselis, S., Qammaz, S., Alevisopoulos, G., and Koutselinis, A. (1983). Percutaneous paraquat intoxication. *J. Toxicol. Cut. Ocular Toxicol.* **2**, 3–5.

Autor, A. P. (1974). Reduction of paraquat toxicity by superoxide dismutase. *Life Sci.* **14**, 1309–1319.

Bagetta, G., Corasaniti, M. T., Iannone, M., Nistico, G., and Stephenson, J. D. (1992). Production of limbic motor seizures and brain damage by systemic and intracerebral injection of paraquat in rats. *Pharmacol. Toxicol.* **71**, 43–448.

Bagetta, G., Iannone, M., Vecchio, I., Rispoli, V., Rotiroti, D., Nistico, G. (1994). Neurodegeneration produced by intrahippocampal injection of paraquat is reduced by systemic administration of the 21-aminoacid U74389F in rats. *Free Rod. Res.* **21**, 85–89.

Baguley, E., Iles, P. B., and Wright, N. (1983). Serial lung function tests in paraquat poisoning. *Human Toxicol.* **2**, 418.

Bainova, A. (1969). Experimental appraisal of the effect of dipyridylium herbicides on skin *Letopisi. HEI* **9**, 25–30.

Bainova, A., and Vulcheva, V. (1977). Lung, changes after chronic paraquat intoxication. *Dokl. Bolg. Akad. Nauk* **30**, 1788–1790.

Bainova, A., Zlateva, M., and Vulcheva, V. I. (1972). Chronic inhalation toxicity of dipyridylium herbicides. *Khig. Zdraveopazvane* **15**, 25–31.

Baldwin, R. C., Pasi, A., MacGregor, J. T., and Hine, C. H. (1975). The rates of radical formation from the dipyridylium herbicides, paraquat, diquat and morfamquat in homogenates of rat lung, kidney and liver: an inhibitory effect of carbon monoxide. *Toxic. Appl. Pharmac.* **32**, 298–304.

Barbeau, A., Cloutier, T., Roy, M., Paris, S., Plasse, L., and Poirier, J. (1985). Ecogenetics of Parkinson's disease: 1—The 4-hydroxylation of debrisoquine. *Lancet* **2**, 1213–1216.

Barbeau, A., Roy, M., Clourier, L., Plasse, L., and Paris, S. (1986). Environmental and Genetic factors in the etiology of Parkinson's disease. *Adv. Neurol.* **45**, 299–306.

Bassett, D. I. P., and Fisher, A. B. (1978). Alterations of glucose metabolism during perfusion of rat lung with paraquat. *Am. J. Physiol.* **234**, E653–E659.

Bateman, D. N. (1987). Pharmacological treatments of paraquat poisoning. *Human Toxicol.* **6**, 57–62.

Baud, F. J., Houze, P., Bismuth, C., Scherrmann, J. M., Jaeger, A., and Keyes, C. (1988). Toxicokinetics of paraquat through the heart lung block six cases of acute human poisoning. *Clin. Toxicol.* **26**, 35–50.

Beebeejaun, A. R., Beevers, G., and Rogers, W. N. (1971). Paraquat poisoning-prolonged excretion. *J. Toxicol. Clin. Toxicol.* **4**, 397–407.

Bennett, P. N., Davies, D. S., and Hawksworth, G. M. (1976). In vivo absorption studies with paraquat and diquat in the dog. *Br. J. Pharmacol.* **58**, 284P.

Berisha, H. L., Pakbaz, H., Absood, A., and Said, S. I. (1994). Nitric oxide as a mediator of oxidant lung injury due to paraquat. *Proc. Natl. Acad. Sci. U.S.A.* **91**, 7445–7449.

Berry, D. J., and Grove, J. (1971). The determination of paraquat 1,1-dimethyl-4,4′-bipyridylium cation in urine. *Clin. Chim. Acta* **34**, 5–11.

Bilinski, T., and Litwinska, J. (1987). On the ideas alternative to the theory of superoxide mediated oxygen toxitity. *Bull. Pol. Acad. Sci. Biol. Sci.* **35**, 25–31.

Binns, C. W. (1976). A deadly cure for lice: a case of paraquat poisoning. *Papua New Guinea Med. J.* **19**, 105–107.

Bismuth, C., Garnier, R., Dally, S., Fournier, P. E., and Scherrman, J. M. (1982). Prognosis and treatment of paraquat poisoning: A review of 28 cases. *Clin. Tox.* **19**, 461–474.

Bismuth, C., Scherrmann, J. M., Garnier, R., Baud, F. J., and Pontal, P. G. (1987). Elimination of paraquat. *Human Toxicol.* **6**, 63–67.

Bismuth, C., Baud, F. J., Garnier, R., Muszinsk, J., and Houze, P. (1988). Paraquat poisoning biological presentation. *J. Toxicol. Clin. Exp.* **8**, 211.

Bismuth, C., Hall, A. H., and Wong, A. (1995). Paraquat ingestion exposure symptomatology and risk. *In* "Paraquat Poisoning" (C. Bismuth and A. H. Hall, eds.), pp. 95–210. Dekker, New York.

Bloch, C. A., and Ausubel, F. M. (1986). Paraquat-mediated selection for mutations in the manganese-superoxide dismutase gene soda. *J. Bacterial.* **168**, 795–798.

Block, E. R. (1979). Potentiation of acute paraquat toxicity by vitamin E deficiency. *Lung* **156**, 195–203.

Bloodworth, L. L., Kershaw, J. B., Stevens, P. E., Alcock, C. J., and Rainford, D. J. (1986). Failure of radiotherapy to reverse progressive pulmonary fibrosis caused by paraquat. *Br. J. Radiol.* **59**, 1037–1038.

Böhler, J., Riegel, W., Keller, E., Logemann, E., Just, H., and Schollmeyer, P. J. (1992). Continuous arteriovenous hemoperfusion for treatment of paraquat poisoning. *Nephrol. Dialysis Transplant.* **7**, 875–878.

Bramley, A., and Hart, T. B. (1983). Paraquat poisoning in the United Kingdom. *Human Toxicol.* **2**, 417.

Brawn, K., and Fridovich, I. (1981). DNA strand scission by enzymatically generated oxygen radicals. *Arch. Biochem. Biophys.* **206**, 414–419.

Brian, R. C., Homer, R. F., Stubbs, J., and Jones, R. L. (1958). A new herbicide, 1:1-ethylene-2,2′-dipyridylium dibromide. *Nature (London)* **181**, 446.

Brigelius, R. (1985). Mixed disulphides: biological functions and increase in oxidative stress. *In* "Oxidative Stress" (H. Sies, ed.), pp. 243–247. Academic Press, London.

Brigelius, R., Dostal, L. A., Horton, J. K., and Bond, J. R. (1986). Alteration of the redox state of NADPH and glutathione in perfused rabbit lung by paraquat. *Toxicol. Ind. Hlth.* **2**, 417–428.

Brigelius, R., Lenzen, R., and Sies, H. (1982). Increase in hepatic mixed disulphide and glutathione disulphide levels elicited by paraquat. *Biochem. Pharmacol.* **31**, 1637–1641.

Brine, D. R., David, K. H., and Wall, M. E. (1981). "Combustion of Paraquat Contaminated Marijuana—Analysis of Paraquat and Its Degradation Products." Final Report, Contract No. 273-79-C-0003, RTI/1755/OF, Research Triangle Institute, Research Triangle Park, NC.

Brooks, R. E. (1971). Ultrastructure of lung lesions produced by ingested chemicals. 1. Effect of the herbicide paraquat on mouse lung. *Lab. Invest.* **25**, 536–545.

Brooke-Taylor, S., Smith, L. L., and Cohen, G. M. (1983). The accumulation of polyamines and paraquat by human peripheral lung. *Biochem. Pharmacol.* **32**, 717–720.

Brown, O. R., Heitkamp, M., and Song, C. (1981). Niacin reduces paraquat toxicity in rats. *Science* **212**, 1510–1512.

Bullivant, C. M. (1966). Accidental poisoning by Paraquat: Report of two cases in man. *Br. Med. J.* **1**, 1272–1273.

Burk, R. F., Lawrence, R. A., and Lane, J. M. (1980). Liver necrosis and lipid peroxidation in the rat as the result of paraquat and diquat administration—Effect of selenium deficiency. *J. Clin. Invest.* **65**, 1024–1031.

Bus, J. S., Aust, S. D., and Gibson, J. E. (1974). Superoxide and singlet oxygen catalysed lipid peroxidation as a possible mechanism for paraquat (methyl viologen) toxicity. *Biochem. Biophys. Res. Commun.* **58**, 749–755.

Bus, J. S., and Gibson, J. E. (1975). Postnatal toxicity of chronically administered paraquat in mice and interactions with oxygen and bromobenzene. *Toxicol. Appl. Pharmacol.* **33**, 461–470.

Bus, J. S., Aust, S. D., and Gibson, J. E. (1976a). Paraquat toxicity: Proposed mechanism of action involving lipid peroxidation. *Environ. Hlth. Perspect.* **16**, 139–146.

Bus, J. S., Preache, M. M., Cagen, S. Z., Posner, H. S., Eliason, B. C., Sharp, C. W., and Gibson, J. E. (1975). Fetal toxicity and distribution of paraquat and diquat in mice and rats. *Toxicol. Appl. Pharmacol.* **33**, 450–460.

Bus, J. S., Cagen, S. Z., Olgaard, M., and Gibson, J. E. (1976b). A mechanism of paraquat toxicity in mice and rats. *Toxicol. Appl. Pharmacol.* **35**, 501–513.

Butler, C. (1975). Pulmonary interstitial fibrosis from paraquat in the hamster. *Arch. Pathol.* **99**, 503–507.

Butler, C., and Kleinerman, J. (1971). Paraquat in the Rabbit. *Br. J. Ind. Med.* **28**, 67–71.

Cadot, R., Descotes, J., Grenot, C., Cuilleron, C. Y., Evreux, J. C. (1985). Increased plasma araquat levels in intoxicated mice following anti-paraquat F(ab′)2 treatment. *J. Immunopharmacol.* **7**, 467–477.

Cagen, S. Z., Janoff, A. S., Bus, J. S., and Gibson, J. E. (1976). Effect of paraquat (methyl viologen) on the liver function in mice. *J. Pharm. Exp. Therap.* **198**, 222–228.

Cagen, S. Z., and Gibson, J. E. (1977). Liver damage following paraquat in selenium deficient and diethyl maleate pretreated mice. *Toxicol. Appl. Pharmacol.* **40**, 193–200.

Calo, M., Iannone, M., Passafaro, M., and Nistico, G. (1990). Selective vulnerability of hippocampal CA3 neurones after microinfusion of paraquat into the rat substantia nigra or into the ventral tegmental area. *J. Comp. Path.* **103**, 73–78.

Campbell, S. (1968). Paraquat poisoning. *Clin. Toxicol.* **1**, 245–249.

Cant, J. S., and Lewis, D. R. H. (1968). Ocular damage due to Paraquat and Diquat. *Br. Med. J.* **3**, 59.

Carson, D. J. L., and Carson, E. D. (1976). The increasing use of Paraquat as a suicide agent. *Forensic Sci.* **7**, 151–160.

Casey, P., and Vale, J. A. (1994). Deaths from pesticide poisoning in England and Wales: 1945–1989. *Hum. Exp. Toxicol.* **13**, 95–101.

Casey, P., Buckley, B. M., and Vale, J. A. (1994). Methemoglobinemia following ingestion of a monolinuron/paraquat herbicide. *J. Toxicol. Clin. Toxicol.* **32**, 185–189.

Castro-Gutierrez, N., McConnell, R., Andersson, K., Pacheco-Anton, F., and Hogstedt, C. (1997). Respiratory symptoms, spirometry and chronic occupational paraquat exposure. *Scand. J. Work Environ. Health* **23**, 421–427.

Cavalli, R. D., and Fletcher, K. (1977). An effective treatment for paraquat poisoning. *In* "Biochemical Mechanisms of Paraquat Toxicity: Proc. 1st Iowa Symp. on Toxic Mechanisms, June 28–29 (1976)" (A. P. Autor, ed.), Chap. 5, pp. 213–230. Academic Press, San Diego.

Chan, B. S. H., Lazzaro, V. A., Seale, J. P., and Duggin, G. G. (1996a). Characterisation and uptake of paraquat by rat renal proximal tubular cells in primary culture. *Human Exp. Toxicol.* **15**, 949–956.

Chan, B. S. H., Lazzaro, V. A., Kirwan, P. D., Seale, J. P., and Duggin, G. G. (1996b). The effect of paraquat on two renal cell lines-LLC-PK$_1$ and MDCK. *Res. Commun. Pharmacol. Toxicol.* **1**, 99–112.

Chan, B. S. H., Seale, J. P., and Duggin, G. G. (1997). The mechanism of excretion of paraquat rats. *Toxicol. Lett.* **90**, 1–9.

Chan, B. S. H., Lazzaro, V. A., Seale, J. P. and Duggin, G. G. (1998). The renal excretory mechanisms and the role of organic cations in modulating the renal handling of paraquat. *Pharmacol. Therap.* **79**, 193–203.

Chen, N., Pond, S. M., and Bowles, M. R. (1992). Competition between paraquat and putrescine for uptake by suspensions of rat alveolar type II cells. *Biochem. Pharmacol.* **44**, 1029–1036.

Chen, N., Bowles, M. R., and Pond, S. M. (1994). Prevention of paraquat toxicity in suspensions of alveolar type II cells by paraquat-specific antibodies. *Human Exp. Toxicol.* **13**, 551–557.

Cheng, W. H., Ho, Y. S., Valentine, B. A., Ross, D. A., Combs, G. F. Jr., and Lei, X. G. (1998). Cellular glutathione peroxidase is the mediator of body selenium to protect against paraquat lethality in transgenic mice. *J. Nutr.* **128**, 1070–1076.

Chester, G., and Ward, R. J. (1984). Occupational exposure and drift hazard during aerial application of paraquat to cotton. *Arch. Environ. Contam. Toxicol.* **13**, 551–563.

Chester, G., and Woollen, B. H. (1981). Studies of the occupational exposure of Malaysian plantation workers to paraquat. *Br. J. Ind. Med.* **38**, 23–33.

Chester, G., Gurunathan, G., Jones, N., and Woollen, B. H. (1993). Occupational exposure of Sri Lankan tea plantation workers to paraquat. *Bull. World Health Org.* **71**, 625–633.

Chui, Y.-C., Poon, G., and Law, F. (1988). Toxicokinetics and bioavailability of paraquat in rats following different routes of administration. *Toxicol. Ind. Health* **4**, 203–219.

Clark, D. G. (1971). Inhibition of the absorption of paraquat from the gastrointestinal tract by absorbents. *Br. J. Ind. Med.* **28**, 186–188.

Clark, D. G., McElligott, T. F., and Weston Hurst, E. (1966). The toxicity of paraquat. *Br. J. Ind. Med.* **23**, 126–132.

Conning, D. A., Fletcher, K., and Swan, A. A. B. (1969). Paraquat and related bipyridyls. *Br. Med. Bull.* **25**, 245–249.

Cooke, N. I., Flenley, D. C., and Matthew, H. (1973). Paraquat poisoning: Serial studies on lung function. *Quart. J. Med.* **62**, 683–692.

Corasaniti, M. T., Defilippo, R., Rodino, P., Nappi, G., and Nistico, G. (1991). Evidence that paraquat is able to cross the blood-brain barrier to a different extent in rats at various ages. *Funct. Neurol.* **6**, 385–391.

Corasaniti, M. T., Bagetta, G., Rodino, P., Gratteri, S., and Nistico, G. (1992). Neurotoxic effects induced by intracerebral and systemic injection of paraquat in rats. *Human Exp. Toxicol.* **11**, 535–539.

Corasaniti, M. T., and Nistico, G. (1993). Determination of paraquat in rat brain by high-performance liquid chromatography. *J. Chromatogr.* **643**, 419–425.

Costantini, P., Petronilli, V., Colonna, R., and Bernardi, P. (1995). On the effects of paraquat on isolated mitochondria. Evidence that paraquat causes opening of the cyclosporin A-sensitive permeability transition pore synergistically with nitric oxide. *Toxicology* **99**, 77–88.

Coxon, R. E., Rae, C., Gallacher, G., and Landon, J. (1988). Development of a simple fluoroimmunoassay for paraquat. *Clin. Chim. Acta* **175**, 297–306.

Cramp, T. P. (1985). Failure of N-acetylcysteine to reduce renal damage due to paraquat in rats. *Human Toxicol.* **4**, 107.

Dabney, B. J. (1995). Genetic, carcinogenic and reproductive effects of paraquat. *In* "Paraquat Poisoning, Mechanisms, Prevention and Treatment" (C. Bismuth and A. H. Hall, eds.), pp. 235–248. Dekker, New York.

Daniel, J. W., and Gage, J. C. (1966). Absorption and excretion of diquat and paraquat in rats. *Br. J. Ind. Med.* **23**, 133–136.

Davies, D. S., Hawksworth, G. M., and Bennett, P. N. (1977). Paraquat poisoning. *Proc. Europ. Soc. Toxicol.* **18**, 21–26.

Davies, D. S., and Connolly, M. E. (1975). Paraquat poisoning—Possible therapeutic approach. *Proc. Royal Soc. Med.* **68**, 442.

Davies, D. S. (1987). Paraquat poisoning: The rationale for current treatment regimes *Human Toxicol.* **6**, 37–40.

Day, B. J., and Crapo, J. D. (1996). A metalloporphyrin superoxide dismutase mimetic protects against paraquat induced lung injury *in vivo*. *Toxicol. Appl. Pharmacol.* **140**, 94–100.

De Gori, N., Froio, F., Strongoli, M. C., De Francesco, A., Calo, M., and Nistico, G. (1988). Behavioural and electrocortical changes induced by paraquat after injection in specific areas of the brain of the rat. *Neuropharmacology* **27**, 201–207.

De Haan, J. B., Bladier, C., Griffiths, P., Kelner, M., O'Shea, R. D., Cheung, N. S., Bronson, R. T., Silverstro, M. J., Wild, S., Zheng, S. S., Beart, P. M., Hertzog, P. J. and Kola, I. (1998). Mice with a homozygous null mutation for the abundant glutathione peroxidase, Gpx1, show increased susceptibility to the oxidative stress-inducing agents paraquat and hydrogen peroxide. *J. Biol. Chem.* **273**, 22528–22536.

Denduyts-Whitehead, A., Hart, T. B., and Volans, G. N. (1985). Effects of the addition of an emetic to paraquat formulations on acute poisoning in man. *J. Toxicol. Clin. Toxicol.* **23**, 422–423.

Department of Health (1996). "Pesticide Poisoning," 2nd ed. Notes for the guidance of medical practitioners (A. Proudfoot, ed.). The Stationary Office, London.

Deveckova, D., and Mydlik, M. (1980). Gramoxone ocular burns. *Cesk. Oftalmol.* **36**, 7–10.

Dey, M. S., Krieger, R. I., and Ritter, R. C. (1987). Paraquat-induced, dose-dependent conditioned task aversions and weight loss mediated by the area postrema. *Toxicol. Appl. Pharmacol.* **87**, 212–221.

Dey, M. S., Breeze, R. G., Hayton, W. L., Karara, A. H., and Krieger, R. I. (1990). Paraquat pharmacokinetics using a subcutaneous toxic low dose in the rat. *Fundam. Appl. Toxicol.* **14**, 208–216.

Dial, C. A. B., and Dial, N. A. (1987). Effects of paraquat on reproduction and mortality in two generations of mice. *Arch. Environ. Contam. Toxicol.* **16**, 759–764.

Dial, C. A. B., and Dial, N. A. (1989). Effects of paraquat on parent generation female and F1 suckling mice using different treatment regimes. *Bull. Environ. Contam. Toxicol.* **43**, 66–73.

Dikshith, T. S. S., Datta, K. K., Raizada, R. B., and Kushwah, H. S. (1979). Effect of paraquat dichloride in male rabbits. *Ind. J. Exp. Biol.* **17**, 926–928.

Dinsdale, D., Preston, S. G., and Nemery, B. (1991). Effects of injury on ^{3}H-putrescine uptake by type I and II cells in rat lung slices. *Exp. Mol. Pathol.* **54**, 218–229.

Douglas, J. F., McGeown, M. G., and McEnvoy, J. (1973). The treatment of paraquat poisoning: Three cases of recovery. *Ulster Med. J.* **42**, 209–212.

Douze, J. M. C., van Dijk, A., Gimbrere, J. S. F., van Heijst, A. N. P., Maes, R., and Rauws, A. G. (1974). Intensive therapy after Paraquat intoxication. *Intensivmedizin* **11**, 241–250.

Douze, J. M. C., and van Heijst, A. N. P. (1977). The paraquat intoxication–Oxygen a real problem. *Acta. Pharmac. Tox.* **41**, 241–245.

Douze, J. M. C., van Dijk, A., Gimbrere, J. S. F., van Heijst, A. N. P., and Maes, R. (1977). Intensive therapy after paraquat intoxication: clinical aspects of paraquat poisoning *RIV. Tossicol. Sper. Clin.* **5**, 333–335.

Draffan, G. H., Clare, R. A., Davies, D. L., Hawksworth, G., Murray, S., and Davies, D. S. (1977). Quantitative determination of the herbicide paraquat in human plasma by gas chromatographic and mass spectrometric methods. *J. Chromat.* **139**, 311–320.

Drew, R., and Gram, T. E. (1979). Vehicle alteration of paraquat lethality in mice. *Toxicol. Appl. Pharmacol.* **48**, 479–487.

Dunbar, J. R., Delucia, A., Acuff, R. V., and Ferslew, K. E. (1988). Prolonged intravenous paraquat infusion in the rat. I. Failure of co-infused putrescine to alternate pulmonary paraquat uptake, paraquat-induced biochemical changes or lung injury. *Toxicol. Appl. Pharmacol.* **94**, 207–220.

Dusinska, M., Kovacikova, Z., Vallova, B., and Collins, A. (1998). Responses of alveolar macrophages and epithelial type II cells to oxidative DNA damage caused by paraquat. *Carcinogenesis* **19**, 809–812.

Dutt, A., Priebe, T. S., Teeter, L. D., Kuo, M. T., and Nelson, J. A. (1992). Postnatal development of organic cation transport and MDR gene expression in mouse kidney. *J. Pharmacol. Exp. Therap.* **261**, 1222–1230.

Ecker, J. L., Gibson, J. E., and Hook, J. B. (1975a). *In vitro* analysis of the renal handling of paraquat. *Toxicol. Appl. Pharmacol.* **34**, 170–177.

Ecker, J. L., Hook, J. B., and Gibson, J. E. (1975b). Nephrotoxicity of paraquat in mice. *Toxicol. Appl. Pharmacol.* **34**, 178–186.

Edmonds, B. K., and Edwards, G. L. (1996). The area postrema is involved in paraquat-induced condition aversion behaviour and neuroendocrine activation of the hypothalamic-pituitary-adrenal axis. *Brain Res.* **712**, 127–133.

Eisenman, A., Armali, Z., Raikhlin-Eisenkraft, B., Bentur, L., Bentur, Y., Guralnik. L., and Enat, R. (1998). Nitric oxide inhalation for paraquat-induced lung injury. *J. Toxicol. Clin. Toxico.l* **36**, 575–584.

Elroy-Stein, O., Bernstei, Y., and Groner, Y. (1986). Overproduction of human Cu/Zn-superoxide dismutase in transfected cells extenuation of paraquat mediated cytotoxicity and enhancement of lipid-peroxidation. *EMBO J.* **5**, 615.

Endo, T., Hara, S., Kano, S., and Kuriiwa, F. (1988). Effects of a paraquat-containing herbicide, Gramoxone, on the central monoamines and acetylcholine in mice. *Res. Comm. Psychol. Psychiatry Behav.* **13**, 261–270.

Ernouf, D., Boussa, N., Legras, A., and Dutertre-Catella, H. (1998). Acute paraquat poisoning: increased toxicity in one case with high alcohol intake. *Human Exp. Toxicol.* **17**, 182–184.

Fairshter, R. D., Rosen, S. M., Smith, W. R., Glasser, F. L., McRae, D. M., and Wilson, A. F. (1976). Paraquat poisoning: New aspects of therapy. *Quart. J. Med.* **45**, 551–565.

Fairshter, R. D., Dubir-Vaziri, N., Smith, W. P., Glauser, F. L., and Wilson, A. F. (1979). Paraquat poisoning: an analytical toxicological study of three cases. *Toxicology* **12**, 259–266.

FAO/WHO (1973). Paraquat. *In* "1972 Evaluations of Some Pesticide Residues in Food." Food and Agricultural Organization of the United Nations, Rome.

FAO/WHO (1986). Paraquat. *In* "1986 Evaluations of Some Pesticide Residues in Food." Food and Agricultural Organisation of the United Nations, Rome.

Farrington, J. A., Ebert, M., Land, E. J., and Fletcher, K. (1973). Bipyridilium quaternary salts and related compounds. V. Pulse radiolysis studies on the reaction of paraquat radical with oxygen, implications for the mode of action of bipyridilium herbicides. *Biochim. Biophys. Acta* **314**, 372–381.

Fennelly, J. J., Gallagher, J. T., and Carroll, R. J. (1968). Paraquat poisoning in a pregnant woman. *Br. Med. J.* **3**, 722–723.

Fennelly, J. J., Fitzgerald, M. X., and Fitzgerald, O. (1971). Recovery from severe Paraquat poisoning following forced diuresis and immunosuppressive therapy. *J. Ir. Med. Ass.* **64**, 69–71.

Ferguson, D. M. (1973). Factors influencing renal excretion of paraquat. *Toxicol. Appl. Pharmacol.* **25**, 486.

Fisher, H. K., Clements, J. A., and Wright, R. R. (1973). Enhancement of oxygen toxicity by the herbicide paraquat. *Am. Rev. Resp. Dis.* **107**, 246–252.

Fisher, H. K., Clements, J. A., Tierney, D. F., and Wright, R. R. (1975). Pulmonary effects of paraquat in the first day after injection. *Am. J. Physiol.* **228**, 1217–1223.

Fisher, A. B., and Reicherter, J. (1984). Pentose pathway of glucose metabolism in isolated granular pneumocytes metabolic regulation and stimulation by paraquat. *Biochem. Pharmacol.* **33**, 1349–1353.

Fitzgerald, G. R., and Barniville, G. (1978). Poisoning by granular paraquat. *J. Irish Phys. Surg.* **7**, 133–136.

Fitzgerald, G. R., Barniville, G., Fitzpatrick, P., Edwards, A., and Silke, B. (1977). Adrenal abnormalities in paraquat poisoning: An indication for corticosteroid therapy? *Irish J. Med. Sci.* **146**, 421–423.

Fitzgerald, G. R., Barniville, G., Black, J., Silke, B., Carmody, M., and O'Dwyer, W. F. (1978a). Paraquat poisoning in agricultural workers. *J. Irish Med. Assoc.* **71**, 336–342.

Fitzgerald, G. R., Cannody, M., Barniville, G., O'Dwyer, W. F., Flanagan, M, and Silke, B. (1978b). The changing pattern of paraquat poisoning: An epidemiologic study. *J. Irish Med. Assoc.* **71**, 103–108.

Fitzgerald, G. R., Barniville, G., Dickstein, K., Cannody, M., and O'Dwyer, W. F. (1979a). Experience with Fuller's Earth in paraquat poisoning. *J. Irish Med. Assoc.* **72**, 149–152.

Fitzgerald, G. R., Barniville, G., Gibney, R. T. N., and Fitzgerald, M. X. (1979b). Clinical, radiological and pulmonary function assessment of 13 long-term survivors of paraquat poisoning. *Thorax* **34**, 414–429.

Florkowski, C. M., Bradberry, S. M., Ching, G. W. K., and Jones, A. F. (1992). Acute renal failure in a case of paraquat poisoning with relative absence of pulmonary toxicity. *Postgraduate Med. J.* **68**, 660–662.

Forman, H. J., Aldrich, T. K., Posner, M. A., and Fisher, A. B. (1982). Differential paraquat uptake and redox kinetics of rat granular pneumocytes and alveolar macrophages. *J. Pharmacol. Exp. Therap.* **221**, 428–433.

Fowler, B. A., and Brooks, R. E. (1971). Effects of the herbicide paraquat on the ultrastructure of the mouse kidney. *Am. J. Path.* **63**, 505–520.

Frank, L. (1983). Superoxide dismutase and lung toxicity. *TIPS* **4**, 124–128.

Frank, L., Neriishi, K., Sio, R., and Pascal, D. (1982). Protection from paraquat-induced lung damage and lethality in adult rats pretreated with clofibrate. *Toxicol. Appl. Pharmacol.* **66**, 269–277.

Frank, L., and Massaro, D. (1979). The lung and oxygen toxicity. *Arch. Intern. Med.* **139**, 347–350.

Fredriksson, A., Fredriksson, M., and Eriksson, P. (1993). Neonatal exposure to paraquat or MPTP induces permanent changes in striatum dopamine and behaviour in adult mice. *Toxicol. Appl. Pharmacol.* **122**, 258–264.

Fukushima, T., Yamada, K., Isobe, A., Shimwaku, K., and Yamane, Y. (1993). Mechanism of cytotoxicity of paraquat I NADH oxidation and paraquat radical formation via complex I. *Exp. Toxic. Pathol.* **45**, 345–349.

Gage, J. C. (1968a). Toxicity of paraquat and diquat aerosols generated by a size selective cyclone: effect of particle size distribution. *Br. J. Ind. Med.* **25**, 304–314.

Gage, J. C. (1968b). The action of paraquat and diquat on the respiration of liver cell fractions. *Biochem. J.* **109**, 757–761.

Garnier, R. (1995). Paraquat poisoning by inhalation and skin absorption. *In* "Paraquat Poisoning" (C. Bismuth and A. H. Hall, eds.), pp. 211–234. Dekker, New York.

Garnier, R., Chataigner, D., Eflhymiou, M. L., Morallion, I., and Bramary, F. (1994). Paraquat poisoning by skin absorption: Report of two cases. *Vet. Human Toxicol.* **36**, 313–315.

Gaudreault, P., Friedman, P. A., and Lovejoy, F. H. (1985). Efficacy of activated charcoal and magnesium citrate in the treatment of oral paraquat intoxication. *Ann. Emerg. Med.* **14**, 123–125.

George, M., and Hedworth-Whitty, R. B. (1980). Non-fatal lung-disease due to inhalation of nebulised paraquat. *Br. Med. J.* **280**, 902.

Gill, R., Qua, S. C., and Moffat, A. C. (1983). High-performance liquid chromatography of paraquat and diquat in urine with rapid sample preparation involving ion-pair extraction on disposable cartridges of octadecyl-silica. *J. Chromat.* **255**, 483–490.

Giri, S. N., Parker, H. R., Spangler, W. L., Misra, H. P., Ishizaki, G., Schiedt, M. J., and Chandler, D. B. (1982). Pharmacokinetics of ^{14}C-paraquat and associated biochemical and pathologic changes in beagle dogs following intravenous administration. *Fund. Appl. Toxicol.* **2**, 261–269.

Golbe, L. J., Farrell, T. M., and Davis, P. H. (1990). Follow-up study of early-life protective and risk factors in Parkinson's disease. *Mov. Dis.* **5**, 66–70.

Gordonsmith, R. H., Brooke-Taylor, S., Smith, L. L., and Cohen, G. M. (1983). Structural requirements of compounds to inhibit pulmonary diamine accumulation. *Biochem. Pharmacol.* **32**, 3701–3709.

Goundar, R. P. (1984). Paraquat poisoning in Fiji. *J. Forensic. Sci. Soc.* **24**, 376.

Grant, H. C., Lantos, P. L., and Parkinson, C. (1980). Cerebral damage in paraquat poisoning. *Histopathology* **4**, 185–195.

Groves, C. E., Morales, M. N., Gandolfi, A. J., Dantzler, W. H., and Wright, S. H. (1995). Peritubular paraquat transport in isolated renal proximal tubules. *J. Pharmacol. Exp. Therap.* **275**, 926–932.

Grundemann, D., Gorboulev, V., Gamabaryan, S., Veyhl, M., and Koepsell, H. (1994). Drug excretion mediated by a new prototype of polyspecific transporter. *Nature* **372**, 549–552.

Grundies, H., Kohmar, D., and Bennhold, I. (1971). Paraquat intoxication. Case report with special reference to hemodialysis. *Dtsch. Med. Wochenschr.* **96**, 588–589.

Hall, A. H. (1995). Paraquat and diquat exposures reported to US Poison Centers 1983–1992. *In* "Paraquat Poisoning" (C. Bismuth and A. H. Hall, eds.), pp. 53–63. Dekker, New York.

Hall, A. H. (1998). Nitric oxide inhalation for paraquat—surviving both poisoning and therapy? *J. Toxicol. Clin. Toxicol.* **36**, 585–586.

Halliwell, B., and Gutteridge, J. M. C. (1984). Oxygen toxicity, oxygen radicals, transition metals and disease. *Biochem. J.* **219**, 1–14.

Hampson, E. C., and Pond, S. M. (1988). Failure of hemoperfusion and hemodialysis to prevent death in paraquat poisoning—A retrospective review of 42 patients. *Med. Toxicol. Adverse Drug Experience* **3**, 64–71.

Hara, S., Iwata, N., Kuriiwa, F., Kano, S., Kawaguchi, N., and Endo, T. (1993). Involvement of opioid receptors in shaking behaviour induced by paraquat in rats. *Pharmacol. Toxicol.* **73**, 146–149.

Hardwick, S.J., Adam, A., Smith, L. L., and Cohen, G. M. (1990). Potentiation of the cell specific toxicity of paraquat by 1,3-bis(2-chloroethyl)-1-nitrosourea (BCNU): Implications for the heterogeneous distribution of glutathione (GSH) in rat lung. *Biochem. Pharmacol.* **39**, 581–589.

Harley, J. B., Grinspan, S., and Root, R. K. (1977). Paraquat suicide in a young women: Results of therapy directed against the superoxide radical. *Yale J. Biol. Med.* **50**, 481–488.

Hart, T. B. (1980). Non-fatal lung disease due to inhalation of nebulised paraquat. *Br. Med. J.* **281**, 63–64.

Hart, T. B. (1984). Letter to the editor: on percutaneous paraquat intoxication. *J. Toxicol.–Cut Ocular Toxicol.* **3**, 239–240.

Hart, T. B, Nevitt, A., and Whitehead, A. (1984). A new statistical approach to the prognostic significance of plasma paraquat concentrations. *The Lancet* **II**, 1222–1223.

Hassan, R. A., Afzal, M., Ali, M., and Gubler, C. J. (1989). Effect of paraquat administered intraperitoneally on the nonpolar lipids of rabbits. *Ecotox. Environ. Saf.* **17**, 47–58.

Hawksworth, G. M., Bennett, P. N., and Davies, D. S. (1981). Kinetics of paraquat elimination in the dog. *Toxicol. Appl. Pharmacol.* **57**, 139–145.

He, P., and Yasumoto, K. (1994). Dietary butylated hydroxytoluene counteracts with paraquat to reduce the rale of hepatic DNA single strand breaks in senescence-accelerated mice. *Mech. Ageing Develop.* **76**, 43–48.

Hearn, C. E. D., and Keir, W. (1971). Nail damage in spray operators exposed to paraquat. *Br. Med. J.* **28**, 399–403.

Hertzman, C., Wiens, M., Bowering, D., Snow, B., and Caine, D. (1990). Parkinson's disease: a case-control study of occupational and environmental risk factors. *Am. J. Ind. Med.* **17**, 349–355.

Hettiarachi, J., and Kodithuwakku, G. C. (1989). Pattern of poisoning in Sri Lanka. *Int. J. Epid.* **18**, 418–422.

Heylings, J. R. (1991). Gastrointestinal absorption of paraquat in the isolated mucosa of the rat. *Toxicol. Appl. Pharmacol.* **107**, 482–493.

Hirai, K., Witschi, H., and Cote, M. G. (1985). Mitochondrial injury of pulmonary alveolar epithelial cells in acute paraquat intoxication. *Exp. Mol. Path.* **43**, 242–253.

Ho, S. C., Woo, I., and Lee, C. M. (1989). Epidemiologic studies of Parkinson's disease in Hong Kong. *Neurology* **39**, 1314–1318.

Ho, Y. S., Magnenat, J. L., Gargano, M., and Cao, J. (1998). The nature of antioxidant defense mechanisms: a lesson from transgenic mice. *Environ. Health Perspec.* **106**, 1219–1228.

Hoet, P. H. M., Dinsdale, D., Lewis, C. P. L., Verbeken, J. M., Lauweryns, J. M., and Nemery, B. (1993). Kinetics and cellular localisation of putrescine uptake in human lung tissue. *Thorax.* **48**, 1235–1241.

Hoet, P. H. M., Lewis, C. P. L., Demedts, M., and Nemery, B. (1994). Putrescine and paraquat uptake in human lung slices and isolated type II pneumocytes. *Biochem. Pharmacol.* **48**, 517–524.

Hoet, P. H. M., Demedts, M., and Nemery, B. (1997). Effects of oxygen pressure and medium volume on the toxicity of paraquat in rat and human type II pneumocytes. *Human Exp. Toxicol.* **16**, 305–310.

Hoffer, E., Tzipiniuk, A., Gal, M., and Taitelman, U. (1989). Skin versus blood distribution of paraquat in experimental animals during percutaneous absorption. *J. Tox. Cut. Ocular Tox.* **8**, 179–182.

Hoffer, E., and Taitelmann, N. (1989). Exposure to paraquat through skin absorption: Clinical and laboratory observations of accidental splashing on healthy skin of agricultural workers. *Human Tox.* **8**, 483–485.

Hoffer, E., Zonis, Z., Tabak, A., and Taitelman, U. (1992). The administration of desferrioxamine to paraquat intoxicated rats. *Vet. Human Toxicol.* **34**, 300–303.

Hoffer, E., Avidor, I., Benjaminar, O., Shenker, L., Tabak, A., Tamir, A., Merzbach, D., and Taitelman, U. (1993). N-Acetylcysteine delays the infiltration of inflammatory cells into the lungs of paraquat intoxicated rats. *Toxicol. Appl. Pharmacol.* **120**, 8–12.

Hogarty, C. (1976). "Exposure of Spray Operators to Paraquat." Internal report Institute for Industrial Research and Chemical Engineering Department, University College, Dublin.

Hong, S. Y., Yang, D. H., and Kim, Y. D. (1996). Successful management of severe paraquat poisoning with free radical scavenger. *Korean. J. Med.* **51**, 99–107.

Hooper, R. G., Bates, P. D., Thomas, A. B., Beechler, C. R., and Kunkle, D. B. (1983). The effect of therapeutic vitamin E and niacin on paraquat toxicity. *Clin. Res.* **31**, A417.

Horton, J. K., Brigelius, R., Mason, R. P., and Bend, J. R. (1986). Paraquat uptake in freshly isolated rabbit lung epithelial cells and its reduction to the paraquat radical under anaerobic conditions. *Mol. Pharmacol.* **29**, 484–488.

Houze, P., Baud, F. I., Mouy, R., Bismuth, C., Bourdon, R., and Scherrmann, J. M. (1990). Toxicokinetics of Paraquat in Humans. *Human Exp. Toxicol.* **9**, 5–12.

Howard, J. K. (1979a). Recent experience with paraquat poisoning in Great Britain—A review of 68 cases. *Vet. Hum. Toxicol.* **21**, 213–216.

Howard, J. K. (1979b). A clinical survey of paraquat formulation workers. *Br. J. Ind. Med.* **36**, 220–223.

Howard, J. K. (1980). Paraquat: A review of worker exposure in normal usage. *J. Soc. Occup. Med.* **30**, 6–11.

Howard, J. K., Sabapathy, N. N., and Whitehead, P. A. (1981). A study of the health of Malayan plantation workers with particular reference to Paraquat spraymen. *Br. J. Ind. Med.* **38**, 110–116.

Howe, D. J. T., and Wright, N. (1965). The toxicity of paraquat and diquat. *In* "Proc. 18th NZ Weed and Pest Control Conference," pp. 105–114.

Hudson, M., Smith, C. C., Patel, S. B., Friend, J. A. R., and Ewen, S. W. B. (1991). Paraquat induced pulmonary fibrosis in three survivors. *Thorax* **46**, 201–204.

Hughes, J. T. (1988). Brain damage due to paraquat poisoning. *Neurotoxicology* **9**, 140.

Hughes, R. D., Millburn, P., and Williams, R. T. (1973). Biliary excretion of some diquaternary ammonium cations in the rat, guinea-pig and rabbit. *Biochem. J.* **136**, 979–984.

Hutchinson, G., Daisley, H., Simmons, V., and Gordon, A. N. (1991). Suicide by poisoning. *West Ind. Med. J.* **40**, 69–73.

Hybertson, B. M., Lampey, A. S., Clarke, J. H., Koh, Y., and Repine, J.'E. (1995). N-acetylcysteine pretreatment attenuates paraquat-induced lung leak in rats. *Redox Rep.* **1**, 337–342.

Iff, H. W., Brewis, R. A. L., Mallick, N. P., Mawer, G. E., Orr, W. McN., and Stern, M. A. (1971). Paraquat poisoning. *Schweiz Med. Wschr.* **101**, 84–88.

Ikebuchi, J., Proudfoot, A. T., Matsubara, K., Hampson, E. O. G. M., Tomita, M., Suzuki, K., Fuke, C., Ijiri, I., Tsunerari, T., Yuasa, I., and Okada, K. (1993). Toxicological index of paraquat: A new strategy for assessment of severity of paraquat poisoning in 128 patients. *Forensic Sci. Int.* **59**, 85–87.

Ilett, K. F., Stripp, B., Menard, R. H., Reid, N. D., and Gillette, J. R. (1974). Studies on the mechanism of the lung toxicity of paraquat: Comparison of tissue distribution and some biochemical parameters in rats and rabbits. *Toxicol. Appl. Pharmacol.* **28**, 216–226.

Ingebrigtsen, K., Nafstad, I., and Andersen, R. A. (1984). Distribution and transplacental transfer of paraquat in rats and guinea-pigs. *Gen. Pharmacol.* **15**, 201–204.

IPCS (1984). "Paraquat and Diqual." Environmental Health Criteria No. 39, World Health Organization, Geneva.

Jaeger, A., Saunder, P., and Scherrmann, J. M. (1995). Mechanisms of paraquat toxicity and therapeutic implications. *In* "Paraquat Poisoning: Mechanisms, Prevention, Treatment" (C. Bismuth and A. H. Hall, eds.), pp. 141–160. Dekker, New York.

Jaros, F., Zuffa, L. M., Kritinova, R., Skakala, I., and Domsova, J. (1978). Acute percutaneous intoxication by Gramoxone. *Pracov. Lek.* **30**, 260–263.

Jarvie, D. R., and Stewart, M. J. (1979). The rapid extraction of paraquat from plasma using an ion pair technique. *Clin. Chim. Acta* **94**, 241–251.

Jenkinson, S. G. (1982). Pulmonary oxygen toxicity. *Clin. Chest Med.* **3**, 109–119.

Joyce, M. (1969). Ocular damage caused by paraquat. *Br. J. Ophthal.* **53**, 688–690.

Kameji, R., Rannels, S. R., Pegg, A. E., and Rannels, D. E. (1989). Spermine uptake by type II pulmonary epithelial cells in primary culture. *Am. J. Physiol.* **256**, C160–167.

Kamholz, S., Veith, F. J., Mollenkopf, F., Montefusco, C., Nehlsen-Cannarella, S., Kaleya, R., Pinsker, K., Tellis, V., Soberman, R., and Sablay, L. (1984). Single lung transplant in paraquat intoxication. *NY State J. Med.* **84**, 82–84.

Karl, P. I., and Friedman, P. A. (1983). Competition between paraquat and putrescine for accumulation by rat lung slices. *Toxicology* **26**, 317–323.

Katopodis, K., Logothetis, E., Noussias, C., and Hadjiconstantinou, V. (1993). Survival of a paraquat poisoned patient despite late (4 days) referral and initiation of conventional haemoperfusion treatment. *Nephrol. Dialysis Transplant.* **8**, 570–571.

Keeling, P. L., Pratt, I. S., Aldridge, W. N., and Smith, L. L. (1981). The enhancement of paraquat toxicity in rats by 85% oxygen-lethality and cell-specific lung damage. *Br. J. Exp. Path.* **62**, 643–654.

Keeling, P. L., and Smith, L. L. (1982). Relevance of NADPH depletion and mixed disulphide formation in rat lung to the mechanism of cell damage following paraquat administration. *Biochem. Pharmacol.* **31**, 3243–3249.

Keeling, P. L., Smith, L. L., and Aldridge, W. N. (1982). The formation of mixed disulphides in rat lung following paraquat administration. Correlation with changes in intermediary metabolism. *Biochem. Biophys. Acta* **716**, 249–257.

Kehrer, I. P., Haschek, W., and Witschi, H. P. (1979). The influence of hyperoxia on the acute toxicity of paraquat and diquat. *Drug Chem. Tox.* **2**, 397–408.

Kelner, M. I., and Bagnell, R. D. (1989). Paraquat resistance associated with reduced NADPH reductase in an energy-dependent paraquat-accumulating cell line. *Arch. Biochem. Biophys.* **274**, 366–374.

Kelner, M. J., Bagnell, R. D., Uglik, S. F., Montoya, M. A., and Mullenbach, G. T. (1995). Heterologous expression of selenium dependent glutathione peroxidase affords cellular resistance to paraquat. *Arch. Biochem. Biophys.* **323**, 40–46.

Kerr, F., Patel, A. R., Scott, P. D. R., and Tompsett, S. L. (1968). Paraquat poisoning treated by forced diuresis. *Br. Med. J.* **3**, 290–291,

Khera, K. S., Whitta, L. L., and Clegg, D. I. (1970). Embryopathic effects of diquat and paraquat in rats. *Ind. Med. Surg.* **37**, 257–261.

Kimbrough, R. D., and Gaines, T. B. (1970). Toxicity of paraquat to rats and its effect on rat lung. *Toxicol. Appl. Pharmacol.* **17**, 679–690.

Kitazawa, K., Kobayashi, T., Shibamoto, T., and Hirai, K. (1988). Effects of methyl prednisolone on acute lung paraquat toxicity in sheep. *Am. Rev. Resp. Dis.* **137**, 173–180.

Kitazawa, Y., Matsubara, M., Takeyama, N., and Tanaka, T. (1991). The role of xanthine oxidase in paraquat intoxication. *Arch. Biochem. Biophys.* **288**, 220–224.

Knepil, J. (1977). A short simple method for the determination of paraquat in plasma. *Clin. Chim. Acta* **79**, 387–390.

Knight, B. A. G., and Tomlinson, T. E. (1967). The interaction of paraquat (1:1′-dimethyl-4,4′-dipyridilium dichloride) with mineral soils. *J. Soil. Sci.* **18**, 233.

Kohen, R., and Chevion, M. (1985). Paraquat toxicity is enhanced by iron and reduced by desferrioxamine in laboratory mice. *Biochemical. Pharmacol.* **34**, 1841–1843.

Kojima, S., Miyazaki, Y., Honda, T., Kiyozumi, M., Shimada, H., and Funakoshi, T. (1992). Effect of L-cystine on toxicity of paraquat in mice. *Toxicol. Lett.* **60**, 75–82.

Koller, W. C. (1986). Paraquat and Parkinsons disease. *Neurology* **36**, 1147.

Koller, W., Vetere-Overfield, B., Gray, C., Alexander, C., Chin, T., Dolezal, J., Hassanein, R., and Tanner, C. (1990). Environmental risk factors in Parkinson's disease. *Neurology* **40**, 1218–1221.

Kopazyk-Locke, K. (1977). *In vitro* and *in vivo* effects of paraquat on rat liver mitochondria. *In* "Biochemical Mechanisms of Paraquat Toxicity" (A. P. Autor, ed.), pp. 93–115. Academic Press, San Diego.

Köppel, C., Wissmann, C. V., Barckow, D., Rossaint, R., Falke, K., Stoltenburg-Didinger, G., and Schnoy, N. (1994). Inhaled nitric oxide in advanced paraquat intoxication. *J. Toxicol. Clin. Toxicol.* **32**, 205–214.

Kornbrust, D. J., and Mavis, R. D. (1980). The effect of paraquat on microsomal lipid peroxidation in vitro and in vivo. *Toxicol. Appl. Pharmacol.* **53**, 323–332.

Krall, J., Bagley, A. C., Mullenbach, G. T., Hallewell, R. A., and Lynch, R. E. (1988). Superoxide mediates the toxicity of paraquat for cultured mammalian cells. *J. Biol. Chem.* **263**, 1910–1914.

Kuo, T. L., and Nanikawa, R. (1990). Effect of ethanol on acute paraquat toxicity in rabbits. *Jpn. J. Legal Med.* **44**, 12–17.

Laithwaitte, J. A. (1975). Paraquat poisoning treated with immunosuppressants and potassium aminobenzoate. *Br. Med. J.* **1**, 266–267.

Lambert, C. E., and Bondy, S. C. (1989). Effects of MPTP, MPP$^+$ and paraquat on mitochondrial potential and oxidative stress. *Life Sci.* **44**, 1277–1284.

Landrigan, P. J., Powell, K. E., James, L. E., and Taylor, P. R. (1983). Paraquat and marijuana—epidemiologic risk assessment. *Am. J. Public Health* **73**, 784–788.

Langston, J. W., Ballard, P., Tetrud, J. W., and Irwin, I. (1983). Chronic Parkinsonism in humans due to a product of mereperidine analog. *Science* **219**, 979–980.

Larsson, B., Oskarsson, J. A., and Tjalve, H. (1977). Binding of paraquat and diquat in melanin. *Exp. Eye Res.* **25**, 353–359.

Larsson, B., Oskarsson, A., and Tjalve, H. (1978). On the binding of the bisquaternary ammonium compound paraquat to melanin and cartilage *in vivo*. *Biochem. Pharmacol.* **27**, 1721–1724.

Lautenschläger, J., Grabensee, B., and Poettgen, W. (1974). Paraquat poisoning and isolated aplastic anaemia. *Dtsch. Med. Wschr.* **99**, 2348–2351.

Lazo, J. S., Kondo, Y., Dellapiazza, D., Michalska, A. E., Choo, K. H. A., and Pitt, B. R. (1995). Enhanced sensitivity to oxidative stress in cultured embryonic cells from transgenic mice deficient in metallothionein I and II genes. *J. Biol. Chem.* **270**, 5506–5510.

Lee, K. Y., and Lee, T. H. (1995). Effect of hemoperfusion on treatment for paraquat intoxication. *Blood Purification* **13**, 60–61.

Lee, S. H., Lee, K. S., Ahn, J. M., Kim, S. H., and Hong, S. Y. (1995). Paraquat poisoning of the lung: thin-section CT findings. *Radiology* **195**, 271–274.

Levin, P. J., Klaff, L. J., Rose, A. G., and Ferguson, A. D. (1979). Pulmonary effects of contact exposure to paraquat: a clinical and experimental study. *Thorax.* **34**, 150–160.

Levitt, T. (1979). Determinations of paraquat in clinical practice using radioimmunoassay. *Proc. Analyt. Div. Chem. Soc.* **161**, 72–76.

Lewin, R. (1984). Trails of ironies to Parkinson's disease. *Science* **224**, 1083–1085.

Lewis, C. P. L. (1989). "The Pulmonary Uptake and Metabolism of Cystamine." Ph.D. Thesis, University of London.

Lewis, C. P. L., Haschek, W. M., Wyatt, I., Cohen, G. M., and Smith, L. L. (1989). The accumulation of cystamine and its metabolism to taurine in rat lung slices. *Biochem. Pharmacol.* **38**, 481–488.

Lheureux, P., Leduc, D., Vanbinst, R., and Askenasi, R. (1995). Survival in a case of massive paraquat ingestion. *Chest* **107**, 285–289.

Licker, M., Schweizer, A., Honn, L., Morel, D. R., and Spiliopoulos, A. (1998). Single lung transplantation from adult respiratory distress syndrome after paraquat poisoning. *Thorax* **53**, 620–621.

Liddle, J. A., Needham, L. L., Rollen, Z. J., Roark, B. R., and Bayse, D. D. (1980). Characterization of the contamination of marijuana with paraquat. *Bull. Environ. Content. Toxicol.* **24**, 49–53.

Lin, J. L., Liu, L., and Leu, M. L. (1995). Recovery of respiratory function in survivors with paraquat intoxication. *Arch. Environ. Health* **50**, 432–439.

Lin, J. L., Wei, M. C., and Liu, Y. C. (1996). Pulse therapy with cyclophosphamide and methylprednisolone in patients with moderate to severe paraquat poisoning: A preliminary report. *Thorax* **51**, 661–663.

Lin, J. L., Leu, M. L., Liu, Y. C., and Chen, G. H. (1999). A prospective clinical trial of pulse therapy with glucocorticoid and cyclophosphamide in moderate to severe paraquat-poisoned patients. *Am. J. Resp. Crit. Care Med.* **159**, 357–360.

Lindquist, N. G., Larsson, B. S., and Lydensokolowski, A. (1988). Autoradiography of C-14 paraquat or C-14 Diquat in frogs and mice—Accumulation in neuromelanin. *Neurosci. Lett.* **93**, 1–6.

Liou, H.-H., Chen, R.-C., Tsai, Y.-F., Chen, W.-P., Chang, Y.-C., and Tsai, M.-C. (1996). Effects of paraquat on the substantia nigra of the Wistar rats: neurochemical, histological and behavioural studies. *Toxicol. Appl. Pharmacol.* **137**, 34–41.

Liou, H. H., Tsai, M. C., Chen, C. J., Jeng, J. S., Chang, Y. C., Chen, S. Y., and Chen, R. C. (1997). Environmental risk factors and Parkinson's disease: A case-control study in Taiwan. *Neurology* **48**, 1583–1588.

Litchfield, M. H., Daniel, J. W., and Longshaw, S. (1973). The tissue distribution of the bipyridylium herbicides, diquat and paraquat in rats and mice. *Toxicology* **1**, 155–165.

Liu, D., Yang, J., Li, L., and McAdoo, D. J. (1995). Paraquat—a superoxide generator—kills neurons in the rat spinal cord. *Free Rod. Biol. Med.* **18**, 861–867.

Lock, E. A. (1979). The effect of paraquat and diquat on renal function in the rat. *Toxicol. Appl. Pharmacol.* **48**, 327–336.

Lock, E. A., Smith, L. L., and Rose, M. S. (1976). Inhibition of paraquat accumulation in rat lung slices by a component of rat plasma and a variety of drugs and endogenous amines. *Biochem. Pharmacol.* **25**, 1769–1772.

Lock, E. A., and Ishmael, J. (1979). The acute effects of paraquat and diquat on the rat kidney. *Toxicol. Appl. Pharmacol.* **50**, 67–76.

Mahieu, P., Hassoun, A., Fautsch, G., Lauwerijs, R., and Tremouroux, J. (1977). Paraquat poisoning: Survival without pulmonary insufficiency after early bleomycin treatment. *Acta Pharmac. Tox.* **41**, 246–248.

Maini, R., and Winchester, J. F. (1975). Removal of paraquat from blood by haemoperfusion over sorbent materials. *Br. Med. J.* **3**, 281–282.

Malcolmson, E., and Beesley, J. (1975). Unsuccessful immunosuppressant treatment of paraquat poisoning. *Br. Med. J.* **3**, 650–651.

Maling, H. M., Saul, W., Williams, M. A., Brown, E. A. D., and Gillette, J. R. (1978). Reduced body clearance as the major mechanism of the potentiation by B_2-adrenergic agonist of paraquat lethality in rats. *Toxicol. Appl. Pharmacol.* **43**, 57–72.

Malone, J. D. G., Carmody, M., Keogh, B., and O'Dwyer, W. F. (1971). Paraquat poisoning—A review of nineteen cases. *J. Irish Med. Ass.* **64**, 59–68.

Markey, S. P., Castagnoli, N., Trevor, A. J., and Kopin, I. J. (eds.) (1986). MPTP: A Neurotoxin Producing a Parkinson Syndrome. Academic Press, New York.

Masek, I., and Richard, R. J. (1990). Interactions between paraquat, endogenous lung amine antioxidants and isolated mouse Clara cells. *Toxicology* **63**, 315–326.

Matkovics, B., Barabas, K., Szabo, L., and Berencsi, G. (1980). In vivo study of the mechanism of protective effects of ascorbic acid and reduced glutathione in paraquat poisoning. *Gen. Pharmac.* **11**, 455–461.

Matsubara, M., Yamagami, K., Kitazawa, Y., Kawamoto, K., and Takana, T. (1996). Paraquat causes S-phase arrest of rat liver and lung cells *in vivo*. *Arch. Toxicol.* **70**, 514–518.

Matthew, H., Logan, A., Woodruff, M. F. A., and Heard, B. (1968). Paraquat poisoning-lung transplantation. *Br. Med. J.* **3**, 759–763.

McArn, G. E., Gee, S. J., and Krieger, R. I. (1980). Ascorbic acid potentiated pathologic and toxicologic effects of paraquat (MV) and n-Propylviologen (PV) in rats. "19th Society of Toxicology," Abstract 14, p. A101.

McCord, J. M., and Da, E. D. (1987). Superoxide dependant production of hydroxyl radical catalysed by iron-EDTA complex. *FEBS Lett.* **86**, 139–142.

McDonah, B. J., and Martin, J. (1970). Paraquat poisoning in children. *Archs. Dis. Child* **45**, 425–427.

McElligott, T. F. (1972). The dermal toxicity of paraquat: Differences due to techniques of application. *Toxicol. Appl. Pharmacol.* **21**, 361–386.

McKean, W. I. (1968). Recovery from Paraquat poisoning. *Br. Med. J.* **3**, 292.

Mehani, S. (1972). The toxic effect of paraquat in rabbits and rats. *Ain. Shams. Med. J.* **23**, 599–601.

Meredith, T. J., and Vale, J. A. (1987). Treatment of paraquat poisoning in man: Methods to prevent absorption. *Human Toxicol.* **6**, 49–55.

Meredith, T., and Vale, J. A. (1995). Treatment of paraquat poisoning: Gastrointestinal decontamination. *In* "Paraquat Poisoning: Mechanisms, Prevention, Treatment" (C. Bismuth and A. H. Hall, eds.), pp. 297–314. Dekker, New York.

Michaelis, L., and Hill, E. S. (1933). Potentiometric studies on semiquinones. *J. Am. Chem. Soc.* **55**, 1481–1494.

Minakata, K., Suzuki, O, Saito, S., and Harada, N. (1996). Effect of dietary paraquat on a rat mutant unable to synthesis ascorbic acid. *Arch. Toxicol.* **70**, 256–258.

Ming, F. K., Chun, C. H., and Khoo, T. K. (1980). Paraquat poisoning is not always fatal. *Singapore Med. J.* **21**, 703–707.

Ministerio de Salud, Division de Saneamiento Ambiental, Depto. Registro y Control de Sustancias Toxicas (1997). Reporte Oficial Intoxicaciones con Plaguicidas, Costa Rica.

Mirchev, N. (1977). Acute poisoning with Gramoxone (Paraquat). *Vetr. Bol.* **16**, 99–101.

Modee, J., Ivemark, B. I., and Robertson, B. (1972). Ultrastructure of the alveolar wall in experimental paraquat poisoning. *Acta. Path. Microbiol. Scand.* **80**, 54–60.

Molck, A.-M., and Friis, C. (1997). The cytotoxic effect of paraquat to isolated renal proximal tubular segments from rabbits. *Toxicology* **122**, 123–132.

Molnar, I. G., and Hayes, W. J. (1971). Distribution and metabolism of paraquat in the rat. *Toxicol. Appl. Pharmacol.* **19**, 405.

Montgomery, M. R., Furry, J., Gee, S. J., and Krieger, R. I. (1982). Ascorbic acid and paraquat: oxygen depletion with concurrent oxygen activation. *Toxicol. Appl. Phartmacol.* **63**, 321–329.

Moody, C. S., and Hassan, H. M. (1982). Mutagenicity of oxygen free radicals. *Proc. Nat. Acad. Sci.* **79**, 2855–2859.

Mullick, F. G., Ishak, K. G., Mahabir, R., and Stomeyer, W. F. (1981). Hepatic injury associated with paraquat toxicity in humans. *Liver* **1**, 209–221.

Murray, R. E., and Gibson, J. E. (1971). Lethality and pharmacokinetics of paraquat in rats. *Toxicol. Appl. Pharmacol.* **19**, Abstr. 115.

Murray, R. E., and Gibson, J. E. (1972). A comparative study of paraquat intoxication in rats, guinea pigs and monkeys. *Exp. Mol. Pathol.* **17**, 317–325.

Murray, R. E., and Gibson, J. E. (1974). Paraquat disposition in rats, guineapigs and monkeys. *Toxicol. Appl. Pharmacol.* **27**, 283–291.

Musson, F. A., and Porter, C. A. (1982). Effect of ingestion of paraquat on a 20-week gestation fetus. *Postgrad. Med. J.* **58**, 731–732.

Nagao, M., Takatori, T., Wu, B., Terazawa, K., Gotouda, H., and Akabane, H. (1989). Immunotherapy for the treatment of paraquat poisoning. *Human Toxicol.* **8**, 121–123.

Nagao, M., Takatori, T., Inoue, K., Shimizu, M., Terazawa, K., and Akabane, H. (1990). Immunohistochemical localisation and dynamics of paraquat in small intestine, liver and kidney. *Toxicology* **63**, 167–182.

Nagao, M., Takatori, T., Wu, B., Terazawa, K., Getouda, H., and Akabane, H. (1991). Immunohistochemical localisation of paraquat in lung and brain. *Med. Sci. Law* **31**, 61–65.

Nagao, M., Zhang, W. D., Itakura, Y., Kobayashi, M., Yamada, Y., Yagi, K., Oono, T., and Takatori, T. (1993). Immunohistochemical localisation and dynamics of paraquat in the stomach and esophagus of rats. *J. Legal Med.* **106**, 142–144.

Nagata, T., Kono, I., Masaoka, T., and Akahori, F. (1992a). Acute toxicological studies on paraquat pathological findings in beagle dogs following single subcutaneous injections. *Vet. Human Toxicol.* **34**, 105–112.

Nagata, T., Kono, I., Masaoka, T., and Akahori, F. (1992b). Subacute toxicity of paraquat in beagle dogs: Clinicopathology and pathologic examination. *Vet. Human Toxicol.* **34**, 15–20.

Nagi, A. H. (1969). Paraquat and adrenal cortical necrosis. *Br. Med. J.* **2**, 669.

Naito, H., and Yamashita, M. (1987). Epidemiology of paraquat in Japan and a new safe formulation of paraquat. *Human Toxicol.* **6**, 87–88.

Naylor, J., Widdowson, P. S., Simpson, M. G., Ellis, M. K., and Lock, E. A. (1995). Studies of systemically administered paraquat on brain penetration and neurotoxicity. *Human Exp. Toxicol.* **14**, 370.

Nemery, B., Smith, L. L., and Aldridge, W. N. (1987). Putrescine and 5-hydroxytryptamine accumulation in rat lung slices: cellular localisation and responses to cell-specific lung injury. *Toxicol. Appl. Pharmacol.* **91**, 107–120.

Nemery, B., Van Lommel, S., Verbeken, E. K., Lauweryns, J. M., and Demedts, M. (1992). Lung injury induced by paraquat, hyperoxia and cobalt chloride: Effects of ambroxol *Pulmonary Pharmacol.* **5**, 53–60.

Nemeth, P., Racz, L., Varga, J., Lang, A., Nemeth, A., and Nemeth, A. (1985). Changes of the serum superoxide dismutase content in gramoxone poisoned patients, measured by anti-SOD monoclonal antibody. *Arch. Toxicol.* **8**, 288.

Newhouse, M., McEvoy, D., and Rosenthal, D. (1978). Percutaneous Paraquat absorption. An association with cutaneous lesions and respiratory failure. *Arch. Dermatol.* **114**, 1516–1519.

Ng, L. L., Naik, R. B., and Polak, A. (1982). Paraquat ingestion with methaemoglobinemia treated with methylene blue. *Br. Med. J.* **284**, 1445–1446.

Nicotera, T. M., Block, A. W., Gibas, Z., and Sandberg, A. A. (1985). Induction of superoxide dismutase, chromosomal aberrations and sister-chromatid exchanges by paraquat in Chinese hamster fibroblasts. *Mutat. Res.* **151**, 263–268.

Nogue, S., Munne, P., Campana, E., Bertran, A., Reig, R., and Rodamilana, M. (1989). Failure of the combination cyclophosphamide-dexamethasone in paraquat poisoning. *Medicina Clinica-Spa.* **93**, 61–63.

Nokata, M., Tanaka, T., Tsuchiya, K., and Yamashita, M. (1984). Alleviation of paraquat toxicity by kayexalate and kalimate in rats. *Acta. Pharmacol. Toxicol.* **55**, 158–160.

Ogata, T., and Manabe, S. (1990). Correlation between lipid peroxidation and morphological manifestation of paraquat-induced lung injury in rats. *Arch. Tox.* **64**, 7–13.

Ohlson, C. G., and Hogstedt, C. (1981). Parkinson's disease and occupational exposure to organic solvents, agricultural chemicals and mercury—a case-referent study. *Scand. J. Work Environ. Health* **7**, 252–256.

Okonek, S., Setyadharma, H., Borchent, A. and Krienke, E.G. (1982). Activated charcoal is as effective as Fullers Earth or bentonite in paraquat poisoning. *Klin. Wochenschr.* **60**, 207–210.

Okonek, S., Baldamus, C. A., Holmann, A., Schister, C. J., Bechstein, P. B., and Zoller, B. (1979). Two survivors of severe paraquat intoxication by "continuous haemoperfusion." *Klin. Wschr.* **57**, 957–959.

Okonek, S., Baldamus, C. A., and Hofmann, A. (1980). Survival despite potentially fatal plasma paraquat concentrations. *The Lancet* **II**, 589.

Okonek, S., Weilemann, L. S., Majdanzic, J., Sethyadarma, H., and Reinecke, H. J. (1982/83). Successful treatment of paraquat poisoning. Activated charcoal per os and "continuous hemoperfusion." *Toxicol. Clin. Toxicol.* **19**, 807–819.

Okonek, S., Wronski, R, Niedermeyer, W., Okonek, M., and Lamer, A. (1983). Near fatal percutaneous paraquat poisoning. *Klin. Wochenschr.* **61**, 655.

Okuda, M., Saito, H., Urakami, Y., Takano, M., and Inui, K. (1996). cDNA cloning and functional expression of a novel rat kidney organic cation transporter, OCT2. *Biochem. Biophys. Res. Commun.* **224**, 500–507.

Omaye, S. T., Reddy, K. A., and Cross, C. E. (1978). Enhanced lung toxicity in selenium deficient rats. *Toxicol. Appl. Pharmacol.* **43**, 237–247.

Ongom, V. I., Owor, R., and Tomusangi, E. T. (1974). Paraquat (Gramoxone) used as a pediculocide. *In* "Uses and Abuses of Drugs and Chemicals in Tropical Africa," pp. 229–233. East Africa Lit. Bureau, Nairobi.

Onyon, L. J., and Volans, G. N. (1987). The epidemiology and prevention of paraquat poisoning. *Hum. Toxicol.* **6**, 19–29.

Oreffo, V. I. C., John, R. A., and Richards, R. J. (1991). Diamine uptake by rat lung type II cells in vitro. *Biochem. Pharmacol.* **41**, 1209–1215.

Oreopoulos, D. G., Soyannwo, M. A., Sinniah, R., Fenton, S. S., and Bruce, J. H. (1968). Acute renal failure in case of paraquat poisoning. *Br. Med. J.* **1**, 749–750.

Osheroff, M. R, Schaich, M. K., Drew, R. T., and Borg, D. C. (1985). Failure of desferrioxamine to modify the toxicity of paraquat in rats. *J. Free Rad. Biol. Med.* **1**, 71–82.

O'Sullivan, M. C., Golding, B. T., Smith, L. L., and Wyatt, I. (1991). Molecular features necessary for the uptake of diamines and related compounds by the polyamine receptor of rat lung slices. *Biochem. Pharmacol.* **41**, 1839–1848.

Palmeira, C. M., Moreno, A. J., and Madeira, V. M. C. (1995). Mitochondrial bioenergetics is affected by the herbicide paraquat. *Biochim. Biophys. Acta* **1229**, 187–192.

Papiris, S. A., Maniati, M. A., Kyriakidis, V., and Constantopoulos, S. H. (1995). Pulmonary damage due to paraquat poisoning through skin absorption. *Respiration* **62**, 101–103.

Park, J., Proudfoot, A. T., and Prescott, L. F. (1975). Paraquat poisoning—A clinical review of 31 cases. *In* "Clinical Aspects of Paraquat Poisoning, Proceedings of an International Meeting." Imperial Chemical Industries Limited, London.

Parkinson, C. (1980). The changing pattern of Paraquat poisoning in man. *Histopathology* **4**, 171–183.

Patterson, C. E., and Rhodes, M. L. (1982). The effect of superoxide dismutase on paraquat mortality in mice and rats. *Toxicol. Appl. Pharmacol.* **62**, 65–72.

Perriens, T., Van der Stuyft, P., Chee, H., and Benimadhos, S. (1989). The epidemiology of paraquat intoxications in Surinam. *Tropical Geographical Med.* **41**, 266–269.

Perriens, J. H., Benimadho, S., Kiauw, I. L., Wisse, J., and Chee, H. (1992). High-dose cyclophosphamide and dexamethasone in paraquat poisoning: A prospective study. *Human Exp. Toxicol.* **11**, 129–134.

Perry, T. L., Yong, V. W., Wall, R. A., and Jones, K. (1986). Paraquat and two endogenous analogues of the neurotoxic substance *N*-methyl-4-phenyl-1,2,3,6-tetrahydropyridine do not damage dopaminergic nigrostriatal neurons in the mouse. *Nenrosci. Lett.* **69**, 285–289.

Peyresblanques, M. J. (1969). Ocular burns caused by Gramoxone. *Bull. Soc. Ophthalmol.* **69**, 928.

Pond, S. M., Rivory, L. P., Hampson, E. C. G. M., and Roberts, M. S. (1993). Kinetics of toxic doses of paraquat and the effects of haemoperfusion in the dog. *J. Toxicol. Clin. Toxicol.* **31**, 229–246.

Proudfoot, A. T. (1982). Methaemoglobinaemia due to monolinuron—not paraquat. *Brit. Med.* **285**, 812.

Proudfoot, A. T., Stewart, M. S., Levitt, T., and Widdop, B. (1979). Paraquat poisoning: significance of plasma paraquat concentrations. *The Lancet* **II**, 330–332.

Proudfoot, A. T., Prescott, L. F., Simpson, D., Buckley, B. M., and Vale, J. A. (1984). Radiotherapy for paraquat lung toxicity. *Br. Med. J.* **289**, 112.

Purser, D. A., and Rose, M. S. (1979). The toxicity and renal handling of paraquat in cynomologus monkeys. *Toxicology* **15**, 31–41.

Ragoucy-Sengler, C., and Pileire, B. (1996a). A biological index to predict patient outcome in paraquat poisoning. *Human Exp. Toxicol.* **15**, 265–268.

Ragoucy-Sengler, C., and Pileire, B. (1996b). Survival after paraquat poisoning in a HIV positive patient. *Human Exp. Toxicol.* **15**, 286–288.

Ragoucy-Sengler, C., Pileire, B., and Daijardin, J. B. (1991). Survival from severe paraquat intoxication in heavy drinkers. *The Lancet* **2**, 1461.

Ramasamy, S., and Nursiah, M. T. A. (1988). A survey of pesticide use and associated incidences of poisoning in Peninsular Malaysia. *J. Pl. Prot. Tropics* **5**, 1–9.

Reddy, K. A., Litov, R. E., and Omaye, S. T. (1977). Effect of pretreatment with anti-inflammatory agents on paraquat toxicity in the rat. *Res. Commun. Chem. Path. Pharm.* **17**, 87–100.

Reddy, K., Omaye, S., Chiu, M., Litov, R., Hasehawa, G., and Cross, C. (1976). Effect of aspirin, indomethacin and hydrocortisone pretreatments on selected aspects of rat lung metabolism before and after paraquat administration. *Am. Rev. Resp. Dis.* **113**, 102.

Redetzki, H. M., Wood, C. D., and Grafton, W. D. (1980). Vitamin E and paraquat poisoning. *Vet. Human Tox.* **22**, 395–397.

Reif, R. M., and Lewinsohn, G. (1983). Paraquat myocarditis and adrenal cortical necrosis. *J. Forensic Sci.* **28**, 505.

Repine, J. E., Pfinninger, O. S., Talmage, D. W., Berger, E. M., and Pettijohn, D. E. (1981). Dimethyl sulphoxide prevents DNA nicking mediated by ionising radiation or iron/hydrogen peroxide-generated hydroxyl radical. *Proc. Natl. Acad Sci. USA* **78**, 1001–1003.

Restuccia, A., Foglini, A., and De Alentis-Nannini, D. (1974). Paraquat toxicity for rabbits. *Vent. Ital.* **25**, 555–565.

Rhodes, M. L., Zavala, D. C., and Brown, D. (1976). Hypoxic protection in paraquat poisoning. *Lab. Invest.* **35**, 496–500.

Ribas, G., Frenzilli, G., Barale, R., and Marcos, R. (1995). Herbicide induced DNA damage in human lymphocytes evaluated by the single cell gel electrophoresis SCGE assay. *Mutat. Res.* **344**, 41–54.

Richards, R. I., Davies, N., Atkins, J., and Oreffo, V. I. C. (1987). Isolation, biochemical characterisation and culture or lung type II cells of the rat. *Lung* **165**, 143–158.

Rios, A. C. C., Salvadori, D. M. F., Oliveira, S. V., and Ribeiro, L. R. (1995). The action of the herbicide paraquat on somatic and germ cells of mice. *Mutat. Res.* **328**, 113–118.

Rose, M. S., Smith, L. L., and Wyatt, I. (1974a). Evidence for the energy-dependant accumulation of paraquat into rat lung. *Nature* **252**, 314–315.

Rose, M. S, Crabtree, H. C., Fletcher, K., and Wyatt, I. (1974b). Biochemical effects of diquat and paraquat: Disturbance of the control of corticosteroid synthesis in rat adrenal and subsequent effects in the control of liver glycogen utilisation. *Biochem. J.* **138**, 437–443.

Rose, M. S., Lock, E. A., Smith, L. L., and Wyatt, I. (1976a). Paraquat accumulation: Tissue and species specificity. *Biochem. Pharmacol.* **25**, 419–423.

Rose, M. S., Smith, L. L., and Wyatt, I. (1976b). The relevance of pentose phosphate pathway stimulation in rat lung to the mechanism of paraquat toxicity. *Biochem. Pharmacol.* **25**, 1763–1767.

Ross, J. H., and Krieger, R. I. (1981). Structure activity correlation's of amines inhibiting active uptake of paraquat (Methyl Viologen) into rat lung slices. *Toxicol. Appl. Pharmacol.* **59**, 238–249.

Sabapathy, N. N. (1995). Paraquat formulation and safety management. *In* "Paraquat Poisoning" (C. Bismuth and A. H. Hall, eds.), pp. 335–347. Dekker, New York.

Saenghirunvattana, S., Sermswan, A., Piratchvej, V., Rochanawutanon, M., Kaojaren, S., and Rattananenya, A. T. (1992). Effect of lung irradiation on mice following paraquat intoxication. *Chest* **101**, 833–835.

Saito, M., Thomas, C. E., and Aust, S. D. (1985). Paraquat and ferritin-dependant lipid peroxidation. *J. Free Rod. Biol. Med.* **1**, 179–185.

Sakai, M., Yamagami, K., Kitazawa, Y., Takeyama, N., and Tanaka, T. (1995). Xanthine oxidase mediates paraquat-induced toxicity on cultured endothelial cell. *Pharmacol. Toxicol.* **77**, 36–40.

Salmona, M., Donnini, M., Perin, L., Diomede, L., Romano, M., Marini, M. G., and Luisetti, M. (1992). A novel pharmacological approach for paraquat poisoning in rat and A549 cell line using ambroxol, a lung surfactant synthesis inducer. *Food Chem. Toxicol.* **30**, 789–794.

Samman, P. D., and Johnston, E. N. M. (1969). Nail damage associated with handling of paraquat and diquat. *Br. Med. J.* **71**, 818–819.

Sandy, M. S., Moldeus, P., Ross, D., and Smith, M. T. (1986). Role of redox cycling and lipid-peroxidation in bipyridyl herbicide cytotoxicity—Studies with a compromised isolated hepatocyte model system. *Biochem. Pharmacol.* **35**, 3095–3101.

Sata, T., Takeshige, K., Takayanagi, R., and Minakami, S. (1983). Lipid peroxidation by bovine heart submitochondrial particles stimulated by 1,1′-dimethyl-4,4-bipyridylium chloride (paraquat). *Biochem. Pharmacol.* **32**, 13–19.

Sato, M., Apostolova, M. D., Hamaya, M., Yamki, J., Choo, K. H. A., Michalaska, A. E., Kodama, N., and Tohyama, C. (1996). Susceptibility of metallothionein-null mice to paraquat. *Env. Tox. Pharm.* **1**, 221–225.

Satoh, M., Naganuma, A., and Imura, N. (1992). Effect of pre-induction of metallothionein on paraquat toxicity of mice. *Arch. Toxicol.* **66**, 145–148.

Saunders, N. A., Rigby, P. J., Ilett, K. F., and Minchin, R. F. (1988). Autoradiographic localisation of putrescine accumulation by type II pneumocytes of rabbit lung slices. *Lab. Invest.* **59**, 380–386.

Saunders, N. R., Alpert, H. M., and Cooper, J. D. (1985). Sequential bilateral lung transplantation for paraquat poisoning—A case report. *J. Thorac. Cardiovasc. Surg.* **89**, 734–742.

Sawada, Y., Yamamoto, I., Hirokane, T., Nagai, Y., Satoh, Y., and Ueyama, M. (1988). Severity index of paraquat poisoning. *The Lancet* **1**, 1333.

Scherrmann, J. M. (1995). Analytical procedures and predictive value of late plasma and urine paraquat concentrations. *In* "Paraquat Poisoning" (C. Bismuth and A. H. Hall, eds.), pp. 285–296. Dekker, New York.

Scherrmann, J. M., Galliot, M., Garnie, R., and Bismuth, C. (1983). Intoxication aigue par le paraquat: Interet prognostique et therapeutique du dosage sanguin. *Toxicol. Eur. Res.* **3**, 141–146.

Scherrmann, J. M., Houze, P., Bismuth, C., and Bourdon, R. (1987). Prognostic value of plasma and urine paraquat concentration. *Human Toxicol.* **6**, 91–93.

Schvartsman, S., Zyngier, S., and Schvartsman, C. (1984). Ascorbic acid and riboflavin in the treatment of acute intoxication by paraquat. *Vet. Human. Toxicol.* **26**, 473–475.

Scott, M. D., Meshnik, S. R., and Eaton, J. W. (1987). Superoxide dismutase-rich bacteria: paradoxical increase in oxidant toxicity. *J. Biol. Chem.* **262**, 3640–3645.

Scott, M. D., and Eaton, J. W. (1996). Superoxide is not the proximate cause of paraquat toxicity. *Redox. Report* **2**, 113–119.

Seidenfeld, J. J., Wycoff, D., Zavala, D. C., and Richerson, H. B. (1978). Paraquat lung injury in rabbits. *Br. J. Ind. Med.* **35**, 245–257.

Seidenfeld, J. J. (1985). Steroid pretreatment does not prevent paraquat pneumonitis in rabbits. *Am. J. Med. Sci.* **289**, 51–54.

Semchuk, K. M., Love, E. J., and Lee, R. G. (1991). Parkinson's disease and exposure to rural environmental factors: A population-based case-control study. *Can. J. Neurol. Sci.* **18**, 279–286.

Senawayake, N., Gurunathan, G., Hart, T. B., Amerasingne, P., Babquille, M., Ellapola, S. B., Udupitille, M., and Basanayake, V. (1993). An epidemiological study of the health of Sri Lankan tea plantation workers associated with long term exposure to paraquat. *Br. J. Ind. Med.* **50**, 257–263.

Shahar, E., Barzilay, Z., and Aladjem, M. (1980). Paraquat poisoning in a child: Vitamin E in amelioration of lung injury. *Arch. Dis. Child* **55**, 830.

Sharp, C. W. M., Ottolenghi, A., and Posner, H. S. (1972). Correlation of paraquat toxicity with tissue concentration and weight loss of the rat. *Toxicol. Appl. Pharmacol.* **22**, 241–251.

Shimada, H., Hirai, K., Simamura, E., and Pan, J. (1998). Mitochondrial NADH-quinone oxidoreductase of the outer membrane is responsible for paraquat cytotoxicity in rat livers. *Arch. Biochem. Biophys.* **351**, 75–81.

Singmaster, J. A., and Liu, L. C. (1998). Low paraquat inhalation exposure for applicators spraying properly with knapsacks. *J. Agric. Univ. PR.* **82**, 97–107.

Shu, H., Talcott, R. E., Rice, S. A., and Wei, E. T. (1979). Lipid peroxidation and paraquat toxicity. *Biochem. Pharmacol.* **28**, 327–331.

Shum, S., Hale, T. W., and Habersang, R. (1982). Reduction of paraquat toxicity by N-acetyl-1-cysteine *Vet. Human Tox.* **24**, 158–160.

Sinow, J., and Wei, E. (1973). Ocular toxicity of paraquat. *Bull. Environ. Contam. Tox.* **9**, 163–168.

Sion, A., Samuni, A., and Chevion, M. (1989). Mechanistic aspects of paraquat toxicity in E. coli. A spin trapping study. *Biochem. Pharmacol.* **38**, 3903–3907.

Smith, J. G. (1988). Paraquat poisoning by skin absorption: A review. *Human. Toxicol.* **7**, 15–19.

Smith, L. L. (1982). The identification of an accumulation system for diamines and polyamines into the lung and its relevance to paraquat toxicity. *Arch. Toxicol.* **5**, 1–14.

Smith, L. L. (1987). Mechanism of paraquat toxicity in the lung and its relevance to treatment. *Human Toxicol.* **6**, 31–36.

Smith, L. L., and Rose, M. S. (1977). A comparison of the effects of paraquat and diquat on the water content of rat lung and the incorporation of thymidine into lung DNA. *Toxicology* **8**, 223–230.

Smith, L. L., Wright, A., Wyatt, I., and Rose, M. S. (1974). Effective treatment for paraquat poisoning in rats and its relevance to the treatment of paraquat poisoning in man. *Br. Med. J.* **4**, 569–571.

Smith, L. L., Lock, E. A., and Rose, M. S. (1976). The relationship between 5-hydroxytryptamine and paraquat accumulation into rat lung. *Biochem. Pharmacol.* **25**, 2485–2487.

Smith, L. L., Wyatt, L., and Rose, M. S. (1978). A comparison of the uptake and elimination of paraquat in rat lung slices with that *in vivo*. *In* "Industrial and Environmental Xenobiotics: *In Vitro* Versus *In Vivo* Biotransformation," pp. 135–140. Publ. Excerpta Medica.

Smith, L. L., and Wyatt, I. (1981). The accumulation of putrescine into slices of rat lung and brain and its relationship to the accumulation of paraquat. *Biochem. Pharmacol.* **30**, 1053–1058.

Smith, L. L., Wyatt, M. S., and Rose, M. S. (1981). Factors affecting the efflux of paraquat from rat lung slices. *Toxicology* **19**, 197–207.

Smith, L. L., Wyatt, I., and Cohen, G. M. (1982). The accumulation of diamines and polyamines into rat lung slices. *Biochem. Pharmacol.* **31**, 3029–3033.

Smith, L. L., and Watson, S. C. (1987). An assessment of the protective effect of cyclophosphamide and dexamethasone in rats. *Human Toxicol.* **6**, 99.

Smith, L. L., Lewis, C. P. L., Wyatt, I., and Cohen, G. M. (1990). The importance of epithelial uptake systems in lung toxicity. *Environ. Health Perspec.* **85**, 25–30.

Smith, N. B., Mathialagen, S., and Brooks, K. E. (1993). Simple and sensitive solid-phase extraction of paraquat using cyanopropyl columns. *J. Anal. Toxicol.* **17**, 143–145.

Smith, P., and Heath, D. (1974a). The ultrastructure and time sequence of the early stages of paraquat lung in rats. *J. Path.* **114**, 177–184.

Smith, P., and Heath, D. (1974b). Paraquat lung: A reappraisal. *Thorax* **29**, 643–653.

Smith, P., and Heath, D. (1975). The pathology of the lung in paraquat poisoning. *J. Clin. Path.* **21**, 81–93.

Smith, P., and Heath, D. (1976). Paraquat. *CRC Crit. Rev. Toxicol.* **4**, 411–445.

Smith, P., Heath, D., and Kay, J. M. (1974). The pathogenesis and structure of paraquat-induced pulmonary fibrosis in rats. *J. Path.* **114**, 57–67.

Sofuni, T., Hatanaka, M., and Ishidate, M. (1985). Chromosomal aberrations and superoxide generating systems. II. Effects of paraquat on Chinese hamster cells in culture. *Mutat. Res.* **147**, 273–274.

Sokol, P. P., Holohan, P. D., Grass, S. M., and Ross, C. R. (1988). Proton-coupled organic cation transport in renal brush-border membrane vesicles. *Biochem. Biophys. Acta* **940**, 209–218.

Staiff, D. C., Comer, S. W., Armstrong, J. F., and Wolfe, H. R. (1975). Exposure to the herbicide paraquat. *Bull. Environ. Contam. Toxicol.* **14**, 334–346.

Steffen, C., and Konder, H. (1979). Absorption of paraquat by rat gut in vitro regional differences. *Arch. Tox.* **43**, 99–103.

Steffen, C., Muliawan, H., and Kappus, H. (1980). Lack of in vivo lipid peroxidation in experimental paraquat poisoning. *Arch. Pharmacol.* **310**, 241–243.

Stephens, D. S., Walker, D. H., Schaffner, W., Kaplovitz, L. G., Brashear, R., Roberts, R., and Spickard, W. A. (1981). Pseudodiptheria: Prominent pharygeal membrane associated with fatal paraquat ingestion. *Ann. Intern. Med.* **94**, 202–204.

Stevens, J. T., and Sumner, D. D. (1991). Herbicides. *In* "Handbook of Pesticide Toxicology" (W. J. Hayes and E. R. Laws, eds.), pp. 1317–1408. Academic Press, San Diego.

Sullivan, T. M., and Montgomery, M. R. (1983). The relationship between paraquat accumulation and covalent binding in rat lung slices. *Drug Metab. Dispos.* **11**, 526–530.

Sullivan, T. M., and Montgomery, M. R. (1984). Ascorbic acid nutritional status does not affect the biochemical response to paraquat. *Fundam. Appl. Toxicol.* **4**, 754–759.

Summers, L. A. (1980). "The Bipyridinium Herbicides." Academic Press, London.

Suntres, Z. E., and Shek, P. N. (1995). Liposomal alpha-tocopherol alleviates the progression of paraquat-induced lung damage. *Drug Targeting* **2**, 493–500.

Suntres, Z. E., and Shek, P. N. (1996). Alleviation of paraquat induced lung injury by pretreatment with bifunctional liposomes containing alpha tocopherol and glutathione. *Biochem. Pharmacol.* **52**, 1515–1520.

Sutton, H. C., Vile, G. F., and Winterbourn, C. C. (1987). Radical driven Fenton reactions evidence from paraquat radical studies for production of tetravalent iron in the presence and absence of ethylenediaminetetraacetic acid. *Arch. Biochem. Biophys.* 462–471.

Suzuki, K., Takasu, N., Arita, S., Maenosono, A., Ishimatsu, S., Nishina, N., Tanaka, S., and Kohama, A. (1989). A new method for predicting the outcome and survival period in paraquat poisoning. *Human Toxicol.* **8**, 33–38.

Suzuki, K., Takasu, N., Okabe, T., Ishimatsu, S., Ueda, A., Tanaka, S., Fukuda, A., Arita, S., and Kohama, A. (1993). Effect of aggressive haemoperfusion on the clinical course of patients with paraquat posioning. *Human Exp. Toxicol.* **12**, 323–327.

Swan, A. A. B. (1967). Paraquat poisoning. *Br. Med. J.* **4**, 551.

Swan, A. A. B. (1969). Exposure of spray operators to paraquat. *Br. J. Ind. Med.* **26**, 322–329.

Sykes, B. I., Purchase, I. F. H., and Smith, L. L. (1977). Pulmonary ultrastructure after oral and intravenous dosage of paraquat to rats. *J. Path.* **121**, 233–241.

Szabo, L., Matkovics, B., Barabas, K., and Oroszlan, G. (1986). Effects of various thiols on paraquat toxicity. *Comp. Biochem. Physiol.* **83**, 149–154.

Tabei, K., Asano, Y., and Hosoda, S. (1982). Efficacy of charcoal hemoperfusion in paraquat poisoning. *Artif. Organs* **6**, 37–43.

Taki, K., Hirahara, K., Tomita, S., and Totoki, S. (1996). Case report: Case of recovery from paraquat poisoning without pulmonary fibrosis. *Therap. Res.* **16**, 521–529.

Talbot, A. R., and Barnes, M. R. (1988). Radiotherapy for the treatment of pulmonary complications of paraquat poisoning. *Human Toxicol.* **7**, 325–332.

Talbot, A. R., Barnes, M. R., and Ting, R. S. (1988a). Early radiotherapy in the treatment of paraquat poisoning. *Br. J. Radiol.* **61**, 405.

Talbot, A. R., Fu, C. C., and Hsieh, M. F. (1988b). Paraquat intoxication during pregnancy: A report of 9 cases. *Vet. Human Toxicol.* **30**, 12–17.

Tanaka, R., and Amano, Y. (1989). Genotoxic effects of paraquat and diquat evaluated by sister chromatid exchange, chromosomal aberration and cell-cycle rate. *Toxicol. In Vitro* **3**, 53–57.

Tanner, C. M., Chen, B., Wang, W., Peng, M., Liu, Z., Liang, X., Kao, L. C., Gilley, D. W., Goetz, C. G., and Schoenberg, B. S. (1989). Environmental factors and Parkinson's disease: A case-control study in China. *Neurology* **39**, 660–604.

Tanner, C. M., Grabler, P., and Goetz, C. G. (1990). Occupation and the risk of Parkinson's disease (PD): A case-control study in young-onset patients. *Neurology* **40**, 422.

Thakar, J. H., and Hassan, M. N. (1988). Effects of 1-methyl-4-phenyl-1,2,3,6-tetrahydro pyridine (MPTP), cyperquat (MPP$^+$) and paraquat on isolated mitochondria from rat striatum, cortex and liver. *Life Sci.* **43**, 143–150.

Thomas, P. D., Thomas, D., Chan, Y.-L., and Clarkson, A. R. (1977). Paraquat poisoning is not necessarily fatal. *Med. J. Aust.* **2**, 564–565.

Thornalley, P. J., and Vasak, M. (1985). Possible role for metallothionein in protection against radiation-induced oxidative stress. Kinetics and mechanism of its reaction with superoxide and hydroxyl radicals. *Biochim. Biophys. Acta* **827**, 36–44.

Tipton, K. F., and Singer, T. P. (1993). Advances in our understanding of the mechanisms of the neurotoxicity of MPTP and related compounds. *J. Neurochem.* **61**, 1191–1205.

Tomita, M. (1991). Comparison of one-electron reduction activity against the bipyridylium herbicides, paraquat and diquat, in microsomal and mitochondrial fractions of liver, lung and kidney (*in vitro*). *Biochem. Pharmacol.* **42**, 303–309.

Tomita, M. (1996). Studies on paraquat toxicity on deoxyribonucleic acid of cultured mammalian cells using flow cytometry. *Redox Report* **2**, 19–24.

Toner, P. G., Vetters, J. M., Spilg, W. G. S., and Harland, W. A. (1970). Fine structure of the lung lesion in a case of paraquat poisoning. *J. Path.* **102**, 182–185.

Trush, M. A., Mimnaugh, E. G., Ginsburg, E., and Gram, T. E. (1981). *In vitro* stimulation by paraquat of reactive oxygen-mediated lipid peroxidation in rat lung microsomes. *Toxicol. Appl. Pharmacol.* **60**, 279–286.

Tsatsakis, A. M., Perakis, K., and Koumantakis, E. (1996). Experience with acute paraquat poisoning in Crete. *Vet. Hum. Toxicol.* **38**, 113–117.

Tsuchiya, T., Yoshida, T., Imaeda, Y. A., Khio, T., and Ukai, S. (1995). Detoxification of paraquat poisoning: Effects of alkylsulfates and alkylsulfonates on paraquat poisoning in mice and rats. *Biol. Pharm. Bulletin* **18**, 523–528.

Tungsanga, K., Israsena, S., Chusilp, S., and Sitprija, V. (1983). Paraquat poisoning: evidence of systemic toxicity after dermal exposure. *Postgrad. Med. J.* **59**, 338.

Turner, C. E., Elsohly, M. A., Cheng, F. P., and Torres, L. M. (1978). Marijuana and paraquat. *JAMA* **240**, 1857.

Ukai, S., Nagai, K., Kiho, T., Tsuchiya, T., and Nochida, Y. (1987). Effectiveness of dextran sulfate on acute toxicity of paraquat in mice and rats. *J. Pharmacobio. Dyn.* **10**, 682–684.

Vale, J. A., Crome, P., Volans, G. N., Widdop, B., and Goulding, R. (1977). The treatment of paraquat poisoning using oral sorbents and charcoal haemoperfusion. *Acta Pharmac. Tox.* **41**, 109–117.

Vale, J. A., Meredith, T. J., and Buckley, B. M. (1987). Paraquat poisoning: Clinical features and immediate general management. *Human Toxicol.* **6**, 41–47.

Van Asbeck, B. S., Hillen, F. C., Boonen, H. C. M., De Jong, Y., Dormans, J. A. M. A., Marx, J. J. M., and Sangster, B. (1989). Continuous intravenous infusion of deferoxamine reduces mortality by paraquat in vitamin E-deficient rats. *Am. Rev. Respir. Dis.* **139**, 769–773.

Van den Bogaerde, J., Schelstraete, J., Colardyn, F., and Heyndrickx, H. (1984). Paraquat poisoning. *Forensic Sci. Int.* **26**, 103–114.

Van der Wal, N. A., Van Oirschot, J. F. L. M., Van Dijk, A., Verhoef, J., and van Asbeck, B. S. (1990). Mechanism of protection of alveolar type II cells against paraquat-induced cytotoxicity by deferoxamine. *Biochem. Pharmacol.* **39**, 1665–1671.

Van der Wal, N. A., Smith, L. L., van Oirschot, J. F., and van Asbeck, B. S. (1992). Effect of iron chelators on paraquat toxicity in rats and alveolar type II cells. *Am. Rev. Resp. Dis.* **145**, 180–186.

Van Dijck, A., Macs, R. A. A., Drost, R. H., Douze, J. M. C., and Van Heyst, A. N. P. (1975). Paraquat poisoning in man. *Arch. Toxicol.* **34**, 129–136.

Van Osten, G. K., and Gibson, J. E. (1975). Effect of paraquat on the biosynthesis of deoxyribonucleic acid, ribonucleic acid and protein in the rat. *Fd. Cosmet. Toxicol.* **13**, 47–54.

Van Wendel de Joode, B. N., De Graaf, I. A. M., Wesseling, C., and Kromhout, H. (1996). Paraquat exposure of knapsack spray operators on banana plantations in Costa Rica. *Int. J. Occup. Environ. Health* **2**, 294–304.

Vargas, E., and Sabapathy, N. N. (1995). "An epidemiology Study on Fatalities from Ingestion and Occupationally-Related Injuries of Agricultural Workers in Costa Rica." Report Series TMF4620B, Zeneca Agrochemicals, Fernhurst, Haslemere, UK.

Vaziri, N. D., Ness, R. L., Fairshter, R. D., Smith, W. R, and Rosen, S. M. (1979). Nephrotoxicity of paraquat in man. *Arch. Intern. Med.* **139**, 172–174.

Vieregge, P., Kömpf, D., and Fassl, H. (1988). Environmental toxins in Parkinson's Disease. *The Lancet* **1**, 362–363.

Vijeyaratnam, G. S., and Corrin, B. (1971). Experimental paraquat poisoning: A histological and electron-optical study of the changes in the lung. *J. Path.* **103**, 123–129.

Vlachos, P., and Kontoes, P. (1987). A study of 30 cases of paraquat inhalation. *Vet. Hum. Toxicol.* **29**, 147.

Waddell, W. J., and Marlowe, C. (1980). Tissue and cellular disposition of paraquat in mice. *Toxicol. Appl. Pharmacol.* **56**, 127–140.

Waight, J. J. (1979). Fatal percutaneous paraquat poisoning. *JAMA* **242**, 472.

Walker, M., Dugard, P. H., and Scott, R. C. (1983). Absorption through human and laboratory animal skins: *In vitro* comparison. *Acta. Pharm. Sci.* **20**, 52–53.

Wasan, S. M., and McElligott, T. F. (1972). An electron microscopic study of experimentally induced interstitial pulmonary fibrosis. *Am. Rev. Resp. Dis.* **105**, 276–282.

Wasserman, B., and Block, E. R. (1978). Prevention of acute paraquat toxicity in rats by superoxide dismutase. *Aviat. Space Environ. Med.* **49**, 805–809.

Watanabe, T., Sakai, K., Toyama, K., Ueno, M., and Watanabe, M. (1979). On three cases of ocular disturbance due to Gramoxone, a herbicide containing 24% paraquat dichloride. *Ganka. Rinsho. Iho.* **73**, 1244–1246.

Webb, D. B. (1983). Nephrotoxicity of paraquat in the sheep and the associated reduction in paraquat secretion. *Toxicol. Appl. Pharmacol.* **68**, 282–289.

Webb, D. B., Williams, M. V., Davies, B. H., and James, K. W. (1984). Resolution after radiotherapy of severe pulmonary damage due to paraquat poisoning. *Br. Med. J.* **288**, 1259–1260.

Wegener, T., Sandhage, B., Chan, K. W., and Saldeen, T. (1988). *N*-acetylcysteine in paraquat toxicity—toxicological and histological evaluation in rats. *Upsala J. Med. Sci.* **93**, 81–89.

Weidel, H., and Russo, M. (1882). Studien uber das pyridin. *Monatsh. Chem.* **3**, 850–885.

Weinbaum, Z., Samuels, S. J., and Schenker, M. B. (1995). Risk factors for occupational illnesses associated with the use of paraquat (1,1′-dimethyl-4,4′-bipyridylium dichloride) in California. *Arch. Environ. Health* **50**, 341–348.

Wesseling, C., Castillo, L., and Elinder, C. G. (1993). Pesticide poisonings in Costa Rica. *Scand. J. Work Environ. Health* **19**, 227–235.

Wesseling, C., Hogstedt, C., Picado, A., and Johansson, L. (1997). Unintentional fatal paraquat poisonings among agricultural workers in Costa Rica: Report of 15 cases. *Am. J. Ind. Med.* **32**, 433–441.

Wester, R. C., and Maibach, H. I. (1985). *In vivo* percutaneous absorption and decontamination of pesticides in humans. *J. Toxicol. Environ. Hlth.* **16**, 25–37.

Wester, R. C., Maibach, H. I., Bucks, D. A., and Aufrere, M. B. (1984). *In vivo* percutaneous absorption of paraquat from hand leg and forearm of humans. *J. Toxicol. Environ. Hlth.* **14**, 759–762.

Whitaker, M. (1989a). The handling and use of paraquat by Malaysian rubber and oil palm smallholders. *J. Pl. Prot. Tropics* **6**, 231–249.

Whitaker, M. (1989b). Normas de manipulation y uso del paraquat por'los pequenos productores de maiz en Centroamerica. *Turrialba* **39**, 260–274.

Whitaker, M., Pitakpaivan, C., and Daorai, A. (1993). The use of paraquat by smallholder maize, cassava, fruit and rubber farmers in Thailand. *Thai. J. Agric. Sci.* **26**, 43–81.

Widdop, B. (1976). Detection of paraquat in urine. *Br. Med. J.* **2**, 1135.

Widdop, B., Medd, R. K., Braithwaite, R. A., and Vale, J. A. (1975). Haemoperfusion in the treatment of paraquat poisoning. *Proc. Europ. Soc. Artific. Organs* **2**, 244–247.

Widdop, B., Medd, R. K., and Braithwaite, R. A. (1977). Charcoal haemoperfusion in the treatment of paraquat poisoning. *Proc. Europ. Soc. Toxicol.* **18**, 156–159.

Widdowson, P. S., Farnworth, M. J., Simpson, M. G., and Lock, E. A. (1996a). Influence of age on the passage of paraquat through the blood-brain barrier in rats: a distribution and pathological examination. *Human Exp. Toxicol.* **15**, 231–336.

Widdowson, P. S., Farnworth, M. J., Upton, R., and Simpson, M. G. (1996b). No changes in behaviour, njgro-strital system neurochemistry or neuronal cell death following toxic multiple oral paraquat administration to rats. *Human Exp. Toxicol.* **15**, 583–591.

Williams, M. V., and Webb, D. B. (1987). Paraquat lung: Is there a role for radiotherapy. *Human Toxicol.* **6**, 75–81.

Winterbourn, C. C., and Sutton, H. C. (1984). Hydroxyl radical production from hydrogen peroxide and enzymatically generated paraquat radicals catalytic requirements and oxygen dependence. *Arch. Biochem. Biophys.* **235**, 116–126.

Witschi, H., Kacew, S., Hirai, K. I., and Cote, M. G. (1977). *In vivo* oxidation of reduced nicotinamide adenine dinucleotide phosphate by paraquat and diquat in rat lung. *Chem. Biol. Interact.* **19**, 143–160.

Wohlfahrt, D. J. (1982). Fatal paraquat poisonings after skin absorption. *Med. J. Aust.* **1**, 512–513.

Wojeck, G. A., Price, J. F., Nigg, H. N., and Stamper, J. H. (1983). Worker exposure to paraquat and diquat. *Arch. Environ. Contam. Toxicol.* **12**, 65–70.

Woollen, B. H., and Mahler, J. D. (1987). An improved spot-test for the detection of paraquat and diquat in biological samples. *Clin. Chim. Acta* **167**, 225–229.

Wright, C. E., Tallan, H. H., Lin, Y. Y., and Gaull, G. E. (1986). Taurine: Biological update. *Am. Rev. Biochem.* **55**, 427–453.

Wright, A. F., Green, T. P., Robson, R. T., Niewola, Z., Wyatt, I., and Smith, L. L. (1987a). Specific polyclonal and monoclonal antibody prevents paraquat accumulation into rat lung slices. *Biochem. Pharmacol.* **36**, 1325–1331.

Wright, A. F., Green, T. P., Daley-Yates, P., and Smith, L. L. (1987b). Monoclonal-antibody does not protect mice from paraquat toxicity. *Vet. Human. Toxicol.* **29**, 102.

Wright, S. H., and Wunz, T. M. (1995). Paraquat 2+/H+ exchange in isolated renal brush-border membrane vesicles. *Biochem. Biophys. Acta* **1240**, 18–24.

Wyatt, I., Doss, A. W., Zavala, D. C., and Smith, L. L. (1981). Intrabronchial instillation of paraquat in rats: Lung morphology and retention study. *Br. J. Ind. Med.* **38**, 42–48.

Wyatt, L., Soames, A. R., Clay, M. F., and Smith, L. L. (1988). The accumulation and localisation of putrescine, spermidine, spermine and paraquat in the rat lung. *Biochem. Pharmacol.* **37**, 1909–1918.

Yamada, K., and Fukushima, T. (1993). Mechanism of cytotoxicity of paraquat. II. Organ specificity of paraquat-stimulated lipid peroxidation in the inner membrane of mitochondria. *Exp. Toxic. Pathol.* **45**, 375–380.

Yamagami, K., Matsubara, M., Kitazawa, Y., Takeyama, N., Tanaka, T., and Kawamoto, K. (1994). Flow cytometric analysis of the direct toxic effects of paraquat on cultured MDCK cells. *J. Appl. Toxicol.* **14**, 155–159.

Yamaguchi, H., Sato, S., Watanabe, S., and Naito, H. (1990). Pre-embarkment prognostication for acute paraquat poisoning. *Human Exp. Toxicol.* **9**, 381–384.

Yamamoto, H. (1993). Protection against paraquat induced toxicity with sulfite or thiosulfate in mice. *Toxicology* **79**, 37–43.

Yamamoto, T., Anno, M., and Sato, T. (1987). Effects of paraquat on mitochondria of rat skeletal muscle. *Comp. Biochem. Physiol.* **86**, 375–378.

Yamashita, M., Naito, H., and Takagi, S. (1987). The effectiveness of a cation resin (kayexalate) as an adsorbent of paraquat: Experimental and clinical studies. *Human Toxicol.* **6**, 89–90.

Yasaka, T., Ohya, I., Matsumoto, J., Shiramizu, T., and Sasaguri, J. (1981). Acceleration of lipid peroxidation in human paraquat poisoning. *Arch. Intern. Med.* **141**, 1169-1171.

Yasaka, T., Okudaira, K., Fujito, H., and Shiramitsu, T. (1986). Further studies of lipid-peroxidation in human paraquat poisoning. *Arch. Intern. Med.* **146**, 681–685.

Yonei, S., Noda, A., Tachibana, A., and Akasaka, S. (1986). Mutagenic and cytotoxic effects of oxygen free radicals generated by methyl viologen (paraquat) on Escherichia Coli with different DNA-repair capacities. *Mutat. Res.* **163**, 15–22.

Yonemitsu, K. (1986). Pharmacokinetic profile of paraquat following intravenous administration to the rabbit. *Forensic Sci. Int.* **32**, 33–42.

Yoshimura, Y., Watanabe, Y., and Shibuya, Y. (1993). Inhibitory effects of calcium channel antagonists on motor dysfunction induced by intracerebroventricular administration of paraquat. *Pharmacol. Toxicol.* **72**, 229–235.

Younes, M., Cornelius, S., and Seigers, C. P. (1985). Iron-supported in vivo lipid peroxidation induced by compounds undergoing redox cycling. *Chem–Biol. Interact.* **54**, 97–103.

Yu, H. Y., Lai, Y. R., Kuo, T. L., and Shen, Y. Z. (1994). Effects of ethanol on pharmacokinetics and intestinal absorption of paraquat in animals. *J. Toxicol. Sci.* **19**, 67–75.

Zavala, D. C., and Rhodes, M. L. (1978). An effect of paraquat on the lungs of rabbits: Its implications in smoking contaminated marijuana. *Chest* **74**, 418–420.

Zayed, J., Ducic, S., Campanella, G., Panisset, J. C., Andre, P., Masson, H., and Roy, M. (1990). Facteurs environnementeaux dans l'etiologie de la maladie de Parkinson. *Can. J. Neurol. Sci.* **17**, 286–291.

Zilker, T., Fogt, F., and von Clarmann, M. (1988). Kein Parkinsonsyndrom nach akuter paraquat intoxikation. *Klin. Wochenschr.* **66**, 1138–1141.

Diquat

Edward A. Lock
Syngenta Central Toxicology Laboratory
Martin F. Wilks
Syngenta Crop Protection AG

71.1 IDENTITY, PROPERTIES, AND USES

71.1.1 CHEMICAL NAME

Diquat is 1,1'-ethylene-2,2'-bipyridyldiylium ion (IUPAC), or 6,7-dihydrodipyrido[1,2-a : 2',1'-c]pyrazinediium (CAS RN [2764-72-9]).

71.1.2 STRUCTURE

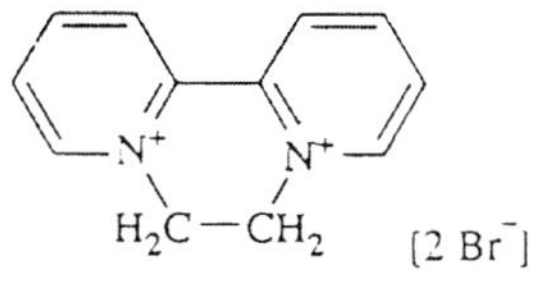

Diquat dibromide

Figure 71.1

71.1.3 SYNONYMS

The common name diquat is in general use (BSI, E-ISO, (m) F-ISO, ANSI, WSSA, JMAF), except in Germany (deiquat) and Russia (reglon). Diquat is formulated as the dibromide salt (CAS NR [85-00-7] and [6385-62-2] for the dibromide monohydrate). A code designation for the material is FB/2. Trade names for diquat dibromide formulations include Desiquat®, Midstream®, Reglone®, and Reglex®. Mixtures of diquat with paraquat are sold under trade names including Actor®, Dukatalon®, Opal®, Pathclear® (also includes simazine and aminotriazole), Preeglox®, Preglone®, Seccatutto®, Spray Seed®, and Weedol®.

71.1.4 PHYSICAL AND CHEMICAL PROPERTIES

The molecular formula of the cation is $C_{12}H_{12}N_2$ with a molecular weight of 184.24. The dibromide salt has the formula $C_{12}H_{12}Br_2N_2$ and a molecular weight of 344.1. Diquat dibromide forms colorless to yellow crystals which decompose above 300°C. With a vapour pressure of <0.013 mPa (monohydrate), it is practically nonvolatile. It is very soluble in water (700 g/l at 20°C), slightly soluble in alcohols and hydroxylic solvents, and insoluble in nonpolar organic solvents. It is stable in neutral and acidic media but readily hydrolyzed in alkaline media. Diquat is photochemically decomposed by ultraviolet radiation.

71.1.5 HISTORY, FORMULATIONS, AND USES

The herbicidal properties of diquat were first described by Brian et al. (1958). Diquat is mainly formulated as an aqueous solution. In some countries, a low-strength granular formulation (also containing paraquat) is available. Diquat is a fast-acting, nonselective contact herbicide and desiccant, absorbed by the foliage with some translocation in the xylem. It is used for preharvest desiccation of cotton, flax, alfalfa, and many other crops, as a defoliant on hops, for destruction of potato haulms, for general weed control on noncrop land, for weed control and tassel inhibition in sugar cane, and for control of emergent and submerged aquatic weeds. Diquat is rapidly deactivated upon contact with the soil and does not leach.

71.2 TOXICITY TO LABORATORY ANIMALS

71.2.1 SIGNS OF TOXICITY

Following a median lethal oral dose of diquat to rats, few signs of toxicity were seen over the first 24 h. Subsequently the animals became lethargic, lost weight, showed slight pupillary dilatation, and excreted mucoid, ropey feces of a characteristic green color which was associated with mild abdominal distension. Renal function was impaired and the animals died 2–14 days after dosing (Clark and Hurst, 1970; Crabtree *et al.*, 1977; Lock, 1979). Similar signs of toxicity were seen in mice, guinea pigs, rabbits, dogs (Clark and Hurst, 1970), and cynomologus monkeys (Cobb and Grimshaw, 1979). Following a single median lethal subcutaneous (sc) injection, rats showed a marked diuresis, became lethargic about 6 h after dosing, and had marked pupillary dilatation which persisted. By 24 h the rats had lost weight and were drinking less, the animals generally became weaker, with deaths occurring between 2 and 10 days, although some animals died as late as 8 weeks. All animals dying after 10 days had grossly distended abdomens due to a grossly swollen caecum. The cause of death is unclear; hypovolaemia and renal tubular necrosis leading to renal shutdown are contributory factors. Histological findings showed injury to the lining of the stomach and gastrointestinal tract but these were not life threatening. A large injection of diquat (four or five times a median lethal dose, sc) to rats produced subdued behavior within a few minutes and labored respiration within 1 h. Muscular twitching then occurred, leading to generalized convulsions and death within a few hours (Clark and Hurst, 1970). Lung injury similar to that seen with paraquat is not a prominent feature with diquat.

71.2.2 SPECIES AND DOSE–RESPONSE RELATIONSHIPS

71.2.2.1 Acute Toxicity

The acute oral toxicity of diquat to a number of species is shown in Table 71.1. The median lethal dose (MLD) of pure diquat dibromide or dichloride expressed as the cation is between 121 to 230 mg/kg in male and female rats. Diquat is, however, more toxic when given by the intraperitoneal (ip) or sc routes. The MLD by injection is about 11 mg/kg, indicating that following oral dosing the compound is poorly absorbed from the gastrointestinal tract. For most other laboratory species the MLD is in the range of 100–200 mg/kg (Table 71.1). Dermal exposure of rabbits to diquat for 24 h produced no ill effects at 400 mg/kg, the maximum dose that could be applied to the skin (Clark and Hurst, 1970). For the mouse and guinea pig the MLD was approximately 400 mg/kg and for the rat about 650 mg/kg (Table 71.2). This finding is consistent with *in vitro* studies showing that diquat is poorly absorbed across the skin of laboratory animals and humans (see later) from an aqueous solution (Scott and Corrigan, 1990). Diquat is not volatile; inhalation exposure of rats to an aerosol of respirable droplets (< 5 μm diameter) at 23 μg/l for 30 min produced no ill effects (Gage, 1968a). The MLD for diquat by inhalation is about 35 μg/l for rats and guinea pigs (Table 71.2) while a value of 83 μg/l was reported for rats by Bainova and Velcheva (1977), the difference presumably being due to particle size or analytical differences. Direct intratracheal administration of diquat to

rats has been shown to produce lung injury and fibrosis (Manabe and Ogata, 1986, 1987).

71.2.2.2 Irritation and Sensitization

A single application of diquat to the skin of mice (Bainova, 1969b) or rabbits (Clark and Hurst, 1970) did not cause local irritation. Diquat is not a skin sensitizer (Bainova, 1969b). Daily applications of diquat at 20 mg/kg/day for 20 days in water to the skin of rabbits provoked some mild erythema, thickening of the skin, and some scabbing at the site of application (Clark and Hurst, 1970). Instillation of one drop of a 20% aqueous solution of diquat into the rabbit eye produced slight conjunctival irritation which persisted for 2 days (Clark and Hurst, 1970). No pupillary dilatation was observed.

71.2.2.3 Subchronic and Chronic Toxicity

The primary target organ for toxicity following prolonged exposure to diquat is the eye, where cataracts develop. Daily oral dosing of rats with diquat at 6.5, 13, and 40 mg/kg/day for 40 days or 2.1 or 4.3 mg/kg/day for 4.5 months produced histological changes in the liver, kidney, lung, and gastrointestinal tract (Bainova, 1969a, 1975). The effects on these organs will be discussed later. Diquat, when administered to rats in their drinking water at 2 and 4 mg/kg/day for up to 2 years, did not increase mortality, although some histological changes were seen in the lungs at the high dose (Bainova and Velcheva, 1978). Daily administration in the diet of rats at 10, 50, 100, 250, 500, or 1000 ppm diquat dichloride for 2 years produced no compound-related deaths. Some reduction in food consumption and body weight gain was seen at 1000 ppm but not at any of the lower doses. Gross and microscopic examination revealed no compound-related changes other than in the eye where cataracts developed in rats receiving 50 ppm and above during the course of the study. The time to onset of cataracts was dose-related. At 1000 ppm partial or complete opacities were present in one or both lenses within six months. Bilateral cataracts were seen at 12 months following 500 ppm (about 25 mg/kg/day), lens opacity was detected in all animals at 250 ppm at 18 months, while at 100 and 50 ppm about 25% of the animals were affected at 2 years. No effects on the eye were seen at 10 ppm (about 0.5 mg/kg/day) for 2 years in any animals (Clark and Hurst, 1970). Rats fed diquat at 500 ppm for 8 weeks and then returned to normal diet for 1 year did not develop cataracts, showing that continuous and prolonged exposure is necessary in the rat for cataract formation (Clark and Hurst, 1970). In a subsequent dietary study, no cataracts were observed when rats were fed 20 ppm diquat dichloride (about 1 mg/kg/day) in their diet for 2 years (FAO/WHO, 1978). Dogs can tolerate doses of 15 mg/kg/day diquat dichloride for 2 years without affecting growth or producing any histological effects, except in the eye. Bilateral cataracts appeared at 15 mg diquat/kg/day after about 10–11 months. However, dogs exposed to 1.7 mg diquat/kg/day for 4 years did not develop cataract (Clark and Hurst, 1970).

Subchronic exposure following dermal application to rabbits at 20 mg/kg/day for 20 days caused some mild erythema,

Table 71.1
Acute Toxicity of Diquat to Laboratory Animals (Data Expressed as mg/kg Diquat Ion)

Species	Sex	Strain	Route of administration	Median lethal dose	Reference
Rat	F	Alderley Park-Wistar	po	231 (194–274)	Clark and Hurst, 1970
Rat	M	Sherman	po	147 (138–155)	Gaines and Linder, 1986
Rat	F	Sherman	po	121 (108–136)	Gaines and Linder, 1986
Rat	M	Alderley Park-Wistar	po	226	Crabtree *et al.*, 1977
Rat	M	Alderley Park-Wistar	sc	11 (5–15)	Clark and Hurst, 1970
Rat	F	Alderley Park-Wistar	sc	11 (9-12)	Clark and Hurst, 1970
Rat			po	281	Verbetskii and Pushkar, 1968
Rat			po	215	Makovskii, 1972
Rat			po	130	Bainova, 1969a
Rat	M	Alderley Park-Wistar	ip	<11	Smith and Rose, 1977
Mouse	M	Alderley Park	po	125 (106–146)	Clark and Hurst, 1970
Dog	F	Alderley Park-beagle	po	100–200	Clark and Hurst, 1970
Guinea pig			po	123	Verbetskii and Pushkar, 1968
Guinea pig	F	Alderley Park	po	approx 100	Clark and Hurst, 1970
Rabbit	F	Albino	po	101 (72–138)	Clark and Hurst, 1970
Cynomolgus monkey	M		po	100–300	Cobb and Grimshaw, 1979

thickening of the skin, and scabbing. Increasing the dose to 40 mg/kg/day caused weight loss and muscular weakness. Four of the six animals in this group died after 8 to 20 applications. The MLD was therefore between 20 and 40 mg/kg/day in the rabbit (Clark and Hurst, 1970). Dermal application of diquat to rats at 5 to 120 mg/kg/day for 20 days, without occluding the skin, produced slight skin irritation at the site of application. An increase in signs of toxicity was observed at 10 mg/kg/day and above, including distension of the abdomen. Mortality was seen at the

Table 71.2
Acute Toxicity of Diquat to Laboratory Animals Following Dermal Application or Inhalation Exposure (Data Expressed as mg/kg Diquat Ion)

Species	Route of administration	Median lethal dose	Reference
Rat	Dermal	650	Makovskii, 1972
Mouse	Dermal	430	Bainova, 1969b
Guinea pig	Dermal	400	Makovskii, 1972
Rabbit	Dermal	>400	Clark and Hurst, 1970
Rat	Inhalation	35 μg/l	Makovskii, 1972
Rat	Inhalation	83 μg/l	Bainova and Velcheva, 1977
Guinea pig	Inhalation	38 μg/l	Makovskii, 1972

higher doses and at toxic doses there was histological evidence of injury to the liver, kidneys, lung, and gastrointestinal tract (Bainova, 1969b). The median lethal dose was 35 mg/kg/day with no effects being seen at 5 mg/kg/day.

Repeated exposure of rats to diquat by inhalation for 6 h per day for 15 days over 3 weeks at 2 μg/l caused signs of respiratory irritation in females. Histological examination showed evidence of irritation with peribronchial lymphoid hyperplasia and slight perivascular oedema. No effects were seen at 0.5 μg/l over the same exposure time (Gage, 1968a). Rats, mice, guinea pigs, rabbits, and a dog exposed to 1.06 μg/l for 15 daily exposures of 6 h remained in good condition during exposure, apart from the rabbits which initially showed signs of rapid, shallow breathing which had recovered at the end of the study (Gage, 1968a). Rats exposed to doses ranging from 0.32 to 1.9 mg/l for 4 or 6 h per day over 4 to 4.5 months showed signs of lung irritation and lung injury at the higher doses. No effects were seen at the lowest doses of 0.32 mg/l for 6 h/day for 4.5 months or at 0.4 mg/l for 4 h/day for 4 months (Bainova *et al.*, 1972; Makovskii, 1972).

Overall, these studies show that following acute and chronic exposure some toxicity is seen in the gastrointestinal tract, liver, kidney, and lung. The major target organ for toxicity following chronic exposure is the eye with the production of cataracts. Dose levels of diquat that do not cause damage in laboratory animals following acute and chronic exposure have been clearly established.

71.2.2.4 Mutagenic and Carcinogenic Potential

Diquat is not carcinogenic in either rats or mice. The activity seen in some short-term assays for mutagenesis is associated with cytotoxicity, believed to arise as a consequence of the redox cycling ability of diquat, leading to superoxide anion formation. Diquat has minimal to no genotoxic activity when evaluated in a wide range of *in vitro* and *in vivo* test systems. Many groups have reported the absence of an effect in the Ames assay (Andersen *et al.*, 1972; Benigni *et al.*, 1979; Levin *et al.*, 1982). Diquat was not mutagenic when tested in the mouse dominant lethal assay (Anderson *et al.*, 1976; Pasi *et al.*, 1974) or in studies including chromosomal aberrations in mice (Selypes *et al.*, 1980). Some positive effects have been observed with gene conversion in *Saccharomyces cerevisiae* (Siebert and Lemperle, 1974), DNA repair in *Salmonella typhimurium*, gene mutation in *Aspergillus nidulans* (Benigni *et al.*, 1979), and sister chromatid exchange in Chinese hamster lung cells (Tanaka and Amano, 1989). These effects were usually associated with cytotoxicity and are believed to arise as a consequence of the redox cycling ability of diquat, leading to the production of superoxide anion (see later). It is well known that DNA damage frequently occurs when cells are exposed to oxidative stress (Brawn and Fridovich, 1981; Repine *et al.*, 1981). Recent studies using the ^{32}P-postlabeling technique showed no differences in DNA adducts in the liver of diquat-treated rats compared to controls (Vulimiri *et al.*, 1995). Importantly diquat did not induce tumors in a 2 year feeding study in rats or mice (Clark and Hurst, 1970; FAO/WHO, 1993) or when given to rats in their drinking water for 2 years (Bainova and Velcheva, 1978).

71.2.2.5 Effects on Reproduction, Embryotoxicity, and Teratogenicity

Diquat has no effect on fertility, is not teratogenic, and only produces fetotoxicity at doses that are maternally toxic. The main finding in the multigeneration study was cataract formation. The testes of male rats dosed orally with diquat dibromide at 6.5 mg/kg/day for 60 days were histologically normal as was the sperm count and sperm motility (Bainova and Velcheva, 1974).

In a multigeneration reproduction study, rats were fed diets containing 0, 16, 80, or 400 ppm diquat for 12 weeks, mated, and then allowed to rear the litters that resulted (F$_{1a}$). The process was repeated with animals selected from the F$_{1a}$ litter, these F$_1$ parents being mated 11 weeks after selection. The dose received by the top dose F1 rats was reduced after 4 weeks to 240 ppm. Diquat had no effect on fertility in either sex; the main finding was cataract formation. Decreased body-weight gain was seen at the top dose in both adults (F$_0$ and F$_1$) and pups. Cataract formation was mostly confined to the top dose although a low incidence was seen at 80 ppm in the F$_1$ female parents. No cataracts were seen at 16 ppm (equivalent to 0.8 mg/kg/day) (FAO/WHO, 1993).

A single ip injection of diquat to rats at 7 mg/kg during days 6–14 of gestation produced a marked reduction in body weight gain and retarded ossification but was not teratogenic. Repeated doses of 0.5 mg/kg/day diquat ip did not produce embryotoxicity (Khera *et al.*, 1970). Bus *et al.* (1975) reported that diquat can cross the rat placenta as fetuses contained [^{14}C] diquat following administration to the mother on days 13, 16, or 21 of gestation. Bus and co-workers also reported that diquat given at 15 mg/kg iv to rats on days 7–21 of gestation resulted in significant fetal reabsorption and maternal death. This is not unexpected as the MLD for diquat given by ip injection is 11 mg/kg (Table 71.1). The embryotoxic effects of high doses of diquat have also been observed in mice receiving 2.7 or 11 mg/kg on days 9, 10, 11, and 12 of gestation. An increase in the number of dead fetuses and postimplantation loss was observed, but no congenital malformations were seen (Selypes *et al.*, 1980). Oral administration of diquat to pregnant rats at doses of 4, 12, or 40 mg/kg diquat cation/day from days 7–16 of gestation resulted in maternal toxicity, reductions in fetal weight and litter weight, as well as fetal defects in ossification at the top dose. No significant effects were seen at 12 mg/kg diquat cation/day (FAO/WHO, 1993). Oral administration of diquat to pregnant rabbits at doses of 1, 3 or 10mg ion/kg/day for days 7–19 of gestation resulted in maternal toxicity at the top dose with some evidence of fetotoxicity in the form of partially ossified sternbrae. No adverse effect on the mother or fetuses was seen at 1 mg/kg/day (FAO/WHO, 1993).

71.2.2.6 Pathology

At postmortem following either oral or sc administration of diquat the most obvious effect is gross distension of the gastrointestinal tract with greenish-yellow fluid. The color is believed to be due to bacterial reduction of diquat. Histological changes to the gastrointestinal tract, liver, kidneys, lungs, and eyes have been reported and these will be discussed later under each target organ.

71.2.2.7 Absorption

The first studies on the absorption and excretion of diquat were conducted by Daniel and Gage (1966) in rats. They showed, following a single oral dose of [^{14}C-ethylene]diquat dibromide or dichloride, that most of the radioactivity was excreted within 48 h, although at the higher doses some appeared in the feces on day 3. Between 6 and 10% of the dose was excreted in the urine over 48 h, the remainder being in the feces. In contrast, when diquat dibromide was given sc the bulk of the radioactivity appeared in the urine within 24 h of dosing, showing that diquat is not completely absorbed across the gastrointestinal tract of the rat. Subsequent studies in rats have reported 5.5% of an oral dose of 60 mg/kg diquat ion excreted in the urine over 1–7 days (Litchfield *et al.*, 1973) and 7.5% of an oral dose of 126 mg/kg diquat ion in 24 h (Lock and Ishmael, 1979). Following oral administration of diquat (126 mg/kg) to rats, the peak plasma concentration occurred before 2 h, the earliest time measured (Rose *et al.*, 1976a), and then remained constant for up to 30 h. Studies in the dog using a tracer dose of 12 μg/kg of [^{14}C-ethylene]diquat did not result in an early plasma peak with only 10–20% of the dose absorbed in 6 h (Bennett and Davies, 1976). The dog appears to absorb a slightly larger percentage of an orally administered dose of diquat than the rat, which is consistent with the greater susceptibility of the dog by this route of administration. Overall, few absorption studies have been reported with diquat. From the available information diquat appears to be rapidly but incompletely absorbed from the gastrointestinal tract of laboratory animals with peak plasma concentrations occurring within a few hours of dosing.

71.2.2.8 Distribution

In the rat after an oral dose of 126 mg/kg, the plasma diquat concentration remained constant between 2 and 30 h after dosing (Rose *et al.*, 1976a). During this time no accumulation into the lung was seen, although the concentration in the adrenal gland and to a lesser extent the liver was higher than that found in the plasma. In no other organs, apart from the kidney, which is the major organ for the excretion of diquat, was the concentration above that found in the plasma (Rose *et al.*, 1976a). Diquat did not appear to enter the brain (Rose *et al.*, 1976a). These findings, plus the earlier observation of Sharp *et al.* (1972) who compared the tissue distribution of diquat and paraquat following 20 mg/kg iv, confirmed that diquat was not retained in the lung. The only organs with higher concentrations of diquat compared to paraquat were the liver and at later times the kidney. Others have subsequently studied the distribution of diquat in the rat following oral or systemic administration with similar findings (Kurisaki and Sato, 1979; Matsuura *et al.*, 1978; Spalding *et al.*, 1989). Following dietary administration of diquat to rats for 2, 4, or 8 weeks at 250 ppm a time-dependent increase in diquat was detected in the kidneys, with lower levels in the liver and lung, while in the brain diquat was at or below the limits of detection (Litchfield *et al.*, 1973).

Whole body autoradiography studies have also provided valuable information on the tissue distribution of diquat. Early studies by Litchfield *et al.* (1973) in mice given iv [^{14}C-ethylene]diquat showed the compound was distributed throughout most tissues 10 min after injection with higher concentrations associated with cartilaginous tissues, the gall bladder, the small intestine, and the urinary bladder. By 1 h the concentration of radioactivity had declined in most tissues apart from the gastrointestinal tract and urinary bladder. By 24 and 48 h excretion was virtually complete apart from some radioactivity present in the gastrointestinal tract. Whole body autoradiography studies have shown that diquat binds to melanin following iv administration to pigmented C57 black mice, but not albino mice. The association of diquat with melanin is probably due to an ionic interaction (Larsson *et al.*, 1977).

71.2.2.9 Metabolism

Diquat is poorly metabolized, the bulk of the material being excreted in the urine and feces unchanged. Daniel and Gage

(1966) and Hughes *et al.* (1973) compared the colorimetric assay for diquat with that found by radiochemical detection in the urine and feces of rats dosed with diquat and showed that they agreed very closely. Incubation of diquat with rat caecal contents for up to 24 h showed up to a 50% loss, indicating microbial metabolism, as the loss was prevented when the contents of the caecum were heat-treated (Daniel and Gage, 1966). However, *in vivo* studies in rats have not shown significant biotransformation, indicating that the *in vitro* studies had overpredicted the likely metabolism.

Hughes *et al.* (1973) reported some unidentified metabolites of diquat in the urine of rabbits and guinea pigs. Subsequent studies in the rat identified diquat monopyridone as a metabolite mainly in the feces, at about 5% of an oral dose, while diquat dipyridone was detected in the urine (FAO/WHO, 1978). Overall these studies indicate that diquat is probably metabolized by gastrointestinal bacteria.

71.2.2.10 Excretion

Whole body autoradiography showed that diquat was present in the gall bladder of mice, indicating biliary excretion (Litchfield *et al.*, 1973). The extent of biliary excretion of diquat was < 5% when dosed to bile cannulated rats, rabbits, or guinea pigs and bile collected over a 3 hour period (Hughes *et al.*, 1973; Spalding *et al.*, 1989).

The major route of diquat elimination from the body is via the kidneys. The renal clearance of diquat is greater than that of inulin in the rat (Lock, 1979), indicating that diquat is actively secreted. Accumulation of the organic cation N^1-methylnicotinamide, but not the organic anion *p*-aminohippuric acid, by slices of rat renal-cortex was reduced by diquat, suggesting that it is actively secreted via a cationic transport system analogous to that for paraquat (Lock and Ishmael, 1979). The renal transport systems for the excretion of organic cations are discussed in detail in the chapter on paraquat toxicology. In the rat *in vivo,* the fractional excretion of diquat was 1.14 at a plasma concentration that may have saturated the transport system analogous to that reported for paraquat (Chan *et al.*, 1998). Thus at low plasma concentrations diquat is probably readily cleared from the body; however, at higher plasma concentrations this system will become saturated and less diquat is cleared. At toxic doses it is well established that diquat can cause renal functional impairment. In rats (Lock, 1979) and monkeys (Cobb and Grimshaw, 1979) given 100 mg diquat cation/kg orally, renal impairment was observed 24 h after dosing (Fig. 71.2).

71.2.2.11 Biochemical Mechanisms of Diquat Toxicity

Diquat can be reduced to form a free radical, which is bright green in color and stable in aqueous solution in the absence of oxygen:

$$DQ^{2+} + e^- \rightarrow DQ^{+\cdot}$$

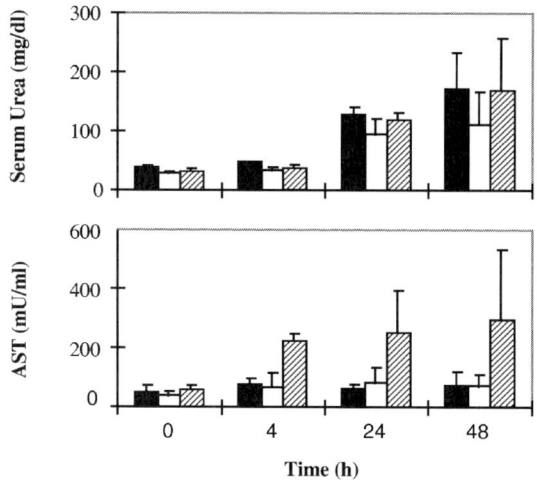

Figure 71.2 The effect of diquat on markers of liver and kidney injury in cynomolgus monkeys following a single oral dose. Results are mean and range for two animals per treatment at 100 and 300 mg/kg and mean ± SE of four animals at 200 mg/kg. 100 mg/kg (■); 200 mg/kg (□) and 300 mg/kg (hatched). From Cobb and Grimshaw (1979).

In the presence of oxygen, in biological systems, the radical will rapidly reoxidize to the cation with the concomitant production of superoxide anion ($O_2^{-\cdot}$).

$$DQ^{+\cdot} + O_2 \rightarrow DQ^{2+} + O_2^{-\cdot}$$

Thus, once diquat enters a cell it will undergo alternate reduction followed by reoxidation, a process known as redox cycling. Gage (1968b) first reported that the diquat cation could be reduced by rat liver NADPH-dependent microsomal flavoprotein reductase to form the radical, with the concomitant oxidation of NADPH. Redox cycling of diquat has also been reported in microsomal preparations of lung, liver, and kidney (Baldwin et al., 1975; Tomita, 1991). Tomita (1991) also demonstrated one electron reduction of diquat by mitochondrial fractions of liver, lung, and kidney with the highest activity in the kidney. Thus, like paraquat, diquat can redox cycle, the major difference being that diquat can more readily accept an electron than paraquat, such that this response is seen at lower intracellular concentrations with diquat. The mechanism is similar to that discussed earlier for paraquat, whereby a cascade of events is triggered, leading to NADPH depletion and lipid peroxidation with the free radical scavenging enzymes such as superoxide dismutase, catalase, and glutathione peroxidase playing a key protective role. The relevance of this mechanism to the toxicity observed in laboratory animals will now be discussed.

71.2.2.12 Effects on the Lung

Diquat is not accumulated into the lung, unlike the situation with paraquat, following oral or systemic administration to rats or mice (Keeling et al., 1981; Litchfield et al., 1973; Rose et al., 1976a; Sharp et al., 1972; Spalding et al., 1989; Witschi et al., 1977). This is consistent with studies using rat lung slices where diquat does not accumulate into the slice (Rose et al., 1974a, 1976a). Although diquat is not accumulated it is able to block

the entry of paraquat into lung cells via the energy-dependent transport system (Rose and Smith, 1977), suggesting it can interact with the transport system but not undergo transport itself. Sufficient diquat can, however, enter lung cells in vitro to undergo redox cycling and thereby stimulate the pentose phosphate pathway (Rose et al., 1976b).

Studies in vivo with toxic oral or systemic doses have shown that diquat **does not** cause histopathological evidence of lung injury, like that seen with paraquat (Clark and Hurst, 1970; Cobb and Grimshaw, 1979). Similarly diquat does not cause pulmonary edema or alter lung function following ip administration, although it does reduce pulmonary cell turnover (Lam et al., 1980; Smith and Rose, 1977). Diquat can, however, stimulate the pentose phosphate pathway in the lung following toxic oral or iv administration (Rose et al., 1976b). Studies by Witschi et al. (1977) showed for the first time that a large dose of diquat (40 mg/kg, iv) produced a marked fall in the NADPH/NADP ratio in the lung, indicative of redox cycling of diquat in lung cells, and further that exposure of these rats to 100% oxygen enhanced the toxicity. These workers also reported damage to type I alveolar epithelial cells, following this large dose of diquat. Subsequent studies by Keeling and Smith (1982) in rats given 20 mg/kg diquat iv did not detect changes in NADPH or NADP in the lung at various times after dosing, although they did find a persistent increase in the total disulphide content of the lung, suggesting redox stress. The finding that diquat in the presence of oxygen can enhance the toxicity to rats has also been confirmed and damage to alveolar type II cells and pulmonary edema may contribute to the death of the animal under these conditions (Keeling et al., 1981; Kehrer et al., 1979). Direct intratracheal administration of diquat to rats can produce lung damage and fibrosis, although much larger doses were required than for paraquat (Manabe and Ogata, 1986, 1987). The early studies of Bainova (1969a), Bainova et al. (1972), Bainova and Velcheva (1978), and Makovskii (1972) also reported lung irritation and injury following subchronic and chronic exposure. Overall these studies indicate that if diquat enters a lung cell it can redox cycle which, if extensive, can overwhelm the defense mechanisms, leading to cell death. However, lung injury is not a contributory factor to the death of animals receiving a MLD and exposed to air.

71.2.2.13 Effects on the Gastrointestinal Tract

The most obvious postmortem observation following diquat administration is distension of the terminal ileum and caecal region of the gastrointestinal tract (Clark and Hurst, 1970; Cobb and Grimshaw, 1979; Crabtree et al., 1977; Pushkar, 1969; Verbetskii and Stolyarchuk, 1967). Following an oral dose, diquat produced a dose-related increase in the water content in the lumen of the gastrointestinal tract (Fig. 71.3), which 24 h after an MLD was about 14 ml/rat. This results in tissue dehydration and hypovolaemia (Fig. 71.3) (Crabtree et al., 1977). The marked decrease in blood volume (Lock, 1979) would be expected to have an effect on peripheral circulation and presumably contributes to the reduced renal function observed

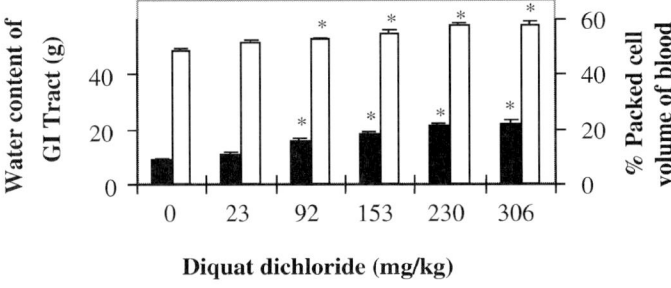

Figure 71.3 Dose response curve for the effect of diquat on the water content of the gastrointestinal tract and the haematocrit values 24 h after a single oral dose to the rat. Results are mean ± SE with * representing statistically significantly different from control. Water content (■) and packed cell volume (□). Adapted from Crabtree *et al.* (1977).

(see later). Whether it contributes to the death of the animal in shock remains to be established. Following sc administration the loss of fluid into the lumen of the gastrointestinal tract is delayed until about 6 days after dosing. An effect on blood volume is seen about 17 h after dosing, which is probably related to the diuretic effect of the compound via this route. At later times the hypovolaemia is less marked than after oral administration (Crabtree *et al.*, 1977). Histological changes in the gastrointestinal tract following oral dosing are minimal, consisting of patchy loss of keratin from the cardiac end of the stomach, edema of the submucosa at the junction of the glandular and nonglandular region, with some dilation of lacteal and submucosal lymphatic vessels of the small intestine and caecum (Clark and Hurst, 1970; Crabtree *et al.*, 1977). In monkeys given toxic doses of diquat, the lining of the stomach was ulcerated and the large and small intestine congested; histological examination revealed large areas of necrosis with exfoliation of the lining epithelium (Cobb and Grimshaw, 1979).

Studies with anaesthetized rats where diquat was added to ligated segments of jejenum or infused into intestinal loops showed that diquat induced a net secretion of fluid into the lumen (Anton *et al.*, 1998; Rawlings *et al.*, 1992). This response is seen at sublethal doses and can be blocked by nitric oxide synthase inhibitors, suggesting a role for nitric oxide in the mechanism of fluid secretion (Anton *et al.*, 1998). The addition of diquat to epithelial cells of the rat small intestine increased the activity of the pentose phosphate pathway and produced NADPH depletion, indicating redox cycling of diquat in these cells. If marked and sustained this may contribute to the fluid loss into the lumen of the gastrointestinal tract (Rawlings *et al.*, 1994).

71.2.2.14 Effects on the Kidney

The major route of elimination for diquat once it has entered the bloodstream is via the kidneys where it is actively secreted by organic cation transport systems (see earlier discussion). At high plasma concentrations diquat produced a mild hydropic change to proximal tubular cells of the Alderley Park rat kidney, which was associated with mild proteinuria and glucosuria (Lock and Ishmael, 1979). More recent studies have shown that

the Fischer 344 rat is more sensitive to diquat-induced liver injury (see later) and this strain is also more sensitive to renal injury (Petry *et al.*, 1992). Renal tubular necrosis was marked in the cynomolgus monkey where a dose-related renal proximal and distal tubular injury was observed, which was associated with a marked elevation in serum urea (Fig. 71.3) (Cobb and Grimshaw, 1979). Oral administration of diquat to rats reduced urine output and glomerular filtration rate and hence the clearance of diquat. This effect may be secondary to hypovolaemia as both total and renal plasma volume were reduced 24 h after treatment (Lock, 1979).

As in other organs, diquat, once it enters a proximal tubular cell, can redox cycle and increase the activity of the pentose phosphate pathway (Lock and Ishmael, 1979), suggesting that if sufficient diquat was concentrated inside the cell it could overwhelm the defense mechanisms, leading to necrosis.

71.2.2.15 Effects on the Eye

Chronic exposure in the diet to diquat produced a dose- and time-dependent appearance of cataracts in both rats and dogs as discussed earlier. This finding was confirmed by Pirie and Rees (1970), who fed rats a diet containing 500 or 750 ppm diquat. They reported that the first change observed in the eye was an irregular "lace-work" of opacity in the posterior cortex, which arose following 4–8 months exposure. The next stage was a clearly defined nuclear cataract that could be seen with the naked eye which progressed to shrinkage and complete opacity. The concentration of diquat that enters the eye at the time of peak blood levels following ip injection is about 0.3–1 nmol/g of lens and 2.7–4.3 nmol/g eye contents, 1 to 3 h after dosing. The concentration in the eye contents resembling that found in the plasma, while that in the lens was much lower than that in the plasma (Pirie and Rees, 1970). Associated with the development of cataract there was a decrease in the concentration of ascorbic acid in ocular fluid, while the glutathione content remained unchanged (Pirie and Rees, 1970). Studies *in vitro* using bovine or rat lens have shown that diquat can catalyze a time-dependent loss of ascorbic acid with the formation of hydrogen peroxide (Pirie *et al.*, 1970) providing evidence that redox cycling of diquat can occur in the eye. Subsequent studies by Bhuyan and Bhuyan (1991, 1994) have provided indirect evidence of diquat-induced production of superoxide anion, hydroxyl radical, and hydrogen peroxide in the rabbit eye following intravitreal injection. Overall, these studies indicate that oxidative stress as a consequence of the redox cycling of diquat is the likely mechanism of cataract formation. Following low dose exposure the onset of cataract will only arise once the defense mechanisms in the eye are overwhelmed.

Following acute sc injection diquat causes a prolonged dilatation of the pupil of the eye, suggesting a sympathomimetic action of the compound after high exposure. This response was less marked after oral dosing and not seen after direct application to the eye, indicating it is a systemic-mediated effect (Clark and Hurst, 1970).

71.2.2.16 Effects on the Liver

Burk and co-workers (1980) reported that diquat was very toxic to selenium deficient rats, and a dose of 5 mg/kg ip produced mortality in 2–3 h. The rats had extensive liver and kidney necrosis and exhaled large quantities of ethane, a marker of lipid peroxidation. By contrast, normal rats given 20 mg/kg ip diquat showed little or no liver injury (Table 71.3). Toxic doses of diquat to cynomolgus monkeys elevated plasma alanine aminotransferase (ALT) and aspartate aminotransferase (AST) (Fig. 71.2) which was associated with minimal histological evidence of hepatic single cell necrosis and sinusoidal congestion (Cobb and Grimshaw, 1979). The discovery that Fischer 344 rats are more susceptible to hepatic necrosis than Sprague–Dawley rats stimulated interest in the mechanism of hepatotoxicity and the role of oxidative stress (Smith *et al.*, 1985). Large ip doses of diquat administered to Fischer 344 rats elevated plasma ALT and AST values (Table 71.3) and produced hepatocyte necrosis. Diquat also increased the biliary efflux of GSSG and decreased hepatic glutathione content at early times after dosing (Smith *et al.*, 1985). Treatment of rats with 1,3-bis(2-chloroethyl)-*N*-nitrosourea (BCNU), an inhibitor of glutathione reductase, followed by diquat increased the efflux of GSSG into bile and potentiated the liver toxicity, relative to control animals, indicating a key role for this enzyme in protecting the liver against oxidative stress (Smith, 1987a). NADPH-cytochrome P-450 reductase catalyzes the reduction of diquat to form a diquat cation radical which can release iron from ferritin both *in vitro* and *in vivo* (Reif *et al.*, 1988; Thomas and Aust, 1986). The availability of free iron presumably contributes to the free radical mediated lipid peroxidation seen in the liver (Burk *et al.*, 1980, 1995; Smith, 1987b;

Wolfgang *et al.*, 1991). Diquat also enhances the biliary excretion of nonhaem iron (Benzick *et al.*, 1994; Gupta *et al.*, 1994. Whether this is a result of intracellular iron overload and hence a clearance mechanism requires further study. Many of the findings reported above with diquat also occur in isolated hepatocytes or liver slices where manipulation of the system has enabled a better understanding of the mechanism of toxicity (DeGray *et al.*, 1991; Eklow-Lastbom *et al.*, 1986; Nakagawa *et al.*, 1992; Rikans and Cai, 1993; Sandy *et al.*, 1986, 1987; Wolfgang *et al.*, 1991). Overall, these studies indicate that high doses of diquat can overwhelm the hepatocytes' defense mechanisms against oxidative stress, leading to necrosis.

71.2.2.17 Effects on Other Organs

Diquat administration to rats prevented the normal depletion of liver glycogen in fasted animals and produced a marked increase in blood glucose that appeared to be mediated by the adrenal gland, since adrenalectomy prevented these changes (Rose *et al.*, 1974b). These effects seen following both diquat and paraquat are thought to be due to catecholamine release and high circulating concentrations of corticosteroids (Rose *et al.*, 1974b). Subsequent studies confirmed that diquat administration to rats produced a dose-related increase in plasma corticosteroid concentration and further confirmed that this could be blocked by pretreating the rats with dexamethasone, which also reduced the concentration of circulating adrenocorticotrophic hormone (ACTH). It was concluded, based on both *in vivo* and *in vitro* studies that the increase in adrenal steroid synthesis was due to the release of ACTH from the pituitary (Crabtree and Rose, 1976). The high circulating corticosteroid concentration may account for the changes reported in the thymus, spleen and

Table 71.3
Liver Injury Produced by High Parenteral Doses of Diquat in Normal and Selenium Deficient Rats

Dietary state	Strain	Dose (mg/kg)	Plasma marker (U/ml)	
			ALT	AST
Normal[a]	Sprague–Dawley[b]	0	41 ± 5	83 ± 8
		26[d]	51 ± 7	199 ± 42
		52[e]	54 ± 18	96 ± 12
Normal[a]	Fischer 344[b]	0	39 ± 3	135 ± 19
		13	$186 \pm 25^*$	105 ± 71
		26[f]	$833 \pm 293^*$	$1063 \pm 388^*$
Normal[a]	Holzmann[c]	20	19 ± 4	
		60[g]	41 ± 5	
Selenium deficient[a]	Holzmann[c]	5[h]	$3490 \pm 1940^*$	

[a] Rats were given a single intraperitoneal injection of diquat and killed 24 h later unless otherwise stated.
[b] Data from Smith *et al.* (1985).
[c] Data from Burk *et al.* (1980).
[d] Mortality 40% at 24 h.
[e] Mortality 80% at 24 h.
[f] Mortality 14% at 24 h.
[g] Animals died within 80 ± 12 minutes of dosing.
[h] Animals died within 150 ± 37 minutes of dosing.
*Statistically significant from control.

adrenal gland of rats after a large sc dose of diquat (Clark and Hurst, 1970) and the observed suppression of cell turnover in the lung and eye at early times after dosing (Pirie and Rees, 1970; Smith and Rose, 1977).

71.2.2.18 Treatment of Poisoning in Animals

Diquat like paraquat binds tightly to diatomaceous clay and hence the treatment is the same as that discussed for paraquat, namely purgation of the gastrointestinal tract with bentonite or Fuller's earth (diatomaceous clay's) along with a cathartic such as magnesium sulphate (Clark, 1971; Smith *et al.*, 1974). See the more detailed discussion on cases of human poisoning.

71.3 TOXICITY TO HUMANS

71.3.1 EXPERIMENTAL EXPOSURE

Following intravenous administration of 1 μCi ^{14}C-labelled diquat to six subjects, $61.2 \pm 16.0\%$ of the dose was excreted in urine over 5 days (Feldmann and Maibach, 1974). In the same study, 4 μg/cm^2 was applied onto the skin, and $0.3 \pm 0.1\%$ (corrected for incomplete urine excretion) of the dose was excreted in urine over 5 days. Diquat was the least absorbed of the 12 pesticides studied. Percutaneous absorption was increased to 1.4% when the site of application was occluded, and to 3.8% when the stratum corneum was removed by successive skin stripping (Wester and Maibach, 1985).

71.3.2 ACCIDENTAL AND INTENTIONAL POISONING

There is a relatively small number of reports on human diquat poisoning in the literature. The first case was reported by Oreopoulos and McEvoy (1969) and involved an 18 year old man who accidentally ingested a mouthful of diquat concentrate which had been decanted into a Coca Cola bottle. This patient survived after treatment with forced diuresis. A further 11 cases of systemic poisoning by ingestion have been reported since then with varying levels of detail (Table 71.4). The overall mortality was 8 out of the 12 cases (67%); however, because of the small number of cases, this figure must be treated with caution. Two of the 3 patients who accidentally ingested diquat survived. The third patient, a 2 1/2 year old boy, died 6 days after ingesting an unknown amount of diquat concentrate which had been decanted into a soft drink bottle. In contrast, 7 of the 9 patients who ingested diquat with suicidal intent died.

In addition, Okonek (1976) mentioned another two fatal diquat intoxication's as a consequence of suicidal ingestion, however, no further information was given regarding these patients. Hall (1995) found that in the 10 year period from 1983–1992 only two diquat-related fatalities were reported by poison control centres in the USA. Table 71.5 gives details of 26 additional diquat poisoning cases where the approximate ingested dose

and the outcome were known, and which were reported to the manufacturer between 1969 and 1996 (Zeneca Agrochemicals, unpublished data). As with the data from the published literature, there is a difference in mortality following accidental ingestion and deliberate ingestion: all 13 patients with accidental or unknown aetiology survived, whereas 11 out of 13 patients with suicidal ingestion died. Most cases of accidental ingestion involved decanting of diquat concentrate from its original container into unmarked drinks bottles.

There are no reports in the literature of systemic illness or fatalities occurring following dermal exposure to diquat.

71.3.3 USE EXPERIENCE

Diquat levels in air after tractor and manual spraying were determined by Makovskii (1972). The application rates were 1.0–1.3 kg diquat/ha. The highest diquat concentrations (mean 0.56 mg/m^3) were found in the tractor cabin when the door was open and spraying was in progress in the direction of the wind. Spraying against the wind and manual spraying resulted in lower concentrations (mean 0.17 and 0.25 mg/m^3, respectively). The diquat concentration in the air decreased rapidly within 10–20 min after completion of the treatment. The dermal exposure of the spraymen ranged from 0.05 mg to 0.08 mg on the face and hands after 2–3 h of daily work. No health effects were reported.

In a study of diquat exposure during aerial application (Sawinsky and Pasztor, 1977), the average diquat concentration in the breathing zone of the pilot was 4.5 μg/m^3. The potential dermal exposure was estimated from filter discs as 61.5 μg/100 cm^2. No diquat was detected in urine samples of pilots who had sprayed diquat for 3 to 4 weeks. In contrast, potential dermal exposure of mechanics and loading personnel ranged from 3.5–8.7 mg/100 cm^2, and average urine concentration of diquat was measured as 6.3 and 19.6 μg/100 ml, respectively.

Wojeck *et al.* (1983) studied the exposure of workers applying diquat by hand-operated sprayer against water hyacinths or using direct injection into the water for hydrilla control. There was no measurable inhalation exposure. Average dermal exposure of spraymen and airboat drivers was 1.82 and 0.20 mg/h, respectively, during the treatment of water hyacinths. Average dermal exposure of spraymen and mixers of diquat for the treatment of hydrilla was 0.17 and 0.47 mg/h, respectively. No diquat could be detected in urine.

Topical effects from exposure to diquat have been described. Inflammation and nose-bleeds were observed in people handling crystalline powder (Clark and Hurst, 1970). Epistaxis in the field has been seen occurring from splashes when mixing the concentrate or prolonged exposure to spray drift. Cases of nail damage from contact with a concentrated paraquat/diquat mixture were first reported by Samman and Johnston (1969). According to Clark and Hurst (1970), contact of the 20% diquat concentrate with the nail base may result in nail growth disturbances, development of coloured spots and white bands,

Table 71.4
Details of Published Cases of Human Diquat Poisoning by Oral Ingestion

Age (years)	Sex	Dose stated[a]	Calculated ingested dose (mg/kg)[b]	Aetiology	Outcome[c]	Reference
18	M	1 mouthful	50	Accident	Survival	Oreopoulos and McEvoy, 1969
25	M	2–3 mouthful	100–150	Suicide	Death (7 days)	Schönborn et al., 1971
43	F	Unknown	—	Suicide	Death (2 days)	Okonek and Hofmann, 1975
53	M	<1 mouthful	<50	Accident	Survival	Fel et al., 1976
45	M	Unknown	—	Suicide	Death (2 days)	Okonek, 1976
33	M	200 ml*	860	Suicide	Death (2 days)	Narita et al., 1978
16	F	50 ml	200	Suicide	Death (1 day)	Vanholder et al., 1981
60	F	20 ml	57	Suicide	Death (5 days)	Vanholder et al., 1981
29	M	1 mouthful	50	Suicide	Survival	Ferguson et al., 1983
23	M	300 ml	860	Suicide	Death (1 day)	McCarthy and Speth, 1983
2.5	M	Unknown	—	Accident	Death (6 days)	Powell et al., 1983
33	M	300 ml	860	Suicide	Survival	Mahieu et al., 1984

[a] Volumes (ml) refer to the 20% liquid concentrate, except * which stated that a 30% concentrate was ingested. A volume of 17.5 ml has been used for "a mouthful."
[b] All doses expressed as mg diquat ion per kg body weight. Where the body weight was not explicitly stated, the following assumptions were used: 3–6 years, 25 kg; 7–11 years, 40 kg; 12–16 years, 50 kg; 17 years and above, 70 kg.
[c] Time interval between ingestion and death indicated in parentheses.

and eventual shedding of the nail. Normal nail growth follows upon cessation of exposure. Concentrated diquat formulations have also been reported to delay the healing of superficial cuts of the hands of spray workers (IPCS, 1984). Perineal and scrotal burns caused by leaking from a knapsack sprayer containing a paraquat/diquat mixture were seen in two patients (Ronnen et al., 1995). The lesions responded well to treatment with topical silver sulfadiazine and oral antibiotics, and the damaged skin healed within a few days without scarring. Ocular damage due to exposure to a concentrated paraquat/diquat mixture has been described by Cant and Lewis (1968). This patient had received a splash in his eye and developed conjunctivitis, uveitis, and corneal epithelial damage. Healing was well progressed after 11 days of treatment. In two cases of eye splashes with a paraquat/diquat mixture reported by Nirep et al. (1993), there were delayed corneal epithelial defects (1–2 weeks) with gradual recovery. It was suggested that the surfactants contained in the concentrate may have contributed to the development of this lesion. Diquat is not known to cause cataract in humans. This may be due to a lack of sufficient exposure, but the absence of any ocular signs in poisoned patients may also indicate a true species difference in susceptibility.

71.3.4 ATYPICAL CASES OF VARIOUS ORIGINS

In a case described by Wood et al. (1976), a 45 year old man was admitted to hospital with confusion, high-grade pyrexia, and a 4 day history of productive cough. Chest x-rays showed areas of pneumonic consolidation. Despite antibiotic treatment the patient's condition continued to deteriorate until he was treated with oral prednisone. Shortly thereafter he improved. An episode of diquat spraying preceded the illness, and the patient described being exposed to a cloud of aerosol from a clogged nozzle. No diquat was measured, and no renal damage was seen. The radiological picture was described as being more typical of Löffler's pneumonia. The absence of any facial, upper airways, or eye irritation as well as the atypical picture make a diagnosis of diquat poisoning very doubtful.

A 24 year old man was admitted to hospital five hours after exposure to diquat (Williams et al., 1986). He stated that he had been spraying the herbicide and had experienced a salty taste on the lips and therefore stopped. Two hours later he developed severe abdominal pain and blurred vision and felt generally unwell. A urine test for diquat was positive. Plasma diquat was 0.56 mg/l upon admission, urinary diquat

Table 71.5
Cases of Human Diquat Poisoning by Oral Ingestion where Dose and Outcome Were Known (Zeneca Agrochemicals, Unpublished Data)

Age (years)	Sex	Dose stated[a]	Calculated ingested dose (mg/kg)[b]	Aetiology	Outcome[c]	Country/ year
36	M	20 ml	57	Unknown	Survival	Japan 1969
Unknown	F	250 ml	715	Suicide	Death	Canada 1974
19	M	200 ml	570	Suicide	Death	Canada 1975
Unknown	M	200 ml	570	Suicide	Death	Japan 1975
Unknown	F	50 ml	140	Accident	Survival	Japan 1977
Unknown	F	300 ml	860	Suicide	Death	Japan 1977
55	M	120 ml	340	Suicide	Death (1 day)	USA 1979
21	M	15 ml	43	Unknown	Survival	UK 1979
44	F	150 ml	430	Suicide	Death (1 day)	N Zealand 1981
21	M	200 ml	570	Suicide	Death (2 days)	France 1981
41	F	30–40 ml	86–115	Suicide	Survival	France 1984
23	M	300 ml	860	Suicide	Died (1 day)	USA 1981
2	F	5 ml	100	Accident	Survival	UK 1984
15	M	15 ml	60	Accident	Survival	USA 1984
2	M	<5 ml	<100	Accident	Survival	USA 1985
29	M	240 ml	685	Suicide	Death (4 days)	USA 1987
21	M	1 mouthful	50	Accident	Survival	USA 1988
39	M	<5 ml	<14	Accident	Survival	USA 1988
Unknown	F	800 ml	2285	Suicide	Death (1 day)	UK 1989
10	?	1 mouthful	88	Accident	Survival	Germany 1989
10	M	1 mouthful	88	Accident	Survival	Ireland 1989
52	M	300 ml	860	Suicide	Survival	UK 1996
5	?	1 mouthful	140	Accident	Survival	USA (year unknown)
20	?	20–30 ml	57–86	Accident	Survival	USA (year unknown)
0.5	?	<5 ml	<100	Accident	Survival	USA (year unknown)
50	F	180 ml	510	Suicide	Death (5 days)	USA (year unknown)

[a] Volumes (ml) refer to the 20% liquid concentrate. A volume of 17.5 ml has been used for "a mouthful."
[b] All doses expressed as mg diquat ion per kg body weight. Where the body weight was not explicitly stated, the following assumptions were used: 0–2 years, 10 kg; 3–6 years, 25 kg; 7–11 years, 40 kg; 12–16 years, 50 kg; and 17 years and above, 70 kg.
[c] Time interval between ingestion and death indicated in parentheses.

was 52 mg/l, and diquat in gastric contents was 74 mg/l. The patient developed a degree of polyuric renal failure which resolved spontaneously. Initial treatment consisted of gastric lavage, Fuller's Earth, activated charcoal, and mannitol. He also received two haemoperfusions. The patient survived and was asymptomatic at follow-up 6 months later. Although he denied that the exposure was intentional, the severity of poi-

soning and the clinical course raise significant doubts on the description of what appeared to be a minor occupational exposure.

A 72 year old farmer with a history of diabetes and transient right-sided hemiparesis developed erythema of the skin with hyperkeratosis and conjunctivitis after exposure of the hands to a 10% diquat solution for about 10 minutes (Sechi *et al.*,

1992). About 10 days later he developed akathisia with moderate hyperexcitability and insomnia. Over a period of 5 days he became dysphonic, bradykinetic, and rigid. Treatment with carbidopa/levidopa and bromocriptine significantly improved his symptoms. An MRI scan 4 months after the onset of the illness showed small, multiple, bilateral, symmetric areas of high signal intensity in the caudate nuclei and putamen and in the white matter near the ventricular wall. The authors suggested a causal relationship to diquat exposure. However, there were no clinical signs suggestive of systemic diquat poisoning, nor has there been anywhere else a description of Parkinson-like illness after diquat exposure.

71.3.5 CLINICAL FINDINGS AND DOSAGE RESPONSE

It is possible from a review of the published literature (Fel *et al.*, 1976; Ferguson *et al.*, 1983; Mahieu *et al.*, 1984; McCarthy and Speth, 1983; Narita *et al.*, 1978; Okonek, 1976; Okonek and Hofmann, 1975; Oreopoulos and McEvoy, 1969; Powell *et al.*, 1983; Schönborn *et al.*, 1971; Vanholder *et al.*, 1981) and unpublished cases to distinguish three categories of severity of diquat poisoning and correlate them to the amount ingested (Table 71.6). This is similar to the situation in paraquat poisoning, however, important differences exist both in terms of the clinical presentation and prognosis. Furthermore, since in the case of diquat poisoning this categorization is based on a relatively small number of cases, the dose–response relationship is less certain.

Following ingestion, nausea, vomiting, abdominal pain, and diarrhea (often bloody), may occur. Ulcerations of mouth, lips, and back of the throat have also been seen as a result of the caustic action of diquat which may lead to oesophageal and intestinal ulceration within 24–48 h after swallowing.

71.3.5.1 Mild Poisoning

In addition to the localized effects on mucous membranes, urea and creatinine may be elevated as a sign of transient renal functional impairment. Patients will make a full recovery regardless of whether treatment is given.

71.3.5.2 Moderate to Severe Poisoning

Depending on the amount ingested, the clinical course can be protracted over several weeks. Although nausea, vomiting, and diarrhea may persist for 2–3 days, there may sometimes be a an asymptomatic period, extending for up to 48 hours (Vanholder *et al.*, 1981). Intestinal paralysis and fluid loss may lead to abdominal distension, tissue dehydration, and hypotensive shock. Within 3–4 days a progressive decline of renal function may occur and continue into complete anuric renal failure. Evidence of reversal may show after 7–10 days. Severe neurologic and neuropsychiatric complications due to brain stem infarction and/or intracranial hemorrhage have been described. In this group of patients, death may occur if treatment is delayed or inadequate.

However, in contrast to paraquat poisoning, pulmonary fibrosis has not been seen after diquat poisoning.

71.3.5.3 Fulminant Poisoning

All organ systems can be affected and death occurs in the majority of patients within 1–2 days. Initial signs are extensive vomiting and diarrhea with massive fluid loss. Typically, patients develop pulmonary edema, acute liver and kidney failure, cardiac arrhythmia, and coma. Death occurs from multiple organ failure.

71.3.6 LABORATORY FINDINGS

In cases of diquat poisoning, laboratory findings are generally nonspecific. The changes seen reflect organ failure, affecting in particular kidneys and liver. A rise in serum creatinine and urea is frequently found, although it is not a very sensitive parameter of renal functional impairment. In a case described by Mahieu *et al.* (1984) a 33 year old man who was said to have ingested about 300 ml of diquat concentrate showed little variation in serum creatinine over the course of 2 weeks. However, evidence of renal damage was seen by a massive increase in albuminuria on day 3 and 4 after the intoxication, accompanied by a rise in urinary excretion of retinol binding protein and beta-2-microglobulin. All parameters had returned to normal by day 15. Increases in liver enzymes such as ALT and AST are a reflection of hepatocellular necrosis which can be seen at autopsy (Schönborn *et al.*, 1971). They also occur after 3–4 days, although maximum values may be delayed as much as 10–12 days (Mahieu *et al.*, 1984). A rise in serum bilirubin is a reflection of intracellular cholestasis.

Thrombopenia without accompanying changes in other blood parameters has been described after diquat poisoning. In the case reported by Schönborn *et al.* (1971) this was severe enough (4000 platelets/mm^3) to cause multiple bleeding and may have contributed to the brain stem hemorrhage which was seen upon autopsy. This patient received hemodialysis, but not hemoperfusion. Mahieu *et al.* (1984) found a reduction in platelet count in their patient to 64,000 mm^3 on day 6 with a return to normal values by day 12. No signs of intoxication were seen.

Many of the analytical methods described for the determination of paraquat are also applicable to diquat. These include the dithionite spot test (Berry and Grove J, 1971; Widdop, 1976) which, although less sensitive than for paraquat, gives a green color in the presence of diquat. The improved spot test using extraction with a silica cartridge gives a detection limit between 0.5 and 2 µg/ml for diquat in plasma (Woollen and Mahler, 1987). A variation of the quantitative method with a spectrophotometric endpoint has been described to determine diquat in plasma (Williams *et al.*, 1986). The high performance liquid chromatography method described by Gill *et al.* (1983) can also be used for measuring diquat. The significance of diquat plasma concentrations in terms of the prognosis has not

Table 71.6
Severity Grade, Aetiology, and Outcome in 38 Cases of Human Diquat Poisoning by Oral Ingestion (Compiled from Tables 71.4 and 71.5)

Severity	Dose (mg/kg)	No. of Cases	Accidents No.	Accidents (%)	Suicides No.	Suicides (%)	Fatalities No.	Fatalities (%)
Mild	≤50	5[a]	3	(60)	1	(20)	0	(0)
Moderate–severe	50–200	15[a]	11	(73)	3	(20)	3	(20)
Fulminant	≥200	18	0	(0)	18	(100)	16	(89)
All cases		38[b]	14	(37)	22	(58)	19	(50)

[a]Includes one case with unknown aetiology.
[b]Includes two cases with unknown aetiology.

been established. However, in two separate studies with a total of 71 patients ingesting a product containing equal levels of paraquat and diquat, the combined plasma concentrations of the two chemicals were above the predictive line established by Proudfoot et al. (1979) in the patients with fatal outcome, and below in the survivors (Ameno et al., 1994; Yoshioka et al., 1992).

71.3.7 ABSORPTION

There is little information on absorption of diquat in humans. There was no difference in serum concentration of paraquat and diquat in the first 24 h after ingestion of a combined herbicide, suggesting a similar absorption of the two cations from the gut (Ameno et al., 1994; Yoshioka et al., 1992). However, after 24 h the plasma concentration of diquat was consistently lower than that of paraquat. It has been suggested that this finding may be related to an increased biliary excretion and possibly metabolism of diquat (Ameno et al., 1994, see below).

71.3.8 DISTRIBUTION

The distribution of diquat and paraquat appears to be similar in humans (Ameno et al., 1994). Following intravenous administration of trace amounts of ^{14}C-labelled diquat to volunteers, the plasma half-life was 4 h (Feldmann and Maibach, 1974). In the case described by Williams et al. (1986), the peak plasma concentration of diquat was measured in the first sample which was taken approximately 5 h after ingestion. Diquat could no longer be detected in plasma 23 h after ingestion. Powell et al. (1983) found a rise in diquat plasma concentrations between 2 and 10 h after ingestion. They also suggested extensive sequestration of diquat in tissues because of a marked rebound of plasma concentrations shortly after the end of haemoperfusion treatments. Tissue levels of diquat in postmortem samples from five patients are shown in Table 71.7. These show marked interindividual differences in tissue distribution which are most likely related to the time interval between ingestion and death. In the patients from the study by Ameno et al. (1994), who died within 48 h, by far the highest concentration of diquat (excluding bile) was measured in the kidneys. In contrast, patients who

died later showed a smaller variation between tissue concentrations (Powell et al., 1983; Schönborn et al., 1971).

71.3.9 METABOLISM

Two metabolites of diquat have been identified in humans (Fuke et al., 1996). Diquat dipyridone and monopyridone were found in both serum and urine following ingestion of a paraquat/diquat mixture in three patients. Serum concentrations of the metabolites accounted for less than 3% of diquat when serum concentrations of diquat were above 10 μg/ml. However, once the diquat concentration had fallen below 1 μg/ml, diquat dipyridone reached up to 20% of diquat in the serum of one patient, with diquat monopyridone being considerably lower. In contrast, urinary excretion of the monopyridone was up to 10 times higher than for the dipyridone. The authors suggested that the monopyridone was the primary metabolite which would also be excreted more rapidly because it remained partially ionized. At high serum diquat concentrations, metabolism would make little difference to the elimination kinetics of the parent compound. However, this would be different at lower serum concentrations, possibly accounting for the more rapid elimination of diquat when compared to paraquat.

71.3.10 EXCRETION

Following intravenous administration of radiolabelled diquat to human volunteers, 37.3% of the administered dose was recovered in urine in the first 4 h (Feldmann and Maibach, 1974). A further 17.0% was excreted in urine between 4 and 24 h after administration with a total of 61.2% of the dose recovered over 5 days. In the case described by Mahieu et al. (1984) most of the amount recovered in urine was found on the first day although trace amounts could be detected until day 13. Ameno et al. (1994) found the biliary concentration of diquat about 3.5 times higher than that of paraquat after ingestion of a product containing equal amounts of the two herbicides. These authors suggested that biliary excretion was a significant route of diquat elimination which could partially explain the significantly lower plasma concentration of diquat compared to paraquat after 24 h following ingestion.

Table 71.7
Diquat Tissue Concentrations in Postmortem Samples of Five Patients (µg/g)

Reference	Schönborn et al., 1971	Powell et al., 1983	Ameno et al., 1994		
			Case 4	Case 5	Case 6
Time after ingestion	7 days	6 days	26 hours	46 hours	18 hours
Brain	—*	0.03	0.23	0.11	0.23
Lung	0.56	0.06	0.32	0.32	1.68
Heart	0.11	<0.01	0.18	—	0.51
Liver	0.33	0.15	0.34	0.12	2.48
Spleen	1.04	—	0.46	0.31	1.20
Pancreas	—	—	0.26	0.05	0.56
Kidney	1.19	0.04	3.36	2.40	4.34
Muscle	—	0.1	0.26	0.07	0.40
Fat	—	—	0.08	0.01	0.15
Blood	—	—	0.09	0.20	0.59
Bile	—	—	28.70	5.56	34.00
Large intestine	0.37	—	—	—	—
Small intestine	0.45	—	—	—	—

*Indicates not determined.

71.3.11 PATHOLOGY

Pathological findings upon autopsy in humans fatalities have been described in a number of cases (McCarthy and Speth, 1983; Powell et al., 1983; Schönborn et al., 1971; Vanholder et al., 1981). Most autopsy reports describe infarction and purpura of the brain stem as a specific complication of diquat intoxication. In particular the pons may show areas of hemorrhage in association with multiple small and sometimes confluent areas of infarction. Necrosis of the capillary walls may be evident. Other cerebral structures appear unaffected.

Depending on the amount of concentrate ingested, the oropharynx, oesophagus, and gastrointestinal tract will show areas of hemorrhagic necrosis, sometimes with pseudomembraneous inflammation. Small and large intestines will be distended with fluid accumulation.

The kidneys are pale and swollen and show signs of acute tubular necrosis with severe degenerative lesions, formation of eosinophilic necrosis, and exfoliation of necrotic cells into the tubular lumen. Perivascular round cell infiltration has been seen in the cortex.

The liver may show fatty generation of the epithelium, lipid storage and vacuolisation of the Kupffer cells, and evidence of intracellular cholestasis.

In contrast to paraquat poisoning, pulmonary findings are of an acute nature, such as hemorrhagic, fibrin-rich edema, localized intraalveolar bleeding, formation of hyaline membranes, and focal bronchopneumonia. Thickening of alveolar walls and accumulation of reactive alveolar epithelial and chronic inflammatory cells may also occur, but the typical fibroblastic proliferation seen in paraquat lung has not ben described after diquat ingestion.

71.3.12 TREATMENT OF POISONING

The therapy of diquat intoxication is based on the same principles as described for paraquat poisoning with prevention of absorption and enhanced elimination being the mainstay of the therapy. Because of the absence of pulmonary fibrosis, no specific pathophysiological therapy has been attempted in most cases of diquat poisoning.

Gastric lavage and the use of Fuller's Earth, Bentonite, or activated charcoal together with administration of a cathartic have been advocated as an early treatment to minimize absorption from the gastrointestinal tract (Vanholder et al., 1981). However, these authors have also pointed out that gastric and intestinal decontamination should be performed cautiously because of the risk of perforation, particularly when therapy is delayed. Adsorbent material should be instilled with care during intestinal paralysis since massive sequestration may occur.

Because of the massive fluid losses into the gastrointestinal tract and its potential circulatory and renal consequences, special attention must be given to adequate hydration of the patient, if possible under control of the central venous pressure (Vanholder et al., 1981). Anticoagulants should be administered with great caution because of the risk of brain stem hemorrhage. However, the use of heparin is often inevitable when hemodialysis or hemoperfusion are needed.

Forced diuresis has been used to enhance the elimination of diquat (Mahieu et al., 1984; Oreopoulos and McEvoy, 1969). However, there is no conclusive evidence of its therapeutic value. Extracorporeal hemodialysis was found to be ineffective in removing diquat from the circulation with an average clearance of 3.17 ml/min and a total removal of 0.84 mg diquat during 11.5 h of dialysis (Okonek and Hofmann, 1975).

Hemoperfusion with activated charcoal has been suggested as a more effective way of lowering the plasma diquat concentration (Okonek, 1976). Powell *et al.* (1983) showed that use of a polystyrene resin cartridge did not remove diquat, but charcoal haemoperfusion achieved clearance rates between 39 and 104 ml/min. However, a slow but marked rebound in diquat concentrations was observed between treatments, indicating extensive tissue sequestration of diquat. Williams *et al.* (1986) suggested that haemoperfusion was probably ineffective in removing significant amounts of diquat in their patient, despite a lowering of the diquat plasma concentration during the treatment.

In conclusion, the treatment of diquat poisoning is directed at preventing gastrointestinal absorption and enhancing elimination from the circulation. There is no conclusive evidence that these therapeutic interventions have contributed significantly to the overall survival of patients. However, in cases of moderate to severe poisoning the prognosis is often favourable, provided the complications of intestinal fluid loss, renal failure and brain stem haemorrhage can be avoided or successfully managed.

Disclaimer   The positions on certain aspects of the toxicology of diquat in this chapter may not be aligned with the Syngenta positions; the latter are derived mainly from internal Syngenta reports many of which have not been published in the open literature.

REFERENCES

Ameno, K., Fuke, C., Shirakawa, Y., and Ogura, S. (1994). Different distribution of paraquat and diquat in human poisoning cases after ingestion of a combined herbicide. *Arch. Toxicol.* **68**, 134–137.

Andersen, K. J., Leighty, E. G., and Takahashi, M. T. (1972). Evaluation of herbicides for possible mutagenic properties. *J. Ag. Fd. Chem.* **20**, 649.

Anderson, D., McGregory, D. B., and Purchase, I. F. H. (1976). Dominant lethal studies with Paraquat and Diquat in male CD-1 mice. *Mutat. Res.* **40**, 347–358.

Anton, P., Theodorou, V., Fioramonti, J., and Bueno, L. (1998). Low-level exposure to diquat induces a neurally mediated intestinal hypersecretion in rats: involvement of nitric oxide and mast cells. *Toxicol. Appl. Pharmacol.* **152**, 77–82.

Bainova, A. (1969a). Chronic oral toxicity of bipyridilium herbicides. *Hig. Zdrav.* **12**, 325–332.

Bainova, A. (1969b). Experimental assessment of the effect of dipyridylium herbicides on the skin. *Letopisi HEI* **9**, 25–30.

Bainova, A., Zlateva, M., and Vulcheva, V. S. (1972). Chronic inhalation toxicity of bipyridilium herbicides. *Hig. Zdrav.* **15**, 25–31.

Bainova, A., and Velcheva, V. S. (1974). Experimental assessment of the effects of dipyridylium on sex glands. *In* "Works of the Research Institute of Hygiene and Laboratory Protection," Vol. 22, pp. 111–122. Sofia, Medzina I Fizkultura.

Bainova, A. (1975). Cumulative action of Gramoxone and Reglone. *In* "Problemi na higiena," Vol. 1, pp. 31–38. Sofia, Medizna I Fizkultura.

Bainova, A., and Velcheva, V. S. (1977). Experimental verification of the maximum allowable concentration of Reglone in the air of the workplace. *Probl. Khig.* **3**, 11–18.

Bainova, A. I., and Velcheva, V. S. (1978). Chronic action of Diquat on lungs. *Dokl. Bolg. Akad. Nauk* **31**, 1369–1372.

Baldwin, R. C., Pasi, A., MacGregor, J. T., and Hine, C. H. (1975). The rates of radical formation from the dipyridylium herbicides, paraquat, diquat and

morfamquat in homogenates of rat lung. Kidney and liver: An inhibitory effect of carbon monoxide. *Toxicol. Appl. Pharmacol.* **32**, 298–304.

Bennett, P. N., and Davies, D. S. (1976). *In vivo* absorption studies with paraquat and diquat in the dog. *Br. J. Pharmacol.* **58**, 284P.

Benigni, R. M., Bignami, A., Carere, P., Comba, G., Conti, L., and Conti, R. (1979). Mutagenicity studies in salmonalla, streptomyces, aspergillus and unscheduled DNA synthesis in eye cells of paraquat and diquat. *Mutat. Res.* **64**, 127–128.

Benzick, A. E., Reddy, S. L., Gupta, S., Rogers, L. K., and Smith, C. V. (1994). Diquat- and acetaminophen-induced alterations of biliary efflux of iron in rats. *Biochem. Pharmacol.* **47**, 2079–2085.

Berry, D. J., and Grove, J. (1971). The determination of PQ 1,1′-Dimethyl-4,4′-bipyridylium cation in urine. *Clin. Chim. Acta* **34**, 5–11.

Bhuyan, K. C., and Bhuyan, D. K. (1991). Oxy radicals in the eye tissues of rabbits after diquat *in vivo*. *Free Rad. Res. Comm.* **12–13**, 621–627.

Bhuyan, D. K., and Bhuyan, K. C. (1994). Assessment of oxidative stress to eye in animal model for cataract. *Methods Enzymol.* **233**, 630–639.

Brian, R. C., Homer, R. F., Stubbs, J., and Jones, R. L. (1958). A new herbicide, 1:1-ethylene-2,2′-dipyridylium dibromide. *Nature (London)* **181**, 446.

Brawn, K., and Fridovich, I. (1981). DNA strand scission by enzymatically generated oxygen radicals. *Arch. Biochem. Biophys.* **206**, 414–419.

Burk, R. F., Lawrence, R. A., and Lane, J. M. (1980). Liver necrosis and lipid peroxidation in the rat as the result of paraquat and diquat administration—Effect of selenium deficiency. *J. Clin. Invest.* **65**, 1024–1031.

Burk, R. F., Hill, K. E., Awad, J. A., Morrow, J. D., Kato, T., Cockell, K. A., and Lyons, P. R. (1995). Pathogenesis of diquat induced liver necrosis in selenium deficient rats: Assessment of the roles of lipid peroxidation and selenoprotein P. *Hepatology* **21**, 561–569.

Bus, J. S., Preache, M. M., Cagen, S. Z., Posner, H. S., Eliason, B. C., Sharp, C. W., and Gibson, J. E. (1975). Fetal toxicity and distribution of paraquat and diquat in mice and rats. *Toxicol. Appl. Pharmacol.* **33**, 450–460.

Cant, J. S., and Lewis, D. R. H. (1968). Ocular damage due to paraquat and diquat. *Br. Med. J.* **3**, 59.

Chan, B. S. H., Lazzaro, V. A., Seale, J. P., and Duggin, G. G. (1988). The renal excretory mechanisms and the role of organic cations in modulating the renal handling of paraquat. *Pharmacol. Therap.* **79**, 193–203.

Clark, D. G., and Hurst, E. W. (1970). The toxicity of diquat. *Br. J. Ind. Med.* **27**, 51–55.

Clark, D. G. (1971). Inhibition of the absorption of Paraquat from the gastrointestinal tract by absorbents. *Br. J. Ind. Med.* **28**, 186–188.

Cobb, L. M., and Grimshaw, P. (1979). Acute toxicity of oral Diquat (1,1′-ethylene-2,2′-bipyridinium) in cynomolgus monkeys. *Toxicol. Appl. Pharmacol.* **51**, 277–282.

Crabtree, H. C., and Rose, M. S. (1976). Early effects of diquat on plasma corticosteroid concentrations in rats. *Biochem. Pharmac.* **25**, 2465–2468.

Crabtree, H. C., Lock, E. A., and Rose, M. S. (1977). Effects of Diquat on the gastrointestinal tract of rats. *Toxicol. Appl. Pharmacol.* **41**, 585–595.

Daniel, J. W., and Gage, J. C. (1966). Absorption and excretion of diquat and paraquat in rats. *Br. J. Ind. Med.* **23**, 133–136.

DeGray, J. A., Rao, D. N. R., and Mason, R. P. (1991). Reduction of paraquat and related bipyridylium compounds to free radical metabolites by rat hepatocytes. *Arch. Biochem. Biophys.* **289**, 145–142.

Eklow-Lastbom, L., Rossi, L., Thor, H., and Orrenius, S. (1986). Effects of oxidative stress caused by hyperoxia and diquat a study in isolated hepatocytes. *Free Radical Res. Commun.* **2**, 57–68.

FAO/WHO (1978). Diquat. *In* "1977 Evaluations of Some Pesticide Residues in Food." Food and Agricultural Organization of the United Nations, Rome.

FAO/WHO (1993). Diquat. *In* "Evaluation 1993, Part II—Toxicology, Pesticide Residues in Food." Food and Agricultural Organization of the United Nations, Rome.

Fel, P., Zela, I., Szule, E., and Varga, L. (1976). Reglone diquat-dibromide poisoning case successfully treated by haemodialysis. *Orv. Hetil.* **117**, 1773–1774.

Feldmann, R. J., and Maibach, H. I. (1974). Percutaneous penetration of some pesticides and herbicides in man. *Toxicol. Appl. Pharmacol.* **28**, 126–132.

Ferguson, A. H., Jacobsen, J. B., and Nielsen, H. (1983). Severe diquat poisoning. *Ex. Med. Toxicol.* **1**, 778.

Fuke, C., Ameno, K., Ameno, S., Kinoshita, H., and Ijiri, I. (1996). Detection of two metabolites of diquat in urine and serum of poisoned patients after ingestion of a combined herbicide of paraquat and diquat. *Arch. Toxicol.* **70**, 504–507.

Gage, J. C. (1968a). Toxicity of paraquat and diquat aerosols generated by a size-selective cyclone. Effect of particle size distribution. *Br. J. Ind. Med.* **25**, 304–314.

Gage, J. C. (1968b). The action of paraquat and diquat on the respiration of liver cell fractions. *Biochem. J.* **109**, 757–761.

Gaines, T. B., and Linder, R. E. (1986). Acute toxicity of pesticides in adult and weanling rats. *Fundam. Appl. Toxicol.* **7**, 299–308.

Gill, R., Qua, S. C., and Moffat, A. C. (1983). High-performance liquid chromatography of paraquat and diquat in urine with rapid sample preparation involving ion-pair extraction on disposable cartridges of octadecyl-silica. *J. Chromat.* **255**, 483–490.

Gupta, S., Rogers, L. K., and Smith, C. V. (1994). Biliary excretion of lysosomal enzymes, iron and oxidised protein in F344 and Sprague-Dawley rats and the effects of diquat and acetaminophen. *Toxicol. Appl. Pharmacol.* **125**, 42–50.

Hall, A. H. (1995). Paraquat and diquat exposures reported to U.S. poison centers 1983–1992. *In* "Paraquat Poisoning" (C. Bismuth and A. H. Hall, eds.), pp. 53–63. Dekker, New York.

Hughes, R. D., Millburn, P., and Williams, R. T. (1973). Biliary excretion of some diquaternary ammonium cations in the rat, guinea-pig and rabbit. *Biochem. J.* **136**, 979–984.

IPCS (1984). "Paraquat and Diquat." Environmental Health Criteria 39, World Health Organization.

Keeling, P. L., Pratt, I. S., Aldridge, W. N., and Smith, L. L. (1981). The enhancement of paraquat toxicity in rats by 85% oxygen-lethality and cell-specific lung damage. *Br. J. Exp. Path.* **62**, 643–654.

Keeling, P. L., and Smith, L. L. (1982). Relevance of NADPH depletion and mixed disulphide formation in rat lung to the mechanism of cell damage following paraquat administration. *Biochem. Pharmacol.* **31**, 3243–3249.

Kehrer, J. P., Haschek, W., and Witschi, H. P. (1979). The influence of Hyperoxia on the acute toxicity of paraquat and diquat. *Drug Chem. Tox.* **2**, 397–408.

Khera, K. S., Whitta, L. L., and Clegg, D. J. (1970). Embryopathic effects of diquat and paraquat in rats. *Ind. Med. Surg.* **37**, 257–261.

Kurisaki, E., and Sato, H. (1979). Tissue distribution of paraquat and diquat after oral administration in rats. *Forensic Sci. Int.* **14**, 165–180.

Lam, H. F., Takezawa, J., Gupta, B. N., and Van Stee, E. W. (1980). A comparison of the effects of paraquat and diquat on lung compliance, lung volumes and single breath diffusing capacity in the rat. *Toxicology* **18**, 111–123.

Larsson, B., Oskarsson, J. A., and Tjalve, H. (1977). Binding of paraquat and diquat in melanin. *Exp. Eye Res.* **25**, 353–359.

Levin, D. E., Hollstein, M., Christman, M. F., and Ames, B. K. (1982). A new salmonella tester strain (TA 102) with A.T. base pairs at the site of mutation detects oxidative mutagens. *Proc. Natl. Acad. Sci.* **79**, 7445–7449.

Litchfield, M. H., Daniel, J. W., and Longshaw, S. (1973). The tissue distribution of the bipyridylium herbicides diquat and paraquat in rats and mice. *Toxicology* **1**, 155–165.

Lock, E. A. (1979). The effect of paraquat and diquat on renal function in the rat. *Toxicol. Appl. Pharmacol.* **48**, 327–336.

Lock, E. A., and Ishmael, J. (1979). The acute effects of paraquat and diquat on the rat kidney. *Toxicol. Appl. Pharmacol.* **50**, 67–76.

Mahieu, P., Bonduelle, Y., Bernard, A., De Cabooter, A., Gala, M., Hassoun, A., Keonig, J., and Lauwerys, R. (1984). Acute diquat intoxication interest of its repeated determination in urine and the evaluation of renal proximal tubule integrity. *J. Toxicol. Clin. Toxicol.* **22**, 363–369.

Makovskii, V. N. (1972). "Toxicological and Hygiene Studies of the Bipyridilium Herbicide Diquat and Paraquat." Ph.D. Thesis, Vinniza, USSR.

Manabe, J., and Ogata, T. (1986). The toxic effect of diquat on the rat lung after intratracheal administration. *Toxicol. Lett.* **30**, 7–12.

Manabe, J., and Ogata, T. (1987). Lung fibrosis induced by diquat after intratracheal administration. *Arch. Toxicol.* **60**, 427–431.

Matsuura, N., Takinami, M., Kurisaki, E., and Satoo, O. (1978). Distribution of paraquat dichloride and diquat dibromide in the living body. *Fukishima Igakkai Zasshi* **28**, 212–215.

McCarthy, L. G., and Speth, C. P. (1983). Diquat intoxication. *Ann. Emerg. Med.* **12**, 294–396.

Nakagawa, Y., Moldeus, P., and Cotgreave, I. (1992). The S-Thiolation of hepatocellular protein thiols during diquat metabolism. *Biochem. Pharm.* **43**, 2519–2525.

Narita, S., Matojuku, M., Sato, J., and Mori, H. (1978). Autopsy in acute suicidal poisoning with diquat dibromide. *Nippon Igakkai Zasshi* **27**, 454–455.

Nirep, M., Hayasaka, S., Nagata, M., Tamap, A., and Tawara, T. (1993). Ocular injury caused by Preeglox-L, a herbicide containing paraquat, diquat and surfactants. *Jpn. J. Ophthalmol.* **37**, 43–46.

Okonek, S. (1976). Poisoning by paraquat or diquat. *Med. Welt.* **27**, 1401–1404.

Okonek, S., and Hofmann, A. (1975). On the question of extracorporeal haemodialysis in diquat intoxication. *Arch. Tox.* **33**, 251–257.

Oreopoulos, D. G., and McEvoy, J. (1969). Diquat poisoning. *Postgrad. Med. J.* **45**, 635–637.

Pasi, A., Embree, J. W., Eisenlord, G. H., and Hine, C. H. (1974). Assessment of the mutagenic properties of diquat and paraquat in the murine dominant lethal test. *Mutat. Res.* **26**, 171–175.

Petry, T. W., Wolfgang, G. H. I., Jolly, R. A., Ochoa, R., and Donarski, W. J. (1992). Antioxidant-dependant inhibition of diquat-induced toxicity *in vivo*. *Toxicology* **74**, 33–43.

Pirie, A., and Rees, J. R. (1970). Diquat cataract in the rat. *Exp. Eye Res.* **9**, 198–203.

Pirie, A., Rees, J. R., and Holmberg, N. J. (1970). Diquat cataract: Formation of the free radical and its reaction with constituents of the eye. *Exp. Eye Res.* **9**, 204–218.

Powell, D., Pond, S. M., Allen, T. B., and Portale, A. A. (1983). Hemoperfusion in a child who ingested diquat and died from pontine infarction and hemorrhage. *J. Toxicol. Clin. Toxicol.* **20**, 405–420.

Proudfoot, A. T., Stewart, M. S., Levitt, T., and Widdop, B. (1979). Paraquat poisoning: Significance of plasma-paraquat concentrations. *Lancet* **II**, 330–332.

Pushkar, M. S. (1969). Morphological changes in the organism under the effect of the herbicide reglone (diquat). *Vrach. Delo.* **9**, 92–96.

Rawlings, J. M., Foster, J. R., and Heylings, J. R. (1992). Diquat-induced intestinal secretion in the anaesthetised rat. *Human Exp. Toxicol.* **11**, 524–529.

Rawlings, J. M., Wyatt, I., and Heylings, J. R. (1994). Evidence for redox cycling of diquat in rat small intestine. *Biochem. Pharmacol.* **47**, 1271–1274.

Reif, D. W., Beales, I. L. P., Thomas, C. E., and Aust, S. D. (1988). Effect of diquat on the distribution of iron in rat liver. *Toxicol. Appl. Pharmacol.* **93**, 506–510.

Repine, J. E., Pfinninger, O. S., Talmage, D. W., Berger, E. M., and Pettijohn, D. E. (1981). Dimethyl sulphoxide prevents DNA nicking mediated by ionising radiation or iron/hydrogen peroxide-generated hydroxyl radical. *Proc. Natl. Acad. Sci. U.S.A.* **78**, 1001–1003.

Rikans, L. E., and Cai, Y. (1993). Diquat-induced oxidative damage in BCNU-pretreated hepatocytes of mature and old rats. *Toxicol. Appl. Pharmacol.* **118**, 263–270.

Ronnen, M., Klin, B., and Suster, S. (1995). Mixed diquat/paraquat-induced burns. *Int. J. Dermatol.* **34**, 23–25.

Rose, M. S., and Smith, L. L. (1977). The relevance of paraquat accumulation by tissues. *In* "Biochemical Mechanisms of Paraquat Toxicity" (A. P. Autor, ed.), pp. 71–91. Academic Press, San Diego.

Rose, M. S., Smith, L. L., and Wyatt, I. (1974a). Evidence for the energy-dependant accumulation of paraquat into rat lung. *Nature* **252**, 314–315.

Rose, M. S., Crabtree, H. C., Fletcher, K., and Wyatt, I. (1974b). Biochemical effects of diquat and paraquat: Disturbance of the control of corticosteroid synthesis in rat adrenal and subsequent effects in the control of liver glycogen utilisation. *Biochem. J.* **138**, 437–443.

Rose, M. S., Lock, E. A., Smith, L. L., and Wyatt, I. (1976a). Paraquat accumulation. Tissue and species specificity. *Biochem. Pharmacol.* **25**, 419–423.

Rose, M. S., Smith, L. L., and Wyatt, I. (1976b). The relevance of pentose phosphate pathway stimulation in rat lung to the mechanism of Paraquat toxicity. *Biochem. Pharmacol.* **25**, 1763–1767.

Samman, P. D., and Johnston, E. N. M. (1969). Nail damage associated with handling paraquat and diquat. *Br. Med. J.* **1**, 818–819.

Sandy, M. S., Moldeus, P., Ross, D., and Smith, M. T. (1986). Role of redox cycling and lipid-peroxidation in bipyridyl herbicide cytotoxicity—Studies with a compromised isolated hepatocyte model system. *Biochem. Pharmacol.* **35**, 3095–3101.

Sandy, M. S., Moldeus, P., Ross, D., and Smith, M. T. (1987). Cytotoxicity of the redox cycling compound diquat in isolated hepatocytes involvement of hydrogen peroxide and transition metals. *Arch. Biochem. Biophys.* **259**, 29–37.

Sawinsky, A., and Pasztor, G. (1977). Study of exposure to Reglone sprayed by aircraft. *Z. Gesamte. Hyg. Ihre. Grenzgeb.* **23**, 845–846.

Schönborn, H., Schuster, H. P., and Kössling, F. K. (1971). Clinical and morphologic findings in an acute oral intoxication with diquat (Reglone). *Arch. Toxicol.* **27**, 204–216.

Scott, R. C., and Corrigan, M. A. (1990). The *in vitro* percutaneous absorption of diquat a species comparison. *Toxicol. In Vitro* **4**, 137–141.

Sechi, G. P., Agnetti, V., Piredda, M., Canu, M., Deserra, F., Omar, H. A., and Rosati, G. (1992). Acute and persistent parkinsonism after use of diquat. *Neurology* **42**, 261–263.

Selypes, A., Nagymajtenyl, L., and Berencsi, G. (1980). Mutagenic and embryotoxic effects of paraquat and diquat. *Bull. Environ. Contam. Toxicol.* **25**, 513–517.

Sharp, C. W. M., Ottolenghi, A., and Posner, H. S. (1972). Correlation of paraquat toxicity with tissue concentration and weight loss of the rat *Toxicol. Appl. Pharmacol.* **22**, 241–251.

Siebert, D., and Lemperle, E. (1974). Genetic effects of herbicides: Induction of mitotic gene conversion in saccharomyces cerevisiae. *Mutat. Res.* **22**, 111–120.

Smith, C. V. (1987a). Effect of BCNU pretreatment on diquat-induced oxidant stress and hepatotoxicity. *Biochem. Biophys. Res. Commun.* **144**, 415–421.

Smith, C. V. (1987b). Evidence for participation of lipid-peroxidation and iron in diquat-induced hepatic-necrosis *in vivo*. *Mol. Pharmacol.* **32**, 417–422.

Smith, L. L., and Rose, M. S. (1977). A comparison of the effects of paraquat and diquat on the water content of rat lung and the incorporation of thymidine into lung DNA. *Toxicology* **8**, 223–230.

Smith, L. L., Wright, A., Wyatt, I., and Rose, M. S. (1974). Effective treatment for paraquat poisoning in rats and its relevance to the treatment of paraquat poisoning in man. *Br. Med. J.* **4**, 569–571.

Smith, C. V., Hughes, H., Lauterbu, B. H., and Mitchell, J. R. (1985). Oxidant stress and hepatic-necrosis in rats treated with diquat. *J. Pharmacol. Exp. Ther.* **235**, 172.

Spalding, D. J. M., Mitchell, J. R., Jaeschke, H., and Smith, C. V. (1989). Diquat hepatotoxicity in the Fischer 344 rat the role of covalent binding to tissue proteins and lipids. *Toxicol. Appl. Pharmacol.* **101**, 319–327.

Tanaka, R., and Amano, Y. (1989). Genotoxic effects of paraquat and diquat evaluated by sister chromatid exchange chromosomal aberration and cell cycle rate. *Toxicol. In Vitro* **3**, 53–57.

Thomas, C. E., and Aust, S. D. (1986). Reductive release of iron from ferritin by cation free radicals of paraquat and other bipyridyls. *J. Biol. Chem.* **261**, 13064–13070.

Tomita, M. (1991). Comparison of one-electron reduction activity against the bipyridylium herbicides, paraquat and diquat, in microsomal and mitochondrial fractions of liver, lung and kidney (*in vitro*). *Biochem. Pharmacol.* **42**, 303–309.

Vanholder, R., Colardyn, F., De Reuck, J., Praet, M., Lameire, N., and Ringoir, S. (1981). Diquat intoxication—Report of two cases and review of the literature. *Am. J. Med.* **70**, 1267–1271.

Verbetskii, V. E., and Stolyarchuk, A. A. (1967). Toxicological and pharmacological properties of herbicides which are bipyridine derivatives—Gramoxone and Reglone. *Vop. Gig. Toksikol. Pestits.* 164–168.

Verbetskii, V. E., and Pushkar, M. S. (1968). Pathological changes in the organs of animals on acute poisoning with the herbicide diquat (Reglone). *In* "Some Questions Concerning Human and Animal Morphology," pp. 51–52. Medizina, Odessa.

Vulimiri, S. V., Gupta, S., Smith, C. V., Moorthy, B., and Randerath, K. (1995). Rapid decrease in indigenous covalent DNA modifications (I-Compounds) of male Fischer-344 rat liver DNA by diquat treatment. *Chem.–Biol. Interact.* **95**, 1–16.

Wester, R. C., and Maibach, H. I. (1985). *In vivo* percutaneous absorption and decontamination of pesticides in humans. *J. Toxicol. Environ. Hlth.* **16**, 25–37.

Widdop, B. (1976). Detection of Paraquat in urine. *Br. Med. J.* **2**, 1135.

Williams, P. F., Jarvie, D. R., and Whitehead, A. P. (1986). Diquat intoxication: Treatment by charcoal haemoperfusion and description of a new method of diquat measurement in plasma. *J. Toxicol. Clin. Toxicol.* **24**, 11–20.

Witschi, H., Kacew, S., Hirai, K. I., and Cote, M. G. (1977). *In vivo* oxidation of reduced nicotinamide adenine dinucleotide phosphate by paraquat and diquat in rat lung. *Chem. Biol. Interact.* **19**, 143–160.

Wojeck, G. A., Price, J. F., Nigg, H. N., and Stamper, J. H. (1983). Worker exposure to paraquat and diquat. *Arch. Environ. Contam. Toxicol.* **12**, 65–70.

Wolfgang, G. H. I., Jolly, R. A., Donarski, W. J., and Petry, T. W. (1991). Inhibition of diquat induced lipid peroxidation and toxicity in precision cut rat liver slices by novel antioxidants. *Toxicol. Appl. Pharmacol.* **108**, 321–329.

Wood, T. E., Edgar, H., and Salcedo, J. (1976). Recovery from inhalation of diquat aerosol. *Chest* **70**, 774–775.

Woollen, B. H., and Mahler, J. D. (1987). An improved spot-test for the detection of paraquat and diquat in biological samples. *Clin. Chim. Acta* **167**, 225–229.

Yoshioka, T., Sugimoto, T., Kinoshita, N., Shimazu, T., Hiraide, A., and Kuwagata, Y. (1992). Effects of concentration reduction and partial replacement of paraquat by diquat on human toxicity. A clinical survey. *Human Exp. Toxicol.* **11**, 241–245.

Phenoxy Herbicides (2,4-D)

Elke Kennepohl and Ian C. Munro
Cantox Health Sciences International

72.1 INTRODUCTION

Phenoxy herbicides have been commercially available for over 50 years and are the most widely used family of herbicides worldwide. 2,4-Dichlorophenoxyacetic acid (2,4-D), the most common of the phenoxy herbicides, is one of the best-studied agricultural chemicals. This chapter focuses primarily on 2,4-D since it is the most widely used herbicide and the majority of the literature on phenoxy herbicides pertains to studies with 2,4-D.

The safety of using phenoxy herbicides was first questioned when a series of case-control studies was published by Lennart Hardell in the late 1970s, in which he hypothesized that the occurrence of three rare forms of cancer (Hodgkin's disease, soft tissue sarcoma, and non-Hodgkin's lymphoma) in workers was related to exposure to these herbicides along with dioxins known to contaminate 2,4,5-trichlorophenoxyacetic acid (2,4,5-T). Since that time, several human and animal studies have been conducted which do not lend support to his hypothesis. As well, several expert panels have been convened to assess the safety of 2,4-D, and all have concluded that there is no evidence to suggest that 2,4-D poses any risk to human health under its intended conditions of use. In fact, 2,4-D has been classified by the U.S. Environmental Protection Agency (EPA) as a Group D (not classifiable as to human carcinogenicity) because "the evidence is inadequate and cannot be interpreted as showing either the presence or absence of a carcinogenic effect."

Because of the vast amount of data available on 2,4-D, this chapter provides a brief summary and overview of the available studies.

72.2 PHYSICAL AND CHEMICAL PROPERTIES

Several phenoxy acids have been used as herbicides, including 2,4,5-T, 4-(2,4-dichlorophenoxy) butyric acid (2,4-DB), 2-(2,4-dichlorophenoxy propionic acid) (dichlorprop), 2-(2-methyl-4-chlorophenoxy) propionic acid (MCPP or mecoprop), 2-methyl-4-chlorophenoxyacetic acid (MCPA), and 2-(2,4,5-trichlorophenoxy) propionic acid (Silvex), with the most commonly and widely used herbicide being 2,4-D. 2,4,5-T and Silvex are no longer manufactured or sold. Figure 72.1 shows the chemical structures of the phenoxy acids.

72.2.1 2,4-D ACID, SALTS, AND ESTERS

The basic form of 2,4-D is the acid, but 2,4-D is often formulated as an inorganic salt, amine, or ester through various manufacturing processes, and is used in many commercial products.

CAS number:	94-75-7
Chemical name:	2,4-dichlorophenoxyacetic acid
Trade names:	Agrotect, Amidox, Amoxone, Aqua-Kleen, Brush-Rhap, Chloroxone, Crop Rider, Crotilin, Dacamine, Dacamine, Ded-weed LV-69, Dicopur, Dinoxol, DMA-4, Dormone, Emulsamine BK, Envert 171, Esteron, Esteron 99C, Estone, Farmco, Fernesta, Fernimine, Fernoxone, Ferxone, Foredex 75, Formula 40, Hedonal, Hebidal, Ipaner, Krotiline, Lawn-Keep, Macrondray, Miracle, Monosan, Moxone, Netagrone, Pennamine, Phenox, Pielik, Planotox, Plantgard, Rhodia, Salvo, Transamine, Tributon, Trinoxol, Vergemaster, Vidon 638, Visko-Rhap, Weed-Ag-Bar, Weedar-64, Weedatul, Weed-B-Gon, Weedez Wonder Bar, Weedone LV4, Weed-Rhap, Weed Tox, Weedtrol
Appearance:	white powder
Empirical formula:	$C_8H_6Cl_2O_3$
Molecular weight:	221.04
Melting point:	140.5°C
Boiling point:	130°C at 1 mm Hg (isopropyl ester)
Water solubility:	900 mg/liter at 25°C (acid)
Vapor pressure:	0.02 mPa at 25°C (acid)
Partition coefficient:	2.81

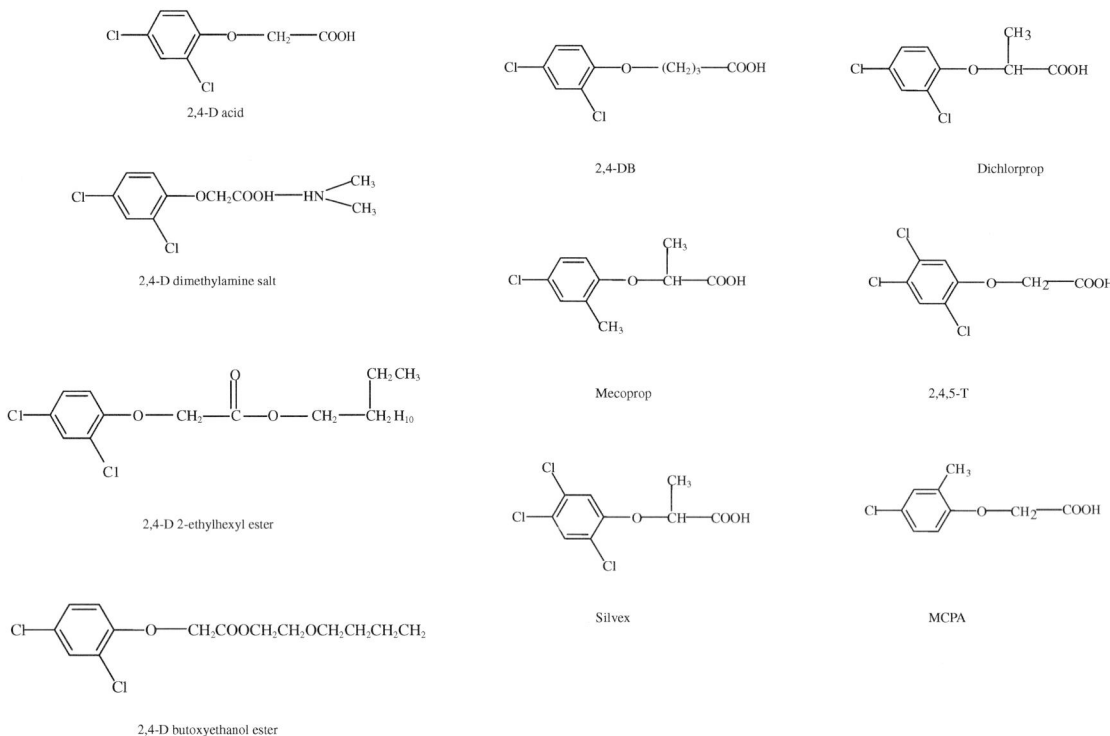

Figure 72.1 Chemical structures of phenoxy acid herbicides.

72.2.2 2,4,5-T

CAS number:	93-76-5
Chemical name:	2,4,5-trichlorophenoxyacetic acid
Trade names:	no longer manufactured or sold
Appearance:	white crystals
Empirical formula:	$C_8H_5Cl_3O_3$
Molecular weight:	255.49
Melting point:	156.6°C (pure acid); 150–151°C (technical acid)
Boiling point:	decomposes
Water solubility:	278 mg/liter at 25°C (acid)
Vapor pressure:	0.022 mm Hg at 25°C

72.2.3 2,4-DB

CAS number:	94-82-6
Chemical name:	4-(2,4-dichlorophenoxy) butyric acid
Trade names:	Butoxone, Butyrac, Butirex, Embutone, Embutox, Legumex, Venceweed
Appearance:	colorless to white crystals
Empirical formula:	$C_{10}H_{10}Cl_2O_3$
Molecular weight:	249.10
Melting point:	117–119°C
Water solubility:	46 mg/liter at 25°C
Vapor pressure:	negligible (acid and salts)

72.2.4 DICHLORPROP (2,4-DP)

CAS number:	120-36-5
Chemical name:	2-(2,4-dichlorophenoxy) propionic acid
Trade names:	Cornox, Hedonal, Weedone, Estaprop
Appearance:	colorless crystals
Empirical formula:	$C_9H_8Cl_2O_3$
Molecular weight:	235.07
Melting point:	117–118°C
Water solubility:	350 mg/liter at 20°C

72.2.5 MECOPROP (MCPP)

CAS number:	7085-19-0
Chemical name:	2-(4-chloro-2-methylphenoxy) propionic acid
Trade names:	Kilprop, Mecopar, Triester-II, MecAmine-D, Triamine-II, Triplet, TriPower, Trimec, Trimec-Encore, U46 KV Fluid
Appearance:	white to light brown crystalline solid
Empirical formula:	$C_{10}H_{11}ClO_3$
Molecular weight:	214.65
Melting point:	93–95°C
Water solubility:	very soluble at 25°C
Vapor pressure:	0.31 mPa at 20°C
Partition coefficient:	1.26 at pH 7

72.2.6 MCPA

CAS number:	94-74-6
Chemical name:	2-methyl-4-chlorophenoxyacetic acid
Trade names:	Agritox, Agroxone, Agrozone, Agsco MXL, Banlene, Blesal MC, Bordermaster, Cambilene, Cheyenne, Chimac Oxy, Chiptox, Class MCPA, Cornox Plus, Dakota, Ded-Weed, Empal, Envoy, Legumex, Malerbane, Mayclene, Mephanac, Midox, Phenoxylene, Rhomene, Rhonox, Sanaphen-M, Shamrox, Selectyl, Tiller, Vacate, Weed-Rhap, Zhelan
Appearance:	colorless crystals
Empirical formula:	$C_9H_9ClO_3$
Molecular weight:	200.62
Melting point:	118–119°C
Water solubility:	825 mg/liter at 25°C (acid)
Vapor pressure:	0.2 mPa at 20°C

72.2.7 SILVEX

CAS number:	93-72-1
Chemical name:	2-(2,4,5-trichlorophenoxy) propionic acid
Trade names:	no longer manufactured or sold
Appearance:	white powder
Empirical formula:	$C_9H_7Cl_3O_3$
Molecular weight:	269.51
Melting point:	181.6°C
Water solubility:	200 mg/liter at 25°C

72.3 HISTORY OF USE

For over 50 years, 2,4-D has been the most commonly and widely used herbicide throughout the world. When applied to plants, 2,4-D is absorbed through the roots and leaves within 4 to 6 hours and is distributed in the plant via the phloem (WHO, 1984). Once absorbed, 2,4-D selectively eliminates broadleaf plants (due to their larger leaf area and hence, greater absorption) by mimicking the effect of auxins (i.e., plant growth-regulating hormones) and stimulating growth, rejuvenating old cells, and overstimulating young cells, leading to an abnormal growth pattern and death in some plants (Mullison, 1987). In addition, 2,4-D affects plant metabolism, which leads to interference with food transport (Mullison, 1987).

2,4-D is primarily used as a herbicide in agriculture, forestry, and lawn care practices, with the majority (>60%) of the total usage in the United States being reported for use as weed control in agriculture (i.e., corn and small grains) (EPA, 1997). 2,4-D is reported to be effective against dandelion, plantain, chickweed, henbit, white clover, heal-all, red sorrel, curly dock, chicory, yellow rocket, speedwell, ground ivy, spurge, oxalis, knotweed, purslane, thistle, wild violet, wild onion, wild garlic, lespedeza, yellow nutsedge, crabgrass, sumac, willow, sagebrush, ragweed, Eurasian water milfoil, and water hyacinth (Lefton *et al.*, 1991; Mullison, 1987; WHO, 1975). To a lesser extent, 2,4-D is used as a growth regulator on various crops ranging from potatoes to citrus fruits (WHO, 1975, 1984).

In the past, 2,4-D was combined with 2,4,5-trichlorophenoxyacetic acid (2,4,5-T) for brush and weed control. Over 10 million gallons of a special concentrated mixture called Agent Orange were applied in the Vietnam War to defoliate trees (Wolfe, 1983).

72.4 FORMULATIONS

2,4-D is formulated into end-use products to facilitate application. Water-soluble salts and amines are usually prepared as aqueous solutions with small amounts of additives such as water conditioners and antifoam agents. The oil-soluble esters are often formulated with petroleum solvents (e.g., kerosene or naphtha) plus emulsifiers. Such formulations are then diluted with relatively large amounts of water to make the final herbicide spray mixture. Several forms of 2,4-D can be combined with dry fertilizer ingredients to form lawn "weed and feed" products.

In the past, concerns arose regarding possible contamination of 2,4-D formulations with dioxins, notably the polychlorinated dibenzo-*p*-dioxins (PCDDs) and more specifically 2,3,7,8-tetrachlorodibenzo-*p*-dioxin (T_4CDD), and nitrosamines. 2,4-D formulations have been reported to contain 2,3,7,8-T_4CDD but only when 2,4,5-T was present (Cochrane *et al.*, 1981, 1982a, 1982b; Woolson *et al.*, 1972). 2,4-D formulations currently sold in the United States contain very few PCDD contaminants. In fact, analytical studies of the more recent formulations have repeatedly shown dioxin levels to be below the limit of quantitation set by the U.S. Environmental Protection Agency (Berry, 1989; Cramer, 1996). In Canada, a limit of 10 ppb per isomer PCDD (nondetectable for 2,3,7,8-T_4CDD at 1 ppb) in 2,4-D formulations has been set (Agriculture Canada, 1983). In an older analysis of 200 samples of various forms of 2,4-D (Cochrane *et al.*, 1981, 1982a, 1982b), all but a few samples tested below the 10-ppb limit.

In the past, there was some possible contamination with nitrosamines formed from nitrates used in preserving metal storage containers; however, plastic or epoxy-lining has replaced the metal used for storage containers and nitrosamine formation no longer presents a concern.

72.5 HUMAN EXPOSURE TO 2,4-D

2,4-D is one of the most commonly used herbicides both domestically and commercially, and exposure to it can occur via inhalation, ingestion, and dermal contact. Respiratory exposure to 2,4-D is less than 2% of total exposure (Grover *et al.*, 1986), and residual levels in foodstuffs or drinking water are essentially nondetectable or only detected in trace amounts (Duggan and Corneliussen, 1972; Duggan and Lipscomb, 1969; Gartrell *et al.*, 1985). By far, dermal contact during use of the product accounts for the greatest potential for exposure, with estimates that approximately 90% of total exposure occurs through dermal exposure (Feldman and Maibach, 1974). Since 2,4-D use is typically seasonal and short-term, the duration of exposure is considered repeated subchronic.

In a 1992 review of 2,4-D, Munro *et al.* (1992) summarized exposures to 2,4-D in a variety of occupational and home-use settings. Based on several epidemiological studies, the highest exposures were obtained in occupational settings, with reported average estimated internal doses ranging from 0.01 to 40 µg/kg body weight/day for forestry workers, and 0.35 to 6.3 µg/kg body weight/day for commercial applicators and farmers (Frank *et al.*, 1985; Grover *et al.*, 1986; Lavy and Mattice, 1984; Lavy *et al.*, 1987; Yeary, 1986). Average estimated internal doses reported to be reached by bystanders or home and garden users were below 0.2 µg/kg body weight/day (Harris *et al.*, 1992; Lavy and Mattice, 1984). Most of the past epidemiological studies do not reflect the growing trend toward using protective apparel when applying herbicides. With an increased awareness of worker safety and the new proposed labeling directions, workers are required to wear protective clothing consisting of eye protection, chemical-resistant gloves, long-sleeved shirt, long pants, socks, and shoes. In addition, following use of 2,4-D, it is recommended that workers thoroughly wash their hands, face, and arms with soap and water and wash any contaminated clothing separately.

72.6 TOXICOLOGICAL STUDIES

72.6.1 ABSORPTION

2,4-D is rapidly absorbed through the gastrointestinal tract following oral exposure, with peak plasma levels being reached in as little as 10 minutes or up to 24 hours depending on the dose and chemical form of 2,4-D (Erne, 1966a; Khanna and Fang, 1966; Knopp and Schiller, 1992; Kohli *et al.*, 1974; Pelletier *et al.*, 1989; Sauerhoff *et al.*, 1977). The rate of absorption is related to dose, with absorption occurring more rapidly at lower doses (i.e., 0.4 mg/kg body weight/day) than at higher doses (i.e., 1 mg/kg body weight/day) (Pelletier *et al.*, 1989). Absorption of 2,4-D esters has been reported to occur more slowly than for acid or salt forms (Erne, 1966a); however, the excretion rates for the various forms are reported to be similar (Khanna and Fang, 1966; Knopp and Schiller, 1992; Pelletier *et al.*, 1989).

Dermal contact is the major route of exposure to 2,4-D. In occupationally exposed humans, dermal absorption was reported to occur rapidly based on the detection of 2,4-D in urine within 4 hours (Feldman and Maibach, 1974), and although the percentage absorbed is variable, it is usually less than 6 % (EPA,

1996; Feldman and Maibach, 1974; Harris and Solomon, 1992). Studies in rats and monkeys showed these percentages to be highly variable and dependent on chemical form, vehicle, and animal species (Grisson *et al.*, 1987; Knopp and Schiller, 1992; Moody *et al.*, 1990, 1991; Pelletier *et al.*, 1989, 1990).

Although no controlled studies have been conducted to assess the absorption rate via inhalation exposure, epidemiological studies of occupationally exposed workers indicate that absorption is rapid by both dermal and inhalation routes (Frank *et al.*, 1985; Kolmodin-Hedman and Erne, 1980).

72.6.2 DISTRIBUTION

2,4-D is highly water soluble and therefore is widely distributed, but does not accumulate, in the body. It also does not readily cross lipid membranes, and at physiological pH, it exists predominately in the ionized form. 2,4-D uses active transport systems to enter tissues and cross the blood/brain barrier (Kim and O'Tuama, 1981; Pritchard, 1980). Another factor which contributes to the extent of tissue distribution of 2,4-D is its ability to bind to serum proteins (Erne, 1966a; Fang and Lindstrom, 1980; Orberg, 1980).

Peak tissue levels in rats have been reported anywhere from 10 minutes to 8 hours depending on the dose administered (0.4 to 240 mg/kg body weight) (Khanna and Fang, 1966; Pelletier *et al.*, 1989). Following exposure, 2,4-D has been detected in liver, kidney, and lung of a variety of animal species (Clark *et al.*, 1975; Erne, 1966a). Levels in brain were reported to account for only a very small percentage of the exposure dose (Erne, 1966a; Tyynela *et al.*, 1990); however, at levels of intoxication (i.e., 300 mg/kg body weight, which is well above the level of renal saturation), levels in brain and cerebrospinal fluid of rats were increased relative to plasma levels (Elo and Ylitalo, 1977, 1979; Tyynela *et al.*, 1990). At these high dose levels, the organic acid transport system responsible for the efflux of 2,4-D out of the brain is inhibited (Kim *et al.*, 1983; Pritchard, 1980; Tyynela *et al.*, 1990; Ylitalo *et al.*, 1990). In addition, vascular damage has been reported in rats administered extremely high doses of 2,4-D (i.e., more than 300 mg/kg body weight) (Elo *et al.*, 1988), which may facilitate an increased influx of 2,4-D through the compromised blood/brain barrier (Elo *et al.*, 1988; Hervonen *et al.*, 1982; Tyynela *et al.*, 1990). Saturation of plasma protein binding also may contribute slightly to the increased brain:blood ratio of 2,4-D reported in rats at these exposure levels (Tyynela *et al.*, 1990; Ylitalo *et al.*, 1990).

2,4-D also has been reported to pass the placental barrier in mice, rats, and pigs, and has been detected in the uterus, placenta, fetus, and intrauterine fluid of exposed animals (Erne, 1966a; Fedorova and Belova, 1974; Lindquist and Ullberg, 1971) but was rapidly eliminated (Lindquist and Ullberg, 1971).

72.6.3 PHARMACOKINETICS

Depending on the chemical form of 2,4-D and the animal species tested, plasma half-lives following oral exposure of

100 mg/kg body weight range from 3.5 to 12 hours (Erne, 1966a). Lower doses (i.e., 3 mg/kg body weight) in rats showed half-lives of 0.5 to 0.8 hours (Khanna and Fang, 1966), indicating that clearance rates are highly dependent on dose. In human studies, plasma clearance of orally administered 2,4-D was found to follow first-order kinetics with urinary excretion half-lives ranging from 10.2 to 28.4 hours (Sauerhoff *et al.*, 1977), which is consistent with the findings (urinary excretion half-life = 18 hours) from a forestry worker who exhibited the highest amount of 2,4-D excretion among two groups exposed over a period of 11 or 18 days (Frank *et al.*, 1985).

The pharmacokinetics of 2,4-D following dermal absorption is apparently different from that following the oral route (Pelletier *et al.*, 1989). Plasma levels tend to reach a plateau and decline more rapidly following oral exposure. In addition, plasma clearance has been reported to follow biphasic kinetics beginning 8 hours post-dosing, with half-lives for various tissues ranging from 0.6 to 2.3 hours for the first phase and 25.7 to 29 hours for the second phase. Furthermore, cumulative urinary excretion of 2,4-D increases more slowly following dermal rather than oral exposure.

72.6.4 METABOLISM

Once absorbed into body fluids and tissues, the salts and esters of 2,4-D undergo acid and/or enzymatic hydrolyzation to form 2,4-D acid. In laboratory animals and humans following oral exposures, the presence of acid-hydrolyzable conjugates has been reported at 0 to 27% of the administered 2,4-D (Erne, 1966b; Grunow and Bohme, 1974; Kohli *et al.*, 1974; Sauerhoff *et al.*, 1977). The available data indicate that 2,4-D is not metabolized to reactive intermediates and is excreted predominately as the parent compound.

72.6.5 EXCRETION

Regardless of the route of exposure, 2,4-D is predominately excreted in the urine (Erne, 1966a; Feldman and Maibach, 1974; Khanna and Fang, 1966; Knopp and Schiller, 1992; Moody *et al.*, 1990, 1991; Pelletier *et al.*, 1989). The rate of urinary excretion is inversely proportional to dose. For example, at oral doses of 3 to 30 mg/kg body weight given to rats, 93 to 96%

of the dose was excreted within 48 hours, whereas at higher doses (i.e., ≥ 60 mg/kg body weight) the percentage of dose excreted within 24 hours decreased linearly with increasing dose (Khanna and Fang, 1966). In rats, $\geq 90\%$ of oral doses of 30 mg/kg body weight or less were excreted in the urine within 24 hours (Khanna and Fang, 1966; Knopp and Schiller, 1992; Pelletier *et al.*, 1989). Similarly, in humans administered an oral dose of 5 mg 2,4-D/kg body weight, 77% of the dose was excreted within 96 hours (Kohli *et al.*, 1974) and 87 to 100% of the dose was excreted in the urine over 6 days (Sauerhoff *et al.*, 1977). 2,4-D is predominately excreted by the kidney using an active transport system. Saturation of renal clearance appears to occur at 50 to 60 mg/kg body weight (Gorzinski *et al.*, 1987; Khanna and Fang, 1966) based on kidney concentrations and urinary excretion rates.

Another significant route of excretion in occupationally exposed workers is perspiration (Sell *et al.*, 1982). Following a 2-hour exposure, 2,4-D was detected in T-shirt extracts (i.e., measure of perspiration) for 2 weeks and in urine for 5 days. 2,4-D also has been reported to be excreted in the milk of lactating rats exposed to 2,4-D (Fedorova and Belova, 1974).

72.6.6 ANIMAL STUDIES

72.6.6.1 Acute Toxicity

Numerous acute toxicological tests have been conducted on the various forms of 2,4-D as summarized in Table 72.1. Overall, oral exposure to 2,4-D shows moderate to low toxicity, whereas dermal and inhalation toxicity are low. Dermal irritation in rabbits was considered slight for the acid form of 2,4-D and minimal for the salt and ester forms. Reported eye irritation in rabbits, on the other hand, is severe for the acid and salt forms, but minimal for the ester.

72.6.6.2 Subchronic Toxicity

Further to the acute toxicity data, numerous subchronic studies have been conducted on a variety of 2,4-D forms, by different exposure routes, and in various animal species. The subchronic studies conducted range from 3-week dermal studies in rabbits to 13-week dietary studies in dogs and rodents. The results of these studies are summarized in Table 72.2. Overall, at doses

Table 72.1
Acute Toxicity[a] Involving Various Chemical Forms of 2,4-D

Form of 2,4-D	Oral LD$_{50}$ (mg/kg bw/d)					Dermal LD$_{50}$ (mg/kg bw/d)		Inhalation LD$_{50}$ (mg/liter)
	Rat	Mouse	Dog	Guinea pig	Chicken	Rat	Rabbit	Rat
Acid	639–980	312–434	25–250	397–553	358–817	na	1400–>2000	1.79
Salt	863–>2000	na	na	na	na	>2000	>2000	>3.8
Ester	440–982	na	na	na	na	na	1829–>2000	>4.6

bw = body weight.
na = not available.
[a]Condensed from Munro *et al.* (1992).

Table 72.2
Summary[a] of Subchronic Studies on 2,4-D Tested in Various Animal Species

Chemical species	Route	Dose (mg/kg bw/d) [in acid equivalents]	NOAEL[b] (mg/kg bw/d)	Reference
13-week: Rat				
2,4-D (100% pure)	diet	0, 15, 60, 100, 150	15 (females only)	Gorzinski *et al.* (1981a)
2,4-D (97.5% pure)	diet	0, 15, 60, 100, 150	15 (females only)	Gorzinski *et al.* (1981b)
2,4-D (97.5% pure)	diet	0, 1, 5, 15, 45	1 (males only)	Serota (1983a)
2,4-D (96.1% pure)	diet	0, 1, 15, 100, 300	15	Charles *et al.* (1996b)
2,4-D ethylhexyl ester	diet	0, 1, 15, 100, 300	15	Charles *et al.* (1996b)
2,4-D dimethylamine salt	diet	0, 1, 15, 100, 300	15	Charles *et al.* (1996b)
2,4-D butoxyethyl ester	diet	0, 1, 15, 100, 300	15	Szabo and Rachunek (1991)
2,4-D triisopropanolamine salt	diet	0, 1, 15, 100, 300	15	Yano *et al.* (1991b)
2,4-D isopropylamine salt	diet	0, 1, 15, 100, 300	15	Yano *et al.* (1991a)
12-week: Rat				
2,4-D sodium salt	intraperitoneal	0, 100, 150	—	Lukowicz-Ratajczak and Krechniak (1988)
13-week: Mouse				
2,4-D acid	diet	0, 5, 15, 45, 90	—	Serota (1983b)
2,4-D acid	diet	0, 1, 15, 100, 300	15	Schulze (1991)
14-day: Mouse				
2,4-D acid	oral intubation	50, 100, 200	—	Kuntz *et al.* (1990)
4-day: Mouse				
2,4-D acid	diet	100	—	Lundgren *et al.* (1987)
13-week: Dog				
2,4-D acid	gelatin capsule	0, 0.3, 1, 3, 10	1	ITF (1990)
2,4-D acid	diet	0, 0.5, 1.0, 3.75, 7.5	1	Charles *et al.* (1996c)
2,4-D dimethylamine salt	diet	0, 1.0, 3.75, 7.5	1	Charles *et al.* (1996c)
2,4-D 2-ethylhexyl ester	diet	0, 1.0, 3.75, 7.5	1	Charles *et al.* (1996c)
21-day: Rabbit				
2,4-D acid	dermal	0, 10, 100, 1000	1000	Schulze (1990a)
2,4-D dimethylamine salt	dermal	0, 10, 100, 300	10	Schulze (1990b)
2,4-D 2-ethylhexyl ester	dermal	0, 10, 100, 1000	10	Schulze (1990c)
2,4-D triisopropanolamine salt	dermal	0, 55, 193, 553	553	Mizell *et al.* (1990b)
2,4-D isopropylamine salt	dermal	0, 39, 98, 275	275	Mizell *et al.* (1990a)
2,4-D butoxyethyl ester	dermal	0, 32, 96, 321	321	Mizell *et al.* (1989)

[a] Adapted from Munro *et al.* (1992).
[b] NOAEL = no-observed-adverse-effect level.

above the threshold of saturation for renal clearance, the key target organs in rats appear to be primarily the kidney and, to some extent, the thyroid. The changes reported in the rat kidney were the loss of epithelial cells in the proximal tubule brush border; the changes in the thyroid were follicular cell hypertrophy in association with a reduction in serum thyroxine levels. These changes were consistent over all forms of 2,4-D tested, with a reported no-observed-adverse-effect level (NOAEL) of 15 mg/kg body weight/day (Charles *et al.*, 1996b; Szabo and Rachunek, 1991; Yano *et al.*, 1991a, 1991b). Some of these findings were reported at lower doses in older rat studies us-

ing the acid form of 2,4-D (Gorzinski *et al.*, 1981a, 1981b); however, the histological effects were not statistically significant at 15 mg/kg body weight/day, which is consistent with the more recent studies. In another older study (Serota, 1983a), other minor histological effects in the kidney were reported in male rats at 5 mg/kg body weight/day and in female rats at 1 mg/kg body weight/day. These effects were not reported in any other of the subchronic studies. Although some thyroid changes have been reported at 15 mg/kg body weight/day in rats (Serota, 1983a), these changes were considered incidental and do not affect the conclusion that the subchronic NOAEL for 2,4-D is 15 mg/kg body weight/day (Munro *et al.*, 1992). Similar results with respect to the kidney have been reported in 13-week dietary mouse studies (Serota, 1983b; Schulze, 1991). In a 13-week dog study in which 2,4-D was administered by gelatin capsules, kidney effects consisting of reduced cytoplasmic eosinophilia of the epithelial cells lining some convoluted tubules were reported at lower doses, resulting in a NOAEL of 1 mg/kg body weight/day (ITF, 1990). Thyroid changes were not reported in the mouse or dog.

72.6.6.3 Reproductive and Developmental Toxicity

Several multigenerational and developmental animal studies have been conducted to assess the potential of 2,4-D to affect reproduction and the developing fetus, and are summarized in Table 72.3. In general, the results of the available studies indicate that 2,4-D is not teratogenic and does not affect reproduction except at maternally toxic doses or those saturating the threshold for renal clearance (i.e., ≥ 50 mg/kg body weight/day). At doses above the maximum tolerated dose (MTD), some developmental effects have been reported in test animals (i.e., decreased fetal weight gain, increased incidence of lumbar ribs and wavy ribs, and delayed ossification of bone). The only teratogenic effect (i.e., cleft palate) reported was in mice, but occurred only at maternally toxic doses.

The potential testicular and ovarian toxicity of 2,4-D has been extensively evaluated in a recent series of subchronic and chronic studies in rats. In rats fed 0, 1, 15, 100, or 300 mg/kg body weight/day of either 2,4-D acid, 2,4-D dimethylamine salt, or 2,4-D 2-ethylhexyl ester for 90 days, only minimal effects were noted in testes at the top dose of 300 mg/kg body weight/day (Charles *et al.*, 1996b). These effects, consisting of decreased testes/body weight ratios accompanied by slight histological evidence of atrophy, occurred only at a dose which exceeded the MTD. The NOAEL for testicular effects was 100 mg/kg body weight/day, while the overall NOAEL for the subchronic studies was 15 mg/kg body weight/day based primarily on minor effects in the kidney. No 2,4-D–induced toxicity was reported in the ovaries at any dose. In a subsequent chronic toxicity/oncogenicity study conducted in rats with 2,4-D acid at doses of 0, 5, 75, or 150 mg/kg body weight/day, no treatment-related effects were reported in testes or ovaries at any dose level (Charles *et al.*, 1996a). The findings from these studies were consistent with observations from a series of earlier 90-day (Gorzinski *et al.*, 1987; Serota, 1983a, b; Serrone *et al.*, 1991; Szabo and Rachunek, 1991; Yano *et al.*, 1991a, 1991b) and chronic studies (Charles *et al.*, 1996a; Serota, 1986) conducted with 2,4-D acid and a variety of salt and ester derivatives.

The testicular and ovarian toxicity of 2,4-D acid and its dimethylamine salt and 2-ethylhexyl ester also have been examined in a recent series of subchronic and chronic studies in beagle dogs. Dogs administered either 0, 1, 3.75, or 7.5 mg/kg body weight/day of 2,4-D acid, 2,4-D dimethylamine salt, or 2,4-D 2-ethylhexyl ester for 13 weeks exhibited decreased testes weights at the two highest dose levels (Charles *et al.*,

1996c). The toxicological significance of these findings is uncertain since the organ weight changes were not accompanied by any corroborative histological changes. In addition, both of the two high-dose group animals exhibited body weight gain depressions of approximately 30 to 85%. No 2,4-D–induced effects were seen in ovaries. A NOAEL of 1.0 mg/kg body weight/day was established from these studies based on effects in the kidneys. In a follow-up 1-year chronic study conducted at dietary doses of 0, 1, 5, or 7.5 mg/kg body weight/day of 2,4-D acid, no testes or ovary alterations were reported (Charles *et al.*, 1996c). The findings from these dog studies were consistent with earlier 13-week (ITF, 1990) and 2-year dog studies (Hansen *et al.*, 1971). The general lack of 2,4-D–associated testicular toxicity is entirely consistent with the failure of 2,4-D to induce changes in reproductive performance.

72.6.6.4 Immunotoxicity

Several subchronic and chronic toxicity studies have provided no evidence from hematological, clinical chemistry, or histopathologic evaluations that 2,4-D is likely to induce immune system dysfunction (Charles *et al.*, 1996a, 1996b, 1996c; Szabo and Rachunek, 1991; Yano *et al.*, 1991a, 1991b). Studies that were conducted specifically to examine the possible impact of 2,4-D on various immune system functional parameters have not provided definitive results (Blakley, 1986; Blakley and Blakley, 1986; Blakley and Schiefer, 1986; Zhamsaranova *et al.*, 1987). These studies are difficult to interpret in that the results (1) were inconsistent when evaluated by different routes of exposure, or by comparison of findings from acute and subchronic test regimes; (2) often not reproducible; and (3) not accompanied by adequate descriptions of the normal range of immune parameter values in the test animal populations (Munro *et al.*, 1992). Dermal exposure to 2,4-D acid, salts, or esters also has not been associated with delayed contact hypersensitivity in guinea pigs (Carreon *et al.*, 1983; Carreon and Rao, 1985; Gargus, 1986; Jeffrey, 1986; Jeffrey and Rao, 1986; Schultz *et al.*, 1990).

72.6.6.5 Neurotoxicity

Overall, it may be concluded that 2,4-D has little, if any, potential to induce adverse effects in the nervous system at doses that do not cause overt systemic toxicity or that do not saturate processes involved with tissue clearance and renal excretion. No lesions or overt clinical signs of central nervous system toxicity were observed in any of the subchronic toxicity studies in rats (Charles *et al.*, 1996b; Szabo and Rachunek, 1991; Yano *et al.*, 1991a, 1991b) or mice (Schulze, 1991), at doses up to 300 to 560 mg/kg body weight/day.

In a chronic rat study designed specifically to investigate the impact of 2,4-D on the nervous system, several neurological parameters were assessed, of which only forelimb grip strength was altered, to a minimal degree, at the highest dose tested, 150 mg/kg body weight/day (Jeffries *et al.*, 1994). Other animal studies have yielded electromyogram results considered indicative of skeletal muscle myotonia following administration of

Table 72.3
Summary of Developmental and Reproductive Toxicity Studies on 2,4-D Tested in Various Animal Species

Chemical species	Route	Exposure duration	Dose (mg/kg bw/d)	NOAEL[a] (mg/kg bw/d)	Reference
Developmental: Rabbit					
2,4-D triisopropanolamine salt	gavage	GD[b] 7–19	0, 10, 30, or 75[c]	10[d]; 75[e]	Liberacki *et al.* (1994), Charles *et al.* (1996a)
2,4-D isopropylamine salt	gavage	GD 7–19	0, 10, 30, or 75[c]	10[d]; 75[e]	Liberacki *et al.* (1994), Charles *et al.* (1996a)
2,4-D butoxyethyl ester	gavage	GD 7–19	0, 10, 30, or 75[c]	10[d]; 75[e]	Liberacki *et al.* (1994), Charles *et al.* (1996a)
2,4-D acid	gavage	GD 6–18	0, 10, 30, or 90	30[d]; 90[e]	Hoberman (1990), Charles *et al.* (1996a)
2,4-D dimethylamine salt	gavage	GD 6–18	0, 10, 30, or 90[c]	30[d]; 90[e]	Martin (1991), Charles *et al.* (1996a)
2,4-D ethylhexyl ester	gavage	GD 6–18	0, 10, 30, or 75[c]	30[d]; 75[e]	Martin (1992a), Charles *et al.* (1996a)
2,4-D diethanolamine	gavage	GD 6–19	0, 10.2, 20.3, or 40.6[c]	10.2[d]; 40.6[e]	
Developmental: Rat					
2,4-D isooctyl ester	oral	GD 6–15	0, 12.5, 25, 50, 75, or 87.5[c]	87.5[d]; 25[e]	Schwetz *et al.* (1971)
2,4-D propylene glycol butyl ether	oral	GD 6–15	0, 12.5, 25, 50, 75, or 87.5[c]	87.5[d]; 25[e]	Schwetz *et al.* (1971)
2,4-D acid	oral	GD 6–15	0, 12.5, 25, 50, 75, or 87.5	87.5[d]; 25[e]	Schwetz *et al.* (1971)
2,4-D isooctyl ester	oral	GD 5–8	0, or 87.5[c]	87.5[d,e]	Schwetz *et al.* (1971)
2,4-D propylene glycol butyl ether	oral	GD 5–8	0, or 87.5[c]	87.5[d,e]	Schwetz *et al.* (1971)
2,4-D isooctyl ester	oral	GD 8–11	0, 50, or 87.5[c]	87.5[d]; <50[e]	Schwetz *et al.* (1971)
2,4-D isooctyl ester	oral	GD 12–15	0, 50, or 87.5[c]	87.5[d,e]	Schwetz *et al.* (1971)
2,4-D isooctyl ester	oral	GD 6–15	0, 50, or 150	150[d]; 50[e]	Khera and McKinley (1972)
2,4-D butyl ester	oral	GD 6–15	0, 50, or 150	150[d]; 50[e]	Khera and McKinley (1972)
2,4-D butoxyethynol	oral	GD 6–15	0, 50, or 150	150[d]; 50[e]	Khera and McKinley (1972)
2,4-D dimethylamine salt (49.5%)	oral	GD 6–15	0, 100, or 300	300[d]; 50[e]	Khera and McKinley (1972)
2,4-D acid	oral	GD 6–15	0, 50, or 100	100[d]; 50[e]	Khera and McKinley (1972)
2,4-D acid	oral	GD 6–15	0, 25, 50, or 100	100[d]; 50[e]	Khera and McKinley (1972)
2,4-D acid	oral	GD 6–15	0, 25, 50, 100, or 150	150[d]; 50[e]	Khera and McKinley (1972)
2,4-D propylene glycol butyl ether	oral	GD 6–15	0, 6.25, 12.5, 25, or 87.5[c]	87.5[d]; 25[e]	Unger *et al.* (1981)
2,4-D isooctyl ester	oral	GD 6–15	0, 6.25, 12.5, 25, or 87.5[c]	87.5[d]; 25[e]	Unger *et al.* (1981)
2,4-D acid	gavage	GD 6–15	0, or 115	<115[d,e]	Chernoff *et al.* (1990)
2,4-D ethylhexyl ester	gavage	GD 6–15	0, 10, 30, or 90[c]	10[d], 30[e]	Martin (1992b), Charles *et al.* (1996a)
2,4-D dimethylamine salt	gavage	GD 6–15	0, 12.5, 50, or 100[c]	12.5[d]; 50[e]	Lochry (1990), Charles *et al.* (1996a)
2,4-D acid	gavage	GD 6–15	0, 8, 25, or 75	75[d,e]	Nemec *et al.* (1983), Charles *et al.* (1996a)
Developmental: Mouse					
2,4-D acid	oral	GD 7–15	0, or 0.56 mM/kg bw	<0.56[d]; 0.56[e]	Courtney (1977)
2,4-D acid	oral	GD 11–14	0, or 0.80 mM/kg bw	<0.80[d,e]	Courtney (1977)
2,4-D acid	oral	GD 12–15	0, or 1 mM/kg bw	<1[d,e]	Courtney (1977)
2,4-D acid	subcutaneous	GD 12–15	0, or 1 mM/kg bw	<1[d,e]	Courtney (1977)
2,4-D isopropyl ester	oral	GD 7–15	0, or 0.56 mM/kg bw	<0.56[d,e]	Courtney (1977)
2,4-D *n*-butyl ester	oral	GD 7–15	0, or 0.56 mM/kg bw	0.56[d,e]	Courtney (1977)
2,4-D *n*-butyl ester	oral	GD 12–15	0, or 1 mM/kg bw	<1[d,e]	Courtney (1977)
2,4-D isooctyl ester	oral	GD 7–15	0, or 0.56 mM/kg bw	<0.56[d,e]	Courtney (1977)
2,4-D propylene glycol butyl ether	oral	GD 7–15	0, or 0.56 mM/kg bw	<0.56[d,e]	Courtney (1977)

(continues)

Table 72.3

(*continued*)

Chemical species	Route	Exposure duration	Dose (mg/kg bw/d)	NOAEL[a] (mg/kg bw/d)	Reference
2,4-D propylene glycol butyl ether	oral	GD 12–15	0, or 1 mM/kg bw	1^{d}; $<1^{e}$	Courtney (1977)
2,4-D acid	oral	GD 8–12	0, or 87.5	$87.5^{d,e}$	Kavlock *et al.* (1987)
2,4-D propylene glycol butyl ether	oral	GD 8–12	0, or 87.5	$87.5^{d,e}$	Kavlock *et al.* (1987)
2,4-D isooctyl ester	oral	GD 8–12	0, or 87.5	$87.5^{d,e}$	Kavlock *et al.* (1987)
2,4-D acid	subcutaneous	GD 6–14	0, or 100	$<100^{d,e}$	Bionetics (1968)
2,4-D acid	subcutaneous	GD 6–14	0, or 98	$<98^{d,e}$	Bionetics (1968)
2,4-D acid	subcutaneous	GD 6–14	0, or 215	$215^{d,e}$	Bionetics (1968)
2,4-D acid	subcutaneous	GD 6–14	0, or 50	$50^{d,e}$	Bionetics (1968)
2,4-D acid	oral	GD 6–14	0, or 100	$<100^{d,e}$	Bionetics (1968)
Developmental: Hamster					
2,4-D	oral	GD 6–10	0, 20, 40, 60, or 100	100^{e}	Collins and Williams (1971)
2,4-D	oral	GD 6–10	0, 40, 60, or 100	100^{e}	Collins and Williams (1971)
2,4-D	oral	GD 6–10	0, 40, 60, or 100	40	Collins and Williams (1971)
Reproductive Toxicity: Rat					
2,4-D acid	diet	2-generation	0, 5, 20, or 80	20^{d}; 5^{e}	Rodwell (1984)

[a]NOAEL = no-observed-adverse-effect level.

[b]GD = gestational days.

[c]2,4-D acid equivalents.

[d]Maternal.

[e]Fetal.

high doses of 2,4-D (50 to 100 mg/kg body weight/day) (Arnold *et al.*, 1991; Beasley *et al.*, 1991; Elo and MacDonald, 1989; Kwiecinski, 1981; Steiss *et al.*, 1987; Toyoshima *et al.*, 1985). In a subchronic toxicity study on 2,4-D 2-ethylhexyl ester, some of the high-dose animals were reported to show clinical signs that could possibly be related to myotonia (e.g., hunched posture, languid behavior, ataxia) (Charles *et al.*, 1996b).

Myotonia induced by high levels of exposure to 2,4-D does not appear to be the result of toxicological action upon the central nervous system (Buslovich and Pichugin, 1983), but appears to be due to effects mediated at the junction of skeletal muscle nerves and muscle tissue. The biochemical mechanism involved in the induction of myotonia in experimental animals is not well understood; however, according to Rudel and Senges (1972), alteration of chloride ion conductance in muscle fibers appears to be involved. Because the development of myotonia in animals exposed to high doses of 2,4-D was not accompanied by any pathological effects, and because the reporting of myotonia is restricted to dose levels greater than the threshold for saturation of renal tubular secretion, the effects reported in animal studies are not considered to be indicative of a potential of 2,4-D to induce peripheral polyneuropathy in humans. In an independent review of the literature, it was concluded that exposure to 2,4-D does not produce polyneuropathy in humans nor does polyneuropathy occur in several animal species exposed to high levels of 2,4-D (Mattsson and Eisenbrandt, 1990).

Using tests of neurobehavioral parameters (such as the Functional Observational Battery), decreased activity levels, behav-

ioral changes, and motor skill abnormalities have been reported in rats at doses greater than 60 mg/kg body weight/day and in rabbits at doses of approximately 30 mg/kg body weight/day (Breslin *et al.*, 1991; de Duffard *et al.*, 1990b; Duffard *et al.*, 1995; Hoberman, 1990; Jeffries *et al.*, 1994; Liberacki *et al.*, 1991; Martin, 1991; Mattsson *et al.*, 1994, 1997; Oliveira and Palermo-Neto, 1993; Rodwell, 1991; Schulze and Dougherty, 1988; Zablotny *et al.*, 1991). In acute studies conducted using beagle dogs, clinical signs of central nervous system depression and/or abnormalities in electroencephalograms were only reported at doses of 175 mg/kg or greater (Arnold *et al.*, 1991).

Rats exposed to high doses of 2,4-D *n*-butyl ester were reported to display alterations in neurotransmitter concentrations in the brain (de Duffard *et al.*, 1990a; Elo and MacDonald, 1989; Oliveira and Palermo-Neto, 1993). These neurochemical alterations have been hypothesized to result from compromise of the blood–brain barrier by high doses of 2,4-D (Elo *et al.*, 1988; Tyynela *et al.*, 1986). These authors reported that doses of 2,4-D greater than 150 mg/kg body weight resulted in extravasation of albumin in various areas of the brain.

Several investigators have reported accumulation of 2,4-D in the brain or cerebrospinal fluid, following administration of high doses (40 to 300 mg/kg body weight) of 2,4-D (Elo and Ylitalo, 1977, 1979; Kim *et al.*, 1988; Oliveira and Palermo-Neto, 1993; Tyynela *et al.*, 1990). Kim *et al.* (1988) suggested that the increased accumulation of 2,4-D in the brain at high doses was likely not the result of increased permeability of the blood–brain barrier since the entry of the organic solute,

2-deoxyglucose, into rabbit brain was unaffected by 2,4-D pretreatment. Instead, it has been hypothesized that reduced elimination of 2,4-D from the brain via the choroid plexus through competitive inhibition of the organic acid transport pathway was likely responsible for the increased accumulation of 2,4-D (Kim *et al.*, 1988; Ylitalo *et al.*, 1990). The organic acid transport pathway normally actively eliminates acidic metabolites from the brain through the blood–brain barrier.

At doses below the capacity of normal renal clearance, there is no evidence in experimental animals to indicate that 2,4-D can have an impact on the nervous system. In fact, no clinically observable adverse effects on the nervous system have been observed in animals at doses below 10 to 30 mg/kg body weight, even in long-term studies.

72.6.6.6 Chronic Toxicity and Carcinogenicity

Several long-term bioassays have been conducted in rats, mice, and dogs (Arkhipov and Kozlova, 1974; Charles *et al.*, 1996a, 1996c; Innes *et al.*, 1969; Hansen *et al.*, 1971; Serota *et al.*, 1986, 1987). There has been no evidence to suggest that 2,4-D acts as a carcinogen in any of these species.

Rats In one older 2-year rat feeding study (Serota *et al.*, 1986), an increase in the incidence of brain astrocytomas was reported in male rats only at the highest dose tested of 45 mg/kg body weight/day; however, the biological characteristics of the tumors were not consistent with chemical carcinogenesis. Moreover, based on the lack of decreased latency, the lack of increased multiplicity, the lack of increased severity, the lack of preneoplastic or target organ effects, the restriction of tumor development to one species and sex, the intergroup variability exhibited among historical controls, the lack of a plausible mechanism of tumorigenesis, the low exposure of the brain to 2,4-D compared to other tissues, and the fact that these tumors have not been reproduced in subsequent studies, it is unlikely that the increased incidence of brain astrocytomas reported by Serota *et al.* (1986) was related to 2,4-D treatment. In another older study (Hansen *et al.*, 1971) in which rats were fed up to 62.5 mg 2,4-D/kg body weight/day for 2 years, an overall increase in the number of randomly distributed tumors was reported to be statistically significant for male rats. As discussed by Munro *et al.* (1992), this study was not considered to provide any evidence that 2,4-D is carcinogenic in the rat since it did not meet the requirements of Good Laboratory Practice (GLP) standards, the dose groups were fairly small, the maximum tolerated dose (MTD) was not achieved, and the microscopic examination was not comprehensive. In a third feeding study (Arkhipov and Kozlova, 1974), rats were fed 10% of the reported LD_{50} (details of dosing not reported) with no significant increase in tumor incidence.

More recently, a 2-year GLP-compliant study in which rats were fed 5 to 150 mg 2,4-D/kg body weight/day was completed without any evidence of carcinogenicity (Charles *et al.*, 1996a). In particular, there was no increased incidence of brain astrocytomas even at the MTD. Noncancer endpoints reported in the animals were very similar to those reported in the subchronic studies (Charles *et al.*, 1996b), and a NOAEL of 5 mg/kg body weight/day was established based on increased thyroid weight.

Mice No evidence of carcinogenicity has been reported in three long-term mouse studies (Charles *et al.*, 1996a; Innes *et al.*, 1969; Serota *et al.*, 1987). In the first study (Innes *et al.*, 1969), mice were orally administered one of three esters of 2,4-D (i.e., isopropyl, butyl, or isooctyl ester) at a dose of 46.4 mg/kg body weight/day for 18 months. No increase in tumor incidence was reported. In the second study (Serota *et al.*, 1987), mice were fed 1 to 45 mg 2,4-D/kg body weight/day for 106 weeks with no evidence of carcinogenicity or other treatment-related effects. In male mice administered the highest two doses (15 and 45 mg/kg body weight/day), an increase in cytoplasmic homogeneity in the renal tubular epithelium was reported. In the third and most recent GLP-compliant study (Charles *et al.*, 1996a), female and male mice were fed 5 to 300 and 5 to 125 mg 2,4-D/kg body weight/day, respectively, for 2 years without any evidence of tumorigenesis. Noncancer effects were limited to slight depression of red blood cell parameters, minor organ weight changes, and histopathological renal effects at the top two doses in both sexes.

Dogs Similar to the results from the rodent studies, there has been no evidence to suggest that 2,4-D has carcinogenic potential in dogs (Charles *et al.*, 1996c; Hansen *et al.*, 1971). The results of the long-term studies in dogs support the results reported in subchronic studies. In the older study by Hansen *et al.* (1971), small groups of beagle dogs were fed 2,4-D in the diet at concentrations reaching 500 ppm over a 2-year period. Following gross and microscopic examinations of several tissues and organs, no lesions related to 2,4-D treatment were reported. The more recent study by Charles *et al.* (1996c) examined the effects of feeding 0, 1, 5, or 7.5 mg 2,4-D/kg body weight/day to beagle dogs for a period of 52 weeks. The reported effects included body weight gain reduction in females, notably at the highest dose, some serum chemistry alterations (i.e., increased urea nitrogen, creatinine, cholesterol, and alanine aminotransferase activity) in the two highest dose groups, and some histopathological alterations (i.e., perivascular chronic active inflammation of the liver and an increase of pigment in tubular epithelium in both sexes in the two highest dose groups, and pigment in the sinusoidal lining cells in the females of the two highest dose groups). Overall, 2,4-D administration was well tolerated and produced no effects on clinical signs, hematology, urinalysis, or gross necropsy. A NOAEL of 1 mg/kg body weight/day was suggested by the authors.

72.6.7 GENOTOXICITY

Numerous *in vitro* and *in vivo* genotoxicity studies have been conducted with 2,4-D. Overall, the results indicate that 2,4-D has very little genotoxic potential. This conclusion has been reached in previous reviews of 2,4-D (CCT, 1987; EPA, 1997; Munro *et al.*, 1992) and is consistent with metabolism studies which have indicated that 2,4-D does not metabolize to reactive intermediates.

With very few exceptions, bacterial mutagenicity tests using *Salmonella typhimurium* and *Escherichia coli* have produced negative results with 2,4-D (Anderson and Styles, 1978; Charles *et al.*, 1996a; Ercegovich and Rashid, 1977; Kappas, 1988; Kappas and Markaki, 1988; Kappas *et al.*, 1984; Mersch-Sundermann *et al.*, 1989; Rashid, 1979; Rashid and Mumma, 1986; Rashid *et al.*, 1984; Simmon *et al.*, 1977; Soler-Niedziela *et al.*, 1988; Styles, 1973; Waters *et al.*, 1980). In yeast cells, mitotic gene conversion and recombination has been reported, but was highly dependent on pH and occurred only at pH 4.3 (Simmon *et al.*, 1977; Waters *et al.*, 1980; Zetterberg, 1978; Zetterberg *et al.*, 1977). Negative or weakly positive results were reported in unscheduled DNA repair and sister chromatid exchange (SCE) assays with mammalian cell systems (Charles *et al.*, 1996a; Clausen *et al.*, 1990; Galloway *et al.*, 1987; Jacobi and Witte, 1991; Styles, 1977; Waters *et al.*, 1980). For the most part, the weakly positive results occurred only in conjunction with cytotoxicity (Clausen *et al.*, 1990; Korte and Jalal, 1982).

Similar to the *in vitro* studies, the majority of *in vivo* studies with animals, using the most accepted and validated procedures, have produced negative results (Munro *et al.*, 1992). Some studies with occupationally exposed individuals provided marginally positive results in lymphocytes but could not be directly correlated with 2,4-D exposure due to various confounding factors (e.g., age, sex, race, lifestyle habits, etc.) (Crossen *et al.*, 1978; Kaye *et al.*, 1985; Yoder *et al.*, 1973). Several other studies have shown that 2,4-D exposure has no effect on chromosomal aberration or SCE frequency (Charles *et al.*, 1996a, b; Hogstedt and Westerlund, 1980; Linnainmaa, 1983a, 1983b, 1984; Mulcahy, 1980; Mustonen *et al.*, 1986, 1989).

72.7 STUDIES IN HUMANS

There has been some concern over a possible association between exposure to 2,4-D and the development of cancer, specifically non-Hodgkin's lymphoma, Hodgkin's disease, and soft tissue sarcoma. In a critical review of over 90 epidemiology studies relating to occupational exposures to various herbicides including 2,4-D, Munro *et al.* (1992) concluded that the epidemiological findings are inconsistent, the evidence for a causal association between 2,4-D and cancer is weak, and that no association between 2,4-D and human cancer has been convincingly documented.

In overview, the majority of the studies were conducted with farmers, forestry workers, and other similar groups of potential users of herbicides. In most of the studies, there were methodological shortcomings in conducting exposure assessments specifically related to 2,4-D. Moreover, the majority of the studies involved occupational exposures to a wide variety of chemical, physical, and biological agents including phenoxy herbicides, and it was difficult to discern specific exposure to 2,4-D. Without specific information regarding exposure to 2,4-D and with the contribution of other confounding factors, the establishment of a dose–response relationship is difficult to ascertain. In cohort studies, exposure to 2,4-D could be reasonably assumed; however, no conclusive evidence was reported to show an association between 2,4-D and cancer. The only positive correlations were reported in three large cohort studies (Saracci *et al.*, 1991; Wigle *et al.*, 1990; Wiklund and Holm, 1986; Wiklund *et al.*, 1987), in which exposures were primarily to 2,4,5-T or were mixed with other herbicides, and none of the reported effects were consistent among the studies. Although there has been a persistent hypothesis that exposure to 2,4-D may be associated with an increased incidence of non-Hodgkin's lymphoma (Hoar *et al.*, 1986; Zahm *et al.*, 1990), the analysis by Munro *et al.* (1992) concluded that the results of these case-control studies did not strongly support the hypothesis based on weaknesses in the methodology employed and lack of control for other possible risk factors for non-Hodgkin's lymphoma (e.g., viruses and immune system modulation).

Other reviews have been conducted since the work by Munro *et al.* (1992). A SAB/SAP Special Joint Committee from the U.S. Environmental Protection Agency (EPA, 1994) reviewed the available data on 2,4-D and concluded that "…the data are not sufficient to conclude that there is a cause and effect relationship between the exposure to 2,4-D and non-Hodgkin's lymphoma" and 2,4-D still remains classified as a Group D (not classifiable as to human carcinogenicity) (EPA, 1997). Similarly, the Joint Meeting of the FAO Panel of Experts on Pesticide Residues in Food and the Environment and the WHO Expert Group on Pesticide Residues reviewed the data on 2,4-D and stated that the results of the available epidemiology studies are inconsistent and that any reported associations are weak (Rowland, 1997). The National Cancer Institute of Canada also convened an Ad Hoc Panel on Pesticides and Cancer which concluded that "it was not aware of any definitive evidence to suggest that synthetic pesticides contribute significantly to overall cancer mortality" (Ritter, 1997).

A few additional studies have been published since the above reviews (Becher *et al.*, 1996; Burns *et al.*, 2001; Fleming *et al.*, 1997; Zahm, 1997). Three of these are mortality studies in factory workers (Becher *et al.*, 1996; Burns *et al.*, 2001) and lawn care workers (Zahm, 1997), and one is a retrospective cohort study in pesticide applicators (Fleming *et al.*, 1997). As with previous epidemiology studies, the findings were inconsistent and did not provide any conclusive evidence of increased cancer risk associated with exposure to 2,4-D. In fact, Fleming *et al.* (1997) reported that in a cohort of 33, 669 pesticide applicators, there were no confirmed cases of soft tissue sarcoma or non-Hodgkins lymphoma and Burns *et al.* (2001) concluded there was "no evidence of causal association between exposure to 2,4-D and mortality due to all causes and malignant neoplasm" and "no significant risk due to NHL was found." In addition, Acquavella *et al.* (1998) conducted a meta-analysis of 37 studies in farmers and concluded that farmers did not have elevated rates of several cancers, with the exception of lip cancer.

In a preliminary study with a small group of farmers, Faustini *et al.* (1996) reported that 2,4-D exposure affected some immunological variables; however, the data were highly variable (i.e., large standard deviations) and the group tested was very small ($n = 10$). There has been some discussion in the literature linking immunosuppressive agents with an increased incidence of non-Hodgkin's lymphoma (Hardell *et al.*, 1998; Hardell and Axelson, 1998), but there has been no clear or consistent evidence in humans indicating that 2,4-D affects the immune system. This is well supported by animal studies.

72.8 SUMMARY

2,4-D is the most common of the phenoxy herbicides and is one of the best-studied agricultural chemicals. It is primarily used as a herbicide in agriculture, forestry, and lawn care practices, and is effective against a wide variety of broadleaf plants. Occupational exposure to 2,4-D is mainly through dermal contact but can also occur, to a lesser extent, via ingestion and inhalation. Studies in humans have shown exposures to be extremely low even in all occupational groups (i.e., <40 μg/kg body weight/day). The extensive database of metabolic, toxicological, and epidemiological studies on 2,4-D has provided no evidence that 2,4-D poses any health risk to humans when used according to label directions.

REFERENCES

Acquavella, J., Olsen, G., Cole, P., Ireland, B., Kaneene, J., Schuman, S., and Holden, L. (1998). Cancer among farmers: A meta-analysis. *Ann. Epidemiol.* **8**(1), 64–74.

Agriculture Canada (1983). "Re: 2,4-D Products Registered Under the Authority of the Pest Control Products Act." (Memorandum to Registrants) No. R-1-216. Agriculture Canada, Food Production and Inspection Branch, Ottawa, Ontario.

Anderson, D., and Styles, J. A. (1978). The bacterial mutation test. *Br. J. Cancer* **37**, 924–930.

Arkhipov, G. N., and Kozlova, I. N. (1974). A study of the carcinogenic potential of a herbicide: 2,4-D amine salt. *Voprosy Pitaniia* **5**, 83–84.

Arnold, E. K., Beasley, V. R., Parker, A. J., and Stedelin, J. R. (1991). 2,4-D toxicosis. II. A pilot study of clinical pathologic and electroencephalographic effects and residues of 2,4-D in orally dosed dogs. *Vet. Hum. Toxicol.* **33**(5), 446–449.

Beasley, V. R., Arnold, E. K., Lovell, R. A., and Parker, A. J. (1991). 2,4-D toxicosis. I. A pilot study of 2,4-dichlorophenoxyacetic acid- and dicamba-induced myotonia in experimental dogs. *Vet. Hum. Toxicol.* **33**(5), 435–440.

Becher, H., Flesch-Janys, D., Kauppinen, T., Kogevinas, M., Steindorf, K., Manz, A., and Wahrendorf, J. (1996). Cancer mortality in German male workers exposed to phenoxy herbicides and dioxins. *Cancer Causes Control* **7**, 312–321.

Bernard, P. A., Toyoshima, E., Eccles, C. U., Mayer, R. F., Johnson, K. P., and Max, S. R. (1985). 2,4-Dichlorophenoxyacetic acid (2,4-D) reduces acetylcholinesterase activity in rat muscle. *Exper. Neurol.* **87**, 544–556.

Berry, D. L. (1989). "Final Report of the Determination of Halogenated Dibenzo-p-dioxins and Dibenzofurans in 2,4-Dichlorophenoxyacetic Acid." No. AL 89-030290. Analytical Sciences Laboratories, The Dow Chemical Company, Midland, MI.

Bionetics Research Laboratory (1968). "Evaluation of Carcinogenic, Teratogenic, and Mutagenic Activities of Selected Pesticides and Industrial Chemicals. Volume I. Carcinogenic Study; Volume II. Teratogenic Study in Mice and Rats." National Cancer Institute (NCI), Bethesda, MD.

Blakley, B. R. (1986). The effect of oral exposure to the *N*-butylester of 2,4-dichlorophenoxyacetic acid on the immune response in mice. *Int. j. Immunopharmacol.* **8**(1), 93–99.

Blakley, B. R., and Blakley, P. M. (1986). The effect of prenatal exposure to the *n*-butylester of 2,4-dichlorophenoxyacetic acid (2,4-D) on the immune response in mice. *Teratology* **33**, 15–20.

Blakley, B. R., and Schiefer, B. H. (1986). The effect of topically applied *n*-butylester of 2,4-dichlorophenoxyacetic acid on the immune response in mice. *J. Appl. Toxicol.* **6**(4), 291–295.

Breslin, W. J., Liberacki, A. B., and Yano, B. L. (1991). "Isopropylamine Salt of 2,4-D: Oral Gavage Teratology Study in New Zealand White Rabbits." Unpublished Report No. M-004725-013. Dow Chemical Company, Midland, MI.

Burns *et al.* (2001).

Buslovich, S. Y., and Pichugin, Y. I. (1983). Electromyographic characteristics of acute poisonings with chlorine derivatives of phenoxy acids. *Farmakologiia i Tosikologiia* **46**(3), 99–101.

Canadian Centre for Toxicology (CCT) (1987). "Panel Report on Carcinogenicity of 2,4-D." Canadian Centre for Toxicology (CCT), Guelph, ON.

Carreon, R., *et al.* (1983). "2,4-Dichlorophenoxyacetic Acid Isopropylamine Salt: Acute Toxicological Properties." Industry Task Force II on 2,4-D Research Data. Unpublished Report, Dow Chemical Company, Midland, MI.

Carreon, R., and Rao, K. S. (1985). "DMA-6 Weed Killer: Dermal Sensitization Potential in the Guinea Pig." Industry Task Force II on 2,4-D Research Data. Unpublished Report, Dow Chemical Company, Midland, MI.

Charles, J. M., Bond, D. M., Jeffries, T. K., Yano, B. L., Stott, W. T., Johnson, K. A., Cunny, H. C., Wilson, R. D., and Bus, J. S. (1996a). Chronic dietary toxicity/oncogenicity studies on 2,4-dichlorophenoxyacetic acid in rodents. *Fund. Appl. Toxicol.* **33**, 166–172.

Charles, J. M., Cunny, H. C., Wilson, R. D., and Bus, J. S. (1996b). Comparative subchronic studies on 2,4-dichlorophenoxyacetic acid, amine and ester in rats. *Fund. Appl. Toxicol.* **33**, 161–165.

Charles, J. M., Dalgard, D. M., Cunny, H. C., Wilson, R. D., and Bus, J. S. (1996c). Comparative subchronic and chronic dietary toxicity studies on 2,4-dichlorophenoxyacetic acid, amine and ester in the dog. *Fund. Appl. Toxicol.* **29**, 78–85.

Chernoff, N., Woodrow Setzer, R., Miller, D. B., Rosen, M. B., and Rogers, J. M. (1990). Effects of chemically induced maternal toxicity on prenatal development in the rat. *Teratology* **42**, 651–658.

Clark, D. E., Palmer, J. S., Radeleff, R. D., Crookshank, H. R., and Farr, F. M. (1975). Residues of chlorophenoxy acid herbicides and their phenolic metabolites in tissues of sheep and cattle. *J. Agric. Food Chem.* **23**(3), 573–578.

Clausen, M., Leier, G., and Witte, I. (1990). Comparison of the cytotoxicity and DNA-damaging properties of 2,4-D and U 46 D fluid (dimethylammonium salt of 2,4-D). *Arch. Toxicol.* **64**, 497–501.

Cochrane, W. P., Singh, J., Miles, W., and Wakeford, B. (1981). Determination of chlorinated dibenzo-p-dioxin contaminants in 2,4-D products by gas chromatography–mass spectrometric techniques. *J. Chromatogr.* **217**, 289–299.

Cochrane, W. P., *et al.* (1982a).

Cochrane, W. P., *et al.* (1982b).

Collins, T. F. X., and Williams, C. H. (1971). Teratogenic studies with 2,4,5-T and 2,4-D in the hamster. *Bulletin Environ. Contamin. Toxicol.* **6**(6), 559–567.

Courtney, K. D. (1977). Prenatal effects of herbicides: Evaluation by the prenatal development index. *Arch. Environ. Contam. Toxicol.* **6**, 33–46.

Cramer, P. H. (1996). "2,4-Dichlorophenoxyacetic Acid: Analysis for Polychlorinated Dibenzo-*p*-dioxins and Dibenzofurans in Acid, Salt, and/or Ester Technical Material." Lab Project ID MRI No. 4199. Midwest Research Institute, Kansas City, MO, for DowElanco, Indianapolis, IN.

Crossen, P. E., Morgan, W. F., Horan, J. J., and Stewart, J. (1978). Cytogenetic studies of pesticide and herbicide sprayers. *N. Zeal. Med. J.* **88**(619), 192–195.

de Duffard, A. M. E., de Alderete, M. N., and Duffard, R. (1990a). Changes in brain serotonin and 5-hydroxyindolacetic acid levels induced by 2,4-dichlorophenoxyacetic butyl ester. *Toxicology* **64**, 265–270.

de Duffard, A. M. E., Orta, C., and Duffard, R. (1990b). Behavioral changes in rats fed a diet containing 2,4-dichlorophenoxyacetic butyl ester. *Neurotoxicology* **11**(4), 563–572.

Duffard, R., Bortolozzi, A., Ferri, A., Garcia, G., and Evangelista de Duffard, A. M. (1995). Developmental neurotoxicity of the herbicide 2,4-dichlorophenoxyacetic acid. *Neurotoxicology* **16**(4), 764.

Duggan and Corneliussen (1972).

Duggan, R. E., and Lipscomb, G. Q. (1969). Dietary intake of pesticide chemicals in the United States (II), June 1966—April 1968. *Pestic. Monit. J.* **2**(4), 153–162.

Elo, H., Hervonen, H., and Ylitalo, P. (1988). Comparative study on cerebrovascular injuries by three chlorophenoxyacetic acids (2,4-D, 2,4,5-T and MCPA). *Comp. Biochem. Physiol.* **90C**(1), 65–68.

Elo, H. A., and Macdonald, E. (1989). Effects of 2,4-dichlorophenoxyacetic acid (2,4-D) on biogenic amines and their acidic metabolites in brain and cerebrospinal fluid of rats. *Arch. Toxicol.* **63**, 127–130.

Elo, H. A., and Ylitalo, P. (1977). Substantial increase in the levels of chlorophenoxyacetic acids in the CNS of rats as a result of severe intoxication. *Acta. Pharmacol. Toxicol.* **41**, 280–284.

Elo, H. A., and Ylitalo, P. (1979).

Environmental Protection Agency (EPA) (1994). "An SAB Report: Assessment of Potential 2,4-D Carcinogenicity. Review of the Epidemiological and Other Data on Potential Carcinogenicity of 2,4-D." U.S. Environmental Protection Agency, Science Advisory Board (SAB), Washington, DC.

Environmental Protection Agency (EPA) (1996). "Toxicology Endpoint Selection Document: 2,4-Dichlorophenoxyacetic Acid." U.S. Environmental Protection Agency, Washington, DC.

Environmental Protection Agency (EPA) (1997). "Pesticides Industry Sales and Usage. 1994 and 1995 Market Estimates," Office of Prevention, Pesticides and Toxic Substances (733-R-97-002). U.S. Environmental Protection Agency, Washington, DC.

Ercegovich, C. D., and Rashid, K. A. (1977). Mutagenesis induced in mutant strains of *Salmonella typhimurium* by pesticides. *Am. Chem. Soc. Abstr. Pap.* 174:PEST (Abstr. No. 43).

Erne, K. (1966a). Distribution and elimination of chlorinated phenoxyacetic acids in animals. *Acta Veterinaria Scandinavica* **7**, 240–256.

Erne, K. (1966b). Studies on the animal metabolism of phenoxyacetic herbicides. *Acta Veterinaria Scandinavica* **7**, 264–271.

Fang, S. C., and Lindstrom, F. T. (1980). *In vitro* binding of (14)C-labeled acidic compounds to serum albumin and their tissue distribution in the rat. *J. Pharmacokinet. Biopharmaceut.* **8**(6), 583–597.

Faustini, A., Settimi, L., Pacifici, R., Fano, V., Zuccaro, P., and Forastiere, F. (1996). Immunological changes among farmers exposed to phenoxy herbicides: Preliminary observations. *Occup. Environ. Med.* **53**, 583–585.

Fedorova and Belova (1974).

Feldman, R. J., and Maibach, H. I. (1974). Percutaneous penetration of some pesticides and herbicides in man. *Toxicol. Appl. Pharmacol.* **28**, 126–32.

Fleming, L. E., Bean, J. A., Rudolph, M., Hamilton, K., Kasl, S., and Stolwijk, J. (1997). Retrospective cohort study of cancer incidence in Florida pesticide applicators. *Amer. J. Epidemiol.* **10**, 249.

Frank, R., Campbell, R. A., and Sirons, G. J. (1985). Forestry workers involved in aerial application of 2,4-dichlorophenoxyacetic acid (2,4-D): Exposure and urinary excretion. *Arch. Environ. Contam. Toxicol.* **14**, 427–435.

Galloway, S. M., Armstrong, M. J., Reuben, C., Colman, S., Brown, B., Cannon, C., Bloom, A. D., Nakamura, F., Ahmed, M., Duk, S., Rimpo, J., Margolin, B. H., Resnick, M. A., Anderson, B., and Zeiger, E. (1987). Chromosome aberrations and sister chromatid exchanges in Chinese hamster ovary cells: Evaluations of 108 chemicals. *Environ. Mol. Mutagen.* **10**(Suppl. 10), 1–175.

Gargus, J. L. (1986). "Dermal Sensitization Study in Guinea Pigs; 2,4-D Acid." Unpublished Report No. 2184-105. Industry Task Force II on 2,4-D Research Data, Hazleton Laboratories America, Inc.

Gartrell, M. J., Craun, J. C., Podrebarac, D. S., and Gunderson, E. L. (1985). Pesticides, selected elements, and other chemicals in infant and toddler total

diet samples, October 1978–September 1979. *J. Assoc. Off. Anal. Chem.* **68**(5), 842.

Gorzinski, S. J., Kociba, R. J., Campbell, R. A., Smith, F. A., Nolan, R. J., and Eisenbrandt, D. L. (1987). Acute, pharmacokinetic, and subchronic toxicological studies of 2,4-dichlorophenoxyacetic acid. *Fund. Appl. Toxicol.* **9**, 423–435.

Gorzinski, S. J., Wade, C. E., Morden, D. C., Keyes, D. G., Dittenber, D. A., Kalnins, R. V., Schuetz, D. J., and Kociba, R. J. (1981a). "Purified 2,4-Dichlorophenoxyacetic Acid (2,4-D): Results of a 13-Week Subchronic Dietary Toxicity Study in the CDF Fischer 344 Rat." Toxicology Research Laboratory, Midland, MI.

Gorzinski, S. J., Wade, C. E., Morden, D. C., Keyes, D. G., Wolfe, E. L., Dittenber, D. A., Kalnins, R. V., Schuetz, D. J., and Kociba, R. J. (1981b). "Technical 2,4-Dichlorophenoxyacetic Acid (2,4-D): Results of a 13-Week Subchronic Dietary Toxicity Study in the CDF Fischer 344 Rat." Toxicology Research Laboratory, Midland, MI.

Grisson, R. E., Brownie, C., and Guthrie, F. E. (1987). *In vivo* and *in vitro* dermal penetration of lipophilic and hydrophilic pesticides in mice. *Bull. Environ. Contam. Toxicol.* **38**, 917–924.

Grover, R., Cessna, A. J., Muir, N. I., Reidel, D., Franklin, C. A., and Yoshida, K. (1986). Factors affecting the exposure of ground-rig applicators to 2,4-D dimethylamine salt. *Arch. Environ. Contam. Toxicol.* **15**, 677–686.

Grunow, W., and Bohme, C.H.R. (1974). Uber den stoffwechsel von 2,4,5-T und 2,4-D bei ratten und mausen. *Arch. Toxicol.* **32**, 217–225.

Hansen, W. H., Quaife, M. L., Habermann, R. T., and Fitzhugh, O. G. (1971). Chronic toxicity of 2,4-dichlorophenoxyacetic acid in rats and dogs. *Toxicol. Appl. Pharm.* **20**, 122–129.

Hardell, L., and Axelson, O. (1998). Environmental and occupational aspects on the etiology of non-Hodgkin's lymphoma. *Oncol. Res.* **10**(1), 1–5.

Hardell, L., Lindstrom, G., Van Bavel, B., Fredrikson, M., and Liljegren, G. (1998). Some aspects of the etiology of non-Hodgkin's lymphoma. *Environ. Health Perspect.* **Suppl 106**(Suppl. 2), 679–681.

Harris, S. A., and Solomon, K. R. (1992). Percutaneous penetration of 2,4-dichlorophenoxyacetic acid and 2,4-d dimethylamine salt in human volunteers. *Fertil. Steril.* **36**, 233–240.

Harris, S. A., Solomon, K. R., and Stephenson, G. R. (1992). Exposure of homeowners and bystanders to 2,4-dichlorophenoxyacetic acid (2,4-D). *J. Environ. Sci. Health (Part B—Pestic. Food Contam. Agric. Wastes)* **B27**(1), 23–38.

Hervonen, H., Elo, H. A., and Ylitalo, P. (1982). Blood-brain barrier damage by 2-methyl-4-chlorophenoxyacetic acid herbicide in rats. *Toxicol. Appl. Pharmacol.* **65**(1), 23–31.

Hoar, S. K., Blair, A., Holmes, F. F., Boysen, C. D., Robel, R. J., Hoover, R., and Fraumers, J. F. (1986). Agricultural herbicide use and risk of lymphoma and soft-tissue sarcoma. *J. Am. Med. Assoc.* **256**(9), 1141–1147.

Hoberman, A. M. (1990). "Developmental Toxicity (Embryo-Fetal Toxicity and Teratogenic Potential) Study of 2,4-Dichlorophenoxyacetic Acid (2,4-D Acid) Administered Orally Via Stomach Tube to New Zealand White Rabbits." Protocol Number: 320–003. Performing Research Laboratories, Inc., Horsham, PA.

Hogstedt, C., and Westerlund, B. (1980). Kohortstudie av dodsorsaker for skogsarbetare med och utan exposition for fenoxisyrapreparat = Cohort studies of cause of death of forest workers with and without exposure to phenoxy acid preparations. **77**(19), 1828–1830.

Innes, J. R. M., Ulland, B. M., Valerio, M. G., Petrucelli, L., Fishbein, L., Hart, E. R., Pallotta, A. J., Bates, R. R., Falk, H. L., Klein, M., Gart, J. J., Mitchell, I., and Peters, J. (1969). Bioassay of pesticides and industrial chemicals for tumorigenicity in mice: A preliminary note. *J. Nat. Cancer Instit.* **42**, 1101–1114.

ITF (1990). "Final Report: Subchronic Toxicity Study in Dogs with 2,4-Dichlorophenoxyacetic Acid." Industry Task Force on 2,4-D Research Data. Hazleton Laboratories America, Inc., Vienna, VA.

Jacobi, H., and Witte, I. (1991). Synergistic effects of U46 D Fluid (dimethylammonium salt of 2,4-D) and $CuCl_2$ on cytotoxicity and DNA repair in human fibroblasts. *Toxicol. Letters* **58**, 159–167.

Jeffrey, N. M. (1986). "2,4-D Butoxyethyl Ester, Technical: Dermal Sensitization Potential in the Hartley Albino Guinea Pig." Unpublished Report No.

K-007722-005. Industry Task Force II on 2,4-D Research Data. Dow Chemical Company, Midland, MI.

Jeffrey, N. M., and Rao, K. S. (1986). "Esteron 6E Herbicide: Dermal Sensitization Potential in the Hartley Albino Guinea Pig." Unpublished Report No. K-007722-005. Industry Task Force II on 2,4-D Research Data. Dow Chemical Company, Midland, MI.

Jeffries, T. K., Yano, B. L., and Orman, J. R. (1994). "2,4-D Chronic Neurotoxicity Study in Fischer 344 Rats." Unpublished Report No. K-002372-064N. Dow Chemical Company, Midland MI.

Kappas, A., Tziolas, V., and Demopoulos, N. (1984). Mutagenicity of herbicides in microbial short-term test systems. *Mutat. Res.* (Abstr. No. II.3B. 3) **130**, 244.

Kappas, A. (1988). On the mutagenic and recombinogenic activity of certain herbicides in *Salmonella typhimurium* and in *Aspergillus nidulans*. *Mutat. Res.* **204**(4), 615–621.

Kappas, A., and Markaki, M. (1988). Genetic activity of herbicides in *Salmonella typhimurium* and *Aspergillus nidulans*. *Mutat. Res.* (Abstr. No. 90) **203**(3), 241.

Kavlock, R. J., Short, R. D., and Chernoff, N. (1987). Further evaluation of an *in vivo* teratology screen. *Terat. Carcin. Mutagen.* **7**, 7–16.

Kaye, C. I., Rao, S., Simpson, S. J., Rosenthal, F. S., and Cohen, M. M. (1985). Evaluation of chromosomal damage in males exposed to Agent Orange and their families. *J. Craniofac. Genet. Develop. Biol. Suppl.* **1**, 259–265.

Khanna, S., and Fang, S. C. (1966). Metabolism of C14-labelled 2,4-dichlorophenoxyacetic acid in rats. *J. Agric. Food Chem.* **14**(5), 500–503.

Khera, K. S., and McKinley, W. P. (1972). Pre- and postnatal studies on 2,4,5-trichlorophenoxyacetic acid, 2,4-dichlorophenoxyacetic acid and their derivatives in rats. *Toxicol. Appl. Pharmacol.* **22**, 14–28.

Kim, C. S., Keizer, R. F., and Pritchard, J. B. (1988). 2,4-Dichlorophenoxyacetic acid intoxication increases its accumulation within the brain. *Brain Res.* **440**, 216–226.

Kim, C. S., and O'Tuama, L. A. (1981). Choroid plexus transport of 2,4-dichlorophenoxyacetic acid: Interaction with the organic acid carrier. *Brain Res.* **224**, 209–212.

Kim, C. S., O'Tuama, L. A., Mann, J. D., and Roe, C. R. (1983). Saturable accumulation of the anionic herbicide 2,4-dichlorophenoxyacetic acid (2,4-D) by rabbit choroid plexus: Early developmental origin and interaction with salicylates. *J. Pharmacol. Exper. Therapeut.* **225**(3), 699–704.

Knopp, D., and Schiller, F. (1992). Oral and dermal application of 2,4-dichlorophenoxyacetic acid sodium and dimethylamine salts to male rats: Investigations on absorption and excretion as well as induction of hepatic mixed-function oxidase activities. *Arch. Toxicol.* **66**, 170–174.

Kohli, J. D., Khana, R. N., Gupta, B. N., Dhar, M. M., Tandon, J. S., and Sircar, K. P. (1974). Absorption and excretion of 2,4-dichlorophenoxyacetic acid in man. *Xenobiotica* **4**(2), 97–100.

Kolmodin-Hedman, B., and Erne, K. (1980). Estimation of occupational exposure to phenoxy acids (2,4-D and 2,4,5-T). *Arch. Toxicol. Suppl.* **4**, 318–321.

Korte, C., and Jalal, S. M. (1982). 2,4-D induced clastogenicity and elevated rates of sister chromatid exchanges in cultured human lymphocytes. *J. Heredity* (**May/June**), 224–226.

Kuntz, D. J., Rao, N. G. S., Berg, I. E., Khattree, R., and Chaturvedi, A. K. (1990). Toxicity of mixtures of parathion, toxaphene and/or 2,4-D in mice. *J. Appl. Toxicol.* **10**(4), 257–265.

Kwiecinski, H. (1981). Myotonia induced by chemical agents. *Crit. Rev. Toxicol.* **8**(4), 279–310.

Lavy, T. L., and Mattice, J. D. (1984). Monitoring human exposure during pesticide application in the forest. *In* "Chemical and Biological Controls in Forestry" (W. Y. Garner and J. Harvey, Jr., eds.), ACS Symposium Series, Vol. 238, pp. 319–330. American Chemical Society, Washington, DC.

Lavy, T. L., Norris, L. A., Mattie, J. D., and Marx, D. B. (1987). Exposure of forestry ground workers to 2,4-D picloram and dichloroprop. *Environ. Toxicol. Chem.* **6**(3), 209–224.

Lefton, J., *et al.* (1991). "Weed Control Recommendations for Turfgrass Areas," AY-40. Pro Series, Purdue University Cooperative Extension Service.

Liberacki, A. B., Yano, B. L., and Breslin, W. J. (1991). "Triisopropanolamine Salt of 2,4-D: Oral Gavage Teratology Study in New Zealand White Rabbits," Unpublished Report K-008876-016. Dow Chemical Company, Midland, MI.

Liberacki, A. B., Zablotny, C. I., Yano, B. L., and Breslin, W. J. (1994). Developmental toxicity studies on a series of 2,4-D salts and esters in rabbits. *Toxicologist* **14**(1), 162.

Lindquist, N. G., and Ullberg, S. (1971). Distribution of the herbicides 2,4,5-T and 2,4,-D in pregnant mice. Accumulation in the yolk sac epithelium. *Experientia* **27**(12), 1439–1441.

Linnainmaa, K. (1983a). Sister chromatid exchanges among workers occupationally exposed to phenoxy acid herbicides 2,4-D and MCPA. *Teratog. Carcinog. Mutagen.* **3**(3), 269–279.

Linnainmaa, K. (1983b). Nonmutagenicity of phenoxy acid herbicides 2,4-dichlorophenoxyacetic acid and 4-methyl-2-chlorophenoxyacetic acid. *In* "Chlorinated Dioxins and Dibenzofurans in the Total Environment" (Choudhary *et al.*, eds.), p. 385. Butterworth Publishers, Woburn, MA.

Linnainmaa, K. (1984).

Lochry, E. A. (1990). "Developmental Toxicity (Embryo-Fetal Toxicity and Teratogenic Potential) Study of 2,4-D Dimethylamine Salt (2,4-D-DMA) Administered Orally via Gavage to Crl:CD®BR VAF/Plus® Presumed Pregnant Rats." Protocol Number: 320-001. Argus Research Laboratories, Inc., Horsham, PA.

Lukowicz-Ratajczak, J., and Krechniak, J. (1988). Effects of sodium 2,4-dichlorophenoxy acetate on renal function in the rat. *Bull. Environ. Contam. Toxicol.* **41**, 815–821.

Lundgren, B., Meijer, J., and Depierre, J. W. (1987). Induction of cytosolic and microsomal epoxide hydrolases and proliferation of peroxisomes and mitochondria in mouse liver after dietary exposure to p-chlorophenoxyacetic acid, 2,4-dichlorophenoxyacetic acid and 2,4,5-trichlorophenoxyacetic acid. *Biochem. Pharmacol.* **36**(6), 815–822.

Martin, T. (1991). "Developmental Toxicity (Embryo-Fetal Toxicity and Teratogenic Potential) Study of 2,4-D Dimethylamine Salt (2,4-D-DMA) Administered Orally via Stomach Tube to New Zealand White Rabbits." Protocol Number: 320-004. Argus Research Laboratories, Inc., Horsham, PA.

Martin, T. (1992a). "Developmental Toxicity (Embryo-Fetal Toxicity and Teratogenic Potential) Study of 2,4-D 2-Ethylhexyl Ester (2,4-D Isooctyl Ester) Administered Orally (Stomach Tube) to New Zealand White Rabbits." Protocol Number: 320-006. Argus Research Laboratories, Inc., Horsham, PA.

Martin, T. (1992b). "Developmental Toxicity (Embryo-Fetal Toxicity and Teratogenic Potential) Study of 2,4-D 2-Ethylhexyl Ester (2,4-D Isooctyl Ester) Administered Orally via Gavage to Crl:CD®BR VAF/Plus® Presumed Pregnant Rats." Protocol Number: 320-005. Argus Research Laboratories, Inc., Horsham, PA.

Mattsson, J. L., Charles, J. M., Yano, B. L., Cunny, H. C., Wilson, R. D., and Bus, J. S. (1997). Single-dose and chronic dietary neurotoxicity screening studies on 2,4-dichlorophenoxyacetic acid in rats. *Fund. Appl. Toxicol.* **40**, 111–119.

Mattsson, J. L., and Eisenbrandt, D. L. (1990). The improbable association between the herbicide 2,4-D and polyneuropathy. *Biomed. Environ. Sci.* **3**, 43–51.

Mattsson, J. L., McGuirk, R. J., and Yano, B. L. (1994). 2,4-D Acute Neurotoxicity Study in Fischer 344 Rats." Unpublished Report K-002372-006. Dow Chemical Company, Midland, MI.

Mersch-Sundermann, V., Hofmeister, A., Muller, G., and Hof, H. (1989). Untersuchungen zur mutagenitat organischer mikrokontaminationen in der umwelt. III. Mitteilung: Die mutagenitat ausgewahlter herbizide und insektizide im SOS-chromotest = Examination of mutagenicity of organic microcontaminations of the environment. III. Communication: The mutagenicity of selected herbicides and insecticides with the SOS-chromotest. *Zentralblatt fur Hygiene und Umweltmedizin (Int. J. Hyg. Environ. Med.)* **189**, 135–146.

Mizell, M. J., Atkin, K. T., and Crissman, J. W. (1990a). "2,4-Dichlorophenoxyacetic Acid Butoxyethyl Ester: 21-Day Dermal Toxicity Study in New Zealand White Rabbits." K-007722-008. The Dow Chemical Company, Midland, MI.

Mizell, M. J., Atkin, K. T., Haut, K. T., and Stebbins, K. E. (1990b). "2,4-D Isopropylamine Salt: 21-Day Dermal Toxicity Study in New Zealand White Rabbits." M-004725-004. The Dow Chemical Company, Midland, MI.

Mizell, M. J., Atkin, K. T., and Stebbins, K. E. (1989). "2,4-D Triisopropanolamine Salt: 21-Day Dermal Toxicity Study in New Zealand White Rabbits." K-008866-004. The Dow Chemical Company, Midland, MI.

Moody, R. P., Franklin, C. A., Ritter, L., and Maibach, H. I. (1990). Dermal absorption of the phenoxy herbicides 2,4-D, 2,4-D amine, 2,4-D isooctyl, and 2,4,5-T in rabbits, rats, rhesus monkeys, and humans: A cross-species comparison. *J. Toxicol. Environ. Health* **29**(3), 237–246.

Moody et al. (1991).

Mulcahy, M. T. (1980). Chromosome aberrations and "Agent Orange." *Med. J. Austral.* **2**(10), 573–574.

Mullison, W. R. (1987). "Environmental Fate of Phenoxy Herbicides. Fate of Pesticides in the Environment." Publication 3320, pp. 121–131. California Agricultural Experiment Station.

Munro, I. C., Carlo, G. L., Orr, J. C., Sund, K. G., Wilson, R. M., Kennepohl, E., Lynch, B. S., Jablinske, M., and Lee, N. L. (1992). A comprehensive, integrated review and evaluation of the scientific evidence relating to the safety of the herbicide 2,4-D. *J. Am. Coll. Toxicol.* **11**(5), 559–664.

Mustonen, R., Kangras, J., Vuojolahti, P., and Linnainmaa, K. (1986). Effect of phenoxyacetic acids on the induction of chromosome aberrations in vitro and in vivo. *Mutagenesis* **1**, 241–255.

Mustonen, R. (1989).

Nemec, M. D., Tasker, E. J., Werchowski, K. M., and Mercieca, M. D. (1983). "A Teratology Study in Fischer 344 Rats with 2,4-Dichlorophenoxyacetic Acid." Industry Task Force on 2,4-D Research Data. No. WIL-81135. Wil Research Laboratories, Inc., Ashland, OH.

Oliveira, G., and Palermo-Neto, J. (1993). Effects of 2,4-dichlorophenoxyacetic acid (2,4-D) on open-field behaviour and neurochemical parameters of rats. *Pharmacol. Toxicol.* **73**(2), 79–85.

Orberg, J. (1980). Effects of low protein consumption on the renal clearance of 2,4-dichlorophenoxyacetic acid (2,4-D) in goats. *Acta. Pharmacol. Toxicol.* **46**, 138–140.

Pelletier, O., Ritter, L., Caron, J., and Somers, D. (1989). Disposition of 2,4-dichlorophenoxyacetic acid dimethylamine salt by Fischer 344 rats dosed orally and dermally. *J. Toxicol. Environ. Health* **28**, 221–234.

Pelletier, O., et al. (1990).

Pritchard, J. B. (1980). Accumulation of anionic pesticides by rabbit choroid plexus in vitro. *J. Pharmacol. Exper. Therapeut.* **212**(2), 354–359.

Rashid, K. A. (1979). The relationship between mutagenic and DNA-damaging activity of pesticides and their potential for carcinogenesis. *Diss. Abstr. Int.* **39**, 4726-B (Abstr. No. 7909115).

Rashid, K. A., Babish, J. G., and Mumma, R. O. (1984). Potential of 2,4-dichlorophenoxyacetic acid conjugates as promutagens in the salmonella/microsome mutagenicity test. *J. Environ. Sci. Health* **B19**(849), 689–701.

Rashid, K. A., and Mumma, R. O. (1986). Screening pesticides for their ability to damage bacterial DNA. *J. Environ. Sci. Health (Part B—Pestic. Food Contam. Agric. Wastes)* **B21**(4), 319–334.

Ritter, L. (1997). Report of a panel on the relationship between public exposure to pesticides and cancer. *Cancer* **80**(10), 2019–2033.

Rodwell, D. (1991). "Teratology Study in Rabbits with Diethanolamine Salt of 2,4-D Acid." Unpublished Report SLS 3229.13. Springborn Laboratories, Inc., OH.

Rodwell, D. E. (1984). "A Dietary Two-Generation Reproduction Study in Fischer 344 Rats with 2,4-Dichlorophenoxyacetic Acid." Project No. WIL-81137. Wil Research Laboratories, Inc., Ashland, OH.

Rowland, J. C. (1997). 2,4-dichlorophenoxyacetic acid (2,4-D). *In* "FAO Panel of Experts on Pesticide Residues, and WHO Expert Group on Pesticides Residues in the Food, and Environment. Pesticide Residues in Food—1996: Toxicological Evaluations." WHO/PCS/97 **1**, 45–96. Food and Agriculture Organization of the United Nations (FAO), Rome, Italy.

Rudel, R., and Senges, J. (1972). Experimental myotonia in mammalian skeletal muscle: Changes in membrane properties. *Pflugers. Arch.* **331**, 324–334. (Cited in Bernard et al., 1985.)

Saracci, R., Kogevinas, M., Bertazzi, P. A., Demesquita, B. H. B., Coggon, D., Green, L. M., Kauppinen, T., Labbe, K. A., Littorin, M., Lynge, E., Mathews, J. D., Neuberger, M., Osman, J., Pearce, N., and Winkelmann, R. (1991). Cancer mortality in workers exposed to chlorophenoxy herbicides and chlorophenols. *Lancet* **338**(8774), 1027–1032.

Sauerhoff, M. W., Braun, W. H., Blau, G. E., and Gehring, P. J. (1977). The fate of 2,4-dichlorophenoxyacetic acid (2,4-D) following oral administration to man. *Toxicology* **8**, 3–11.

Schultz, S. K., Brock, A. W., and Killeen, J. C. (1990). "Dermal Sensitization Study (Closed Patch Repeated Insult) in Guinea Pigs, Rabbits with Diethanolamine Salt of 2,4-D." Unpublished Report 90-165. Industry Task Force II on 2,4-D Research Data. Ricerca Inc., Painesville, OH.

Schulze, G. E. (1990a). "21-Dermal Irritation and Dermal Toxicity Study in Rabbits with 2,4-Dichlorophenoxyacetic Acid." HLA Study No. 2184-109. Hazleton Laboratories America Inc., Vienna, VA.

Schulze, G. E. (1990b). "21-Dermal Irritation and Dermal Toxicity Study in Rabbits with Dimethylamine Salt of 2,4-Dichlorophenoxyacetic Acid." HLA Study No. 2184-111. Hazleton Laboratories America Inc., Vienna, VA.

Schulze, G. E. (1990c). "21-Dermal Irritation and Dermal Toxicity Study in Rabbits with 2,4-Dichlorophenoxyacetic Acid-2-Ethylhexyl Ester." HLA Study No. 2184-110. Hazleton Laboratories America Inc., Vienna, VA.

Schulze, G. E. (1991). "Final Report: Subchronic Toxicity Study in Mice with 2,4-Dichlorophenoxyacetic Acid." Industry Task Force II on 2,4-D Research Data. Hazleton Laboratories America, Inc., Vienna, VA.

Schulze, G. E., and Dougherty, J. A. (1988). Neurobehavioral toxicity of 2,4-D-n-butyl ester (2,4-D ester): Tolerance and lack of cross-tolerance. *Neurotoxicol. Teratol.* **10**, 75–79.

Schwetz, B. A., Sparschu, G. L., and Gehring, P. J. (1971). The effect of 2,4-dichlorophenoxyacetic acid (2,4-D) and esters of 2,4-D on rat embryonal, foetal and neonatal growth and development. *Fd. Cosmet. Toxicol.* **9**, 801–817.

Sell, C. R., Maitlen, J. C., and Aller, W. A. (1982). Perspiration as an important physiological pathway for the elimination of 2,4-dichlorophenoxyacetic acid from the human body. *Am. Chem. Soc. Abstr. Pap.* **183**, PEST #74.

Serota, D. G. (1983a). "Subchronic Toxicity Study in Rats with 2,4-D Acid." Unpublished Report 2184-102. Industry Task Force II on 2,4-D Research Data. Hazleton Laboratories America, Inc., Vienna, VA.

Serota, D. G. (1983b). "Subchronic Toxicity Study in Mice with 2,4-D Acid." Unpublished Report 2184-100. Industry Task Force II on 2,4-D Research Data. Hazleton Laboratories America, Inc., Vienna, VA.

Serota, D. G. (1986). "Combined chronic toxicity and oncogenicity study in rats with 2,4-D acid." Unpublished Report 2184-103. Industry task Force II on 2,4-D Research Data. Hazleton Laboratories America, Inc., Vienna, VA.

Serota, D. G., et al. (1986). "Combined Chronic Toxicity and Oncogenicity Study in Rats with 2,4-D Acid." Unpublished Report 2184-102. Hazleton Laboratories America, Inc., Vienna, VA.

Serota, D. G., et al. (1987). "Oncogenicity Study in Mice with 2,4-D Acid." Unpublished Report 2184-101. Hazleton Laboratories America, Inc., Vienna, VA.

Serrone, D. M., Killeen, J. C., and Benz, G. (1991). "A Subchronic Toxicity Study in Rats with the Diethanolamine Salt of 2,4-Dichlorophenoxyacetic Acid." Unpublished Report 90-0186. Ricera Inc., Painesville, OH.

Simmon, V. F., Kauhanen, K., and Tardiff, R. G. (1977). Mutagenic activity of chemicals identified in drinking water. *In* "Progress in Genetic Toxicology" (B. A. Bridges Scott and F. H. Sodels, eds.), Vol. 2, pp. 249–258. Elsevier/North-Holland, Amsterdam.

Soler-Niedziela, L., Ong, T., Nath, J., and Zeiger, E. (1988). Mutagenicity studies of dioxin and related compounds with the Salmonella arabinose resistant assay system. *Toxic. Assess.* **3**(2), 137–145.

Steiss, J. E., Braund, K. G., and Clark, E. G. (1987). Neuromuscular effects of acute 2,4-dichlorophenoxyacetic acid (2,4-D) exposure in dogs. *J. Neurol. Sci.* **78**, 295–301.

Styles, J. A. (1973). Cytotoxic effects of various pesticides *in vivo* and *in vitro*. *Mutat. Res.* **21**(1), 50–51.

Styles, J. A. (1977). Mammalian cell transformation *in vitro*. *Br. J. Cancer* **37**, 931–936.

Szabo, J. R., and Rachunek, B. L. (1991). "2,4-D, Butoxyethyl Ester: 13-Week Dietary Toxicity Study in Fischer Rats." ID. DECO-TXT:K-007722-015. DowElanco: Indianapolis, IN.

Toyoshima, E., Mayre, R. F., Max, S. R., and Eccles, C. (1985). 2,4-Dichlorophenoxyacetic acid (2,4-D) does not cause polyneuropathy in rats. *J. Neurol. Sci.* **70**, 225–229.

Tyynela, K., Elo, H. A., and Ylitalo, P. (1990). Distribution of three common chlorophenoxyacetic acid herbicides into the rat brain. *Arch. Toxicol.* **64**(1), 61–65.

Tyynela, K., Elo, H., Ylitalo, P., and Hervonen, H. (1986). The central nervous system toxicity of chlorophenoxyacetic acid herbicides. *Arch. Toxicol.* **(Suppl. 9)**, 355.

Unger, T. M., Kliethermes, J., Van Goethem, D., and Short, R. D. (1981). "Teratology and Postnatal Studies in Rats of the Propylene Glycol Butyl Ether and Isooctyl Esters of 2,4-Dichlorophenoxyacetic Acid." PB81-191140. U.S. Environmental Protection Agency, Research Triangle Park, NC.

Waters, G. D., Simmon, V. F., Mitchell, A. D., Jorgenson, T. A., and Valencia, R. (1980). An overview of short-term tests for the mutagenic and carcinogenic potential of pesticides. *J. Environ. Sci. Health.* **B15**(6), 867–906.

Wigle, D. T., *et al.* (1990). Mortality study of Canadian male farm operators: Non-Hodgkin's lymphoma mortality and agricultural practices in Saskatchewan. *J. Nat. Cancer Inst.* **82**(7), 575–582.

Wiklund, K., and Holm, L. E. (1986). Soft tissue sarcoma risk in Swedish agricultural and forestry workers. *J. Nat. Cancer Inst.* **76**(2), 229–234.

Wiklund, K., *et al.* (1987). Soft tissue sarcoma risk among agricultural and forestry workers in Sweden. *Chemosphere* **16**(8/9), 2107–2110.

Wolfe, W. H. (1983). The epidemiology and toxicology of Agent Orange. *In* "Proceedings of the 14th Conference on Environmental Toxicology," Dayton, OH.

Woolson, E. A., Thomas, R. F., and Ensor, P. D. J. (1972). Survey of polychlorodibenzo-p-dioxin content in selected pesticides. *J. Agr. Food Chem.* **20**(2), 351–354.

World Health Organization (WHO) (1975). "Evaluations of Some Pesticides in Food," The Monographs, WHO Pesticide Series No. 4, pp. 159–183. World Health Organization, Geneva.

World Health Organization (WHO) (1984). "2,4-Dichlorophenoxyacetic Acid (2,4-D)." Environmental Health Criteria 29, pp. 1–151. IPCS International Programme on Chemical Safety, United Nations Environment Programme, International Labour Organisation, and the World Health Organisation.

Yano, B. L., Cosse, P. F., Atkin, L., and Corley, R. A. (1991a). "2,4-D Isopropylamine Salt (2,4-D IPA): A 13-Week Dietary Toxicity Study in Fischer 344 Rats." ID. HET m-004725-006. Dow Elanco, Indianapolis, IN.

Yano, B. L., Cosse, P. F., Markham, D. A., and Atkin, L. (1991b). "2,4-D Triisopropanolamine Salt (2,4-D IPA): A 13-Week Dietary Toxicity Study in Fischer 344 Rats." ID. K-008866-006. DowElanco, Indianapolis, IN.

Yeary, R. A. (1986). Urinary excretion of 2,4-D in commercial lawn specialists. *Appl. Ind. Hyg.* **(1)**3, 119–121.

Ylitalo, P., Narhi, U., and Elo, H. A. (1990). Increase in the acute toxicity and brain concentrations of chlorophenoxyacetic acids by probenicid in rats. *Gen. Pharmacol.* **21**(5), 811–814.

Yoder, J., Watson, M., and Benson, W. W. (1973). Lymphocyte chromosome analysis of agricultural workers during extensive occupational exposure to pesticides. *Mutat. Res.* **21**, 335–340.

Zablotny, C. L., Yano, B. L., and Breslin, W. J. (1991). "2,4-D Triisopropanolamine Salt (2,4-D TIPA): A 13-Week Dietary Toxicity Study in Fischer 344 Rats." Unpublished Report No. K-008866-006.

Zahm, S. H., *et al.* (1990). A case-control study of non-Hodgkin's lymphoma and the herbicide 2,4-dichlorophenoxyacetic acid (2,4-D) in eastern Nebraska. *Epidemiology* **1**(5), 349–356.

Zahm, S. H. (1997). Mortality study of pesticide applicators and other employees of a lawn care service company. *J. Occup. Environ. Med.* **39**(11), 1055–1067.

Zetterberg, G. (1978). Genetic effects of phenoxy acids on microorganisms. *Ecol. Bull.* **27**, 193–204.

Zetterberg, G., Busk, L., Elovson, R., Starec-Nordenhammar, I., and Ryttman, H. (1977). The influence of pH on the effects of 2,4-D (2,4-dichlorophenoxyacetic acid, Na salt) on the *Saccharomyces cerevisiae* and *Salmonella typhimurium. Mutat. Res.* **42**, 3–18.

Zhamsaranova, S. D., Lebedeva, S. N., and Lyashenko, V. A. (1987). The immunodepressive effects of the herbicide 2,4-D in mice. *Gig. I. Sanit.* **5**, 80–81.

CHAPTER

73

Dicamba

Paul Harp
Virginia Polytechnic State University

Chemical name: 3, 6-dichloro–2–methoxybenzoic acid or 3,6-dichloro–*o*–anisic acid.

Structure:

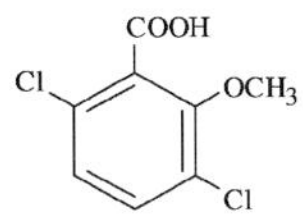

73.1 SYNONYMS

Common names are dicamba (ANSI, BSI, ISO, WSSA) and dianat (USSR). Code numbers include CAS 1918-00-9, CAS 1982-69-0 (for the sodium salt), CAS 2300-66-5 (dicamba dimethylammonium), SHA 029801, and Velsicol 58-CS-11. Trade names include Banfel®, Banvel®, Banvel® 4S, Banvel® CST, Banvel® D, Banvel® S, Banvel® XG, Clarity® 4S, Metambane®, Veteran® 10G, and Veteran® CST. Combinations of dicamba and other herbicides are marketed in products such as Banlene Plus®, Banlene Solo®, Brushmaster®, Celebrity®, Diptyl®, Distinct®, Docklene®, Durtok® 540, Durtok® Amina 270, Fallowmaster®, Field Marshall®, Grassland Herbicide®, Marksman®, Northstar®, Novertex® gazons H, OpTill®, Resolve®, Selectone G®, Trimec® 992, Trimec® Bentgrass, Trimec® Brush Killer, Trimec® Classic, Trimec® Encore, Trimec® Plus, Trimec® S.I., Trimec® Southern, Trimonal®, Tri-Power®, Veteran® 720, Veteran® 2010, Wallop®, and Weedmaster®.

73.2 PHYSICAL AND CHEMICAL PROPERTIES

Dicamba in pure form is an odorless white crystalline solid with a melting point of 114–116°C and a vapor pressure at 100°C of 3.75×10^{-3} mm Hg. The chemical formula is $C_8H_6Cl_2O_3$ and the molecular weight is 221.04. Technical grade dicamba (80–90% purity) is a crystalline solid with a pale buff color. Dicamba is soluble in water and is resistant to hydrolysis and oxidation under normal environmental conditions.

73.3 FORMULATIONS AND USES

Dicamba is a benzoic acid herbicide that acts by mimicking the effects of auxins (i.e., natural plant growth hormones), causing enhanced but uncontrolled growth rates, alterations in plant function homeostasis, and death. Liquid, pellet, and granule formulations are available that contain either the acid or one of several salts (diglycolamine, dimethylamine, dimethylammonium, isopropylamine, potassium, or sodium). As indicated in Section 73.1, dicamba is often combined with one or several other herbicidal agents including 2,4-D, 2,4-DP, atrazine, glyphosate, imazethapyr, ioxynil, MCPA, and mecoprop. It is used to control a wide spectrum of annual and perennial broadleaf weeds and is effective in both pre- and post-emergence applications. A primary agricultural use is weed reduction in grain/cereal crops. Industrial/commercial applications include maintenance of pastures, forest lands, fence rows, and transportation and utility rights-of-way.

73.4 TOXICOKINETICS

Dicamba is readily absorbed following ingestion, but only minimal absorption occurs after dermal exposure. Following ingestion, dicamba appears to be rapidly and nonselectively distributed to most organ systems. Most animal studies indicate greater than 90% of the original dose ultimately undergoes urinary excretion. Small amounts of dicamba are excreted in the feces and have been shown to represent both true elimination (indicated after subcutaneous administration) and excretion of unabsorbed herbicide (following oral exposure). Dicamba is excreted mostly in unmetabolized form but may also be conjugated with glucuronic acid or glycine. Elimination occurs rapidly, and there is no evidence of bioaccumulation in mammalian systems.

73.5 TOXICITY TO LABORATORY ANIMALS

Dicamba has a low mammalian toxicity, with reported oral LD_{50} values in rats ranging from 757 to 2629 mg/kg. Mouse oral LD$_{50}$ values are greater than 1000 mg/kg, and values ranging from 566 to 3000 mg/kg have been reported for rabbits and guinea pigs. Dermal LD$_{50}$ values in rabbits are greater than 2000 mg/kg.

73.6 TOXICITY TO HUMANS

Evaluation of the specific adverse effects of dicamba in humans has been confounded by the relatively small amount of data available from exposures exclusively to dicamba. Many of the documented exposures have been to products containing a combination of herbicidal agents. Signs of dicamba intoxication include vomiting, bradycardia, shortness of breath, cyanosis, depression, incontinence, muscular weakness/exhaustion subsequent to muscle spasms (myotonia), and death. Survivors usually recover quickly (within 2–3 days) with no long-term effects. Dicamba is a mildly corrosive sensitizing agent, and skin irritation or burns can follow dermal exposure. Eye contact can result in a temporary clouding of the cornea that may persist for 5 to 7 days. However, more severe or permanent ocular damage is possible and appropriate eye protection should be used, especially when working with concentrated solutions.

A study of circulating cholinesterase activity in pesticide applicators has suggested an anticholinesterase action of dicamba (Potter *et al.*, 1993). Of the 14 herbicide appliers in the study that worked with dicamba, six had significant reductions (>20%) in red blood cell (RBC) acetylcholinesterase (AChE) activity. The six workers applied an average seasonal volume of 191 gallons of dicamba, while the eight workers without significant AChE inhibition applied an average of only 17 gallons. None of the workers had reductions in plasma butyrlcholinesterase, however, even though *in vitro* experiments with commercial-grade dicamba showed significant inhibition of both RBC and plasma cholinesterase [IC$_{50}$ ≈ 70 ppm (Potter *et al.*, 1993)]. Contamination of the commercial-grade dicamba with impurities capable of inhibiting cholinesterase could explain the apparent anticholinesterase activity of dicamba. Conversely, the structural similarity to a group of amphiphilic agents known to inhibit RBC AChE may indicate an ability of dicamba to alter the conformational state of the membrane-bound enzyme.

73.7 REPRODUCTIVE EFFECTS

No adverse effects were measured in a three-generation study in rats treated with dicamba.

73.8 GENOTOXIC EFFECTS

Dicamba has been examined for possible carcinogenic or mutagenic activity with somewhat contradictory and inconclusive results. In early studies, rats chronically exposed to dicamba (25 mg/kg/day for 2 years) did not exhibit an increase in tumor formation (U.S. EPA, 1988). Perocco and co-workers (1990), however, reported a DNA-damaging potential of dicamba based on an enhanced unwinding rate of rat liver DNA following *in vivo* dicamba administration. Using *in vitro* experiments with human peripheral blood lymphocytes, dicamba induced unscheduled DNA synthesis and slightly increased the frequency of sister chromatid exchange. Conversely, several studies prior to the work of Perocco *et al.* (1990) reported negative results for mutagenicity using various non-mammalian-based assay systems. More recent work (Hrelia *et al.*, 1994) with mammalian tissue also failed to detect any clastogenic activity of dicamba, but the difference in results compared with Perocco *et al.* (1990) may reflect differences associated with exposure route (*in vivo* versus *in vitro*).

Dicamba has been shown to induce peroxisomal enzymes in rat liver and cause transcriptional upregulation of the peroxisome proliferator-activated receptor (Espandiari *et al.*, 1995). Although tumorigenic effects of dicamba have not been reported, long-term exposure to peroxisome proliferators has been associated with increased hepatic tumor frequency in rodents. Further investigation also revealed activation of hepatic nuclear factor-κB, a transcription factor that may be involved in the hepatocarcinogenic action of certain peroxisome proliferators (Espandiari *et al.*, 1998). The exact implications of these findings are unclear and may represent actions of dicamba that require further study in order to fully understand any possible long-term consequences of chronic exposure to the herbicide.

73.9 TREATMENT OF POISONING

Treatment is symptomatic and supportive. No specific antidote is available.

REFERENCES

Espandiari, P., Ludewig, G., Glauert, H. P., and Robertson, L. W. (1998). Activation of hepatic NF-κB by the herbicide dicamba (2-methoxy-3,6-dichlorobenzoic acid) in female and male rats. *J. Biochem. Mol. Toxicol.* **12**, 339–344.

Espandiari, P., Thomas, V. A., Glauert, H. P., O'Brien, M., Noonan, D., and Robertson, L. W. (1995). The herbicide dicamba (2-methoxy-3,6-dichlorobenzoic acid) is a peroxisome proliferator in rats. *Fundam. Appl. Toxicol.* **26**, 85–90.

Hrelia, P., Vigagni, F., Maffei, F., Morotti, M., Colacci, A., Perocco, P., Grilli, S., and Cantelli-Forti, G. (1994). Genetic safety evaluation of pesticides in different short-term tests. *Mutat. Res.* **321**, 219–228.

Perocco, P., Ancora, G., Rani, P., Valenti, A. M., Mazzullo, M., Colacci, A., and Grilli, S. (1990). Evaluation of genotoxic effects of the herbicide dicamba using in vivo and in vitro test systems. *Environ. Mol. Mutagen.* **15**, 131–135.

Potter, W. T., Garry, V. F., Kelly, J. T., Tarone, R., Griffith, J., and Nelson, R. L. (1993). Radiometric assay of red cell and plasma cholinesterase in pesticide appliers from Minnesota. *Toxicol. Appl. Pharmacol.* **119**, 150–155.

U.S. Environmental Protection Agency (1988). "Dicamba: Health Advisory." Office of Drinking Water, U.S. EPA, Washington, DC.

Imidazolinones*

Frederick G. Hess and Jane E. Harris
BASF Corporation
Kimberly Pendino
Hoffman-La Roche, Inc.
Kathryn Ponnock
Middlesex County Community College

74.1 IDENTITY, PROPERTIES, AND USES

74.1.1 CHEMICAL NAMES

Imazapyr (Arsenal® herbicide): 2-(4-isopropyl-4-methyl-5-oxo-2-imidazolin-2-yl) nicotinic acid.

Imazamethabenz-methyl (Assert® herbicide): methyl 2-(4-isopropyl-4-methyl-5-oxo-2-imidazolin-2-yl)-p-toluate mixed with methyl 6-(4-isopropyl-4-methyl-5-oxo-2-imidazolin-2-yl)-m-toluate (3:2).

Imazapic (Cadre® herbicide): 2-(4-isopropyl-4-methyl-5-oxo-2-imidazolin-2-yl)-5-methylnicotinic acid.

Imazethapyr (Pursuit® herbicide): 5-ethyl-2-(4-isopropyl-4-methyl-5-oxo-2-imidazolin-2-yl) nicotinic acid.

Imazamox (Raptor® herbicide): 2-(4-isopropyl-4-methyl-5-oxo-2-imidazolin-2-yl)-5-(methoxymethyl) nicotinic acid.

Imazaquin (Scepter® herbicide): 2-(4-isopropyl-4-methyl-5-oxo-2-imidazolin-2-yl)-3-quinoline carboxylic acid.

74.1.2 PHYSICAL AND CHEMICAL PROPERTIES

The physical and chemical properties of the six imidazolinone herbicides (technical products) are presented in Table 74.1. The

*The summaries and evaluations contained in this chapter are, in most cases, based on unpublished proprietary data. A registration authority should not grant a registration on the basis of this information unless it has first received authorization for such use from the owner of the data or has received the data on which these summaries are based, either from the owner of the data or from a second party that has obtained permission from the owner of the data for this purpose.

respective empirical formulas, molecular weights (range from 261–311), physical state (off-white to tan powders), melting points (range from 144–222°C), and vapor pressures ($<1 \times 10^{-7}$ mm Hg) are very similar. One might expect that such close similarities in physical properties would be reflected in similarities of toxicological profiles, as discussed in Section 74.2.

The very low vapor pressures of the imidazolinones indicate a low potential to volatilize. With the exception of imazamethabenz-methyl, which is an ester, the imidazolinones have pK_a values (dissociation constants) for the carboxylic acid group that range from 3.0 to 3.5. Based on these dissociation constants, both the water solubility and n-octanol/water partition coefficients are pH dependent. For example, if the localized pH is above approximately 3.5, the amount of the imidazolinone in ionized form increases, which consequently increases water solubility and decreases the n-octanol/water partition coefficients. In contrast, if the local pH is below approximately 3.0, the amount of the imidazolinone in ionized form decreases, which consequently decreases water solubility and increases the n-octanol/water partition coefficients. In addition, the imidazolinone herbicides demonstrate other dissociation constants at approximately 2 and 11, which, in turn, alter the specific water solubility and n-octanol/water partition coefficients.

74.1.3 STRUCTURE

The chemical structures of the respective imidazolinone herbicides bear a close resemblance to each other, as presented in Fig. 74.1. The active molecule of each compound has an identical imidazolinone ring structure with a carboxylic acid group, or specifically a carboxylic ester group for imazamethabenz-methyl, attached to respective backbone groups, such as a pyridine ring.

Table 74.1

Comparison of the Physical and Chemical Properties of the Imidazolinone Herbicides

Properties	Technical herbicide					
	Imazapyr	Imazamethabenz-methyl	Imazapic	Imazethapyr	Imazamox	Imazaquin
Empirical formula	$C_{13}H_{15}N_3O_3$	$C_{16}H_{20}N_2O_3$	$C_{14}H_{17}N_3O_3$	$C_{15}H_{19}N_3O_3$	$C_{15}H_{19}N_4O_3$	$C_{17}H_{17}N_3O_3$
Molecular weight	261	288	275	289	305	311
Physical state	White-to-tan powder	Off-white powder	Off-white-to-tan powder	Light-tan powder	Off-white powder	Light-tan powder
Melting point	169–173°C	144–153°C	204–206°C	177–179°C	166–167°C	219–222°C
Vapor pressure	$<1 \times 10^{-7}$ mmHg at 60°C	1.13×10^{-8} mmHg at 25°C	$<1 \times 10^{-7}$ mmHg at 60°C	$<1 \times 10^{-7}$ mmHg at 60°C	$<1 \times 10^{-7}$ mmHg at 60°C	$<2 \times 10^{-8}$ mmHg at 45°C

Several of the compounds show very similar structure–activity relationships. For instance, imazapic, imazethapyr, imazamox, and imazaquin differ only by the respective substituent groups that are attached to the pyridine ring (Fig. 74.1). Imazapic has a methyl group, whereas imazethapyr has an ethyl group, imazamox has a methoxymethyl group, and imazaquin has a benzene ring fused to the pyridine ring. One might expect that such close resemblance in chemical structures would be reflected in similarities of toxicological profiles, as discussed in Section 74.2.

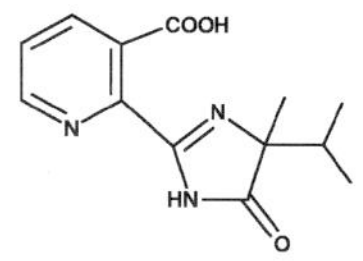

74.1.4 HISTORY AND USES

The unique class of synthetic chemical compounds called the imidazolinone herbicides was discovered in the 1970s, with the first U.S. patent awarded in 1980 for imazamethabenz-methyl (Assert®). Other imidazolinones in the series, imazapyr (Arsenal®), imazapic (Cadre®), imazethapyr (Pursuit®), and imazaquin (Scepter®), received U.S. patents in 1989. More recently, imazamox (Raptor®) received a U.S. patent in 1994.

The active ingredients of the imidazolinone herbicides are effective for selective postemergent weed control for the following crops: cereals, including wheat and barley (imazamethabenz-methyl); peanuts (imazapic); soybeans (imazamox, imazaquin, and imazethapyr); and other legumes, including peas, beans, and alfalfa (imazamox and imazethapyr). In addition, imazapyr is a broad-spectrum herbicide that is effective for noncrop uses for total vegetation control on industrial sites and railroad, highway, and utility rights-of-way and for forestry applications.

Most recently, the imidazolinone herbicides have shown specificity for postemergent weed control on imidazolinone-tolerant corn called Imi-Corn® (imazethapyr and imazapyr), Smart™ canola (imazethapyr and imazamox), imidazolinone-tolerant rice (imazethapyr), imidazolinone-tolerant sugar beet (imazamox), and imidazolinone-tolerant wheat (imazamox).

After application, each imidazolinone herbicide is taken up by the foliage and/or roots of the susceptible weed, and subsequently, becomes translocated throughout the plant. Susceptible weeds stop growing and competing with the specific crop shortly after translocation; the weeds die within several weeks postapplication.

imazapyr
(ARSENAL® herbicide)
(BAS 693 H)

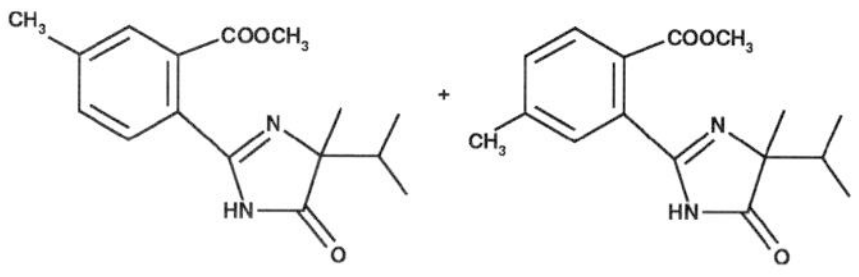

imazamethabenz-methyl
(ASSERT® herbicide)
(BAS 712 H)

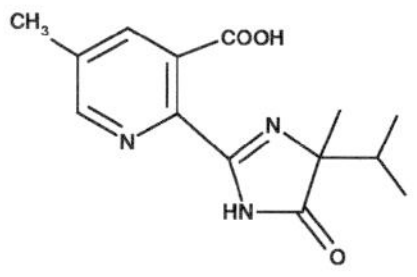

imazapic
(CADRE® herbicide)
(BAS 715 H)

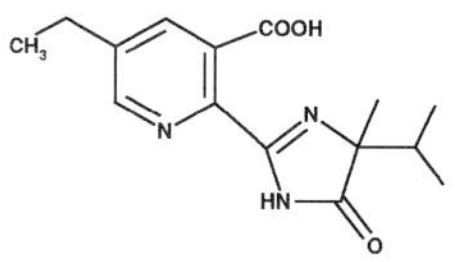

imazethapyr
(PURSUIT® herbicide)
(BAS 685 H)

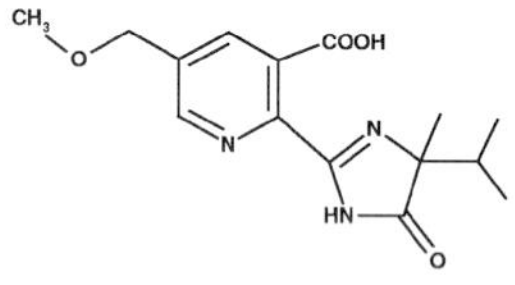

imazamox
(RAPTOR® herbicide)
(BAS 720 H)

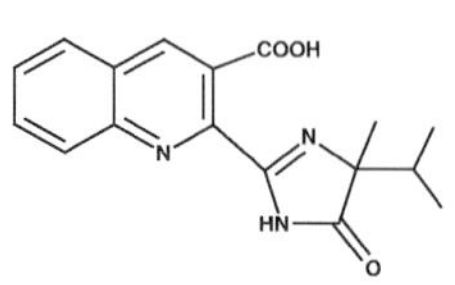

imazaquin
(SCEPTER® herbicide)
(BAS 725 H)

® Registered Trademark of BASF Corporation

Figure 74.1 Chemical structures of the imidazolinone herbicides.

74.2 TOXICITY TO LABORATORY ANIMALS

Following extensive testing in the required mammalian toxicity studies, the six imidazolinone herbicides demonstrate a low toxicological potential. The results of these studies with the respective technical products are presented in Table 74.2.

The imidazolinone herbicides demonstrate this very low toxicity profile in mammals because their herbicidal activity relies on their mode of action, that is, the inhibition of the specific plant enzyme, acetohydroxyacid synthase (AHAS). AHAS is an important biosynthetic enzyme in the formation of three branched-chain aliphatic amino acids, namely, isoleucine, leucine, and valine, and is found in plant but not mammalian tissues. This inhibition of AHAS disrupts protein synthesis and subsequently interferes with DNA synthesis and cell growth, eventually leading to cell death in the specific weed, as described in Section 74.1.

74.2.1 BASIC FINDINGS

74.2.1.1 Acute Toxicity Studies

The results of the acute toxicity tests indicate that the technical products of the imidazolinone herbicides are generally relatively nontoxic (U.S. EPA Toxicity Category IV) by the oral and inhalation routes of administration and only slightly toxic (Category III) by the dermal route, according to the respective LD_{50} and LC_{50} values presented in Table 74.2. Further, the technical products of this class of chemical compounds are either nonirritating or only slightly irritating in the rabbit primary skin irritation studies. The skin sensitization studies in guinea pigs, conducted according to the method of Buehler, demonstrate that the technical products of the six imidazolinone herbicides are nonsensitizers (Table 74.2).

Results from the rabbit primary eye irritation studies with the technical products of the imidazolinone herbicides ranged from no irritation (imazaquin) to slightly irritating (imazamethabenz-methyl and imazamox) to moderately irritating (imazapic and imazethapyr), showing complete recovery by day 7 postdosing. Consequently, these five imidazolinone herbicides are classified into U.S. EPA Toxicity Category III or IV. Finally, the rabbit primary eye irritation study with imazapyr demonstrated irreversible irritation (Category I) based on two out of six animals with scattered opacities at day 21. Thus, the labels for imazapyr's formulated products recommend protective eyewear, which should mitigate any potential for eye irritation during mixing/loading and application.

74.2.1.2 Short-Term/Subchronic Toxicity Studies

21-Day Dermal Studies in the Rabbit All six imidazolinone herbicides showed no dermal or systemic toxicity following 21 days of dermal exposure (6 hours per day, 5 days per week) at the highest doses tested, supporting no observable effect levels (NOELs) at the highest doses tested. Specifically, these no-effect levels were 1000 mg/kg body weight/day for imazapic, imazethapyr, imazamox (28-day study), and imazaquin; and 400 and 200 mg/kg body weight/day for imazapyr and imazamethabenz-methyl, respectively.

90-Day Dietary Toxicity Studies in the Dog Subchronic (90-day) feeding studies were conducted in dogs with imazapyr, imazethapyr, and imazamox. For these subchronic (90-day) feeding studies, the imidazolinone herbicides showed no systemic toxicity at the highest concentrations tested. Specifically, the NOELs were 10,000 ppm for imazapyr and imazethapyr and 40,000 ppm for imazamox. These highest dietary concentrations are equivalent to approximately 250 mg/kg body weight/day for imazapyr and imazethapyr, and equivalent to an approximate daily intake value of 1370 mg/kg body weight/day for imazamox, as calculated from food consumption data.

90-Day Dietary Toxicity Studies in the Rat For the subchronic (90-day) feeding studies in rats, most of the imidazolinone herbicides showed no systemic toxicity when tested at very high dietary concentrations of 20,000 ppm (imazapyr, imazapic, and imazamox) or 10,000 ppm (imazethapyr and imazaquin). Moreover, these highest dietary concentrations are equivalent to approximate daily intake values of 1740 mg/kg body weight/day (imazapyr), 1625 mg/kg body weight/day (imazapic), 1660 mg/kg body weight/day (imazamox), 820 mg/kg body weight/day (imazethapyr), and 830 mg/kg body weight/day (imazaquin), as calculated from food consumption data.

Only imazamethabenz-methyl induced several mild treatment-related effects following 90 days of dietary exposure at the two highest concentrations tested, 5000 and 10,000 ppm. Specifically, slight but consistent decreases in mean body weight occurred for males and females at 5000 and 10,000 ppm, as compared to controls. These reductions in body weights resulted in decreases in overall body weight gain of 8% and 6% for males at 5000 and 10,000 ppm, respectively. For females at both 5000 and 10,000 ppm, overall body weights were decreased by 5%, as compared to controls. No effects on mean body weight or body weight gain were noted for males or females at 1000 ppm, the lowest dietary concentration tested. In addition, statistically significant increased relative (to body weight) liver weights were observed for males at 10,000 ppm, as compared to controls. Increased incidences of hepatocellular hypertrophy were noted for male rats at 5000 ppm (14/19) and 10,000 ppm (20/20), as compared to controls (0/20). The microscopic change of hepatocellular hypertrophy may represent an adaptive response in the liver, that is, induction of microsomal enzymes, which is generally not considered to be a toxic effect (Popp and Cattley, 1991). It is known that this morphological change and associated enzyme induction are reversible following withdrawal of chemical treatment (Popp and Cattley, 1991). In conclusion, for the 90-day dietary toxicity study in rats with imazamethabenz-methyl, the no-effect level was the lowest concentration tested, 1000 ppm (equivalent to approx-

Table 74.2

Comparison of Mammalian Toxicity Data and Genotoxicity Data for the Imidazolinone Herbicides

Study	Technical herbicide					
	Imazapyr	Imazamethabenz-methyl	Imazapic	Imazethapyr	Imazamox	Imazaquin
Acute toxicity						
Acute oral toxicity (rat) LD_{50}	>5000 mg/kg (relatively nontoxic) (Category IV)	>5000 mg/kg (relatively nontoxic) (Category IV)	>5000 mg/kg (relatively nontoxic) (Category IV)	>5000 mg/kg (relatively nontoxic) (Category IV)	>5000 mg/kg (relatively nontoxic) (Category IV)	>5000 mg/kg (relatively nontoxic) (Category IV)
Acute dermal toxicity (rabbit) LD_{50}	>2000 mg/kg (slightly toxic) (Category III)	>2000 mg/kg (slightly toxic) (Category III)	>2000 mg/kg (slightly toxic) (Category III)	>2000 mg/kg (slightly toxic) (Category III)	>4000 mg/kg (slightly toxic) (Category III)	>2000 mg/kg (slightly toxic) (Category III)
Acute inhalation toxicity (rat) LC_{50} (analytical)	>1.3 mg/l (slightly toxic) (Category III)	>1.4 mg/l (slightly toxic) (Category III)	>4.8 mg/l (relatively nontoxic) (Category IV)	>3.3 mg/l (relatively nontoxic) (Category IV)	>6.3 mg/l (relatively nontoxic) (Category IV)	>5.7 mg/l (relatively nontoxic) (Category IV)
Primary dermal irritation (rabbit)	Slight irritation (Category III)	Nonirritating (Category IV)	Slight irritation (Category IV)	Slight irritation (Category IV)	Slight irritation (Category IV)	Slight irritation (Category III)
Primary eye irritation (rabbit)	Irreversible irritation (Category I)	Slight irritation (Category III)	Moderate irritation (Category III)	Moderate irritation (Category III)	Slight irritation (Category III)	Nonirritating (Category IV)
Dermal sensitization (guinea pig) (Buehler method)	Nonsensitizer	Nonsensitizer	Nonsensitizer	Nonsensitizer	Nonsensitizer	Nonsensitizer

(continues)

Table 74.2
(*continued*)

Study	Technical herbicide					
	Imazapyr	Imazamethabenz-methyl	Imazapic	Imazethapyr	Imazamox	Imazaquin
Short-term/ subchronic toxicity						
21-day dermal (Rabbit) No observable effect level	400 mg/kg b.w./day (HDT)	200 mg/kg b.w./day (HDT) (HDT)	1000 mg/kg b.w./day (HDT)	1000 mg/kg b.w./day (HDT) (HDT)	1000 mg/kg b.w./day (HDT) (28-day dermal)	1000 mg/kg b.w./day (HDT)
90-day dietary (dog) No observable effect level	10,000 ppm (HCT) (≈250 mg/kg b.w./day)	—	—	10,000 ppm (HCT) (≈250 mg/kg b.w./day)	40,000 ppm (HCT) (1370 mg/kg b.w./day) (based on FC data)	—
90-day dietary (rat) No observable effect level	20,000 ppm (HCT) (1740 mg/kg b.w./day) (based on FC data)	1000 ppm (87.5 mg/kg b.w./day) (based on FC data)	20,000 ppm (HCT) (1625 mg/kg b.w./day) (based on FC data)	10,000 ppm (HCT) (820 mg/kg b.w./day) (based on FC data)	20,000 ppm (HCT) (1660 mg/kg b.w./day) (based on FC data)	10,000 ppm (HCT) (830 mg/kg b.w./day) (based on FC data)
Chronic toxicity						
1-year dietary (dog) No observable effect level	10,000 ppm (HCT) (≈250 mg/kg b.w./day)	1000 ppm (≈25 mg/kg b.w./day)	No observable adverse effect level = 5000 ppm (135 mg/kg b.w./day) (based on FC data)	1000 ppm (≈25 mg/kg b.w./day)	40,000 ppm (HCT) (1165 mg/kg b.w./day) (based on FC data)	1000 ppm (≈25 mg/kg b.w./day)

(*continues*)

Table 74.2
(*continued*)

Study	Technical herbicide					
	Imazapyr	Imazamethabenz-methyl	Imazapic	Imazethapyr	Imazamox	Imazaquin
Chronic toxicity/ oncogenecity 18-month dietary (mouse)						
Systemic toxicity No observable effect level	10,000 ppm (HCT) (≈1500 mg/kg b.w./day)	No observable Adverse effect level = 525 ppm (≈79 mg/kg b.w./day)	7000 ppm (HCT) (1135 mg/kg b.w./day) (based on FC data)	5000 ppm (≈750 mg/kg b.w./day)	7000 ppm (HCT) (1200 mg/kg b.w./day) (based on FC data)	1000 ppm (≈150 mg/kg b.w./day)
Oncogenicity No observable effect level	10,000 ppm (HCT) (≈1500 mg/kg b.w./day)	2100 ppm (HCT) (≈315 mg/kg b.w./day)	7000 ppm (HCT) (1135 mg/kg b.w./day) (based on FC data)	10,000 ppm (HCT) (≈1500 mg/kg b.w./day)	7000 ppm (HCT) (1200 mg/kg b.w./day) (based on FC data)	4000 ppm (HCT) (≈600 mg/kg b.w./day)
2-year dietary (rat)						
Systemic toxicity No observable effect level	10,000 ppm (HCT) (500 mg/kg b.w./day — males; 640 mg/kg b.w./day — females) (based on FC data)	250 ppm (≈12.5 mg/kg b.w./day)	20,000 ppm (HCT) (1030 mg/kg b.w./day) (based on FC data)	10,000 ppm (HCT) (≈500 mg/kg b.w./day)	20,000 ppm (HCT) (1165 mg/kg b.w./day) (based on FC data)	10,000 ppm (HCT) (≈500 mg/kg b.w./day)
Oncogenicity No observable effect level	10,000 ppm (HCT) (500 mg/kg b.w./day — males; 640 mg/kg b.w./day — females) (based on FC data)	4000 ppm (HCT) (≈200 mg/kg b.w./day)	20,000 ppm (HCT) (1030 mg/kg b.w./day) (based on FC data)	10,000 ppm (HCT) (≈500 mg/kg b.w./day)	20,000 ppm (HCT) (1165 mg/kg b.w./day) (based on FC data)	10,000 ppm (HCT) (≈500 mg/kg b.w./day)

(*continues*)

Table 74.2
(*continued*)

	Technical herbicide					
Study	Imazapyr	Imazamethabenz-methyl	Imazapic	Imazethapyr	Imazamox	Imazaquin
Developmental and reproductive toxicity						
Teratology (rabbit)						
Maternal No observable effect level	400 mg/kg b.w./day (HDT)	500 mg/kg b.w./day	500 mg/kg b.w./day	300 mg/kg b.w./day	300 mg/kg b.w./day	250 mg/kg b.w./day
Developmental No observable effect level	400 mg/kg b.w./day (HDT)	500 mg/kg b.w./day	700 mg/kg b.w./day (HDT)	1000 mg/kg b.w./day (HDT)	900 mg/kg b.w./day (HDT)	500 mg/kg b.w./day (HDT)
Teratology (rat)						
Maternal No observable effect level	300 mg/kg b.w./day	No observable adverse effect level = 1000 mg/kg b.w./day (HDT)	1000 mg/kg b.w./day (HDT)	375 mg/kg b.w./day	500 mg/kg b.w./day	500 mg/kg b.w./day
Developmental No observable effect level	1000 mg/kg b.w./day (HDT)	1000 mg/kg b.w./day (HDT)	1000 mg/kg b.w./day (HDT)	1125 mg/kg b.w./day (HDT)	1000 mg/kg b.w./day (HDT)	500 mg/kg b.w./day
Reproduction (multigeneration) (rat) Reproductive Toxicity No observable effect level	10,000 ppm (HCT) (800 mg/kg b.w./day — males; 980 mg/kg b.w./day – females) (based on FC data)	4000 ppm (HCT) (≈320 mg/kg b.w./day)	20,000 ppm (HCT) (1600 mg/kg b.w./day) (based on FC data)	10,000 ppm (HCT) (≈800 mg/kg b.w./day)	20,000 ppm (HCT) (1640 mg/kg b.w./day) (based on FC data)	10,000 ppm (HCT) (≈800 mg/kg b.w./day)
Genotoxicity [Gene mutations (Ames and mammalian cell); *in vitro* structural chromosomal aberrations; *in vivo* cytogenetics (mouse micronucleus assay)]	Not mutagenic or genotoxic	Not mutagenic or genotoxic	Not mutagenic or genotoxic	Not mutagenic or genotoxic	Not mutagenic or genotoxic	Not mutagenic or genotoxic

Categories are EPA Toxicity Categories.

b.w., body weight; HDT, highest dose tested; HCT, highest concentration tested; ≈, approximately equal to; FC, food consumption.

imately 87.5 mg/kg body weight/day, as based on actual food consumption data).

74.2.1.3 Chronic Toxicity Studies

1-Year Dietary Toxicity Study in the Dog For the 1-year chronic dog studies, imazapyr and imazamox demonstrated no treatment-related effects following dietary exposure at the highest concentration tested (HCT), namely: 10,000 ppm (equivalent to approximately 250 mg/kg body weight/day) for imazapyr and 40,000 ppm (approximately 1165 mg/kg body weight/day, as based on food consumption data) for imazamox (see Table 74.2). For the other imidazolinone herbicides, imazethapyr, imazapic, imazaquin, and imazamethabenz-methyl, slight treatment-related effects were observed in the respective 1-year chronic dog studies.

Specifically, for the 1-year chronic feeding study in dogs with imazethapyr using dietary concentrations of 1000, 5000, and 10,000 ppm, the only treatment-related effects were indicative of a slight anemia, that is, decreased red cell parameters [statistically significant decreases in hematocrit, hemoglobin, red blood cell (RBC) count, mean corpuscular hemoglobin (MCH), mean corpuscular volume (MCV), and mean corpuscular hemoglobin concentration (MCHC)], which were observed at weeks 26 and 52 for females at the mid-concentration (5000 ppm) and the high concentration (10,000 ppm). For this chronic dog study with imazethapyr, no treatment-related histopathological lesions were observed at any dietary concentration, including the highest concentration tested (10,000 ppm). The no observable effect level for the study was 1000 ppm (equivalent to approximately 25 mg/kg/day).

Similar effects indicative of anemia were observed in the 1-year chronic dietary dog study with imazapic. In this study, the anemia occurred in both sexes and at higher dietary concentrations of 20,000 and 40,000 ppm. At the highest concentration tested (40,000 ppm), decreased red blood cell parameters (statistically significant decreases in hematocrit, hemoglobin, RBC count, MCH, MCV, and MCHC) were observed at weeks 5, 6, 13, 26, and 52 for males and females with accompanying statistically significant increased numbers of normoblasts and reticulocytes, as compared to controls. In addition, in the 40,000 ppm treatment group, increased incidences of erythropoiesis were observed microscopically in the bone marrow (5 of 6 males, 6 of 6 females) and spleen (4 of 6 males, 2 of 6 females), as compared to controls (0 of 6 males, 0 of 6 females for both bone marrow and spleen). For male and female dogs at 20,000 ppm, only transient statistically significant decreases in red blood cell parameters were observed at sporadic time points throughout the study. At the terminal sacrifice, generally slightly increased incidences of erythropoiesis were diagnosed microscopically in the bone marrow of both sexes (2 of 6 males, 1 of 6 females) and spleen of males (1 of 6 males, 0 of 6 females), as compared to controls (0 of 6 males, 0 of 6 females). For male and female dogs at 5000 ppm, no treatment-related effects indicative of anemia were observed.

Further, for most dogs (4 of 5 males and 5 of 6 females) at the 40,000-ppm concentration in the chronic dog study

with imazapic, slight-to-moderate skeletal muscle myopathy was diagnosed microscopically at the terminal sacrifice of 52 weeks, which was preceded by transient increases (beginning at week 5) in the blood serum of the following enzymes contained in skeletal muscle: creatine kinase, aspartate aminotransferase, and lactate dehydrogenase. In addition, one male dog at 40,000 ppm, that died during the study (week 33) with nontreatment-related bronchopneumonia, showed moderate-to-marked skeletal muscle degeneration on microscopic examination.

In contrast, only a limited presence of skeletal myopathy of minimal severity was diagnosed at 20,000 ppm (5 of 6 males and 2 of 6 females) and at 5000 ppm (5 of 6 males and 1 of 6 females). The skeletal myopathy observed at both 5000 and 20,000 ppm was not considered to be adverse because the limited presence of minimal skeletal myopathy at both concentrations was evidenced by only a few fibers out of hundreds evaluated per section per animal. Furthermore, these focal myopathies of minimal severity were not consistently diagnosed in all skeletal muscle sites examined per dog (i.e., vastus and abdominal muscles, diaphragm, and esophagus). Moreover, none of the dogs on study, including the 6 males and 6 females at 40,000 ppm, showed any clinical observations during the 1-year study to indicate any muscle dysfunction. Finally, at the 5000- and 20,000-ppm dietary concentrations, no statistically or biologically significant elevations occurred during the course of the 1-year study in serum enzymes that are normally increased with skeletal muscle myopathy (i.e., creatine kinase, aspartate aminotransferase, or lactate dehydrogenase). For the reasons given previously, the minimal myopathy diagnosed histologically at 5000 and 20,000 ppm was not considered to impair or adversely affect the functional capacity of the affected skeletal muscles. Thus, based on the slight anemia observed at the mid-concentration (20,000 ppm), the lowest dietary concentration (5000 ppm) was regarded as the no observable adverse effect level (NOAEL), equivalent to 135 mg/kg body weight/day, as calculated from actual food consumption data.

Similar skeletal muscle myopathies were observed for another imidazolinone herbicide, imazaquin, having similar structure–activity relationships to imazapic and imazethapyr, as mentioned in Section 74.1. For the 1-year chronic feeding study in dogs with imazaquin, the dietary concentration of 5000 ppm (highest concentration tested) induced slight anemia as evidenced by bone marrow hyperplasia (erythropoiesis), observed microscopically in 2 of 8 males and 4 of 8 females, and slight skeletal myopathy, observed microscopically in 7 of 8 males and 3 of 8 females. In addition, decreased red blood cell parameters indicative of anemia (statistically significant decreases in hematocrit, hemoglobin, RBC count, MCH, MCV, and MCHC) were observed at weeks 13, 26, and 52 for males and females. Additionally, at 5000 ppm, clinical chemistry parameters indicative of slight skeletal myopathy included statistically significant increased mean serum enzyme levels of creatine kinase, aspartate aminotransferase, and lactate dehydrogenase at weeks 13, 26, and/or 52 for males and females. The NOEL for systemic toxicity for this chronic dog study with imazaquin was the mid-concentration of 1000 ppm (equivalent to approximately 25 mg/kg body weight/day), which is the same NOEL in the 1-year dog study with imazethapyr.

Finally, for the 1-year chronic toxicity study in dogs with imazamethabenz-methyl, males and females were fed dietary concentrations of 0, 250, 1000, or 4000 ppm. Body weights at the highest concentration were consistently, but not statistically, lower than the controls for males throughout the study and for females from weeks 1–28. This reduction in body weight resulted in an 11% decrease in overall body weight gain for males at 4000 ppm. There were no treatment-related effects on hematology or clinical chemistry parameters and no treatment-related gross necropsy or microscopic findings. Slight but statistically significant increases in absolute and relative (to body weight) liver weights were noted for females at 4000 ppm, as compared to controls. However, these slight increases in absolute and relative (to body weight) liver weights for females at 4000 ppm are considered to be equivocal because of the absence of statistically significant increases in relative (to brain) liver weights for females at 4000 ppm and the lack of treatment-related histopathological findings in the liver of males or females at 4000 ppm. The absence of hepatocellular hypertrophy in the liver of dogs at 4000 ppm suggests that the small increase in liver weight may not be treatment related. Based on the slight decreases in mean body weights and an 11% decrease in overall body weight gain for males at 4000 ppm, the no observable effect level was 1000 ppm (equivalent to approximately 25 mg/kg body weight/day).

74.2.1.4 Chronic Toxicity/Oncogenicity Studies

18-Month Chronic Toxicity/Oncogenicity Studies in the Mouse For the 18-month mouse feeding studies, all six of the imidazolinone herbicides showed no evidence of potential oncogenicity at the highest dietary concentrations of technical materials tested, namely, 10,000 ppm (imazapyr and imazethapyr), 7000 ppm (imazapic and imazamox), 4000 ppm (imazaquin), and 2100 ppm (imazamethabenz-methyl). Furthermore, three of the imidazolinone herbicides showed no systemic toxicity at the highest dietary concentrations tested, namely, imazapyr (at 10,000 ppm) and both imazapic and imazamox (at 7000 ppm).

The other three imidazolinones showed mild systemic toxicity in the 18-month mouse studies. Specifically, imazamethabenz-methyl was tested in the mouse at dietary concentrations of 0, 130, 525, and 2100 ppm. Mean body weights for females at 2100 ppm were statistically significantly lower than the controls during the first 8 weeks of the study, which resulted in a 7% decrease in overall body weight gain. At terminal sacrifice, mean absolute and relative (to body weight) thyroid/parathyroid weights were slightly but statistically significantly increased for females at 525 ppm and for both males and females at 2100 ppm, as compared to controls. In addition, mean absolute and relative (to body weight) adrenal gland weights were slightly but statistically significantly increased for males at 2100 ppm. However, these slight organ weight changes are not

considered to be adverse because no correlating histopathological changes were noted in the adrenal, thyroid, or parathyroid glands at any dietary concentration in the study. Based on decreased mean body weights and body weight gain for females at 2100 ppm, the no observable adverse effect level (NOAEL) for systemic toxicity was 525 ppm (equivalent to approximately 79 mg/kg body weight/day).

Imazethapyr was tested in the mouse for 18 months at dietary concentrations of 0, 1000, 5000, and 10,000 ppm. The only treatment-related effect occurred at the highest concentration tested (10,000 ppm); that is, decreased overall mean body weight gain was noted in both sexes (14% for males and 24% for females) at 10,000 ppm, as compared to controls. Therefore, the NOEL for systemic toxicity was 5000 ppm (equivalent to approximately 750 mg/kg body weight/day).

Lastly, imazaquin was tested in the mouse for 18 months at dietary concentrations of 0, 250, 1000, and 4000 ppm. The only treatment-related effect occurred at the highest concentration tested (4000 ppm); that is, decreased mean body weights were noted at 4000 ppm, as compared to controls. Specifically, mean body weights of males at 4000 ppm were statistically significantly decreased during the first 12 weeks of the study, resulting in an 8% decrease in body weight gain for weeks 1–12, as compared to control males. In addition, mean body weights of females at 4000 ppm were statistically significantly lower than controls throughout the study, resulting in a decrease in overall mean body weight gain of 15%, as compared to control females. Therefore, the NOEL for systemic toxicity was 1000 ppm (equivalent to approximately 150 mg/kg body weight/day).

2-Year Chronic Toxicity/Oncogenicity Studies in the Rat In chronic studies performed at high dietary concentrations for 2 years in the rat, all six of the imidazolinone herbicides showed no evidence of potential oncogenicity/carcinogenicity. Specifically, no treatment-related increased incidences of benign or malignant tumors were induced by the imidazolinones at the highest concentrations tested, namely, 20,000 ppm (imazapic and imazamox), 10,000 ppm (imazapyr, imazethapyr, and imazaquin), and 4000 ppm (imazamethabenz-methyl). Furthermore, five of the six imidazolinone herbicides showed no systemic toxicity at the highest dietary concentrations tested, namely, imazapic and imazamox (at 20,000 ppm) and imazapyr, imazethapyr, and imazaquin (at 10,000 ppm).

Only imazamethabenz-methyl showed mild systemic toxicity in the 2-year rat feeding study. Specifically, imazamethabenz-methyl was tested in the rat at dietary concentrations of 0, 250, 1000, and 4000 ppm. Mean body weights were slightly but consistently decreased for males and females at 4000 ppm, and for females at 1000 ppm, as compared to controls. For males at 4000 ppm a decreased overall mean body weight gain of 6% was noted, as compared to controls. For females at 1000 and 4000 ppm, respective decreased overall mean body weight gains of 6% and 11% were noted, as compared to controls. There were no treatment-related microscopic lesions with the exception of a statistically significant increased incidence of thymic epithelial hyperplasia in females at 4000 ppm (21/53), as compared to controls (7/49). However, for this 2-year (lifetime) rat study with imazamethabenz-methyl, the thymic hyperplasia did not progress to a neoplastic lesion nor has such a progression been described in the literature. Therefore, for this reason, this hyperplastic change in females at 4000 ppm appears to have only an equivocal toxicologic significance. In conclusion, based on the results from this study, the NOEL for systemic toxicity was 250 ppm (equivalent to approximately 12.5 mg/kg body weight/day).

For imazamethabenz-methyl, the increased incidence of hepatocellular hypertrophy in the liver of male rats at both 5000 and 10,000 ppm, which was noted at termination of the 90-day dietary toxicity study, was not observed at either the 12-month interim sacrifice or the terminal sacrifice of the 2-year chronic rat study at dietary concentrations up to and including 4000 ppm. The absence of this microscopic finding indicates that adaptation probably occurred in the liver following prolonged exposure.

In conclusion, the collective results from the oncogenicity studies in both the rat and the mouse indicate a lack of oncogenic/carcinogenic potential for all six imidazolinone herbicides.

74.2.2 ABSORPTION, DISTRIBUTION, METABOLISM, AND EXCRETION

In the rat metabolism studies with five of the six imidazolinone herbicides, only minimal metabolism is demonstrated. Following single oral gavage doses of imazapyr, imazapic, imazethapyr, imazamox, or imazaquin, these imidazolinone herbicides are rapidly absorbed and excreted, as evidenced by the presence of greater than 70% of unchanged parent compound in the urine within 24–48 h. Although imazamethabenz-methyl is also rapidly absorbed in the rat, greater than 60% becomes metabolized via hydrolysis of the ester to imazamethabenz acid, which is rapidly excreted in the urine within 24 h. The presence of a significant amount of unchanged parent or metabolite in the urine within 24–48 h, indicates rapid absorption of the imidazolinone herbicides from the gastrointestinal tract following a single oral gavage dose, as well as a low potential for bioaccumulation of parent compound or acid metabolite in mammalian tissues.

74.2.3 EFFECTS ON ORGANS AND TISSUES

The only consistent treatment-related effects that were observed in the extensive toxicological profile of the imidazolinone herbicides were slight-to-moderate skeletal myopathy and/or slight anemia in dogs, occurring in the 1-year dietary toxicity studies with three structurally similar imidazolinones (imazapic, imazaquin, and imazethapyr). Specifically, both of these treatment-related effects were seen in male and female dogs treated with imazapic. Slight anemia at 20,000 ppm (mid-concentration) and 40,000 ppm (highest concentration

tested) was noted by decreases in hematological parameters and by histopathological examination, whereas slight-to-moderate skeletal myopathy at 40,000 ppm was determined by clinical chemistry evaluation and histopathological examination. Similarly, both of these treatment-related effects were seen in male and female dogs treated with imazaquin. Slight anemia at 5000 ppm (highest concentration tested) was noted by decreases in hematological parameters and by histopathological examination, whereas slight skeletal myopathy at 5000 ppm was determined by clinical chemistry evaluation and histopathological examination. In contrast, only slight anemia was observed by hematological parameters in female dogs with imazethapyr at both 5000 ppm and 10,000 ppm (highest concentration tested).

There was no evidence of potential carcinogenicity in gross necropsy observations or in microscopic examinations of the full battery of tissues in the rat or mouse for any of the imidazolinone herbicides.

74.2.4 EFFECTS ON REPRODUCTION

Results from the reproductive and developmental toxicity studies indicate that the six imidazolinone herbicides are not reproductive toxicants, developmental toxicants, or teratogens (Table 74.2). Specifically, in the multigeneration reproductive toxicity studies conducted in rats, the imidazolinone herbicides did not affect reproductive performance, nor was there evidence of any significant prenatal or postnatal effects. All six reproduction studies support reproductive NOELs at the highest concentrations tested, namely, 20,000 ppm (imazapic and imazamox), 10,000 ppm (imazapyr, imazethapyr, and imazaquin), or 4000 ppm (imazamethabenz-methyl). These highest dietary concentrations are equivalent to approximate daily intake values of 1600 mg/kg body weight/day (imazapic), 1640 mg/kg body weight/day (imazamox), and 800 mg/kg body weight/day for males and 980 mg/kg body weight/day for females (imazapyr), as calculated from food consumption data. The preceding doses are equivalent to approximately 800 mg/kg body weight/day (imazethapyr and imazaquin) or 320 mg/kg body weight/day (imazamethabenz-methyl).

Further, the teratology studies, which evaluated potential developmental toxicity of the six imidazolinone herbicides in rabbits and rats, revealed no evidence of developmental toxicity or teratogenic effects for fetuses of either species. All six imidazolinones, as tested in rabbits and rats, showed developmental NOELs equal to or higher than the maternal NOEL/NOAELs. For the rabbit teratology studies, the developmental NOELs were 1000 mg/kg body weight/day, the highest dose tested (HDT) for imazethapyr; 900 mg/kg body weight/day (HDT) for imazamox; 700 mg/kg body weight/day (HDT) for imazapic; 500 mg/kg body weight/day for imazamethabenz-methyl, 500 mg/kg body weight/day (HDT) for imazaquin; and 400 mg/kg body weight/day (HDT) for imazapyr. For these rabbit studies, the maternal NOELs were either the same dose level as the developmental no-effect level (e.g., 500 mg/kg body weight/day for imazamethabenz-methyl; 400 mg/kg body weight/day for imazapyr) or lower dose levels of 500 mg/kg body weight/day for imazapic, 300 mg/kg body weight/day for imazethapyr and imazamox, or 250 mg/kg body weight/day for imazaquin. Importantly, for all six imidazolinone herbicides, no treatment-related teratogenic effects were observed in the rabbit fetuses.

For the rat teratology studies, the developmental NOELs were 1000 mg/kg body weight/day, the HDT for imazapyr, imazamethabenz-methyl, imazapic, and imazamox; 500 mg/kg body weight/day (imazaquin); and 375 mg/kg body weight/day (imazethapyr). For these rat studies, the maternal NOEL/ NOAELs were either the same dose level as the developmental no effect level (e.g., 1000 mg/kg body weight/day for imazamethabenz-methyl and imazapic; 500 mg/kg body weight/day for imazaquin) or lower dose levels of 500 mg/kg body weight/day for imazamox, 375 mg/kg body weight/day for imazethapyr or 300 mg/kg body weight/day for imazapyr. Importantly, for all six imidazolinone herbicides, no treatment-related teratogenic effects were observed in the rat fetuses.

In conclusion, based on the results given previously for the multigeneration reproduction studies and the rabbit and rat teratology studies, the imidazolinone herbicides demonstrate a lack of reproductive toxicity and are neither selective developmental toxicants nor teratogens in either the rabbit or the rat.

74.2.5 PATHOLOGY

The only consistent treatment-related effects that were observed microscopically in the extensive toxicological profile of the imidazolinone herbicides were slight anemia and slight-to-moderate skeletal myopathy in dogs, occurring in the 1-year dietary toxicity studies with two structurally similar imidazolinones (imazapic and imazaquin). Specifically, both of these treatment-related effects were seen in male and female dogs treated with imazapic. Slight anemia was noted by histopathological examination (erythropoiesis in the bone marrow and spleen) at 20,000 ppm (mid-concentration) and 40,000 ppm (highest concentration tested). Slight-to-moderate skeletal myopathy was also diagnosed by histopathological examination (skeletal muscle degeneration) at 40,000 ppm (terminal sacrifice). Similarly, both of these treatment-related effects were seen in male and female dogs treated with imazaquin. Slight anemia (erythropoiesis in the bone marrow) was diagnosed at 5000 ppm (highest concentration tested). In addition, slight skeletal myopathy (skeletal muscle degeneration) was observed at 5000 ppm by histopathological examination.

There was no evidence of potential carcinogenicity for any of the imidazolinone herbicides from evaluations of the gross necropsy observations or the microscopic findings of the full battery of tissues in the rat or mouse.

74.2.6 GENOTOXICITY STUDIES

As presented in Table 74.2, based on the battery of *in vitro* and *in vivo* assays, the imidazolinone herbicides show a lack of potential genotoxic activity. This series of tests comprised the genotoxicity testing data requirements for all three categories [i.e., gene mutations (Ames and mammalian cell), *in vitro* structural chromosomal aberrations, and *in vivo* abnormal cytogenetics such as detected in the mouse micronucleus assay using bone marrow cells].

74.3 TOXICITY TO HUMANS

74.3.1 USE EXPERIENCE

There are no incident reports attributable to the active ingredients for workers involved in the manufacturing process of the imidazolinone herbicides or for workers involved in mixing/loading/applying the end-use products of the imidazolinone herbicides for crop or noncrop uses. Results from the acute dermal and oral toxicity data, as cited in Section 74.2, indicate that the imidazolinone herbicides do not pose any acute dermal or dietary risks.

Furthermore, because of their relatively low toxicity to mammals, the imidazolinone herbicides demonstrated relatively high no observable effect levels for potential systemic toxicity in the long-term studies, as cited in Section 74.2. In the absence of genotoxic, carcinogenic, reproductive, or teratogenic effects, a safety factor of 100 ($10\times$ for interspecies differences, $10\times$ for intraspecies differences) is appropriate to calculate the acceptable daily intake (ADI) for chronic human exposure. Applying a low (100-fold) safety factor to these relatively high systemic NOELs from the long-term studies with the imidazolinone herbicides results in ADIs that are relatively high. These relatively high ADIs suggest that this class of compounds does not pose a concern for chronic dietary exposure to humans.

74.3.2 TREATMENT OF POISONING

There are no known cases of accidental or deliberate poisonings in humans. Because of their low toxicity profile and rapid excretion rate (see preceding discussion), the development of any physiological antidotes for the imidazolinone herbicides appears unnecessary. For formulated products, it is advisable to consult the specific material safety data sheet (MSDS) for emergency and first-aid procedures.

REFERENCES

Popp, J. A., and Cattley, R. C. (1991). Hepatobiliary system. *In* "Handbook of Toxicologic Pathology" (W. M. Haschek and C. G. Rousseaux, eds.), pp. 279–314. Academic Press, San Diego.

Toxicology of Triazolopyrimidine Herbicides

Thomas R. Hanley, Jr., and Richard Billington
Dow AgroSciences, LLC

75.1 INTRODUCTION

The triazolopyrimidines are herbicides used for the preemergent and postemergent control of broadleaf weeds in a variety of crops. The general structure of this class is a substituted triazolopyrimidine connected to a substituted phenyl ring through a sulfonamide bridge as presented in Fig. 75.1. The substituents of the various members of this class are presented in Table 75.1. The mode of action is through inhibition of acetolactate synthase (ALS) in plants, though the mechanism appears to be different from that of sulfonylureas. Acetolactate synthase (EC 4.13.18), also known as acetohydroxyacid synthase, is a key enzyme in the synthesis of the branched-chain aliphatic amino acids leucine, isoleucine, and valine. Inhibition of this enzyme in plants results in cessation of cell growth and division, leading to the death of susceptible plants. However, this enzyme is lacking in humans and other animals, which accounts for the low mammalian toxicity of these materials.

Extensive toxicological testing has been conducted with these compounds according to standard test guidelines as published by the U.S. Environmental Protection Agency (EPA), the Organization for Economic Cooperation and Development (OECD), the European Union (EU) and the Japanese Ministry of Agriculture, Forestry and Fisheries (JMAFF) to determine potential health effects. The results of these studies have been evaluated in conjunction with use rates and exposure and residue data to provide comprehensive risk assessments. In general, these materials have low acute toxicity, have low chronic toxicity, and have been negative in tests for mutagenicity. The kidneys and, to a lesser extent, the liver are the primary organs affected by repeated exposure, and in most cases the histologic changes represent adaptive responses. Absorption is rapid, as is excretion, with no evidence of accumulation, and these materials appear, for the most part, to be metabolically stable in mammals. The mammalian toxicity of these materials is reviewed in this chapter.

75.2 CLORANSULAM-METHYL

75.2.1 IDENTITY, PROPERTIES, AND USES

Chemical Name The chemical name for cloransulam-methyl is N-(2-carboxymethyl-6-chlorophenyl)-5-ethoxy-7-fluoro-(1,2,4)triazolo(1,5c)pyrimidine-2-sulfonamide.

Structure See Fig. 75.1 and Table 75.1.

Synonyms Cloransulam-methyl is also known as XR-565, or XDE-565, and is sold as FirstRate® herbicide in the United States, and as PACTO® and SUPRA® herbicides in South America. (All trade names used in this chapter are registered trademarks of Dow AgroSciences, LLC.) The Chemical Abstract Service (CAS) registry number is 147150-35-4.

Physical and Chemical Properties The empirical formula for cloransulam-methyl is $C_{15}H_{13}ClFN_5O_5S$, with a molecular weight of 429.8. It is a solid at room temperature, with a low vapor pressure (3×10^{-16} mm Hg at 25°C). The water solubility is pH dependent, with values of 2.96 mg/l at pH 5, 184 mg/l at pH 7, and 3430 mg/l at pH 9 (20°C). The log K_{ow} is estimated at 3.7; the pK_a is 4.81.

Uses Cloransulam-methyl is used as a soil-applied or incorporated preemergence or postemergence broadleaf herbicide in soybeans at maximum label rates of 44 g per hectare soil applied and 18 g per hectare postemergence.

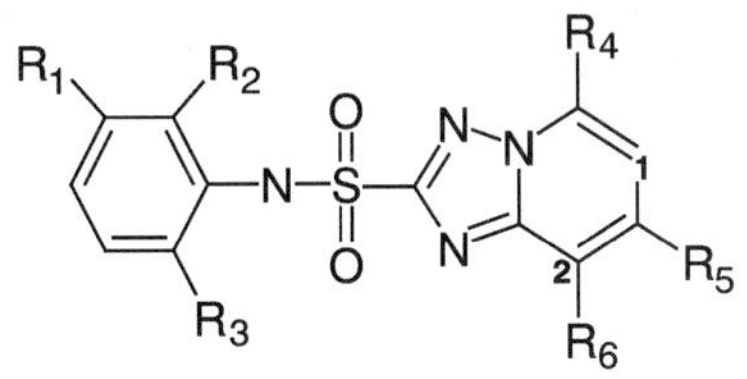

Figure 75.1 Generic structure of the triazolopyrimidine herbicides.

Table 75.1
Substituents of Triazolopyrimidine Sulfonamide Herbicides

	1	2	R_1	R_2	R_3	R_4	R_5	R_6
(1,5c)								
Clorasulam-methyl	N	C	H	CO_2CH_3	Cl	CO_2CH_3	F	H
Diclosulam	N	C	H	Cl	Cl	OCH_2CH_3	F	H
Florasulam	N	C	H	F	F	OCH_3	H	F
(1,5a)								
Flumetsulam	C	N	H	F	F	H	CH_3	—
Metosulam	C	N	CH_3	Cl	Cl	OCH_3	OCH_3	—

75.2.2 TOXICITY TO LABORATORY ANIMALS

Acute Exposure The acute toxicity of cloransulam-methyl was low. The acute oral LD_{50} in the rat was greater than 5000 mg/kg in both males and females and the dermal LD_{50} in the rabbit was greater than 2000 mg/kg. The 4-hr inhalation LC_{50} in the rat was greater than 3.77 mg per liter of air, which was the highest attainable respirable aerosol concentration. Cloransulam-methyl produced no indications of dermal irritation in rabbits or sensitization in the guinea pig, and only slight transient eye irritation in the rabbit following acute exposure (EPA, 1997a, b).

Repeated Exposure Cloransulam-methyl was evaluated in subacute and subchronic dietary studies in rats, mice, and dogs. The primary target organs identified in these studies were the kidneys (rat and mouse), the liver (rat, mouse, and dog), and thyroid (rat).

In the Fischer 344 (F344) rat, dosages of 100–1000 mg/kg/day for 2 weeks produced slight decreases in red blood cell parameters and urine specific gravity in males, and slightly increased cecal and liver weights in females at 1000 mg/kg/day. The no-observed-effect level (NOEL) was 500 mg/kg/day. Dosages of 100–1000 mg/kg/day for 13 weeks produced treatment-related kidney changes consisting of very slight to moderate hypertrophy of collecting tubule epithelial cells and/or slight vacuolation of the renal proximal tubular epithelium consistent with fatty changes in all dosage groups. Decreased body weight gain and feed consumption, very slight hepatocellular vacuolation, and slight thyroid follicular hypertrophy were also seen at 500 and 1000 mg/kg/day (Haut *et al.*, 1991, 1992a; Stebbins and Haut, 1994).

Dosages of 100, 500, or 1000 mg/kg/day fed to B6C3F1 mice for 2 weeks produced slight hepatocellular hypertrophy at 500 mg/kg/day and above in males, and at 1000 mg/kg/day in females. The NOEL was 100 mg/kg/day. Dosages ranging from 50 to 1000 mg/kg/day given for 13 weeks produced slight centrilobular and midzonal hepatocellular hypertrophy at 100 mg/kg/day and above in males, and at 500 mg/kg/day and above in females. Electron microscopy characterized the hypertrophy as an increase in rough endoplasmic reticulum (RER) with a decrease in cytoplasmic glycogen content. Kidney effects in mice consisted of decreased vacuolation of the renal tubules, consistent with decreased cytoplasmic lipid, accompanied by lower kidney weights at 500 mg/kg/day and higher. The subchronic lowest observed effect level (LOEL) and NOEL values in mice were 100 and 50 mg/kg/day, respectively (Haut *et al.*, 1992b; Stebbins and Haut, 1993).

Cloransulam-methyl, when fed to dogs for 2 weeks at dosages of 500 mg/kg/day or higher, produced hepatic inflammation, degeneration, and necrosis. No effects were seen at dosages of 200 mg/kg/day or lower. In a subchronic study, dogs exhibited a taste aversion to this material at dosages of 200 mg/kg/day and above, which resulted in a combination of impaired nutritional status and toxicity of the material. A dosage of 40 mg/kg/day resulted in lower body weight gains. Histologic examination did not identify a target organ, though a subsequent chronic study in dogs identified the liver as the primary target organ. Based on decreased body weights, a subchronic NOEL was not established in dogs (Stebbins *et al.*, 1996; Szabo *et al.*, 1992).

In a 21-day repeated dermal application study in rabbits, cloransulam-methyl at dosages of 100, 500, or 1000 mg/kg/day produced slight anemia in female rabbits at the highest dosage. Male rabbits were unaffected at 1000 mg/kg/day and the NOEL in females was 500 mg/kg/day (Gilbert and Yano, 1995a).

Chronic Toxicity and Carcinogenicity The chronic toxicity of cloransulam-methyl has been evaluated in rats, mice, and dogs. In a 2-year study, Fischer 344 rats were fed cloransulam-methyl at dosages of 10–325 mg/kg/day. Body weight gain was decreased at the highest dosage. Treatment-related histologic effects were limited to the kidneys and thyroid. Hypertrophy of a population of renal collecting duct epithelial cells identified as α-intercalated cells was reported in males and females fed 325 mg/kg/day. (A similar histologic change noted in rats, mice, and dogs following exposure to florasulam will be discussed later in this chapter.) Vacuolation of the proximal tubules (consistent with fatty changes) in males fed cloransulam-methyl at 325 mg/kg/day, and females fed 75 or 325 mg/kg/day, and an increase in the incidence of mineralization of the renal pelvis in males fed 75 or 325 mg/kg/day also were present. Thyroid changes were confined to the high-dosage males (325 mg/kg/day) and consisted of hyperplasia and hypertrophy of follicular epithelium. The NOEL in this study was 10 mg/kg/day (Jeffries *et al.*, 1995a).

B6C3F1 mice were fed diets containing cloransulam-methyl at dosages of 10–1000 mg/kg/day for 2 years. As was seen in subchronic studies, the liver was the primary target organ in mice, with effects also noted in the kidneys. Increases in liver weights in males at ≥100 mg/kg/day and females at 1000 mg/kg/day, and centrilobular hypertrophy in males at ≥ 100 mg/kg/day were the only treatment-related effects noted in the liver. Kidney weights were decreased in males at 1000 mg/kg/day and females at ≥100 mg/kg/day. In the kidneys, depletion of the normal epithelial cytoplasmic vacuoles, and decreases in the incidence of renal mineralization and renal tubular degeneration were noted in males at ≥100 mg/kg/day. All of these histologic changes were interpreted to be either incidental or adaptive–physiologic responses to the test material rather than adverse effects. The NOEL in mice following chronic exposure was 10 mg/kg/day (Jeffries *et al.*, 1995b).

There was no evidence of a tumorigenic or carcinogenic response in either mice or rats following long-term exposure.

In a 1-year chronic toxicity study, beagle dogs were fed dosages of 5–50 mg/kg/day. The only treatment-related effects were in the liver and consisted of a slight-to-moderate increase in accumulation of pigment in Kuppfer cells and hepatocytes, and slight centrilobular and midzonal hepatocellular hypertrophy at ≥10 mg/kg/day, with changes in hepatic-related serum chemistry parameters at 50 mg/kg/day (Szabo and Davis, 1994). The U.S. EPA considered 10 mg/kg/day the NOEL in this study (EPA, 1997a).

Mutagenicity In a battery of genotoxicity tests, cloransulam-methyl showed no evidence of mutagenic potential. These tests included a bacterial reverse mutation assay (Ames test), an *in vitro* cytogenetic assay in Chinese hamster ovary cells (CHO/HGPRT assay), an *in vitro* chromosomal aberration assay in rat lymphocytes, and an *in vivo* cytogenetic assay in mouse bone marrow cells (EPA, 1997a, b).

Neurotoxicity The neurotoxic potential of cloransulam-methyl was evaluated in specialized studies. No neurotoxicologic effects were observed in rats following acute gavage exposure of up to 2000 mg/kg (highest dose tested). A complete battery of neurologic tests including functional observations (handheld and open field observations, grip strength, and landing foot splay), motor activity, and detailed neurohistopathology was conducted following 13-week exposure via the diet to dosages up to 1000 mg/kg/day. No treatment-related neurotoxic effects were observed in any of these measures (Shankar *et al.*, 1993; Spencer *et al.*, 1995).

Reproductive Toxicity Cloransulam-methyl had no effect on reproduction or fetal development. In a multigeneration reproduction study in Sprague-Dawley (SD) rats, dosages of 100 mg/kg/day and above produced kidney and thyroid effects in the adults consistent with effects seen in subchronic and chronic studies. The NOEL for parental animals was 10 mg/kg/day. No

effects on reproductive performance or neonatal survival were seen even at the high dosage of 500 mg/kg/day. In a developmental toxicity study in SD rats, gavage dosages of up to 1000 mg/kg/day (limit test) on gestation days 6–15 produced no maternal or developmental toxicity. In a developmental toxicity study in New Zealand White rabbits administered gavage dosages of 0, 30, 100, or 300 mg/kg/day on gestation days 7–19, maternal weight gain and feed consumption were affected only at 300 mg/kg/day. No adverse embryonal or fetal effects were noted at any dose level (Vedula *et al.*, 1992; Zablotny *et al.*, 1993, 1994).

Absorption, Distribution, Metabolism, and Excretion Metabolism studies were conducted with ^{14}C-radiolabeled cloransulam-methyl in the F344 rat using dose levels of 5 or 1000 mg/kg. At 5 mg/kg, over 90% of either a single dose or repeated (15 days) doses was absorbed. At 1000 mg/kg, only 28–30% of a single dose was absorbed. Urinary elimination was rapid in both cases with half-lives of approximately 6–9 hr. A higher percentage of the 5-mg/kg dose was excreted in the urine by females (68–80%) than by males (40–50%) and these sex-dependent differences in disposition of the 5-mg/kg dose were attributed to more efficient elimination of unchanged cloransulam-methyl in the female versus male kidney. Analyses of urine and fecal extracts indicated that parent cloransulam-methyl accounted for the majority of the excreted radiolabled material. The only metabolite present at amounts greater than 5% was identified as the 4-OH phenyl derivative of cloransulam-methyl. Other minor metabolites included a hydroxylation of the pyrimidine ring, though the position of hydroxylation was not identified, and an *N*-acetyl cysteine conjugate of the parent material. Due to rapid elimination, cloransulam-methyl has little potential to accumulate upon repeated administration (Domoradzki *et al.*, 1995; Nolan *et al.*, 1995).

75.2.3 TOXICITY TO HUMANS

No data are available on accidental human exposures. However, the risk to humans from exposure to cloransulam-methyl following normal use patterns is low. No detectable residues were found either in soybeans or, in most cases, in soybean forage or hay at a limit of detection of 0.005 ppm, and accumulation is unlikely based on plant and animal data. Tolerance levels of 0.02 ppm in soybean, 0.1 ppm for soybean forage, and 0.2 ppm for soybean hay have been established (EPA, 1997a). Using conservative estimates which assume 100% of crops contain the tolerance limit, and a reference dose (RfD) of 0.10 mg/kg/day (based on the NOEL from the chronic dog study), the calculated maximum potential average daily dose from all sources indicate use of less than 0.22% of the RfD in the subgroup with the highest aggregate exposure (nonnursing infants). The EPA estimated the margin of exposure (MOE) for occupational exposure to cloransulam-methyl to be between 2500 and 14,000, based on the use of a NOEL of 10 mg/kg/day (EPA, 1997a).

75.3 DICLOSULAM

75.3.1 IDENTITY, PROPERTIES, AND USES

Chemical Name The chemical name for diclosulam is N-(2,6-dichlorophenyl)-5-ethoxy-7-fluoro-(1,2,4)triazolo(1,5c)pyrimidine-2-sulfonamide.

Structure See Fig. 75.1 and Table 75.1.

Synonyms Diclosulam is also known as XR-564 or XDE-564 and is sold primarily in the United States and South America under the trade names Strongarm®, SPIDER®, and CROSSER® herbicides. The CAS registry number is 145701-21-9.

Physical and Chemical Properties The empirical formula of diclosulam is $C_{13}H_{10}Cl_2FN_5O_3S$, with a molecular weight of 406.2. Diclosulam is a solid, with a burnt vanilla odor, though the vapor pressure is low (5×10^{-15} mm Hg at 25°C). The water solubility is pH dependent and increases with increasing pH, from 117 mg/l at pH 5 to 4290 mg/l at pH 9, and the log K_{ow} values are −0.047 at pH 7 and −0.448 at pH 9.

Uses Diclosulam is a soil-applied, preplanting broadleaf herbicide for use in soybeans and peanuts at maximum label rates 35 and 26 g per hectare, respectively.

75.3.2 TOXICITY TO LABORATORY ANIMALS

Acute Exposure The acute toxicity of diclosulam was low. The acute oral LD_{50} in the rat was greater than 5000 mg/kg, the dermal LD_{50} in the rabbit was greater than 2000 mg/kg, and the 4-hr inhalation LC_{50} in the rat was greater than 5.04 mg/l of air. Diclosulam produced no indications of dermal irritation in rabbits or sensitization in the guinea pig, and only very slight transient eye irritation in the rabbit following acute exposure (EPA, 1998).

Repeated Exposure The primary target organs identified in dietary toxicity studies were the kidneys (rat) and the liver (rat, mouse, and dog).

In the F344 rat, dosages of 500 and 1000 mg/kg/day for 2 weeks resulted in increased liver weights and enlarged ceca in males with no histopathologic changes. The NOEL was 100 mg/kg/day in males and 1000 mg/kg/day in females. Rats were given dietary dosages of 50–1000 mg/kg/day for 13 weeks. At 500 and 1000 mg/kg/day, body weights were decreased, and kidney and liver weights were increased. Very slight-to-moderate treatment-related hepatocellular hypertrophy was observed in males at 100 mg/kg/day and above, and in females at 1000 mg/kg/day. Kidney changes characterized as slightly to moderately decreased intracellular protein in the proximal tubule epithelium were seen in male rats at 500 mg/kg/day and

above, secondary to slightly lower feed consumption in these animals. Slight decreases in red blood cell parameters were noted at 100 mg/kg/day and above. The NOEL from this study was 50 mg/kg/day (Stewart et al., 1992a; Szabo and Davis, 1993a).

Dietary exposure of B6C3F1 mice to dosages of 100–1000 mg/kg/day for 2 weeks resulted in slightly decreased kidney weights in both males and females at the high dosage (1000 mg/kg/day), and slightly decreased hepatocellular vacuolation (consistent with decreased glycogen content) in females at 500 mg/kg/day and above. The NOEL was 500 mg/kg/day in males and 100 mg/kg/day in females. Dosages of 100–1000 mg/kg/day were given to B6C3F1 mice for 13 weeks. Significant body weight effects were seen in males at 1000 mg/kg/day and in females at 500 and 1000 mg/kg/day, and slight-to-moderate hepatocellular hypertrophy was the primary histopathologic change noted at 500 and 1000 mg/kg/day in males and females, respectively. Kidney weights were lower in males and females at 500 mg/kg/day and above, but there were no correlative changes in clinical chemistry or histopathologic parameters. The NOEL for subchronic exposure in the mouse was 100 mg/kg/day (Grandjean and Szabo, 1993; Stewart et al., 1992b).

Beagle dogs were given diclosulam at dosages of 50–500 mg/kg/day for 2 weeks. Dosages of 250 mg/kg/day and above were unpalatable and resulted in severely decreased weight gain or actual weight loss, degenerative changes in the kidneys, and hepatocellular necrosis. A dosage of 50 mg/kg/day produced microfocal hepatocellular necrosis in males, but no effects in females. In a subchronic study, dogs were given dosages of 0, 5, 25, or 100 mg/kg/day for 13 weeks. Slight, diffuse centrilobular hepatocellular hypertrophy was observed at 25 mg/kg/day. Higher dosages proved to be unpalatable, with secondary toxicity associated with inanition superimposed on the effects of diclosulam on the liver. The subchronic NOEL for the dog was 5 mg/kg/day (Swaim and Szabo, 1992; Szabo and Rachunek, 1992).

In a 21-day repeated dermal application study in rabbits, no dermal or systemic effects were seen at 1000 mg/kg/day, the highest dosage tested (Redmond and Kociba, 1996).

Chronic Toxicity and Carcinogenicity Chronic studies in rodents with diclosulam produced adaptive changes in the kidney as the primary effect. In a 2-year study in Fischer 344 rats, decreased body weight and weight gain were observed at 400 mg/kg/day, along with changes in hematology, clinical chemistry, and urinalysis parameters associated with the decreased body weight. Histologically, a slight alteration in tubular morphology, mostly within the corticomedullary junction, was observed in the kidneys at 100 and 400 mg/kg/day. This subtle change in the cytologic character and architecture was considered a slight alteration of the normal physiologic state, rather than a pathologic effect indicative of a toxic injury. No effects were noted in rats at 5 mg/kg/day (Minnema, 1996a).

Chronic dietary exposure of B6C3F1 mice to dosages of 50–500 mg diclosulam/kg/day for two years produced no treatment-related effects on survival, body weights, feed consumption, or clinical observations. The primary histologic change noted in male mice was a reduced vacuolation of the kidney tubular epithelium at all dose levels at the interim and terminal sacrifices, which correlated with decreased absolute and relative kidney weights. In female mice, minimal focal dilation with hyperplasia of the lining epithelium of renal cortical tubules was seen at 100 mg/kg/day and above. In males, this same focal dilation was seen spontaneously across all groups, including controls. There appeared to be no biologic or toxicologic significance to these microscopic changes. The no-observed-adverse-effect level (NOAEL) in mice following chronic exposure was 50 mg/kg/day (Minnema, 1996b). There was no evidence of tumorigenicity or carcinogenicity in either mice or rats.

In beagle dogs fed dosages of 2–25 mg diclosulam/kg/day for 1 year, only slight elevations in mean alkaline phosphatase and creatinine levels in dogs given 25 mg/kg/day were observed. These slight elevations, however, were considered reflective of the normal variability in this species, and 25 mg/kg/day was the NOEL (Walker, 1996).

Mutagenicity   In a battery of genotoxicity tests, diclosulam showed no evidence of mutagenicity. These tests included a bacterial reverse mutation assay (Ames test), an *in vitro* cytogenetic assay in Chinese hamster ovary cells (CHO/HGPRT assay), an *in vitro* chromosomal aberration assay in rat lymphocytes, and an *in vivo* cytogenetic assay in mouse bone marrow (EPA, 1998).

Neurotoxicity   No neurotoxicologic effects were noted in rats following acute gavage exposure to up to 2000 mg/kg (highest dose tested) or in a complete battery of neurologic tests including detailed histopathologic examination following 1 year of exposure via the diet to dosages up to 400 mg/kg/day (Mattsson *et al.*, 1996; Minnema, 1996c).

Reproductive Toxicity   Treatment with diclosulam had no effect on reproduction or fetal development. In a multigeneration reproduction study in Sprague-Dawley rats at dietary dosages up to 1000 mg/kg/day, no indications of parental or reproductive toxicity were seen. Gavage dosages of up to 1000 mg/kg/day to pregnant Sprague-Dawley rats on gestation days 6–15 produced no maternal or developmental toxicity. In New Zealand White rabbits, no developmental effects were noted even at gavage dosages up to 650 mg/kg/day on gestation days 7–19, which severely affected maternal feed consumption and weight gain. The maternal NOEL in rabbits was 65 mg/kg/day, whereas the developmental NOEL was 650 mg/kg/day (Morseth, 1994; Zablotny, 1996; Zablotny *et al.*, 1996).

Absorption, Distribution, Metabolism, and Excretion   Metabolism studies conducted with ^{14}C-diclosulam in the F344 rat using dose levels of 5 or 500 mg/kg revealed that approximately 80% of a single or repeated (15 days) low doses was absorbed

by both males and females. At 500 mg/kg, only 15–20% of a single dose was absorbed. Urinary elimination was rapid in both cases with half-lives of approximately 7–12 hr. A higher percentage of the 5-mg/kg dose was excreted in the urine by females (62–68%) than by males (39–43%), with the remainder of the absorbed dose eliminated in the feces. At 500 mg/kg, the majority of the administered dose (82–85%) was found in the feces, with only 6–12% eliminated via the urine in both males and females. Within 72 hr, less than 3% of the dose remained in the tissues and carcass in all dose groups. The primary urinary and fecal excretion products were identified as unchanged diclosulam and an OH-phenyl oxidation product. In addition, the *N*-acetyl cysteine conjugate of diclosulam, and the *S*-oxide of the *N*-acetyl cysteine conjugate were excreted in the urine of males and females, whereas the sulfate and/or glucuronide conjugate of the OH-phenyl metabolite was seen only in the urine of male rats. Based on rapid elimination, diclosulam has little potential to accumulate upon repeated administration (Stewart *et al.*, 1996).

75.3.3 TOXICITY TO HUMANS

Risk assessments using conservative assumption indicate high margins of safety with diclosulam. Residue studies indicated no detectable residues at a limit of detection of 0.003 ppm, and no likelihood for accumulation. A tolerance level of 0.02 ppm, based on a limit of quantitation of 0.01 ppm, and a reference dose of 0.05 mg/kg/day based on the lowest NOEL (5 mg/kg/day from the chronic rat study) have been proposed (EPA, 1998). Calculation of a maximum potential average daily dose assuming 100% of proposed crops with residues equal to the tolerance level indicates theoretical exposure to only 0.1% of the RfD in the population with the highest potential exposure (nonnursing infants under 1 year old). The MOE for occupational exposure to diclosulam, calculated using exposure estimates from the U.S. EPA Pesticide Handlers Exposure Database (PHED), is estimated to be greater than 1000 based on the NOEL from the chronic dog study and assuming 100% absorption.

75.4 FLORASULAM

75.4.1 IDENTITY, PROPERTIES, AND USES

Chemical Name   The chemical name for florasulam is *N*-(2,6-difluorophenyl)-5-methoxy-8-fluoro-(1,2,4)triazolo(1,5c)pyrimidine-2-sulfonamide.

Structure   See Fig. 75.1 and Table 75.1.

Synonyms   Florasulam is also known as XR-570, XDE-570, or DE-570 and is sold either alone or in combination under the registered trade names PRIMUS®, DERBY®, KANTOR®, and MUSTANG® herbicides. The CAS registry number is 145701-23-1.

Physical and Chemical Properties Florasulam is a light colored solid with an empirical formula of $C_{12}H_8F_3N_5O_3S$ and a molecular weight of 359.3. It has a low vapor pressure (7.5 × 10^{-8} mm Hg at 25°C) and decomposes at 193.5–230.5°C. The solubility increases with increasing pH, ranging from 84 mg/l at pH 5 to 9400 mg/l at pH 9. Florasulam is highly soluble in acetone (123 g/l) and acetonitrile (72 g/l), but substantially less soluble in octanol (0.18 g/l) and xylene (0.23 g/l). It has a pK_a of 4.54 and log K_{ow} values ranging from 1.00 at pH 4 to −2.06 at pH 10.

Uses Florasulam is a highly effective postemergence broadleaf herbicide for use in cereals, grassland, and turf. Maximum label use rate for the various crops range from 5 to 10 g per hectare.

75.4.2 TOXICITY TO LABORATORY ANIMALS

Acute Exposure Florasulam was essentially nonhazardous by the oral, dermal, and inhalation routes, was nonirritating to skin and eyes, and did not induce delayed contact hypersensitivity in either a modified Buehler test or a Magnusson and Kligman maximization study. The oral LD_{50} was greater than 6000 mg/kg in the rat and 5000 mg/kg/day in the mouse, the dermal LD_{50} in the rabbit was greater than 2000 mg/kg, and the 4-hr inhalation LC_{50} in the rat exceeded 5 mg/l (Brooks, 1997; Clements and Cieszlak, 1995; Gilbert, 1995a, b, c, d; Gilbert and Yano, 1995b; Johnson, 1996).

Repeated Exposure In dietary studies of 2- to 13-week duration, the kidney was identified as a target organ in rats, mice, and dogs, whereas the liver was a target organ in dogs.

In F344 rats, subacute exposure to dosages of 500 mg/kg/day and above was associated with karyomegaly and anisokaryocytosis in proximal tubular epithelial cells in males and females, and tubular degeneration with regeneration in females. Individual proximal tubular cell necrosis was also seen in both sexes at 1000 mg/kg/day. The NOEL was 100 mg/kg/day. Subchronic studies were conducted in F344 and Sprague-Dawley rats at dosages up to 1000 mg/kg/day. Dosages of 500 or 1000 mg/kg/day produced necrosis with regeneration in descending proximal tubules and a marginally increased incidence of degeneration with regeneration of renal tubules in females. Papillary mineralization (tubular debris) and papillary necrosis were reported at the highest dosages (≥800 mg/kg/day). Other high-dosage effects included acidic urine (males only), increased kidney weight, perineal soiling, reduced body weight gain and feed consumption (due, at least in part, to reduced palatability of the diet), and reduced red blood cell indices. With the exception of mineralized debris in renal papillae and degeneration and regeneration of cortical tubules, all effects partially or completely resolved by the end of a 4-week recovery period. The subchronic NOEL in rats was 100 mg/kg/day (Liberacki et al., 1996; Redmond and Johnson, 1996a; Szabo and Davis, 1993b).

In B6C3F1 mice, subacute exposure to dosages up to 1000 mg/kg/day was without effect (Szabo and Davis, 1992). The only response to subchronic exposure to dosages up to 1000 mg/kg/day was hypertrophy of renal collecting duct epithelial cells at 500 mg/kg/day and above. The subchronic NOEL in mice was 100 mg/kg/day (Redmond and Johnson, 1996b).

In Beagle dogs, subacute exposure to a nominal dosage of 450 mg/kg/day was associated with reduced body weight gain and reduced feed consumption (due, at least in part, to reduced palatability of the diet). Hepatic changes characterized by increased liver weight and bile duct hyperplasia in males and females, and bile stasis and hepatocellular necrosis in males were observed in this group. At 150 mg/kg/day, effects were limited to increased liver weight and bile duct hyperplasia. Serum alkaline phosphatase (AP) activity, probably of hepatic origin, was elevated at all dosages, including the low dosage of 50 mg/kg/day. The increase in serum AP at the low dosage was without histopathological correlate. Therefore, 50 mg/kg/day was considered a subacute NOAEL. Liver effects were not exacerbated by an extended treatment period, but renal hypertrophy (not seen after 4 weeks of exposure) similar to that reported in rats and mice was evident in dogs after subchronic exposure to 50 mg/kg/day (Sullivan and Cronin-Singleton, 1995; Sullivan and Singleton, 1995).

Repeated dermal exposure to dosages up to 1000 mg/kg/day for 4 weeks produced only transient dermal irritation in rats during the last week of treatment, with no systemic effects (Scortichini and Kociba, 1997).

Chronic Toxicity and Carcinogenicity In chronic dietary studies (1- to 2-year duration), hypertrophy of a population of renal collecting duct cells identified as α-intercalated cells remained the most sensitive morphological effect in all species. Hypertrophy was present at 50 mg/kg/day in dogs, 125 and 250 mg/kg/day and above in male and female rats, respectively, and 500 mg/kg/day and above in mice.

In F344 rats, 2-year dietary exposure to dosages between 10 and 500 mg/kg/day identified the kidney as the only target organ. At the high dosage (250 mg/kg/day in females and 500 mg/kg/day in males), very slight to slight hypertrophy of renal collecting duct epithelial cells was evident after 1 year. After 2 years, this change had progressed to a moderate degree in some males. Other effects at this dosage included reduced body weight gain, reduced urinary pH, perineal soiling, reduced red blood cell indices, and renal changes similar to effects seen following subchronic exposure to high dose levels. At the next dosage (125 mg/kg/day in females and 250 mg/kg/day in males), very slight to slight hypertrophy of renal collecting duct epithelial cells was evident in males after 1 year, and in males and females after 2 years. Reduced body weight gain, renal papillary mineralization (males), decreases in spontaneous chronic renal disease, reduced urinary pH, and perineal soiling were also seen in these animals. No effects occurred at 10 mg/kg/day and there was no treatment-related tumorigenicity or carcinogenicity (Johnson et al., 1997).

In B6C3F1 mice, 2-year dietary exposure to dosages up to 1000 mg/kg/day identified the kidney as the only target organ with hypertrophy of intercalated cells, decreased renal epithelial cell cytoplasmic lipid-like microvacuoles, and a decreased incidence of spontaneous chronic renal disease at 1000 mg/kg/day. Reduced body weights accompanied by minor changes in serum cholesterol and triglycerides also were present at 1000 mg/kg/day. At 500 mg/kg/day, very slight hypertrophy of renal collecting duct epithelial cells occurred in most males and females along with decreases in cytoplasmic lipid-like microvacuoles and spontaneous chronic renal disease (females only) of renal tubules. No effects occurred at 50 mg/kg/day, and there was no treatment-related tumorigenic or carcinogenic response at any dosage (Quast *et al.*, 1997).

In Beagle dogs, 1-year dietary exposure to florasulam revealed kidneys, liver, and adrenal glands as target organs. In the subchronic study, renal hypertrophy and modest elevations of serum alkaline phosphatase and liver weight were the only treatment-related effects seen at 100 mg/kg/day. However, treatment beyond 13 weeks resulted in reduced food consumption and body weight gain in some animals, and significant elevations in serum enzyme activities associated with liver toxicity. The original high dosage of 100 mg/kg/day was therefore reduced to 50 mg/kg/day on Day 105. Thereafter, food consumption and body weight gain improved and red blood cell indices in females and serum transaminases in both sexes returned to normal. Serum alkaline phosphatase remained elevated to the end of the study. Slight hypertrophy of renal collecting duct epithelial cells and slight vacuolization of the zona reticularis and zona fasciculata of adrenal glands were detected histologically in this high dosage group. The fatty change in the adrenals of dogs represented a slight exacerbation of a spontaneous lesion, not associated with inflammation, necrosis, or clinical chemistry changes, and was considered of uncertain toxicological importance. No histopathological lesions were evident in the liver. The NOEL was 5 mg/kg/day (Stebbins and Haut, 1997).

Histological and ultrastructural evaluation of the affected renal collecting duct cells characterized the hypertrophy as a mitochondrial proliferation of α-intercalated cells, which functionally are involved in acid–base regulation and contain high levels of H^+-ATPase and H^+K^+-ATPase in the apical membrane (Brown *et al.*, 1988; Garg, 1991; Hamm and Hering-Smith, 1993; Madsen and Tisher, 1986; Stokes, 1993; Verlander *et al.*, 1991). Hypertrophy of intercalated cells has been reported as a physiological response to several factors affecting acid–base homeostasis, including respiratory acidosis, metabolic acidosis, hypokalemia, and altered serum adrenal mineralocorticoid levels (Ahn *et al.*, 1996a, b; DeFronzo, 1980; Eiam-ong *et al.*, 1994; Hansen *et al.*, 1980; Madsen *et al.*, 1991; Tsuruoka and Schwartz, 1996a, b; Verlander *et al.*, 1994; Weiner and Wingo, 1997; Wingo and Cain, 1993). However, none of these factors was found to be adversely affected by florasulam (Weiner, 1997). The lack of any adverse sequelae associated with this change suggests that it is an adaptive rather than an adverse response to florasulam.

Mutagenicity   In a battery of genotoxicity tests, florasulam showed no evidence of mutagenic potential. These tests included an *in vitro* bacterial reverse mutation assay (Ames test), an *in vitro* cytogenetic assay in Chinese hamster ovary cells (CHO/HGPRT assay), an *in vitro* chromosomal aberration assay in rat lymphocytes, and an *in vivo* cytogenetic assay in mouse bone marrow cells (Lawlor, 1995; Lick *et al.*, 1995; Linscombe *et al.*, 1995a, b).

Neurotoxicity   Acute gavage and chronic (1-year dietary) neurotoxicity studies in Fischer 344 rats revealed only nonspecific findings. In both acute and chronic neurotoxicity studies with florasulam, perineal urine staining at the highest dosages was the only treatment-related effect. No other effects were seen following an extensive battery of neurologic tests and neurohistopathological examinations (Mattsson and McGuirk, 1997; Shankar and Johnson, 1996).

Reproductive Toxicity   In developmental toxicity studies, there were no adverse effects on intrauterine development or prenatal survival in rats or rabbits administered gavage dosages as high as 600–750 mg/kg/day. Maternal effects on survival, feed consumption, and/or weight gains occurred at these high dosages. In SD rats, the embryo–fetal NOEL was 750 mg/kg/day, whereas the maternal NOEL was 250 mg/kg/day. In New Zealand White rabbits, the NOEL for both maternal and embryo–fetal effects was 500 mg/kg/day. In a two-generation dietary reproduction study in SD rats at dosages of 10–500 mg/kg/day, parental effects (weight gain, feed consumption, renal changes) were seen only at the highest dosage, with no effects on any reproductive parameter. Transient decreases in neonatal body weights, secondary to decreases in maternal feed consumption, were seen at 500 mg/kg/day. The parental NOEL was 100 mg/kg/day, whereas the NOEL for reproductive effects was 500 mg/kg/day (Liberacki and Carney, 1997; Liberacki *et al.*, 1997; Zablotny and Carney, 1997).

Absorption, Distribution, Metabolism, and Excretion   In metabolism studies in F344 rats, single oral doses of 10–500 mg ^{14}C-florasulam per kilogram were readily and extensively absorbed (>90% of a 10-mg/kg dose within 24 hr) and rapidly eliminated (plasma $t_{1/2} = 8$–10 hr) primarily in the urine (>85% of administered dose). The feces contained small amounts of the administered radioactivity (5–17%) depending on dose. More than 75% of the ^{14}C activity in urine was found to be unchanged florasulam. Two minor metabolites, identified as a free and a conjugated (sulfated) hydroxyphenyl derivative of florasulam, were found. Feces contained unchanged florasulam and the free hydroxyphenyl-derivative. There was no evidence of hydrolysis of the sulfonamide bridge based on the metabolites found in the urine and feces. The rapid elimination of florasulam from tissues indicated no potential to accumulate upon repeated administration (Dryzga *et al.*, 1996; Hansen, 1997). Absorption following *in vivo* dermal exposure of rats to a concentrated suspension formulation containing ^{14}C-florasulam was minimal (mean <0.5% over 72 hr). Results obtained from *in vitro* studies were similar to those obtained from the *in vivo* study (Bounds, 1997; Perkins and Billington, 1998).

75.4.3 TOXICITY TO HUMANS

Risk assessment calculations for the general population and for pesticide handlers indicate a low-risk estimate. Residue studies have indicated no detectable levels in cereal gains at the limit of quantitation. Maximum residue limits (MRLs) of 0.01 ppm in grains, and 0.05 ppm whole plants and straw based on the limit of detection, and an acceptable daily intake (ADI) of 0.05 mg/kg/day on the basis of a chronic NOEL of 5 mg/kg/day in dogs have been proposed. The theoretical dietary intake of florasulam from all routes has been estimated to account for <0.5% of the ADI even in infants, the most susceptible subpopulation. Margins of exposure of >2000 have been calculated for pesticide handlers using the PHED and an NOEL of 5 mg/kg/day.

75.5 FLUMETSULAM

75.5.1 IDENTITY, PROPERTIES, AND USES

Chemical Name   The chemical name for flumetsulam is *N*-(2,6-difluorophenyl)-5-methyl-(1,2,4)triazolo(1,5-a)pyrimidine-2-sulfonamide.

Structure   See Fig. 75.1 and Table 75.1.

Synonyms   Flumetsulam (also known as XRD-498) is the generic name for this material which is sold globally as BROADSTRIKE®, PYTHON®, PRESIDE®, and SCORPION® herbicides. The CAS registry number is 98967-40-9.

Physical and Chemical Properties   The empirical formula of flumetsulam is $C_{12}H_9F_2N_5O_2S$, with a molecular weight of 325.3. Flumetsulam is a light colored powder at room temperature, with a melting point of 252.9°C, a vapor pressure of 2.8×10^{-15} mm Hg at 25°C, a K_{ow} of 1.62 at pH 3.44, and a pK_a of 4.60. Flumetsulam is soluble in water at 5.65 g/l at pH 7 and 25°C, but solubility decreases with decreasing pH, and it is less soluble in organic solvents.

Uses   Flumetsulam is a broad-spectrum, season-long herbicide used in the control of broadleaf weeds in soybeans, corn, and other major crops. Flumetsulam is applied as a soil-incorporated preplanting, preemergence, or postemergence herbicide depending on the formulation, at a maximum use rate of 80 g per hectare.

75.5.2 TOXICITY TO LABORATORY ANIMALS

Acute Exposure   Flumetsulam has been examined in a complete battery of toxicologic studies to evaluate potential mammalian toxicity. Flumetsulam was relatively nontoxic following acute exposure, with an acute oral LD_{50} greater than 5000 mg/kg, a dermal LD_{50} greater than 2000 mg/kg, an acute 4-hr inhalation LC_{50} above the highest attainable aerosol concentration of 1.2 mg/l of air, and only slight, transient eye irritation. No signs of dermal irritation were observed in rabbits following acute exposure, nor was there any evidence of dermal sensitization in guinea pigs (EPA, 1993).

Repeated Exposure   Subchronic toxicity studies in rats, mice, and dogs have indicated a low degree of toxicity following repeated oral exposure. In rats, dietary exposure to concentrations of up to 5% (approximately 6000 mg/kg/day) for 2–4 weeks identified the kidney as the primary target organ. Effects in the kidneys consisted of focal necrosis and inflammation of the papilla(e), and tubular epithelial cell degeneration and regeneration, with secondary effects on urinalysis parameters at the highest dosage. The only effect reported at 1000 mg/kg/day was cecal enlargement in males. However, the ceca were normal histologically, and 1000 mg/kg/day was considered the NOAEL following 2–4 weeks of exposure. Rats fed diets containing flumetsulam at dosages of 250–2500 mg/kg/day for 13 weeks exhibited dose-dependent changes similar to those seen after 4 weeks of exposure. The NOAEL in rats following subchronic exposure was 25 mg/kg/day (Yano *et al.*, 1987, 1988 ; Zempel *et al.*, 1988).

In B6C3F1 mice fed flumetsulam for 2 weeks, decreased kidney weights were reported in males at dietary concentrations of 1.5 and 3.0% and in females given 3.0%, which corresponded to dosages >3500 mg/kg/day. The NOEL in mice was 0.5% (approximately 1150–1365 mg/kg/day). B6C3F1 mice given dosages of 100–5000 mg/kg/day for 13 weeks displayed only a minimal increase in centrolobular-to-midzonal hepatocellular eosinophilia at the highest dosage, and decreased vacuolation of renal proximal tubular epithelium which is of doubtful toxicologic significance. The NOEL for mice was 1000 mg/kg/day, and 5000 mg/kg/day was considered a NOAEL (Bond *et al.*, 1987; Stott *et al.*, 1986). In both rats and mice, the increases in the size and weight of the cecum, observed only at high dosages and unassociated with any histologic changes, were considered adaptive in nature, most likely secondary to the effects of flumetsulam on the microenvironment within the cecum.

Beagle dogs were fed flumetsulam at nominal dosages of 100–1000 mg/kg/day (males) or 1500 or 2500 mg/kg/day (females) for 2 weeks. In females, degeneration and regeneration of the renal tubular epithelial cells, and lymphocytic infiltration of hepatic sinusoids were reported. The NOEL in dogs was approximately 800 mg/kg/day (nominally 1000 mg/kg/day). In dogs given a dosage of 1000 mg/kg/day for 13 weeks, degenerative microscopic changes in the renal papilla, slight biliary stasis, and hepatocellular necrosis were observed. At 500 mg/kg/day, slight renal papillary degeneration was noted microscopically in males, and increases in serum AP and globulin levels and decreased serum albumin levels, with no histopathologic correlates, were reported in both males and females. A dosage of 500 mg/kg/day was considered the NOAEL in females (Cosse *et al.*, 1989).

Repeated dermal exposure to dosages of ≥100 mg/kg/day for 21 days produced very slight epidermal hyperplasia, but no indications of any systemic effects (Stebbins *et al.*, 1990).

Chronic Toxicity and Carcinogenicity Flumetsulam was fed to F344 rats and B6C3F1 mice for 2 years at dosages of 100–1000 mg/kg/day. No treatment-related adverse effects were noted in mice (Bond *et al.*, 1991). In rats, atrophy of the renal papilla(e) with secondary hyperplasia and/or mineralization of the pelvic epithelium were noted in males given 1000 mg/kg/day, but not in females, and the NOEL was 500 mg/kg/day (Stott *et al.*, 1991). As was noted following subchronic exposure, cecal enlargement with no accompanying histopathologic changes was observed in both rats and mice following chronic exposure.

There was no evidence of a tumorigenic or carcinogenic response in either rats or mice at dosages up to 1000 mg/kg/day.

The dog appeared to be the most sensitive species to long-term exposure to flumetsulam. Administration of dosages of 500 mg/kg/day in the diet for 1 year produced inflammatory and atrophic changes in the kidney, accompanied by calculi in females. At 100 mg/kg/day, only increased alkaline phosphatase activity and decreased serum albumin were reported, with no histologic changes in any organs. The chronic NOEL in dogs from this study was 20 mg/kg/day, whereas the NOAEL was 100 mg/kg/day (Yano *et al.*, 1991).

Mutagenicity Flumetsulam was negative for mutagenic activity in an *in vitro* bacterial reverse mutation assay (Ames test), an *in vitro* cytogenetic assay in Chinese hamster ovary cells (CHO/HGPRT assay), an *in vitro* rat hepatocyte unscheduled DNA synthesis (UDS) assay, and an *in vivo* cytogenetic assay in mouse bone marrow cells (EPA, 1993).

Reproductive Toxicity Flumetsulam did not affect development or reproduction in either rats or rabbits. No evidence of maternal toxicity, embryo–fetotoxicity or teratogenicity was observed in rats following exposure of pregnant females to 1000 mg/kg/day in the diet, though the weights of the ceca were increased, consistent with effects noted in previous dietary studies. No parental toxicity or alterations in reproductive performance occurred in rats given up to 1000 mg/kg/day over two generations. Gavage administration of flumetsulam to pregnant rabbits at dosages of 500–700 mg/kg/day produced dose-related episodes of anorexia, with sequelae secondary to the altered nutritional status (deteriorated clinical condition, mortality, stomach erosions, etc.), but no embryo–fetotoxicity or teratogenicity accompanied these maternal effects. The maternal NOEL from this study was 100 mg/kg/day, whereas the NOEL for

embryo–fetal development was 700 mg/kg/day (Hanley *et al.*, 1989; Zempel *et al.*, 1990; Zielke *et al.*, 1988).

Absorption, Distribution, Metabolism, and Excretion Flumetsulam was rapidly, though incompletely, absorbed in mice and rats, with absorption half-lives of less than 1 hr following oral administration of doses of either 5 or 1000 mg/kg. Excretion was also rapid, with a urinary half-life of approximately 5–7 hr. Following oral administration of ^{14}C-flumetsulam, approximately 50–75% of the administered radiolabel was excreted in the urine primarily as unchanged parent material, though two minor (<20% of urinary radiolabel) metabolites, believed to be conjugates of parent flumetsulam, were found in the urine of mice. Approximately 20–35% of the dose was found in the feces, which represented apparently unabsorbed flumetsulam (based on almost total elimination in the urine of an intravenous dose to rats) and tissue levels of ^{14}C accounted for less than 1.5% of the administered dose. There were no differences in absorption, distribution or elimination based on sex, though slight differences were seen with increasing dose (Pottenger *et al.*, 1991; Timchalk *et al.*, 1988).

75.5.3 TOXICITY TO HUMANS

Risk assessment indicates a low potential risk from normal use of flumetsulam. Residue tolerances of 0.05 ppm have been set by the U.S. EPA for soybeans and for corn grain, fodder, and forage. However, no residues were detected in soybeans even after postemergent application of six times the maximum label rate. A reference dose of 1 mg/kg/day was established on the basis of a NOAEL of 100 mg/kg/day from a 1 year study in dogs. Dietary risk evaluation assuming 100% of crops are treated and residues are at the established tolerance levels indicates only 0.013% of the RfD is used even by the highest exposed subgroup, nonnursing infants less than 1 year old (EPA, 1993). Based on the use rates, and the NOEL from the chronic dog study, the MOE for worker exposure is greater than 1000.

75.6 METOSULAM

75.6.1 IDENTITY, PROPERTIES, AND USES

Chemical Name The chemical name for metosulam is *N*-(2,6-dichloro-3-methylphenyl)-5,7-dimethoxy-(1,2,4) triazolo(1,5a)pyrimidine-2-sulfonamide.

Structure See Fig. 75.1 and Table 75.1.

Synonyms Metosulam is also known as methoxsulam, XRD-511, XDE-511, and DE-511, and is sold either alone or in combination, under a variety of registered trade names including TACCO®, SANSAC®, ECLIPSE®, ATOL®, KOMPAL®, and SINAL® herbicides. The CAS number is 139528-85-1.

Physical and Chemical Properties Metosulam is a cream to tan colored powder with a low vapor pressure (7.5×10^{-15} mm Hg at 25°C). The empirical formula is $C_{14}H_{13}Cl_2N_5O_4S$, and the molecular weight is 418.3. The solubility of metosulam in water at 20°C and pH 7 is 700 mg/l. Given a pK_a of 4.8, the solubility is pH dependent, with values of 100 mg/l at pH 5 and 5600 mg/l at pH 9 (at 20°C), and the log K_{ow} is 2.12 at pH 5.

Uses Metosulam is a broad-spectrum, postemergence broadleaf herbicide intended for use in cereals, maize, pasture, alfalfa, and rice. Maximum label use rates for the various crops range from 5 to 30 g per hectare.

75.6.2 TOXICITY TO LABORATORY ANIMALS

Acute Exposure The acute toxicity of metosulam was very low. The LD_{50} values of metosulam given orally to Fischer 344 rats and CD-1 mice were both greater than 5000 mg/kg. No toxicity, including histopathological changes of eyes and kidneys, was evident in beagle dogs given one to five daily doses of 2000 mg/kg, by gelatine capsule. The dermal LD_{50} in the rabbit was greater than 2000 mg/kg. The 4-hr inhalation LC_{50} in the rat was greater than the highest attainable concentration of 1.9 mg/l of air. Metosulam, when applied to the intact skin of rabbits, produced no signs of irritation. Following instillation into rabbit eyes, slight conjunctival redness developed within 1 hr of treatment, but all treated eyes were normal within 1 day of treatment. There was no indication of contact sensitization in guinea pigs exposed to metosulam using either a Magnusson and Kligman maximization test or a modified Buehler topical patch method (UK Ministry of Agriculture, Fisheries, and Food, 1996).

Repeated Exposure Repeated exposure toxicity studies were conducted with metosulam in rats, mice, dogs, rabbits, and monkeys. In rats, dietary administration of dosages of 500–5000 mg/kg/day for 2 weeks to Sprague-Dawley rats resulted in lower body weights associated with unpalatability and the NOEL was 100 mg/kg/day. No significant effects were reported in Long Evans rats administered dosages of up to 2000 mg/kg/day for 2 weeks. Following subchronic exposure, the kidney was identified as the major target organ. In a 13-week dietary study, the primary toxicological effects were renal alterations characterized as hypertrophy and nuclear pleomorphism of cells lining the proximal convoluted tubules at 100 mg/kg/day and above. After 4 weeks on control diet, hypertrophy of renal tubular cells had resolved, and nuclear pleomorphism was markedly decreased. The NOEL for subchronic dietary administration of metosulam in rats was 10 mg/kg/day.

CD-1 mice administered metosulam in the diet at 100–5000 mg/kg/day for 2 weeks exhibited centrilobular hepatocellular necrosis and decreased vacuolation in the liver only at 2000 mg/kg/day and above. The NOEL was 1000 mg/kg/day. The only effect observed in a 13-week dietary study at dosages up to 2000 mg/kg/day, was mild hepatocellular hypertrophy and the NOEL was 250 mg/kg/day.

The kidney was identified as the most sensitive target organ in the dog (similar to the rat). In addition, ocular toxicity in the form of retinal damage unique to this species was also observed. Dietary administration of metosulam to Beagle dogs at dosages of 100–1000 mg/kg/day for 14 days proved unpalatable and produced dose-related decreases in feed consumption and body weights; retinal degeneration, necrosis, and detachment; and degeneration or focal necrosis of distal renal collecting tubules and collecting ducts. The NOEL in this study was 25 mg/kg/day. Metosulam was fed to dogs at dosages of 5, 25, and 50 mg/kg/day for 13 weeks. Clinical signs of blindness occurred as early as 6 weeks in all dogs administered 50 mg/kg/day. Microscopic examination of the eyes from these dogs showed retinal degeneration with detachment. Choroidal structures (tapetum lucidum, pigmented epithelium, and choroidal blood vessels) and other ocular structures were normal. Ocular tissues from dogs administered 5 mg/kg/day were normal. In the kidneys, very slight to moderate degeneration of the distal convoluted tubules and collecting ducts of dogs administered 25 mg/kg/day and above was reported, and the NOEL was 5 mg/kg/day.

Male and female Cynomolgus monkeys exposed to oral dosages of 0 or 100 mg/kg/day for 6 weeks showed no renal or ocular toxicity after detailed examination which included an extensive histopathologic evaluation. Repeated dermal exposure of New Zealand White rabbits to dosages of up to 1000 mg/kg/day for 21 days produced no signs of dermal irritation or systemic effects (UK Ministry of Agriculture, Fisheries, and Food, 1996).

Chronic Toxicity and Carcinogenicity Following chronic (2-yr) exposure in Sprague-Dawley rats at dosages of 5–100 mg/kg/day, the primary effects were confined to the kidneys, consistent with the findings following subchronic exposure, and the effects were more severe in male than in female rats. At 100 mg/kg/day, nuclear pleomorphism and hyperplasia of cells of the proximal tubules as well as basophilic adenomas and adenocarcinomas of the renal cortex were observed. At 30 mg/kg/day, nuclear pleomorphism of proximal tubular cells was present and only a single renal cortical adenocarcinoma, which was within the historical control incidence for this tumor (Charles River Breeding Laboratories, 1987), was observed in this group. Short-term exposure studies demonstrated the presence of mitotic figures and nuclear pleomorphism in the renal cortex of male rats following as little as 1 week of dietary exposure to 100 mg metosulam/kg/day. Increased mitotic activity measured by BrdU incorporation correlated with the renal tubular epithelial changes noted histologically (UK Ministry of Agriculture, Fisheries, and Food, 1996). This suggested a nongenotoxic mechanism of repeated injury as described by Dietrich and Swenberg (1991) as the probable origin of the renal tumors in the chronic study with metosulam.

In CD-1 mice fed dose levels of metosulam of up to 1000 mg/kg/day for 18 months, there was no evidence of any increase in tumor incidence and no effects were noted in any other parameter.

Metosulam administered to Beagle dogs at dosages of 3–37.5 mg/kg/day for 12 months produced effects in the eyes and kidneys consistent with the findings of the subchronic study. At 37.5 mg/kg/day, variable retinal degeneration with detachment, beginning with diminished or absent pupillary light reflex, increased tapetal reflectivity, and progressive retinal deterioration, were observed. Degenerative lesions of the distal convoluted tubules and collecting ducts were also observed at 37.5 mg/kg/day. No effects were observed at lower levels, and the NOEL was 10 mg/kg/day (UK Ministry of Agriculture, Fisheries, and Food, 1996).

The sensitivity of the dog eye to metosulam appears to be unique to this species. The pathology involved the loss of the photoreceptor layer and its nuclei, together with a collapse of the outer and inner plexiform layers and inner nuclear layer. No retinopathy was associated with the pigmented epithelial layer or in the tapetal cells. The pathologic changes were not consistent with either inherited retinal degeneration or nutritional deficiencies as an etiology. It is important to note that retinal pathologies were not detected with metosulam in any other species. Dosages of 300 mg/kg/day for 12 days in rabbits, and up to 1000 and 2000 mg/kg/day for 13 weeks in rats and mice, respectively, were not associated with any retinal changes. Exposure of mice to 1000 mg/kg/day for 18 months or rats to 100 mg/kg/day for 2 years likewise induced no retinal pathology. Significantly, dosages of 100 mg/kg/day for 6 weeks in the nonhuman primate, the species most closely resembling human ocular anatomy and physiology, also produced no evidence of retinal toxicity. Pharmacokinetic studies using radiolabeled metosulam indicated metosulam localized over the outer layer of the retina in the dog, but no selective localization was detected in the rat or mouse (see below) (UK Ministry of Agriculture, Fisheries, and Food, 1996).

Mutagenicity A battery of mutagenicity tests which included an *in vitro* bacterial assay (Ames test), *in vitro* assays using mammalian cells (CHO/HGPRT, RLCAT, and UDS assay), and an *in vivo* mouse bone marrow micronucleus test were all negative (UK Ministry of Agriculture, Fisheries, and Food, 1996).

Reproductive Toxicity Metosulam did not produce any adverse reproductive or developmental effects when tested in rats and rabbits. There were no effects on maternal or developmental parameters in a conventional teratogenicity study in the SD rat at dietary levels up to 1000 mg/kg/day. In New Zealand White rabbits, maternal effects were noted at oral gavage dosages of 100 or 300 mg/kg/day and the maternal NOEL in rabbits was 30 mg/kg/day, but there was no indication of developmental effects at 300 mg/kg/day. In a two-generation reproduction study in Sprague-Dawley rats at dosages of 5–100 mg/kg/day, renal toxicity was observed among the parental rats at 100 mg/kg/day consistent with the effects noted

following chronic exposure, but reproductive performance was unaffected. The NOEL for parental toxicity from this study was 30 mg/kg/day, whereas the NOEL for reproductive effects was 100 mg/kg/day (UK Ministry of Agriculture, Fisheries, and Food, 1996).

Absorption, Distribution, Metabolism, and Excretion The metabolic fate of ^{14}C-metosulam in rats, mice, and dogs following single or multiple oral administrations was evaluated. ^{14}C-Metosulam was absorbed rapidly ($t_{1/2} < 1$ hr) in all three species, though the extent of absorption was significantly higher in the rat ($>70\%$) than in the dog and mouse ($\sim20\%$). The rate of ^{14}C elimination in mice and rats was comparable ($t_{1/2} = 54$–60 hr), whereas the elimination rate in dogs was slightly slower ($t_{1/2} = 73$ hr). In all three species, ^{14}C-metosulam and metabolites were excreted in the urine. HPLC analysis of urine samples revealed extensive metabolism in both mice and rats, but much less pronounced metabolism in dogs. Analysis of ^{14}C activity of the dog eyes indicated that this organ, a target for toxicity in the dog, exhibited an affinity for the radiotracer not seen in other species. Histoautoradiographic sections of dog eyes revealed radioactivity localized regionally over the outer layer of the retina, whereas analysis of tissues from rats and mice for ^{14}C activity and histoautoradiography indicated a lack of selective affinity for any ocular tissues (Timchalk *et al.*, 1996). The major metabolites were an oxidation product of the 3-methyl moiety of the phenyl ring and a demethylation of the 3-methoxy moiety of the pyrimidine ring. In studies performed in male rats with ^{14}C-metosulam labelled in either the phenyl or pyrimidine ring, no evidence of cleavage of the sulfonamide bridge was seen (UK Ministry of Agriculture, Fisheries, and Food, 1996).

In vitro dermal penetration studies using rat (Sprague-Dawley) and fresh human skin demonstrate that less than 1% of the applied metosulam actually penetrated the skin (UK Ministry of Agriculture, Fisheries, and Food, 1996).

75.6.3 TOXICITY TO HUMANS

Risk assessment calculations for the general population and for pesticide handlers indicate acceptable risk estimates. Residue studies have indicated no detectable levels in cereal grains at the limit of quantitation. Maximum residue limits of 0.1 ppm in grains based on the limit of quantitation, and an acceptable daily intake (ADI) of 0.01 mg/kg/day on the basis of the chronic NOEL of 5 mg/kg/day in rats and a conservative safety factor of 500 have been proposed. Using these values, the maximum theoretical dietary intake (MTDI) of metosulam from all routes of exposure has been estimated to account for $<5\%$ of the ADI. An acceptable operator exposure level (AOEL) of 0.04 mg/kg/day has been calculated using a NOEL of 10 mg/kg/day and a safety factor of 250 (UK Ministry of Agriculture, Fisheries, and Food, 1996).

REFERENCES

Ahn, K. Y., Park, K. Y., Kim, K. K., and Kone, B. C. (1996a). Chronic hypokalemia enhances expression of the H^+K^+-ATPase α_2-subunit gene in renal medulla. *Am. J. Physiol.* **217**, F314–321.

Ahn, K. Y., Turner, P. B., Madsen, K. M., and Kone, B. C. (1996b). Effects of chronic hypokalemia on renal expression of the "gastric" H^+K^+-ATPase α-subunit gene. *Am. J. Physiol.* **270**, F557–566.

Bond *et al.* (1987). Dow AgroSciences, LLC, unpublished data.

Bond *et al.* (1991). Dow AgroSciences, LLC, unpublished data.

Bounds (1997). Dow AgroSciences, LLC, unpublished data.

Brooks (1997). Dow AgroSciences, LLC, unpublished data.

Brown, D., Hirsch, S., and Gluck, S. (1988). Localization of a proton-pumping ATPase in rat kidney. *J. Clin. Invest.* **82**, 2114–2126.

Charles River Breeding Laboratories (1987). "Spontaneous Neoplastic Lesions in the Crl:CD BR Rat." Charles River Breeding Laboratories.

Clements and Cieszlak (1995). Dow AgroSciences, LLC, unpublished data.

Cosse *et al.* (1989). Dow AgroSciences, LLC, unpublished data.

DeFronzo, R. A. (1980). Hyperkalemia and hyporeninemic hypoaldosteronism. *Kidney Int.* **17**, 118–134.

Dietrich, D. R., and Swenberg, J. A. (1991). Preneoplastic lesions in rodent kidney induced spontaneously or by non-genotoxic agents: Predictive nature and comparison to lesions induced by genotoxic carcinogens. *Mutat. Res.* **248**, 239–269.

Domoradzki *et al.* (1995). Dow AgroSciences, LLC, unpublished data.

Dryzga *et al.* (1996). Dow AgroSciences, LLC, unpublished data.

Eiam-ong, S., Laski, M. E., Kurtzman, N. A., and Sabatini, S. (1994). Effect of respiratory acidosis and respiratory alkalosis on renal transport enzymes. *Am. J. Physiol.* **267**, F390–399.

Environmental Protection Agency (EPA) (1993). Pesticide tolerance for flumetsulam. 40 CFR 180, *Federal Register* **58**(207), 57966 (Thursday, October 28, 1993).

Environmental Protection Agency (EPA) (1997a). Cloransulam-methyl: Pesticide fact sheet. OPPTS 7501C (available at http://www.epa.gov/opprd001/factsheets/cloransu.html).

Environmental Protection Agency (EPA) (1997b). Cloransulam-methyl: Pesticide tolerances. 40 CR 180, *Federal Register* **62**(182), 49158 (Friday, September 19, 1997) (available at http://www.epa.gov/fedrgstr/EPA-PEST/1997/September/Day-19/p24939.htm).

Environmental Protection Agency (EPA) (1998). Diclosulam: Notice of filing of pesticide petitions. 40 CR 180, *Federal Register* **63**(224), 64484 (Friday, November 20, 1998) (available at http://www.epa.gov/fedrgstr/EPA-PEST/1998/November/Day-20/p31066.htm).

Garg, L. C. (1991). Respective role of H-ATPase and H-K-ATPase in ion transport in the kidney. *J. Am. Soc. Nephrol.* **2**, 949–960.

Gilbert (1995a). Dow AgroSciences, LLC, unpublished data.

Gilbert (1995b). Dow AgroSciences, LLC, unpublished data.

Gilbert (1995c). Dow AgroSciences, LLC, unpublished data.

Gilbert (1995d). Dow AgroSciences, LLC, unpublished data.

Gilbert and Yano (1995a). Dow AgroSciences, LLC, unpublished data.

Gilbert and Yano (1995b). Dow AgroSciences, LLC, unpublished data.

Grandjean and Szabo (1993). Dow AgroSciences, LLC, unpublished data.

Hamm, L. L., and Hering-Smith, K. S. (1993). Acid–base transport in the collecting duct. *Semin. Nephrol.* **13**, 246–255.

Hanley *et al.* (1989). Dow AgroSciences, LLC, unpublished data.

Hansen (1997). Dow AgroSciences, LLC, unpublished data.

Hansen, G. P., Tisher, C. C., and Robinson, R. R. (1980). Response of the collecting duct to disturbances of acid–base and potassium balance. *Kidney Int.* **17**, 326–337.

Haut *et al.* (1991). Dow AgroSciences, LLC, unpublished data.

Haut *et al.* (1992a). Dow AgroSciences, LLC, unpublished data.

Haut *et al.* (1992b). Dow AgroSciences, LLC, unpublished data.

Jeffries *et al.* (1995a). Dow AgroSciences, LLC, unpublished data.

Jeffries *et al.* (1995b). Dow AgroSciences, LLC, unpublished data.

Johnson (1996). Dow AgroSciences, LLC, unpublished data.

Johnson *et al.* (1997). Dow AgroSciences, LLC, unpublished data.

Lawlor (1995). Dow AgroSciences, LLC, unpublished data.

Liberacki and Carney (1997). Dow AgroSciences, LLC, unpublished data.

Liberacki *et al.* (1996). Dow AgroSciences, LLC, unpublished data.

Liberacki *et al.* (1997). Dow AgroSciences, LLC, unpublished data.

Lick *et al.* (1995). Dow AgroSdences, LLC, unpublished data.

Linscombe *et al.* (1995a). Dow AgroSciences, LLC, unpublished data.

Linscombe *et al.* (1995b). Dow AgroSciences, LLC, unpublished data.

Madsen, K. M., and Tisher, C. C. (1986). Structural–functional relationship along the distal nephron. *Am. J. Physiol.* **250**, F1–15.

Madsen, K. M., Verlander, J. W., Kim, J., and Tisher, C. C. (1991). Morphological adaptation of the collecting duct to acid–base disturbances. *Kidney Int. Suppl.* **33**, S57–63.

Mattsson *et al.* (1996). Dow Dow AgroSciences, LLC, unpublished data.

Mattsson and McGuirk (1997). Dow AgroSciences, LLC, unpublished data.

Minnema (1996a). Dow AgroSciences, LLC, unpublished data.

Minnema (1996b). Dow AgroSciences, LLC, unpublished data.

Minnema (1996c). Dow AgroSciences, LLC, unpublished data.

Morseth (1994). Dow AgroSciences, LLC, unpublished data.

Nolan *et al.* (1995). Dow AgroSciences, LLC, unpublished data.

Perkins, J. M., and Billington, R. (1998). *In vitro/in vivo* correlation for skin absorption of a spray solution of the herbicide florasulam. *In* "Sixth Int. Conf. on the Perspectives in Percutaneous Penetration," Leiden, Holland.

Pottenger *et al.* (1991). Dow AgroSciences, LLC, unpublished data.

Quast *et al.* (1997). Dow AgroSciences, LLC, unpublished data.

Redmond and Johnson (1996a). Dow AgroSciences, LLC, unpublished data.

Redmond and Johnson (1996b). Dow AgroSciences, LLC, unpublished data.

Redmond and Kociba (1996). Dow AgroSciences, LLC, unpublished data.

Scortichini and Kociba (1997). Dow AgroSciences, LLC, unpublished data.

Shankar and Johnson (1996). Dow AgroSciences, LLC, unpublished data.

Shankar *et al.* (1993). Dow AgroSciences, LLC, unpublished data.

Spencer *et al.* (1995). Dow AgroSciences, LLC, unpublished data.

Stebbins and Haut (1993). Dow AgroSciences, LLC, unpublished data.

Stebbins and Haut (1994). Dow AgroSciences, LLC, unpublished data.

Stebbins and Haut (1997). Dow AgroSciences, LLC, unpublished data.

Stebbins *et al.* (1990). Dow AgroSciences, LLC, unpublished data.

Stebbins *et al.* (1996). Dow AgroSciences, LLC, unpublished data.

Stewart *et al.* (1992a). Dow AgroSciences, LLC, unpublished data.

Stewart *et al.* (1992b). Dow AgroSciences, LLC, unpublished data.

Stewart *et al.* (1996). Dow AgroSciences, LLC, unpublished data.

Stokes, J. B. (1993). Ion transport by the collecting duct. *Semin. Nephrol.* **13**, 202–212.

Stott *et al.* (1986). Dow AgroSciences, LLC, unpubliahed data.

Stott *et al.* (1991). Dow AgroSciences, LLC, unpubliahed data.

Sullivan and Cronin-Singleton (1995). Dow AgroSciences, LLC, unpubliahed data.

Sullivan and Singleton (1995). Dow AgroSciences, LLC, unpublished data.

Swaim and Szabo (1992). Dow AgroSciences, LLC, unpublished data.

Szabo and Davis (1992). Dow AgroSciences, LLC, unpublished data.

Szabo and Davis (1993a). Dow AgroSciences, LLC, unpublished data.

Szabo and Davis (1993b). Dow AgroSciences, LLC, unpublished data.

Szabo and Davis (1994). Dow AgroSciences, LLC, unpublished data.

Szabo and Rachunek (1992). Dow AgroSciences, LLC, unpublished data.

Szabo *et al.* (1992). Dow AgroSciences, LLC, unpublished data.

Timchalk *et al.* (1988). Dow AgroSciences, LLC, unpublished data.

Timchalk, C., Dryzga, M. D., Johnson, K. A., Eddy, S. L., Freshour, N. L., Kropscott, B. E., and Nolan, R. J. (1996). Comparative pharmacokinetics of [^{14}C]metosulam (N[2,6-dichloro-3-methylphenyl]-5,7-dimethoxy-1,2,4-triazolo-[1,5a]-pyrimidine-2-sulfonamide) in rats, mice and dogs. *J. Appl. Toxicol.* **17**, 9–21.

Tsuruoka, S., and Schwartz, G. J. (1996a). Adaptation of rabbit cortical collecting duct HCO_3^- transport to metabolic acidosis *in vitro*. *J. Clin. Invest.* **97**, 1076–1084.

Tsuruoka, S., and Schwartz, G. J. (1996b). Metabolic acidosis stimulates H^+ secretion in the perfused rabbit outer collecting duct of the inner stripe. *J. Am. Soc. Nephrol.* **7**, 1262.

UK Ministry of Agriculture, Fisheries, and Food (1996). "Evaluation of Fully Approved or Provisionally Approved Products. Evaluation on: Metosulam."

Pesticide Safety Directorate, Issue 13, No. 148, Ministry of Agriculture, Fisheries, and Food.

Vedula *et al.* (1992). Dow AgroSciences, LLC, unpublished data.

Verlander, J. W., Madsen, K. M., and Tisher, C. C. (1991). Structural and functional features of proton and bicarbonate transport in the rat collecting duct. *Semin. Nephrol.* **11**, 465–477.

Verlander, J. W., Madsen, K. M., Cannon, J. K., and Tisher, C. C. (1994). Activation of acid-secreting intercalated cells in rabbit collecting duct with ammonium chloride loading. *Am. J. Physiol.* **266**, F633–645.

Walker (1996). Dow AgroSciences, LLC, unpublished data.

Weiner (1997). Dow AgroSciences, LLC, unpublished data.

Weiner, I. D., and Wingo, C. S. (1997). Hypokalemia—consequences, causes and correction. *J. Am. Soc. Nephrol.* **8**, 1179–1188.

Wingo, C. S., and Cain, B. D. (1993). The renal H-K-ATPase: Physiological significance and role in potassium homeostasis. *Ann. Rev. Physiol.* **55**, 323–347.

Yano *et al.* (1987). Dow AgroSciences, LLC, unpublished data.

Yano *et al.* (1988). Dow AgroSciences, LLC, unpublished data.

Yano *et al.* (1991). Dow AgroSciences, LLC, unpublished data.

Zablotny (1996). Dow AgroSciences, LLC, unpublished data.

Zablotny and Carney (1997). Dow AgroSciences, LLC, unpublished data.

Zablotny *et al.* (1993). Dow AgroSciences, LLC, unpublished data.

Zablotny *et al.* (1994). Dow AgroSciences, LLC, unpublished data.

Zablotny *et al.* (1996). Dow AgroSciences, LLC, unpublished data.

Zempel *et al.* (1988). Dow AgroSciences, LLC, unpublished data.

Zempel *et al.* (1990). Dow AgroSciences, LLC, unpublished data.

Zielke *et al.* (1988). Dow AgroSciences, LLC, unpublished data.

Inhibitors of Aromatic Acid Biosynthesis

Donna Farmer
Monsanto Company

76.1 INTRODUCTION

Glyphosate is a broad-spectrum, postemergent systemic herbicide with activity on essentially all annual and perennial plants. Glyphosate-based formulations are used worldwide in virtually every phase of agricultural, industrial, silvicultural, and residential weed control. Due to low solubility in water, glyphosate is typically formulated into commercial products in the form of a salt. Glyphosate is poorly absorbed both dermally and via oral exposure and it is not biotransformed. It has been shown that glyphosate does not bioaccumulate. Animal studies indicate that glyphosate is essentially nontoxic via acute oral and dermal exposure, and that glyphosate salts are nonirritating to the eyes and skin. Glyphosate does not produce dermal sensitization in guinea pigs. In repeated dose studies in laboratory animals, treatment-related effects included reduced body weight gain, increased liver weights, degenerative ocular lens changes, and microscopic liver changes but only at very high dose levels (approximately 2–3% of the diet). No treatment-related tumors have been found in multiple carcinogenicity studies. Glyphosate has consistently produced negative results in standard mutagenicity assays conducted according to international guidelines. Regulatory agencies and other scientific organizations have concluded that glyphosate is neither carcinogenic nor mutagenic. The U.S. Environmental Protection Agency (U.S. EPA) USEPA has classified glyphosate in Category E ("Evidence of Non-Carcinogenicity in Humans"). There is no evidence of developmental or reproductive effects resulting from glyphosate exposure. In humans, accidental exposure to glyphosate formulations may result in minor, transient ocular and dermal irritation, but serious effects have not been observed.

76.2 GLYPHOSATE

76.2.1 IDENTITY, PROPERTIES, AND USES

Chemical name Glyphosate is *N*-(phosphonomethyl) glycine.

Structure The structure of glyphosate is shown in Fig. 76.1.

Synonyms The common name glyphosate is in general use. Trade names include Roundup®, RoundupUltra®, RoundupPro®, Landmaster®, Rodeo®, Accord®, Spark®, Vision®, and Biactive®. The CAS registry number for the acid is 1071-83-6.

Physical and Chemical Properties Glyphosate acid is typically referred to as the technical grade material and has the empirical formula $C_3H_8NO_5P$. It is a white, odorless, crystalline powder with a melting point of 184.5°C, a molecular weight of 169.1, and a specific gravity of 1.704. Glyphosate is not flammable, is not explosive and has a vapor pressure of 1.84×10^{-7} mm Hg at 45°C. Glyphosate is a relatively strong acid with a pH of 2 in 1% aqueous solution. The solubility of glyphosate in water is 1.2 wt% at 25°C and approximately 6 wt% at 100°C. It is slightly soluble in a few strong organic acids but relatively insoluble in most organic solvents. Because of its limited solubility in water, commercial herbicide formulations contain glyphosate in the form of a salt (i.e., isopropylamine, ammonium, phosphonium, etc.) (Franz *et al.*, 1997).

History, Formulations, and Uses Glyphosate is a broad-spectrum, nonselective, postemergent, systemic herbicide with activity on essentially all annual and perennial plants. The herbicidal properties of glyphosate were discovered by Monsanto in 1970, and the first commercial formulations were introduced in 1974 under the Roundup brand name. Today, glyphosate-based formulations are used in over 100 countries in virtually every phase of agricultural, industrial, silvicultural, and residential weed control, making it one of the most important weed-pest control tools ever introduced. Agricultural use of

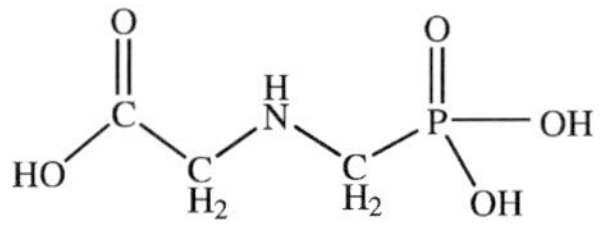

Figure 76.1 Glyphosate acid.

1667

glyphosate continues to expand. It has contributed significantly to the growing worldwide adoption of conservation and reduced tillage techniques as well as applications involving genetically modified plant varieties which can tolerate glyphosate treatment.

76.2.2 TOXICITY TO LABORATORY ANIMALS

Standard toxicity studies have been performed with technical grade glyphosate (averaging 96% purity on a dry weight basis). The results have been summarized in the reregistration eligibility decision (RED) document issued by the United States Environmental Protection Agency (U.S. EPA, 1993), the World Health Organization (WHO, 1994), and Williams *et al.* (2000). These results demonstrate that glyphosate has very low acute toxicity and is not mutagenic, teratogenic, carcinogenic, or a reproductive toxicant.

Acute Studies The oral LD_{50} in rats is >5000 mg/kg and the dermal LD_{50} in rabbits is >5000 mg/kg (WHO, 1994). An acute rat inhalation study has not been conducted with glyphosate technical because it is a nonvolatile solid material which would not generate a respirable vapor or particulate under circumstances of normal use. However, a 4-hour LC_{50} for an aqueous solution of the isoproplyamine salt of glyphosate was shown to be greater than the highest attainable atmospheric concentration of 1.3 mg/l (Dudek, 1987).

Irritation and Sensitization Studies Glyphosate technical produced mild skin irritation after a single 4-hour exposure. However, glyphosate did not produce dermal sensitization in guinea pigs (U.S. EPA, 1993). Glyphosate, when applied undiluted and without a wash, was severely irritating to the eyes (WHO, 1994). In contrast, the neutral pH isoproplyamine and monosodium salts are nonirritating to the eyes (Branch, 1981; Busch, 1987).

Dose Studies Several subchronic and chronic toxicology studies have been conducted on glyphosate, and the results of these investigations have been reported by the U.S. EPA (1993), WHO (1994), and Williams *et al.* (2000). The major findings of these studies are summarized in this chapter. In a 3-month feeding study with Sprague-Dawley rats, the no-observed-effect level (NOEL) was 20,000 ppm (approximately 1445 mg/kg/day), the highest dose tested. Administration of glyphosate to CD-1 mice for 3 months at dietary levels of 0, 5000, 10,000, and 50,000 ppm resulted in reduced body weight gains in high-dose animals. The NOEL was 10,000 ppm (approximately 2300 mg/kg/day). Glyphosate was applied to the shaven intact and abraded skin of New Zealand white rabbits for 6 hour per day, 5 days per week for 3 weeks at dose levels of 0, 100, 1000, and 5000 mg/kg/day. A slight degree of dermal irritation was observed at the site of application in the high-dose group. No adverse effects were noted in the hematologic, biochemical, and histopathological evaluations. The systemic NOEL was considered to be 5000 mg/kg/day. Glyphosate was given to beagle dogs via oral capsule at dosages of 0, 20, 100, or 500 mg/kg/day for 1 year. No treatment-related effects were noted even at the highest dose tested; therefore, the NOEL was considered to be 500 mg/kg/day. Brahman-cross heifers received daily dosages of the isopropylamine salt of glyphosate via stomach tube for seven consecutive days at dosages of 0, 540, 830, 1290, and 2000 mg/kg/day. Mortality was observed only at the two highest doses. Other effects, including body weight loss, diarrhea, serum chemistry changes, and histopathological findings were observed at or above 830 mg/kg/day. Changes in several hematologic parameters observed at 1290 mg/kg/day and above were considered secondary to fluid and blood volume alterations resulting from the diarrhea. The NOEL was considered to be 540 mg/kg/day. Three rodent bioassays were conducted with glyphosate. In the first of two long-term feeding studies conducted in Sprague-Dawley rats, glyphosate was administered in the diet at concentrations of 0, 60, 200, and 600 ppm for approximately 26 months. The NOEL was considered to be >600 ppm (32 mg/kg/day) because no tumors or other adverse effects related to treatment were noted at any dose level. In the second chronic study, rats were fed glyphosate in the diet at concentrations of 0, 2000, 8000, and 20,000 ppm for approximately 2 years. No tumors related to treatment were observed. The only effects considered related to treatment were observed in high-dose animals and included decreased body weight gain in females and degenerative ocular lens changes, increased liver weights, and elevated urine pH or specific gravity in males. The NOEL in this study was concluded to be 8000 ppm (409 mg/kg/day). Glyphosate was fed to CD-1 mice in the diet at concentrations of 0, 100, 5000, or 30,000 ppm. No treatment-related tumors were observed. The NOEL in this study was concluded to be 5000 ppm (750 mg/kg/day) based upon reduced body weight gains in high-dose males and females and microscopic liver changes (central lobular hepatocyte hypertrophy and hepatocyte necrosis) in high-dose males.

Absorption, Distribution, Metabolism, and Excretion Absorption of glyphosate across skin and gastrointestinal membranes is minimal. *In vitro* absorption of glyphosate through human skin was no more than 2% of applied dose (Wester *et al.*, 1991). Wester *et al.* (1991) also reported the *in vivo* dermal absorption of glyphosate in the rhesus monkey to be 2.2% at a high dose of 5400 $\mu g/cm^2$. The results of several studies show that there is rapid elimination, no biotransformation, and minimal tissue retention of glyphosate in various species, including mammals, birds, and fish (U.S. EPA, 1993; WHO, 1994). Greater than 90% of an orally administered dose of glyphosate is rapidly eliminated in 72 hours (National Toxicology Program, 1992). Typically, approximately 70% of the administered dose is eliminated in the feces, with the remainder eliminated in the urine. In all cases, less than 0.5% of the administered dose is found in the tissues and organs, demonstrating that glyphosate does not bioaccumulate in edible tissues. Studies of the metabolism of glyphosate in experimental animals (rats, rabbits, lactating goats, and chickens) indicate that it is not biotransformed, with essentially all the administered dose excreted as unchanged parent molecule (Bodden, 1988; Colvin and Miller, 1973; Ridley and Mirly, 1988).

Genotoxicity Studies Glyphosate was negative in well-validated mutagenicity assays performed for regulatory purposes conducted according to international guidelines under good laboratory practices (U.S. EPA, 1993; WHO, 1994). These assays assessed a variety of end points both *in vitro* and *in vivo* and included the following: *Salmonella typhimurium* (Ames assay), *Escherichia Coli* WP-2 reverse mutation, rec-assay with *Bacillus subtilis*, CHO/HGPRT, *in vivo* mouse bone marrow micronucleus, and *in vitro* hepatocyte primary culture–DNA repair assay. Williams *et al.* (2000), in a review on glyphosate, employed a weight-of-evidence evaluation of the many genotoxicity assays including those submitted for regulatory purposes as well as others in the published scientific literature. It was concluded that glyphosate is neither mutagenic nor clastogenic. A limited number of studies in the literature have reported positive results regarding the genotoxic potential of glyphosate; review by these authors found that these assays used toxic dose levels, irrelevant routes of exposure, end points, and test systems, and/or deficient testing methodology.

Carcinogenicity Studies Regulatory agencies and other scientific organizations have concluded that glyphosate is neither carcinogenic nor mutagenic. In June of 1991, the U.S. EPA following a thorough review of all toxicology data available concluded that glyphosate should be classified in Category E ("Evidence of Non-Carcinogenicity in Humans"). This classification was based upon the observation of no treatment-related tumors at any dose level with glyphosate tested up to the limit dose in rats and up to levels higher than the limit dose in mice, and upon the lack of evidence for mutagenicity with glyphosate (U.S. EPA, 1992).

Mode of Action Glyphosate's mode of action has been previously described in detail (Franz *et al.*, 1997). Glyphosate inhibits plant growth through competitive inhibition of the enzyme 5-enolpyruvoylshikimate 3-phosphate synthase (EPSPS). This enzyme plays a key role in the biosynthesis of the intermediate, chorismate, necessary for the synthesis of the essential amino acids phenylalanine, tyrosine, and tryptophan. This aromatic amino acid biosynthetic pathway (shikimic acid pathway) is found in plants as well as some fungi and bacteria but not in insects, birds, fish, mammals, and humans, thus providing a specific selective toxicity to plant species.

Developmental and Reproduction Studies The reproductive and developmental toxicity data base has been evaluated by the U.S. EPA (1999). This assessment was conducted under the Federal Food, Drug, and Cosmetic Act, as amended by the Food Quality Protection Act (FQPA). The FQPA was enacted by the U.S. Congress in 1996 with provisions that support the governments focus on children's environmental health risks. It requires the U.S. EPA to more carefully consider the risks posed to infants and children by pesticide residues on food when setting acceptable residue levels and tolerances. The U.S. EPA is required to apply an additional 10-fold safety factor to ensure the protection of infants and children unless a determination can be made on the basis of reliable data that a lesser margin of safety is protective. As a result of their assessment, the EPA may also require additional testing to detect potential developmental neurotoxic effects. Regarding glyphosate, EPA has concluded that there is a complete toxicity data base and exposure data is complete or can be estimated based on data that reasonably accounts for potential exposures. It was concluded there is no indication that the developing fetus or neonate is more sensitive than adult animals. Consequently no developmental neurotoxicity studies were required. The EPA believes that reliable data support the use of the standard 100-fold uncertainty factor and concluded that there is a reasonable certainty that no harm will result to infants and children from aggregate exposure to glyphosate residues. The studies supporting these conclusions are summarized next.

Sprague-Dawley rats were dosed by gavage at doses of 0, 300, 1000, or 3500 mg/kg/day during days 6–19 of gestation. At 3500 mg/kg/day, the following signs of toxicity were observed: increased mortality (6 of 25 dams died) and other clinical signs of toxicity, decreased fetal weights, increased incidence of early resorptions, decreases in total number of implantations and the number of viable fetuses, and increased number of fetuses with reduced ossification of sternebrae. At the lower dose levels these effects were absent. There was no evidence of teratogenicity at any dose level. The NOEL for both maternal and developmental toxicity was 1000 mg/kg/day. In Dutch belted rabbits, glyphosate was tested at dose levels of 0, 75, 175, or 350 mg/kg/day from days 6 through 27 of gestation. The maternal NOEL was determined to be 175 mg/kg/day based on maternal signs of toxicity seen only at the highest dose tested. These effects included death (10 of 16 does died), diarrhea, and nasal discharge. Excessive maternal mortality resulted in an inadequate number of fetuses for evaluation at 350 mg/kg/day. Therefore, although no developmental toxicity was observed at any dose level, the developmental NOEL was considered to be 175 mg/kg/day.

Glyphosate was administered to Sprague-Dawley rats in the diet at dosages of 3, 10, and 30 mg/kg/day for three successive generations (2 litters per generation). There were no treatment-related effects on mating, fertility, or other reproductive parameters. An equivocal increase was noted for the incidence of unilateral renal tubular dilation in male pups of the F3b generation in the high-dose group. The small increase in incidence was not considered related to treatment. This conclusion is supported by the absence of a similar effect in a more recent study which evaluated substantially more animals and used significantly higher dose levels (3% of the diet). In the more recent reproduction study, Sprague-Dawley rats were administered glyphosate in the diet at dosages of 0,

2000, 10,000, and 30,000 ppm (equivalent to 0, 100, 500, and 1500 mg/kg/day). There was no effect on the ability of treated rats to mate, conceive, carry, or deliver normal offspring. The systemic NOEL was 10,000 ppm based on soft stools and decreased body weights and pup weights during the second and third weeks of lactation. The reproductive NOEL was the highest dose tested, 30,000 ppm.

76.2.3 HUMAN EXPERIENCE

No evidence was observed for the induction of photoirritation nor of allergic or photoallergic contact dermatitis when Roundup herbicide (41% IPA salt of glyphosate, water, and a surfactant) was evaluated in 346 volunteers (Maibach, 1986). Roundup was less irritating than a standard dishwashing detergent and a general all-purpose cleaner and was no different than baby shampoo.

Acquavella *et al.* (1999) evaluated effects from 1513 human ocular exposures to various Roundup formulations reported to an American Association of Poison Control Centers (AAPCC) certified regional poison control center during the years 1993 through 1997. The majority of the reported exposures were judged by the poison center specialists to result in either no injury (21%) or transient minor symptoms (70%). In no case did exposure result in permanent change to the structure or function of the eye.

The exposure potential of the general population and applicators to glyphosate have been reviewed by Williams *et al.* (2000). Exposure of the general population to glyphosate is very low and occurs primarily from the diet. Glyphosate has been registered for use in food crops for over 20 years, and glyphosate is now used in a wide range of crops. The initial uses for glyphosate were for preplanting or preemergence applications and resulted in negligible residues in the crops. Later uses have included applications when the crops are present, either using directed spray techniques, applications close to harvest, or herbicide-tolerant crops. These uses can result in residues in edible commodities, although they are still at very low levels. The reference dose (RfD) for glyphosate based on the developmental toxicity study with rabbits (NOEL of 175 mg per kilogram of body weight per day) and using a 100-fold safety factor is calculated to be 2.0 mg(kg body weight)day (U.S. EPA, 1999). The RfD represents the level at or below which daily aggregate dietary exposure over a lifetime will not pose appreciable risks to human health. The U.S. EPA generally has no concern for exposures below 100% of the RfD. The theoretical maximum residue contributions (TMRC) and percentage of RfDs for the U.S. population was estimated to be 0.029960 or 1.5% of the RfD and 0.064388 or 3.2% or the RfD for children (1–6 years old) (U.S. EPA, 1999). Because the qualitative nature of glyphosate residues is well understood and the aggregate exposure is not expected to exceed 100% of the RfD, the U.S. EPA concludes that there is reasonable certainty that no harm will result from aggregate exposure to glyphosate residues.

Dermal contact is the most likely route of exposure for applicators; activities such as mixing and loading of glyphosate and extended applications using hand sprayers have the highest potential for exposure. Inhalation is considered to be a minimal route of exposure under most circumstances because of glyphosate's extremely low vapor pressure. Biological measurements estimating the amount of pesticide that has penetrated into the body, the internal dose, provide the most relevant information for safety assessments. Lavy *et al.* (1992) found that, of 355 daily urine samples analyzed from silvicultural workers, none contained quantifiable levels of glyphosate, with a limit of quantification of 10 ppb. Cowell and Steinmetz (1990) found that, of 96 urine samples analyzed from silvicultural workers, only 5 contained quantifiable levels of glyphosate. The highest measurement was 14 ppb. In a recent pilot study with three farmers and their families, there were no quantifiable residues of glyphosate in the study except one farmer with a urinary glyphosate measurement of 12 ppb on the day of a 5-hour, hand-wand sprayer application to weeds along a fence line (Alexander *et al.*, 1999). This application method is similar to those in the previous silvicultural studies. In a worst case analysis, Williams *et al.* (2000) estimated that an adult worker's peak acute exposure to glyphosate during application was 56.2 μg(kg body weight)day and, for a 5-day working week, the chronic applicator exposure was 8.5 μg(kg body weight)day. Comparison of these values to lowest relevant NOEL of 175 mg/kg/day in a the rabbit developmental toxicity study produced margins of exposure (MOEs) of 3114 and 20,588 in acute and chronic exposure, respectively. Actual exposures are anticipated to be significantly less. Jauhiainen *et al.* (1991), in addition to biological and inhalation monitoring of glyphosate of forestry workers during application, had each worker receive a medical examination on the first and last days that Roundup® herbicide was applied and a follow-up examination 3 weeks after the last application day. No changes were noted in hematology, clinical chemistry, electrocardiogram, pulmonary function, blood pressure, or heart rate.

Accidental exposures to small volumes of glyphosate have not produced serious effects. In spite of this experience, it has been stated that glyphosate is a leading cause of pesticide poisoning in California. California's Department of Pesticide Regulation (CDPR) pesticide incident program accepts telephone inquiries from physicians, who are required to report pesticide incidents, as well as from the general public. Although many calls are purely informational or report effects limited to topical irritation, all telephone calls are recorded as "poisonings," incorrectly suggesting some degree of systemic illness. In 1994, CDPR reported only 13 "definite" or "probable" calls related to glyphosate exposure alone among the 1995 total calls received (California Environmental Protection Agency, 1996). Eleven of these 13 cases reported only minor and reversible eye irritation likely due to accidental overexposure. Of the remaining two cases, one involved a worker who reported a headache in addition to eye irritation. The other case involved symptoms related to ingestion and/or aspiration of hydrocarbon solvent. The latter case cannot be related to glyphosate itself or to a marketed formulation, because commercial preparations of glyphosate are not formulated using hydrocarbon solvents. The

CDPR noted in its 1994 Pesticide Illness Surveillance Report that greater than 80% of the people affected by glyphosate experienced only irritant effects and that, of the 515 pesticide-related hospitalizations recorded over the 13 years on file, none was attributed to glyphosate. Statements to the effect that glyphosate is a major cause of clinical poisoning in California are clearly not substantiated by the available data.

It has become customary to generically refer to any organic compound containing phosphorous as an "organophosphate." However, there are actually different classes of "organic phosphate" compounds that are determined by the atoms attached to the phosphorus. The phosphorus atom of a true organophosphate is attached only to oxygen atoms (O'Brien, 1967). The structure of glyphosate is different in two important respects. First, the phosphorus atom is attached to the remainder of the molecule by a carbon atom, not an oxygen. This classifies the glyphosate molecule as an organophosphonate (O'Brien, 1967). Second, there are no other side chains attached to the phosphorus atom. Glyphosate consists of a glycine moiety and a phosphonomethyl moiety. These distinctions are important for the following reason. The nature of the groups attached to the phosphorous determine how strongly the molecule will interact with the enzyme cholinesterase (O'Brien, 1967). The groups attached to the phosphorus of a true organophosphate allow it to be readily hydrolyzed by cholinesterase. In contrast, the carbon–phosphorus bond of an organophosphonate is not easily broken (Roberts and Caserio, 1965). This interaction is responsible for the subsequent inhibition of the enzyme and disruption of normal nerve function. The phosphorus of an organophosphonate such as glyphosate, on the other hand, does not react with or inhibit cholinesterase. Thus, this type of molecule does not interfere with normal nerve function (Williams *et al.*, 2000).

Large amounts of glyphosate-based herbicides are occasionally deliberately ingested to attempt suicide and may result in serious gastrointestinal, cardiovascular, pulmonary, and renal effects and possibly death. Aggressive supportive care is recommended (Tominack *et al.*, 1989). Glyphosate is sometimes mistakenly referred to as an organophosphate, thus contributing to the incorrect perception that glyphosate is a cholinesterase inhibitor similar to the organophosphate insecticides. As a result, some patients who have ingested glyphosate-based herbicides have received inappropriate medical treatment which may have worsened their condition. Atropine or 2-PAM (Pralidoxime) are not indicated in the treatment of glyphosate exposure.

REFERENCES

Acquavella, J. F., Weber, J. A., Cullen, M. R., Cruz, O. A., Martens, M. A., Holden, L. R., Riordan, S., Thompson, M., and Farmer, D. R. (1999). Human ocular effects from self-reported exposure to Roundup herbicides. *Hum. Expl. Toxicol.* **18**, 479–486.

Alexander, B. H., Mandel, J. S., Baker, B. A., and Honeycutt, R. (1999). "The Farm Family Exposure Pilot Study." Unpublished draft final report.

Bodden, R. M. (1988). "Metabolism Study of Synthetic ^{13}C/^{14}C-Labeled Glyphosate and Aminomethylphosphonic Acid in Laying Hens." Unpublished report, Hazleton Laboratories America, Inc., Madison, WI.

Branch, D. K. (1981). "Primary Eye Irritation of Isopropylamine Salt of Glyphosate to Rabbits Eyes." Unpublished report, Monsanto Environmental Health Laboratory, St. Louis, MO.

Busch, B. (1987). "Primary Eye Irritation Study of Monosodium Salt of Glyphosate in New Zealand White Rabbits." Unpublished report, Food and Drug Research Laboratories, Inc., Waverly, NY.

California Environmental Protection Agency (1996). "California Pesticide Illness Surveillance Program Summary Report 1994." Department of Pesticide Regulation, California Environmental Protection Agency, Sacramento.

Colvin, L. B., and Miller, J. A. (1973). "Residue and Metabolism—The Gross Distribution of N-Phosphonylmethylglycine-^{14}C in Rabbits." Unpublished report, Monsanto Company, St. Louis, MO.

Cowell, J. E., and Steinmetz, J. R. (1990). "Assessment of Forest Worker Exposures to Glyphosate During Backpack Foliar Applications of Roundup® Herbicide." Unpublished report, Monsanto Company, St. Louis, MO.

Dudek, B. R. (1987). "Acute Toxicity of Rodeo® Herbicide Administered by Inhalation to Male and Female Sprague-Dawley Rats." Unpublished report, Monsanto Environmental Health Laboratory, St. Louis, MO.

Franz, J. E., Mao, M. K., and Sikorski, J. A. (1997). "Glyphosate: A Unique Global Herbicide," ACS Monograph No. 189. Am. Chem. Soc., Washington, D.C.

Jauhiainen, A., Rasanen, K., Sarantila, R., Nuntineg, J., and Kangas, J. (1991). *Am. Ind. Hyg. Assoc. J.* **52**, 61–64.

Lavy, T. L., Cowell, J. E., Steinmetz, J. R., and Massey, J. H. (1992). Conifer seedling nursery worker exposure to glyphosate. *Arch. Environ. Contam. Toxicol.* **22**, 6–13.

Maibach, H. I. (1986). Irritation, sensitization, photoirritation, and photosensitization assays with a glyphosate herbicide. *Contact Dermatitis* **15**, 152–156.

National Toxicology Program (1992). "Technical Report on Toxicity Studies of Glyphosate (CAS No. 1071-83-6) Administered in Dosed Feed to F344/N Rats and B6C3F, Mice." Toxicity Report Series Number 16, NIH Publication 92-3135, July 1992, National Toxicology (NTP), U.S. Department of Health and Human Services, Research Triangle Park, NC.

O'Brien, R. D. (1967). Organophosphates: Chemistry and inhibitory activity. *In* "Insecticides: Action and Metabolism," pp. 32–54. Academic Press, New York.

Ridley, W. P., and Mirly, K. (1988). "The Metabolism of Glyphosate in Sprague-Dawley Rats. I. Excretion and Tissue Distribution of Glyphosate and Its Metabolites Following Intravenous and Oral Administration." Unpublished report, Monsanto Environmental Health Laboratory, St. Louis, MO.

Roberts, J. D., and Caserio, M. S. (1965). Organophosphorus compounds. *In* "Basic Principles of Organic Chemistry," pp. 1194–1215. Benjamin, New York.

Tominack, R. L., Conner, P., and Yamashita, M. (1989). Clinical management of Roundup herbicide exposure. *Jpn. J. Toxicol.* **2**, 187–192.

U.S. Environmental Protection Agency (U.S. EPA) (1992). Pesticide tolerance proposed rule. *Fed. Reg.* **57**, 8739–8740.

U.S. Environmental Protection Agency (U.S. EPA) (1993). "Re-registration Eligibility Decision (RED): Glyphosate." Office of Prevention, Pesticides and Toxic Substances, U.S. Environmental Protection Agency, Washington, D.C.

U.S. Environmental Protection Agency (U.S. EPA) (1999). Glyphosate: Pesticide tolerance, Final Rule—40 CFR, Part 180 [Opp-300835; FRL-6073-5]. *Fed. Reg.* **64**(71), 18360–18367.

Wester, R. C., Melendres, J., Sarason, R., McMaster, J., and Maibach, H. I. (1991). Glyphosate skin binding, absorption, residual tissue distribution, and skin decontamination. *Fundam. Appl. Toxicol.* **16**, 725–732.

World Health Organization (WHO) (1994). "Glyphosate," Environmental Health Criteria No. 159. International Programme of Chemical Safety (IPCS), World Health Organization, Geneva.

Williams, G. M., Kroes, R., and Munro, I. C. (2000). Safety evaluation and risk assessment of the herbicide roundup and its active ingredient, glyphosate, for humans. *Regul. Toxicol. Pharmacol.* **31**, 117–165.

CHAPTER

77

Inhibitors of DNA Biosynthesis–Mitosis: Benzimidazoles—The Benzimidazole Fungicides Benomyl and Carbendazim

Ronald L. Mull

RLM Strategies, Inc.

Leon W. Hershberger

DuPont Agricultural Products

77.1 AGRICULTURAL USE AND SCIENTIFIC INTEREST

The benzimidazole fungicides benomyl and carbendazim are extensively used worldwide on a variety of crops (vegetables, fruits, nuts, cereals, cotton, ornamentals, mushrooms, and others) for numerous fungal pests. They have been in use for approximately 30 years with an excellent safety record. They are toxicologically very similar because benomyl is rapidly converted to carbendazim. Therefore, it is advisable to consider information available from both products to have a complete understanding of the toxicity of benomyl. Studies with both benomyl and carbendazim are considered in this chapter.

A complete contemporary toxicology database exists to support the widespread registration of these products. Relatively little of this data has been published in the open literature by the pesticide manufacturers, but most of the available data have been reviewed and commented upon by panels of experts and are available to the public. The World Health Organization (WHO) *Environmental Health Criteria* (EHC) *148* (benomyl) and *149* (carbendazim) were published in 1993 (WHO, 1993a, b); the Food and Agriculture Organization (FAO) and WHO published the Joint FAO/WHO Meeting on Pesticide Residues (JMPR) 1995 evaluation of benomyl and carbendazim toxicology in 1996 (FAO/WHO, 1996a, b) and 1998 evaluation of residues in 1999 (FAO/WHO, 1999a, b). These documents will serve as excellent resources for the reader wishing to probe further than is done here. References in this chapter to un-

published work may be found in the WHO and FAO/WHO documents, along with summaries of individual studies.

Benomyl and carbendazim are of low acute toxicity and present little likelihood of acute systemic illness from their use in agriculture; in fact, none have been reported from either product after years of widespread use. However, both have been extensively studied because of reproductive and developmental effects seen in laboratory animals given high oral doses and because they cause aneuploidy (numerical chromosome aberrations) in mammalian cells both *in vitro* and *in vivo*. Studies employing new techniques have demonstrated thresholds for the aneugenic effects. Their fungicidal activity is due to the ability to bind to tubulin and disrupt microtubule assembly during cell replication. Studies have shown that mammalian cells have a much lower capacity for binding in comparison to fungal tubulin.

Benomyl, but not carbendazim, is presently registered in the United States; however, both products are registered and sold in many countries throughout the rest of the world. Benomyl is sold only as a wettable powder formulation whereas carbendazim is sold in several formulation types. Outside the United States, both are sold alone and as mixtures with other fungicides. These mixtures aid in preventing the resistance that such site-specific pesticides are prone to cause. In the United States, benomyl is commonly mixed in the spray tank with other fungicides.

Exposure of the general population is likely limited to residues in the diet whereas the skin is the primary exposure route for persons using these fungicides in agriculture, with limited exposure from inhalation. Extensive available data show that a wide margin of safety exists between potential environmental and occupational exposures and those that cause mammalian toxicity. There are no reports of human ingestion of large amounts of benomyl or carbendazim in cases of accident or suicide.

77.2 POTENTIAL FOR HUMAN HEALTH EFFECTS

Benomyl and carbendazim present low potential risk for causing acute illness. They are of relatively low toxicity in all mammalian species tested. Both are well absorbed after oral exposure, but poorly absorbed by dermal exposure. Illness following acute exposure has not been reported except for skin irritation. Benomyl, but not carbendazim, has been implicated in skin sensitization in humans. Given the expected low exposures and the poor absorption through the skin, it is not likely that the exposures of either the general population or agricultural users will result in systemic illness.

Exposure of the general population is most likely to occur through residues on food. Estimates of dietary exposure based on regional or national food consumption patterns have been made in Europe, the United States, and elsewhere. These estimates indicate exposures well below the acceptable daily intake (ADI) established by the World Health Organization in 1993 (WHO, 1993a, b). Regulatory bodies and the WHO have concluded that the exposures likely to result from use of these fungicides in agriculture pose little risk of human health effects (FAO/WHO, 1996a, b, 1999a, b; WHO, 1993a, b).

Benomyl and carbendazim cause reproductive and developmental effects when given to certain laboratory animals in high oral doses. In laboratory studies, developmental toxicity was demonstrated when benomyl or carbendazim was given by gavage administration. Similar developmental toxicity was not observed in dietary exposure studies. Bolus dose exposures, similar to the gavage laboratory animal dosing, are not expected to occur in humans, and the dietary experiments represent the more likely approximation of any human effects from exposure.

These compounds are not directly mutagenic, but have been widely studied because they induce numerical chromosome aberrations (aneuploidy). Disruption of microtubule assembly in the actively dividing cell results in aneuploidy, an effect which has a demonstrable no-observed-effect level (NOEL) and threshold doses below which effects are not seen (Bentley et al., 2000). Their fungicidal activity is thought to be due to the ability to bind to tubulin during cell replication, causing nondisjunction and cell death. Studies have shown that mammalian cells have less affinity for this binding than do fungal cells, and human cells have a low capacity for binding.

Benomyl and carbendazim were not carcinogenic after lifetime dietary exposures in rats and up to 2 years of feeding in dogs. However, benign liver tumors have been shown following lifetime feeding in mouse strains having high background incidences of these tumors. Tumors were not seen in a mouse strain with a low background incidence of liver tumors, suggesting that the relevance of the mouse liver tumors to other species is questionable. Efforts to better understand the propensity of the mouse to develop liver tumors continue (Fox and Gonzalez, 1996).

Both have been thoroughly evaluated in acute, subchronic, and chronic studies in rats, mice, rabbits, and dogs. In extended feeding studies, the dog was the most sensitive species tested. The 2-year NOEL for benomyl was 13 mg/kg/day (females) and 14 mg/kg/day (males). In carbendazim studies, the NOELs were similar to those of the benomyl dog studies, if adjusted for the molecular weight difference. Based on the 2-year benomyl dog study and applying a 100-fold safety factor, the ADI for benomyl would be 0.1 mg/kg. Based on the 2-year carbendazim dog study and applying a 100-fold safety factor, the ADI for carbendazim would be 0.03 mg/kg/day (FAO/WHO, 1996a, b).

The potential dietary exposure of humans to benomyl residues was estimated to be 0.000218 mg/kg/day in the United States (Eickhoff et al., 1989). This is considerably lower than the Environmental Protection Agency (EPA) reference dose (0.05 mg/kg/day). Because postharvest usages of benomyl were removed from the Benlate® fungicide label in 1989, this value is likely to represent an overestimate of current dietary intake. The potential benomyl and carbendazim dietary exposure was evaluated for five different geographic regions by the 1998 JMPR meeting. The international estimated daily intake (EIDI) ranged between 1 and 14% of the WHO ADI (0.03 mg/kg/day) (FAO/WHO, 1999b).

Agricultural usage results in primarily dermal exposure to the sprayers or other agricultural workers. Studies of dermal absorption of benomyl and carbendazim, both in vivo and in vitro, show them to be poorly absorbed by this route. Topical effects such as skin irritation and sensitization are the primary complaints from agricultural use. Mild eye irritation is also possible. Inhalation exposure is limited due to the low vapor pressure and to the size of the airborne droplets from spray application, which is generally well above the respirable range. No systemic toxicities in humans have been shown to result from either benomyl or carbendazim exposure.

The exposure levels from studies on occupational exposure to benomyl vary. Procedures such as mixing operations that involve the direct handling of fungicide formulations have the highest potential to cause exposure. Average values of potential dermal deposition during mixing, during field reentry and harvesting, and during simulated use on home gardens were 26 mg per mixing cycle, 12 mg on reentry, 5.9 mg per hour of harvesting, and <1 mg per application cycle, respectively (Everhart and Holt, 1982). Similar results for harvesting were reported by Zweig et al. (1983), who found that benomyl exposures averaged 5.39 mg/hour for strawberry pickers. All values were calculated for "worst case" situations in which no protective clothing would be worn. These estimated exposures must be reduced by the limited degree of skin absorption, to judge potential systemic exposures.

To determine potential dermal exposure from contact with foliage during reentry, Liesivuori et al. (1988) studied dissipation rates for benomyl following applications in three rose greenhouses. The mean half-lives for benomyl and carbendazim were 44 and 53 hours, respectively. When benomyl was sprayed on apples, foliage residues dissipated quickly during the first 3–7 days, but at least 15% of the original deposit remained after 12 days.

Exposure by inhalation is potentially greatest in manufacturing operations where handling takes place in an enclosed area on a daily basis. Industrial hygiene surveys in manufacturing facilities over a 4.5-year period (1974–1979) reported Benlate dust concentrations averaged 0.708 mg/m^3 [6–8 hour time-weighted average (TWA); range is 0–2.01 mg/m^3] (DuPont, 1979).

In an agricultural setting, potential human exposure to benomyl via inhalation was calculated to be 0.08 mg per work cycle for the mixing and loading of formulations for aerial spraying; 0.003 mg for field reentry; 0.002 mg/hour for hand-harvesting; and 0.003 mg per application for simulated home use (Everhart and Holt, 1982). No inhalation exposure to benomyl could be detected among lawn-care workers (limit of detection equivalent to 0.004 mg/m^3) (Leonard and Yeary, 1990).

More recent investigations (Hoekstra et $al.$, 1996; Lavy et $al.$, 1993; NIOSH, 1994) have utilized measurements of dermal deposition, inhalation, and excretion of the urinary metabolites 4-hydroxy-2-benzimidazole carbamate (4-HBC) and methyl-5-hydroxy-2-benzimidazole carbamate (5-HBC) to obtain a more refined estimate of systemic exposure. Lavy et $al.$ conducted a year-long monitoring study of tree nursery workers engaged in varying tasks and have estimated the exposures to benomyl based on urinary excretion of 4-HBC and 5-HBC. They estimated the margins of safety to be from 14,000 to 69,400 for a 10-day exposure period and even greater margins of safety for a 30-day period. Hoekstra et $al.$ also found low levels of exposure for greenhouse nursery workers involved in typical operations in Florida. The systemic exposure was estimated from urinary excretion of 5-HBC, and they found the highest average concentration in the urine to be 23.8 μmol 5-HBC per mole of creatinine. Additionally, inhalation exposure to both benomyl and BIC (bulylisocyanate) was measured and found to be quite low, the highest average for benomyl being 32.8 μg/m^3 and for BIC, 6.6 ppb.

The American Council of Governmental and Industrial Hygienists (ACGIH) has recommended an 8-hour TWA threshold limit value (TLV) of 10 mg/m^3 for benomyl and carbendazim. The Occupational Safety and Health Administration (OSHA) permissible exposure limit (PEL) is 10 mg/m^3 (total dust) and 5 mg/m^3 (respirable dust).

77.2.1 MEDICAL SURVEILLANCE AND TESTING

The primary adverse health consequence associated with exposure to benomyl or carbendazim is contact dermatitis. Patch testing with benomyl confirmed positive dermal reactions in a number of patients (Fregert, 1973; Kuehne et $al.$, 1985; Savitt,

1972; Schuman and Dobson, 1985; van Joost et $al.$, 1983; van Ketel, 1976). One report also suggests the possibility of false negative readings for an individual tested with benomyl (Larsen et $al.$, 1990). Despite the widespread use of benomyl and carbendazim, adverse skin effects are relatively rare (Cronin, 1980; Lisi et $al.$, 1986; van Joost et $al.$, 1983). Some researchers have suggested that allergic effects attributed to benomyl may be cross-reactions to other pesticides (Larsen et $al.$, 1990; Matsushita and Aoyama, 1981).

Fertility in male workers was studied due to early animal study results that implicated the testes as a target of toxicity. A group of 286 male workers with potential exposure to benomyl and carbendazim were studied for fertility patterns by assessing the birth rates among their spouses. Workers were divided into three exposure categories: average exposure, below-average exposure, and varied exposures. Birth rates for each group were at or above expected levels when compared to control populations, and it was concluded that benomyl exposure had no adverse effect on fertility rates among exposed workers (Gooch, 1978).

Media allegations of a relationship between exposure to benomyl and the occurrence of birth defects prompted investigators in several countries to undertake epidemiology studies. A study was conducted in Italy to look at cases of anophthalmia and their relationship to benomyl exposure. Parental exposure to benomyl did not appear to be a factor, and the authors concluded that an association between benomyl use and congenital microphthalmia and anophthalmia appears unlikely (Spagnolo et $al.$, 1994). In another study of farm workers in Norway investigators found no association between exposure to benomyl and cases of children born with anophthalmia (Kristensen and Irgens, 1994). A third study in England found no clustering of cases of anophthalmia or microphthalmia in any region in England, refuting media allegations of clusters in farming areas where benomyl may have been used (Dolk et $al.$, 1988).

77.2.2 EXPOSURE-RELATED ILLNESS

The products may cause a temporary contact dermatitis. However, no specific human symptoms of benomyl or carbendazim toxicity are known. In a practical sense, exposures are likely to be from benomyl or carbendazim plus a mixture partner so it is important for the medical provider to try to determine the probable constituents of the mixture. Treatment for overexposure should be symptomatic and supportive.

77.3 PHYSICAL AND CHEMICAL PROPERTIES

The structures of benomyl and carbendazim are shown in Fig. 77.1. The physical properties are given in table from Fig. 77.1.

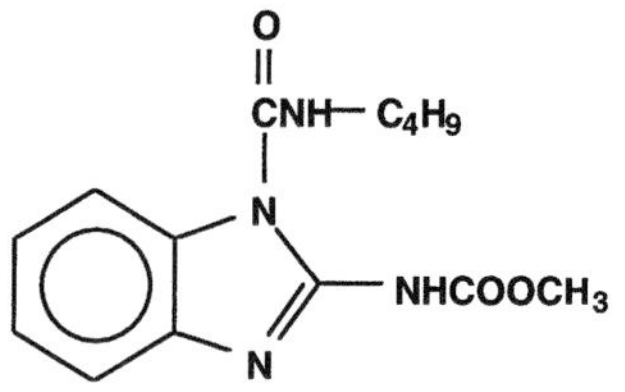

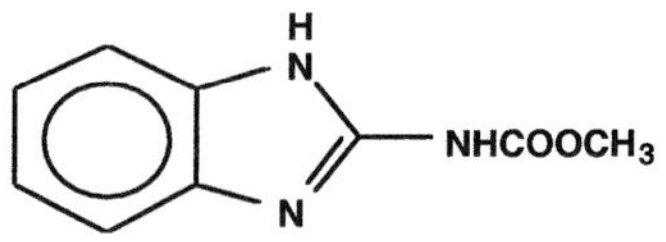

Name	benomyl	carbendazim
Common	Benomyl	Carbendazim
IUPAC	methyl 1-(butylcarbamoyl)-benzimidazol-2-ylcarbamate	methyl benzimidazol-2-ylcarbamate
CAS	Methyl [1-[(butylamino)carbonyl]-1*H*-benzimidazol-2-yl]carbamate	methyl 1*H*-benzimidazol-2-ylcarbamate
CAS number	17804-35-2	10605-21-7
Empirical Formula	$C_{14}H_{18}N_4O_3$	$C_9H_9N_3O_2$
Molecular Weight	290.62	191.19
Physical State	Colorless crystal	Colorless crystal

Physical Properties	Benomyl	Carbendazim
Melting Point (°C)	Decomposes shortly after starting to melt at about 100°C.	302-307°, with decomposition
Aqueous Solubility (at 25 °C)	at pH 5: 3.6 mg/L at pH 7: 2.9 mg/L at pH 9: 1.9 mg/L	at pH 4: 28 mg/L at pH 7: 8 mg/L at pH 8: 7 mg/L
Vapor Pressure	$<5.0 \times 10^{-6}$ Pa @ 25° C	6.5×10^{-8} Pa @ 20° C
Henry's Law Constant[a]	at pH 5: $<4.0 \times 10^{-4}$ Pa-m^3/mol at pH 7: $<5.0 \times 10^{-4}$ Pa-m^3/mol at pH 9: $<7.7 \times 10^{-4}$ Pa-m^3/mol	at pH 4: 4.42×10^{-7} Pa-m^3/mol at pH 7: 1.55×10^{-6} Pa-m^3/mol at pH 8: 1.77×10^{-6} Pa-m^3/mol
Octanol/Water Partition Coefficient	23.4 (from unbuffered water)	at pH 5: 24 at pH 7: 32 at pH 9: 31
Dissociation Constant (pK$_a$)		4.48

[a]   Henry's law constant was calculated from the vapor pressure and aqueous solubility data. Thus for carbendazim it was calculated using a vapor pressure determined at 20°C and a solubility determined at 25°C.

Figure 77.1   Structures of benomyl and carbendazim.

77.4 ABSORPTION, DISTRIBUTION, METABOLISM, AND EXCRETION

The metabolism and toxicokinetics of benomyl and carbendazim have been reviewed by WHO (1993a, b) and JMPR (FAO/WHO, 1996a, b); more recently, the metabolism has been reviewed by Anderson (1999). In general, both benomyl and carbendazim are well absorbed following oral administration (80–85%) but poorly absorbed following dermal administration (1–2%). After oral and intravenous treatment of rats with benomyl low levels of residues were found in blood and some tissues with minimal bioaccumulation potential.

Benomyl is primarily metabolized in animals to carbendazim through the loss of the *n*-butylcarbamoyl side chain prior to further metabolism (Gardiner *et al.*, 1974). Carbendazim then undergoes aryl hydroxylation–oxidation of the benzimidazole ring at the 5 and 6 positions followed by sulfate or glucuronide conjugation as the primary metabolic pathway in dogs and rats (Anderson, 1999). The hydrolysis of carbendazim to 2-aminobenzimidazole is another significant pathway in rats (Krechniak and Klosowska, 1986).

Krupka (1974) has shown that benomyl does not inhibit either acetyl or butyryl cholinesterase *in vitro*, as did Belasco (1979a), who examined *in vitro* inhibition of acetylcholinesterase using bovine red blood cells.

Absorption Benomyl and carbendazim were shown to be well absorbed following oral administration to rats, mice, dogs, and hamsters (Belasco, 1969; Culik, 1981a, b; Douch, 1973; Monson, 1990). Benomyl, or its metabolites, appeared in rat blood within one hour following a single oral gavage dose of ^{14}C-benomyl in peanut oil or when benomyl was administered mixed with ground chow at a dose level of 1000 mg per kilogram of body weight (Belasco *et al.*, 1969).

Krechniak and Klosowska (1986) measured urinary excretion of radiolabeled carbendazim and its metabolites 5-HBC and 2-AB (z-amine-1H-benzimidazole) following oral dosing of male rats with radiolabled carbendazim in diethyl glycol–ethanol. Total absorption was found to be about 85% based on the degree of urinary excretion of the metabolites. In another study, carbendazim was rapidly absorbed (80–85%) in both male and female rats following oral dosing. With absorption of carbendazim being so rapid, the urinary excretion half-life for both males and females was approximately 12 hours, with over 40% of the dose eliminated within the first 12-hour collection interval (Monson, 1990).

A dermal absorption study was done with a radiolabeled benomyl formulation (50% wettable powder) in male rats, with four rats killed at each of 0.5-, 1-, 2-, 4-, and 10-hour intervals. A dose of 0.1, 1, 10, or 100 mg of benomyl was applied to a shaved area approximating 16% of the animals' skin. Blood levels of radioactivity peaked between 2 and 4 hours postapplication, reaching 0.05 mg/l in the low dose at 2 hours and 0.1 mg/l at the high dose in 4 hours (Belasco, 1979b). An *in vitro* study of the penetration through human skin of a similar benomyl formulation applied at a spray-tank dilution showed poor penetration. Even less penetration occurred when the benomyl was applied to the skin dry (Ward and Scott, 1992). Percutaneous absorption of carbendazim was also shown to be very low in rats, with only 0.03% of a 60-mg/rat applied dose excreted after 24 hours (Dorn and Keller, 1980).

Distribution In rats exposed orally or intravenously, benomyl and its metabolites were cleared rapidly from blood and exhibited minimal potential for bioaccumulation (Han, 1979; Monson, 1990). Rats examined 24 hours after a single oral dose of radiolabeled ^{14}C-benomyl (1000 mg per kilogram of body weight) had radiolabel levels of 3–13 ppm in blood and 2–4 ppm in the testes (Belasco, 1969). However, no residues of benomyl, carbendazim, 5-HBC, or 4-HBC were detected 24 hours after the last of 10 oral benomyl doses (200 mg/kg/day). This was further confirmed in a study where blood from rats fed a diet containing 2500 ppm benomyl for 1 year had no

detectable amounts of benomyl, carbendazim, or 4-HBC. Although traces of 5-HBC were present (0.2 ppm), no 5-HBC was found in the testes (Belasco, 1969). Studies were reported by Krechniak and Klosowska (1986) in which similar results were seen with carbendazim-treated rats.

Metabolism The metabolic pathways for benomyl and carbendazim are shown in Fig. 77.2. Studies show that benomyl is extensively hydrolyzed to carbendazim, which is then further metabolized. A possible route under certain conditions is the conversion of benomyl to STB (3-butyl-1,3,5triazine (1,29)benzimidozol 2,4(1H,3H)dione).

Investigations using rats exposed to benomyl by intravenous (Han, 1979), dermal (Belasco, 1979b), and inhalation (WHO, 1993a) routes have shown that 5-HBC is the major urinary metabolite, with some carbendazim also found. The proposed metabolic pathway for metabolism in mammals is shown in Fig. 77.2. There are two divergent pathways in the biotransformation of benomyl: the release and subsequent degradation of the *n*-butylcarbamoyl moiety at N1 of benomyl, and the metabolism of the remaining carbendazim molecule.

The products of benomyl and carbendazim metabolism containing a hydroxyl functional group typically underwent conjugation reactions. Conjugation products were often more polar and more readily excreted than their parent compounds. Production and conjugation of 5-HBC appeared to be the primary path of elimination from mammalian systems. Parent compound accounted for less than 5% of the urinary radiolabel. When the metabolism of carbendazim was compared in rats and mice, only quantitative differences were evident (Dorn *et al.*, 1983). Almost all of the urinary metabolites were in the form of glucuronide and sulfate conjugates, cleavage of which liberated 5-HBC.

Excretion Benomyl, carbendazim, and their metabolites were rapidly eliminated in the urine and feces in all mammalian test systems examined. Greater than 98% of the administered radiolabel appeared in the urine or feces of rats within 72 hours following treatment with ^{14}C-carbendazim by using a variety of dosing regimens. Groups of Sprague-Dawley rats were gavaged with a single dose of 50 mg/kg, 14 days preconditioning with gavage dosing of unlabeled carbendazim followed by a single dose of 50 mg/kg of the radiolabeled material or a single gavage dose of 1000 mg/kg (Monson, 1990). Urinary excretion, which was dose dependent, accounted for 41–66% of the dose. The remainder of the radioactivity was virtually all found in the feces, with only traces of radiolabel found in the expired air.

Results similar to those in rats were obtained with mice and hamsters (Han, 1978). In mice, 64% of the dose (^{14}C-benomyl) was eliminated in the urine and 11.7% in the feces during the first 24 hours after dosing. In hamsters, 44.3% was eliminated in the urine and 14.8% in the feces over the same 24-hour period. By 72 hours postdose, 92.7 and 97% had been eliminated in mice and hamsters, respectively. Urinary elimination was by far the major pathway of clearance. However, in the dog this was

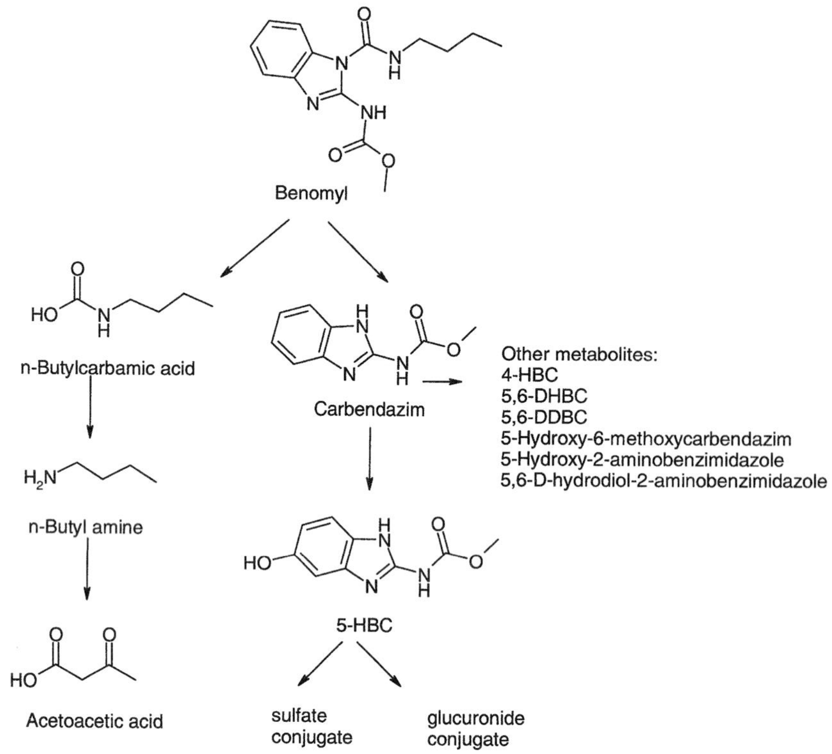

Figure 77.2 Metabolism of benomyl and carbendazim in mammals.

not the case. A beagle dog was fed a diet supplemented with unlabeled benomyl for 7 weeks (2500 ppm) and then administered an equivalent ^{14}C-labeled dose via capsule. The majority of the dose (83.4%) was eliminated in the feces with only 16.2% of the dose eliminated in the urine over the following 72-hour collection interval. The reason for such a high level of radiolabel in dog feces cannot be reliably commented on without further characterization of the radiolabeled material found in the feces.

Urinary excretion of metabolites was measured following intravenous dosing of radiolabeled carbendazim in albino rats. Twelve hours postdosing the urinary metabolite composition was found to be 94% 5-HBC, 3% 2-AB, and 3% carbendazim (Krechniak and Klosowska, 1986).

77.5 MAMMALIAN TOXICITY

77.5.1 SUMMARY

Benomyl and carbendazim have low toxicity in acute toxicity studies. The results were consistent in oral (LD$_{50}$ > 1000 mg/kg in the dog to >10,000 mg/kg in the rat), dermal (LD$_{50}$ > 10,000 mg/kg), and inhalation (LC$_{50}$ > 5.9 mg/l) studies in several animal species. Benomyl, but not carbendazim, caused dermal sensitization in guinea pigs by the maximization test but not by the Buehler method. They are mild to moderate irritants to both the eye and skin.

Subchronic toxicity studies showed the gastrointestinal tract, testes, liver, and bone marrow as target organs following high oral doses of benomyl or carbendazim. The liver was a primary target of toxicity in feeding studies with these fungicides. Mechanistic studies have shown that xenobiotic metabolizing enzymes in the liver are induced. Hepatotoxicity is indicated by changes in serum enzymes, elevated organ weights, or histopathological effects.

Following subchronic inhalation exposures to benomyl, rats had localized nasal irritation and degeneration of the olfactory epithelium at high doses although no systemic effects were observed. Later study showed these changes to be specific to the route of exposure (Hurtt *et al.*, 1993). The NOEL for rats exposed to benomyl by inhalation for 90 days was 10 mg per cubic meter of air.

Genetic toxicity studies indicate that benomyl and carbendazim do not induce gene mutations or DNA damage and repair. In addition, neither compound causes structural chromosome aberrations *in vivo* in somatic or germ cells. However, consistent with their mode of action, these fungicides are positive in tests that assess numerical chromosome aberrations (aneuploidy) in mammalian cells *in vitro* and in somatic and germ cells *in vivo*. This activity is observed only when the compounds are administered at relatively high doses. Studies utilizing more sophisticated techniques have shown a threshold for induction of aneuploidy.

In chronic feeding studies, rats fed diets that contained up to 2500 ppm of benomyl for 2 years had no signs of chronic toxicity. Rats fed up to 10,000 ppm of carbendazim had body weight, blood, and liver effects. There was no evidence of increased tumor incidence.

Mice fed benomyl or carbendazim in long-term studies had notable liver effects. In multiple studies, mice that ingested diets that contained 500 ppm of either fungicide had nonneoplastic lesions in the liver as well as an increased incidence of benign liver tumors. These long-term studies were conducted with CD-1 mice, a strain that has a high incidence of spontaneous liver tumors. When carbendazim was fed to a strain of mice with a low incidence of spontaneous tumors, no compound-induced neoplasms were observed. These compounds are known to induce liver enzymes, and the tumor increases in mice are believed to result from induction of cytochrome P450 enzymes and modulation of the growth of spontaneous neoplasms.

Liver injury (primarily increases in serum enzyme activities and cholesterol levels) was evident in long-term dog studies with benomyl or carbendazim. Decreased protein and albumin-to-globulin ratio in the blood and increased pituitary and thyroid weights were also noted at high doses. The lowest NOEL for 2 years of chronic oral exposure in dogs was 500 ppm, based on clinical and microscopic evidence of liver injury at 2500 ppm.

Reproductive toxicity studies in rats showed that benomyl and carbendazim cause effects on the reproductive system. Decreased sperm counts, decreased testicular weights, and histopathological changes occurred at higher dose levels. Reproductive changes in rats occurred at approximately the same or at higher doses than those resulting in general toxicity. Accordingly, benomyl and carbendazim are not selective reproductive toxins.

The potential for benomyl and carbendazim to cause developmental toxicity was assessed in studies in pregnant rats and rabbits. They are toxic if administered in a single large oral dose but not when given in the diet because of the resulting higher blood levels after bolus dosing. Developmental effects included reduced fetal weight and anomalies of the eyes, skull, and head. In feeding studies, toxic effects to the dams (reduced food consumption and body weight gain) occurred at lower doses than those which produced fetal effects (reduced fetal weights). Results from feeding studies are believed to be more appropriate than gavage studies in determining human risk from daily ingestion or dermal exposure. When benomyl is administered by gavage, some studies show that toxicity to the developing fetus occurs at a lower dose than that causing toxicity to the dam. However, in a more recent expanded rabbit gavage study of benomyl, no fetal effects occurred at levels below maternal toxicity.

Both benomyl and carbendazim were found to be negative when evaluated for neurotoxic potential in traditional hen studies. Additionally, no evidence of mammalian neurotoxicity was seen when rats were dosed with benomyl, either in acute doses or in the feed for 90 days. NOELs were based on general toxicity. The NOEL in rats for neurotoxicity from acute exposure to benomyl was 2000 mg/kg, the highest dose tested. In other tests, both compounds were shown not to inhibit acetylcholinesterase.

77.5.2 ACUTE TOXICITY

Benomyl and carbendazim as well as formulations made from them were investigated in acute studies in several animal species over the years. They are generally of low oral toxicity, quite low dermal toxicity, and low toxicity by inhalation. They are not classified as irritating to either the skin or the eye. Benomyl was found not to be a sensitizer by the Buehler method whereas it was found to be a sensitizer by the maximization method (Matsushita *et al.*, 1977). Ford (1981) studied technical carbendazim and a 75% wettable powder in male guinea pigs, finding no evidence of dermal sensitization. Martin *et al.* (1987) assessed a 50% carbendazim formulation in both male and female guinea pigs and found no evidence of sensitization. Carbendazim is not a dermal sensitizer.

Numerous acute toxicity studies were summarized and reported in WHO (1993a, b) and FAO/WHO (1996a, b). Studies representing the range of findings are presented in Table 77.2. Benomyl has an oral LD_{50}(rat) > 10,000 mg/kg and an inhalation LD_{50}(rat) of >4 mg/l. Oral LD_{50}s were determined in rats dosed with the minor metabolites 2-AB (>3400 mg/kg), 5-HBC (>7500 mg/kg), BUB (2-(3-butylureido)benzimidazole) (>17,000 mg/kg), and STB (>17,000 mg/kg). Carbendazim (the major metabolite) has been shown to have a similar range of acute toxicity to that of benomyl.

The dermal irritation potential of benomyl and carbendazim or their formulations has been assessed. Results varied from "mild irritation" to "not an irritant" (Vick and Brock, 1987a, b).

The potential for eye irritation by benomyl and carbendazim and their formulations has been evaluated in rabbits. Edwards (1974a), Vick and Valentine (1987), and have assessed the eye irritation and found them to be mild to moderate irritants. Others studied both technical benomyl and 50% wettable powder formulation as well as a suspension in mineral oil, finding mild conjunctival irritation and minor, transitory corneal opacity (WHO, 1993a).

77.5.3 SUBCHRONIC TOXICITY

77.5.3.1 Oral

Several studies of 10 days to 3 months of repeated dosing by both gavage and feeding have been reviewed (Table 77.3). Feeding at the higher doses caused liver changes in rats, dogs, and mice whereas high gavage doses have also resulted in changes in the testis, bone marrow, or gastrointestinal tract.

In early studies, both benomyl and carbendazim were given to rats gavaged daily for 5 days/week for 2 weeks. The technical material was given at doses of 0, 200, and 3400, and with carbendazim, 5000 mg/kg/day (Sherman, 1965; Sherman and Krauss, 1966). With benomyl, mortality occurred at 3400 (four of six rats) and with carbendazim, two of six rats died at 3400. Slight testicular changes were noted at the 200 mg/kg dose. Testicular effects, including degeneration of germinal epithelium

Table 77.2
Summary of Acute Toxicity Studies

Route and species	Sex (No./dose)	Material tested	Vehicle	Results	Reference
Oral, rat	Male (10) Female (10)	Benomyl	Peanut oil	$LD_{50} > 10,000$ mg/kg	Sherman (1969a)
Oral, guinea pig	Male (10)	Carbendazim	Corn oil suspension	$LD_{50} > 5000$ mg/kg	Davidse (1975)
Oral, mouse	Male (10)	Carbendazim	Propylene glycol	$LD_{50} > 15,000$ mg/kg	
Oral, rat	Male (10)	Benlate OD (50% benomyl)	Corn oil	$LD_{50} > 12,000$ mg/kg	Hostetler (1977)
Oral, rat	Male/female (10)	Carbendazim	Sesame oil	$LD_{50} > 15,000$ mg/kg	Kramer and Weigand (1971)
Dermal, rabbit	Male (10)	Carbendazim	Aqueous paste	$LD_{50} > 10,000$ mg/kg	Edwards (1974a)
Dermal, rabbit	Male/female (5)	Benlate C (50%WP, carbendazim)	Aqueous paste	$LD_{50} > 2000$ mg/kg	Vick and Brock (1987c)
Dermal, rabbit	Male/female (4)	Fungicide 1991 (benomyl)	50% wettable powder	$LD_{50} > 10,000$ mg/kg	Busey (1968a)
Dermal, rabbit	Male/female (10)	Benlate PNW (benomyl)	50% wettable powder	$LC_{50} > 2000$ mg/kg	Gargus and Zoetis (1983c)
Inhalation, rat	Male (6)	Fungicide 1991 (benomyl)	50% wettable powder	$LC_{50} > 4.01$ mg/L	Busey (1968b)
Inhalation, dog	Male (10)	Fungicide 1991 (benomyl)	50% wettable powder	$LC_{50} > 1.65$ mg/L	Littlefield and Busey (1969)
Inhalation, rat	Male/female (10)	Carbendazim, 75% WP	Dust	$LC_{50} > 5$ mg/L	Nash and Ferenz (1982)
Inhalation, rat	Male (6)	Carbendazim	Particulate in air	LC_{50} (1 hr) > 5.9 mg/l	Sarver (1975)

and reduction or lack of sperm, erosion and thickening of the gastric mucosa as well as liver changes were seen at the higher doses.

Janardhan *et al.* (1987) conducted a 90-day gavage study of carbendazim in rats dosed daily at 0, 16, 32, or 64 mg/kg. They reported numerous hematological and clinical chemistry effects in all dose groups. However, reported alterations were minimal, were out of the expected ranges in the control animals, and did not show a dose response. Absence of raw data and the variability of the results confound interpretation of the results of the study.

Ninety-day feeding studies have been conducted in rats with both benomyl and carbendazim. Except for the increased liver weights seen in rats fed benomyl, there were no remarkable differences in the effects noted. In male and female rats fed benomyl diets for 90 days at levels of 0, 100, 500, and 2500 ppm, there was no clinical evidence of toxicity and there were no effects on blood or urine parameters. Female rats fed 2500-ppm diets had slightly elevated liver weights, but no microscopic abnormalities. At the end of the 90–103-day feeding period, 10 of 16 males and females from each dose group were killed and evaluated. The remaining 6 males and females from each group were used in a one-generation reproduction study. No compound-related effects were noted in reproduc-

tive parameters. Gross and microscopic evaluation of tissues and organs showed no significant effects at dietary levels of up to 2500 ppm, equivalent to 198 mg/kg/day for males and 215 mg/kg/day for females (Sherman, 1967).

In a similarly designed 90-day feeding study in rats with carbendazim also fed at dietary levels of 0, 100, 500, and 2500 ppm), no compound-related effects were seen during clinical observations, blood or urine analyses, or gross and microscopic examinations. No reproductive effects were found in the subset of animals used for a one-generation reproduction study. The liver-to-body-weight ratio was slightly increased over controls in females in the top dose group. No significant compound-related effects were seen in this study at the highest dose tested, 2500 ppm, equivalent to 197 mg/kg/day for male and 210 mg/kg/day for female rats (Sherman, 1968).

Ninety-day feeding studies of benomyl and carbendazim were also conducted in dogs. The pattern of toxicity was similar and indications of liver effects were seen with both compounds. Male and female beagle dogs were fed diets containing 0, 100, 500, or 2500 ppm of benomyl. Clinical chemistry results indicative of compound-related liver effects, which included a slight increase in the activity of alkaline phosphatase and glutamic pyruvic transaminase and a decrease in the albumin-to-globulin ratio, were seen at the top dose. There were no

Table 77.3
Summary of Subchronic Toxicity Studies

Study	Material tested	Dose levels	NOEL ppm	NOEL mg/kg/day	NOAEL	Reference
90-Day feeding study in rats	Benomyl formulation	0, 100, 500, 2500 ppm	500	41 (M) 44 (F)	2500 ppm (198–215 mg/kg/day)	Sherman (1967)
90-Day feeding study in rats	Carbendazim formulation	0, 100, 500, 2500 ppm	2500	197 (M) 210 (F)	2500 ppm	Sherman (1968)
90-Day feeding study in dogs	Benomyl formulation	0, 100, 500, 2500 ppm	500	18 (M) 19 (F)	500 ppm	Sherman (1968)
90-Day feeding study in dogs	Carbendazim formulation	0, 100, 500, 1500–2500 ppm	100	2.7 (M&F)	500 ppm [14.4 mg/kg/day (M) and 11.3 mg/kg/day (F)]	Sherman (1970a)
90-Day feeding study in dogs	Carbendazim formulation	0, 100, 300, or 1000 ppm (increased to 2000 after 6 weeks)	300	7.5 (M&F)	300 ppm	Til *et al.* (1972)
15-Dose dermal study in rabbits	Benomyl formulation	0, 1000 mg/kg	NA[a]	None	None	Busey (1968d)
15-Dose dermal study in rabbits	Benomyl formulation	0, 50, 250, 500, 1000, 5000 mg/kg/day	NA	250	250 mg/kg/day	Hood (1969)
90-Day inhalation study in rats	Benomyl technical	0, 10, 50, 200 mg/m^3	NA	10 mg/m^3	10 mg/m^3	Warheit *et al.* (1989)
14-Day gavage study in rats	Benomyl technical	0, 200, 3400 mg/kg/day	NA	200	200 mg/kg/day	Sherman and Krauss (1966)
14-Day gavage study in rats	Carbendazim technical	0, 200, 3400, or 5000 mg/kg/day	NA	None	None	Sherman (1965)
10-Dose dermal study in rabbits	Carbendazim technical	0, 2000 mg/kg	NA	None (local skin effects at treatment sites)	None	Dashiell (1974)
Enzyme induction in rats and mice (28-day feeding study)	Carbendazim and benomyl	0, 10, 30, 100, 300, 1000, 3000 ppm			Epoxide hydrolase induced at 1000 ppm (NOEL 300 ppm) Glutathione-5-transferase induced at 3000 ppm (NOEL 1000 ppm)	Guengerich (1981)

[a]NA, not applicable.

histopathological abnormalities in any dogs fed test material and no other evidence of toxicity was observed. The NOEL was 500 ppm benomyl, approximately 18 mg/kg/day for male dogs and 19 mg/kg/day for females (Sherman, 1968).

Dogs were also fed carbendazim in other 90-day feeding studies. In a study by Sherman (1970a) original dietary carbendazim concentrations of 0, 100, 500, and 2500 ppm were changed to a top dose of 1500 ppm because of reduced food intake at 2500 ppm. There was histological evidence of liver injury in dogs in the 1500-ppm group. The study NOEL was considered to be 500 ppm, a daily dosage equivalent to 14.4 mg/kg/day for males and 11.3 mg/kg/day for females. Til *et al.* (1972) fed dogs carbendazim at dietary levels of 0, 100, 300, and 1000 ppm for 13 weeks. The top dose was raised to 2000 ppm after 6 weeks of feeding. There were no clinical signs of toxicity or changes in body weight, hematological parameters, and kidney or liver function. Slight increases were seen in relative liver and thyroid weights with a decrease in

relative heart weights at the top dose, but histopathologic evaluation showed no compound-related changes. The NOEL was judged to be 300 ppm, equivalent to 7.5 mg/kg/day of carbendazim.

Twenty-eight-day feeding studies were done to investigate hepatic toxicity and enzyme induction with benomyl or carbendazim in mice and rats of both sexes fed dietary concentrations of 0, 10, 30, 100, 300, 1000, and 3000 ppm. Rats were found to have increased liver weights. These effects were noted in animals fed carbendazim diets at 1000 and 3000 ppm and benomyl diets at 3000 ppm. Both benomyl and carbendazim induced hepatic epoxide hydrolase (EPH) in a dose-dependent fashion in mice and rats, with females of both species exhibiting a greater sensitivity to induction. Glutathione-s-transferase (GST) induction was qualitatively similar to EPH induction; however, the extent of induction was not as great. Significant induction occurred in rats and mice that received a dietary concentration of 3000 ppm (Guengerich, 1981).

77.5.3.2 Dermal

The repeated-dose dermal toxicity of benomyl and carbendazim was studied in rabbits. Applications of a 50% benomyl formulation to either intact or abraded abdominal skin sites were made 5 days/week for 3 weeks at a dose rate of 1000 mg per kilogram of body weight. Slight edema, erythema, and atonia were noted at all skin sites as well as some desquamation. Compound-related changes in body weight or organ weights were not seen. Microscopic evaluation of the testes showed degenerative changes in the spermatogenic elements of the seminiferous tubules (Busey, 1968d). A more extensive study of the benomyl formulation was done by Hood (1969), applying doses of 0, 50, 250, 500, 1000, and 5000 mg/kg to nonoccluded abraded dorsal skin sites for 6 hours per day, 5 days/week for 3 weeks. Decreased body weight gains and diarrhea, oliguria, and hematuria were seen in both males and females at the top two doses. Mild to moderate skin irritation was most notable at the top dose. Average testicular weights and testes-to-body-weight ratio changes were only noted at the 1000-mg/kg dose. Histopathologic changes were not reported. Technical carbendazim in a 50% aqueous paste was applied to shaved, intact dorsal skin sites of rabbits daily, 6 hours/day, for 10 days at doses of 0 or 1000 mg/kg. No adverse effects were reported on body weight, clinical signs, organ weights, gross pathology, or histopathology of selected organs. Focal epidermal necrosis and polymorphonuclear cell infiltration was noted in five of the six rabbits (Dashiell, 1975).

77.5.3.3 Inhalation

Effects observed in rats exposed to benomyl by inhalation were localized to the respiratory tract. A 90-day study was conducted in rats with a dust of benomyl technical. Groups of 20 male and 20 female rats were exposed, nose-only, 6 hours/day, 5 days/week. Particle sizes were within range of respirability for the rat. Male rats exposed to 200 mg/m^3 had low mean body weights and low food consumption. Male and female rats exposed to 200 mg/m^3 and male rats exposed to 50 mg/m^3 had degeneration of the olfactory epithelium. No other pathological abnormalities were observed. The study NOEL was 10 mg/m^3, based on the respiratory tract toxicity (Warheit *et al.*, 1989). Hurtt *et al.* (1993) have utilized both respiratory and oral exposures of rats to demonstrate that the effects on the nasal epithelium are only seen when exposure is by inhalation.

77.5.4 CHRONIC TOXICITY

Feeding studies were conducted in rats and mice to evaluate the chronic toxicity and carcinogenicity of benomyl and carbendazim. Dogs were also fed the respective chemicals to evaluate chronic toxicity in a nonrodent species (Table 77.4). The liver was the primary target for chronic toxicity, and a subchronic study conducted to address hepatic enzyme induction was previously described.

Table 77.4
Summary of Chronic Toxicity Studies

Study	Material tested	Dose (ppm)	NOEL ppm	NOEL mg/kg/day	NOAEL (ppm)	Reference
Two-year feeding study in rats	Benomyl (formulation)	0, 0, 100, 500, 2500	2500	109 (M) 128 (F)	2500	Sherman (1969c)
Two-year feeding study in rats	Carbendazim (formulation)	0, 0, 100, 500, 2500–10,000, 5000	500	21.6 (M) 24.5 (F)	500	Sherman (1972)
Two-year feeding study in mice	Benomyl (technical)	0, 500, 1500, 5000–7500	None	NA	None	Weichman (1982) Peer review: Hardisty (1990); Frame and Van Pelt (1990)
Two-year feeding study in mice	Carbendazim (technical)	0, 500, 1500, 3750–7500	500; none[a]	81 (M) 125 (F)	500; none[a]	Wood (1982) Peer review: Hardisty (1990); Frame and Van Pelt (1990)
Two-year feeding study in NMRKf mice	Carbendazim	0, 50, 150, 300, or 5000	300	34.4 (M) 41.9 (F)	Same as NOEL	
One-year feeding study in dogs	Carbendazim (technical)	0, 100, 200, 500	200	6.4 (M) 7.2 (F)	500 [16.5 mg/kg/day (M) and 17.1 mg/kg/day (F)]	Stadler (1986)
Two-year feeding study in dogs	Carbendazim	0, 150, 300, or 2000	300		300	Reuzel *et al.* (1976)
Two-year feeding study in dogs	Carbendazim	0, 100, 500, 1500	100	2.6	100	Sherman (1972)

[a] NOEL set by peer review pathologists.

77.5.4.1 Rats

In long-term studies with male and female rats, no compound-related toxicity was observed with benomyl. With carbendazim, effects on body weight, blood, and liver were noted. There was no evidence of carcinogenicity with either compound in rats.

Groups of 36 male and 36 female weanling rats were fed diets for 2 years that contained benomyl at dietary concentrations of 0, 100, 500, and 2500 ppm. During the study, there were no compound-related effects on mortality, body weight, food consumption, or clinical signs. There were no changes in blood or urine parameters, no organ weight effects at the 1- or 2-year sacrifice, and no histopathological lesions of note. The study NOEL was the highest dose tested, 2500 ppm of benomyl, 109 mg per kilogram body weight per day for male rats and 128 mg per kilogram body weight per day for females (Lee, 1977; Sherman, 1969c).

Carbendazim was fed to groups of 36 male and 36 female Sprague-Dawley rats in a study of similar design. Initial doses contained 0, 100, 500, 2500, or 5000 ppm of carbendazim. The dietary concentration for the 2500-ppm group was raised to 7500 ppm at 18 weeks, then raised again after two weeks to 10,000 ppm for the remainder of the study. In the study, male and female rats fed 2500–10,000-ppm and female rats fed 5000-ppm diets had a low body weight gain. There were no effects on food consumption, food efficiency, clinical signs, or mortality. During the last 6 months of the study, female rats fed 10,000-ppm diets were anemic. There were also increases in alkaline phosphatase and glutamic pyruvic transaminase (GPT) activities in high-dose rats. None of the histopathological changes were related to carbendazim intake. A review of tissues confirmed that there was no evidence of histopathological effects on the testes. The NOEL was 500 ppm, an average dose of 22 mg per kilogram body weight per day for male rats and 25 mg/kg/day for female rats (Sherman, 1972).

The results in these studies were similar to those in another chronic study in which groups of 60 male and 60 female Wistar-derived rats were fed carbendazim diets at concentrations of 0, 150, 300, and 2000 ppm for 2 years. The 2000-ppm concentration was increased to 5000 ppm after 1 week and to 10,000 ppm after 2 weeks for the rest of the study. Decreased body weights, and blood and liver effects occurred in rats fed the high-dose diets, but there were no carcinogenic or other effects from the dietary intake of carbendazim. Except for an increased incidence of diffuse proliferation of parafollicular cells of the thyroid in the high-dose females (Til *et al.*, 1976a). The NOEL was 300 mg/kg, a dosage equivalent to approximately 15 mg/kg/day. Because the molar ratio (on a weight basis) of benomyl to carbendazim is approximately 1.5:1, it is not surprising that studies with carbendazim can result in a somewhat lower NOEL than studies with benomyl.

77.5.4.2 Mice

In contrast to studies in rats, there was an increased incidence of benign liver tumors in long-term studies in mice with either benomyl or carbendazim. The data and slides from the original evaluation of liver tumors were subsequently peer-reviewed by a panel of pathologists, who concluded that there was in increase in benign but not malignant liver tumors. The mechanism of tumor induction appears to be an indirect effect that promotes the growth of spontaneous tumors in CD-1 mice rather than a direct genotoxic effect of the test compound.

Groups of 80 male and 80 female CD-1 mice were fed diets that contained benomyl at concentrations of 0, 500, 1500, and 5000 ppm for two years (the highest concentration was reduced from 7500 to 5000 mg/kg after 37 weeks because the mice experienced marked reductions in body weight). The body weights of mice in the low- and intermediate-dosage groups were not affected. There were no effects in clinical signs, mortality, or hematological parameters; however, there were a number of significant findings from histopathological evaluation of animal tissues. Increased liver weights in the 1500- and 5000–7500 mg/kg groups and decreased testicular weights in the 5000–7500 mg/kg males were noted. Significant increases in the incidence of hepatocellular carcinomas and combined neoplasms were also reported initially at the 500 and 1500 but not 7500 ppm. It was noted, however, that there were no differences between control and treated groups with respect to time-to-tumor or histomorphological appearance of the tumors. There was not a no-effect level in the study (Weichman, 1982).

In a similar 2-year study, groups of 80 male and 80 female CD-1 mice were fed diets containing carbendazim at concentrations of 0, 500, 1500, and 7500 ppm for 2 years. Because of early mortality, the concentration of high-dose diets given to male mice was reduced from 7500 to 3750 ppm. Mortalities continued and the group was terminated at 73 weeks. Increased mortality also occurred among males fed 1500-ppm diets. Female mice continued to receive 7500-ppm diets. There were no compound-related effects on clinical signs or hematological parameters. At necropsy, there were increased liver weights in females in the 7500-ppm group. Notable histopathological changes were initially reported to include an increased incidence of nonneoplastic liver lesions as well as hepatocellular carcinomas, hepatocellular adenomas, and combined hepatocellular neoplasms. Tumor incidences were elevated in mice from all carbendazim dietary groups (Wood, 1982).

A subsequent independent peer review of the slides and data for both the benomyl and the carbendazim mouse studies by three pathologists concluded that both compounds produced benign, but not malignant, hepatocellular neoplasms. There were also an increased incidence of multiple hepatocellular adenomas and a slight increase in the incidence of focus or foci of cellular alteration. A NOEL could not be established for histopathological lesions in either study (Frame and Van Pelt, 1990; Hardisty, 1990).

There are two additional reports on long-term effects of carbendazim in the mouse. An 80-week study was conducted with groups of 100 male and 100 female Swiss (SBF) mice fed diets containing carbendazim at concentrations of 0, 150, 300, and 5000 ppm. Increased liver weights, an increased incidence of liver adenomas and carcinomas, and an increased incidence of liver nodules were present (Beems *et al.*, 1976; Mohr, 1977). Another study to confirm the findings of the first was conducted with HOE NMRKf (SPF-71) mice, a strain with a low incidence of spontaneous tumors. The dietary concentrations were 50, 150, 300, and 5000 ppm. Although there histopathological effects were observed in livers of mice fed the 5000-mg/kg diets, there was no compound-related effect on the incidence or time of onset of tumors, and the total number of benign and malignant tumors was comparable among the groups of mice. There was no evidence of carcinogenicity at any dose tested (Donaubauer *et al.*, 1982).

It appears that benomyl and carbendazim are not directly carcinogenic, but act to promote a common tumor type in CD-1 mice. It is likely that adaptive metabolic responses rather than a genotoxic insult cause the tumors. Several observations support this conclusion: (1) There is no evidence that benomyl or metabolites interact directly with DNA. (2) The absence of a decreased latency period indicates that benomyl is not acting as a classical tumor promoter. (3) There have been no significant differences identified between rats and mice in the metabolism of benomyl that would explain the different sensitivities to tumor formation. (4) The different results between the rat and mouse lifetime studies, and between the NMRKf mice and other strains, indicate that mice having high rates of spontaneous liver tumor formation are uniquely affected by benomyl or carbendazim. Viewed together, study results indicate that increased incidence of hepatic neoplasia in mice fed benomyl or carbendazim does not indicate risk of carcinogenicity in other mammalian species.

77.5.4.3 Dogs

Dogs were fed benomyl or carbendazim to evaluate chronic toxicity in a nonrodent species. In all studies, evidence of liver injury was noted after extended intake of test material.

Dogs (five per sex per group) were fed diets with carbendazim concentrations of 0, 100, 200, and 500 ppm in a 1-year study. There were no compound-related effects on body weight, food consumption, clinical observations, or organ weights. The

concentrations of serum cholesterol were slightly elevated in dogs in the 500-ppm group. One dog had a rare thyroid follicular cell adenoma, but the tumor was considered a chance finding. No histopathological lesions resulted from intake of carbendazim. The NOEL was 500 ppm, a mean daily intake of approximately 16.5 mg/kg/day for male dogs and approximately 17.1 mg/kg/day for females (Stadler, 1986).

In an earlier study, dogs were fed 0, 100, 500, or 1500–2500 ppm of carbendazim in the diets for 2 years. Albumin concentration was decreased in dogs fed the high-concentration carbendazim diets. Evidence of hepatic cirrhosis and/or mild chronic toxic hepatitis was seen in dogs from the 500-ppm and 1500–2500-ppm carbendazim groups. These effects were attributed to compound intake. Testicular changes in two dogs that were fed 100 ppm were not attributed to carbendazim, because similar effects were not seen at 500 ppm. The NOEL was 100 mg/kg of carbendazim (Sherman, 1972).

In another 2-year study with carbendazim, dogs received diets containing 0, 150, 300, or 2000–5000 ppm. Biochemical evidence of liver effects and increases in weights of livers, pituitary, and thyroid were noted in the high-dose animals. The NOEL was 300 ppm (Reuzel *et al.*, 1976).

Although sporadic findings were noted in dogs fed benomyl or carbendazim, the common target organ in these studies was the liver. The no-effect levels ranged from 100 to 500 ppm based primarily on biochemical markers of liver effects rather than overt toxicity due to test material.

77.5.5 NEUROTOXICITY

Neurotoxicity studies have been conducted in hens and mammals (Table 77.5). Two rat neurotoxicity studies have been summarized (FAO/WHO, 1996a, b) and an acute study was reported earlier (Desi, 1983). A number of earlier studies conducted in hens with benomyl or carbendazim were also reported (Goldenthal, 1978; Jessup, 1979; Jessup and Dean, 1979). *In vitro* studies by Belasco (1979a) and Krupka (1974) demon-

Table 77.5
Summary of Neurotoxicity Studies

Study	Material tested	Dose levels	NOEL or NOAEL	References
Acute oral in rats (gavage)	Benomyl	0, 500, 1000, or 2000 mg/kg	Neurotoxicity >2000 mg/kg; other, none	Foss (1993)
90-Day oral in rats (feeding)	Benomyl	0, 100, 2500, or 7500 ppm	Neurotoxicity >7500 ppm; other 2500 ppm	Foss (1994)
Neurotoxicity in hens	Benomyl	500, 2500, or 5000 mg/kg	Neurotoxicity >5000 mg/kg	Goldenthal (1978)
Acute delayed neurotoxicity in chickens	Benomyl	500, 2500, or 5000 mg/kg	Neurotoxicity >5000 mg/kg	Jessup (1979)
Neurotoxicity in hens	Carbendazim	500 or 2500 mg/kg	Neurotoxicity >2500 mg/kg	Jessup and Dean (1979)

strated that benomyl did not inhibit either acetyl cholinesterase or butyryl cholinesterase.

In an acute neurotoxicity study, rats were given single oral doses of benomyl at doses up to 2000 mg/kg. Doses of 500 mg/kg and above affected body weight and feed consumption. Motor activity was reduced in the female group dosed with 2000 mg/kg on the day of dosing; however, the reduced activity was associated with general toxicity and not with specific neurotoxicity. Neither the FOB parameters nor the neurohistological evaluation showed evidence of any neurotoxicity due to benomyl (Foss, 1993).

In a 90-day study, rats exhibited reduced body weight and feed consumption and increased motor activity in the groups fed 7500 ppm in the diet. There were no specific neurotoxic end points identified for rats fed benomyl, because all FOB (functional observational battery) measurements and histopathological evaluations were similar to control parameters (Foss, 1994). The study NOEL was set at 2500 ppm, a dose equivalent to 126–266 mg/kg/day, based on end points of general toxicity. The NOEL for neurotoxicity resulting from administration of benomyl in the feed is 7500 ppm.

The mammalian neurotoxicity studies indicate that benomyl is not a specific neruotoxicant. The significant effects on motor activity parameters (reduced in the acute study and increased in the subchronic study) appear to be related to general toxicity in animals that received high doses. In another rat study, no effects on electroencephalogram (EEG), behavior, or cholinesterase activity in the cerebellum, brain stem, white matter, or cerebral cortex were detected after daily oral doses of 250 or 500 mg/kg for 90 days (Desi, 1983).

Similar conclusions were reached in early neruotoxicity studies conducted with benomyl and carbendazim in hens (Goldenthal, 1978; Jessup, 1979; Jessup and Dean, 1979). Transient ataxias in hens treated with benomyl were related to acute toxicity and not to any specific neurotoxic action. One benomyl study noted demyelination and axonal degeneration in all treated hens as well as in positive and negative control groups. These lesions were found to be due to Marek's disease, which was present in birds throughout the study. Similar ataxias were seen in hens treated with carbendazim.

77.5.6 GENOTOXICITY

Benomyl and carbendazim have long been recognized for their ability to cause numerical chromosome aberrations (aneuploidy) both *in vitro* and *in vivo* because of their ability to bind tubulin and to disrupt microtubule assembly during cell division. They inhibit fungal growth by binding to tubulin (Davidse, 1975; Davidse and Flach, 1976b) and can also bind to mammalian tubulin (Albertini *et al.*, 1988; De Brabander *et al.*, 1976b) but with much less affinity (Albertini *et al.*, 1993; Ireland *et al.*, 1979; Russell *et al.*, 1992). Studies selected to show the range of testing done are presented in Tables 77.6–77.8.

These substances do not interact directly with DNA and have given negative results for gene mutations, structural chromosome aberrations (clastogenicity), and DNA damage and repair

in the majority of studies conducted (Bentley *et al.*, 2000). Many studies using various test systems have been conducted to define the mutagenic potential of these chemicals both *in vitro* and *in vivo*, including studies in nonmammalian cells and in mammalian somatic and germ cells. This has resulted in the predictable situation of having apparently conflicting results in some cases. WHO expert panels reviewed the available studies, both public and proprietary, for both compounds in 1993 (WHO, 1993a, b). They provided a service for those interested in this data by tabulating those studies that presented "sufficient detail to evaluate the reasons for the conflicting data". A similar presentation is available in the FAO/WHO (1996a, b) JMPR publications.

One of the reasons for some of the conflicting data was the presence of phenazine contaminants [2-amino-3-hydroxyphenazine (AHP) and 2,3-diaminophenazine (DAP)] in some of the carbendazim test samples produced prior to the mid-1980s. These contaminants were shown to be quite effective in inducing gene mutations in the *Salmonella typhimurium* Ames test whereas pure carbendazim or benomyl was negative. These contaminants are mutagenic at very low concentrations in the Ames test. Concentrations of >5 ppm DAP and 10 ppm AHP in carbendazim test samples resulted in positive test results (Sarrif *et al.*, 1994a). Since that time, most of the carbendazim manufacturers have changed the process to reduce the level of these impurities to below 0.5 ppm for DAP and 3.5 ppm for AHP, and technical carbendazim has been demonstrated to be nonmutagenic in subsequent Ames tests. These contaminants are not produced when benomyl is metabolized to carbendazim.

Cytotoxicity and, with benomyl, toxicity resulting from the release of the *n*-butylcarbamoyl moiety also contributed to the conflicting results (Sarrif *et al.*, 1994a). Toxicity relating to the *n*-butylcarbamoyl moiety is likely to be responsible for the reported positives in the mouse lymphoma assay with benomyl because no such activity is reported in similar assays using purified carbendazim. In two *in vitro* studies evaluating numerical chromosome aberrations, structural chromosome aberrations were observed at benomyl concentrations greater than those causing aneuploidy or polypoloidy. This observation supports the view that the clastogenic effects produced by benomyl resulted from cytotoxicity due to the *n*-butylcarbamoyl moiety rather than direct interaction with DNA. However, the positive clastogenic finding in these studies with benomyl appears to have little significance *in vivo* because structural chromosome aberrations have not been observed in animal studies (Sarrif *et al.*, 1994b).

A number of additional studies have been reported since the WHO reviews in 1993 and the FAO/WHO reviews in 1995. Those using newer techniques of antikinetichore antibodies and fluorescence *in situ* hybridization (FISH) have provided conclusive evidence of the lack of direct interaction with DNA and the existence of thresholds for the aneugenic effects of benomyl and carbendazim (Bentley *et al.*, 2000; Bjorge *et al.*, 1996; Elhajouji *et al.*, 1995; Elhajouji *et al.*, 1997; Jeffay *et al.*, 1996; Mailhes and Aardema, 1992; Sarrif *et al.*, 1994b; WHO, 1993a, b).

Table 77.6
Summary of *In Vitro* Genotoxicity Studies

Test	Test organism	Material tested	Concentration range	Result	Reference
Salmonella–Ames assay	*Salmonella typhimurium*	Benomyl (technical)	0–10,000 µg/plate	Negative	Russell (1978a, b); Rickard (1986); Arce (1984a)
		2-Amino-3-hydroxy-phenazine	0–0.1 µg/plate (with S9)	Positive ≥0.02 µg/plate	
		2,3-Phenazine-diamine	0–0.1 µg/plate (with S9)	Positive ≥0.01 µg/plate	Arce (1984b)
CHO/HPRT assay	Chinese hamster ovary (CHO) cells	Benomyl (technical)	0–172 µM (with S9) 0–120 µM (without S9)	Negative	Fitzpatrick (1980)
Mouse lymphoma assay	L5178Y cells	Benomyl (technical)	0–25 µM (with S9) 0–15 µM (without S9)	Positive at 10 and 12.5 µM (without S9)	McCooey *et al.* (1983a)
		Carbendazim (purified technical)	0–200 µM (with & without S9)	Negative	McCooey *et al.* (1983b)
Unscheduled DNA synthesis	Rat hepatocytes	Carbendazim (technical)	0–125 µg/ml (654 µM)	Negative	Tong (1981b)
	Mouse hepatocytes	Benomyl (technical)	0–500 µg/ml (1722 µM)	Negative	Tong (1981a)
	Mouse hepatocytes	Carbendazim (technical)	0–125 µg/ml (654 µM)	Negative	Tong (1981c)

Note: Concentrations given in parentheses are the µM equivalent of the concentrations given in the original report.

As noted previously, inhibition of microtubular function by benomyl and carbendazim results from the interaction with a non-DNA target (tubulin). Therefore, it is reasonable to expect that a "threshold" can be demonstrated for the aneugenic effect (Dellarco *et al.*, 1985; Parry *et al.*, 1994) where a critical number of target sites must be occupied before aneuploidy is expressed. Studies designed to demonstrate the presence of thresholds utilizing new and more sensitive techniques for the detection of aneuploidy at low concentrations have been reported. Elhajouji *et al.* (1995), Marshall *et al.* (1996), and Bentley *et al.* (2000) have employed fluorescent DNA probes and fluorescence *in situ* hybridization techniques to demonstrate clear thresholds for benomyl and carbendazim in cultured human lymphocytes. Bentley *et al.* (2000) evaluated the threshold for both benomyl- and carbendazim-induced aneuploidy using cultured binucleate human lymphocytes to track numerical chromosome abnormalities for six chromosomes. The results showed that there were similar dose responses for each chromosome and equimolar threshold concentrations for benomyl and carbendazim.

Table 77.7
Summary of *In Vitro* Chromosome Aberration Studies

Test organism	Material tested	Concentration range	Result	NOEL	Reference
R3-5 human–mouse hybrid cell line	Benomyl (technical)	0, 1.5, 3.0, 7.5, and 15 µg/ml	Aneuploidy Polyploidy Clastogenicity	Effect at all concs. 1.5 µg/ml 7.5 µg/ml	Athwal and Sandhu (1985); Sandhu *et al.* (1988)
Chinese hamster ovary (CHO) cells	Benomyl (technical)	0, 1.4, 2.8, 5.7, 11.3, and 22.7 µg/ml (without S9)	Polyploidy Clastogenicity	1.4 µg/ml 11.3 µg/ml	Sasaki (1988)
		0, 3.1, 6.2, 12.5, 22.7, 49.9, and 90.6 µg/ml (with S9)	Polyploidy Clastogenicity	Not induced 22.7 µg/ml	

Table 77.8
Summary of *In Vivo* Genotoxicity Studies

Test	Test species	Material tested	Dose levels	Result	Reference
Bone marrow chromosome aberrations	Mouse	Benomyl (technical)	0, 625, 1250, 2500, 5000 mg/kg by gavage	Negative	Stahl (1990)
Bone marrow micronucleus assay	Mouse	Benomyl (technical)	0, 1250, 2500, 5000 mg/kg by gavage	Positive $\geq$2500 mg/kg	Sasaki (1990)
	Mouse	Benomyl (technical)	0, 100, 2500, 5000 mg/kg by gavage	Positive $\geq$2500 mg/kg	Bentley (1992a)
	Mouse	Carbendazim (technical)	0, 66, 1646, 3293 mg/kg by gavage	Positive $\geq$1646 mg/kg	Bentley (1992b)
Dominant lethal assay	Rat	Benomyl (formulation)	0, 500, 2500, 5000 ppm in feed 7 days	Negative	Culik (1974)

Some investigators have reported possible increases in chromosomal aberrations (Carbonell *et al.*, 1990) and sister chromatid exchanges (Lander and Ronne, 1995) in workers exposed to multiple pesticides. Others have found either lack of genotoxicity (Dolara *et al.*, 1993) or possible effects (Dolara *et al.*, 1994) from such exposures. Benomyl and carbendazim are often included in these types of studies because of their widespread use. However, there is no conclusive evidence of cytogenetic effects in humans from exposure to these two compounds.

The weight of extensive available evidence is that benomyl and carbendazim do not directly interact with cellular DNA and do not induce either point mutations or chromosome aberrations. This has been demonstrated in both mammalian and nonmammalian systems *in vitro* and *in vivo*, and in somatic cells as well as in germ cells (Bentley *et al.*, 2000; FAO/WHO, 1996a, b; Sarrif *et al.*, 1994b; WHO, 1993a, b).

77.5.7 REPRODUCTIVE AND DEVELOPMENTAL TOXICITY

Because of their mechanism of action on the dividing cell, these compounds have been thoroughly studied in various studies of reproductive and developmental toxicity (Tables 77.9–77.12). In early testing of benomyl, it was learned that high doses by gavage could cause testicular effects. Biotransformation studies showed the rapid conversion of benomyl to carbendazim so many studies were conducted with carbendazim rather than benomyl. It is clear that, despite extensive study, benomyl and carbendazim continue to hold interest for those investigating reproductive and developmental effects of chemicals.

It was also recognized early in testing of benomyl that teratogenic effects seen with bolus (gavage) dosing in rats were not seen in feeding studies with either rats or rabbits. This is important in assessment of risk of health effects in humans, be-

Table 77.9
Studies of Reproductive Effects via Dietary Exposure

Species	Sex	Dosing duration	Doses given	Results and comments	Reference	Chemical
Rat, Sprague-Dawley	M/F	2 generations	0, 100, 500, 3000, or 10,000 ppm of diet	Decreased body weights in parents and fewer, smaller pups at 10,000; sperm count decreased with testicular changes at 3000 and 10,000 ppm; no effect on mating or fertility indexes	Mebus (1990)	Benomyl
Rat, Sprague-Dawley	M/F	3 generations	0, 100, 500, 5000, or 10,000 ppm of diet	Lower avg. litter weights at 5000 and 10,000; no effects on fertility, gestation, lactation, or pup viability	Sherman (1972)	Carbendazim
Rat, Wistar	M/F	3 generations	0, 150, 300, or 2000 ppm of diet	No reproductive or teratogenic effects at up to 2000 ppm of diet	Koeter *et al.* (1976a, b)	Carbendazim
Rat, Wistar	M	70 days on and 70 days off feed	0, 1, 6.3 or 203 mg/kg	Decreased sperm count, testicle weight; reversal of all effects at end of recovery phase	Barnes *et al.* (1983)	Benomyl

Table 77.10
Studies of Developmental Toxicity Effects via Dietary Exposure

Species	Dosing duration[a]	Doses given	Results and comments	Reference	Chemical
Rat, Sprague-Dawley	g.d. 6–15	0, 9, 44, 210, or 373 mg/kg body weight	No significant maternal or fetal effects		Benomyl
Rat, Wistar	g.d. 7–16	0, 169, 298, or 505 mg/kg body weight	Decreased fetal weight at top dose but no major malformations or anomalies	Kavlock et al. (1982)	Benomyl
Rat, Sprague-Dawley	g.d. 6–15	0, 9, 46, 218, 432, or 626 mg/kg body weight	No adverse maternal or fetal effects		Carbendazim
Rat, Wistar	g.d. 6–15	0, 600, 2000, or 6000 ppm of diet	Maternal body weight decrease at top dose; no evidence of teratogenicity	Koeter (1975a)	Carbemdazim
Rabbit, New Zealand	g.d. 8–16	0, 100, or 500 ppm of diet	No developmental toxicity but inadequate pups or litters for full evaluation	Busey (1968c)	Benomyl
Rabbit, New Zealand	g.d. 6–18	0, 600, 2000, or 6000 ppm of diet	Delayed ossification and increased supernumerar ribs and skull bones at top dose; inadequate data for full evaluation	Koeter (1975b)	Carbendazim

[a] g.d. = gestation day(s).

cause it is unlikely that anyone will unintentionally receive a large oral dose of these fungicides.

77.5.7.1 Reproductive Toxicity Studies

Reproduction studies of varying designs have been conducted in rats, mice, and hamsters. Comprehensive multigeneration feeding studies have been reported with both benomyl and carbendazim. Gavage dosing and, in one case, intraperitoneal and intratesticular injection have also been used (Lim and Miller, 1997).

Feeding Studies of Reproductive Toxicity   Reproduction feeding studies are summarized in Table 77.9. A two-generation reproduction study in Sprague-Dawley rats was done to recent international guidelines with benomyl at dietary concentrations of 0, 100, 500, 3000, and 10,000 ppm (Mebus, 1990). Parental rats were fed the treated diets for 71 days before breeding to produce the F1 offspring. Selected F1 rats were fed diets with the same concentrations of benomyl for at least 105 days after weaning and were mated to produce the F2a generation. The F1 females were mated again, to nonsibling males, to produce the F2b litters. Indices of reproductive function assessed for the F0 and F1 adults included mating, fertility, gestation, viability, lactation, percentage of pups born alive, and percentage litter survival. Clinical observations were recorded and body weight parameters, food consumption, and food efficiency were measured. Parental rats were killed after litter production and subjected to gross and microscopic pathology evaluation. Selected weanlings were also examined grossly.

Effects were observed in both parents and offspring fed the two highest dietary concentrations. No increase in parental mortality was seen at any dose; however, body weight pa-

rameters and overall food consumption by F0 and F1 rats were decreased at 10,000 ppm. The number of F2a and F2b pups alive before culling on day 4 was decreased, and the offspring of this dose group had low body weights at birth. Offspring of rats treated with 3000 ppm of benomyl also had decreased body weights at some evaluations during lactation. Decreased testicular weight, histopathologic changes, and depressed sperm counts were seen in F0 and F1 male rats at 3000 and 10,000 ppm. Histopathologic changes included atrophy and degeneration of the seminiferous tubules in the testes of rats at 3000 and 10,000 ppm and oligospermia in the epididymides of F0 rats at 10,000 ppm and of F1 rats at 3000 and 10,000 ppm. There were no compound-related differences in mating indices, fertility indices, or gestation length. The NOEL for adults and offspring was 500 ppm, equivalent to about 37 mg/kg/day.

A three-generation feeding study was conducted in Sprague-Dawley rats with carbendazim at doses of 0, 100, 500, 5000, and 10,000 ppm of diet (Sherman, 1972). Parental rats were fed the diets for approximately 80 days and mated to produce the F1 generation. The number of matings, of pregnancies, and of pups per litter at birth were recorded. Litter body weights and number alive were recorded during lactation. The parents were again mated to produce the F1b litters. Subsequent matings produced F2a, F2b, F3a, and F3b litters. Selected rats from the control, and the 5000- and 10,000-ppm groups were examined for gross and histologic lesions. No carbendazim-related effect was apparent on fertility, gestation, viability, or lactation. Average litter weights at weaning were decreased in all generations fed 5000 and 10,000 ppm. The NOEL was 500 ppm, the same as found in the two-generation study with benomyl.

Another three-generation feeding study was conducted with Wistar rats, at carbendazim dietary levels of 0, 150, 300, and

Table 77.11
Studies of Reproductive Effects via Gavage Exposure

Species	Sex	Dosing duration	Doses given	Results and comments	Reference	Chemical
Rat, Sprague-Dawley	M	10 days	0 or 200 mg/kg	Killed at various days after treatment ended; no treatment-related effects	Carter (1982)	Benomyl
Rat, Sprague-Dawley	M	10 days	0, 200, or 400 mg/kg	Done to evaluate sperm effects; found effects on all stages at 400 mg/kg	Carter and Laskey (1982)	Benomyl
Rat, Wistar	M	62 days	0, 1, 5, 15, or 45 mg/kg	No hormonal or reproductive effects; testicular effects at 45	Linder *et al.* (1988)	Benomyl
Rat, Sprague-Dawley	M	Single dose	0, 25, 50, 100, 200, 400, or 800 mg/kg	Germ cell sloughing at 100 and higher; no long-term effects at 25 and 50	Hess *et al.* (1991)	Benomyl
Rat, Sprague-Dawley	M/F	10 days	400 mg/kg	Serial breeding protocol, 75% infertile at 5th week; 50% still infertile at 32 weeks	Carter *et al.* (1987)	Carbendazim
Rat	M/F	1 generation	0, 50, 100, 200, or 400 mg/kg	Reproductive effects at 200 and 400; sperm effects at 50 and above	Gray *et al.* (1988, 1990)	Carbendazim
Hamster	M//F	1 generation	0, 50, 100, 200, or 400 mg/kg	No reproductive effects; testicular and sperm effects at 400	Gray *et al.* (1988, 1990)	Carbendazim
Rat, Holtzman	F	g.d. 1–8[a]	0, 25, 50, 100, 200, 400, or 1000 mg/kg	Toxicity at 1000 with decreased serum LH (luteinizing hormone) and increased serum estradiol		Carbendazim
Rat	F	8 days	0 or 400 mg/kg	Induced pseudopregnancy; reported reduced uterine competency		Carbendazim
Mouse	M	5 days	0, 250, 500, or 1000 mg/kg	Sperm quality study; found decreased testicular weight and sperm effects at 1000	Evanson *et al.* (1987)	Carbendazim
Hamster	F	Single dose	0, 250, 500, 750, or 1000 mg/kg; then 0 or 1000 in follow-up study	Reduced pregnancy rate and number of live pups at 750 and 1000; early pregnancy loss at 1000 given during microtubule sensitive meiotic stage	Perrault *et al.* (1992)	Carbendazim
Rat, Sprague-Dawley	M	Single dose	0 or 400 mg/kg	Time and testicular effects; saw various adverse effects on sperm and testicles	Nakai *et al.* (1992)	Carbendazim
Rat, Sprague-Dawley	M	Single dose	0, 50, 100, 200, 400, or 800 mg/kg	Follow-up time and testicular effects; found dose-dependent adverse effects on spermatids and seminiferous tubules at doses of 100 and above	Nakai *et al.* (1992)	Carbendazim
Dog	M	4-hr inhalation	0.065 and 1.65 mg/l	Reduced spermatogonic activity at 14 days but not 28 days postexposure at 1.65 mg/l	Littlefield and Busey (1969)	Benomyl
Rat, Sprague-Dawley	M	Single dose	100 mg/kg	Electromagnetic and light microscopy for study of morphologic changes in spermatids; concluded that abnormalities seen are in common with those reported in testes with several chemicals and in mutant animals	Nakai *et al.* (1997)	Carbendazim
Hamster		Single dose	1000 mg/kg	Direct oocyte effect, not endocrine effect; oocyte aneuploidy results in early pregnancy loss	Jeffay *et al.* (1996)	Carbendazim

(*continues*)

Table 77.11
(*continued*)

Species	Sex	Dosing duration	Doses given	Results and comments	Reference	Chemical
Rat, Sprague-Dawley	M	Single dose	100 mg/kg	Found rapid direct effects on spermatids aside from effects caused by tubular blockage from sloughing	Naki and Hess (1997)	Carbendazim
Rat, Sprague-Dawley	M	ip and testicular injection[a]	ip, 250 (ben) and 164 (mbc) mg/kg[a] testicular injection, 400 (ben) and 262 (mbc) µg/kg	Compared benomyl and mbc effects; concluded that all of benomyl-related testicular damage and microtubule-assembly disruption could be explained by the mbc contribution	Lim and Miller (1997)	Benomyl and carbendazim
Rat, Wistar	F	OECD screen protocol	0, 10, 30, 90 mg/kg	No malformations, only reproductive effects	Piersma *et al.* (1995)	Benomyl

[a] g.d. = gestation day(s); ip = intraperitoneal; ben = benomyl; mbc = carbendazim.

2000 ppm (Koeter *et al.*, 1976a, b). In a slightly different study design, the F1a and F2a litters were discarded at weaning and the F1b and F2b litters used to produce succeeding generations. F3a pups were used for a teratology study and the F3b pups were used in a 4-week toxicology study. Body weight gain was unaffected, but all generations in the treated groups weighed more than the controls. There was no effect on fertility, survival, litter size, or lactation. Necropsy of rats from the 4-week toxicity study showed increased relative liver weights and decreased relative spleen weights in females fed 2000 ppm as well as decreased relative ovarian weights in all treated groups. Histopathologic evaluation of the livers failed to show any compound-related changes. There were no apparent carbendazim-related effects on reproduction and no teratogenic effects at doses of carbendazim of up to 2000 ppm of the diet.

A feeding study was done in male Wistar rats to assess effects on testicular function and recovery after cessation of exposure to benomyl (Barnes *et al.*, 1983). The treated diets provided doses of approximately 0, 1, 6, and 203 ppm. The test groups were split into two groups each to be killed after 70 days of feeding or after 70 days of recovery. Decreased relative testicular weights and slightly lower fertility index were found in all treated groups, with ejaculated sperm counts down in the top dose group. Copulatory behavior was unaffected and dominant lethal mutation was not induced by treatment with benomyl. Plasma testosterone and gonadotropin levels were unchanged. Studies of the recovery group showed that all changes had reversed.

Gavage Studies of Reproductive Toxicity Numerous studies ranging from single doses to daily dosing for one generation have been done with rats, mice, and hamsters to investigate various aspects of reproductive function (Table 77.11). A single dose of 100 mg/kg or more is genera!ly required for any effect to be seen with either benomyl or carbendazim. Multiple doses similarly are generally without effect at doses lower

than 100 mg/kg/day, although Gray *et al.* (1988) reported some effects on sperm at 50 mg/kg and above of carbendazim in a one-generation reproduction study. A similar study done in hamsters by the same group found no effects at up to 400 mg/kg.

Male reproductive effects of benomyl and carbendazim in rats have been extensively studied. Naki and Hess (1997) found that carbendazim has a direct effect on spermatids, in addition to the effects caused by tubular blockage from sloughing of spermatids. Lim and Miller (1997) used intraperitoneal and direct testicular injection of benomyl and carbendazim to compare the degree of effects at measured testicular concentrations of both. They concluded that all of the testicular damage and microtubule disruption seen after treatment with benomyl can be explained by the carbendazim released from the benomyl rather than benomyl itself.

Effects on female reproductive organs have also been studied. Although numerous authors have listed benomyl with other pesticides in suggesting that it may have endocrine activity, none of the studies conducted to date have shown direct or indirect evidence of hormonal activity. Spencer *et al.* (1996) showed that benomyl and carbendazim affected uterine weight without producing effects on hormone activity. Jeffay *et al.* (1996) concluded that the effects seen on oocytes is direct and not mediated by endocrine changes. The aneugenic effect on the oocyte results in early pregnancy loss.

77.5.7.2 Developmental Toxicity Studies

The developmental toxicity of benomyl and carbendazim has been shown to be similar in the rather extensive testing which has been reported in rabbits, rats, mice, and hamsters. There appears to be no contribution from the *n*-butylcarbamoyl moiety to the effects noted.

Feeding Studies of Developmental Toxicity (See Table 77.10.) Sherman *et al.* (1970a) fed carbendazim to rats during

Table 77.12
Studies of Developmental Toxicity Effects via Gavage Exposure

Species	Dosing duration	Doses given	Results and comments	Reference	Chemical
Mouse, CD-1	g.d. 7–17[a]	0, 50, 100, or 200 mg/kg	No maternal toxicity; increased fetal abnormalities at 100 and 200 mg/kg	Kavlock et al. (1982)	Benomyl
Rat, Sprague-Dawley	g.d. 7–16	0, 3, 10, 30, 62.5, or 125 mg/kg	No maternal toxicity; decreased fetal weight and increased mortality at 125 mg/kg, increased skeletal variations at 62.5; microphthpalmia seen in few fetuses	Staples (1980)	Benomyl
Rat, Sprague-Dawley	g.d. 7–16	0, 3, 6.25, 10, 20, 30, or 62.5 mg/kg	Follow-up to better define microphthalmia; only 2 fetuses with malformations, both in top dose group, 1 with microphthalmia; no teratogenicity seen at lower doses	Staples (1982)	Benomyl
Rat, Wistar	g.d. 7–16	0, 15.6, 31.2, 62.5, or 125 mg/kg	Lower maternal body weight at top dose, some anomalies at top 2 doses, including microphthalmia	Kavlock et al. (1982)	Benomyl
Rat, Wistar	g.d. 7 to lactation day 15	0, 15.6, or 31,2 mg/kg	No effects at 100 days after birth except for reduction in testes and seminal vesicle weights at top dose	Kavlock et al. (1982)	Benomyl
Rat	g.d. 7–21	0, 31.2, or 62.4 mg/kg	Ocular and craniocerebral malformations at both doses with protein-deficient diet	Zeman et al. (1986)	Benomyl
Rat	g.d. 7–21	0, 31.2, or 62.4 mg/kg	Ocular and craniocerebral malformations at both doses with protein-deficient diet	Hoogenboom et al. (1991)	Benomyl
Rat, Holtzman	g.d. 1–8	0, 100, 200, 400, or 600 mg/kg	Killed at g.d. 11 or 20; no maternal toxicity; saw developmental delays and embryo or fetal toxicity at 200 and above, decreased fetal weight, litter size, and delayed ossification at all doses	Cummings et al. (1992)	Carbendazim
Rat, Sprague-Dawley	g.d. 7–16 (guideline study)	0, 5, 10, 20, or 90 mg/kg	Maternal toxicity at top dose; malformations at top dose; fetal toxicity at 20 and 90; NOEL 20 (maternal) and 10 (fetal)	Alvarez (1987)	Carbendazim
Rat, Sprague-Dawley	g.d. 8–15	19.1 mg/kg	11 rats, one dose; reported fetal toxicity and malformations	Delatour and Besse (1990)	Carbendazim
Rat, Wistar	g.d. 6–15	0, 20, 40, or 80 mg/kg	No malformations; embryo or fetal toxicity at two top doses	Janardhan et al. (1984)	Carbendazim
Rabbit	g.d. 8–16	0, 40, 80, or 160 mg/kg	No malformations; dose-related increase in fetal toxicity	Janardhan et al. (1984)	Carbendazim
Rabbit, New Zealand	g.d. 7–19 (guideline study)	0, 10, 20, or 125 mg/kg	Maternal toxicity at top dose; malformations at top dose; fetal toxicity at 20 and 125; NOEL 20 (maternal) and 10 (fetal)	Christian et al. (1985)	Carbendazim
Rabbit, New Zealand	g.d. 7–28 (guideline study)	0, 15, 30, 90, or 180 mg/kg	Maternal toxicity at top dose; fetal toxicity and variations at top dose; NOEL 90 mg/kg for both maternal and fetal toxicity	Munley (1995)	Benomyl
Hamster	Single dose, g.d. 10	0, 15, 30, 75, or 150 mg/kg	NOEL 30 mg/kg; malformations, embryotoxicity, resorptions at higher doses	Minata and Biernacki (1982)	Carbendazim

(continues)

Table 77.12
(*continued*)

Species	Dosing duration	Doses given	Results and comments	Reference	Chemical
Rat, Sprague-Dawley	g.d. 6–15	0, 10, 30, 60, 100, 300, 1000, or 3000 mg/kg	Malformations at 60 and 100, all resorbed (early) at 300, 1000, and 3000; NOEL 10 mg/kg	Hofmann and Peh (1987a, b)	Carbendazim
Rat, Wistar	14 days prior to mating to postnatal day 6	10, 30, or 90 mg/kg	No malformations, reproductive effects only	Piersma *et al.* (1995)	Benomyl
Rat, Wistar	g.d. 6–15	90 and 270 mg/kg	Malformations and reproductive effects	Piersma *et al.* (1995)	Benomyl
Rat, Holtzman	g.d. 1–8	≥100 mg/kg	Embryotoxicity, decreased growth, malformations	Cummings *et al.* (1992)	Carbendazim
Rat, Wistar	g.d. 6–15	0, 40, 60, 80, 100 mg/kg	NOEL 20 mg/kg; all embryos dead at 100; malformations at 40, 60, and 80 mg/kg	Lu *et al.* (1995)	Carbendazim

[a] g.d. = gestation day(s).

gestation days 6–15 at dietary concentrations providing doses of approximately 0, 9, 46, 218, 432, 626, and 747 mg/kg/day. No mortality, effects on body weight, or clinical signs of toxicity were seen. Food intake was reduced at the top dose during the period of dosing but returned to control afterward. There was no reduction in implantation sites, increase in resorptions, or differences in live to dead fetuses. A repeat of this study design using benomyl at dietary concentrations providing doses of approximately 0, 9, 44, 210, and 373 mg/kg/day gave results identical to those of the earlier carbendazim study, with the exception that three litters in the top dose group had some fetuses with hydronephrosis and retarded ossification. A later benomyl study of similar design fed rats dietary concentrations providing daily doses of 0, 169, 298, or 505 mg/kg/day on gestation days 7–16. A decrease in fetal body weight was seen at the top dose, but no major malformations or abnormalities were noted (Kavlock *et al.*, 1982).

An early feeding study in rabbits fed benomyl at dietary concentrations of 0, 100, and 500 ppm during gestation days 8–16 showed no evidence of developmental toxicity or malformations. However, there were inadequate numbers of litters or pups available for examination (Busey, 1968c) to fully evaluate this study. Carbendazim was fed to rabbits in a later study at dietary concentrations of 0, 600, 2000, and 6000 ppm during gestation days 6–18 (Koeter, 1975b). A significant increase was found in the number of supernumerary ribs and skull bones at the top dose and ossification was delayed or absent in these fetuses. Some study design deficiencies and lack of adequate data presented prevent the clear understanding of the developmental toxicity potential of carbendazim (WHO, 1993b).

Gavage Studies of Developmental Toxicity (See Table 77.12.) Studies utilizing gavage administration were done in rabbits, mice, rats, and hamsters with benomyl or carbendazim. It appears that, when such bolus exposure of the dam is utilized, the fetus is sometimes somewhat more sensitive than is the dam. However, the comprehensive studies that have been done allow one to identify a NOEL for the fetus which may be used in risk assessment. Additionally, in the most recent study of benomyl in rabbits done to the current expanded testing protocol no fetal effects were shown at doses below those causing maternal effects.

In a standard Segment II study, benomyl was given to Sprague-Dawley rats by gavage at doses of 0, 3, 10, 30, 62.5, and 125 mg/kg/day on gestation days 7–10. Test animals were observed daily for clinical signs of toxicity or changes in behavior. No clinical signs of toxicity were seen in any dose group. Body weight gain and incidences of pregnancy, corpora lutea, implantation sites, and sex ratios were unchanged compared to controls. Fetal body weight was decreased at 62.5 and 125 mg/kg and there was an increase in fetal mortality at 125 mg/kg. Malformations noted included microphthalmia, anophthalmia, and hydrocephaly. These appeared possibly treatment related at the higher dose levels. Histopathologic evaluation of the fetal eyes showed irregularities in fetuses from the two top doses. Major skeletal malformations were seen at the top dose and other skeletal variations were increased at both doses (Staples, 1980).

A follow-up study was done to better determine a NOEL for the microphthalmia and hydrocephaly (Staples, 1982). Groups of rats from the same strain and the same supplier were given doses of 0, 3, 6.25, 10, 20, 30, and 62.5 mg/kg from gestation days 7–16. Following a gross pathologic evaluation, reproductive status was determined on a litter basis. The number of implantation sites, resorptions and dead, live, and stunted fetuses as well as the mean weight of live fetuses per litter were determined. Microscopic examination was done of fetal heads.

At the top dose, mean fetal body weight was decreased. Two fetuses had malformations; both were from the 62.5-mg/kg dose group and from different litters. One had unilateral microphthalmia and the other showed internal hydrocephaly. No malformations were seen at the lower doses.

Kavlock *et al.* (1982) evaluated the teratologic potential of Wistar rats given daily doses of 0, 15.6, 31.2, 62.5, or

125 mg/kg during gestation days 7–16. Maternal toxicity was seen in decreased body weight at 125 mg/kg. Developmental toxicity was evident as increased incidence of fetal abnormalities at the top two doses. These included microphthalmia, hydrocephaly, encephaloceles, fused vertebrae, and fused ribs. The lower two doses were without adverse effect on the fetus.

Kavlock *et al.* (1982) also evaluated the postnatal effects of benomyl on pups. Dams were given benomyl at daily doses of 0, 15.6, or 31.2 mg/kg from gestation day 7 to lactation day 15 and pups were evaluated periodically for 100 days after birth. At 100 days of age, organs weighed included adrenals, liver, kidney, ovaries, testes, and ventral prostate plus seminal vesicles. Organ weights were not affected by benomyl exposure except that weight of the testes and the ventral prostate and seminal vesicles was reduced at the top dose. There were no compound-related effects on litter size at birth or weaning, fetal body weight, growth, survival, or locomotor activity.

Additionally, Kavlock *et al.* (1982) studied the effects of benomyl given to CD-1 mice at doses of 0, 50, 100, and 200 mg/kg on gestation days 7–17. Pups were delivered (by Cesarean section) on day 18 and the number of live, dead, and resorbed fetuses determined. Fetuses were examined grossly for abnormalities. Maternal toxicity was not noted at any dose. Fetal developmental toxicity appeared to be shown at all doses by a significant dose–response trend for increased incidence of subnormal vertebrae and supernumerary ribs as well as a significant increase in enlarged renal pelvises in pups from the top-dose dams. The number of abnormal litters and fetuses was also significantly increased at the top two doses and fetal weights were decreased.

Zeman *et al.* (1986) and Hoogenboom *et al.* (1991) studied the effects of benomyl on Sprague-Dawley rats given doses of 31.2 and 62.4 ml/kg on gestation days 7–21. Ocular abnormalities were seen in 43% of the fetuses from the top dose group. These abnormalities increased in incidence to 63% when the dams were fed a protein-deficient diet and 62.4 mg/kg of benomyl. Craniocerebral abnormalities (primarily hydrocephaly) were found in fetuses from dams given protein-deficient diets plus 31.2 mg/kg of benomyl.

In a standard Segment II study, Sprague-Dawley rats were given daily doses of 0, 5, 10, 20, or 90 mg/kg of carbendazim on gestation days 7–16. Maternal toxicity was seen at the top dose as decreased body weight, increased mean liver weight, and decreased pregnancy rate. Fetal body weight was reduced at the top two doses and malformations were increased in incidence at the top dose. The malformations included hydrocephaly, microphthalmia, anophthalmia, malformed scapulae, and axial skeletal malformations (vertebral, rib, and sternal fusions, exencephaly, hemivertebrae, and rib hyperplasia). The NOEL was found to be 20 mg/kg for the dams and 10 mg/kg for the fetus (Alvarez, 1987).

Cummings *et al.* (1992) dosed Holtzman rats daily at rates of 0, 100, 200, 400, and 600 mg/kg of carbendazim on gestation days 1–8. Dams were killed on day 11 or 20. Maternal toxicity was not noted. Crown–rump length, head length, number of somites, and number of embryos per dam were reduced at

doses of 200 mg/kg and greater at day 11. Increased resorptions, decreased live litter size and decrease fetal body weight, and delayed ossification were seen at day 20 in all treated groups. Delatour and Besse (1990) dosed 11 Sprague-Dawley rats at 19.1 mg/kg on gestation days 1–15. They reported an increase in dead fetuses and fetal skeletal and external malformations with a decrease in fetal body weight in the treated group.

Janardhan *et al.* (1984) studied rats and rabbits to determine effects of carbendazim on fetal survival and development. Wistar rats were given daily doses of 0, 20, 40, or 80 mg/kg on gestation days 6–15. Half of the animals were killed on day 21 and half were allowed to have normal deliveries. Rabbits were dosed at 0, 40, 80, or 160 mg/kg on gestation days 6–18 and killed on day 31. There was a dose-related increase in dead and resorbed fetuses in rats killed at day 21 and in rabbits. There was no effect on mean fetal weight and no malformations were seen. In rats allowed to deliver, there appeared to be a dose-related reduction in pups per litter and mean fetal weight was increased in the top two dose groups. Mortality at 21 days postpartum was 3–3.5 times greater at these doses also as compared with controls.

Christian *et al.* (1985) studied the developmental toxicity of carbendazim in a typical Segment II study. New Zealand rabbits were given daily doses of 0, 10, 20, or 125 mg/kg on gestation days 7–19. Maternal toxicity and fetal malformations were noted at the top dose. Fetal toxicity and variations were noted at 20 and 125 mg/kg. The NOEL was 20 for the dam and 10 for the fetus.

Munley (1995) did a more recent, contemporary, expanded Segment II study of New Zealand rabbits dosed with benomyl at doses of 0, 15, 30, and 180 mg/kg on gestation days 7–28. Maternal toxicity and fetal toxicity and variations were seen at the top dose. The NOEL for both maternal and fetal toxicity was determined to be 90 mg/kg.

Hamsters were given a single dose of carbendazim at 0, 15, 30, 75, or 150 mg/kg on gestation day 10. An increase in malformations and embryotoxicity was seen at 75 and 150 mg/kg (Hofmann and Peh, 1987a, b).

Piersma *et al.* (1995) used benomyl in a proposed Organization for Economic Cooperation and Development (OECD) screening protocol for reproductive toxicology. Male and female Wistar rats were gavaged daily at doses of 0, 10, 30, and 90 mg/kg from 14 days prior to mating onward. Males were killed after 28 days of exposure and females were killed after 4–6 days of lactation, approximately 54 days of exposure. Adults and pups were necropsied and evaluated. Male rats showed the expected testicular degeneration after 28 days at the top dose. Dams in the high-dose group had decreased body weights, and pup weights were decreased as well. However, there was no increase in pup mortality and, unexpectedly, no malformations were found.

The investigators then proceeded to conduct a typical developmental toxicity study, giving dams daily doses of 0, 90, or 270 mg/kg of benomyl during gestation days 6–15 for comparison with the earlier results. Body weight gain was reduced at both 90 and 270 mg/kg. Postimplantation loss and total litter resorptions were increased in both groups as well. Ophthalmic abnormalities were increased in a dose-related fashion. The authors note that the developmental toxicity study has 10 exposure days whereas the OECD protocol exposes the females for 54 days. They speculate that changes in maternal metabolism during the premating phase exposure may somehow protect against fetal malformations.

Lu *et al.* (1995) have reported exposure of female rats to carbendazim at daily doses of 0, 20, 40, 60, 80, or 100 mg/kg during gestation days 6–15. Complete embryo mortality was seen at the top dose, with increased malformations at 40, 60, and 80 mg/kg. The dams in all treated groups showed reduction in body weight gains and liver weights were increased in all but the 20-mg/kg group. The NOEL would appear to be 20 mg/kg for both dam and fetus.

REFERENCES

Unpublished references that are dealt with in WHO (1993a) are marked with an asterisk (∗). Those dealt with in WHO (1993b) are marked with a dagger (†). Unpublished references that are dealt with in FAO/WHO (1996a) are marked with a double dagger (‡). Those dealt with in FAO/WHO (1996b) are marked with a section symbol (§).

Albertini, S., Brunner, M., and Wurgler, F. E. (1993). Analysis of the six additional chemicals for in vitro assays of the European Economic Communities' EEC Aneuploidy Programme using *Saccharomyces cerevisiae* D61. M and the *in vitro* porcine brain tubulin assembly assay. *Environ. Mol. Mutagen.* **21**, 180–192.

Albertini, S., Friedreich, U., Holderegger, C., and Wurgler, F. E. (1988). The *in vitro* porcine brain tubulin and assembly assay: Effects of a genotoxic carcinogen (aflatoxin B1), eight tumor promotors and nine miscellaneous substances. *Mutat. Res.* **201**, 283–292.

†Alvarez, L. (1987). "Teratogenicity Study of INE-965 (carbendazim) in Rats." Unpublished report HLR 281-87, E. I. du Pont de Nemours and Co., Inc., Haskell Laboratory, Newark, DE.

†Anderson (1999).

†Arce, G. T. (1984a). "Mutagenicity Evaluation in *Salmonella typhimurium*." Unpublished report HLR 72-84, E. I. du Pont de Nemours and Co., Inc., Haskell Laboratory, Newark, DE.

†Arce, G. T. (1984b). "Mutagenicity Evaluation in *Salmonella typhimurium*." Unpublished report HLR 71-84, E. I. du Pont de Nemours and Co., Inc., Haskell Laboratory, Newark, DE.

Athwal, R. S., and Sandhu S. S. (1985). Use of human × mouse hybrid cell line to detect aneuploidy induced by environmental chemicals. *Mutat. Res.* **149**, 73–81.

Barnes, T. B., Verlangieri, A. J., and Wilson, M. C. (1983). Reproductive toxicity of methyl-1-(butylcarbamoyl)-2-benzimidazole carbamate (benomyl) in male Wistar rats. *Toxicology* **28**, 103–115.

†Beems, R. B., Til, H. P., and van der Heijden, C. A. (1976). "Carcinogenicity Study with Carbendazim (99% MBC) in Mice." Central Institute for Nutrition and Food Research (TNO), The Hague. (Unpublished summary report A08129, Hoechst AG, Frankfurt, and BASF AG, Ludwigshafen, Germany.)

Belasco, I. J. (1969).

Belasco, I. J. (1970).

∗Belasco, I. J. (1979a). "Study Showing the Absence of Acetylcholinesterase Inhibition with a Wettable Powder Formulation (50% Benomyl)." Unpublished report B/TOX 4, E. I. du Pont de Nemours and Co., Inc., Wilmington, DE.

∗Belasco, I. J. (1979b). "2-^{14}C-Benomyl (50 WP) Adsorption through Rat Skin. Part II. Effect of Time and Dose Applied, with Supplement." Unpublished report B/ME 47 and supplement HLR 117-79, E. I. du Pont de Nemours and Co., Inc., Wilmington, DE.

∗Belasco, I. J., Kirkland, J. J., Pease, H. L., and Sherman, H. (1969). "Studies with 2-^{14}C-Labelled Methyl-l-(butylcarbamoyl)-2-benzimidazolecarbamate (Benomyl) in Rats." Unpublished report B/ME 36, E. I. du Pont de Nemours and Co., Inc., Biochemical Department, Research Division, Experimental Station, Wilmington, DE.

∗Bentley, K. S. (1992a). "Classification of DPX-T1991-529 (Benomyl)-Induced Micronuclei in Mouse Bone Marrow Erythrocytes using Immunofluorescence Antikinetochore Antibodies." Unpublished report HLR 568-92, E. I. du Pont de Nemours and Co., Inc., Haskell Laboratory, Newark, DE.

∗Bentley, K. S. (1992b). "Classification of DPX-E965-299 (Carbendazim, MBC)-Induced Micronuclei in Mouse Bone Marrow Erythrocytes using Immunofluorescent Antikinetochore Antibodies." Unpublished report HLR 569-92, E. I. du Pont de Nemours and Co., Inc., Haskell Laboratory, Newark, DE.

Bentley, K. S., Kirkland, D., Murphy, M., and Marshall, R. (2000). Evaluation of thresholds for benomyl- and carbendazim-induced aneuploidy in cultured human lymphocytes using fluorescence *in situ* hybridization. *Mutat. Res.* **464**, 41–51.

Bjorge, C., Brunborg, G., Wiger, R., Holme, J. A., Scholz, T., Dybing, E., and Soderlund, E. J. (1996). A comparative study of chemically induced DNA damage in isolated human and rat testicular cells. *Reprod. Toxicol.* **10(6)**, 509–519.

∗Busey, W. M. (1968a). "Acute Dermal LD. Test and Dermal Irritation Test on Rabbits Using a Wettable Powder Formulation (50% Benomyl) with Histological Addendum." Hazelton Laboratories, Inc., Falls Church, VA. (Unpublished report MRO 581-239, E. I. du Pont de Nemours and Co., Inc., Wilmington, DE.)

∗Busey, W. M. (1968b). "Acute Inhalation Exposure Test in Rats Using a Wettable Powder Formulation (50% Benomyl)." Hazelton Laboratories, Inc., Falls Church, VA. (Unpublished report MRO 1126-1, E. I. du Pont de Nemours and Co., Inc., Wilmington, DE.)

∗Busey, W. M. (1968c). "Teratology Study in Rabbits Using a Wettable Powder Formulation (50% Benomyl)." Hazelton Laboratories, Inc., Falls Church, VA. (Unpublished report MRO 1079, E. I. du Pont de Nemours and Co., Inc., Wilmington, DE.)

∗Busey, W. M. (1968d). "Repeated Dermal Application Test on Rabbits Using a Wettable Powder Formulation (50% Benomyl)." Hazelton Laboratories, Inc., Falls Church, VA. (Unpublished report HLO 298-68, E. I. du Pont de Nemours and Co., Inc., Wilmington, DE.)

Carbonell, E., Puig, M., Zamela, N., Creus, A., and Marcos, R. (1990). Sister chromatid exchange in lymphocytes of workers exposed to pesticides. *Mutagenesis* **5**, 403–405.

Carter, S. D. (1982). "Effect of Benomyl on the Reproductive Development in the Prepubertal Male Rat." Thesis, North Carolina State University, Raleigh.

Carter, S. D., and Laskey, J. W. (1982). Effect of benomyl on reproduction in the male rat. *Toxicol. Lett.* **11**, 87–94.

Carter, S. D., Hess, R. A., and Laskey, J. W. (1987). The fungicide methyl 2-benzimidazolecarbamate causes infertility in male Sprague-Dawley rats. *Biol. Reprod.* **37(3)**, 709–718.

†Christian, M. S., Hoberman, A. M., and Feussner, E. L. (1985). "Developmental Toxicity Study of Carbendazim Administered via Gavage to New Zealand White Rabbits." Argus Research Laboratories, Inc., Horsham, PA. (Unpublished report HLO 515-85, E. I. du Pont de Nemours and Co., Inc., Wilmington, DE.)

∗Colburn, C. W. (1969). "Skin Irritation and Sensitization Tests on Guinea Pigs Using Technical Benomyl (>95% Benomyl)." Unpublished report HLR 84-69, E. I. du Pont de Nemours and Co., Inc., Haskell Laboratory, Newark, DE.

Cronin, E. (1980). *In* "Contact Dermatitis," pp. 391–398. Churchill–Livingstone, London.

Culik, R. (1974).

∗Culik, R. (1981a). "Determination of Benomyl/methyl-2-benzimidazole Carbamate (MBC) Concentrations in Maternal Blood and in the Concepti of Rats Exposed to Benomyl and Benlate by Diet." Unpublished report HLR 916-80, E. I. du Pont de Nemours and Co., Inc., Haskell Laboratory, Newark, DE.

*Culik, R. (1981b). "Determination of Benomyl/methyl-2-benzimidazolecar-bamate (MBC) 4OH MBC and 5-OH MBC Concentrations in Maternal Blood and in the Concepti of Rats Exposed to Benomyl by Gavage." Unpublished report HLR 970-80, E. I. du Pont de Nemours and Co., Inc., Haskell Laboratory, Newark, DE.

*Culik, R., and Gibson, J. R. (1974). "Benlate' Dominant Lethal Study in Male Rats with Supplemental Statistical Report (22-77)." Unpublished report HLR 72-74, E. I. du Pont de Nemours and Co., Inc., Haskell Laboratory, Newark, DE.

Cummings, A. M., Ebron-McCoy, M. T., Rogers, J. M., Barbee, B. D., and Harris, S. T. (1992). Developmental effects of methyl benzimidazole carbamate following exposure during early pregnancy. *Fundam. Appl. Toxicol.* **18**, 288–293.

Cummings, A. M., Harris, S. T., and Rehnberg, G. L. (1990). Effects of methyl benzimidazole carbamate during early pregnancy in the rat. *Fundam. Appl. Toxicol.* **15**, 528–535.

*Dashiell, O. L. (1972). "Acute Oral Test (Benzimidazole, 2-(3-butylureido))." Unpublished report HLR 456-72, E. I. du Pont de Nemours and Co., Inc., Haskell Laboratory, Newark, DE.

*Dashiell, O. L. (1974). "Ten-Day Sub-acute Exposure of Rabbit Skin to 2-Benzimidazolecarbamic Acid, Methyl Ester." Unpublished report HLR 826-74, E. I. du Pont de Nemours and Co., Inc., Wilmington, DE.

†Dashiell, O. L. (1975). "Oral LD50 Test in Guinea Pigs (Carbendazim)." Unpublished report HLR 846-74, E. I. du Pont de Nemours and Co., Inc., Haskell Laboratory, Newark, DE.

Davidse, L. C. (1975). Antimitotic activity of methyl benzimidazol-2-yl-carbamate in fungi and its binding to cellular protein. *In* "Microtubules and Microtubule Inhibitors" (M. Borgers and M. de Brabander, eds.), pp. 483–495. Elsevier, Amsterdam/New York.

Davidse, L. C., and Flach, W. (1977). Differential binding of methyl benzimidazol-2-yl carbamate to fungal tubulin as a mechanism of resistance to this antimitotic agent in mutant strains of *Aspergillus nidulans. J. Cell Biol.* **72**, 174–193.

Davidse, L. C., and Flach, W. (1976b). Differential binding of methyl benzimidazol-2-yl carbamate to fungal tubulin as a mechanism of resistance to this antimitotic agent in mutant strains of *Aspergillus nidulans. J. Cell Biol.* **72**, 174–193.

De Brabander, M., Van de Veire, R., Aerts, F., Geuens, S., and Hoebeke, J. (1976a). A new culture model facilitating rapid quantitative testing of mitotic spindle inhibition in mammalian cells. *J. Natl. Cancer Inst.* **56**, 357–363.

De Brabander, M., Van de Veire, R., Aerts, F., Brogers, M., and Janssen, P. A. J. (1976b). The effect of methyl 5(2-thienylcarbonyl)-1H-benzimidazol-2-yl-carbamate (RI7934;NSC238159), a new synthetic antitumoral drug interfering with microtubules, on mammalian cells cultured in vitro. *Cancer Res.* **36**, 905–916.

Delatour, P., and Besse, S. (1990). Benzimidazole carbamate d'ethyle: Effet teratogene et présence dans le lait de vache après administration de thiophanate. *Ann. Rech. Vet.* **21**, 87–92.

Dellarco, V. L., Mavournin, K. H., and Tice, R. R. (1985). Aneuploidy and health risk assessment: Current status and future directions. *Environ. Mol. Mutagen.* **7**, 405–424.

Desi, L. (1983). Neurotoxicological investigation of pesticides in animal experiments. *Neurobehav. Toxicol. Teratol.* **5**, 503–515.

Desi, L., Dura, G., Szlobodnyik, J., and Csuka, L. (1977). Testing of pesticide toxicity in tissue culture. *J. Toxicol. Environ. Health* **2**, 1053–1066.

Dolara, P., Torricelli, F., and Antonelli, N. (1994). Cytogenetic effects on human lymphocytes of a mixture of fifteen pesticides commonly used in Italy. *Mutat. Res.* **325**, 47–51.

Dolara, P., Vezani, A., Caderni, G., Coppi, C., and Torricelli, F. (1993). Genetic toxicity of a mixture of fifteen pesticides commonly found in the Italian diet. *Cell. Biol. Toxicol.* **9(4)**, 333–343.

Dolk, H., Busy, A., Amstron, B. G., and Walls, P. H. (1988). Geographical variation in anophthalmia and microphthalmia in England, 1988–94. *Br. Med. J.* **317**, 905–909.

†Donaubauer, H. H., Schuetz, E., Weigand, W., and Kramer, M. (1982). "Repeated Dose (24 Month) Feeding Study for Determination of the Carcinogenic Effect of HOE 17411 OFAT204 (Carbendazim) in Mice." Unpublished report A24749, Hoechst AG, Pharmaceuticals Research, Toxicology Section, Frankfurt, Germany.

§Dorn, E., and Keller, H. M. (1980). "Carbendazim (60% Wettable Powder) Absorption via the Skin in Rats." Unpublished report A48605, Hoechst AG, Frankfurt.

†Dorn, E., Schmidt, E., Kellner, H. M., and Leist, K. H. (1983). "HOE 017441-14-C (Carbendazim-14C) Metabolic Fate in Rats and Mice, a Comparison." Unpublished report A26222, Hoechst AG, Frankfurt, Germany.

Douch, P. G. C. (1973). The metabolism of benomyl fungicide in mammals. *Xenobiotica* **3**, 367–380.

‡DuPont (1979). "Benlate Dust Exposure Survey—Blood Profile Analysis." Unpublished report B/TOX 5, E. I. duPont de Nemours & Co., Haskell Laboratory, Newark, DE.

†Edwards, D. F. (1974a). "Skin Absorption LD50 (Carbendazim)." Unpublished report HLR 798-74, E. I. du Pont de Nemours and Co., Inc., Haskell Laboratory, Newark, DE.

†Edwards, D. F. (1974b). "Federal Hazardous Substances Act—Eye Irritation Test in Rabbits (Carbendazim)." Unpublished report HLR 799-74, E. I. du Pont de Nemours and Co., Inc., Haskell Laboratory, Newark, DE.

*Eickhoff, J., Petersen, B., and Chaisson, C. (1989). "Anticipated Residues of Benomyl in Food Crops and Potential Dietary Exposure and Risk Assessment." Technical Assessment Systems, Inc., Washington, D.C. (Unpublished report TAS 000-005, E. I. du Pont de Nemours and Co., Inc., Wilmington, DE.)

Elhajouji, A., Tibaldi, F., and Kirsch-Volders, M. (1997). Indication for thresholds of chromosome non-disjunction versus chromosome lagging induced by spindle inhibitors *in vitro* in human lymphocytes. *Mutagenesis* **12**, 133–140.

Elhajouji, A., Van Hummelen, P., and Kirsch-Volders, M. (1995). Indications for a threshold of chemically induced aneuploidy *in vitro* in human lymphocytes. *Environ. Mol. Mutagen.* **26**, 292–304.

Ellis, W. G., De Roos, F., Kavlock, R. J., and Zeman, F. (1988). Relationship of periventricular overgrowth to hydrocephalus in brains of fetal rats exposed to benomyl. *Teratog. Carcinog. Mutagen.* **8**, 377–391.

Ellis, W. G., Semple, J. L., Hoogenboom, E. R., Kavlock, R. J., and Zeman, F. (1987). Benomyl induced craniocerebral anomalies in fetuses of adequately nourished and protein-deprived rats. *Teratog., Carcinog., Mutagen.* **7**, 357–375.

Evanson, D. P., Janca, F. C., and Jost, L. K. (1987). Effects of the fungicide methyl-benzimidazol-2-yl carbamate (MBC) on mouse germ cells as determined by flow cytometry. *J. Toxicol. Environ. Health* **20**, 387–399.

Everhart, L. P., and Holt, R. F. (1982). Potential Benlate fungicide exposure during mixer/loader operations, crop harvest and home use. *J. Agric. Food Chem.* **30**, 222–227.

*Fitzpatrick, K. (1980). "Chinese Hamster Ovary Cell Assay for Mutagenicity." Unpublished report HLR 438-80, E. I. du Pont de Nemours and Co., Inc., Haskell Laboratory, Newark, DE.

Food and Agriculture Organization–World Health Organization (FAO/WHO) (1996a). Pesticide residues in food—1995 (benomyl). *In* "Joint FAO/WHO Meeting on Pesticide Residues, Evaluations 1995 Part II—Toxicological and Environmental." International Programme on Chemical Safety, Geneva.

Food and Agriculture Organization–World Health Organization (FAO/WHO) (1996b). Pesticide residues in food—1995 (carbendazim). *In* "Joint FAO/WHO Meeting on Pesticide Residues, Evaluations 1995 Part II—Toxicological and Environmental." International Programme on Chemical Safety, Geneva.

Food and Agriculture Organization–World Health Organization (FAO/WHO) (1999a). Pesticide residues in food—1998 (benomyl). *In* "Joint FAO/WHO Meeting on Pesticide Residues, Evaluations 1998 Part I—Residues." International Programme on Chemical Safety, Geneva.

Food and Agriculture Organization–World Health Organization (FAO/WHO) (1999b). Pesticide residues in food—1998 (carbendazim). *In* "Joint FAO/WHO Meeting on Pesticide Residues, Evaluations 1998 Part I—Residues." International Programme on Chemical Safety, Geneva.

†Ford, L. S. (1981). "Primary Skin Irritation and Sensitization on Guinea Pigs." Unpublished report HLR 729-81, E. I. du Pont de Nemours and Co., Inc., Haskell Laboratory, Newark, DE.

‡Foss, J. A. (1993). "Acute Neurotoxicity Study of DPX-T1991-529 (Benomyl) Administered Orally via the Diet to Crl: CD BR VAF/Plus Rats." Unpublished report HLO 825-92, E. I. du Pont de Nemours and Co., Haskell Laboratory, Newark, DE.

‡Foss, J. A. (1994). "Subchronic Neurotoxicity Study of DPX-T1991-529 (Benomyl) Administered Orally via the Diet to Crl: CD BR VAF/Plus Rats." Unpublished report HLO 551-93, E. I. du Pont de Nemours and Co., Haskell Laboratory, Newark, DE.

Fox, T. R., and Gonzalez, A. J. (1996). Cell cycle controls as potential targets for the development of chemically induced mouse liver cancer. *CIIT Activities* July 1996.

*Frame, S. R., and Van Pelt, C. S. (1990). "Oncogenicity Studies with Benomyl and MBC in Mice: Supplemental Peer Review." Unpublished report HLR 20-82 and supplement HLR 70-82, E. I. du Pont de Nemours and Co., Inc., Haskell Laboratory, Newark, DE.

Fregert, S. (1973). Allergic contact dermatitis from two pesticides. *Contact Derm. Newsletter* 13, 367.

Gardiner, J. A., Kirkland, J. J., Klopping, H. L., and Sherman, H. (1974). Fate of benomyl in animals. *J. Agric. Food Chem.* 22(3), 419–427.

*Gargus, J. L., and Zoetis, T. (1983a). "Primary Irritation Study in Rabbits (Benlate PNW)." Hazelton Laboratories, Inc., Vienna, VA. (Unpublished report HLO 510-83, E. I. du Pont de Nemours and Co., Inc., Wilmington, DE.)

*Gargus, J. L., and Zoetis, T. (1983b). "Eye Irritation Test in Rabbits (EPA Pesticide Registration Benlate PNW)." Hazelton Laboratories, Inc., Vienna, VA. (Unpublished report HLO 511-83, E. I. du Pont de Nemours and Co., Inc., Wilmington, DE.)

*Gargus, J. L., and Zoetis T. (1983c). "Acute Skin Absorption LD50 Test on Rabbits (EPA Pesticide Registration Guidelines—Benlate PNW)." Hazelton Laboratories, Inc., Vienna, VA. (Unpublished report HLO 512-83, E. I. du Pont de Nemours and Co., Inc., Wilmington, DE.)

*Gargus, J. L., and Zoetis, T. (1984). "Primary Skin Irritation and Sensitization Test on Guinea Pigs (Benlate PNW)." Hazelton Laboratories, Inc., Vienna, VA. (Unpublished report HLO 67-84, E. I. du Pont de Nemours and Co., Inc., Wilmington, DE.)

*Goldenthal, E. I. (1978). "Neurotoxicity Study in Hens [Using Technical Benomyl (<95% Benomyl)." International Research and Development Corporation, Mattawan, MI. (Unpublished report and addendum HLO 28-79, E. I. du Pont de Nemours and Co., Inc., Wilmington, DE.)

*Gooch, J. J. (1978). "Fertility of Workers Potentially Exposed to Benomyl." Unpublished report B/TOX 7, E. I. du Pont de Nemours and Co., Inc., Wilmington, DE.

†Goodman, N. C. (1974). "Intraperitoneal LD50 Test [in Rats Using Technical Carbendazim (Less than 98%)]." Unpublished report HLR 845-74, E. I. du Pont de Nemours and Co., Inc., Haskell Laboratory, Newark, DE.

Goodman, N. C. (1975).

*Goodman, N. C. (1979). "Intraperitoneal LD50 Test in Rats." Unpublished report HLR 847-74, E. I. du Pont de Nemours and Co., Inc., Haskell Laboratory, Newark, DE.

†Goodman, N. C., and Sherman, H. (1975). "Oral LD50 Tests (Fasted Male and Female Rats)." Unpublished report HLR 847-74, E. I. du Pont de Nemours and Co., Inc., Haskell Laboratory, Newark, DE.

Gray, L. E., Ostby, J., Sigmon, R., Ferrell, J., Rehnberg, G., Linder, R., Cooper, R., Goldman, J., and Laskey, J. (1988). The development of a protocol to assess reproductive effects of toxicants in the rat. *Reprod. Toxicol.* 2, 281–287.

Gray, L. E., Ostby, J., Linder, R., Goldman, J., Rehnberg, G., and Cooper, R. (1990). Carbendazim induced alterations of reproductive development and function in the rat and hamster. *Fund. Appl. Toxicol.* 15, 281–297.

*Guengerich, F. P. (1981). "Enzyme Induction with Du Pont Compounds H11,202-02 and HIO, 962-02." School of Medicine, Vanderbilt University, Nashville, TN. (Unpublished report HLO 850-81, E. I. du Pont de Nemours and Co., Inc., Wilmington, DE.)

*Han, J. C. Y. (1978). "Metabolism of ^{14}C-Labeled Benomyl in the Mouse and Hamster." Unpublished report B/ME 65, E. I. du Pont de Nemours and Co., Inc., Biochemicals Department, Wilmington, DE.

*Han, J. C. Y. (1979). 2-^{14}C-Benomyl (50% WP) Rat Study—Intravenous Injection." Unpublished report B/ME 41, E. I. du Pont de Nemours and Co., Inc., Biochemicals Department, Wilmington, DE.

*Hardisty, J. F. (1990). "Oncogenicity Studies with Benomyl and MBC in Mice. Peer-Review of Liver Neoplasms." Experimental Pathology Laboratories, Inc., Research Triangle Park, NC. (Unpublished report 129-012, E. I. du Pont de Nemours and Co., Inc., Wilmington, DE.)

Hess, R. A., Moore, B. J., Forrer, J., Linder, R. E., and Abuel-Atta, A. A. (1991). The fungicide benomyl (methyl) 1-(butylcarbomyl)-2-benzimidazole carbamate causes testicular dysfunction by inducing the sloughing of germ cells and occlusion of efferent ductules. *Fundam. Appl. Toxicol.* 17, 733–745.

Hoekstra, E. J., Kiefer, M., and Tepper, A. (1996). Monitoring of exposure to benomyl in nursery workers. *JOEM* 38(8), 775–781.

§Hofmann, H. T., and Peh, J. (1987a). "Report on the Study to Determine the Prenatal Toxicity of Methyl Benzamidazole-2-carbamate (MBC) in Rats." Unpublished report A52505, BASF AG, Ludwigshafen, Germany.

§Hofmann, H. T., and Peh, J. (1987b). "Report on the Study to Determine the Prenatal Toxicity of Methyl Benzamidazole-2-carbamate (MBC) in Rats." Unpublished report A52506, BASF AG, Ludwigshafen, Germany.

*Hood, D. B. (1969). "Fifteen Exposure Dermal Tests on Rabbits Using a Wettable Powder Formulation (50% Benomyl)." Unpublished report HLR 211-69, E. I. du Pont de Nemours and Co., Inc., Haskell Laboratory, Newark, DE.

Hoogenboom, E. R., Ransdell, J. F., Ellis, W. G., Kavlock, R. J., and Zeman, F. J. (1991). Effects on the fetal rat eye of maternal benomyl exposure and protein malnutrition. *Curr. Eye Res.* 10, 601–612.

*Hostetler, K. H. (1977). "Oral LD50 Test (Benlate OD)." Unpublished report HLR 527-77, E. I. du Pont de Nemours and Co., Inc., Haskell Laboratory, Newark, DE.

Hurtt, M. E., Mebus, C. A., and Bogdanffy, M. S. (1993). Investigation of the effects of benomyl on rat nasas mucosa. *Fundam. Appl. Toxicol.* 21, 253–255.

Ireland, C. M., Gull, K., Gutteridge, W. E., and Pogson, C. I. (1979). The interaction of benzimidazole carbamates with mammalian microtubule protein. *Biochem. Pharmacol.* 28, 2680–2682.

Janardhan, A., Rao, A. B., and Sisodia, P. (1987). Sub-chronic toxicity of methyl benzimidazole carbamate in rats. *Bull. Environ. Contam. Toxicol.* 38(5), 890–898.

Janardhan, A., Sattur, P. B., and Sisodia, P. (1984). Teratology of methyl benzimidazole carbamate in rats and rabbits. *Bull. Environ. Contam. Toxicol.* 33(3), 257–263.

Jeffay, S., Libbus, B., Barbee, R., and Perreault, S. (1996). Acute exposure of female hamsters to carbendazim (mbc) during meiosis results in aneuploid oocytes with subsequent arrest of embryonic cleavage and implantations. *Reprod. Toxicol.* 10(3), 183–189.

*Jessup, C. D. (1979). "Acute Delayed Neurotoxicity Study in Chickens Using Technical Benomyl (>95% Benomyl)." International Research and Development Corporation, Mattawan, MI. (Unpublished report HLO 674-79, E. I. du Pont de Nemours and Co., Inc., Wilmington, DE.)

*Jessup, D. C., and Dean, W. (1979). "Acute Delayed Neurotoxicity Study in Chickens Using Technical Benomyl (Less than 95% Benomyl)." International Research and Development Corporation, Mattawan, MI. (Unpublished report HLO 29-79, E. I. du Pont de Nemours and Co., Inc., Wilmington, DE.)

Kavlock, R. J., Chernoff, N., Gray, L. E., Gray, J. A., and Whitehouse, D. (1982). Teratogenic effects of benomyl in the Wistar rat and CD-1 mouse, with emphasis on the route of administration. *Toxicol. Appl. Pharmacol.* 62, 44–54.

Kilmartin, J. V. (1981). Purification of yeast tubulin by self-assembly *in vitro*. *Biochemistry* 20, 3629–3633.

†Koeter, H. B. W. M. (1975a). "Effect of HOE 17411F (=BAS 3460F) on Pregnancy of the Rat." Central Institute of Nutrition and Food Research

(TNO), The Hague. (Unpublished report A04120, Hoechst AG, Frankfurt, and BASF AG, Ludwigshafen, Germany.)

†Koeter, H. B. W. M. (1975b). "Effect of HOE 17411F (=BAS 3460F) on Pregnancy of the New Zealand White Rabbit." Central Institute for Nutrition and Food Research (TNO), The Hague. (Unpublished report A09804, Hoechst AG, Frankfurt, and BASF AG, Ludwigshafen, Germany.)

†Koeter, H. B. W. M., *et al.* (1976a).

†Koeter, H. B. W. M., *et al.* (1976b).

†Kramer, M., and Weigand, W. (1971). "(HOE 17411 O.F.) Toxicological Examination." Unpublished report A00936, Hoechst AG, Pharmaceuticals Research, Toxicology Section, Frankfurt, Germany.

Krechniak, J., and Klosowska, B. (1986). The fate of 14-C-carbendazim in rat. *Xenobiotica* **16**(9), 809–815.

Kristensen, P., and Irgens, L. (1994). Clusters of anophthalmia. *Br. Med. J.* **206**, 308–309.

Krupka, R. M. (1974). On the anti-cholinesterase activity of benomyl. *Pestic. Sci.* **5**, 211–216.

Kuehne, G., Heise, H., Plottke, B., and Puskeiler, T. (1985). Dermatitis after Benlate contact. *Z. Gesamte. Hyg., Grenzgeb.* **31**, 710–711.

Lander, F., and Ronne, M. (1995). Frequency of sister chromatid exchange and hematological effects in pesticide-exposed greenhouse sprayers. *Scand. J. Work Environ. Health* **21**, 283–288.

Larsen, A. I., Larsen, A., Jepsen, J. R., and Jorgensen, R. (1990). Contact allergy to the fungicide benomyl? *Contact Dermatitis* **22**, 278–281.

Lavy, T. L., Mattice, J. D., Massey, J. H., and Skulman, B. W. (1993). Measurements of year-long exposure to tree nursery workers using multiple pesticides. *Arch. Environ. Contam. Toxicol.* **24**, 123–144.

*Lee, K. P. (1977). "The Two-Year Feeding Study in Rats with Benomyl with Supplemental Pathology Report." Unpublished report HLR 66-77, E. I. du Pont de Nemours and Co., Inc., Haskell Laboratory, Newark, DE.

Leonard, J. A., and Yeary, R. A. (1990). Exposure of workers using hand-held equipment during urban application of pesticides to trees and ornamental shrubs. *Am. Ind. Hyg. Assoc. J.* **50**, 605–609.

Liesivuori, J., Liukkonen, S., and Pirhonen, P. (1988). Reentry intervals after pesticide application in greenhouses. *Scand. J. Work Environ. Health* **14**(Suppl. 1), 35–36.

Lim, J., and Miller, M. (1997). The role of the benomyl metabolite carbendazim in benomyl-induced testicular toxicity. *Toxicol. Appl. Pharmacol.* **142**, 401–410.

Linder, R. E., Rehnberg, G. L., Strader, L. F., and Diggs, J. P. (1988). Evaluation of reproductive parameters in adult male Wistar rats after subchronic exposure. *J. Toxicol. Environ. Health* **25**, 285–298.

Lisi, P., Caraffini, S., and Assalve, D. (1986). A test series for pesticide dermatitis. *Contact Dermatitis* **15**, 266–269.

*Littlefield, N. A., and Busey, W. M. (1969). "Four-Hour Acute Inhalation Exposure Test in Dogs Using a Wettable Powder Formulation (50% Benomyl)." Hazelton Laboratories, Inc., Falls Church, VA. (Unpublished report HLR 192-69, E. I. du Pont de Nemours and Co., Inc., Wilmington, DE.)

Lu, S. Y., Hong-Wei, L., and Shun-Cheng, W. (1995). Taiwan Agricultural Chemicals and Toxic Substance Research Institute. *Plant Protection Bulletin (Taichung)* **37**(3), 331–338.

Mailhes, J. B., and Aardema, M. J. (1992). Benomyl-induced aneuploidy in mouse oocytes. *Mutagenesis* **7**, 303–309.

Marshall, R. R., Murphy, M., Kirkland, D. J., and Bentley, K. S. (1996). Fluorescence *in situ* hybridisation with chromosome-specific centromeric probes: A sensitive method to detect aneuploidy. *Mutat. Res.* **372**, 233–245.

†Martin, D. A., Henry, J. E., and Brock, W. J. (1987). "Closed-Patch Repeated Insult Dermal Sensitization Study (Buehler Method) with Benlate C Fungicide in Guinea-Pigs." Unpublished report HLR 510-87, E. I. du Pont de Nemours and Co., Inc., Haskell Laboratory, Newark, DE.

Matsushita, T., and Aoyama, K. (1981). Cross reactions between some pesticides and the fungicide benomyl in contact allergy. *Ind. Health.* **19**, 77–83.

Matsushita, T., Yoshioka, M., Aoyama, K., Aritmatsu, Y., and Nomura, S. (1977). Experimental study on contact dermatitis caused by fungicides benomyl and thiophanate-methyl. *Ind. Health* **15**, 141.

*McCooey, K. T., Arce, G. T., Sarrif, A. M., and Krahn, D. F. (1983a). "L5178Y Mouse Lymphoma Cell Assay for Mutagenicity." Unpublished

report HLR 86-83, E. I. du Pont de Nemours and Company, Haskell Laboratory, Newark, DE.

*McCooey, K. T., Arce, G. T., Sarrif, A. M., and Krahn, D. F. (1983b). "L5178Y Mouse Lymphoma Cell Assay for Mutagenicity." Unpublished report HLR 253-83, E. I. du Pont de Nemours and Company, Haskell Laboratory, Newark, DE.

*Mebus, C. A. (1990). "Reproductive and Fertility Effects with DPX-1991-529 (Benomyl). Multigeneration Reproduction Study in Rats." Unpublished report HLR 765-90, E. I. du Pont de Nemours and Co., Inc., Haskell Laboratory, Newark, DE.

Minata, M., and Biernacki, B. (1982). Embryotoxicity of carbendazim in rats, rabbits and hamsters. *Bull. Vet. Inst. Pulaway* **2**, 42–52.

†Mohr, U. (1977). "Review of Liver Sections from Mice and Rats Fed with Carbendazim." Department of Experimental Pathology, Medical School, Hannover, Germany. (Unpublished report MBC/TOX 6 from Hoechst AG, Frankfurt, and BASF AG, Ludwigshafen, Germany.)

*Monson, K. D. (1990). "Metabolism of [phenyl(U)-^{14}C]Carbendazim in Rats." Unpublished report AMR 1141-88, E. I. du Pont de Nemours and Co., Inc., Wilmington, DE.

‡Munley, S. M. (1995). "Developmental Toxicity Study of DPX-T1991-529 (Benomyl)." Unpublished report HLR 164-95, E. I. du Pont de Nemours and Co., Haskell Laboratory, Newark, DE.

Nakai, M., Hess, R. A., Moore, B. J., Guttroff, R. F., Strader, L. F., and Linder, R. E. (1992). Acute and long-term effects of the fungicide carbendazim (methyl 2-benzimidazole carbamate; mbc) on the male reproductive system in the rat. *J. Androl.* **13**, 507–518.

Nakai, M., *et al.* (1997).

Naki, M., and Hess, R. A. (1997). Effects of carbendazim (methyl 2-benzimidazole carbamate; mbc) on meiotic spermatocytes and subsequent spermatogenesis in the rat testis. *Anat. Rec.* **247**, 379–387.

Naki, M., Hess, R. A., Matsuo, F., Gotoh, Y., and Nasu, T. (1996). Further observations on carbendazim-induced abnormalities of spermatid morphology in rats. *Tissue Cell* 477–485.

†Nash, S. D., and Ferenz, R. (1982). "Inhalation Median Lethal Concentration (LC50) in Rats—EPA Protocol (Carbendazim 75% Wettable Powder)." Unpublished report HLR 365-82, E. I. du Pont de Nemours and Co., Inc., Haskell Laboratory, Newark, DE.

NIOSH (1994). "Ornamental Plant Nurseries, Florida." NIOSH Hazard Evaluation and Technical Assistance Report No. 92-0381-2445.

Parry, J. M., Fielder, R. J., and McDonald, A. (1994). Thresholds for aneuploidy-inducing chemicals. *Mutagenesis* **9**, 503–504.

Perrault, S. D., Jeffay, S., Poss, P., and Laskey, J. W. (1992). Use of the fungicide carbendazim as a model compound to determine the impact of acute chemical exposure during oocyte maturation and fertilization on pregnancy outcome in the hamster. *Toxicol. Appl. Pharmacol.* **114**, 225–231.

Piersma, A. H., Verhoef, A., and Dortant, P. M. (1995). Evaluation of the OECD 421 Reproductive Toxicity Screening Test Protocol using 1-(butylcarbamoyl)-2-benzimidazole carbamate (benomyl). *Teratog. Carcinog., Mutagen.* **15**, 93–100.

†Reuzel, P. G. J., Hendriksen, C. F. M., and Til, H. P. (1976). "Long-Term (Two-Year) Toxicity Study with Carbendazim in Beagle Dogs." Central Institute for Nutrition and Food Research (TNO), The Hague. (Unpublished report A06583, BASF AG, Ludwigshafen, and Hoechst AG, Frankfurt, Germany.)

*Rickard, L. B. (1983a). "Mutagenicity Evaluation in *Salmonella typhimurium*." Unpublished report HLR 97-83, E. I. du Pont de Nemours and Co., Inc., Haskell Laboratory, Newark, DE.

*Rickard, L. B. (1983b). "Mutagenicity Evaluation in *Salmonella typhimurium*." Unpublished report HLR 98-83, E. I. du Pont de Nemours and Co., Inc., Haskell Laboratory, Newark, DE.

*Rickard, L. B. (1986).

*Russell, J. F. (1978a). "Mutagenic Activity of 2-Benzimidazolecarbamic Acid, 1(Butylcarbamoyl)-methyl Ester in the Salmonella/Microsome Assay." Unpublished report HLR 18-78, E. I. du Pont de Nemours and Co., Inc., Haskell Laboratory, Newark, DE.

*Russell, J. F. (1978b). "Mutagenic Activity of 2-Benzimidazolecarbamic Acid, 1(Butylcarbamoyl)-methyl Ester in the Salmonella/Microsome Assay." Unpublished report HLR 31-78, E. I. du Pont de Nemours and Co., Inc., Haskell Laboratory, Newark, DE.

*Russell, J. F., *et al.* (1992).

§Russell, L. D. (1992). "Review of Prof. Hilscher's Report 'Effects of Carbendazim on Spermatogenesis'." Unpublished report, University of Illinois. (Unpublished report A49229, Hoechst AG, Frankfurt.)

Sandhu, S. S., Gudi, R. D., and Athwal, R. S. (1988). A monochromosomal hybrid cell assay for evaluating the genotoxicity of environmental chemicals. *Cell. Biol. Toxicol.* **4**, 495–506.

Sarrif, A. M., Arce, G. T., Krahn, D. F., O'Neil, R. M., and Reynolds, V. L. (1994a). Evaluation of carbendazim for gene mutations in the *Salmonella*/Ames plate-incorporation assay: The role of aminophenazine impurities. *Mutat. Res.* **321**, 43–56.

Sarrif, A. M., Bentley, K. S., Fu, L. J., O'Neil, R. M., Reynolds, V. L., and Stahl, R. G. (1994b). Evaluation of benomyl and carbendazim in the *in vivo* aneuploidy/micronucleus assay in BDF1 mouse bone marrow. *Mutat. Res.* **310**, 143–149.

†Sarver, J. W. (1975). "Acute Inhalation Toxicity—One Hour Head Only (Carbendazim)." Unpublished report HLR 58-75, E. I. du Pont de Nemours and Co., Inc., Haskell Laboratory, Newark, DE.

Sasaki, Y. F. X. (1988). Benomyl in-vitro cytogenetics test. IET-88-0043. The Institute of Environmental Toxicology, Kodiara Laboratories, Suzuki-cho 2-772, Kodaira, Tokyo 187, Japan.

*Sasaki, Y. F. X. (1990). "Benomyl: Micronucleus Test in Mice." Kodaira Laboratories, Institute of Environmental Toxicology, Tokyo (Unpublished report IET 89-0046, E. I. du Pont de Nemours and Co., Inc., Wilmington, DE.)

Savitt, L. E. (1972). Contact dermatitis due to benomyl (letter). *Arch. Dermatol.* **105**, 926–927.

Schuman, S. H., and Dobson, R. L. (1985). An outbreak of contact dermatitis in farm workers. *J. Am. Acad. Dermatol.* **13**, 220–223.

†Sherman, H. (1965). "Acute Oral Test." Unpublished report HLR 125-65, E. I. du Pont de Nemours and Co., Inc., Haskell Laboratory, Newark, DE.

Sherman, H. (1967).

*Sherman, H. (1968). "Three-Month Feeding Study in Dogs Using a Wettable Powder Formulation (50% Benomyl)." Unpublished report HLR 269-68, E. I. du Pont de Nemours and Co., Inc., Haskell Laboratory, Newark, DE.

*Sherman, H. (1969a). "Acute Oral LD50, Test in Rats Using Technical Benomyl (>95% Benomyl) and a Wettable Powder Formulation (50% Benomyl)." Unpublished report HLR 17-69, E. I. du Pont de Nemours and Co., Inc., Haskell Laboratory, Newark, DE.

*Sherman, H. (1969b). "Acute Oral ALD Test in a Dog Using Technical Benomyl (>95% Benomyl)." Unpublished report HLR 168-69, E. I. du Pont de Nemours and Co., Inc., Haskell Laboratory, Newark, DE.

*Sherman, H. (1969c). "Long Term Feeding Study in Rats with 1-Butylcarbamoyl-2-benzimidazolecarbamic Acid, Methyl Ester (INT-1991)." Unpublished report HLR 232-69, E. I. du Pont de Nemours and Co., Inc., Haskell Laboratory, Newark, DE.

†Sherman, H. (1970a). "Three-Month Feeding Study in Dogs Using a Wettable Powder Formulation (50% MBC)." Unpublished report HLR 283-70, E. I. du Pont de Nemours and Co., Inc., Haskell Laboratory, Newark, DE.

*Sherman, H. (1970b). "Long-Term Feeding Study in Dogs with 1-Butycarbamoyl-2-benzimidazolecarbamic Acid, Methyl Ester (INT-1991)." Unpublished report HLR 48-70, E. I. du Pont de Nemours and Co., Inc., Haskell Laboratory, Newark, DE.

*, †Sherman, H. (1972). "Long-Term Feeding Studies in Rats and Dogs with 2-Benzimadazolecarbamic Acid, Methyl Ester (INE-965) (50% and 70% MBC Wettable Powder Formulations): Parts I and II." Unpublished report HLR 195-72, E. I. du Pont de Nemours and Co., Inc., Haskell Laboratory, Newark, DE.

*Sherman, H., and Krauss, W. C. (1966). "Acute Oral Test [Benomyl]." Unpublished report HLR 100-66, E. I. du Pont de Nemours and Co., Inc., Haskell Laboratory, Newark, DE.

*Sherman, H., Barnes, J. R., and Krauss, W. C. (1967). "Ninety-Day Feeding Study with 1-Butylcarbamoyl-2-benzimidazolecarbamic Acid, Methyl Ester (INT-1991)." Unpublished report HLR 11-67, E. I. du Pont de Nemours and Co., Inc., Haskell, Laboratory, Newark, DE.

Sherman, H., Culik, R., and Jackson, R. A. (1975). Reproduction, teratogenic and mutagenic studies with benomyl. *Toxicol. Appl. Pharmacol.* **32**, 305–315.

Sherman, H. *et al.* (1970a).

Spagnolo, A., Bianchi, F., Calabro, A., Calzolari, E., Clementi, M., Mastroiacovo, P., Meli, P., Petrelli, G., and Tenconi, R. (1994). Anophthalmia and benomyl in Italy: A multicenter study based on 940,615 newborns. *Reprod. Toxicol.* **8**, 397–403.

Spencer, F., Chi, L., and Zhu, M. (1996). Effect of benomyl and carbendazim on steroid and molecular mechanisms in uterine decidual growth in rats. *J. Appl. Toxicol.* **16**, 211–214.

§Stadler, J. C. (1986). "One-Year Feeding Study in Dogs with Carbendazim." Unpublished report HLR 291-86, E. I. du Pont de Nemours and Co., Inc., Haskell Laboratory, Newark, DE.

*Stahl, R. G., Jr. (1990). "*In Vivo*" Evaluation of INT-1991-259 for Chromosome Aberrations in Mouse Bone Marrow." Unpublished report HLR 401-90, E. I. du Pont de Nemours and Co., Inc., Haskell Laboratory, Newark, DE.

*Staples, R. E. (1980). "Teratogenicity Study in the Rat after Administration by Gavage of Technical Benomyl (>95% Benomyl): Parts I, II and III." Unpublished report HLR 649-80, E. I. du Pont de Nemours and Co., Inc., Haskell Laboratory, Newark, DE.

*Staples, R. E. (1982). "Teratogenicity Study in the Rat Using Technical Benomyl (>95% Benomyl) Administered by Gavage and Supplement with Individual Animal Data." Unpublished report HLR 587-82, E. I. du Pont de Nemours and Co., Inc., Haskell Laboratory, Newark, DE.

Til, H. P., Beems, R. B., and Grout, A. P. (1981). Determination of the acute oral toxicity of carbendazim in mice. The Hauge, Central Institute for Nutrition and Food Research (TNO), Unpublished report No. A-21604, prepared for BASFAG, Ludwigshafen, Germany.

†Til, H. P., Koellen, C., and van der Heijden, C. A. (1976a). "Combined Chronic Toxicity and Carcinogenicity Study with Carbendazim in Rats." Central Institute for Nutrition and Food Research (TNO), The Hague. (Unpublished report A08128, BASF AG, Ludwigshafen, and Hoechst AG, Frankfurt, Germany.)

†Til, H. P., Koeter, H. B. W. M., and van der Heijden, C. A. (1976b). "Multigeneration Study with Carbendazim in Rats." Central Institute for Nutrition and Food Research (TNO), The Hague. (Unpublished report A10295, Hoechst AG, Frankfurt.)

†Til, H. P., van den Muelen, H. C., Feron, V. J., Seinen, W., and de Groot, A. P. (1972). "Sub-chronic (90 Day) Toxicity Study with W 17411 in Beagle Dogs." Central Institute for Nutrition and Food Research (TNO), The Hague. (Unpublished report A00292, Hoechst AG, Frankfurt.)

*Tong, C. (1981a). "Hepatocyte Primary Culture/DNA Repair Assay on Compound 10,962-02 (Benomyl) Using Mouse Hepatocytes in Culture." Naylor Dana Institute, Valhalla, NY. (Unpublished report HLO 741-81 from E. I. du Pont de Nemours and Co., Inc., Wilmington, DE.)

†Tong, C. (1981b). "The Hepatocyte Primary Culture/DNA Repair Assay on Compound 11,201-01 Using Rat Hepatocytes in Culture." Naylor Dana Institute, Valhalla, NY. (Unpublished report HLO 743-81, E. I. du Pont de Nemours, Inc., Wilmington, DE.)

†Tong, C. (1981c). "The Hepatocyte Primary Culture/DNA Repair Assay on Compound 11,201-01 Using Mouse Hepatocytes in Culture." Naylor Dana Institute, Valhalla, NY. (Unpublished report HLO 744-81, E. I. du Pont de Nemours, Inc., Wilmington, DE.)

*Turney, R. T. (1979). "Rat Inhalation Study—Benlate." Unpublished report HLR 116-79, E. I. du Pont de Nemours and Co., Inc., Haskell Laboratory, Newark, DE.

Van Joost, T. H. *et al.*(1983). "Benomyl."

Van Joost, T. H., Naafs, B., and van Ketel, W. G. (1983). Sensitization to benomyl and related pesticides. *Contact Dermatitis* **9**, 153–154.

Van Ketel, W. G. (1976). Sensitivity to the pesticide benomyl. *Contact Dermatitis* **2**, 290–291.

*Vick, D. A., and Brock, W. J. (1987a). "Primary Dermal Irritation Study with Benlate 50 DF Fungicide in Rabbits." Unpublished report HLR 300-87, E. I. du Pont de Nemours and Co., Inc., Haskell Laboratory, Newark, DE.

†Vick, D. A., and Brock, W. J. (1987b). "Primary Dermal Irritation Study with Benlate C Fungicide in Rabbits." Unpublished report HLR 299-87, E. I. du Pont de Nemours and Co., Inc., Haskell Laboratory, Newark, DE.

†Vick, D. A., and Brock, W. J. (1987c). "Acute Dermal Toxicity Study of Benlate C Fungicide in Rabbits." Unpublished report HLR 303-87, E. I. du Pont de Nemours and Co., Inc., Haskell Laboratory, Newark, DE.

Vick, D. A., and Valentine, R. (1987). "Primary Eye Irritation Study with Benlate C Fungicide in Rabbits." Unpublished report HLR 287-87, E. I. du Pont de Nemours and Co., Inc., Haskell Laboratory, Newark, DE.

*Ward, R. S., and Scott, R. C. (1992). "Benomyl: *In Vitro* Absorption of a 500 g kg-1 WP Formulation through Human Epidermis." Imperial Chemical Industries (ICI), Fernhurst, Naslemer, Surrey, UK. (Unpublished report CTL/P/3659, E. I. du Pont de Nemours and Co., Inc., Wilmington, DE.)

Warheit, D. B., Kelly, D. P., Carakostas, M. C., and Singer, A. W. (1989). A 90-day inhalation toxicity study with benomyl in rats. *Fundam. Appl. Toxicol.* **12**, 333–345.

*, ‡Weichman, B. E. (1982). "Long Term Feeding Study with Methyl 1-(Butylcarbamoyl)-2-benzimidazolecarbamate in Mice (INT-1991; >95% Benomyl): Parts I, II and III." Unpublished report HLR 20-82, E. I. du Pont de Nemours and Co., Inc., Haskell Laboratory, Newark, DE.

†Wood, C. K. (1982). "Long-Term Feeding Study with 2-Benzimidazole-carbamate, Methyl Ester (<99% MBC, INE-965) in Mice. Parts I and II." Unpublished report HLR 70-82, E. I. du Pont de Nemours and Co., Inc., Haskell Laboratory, Newark, DE.

World Health Organization (WHO) (1993a). "Environmental Health Criteria. 148. Benomyl." World Health Organization, Geneva.

World Health Organization (WHO) (1993b). "Environmental Health Criteria. 149. Carbendazim." World Health Organization, Geneva.

Zelesco, P. A., Barbieri, I., and Graves, J. A. M. (1990). Use of a cell hybrid test system to demonstrate that benomyl induces aneuploidy and polyploidy. *Mutat. Res.* **242**, 329–335.

Zeman, F. J., Hoogenboom, E. R., Kavlock, R. J., and Semple, J. L. (1986). Effects on the fetus of maternal benomyl exposure in the protein-derived rat. *J. Toxicol. Environ. Health* **17**, 405–417.

Zweig, G., Gao, R., and Popendorf, W. (1983). Simultaneous dermal exposure to captan and benomyl by strawberry harvesters. *J. Agric. Food Chem.* **31**, 1109–1113.

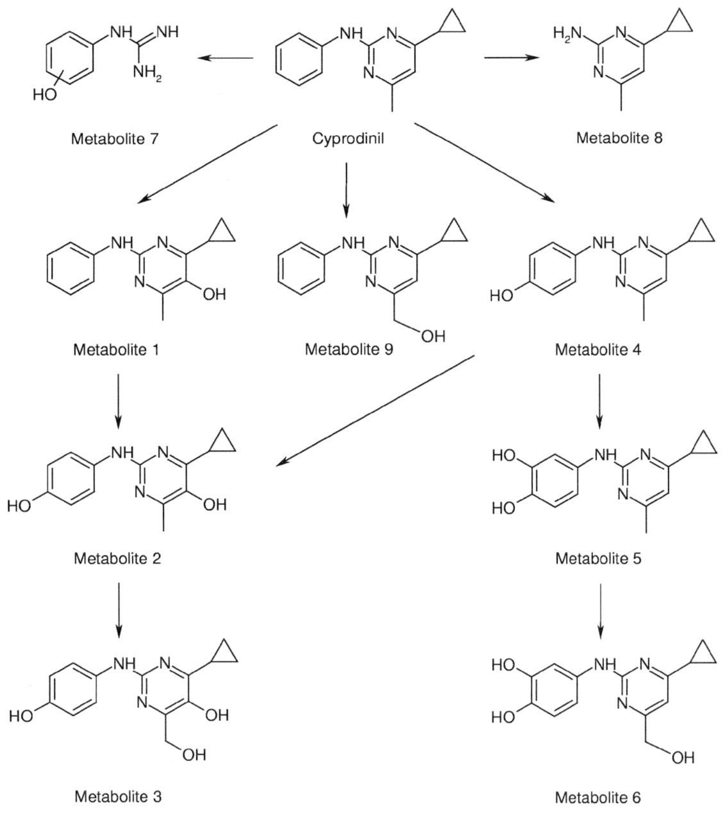

Figure 78.2   Phase 1 metabolism of Cyprodinil in the rat.

(metabolite 2). This metabolite was excreted in the urine as β-glucuronic acid conjugate as well as mono- and disulfuric acid conjugates. Although female rats formed the monosulfate almost exclusively, the males excreted equal amounts of the mono- and disulfate. Further oxidation of the methyl group led to the formation of 4-cyclopropyl-5-hydroxy-6-hydroxymethyl-N-(4-hydroxy)-phenyl-2-pyrimidinamine (metabolite 3), which was excreted in the urine in unconjugated form.

Alternative pathways proceeded either by sequential oxidation of the phenyl ring to the 4-hydroxy and 3,4-dihydroxy derivatives (metabolites 4 and 5), followed by oxidation of the methyl group (metabolite 6), or started with hydroxylation of the methyl group as the first oxidation step (metabolite 9). Urinary and biliary metabolites were found to be conjugated with β-glucuronic acid and sulfuric acid.

The major metabolites identified in feces were the 5-hydroxypyrimidine derivative of Cyprodinil (metabolite 1) and metabolite 4. Metabolites 1 and 4 also were present in conjugated form in urine and bile.

In addition, liver and kidney tissue residues were analyzed for metabolites 12 h after single oral administration of [2-^{14}C]pyrimidyl-Cyprodinil at 100 mg/kg to male rats. During this period, 17.0% of the total applied dose was eliminated via urine. The identified liver and kidney metabolites essentially confirmed the metabolic pathways proposed upon analysis of metabolites isolated from excreta. However, two additional metabolites were found in liver and/or kidney tissue, but not in excreta. Metabolite 7 was identified as ring-hydroxylated N-phenyl-guanidine, a breakdown product of the pyrimidine ring moiety. Metabolite 8 (i.e., 4-cyclopropyl-6-methyl-pyrimidine-2-ylamine) demonstrated a cleavage of the parent molecule between the pyrimidine and the phenyl ring. Metabolite 7 was found exclusively in the liver, where it represented the major metabolite. Minor amounts of metabolite 8 were found in the liver and kidneys.

78.4.3 TOXICOKINETICS AND METABOLISM IN LACTATING GOATS

[U-^{14}C]phenyl or [2-^{14}C]pyrimidyl labelled Cyprodinil were orally administered in gelatin capsules once daily to lactating goats for four consecutive days at dose levels of about 0.2 and 10 mg/kg. The absorption and excretion of radioactivity were measured over 78 h. Six hours after the last dose, the animals were sacrificed and the tissue residues were determined.

Independent of the label and the dose administered, Cyprodinil was absorbed in goats to a lesser extent and more slowly than in rats. The major route of excretion was in urine and feces, whereas excretion via the milk was minimal. Residues of radioactivity in edible tissues were generally low. The metabolic pathways of Cyprodinil in lactating goats were similar to those observed in the rat.

78.4.4 TOXICOKINETICS AND METABOLISM IN LAYING HENS

[U-^{14}C]phenyl or [2-^{14}C]pyrimidyl labelled Cyprodinil were orally administered in gelatin capsules to laying hens once daily for 4 consecutive days at dose levels of about 0.4 and 19 mg/kg. The excretion of radioactivity was measured over 78 h. Six hours after the last dose, the animals were sacrificed and the tissue residues were determined.

In laying hens, Cyprodinil was rapidly and completely eliminated. Residues of radioactivity in eggs and edible tissues were very low. The distribution and excretion pattern was independent of the dose and the site of labelling. The metabolic pathways of Cyprodinil in laying hens were similar to those observed in the rat.

78.5 TOXICITY TO LABORATORY ANIMALS

78.5.1 ACUTE TOXICITY

The acute toxicity profile of Cyprodinil is summarized in Table 78.1. According to these data, Cyprodinil is unlikely to present an acute hazard in normal use (Class III, according to the WHO hazard classification scheme). Cyprodinil is nonirritant to skin and eye when classified according to the EC Directive 83/467, but it may cause sensitization by skin contact.

78.5.2 SUBCHRONIC TOXICITY

The following subchronic toxicity studies were performed:

Table 78.1
Acute Toxicity of Cyprodinil

Parameter	Species, strain, number, and sex	Result
Acute oral LD$_{50}$	Rat, Tif RAIF (SPF), 5m+5f	Greater than 2000 mg/kg
	Mouse, Tif MAG (SPF), 5m+5f	Greater than 5000 mg/kg
Acute dermal LD$_{50}$	Rat, Tif RAIf (SPF), 5m+5f	Greater than 2000 mg/kg
Acute inhalation LC$_{50}$	Rat, Tif RAIf (SPF), 5m+5f	Greater than 1200 mg/m^{3a}
Skin irritation	Rabbit, New Zealand White, 3f	Nonirritant[b]
Eye irritation	Rabbit, New Zealand White, 3m	Nonirritant[b]
Sensitization (maximization test)	Guinea pig, Pirbright White, 10m+10f	Sensitizing[b]

[a]Maximum attainable concentration.
[b]Classified according to EC Directive 83/467.

- Rat, 28-day gavage
- Rat, 28-day dermal
- Rat, 90-day feeding
- Mouse, 90-day feeding
- Dog, 90-day feeding
- Dog, 12-month feeding

Rat, 28-Day Gavage Cyprodinil was administered by gastric intubation at 0, 10, 100, and 1000 mg/kg to groups of 10 male and female Tif:RAIf (SPF) rats for 5 days per week for 4 weeks. The main findings in both sexes were a hepatomegaly, as expressed by increased liver weight at 100 and 1000 mg/kg with a corresponding hepatocellular hypertrophy, and increased thyroid weights associated with follicular cell hypertrophy at 1000 mg/kg. The findings in the thyroid were considered to be secondary to liver stimulation. Further changes at 1000 mg/kg included decreased body weight development and food consumption, hypochromasia, and increased serum concentrations of albumin, globulin, bilirubin, phospholipids, and cholesterol.

Rat, 28-Day Dermal Groups of five male and female Tif: RAIf (SPF) rats were dermally treated with Cyprodinil at doses of 0, 5, 25, 125, and 1000 mg/kg for 6 h per day, 5 days per week for 4 weeks (OECD Guideline 410). Except for some clinical observations of doubtful relationship to treatment (piloerection, dyspnea, hunched posture) and pathological changes at the application site, which were attributed to the application procedure, no effects of treatment were observed. In particular, Cyprodinil did not induce local irritations or effects on clinical chemistry parameters.

Rat, 90-Day Feeding Groups of 10 male and female Tif:RAIf (SPF) rats received Cyprodinil at dietary concentrations of 0, 50, 300, 2000 and 12,000 ppm for 90 days. An additional control and high dose group was kept for a 4-week recovery period. Treatment resulted in partially reversible reduction of body weight development and food consumption at 12,000 ppm. Elevated serum concentrations of cholesterol and phospholipids occurred in both sexes treated at 2000 and 12,000 ppm, and increased serum activities of hepatic enzymes (alkaline phosphatase, γ-glutamyltranspeptidase) were noted at 12,000 ppm. These changes were completely reversible after 4 weeks of recovery. Slightly elevated weights were found for liver, kidneys, and thyroid gland in both sexes treated at 2000 and 12,000 ppm. In the recovery group, only the thyroid weights remained slightly elevated. Histopathology revealed treatment-related effects in the kidneys (chronic tubular lesion) as well as in the liver (hepatocellular hypertrophy, foci of necrotic hepatocytes, hepatocellular inclusion bodies), thyroid (hypertrophy of thyroid follicles), and pituitary gland (hypertrophy of pituitary cells). The changes in the thyroid and pituitary gland might be related to liver stimulation. Except for the renal lesions, all changes were at least partially reversible within the 4-week recovery period.

The elevated serum concentrations of cholesterol and phospholipids, seen after treatment with Cyprodinil for 90 days in rats, are different from those reported by Terada *et al.* (1998a, b) for the structurally closely related anilinopyrimidine Mepanipyrim. Treatment of male rats at 4000 ppm Mepanipyrim for 3 weeks decreased the serum cholesterol, triglyceride, and phospholipid levels (Terada *et al.*, 1998b). In addition, these authors reported hepatocellular fatty vacuolation after treatment for 13 weeks at 200 ppm and above (Terada *et al.*, 1998a), an effect that did not occur in Cyprodinil-treated rats at doses up to 12,000 ppm.

Mouse, 90-Day Feeding Cyprodinil was administered to groups of 10 male and female Tif:MAGf (SPF) mice over 90 days at dietary concentrations of 0, 500, 2000, and 6000 ppm. The animals tolerated the subchronic dietary administration without mortality or overt clinical signs. Body weight gain, food consumption, and hematological profile remained unaffected by the treatment. The liver was the main target organ of toxicity. Treatment of males at 6000 ppm caused increased absolute and relative liver weight. Histopathological changes at 2000 ppm and above comprised single cell necroses in males and depletion of glycogen in females. Clinical chemistry parameters were not investigated.

Dog, 90-Day Feeding Groups of four male and females beagle dogs received Cyprodinil at dietary concentrations of 0, 200, 1500, 7000, and 20,000 ppm for 90 days (OECD Guideline 409). Treatment with Cyprodinil was well tolerated even at very high dose levels. The animals reacted to the treatment mainly by reduced food consumption and reduced body weight gain. In addition, increased numbers of blood platelets were recorded in the males treated at the top dose level of 20,000 ppm. The laboratory examinations indicated no deviations of possible toxicological significance. In particular, the treatment did not affect the plasma concentrations of cholesterol. This observation is in line with the lack of changes in clinical chemistry parameters in Mepanipyrim-treated dogs (Terada *et al.*, 1998a). The lipofuscin deposition in Kupffer cells and hepatocytes, as observed with Mepanipyrim (Terada *et al.*, 1998a), was not seen with Cyprodinil.

Dog, 12-Month Feeding Groups of four male and female beagle dogs received Cyprodinil at dietary concentrations of 0, 25, 250, 2500, and 15,000 ppm (OECD Guideline 452). The animals tolerated the treatment without clinical signs or mortality and no effects on laboratory parameters were encountered. Reactions to the treatment mainly consisted of reduced body weight gain and food consumption. In addition, the livers of the male dogs contained minor amounts of lipofuscin-like pigments. Lipofuscinosis also has been reported upon treatment of dogs with Mepanipyrim (Terada *et al.*, 1998a).

78.5.3 CHRONIC TOXICITY AND ONCOGENICITY

The following chronic toxicity and oncogenicity studies were performed:

- Mouse, 18-month feeding
- Rat, 24-month feeding

Mouse, 18-Month Feeding Cyprodinil was administered to groups of 60 male and female Tif:MAGf (SPF) mice over 18 months at dietary concentrations of 0, 10, 150, 2000, and 5000 ppm (OECD Guideline 451). The animals tolerated the chronic treatment without clinical signs. Most probably due to a reduced body weight development, survival was slightly increased in the top dose group. Slightly increased liver and kidney weights were noted in the top dose group animals. Histopathological examinations revealed increased incidences of slight to moderate hyperplasia of the exocrine pancreas in the top dose group males. The incidence and distribution of neoplastic changes was similar in treated and untreated control groups, and remained within the range of the historical controls.

Rat, 24-Month Feeding Cyprodinil was administered to groups of 80 male and female Tif:RAIf (SPF) rats at dietary concentrations of 0, 5, 75, 1000, and 2000 ppm over 24 months (OECD Guideline 453). The chronic dietary administration of Cyprodinil was tolerated without clinical signs or treatment-related mortality. Hematological examinations revealed a slight prolongation of the prothrombin time in the top dose group males. At the 12-month interim sacrifice, higher kidney to body weight ratios were observed for both sexes at 2000 ppm. At terminal sacrifice, males showed increased absolute and relative liver weights at the top dose level and hepatic sinusoidal cystic dilatation at 1000 ppm and above. The incidence and distribution of neoplastic lesions gave no indication of a carcinogenic effect. In particular, there was no induction of thyroid follicular cell tumors, which were found to be elicited in rats by treatment with the structurally closely related anilinopyrimidine Pyrimethanil (Hurley, 1998). Enhancement of hepatic thyroid hormone metabolism and excretion are considered to be the mode of action of thyroid tumorigenesis (Hurley, 1998).

78.5.4 EFFECTS ON LIVER XENOBIOTIC METABOLIZING ENZYMES IN THE RAT

In subchronic oral toxicity studies in the rat, Cyprodinil caused increased liver weights and hepatocellular hypertrophy. Its possible effects on hepatic xenobiotic metabolizing enzymes were investigated in an explorative 28-day study where male Tif RAIf (SPF) rats were treated by oral intubation at dose levels of 0, 100, and 1000 mg/kg per day (Table 78.2). The treatment was without effect on body weight, but caused increased liver weights to 123 and 160% of control at 100 and 1000 mg/kg, respectively.

Increased microsomal protein and cytochrome P450 contents at 1000 mg/kg were accompanied by an induction of the investigated cytochrome P450 dependent monooxygenase activities, that is, ethoxyresorufin *O*-deethylase and pentoxyresorufin *O*-depentylase as well as lauric acid 11- and 12-hydroxylase. The most prominent effect was a nearly 30-fold

Table 78.2
Effects of Cyprodinil on Liver Xenobiotic Metabolizing Enzymes in the Male Rat[a]

Parameter	Dose (mg/kg body weight/day)		
	0	100	1000
Final body weight (g)	341	357	330
	(10)	(11)	(26)
Absolute liver weight (g)	10.1	12.5**	16.2***
	(0.5)	(0.9)	(1.7)
Microsomal protein (mg/g liver)	25.9	25.3	35.0*
	(1.3)	(4.6)	(5.0)
Cytosolic protein (mg/g liver)	127	123	114***
	(5)	(5)	(3)
Cytochrome P450 (nmol/g liver)	20.6	18.1	46.6***
	(2.7)	(3.3)	(11.3)
Ethoxyresorufin O-deethylase	4.40	9.40**	43.5***
(nmol/min g^{-1} liver)	(1.25)	(3.86)	(10.1)
Pentoxyresorufin O-depentylase	1.18	3.56**	33.6***
(nmol/min g^{-1} liver)	(0.12)	(1.92)	(6.95)
Lauric acid 11-hydroxylase	22.5	22.8	46.0***
(nmol/min g^{-1} liver)	(1.8)	(5.4)	(8.8)
Lauric acid 12-hydroxylase	14.9	21.0*	45.7***
(nmol/min g^{-1} liver)	(2.6)	(5.2)	(7.1)
Glutathione S-transferase	87.4	184**	305***
(μmol/min g^{-1} liver)	(32.3)	(49)	(36)
Fatty acid β-oxidation	1034	1129	1139
(nmol/min g^{-1} liver)	(204)	(128)	(160)

[a] Mean values; standard deviations are given in parentheses. Asterisks indicate statistical significant difference:
* $p < 0.05$, ** $p < 0.01$, *** $p < 0.001$. Five animals were used in each dosage group.

induction of pentoxyresorufin O-depentylase, a marker enzyme activity for phenobarbitone-inducible cytochrome P450 isoenzyme CYP2B1 (Whitlock and Denison, 1994). Cytosolic glutathione S-transferase activity toward 2,4-dinitrochlorobenzene was induced 2- and 3.5-fold at the lower and higher dose level, respectively, whereas cyanide insensitive fatty acyl CoA β oxidation, a marker for hepatic peroxisome proliferation (Lake and Lewis, 1993), was not affected. According to these data, the hepatomegaly induced by Cyprodinil in the rat can be interpreted as an adaptation to a functional load.

78.5.5 EFFECTS ON LIVER AND PLASMA LIPIDS IN THE RAT

Upon subchronic feeding to rats, Cyprodinil caused increased plasma concentrations of cholesterol and phospholipids. In an exploratory study, male Tif:RAIf (SPF) rats were treated with Cyprodinil for 28 days by oral intubation at dose levels of 0, 100, and 1000 mg/kg per day. After a 20-h fasting period, the animals were sacrificed and analyzed for the content of liver free cholesterol and cholesterol esters and for the concentration of serum total cholesterol, as well as for the concentration of cholesterol bound to high density lipoprotein (HDL), low density lipoprotein (LDL), and very low density lipoprotein (VLDL) (Table 78.3).

In the liver, the concentration of free cholesterol level remained unaffected and the cholesterol ester concentration was, if at all, slightly reduced in both treatment groups. In the rat, cholesterol is mainly transported by HDL and to a lower extent also by LDL, whereas VLDL is of minor importance (Carroll and Feldman, 1989). Serum total cholesterol concentration was increased by a factor of about 2 at 1000 mg/kg. As expected, cholesterol concentrations were increased in all three serum lipoprotein fractions of animals treated with 1000 mg/kg, whereby the higher total serum cholesterol level could largely be attributed to increased HDL and LDL levels.

These data confirm that, upon subchronic administration to rats, Cyprodinil interacts with lipid homeostasis. In special investigations, the structurally related anilinopyrimidine Mepanipyrim was also shown to interfere with lipid homeostasis in the rat (Terada et al., 1998b). However, the effects elicited by the two anilinopyrimidines are quite different (Table 78.4). Mepanipyrim caused fatty liver that comprised increased liver cholesterol, phospholipid, and triglyceride con-

Table 78.3
Effects of Cyprodinil on Liver Free Cholesterol, Liver Cholesterol Esters, and Serum Cholesterol in the Male Rat[a]

Parameter	Dose (mg/kg body weight/day)		
	0	100	1000
Liver free cholesterol	8.3	7.7	8.2
(μg/mg homogenate protein)	(0.5)	(0.5)	(0.5)
Liver cholesterol esters	1.8	1.4	1.3
(μg/mg homogenate protein)	(0.2)	(0.2)	(0.2)
Serum total cholesterol	1.78	1.90	3.89***
(μmol/ml serum)	(0.22)	(0.30)	(0.74)
High density lipoprotein cholesterol	1.24	1.36	2.23***
(μmol/ml serum)	(0.09)	(0.24)	(0.42)
Low density lipoprotein cholesterol	0.64	0.67	1.86***
(μmol/ml serum)	(0.16)	(0.15)	(0.34)
Very low density lipoprotein cholesterol	0.020	0.036	0.128
(μmol/ml serum)	(0.021)	(0.014)	(0.110)

[a]Mean values; standard deviations are given in parentheses. Asterisks indicate statistical significant difference:
* $p < 0.05$, ** $p < 0.01$, *** $p < 0.001$. Five animals were used in each dosage group.

centrations. Cyprodinil was without an effect on liver cholesterol concentration (liver phospholipid and triglycerides were not measured) and did not cause fatty liver. In blood, Mepanipyrim decreased cholesterol and high-density lipoprotein cholesterol, phospholipid, and triglyceride concentrations, whereas Cyprodinil caused increased cholesterol concentration, cholesterol concentrations in high-, low-, and very low-density lipoprotein fractions, and phospholipid concentrations. It was suggested that the fatty liver induced by Mepanipyrim in the rat is the result of an inhibition of intracellular transport of very low-density lipoproteins from the Golgi apparatus to the cell surface (Terada *et al.*, 1999). This hypothesis is in accordance with its presumed mode of action in pathogenic fungi, where the compound was shown to block intracellular trafficking and secretion of plant cell-wall digesting enzymes (Miura *et al.*, 1994).

The mechanism by which Cyprodinil induces increased blood cholesterol and phospholipid concentrations in the rat is not known. However, *in vitro* investigations with Cyprodinil in primary cultured rat hepatocytes showed that the hypercholesterolemia observed with this compound was neither due to increased hepatic cholesterol synthesis nor a consequence of inhibition of bile acid synthesis or bile acid transport (data not shown).

Table 78.4
Cyprodinil and Mepanipyrim: Comparison of Effects on Selected Lipid Parameters in Liver and Blood Following Subchronic Treatment of Rats

Parameter	Cyprodinil[a]	Mepanipyrim[b]
Liver free cholesterol	No effect	No effect
Liver cholesterol esters	No effect	↑
Liver total cholesterol	No effect	↑
Liver phospholipid	Not measured	↑
Liver triglyceride	Not measured	↑
Plasma or serum total cholesterol[c]	↑	↓
Plasma or serum phospholipid[c]	↑	↓
Serum high-density lipoprotein cholesterol	↑	↓

[a]Cyprodynil was administered to Tif:RAIf (SPF) male rats via gavage for 4 weeks at a rate of 1000 mg/kg per day.
[b]Mepanipyrim was administered to F344/DuCrj male rats via diet for 3 weeks at a rate of 4000 ppm. Data from Terada *et al.* (1998b).
[c]Cyprodinil: plasma; Mepanipyrim: serum.

78.5.6 EFFECTS ON REPRODUCTION AND DEVELOPMENT

Possible effects of Cyprodinil on reproduction and development were investigated in the following studies:

- Rat, teratogenicity
- Rabbit, teratogenicity
- Rat, two-generation reproduction

Rat, Teratogenicity Cyprodinil was orally administered by gastric intubation to groups of 20–22 pregnant Tif:RAIf (SPF) rats from day 6 to day 15 of gestation at daily doses of 0, 20, 200, and 1000 mg/kg per day. The dams were sacrificed on day 21 of gestation and the fetuses were removed, weighed, sexed, examined for external malformations, and subjected to visceral and skeletal examination.

In the dams, no treatment-related mortality occurred and no clinical signs of possible relevance were noted. Body weight development and food consumption were significantly reduced in the top dose animals. No treatment-related changes were noted upon necropsy. No treatment-related effects were observed on pregnancy rate, corpora lutea, implantations, early or late resorptions, sex or number of fetuses. Weight reduction and reduced ossification of digits and metacarpalia were observed in the top dose group. These findings were considered to be a consequence of the observed maternal toxicity at top dose treatment. In conclusion, the results of this study gave no indication of teratogenic effects.

Rabbit, Teratogenicity Groups of 17–18 pregnant Russian rabbits were orally treated by gavage from day 7 to day 19 of gestation at daily doses of 0, 5, 30, 150, and 400 mg/kg per day. The does were sacrificed on day 29 of gestation and the fetuses were removed by hysterectomy, weighed, sexed, examined for external malformations, and subjected to visceral and skeletal examination.

Neither mortality nor treatment-related clinical signs occurred in the does. The body weight development and the food consumption of the top dose animals was reversibly reduced during the treatment period. No treatment-related changes were noted upon necropsy. No treatment-related effects were observed on pregnancy rate, corpora lutea, implantations, early or late resorptions, sex, or number of fetuses. The fetal weights were similar in treated and untreated animals, and the external, visceral, and skeletal examinations of the fetuses revealed no treatment-related effects. In conclusion, the results of this study gave no indication of teratogenic effects.

Rat, Two-Generation Reproduction Cyprodinil was administered to groups of 30 male and female Tif:RAIf (SPF) rats at dietary doses of 0, 10, 100, 1000 and 4000 ppm over two generations. In the F0 generation, no treatment-related clinical signs or mortality were noted, but slight changes in body weight gain and food consumption were observed in the top dose group.

The parameters of fertility and reproduction showed no significant intergroup differences. At necropsy, slightly higher organ weights (liver, kidney, adrenal gland) and renal tubular basophilia were observed.

The F1 litter sizes were not affected by treatment and the average pup weight at birth was similar in all groups. The body weight development of the top dose group pups was significantly reduced during the lactation period, but the pups reached all milestones of physiological development at the same time as the untreated animals. The parameters of fertility and reproduction were similar in treated and untreated groups. At necropsy, increased liver weights were noted, but the histopathological examination revealed no changes of toxicological significance.

In the F2 litters of the top dose group, the mean pup weight at birth was slightly lower than the control value. All litters reached the milestones of physical development at similar time points.

In conclusion, the results of this study gave no indication of effects on reproduction or fertility.

78.5.7 NEUROTOXIC EFFECTS

The neurotoxic potential of Cyprodinil was investigated in the following studies:

- Rat, single oral dose
- Rat, 90-day feeding

Rat, Single Oral Dose Groups of 10 male and female Tif:RAIf (SPF) rats received a single oral dose of 0, 200, 600, or 2000 mg/kg. The study included a functional observational battery that covered central nervous system (CNS) activity, CNS excitation, and sensorimotor, autonomic, and physiological functions. Neurological examinations covered sensorimotor functions, autonomic functions, and sensorimotor coordination. Motor activity was assessed and neuropathological examinations included different areas of the brain, the spinal cord, peripheral nerves, and muscles. The time of peak effect, determined in a range-finding test, was found to be approximately 2 h after treatment. There was no effect of treatment on mortality, body weight, or food consumption.

Observations and functional tests showed relevant changes mainly at the time of peak effect. In females of the intermediate and high dose groups, reduced activity, hunched posture, piloerection, and increased responsiveness to sensory stimuli were observed; hunched posture was seen also in a few low dose females. In females of the two higher dose groups, signs lasted up to test day 4 and were considered to indicate toxicity. In addition, a dose-related decrease in body temperature was observed. Changes in motor activity parameters were limited to the time of peak effect. In high dose males and in females of the two higher dose groups, horizontal and vertical activity parameters were reduced.

Macroscopic and microscopic examinations of the multiple areas of the central and peripheral nervous system, the eyes, optic nerves, and skeletal muscle of the male and female control and high dose animals did not reveal treatment-related neuropathologic changes. The results of this study gave no indication of neurotoxic effects.

Rat, 90-Day Feeding Groups of 10 male and female Tif:RAIf (SPF) rats received Cyprodinil at dietary concentrations of 0, 80, 800, and 8000 ppm for 90 days. The study included a functional observational battery, covering CNS activity, CNS excitation, and sensorimotor, autonomic, and physiological functions. Neurological examinations covered sensorimotor functions, autonomic functions, and sensorimotor coordination. Motor activity was assessed and neuropathological examinations included different areas of the brain, the spinal cord, peripheral nerves, and muscles.

There was no effect on mortality and clinical signs. In high dose animals, a moderately reduced body weight gain was seen throughout the treatment period. In high dose animals, absolute and relative liver weights were increased in both sexes and kidney weights were elevated in females. Microscopic examination revealed hepatocellular hypertrophy in the liver of high dose animals. In addition, chronic tubular lesions combined with tubular casts and single cystic changes in the kidneys, and hypertrophy of the follicular epithelial cells in the thyroid gland were seen in these animals.

Observations and functional tests showed no effect of toxicological significance and no treatment-related effects on the different motor activity parameters. Neuropathologic examination of the eyes, optic nerves, and multiple areas of the central and peripheral nervous system of the male and female control and high dose animals revealed no treatment-related neuropathologic changes. The results of this study gave no indication of neurotoxic effects.

78.5.8 PHARMACOLOGICAL EFFECTS

General pharmacological studies were performed with male ICR mice, male Wistar rats, and male Hartley guinea pigs. Single dose levels of 0, 150, 500, 1500, and 5000 mg/kg Cyprodinil were orally administered. In the *in vitro* experiments, the test material was dissolved in ethanol and applied at concentrations of 0, 0.1, 1.0, and 10 µg/ml.

Mouse, General Behavior and CNS Tests No animals died at any dose level. At 1500 mg/kg, slightly decreased spontaneous motor activity, slightly dilated pupil size, and slightly narrowed palpebral opening were observed within the first few hours. All signs disappeared by 6 h after treatment. At 5000 mg/kg, slight piloerection and abnormalities of body and limb position were seen in addition. All signs disappeared within 24 h in this dose group. Doses of 1500 mg/kg or higher prolonged hexobarbital-induced sleeping time. No effects on tonic extensor, clonic convulsions, or coma in electrically stimulated mice were noted at any dose level.

Rat, Body Temperature Body temperature was not affected in any dosage group.

Rat, Cardiovascular System Treatment with Cyprodinil had no effect on the systolic blood pressure. At 5000 mg/kg, the heart rate was significantly decreased at 1 h after dosing.

In Vitro, **Autonomic Nervous System** Cyprodinil inhibited the induced contractions of isolated guinea pig ileum at concentrations of 10 µg/ml. No effects were noted at lower concentrations.

Mouse, Gastrointestinal System No effect was seen on intestinal transport at any dose level.

Mouse, Skeletal Muscle System No effect was seen in the traction test at any dose level.

Rat, Hematology No effects on prothrombin time or activated partial thromboplastin time were seen at any dose level. No hemolytic effects were noted.

78.6 MUTAGENICITY

The mutagenic potential of Cyprodinil was investigated in five independent studies that covered different end points in eukaryotes and prokaryotes *in vivo* and *in vitro*. No induction of back mutations was noted in four strains of *Salmonella typhimurium* (TA 98, TA 100, TA 1535, and TA 1537) or in *Escherichia coli* WP2 uvrA. The compound was tested in the presence and in the absence of an extrinsic metabolic activation system (rat liver S9 fraction), covering a concentration range of 20–5000 µg/plate.

The induction of gene mutations was further investigated at the hprt gene of Chinese hamster V79 cells. Concentrations up to the limit of toxicity of 96 and 30 µg/ml were tested in the presence and in the absence of rat liver S9 fraction, respectively. No increased incidence of gene mutations was detected in this *in vitro* system.

Chinese hamster CHO cells were used for the detection of chromosome aberrations *in vitro*. Three experiments in the presence and in the absence of rat liver S9 fraction were performed by applying different exposure scenarios. Concentrations higher than 50 µg/ml could not be investigated due to cytotoxicity. In none of the experiments was an increased incidence of metaphases containing chromosome aberrations seen.

Primary cultures of rat hepatocytes were treated with Cyprodinil at concentrations up to 80 µg/ml to investigate DNA damaging effects. Higher concentrations caused cytotoxicity. None of the tested concentrations caused enhanced unscheduled DNA synthesis, which would be indicative of the DNA damaging activity of the compound.

The formation of micronuclei was investigated in bone marrow cells of Tif:MAGf (SPF) mice. Single oral doses of up to 5000 mg/kg body weight were administered 16, 24, and 48 h before preparation of bone marrow. No cytotoxicity was observed at any dose level and the incidence of micronucleated polychromatic erythrocytes was not affected. Therefore, there is no evidence for a clastogenic or aneugenic activity of Cyprodinil in somatic cells *in vivo*.

78.7 TOXICITY TO HUMANS

78.7.1 DIRECT OBSERVATIONS AND HEALTH RECORDS

Three cases of moderate, reversible local irritation (erythema, swelling of eyelids) occurred among laboratory personnel during formulation development. No further complaints were noted.

78.7.2 DIAGNOSIS OF POISONING

In animal studies, symptoms of acute intoxication were unspecific and transient only. The same can be expected for humans. However, no case of intoxication with Cyprodinil has yet been observed.

78.7.3 SENSITIZATION OBSERVATIONS

No cases of skin sensitization were recorded in humans.

78.7.4 PROPOSED TREATMENT

Whereas no specific antidote is known, symptomatic therapy is to be applied on persons who show symptoms after exposure to Cyprodinil.

REFERENCES

Carroll, R. M., and Feldman, E. B. (1989). Lipids and lipoproteins. *In* "The Clinical Chemistry of Laboratory Animals" (W. F. Loeb and F. W. Quimby, eds.), pp. 95–116. Pergamon, New York.

Fritz, R., Lanen, C., Colas, V., and Leroux, P. (1997). Inhibition of methionine biosynthesis in *Botrytis cinerea* by the anilinopyrimidine fungicide pyrimethanil. *Pestic. Sci.* **49**, 40–46.

Heye, U. J., Speich, J., Siegle, H., Steinemann, A., Forster, B., Knauf-Beiter, G., Herzog, J., and Hubele, A. (1994). CGA 219417: A novel broad-spectrum fungicide. *Crop Protection* **13**, 541–549.

Hurley, P. M. (1998). Mode of carcinogenic action of pesticides inducing thyroid follicular cell tumors in rodents. *Environ. Health Perspect.* **106**, 437–445.

Lake, B. G., and Lewis, D. F. V. (1993). Structure–activity relationships for chemically induced peroxisome proliferation in mammalian liver. *In* "Peroxisomes: Biology and Importance in Toxicology and Medicine" (G. Gibson and B. Lake, eds.). Taylor and Francis, London.

Masner, P., Muster, P., and Schmid, J. (1994). Possible methionine biosynthesis inhibition by pyrimidinamine fungicides. *Pestic. Sci.* **42**, 163–166.

Milling, R. J., and Richardson, C. J. (1995). Mode of action of the anilinopyrimidine fungicide pyrimethanil. 2. Effects on enzyme secretion in *Botrytis cinerea*. *Pestic. Sci.* **45**, 43–48.

Miura, I., Kamakura, T., Maeno, S., Hayashi, S., and Yamaguchi, I. (1994). Inhibition of enzyme secretion in plant pathogens by mepanipyrim, a novel fungicide. *Pestic. Biochem. Physiol.* **48**, 222–228.

Terada, M., Mizuhashi, F., Tomita, T., Inoue, H., and Murata, K. (1998a). Mepanipyrim induced fatty liver in rats but not in mice and dogs. *J. Toxicol. Sci.* **23**, 223–234.

Terada, M., Mizuhashi, F., Tomita, T., and Murata, K. (1998b). Effects of mepanipyrim on lipid metabolism in rats. *J. Toxicol. Sci.* **23**, 235–241.

Terada, M., Mizuhashi, F., Murata, K., and Tomita, T. (1999). Mepanipyrim, a new fungicide, inhibits intracellular transport of very low density lipoprotein in rat hepatocytes. *Toxicol. Appl. Pharmacol.* **154**, 1–11.

Whitlock, J. P., and Denison, M. S. (1994). Induction of cytochrome P450 enzymes that metabolize xenobiotics. *In* "Cytochrome P450: Structure, Mechanism, and Biochemistry" (R. Ortiz de Montellano, ed.), 2nd ed., pp. 367–390. Plenum, New York

Yamagata, S. (1989). Roles of *O*-acetyl-*L*-homoserine sulfhydrylase in microorganisms. *Biochimie* **71**, 1125–1143.

Captan and Folpet

Elliot B. Gordon
Makhteshim-Agan of North America, Inc.

79.1 INTRODUCTION

Captan and folpet are fungicides that have been in use for over 50 years. During this period there have been no reports of systemic toxicity and only a very low incidence of skin sensitization. This record of safe use is consistent with the toxicological data base developed for these compounds. Adverse findings in laboratory test systems consist of mutagenicity, carcinogenicity, and eye irritation. The first two outcomes resulted in the EPA classifications of captan and folpet as "probable human carcinogens"; the latter outcome resulted in reentry restrictions on farm workers.

Analysis of the oncogenic findings has demonstrated that the etiology of this effect is compensatory proliferation of duodenal crypt cells following damage to duodenal villi caused by high dietary exposure. Analysis of mutagenicity delineates a clear distinction between positive *in vitro* and negative *in vivo* effects. This paradox is explained by rapid degradation in blood: captan degrades with a half-life of less than 1 s; folpet has a half-life of less than 5 s.

Using a margin of exposure (MOE) analysis for human cancer, dietary exposure has a MOE of 1,000,000. The EPA's proposed 1996 cancer guidelines characterize this exposure level as "not likely at all to cause cancer in humans at low doses." In practical terms, this means that neither captan nor folpet is a human carcinogen.

Draize rabbit studies show that these compounds are severe ocular irritants. Extensive experience, however, particularly with reentry operations, has shown that this laboratory phenomenon is not predictive of human experience. Captan and folpet remain highly valued, low risk fungicides.

79.1.1 OVERVIEW

Captan and folpet are broad-spectrum protectant fungicides whose mode of action centers on their reaction with thiols. These compounds along with a third, captafol, are collectively called chloroalkylthio fungicides due to the presence of side chains that contain chlorine, carbon, and sulfur. Of the chloroalkylthio fungicides, captan and folpet predominate in agronomic practice today; captafol registrations in the United States were withdrawn in 1988. Related compounds associated with this fungicide class, but never registered in the United States, are dichlofluanid and tolylfluanid. These later two compounds have a fluorine atom substituted for one of the terminal chlorine atoms.

Early investigations on captan and folmet focused on their mutagenicity. These assays, conducted *in vitro*, showed captan and folpet to be active. This led regulators to ascribe a genotoxic basis to the duodenal tumors that occur in mice, resulting in a linear low-dose extrapolation for cancer risk assessment. Teratogenicity studies of folpet were conducted following the perceived association of folpet's phthalimide moiety with the human teratogen *S*-thalidomide; these structures have since been shown to be toxicologically unrelated. Captan and folpet show developmental toxicity at maternally toxic doses; neither compound is teratogenic. A number of reviews have addressed the toxicology of the chloroalkylthio fungicides (Ecobichon, 1996; Edwards *et al.*, 1991; Elder, 1989; IARC, 1983; Saunders and Harper, 1994; Trochimowicz *et al.*, 2001; U.S. EPA, 1975). Data now show that a threshold-based nonmutagenic mode of action exists for the development of tumors in mice. Captan and folpet are not carcinogenic to farm workers because systemic exposure is absent; they will not cause tumors in consumers because the margin of exposure from dietary intake is approximately 1 million. The U.S. Environmental Protection Agency (U.S. EPA) has reviewed captan and folpet under some of the provisions of the Food Quality Protection Act (FQPA) of 1996 (U.S. Congress, 1996), but has not reevaluated them under the proposed new carcinogen risk assessment guidelines (U.S. EPA, 1996).

This chapter identifies the hazards associated with captan and folpet, and assesses risks for both cancer and noncancer endpoints. Controversy continues to surround their cancer risk characterization. The EPA classified these compounds as B2 carcinogens over 15 years ago (Engler, 1986; U.S. EPA, 1986a) and has yet to review the initial classification using the 1996 draft guidelines (U.S. EPA, 1999a, b).

79.1.2 HISTORY AND USE

Captan was first registered in the United States on March 8, 1949 as a fruit tree spray (NPIRS, 1999a) and its properties were described in 1953 (Kittleson, 1953). This compound proved extremely efficacious, spurring chemists to turn out a series of analogs in an attempt to capitalize on the fungicidal properties of the trichloromethylthio moiety (Horsfall and Rich, 1957; Kittleson, 1953; Lukens, 1966). Folpet was synthesized after captan; captafol was the last to be developed. As preventative fungicides, they are efficacious when applied prior to the establishment of pathogenic fungi. Captan and folpet are often used in integrated pest management (IPM) programs in conjunction with other fungicides. Registrations cover both agricultural and industrial uses (NPIRS, 1999b; U.S. EPA, 1985b). Captan is also efficacious as a bacteriostat in cosmetics (Elder, 1989).

The U.S. EPA issued registration standards for captan (U.S. EPA, 1986b), folpet (U.S. EPA, 1987), and captafol (U.S. EPA, 1984a). A special review for captafol (U.S. EPA, 1985a) concluded in 1988 with the voluntary withdrawal of registrations. A special review for captan was completed in 1989 with the issuance of Position Document 4 (U.S. EPA, 1989). Reregistration Eligibility Decision documents (REDs) have now been promulgated for captan and folpet (U.S. EPA, 1999a, b).

79.1.3 TOXICOLOGICAL OVERVIEW

The principle governing the toxicity of captan and folpet centers on their rapid reaction with thiol groups (i.e., sulfhydryl, −SH groups). This reaction results in degradation of the parent compound. Thiophosgene is a key degradation product that also reacts with thiols as well as other functional groups. It is reactive and short-lived. The net result of these chemical interactions is that both captan and folpet elicit primary toxicological effects locally at the site of initial contact. In mice, dietary exposure results in local irritation of the gastrointestinal tract, predominantly in the duodenum. It is solely at this site that tumors eventually develop. Continued administration of high doses often leads to secondary effects such as decreased body weight or developmental retardation in fetuses and pups.

Pursuant to the Food Quality Protection Act and subsequent guidance by the EPA, captan and folpet have been found to share a common mechanism of toxicity with regard to the development of duodenal tumors in mice (see discussion in Section 79.4). Although this finding requires that both compounds be considered for cumulative risk assessment, it affords the toxicologist the opportunity to combine mechanistic data for each into one unified data base. Captafol, in contrast, was found not to share a common mechanism of toxicity with captan or folpet.

The paradigm that details the methods for conducting cumulative risk assessments are under development at EPA. The FQPA also requires consideration of the special sensitivities to infants and children, and the potential for endocrine disruption. There is no indication that captan or folpet shows disproportionate toxicity to infants or children. The mechanism by which these compounds exert their toxicity would make such a distinction unexpected. The EPA has recognized this for captan but currently has assigned an additional threefold safety factor for folpet (see Section 79.3.4; U.S. EPA, 1999a, b). Captan or folpet shows no evidence of being endocrine disruptors. The EPA, however, is still developing its approach to identify endocrine disruptors.

Captan and folpet induce mutagenic and clastogenic effects in a variety of *in vitro* assays. Mutagenic activity *in vivo*, however, does not occur. This paradox is explained by the extremely rapid degradation of these compounds in the intact animal. Whereas the delivered dose is negligible, captan and folpet are classic examples of the adage, "the (delivered) dose makes the poison." Despite the obvious potential for mutagenic events, the dose at sensitive targets in the intact animal, such as cellular DNA, is essentially zero.

Although these fungicides have low acute toxicity, their interaction with biological tissues can cause irritation. Thus, a low percentage of exposed people exhibit ocular or respiratory irritation or dermal sensitization reactions. Persons handling these materials should also avoid inhalation due to their irritant properties. The compounds are not considered teratogens, reproductive toxins, or selective developmental toxins.

The appearance of duodenal tumors in mice fed diets admixed with captan or folpet is a key toxicological finding that has heretofore been one of the central issues for the regulation of these compounds. Data show that a mode of action based on increased rates of cell proliferation, a threshold phenomenon, accounts for the incidence of tumors seen. This proliferative pressure is thought to promote nascent tumor cells that are normally resident within the duodenal crypt compartment. The EPA, however, continues to classify both compounds, under the 1986 Carcinogen Risk Assessment Guidelines, as probable human carcinogens (U.S. EPA, 1984b, 1986a).

Human cancer risk assessments of captan and folpet show that farm workers are at no cancer risk because there is no systemic exposure. Persons exposed to residues in their food are not at risk because the margins of safety for both compounds are approximately 1 million (see Section 79.5).

79.2 PHYSICAL PROPERTIES AND CHEMICAL REACTIONS

79.2.1 OVERVIEW

The toxicology of the chloroalkylthio fungicides is dependent on their physical properties and chemical reactions. The structures of captan and folpet along with typical ring degradates are shown in Figs. 79.1 and 79.2. The chemical identity and physical properties are noted in Table 79.1, and the rates of selected chemical reactions are shown in Table 79.2. The characteristic chemical moiety for captan and folpet is the trichloromethylthio side chain that is connected to an imide ring structure by way of a nitrogen–sulfur bond. Captan's ring is tetrahydrophthalimide (THPI) and folpet's is phthalimide. This ring imparts certain

Chemical	Structure
Captan	
4,5-cyclohexene-1,2-dicarboximide (THPI)	
4,5-epoxy-1,2-dicarboximide (THPI expoxide)	
4,5-dihydroxy-1,2-dicarboximide (4,5-diOH THPI)	
7-hydroxy-4,5-cyclohexene-1,2-dicarboximide (*ci/trans*-3-OH THPI)	
6-hydroxy-4,5-cyclohexene-1,2-dicarboximide (*cis/trans*-5-OH THPI)	
1-amido-2-carboxy-4,5-cyclohexene (*cis/trans*-THPAM)	
6-hydroxy-1-amido-2-carboxy-4,5-cyclohexene (3-OH THP-amic acid)	

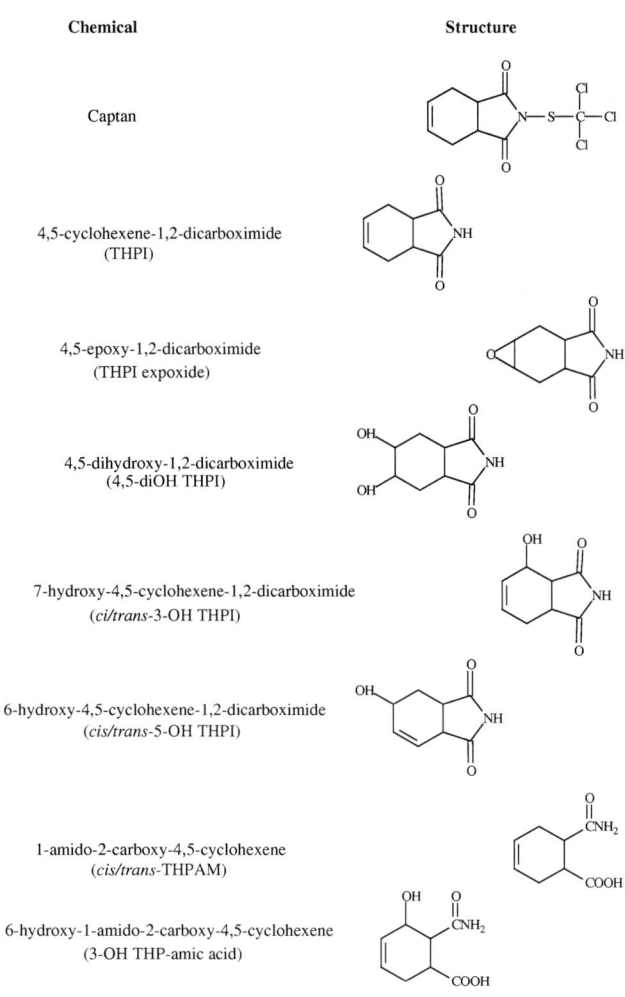

Figure 79.1 Captan and its ring metabolites.

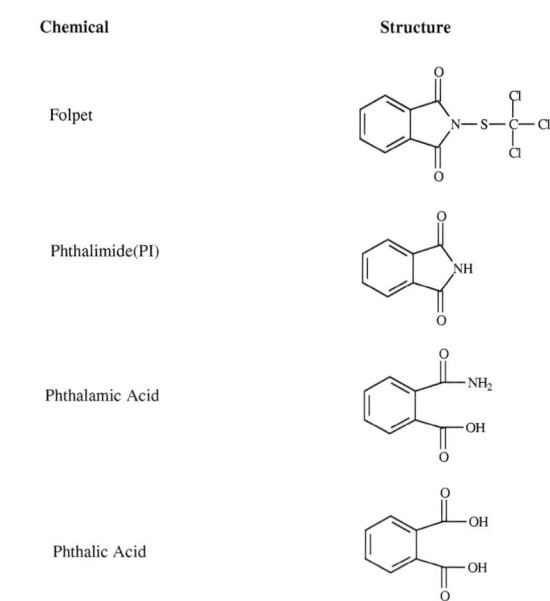

Chemical	Structure
Folpet	
Phthalimide(PI)	
Phthalamic Acid	
Phthalic Acid	

Figure 79.2 Folpet and its ring metabolites.

physical properties to the molecule, but is subordinate to the side chain with regard to the fungicide's toxicological properties. The phthalimide ring is aromatic and, as such, is a resonance structure; THPI has one double bond between carbons 3 and 4. This hexene imide, unlike phthalimide, is nonplanar (Fickentscher *et al.*, 1977).

79.2.2 PHYSICAL PROPERTIES

Captan and folpet have similar physical properties. They have low water solubility, low volatility, and melt at approximately the same temperature. Octanol–water coefficients are high for both, although folpet's K_{ow} is somewhat higher than that of captan.

79.2.3 CHEMICAL REACTIONS

Captan and folpet are unstable in aqueous solution, but the rate of hydrolysis is slow compared to their reaction with thiols. The key to their fungicidal efficacy is the balance between the reactivity of the trichloromethylthio moiety and the stability of

the nitrogen–sulfur bond linking this moiety to the imide ring. Analogs with very stable bonds prove to be ineffective fungicides, whereas analogs with bonds that are overly labile degrade spontaneously (Horsfall and Rich, 1957; Lukens, 1966, 1967). The hydrolytic and thiol reactions serve to degrade the parent molecule and thus influence the toxicology outcome by effectively reducing or eliminating exposure.

79.2.3.1 Hydrolysis

The rates of aqueous hydrolysis increase in alkaline conditions and are more rapid for folpet than captan at comparable pH values (Table 79.2). At pH 5, for instance, captan is approximately eight times more stable than folpet; thus, in the acid conditions of the stomach, it would be expected that relatively more folpet degradation products would be present compared to captan. The higher hydrolytic rates for folpet are related to the higher standard free energy of the phthalimide ring structure compared to the THPI ring (Lukens, 1966).

79.2.3.2 Reaction with Thiols

As previously noted, reactions with thiol groups are central to the fungicidal and toxicological properties of captan and folpet. This reaction has been studied with glutathione (GSH), proteins, and other thiol-containing compounds. In general, the thiol group is oxidized (e.g., GSH → GSSG and cysteine → cystine). Common to both captan and folpet is the generation of thiophosgene during degradation. This chemical entity appears to be a contributing toxicophore in that it rapidly reacts with a variety of functional groups in addition to thiols (Lukens, 1969; Lukens and Sisler, 1958b; Sharma, 1986). A general scheme of degradation for captan and folpet is shown in Fig. 79.3.

The rate of hydrolysis is faster for folpet than for captan, whereas the reverse is true for thiol-mediated degradation.

Table 79.1
Physical Properties of Captan and Folpet

Parameter	Captan	Folpet
CAS number	133-06-2	133-07-3
Molecular weight	300.61	296.56
Formula A	$C_9H_8Cl_3NO_2S$	$C_9H_4Cl_3NO_2S$
Formula B	$C_6H_8(C=O)_2N-SCCl_3$	$C_6H_4(C=O)_2N-SCCl_3$
IUPAC name	1,2,3,6-Tetrahydro-N-(trichloromethyl thio) phthalimide	N-(trichloromethyl thio) phthalimide
CA name	3a,4,7,7a-Tetrahydro-2-[(trichloromethyl) thio]-1H-isoindole-1,3(2H)-dione	2-[(Trichloromethyl) thio]-1H-isoindol-1,3(2H)-dione
Physical form	Crystals	Crystals
Melting point	178°C	177°C
Solubility, water	3.3 mg/liter at 25°C	1 mg/liter at 20°C
Solubility, acetone	3.0 g/100 ml	3.4 g/100 ml
log K_{ow}	2.35	2.85

The reaction of captan and folpet with cysteine results in the formation of thiazolidine-2-thione-4-carboxylic acid (TTCA; Lukens and Sisler, 1958a). This compound is seen in mammalian metabolism studies (DeBaun et al., 1974) and has been suggested for use as a biological marker for human exposure assessment (Krieger and Thongsinthusak, 1993; van Welie et al., 1991).

The fate of captan and folpet in human and rabbit blood has been investigated (Crossley, 1967a, b). Crossley added captan and folpet to human blood and measured the decline of the parent with time and, concurrently, the increase of the imide ring (THPI or phthalimide). At initial concentrations of 1 μg/ml, captan degraded with a half-life of 18 s. The degradation of folpet was three times slower, with a half-life of 54 s. By measuring the generation of the imide rings, it was shown that the parent compounds actually degraded rather than complexed with blood constituents. These investigations were carried out at 22°C with unlabeled materials.

Recent investigations of degradation rates employed radiolabeled captan and folpet and physiological temperatures (37°C).

As predicted by the Q_{10} (Purves et al., 1992), increased temperature results in a higher rate of degradation. The new data demonstrate that at physiological temperatures, captan degrades rapidly in human blood, having a $t^{1/2}$ of 0.97 s, whereas folpet degrades somewhat slower but still quite rapidly (i.e., $t^{1/2}$ = 4.9 s; Gordon et al., 2001). These data, which demonstrate the rapid degradation of the two compounds, are of course a critical component in any exposure assessment and risk evaluation modeling. With oral exposure, it is unlikely that captan, folpet, or thiophosgene would survive long enough to reach systemic targets such as the liver, uterus, or testes. With dermal exposure and subsequent low absorption, captan will be eliminated in less than 7 s and folpet in less than 35. This determination follows from the notion that compounds are considered to be essentially gone in seven half-lives (Medinsky and Klaassen, 1996).

79.2.3.3 Reaction with Proteins

Investigations on the effects of captan and folpet with proteins generally have been carried out *in vitro*. Such studies identify potential interactions that may occur in the living animal; how-

Table 79.2
Rates of Chemical Reactions of Captan and Folpet

Parameter	Captan	Folpet	Reference
Aqueous Hydrolysis			
pH 5	18.8 h	2.6 h	Captan: Pack (1987)
pH 7	4.9 h	1.1 h	Folpet: Ruzo and Ewing
pH 9	8.3 min	1.5 min	(1988)
Reaction with blood thiols	18 s, 22°C	51 s, 22°C	Captan: Crossley (1967a)
			Folpet: Crossley (1967b)
Degradation half-life (acid conditions to minimize hydrolysis)	0.97 s, 37°C	4.9 s, 37°C	Gordon et al. (2001)
Decolorization of dithionitrobenzoic acid (DTNB)–thiol complex in blood	1 min	3 min	Liu and Fishbein (1967)

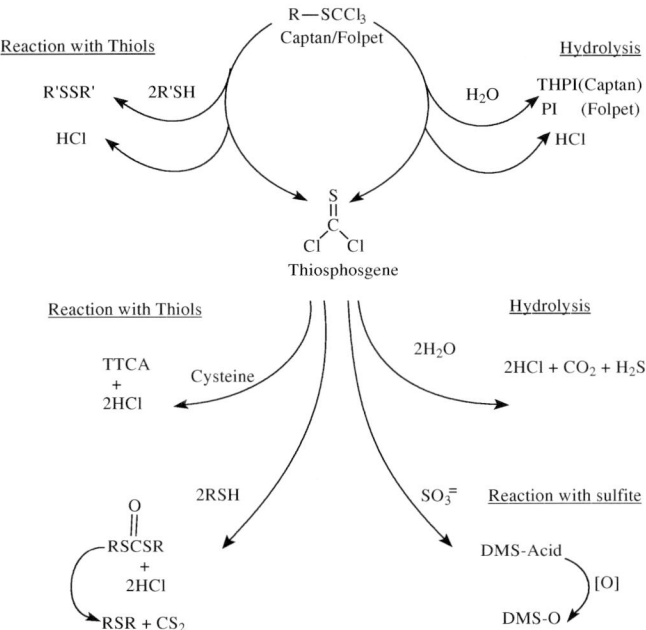

Figure 79.3 General degradation scheme. For captan, R = THPI (Tetrahydrophthalimide); for folpet, R = PI (phthalimide); TTCA: thiazolidine-2-thione-4-carboxylic acid; DMS-Acid: dithio-bis-methanesulphonic acid; DMS-O: monosulfoxide of dithio-bis-methanesulphonic acid.

ever, for captan and folpet, the rapid degradation of reactive species and the resultant limitation in exposure prevent many of these reactions from resulting in *in vivo* toxicological phenomena. Folpet reacts with thiol-containing proteins (e.g., glyceraldehyde 3-phosphate; Siegel, 1971a), non-thiol-containing proteins (e.g., α-chymotrypsin; Siegel, 1971b), and nuclear histones (Couch and Siegel, 1972, 1977). These reactions are often pH dependent.

79.2.3.4 Reaction with DNA

The reactions of captan and folpet with DNA are not well characterized. Captan and folpet induce point mutations and clastogenic changes *in vitro*, but the mechanism by which such effects are induced has not been elucidated. When ^{35}S-captan was incubated with calf thymus DNA in buffer at pH 7.5 or 9.0, binding of appreciable amounts of radioactivity could not be demonstrated (Couch and Siegel, 1977). Captan reacts with guanine *in vitro* to produce 7-(trichloromethylsulfenyl) guanine (Elder, 1989) as reported by FAO/WHO (1990). *In vivo* DNA binding studies are discussed in Section 79.3.5.5.

79.2.3.5 Miscellaneous Chemical Reactions

Because captan and folpet are reactive, there are unlimited opportunities for chemical reactions in isolation. Absent data that indicate exposure *in vivo* or relevance to the intact animal, these observations remain ancillary, reflecting their chemical reactivity, but having little bearing on mammalian toxicity.

Captan and folpet react with *p*-nitrothiophenol via the thiol group (Liu and Fishbein, 1967). This differential rate of reac-

tion was measured at 25°C and was 1.9×10^4 liter/(mol min) for captan and 1.5×10^4 liter/(mol min) for folpet.

Other effects include the inhibition of *Escherichia coli* RNA polymerase (Elder, 1989), the inhibition of RNA synthesis by intact bovine nuclei (Elder, 1989), the inhibition of microsomal cytochrome P-450 benzphetamine *N*-demethylase and aniline hydroxylase after intraperitoneal dosing (Dalvi, 1988, 1989), the inhibition of the Ca^{2+} transport ATPase in human erythrocytes (Janik, 1986), and the inhibition of oxidative phosphorylation in rat liver mitochondria, correlated to mitochondrial swelling (Elder, 1989). Captan also disrupted the differentiation of cultured cells from the midbrains and limb buds of 34–36 somite rat embryos *in vitro* (Flint and Ortaon, 1984) and inhibited the attachment of tumor cells to polyethylene disks that were coated with concanavalin (Braun and Horowicz, 1983).

79.2.3.6 Thiophosgene

Thiophosgene (CAS 463-71-8) is a very short-lived compound that has a broad spectrum of reactions with a variety of functional groups (Sharma, 1978, 1986). Although this compound hydrolyzes at a slower rate than its oxygen analog, phosgene, the rate is sufficient to eliminate mutagenic activity in *Salmonella typhimurium* TA 100 when dimethyl sulfoxide (DMSO) is the solvent (Schuphan *et al.*, 1981).

Thiophosgene is a toxicophore of captan and folpet, although its role in their fungicidal properties has been questioned (Lien, 1969). It is volatile and reacts with water to form carbonyl sulfide (COS) and two molecules of hydrogen chloride. The carbonyl sulfide then reacts with another water molecule to form hydrogen sulfide and carbon dioxide (Fig. 79.3). Thiophosgene has two reactive sites associated with the carbon atom. Whereas both chlorine atoms are electronegative, the carbon atom becomes positively charged, thus creating an electrophile. The reaction with cysteine is shown in Fig. 79.4.

79.2.4 METABOLISM

The fate of captan and folpet in mammalian systems is determined by an amalgam of nonenzymatic chemical reactions with thiols and subsequent enzyme-mediated metabolism that predominately involve the generation of ring metabolites. In the intestine, both hydrolysis and thiol-mediated reactions occur. The rate of hydrolysis is particularly sensitive to pH, and the transition from the acid environment of the stomach to the neutral or basic conditions of the duodenum promotes the hydrolytic breakdown of these materials. These fungicides undergo a similar pattern of degradation (Fig. 79.3). The side chain is either fully mineralized or forms by-products such as TTCA with cysteine. The respective imides, THPI and phthalimide, are initially formed either through hydrolysis or through reaction with thiols. These are subsequently metabolized to secondary products; the THPI hexene structure of captan is more extensively metabolized than the phthalimide structure of folpet (Figs. 79.1 and 79.2).

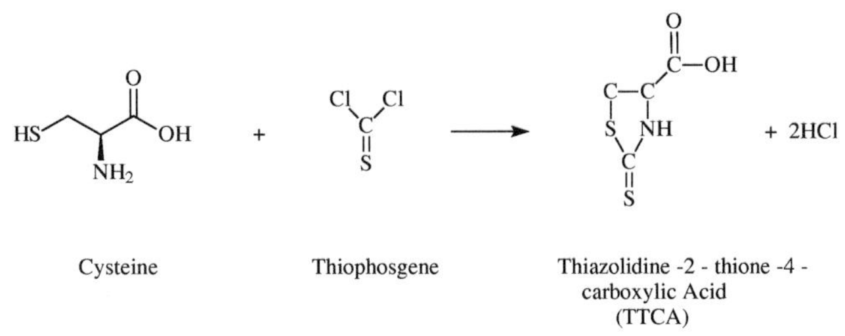

Cysteine   Thiophosgene   Thiazolidine -2 - thione -4 - carboxylic Acid (TTCA)

Figure 79.4 Reaction of cysteine with thiophosgene.

79.2.4.1 Rat Metabolism

Captan and folpet are rapidly eliminated when administered either orally or intraperitoneally. Multiple doses of captan or folpet do not alter subsequent excretory patterns, suggesting that liver enzymes are not induced by repeated exposure. This finding was expected because the parent molecules are not likely to reach the liver. There is no sex difference in the way these fungicides are metabolized. A 10-mg/kg dose of ring-labeled captan is rapidly excreted in the urine. After 24 h, approximately 75% of the administered dose is excreted in the urine and 6.5% is excreted in the feces. Nearly all radioactivity is excreted by 36 h (Trivedi, 1990a). Fourteen repeated single doses of 10 mg/kg followed by a dose of radiolabeled captan produced a similar excretory profile (Bratt, 1990). A dose of 6-mg/kg ^{35}S-captan given intraperitoneally to male rats was effectively eliminated within 72 h (Couch *et al.*, 1977).

Captan at 500-mg/kg dose resulted in a similar profile except that relatively more material was excreted via the feces. In 96 h, 68.8 and 23.1% was excreted via the urine and feces in males and 73.4 and 25.0% was excreted, respectively, in females (Trivedi, 1990b).

Folpet demonstrates a similar pattern. Administration of 10 mg/kg results in approximately 96% of the radioactivity being excreted by 24 h (90% in urine; 6% in feces). With doses 50 times higher, only approximately 69% of the administered dose is cleared by 24 h (47% in urine; 22% in feces). The imide ring is relatively stable and is excreted along with additional ring metabolites. The side chain is unstable and reacts with thiols to form mineralized products such as CO_2, HCl, and H_2S. In addition, products of the reaction also include TTCA, dithiobis(methanesulfonic acid) and its disulfide monoxide derivative. The reactions of captan and folpet are identical with regard to the −[trichloromethylthio] side-chain reactions. The THPI generated from captan is more easily metabolized than the phthalimide from folpet. This is due to the carbonyl groups of captan that draw electrons away from the hexene double bond, creating a δ^+ charge at this site, thereby promoting substitutions.

Administration of phthalimide results in metabolism to phthalamic acid ($\cong$79%, in females) and phthalic acid ($\cong$7%). Less than 1% of the original phthalimide is recovered in the urine (Chasseaud *et al.*, 1974). Phthalamic acid accounts for 80% of the original dose when ^{14}C-[carbonyl] folpet is given to rats (Chasseaud, 1980).

79.2.4.2 Effect on Glutathione Levels in the Duodenum

Sulfhydryl groups are intimately involved with the degradation of captan and folpet. It is therefore of interest to see their effect on GSH. Swiss Webster mice fed captan at 4000, 8000, and 16,000 ppm for 35 days had GSH levels ("soluble thiols") elevated by day 1 (Miaullis *et al.*, 1980). The percent increase over controls ranged from 146 to 227%. Gavage treatment at a relatively high dose of captan (2000 mg/kg) induced an increase in GSH levels that was observable within 2 h of treatment, whereas a smaller dose (20 mg/kg) induced a measurable increase at 4 h (Katz *et al.*, 1982; Sauerhoff *et al.*, 1982).

Folpet induced increased GSH levels were demonstrated after both dietary administration and gavage (Chasseaud *et al.*, 1991). Folpet, administered by gavage (7.6, 72, and 668 mg/kg) initially induced a decrease (30 and 60 min), which subsequently rebounded to a higher than normal level. The decrease was statistically significant for the 72-mg/kg dose: levels of 76, 54, 82, 155, and 130% (of control values) were observed at 0.5, 1, 2, 6, and 24 h, respectively. This rebound effect was also seen at 668 mg/kg: 72, 52, 94, 143, and 178% at the same time periods. Diethylmaleate produced a similar pattern of GSH loss and rebound. These data demonstrate that captan and folpet cause an initial lowering of GSH levels followed by an increase due to a homeostatic rebound. The generative process for GSH exceeds the loss, and a steady state of higher GSH levels is quickly reached.

79.2.4.3 Goat Metabolism

Ring labeled (^{14}C)captan was administered to goats in gelatin capsules three times per day for 4 days. The total daily dose equaled approximately 50 ppm (Cheng, 1980). Most of the radioactivity was excreted in the urine, and the next highest excretion was via the feces. Five biochemical reactions were noted from this study:

1. Cleavage of the N−S linkage in the captan molecule to form THPI, either by hydrolysis or reaction with SH compounds.
2. Ring hydroxylation of THPI to form 3-OH THPI.
3. Isomerization of the 3-OH THPI to form 5-OH THPI.
4. Epoxidation of THPI to form THPI-epoxide, which is subsequently hydrolyzed to form 4,5-diOH HHPI.
5. Hydrolysis of THPI and/or its hydroxylated derivatives to form their corresponding THP-amic acid derivatives.

When radiolabeled folpet [^{14}C-labeled on the trichloromethylthio side chain (TCM)] was administered via capsules to goats, radioactivity was recovered as expired ^{14}CO$_2$ ($\cong$31%; reflecting the breakdown of the TCM), in the feces ($\cong$21%), and in the urine ($\cong$10%; Corden, 1997). Recovered ^{14}CO$_2$ from the expired air (ca. 31%) reflected the breakdown of the trichloromethylthio moiety to CO_2. In contrast, administration of ring-labeled folpet showed the same excretion pattern as discussed for captan [i.e., more excretion via the urine ($\cong$58%)

than the feces ($\cong$35%), with the major urinary metabolite being phthalamic acid ($\cong$49% of the dose)].

79.2.4.4 Hen Metabolism

Laying hens metabolize captan in a similar way as mammals (Daun, 1988a, b). When tagged with ^{14}C on the imide ring, the identified metabolites were THPI (15.8–68.9% of the tissue radioactivity), and 3-OH, and 5-OH-THPI, which represented 2.4–26% of the radioactivity. When tagged with ^{14}C on the trichloromethylthio moiety TTCA, dithiobis-methanesulfonic acid and its monosulfoxide were seen. Parent captan was not present in the eggs or tissues.

79.2.4.5 Dermal Absorption

Dermal absorption of captan and folpet, as subsequently noted, is estimated at no greater than 0.5% per hour. Captan penetration of skin has been measured *in vitro*, comparing rat to human, and *in vivo*, using rats. The rat study measured absorption at 1, 2, 4, and 8 h at 19.4 μg/cm^2 (0.5 mg/kg) and 194 μg/cm^2 (5 mg/kg; Adir *et al.*, 1982), and the data have been interpreted as indicating from 0.4% per hour absorption (Ghali, 1997) to 1.5% per hour (11.7% per 8 h; Thongsinthusak *et al.*, 1999). The 11.7% per 8-h rate has been noted as overly conservative because the test sites were not occluded, allowing contamination of the urine and feces samples. Additionally, the absorption rate did not consider the difference between rat and human skin permeability (Fletcher *et al.*, 1995). The *in vitro* rat/human comparisons showed that human skin was consistently less permeable than rat skin, but that the ratio of permeability was partly dependent on the concentration of captan applied and the solvent used.

A study with ^{14}C-folpet 50 WP in rats indicated a systemic absorption of 0.27% per hour (6.5% in 24 h; Wilson and Wright, 1990). This calculation was based on a least square analysis of 24-h urinary excretion at dose levels of 49, 460, and 4800 μg/cm^2 (13.2, 3.5, and 1.3%, respectively), matching the excretion to the approximate dermal exposure of 2400 μg/cm^2, based on the 50WP formulation concentration. There was rapid uptake of folpet into the skin and 95 and 94% for dose levels 4800 and 460 μg/cm^2, respectively, were retained there at 24 h. The amount still in the skin after 24 h for the low dose was approximately 85% of the applied dose.

A comparison with ring-labeled captan and side-chain-labeled folpet showed no difference in absorption between adult and young Fischer 344 rats, but a lesser amount of folpet was absorbed compared to captan (Shah *et al.*, 1987). At 0.54 and 2.68 μm/cm^2, captan penetration in adult rats was 3.7 and 3.6%, whereas folpet penetration was 2.7 and 1.1%, respectively. These data were interpreted by EPA to suggest 0.4% per hour (4.29% in 10 h) dermal absorption for folpet (Ghali, 1997; Levy *et al.*, 1997). These data show high dermal adsorption, but low penetration rates for captan and folpet. There are differing interpretations of these data, but it is reasonable to conclude that the hourly dermal penetration rate is no greater than 0.5%. The

normal sloughing of the stratum corneum serves to deplete the amount available for absorption.

79.2.4.6 Human Metabolism

Humans appear to metabolize captan in a similar manner to other mammals (Krieger and Thongsinthusak, 1993). Both THPI and TTCA have been recovered after oral and dermal dosing. Comparable human studies with folpet have not been conducted, but are expected to yield similar results except for the imide ring recovered.

79.2.5 SUMMARY

Captan and folpet are extensively altered in mammalian and avian systems through a combination of enzymatic as well as nonenzymatic chemical reactions. Two complementary processes, hydrolysis and thiol interactions, initially split the fungicides into their respective imide rings and trichloromethylthio complexes. Subsequent reactions, some of which may be enzymatic, produce a series of imide-based degradates and thiophosgene-mediated products. The reactions are rapid and nearly all material is eliminated from the animal within 24–48 h; there is no accumulation of either imide or side chain. Urinary metabolites from the rings differ between captan and folpet, but those associated with the trichloromethylthio side chain are common [e.g., TTCA and dithiobis(methanesulfonic acid)]. Captan or folpet do not survive in the systemic circulation, thus limiting their primary effects to areas of initial contact. Due to this rapid elimination, meat, milk, or eggs from livestock that might have consumed feed with residues of captan or folpet present would be devoid of the parent materials.

79.3 TOXICOLOGY

79.3.1 ACUTE TOXICOLOGY

79.3.1.1 Overview

Both captan and folpet have low acute toxicity, except for the intraperitoneal route (Table 79.3). The reactivity to mucus membranes is high and the severe eye irritant finding is consistent with this property. When single 0.5-g doses are applied to the skin, the results show mild to low irritancy. Results of guinea pig sensitization studies give both positive and negative results; however, experience with handlers of these materials suggest that some persons (less than 10% of the population) are susceptible to sensitization.

79.3.1.2 Acute Oral Toxicity

The low acute oral toxicity of captan and folpet reflects the rapid degradation of the fungicides once ingested and the absence of intact fungicide at sensitive biochemical targets. The LD$_{50}$ values are above 5 g/kg for both technical and formulated

Table 79.3
Acute Toxicity of Captan and Folpet[a]

Parameter	Captan	Reference	Folpet	Reference
Oral LD$_{50}$, rat	>5 g/kg	Gaines and Linder (1986)	>5 g/kg	Gaines and Linder (1986)
	8 g/kg 50W formulation	Ben-Dyke *et al.* (1970)	>10 g/kg 50W formulation	Ben-Dyke *et al.* (1970)
Intraperitoneal LD$_{50}$, rat	40 mg/kg, M 35 mg/kg, F	Copley (1985)	48–52.5 mg/kg	Dickhaus and Heisler (1983)
Dermal LD$_{50}$, rabbit	>2000 mg/kg	Thoa and Redden (1995)	>5000 mg/kg	Korenaga (1982)
Irritation, eye	Severe	Thoa and Redden (1995)	Severe	U.S. EPA (1987)
Skin	Minimal	U.S. EPA (1975)	Minimal	U.S. EPA (1987)
Inhalation LC$_{50}$, rat, 4 h exposure	0.72–0.87 mg/liter	Thoa and Redden (1995)	1.89 mg/liter	Cracknell (1993)
Sensitization, guinea pig	Moderate	Thoa and Redden (1995)	Moderate	U.S. EPA (1987)

[a]M, males; F, females.

products, placing them in Toxicity Category IV for EPA regulatory purposes. The captan 50W formulation LD$_{50}$ is 8.4 g/kg, whereas the comparable folpet formulation LD$_{50}$ is greater than 10 g/kg (Ben-Dyke *et al.*, 1970). Results from other investigators consistently show LD$_{50}$ values above 5 g/kg for both compounds (Boyd and Krijnen, 1968; Nelson, 1949).

The imide ring degradates of captan and folpet, THPI and phthalimide, respectively, are stable compared to the parent compounds. Accordingly, some measure of their acute toxicity is in order. Both these compounds have low acute oral toxicity in mammals. The LD$_{50}$ of THPI is 2 g/kg (Cavalli, 1970); for phthalimide it is greater than 8 g/kg (U.S. EPA, 1974). In contrast to mammals, aquatic organisms are particularly sensitive to captan and folpet, and offer a useful test system to compare the toxicity of parent and degradate. Comparative toxicity in trout show THPI to be approximately 3500-fold less toxic than captan (captan LC$_{50}$ = 34 ppb versus THPI LC$_{50}$ > 120,000 ppb; U.S. EPA, 1999a). A similar comparison for folpet shows a 3267-fold difference (folpet LC$_{50}$ = 15 ppb versus phthalimide LC$_{50}$ = 49,000 ppb; U.S. EPA, 1999b).

79.3.1.3 Acute Intraperitoneal Toxicity

Intraperitoneal administered acute toxicity studies are not generally required for regulatory purposes because this route of entry affords little information for human risk assessment. The intraperitoneal route bypasses the intestine, although materials are still primarily absorbed by the portal system (Rozman and Klaassen, 1996). In the case of oral administration of captan or folpet, only trace amounts of parent material would enter the portal system and would be rapidly degraded. Intraperitoneal administration bypasses this degradation and thus affords an observation into the inherent toxicity of the materials.

Male and female SPF Wistar rats treated with 92.7% captan administered by injection in 1% methylcellulose had LD$_{50}$ values approximately 40 mg/kg for males and 35 mg/kg for females (Copley, 1985). This LD$_{50}$, lower by over 100-fold compared to oral administration, indicates the inherent toxicity of captan. It also demonstrates the effective barrier provided by the intestine .

Male and female Wistar rats injected with 87.5% folpet in 1% methylcellulose had a 24-h LD$_{50}$ of 48.0–52.5 mg/kg. Deaths occurred between 24 h and 7 days, resulting in a 7-day LD$_{50}$ of 36–40 mg/kg. There was a steep dose–response curve: at 30 mg/kg, 1 in 10 deaths were seen, but at 60 mg/kg, 10 in 10 deaths occurred by day 7 (Dickhaus and Heisler, 1983). The intraperitoneal LD$_{50}$ values for captan and folpet are similar and reflect the rule that governs their toxicological profile: hazard in the absence of exposure limits adverse effects.

79.3.1.4 Acute Dermal Toxicity

Captan and folpet pose little hazard of acute toxicity from dermal exposure. Limit doses of 2 g/kg are without effect in rabbits (Foster and Morgan, 1984; Gaines and Linder, 1986). A study with Phaltan (folpet 50%) showed that the LD$_{50}$ was greater than 22.6 g/kg (Kay and Calandra, 1960).

79.3.1.5 Eye Irritation

Captan and folpet irritate mucus membranes and there is the potential for damage when they contact the eyes. Bioassays, however, vary in their estimation of this hazard. Captan eye irritation studies show variable results. Minimal damage, as noted by no corneal or iris involvement, and low redness and swelling to the eyelids, has been reported (Harris, 1976). Conversely, severe damage, including corneal opacity, has also been reported

(Rosenfeld, 1984). Washing the treated eyes after instillation of test material reduces irritation, as was observed in a study that employed a captan 50W formulation (Sauer and Seaman, 1980). An additional study employed a combination formulation that included captan (8%), folpet (44%), and captafol (8%), and showed conjunctival irritation, but no corneal involvement (Cisson *et al.*, 1983).

Folpet Technical, in unwashed eyes, induced transient corneal opacity that progressed to vascularization of the cornea in two of six rabbits (Dreher, 1992a). A 100-mg instillation of Folpet Technical caused corneal opacity in some unwashed eyes and no opacity in eyes that were washed 30 s after instillation (Cisson *et al.*, 1982). All eyes returned to normal by 7 days (washed) or 10 days (unwashed). Phaltan 500 Flowable formulation (50% folpet) instilled in rabbit eyes, followed by a 30 s wash after 30 s, resulted in no corneal opacity and minimal redness and swelling (Mercier, 1988). By 72 h, all swelling had subsided, but there was some residual redness and congestion.

79.3.1.6 Skin Irritation

Both captan and folpet elicit very little irritation when applied as a single dose to either intact or abraded skin. Captan Technical applied to rabbit skin at 0.5 g showed no redness or edema at either 24 or 48 h for both intact and abraded test sites (Harris, 1976). Folpet Technical applied to rabbit skin at 0.5 g showed no redness or edema at observation periods up to 72 h (Rees, 1993). Doses of folpet as high as 22.6 g/kg produced only transient redness in rabbits (Kay and Calandra, 1960).

79.3.1.7 Acute Inhalation Toxicity

Acute toxicity via the inhalation route of exposure varies somewhat with the specific formulation tested. For captan, the 4-h LC_{50} was 1.21 mg/liter for males and 1.05 mg/liter for females (Cummins, 1995). An earlier study reported these values as 0.90 mg/liter for males and 0.67 mg/liter for females (Blagden, 1991). For folpet, the 4-h LC_{50} for males and females was 1.89 mg/liter (95% confidence limits 1.47–2.31 mg/liter; Cracknell, 1993). The particle size mass median equivalent aerodynamic diameter was 4.6–5.2 μm. Males were slightly more susceptible than females. The mortality for males was 0 in 5, 3 in 5, and 4 in 5 for dose levels 0.80, 1.60, and 1.99 mg/liter, respectively. Females at these respective doses showed mortality of 0 in 5, 1 in 5, and 1 in 5.

79.3.1.8 Skin Sensitization

Guinea pig bioassays show that both captan and folpet have the potential to induce delayed contact hypersensitivity reactions. Captan Technical was positive in the Magnusson and Kligman maximization guinea pig assays (Dreher, 1992b). Folpet Technical was tested using the Magnusson and Kligman protocol in which a 10% w/v preparation in propylene glycol was injected by the intradermal route along with a 1:1 preparation of Freund's Complete Adjuvant. Subsequent topical inductions were made with 50% w/v folpet. Challenge with either 10 or 50%

w/v folpet in propylene glycol resulted in positive reactions (LSR, 1993).

79.3.1.9 Human Experience

Reports of adverse effects are limited to incidences of skin irritation or sensitization reactions (Guo *te al.*, 1996; Peluso *et al.*, 1991; U.S. EPA, 1989). In human patch tests, 9 in 205 (4.4%) subjects showed a positive Draize reaction (Marzulli and Maibach, 1973), 8 in 150 (5.3%) were sensitized by 1% topically applied captan (Jordan and King, 1977), and 24 in 200 were positive to chemicals in the fungicide category, predominantly the thiophthalimides (Lisi *et al.*, 1986). Additionally, a case of urticaria was associated with use of a captan-formulated product (Croy, 1973). However, a powder blush that contained 0.3% captan failed to sensitize any of 25 adult volunteers on which it was tested. This was in spite of the study design, which included repeated doses (five consecutive 300-mg induction exposures to the forearms) and occlusion of the application site for 48 h after each dose. The individuals were challenged 10 days later and all individuals were negative (Ivy Research Laboratories, 1981).

Regular exposure to captan, formulated in a shampoo at 7%, appears to be well tolerated (Guo, 2001). Although there is potential for eye irritation, based on laboratory studies, there are no reports in the literature of adverse effects (NLM, 2001). Likewise, eye injuries in agricultural workers who carry out reentry activities do not appear to be problematic (Krieger, 2001).

79.3.1.10 Summary

Adverse skin reactions to captan and folpet due to delayed contact hypersensitivity are possible for mixers, loaders, and applicators, and may occur in low incidence. The potential for eye irritation exists, but extensive use experience suggests this problem is minimal. There is little acute risk from oral ingestion or dermal exposure to either product. The World Health Organization has classified folpet as unlikely to present an acute hazard in normal use (FAO/WHO, 1996).

79.3.2 SUBCHRONIC TOXICITY

Mechanistic studies in mice have focused on changes to the duodenum and illuminate the mode of action for tumor formation. These studies confirm the irritant properties of captan and folpet, the effects of irritation to the duodenum, and the reversibility of these effects upon cessation of treatment. Other observations in the mouse include reduced weight gain and depressed food intake at high doses; this is also seen as a general secondary effect in rat studies. Observations in rats also include hyperkeratosis and acanthosis of the esophagus and stomach, particularly for folpet. Dogs do not tolerate capsule-administered captan or folpet well; emesis is always seen. Rabbits administered folpet dermally show marked skin irritation, and rats respond to repeated dermal application of folpet with severe skin irritation.

79.3.2.1 Mice

Mechanistic Studies Male CD-1 mice (four or five per group) treated with 3000-ppm captan for 1, 3, 7, 14, or 28 days showed shortened duodenal villi due to damage by captan. This effect was observable in the crypts within 3 days of treatment initiation (Tinston, 1996). Immature cells were observed at the villi tips from day 7 onward, indicating a higher turnover of cells. There was some focal gastritis and parakeratosis noted in one mouse. When captan is fed to mice at 6000 ppm for 28–90 days, villus atrophy occurs, together with a crypt hypertrophy and crypt cell hyperplasia (Tinston, 1995).

CD-1 mice administered captan for 56 days as 0, 400, 800, 3000, or 6000 ppm were evaluated for proliferative changes in the duodenum (Tinston, 1995). An assessment of the duodenum was made using histopathology and a bromodeoxyuridine-labeling index to measure crypt cell proliferation. Captan induced hyperplasia of the crypt cells, an increase in the crypt cell labeling index, and an increase in the number of cells in the crypt cell population. At 3000 ppm, the villus-to-crypt height ratio decreased from 5.4 in males and 5.9 in females to 1.4 and 2.6, respectively. These observed changes are consistent with an irritant action of captan on the duodenum. The no observed effect limit (NOEL) for duodenal hyperplasia is 400 ppm.

Male CD-1 mice treated with 5000-ppm folpet for 28 days (Waterson, 1995) were observed to have proliferative changes in the duodenum proximal to the pyloric sphincter. An inflammatory response, similar to that noted with captan, was not seen. Treatment of CD-1 mice with folpet at 0, 150, 450, and 5000 ppm for 28 days resulted in duodenum proliferative effects (Milburn, 1997). Villi length was reduced and crypt compartments were expanded, reducing the villi-to-crypt ratio. The NOEL for hyperplasia in the duodenum for males was 450 ppm (69 mg/kg per day) and the NOEL for females was 150 ppm (29 mg/kg per day).

Subchronic Study B6C3F1 mice were fed folpet at 0, 1000, 5000, or 10,000 ppm for 4 weeks (Rubin, 1981). There was reduced food intake and body weight gain at 5000 ppm.

79.3.2.2 Rats

Oral Wistar rats treated for 4 weeks with captan at 0, 2000, 4000, 8000, or 12,000 ppm were observed to have a dose-related decrease in body weight gain and food intake (Til and Beems, 1979). At the top two doses, there were increases in basophilia of hepatocytes in the periportal area of the liver accompanied by increases in relative liver weight. A similar finding was observed in the females at the next lower dose (4000 ppm). The relative organ to body kidney weights were statistically increased at all doses.

Folpet Technical admixed in the diet at 0, 2000, 4000, and 8000 ppm, and fed to Fischer rats for 13 weeks produced a treatment and dose-related decrease in body weight gain and hyperkeratosis/acanthosis of the esophagus and nonglandular stomach (Sela, 1982). The NOEL for decreased weight gain was 2000 ppm in males (136 mg/kg per day) and 4000 ppm

in females (291 mg/kg per day). Irritation to the esophagus and forestomach occurred at all doses and in both sexes. A variety of hematological and clinical chemistry changes were noted, but the incidence and pattern did not indicate a clear target.

Folpet Technical admixed in the diet at 0, 300, 100, 3000, or 10,000 ppm and fed to Sprague–Dawley rats for 13 weeks, followed by a 2-week recovery showed similar signs of irritation in the forestomach, primarily at 10,000 ppm, but no irritation of the esophagus (Reno et al., 1981). Following a 2-week recovery period during which the rats received control diet, the forestomach histology returned to normal.

Folpet Technical fed to B6C3F1 mice for 28 days at levels of 0, 1000, 5000, and 10,000 ppm induced a reduced body weight gain in the top two doses (Crown, 1981).

Dermal A 28-day rat study with Folpet Technical applied in mineral oil at 0, 1, 10, 20, and 30 mg/kg per day to the backs of Sprague–Dawley rats 6 h per day, five days per week. All dose levels elicited irritation that was more severe in males than females and resulted in decreased weight gain (Dougherty, 1988). The irritation was so severe in the 30-mg/kg per day male group, that application was terminated after 10 days. All adverse effects noted were related to the skin irritation induced by folpet.

Inhalation Captan has been tested in Wistar rats by nose-only inhalation at nominal dose levels of 0.1, 0.5, 5, and 15 µg/liter for 13 weeks (Hext, 1989). There were deaths in males at the high dose and dose-related effects on the larynx (e.g., squamous metaplasia, squamous hyperplasia, vacuolar degeneration of squamous epithelium). The no observed effect concentration (NOEC) for toxic effects (other than generalized irritation) was 0.6 µg/liter (measured).

79.3.2.3 Rabbits

A 21-day dermal study with captan in rabbits at 0, 12.5, 110, or 1000 mg/kg per day (6-h exposure per day) resulted in a dose-related desquamation of the skin by day 21, erythema and edema at the high dose, and acanthosis and hyperkeratosis of the treated skin at all doses (Johnson, 1987).

79.3.2.4 Dogs

Beagles, two per sex per treatment group, were administered captan at 0, 30, 100, 300, 600, or 1000 mg/kg per day for 4 weeks. The results included treatment-related emesis and a dose-related decrease in food intake and body weight gain (Blair, 1987). There was an increase in relative liver weight in males at 600 and 1000 mg/kg per day and relative kidney weight in females at 1000 mg/kg per day. Some fatty changes were seen in the kidney and liver of one male at 1000 mg/kg per day.

Folpet administered to two beagle dogs per sex per group at 0, 20, 60, 180, and 540 mg/kg per day for 4 weeks induced emesis (Daly, 1983). Food intake and body weights were reduced in a dose-related manner. There were, however, no histopathologic changes noted.

Folpet was administered to four beagles per sex at 0, 790, 1800, and 4000 mg/kg per day for 13 weeks with gelatin capsules (Barel *et al.*, 1985). Daily doses of 4 g/kg were well above the maximum tolerated dose and resulted in severe deterioration of the males, all of which were killed for humane reasons. One of the females at the high dose was also terminated in moribund condition. Vomiting and diarrhea were noted clinical signs and both food intake and body weight gains were reduced in a dose-related fashion. Treatment resulted in irritation of the gastric mucosa, atrophied testes, thyroid degeneration, and muscular dystrophy.

79.3.2.5 Miscellaneous Studies

Rats and mice administered 3000-ppm captan had reduced immune function as measured by sheep red blood cell antibody formation after treatment for 42 days (LaFarge-Frayssinet and Decloitre, 1982). Captan was reported to suppress both B- and T-cell function in mice. Wistar rats had depressed lymphocyte count and lower relative thymus weight after 3 weeks of dietary administration of captan at 1000 ppm [50 mg/kg body weight (bw) per day], initiated as weanlings (Vos and Krajnc, 1983). Additionally, rats administered pre- and postnatal captan at 750 and 2000 ppm (37.5 and 100 mg/kg bw per day) showed a decrease in secondary IgG response to tetanus toxoid in the high-dose animals (Vos and Krajnc, 1983). Evaluation of these studies by Joint Meeting on Pesticide Residues (JMPR) concluded that captan may be an immunodepressant (FAO/WHO, 1990). These dose levels, however, are high and may not be relevant to anticipated human exposure scenarios.

79.3.3 CHRONIC TOXICITY

One mechanistic study was conducted in mice with captan. These data are also relevant for folpet because both share a common mechanism of toxicity. Duodenal tumors in mice were seen in both chronic and oncogenic studies (discussed later). Chronic administration of folpet produced evidence of irritation to the esophagus and stomach in rats.

79.3.3.1 Mice

In a mechanistic study, male CD-1 mice were administered captan at dietary doses of 0 and 6000 ppm for 3, 6, 9, 12, 18, or 20 months (Pavkov and Thomasson, 1985). Mice were examined at the end of each dosing period and, in addition, various recovery periods were evaluated (Table 79.4). One group dosed with 6000 ppm for 6 months was held for an additional 6-month recovery period; another was held for a 12-month recovery period. One group dosed with 6000 ppm for 12 months was followed after a 6- and 8-month recovery. The most characteristic pathologic findings consisted of necrotizing and proliferative changes in the nonglandular portion of the stomach (after 3 months), dilation of the small intestine, and focal epithelial

Table 79.4
Captan Mechanistic Study Design[a]

Dose (ppm)	Time (months)					
	3	6	9	12	18	20
0	S	S	S	S	S	S
6000	T, S					
6000	T	T, S		RS	RS	
6000	T	T	T	T, S	RS	RS
6000	T	T	T	T	T, S	
6000	T	T	T	T	T	T, S

[a]Reproduced with permission from Pavkov and Thomasson (1985). T = treatment; S = sacrifice; RS = recovery sacrifice.

hyperplasia in the proximal part of the small intestine. Focal epithelial hyperplasia was also found in controls, but the incidence was lower compared to that of the treated animals, and the localization of these foci was more caudal than was the case for captan-administered mice. Diffuse hyperplasia was found only in treated mice and was not considered prerequisite for the development of focal hyperplasia. Adenomas and adenocarcinomas also developed in the small intestines of treated mice with localization in the proximal 7 cm of the small intestine; the area of localization was the same as for the focal hyperplasia.

Removal of captan from the diet resulted in a significant reduction in the incidence of focal epithelial hyperplasia as compared to the incidence in concurrent lifetime-treated mice, and was no greater than that in concurrent controls. The incidence of neoplasia, however, in mice in the recovery group was not significantly different from that of concurrent lifetime-treated mice, but increased in mice treated for 6 months with a recovery period of 6 months and in mice treated for 12 months with a recovery period of 6–8 months, respectively, when compared to controls. The latter increase was not found in mice treated for 6 months with a recovery period of 12 months.

79.3.3.2 Rats

Rats were administered folpet at dietary concentrations of 0, 250, 1500, and 5000 ppm (Crown *et al.*, 1989). Body weight gain and food intake were decreased at 5000 ppm. The incidence and severity of diffuse hyperkeratosis in the esophagus and nonglandular epithelium of the stomach were increased in both sexes at 5000 ppm. The stomach was also affected at 1500 ppm. The NOEL was 250 ppm (12 and 15 mg/kg per day, males and females, respectively).

A folpet combined chronic toxicity/oncogenicity study from which the EPA derived a NOEL for use in chronic dietary risk assessment employed dietary dose levels of 0, 200, 800, or 3200 ppm (Cox *et al.*, 1985). The EPA selected the 200-ppm level (9 mg/kg per day) as the NOEL for conducting chronic dietary risk assessments, based on hyperkeratosis/acanthosis and ulceration/erosion of the nonglandular stomach at 800 ppm (equivalent to 35 mg/kg per day; U.S. EPA, 1999b).

79.3.3.3 Dogs

Dogs were treated with captan at 0, 12.5, 60, and 300 mg/kg per day for 1 year (Blair, 1988). Only the high-dose animals differed from control in increased incidence of emesis and soft stool, increased relative liver weight, and decreased total serum protein and albumin. There were two 1-year dog studies conducted with folpet: the first at 0, 10, 60, and 140/120 mg/kg per day (Daly and Knezevich, 1986) and the second at 0, 325, 650, and 1300 mg/kg per day (Waner, 1988). In the first study, the 140 mg/kg per day was reduced to 120 mg/kg per day on day 50 due to unacceptable decreases in body weight gain and food intake. A NOEL was selected for the study at 10 mg/kg per day based on lowered body weight gain and food intake at 60 and 120 mg/kg per day. There were no clinical signs of toxicity noted, but clinical chemistry values showed a treatment-related decrease in total plasma protein parameters and cholesterol. Organ weights were not affected by treatment nor was there evidence of macroscopic or microscopic changes as a result of treatment.

In the second study, folpet induced incidences of diarrhea, vomiting, and salivation that were associated with reduced food intake and reduced body weight gain. Testes weights were reduced in males administered 1300 mg/kg per day when compared to controls on an absolute basis, but were similar to controls when measured on a relative body weight basis. The NOEL for this study was 325 mg/kg per day, based on decreased body weight gain. The WHO acceptable daily intake (ADI) is 0.1 mg/kg per day for both captan (FAO/WHO, 1990) and folpet (FAO/WHO, 1996).

79.3.4 DEVELOPMENTAL AND REPRODUCTIVE TOXICITY

79.3.4.1 Developmental Studies

Rats Captan administered to Sprague–Dawley CD rats at 0, 18, 90, and 450 mg/kg per day resulted in decreased maternal weight gain and decreased food consumption at the high dose (Rubin, 1987). There were no effects on postimplantation loss or fetal survival. Fetal body weight was reduced and the incidence of "small" fetuses (<3.0 g) was increased at the high dose. There were no increases in incidences of treatment-related malformations. The incidence of minor skeletal variations, including the presence of a fourteenth (lumbar) rib, incomplete fusion of vertebral hemicentra fusion, and reduced ossification of the pubes was increased at 450 mg/kg per day. The NOELs for maternal and developmental toxicity in this study were 18 and 90 mg/kg per day.

In another study, folpet was administered by gavage to Sprague–Dawley CD rats at 0, 150, 550, or 2000 mg/kg per day from gestation days 6–15. Maternal toxicity in the form of decreased food intake and body weight gain was observed at the mid- and high dose. Fetuses showed slight developmental retardation at 150 mg/kg per day, suggesting the NOEL was slightly below this level (Rubin, 1983). Pups from rats treated with 400

mg/kg per day from gestation days 8–10 were normal (Kennedy et al., 1968) as were rats treated with 360 mg/kg per day from gestation days 6–19 (Hoberman et al., 1983).

Rabbits Captan did not induce any teratogenic effects when administered to New Zealand White (NZW) rabbits at 0, 10, 40, and 160 mg/kg per day from gestation days 7–19 (Rubin and Nyska, 1987). The highest dose was toxic to both dams and fetuses. An increased incidence of minor skeletal variations was seen at this dose. In another study, captan was administered to New Zealand White rabbits at 0, 10, 30, or 100 mg/kg per day (Tinston, 1991). The developmental NOEL was 10 mg/kg per day based on increased postimplantation loss, reduced mean fetal weight, and increased skeletal defects in fetuses (27 presacral vertebrae) at the maternally toxic dose of 30 mg/kg per day.

Folpet was tested in both Dutch Belted and NZW rabbits for potential developmental toxicity. The original studies (Fabro et al., 1966; Kennedy et al., 1968; McLaughlin et al., 1969) were performed at high doses ranging from 75 to 150 mg/kg per day during gestation days 7–12, 6–16, or 6–18. These studies consistently demonstrated the absence of adverse effects. One study reported five incidences of hydrocephaly at doses that were maternally toxic (Feussner et al., 1984; one at 20 mg/kg per day and four at 60 mg/kg per day). A second study in which doses of folpet were "pulsed" failed to replicated this finding (Feussner, 1985). The most recent study employed doses of 10, 40, and 160 mg/kg per day, and confirmed the absence of folpet-induced developmental effects (Rubin, 1985b). Although a weight-of-evidence (WOE) analysis concluded folpet is not a developmental toxin, the EPA has assigned this compound an FQPA uncertainty factor of 3 based on the initial Feussner study.

Although the EPA pointed to one study where hydrocephaly occurred at maternally toxic doses of 20 (one instance) and 60 mg/kg per day (three fetuses in two litters; Feussner et al., 1984), a second "pulse dose" study (Feussner, 1985) failed to replicate this finding and other developmental studies in NZW rabbits showed no evidence of teratogenicity or hydrocephaly (Fabro et al., 1966; Kennedy et al., 1968; McLaughlin et al., 1969; Rubin, 1985b). The EPA cited the Feussner study as the basis for assigning an FQPA three-fold uncertainty factor (U.S. EPA, 1999b), although a WOE analysis concluded that folpet is not a selective developmental toxin (Neal, 2000).

Mice CD-1 mice administered folpet by gavage, subcutaneously (100 mg/kg per day), or by inhalation at (624 μg/m^3) showed no developmental abnormalities (Courtney et al., 1983). BL6 mice treated subcutaneously and orally with folpet at 100 mg/kg per day and AKR mice treated subcutaneously at 100 mg/kg per day were judged to have not adverse developmental findings (Bionetics Research Laboratories, 1968).

Other Species Captan is not teratogenic in beagles when administered in the diet at 60 mg/kg per day either throughout gestation or throughout gestation plus lactation (Kennedy *et al.*, 1975b). Folpet was studied in Rhesus and stump-tailed macaques as part of research on thalidomide (Vondruska, 1969). There were no malformations with folpet at doses up to 75 mg/kg per day. Thalidomide at 10 mg/kg per day produced limb defects.

79.3.4.2 Reproductive Studies

In a three-generation study, COBS CD rats were treated with captan at 25, 100, 250, and 500 mg/kg per day (Schardein *et al.*, 1982). Nonreproductive parental toxicity was seen at 100 mg/kg per day and above in the absence of reproductive effects. Pup weights were lower by 7% compared to controls at 25 mg/kg per day. A subsequent one-generation study at 0, 6, 12.5, and 25 mg/kg per day showed no effect on pup weights at 25 mg/kg per day. The NOEL selected by the EPA for use in risk assessment was 12.5 mg/kg per day, based on the weight gain depression in the three-generation study (Ghali, 1997; Schardein and Aldridge, 1982). The reference dose employed by the EPA, 0.13 mg/kg per day, is based on this NOEL and the use of a 100-fold safety factor.

Folpet administered to rats at 0, 250, 1500, and 5000 ppm showed diffuse hyperkeratosis of the nonglandular epithelium of the stomach (Rubin, 1986). The NOEL for this study was 250 ppm, which averaged 24 mg/kg per day. There were no reproductive effects noted. Other two- or three-generation studies in rats with folpet also showed no adverse reproductive effects (Hardy, 1985; Kennedy, 1967).

79.3.5 MUTAGENICITY

79.3.5.1 Overview

The issue of mutagenicity is controversial. Throughout this chapter, the rapid degradation of captan and folpet in living systems has been central to understanding their toxicology. The pattern of mutagenicity is consistent with this degradation and provides examples of how such degradation diminishes adverse effects. Interest in the mutagenicity of captan and folpet has produced many mutagenicity studies. *In vitro* studies showed clear evidence that both are mutagenic, captan is more potent compared to folpet, and their activity is inversely proportional to the presence of thiols in the reaction vessels. Once thresholds for complete degradation are reached, *in vitro* activity is abolished. The large reserves of thiols present in the intact animal and the near instantaneous reaction of captan and folpet with the thiols serves to ensure complete elimination of captan and folpet before they reach sensitive DNA targets. The net result of this rapid degradation is the absence of mutagenicity *in vivo*.

The mechanism by which captan and folpet effect their mutagenicity is not clear; however, data suggest that thiophosgene, in addition to the parent compounds, is mutagenic (Arlett *et al.*, 1975). For *in vitro* systems, both frame-shift and base-pair substitutions are seen. Cytogenetic effects are seen *in vitro*, but positive results are not as ubiquitous as point mutations. These clastogenic effects are reduced when enzyme enhanced rat liver extract (S-9) is present and are generally absent *in vivo*. The weight of evidence shows that although captan and folpet possess inherent mutagenic potential, they are not mutagenic *in vivo*.

79.3.5.2 Mutations

In Vitro **Assays**   Table 79.5 shows results from representative *in vitro* assays with *S. typhimurium*, strain TA 100, a prokaryote organism. The greater potency of captan relative to folpet is noted. Other *S. typhimurium* strains showed similar results. A mutation index (the ratio between induced versus spontaneous revertants) of 7.3 for captan and 6.3 for folpet was seen for strain 104 (Barrueco and de la Pena, 1988). Positive findings were generally seen with strains 98, 1535, 1537, and 1538 (Carere *et al.*, 1978; Shiau *et al.*, 1981; Shirasu *et al.*, 1976), but negative findings were seen with strain 1536 (Shiau *et al.*, 1981). Where there were marginally positive results with captan, folpet was usually negative. Strain WP2 try⁻hcr⁺ of *E. coli*

Table 79.5

Prokaryote Reverse Mutation: *Salmonella typhimurium,* Strain TA 100

Compound	Results[a]	Reference
Captan	26.7 revertants per 10^8 cells/nmol, −S-9	Shiau *et al.* (1981)
	++ @ 50 μg/plate (167 nmol), +S-9	
	+ @ 50 μg/plate (167 nmol), +S-9	
Folpet	7.7 revertants per 10^8 cells/nmol, −S-9	Shiau *et al.* (1981)
	+ @ 50 μg/plate (167 nmol), −S-9	
	− @ 50 μg/plate (167 nmol), +S-9	
Captan	26 revertants/nmol, −S-9	De Flora *et al.* (1984)
Folpet	8 revertants/nmol, −S-9	
Captan	93.7 revertants/nmol, −S-9	Moriya *et al.* (1983)
Folpet	15.0 revertants/nmol, −S-9	

[a] +S-9: Rat liver homogenate included for "metabolism" of test material. −S-9: Incubation without rat liver homogenate.

Table 79.6
In Vitro Eukaryote Mutation Assays

Assay	Compound	Results	Reference
Chinese hamster V79/Hgprt	Captan	Positive only in the absence of serum from the culture media Mean number of resistant colonies: 0.3 and 0.6 at 5 and 10 μg/ml captan; vapor emitted from sodium bicarbonate activated captan impregnated on filter paper above the test system also induced mutations	Arlett *et al.* (1975)
Chinese hamster CHO/Hgprt	Captan and Folpet	Both compounds were positive in the absence of S-9	O'Neill *et al.* (1981)
Mouse lymphoma L5178Y/TK	Captan	Positive in the absence of S-9	Oberly *et al.* (1984)

showed a strong response to captan and a negative response to folpet (Nagy *et al.*, 1975) or, where both were positive, the revertants per plate were greater for captan than for folpet (Shirasu *et al.*, 1976). Both were positive with the WP2 try⁻hcr⁻ strain (Nagy *et al.*, 1975; Shirasu *et al.*, 1976) as well as other tests with the WP2 strain (Bridges *et al.*, 1972; Simmon *et al.*, 1976). Tests with *Bacillus subtilis* strains TK 6321 and 5211 were positive for both compounds: captan showed a greater mutagenic response than folpet (Shiau *et al.*, 1981). Captan also induced point mutations in *Aspergillus nidulans* (Martinez-Rossi and Azevedo, 1987).

Assays with eukaryote organisms such as Chinese Hamster cells and mouse lymphoma cells are shown in Table 79.6. These data show that captan and folpet induce mutations when measured *in vitro*. THPI was tested with *S. typhimurium* strains TA 98, 100, 1535, and 1202 as well as *E. coli* WP2 uvrA, and

was negative (Carver, 1985). Phthalimide is inactive in *S. typhimurium* as well (Rideg, 1982).

Effect of Exogenous Thiols on Mutagenicity Assays   The rat liver S-9 fraction is added to *in vitro* systems to simulate the metabolic capability of intact organisms. In this way compounds that are mutagenic only after they are metabolized by cell enzyme systems are detected. Metabolism, however, appears to play no role in the expression of mutagenicity of captan or folpet; on the contrary, the addition of S-9 serves to diminish mutagenic potency. The reduced mutagenic activity following the addition of S-9 is an example of the general phenomenon of thiol-related degradation of captan and folpet. The presence of sufficient thiols abolishes mutagenic activity. The addition of S-9 or rat blood prior to the addition of captan or folpet reduces or abolishes activity (Table 79.7).

Table 79.7
Comparison of Captan and Folpet Mutagenicity with the Addition of Exogenous Protein[a]

Strain and Dose	Component	Captan (rev/plate)	Folpet (rev/plate)	Comment[b]
E. coli	None	3200	1320	Captan is more active than folpet
WP2 hcr	S-9	30	50	S-9 decreases activity
0.15μ M/plate	S-9 fraction	111	60	S-9 fraction decreases activity
(45 μg/plate)	20-mM cysteine	19	21	Cysteine abolishes activity (control rev/plate < 30)
	Rat blood	32	19	Blood abolishes activity
S. typhimurium	None	268	219	Captan is more active than folpet
	S-9	6	8	S9 abolishes activity (control rev/plate <17)
TA 1535	S-9 fraction	31	35	S-9 fraction decreases activity
0.15 μM/plate	20 mM cysteine	4	6	Cysteine abolishes activity
(45 μg/plate)	Rat blood	6	14	Blood abolishes activity

[a]Reproduced from Moriya *et al.* (1978).
[b]Captan (0.1 ml of 1.5 μM/ml) or folpet (0.2 ml of 0.75 μM/ml) was incubated for 10 min at 37°C with 0.5 ml of one of the following: S-9 (containing 0.3 ml S-9/ml), S-9 fraction (S-9 mix minus cofactors), 20-mM cysteine, or rat blood diluted twice with phosphate buffer or water as control. After incubation the tester strains (0.1 ml) and agar (2 ml) were added to the test tubes and plated out. Revertants/plate were read after incubation at 37°C for 2 days.

Table 79.8
In Vivo Mutagenicity Assays

Assay	Compound	Results	Reference
Somatic cell mutation	Captan	Negative, oral	Nguyen (1981)
(mouse spot test)	Captan	2.2% frequency after intraperitoneal dose of 15 mg/kg	Imanishi *et al.* (1987)
	Folpet	Negative, oral	Moore (1985)
Somatic mutation and recombination (Drosophila SMART test)	Captan	Negative	Mollet and Wurgler (1974)
Mouse heritable translocation assay	Captan	Negative	Simmon *et al.* (1977)
Drosophila sex-linked	Captan	Negative	Kramers and Knaap (1973)
recessive lethal assay	Folpet	Negative	
	Captan	Negative	Mollet (1973)
	Captan	Weakly mutagenic	Valencia (1981)
	Folpet	Weakly mutagenic	
	Folpet	Negative	Vogel and Chandler (1974)
Mouse dominant	Captan	Negative	Jorgenson *et al.* (1976)
lethal assay	Folpet	Negative	
	Captan	Negative	Kennedy *et al.* (1975a)
	Folpet	Negative	
	Captan	Negative	Rideg (1982)
	Folpet	Negative	
	Folpet	Negative	Epstein *et al.* (1972)
	Captan	Negative	Simmon *et al.* (1977)
Rat dominant	Captan	Positive	Collins (1972a)
lethal assay	Folpet	Positive	Collins (1972b)
	Folpet	Negative	Bradfield (1980)

When cysteine is added to either captan or folpet in varying ratios, the mutagenic activity declines as the ratio increases from 0.5 to 2.5. At a ratio of 5-μm cysteine to 1-μm captan or folpet mutagenic activity is abolished (Moriya *et al.*, 1978). Glutathione provided similar protective actions when added to assay vessels in ratios of 1 or higher compared to the fungicide (Rideg, 1982). Adverse toxicity as well as mutagenicity in Chinese hamster V79 cells is reduced when 10% fetal calf serum is used in the standard V79/Hgprt assay (Arlett *et al.*, 1975).

***In Vivo* Assays**   Armed with knowledge of how these compounds degrade, it is not surprising that mutagenicity is absent *in vivo* (Table 79.8).

79.3.5.3 Cytogenetic Effects

The effects on chromosomes mirror the pattern of activity for mutations: clastogenic findings are seen *in vitro* but are generally absent *in vivo*.

***In Vitro* Assays**   Table 79.9 lists representative *in vitro* cytogenetic studies with captan or folpet. The addition of S-9

to assay vessels serves to detoxify captan and folpet as it does in the mutation assays. This action is expressed by a decrease in cytotoxicity with a resulting increase in tolerated dose levels. At some point it is expected that the threshold for detoxification is exceeded and the remaining captan or folpet can act to affect the chromosomes. These data are mixed in that some positive and some negative findings are reported.

***In Vivo* Assays**   Table 79.10 lists representative *in vivo* cytogenetic studies with captan or folpet. Micronucleus assays were conducted in CD-1 mice with both compounds and yielded negative results. Captan was administered at 40, 200, and 1000 mg/kg (Jacoby, 1985b) and folpet was administered at 10, 50, and 250 mg/kg (Jacoby, 1985a). Chlorambucil, the positive control, resulted in a significant increase in micronuclei. These negative results contrast with positive findings by Chinese investigators who treated mice with captan (96.5% purity) at 10, 50, 100, 400, and 800 mg/kg by gavage and reported a dose-related increase in micronuclei (Feng and Lin, 1987). These same investigators also reported effects on chromosomal aberrations at 400 mg/kg and above. The results remain unexplained.

Table 79.9

In Vitro Cytogenetic Assays

Assay	Compound	Results	Reference
Chinese hamster V79	Captan	Positive for sister chromatid exchange and chromosomal aberrations	Tezuka *et al.* (1980)
Chinese hamster lung fibroblasts	Captan, Folpet	Positive in the absence of S-9	Ishidate *et al.* (1981)
Chinese hamster ovary (CHO)	Folpet	Positive, but higher concentrations required with S-9	Loveday (1989)
Human blood lymphocytes	Captan	Negative	Pilinskaya (1983)
	Folpet	Negative (5 µg, 2-h exposure)	Bootman *et al.* (1987)
Human lymphoid cell line	Captan	Positive in the absence of S-9	Sirianni and Huang (1978)
Human diploid fibroblast cell line	Captan	Negative	Sasaki *et al.* (1980); Tezuka *et al.* (1978)
Human embryonic lung and rat kangaroo cell lines	Captan	Positive	Legator (1969)

The work by Chidiac (Chidiac, 1985; Chidiac and Goldberg, 1987) provides valuable information with regard to the genotoxicity of these compounds. The basis for this work drew upon evidence of mutagenicity and the tumorigenic effect captan has on the mouse duodenum. It was postulated that evidence of cytogenetic damage would be seen in the duodenum after exposure to captan. This mouse bioassay was validated with known carcinogens and noncarcinogens. Nuclear aberrations (NA) consisted of micronuclei and apoptotic bodies in the crypt cells of the duodenal epithelium. X-irradiation, 1,2-dimethylhydrazine, benzo(*a*)pyrene (B(*a*)P), and *N*-methyl-*N*-nitrosourea (MNU) induced tumors in the small intestine. Each led to a dose-related increase in the incidence of NA 24 h after administration to mice. Benzo(*e*)pyrene and methylurea, which are noncarcinogenic structural analogs of B(*a*)P and MNU, did not induce NA. Cells of the duodenum were harvested and examined for the presence of NA

after a variety of captan dose regimens. Captan as well as THPI consistently failed to induce NA. Captan was administered to male CD-1 mice using a number of regimens, including a single bolus dose of 4000 mg/kg, dietary dose levels of 4000 and 16,000 ppm, and five repetitive doses totaling 5000 mg/kg (Table 79.11). In all cases, including pretreatment with L-buthionin-*S*,*R*-sulfoximine (an inhibitor of glutathione synthesis), the investigators noted an absence of the expected signs of DNA damage.

Folpet was recently tested in a study that replicated the Chidiac experimental design (Gudi and Krsmanovic, 2001). Mice were administered five consecutive daily oral doses of folpet at 2000 mg/kg per day. Nuclear aberrations in the duodenal crypt compartment were absent in folpet-treated mice, whereas mice administered a single dose (65 mg/kg) of dimethylhydrazine showed both apoptotic cells and micronuclei in the crypts.

Table 79.10

In Vivo Cytogenetic Assays

Assay	Compound	Results	Reference
Micronucleus	Captan	Negative	Jacoby (1985b)
		Positive	Feng and Lin (1987)
	Folpet	Negative	Jacoby (1985a)
Chromosomal aberration	Captan	Negative	Tezuka *et al.* (1978)
		Negative	Fry and Fiscor (1978)
		Negative (see Table 22)	Chidiac and Goldberg (1987)
		Positive	Feng and Lin (1987)
	Folpet	Negative	Esber (1983)
Heritable translocation	Captan	Negative	Jorgenson *et al.* (1976)

Table 79.11
Nuclear Aberration Study with Captan[a]

Treatment	Dose levels		Results
Single bolus dose	0 and 4000 mg/kg		Negative
Single bolus dose after pretreatment with BSO[b]	0 and 4000 mg/kg		Negative
Dietary administration, 7 days	0, 8000, and 16,000 ppm		Negative
Five daily doses	Single	Cumulative	Negative
	0	0	
	20	100	
	200	1000	
	1000	5000[c]	

[a]Reproduced with permission from Chidiac and Goldberg (1987).
[b]BSO: L-buthionin-S,R-sulfoximine, an inhibitor of glutathione synthesis.
[c]Doses: Day 1, 2000 mg/kg; day 2, dosing suspended due to toxicity; days 3–5, 1000 mg/kg.

79.3.5.4 Dominant Lethal Assays

Dominant lethal assays have generally been negative (Table 79.7). However, positive findings for both compounds have been reported (Collins, 1972a, b). In spite of these positive findings, it appears that the compounds do not induce dominant lethal effects. This conclusion is based on (1) the absence of positive micronucleus assays [with the noted exception of Feng and Lin (1987)]; (2) the absence of adverse effects in two-generation rat reproductive studies; (3) the lack of negative dominant lethal effects in other studies [captan: Kennedy *et al.* (1975a), Rideg (1982), Shirasu *et al.* (1978), Tezuka *et al.* (1978); folpet: Bradfield (1980), Calandra (1971), Kennedy *et al.* (1975a), Rideg (1982)], and (4) the consistency of the findings with the rapid degradation of these compounds. A less than 1-s (captan) or less than 5-s (folpet) half-life in blood argues against the possibility of parent molecules reaching the testes. Thiophosgene is considered to be more reactive than captan or folpet, but also would not reach the testes.

79.3.5.5 DNA Interaction

Captan was negative for inducing unscheduled DNA synthesis (UDS) in human diploid fibroblasts *in vitro* (Mitchell, 1975). It was also negative for UDS in primary liver cells (Probst *et al.*, 1981; Rocchi *et al.*, 1980).

The nature of the captan and folpet molecules imparts difficulties in conducting *in vivo* DNA binding studies. Two approaches, using radiolabeled test material, have sought to determine if captan covalently binds with duodenal DNA of the mouse. In both cases, the trichloromethylthio side chain was labeled because it is the chemically active portion of the molecule and is expected to participate in DNA binding if it occurs. The first study used ^{14}C-captan (Selsky and Matheson, 1981); the second study used ^{35}S-captan (Provan *et al.*, 1995).

When the carbon atom of the trichloromethylthio moiety is labeled, it enters the C-1 carbon pool via CO_2 that is formed as the molecule degrades. As such, a low level of ubiquitous labeling appears throughout the mouse. When the sulfur atom

of the trichloromethylthio moiety is labeled, sulfur exchange occurs, resulting in a low level of incorporation of ^{35}S into proteins. Histones, in turn, are associated with DNA and result in a low level of associated radioactivity (Provan *et al.*, 1995). Investigators have concluded that covalent binding of captan to DNA has not been demonstrated (Pritchard and Lappin, 1991; Provan *et al.*, 1992, 1993; Selsky and Matheson, 1981). An experimental design that "proves the negative," however, has not been achieved and the EPA holds that *in vivo* DNA binding has not been ruled out (Hsu and McCarroll, 1998).

The polyps, adenomas, and adenocarcinomas that develop in the mouse duodenum as a result of continuous oral administration of captan or folpet arise from the crypt cell compartment. Figure 79.5 depicts a much simplified anatomy of the duodenum. Should mutagenicity play a role in the development of these tumors, it must be consistent with this anatomy and the nature of the chemical reactions associated with these compounds. There are two factors that suggest mutagenicity cannot be involved in the etiology of these tumors: first, nearly all absorption takes place through the villi; second, the degradation rates of captan and folpet prevent them from reaching the crypt compartment through diffusion. Material that is absorbed through the villi enters blood or lacteal vessels and is transported away from the crypts. Crypt cells receive blood supply from arterial vessels rather than the portal system. The remaining molecules that start to diffuse down to the crypt compartment must first pass through mucus and then diffuse through approximately 16 epithelial cells before reaching the stem cells located in position T4 from the base of the crypt (Potten and Loeffler, 1990). Mutational events in cells distal to the stem cells (some of which may still be dividing) are of no import because these cells migrate up the villi and are shed within 2–4 days. The duodenal mucosal cells are rich in glutathione, having a concentration of approximately 8 mmol in CD-1 mice (Chasseaud *et al.*, 1991); thus, the degradation of parent molecules is promoted. Whereas the half-lives of captan and folpet are very short, the exponential loss of captan virtually eliminates all molecules in short order.

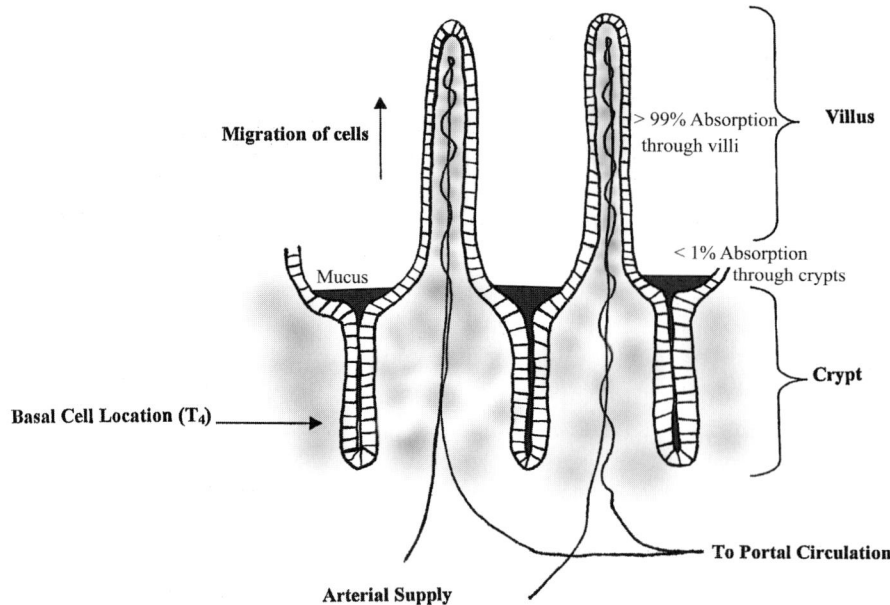

Figure 79.5 Schematic of duodenal villi and crypts.

In summary, captan and folpet are chemically active molecules that can induce mutations and cytogenetic effects if they are positioned to interact with sensitive targets. The very nature of this reactivity coupled with mammalian anatomy, however, precludes such interaction *in vivo*. This conclusion is supported by the weight of evidence (including chemical fate), although instances of positive results *in vivo* have been reported. Captan and folpet are judged not to act as mutagens or genotoxins in the intact animal.

79.3.6 CARCINOGENICITY

79.3.6.1 Overview

Carcinogenicity joins mutagenicity as a controversial topic with captan and folpet. Both compounds induce the development of duodenal tumors in mice when fed at high doses. This observation is cited by governmental agencies and has become the focus of regulatory actions. Rodent bioassay data are robust: there is a treatment and dose relationship of tumor incidence in mice, but such a relationship is absent in rats. Rat studies, however, have shown increased incidences of some tumors, but these are judged to be not treatment related (Gordon *et al.*, 1994).

This finding is not embraced by the EPA (Quest *et al.*, 1993; U.S. EPA, 1999a, b). At issue is the regulatory classification of captan and folpet. The current B2 classification held by the EPA characterizes these fungicides as "probable human carcinogens" (U.S. EPA, 1984b, 1986a, 1989). The framework around which the EPA analyzes captan and folpet carcinogenicity data is the 1986 carcinogen risk assessment guidelines (U.S. EPA, 1986c). The proposed new cancer guidelines (U.S. EPA, 1996) provide an opportunity for fresh evaluation that incorporates both mechanistic and chemical property data. Studied in

this light, both captan and folpet are judged not to pose a carcinogenic risk to humans and should be classified as "not likely to cause tumors at low doses." The practical meaning of such a classification is that captan and folpet are not human carcinogens.

79.3.6.2 Mouse Bioassays

An early captan study combined both gavage and dietary administration (Innes *et al.*, 1969). These investigators dosed neonatal F_1 hybrid mice by gavage with 215 mg/kg per day for 3 weeks and followed by dietary administration of 560 ppm for 18 months. This study was negative. However, the dietary concentration, in hindsight, appears to be below the threshold necessary for tumor induction. The National Cancer Institute administered captan to $B_6C_3F_1$ mice at 8000 and 16,000 ppm for 80 weeks (NCI, 1977). Duodenal tumors were evident at the high dose (3 in 46 males; 3 in 48 females). There was 1 in 43 males at the 8000 ppm that also had a tumor. Two other studies confirmed the treatment relationship of captan and duodenal tumors (Daly and Knezevich, 1983; Wong *et al.*, 1981). The tumor incidence is shown in Table 79.12. The NOEL for duodenal tumors in mice (based on proliferative changes in the duodenum) is 400 ppm.

Captan has also been evaluated by intraperitoneal and dermal administration. A study that treated two different "strain A" mice intraperitoneally with captan (along with 64 other chemicals previously tested by the National Cancer Institute) indicated a slight increase in lung tumors in males in one strain (Maronpot *et al.*, 1986), but the significance of these data was questioned due to lack of interlaboratory consistency and lack of correlation to the standard rodent bioassays (FAO/WHO, 1990). A dermal study using the two-stage carcinogenesis model concluded that captan was neither a complete skin car-

Table 79.12
Captan Duodenal Tumor Incidence in Mice[a]

	Dose (ppm and mg/kg/day)								
	0	100	400	800	6000	8000	10,000	16,000	
	0	15	61	123	925	NC	NC	NC	Reference
Males									
Adenoma	2/91	3/83	0/93	1/87	4/84				Daly and Knezevich
Carcinoma	0/91	0/83	0/93	0/87	2/84				(1983)[a]
Adenocarcinoma	0/9					3/43		5/46	NCI (1977)
Duodenal									Wong et al. (1981)[b]
neoplasms	2/74				20/73		21/72	39/75	
	0	100	400	800	6000	8000	10,000	16,000	
	0	18	70	142	1043	NC	NC	NC	
Females									
Adenoma	3/85	1/82	1/83	7/81	3/91				Daly and Knezevich
Carcinoma	0/85	0/83	0/83	0/81	1/91				(1983)[c]
Adenocarcinoma	0/9					0/49		3/48	NCI (1977)
Duodenal									Wong et al. (1981)[b]
neoplasms	2/72				24/78		19/76	26/76	

[a] NC: not calculated.
[b] Incidence reported reflects pathology reevaluation of slides (Robinson, 1993).
[c] The total tumor incidence combines both benign and malignant tumors.

cinogen nor a promoter, although at high doses (450 mg/kg three times per week for 3 weeks, followed by croton oil factor A₁ three times per week for 51 weeks) there was some evidence it may act as a weak initiator (Antony and Mehrota, 1994). Tissue damage rather than mutagenic effect might account for this finding, however, because the control, DMSO, did not replicate the irritation effects of captan.

The carcinogenic effect of folpet on the mouse duodenum is similar to that of captan (Table 79.13). The first two bioassays had doses of 1000, 5000, and 10,000 ppm (Rubin, 1985a), and 1000, 5000, and 12,000 ppm (Wong *et al.*, 1982). In both cases there was a low incidence of tumors at 1000 ppm. This finding triggered a third study with lower doses (East, 1994). The NOEL for tumors in the third study was established at 450 ppm. Although the primary site of gastrointestinal tumors is the duodenum in mice, a low incidence of tumors is seen in the stomach with folpet. There were some tumors noted with captan, but the incidence was low, not dose related, and not obviously treatment related. The differential aqueous stability in acid conditions of the stomach between captan and folpet may account for this finding. Captan elicits effects in the stomach, but these are restricted to polyp formation.

The blockage from the stomach to the duodenum seen in some mice that resulted from the presence of polyps and tumors located just after the pyloric sphincter was suggested as a contributing cause of stomach tumors (Nyska *et al.*, 1990). This blockage was thought to result in an increased concentration of folpet and folpet degradates in the stomach. Stomach tumors were evident, however, where no blockage was apparent and thus argue against this hypothesis (East, 1994).

79.3.6.3 Rat Bioassays

In contrast to mice, there is no consistent tumor response across studies with rats (Table 79.14). Evaluation of captan tumor incidence data for kidney and uterine tumors using appropriate statistics and proper tumor grouping shows no treatment effect (Foster and Elliott, 2000; Gordon *et al.*, 1994). It is unlikely the kidney tumors are related to treatment with captan because there is no increase in malignant tumors (carcinomas), there is a small increase (in a single animal) in benign tumors (adenomas) only, there is no statistically significant increase or trend in kidney adenomas, and the finding of kidney adenomas is seen in one out of four rat bioassays with captan and one out of seven bioassays with both captan and folpet.

It is unlikely the uterine sarcoma tumors are related to treatment with captan because there is no statistical significance when tumors and polyps are considered together, a consideration dictated by the etiology of uterine sarcomas (Leininger and Jokinen, 1990). The four tumors noted are comprised of three different cell types and this finding was not consistent with the other bioassay results. In evaluating this study, the JMPR found "no other effects" in addition to depression of food intake and body weight gain at 2000 ppm and a slight increase in relative liver weight in males (FAO/WHO, 1990). With folpet, the study director concluded that the incidence for mammary glands and thyroid tumors were not related to treatment (Crown *et al.*, 1985, 1989). The EPA, however, continues to cite the rat tumor data as supportive of their B2 classification of captan (U.S. EPA, 1985a) and folpet (U.S. EPA, 1995b).

Table 79.13
Folpet Duodenal Tumor (Adenoma/Carcinoma) Incidence in Mice

	Dose (ppm and mg/kg/day)								
	0	150	450	1000	1350	5000[a]	10,000[a]	12,000	
	0	16	47	93[b]	151	502[b]		1282	Reference
Males	0/52			4/52		17/52	25/52		Rubin (1985a)
	1/87			2/61		8/67		38/71	Wong *et al.* (1982)
	0/89	0/48	0/42		0/44				East (1994)
	0	150	450	1000	1350	5000[a]	10,000[a]	12,000	
	0	16	51	96[b]	154	515[b]		1284	
Females	1/51			2/52		10/52	19/52		Rubin (1985a)
	0/88			1/63		7/67		38/73	Wong *et al.* (1982)
	0/96	0/49	0/49		1/50				East (1994)

[a]Dose levels for the Rubin study were 5000 and 10,000 ppm for the first 21 weeks and then adjusted down to 3500 and 7000 ppm.
[b]Wong *et al.* (1982).

79.3.6.4 Comparison of Rat and Mouse Response to Folpet

A stark difference between mice and rats exists when comparing their tumor response to captan and folpet. All strains of mice tested show a treatment and dose-related incidence of duodenal tumors. All strains of rats show neither duodenal tumors nor proliferative changes. This suggests that the physiology of the mouse and rat differ in specific toxicokinetic and/or toxicodynamic ways that account for this difference. A series of comparative studies in the CD-1 mouse and Sprague–Dawley rat were conducted with folpet at 50 and 5000 ppm in an attempt to uncover the reason or reasons for this difference (Chasseaud *et al.*, 1991). Areas investigated included respective milligrams per kilogram per day doses, transit times through the gut, glutathione changes with dosing, effects on enzymes, pH changes, GSH levels, and binding of ^{14}C-folpet to intestinal components. There were a variety of quantitative differences between rats and mice; however, none appeared to account for the qualitative difference seen in tumor response. Had a "smoking gun" been elucidated, that is, had the precise basis for the rat being refractory and the mouse being susceptible been determined, then this factor in humans could be compared with these two species.

79.3.6.5 Relevance of Mutagenicity to Mouse Tumors and Human Risk Assessment

The presence or absence of a mutagenic component in the etiology of mouse duodenal tumors determines the paradigm used to assess risk to humans. Mutagenic carcinogens are thought to confer some increased risk at all dose levels, whereas chemicals that induce tumors through epigenetic means have thresholds. The paradigm for the mutagenic (nonthreshold) carcinogens assumes an increased risk at any dose above zero and is reflected by such mathematical paradigms as the linear multistage model (Pitot and Dragan, 1996) that determines the q_1^*, the slope of the 95% upper bound of the curve that describes increased risk. The procedure for assessing risk for threshold carcinogens is the MOE paradigm. MOE calculates the difference between the no effect level (NOEL) in rodent bioassays and the expected exposure to humans. An MOE of 100 or greater (NOEL/exposure > 100) is generally considered to provide sufficient safety.

Section 79.3.5 concluded that captan and folpet are not *in vivo* mutagens. This view was also reflected by the EPA in its PD4 document on captan: "The studies on the mutagenicity of captan lend significant support to its classification as an oncogen, but there is little or no risk of its producing mutagenic effects in humans" (U.S. EPA, 1989, p. 8126). Absent this mutagenic component, a plausible alternative explanation for these tumors must be advanced. This explanation must account for the development of tumors without requiring genetic damage such as alkylation of DNA or cross-linking of DNA to proteins. Mechanistic studies have provided these data.

79.3.6.6 Mode of Action Leading to Duodenal Tumors in the Mouse

There is a preponderance of data that point unambiguously to a proliferation-based nongenotoxic mode of action for captan and folpet. This mode of action is consistent with the chemical and physical properties of captan and folpet, and the effect these compounds produce with high dietary exposure in the mouse. A key component of this mode of action is that it is threshold-based; that is, at dietary doses below the threshold, tumors will not develop.

The physical and chemical properties include the instability of captan and folpet in aqueous solution at physiological pH, the reaction of captan and folpet with thiols, the generation of thiophosgene from both hydrolysis and thiol interactions, the transient nature of thiophosgene due to its chemical reactivity,

Table 79.14
Rat Bioassays with Captan and Folpet

Test material	Experimental design	Findings[a]	Reference
Captan	Osborne–Mendel	Negative	NCI (1977)
	0, 2525, 6060 ppm (TWA)[b]		
	mg/kg/day not calculated		
	Wistar (Cpb:WU)	Negative (uterus)	Til *et al.* (1983)
	0, 125, 500, 2000 ppm		
	0, 6.25, 24, 98 mg/kg/day		
	Charles River CD1	Negative (kidney)	Goldenthal *et al.* (1982)
	0, 500, 2000, 5000 ppm		
	0, 25, 100, 250 mg/kg/day		
	0, 1000, 5000, 10,000 ppm	Negative	Hazleton (1956)
	mg/kg/day not calculated		
Folpet	Fischer (chronic toxicity study)	Negative	Crown *et al.* (1989)
	0, 250, 1500, 5000 ppm		
	0, 12.5, 75, 250 mg/kg/day		
	CD	Negative (thyroid, testes)	Cox *et al.* (1985)
	0, 200, 800, 3200 ppm		
	0, 10, 40, 160 mg/kg/day		
	Fischer	Negative (mammary glands, thyroid, lymphoma)	Crown *et al.* (1985)
	0, 500, 1000, 2000 ppm		
	0, 25, 50, 100 mg/kg/day		

[a] The EPA notes the incidence of tumors (in tissues) "associated" with treatment in organs listed in support of B2 cancer classification for both captan and folpet (Quest *et al.*, 1993). Weight of evidence analysis shows captan is not a rat carcinogen (Foster and Elliott, 2000) nor is folpet (Study Director conclusions).
[b] TWA: time weighted average.

and the comparatively low toxicity of THPI and phthalimide. The mode of action for mouse duodenal tumors must be consistent with these properties and effects. It must also be supported by generally accepted principles of carcinogenicity.

Mouse duodenal tumors develop with oral administration above a threshold if maintained for at least 6 months (Pavkov and Thomasson, 1985). Histopathological analysis shows that tumors arise from the crypt compartment and show a continuum from hyperplasia to polyps, adenomas, and adenocarcinomas (Tinston, 1995, 1996). Histologic and proliferation studies have characterized the changes to the duodenum with exposure to captan and show two sequential events (Allen, 1994; Foster, 1994). First, epithelial cells that comprise the villi are damaged by exposure to captan and sloughed off into the intestinal lumen at an increased rate. The villi height is shortened. Second, basal cells in the crypt compartment that normally divide at a rate commensurate with the normal loss of villi cells from the tips of the villi increase their rate of proliferation to a hyperphysiologic state. Crypt depth is subsequently increased and the villi-to-crypt ratio (measured by their respective sizes) decreases.

A small number of transformed cells exist in the duodenum as evidenced by a low incidence of duodenal tumors in bioassay control (Tables 79.12 and 79.13) and historical control mice (Bomhard and Mohr, 1989; Chandra and Frith, 1992; Lang, 1995; Maita *et al.*, 1988; Ward *et al.*, 1979). It is postulated

that these transformed cells are subject to proliferative pressure and, as a result of this continued pressure for at least 6 months, progress to tumors. The basis for this postulation is the body of data that show abnormally high cell proliferation, which is not carcinogenic *per se*, but does play a role in tumor development (Butterworth *et al.*, 1992; Ledda-Columbano *et al.*, 1989; Pitot *et al.*, 1991). The role of proliferation in thyroid tumors is well established (Chhabra *et al.*, 1992) and the influence of proliferation on initiated liver cells is also known (Solt *et al.*, 1977). Classically, the two-stage carcinogenesis model in the skin points to the importance of sustained proliferation in the promotion of initiated cells to tumors (Berenblum and Armuth, 1977).

In addition to promoting the clonal expansion of nascent tumor cells *in situ*, abnormally high proliferation may increase fixation and expression of premutagenic DNA lesions, increase the number of spontaneously initiated cells during replication, perturb checkpoints in the cell cycle leading to mutagenic events, and increase the number of spontaneously initiated cells by blocking cell death/elimination (Ledda-Columbano *et al.*, 1989). Thus, there are two avenues for duodenal tumors to develop: promotion of nascent tumors cells and initiation of normal basal cells through disruptions in normal DNA replication.

The progression to tumors under this mode of action is depicted schematically in Fig. 79.6. A genetic component is nei-

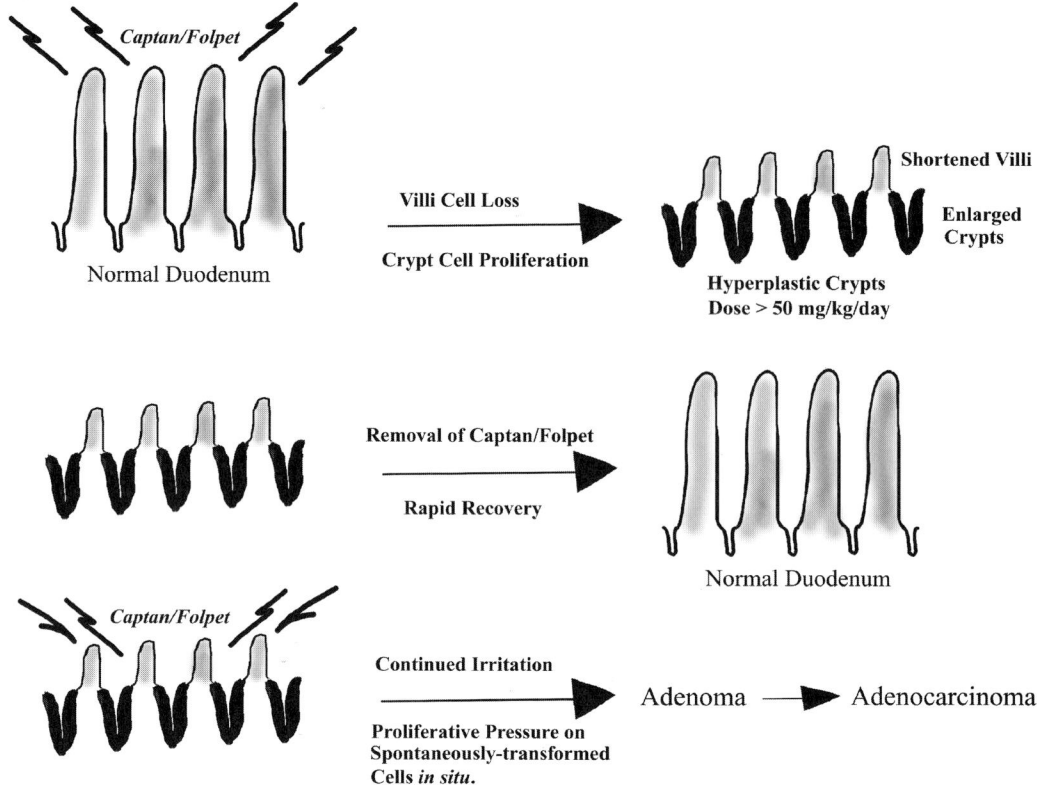

Figure 79.6 Mode of action for captan and folpet in the mouse duodenum.

ther required nor plausible. Thresholds have been established for the initial cellular response to captan or folpet administration: villi damage and crypt cell hyperplasia. The NOELs for captan and folpet are similar: 400 ppm (60 mg/kg per day) for captan and 450 (69 mg/kg per day; males) or 150 ppm (29 mg/kg per day; females) for folpet. Administration of captan or folpet below these thresholds will not lead to tumors, because the basis for tumor progression (hyperphysiologic cell division rate) is absent. This mode of action requires that the appropriate paradigm for assessing carcinogenic risk in humans is margin of exposure not linear low-dose extrapolation (q_1^*).

79.3.6.7 Epidemiology

In a limited retrospective cohort mortality study, 138 workers in a captan manufacturing plant who were employed for a minimum of 3 months during a 23-year period beginning in 1954 were followed for 30 years (Palshaw, 1980). These workers were exposed to captan at estimated air concentrations ranging from 0.83 mg/m^3 for THPI operators to 1.54 mg/m^3 for captan operators. Other workers had little or no exposure (originally ranked as 0, 1, 2, or 3 for none, low, moderate, or high, respectively). These data showed there were no increased deaths that resulted from captan exposure.

79.3.6.8 Summary

Captan and folpet at sufficiently high doses act locally on the duodenal mucosa and result in damage to villi. Epithelial cells

of the villi are lost and the homeostatic feedback mechanism increases cell proliferation in an attempt to make up this loss. Transformed cells that reside in the crypt compartment are sensitive to this proliferative pressure and are promoted to frank tumors (Fig. 79.6). This mode of action has no mutagenic component and has a clear threshold for the first event that leads to tumors: increased proliferation/hyperplasia of the duodenal crypt compartment.

79.4 COMMON MECHANISM OF TOXICITY

79.4.1 CAPTAN AND FOLPET

Captan and folpet show obvious similarities in structure and effects. The Food Quality Protection Act (U.S. Congress, 1996) formally recognized the existence of such similarities and mandated that the EPA consider common mechanisms of toxicity when conducting risk assessments. The EPA issued guidance on how to determine the presence of a common mechanism for two or more pesticides (U.S. EPA, 1999c). Their criteria include structure, adverse effects, and mode of action. Captan and folpet share sufficient common characteristics to conclude that they have a common mechanism of toxicity (Bernard and Gordon, 2000). This finding is specific to the key toxicological endpoint, duodenal tumors in mice, but may apply as well to other nonspecific endpoints. The finding that a common mechanism of toxicity exists for captan and folpet is supported by the following determinations:

1. Structural similarity. The active side chains, $-SCCl_3$, are identical.
2. Site of action. Toxicity is expressed at the site of contact for both chemicals (that is, they are local irritants as opposed to systemic toxicants).
3. Reactivity with thiols. Both react with thiols to produce similar degradates. Differences in rates of reaction are attributable to physical/chemical properties of the two compounds and do not serve to diminish their commonality.
4. Mechanism of pesticidal action. Toxicity to fungi is mediated through reactions with both soluble and insoluble thiols in fungal conidia. These same reactions account for expression of the common toxic endpoint in mammals.
5. Common toxic endpoint. Gastrointestinal tumors in mice that generally are specific to the duodenum.
6. Mode of action. Both captan and folpet express their common toxic endpoint through a nongenotoxic compensatory proliferation mechanism.
7. Specificity of action. For both materials, the majority of tumors appear in the duodenum, but with folpet, some tumors are noted in the stomach. The hydrolytic rate of folpet is approximately 8 times faster than that of captan at pH 5 and may promote the presence of active metabolites in the acid environment of the stomach. Tumors are restricted to the mouse; rats are refractory.
8. Other toxic endpoints. Both captan and folpet show a similar pattern of toxicity for mutagenicity and skin sensitization. Both compounds show nonspecific secondary endpoints such as developmental toxicity manifested as decreased fetal weights and ossification defects at maternally toxic doses.

Finding a common mechanism of toxicity for captan and folpet will influence the way the EPA regulates these two fungicides under FQPA. It also will afford toxicologists an opportunity to integrate data from the individual compounds to generate a more robust data base, which is particularly valuable for evaluation of noncarcinogenicity in rats and elucidation of the mode of action of carcinogenicity in mice.

79.4.2 CAPTAFOL

Captafol (CAS 2939-80-2, Fig. 79.7) differs from captan and folpet in a number of areas. The side chain differs in structure as well as chemical activity. The two-carbon tetrachloro moiety of captafol is able to produce an episulfonium ion that can act as a systemic alkylating agent (Fig. 79.8). This ion, absent with captan and folpet, is able to enter the systemic circulation and may be carcinogenic (Williams, 1992). The spectrum of tumors in rodent bioassays is broad and affects both mice (Ito *et al.*, 1984) and rats (Nyska *et al.*, 1989; Quest *et al.*, 1993), whereas the tumor spectrum of captan and folpet is narrow, focusing on

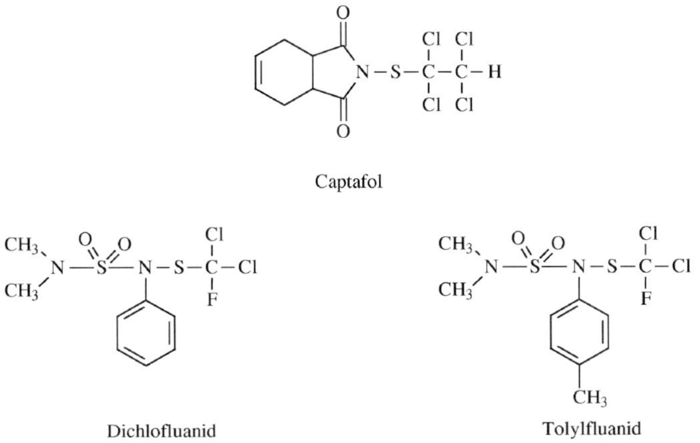

Figure 79.7 Captafol, dichlofluanid, and tolylfluanid.

the mouse duodenum (Gordon *et al.*, 1994). Mutagenic results in some assays show a differing pattern of activity. For example, when tested in *S. typhimurium*, TA 102 and TA 104, captan was negative in strain TA 102 and positive in strain TA 104, whereas captafol was negative for TA 104 and positive for TA 102 (Barrueco and de la Pena, 1988). In *S. typhimurium* strains TA 100, TA 98, TA 1535, TA 1537, and TA 1538 as well as *E. coli* strain WP2 *hcr*, captan and folpet were positive in all systems, whereas captafol was positive only in WP2 *hcr* and was "doubtful" in TA 100 (Moriya *et al.*, 1983).

Two results follow from the finding that captafol does not share a common mechanism of toxicity with captan and folpet. First, under FQPA, residues will not be combined for a cumulative risk assessment. Second, the "structural similarity" (Quest *et al.*, 1993) of captafol should not be referenced when evaluating the carcinogenicity of captan or folpet. The first point is moot, because captafol is not registered in the United States; the second point avoids confounding comparisons.

79.4.3 DICHLOFLUANID AND TOLYLFLUANID

Dichlofluanid (CAS 1085-98-9) and tolylfluanid (CAS 731-27-1) do not share a common mechanism of toxicity with captan or folpet with regard to mouse duodenal tumors, principally because they do not induce these tumors. Both compounds have a fluorine atom substituted for one of the three chlorine atoms on the trichloromethylthio moiety (Fig. 79.7). They differ from one another by the addition of a methyl group on

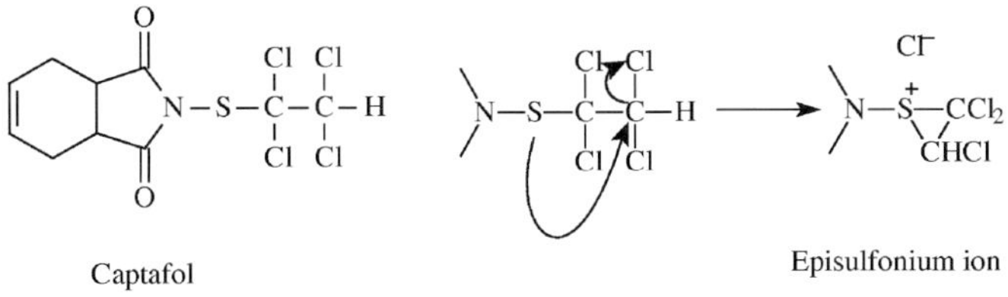

Figure 79.8 Episulfonium ion formation by captafol.

the benzene ring. Like captan and folpet, these compounds react with sulfhydryl groups (Schuphan *et al.*, 1981). The monofluorodichloromethylthio moiety conveys more chemical reactivity to the parent as measured by the reaction rate with 4-nitrothiophenol compared to the trichloromethylthio moiety. The reaction rate of dichlofluanid is over twice that of captan and folpet, but the trichloro dichlofluanid analog is less reactive than either captan or folpet. Dichlofluanid and its bis(fluorodichloromethyl) disulfide degradate were reported to be negative for mutagenicity in *S. typhimurium* TA100, whereas the bis-(trichloromethyl) disulfide from captan and folpet was positive (Schuphan *et al.*, 1981). The presence of the fluorine atom apparently lessens the mutagenicity of these compounds. Thiophosgene and its monofluorine analog are postulated to be degradates of dichlofluanid. Either compound reacts with cysteine to form TTCA in a similar way as it is formed with captan or folpet.

These compounds have been reviewed by the Joint Meeting of the FAO Panel of Experts on Pesticide Residues in Food and the Environment and the WHO Expert Group on Pesticide Residues (FAO/WHO, 1984, 1989). Dichlofluanid was negative for carcinogenicity when tested in mice at 5000 ppm. The levels that cause no toxicological effect in rats and dogs are 500 (30 mg/kg bw per day) and 1000 ppm (25 mg/kg bw per day), respectively. For tolylfluanid, the levels that cause no toxicological effect in rats and dogs are 300 ppm (15 mg/kg bw per day) and 12.5 mg/kg bw per day, respectively. The absence of duodenal tumors in mice suggests that the ability to induce these tumors is not a general property of the chloroalkylthio fungicides.

79.5 HUMAN RISK ASSESSMENT

79.5.1 CANCER

In contrast to the relatively high background duodenal tumor incidence seen in mice, the incidence in humans (Parkin *et al.*, 1992) and rats (Goodman *et al.*, 1979; Maekawa *et al.*, 1983; Maita *et al.*, 1987; McMartin *et al.*, 1992) is low. This suggests that humans are closer to rats; that is, humans are refractory to tumors with captan or folpet because the number of transformed cells *in situ* is low. Nonetheless, prudence dictates that humans be considered similarly to the mouse for risk assessment purposes.

The no effect levels for duodenal crypt cell proliferation, the prerequisite for tumor formation, are 400 ppm for captan and 150–450 ppm for folpet. The approximate equivalent doses are 30–60 mg/kg per day. For this assessment we used a NOEL of 50 mg/kg per day.

Humans are exposed to captan and folpet predominantly by two routes: oral and dermal. Exposure via the oral route occurs through consumption of food that contains residues; exposure via the dermal route occurs through the use of products that contain these fungicides. Exposure from food is low and there are no contributions from water. Milk, which is both aqueous

based and metabolically produced, was shown to have no captan or degradates present. A national milk survey for captan that was conducted over the course of 1 year and analyzed 224 samples from a statistically derived paradigm across four regions of the United States (North East, North Central, West, and South) found no detectable levels (LOQ = 0.005 ppm) of captan, THPI, 3-OH-THPI, or 5-OH-THPI (Slesinski and Wilson, 1992).

Exposure to oral residues only is considered relevant for human cancer risk assessment. Dermal exposure is not relevant for human cancer risk assessment, because dermal contact does not result in systemic exposure and captan has been found not to be a skin carcinogen (Antony and Mehrota, 1994). For both captan and folpet, the EPA has calculated the estimated exposure for cancer risk purposes as 0.00005 mg/kg per day (U.S. EPA, 1999a, b).

The MOE for each of these fungicides, based on a NOEL for duodenal crypt cell proliferation of 50 mg/kg per day is 1,000,000. These MOEs suggest virtually no risk of cancer to persons who consume produce treated with either captan or folpet. It is unlikely that both compounds would be present on the same commodity at the same time because the uses of captan in the United States do not overlap those of folpet. Additionally, normal agronomic practice usually relies on one or the other, not both. Nonetheless, if the expected residues are combined for a cumulative risk assessment, the MOE is still satisfactory.

This analysis shows that humans are not at risk for duodenal tumors from these fungicides. This level of risk would be characterized as "not likely at oral low doses" and "not likely by dermal exposure" according to the proposed cancer risk assessment guidelines (U.S. EPA, 1996). In contrast to the EPA B2 classification, the practical meaning of this assessment, based on the mode of action of captan and folpet is that they are not human carcinogens. This assessment is particularly relevant for reentry workers such as strawberry harvesters who might be exposed to captan residues.

79.5.2 NONCANCER

For noncancer risks, captan and folpet present an interesting challenge for risk assessors. The transient nature of these molecules coupled with their inherent low toxicity make it difficult to assign meaningful endpoints. Noncancer endpoint risk characterization requires the selection of relevant endpoints for nondietary and dietary exposure, and that NOELs be determined for both acute and chronic exposure. Nondietary exposure, in turn, comprises dermal exposure (including eye exposure) and inhalation.

Three nondietary hazards associated with captan and folpet that are relevant to human safety are skin sensitization, eye irritation, and lung irritation. Only one of these, skin sensitization, appears to effect persons who come in contact with these materials. The incidence of sensitization reactions is below 10% in trials with captan and well below this incidence in actual use

(Krieger, 2001). Systemic toxicity from dermal exposure is not possible due to the labile nature of these molecules in the blood. Skin irritation from single instance contact with captan or folpet is not expected. Repetitive dermal exposure, however, might induce progressive skin irritation, although it is not evident with people who repeatedly use a shampoo containing 7% captan (Guo, 2001).

Inhalation is a potential avenue for adverse effects, although the absence of adverse reports suggest that this is not an issue. The AIHGH has assigned a threshold limit value of 5 mg/m^3 for captan (ACGIH, 1998) and the same value has been suggested as appropriate for folpet (Seifried, 1996).

For acute dietary risk, the EPA has used the NOEL from developmental studies for both captan (U.S. EPA, 1995a) and folpet (Levy *et al.*, 1997). For captan, this is 10 mg/kg per day, based on effects at 30 mg/kg per day (a maternally toxic dose) in a rabbit study. For folpet, this is 10 mg/kg per day, based on effects at 20 mg/kg per day in a rabbit study. This "default" selection is not ideal because the NOEL is based on multiple doses, it is based on effects on the fetus not the individual, and it is specific for a subgroup (women of childbearing age) that comprises only part of the general population. A meaningful acute dietary risk assessment is dependent on an appropriately designed single exposure oral toxicity study; such data are not currently at hand.

Captan acute dietary exposure at the 99th percentile is estimated for the general U.S. population at 0.009512 mg/kg per day (Kidwell and Watters, 1999); the exposure for folpet is estimated at 0.00046 mg/kg per day (Guo, 2001; Petersen, 1997). The EPA estimates these acute dietary exposures at 0.036 mg/kg per day for captan at the 99.9th percentile (U.S. EPA, 1999a) and at 0.001532 mg/kg per day for folpet at the 99th percentile (U.S. EPA, 1999b). For chronic EPA estimates, the dietary exposure for the general population in the United States is at 0.000664 mg/kg per day for captan and at 0.000053 mg/kg per day for folpet (U.S. EPA, 1999a, b). For chronic dietary risk assessment, the captan NOEL of 12.5 mg/kg per day and the folpet NOEL of 9 mg/kg per day are used. Margins of exposure (NOEL ÷ exposure) for captan are 18,825 and for folpet are 169,811. The WHO ADI is 0.1 mg/kg per day for both captan (FAO/WHO, 1990) and folpet (FAO/WHO, 1996). This is approximately equal to the EPA's cPAD for captan, 0.13 mg/kg per day, and the EPA's PAD (without the threefold FQPA safety factor) for folpet, 0.09 mg/kg per day.

79.6 CONCLUSION

Captan and folpet are structurally similar molecules that act through a common mechanism with regard to their ability to induce duodenal tumors in mice. The mode of action has been elucidated for these tumors and is dependent on irritation to and cell loss from the intestinal villi, followed by a compensatory increase in proliferation within the crypt compartment. This proliferative pressure, with time, promotes transformed cells that are normally resident *in situ*.

The mode of action is not dependent on a mutagenic component nor are mutations within basal cells of the crypts a plausible occurrence. Captan and folpet are, however, mutagenic when tested in a variety of *in vitro* systems, and this observation has challenged investigators to solve the paradox that exists between *in vitro* and *in vivo* test results. The solution to this question is the finding that these compounds degrade extremely rapidly when thiols are present. In human blood, captan's $t^{1/2}$ is less than 1 s and folpet's is less than 5 s. Thiophosgene, the reactive degradate that is formed from the trichloromethylthio side chain, reacts not only with thiols, but with other functional groups as well and is also rapidly lost.

The import of this rapid degradation is that systemic exposure to captan, folpet, or their common degradate, thiophosgene, is absent. This, along with the low estimated dermal absorption rate of 0.5% per hour, assures that adverse systemic risk in agricultural workers is absent. Local effects due to irritation, however, may occur. These include eye and skin irritation, skin sensitization, and irritation of the airways. Oral exposure at sufficient doses will irritate the mucus membranes of the gastrointestinal tract.

Systemic effects noted in laboratory studies such as depressed weight gain or delayed development of fetuses and pups are secondary effects that result from the primary irritation of the gastrointestinal tract. Thus, captan and folpet, when used in the agricultural setting are characterized as follows:

- They have low acute toxicity.
- They are not carcinogenic, mutagenic, or teratogenic.
- They are neither selective developmental toxins nor are they reproductive toxins.

Relevant hazards are the following:

- Irritation of mucus membranes.
- Sensitization after repeated exposure.
- Irritation of the skin after repeated exposures (specifically for folpet).
- Irritation of the airways.

These products have been in use for over 50 years and experience shows that eye irritation and sensitization reactions, particularly with reentry operations, are not problematic. In addition, a limited survey of persons using a 7% captan-based shampoo indicates that repeated use does not cause skin irritation or skin sensitization reactions.

The risks of captan and folpet are low; the benefits to the agricultural community are high. Captan and folpet remain valuable fungicides.

REFERENCES

Reports with MRID numbers are available from U.S. Environmental Protection Agency, Freedom of Information Office, Ariel Rios Building, 1200 Pennsylvania Avenue, N.W., Washington, DC 20460.

ACGIH (1998). "Threshold Limit Values (TLVs) for Chemical Substances and Physical Agents and Biological Exposure Indices (BEIs)." American Conference of Governmental Industrial Hygienists, Cincinnati, OH.

Adir, J., Chin, T., and Ruch, G. (1982). "Captan 50-WP: A Dermal Absorption Study in Rats." Report T-11008, Stauffer Chemical Company (MRID 00117083).

Allen, S. L. (1994). "Captan: Investigation of Duodenal Hyperplasia in Mice." Report CTL/L/5674, Central Toxicology Laboratory, Cheshire, UK (MRID 43393503).

Antony, M. Y. S., and Mehrota, N. K. (1994). Preliminary carcinogenic and cocarcinogenic studies on captan following topical exposure in mice. *Bull. Environ. Contam. Toxicol.* **52**, 203–211.

Arlett, C. F., Turnbull, D., Harcourt, S. A., Lehman, A. R., and Colella, C. M. (1975). A comparison of the 8-azaguanine and ouabain-resistance systems for the selection of induced mutant Chinese hamster cells. *Mutat. Res.* **33**, 261–278.

Barel, Z., Nyska, A., and Waner, T. (1985). "Folpan, 90-Day Preliminary Toxicity Study in Beagle Dogs." Report MAK/061/FOL, Life Science Research Israel, Ness Ziona, Israel (MRID 00147135).

Barrueco, C., and de la Pena, E. (1988). Mutagenic evaluation of the pesticides captan, folpet, captafol, dichlofluanid and related compounds with the mutants TA102 and TA104 of *Salmonella typhimurium*. *Mutagenesis* **3**(6), 467–480.

Ben-Dyke, R., Sanderson, D. M., and Noakes, D. N. (1970). Acute toxicity data for pesticides. *World Rev. Pest Control* **9**, 119–127.

Berenblum, I., and Armuth, V. (1977). Effect of colchicine injection prior to the initiating phase of two-stage skin carcinogenesis in mice. *Br. J. Cancer* **35**, 615–620.

Bernard, B. K., and Gordon, E. B. (2000). An evaluation of the common mechanism approach to the Food Quality Protection Act: Captan and four related fungicides, a practical example. *Int. J. Toxicol.* **19**(1), 43–61.

Bionetics Research Laboratories (1968). "Evaluation of Carcinogenic, Teratogenic, and Mutagenic Activities of Selected Pesticides and Industrial Chemicals. Vol. II: Teratogenic Study in Mice and Rats." Report NCI-DCCP-CG-1973-1-2, National Cancer Institute.

Blagden, S. M. (1991). "Captan Technical: Acute Inhalation Toxicity Study. Four-Hour Exposure (Nose Only) in the Rat." Report 306/102, SafePharm Laboratories Limited, Derby, UK.

Blair, M. (1987). "Four Week Oral Range-Finding Study in Beagle Dogs with Captan." Report 153-197, International Research and Development Corporation, Northbrook, IL.

Blair, M. (1988). "One Year Oral Toxicity Study in Dogs with Captan Technical." Report 153-198, International Research and Development Corporation, Northbrook, IL (MRID 40893604).

Bomhard, E., and Mohr, U. (1989). Spontaneous tumors in NMRI mice from carcinogenicity studies. *Exp. Pathology* **36**(3), 129–145.

Bootman, J., Dance, C. A., and Hodson-Walker, G. (1987). "*In Vitro* Assessment of the Clastogenic Activity of Folpan Technical in Cultured Human Lymphocytes." Report 87/MAK053/031, Life Science Research, Eye, England (MRID 42122015).

Boyd, E. M., and Krijnen, C. J. (1968). Toxicity of captan and protein-deficient diet. *J. Clin. Pharmacol.* 225–234.

Bradfield, L. G. (1980). "Dominant Lethal Study of Phaltan Technical (folpet)." Report SOCAL 1355, Chevron Environmental Health Center, Richmond, CA (MRID 00029462).

Bratt, N. (1990). "Captan: Repeat Dose Study (10 mg/kg) in the Rat." Report CTL/P/2958, ICI Central Toxicology Laboratory, Alderley Park, Macclesfield, England (MRID 41505404).

Braun, A. G., and Horowicz, P. B. (1983). Lictin-mediated attachment assay for teratogens: Results with 32 pesticides. *J. Toxicol. Environ. Health* **11**(2), 275–286.

Bridges, B. A., Mottershead, R. P., Rothwell, M. A., and Green, M. H. L. (1972). Repair-deficient bacterial strains suitable for mutagenic screening: Tests with the fungicide captan. *Chem.-Biol. Interact.* **5**, 77–84.

Butterworth, B. E., Popp, J. A., Conolly, R. B., and Goldsworthy, T. L. (1992). Chemically induced cell proliferation in carcinogenesis. *IARC Sci. Publ.* **116**, 279–305.

Calandra, J. (1971). "Phaltan Mutagenic Study in Mice (Albino). Bateman Dominant Lethal Gene Test." Report 99447, Industrial Bio-Test Laboratories, Inc.

Carere, A., Ortali, V. A., Cardamone, G., Torracca, A. M., and Raschetti, R. (1978). Microbiological mutagenicity studies of pesticides in vitro. *Mutat. Res.* **57**, 277–286.

Carver, J. H. (1985). "Microbial/Mammalian Microsome Mutagenicity Plate Incorporation Assay with Tetrahydrophthalimide." Report CEHC 2618, Chevron Environmental Health Center, Richmond, CA.

Cavalli, M. S. (1970). "Acute Oral Toxicity of Tetrahydrophthalimide." Report SOCO 163/IV:5, Standard Oil Company of California.

Chandra, M., and Frith, C. H. (1992). Spontaneous neoplasms in aged CD-1 mice. *Toxicol. Lett.* **61**, 67–74.

Chasseaud, L. (1980). "(Carbonyl-14C) Folpet Metabolism in Rats." Report DPBP 51202, Huntingdon Research Centre Ltd., Huntingdon, England.

Chasseaud, L., Hawkins, D. R., Franklin, E. R., and Weston, K. T. (1974). "The Metabolic Fate of ^{14}C-Folpet (Phaltan) in the Rat (Folpet)." Report CHR1/74482, Huntingdon Research Centre Ltd., Huntingdon, England.

Chasseaud, L. F., Hall, M., and McTigue, J. J. (1991). "Comparative Metabolic Fate and Biochemical Effects of Folpet in Male Rats and Mice." Report NRC/MBS 32/90110, Huntingdon Research Centre Ltd., Cambridgeshire, England (MRID 42122016).

Cheng, H. M. (1980). "Metabolism of [Carbonyl-^{14}C]-Captan in a Lactating Goat." Report File 721.14, Agricultural Chemicals Division, Research and Development Department, Chevron Chemical Company, Richmond, CA (MRID 00058940).

Chhabra, R. S., Eustis, S., Haseman, J. K., Kurtz, P. J., and Carlton, B. D. (1992). Comparative carcinogenicity of ethylene thiourea with or without perinatal exposure in rats and mice. *Fundam. Appl. Toxicol.* **18**, 405–417.

Chidiac, P. (1985). "Genotoxicity of Captan in Murine Duodenum." Thesis, University of Guelph, Ontario, Canada.

Chidiac, P., and Goldberg, M. T. (1987). Lack of induction of nuclear aberrations by captan in mouse duodenum. *Environ. Mutagen.* **9**, 297–306.

Cisson, C. M., Bullock, C. H., and Wong, Z. A. (1982). "Eye Irritation Potential of Phaltan Technical (PN 2623)." Report SOCAL 1907, Environmental Health & Toxicology, Standard Oil Company of California, Richmond, CA.

Cisson, C. M., Bullock, C. H., and Wong, Z. A. (1983). "The Acute Eye Irritation Potential of Codicap W. P." Report SOCAL 2119, Environmental Health & Toxicology, Standard Oil Company of California.

Collins, T. F. X. (1972a). Dominant lethal assay: I. Captan. *Food Cosmet. Toxicol.* **10**, 353–361.

Collins, T. F. X. (1972b). Dominant lethal assay: II. Folpet and Difolatan. *Food Cosmet. Toxicol.* **10**, 363–371.

Copley, M. P. (1985). EPA Data Evaluation "Acute Toxicological Study of Captan after Intraperitoneal Application to the Rat." EPA Data Evaluation Report DER 004451, Environmental Protection Agency [MRID (Accession No.) 252585].

Corden, M. T. (1997). "14C-Folpet—Metabolism in the Lactating Goat. Part A. 14C-Trichloromethyl Folpet: Material Balance of Dosed Radioactivity." Report MBS 72a/972856, Huntingdon Life Sciences Ltd., Huntingdon, England (MRID 44807701).

Couch, R., and Siegel, M. R. (1972). Reactions of the trichloromethyl sulfenyl fungicides with histones. *Phytopathology* **62**(8), 802.

Couch, R. C., and Siegel, M. R. (1977). Interaction of captan and folpet with mammalian DNA and histones. *Pestic. Biochem. Physiol.* **7**, 531–546.

Couch, R. C., Siegel, M. R., and Dorough, H. W. (1977). Fate of captan and folpet in rats and their effects on isolated liver nuclei. *Pestic. Biochem. Physiol.* **7**, 547–558.

Courtney, K. D., Andrews, J. E., Stevens, J. T., and Farmer, J. D. (1983). "Inhalation Teratology Studies of Captan and Folpet in Mice." Report EPA-

600/1-83-017, Health Effects Research Laboratory, U.S. Environmental Protection Agency, Springfield, VA.

Cox, R. H., Marshall, P. M., Voelker, R. W., Vargas, K. J., Alsaker, R. D., and Dudeck, L. E. (1985). "Combined Chronic Oral Toxicity/Oncogenicity Study in Rats with Chevron Folpet Technical (SX-1388)." Report, Project 2107-109, Hazleton Labs America, Inc., Vienna, VA (MRID 00151560).

Cracknell, S. (1993). "Folpet Technical (Micronized): Acute Inhalation Toxicity Study in the Rat." Report 93/MAK139B/0507, Pharmaco-LSR Ltd., Eye, Suffolk, England (MRID 44286301).

Crossley, J. (1967a). "The Stability of Captan in the Blood." Report File 721.11, Chevron Chemical Company (MRID 00025128, 00043382).

Crossley, J. (1967b). "The Stability of Folpet in Human Blood." Report File 721.11, Chevron Chemical Company (MRID 70970).

Crown, S. (1981). "Folpet Technical: Pilot 28 Day Study in Mice with Folpet." Report R-1777, Life Science Research Israel, Ltd., Ness Ziona, Israel.

Crown, S., Nyska, A., and Waner, T. (1985). "Folpan Carcinogenicity Study in the Rat." Report MAK/022/FOL, Life Science Research Israel, Ltd., Ness Ziona, Israel (MRID 00157493).

Crown, S., Nyska, A., Waner, T., and Kenan, G. (1989). "Folpan: Toxicity by Dietary Administration to Rats for Two Years." Report MAK/053/FOL, Life Science Research Israel, Ness Ziona, Israel (MRID 43640201, 00124023).

Croy, I. (1973). Etiology of urticaria due to captan based antifungal agents: Case report. *Z. Gesamte Hyg. Ihre Grenzgeb* **19**, 710–711.

Cummins, H. A. (1995). "Merpan (Captan) Technical: Acute Inhalation Toxicity Study in the Rat." Report 94/MAK261/1087, Pharmaco–Life Science Research Ltd., Eye, England.

Dalvi, R. R. (1988). Involvement of glutathione in the reduction of captan-induced *in vivo* inhibition of mono-oxygenases and liver toxicity in the rat. *J. Environ. Sci. Health* **23**(2), 171–180.

Dalvi, R. R. (1989). Metabolism of captan and its hepatoxic implications: A review. *J. Environ. Biol.* **10**(1), 81–86.

Daly, I. W. (1983). "A Four-Week Pilot Oral Toxicity Study in Dogs with Folpet Technical." Report 82-2664, BioDynamics Laboratories, East Millstone, NJ (MRID 161314).

Daly, I. W., and Knezevich, A. (1983). "A Lifetime Oral Oncogenicity Study of Captan in Mice." Report 80-2491, BioDynamics Laboratories, East Millstone, NJ (MRID 00126845).

Daly, I. W., and Knezevich, A. L. (1986). "A One-Year Oral Toxicity Study in Dogs with Folpet Technical." Report 82-2677, BioDynamics Laboratories, East Millstone, NJ (MRID 00161315).

Daun, R. J. (1988a). "[Cyclohexene-1,2^{14}C]Captan: Nature of the Residue in Livestock—Laying Hens." Report HLA 6183-104, Hazleton Laboratories America, Inc., Madison, WI (MRID 4065004).

Daun, R. J. (1988b). "[Trichloromethyl-14C]Captan: Nature of Residue in Livestock—Laying Hens." Report HLA 6183-106, Hazleton Laboratories America, Inc., Madison, WI (MRID 40658003).

DeBaun, J. R., B., M. J., Knarr, J., Mihailovski, A., and Menn, J. J. (1974). The fate of *N*-trichloro[^{14}C]methylthio-4-cyclohexene-1,2-dicarboximide ([^{14}C]Captan) in the rat. *Xenobiotica* **4**(2), 101–119.

De Flora, S., Zannacchi, P., Camoirano, A., Bennicelli, C., and Badolati, G. S. (1984). Genotoxic activity and potency of 135 compounds in the Ames reversion test and in a bacterial DNA-repair test. *Mutat. Res.* **133**, 161–198.

Dickhaus, S., and Heisler, E. (1983). "Acute Toxicological Study of Folpet after Intraperitoneal Application to the Rat." Report E.H./P. 1-4-113-83, Pharmatox Forschung und Beratung GmbH, W. Germany (MRID 00137699).

Dougherty, K. K. (1988). "Four-Week Repeated-Dose Dermal Toxicity Study in Rats with Folpet Technical (SX-1388)." Report, Laboratory Project S-3076, Chevron Environmental Health Center, Richmond, CA (MRID 40750802).

Dreher, D. M. (1992a). "Folpet Technical: Acute Eye Irritation in Rabbits." Report R-6511, SafePharm Laboratories Ltd., Derby, UK.

Dreher, D. M. (1992b). "Merpan 80 WDG: Acute Oral Toxicity (Limit Test) in the Rat." Report, Project 306/158, SafePharm Laboratories Ltd., Derby, UK.

East, P. W. (1994). "Folpet: Oncogenicity Study by Dietary Administration to CD-1 Mice for 104 Weeks." Report MAK/117, Huntingdon Research Centre Ltd., Huntingdon, England (MRID 44316501).

Ecobichon, D. J. (1996). Toxic Effects of Pesticides. *In* "Casarett & Doull's Toxicology, The Basic Science of Poisons" (C. D. Klaassen, ed.), pp. 678–679. McGraw–Hill, New York.

Edwards, I. R., Ferry, D. G., and Temple, W. A. (1991). Fungicides and related compounds. *In* "Handbook of Pesticide Toxicology" (W. J. Hayes and E. R. Laws, eds.), Vol. 3, pp. 1409–1470. Academic Press, San Diego.

Elder, R. L. (1989). Safety assessment of cosmetic ingredients: Final report on the safety assessment of captan. *J. Am. College Toxicol.* **8**(4), 643–680.

Engler, R. (1986). "Peer Review of Captan, Caswell No. 159." Report TS-769C, Carcinogenicity Peer Review Committee, Health Effects Division, Environmental Protection Agency, Washington, DC.

Epstein, S. S., Arnold, E., Andrea, J., Bass, W., and Bishop, Y. (1972). Detection chemical mutagens by the dominant lethal assay in the mouse. *Toxicol. Appl. Pharmacol.* **23**, 288–325.

Esber, H. J. (1983). "In-Vivo Cytogenetics Study in Rats with Chevron Folpet Technical." Report 2-225, EG&G Mason Research Institute (MRID 160445).

Fabro, S., Smith, R. L., and Williams, R. T. (1966). Embryotoxic activity of some pesticides and drugs related to phthalimide. *Food Cosmet. Toxicol.* **3**, 587–590.

FAO/WHO (1984). "Pesticide Residues in Food—1983 (Dichlofluanid)." Food and Agriculture Organization/World Health Organization, United Nations.

FAO/WHO (1989). "Pesticide Residues in Food—1988 (Tolylfluanid)." Report 324, Food and Agriculture Organization/World Health Organization, United Nations.

FAO/WHO (1990). "Pesticide Residues in Food—1989 (Captan)." Food and Agriculture Organization/World Health Organization, United Nations.

FAO/WHO (1996). "Pesticide Residues in Food—1995 (Captan; Folpet)." Food and Agriculture Organization/World Health Organization, United Nations.

Feng, J. Y., and Lin, B. Y. (1987). Cytogenetic effects of an agricultural antibiotic, captan, on mouse bone marrow and testicular cells. *Environ. Res.* **43**(2), 359–363.

Feussner, E. (1985). "Teratology Study in Rabbits with Folpet Technical Using a "Pulse-Dosing" Regimen." Report 303-004, Argus Research Laboratories, Horsham, PA (MRID 00151490).

Feussner, E., Hoberman, A. M., Johnson, D. M., and Christian, M. S. (1984). "Teratology Study in Rabbits with Folpet Technical." Report, Project 303-002, Argus Research Laboratories, Inc., Horsham, PA (MRID 00160432).

Fickentscher, K., Kirfel, A., Will, G., and Köhler, F. (1977). Stereochemical properties and teratogenic activity of some tetrahydrophthalimides. *Mol. Pharmacol.* **13**, 133–141.

Fletcher, A. L., Elliott, B., Rhodes, M. E., and Sargent, D. E. (1995). "Captan Task Force Response to the Draft HED Chapter of the Reregistration Eligibility Decision Document (RED) for Captan, *N*-Trichloro-methylthio-4-cyclohexene-1,2-dicarboximide, Case #0120, Chemical Code 081301; Reg. Group A (Dated 2/21/95)." Report 95 ALF202, Captan Task Force (MRID 43875601).

Flint, O. P., and Ortaon, T. C. (1984). An in vitro assay for teratogens with cultures of rat embryo midbrain and limb bud cells. *Toxicol. Appl. Pharmacol.* **76**, 383–395.

Foster, J. R. (1994). "Captan: Second Investigation of Duodenal Hyperplasia in Mice." Report CTL/L/6022, Central Toxicology Laboratory, Zeneca Inc., Cheshire, UK (MRID 43393504).

Foster, J. R., and Elliott, B. (2000). "The Significance of the Increased Incidence of Rat Tumors on the Long Term Studies with Captan." Position Paper, Report CTL/R/1461, Central Toxicology Laboratory, AstraZeneca, Alderley Park, Macclesfield, England (MRID 45071801).

Foster, T. L., and Morgan, R. L. (1984). "Acute Toxicity of Captan Technical (AOT, ADT, Skin Irritation)." Report T-11474, Richmond Toxicology Laboratory, Richmond (MRID 00164356).

Fry, S. M., and Fiscor, G. (1978). Cytogenetic test of captan in mouse bone marrow. *Mutat. Res.* **58**, 111–114.

Gaines, T. B., and Linder, R. E. (1986). Acute toxicity of pesticides in adult and weanling rats. *Fundam. Appl. Toxicol.* **7**, 299–308.

Ghali, G. Z. (1997). "Captan: Hazard Identification Committee Report." Hazard Identification Committee, Health Effects Division (7509C), U.S. Environmental Protection Agency, Washington, DC.

Goldenthal, E., Warner, M., and Rajasekaran, D. (1982). "Two Year Oral Toxicity/Carcinogenicity Study of Captan in Rats." Report 153-097, International Research and Development Corporation, Northbrook, IL (MRIDs 00120316, 00129163, 00129164, 00132742).

Goodman, D. G., Ward, J. M., Squire, R. A., Chu, K. C., and Linhart, M. S. (1979). Neoplastic and nonneoplastic lesions in aging F344 rats. *Toxicol. Appl. Pharmacol.* **48**, 237–248.

Gordon, E. B., Foster, J. R., Bernard, B. K., and Middleton, M. (1994). "Response to 59 FR 33941 Summarizing Data Concluding Captan Is Not a Human Carcinogen." Report CTF/94/1, Captan Task Force (MRID 43405101).

Gordon, E. B., Mobley, S. C., Ehrlich, T., and Williams, M. (2001). Measurement of the reaction between the fungicides captan or folpet and blood thiols. *Toxicol. Methods* **11**(3), in press.

Gudi, R., and Krsmanovic, L. (2001). "Nuclear Aberration Test in the Mouse Duodenum (Folpet)." Report AA31SK.123005.BTL, BioReliance Corporation, Rockville, MD.

Guo, Y.-J. (2001). "Survey of Users: *Dare to Wear Black Shampoo* Containing 7% Captan." AUTOGRAF Specialty Hair Care Products.

Guo, Y. L., Wang, B. J., Lee, C. C., and Wang, J. D. (1996). Prevalence of dermatoses and skin sensitisation associated with use of pesticides in fruit farmers of southern Taiwan. *Occup. Environ. Med.* **53**(6), 427–431.

Hardy, L. (1985). "Two Generation (Two Litter) Reproduction Study in Rats with Folpet." Report SOCAL 2140, Chevron Environmental Health Center, Richmond, CA (MRID 00151489).

Harris, D. (1976). "Analysis for Skin Irritation, Eye Irritation, and Inhalation in Albino Rabbits." Report 6051094, WARF Institute, Inc., Madison, WI.

Hazleton (1956). "Chronic Toxicity Study in Rats." Hazleton Laboratories America, Inc., Vienna, VA (MRID 250921–250924).

Hext, P. (1989). "90-Day Inhalation Toxicity in the Rat." Report CTL/P/2543, Central Toxicology Laboratory, Alderley Park, Macclesfield, England (MRID 41234402).

Hoberman, A., Christian, M., and Sica, E. (1983). "Teratology Study in Rats with Folpet Technical." Report 303-001, Argus Research Laboratories, Horsham, PA (MRID 00132457).

Horsfall, J. G., and Rich, S. (1957). Structure–activity relationships in captan derivatives. *Phytopathology* **47**, 17.

Hsu, C.-H., and McCarroll, N. (1998). "*In Vivo* Mammalian DNA Binding in the Mouse." Data Evaluation Record, Report 012863, Toxicology Branches 1 and 2, Health Effects Division, U.S. Environmental Protection Agency, Washington, DC.

IARC (1983). "Monographs on the Evaluation of the Carcinogenic Risk of Chemicals to Humans: Miscellaneous Pesticides: Captan." International Agency for Research on Cancer, Lyon, France.

Imanishi, H., Sasaki, Y. F., Watanabe, M., Moriya, M., Sjirasu, Y., and Tutikawa, K. (1987). "Mutagenicity evaluation of pesticides in the mouse spot test." *Mutat. Res.*

Innes, J. R. M., Ulland, B. M. G., V. M., Petrucelli, L. L. F., Hart, E. R., Palotta, A. J., Bates, R. R., Falk, H. L., Gart, J. J., Klein, M., Mitchell, I., and Peters, J. (1969). Bioassay of pesticides and industrial chemicals for tumorigenicity in mice: A preliminary note. *J. Natl. Cancer Inst.* **42**(6), 1101–1114.

Ishidate, M. J., Sofuni, T., and Yoshikaw, K. (1981). Chromosomal aberration tests *in vitro* as a primary screening tool for environmental mutagens and/or carcinogens. *Gann Monogr. Cancer Res.* **27**, 95–108.

Ito, N., Ogiso, T., Fukushima, S., Shibata, M., and Hagiwara, A. (1984). Carcinogenicity of captafol in B6C3F1 mice. *Gann* **75**(10), 853–865.

Ivy Research Laboratories (1981). "Report on the Appraisal of the Contact Sensitizing Potential of Four Materials by Means of the Maximization Study." Cosmetic, Toiletries and Fragrance Association, Washington, DC.

Jacoby, O. (1985a). "Folpan Mouse Micronucleus Test." Report MAK/071/FOL, Life Science Research Israel, Ltd., Ness Ziona, Israel (MRID 150558).

Jacoby, O. (1985b). "Merpan Mouse Micronucleus Test." Report MAK/072/MER, Life Science Research Israel, Ltd., Ness Ziona, Israel.

Janik, F. (1986). Effects of biocides on the Ca2+-transport-ATPase activity of human erythrocytes. *Naunyn–Schmiedeberg's Arch. Pharmacol.* **334**(Suppl.), R20.

Johnson, D. (1987). "Twenty-One Day Dermal Toxicity Study in Rabbits with Technical Captan." Report 415-046, International Research and Development Corp., Northbrook (MRID 40273201).

Jordan, W. P., and King, S. E. (1977). Delayed hypersensitivity in females. The development of allergic contact dermatitis in females during the comparison of two predictive patch tests. *Contact Dermatitis* **3**(1), 19–26.

Jorgenson, T. A., Rushbrook, C. J., and Newell, G. W. (1976). *In vivo* mutagenesis investigations of ten commercial pesticides. *Toxicol. Appl. Pharmacol.* **37**(1), 109.

Katz, A., Sauerhoff, M., Zwicker, G. M., and Freudenthal, R. I. (1982). "The Effect of Captan on Duodenal Sulfhydryl Levels in Rats." Report T-10832, Stauffer Chemical Company, Farmington, CT.

Kay, J. H., and Calandra, J. C. (1960). "Acute Percutaneous and Eye Irritation Studies on Phaltan." Industrial Bio-Test Laboratories, Inc., Northbrook, IL (MRID 00062612).

Kennedy, G. (1967). "Three-Generation Reproduction Study in Albino Rats—Phaltan: Results of All Three Generations." Report B 3566, Industrial Bio-Test Laboratories, Inc., Northbrook, IL (MRIDs 00065143, 00081262).

Kennedy, G., Fancher, O. E., and Calandra, J. C. (1968). An investigation of the teratogenic potential of captan, folpet, and difolatan. *Toxicol. Appl. Pharmacol.* **13**(3), 420–430.

Kennedy, G. L., Arnold, D. W., and Keplinger, M. L. (1975a). Mutagenicity studies with captan, captafol, folpet and thalidomide. *Food Cosmet. Toxicol.* **18**, 55–64.

Kennedy, G. L., Fancher, O. E., and Calandra, J. C. (1975b). Nonteratogenicity of captan in beagles. *Teratology* **11**(2), 223–225.

Kidwell, J. L., and Watters, J. L. (1999). "Acute Dietary Exposure and Risk Assessment for Captan Residues in Foods." Report Captan 99-01, Novigen Sciences, Inc., Washington, DC (MRID 44737601).

Kittleson, A. R. (1953). Preparation and some properties of *N*-trichloromethylthiotetrahydrophthalimide. *Agricultural Food Chem.* **1**(10), 677–679.

Korenaga, G. (1982). "The Acute Dermal Toxicity of Chevron Folpet Technical (SX-1346) in Adult Male and Female Rabbits." Report S-2152, Chevron Environmental Health Center, Richmond, CA (MRID 00131728).

Kramers, P. G. N., and Knaap, A. G. A. C. (1973). Mutagenicity tests with captan and folpet in drosophila melanogaster. *Mutat. Res.* **21**, 149–154.

Krieger, R. I. (2001). Personal communication.

Krieger, R. I., and Thongsinthusak, T. (1993). Captan metabolism in humans yields two biomarkers, tetrahydrophthalimide (THPI) and thiazolidine-2-thione-4-carboxylic acid (TTCA) in urine. *Drug Chem. Toxciol.* **16**(2), 207–225.

LaFarge-Frayssinet, C., and Decloitre, F. (1982). Modulatory effect of the pesticide captan on the immune response in rats and mice. *J. Immunopharmacol.* **4**(1-2), 43–52.

Lang, P. (1995). "Spontaneous Neoplastic Lesions in the Crl:CD-1 BR Mouse." Tech. Bull. Charles River Laboratories.

Ledda-Columbano, G. M., Columbano, A., Curto, M., Ennas, M. G., Coni, P., Sarma, D. S. R., and Pani, P. (1989). Further evidence that mitogen-induced cell proliferation does not support the formation of enzyme-altered islands in rat liver by carcinogens. *Carcinogenesis* **10**(5), 847–850.

Legator, X. X. (1969). Mutagenic effects of captan. *Ann. N.Y. Acad. Sci.* **160**, 344–351.

Leininger, J. R., and Jokinen, M. P. (1990). Oviduct, uterus, and vagina. *In* "Pathology of the Fischer Rat, Reference and Atlas," pp. 443–459. Academic Press, San Diego.

Levy, A. C., Rowland, J. C., and Ioannou, Y. M. (1997). Meeting Minutes, April 3. Toxicology Endpoint Selection Document, Toxicology Endpoint Selection Committee, Health Effects Division (7509C), U.S. Environmental Protection Agency, Washington, DC.

Lien, E. J. (1969). Structure–activity correlations in fungitoxicity of imides and their imide-SCCl3 compounds. *J. Agric. Food Chem.* **17**(6), 1265–1268.

Lisi, P., Caraffini, S., and Assalve, D. (1986). A test series for pesticide dermatitis. *Contact Dermatitis* **15**(5), 266–269.

Liu, M. K., and Fishbein, L. (1967). Reactions of captan and folpet with thiols. *Experientia* **23**(2), 81–82.

Loveday, K. (1989). "*In Vitro* Chromosomal Aberration Assay on Folpet Technical." Report 61565-00, A. D. Little Company, Cambridge, MA (MRID 42122014).

LSR (1993). "Folpet Technical: Micronized-Hypersensitivity in Guinea Pigs." Pharmaco-Life Science Research Ltd., Eye, Suffolk, England.

Lukens, R. J. (1966). The fungitoxicity of compounds containing a trichloromethylthio-group. *J. Agric. Food Chem.* **14**(4), 365–367.

Lukens, R. J. (1967). Heterocyclic nitrogen compounds. *In* "Fungicides, An Advanced Treatise" (D. C. Torgeson, ed.), Vol. II, pp. 396–435. Academic Press, New York.

Lukens, R. J. (1969). Fungitoxic action of nonmetallic organic fungicides. *In* "Biodeterioration of Materials," p. 486. Elsevier, Barking, England.

Lukens, R. J., and Sisler, H. D. (1958a). 2-Thiazolidinethione-4-carboxylic acid from the reaction of captan with cysteine. *Science* **127**, 650.

Lukens, R. J., and Sisler, H. D. (1958b). Chemical reactions involved in the fungitoxicity of captan. *Phytopathology* **48**(5-1), 235–244.

Maekawa, A., Kurokawa, Y., Takahashi, M., Kobubo, T., Ogiu, T., and Hayashi, Y. (1983). Spontaneous tumors in F-344/Ducrj rats. *Gann* **74**, 365.

Maita, K., Hirano, M., Harada, T., Mitsumori, K., Yoshida, A., Takahashi, K., Nakashima, N., Kitazawa, T., Enomoto, A., Inui, K., and Shirasu, Y. (1987). Spontaneous tumors in F344/DuCrj rats from 12 control groups of chronic and oncogenicity studies. *J. Toxicol. Sci.* **12**, 111–126.

Maita, K., Hirano, M., Harada, T., Mitsumori, K., Yoshida, A., Takahashi, K., Nakashima, N., Kitazawa, T., Enomoto, A., Inui, K., and Shirasu, Y. (1988). Mortality, major cause of morbundity and spontaneous tumours in CD-1 mice. *Toxicol. Pathol.* **16**, 340–350.

Maronpot, R. R., Shimkin, M. B., Witschi, H. P., Smith, L. H., and Cline, J. M. (1986). Strain A mouse pulmonary tumour test results for chemicals previously tested in the National Cancer Institute carcinogenicity tests. *J. Natl. Cancer Inst.* **76**(6), 1101–1112.

Martinez-Rossi, N. M., and Azevedo, J. L. (1987). Detection of point-mutation mutagens in *Aspergillus nidulans*: Comparison of methionine suppressors and arginine resistance induction by fungicides. *Mutat. Res.* **176**(1), 29–35.

Marzulli, F. N., and Maibach, H. I. (1973). Antimicrobials: Experimental contact sensitization in man. *J. Soc. Cosmet. Chemists* **24**(7), 399–421.

McLaughlin, J., Jr., Reynaldo, E. F., Lamar, J. K., and Marliac, J.-P. (1969). Teratology studies in rabbits with captan, folpet, and thalidomide. *Toxicol. Appl. Pharmacol.* **14**, 641.

McMartin, D. N., Sahota, P. S., Gunson, D. E., Hsu, H. H., and Spaet, R. H. (1992). Neoplasms and related proliferative lesions in control Sprague–Dawley rats from carcinogenicity studies. Historical data and diagnostic considerations. *Toxicol. Pathol.* **20**(2), 212–225.

Medinsky, M. A., and Klaassen, C. D. (1996). Toxicokinetics. *In* "Casarett and Doull's Toxicology, The Basic Science of Poisons" (C. D. Klaassen, ed.). McGraw–Hill, New York.

Mercier, O. (1988). "Phaltan 500 Flowable (SXE 29): Test to Evaluate the Acute Cutaneous Primary Irritation and Corrosivity in the Rabbit and the Acute Occular Irritation and Corrosivity in the Rabbit." Report 804377, Hazleton–IFT, Paris.

Miaullis, J. B., Quale, D. C., Vispetto, A. R., and DeBaun, J. R. (1980). "Effect of Dietary Captan of Soluble Thiol Content of Liver and Duodenal Tissues." Reports MRC-B-109, MRC-80-04, Mountain View Research Center, Mountain View, CA (MRID 00153291).

Milburn, G. M. (1997). "Folpet: Study of Hyperplasia in the Mouse Duodenum." Report CTL/P/5577, Central Toxicology Laboratory, Alderley Park, Macclesfield, England (MRID 44866402).

Mitchell, J. T. (1975). Comparative teratogenic effects of malathion, captan and thalidomide in the embryo of the common snapping turtle, *Chelydra serpentine. Anat. Rec.* **181**, 428–426.

Mollet, P. (1973). Mutagenicity and toxicity testing of captan in drosophila. *Mutat. Res.* **21**, 137–148.

Mollet, P., and Wurgler, F. E. (1974). Detection of somatic recombination and mutation in *Drosophila*: A method for testing genetic activity of chemical compounds. *Mutat. Res.* **25**, 421–424.

Moore, M. (1985). "Evaluation of Chevron Folpet Technical in the Mouse Somatic Cell Mutation Assay." Report, Study 20994, Litton Bionetics, Inc. (MRID 00148625).

Moriya, M., Kato, K., and Shirasu, Y. (1978). Effects of cysteine and a liver metabolic activation system on the activities of mutagenic pesticides. *Mutat. Res.* **57**, 259–263.

Moriya, M., Ohta, T., Watanabe, K., Miyazawa, T., Kato, K., and Shirasu, Y. (1983). Further mutagenicity studies on pesticides in bacterial reversion assay systems. *Mutat. Res.* **116**, 185–216.

Nagy, Z., Mile, I., and Antoni, F. (1975). The mutagenic effect of pesticides on *Escherichia coli* WP try. *Acta Microbiol. Acad. Sci. Hung.* **22**, 309–314.

NCI (1977). "Bioassay of Captan for Possible Carcinogenicity." Carcinogenesis Technical Report Series. Report NCI-CG-TR-15, Gulf South Research Institute.

Neal, B. (2000). "Analyses of Developmental and Reproductive Toxicity of Folpet and Justification for Removal of the FQPA 3× Safety Factor." Folpet RED Response, Jellinek, Schwartz and Connolly, Inc., Arlington, VA.

Nelson, N. (1949). "A Preliminary Toxicological Study of SR-406, a Fungicide." Report, Bull. Inst. Indust. Med., Laboratory of Industrial Toxicology, New York University, Bellevue Medical Center, New York (MRID 00054789).

Nguyen, T. D. (1981). "Mutagenicity Evaluation of Captan in the Somatic Cell Mutation Assay." Report, Project 20951, Litton Bionetics Research Laboratories, Rockville, MD (MRID 251576).

NLM (2001). Medline/Toxline on-line Search: "Captan" or "folpet" and "eye damage" or "eye" for the years 1981–2001. National Library of Medicine, Bethesda, MD.

NPIRS (1999a). "Federal Data: New Products Containing Captan as the Ingredient." Product Search Summary, National Pesticide Information Retrieval System, Center for Environmental & Regulatory Information Systems, West Lafayette, IN.

NPIRS (1999b). "Registered Uses of Captan and Folpet." Federal Data Search Summary, National Pesticide Information Retrieval System, Center for Environmental & Regulatory Information Systems, West Lafayette, IN.

Nyska, A., Waner, T., Pirak, M., Gordon, E., Bracha, P., and Klein, B. (1989). The renal carcinogenic effect of Merpafol in the Fisher 344 rat. *Isr. J. Med. Sci.* **25**(8), 428–432.

Nyska, A., Waner, T., Paster, Z., Bracha, P., Gordon, E. B., and Klein, B. (1990). Induction of gastrointestinal tumors in mice fed the fungicide folpet: Possible mechanisms. *J. J. Can. Res.* **81**(6-7), 545–549.

Oberly, T. J., Bewsey, B. J., and Probst, G. S. (1984). An evaluation of the L5178Y TK (+/−) mouse lymphoma forward mutation assay using 42 chemicals. *Mutat. Res.* **125**, 291–306.

O'Neill, J. P., Forbes, N. L., and Hsie, A. W. (1981). Cytotoxicity and mutagenicity of the fungicides captan and folpet in cultured mammalian cells (CHO/HGPRT system). *Environ. Mutagenesis* **3**, 233–237.

Pack, D. E. (1987). "[Trichloromethyl-C-14] Captan Hydrolysis Products." Report MEF-0002,8702383, Ortho Research Center, Metabolism Laboratories (MRID 40208101).

Palshaw, M. W. (1980). "An Epidemiologic Study of Mortality within a Cohort of Captan Workers." Stauffer Chemical Company (MRID 00153294).

Parkin, D. M., Muir, C. S., Whelan, S. L., Gao, Y.-T., Ferlay, J., and Powell, J. (1992). "Cancer Incidence in Five Continents," Vol. VI. IARC Scientific Publications 120, pp. 922–923. International Agency for Research on Cancer, Lyon, France.

Pavkov, K. L., and Thomasson, R. W. (1985). "Identification of a Pre-neoplastic Alteration Following Dietary Administration of Captan Technical to CD-1 Mice." Report T-11007, Environmental Health Center, Stauffer Chemical Company (MRID 00151472).

Peluso, A. M., Tardio, M., Adamo, F., and Venturo, N. (1991). Multiple sensitization due to bis-dithiocarbamate and thiophthalidimide pesticides. *Contact Dermatitis* **25**(5), 327.

Petersen, B. J. (1997). "Dietary Exposure to Folpet." Report Folpet 97-01, Novigen Sciences, Inc., Washington, DC (MRID 44354804).

Pilinskaya, M. A. (1983). Investigation of the cytogenetic effects of the pesticides captan and benomyl in a culture of human peripheral blood lymphocytes with and without metabolic activation. *Tsitologiya i Genetika* **17**(1), 30–34.

Pitot, H. C., III, and Dragan, Y. P. (1996). Chemical carcinogenesis. *In* "Casarett and Doull's Toxicology, The Basic Science of Poisons" (C. D. Klaassen, M. O. Amdur, and J. Doull, eds.), pp. 201–267. McGraw–Hill, New York.

Pitot, H. C., Dragan, Y. P., Nevsu, M. J., Rizvi, T. A., Hully, J. R., and Campbell, H. A. (1991). Chemical, cell proliferation, risk estimation, and multistage carcinogenesis. *In* "Chemically Induced Cell Proliferation: Implications for Risk Assessment" (B. E. Butterworth, T. J. Slaga, W. Farland, and M. McClain, eds.), pp. 517–532. Wiley–Liss, New York.

Potten, C. S., and Loeffler, M. (1990). Stem cells: Attributes, cycles, spirals, pitfalls and uncertainties. Lessons for and from the crypt. *Development* **110**, 1001–1020.

Pritchard, D. J., and Lappin, G. J. (1991). "Captan: DNA Binding Study in the Mouse." Report CTL/P/3380, ICI Americas, Inc. (MRID 43405102).

Probst, G. S., McMahon, R. E., Hill, L. E., Thompson, C. Z., Epp, J. K., and Neal, S. B. (1981). Chemically-induced unscheduled dna synthesis in primary rat hepatocyte cultures: A comparison with bacterial mutagenicity using 218 compounds. *Environ. Mutagenesis* **3**, 11–32.

Provan, W. M., Eyton-Jones, H., and Green, T. (1992). "The Potential of Captan to React with DNA." Report CTL/R/1131, ICI Central Toxicology Laboratory (MRID 43393501).

Provan, W. M., Eyton-Jones, H., and Green, T. (1993). "First Revision to the Potential of Captan to React with DNA." Report CTL/R/1131, Central Toxicology Laboratory (MRID 43393501).

Provan, W. M., Eyton-Jones, H., Lappin, G., Pritchard, D., Moore, R. B., and Green, T. (1995). The incorporation of radiolabelled sulphur from captan into protein and its impact on a DNA binding study. *Chem.-Biol. Interact.* **96**, 173–184.

Purves, W. K., Orians, G. H., and Heller, H. C. (1992). Physiology, homeostasis, and the regulation of body temperature. *In* "Life, The Science of Biology," pp. 749. Freeman, Salt Lake City.

Quest, J. A., Fenner-Crisp, P. A., Burnam, W., Copley, M., Dearfield, K. L., Hamernik, K. L., Saunders, D. S., Whiting, R. J., and Engler, R. (1993). Evaluation of the carcinogenic potential of pesticides. 4. Chloroalkylthiodicarboximide compounds with fungicidal activity. *Regulatory Toxicol. Pharmacol.* **17**(1), 19–34.

Rees, P. B. (1993). "Folpet Technical (Micronized): Acute Dermal Irritation Test in the Rabbit." Report 93/MAK175/0759, Life Science Research, Eye, England.

Reno, F. E., Burdock, G., and Serota, D. (1981). "Subchronic Toxicity Study in Rats: Phaltan (Folpet)." Report: 2107-100, Hazleton Laboratories America, Inc., Vienna, VA (MRID 00115269).

Rideg, K. (1982). Genetic toxicology of phthalimide-type fungicides. *Mutat. Res.* **97**(3), 217.

Robinson, M. (1993). "Captan: A CTL Re-examination of Duodenal Sections from a Lifetime Oral Oncogenicity Study in Mice (BioDynamics Project 80-2491)." Report CTL/T/2829, Central Toxicology Laboratory (MRID 43393502).

Rocchi, D., Perocco, P., Alberghini, W., Fini, A., and Prodi, G. (1980). Effect of pesticides on scheduled and unscheduled DNA-synthesis of rat thymocytes and human lymphocytes. *Arch. Toxicol.* **45**, 101–108.

Rosenfeld, G. (1984). "Captan Technical 94%: Primary Eye Irritation Study in Rabbits." Report 1194D, Cosmopolitan Safety Evaluation, Inc., Lafayette, NJ (Inc. MRID 00148315).

Rozman, K. K., and Klaassen, C. D. (1996). Absorption, distribution, and excretion of toxicants. *In* "Casarett and Doull's Toxicology, The Basic Science of Poisons" (C. D. Klaassen, M. O. Amdur, and J. Doull, eds.), pp. 91–112. McGraw–Hill, New York.

Rubin, Y. (1981). "Folpan: Four Week Range-Finding Study in Dietary Administration to Mice." Report MAK/020/FOL, Life Science Research Israel, Ltd., Ness Ziona, Israel.

Rubin, Y. (1983). "Folpan: Teratology Study in the Rat." Report MAK/049/FOL, Life Science Research Israel Ltd., Ness Ziona, Israel (MRIDs 00134026, 00115617).

Rubin, Y. (1985a). "Folpan: Oncogenicity Study in the Mouse." Report MAK/015/FOL, Life Science Research Israel, Ltd., Ness Ziona, Israel (MRIDs 259873–259877).

Rubin, Y. (1985b). "Folpan: Teratology Study in the Rabbit." Report MAK/051/FOL, Life Science Research Israel, Ltd., Ness Ziona, Israel (MRID 00156636).

Rubin, Y. (1986). "Folpan: Two-Generation Reproduction Study in the Rat." Report MAK/052/FOL, Life Science Research Israel, Ltd., Ness Ziona, Israel (MRID 40135901).

Rubin, Y. (1987). "Captan: Teratology Study in the Rat." Report MAK/097/CAP, Life Science Research Israel, Ltd., Ness Ziona, Israel.

Rubin, Y., and Nyska, A. (1987). "Captan: Teratology study in the rabbit." Report MAK/099/CAP, Life Science Research Israel Ltd., Ness Ziona, Israel.

Ruzo, L. O., and Ewing, A. D. (1988). "Hydrolysis of [^{14}C]-Folpet." Report PTRL 124, PTRL West, Inc., Richmond, CA (MRID 40818801).

Sasaki, M., Sugimura, K., Yoshida, M., and Abe, A. (1980). Cytogenetic effects of 60 chemicals on cultured human and Chinese hamster cells. *Sensoshuktai* **20**, 574–584.

Sauer, C., and Seaman, L. R. (1980). "Primary Eye Irritation Study in Rabbits. Test Article: Merpan 50 WP." Report 0414D, Cosmopolitan Safety Evaluation, Inc., Somerville, NJ (MRID 00045688).

Sauerhoff, M. W., DeBaun, J., Miaullis, J. B., and Freudenthal, R. I. (1982). The influence of captan on levels of reduced sulfhydryls in the duodenum of mice. *Toxicologist* **2**(1), 425.

Saunders, D. S., and Harper, C. (1994). Pesticides. *In* "Principles and Methods of Toxicology" (A. W. Hayes, ed.), pp. 389–415. Raven Press, New York.

Schardein, J., and Aldridge, D. (1982). "One Generation Reproduction Study in Rats with Captan." Report 153-190; T-10486, International Research and Development Corporation (MRID 00120315).

Schardein, J., Schwartz, C., and Thorstenson, J. (1982). "Three Generation Reproduction Study in Rats." Report 153-096, International Research and Development Corporation (MRID 00125293).

Schuphan, I., Westphal, D., Haque, A., and Ebing, W. (1981). Biological and chemical behavior of perhalogen methylmercapto fungicides: Metabolism and *in vitro* reactions of dichlofluanid in comparison with captan. *Am. Chem. Soc. Symp. Ser.* **158**, 85–96.

Seifried, H. (1996). "Folpet: Threshold Limit Value." Industrial Hygiene Consultant, Bethesda, MD.

Sela, J. (1982). "Folpan Toxicity in Dietary Administration to Rats for 13 Weeks." Report MAK/021/FOL, Life Science Research, Stock, England.

Selsky, C. A., and Matheson, D. W. (1981). "The Association of Captan with Mouse and Rat Deoxyribonucelic Acid." Report T-10435, Environmental Health Center, Richmond, CA (MRID 00093759).

Shah, P. V., Fisher, H. L., Sumler, M. R., Monroe, R. J., Chernoff, N., and Hall, L. L. (1987). Comparison of the penetration of 14 pesticides through the skin of young and adult rats. *J. Toxicol. Environ. Health* **21**.

Sharma, S. (1978). Thiophosgene in Organic Synthesis. *Int. J. Methods Synth. Organic Chem.* 803–820.

Sharma, S. (1986). "The Chemistry of Thiophosgene" (A. Senning, ed.), Sulfur Reports, Vol. 5. Harwood, London.

Shiau, S. Y., Huff, R. A., and Falkner, I. C. (1981). Pesticide mutagenicity in *Bacillus subtilis* and *Salmonella typhimurium* detectors. *J. Agric. Food Chem.* **29**, 268–271.

Shirasu, Y. (1978). Cytogenic and dominant-lethal studies on captan. *Mutat. Res.* **54**, 227–228.

Shirasu, Y., Moriya, M., Kato, K., Furuhashi, A., and Kada, T. (1976). Mutagenicity screening of pesticides in the microbial system. *Mutat. Res.* **40**, 19–30.

Siegel, M. R. (1971a). Reaction of the fungicide folpet (*N*-trichloromethylthio phthalimide) with a thiol protein. *Pestic. Biochem. Physiol.* **1**, 225–233.

Siegel, M. R. (1971b). Reactions of the fungicide folpet (*N*-trichloromethyl-thio)phthalimide with a nonthiol protein. *Pestic. Biochem. Physiol.* **1**, 234–240.

Simmon, V. F., Poole, D. C., and Newell, G. W. (1976). *In vitro* mutagenesis investigations of twenty pesticides. *Toxicol. Appl. Pharmacol.* **37**(1), 109.

Simmon, V., Mitchell, A., and Jorgenson, T. (1977). "Evaluation of Selected Pesticides as Chemical Mutagens: *In vitro* and *in vivo* Studies." Health

Effects Research Series, EPA-600/1-77-028, Health Effects Research Laboratory, Stanford Research Institute, Research Triangle Park, NC (MRID 132582).

Sirianni, S. R., and Huang, C. C. (1978). Effect of the fungicide folpet on growth and chromosomes of human lymphoid cell lines. *Can. J. Genet. Cytol.* **20**, 193–197.

Slesinski, R. S., and Wilson, A. E. (1992). "National Milk Survey." Report Captan 91-01, Technical Assessment Systems, Inc., Washington, DC (MRID 42458801).

Solt, D. B., Medline, A., and Farber, E. (1977). Rapid emergence of carcinogen-induced hyperplastic lesions in a new model for the sequential analysis of liver carcinogenesis. *Am. J. Pathol.* **88**, 595–618.

Tezuka, H., Teramoto, S., Kaneda, M., Henmi, R., Murakami, N., and Shirasu, Y. (1978). Cytogenic and dominant lethal studies on captan. *Mutation Research* **57**, 201–207.

Tezuka, H., Ando, N., Suzuki, R., Terahata, M., Moriya, M., and Shirasu, Y. (1980). Sister-chromatid exchanges and chromosomal aberrations in cultured Chinese hamster cells treated with pesticides positive in microbial reversion assays. *Mutat. Res.* **78**, 177–191.

Thoa, N. B., and Redden, J. C. (1995). "The HED Chapter of the Reregistration Eligibility Decision Document (RED) for Captan." Risk Characterization and Analysis Branch, Health Effects Division, U.S. Environmental Protection Agency, Washington, DC.

Thongsinthusak, T., Haskell, D., and Ross, J. H. (1999). "Dermal Absorption of Propargite, Bensulfuron-methyl, Captan, and Maneb in Rats." Technical Report HS-1792, Worker Health and Safety Branch, California Department of Pesticide Regulation, Sacramento, CA.

Til, H. P., and Beems, R. B. (1979). "Sub-acute (4-Week) Oral Toxicity Study with Merpan (Captan) in Rats." Report R-6241, Central Institute for Nutrition and Food Research TNO (MRID 00054467).

Til, H., Kuper, C. F., and Folke, H. E. (1983). "Life-span Oral Carcinogenicity Study of Merpan in Rats." Report B80-0153, Netherlands Organization for Applied Scientific Research TNO, Zeist, Netherlands (MRID 00161230).

Tinston, D. J. (1991). "Captan: Teratogenicity Study in the Rabbit." Report CTL/P/3039, ICI Central Toxicology Laboratory, Alderley Park, Macclesfield, UK (MRID 41826901).

Tinston, D. J. (1995). "Captan: Investigation of Duodenal Hyperplasia in Mice." Report CTL/P/4532, Central Toxicology Laboratory, Alderley Park, Macclesfield, England (MRID 43875602).

Tinston, D. J. (1996). "Captan: A Time Course Study of Induced Changes in the Small Intestine and Stomach of the Male CD-1 Mouse." Report CTL/P/4893, Central Toxicology Laboratory, Alderley Park, Macclesfield, England (MRID 43982201).

Trivedi, S. (1990a). "Captan: Excretion and Tissue Retention of a Single Oral Dose (10 mg/kg) in the Rat." Report CTL/P/2820, ICI Central Toxicology Laboratory, Alderley Park, Macclesfield, England (MRID 41505401).

Trivedi, S. (1990b). "Captan: Excretion and Tissue Retention of a Single Oral Dose (500 mg/kg) in the Rat." Report CTL/P/2862, ICI Central Toxicology Laboratory, Alderley Park, Macclesfield, England (MRID 41505402).

Trochimowicz, H. J., Kennedy, G. L., Jr., and Krivanek, N. D. (2001). Aliphatic and aromatic nitrogen compounds. *In* "Patty's Toxicology" (B. Bingham, C. Cohrssen, and C. Powell, eds.), Vol. 4, pp. 1163–1171. Wiley, New York.

U.S. Congress (1996). "Food Quality Protection Act of 1996." Pub. Law No. 104-170, 110 Stat. 1989. August 3, 1996.

U.S. EPA (1974). "Acute Toxicity Screen on PVI Materials and Intermediates." OTS Public Files, Record number 35097, Fiche number: 0000346-0, Document number FYI-OTS-1084-0346, Younger Labs (TSCATS Accession Number 16707).

U.S. EPA (1975). "Initial Scientific and Minieconomic Review of Captan." Report EPA/540/1-75-012, Office of Pesticide Programs, Criteria and Evaluation Division, U.S. Environmental Protection Agency, Washington, DC.

U.S. EPA (1984a). "Guidance for the Reregistration of Pesticide Products Containing Captafol as the Active Ingredient." Registration Standard, U.S. Environmental Protection Agency, Office of Pesticide Programs, Washington, DC.

U.S. EPA (1984b). "Weight of Evidence Classification of Captan as B2." Report 46, Fed. Reg. 46294, U.S. Environmental Protection Agency, Washington, DC.

U.S. EPA (1985a). "Captafol: Notice of Special Review." Report 49, Fed. Reg. 1103, U.S. Environmental Protection Agency, Washington, DC.

U.S. EPA (1985b). "Captan Position Document 2/3." Report 50, Fed. Reg. 25885, Office of Pesticides and Toxic Substances, U.S. Environmental Protection Agency, Washington, DC.

U.S. EPA (1986a). "Classification of Folpet as B2." Report 51, Fed. Reg. 33992, U.S. Environmental Protection Agency, Washington, DC.

U.S. EPA (1986b). "Guidance for the Reregistration of Pesticide Products Containing Captan as the Active Ingredient (EPA Case Number 0120)." U.S. Environmental Protection Agency, Washington, DC.

U.S. EPA (1986c). "Guidelines for Carcinogen Risk Assessment." Report 51, Fed. Reg. 33992-34003, U.S. Environmental Protection Agency, Washington, DC.

U.S. EPA (1987). "Guidance for the Registration of Pesticide Products Containing Folpet as the Active Ingredient (Case Number 0630)." U.S. Environmental Protection Agency, Washington, DC.

U.S. EPA (1989). "Captan; Intent to Cancel Registrations; Conclusion of Special Review (PD4)." Report 54, Fed. Reg. 8116-8150, Office of Prevention, Pesticides and Toxic Substances, U.S. Environmental Protection Agency, Washington, DC.

U.S. EPA (1995a). "The HED Chapter of the Re-registration Eligibility Decision Document (RED) for Captan." Health Effects Division, Office of Pesticide Programs, U.S. Environmental Protection Agency, Washington, DC.

U.S. EPA (1995b). "The HED Chapter of the Re-registration Eligibility Decision Document (RED) for Folpet." Health Effects Division, Office of Pesticide Programs, U.S. Environmental Protection Agency, Washington, DC.

U.S. EPA (1996). "Proposed Guidelines for Carcinogen Risk Assessment." Report 61, Fed. Reg. 17960-18011, U.S. Environmental Protection Agency, Washington, DC.

U.S. EPA (1999a). "Captan: Reregistration Eligibility Decision (RED)." Report 738-R-99-015, Prevention, Pesticides and Toxic Substances (7508C), U.S. Environmental Protection Agency, Washington, DC.

U.S. EPA (1999b). "Folpet: Reregistration Eligibility Decision (RED)." Report 738-R-99-011, Prevention, Pesticides and Toxic Substances (7508C), U.S. Environmental Protection Agency, Washington, DC.

U.S. EPA (1999c). "Guidance for Identifying Pesticide Chemicals that Have a Common Mechanism of Toxicity, for Use in Assessing the Cumulative Toxic Effects of Pesticides." Report 6055, U.S. Environmental Protection Agency, Washington, DC.

Valencia, R. (1981). "Mutagenesis Screening of Pesticides Using Drosophila." Report 600/1-81-017, U.S. Environmental Protection Agency, Washington, DC.

van Welie, R., T. H., van Duyn, P., Lamme, E. K., Jäger, P., van Baar, B. L. M., and Vermeulen, N. P. E. (1991). Determination of tetrahydrophthalimide and 2-thiothiazolidine-4-carboxylic acid, urinary metabolites of the fungicide captan, in rats and humans. *Int. Arch. Occup. Environ. Health* **63**(3), 181–186.

Vogel, E., and Chandler, J. L. R. (1974). Mutagenicity testing of cyclamate and some pesticides in *Drosophila melanogaster*. *Experientia* **30**(6), 621–623.

Vondruska, J. F. (1969). "Teratologic Investigation of Captan in *Macaca mulatta* (Rhesus monkey) and *Macac arctoides* (Stumptailed macaque)." Report M5519, Industrial Bio-Test Laboratories, Inc. (MRID 00043398).

Vos, J. G., and Krajnc, E. I. (1983). Immunotoxicity of pesticides. *Dev. Sci. Practice Toxicol.* **11**, 229–240.

Waner, T. (1988). "Folpan: Chronic Oral Study in Beagle Dogs for 52 Weeks." Report MAK.062/FOL, Life Science Research Israel, Ltd., Ness Ziona, Israel.

Ward, J. M., Goodman, D. G., Squire, R., Chu, A., and Linhart, M. S. (1979). Neoplastic and nonneoplastic lesions in aging (C57BL/6N x C3H/HeN)F1 (B6C3F$_1$) mice. *J. Natl. Cancer Inst.* **63**, 849–854.

Waterson, L. (1995). "Folpet: Investigation of the Effect on the Duodenum of Male Mice after Dietary Administration for 28 Days with Recovery." Report MBS 45/943003, Huntingdon Research Centre Ltd. (MRID 44286303).

Williams, G. M. (1992). DNA reactive and epigenetic carcinogens. *Exp. Toxicol. Pathol.* **44**, 457–464.

Wilson, A., and Wright, A. (1990). "A Study of Dermal Penetration of Carbon 14-Folpet in the Rat." Report MAG/1/PH, Toxicol Laboratories, Inc. (MRID 42122018).

Wong, Z. A., Bradfield, L. G., and Akins, B. J. (1981). "Lifetime Oncogenic Feeding Study of Captan Technical (SX-944) in CD-1 Mice (ICR Derived)." Report SOCAL 1150, Chevron Environmental Health Center, Richmond, CA (MRID 00068076).

Wong, Z. A., Eisenlord, G. H., and MacGregor, J. (1982). "Lifetime Oncogenic Feeding Study of Phaltan Technical (SX-946) in CD-1 (ICR Derived) Mice." Report SOCAL 1331, Chevron Environmental Health Center, Richmond, CA (MRID 125718).

Mammalian Toxicokinetics and Toxicity of Chlorothalonil

P. P. Parsons

Syngenta

80.1 IDENTITY AND USES OF CHLOROTHALONIL

Chlorothalonil is a halogenated benzonitrile fungicide with broad spectrum activity against vegetable, ornamental, orchard, and turf diseases. It was first registered for use as an agrochemical in the United States in 1966. Chlorothalonil is available in a wide variety of formulations including suspension concentrates, wettable powders, and water dispersible granules. Its mode of fungicidal action is to bind to sulfhydryl groups of amino acids, proteins, and peptides and, in doing so, it ties up free glutathione in fungal cells, thereby blocking glycolytic and respiratory enzyme pathways. This action prevents the ability of fungal cells to infect plants and results in death of the fungus. Chlorothalonil's multisite mode of action has meant that no significant problem with fungal resistance has been encountered. In addition to its use as an agricultural fungicide, chlorothalonil also has wider biocidal applications, for example in paints and lubricating fluids.

80.1.1 PHYSICAL AND CHEMICAL PROPERTIES

80.1.1.1 Structure

80.1.1.2 Chemical Identity

Common name	chlorothalonil
CAS No.	1897-45-6
EINECS	217-588-1
Chemical name	2,4,5,6-tetrachloroisophthalonitrile

Chemical class	halogenated benzonitrile
Empirical formula	CCl_4N_2
Synonyms and trade names	Bravo®, Daconil®, Tuffcide®, Acticide®

80.1.1.3 Physical Properties

Physical appearance	grey/white crystalline solid, odorless in pure form
Solubility (at 25°C)	practically insoluble in water (0.6–0.8 mg/l) xylene—80 g/l acetone—20 g/l cyclohexane—30 g/l
Vapor pressure	7.62×10^{-5} Pa at 25°C
Molecular weight	265.9
Melting point	250–251°C
log Po/w	2.94 at 25°C

80.2 MAMMALIAN TOXICOKINETICS

An overview of the available metabolism and pharmacokinetic data for chlorothalonil has been published by Wilkinson and Killeen (1996).

80.2.1 ORAL ADMINISTRATION

In rats, given a single, oral low dose (1.5 mg/kg) of chlorothalonil, around 20–22% of the absorbed dose is excreted in bile and around 10% in urine (Marciniszyn *et al.*, 1985a, b, 1986a). At higher doses (200 mg/kg) a considerably lower proportion (8%) of the absorbed dose is excreted in bile, indicating that this is a saturable process. These data indicate that overall absorption from the G.I. tract is in the order of 30–32% of the administered dose. The majority of radiolabel is excreted in feces with at least 80% of administered dose excreted by this route within 96 h. Approximately 90% of the administered dose was excreted within 24–48 h although excretion was less rapid at doses of 50 mg/kg and above. Highest tissue concentrations were observed in the kidney, approximately 0.1% of the dose. A similar metabolic profile was seen on repeated dosing and there was no evidence for bioaccumulation (Savides *et al.*, 1986a, b). Thiol-derived metabolites were identified in urine. Following administration of similar doses of chlorothalonil to germ-free rats, only 3% of the dose appeared in urine with lower proportions excreted as thiol-derived metabolites, indicating that gut microflora may play a role in the disposition and metabolism of chlorothalonil in the rat. Bile cannulation studies have confirmed that chlorothalonil undergoes enterohepatic circulation in the rat (Marciniszyn *et al.*, 1986b).

In dogs, approximately 6% of an oral dose of 50 mg/kg was excreted within 48 h (1% in urine and 5% in bile). As with the rat, absorption and subsequent excretion were rapid with around 89% of an administered dose recovered within 48 h. The extent of urinary thiol-derived metabolite excretion in dogs was lower than that seen in rats. At necropsy at 48 h approximately 0.1% of the administered dose was present in the liver and kidneys with <0.01% in other tissues (Savides *et al.*, 1995).

Limited data for the monkey show that, following a single oral dose of 50 mg/kg, 1.8–4.1% of the dose appeared in urine with very low levels of thiol-derived metabolites appearing in urine. Fecal excretion predominated with around 92% of the dose eliminated via this route over 96 h. Absorption and excretion were rapid and there was no evidence of bioaccumulation (Savides *et al.*, 1990).

There are limited data concerning the disposition and excretion of chlorothalonil in the mouse with no metabolism data in this species. Low levels of radioactivity were found in the tissues and urinary excretion indicated that at least 10% of the dose was absorbed with the majority (70–80%) of the dose excreted in faeces (Ribovich *et al.*, 1982).

Comparison of the differences in urinary metabolite excretion profile between species suggests that the ability to excrete thiol-derived metabolites may be correlated with the observed species differences in susceptibility to renal toxicity.

Mechanistic studies have been conducted to determine if a relationship exists between the ability to excrete urinary thiol-derived metabolites of chlorothalonil and the potential to induce renal toxicity. Inhibition of γ-glutamyltranspeptidase using Acivicin (Savides *et al.*, 1985) and renal organic anion transport using probenecid (Marciniszyn *et al.*, 1986b) decreased urinary thiol-derived metabolite excretion in rats. Administration of the monoglutathione conjugate to rats was shown to produce a qualitatively similar pattern of metabolite excretion to that seen following administration of chlorothalonil itself (Mead *et al.*, 1987a, b). These studies indicate that excretion of thiol-derived metabolites of chlorothalonil requires glutathione conjugation and then subsequent enzymatic processing of glutathione-derived conjugates that are selectively accumulated within the kidney. By analogy with other chemicals that undergo extensive glutathione conjugation, it is reasonable to presume that metabolism proceeds via cysteine conjugates and *N*-acetyl cysteine conjugates ("mercapturates") as outlined in Fig. 80.1.

In conclusion, data from a variety of species demonstrate that, following oral administration, chlorothalonil is rapidly absorbed with fecal excretion predominating. The toxicokinetic profile is similar on repeated dosing with no evidence for bioaccumulation. Glutathione conjugation plays a central role

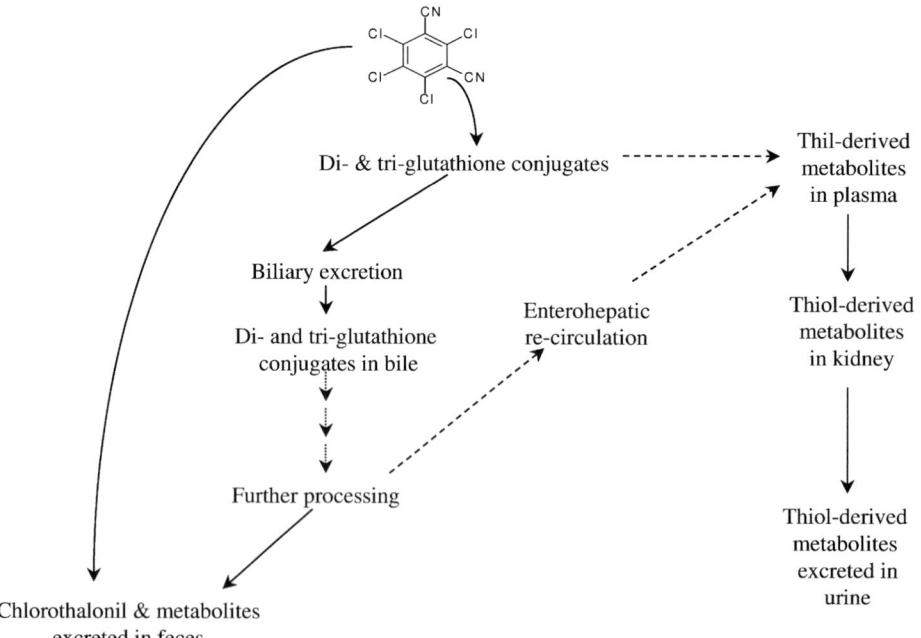

Figure 80.1 Diagram illustrating proposed metabolism of chlorothalonil following oral administration to rats. Broken lines indicate multistage events involving several enzymatic steps and transport processes.

in the metabolism of chlorothalonil and subsequent complex metabolic processing of these conjugates results in selective renal uptake and urinary excretion of thiol-derived metabolites. Knowledge from the metabolism of other chemicals that undergo extensive glutathione conjugation implicates a role for mercapturic acid-mediated metabolism for chlorothalonil.

80.2.2 DERMAL ADMINISTRATION

Studies have been conducted to determine the nature of metabolites appearing after dermal administration of chlorothalonil to the rat and monkey. Separate *in vitro* and *in vivo* studies have been conducted to determine the extent to which chlorothalonil undergoes percutaneous absorption.

80.2.2.1 Urinary Metabolite Profile Following Dermal Exposure

Limited studies have been conducted in the rat and the monkey to investigate the profile of urinary metabolite excretion after dermal administration of chlorothalonil. In rats, a maximum of 3.1% of the applied dose was excreted in urine of which around 0.1–1% constituted thiol-derived metabolites (Savides *et al.*, 1989). Fecal excretion of radiolabel was similarly low. A high proportion (20–40%) of administered dose was retained in skin at the application site. The low level of thiol-derived metabolites excreted in urine following dermal administration of chlorothalonil may explain the absence of renal toxicity seen in the subchronic toxicity studies using this route. In monkeys, only 1.2% of the dose was excreted in urine and similar amounts in feces. Around 2–4% of the dose was retained in skin at the application site after a 48 h exposure and no thiol metabolites could be detected in urine (Magee *et al.*, 1990).

80.2.2.2 Percutaneous Absorption

A number of percutaneous absorption studies have been conducted with chlorothalonil using both *in vitro* and *in vivo* approaches. These studies used either acetone or formulation blank as the vehicle.

***In Vitro* Studies** Two *in vitro* studies have been conducted using human abdominal epidermis. In one study, the chlorothalonil was used either neat (no vehicle) or as a solution in acetone (Ward, 1989a). The mean absorption rate observed in this study over a 48 to 55 h exposure interval was 0.034 ± 0.020 $\mu g/cm^2/h$, equating to 0.085% of the applied dose. No radiolabel was detected in the receptor chamber fluid until 48 h after application using either neat or diluted material. In a separate study (Ward, 1989b), chlorothalonil was applied as a suspension in a commercial formulation base either as a concentrate or as a spray-strength dilution under both occluded and nonoccluded conditions.

The mean absorption rate per hour was higher with the occluded application than with the nonoccluded application (0.18 vs 0.005 $\mu g/cm^2/h$). Approximately 0.094% of the applied dose was absorbed over a 10 h period with the nonoccluded application.

These data indicate that the absorption of chlorothalonil through the human epidermis is considerably lower than 1% of the applied dose.

***In Vivo* Studies** A study was conducted in the rat which investigated the percutaneous absorption of chlorothalonil using acetone and a blank commercial formulation as dosing vehicles (Andre *et al.*, 1991a). Absorption values ranging from 6 to 26% were obtained taking into account the radiolabelled material bound to skin at the application site. A more realistic indication of systemic absorption is obtained when skin bound material is discounted. Using this approach, percutaneous absorption at 10 h postapplication in formulation blank was 2.2, 3.6, and 0.4% of the applied using applications of 0.1, 0.5, and 5.0 mg/kg, respectively. These values are consistent with the absorption profile seen *in vitro*.

Thus, the available data indicate that chlorothalonil is a poor skin penetrant. This view is supported by the estimation of percutaneous absorption by comparison of the ability of chlorothalonil to induce toxicity within the key target organ (kidney) following dermal and oral administration to rats. Such a comparison is based on the findings of the 21 day dermal toxicity study (see Section 80.5.2) with the interim findings after a similar dosing period in a 90 day subchronic oral toxicity study (see Section 80.5.1). In these respective studies, the NOAELs for the induction of renal tubular hyperplasia were 600 mg/kg/d (the highest dose) and 3 mg/kg/d. Toxicokinetic studies in rats indicate that approximately 32% of an oral dose of chlorothalonil is absorbed from the G.I. tract. Therefore, the NOAEL for renal hyperplasia after 6 weeks in the 90 day oral rat study of 3 mg/kg/d equates to a systemic dose of 0.96 mg/kg/d (i.e., 0.32×3). Since the application of 600 mg/kg/d of chlorothalonil to rat skin did not result in any kidney toxicity, it can be deduced that that approximately 0.16% of the applied dermal dose was absorbed systemically (i.e., $0.96/600 \times 100\%$).

80.3 ACUTE TOXICITY

80.3.1 ORAL

Chlorothalonil is not acutely toxic by the oral route having a maximum lethal dose (MLD) > 5000 mg/kg in the rat with no deaths at 5000 mg/kg in carbosa methyl cellulose (Moore, 2000). The only clinical signs of toxicity were congenital staining, soft feces, and/or occurred on the day of dosing and the day following dosing.

80.3.2 DERMAL

The dermal MLD was >10,000 mg/kg in rabbits with no deaths observed at this dose. In this study, chlorothalonil was applied to abraded skin for 24 h (Shults *et al.*, 1981b). Slight edema and yellow discoloration were observed at the application site and eye irritation was also seen. At necropsy, pale areas were observed in the liver. Chlorothalonil is not systemically toxic by the dermal route.

80.3.3 INTRAPERITONEAL

The intraperitoneal MLD has been estimated to be 3.2 mg/kg in the rat. Clinical signs of toxicity were not reported. Pathological findings were generally consistent with injection of an irritant substance into the peritoneal cavity with chronic fibrinous peritonitis, enlarged and congested mesenteric lymph nodes, intestinal edema, and red foci on the kidneys and lungs (Wazeter and Lucas, 1971).

80.3.4 INHALATION

Acute inhalation exposure (whole body) of rats to an atmosphere containing chlorothalonil dust resulted in a 4 h MLC of 0.1 mg/l (Shults *et al.*, 1993). Mortality was dose-related with deaths at 0.08, 0.14, and 0.21 mg/l (4, 6, and 9/10 animals, respectively) occurring from 10 minutes to 2 days postexposure. Clinical signs of toxicity included gasping, eye closure, and exaggerated breathing observed during exposure. Recovery was evident from day 4 onward and the majority of animals were normal by day 9. Congestion of the lungs and white frothy fluid in the trachea were observed in those animals that died with no abnormal pathology in surviving animals. The MMAD was 2.5–3.6 μm with 25% of particles <2 μm in diameter.

In a separate study (Shults *et al.*, 1981c), rats were exposed (whole body) to a dust atmosphere containing chlorothalonil at concentrations of 0.07–0.22 mg/l for 4 h. The MMAD was 1.35–5.5 μm with 90% of particles of <10 μm in diameter. The MLC was estimated to be 0.09 mg/l with a dose-related incidence of mortality (1/20 at 0.7 mg/l vs 19/20 at 0.22 mg/l). Clinical signs of toxicity included rales and a bloody nasal discharge. Pulmonary congestion was observed in animals that died during the study. Hepatic necrosis and deposition of eosinophillic material were observed at the top dose. A high incidence of respiratory mycoplasmosis was seen in all animals in this study. Although the study is compromised by the presence of concomitant infection, the 4 h MLC was in agreement with that observed in the study above.

It is concluded that chlorothalonil is toxic by inhalation causing death by asphyxiation secondary to pulmonary edema. In standard regulatory studies, the clinical signs of toxicity and pathological findings are consistent with exposure to a substance that causes pulmonary irritation to the lungs and respiratory tract.

80.3.5 SKIN IRRITATION

Technical chlorothalonil is not a skin irritant in rabbits (Shults *et al.*, 1981d). In this study, a prolonged exposure period of 24 h

was used and effects were studied using both abraded and intact skin. Although the study conditions were designed to maximize the potential to induce skin irritation, the only effects observed were isolated signs of mild irritation.

In contrast, prolonged and/or repeated dermal exposure to chlorothalonil has been shown to produce significant signs of skin irritation in acute and subchronic dermal toxicity studies in the rat and rabbit (see Section 80.5.2). It is concluded that, while chlorothalonil is not a skin irritant in standard studies for assessment of this endpoint, it does display potential to cause skin irritation in other dermal toxicity studies involving prolonged or repeated dermal application.

Chlorothalonil has been shown to cause dermal reactions in humans who have been occupationally exposed to chlorothalonil, although it has not always been apparent if this constitutes and irritation or sensitization response (see Section 80.11.1).

80.3.6 EYE IRRITATION

In a standard rabbit eye irritation study, chlorothalonil caused irreversible ocular lesions in rabbits with corneal opacity persisting for up to 14 days postinstillation. Effects also persist in the iris and conjunctiva (Wilson, 1977a). A further four studies have been conducted with technical chlorothalonil and each of these studies demonstrated irreversible corneal opacity (Francis *et al.*, 1973; O'Meara and Laveglia, 1995; Wilson, 1977b, c). The severity and persistence of these eye lesions indicates that chlorothalonil has potential to cause serious damage to eyes. The effect of washing the eyes postcompound instillation has not been investigated using the technical material itself, although studies with high strength formulations have shown that postinstillation washing ameliorates these effects. This observation is relevant to the recommended treatment of individuals following accidental ocular exposure. Experience from accidental human exposure indicates that chlorothalonil causes ocular pain and is also irritating to the human eye (see Section 80.11.2). However, the severe and irreversible eye lesions seen in the rabbit have not been documented in humans.

80.3.7 SUMMARY OF ACUTE TOXICITY

Chlorothalonil has very low acute toxicity by the oral and dermal routes although it is very toxic by inhalation. Many of the effects seen following acute exposure are consistent with irritation at the initial site of contact. However, chlorothalonil was not irritating to skin when tested in a standard skin irritation study although dermal irritation has been observed in acute and subchronic toxicity studies in the rat and rabbit, indicating the potential for chlorothalonil to cause skin irritation following repeated or prolonged exposure. Chlorothalonil causes irreversible and severe ocular lesions in rabbits. The acute toxicity of chlorothalonil is summarized in Table 80.1.

Table 80.1
Acute Toxicity of Chlorothalonil

Study	Species	Result
Oral toxicity	Rat	MLD > 10,000 mg/kg
Dermal toxicity	Rabbit	MLD > 10,000 mg/kg
Inhalation toxicity	Rat	4 h MLC 0.1 mg/l
	Rat	4 h MLC 0.09 mg/l
	Rat	1 h MLC 0.52 mg/l
Intraperitoneal toxicity	Rat	MLD 3.2 mg/kg
	Rat	MLD 8 mg/kg
	Mouse	MLD 12 mg/kg
Skin irritation	Rabbit	[a]Not a skin irritant
Eye irritation	Rabbit	Irreversible corneal opacity
	Rabbit	Irreversible corneal opacity
	Rabbit	Irreversible corneal opacity
	Rabbit	Irreversible corneal opacity
	Rabbit	Irreversible corneal opacity

[a]Potential skin irritant with prolonged or repeated dermal exposure.

80.4 SENSITIZATION

80.4.1 SKIN SENSITIZATION

The potential for chlorothalonil to induce skin sensitization has been investigated in guinea pigs using a number of different study designs (see Table 80.2). Although these studies provide an inconsistent profile with regard to skin sensitization potential, the data are supportive of the view that chlorothalonil is a skin sensitizer of relatively low potency. It appears that a concentration of at least 40% w/v technical chlorothalonil is required for the induction of sensitization in guinea pigs. It is concluded that chlorothalonil is a weak skin sensitizer in guinea pigs.

In addition to these data in animals, information is available concerning the potential of chlorothalonil to cause skin sensitization in humans following dermal exposure in the occupational setting (see Section 80.11.1).

80.4.2 RESPIRATORY SENSITIZATION

There are no animal data concerning the potential for chlorothalonil to induce respiratory sensitization.

80.5 SUBCHRONIC TOXICITY

80.5.1 ORAL

In rats, dietary administration of chlorothalonil for 28 days caused clinical signs of toxicity, decreased body weight, and decreased hematological parameters at doses of ≥375 mg/kg/d. One death occurred at the top dose (1500 mg/kg/d). Absolute kidney weight was increased at ≥175 mg/kg/d. No effects were observed at 80 mg/kg/d but this cannot reliably be considered

as a NOEL as histopathological examination was not conducted in this study and longer term studies suggest that hyperplasia of the forestomach and proximal tubular epithelium can occur at this dose level (Wilson *et al.*, 1982b).

The principal lesions observed following dietary administration of chlorothalonil to rats and mice for up to 90 days were hyperplasia and hyperkeratosis of the forestomach and hyperplasia of the proximal tubular epithelium of the kidney (Shults *et al.*, 1983, 1985; Wilson *et al.*, 1983a, b, 1984, 1985a, b). No treatment-related mortality was observed in these studies at doses up to 1500 mg/kg/d and there were only limited clinical signs of toxicity. Renal hyperplasia only occurred at a low incidence at the top dose tested in male mice with no effect in females. Other effects included decreased plasma ALT activity and increased kidney weight. The overall NOELs in these studies were 1.5 mg/kg/d for rats and 2.8 mg/kg/d for mice with respective LOELs of 3.0 and 9.2 mg/kg/d.

The NOEL for hyperplasia of the forestomach was 3 mg/kg/d in both species with LOELs of 10 mg/kg/d in the rat and 9 mg/kg/d in the mouse. The forestomach lesions were fully reversible after a 13 week recovery period in rats but were not investigated in mice.

The NOAEL for proximal tubular hyperplasia after 6 weeks dosing was 3 mg/kg/d in rats with a clear increase in the incidence of hyperplasia at ≥40 mg/kg/d in animals necropsied at 13 weeks. Proximal tubular hyperplasia was evident in 2/5 animals at 6 weeks at 10 mg/kg/d. In male mice, the NOEL for renal hyperplasia was 48 mg/kg/d with a LOEL of 130 mg/kg/d.

Further investigative studies have been conducted in the rat. Vacuolar degeneration has been shown to be present in the proximal tubular epithelium after only two daily doses of chlorothalonil at 175 mg/kg/d (Ford *et al.*, 1988). In 28 day (Hironaka *et al.*, 1996) and 90 day (Mizens *et al.*, 1996) studies, chlorothalonil has also been shown to increase cell proliferation in the forestomach (BrdU) and proximal tubule (PCNA) of rats. Significant increases in labelling indices were evident from day 7 of dosing through to days 28 or 90 respectively at doses of ≥15 mg/kg/d. The NOEL for increased labelling indices in both tissues was 1.5 mg/kg/d.

Similar morphological lesions were seen in the renal proximal tubular epithelium following gavage administration of equivalent doses of the monoglutathione conjugate of chlorothalonil (150 mg/kg/d) or parent compound (75 mg/kg/d), although in these animals no hyperplastic changes were seen in the forestomach (Mead, 1987b). This finding implicates glutathione conjugation in the metabolism of chlorothalonil-induced renal toxicity and demonstrates that it is the parent compound that causes toxicity in the rodent forestomach.

In dogs, administration of chlorothalonil for 90 days caused a decrease in body weight gain at 150 and 500 mg/kg/d with one death seen at the top dose (Fillmore *et al.*, 1993). There was some indication of a decrease in mean body weight throughout the study in both sexes at 15 mg/kg/d, but this was not considered to be toxicologically significant. Some changes in clinical chemistry were seen at these dose levels with plasma ALT decreased at all dose levels. The NOAEL was 15 mg/kg/d

Table 80.2
Summary of Skin Sensitization Studies Conducted in Guinea Pigs

Test method (date)	Induction concentration	Challenge concentration	Conclusion	Reference
9 induction Buehler (1974)	10% in water	10% in water	Not a sensitizer	CTL/C/3873
9 induction Buehler (1985)	100%	10% in saline	[a] Sensitizer	Shults and Wilson, 1985
9 induction Buehler (1985)	100%	100%	[a] Not a sensitizer	CTL/C/3573
Maximization (1986)	i.d.—0.5% in acetone topical—1% in acetone	0.001% in acetone	[a] Not a sensitizer	Tucker, 1986
Maximization (1986)	i.d.—5% in propylene glycol topical—1% in acetone	0.0125% in acetone	Sensitizer	Tucker, 1986
20 induction open cutaneous (1986)	0.01, 0.1, or 1%	0.0025, 0.0075 or 0.025%	Sensitizer	Tucker, 1986
10-induction Buehler (1982)	100%	100%	Not a sensitizer	Wilson et al., 1982a
Maximization (1988)	Acetone vehicle	Acetone vehicle	Equivocal	Wilson et al., 1988a
Buehler	Acetone vehicle	Acetone vehicle	Sensitizer	Wilson et al., 1988b
Maximization	Acetone vehicle	Acetone vehicle	Sensitizer	Wilson et al., 1988c

[a] Result confirmed by rechallenge.

as effects on ALT were not considered adverse. No lesions were observed in the stomach or the kidney, indicating that the dog has a different toxicity profile to rodents.

80.5.2 DERMAL

Subchronic (21 day) dermal toxicity studies have been conducted in rats and rabbits.

In rabbits, no systemic effects were observed that were associated with chlorothalonil administration at doses up to 50 mg/kg/d (Shults et al., 1986). However, histopathological examination revealed evidence of parasitic infection in all animals which compromises the value of this study. The NOEL for local effects in the skin was 0.1 mg/kg/d based on the observation of erythema and skin thickening at ≥2.5 mg/kg/d.

In rats, decreases in body weight gain were observed over the 21 day study period along with simultaneous decreases in food consumption (Mizens et al., 1986a). The decrease in weight gain was more prominent early in the study with increasing weight gain observed toward the end of the study. Plasma ALT activity was decreased at all dose levels. No histopathological effects were observed in the kidney, indicating that the NOEL for renal effects following dermal application was >600 mg/kg/d. Erythema, hyperkeratosis, and squamous epithelial cell hyperplasia where observed at the site of application

at all dose levels, indicating the potential for chlorothalonil to cause dermal irritation with repeated exposure.

80.5.3 INHALATION

No repeat-dose inhalation toxicity studies have been conducted with technical chlorothalonil. However, the symptoms and pathological findings seen after acute inhalation exposure are confined to the respiratory tract with no evidence of systemic toxicity. It is therefore anticipated that toxicity in a repeat-dose inhalation study would be expected to manifest as local irritation with the NOAEL being driven by site-of-contact toxicity within the lungs and respiratory tract as opposed to systemic toxicity.

The subchronic toxicity of chlorothalonil is summarized in Table 80.3.

80.6 CHRONIC TOXICITY

The chronic oral toxicity of chlorothalonil has been determined in the rat and mouse with two long-term studies available in each species. The initial studies on chlorothalonil (Wilson et al., 1983c, 1985c) were conducted at relatively high dose levels and failed to demonstrate NOELs, so the studies were repeated (Wilson et al., 1987, 1989) using lower doses. The

Table 80.3
Summary of Subchronic Toxicity Data

Species	Route	Duration (days)	NOEL (mg/kg/d)	LOEL (mg/kg/d)
Rat	Oral diet	90	None	40 (hyperplasia of forestomach and kidney)
Rat	Oral diet	90	1.5	3 ($\uparrow$ kidney weight, $\downarrow$ ALT)
			3	10 (hyperplasia of forestomach)
			10	40 (hyperplasia of kidney)
Mouse	Oral diet	90	3	9 ($\uparrow$ kidney weight, $\downarrow$ ALT)
			3	9 (hyperplasia of forestomach)
			48	130 (hyperplasia of kidney)
Dog	Oral—capsule	90	15	150 ($\downarrow$ weight gain)
Rabbit	Dermal	21	0.1	2.5 local effects
			50	2.6 no systemic effects
Rat	Dermal	21	None	60 local effects
			600	No renal histopathology observed at top dose—600

findings in the chronic rat and mouse studies were consistent with those seen in the subchronic studies with hyperplasia of the forestomach and proximal tubular epithelium being the most prominent effects. The hyperplastic changes in the proximal tubular epithelium were associated with an increase in absolute kidney weight. The NOELs for hyperplasia and hyperkeratosis of the forestomach were 1.8 and 1.6 mg/kg/d for rats and mice respectively and the NOELs for hyperplastic changes in the proximal tubular epithelium were 1.8 mg/kg/d for rats and 5.4 mg/kg/d for mice. In addition to the hyperplastic lesions in the kidney and forestomach, some minor changes were seen in clinical chemistry, hematology, and urinalysis. There was no evidence of systemic toxicity in organs other than the kidney and forestomach. Although changes occurred in some organ weight : body weight ratios, these were attributable to decreases in body weight.

In beagle dogs, 1 year administration of chlorothalonil caused a significant decrease in body weight gain at 500 mg/kg/d with increases in absolute liver and kidney weights at $\geq$150 mg/kg/d (Mizens and Laveglia, 1994). No histopathological findings were seen in association with the organ weight changes. Changes in clinical chemistry were seen but only at one time point (27 weeks) and with no relationship to dose. Increased pigmentation of the kidney was observed at 150 and 500 mg/kg/d. The severity of this effect was similar at both dose levels and minimal pigmentation was seen in control and low dose animals. Due to its presence in control animals and lack of relationship to dose, the renal pigmentation was not considered to be of toxicological significance. Moreover, this observation was clearly distinct from the hyperplastic lesion seen in the renal proximal tubular epithelium of rodents. This indicates that there are species-specific differences in susceptibility to the renal toxicity of chlorothalonil.

Although dogs do not possess an anatomical equivalent of the rodent forestomach, the stomachs from this study were examined to determine if there was any evidence of cell proliferation using PCNA labelling. There was no increase in labelling index in any treated group when compared to concurrent controls, providing reassurance that chlorothalonil is not toxic to the gastric mucosa of dogs. The overall NOAEL for this study was 150 mg/kg/d.

The chronic toxicity findings are summarized in Table 80.4.

80.7 GENOTOXICITY

80.7.1 *IN VITRO* GENOTOXICITY STUDIES

An extensive range of tests have been conducted to assess the genotoxic potential of technical chlorothalonil. *In vitro* studies were mostly negative including Ames tests using renal and hepatic metabolic activation systems. Up to 17 metabolites of chlorothalonil have also been tested and shown to give gave negative results using rat kidney S9. Two nonstandard bacterial DNA repair assays have been performed, one of which was positive and the other negative.

A significant increase in the incidence of chromosomal aberrations has been observed in Chinese hamster ovary cells although this was only evident in the absence of auxiliary metabolic activation (Mizens *et al.*, 1986b). In the absence of S9, increases in structural aberrations over control values were observed only at the top two concentrations which approached cytotoxic levels. These data indicate that chlorothalonil has clastogenic activity *in vitro* in the absence of S9. The effect was not observed in the presence of S9, even at dose levels some 20 times higher. However, given the lack of genotoxicity observed in other *in vitro* test systems (e.g., the Ames test) and the known

Table 80.4
Summary of Chronic Toxicity Data

Duration of study	Species	NOAEL (mg/kg bwt/day)	LOEL (mg/kg bwt/day)
2 years	Rat	None	40
2 years	Rat	3.8	15 (kidney tumors)
		1.8	3.8 (kidney hyperplasia)
		1.8	3.8 (stomach mucosal tumors)
		1.8	3.8 (stomach squamous cell tumors)
2 years	Mouse	None	125
2 years	Mouse	5.4	23 (kidney hyperplasia)
		23	100 (stomach mucosal tumors)
		1.6	5.4 (stomach squamous cell tumors)
1 year oral	Dog	150	500 (decreased body weight gain)

reactivity of chlorothalonil, a rationale for such a profile is possible.

Chlorothalonil can be viewed as a reactive molecule insofar as it is known to be reactive towards thiol (-SH) groups. It can be considered as a soft electrophile with a preference for sulphur nucleophiles rather then nitrogen/oxygen nucleophiles. Such chemicals tend to show reactivity toward protein (contains critical S electrophiles) rather than toward DNA (contains critical O and N nucleophiles). The profile of activity in genotoxicity assays is that such material displays negative findings in the Ames test but apparent positive findings in the *in vitro* cytogenetics assay, usually in the absence of exogenous metabolic activation.

The activity of chlorothalonil in the IVC assay is likely to be through reactivity with protein (not DNA), and with the protein dependency of the chromosomal structure allowing visualization as a structural aberration. Such an activity would not be expected to produce genotoxicity *in vivo*, as reaction with inter- and intracellular thiols would dissipate the activity. This is supported by the observation that the *in vitro* activity of chlorothalonil in the IVC assay is removed by the addition of S9, and also by the fact that *in vivo* metabolism/distribution studies have confirmed that chlorothalonil reacts very rapidly with thiols. The clastogenic response observed *in vitro* in the IVC assay is therefore considered to be of no real significance regarding possible genotoxicity *in vivo* especially when considered in light of the findings of the *in vivo* cytogenetic studies with chlorothalonil.

80.7.2 *IN VIVO* GENOTOXICITY STUDIES

Several *in vivo* bone marrow cytogenetic studies have been conducted with chlorothalonil using single or repeated dosing schedules in three different species (rat, mouse, and Chinese hamster). Most of these studies used high doses of chlorothalonil (up to 5000 mg/kg) which resulted in some mortality. All of these *in vivo* cytogenetic studies were negative indicating that the clastogenicity seen with chlorothalonil *in vitro*

is not manifest *in vivo*. Further reassurance for lack of genotoxic activity *in vivo* comes from a study which demonstrated that intraperitoneal administration of radiolabelled chlorothalonil to the rat did not result in any labelled material binding covalently to rat kidney DNA. It is therefore concluded that chlorothalonil is not genotoxic *in vivo*.

The results of the genotoxicity studies conducted with chlorothalonil are summarized in Table 80.5.

80.8 CARCINOGENICITY

Treatment-related increases in the incidence of renal tubular adenoma and carcinoma were observed in rats and male mice (Wilson *et al.*, 1983c, 1985c, 1987, 1989). Squamous cell adenomas and carcinomas were also observed in the forestomach of both species. In dogs, there was no evidence of neoplastic development nor was there any evidence for the occurrence of preneoplastic lesions in the kidney or stomach after administration of chlorothalonil for up to 1 year. The NOEL for mucosal cell tumors of the forestomach was 1.8 mg/kg/d in rats and 23 mg/kg/d in mice. In rats, the NOEL for tumors of the proximal tubular epithelium was 3.8 mg/kg/d in males and 15 mg/kg/d in females.

In the first mouse carcinogenicity study, renal tubular adenomas and carcinomas were observed at all dose levels in males including the lowest dose of 125 mg/kg/d. In a subsequent study using the same strain of male mice, there were no treatment-related increases in the incidence of renal tumors up to a dose level of 100 mg/kg/d. Table 80.6 summarizes the key NOAELs observed in these studies.

80.8.1 MODE OF CARCINOGENIC ACTION

A mechanistic interpretation for the carcinogenicity of chlorothalonil has been published by Wilkinson and Killeen (1996).

Table 80.5
Summary of Genotoxicity Data

Test	Study type	Result	Reference
In vitro	Ames test (hepatic activation)	Negative ($\pm$ activation)	Banzer and Kouri, 1977
	Ames test (renal activation)	Negative ($\pm$ activation)	Jones *et al.*, 1984
	Chromosomal aberration assay (CHO)	Negative (+ activation) Positive ($-$ activation)	Mizens *et al.*, 1986b
	Gene mutation assay (Chinese hamster V-79 cells & mouse fibroblast BALB/3T3 cells)	Negative ($\pm$ activation)	Kouri, 1977
	DNA repair test (*S. typhimurium*)	Positive	Auletta and Kouri, 1977
	DNA repair test (*B. subtilus*)	Negative	Shirasu, 1978
	Cell transformation assay (F1706 P95 and H4536 P97 cells)	Negative	Price and Ballee, 1979
In vivo	Micronucleus test	Negative (rat) Negative (mouse) Negative (Chinese hamster)	Killeen and Siou, 1983
	Chromosome aberration test	Negative (rat) Negative (mouse) Negative (Chinese hamster)	Killeen, 1983
	Chromosome aberration test (Chinese hamster)	Acute study—negative Subchronic study—negative	Siou *et al.*, 1985
	Covalent binding to DNA	Negative (rat)	Savides *et al.*, 1987
	Chromosome aberration test	Negative (Chinese hamster)	Proudlock, 1995

Table 80.6
Summary of Carcinogenicity Findings

Duration of study	Species	NOAEL (mg/kg bwt/day)	LOEL (mg/kg bwt/day)
2 years	Rat	None	40
2 years	Rat	3.8	15 (kidney tumors)
		1.8	3.8 (kidney hyperplasia)
		1.8	3.8 (stomach mucosal tumors)
2 years	Mouse	None	125
2 years	Mouse	5.4	23 (kidney hyperplasia)
		23	100 (stomach mucosal tumors)
1 year oral	Dog	150	500 (decreased body weight gain)

80.8.1.1 Forestomach Tumors

Repeated administration of chlorothalonil causes hyperplasia in the forestomach of rats and mice. The data are consistent with a temporal sequence of events starting with increased cell proliferation, multifocal ulceration and erosion of the forestomach mucosa, regenerative hyperplasia and hyperkeratosis, ultimately progressing to the formation of gastric tumors within the forestomach. Clear thresholds have been demonstrated for the induction of hyperplasia and neoplasia in both species. The fact that chlorothalonil is not genotoxic provides reassurance that these tumors occur as a secondary consequence of local irritation within the rodent forestomach. Oral subchronic studies with the monoglutathione conjugate of chlorothalonil, failed to induce any toxicity in the rat forestomach, indicating that it is parent chlorothalonil, and not a metabolite, that is the toxic agent at this site.

In contrast to the findings in the rat, there was no evidence of preneoplastic stomach lesions in dogs orally administered chlorothalonil for up to 1 year at dose up to 500 mg/kg/d, a dose level considerably higher than that which causes hyperkeratosis and hyperplasia in the rodent forestomach (approximately 4 mg/kg/d in the rat). The absence of any evidence of increased cell proliferation in the dog stomach was confirmed by PCNA labelling of tissue obtained at the termination of this study. The absence of stomach lesions in the dog is attributable to the anatomical differences between rodents and dogs in that dogs do not possess a forestomach. Similarly, humans are like the dog in that they do not possess an anatomical equivalent of the rodent forestomach. It is therefore concluded that the rodent forestomach tumors induced by chlorothalonil are not indicative of a carcinogenic risk to humans.

80.8.1.2 Renal Tumors

The experimental data show a temporal sequence of events that lead to the formation of renal tumors in rats and male mice. Vacuolar degeneration of the renal proximal tubular epithelium has been shown to occur after two daily doses of chlorothalonil and cytotoxicity and degeneration of tubular epithelial cells can be seen after only 2 days treatment. Continued administration of chlorothalonil leads to the development of a regenerative hyperplasia within the renal proximal tubular epithelium. Continued regenerative hyperplasia ultimately results in progression of the kidney lesion to tubular adenoma and carcinoma. Thus, the data clearly show that initial cytotoxicity and regenerative hyperplasia within the proximal tubular epithelium are essential prerequisites for subsequent tumor development. Clear thresholds have been demonstrated for this nongenotoxic secondary mode of action which is a direct consequence of chronic stimulation of cell proliferation. Doses of chlorothalonil below the threshold for the induction of these preneoplastic lesions would not be expected to be carcinogenic.

Studies have been conducted investigating the role of the glutathione conjugation pathway and subsequent formation of urinary thiol-derived metabolites in renal tumor formation. The central role of glutathione in the metabolism and subsequent toxicity of chlorothalonil has been shown by studies with a monoglutathione conjugate of chlorothalonil. Knowledge of the metabolism of other chemicals that undergo extensive glutathione conjugation implicates a role for mercapturic acid-mediated metabolism for chlorothalonil.

Maneuvers that inhibit key enzymes in this metabolic process, such as inhibition of the activity of γ-glutamyltranspeptidase or the renal organic anion transporter, decrease the urinary excretion of thiol-derived metabolites in the rat. Administration of a monoglutathione conjugate to rats caused similar lesions in the kidney to parent chlorothalonil although no effects were seen in the forestomach. Studies undertaken *in vitro* using isolated kidney mitochondria have shown that respiration is inhibited in the presence of synthetic mono- and dithiol conjugates derived from chlorothalonil (Andre *et al.*, 1991b; Savides *et al.*, 1988). Furthermore, a correlation appears

to exist between the interspecies differences in susceptibility to renal toxicity and the differences in capacity to produce these thiol-derived metabolites as rats excrete more thiol-derived metabolites than dogs. The proposed mode of action for the induction of renal toxicity in rodents is outlined in Fig. 80.2.

It is concluded that chlorothalonil is a nongenotoxic kidney carcinogen in rats and mice and the NOAELs observed for both tumors and the precursor lesions indicate that it is appropriate to assume that a threshold exists for carcinogenicity. The species differences in metabolism are reflected in the different toxicity profiles seen in rodents and dogs and suggest that the dog is the most appropriate species for human health risk assessment and that these tumors are highly unlikely to develop in humans exposed to chlorothalonil.

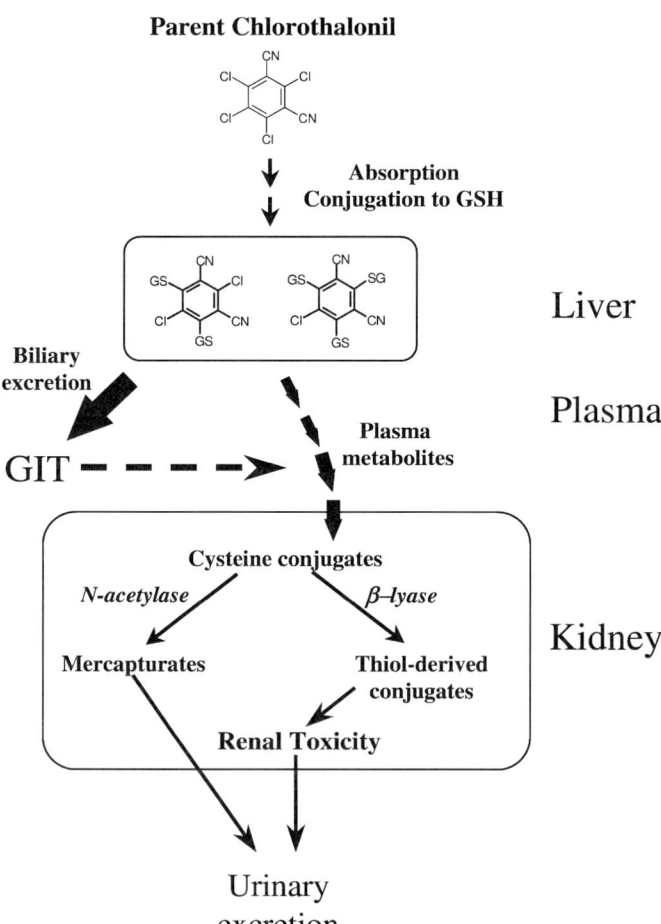

Figure 80.2 Schematic outlining potential pathways of chlorothalonil metabolism in the rat that lead to formation of toxic metabolites within the kidney. Following absorption from the gastrointestinal tract, chlorothalonil is conjugated to glutathione in the liver. Further metabolic processing results in the formation of cysteine conjugates that may be detoxified via *N*-acetylase or activated to toxic thiol-derived species. GSH = glutathione, GIT = gastrointestinal tract.

80.9 REPRODUCTIVE TOXICITY

80.9.1 DEVELOPMENTAL TOXICITY

The potential for chlorothalonil to induce developmental toxicity has been investigated in the rat and rabbit. In rabbits, maternal toxicity was evident at 20 mg/kg/d with body weight loss and decreased food consumption observed at this dose (Wilson *et al.*, 1988d). One death occurred in each of the mid and high dose groups. There were no adverse effects on the fetus and no treatment-related effects on the incidence of skeletal or visceral malformations. The NOEL for maternal toxicity was 10 mg/kg/d and the NOEL for developmental toxicity was 20 mg/kg/d.

In rats, chlorothalonil was maternally toxic at 400 mg/kg/d with mortality, decreased body weight gain, and decreased food consumption at this dose (Mizens *et al.*, 1983). Food consumption was significantly decreased at all doses during days 6–9 of gestation and at the top dose on days 9–15. Food consumption returned to normal values on cessation of treatment with a compensatory increase seen at 25 and 100 mg/kg/d. There was a significant increase in the incidence of postimplantation loss due to early embryonic death at 400 mg/kg/d with a corresponding decrease in viable litter size. One rat at this dose level had reabsorbed 16 out of 17 implantation sites. However, exclusion of this animal from the statistical analysis still resulted in a significant increase in postimplantation loss compared to concurrent and historical controls. The NOELs for maternal and developmental toxicity were 100 mg/kg/d.

It is concluded that chlorothalonil is not a developmental toxicant when tested up to doses that cause significant maternal toxicity and maternal death.

80.9.2 FERTILITY

In a two-generation reproductive toxicity study (Lucas *et al.*, 1990), chlorothalonil caused a dose-related decrease in body weight gain which was evident at all doses in F0 and F1 parental generations although achieving statistical significance at 1500 and 3000 ppm (68 and 145 mg/kg/d). No mortalities or clinical signs of toxicity were observed in this study. Hyperplasia of the forestomach and kidney was observed at all doses in both parental generations with more marked effects in the F1 generation. Thus, a NOEL could not be established for parental toxicity.

There were no adverse effects on reproductive performance or development including fertility indices, gestation length, litter size, number of live pups and stillborn pups, and pup survival. No gross malformations were observed which could be considered as treatment-related. There was a significant decrease in mean pup body weight on day 21 postpartum at 1500 (68 mg/kg/d) and 3000 ppm (145 mg/kg/d). This was only seen in the F1b litter at 1500 ppm but was seen consistently across all litters at 3000 ppm. Therefore, NOAEL for fetotoxicity is considered to be 1500 ppm (68 mg/kg/d). The NOEL for reproductive performance was 145 mg/kg/d with no effects at the top dose.

It is concluded that chlorothalonil is not a reproductive toxicant. There was no evidence of reproductive toxicity in the absence of maternal toxicity. Therefore, the data are consistent with the view that the fetus and developing animal are not uniquely sensitive to chlorothalonil. Table 80.7 presents a summary of the reproductive toxicity studies.

The key NOAELs for all toxicological endpoints are summarized in Table 80.8.

80.10 INVESTIGATIVE TOXICITY STUDIES

80.10.1 ACUTE EFFECTS ON HEPATIC AND RENAL GLUTATHIONE CONTENT

This study was designed to investigate and compare the time course effect of the acute oral administration of chlorothalonil on hepatic and renal glutathione (nonprotein sulfhydryl) content (Sadler and Ignatoski, 1985). At 5000 mg/kg chlorothalonil caused an decrease in body weight gain and liver weight which were evident 18 h after treatment. Within 9 h of treatment, hepatic glutathione levels were decreased and renal glutathione

Table 80.7

Summary of Reproductive Toxicity of Chlorothalonil

Study	Species	NOAEL (mg/kg bwt/day)
Developmental	Rat	Maternal and developmental toxicity—100 (decreased maternal weight gain and increased incidence of resorptions at 400 mg/kg/d)
Developmental	Rabbit	Maternal—10 (decreased weight gain at 20 mg/kg/d)
		Developmental—20 (top dose)
Two-generation reproduction	Rat	Parental—none (renal and forestomach lesions at all doses; LOAEL was 23 mg/kg/d)
		Developmental—68 (decreased pup weight at day 21 at 145 mg/kg/d)
		Reproductive—145 (no effects at top dose)

Table 80.8
Summary of Key Toxicological Endpoints

Study	Endpoint	NOEL (mg/kg/d)	LOEL (mg/kg/d)
90 day rat diet	Increased kidney weight	1.5	3
	Hyperplasia of forestomach	3	10
	Renal hyperplasia	10	40
90 day mouse diet	Increased kidney weight	3	9
	Hyperplasia of forestomach	3	9
	Renal hyperplasia	48	130
90 day dog (capsule)	Decreased body weight gain	15	150
1 year dog (capsule)	Decreased body weight gain	150	500
2 year rat diet	Renal hyperplasia	1.8	3.8
	Renal tumors	3.8	15
	Forestomach hyperplasia	1.8	3.8
	Forestomach tumors	1.8	3.8
2 year mouse oral	Renal hyperplasia	5.4	23
	Renal tumors	99 (top dose)	None
	Forestomach hyperplasia	1.6	5.4
	Forestomach tumors (squamous cell)	1.6	5.4
21 day dermal—rat	Local effects in skin	None	60 (lowest dose)
	Systemic toxicity	None—but NOEL for renal hyperplasia of 600	60 (23% decrease in body weight gain at lowest dose)
Rat reproductive toxicity	Parental NOEL (renal and forestomach hyperplasia)	None	23 (lowest dose)
	Developmental (decreased pup weight at day 21)	68	145
Developmental toxicity	Rat:		
	Maternal (decreased weight gain)	100	400
	Developmental (increased resorptions)	100	400
	Rabbit:		
	Maternal (decreased weight gain)	10	20
	Developmental	20	None

levels were elevated. The depletion of hepatic glutathione is considered a direct consequence of glutathione conjugation within the liver utilizing tissue resources. The increase in renal glutathione content is more difficult to explain but may be a consequence of urinary excretion of glutathione conjugates.

80.10.2 EFFECT OF DIETARY VS GAVAGE DOSING ON RENAL TOXICITY IN THE RAT

A study was conducted that was designed to compare the early morphological changes in the rat kidney following oral administration of chlorothalonil by gavage with those following dietary administration (Ford *et al.*, 1988). Chlorothalonil was administered by gavage at 175 and 1750 mg/kg in the diet (equivalent to 88 mg/kg bw). Effects in the kidney were determined at 24, 48, 73, and 96 h postadministration.

At the 48 h postadministration time point, vacuolar degeneration of the proximal tubular epithelium was observed in 2/3 animals that were gavaged. After 96 h all animals (gavage and diet) exhibited vacuolar degeneration of proximal tubular epithelium although the incidence of affected tubules was higher in gavaged animals than in those administered chlorothalonil in diet.

80.11 HUMAN DATA

Most information concerning the effects of chlorothalonil in humans has been obtained from exposures arising in the manufacture and production and chlorothalonil. Health screening programs in such facilities have shown that the majority of effects documented following exposure to chlorothalonil were attributable to the irritant nature of the substance and included irritation to the skin, eyes, and respiratory tract.

80.11.1 DERMAL EFFECTS

There are a number of case reports in the published literature documenting occupational dermatitis in workers exposed to technical chlorothalonil. Skin reactions have also been documented in patch test studies with human volunteers. The main criticism of these reports is that they do not clearly discriminate between effects that may be a consequence of skin irritation and those that may represent a true sensitization response. Nevertheless, the weight of evidence suggests that chlorothalonil is a weak skin sensitizer in humans.

Special skin surveys were conducted at the main chlorothalonil manufacturing plant to compare dermal findings in 1978 and 1979. In 1978, 60% of the employees had some type of skin abnormality including 19 cases of contact dermatitis (McAmis, 1994a). In 1979, following the initiation of improved industrial hygiene measures in late 1978, there were no cases of contact dermatitis and only 21% of the workers had some kind of skin abnormality. The most common abnormality was skin drying which was seen in 19 of the 26 employees with skin abnormalities (Chelsky, 1980a, b). A delayed irritant dermatitis has been documented which may occur up to 72 h after exposure and, although photosensitization reactions may occur, they are very rare events.

80.11.2 OCULAR EFFECTS

A review of clinical cases from employees exposed to chlorothalonil, at a packaging plant where the exposure was described as infrequent and light, was conducted in 1990 (Chelsky, 1990a). The purpose of this review was to assess the effects of chlorothalonil on the human eye. All of the ocular exposures to chlorothalonil involved intense pain with mild to moderate conjunctivitis and irritation of the corneal surface. Ocular edema was also seen in more extensive exposures. With lesser exposures, complete recovery occurred within 24 h. Recovery took slightly longer with following extensive exposure. In no instance was corneal opacity observed.

80.11.3 RESPIRATORY EFFECTS

Where respiratory effects have been noted these are generally consistent with the irritant properties noted in animal studies, although of a much less severe nature. In a review of medical records from workers at an independent facility used to grind technical chlorothalonil (Chelsky, 1990b, 1992; McAmis, 1994b), it was noted that, even in a workplace described as "dusty" and with workers wearing little protective clothing, ocular and dermal effects predominated, although a few cases of nasal and pharyngeal pain, burning, and soreness were noted. In a study conducted at another manufacturing facility, workers exposed to chlorothalonil showed a lower forced expiratory volume and higher incidences of nose and throat irritation, coughing phlegm, and shortness of breath than reference workers (Huang et al., 1995). Thus, the information available from animal and human exposure indicates that chlorothalonil is irritating to the respiratory tract; a finding that is entirely consistent with the local site-of-contact toxicity seen in other epithelial tissues.

80.11.4 CLINICAL CASES AND POISONING INCIDENTS

Considering that chlorothalonil has been a commercial fungicide for over 25 years, there have been few reports of adverse effects in humans resulting from its use. The majority of the reported human effects have been related to the irritant properties of chlorothalonil. Of the reported skin effects, contact dermatitis is the most frequent diagnosis and this finding is almost exclusively in individuals exposed to chlorothalonil for prolonged periods (over 8 h) in an occupational environment.

In summary, there have been a few reports in the literature of humans suffering adverse health effects following exposure to chlorothalonil (McAmis, 1995). Considering that chlorothalonil has been marketed for more than 25 years as a fungicide in agriculture, forestry, nursery plants, paints, and stains, the reports of adverse effects are very rare. The reported effects are associated with the irritant properties of the technical material.

REFERENCES

Andre, J. C., et al. (1991a). "Comparison of the Effects of Dose Level and Vehicle on the Dermal Absorption of ^{14}C-Chlorothalonil by Male Rats." Unpublished Syngenta study, Rep. 1698-88-0007-AM-001.

Andre, J. C., et al. (1991b). "Evaluation of Mitochondrial Function in the Presence and Absence of Sulfur-Containing Analogs of Chlorothalonil." Unpublished Syngenta study, Rep. 3113-88-0107-AM-001.

Auletta, A., and Kouri, R. (1977). "Activity of DTX-77-0033 in a Test for Differential Inhibition of Repair Deficient and Repair Competent Strains of Salmonella typhimurium." Unpublished Syngenta study, Rep. 000-5TX-77-0033-002.

Banzer, C. B., and Kouri, R. E. (1977). "Activity of Chlorothalonil in the Salmonella Microsomal Assay for Bacterial Mutagenicity." Unpublished Syngenta study, Rep. 000-5TX-77-0035-001.

Chelsky, M. (1980a). "Special Skin Surveys of Green's Bayou Plant Employees, 1978 and 1979." Confidential company medical report originally generated by Diamond Shamrock Corp.

Chelsky, M. (1980b). "Skin Rashes among Green's Bayou Plant Employees." Confidential company medical report originally generated by Diamond Shamrock Corp.

Chelsky, M. (1990a). "Study of Chlorothalonil Plant Workers 1990. Evaluation of Potential for Persistent Effects on Eyes of Workers." Confidential company medical report originally generated by Diamond Shamrock Corp.

Chelsky, M. (1990b). "Annual Employee Health Screening Greens Bayou Plant, 1986–1990. Special Reference to Chlorothalonil Workers and the Respiratory System." Confidential company medical report originally generated by Diamond Shamrock Corp.

Chelsky, M. (1992). "Annual Employee Health Screening Reports, Greens Bayou Plant, 1986–1991. Special Reference to Chlorothalonil Workers and the Respiratory System." Confidential company medical report originally generated by Diamond Shamrock Corp.

Fillmore, G., et al. (1993). "A 90-Day Oral Toxicity Study in Dogs with Chlorothalonil." Unpublished Syngenta study, Rep. 5210-92-0103-TX-003.

Ford, W. H., et al. (1988). A 4-Day Study in Rats with Technical Chlorothalonil." Unpublished Syngenta study, Rep. 1095-86-0091-TX-002.

Francis et al. (1973). "Daconil Technical Air Milled, Eye Irritation in the Albino Rabbit." Unpublished Syngenta study, Rep. 7948-95-3.

Hironaka, M., et al. (1996). "Analysis of Hyperplastic Changes in the Stomach and Kidney of Male Rats after 28-day Induction by Chlorothalonil Technical." Unpublished Syngenta study, Rep. 3561.

Huang, J., et al. (1995). Respiratory effects and skin allergy in workers exposed to tetrachloroisophthalonitrile. *Bull. Environ. Contam. Toxicol.* **55**, 320–324.

Jones, R. E., et al. (1984). "*Salmonella*/Mammalian-Microsome Plate Incorporation Assay (Ames Test) with and without Renal Activation with Technical Chlorothalonil." Unpublished Syngenta study, Rep. 694-5TX-84-0064-002.

Killeen, J. C., Jr. (1983). "Research on the Possible Mutagenic Potentiality of Chlorothalonil by the Detection of Chromosomal Alteration in the Rat (Rat, Mouse and Hamster)." Unpublished Syngenta study, Rep. 000-5TX-81-0025-001.

Killeen, J. C., Jr., and Siou, G. (1983). "The Micronucleus Test in the Rat, Mouse and Hamster Using Chlorothalonil." Unpublished Syngenta study, Rep. 000-5TX-81-0024-004.

Kouri (1977).

Lucas, F., et al. (1990). "A Two Generation Reproduction Study in Rats with Technical Chlorothalonil." Unpublished Syngenta study, Rep. 1722-87-0121-TX-003.

Magee, T. A., et al. (1990). "Study to Evaluate the Urinary Metabolites of Chlorothalonil Following Dermal Application to Male Rhesus Monkeys." Unpublished Syngenta study, Rep. 3382-89-0214-AM-001.

Marciniszyn, J. P., et al. (1985a). "Pilot Study of the Biliary Excretion of Radioactivity Following Oral Administration of Chlorothalonil (^{14}C-DS-2787) to Sprague–Dawley Rats." Unpublished Syngenta study, Rep. 633-4AM-83-0062-002.

Marciniszyn, J. P., et al. (1985b). "Study of the Distribution of Radioactivity Following Oral Administration of ^{14}C-Chlorothalonil (^{14}C-SDS-2787)." Unpublished Syngenta study, Rep. 631-4AM-84-0078-002.

Marciniszyn, J. P., et al. (1986a). "Study of the Biliary Excretion of Radioactivity Following Oral Administration of ^{14}C-Chlorothalonil (^{14}C-DS-2787) to Male Sprague–Dawley Rats." Unpublished Syngenta study, Rep. 633-4AM-85-0012-002.

Marciniszyn, J. P., et al. (1986b). "Pilot Study of the Effect of the Gamma-Glutamyl Transpeptidase Inhibitor, AT-125 on the Metabolism of ^{14}C-Chlorothalonil." Unpublished Syngenta study, Rep. 1376-86-0072-AM-002.

McAmis, R. J. (1994a). "Review of Dermal Chlorothalonil Exposures in Humans." Confidential company medical report originally generated by Diamond Shamrock Corp.

McAmis, R. J. (1994b). "Review of Respiratory Chlorothalonil Exposures in Humans." Confidential company medical report originally generated by Diamond Shamrock Corp.

McAmis, R. J. (1995). "Diagnosis of Poisoning, Specific Signs of Poisoning, Clinical Tests." Confidential company medical report originally generated by Diamond Shamrock Corp.

Mead, R. L., et al. (1987a). "Analysis of Urine Samples from a 90-Day Feeding Yes No Study in Rats with the Monoglutathione Conjugate of Chlorothalonil (T-117-11)." Unpublished Syngenta study, Rep. 1108-85-0078-TX-006.

Mead, R. L., et al. (1987b). "Analysis of Urine Samples from a 90-Day Feeding Study in Rats with Chlorothalonil (T-117-11)." Unpublished Syngenta study, Rep. 1115-85-0079-TX-005.

Mizens, M., and Laveglia (1994). "A Chronic (12-Month) Oral Toxicity Study in Dogs with Technical Chlorothalonil." Unpublished Syngenta study, Rep. 92-0457.

Mizens, M., et al. (1983). "A Teratology Study in Rats with Technical Chlorothalonil." Unpublished Syngenta study, Rep. 517-5TX-82-0011-003.

Mizens, M., et al. (1986a). "A 21-Day Repeated Dose Dermal Toxicity Study Rats with Technical Chlorothalonil." Unpublished Syngenta study, Rep. 68-59-96-0113-TX-02.

Mizens, M., et al. (1986b). "*In Vitro* Chromosomal Aberration Assay in Chinese Hamster Ovary (CHO) Cells with Technical Chlorothalonil." Unpublished Syngenta study, Rep. 1109-85-0082-TX-002.

Mizens, M., et al. (1996). "A 90-Day Pilot Study for the Evaluation Proliferation in the Kidneys of Male Rats Following the Oral Administration of Technical Chlorothalonil." Unpublished Syngenta study, Rep. 6704-96-0010-TX-003.

O'Meara, H. O., and Laveglia, J. (1995). "Eye Irritation Study in Albino Rabbits with Technical Chlorothalonil." Unpublished Syngenta study, Rep. 6300-95-0083-TX-001.

Moore (2000).

Price, P., and Ballee, D. (1979). "Analyses of Samples from Cell Transformation Studies for 2,4,5,6-Tetrachloroisophthalonitrile (Chlorothalonil, DS-2787) and 4-Hydroxy-2,5,6-Trichloroiso-Phthalonitrile (DS-3701) (DTX-77-0037 and DTX-77-0041)." Unpublished Syngenta study, Rep. 041-5TX-79-0021-001.

Proudlock, R. J. (1995). "*In Vivo* Bone Marrow Chromosomal Analysis in Chinese Hamsters Following Multiple Dose Administration of Technical Chlorothalonil." Unpublished Syngenta study, Rep. 6005-94-0047-TX-003.

Ribovich, M. L., et al. (1982). "Balance Study of the Distribution of Radioactivity Following Oral Administration of ^{14}C-Chlorothalonil (^{14}C-DS-2787) to Male Mice." Unpublished Syngenta study, Rep. 613-4AM-82-0178-001.

Sadler, E. M., and Ignatoski, J. A. (1985). "Time Course of the Acute Effect of Technical Chlorothalonil on Hepatic and Renal Glutathione Content in Male Rats." Unpublished Syngenta study, Rep. 751-5TX-85-0032-001.

Savides, M. C., et al. (1985). "Pilot Study for the Determination of the Effects of Probenecid Pre-treatment on Urinary Metabolites and Excretion of ^{14}C-Chlorothalonil (^{14}C-SDS-2787) Following Oral Administration to Male Sprague–Dawley Rats." Unpublished Syngenta study, Rep. 621-4AM-85-0035-001.

Savides, M. C., et al. (1986a). "Study of the Distribution of Radioactivity Following Repeated Oral Administration of ^{14}C-Chlorothalonil to Male Sprague–Dawley Rats." Unpublished Syngenta study, Rep. 1173-84-0079-AM-003.

Savides, M. C., et al. (1986b). "Identification of Metabolites in Urine and Blood Following Oral Administration of ^{14}C-Chlorothalonil to Male Rats: Effects of Multiple Dose Administration on the Excretion of Thiol Metabolites in Urine." Unpublished Syngenta study, Rep. 621-4AM-83-0061-002.

Savides, M. C., et al. (1987). "Determination of the Covalent Binding of Radiolabel to DNA in the Kidneys of Male Rats Administered ^{14}C-Chlorothalonil (^{14}C-SDS-2787)." Unpublished Syngenta study, Rep. 1173-86-0096-AM-002.

Savides, M. C., et al. (1988). "A Study to Evaluate the Effects of Sulfur-Containing Analogs of Chlorothalonil on Mitochondrial Function." Unpublished Syngenta study, Rep. 1479-87-0037-AM-001.

Savides, M. C., et al. (1989). "Study to Determine the Metabolic Pathway for Chlorothalonil Following Dermal Application to Rats." Unpublished Syngenta study, Rep. 1625-87-0057-AM-001.

Savides, M. C., et al. (1990). "Study to Evaluate the Urinary Metabolites of Chlorothalonil from Male Rhesus Monkeys." Unpublished Syngenta study, Rep. 3349-89-0179-AM-001.

Savides, M. C., et al. (1995). "Study to Determine the Extent and Nature of Yes No Biliary Excretion of Chlorothalonil and/or Metabolites in the Dog." Unpublished Syngenta study, Rep. 5521-93-0319-AM-001.

Shirasu, Y. (1978). "Mutagenicity Testing on Daconil in Microbial Systems." Unpublished Syngenta study, Rep. 000-5TX-61-0002-001.

Shults and Wilson (1985). "Dermal Sensitisation Study (Closed Patch Repeated Insult) in Guinea Pigs with Chlorothalonil 90DG Formulation." Unpublished Syngenta study, Rep. 707-5TX-84-0126-002.

Shults, S. K., *et al.* (1981a). "Acute Oral Toxicity (LD$_{50}$) Study in Rats with Technical Chlorothalonil." Unpublished Syngenta study, Rep. 296-5TX-80-0092-002.

Shults, S. K., *et al.* (1981b). "Acute Dermal Toxicity (LD$_{50}$) Study in Albino Rabbits with Technical Chlorothalonil." Unpublished Syngenta study, Rep. 296-5TX-80-0093-002.

Shults, S. K., *et al.* (1981c). "Acute Inhalation Toxicity Study (Four Hour Exposure) in Rats with Technical Chlorothalonil (SDS-2787)." Unpublished Syngenta study, Rep. 296-5TX-80-0096-002.

Shults, S. K., *et al.* (1981d). "Primary Dermal Irritation Study in Albino Rabbits with Technical Chlorothalonil." Unpublished Syngenta study, Rep. 296-5TX-80-0094-002.

Shults, S. K., *et al.* (1983). "A 90 Day Feeding Study in Mice with 2,4,5,6-Tetrachloroisophthalonitrile (Chlorothalonil)." Unpublished Syngenta study, Rep. 618-5TX-83-0007-004.

Shults, S. K., *et al.* (1985). "Histopathologic Re-evaluation of Renal Tissue from a 90-Day Feeding Study in Mice with Technical Chlorothalonil." Unpublished Syngenta study, Rep. 753-5TX-85-0053-002.

Shults, S. K., *et al.* (1986). "21-Day Repeated Dose Dermal Toxicity Study in Albino Rabbits with Technical Chlorothalonil." Unpublished Syngenta study, Rep. 754-5TX-85-0023-007.

Shults, S. K., *et al.* (1993). "Acute (Four-Hour) Inhalation Toxicity (LC$_{50}$) Study in Rats with Hammer-Milled Technical Chlorothalonil." Unpublished Syngenta study, Rep. 5290-92-0160-TX-002.

Siou, G., *et al.* (1985). "Acute and Subchronic *In Vivo* Bone Marrow Chromosomal Aberration Assay in Chinese Hamsters with Technical Chlorothalonil." Unpublished Syngenta study, Rep. 625-5TX-83-0014-003.

Tucker, S. B. (1986). "Skin Sensitisation Studies with Chlorothalonil Conducted at the Department of Occupational Dermatology, University of Texas." Unpublished Syngenta studies, Reps. 5TX-84-0023, 5TX-84-0027, 5TX-84-0012, 1094-84-0012-DA002, 5TX-84-0044, 5TX-84-0076, and 5TX-84-0045.

Ward, R. J. (1989a). "Chlorothalonil: *In Vitro* Absorption from Technical Material through Human Epidermis." Unpublished Syngenta study, Central Toxicology Laboratory, Rep. CTL/P/2640.

Ward, R. J. (1989b). "Chlorothalonil: *In Vitro* Absorption from Bravo 720 Formulation through Human Epidermis." Unpublished Syngenta study, Central Toxicology Laboratory, Rep. CTL/P/2880.

Wazeter and Lucas (1971). "Acute Intraperitoneal Toxicity (LD$_{50}$) in Male Albino Rats of Technical Chlorothalonil." Unpublished Syngenta studies, Rep. 000-5TX-71-0006-001.

Wilkinson, C. F., and Killeen, J. C. (1996). A mechanistic interpretation of the oncogenicity of chlorothalonil in rodents and an assessment of human relevance. *Regulatory Toxicol. Pharmacol.* **24**, 69–84.

Wilson, P. D. (1977a). "Primary Eye Irritation Study in Rabbits." Unpublished Syngenta study, Rep. DTX-77-0075.

Wilson, P. D. (1977b). "Primary Eye Irritation Study in Rabbits." Unpublished Syngenta study, Rep. DTX-77-0059.

Wilson, P. D. (1977c). "Primary Eye Irritation Study in Rabbits." Unpublished Syngenta study, Rep. DTX-77-0069.

Wilson, N. H., *et al.* (1982a). "Dermal Sensitisation Study in Hartley-Derived Guinea Pigs with Technical Chlorothalonil." Unpublished Syngenta study, Rep. 394-5TX-81-0132-002/7020.

Wilson, N. H., *et al.* (1982b). "Four Week Dietary Range-Finding Study in Rats with Technical Chlorothalonil." Unpublished Syngenta study, Rep. 099-5TX-81-0174-003.

Wilson, N. H., *et al.* (1983a). "A 90-Day Toxicity Study of Technical Chlorothalonil in Rats." Unpublished Syngenta study, Rep. 099-5TX-80-0200-006.

Wilson, N. H., *et al.* (1983b). "A Subchronic Toxicity Study of Technical Chlorothalonil in Rats." Unpublished Syngenta study, Rep. 562-5TX-81-0213-004.

Wilson, N. H., *et al.* (1983c). "A Chronic Dietary Study in Mice with Technical Chlorothalonil." Unpublished Syngenta study, Rep. 108-5TX-79-0102-004.

Wilson, N. H., *et al.* (1984). "A Subchronic Toxicity Study of Technical Chlorothalonil in Rats (Electron Light Microscopy of Kidneys)." Unpublished Syngenta study, Rep. 562-5TX-8-0213-004-001.

Wilson, N. H., *et al.* (1985a). "Histopathologic Re-evaluation of Renal Tissue from a 90-Day Toxicity Study in Rats with Technical Chlorothalonil." Unpublished Syngenta study, Rep. 753-5TX-85-0055-002.

Wilson, N. H., *et al.* (1985b). "Histopathologic Re-evaluation of Renal Tissue from a Subchronic Toxicity Study of Technical Chlorothalonil in Rats." Unpublished Syngenta study, Rep. 753-5TX-85-0056-002.

Wilson, N. H., *et al.* (1985c). "A Tumourgenicity Study of Technical Chlorothalonil in Rats." Unpublished Syngenta study, Rep. 099-5TX-80-0234-008.

Wilson, N. H., *et al.* (1987). "A Tumourgenicity Study of Technical Chlorothalonil in Male Mice." Unpublished Syngenta study, Rep. 1099-84-0077-TX-006.

Wilson, N. H. (1988a). "Guinea Pig Maximization Test with Technical Chlorothalonil (T-117-11)." Unpublished Syngenta study, Rep. 1094-84-0044-TX-001.

Wilson, N. H. (1988b). "Guinea Pig Epicutaneous Test Involving Chlorothalonil in Acetone." Unpublished Syngenta study, Rep. 1094-84-0045-TX-001.

Wilson, N. H. (1988c). "Guinea Pig Maximization Test with Technical Chlorothalonil (T-117-11)." Unpublished Syngenta study, Rep. 1094-84-0076-TX-001.

Wilson, N. H., *et al.* (1988d). "A Teratology Study in Rabbits with Technical Chlorothalonil." Unpublished Syngenta study, Rep. 1544-87-0060-TX-002.

Wilson, N. H., *et al.* (1989). "A Tumourgenicity Study of Technical Chlorothalonil in Rats." Unpublished Syngenta study, Rep. 1102-84-0103-TX-007.

Dialkyldithiocarbamates (EBDCs)

Susan Hurt, Janet Ollinger

Rohm and Haas Company

Gail Arce

Griffin LLC

Quang Bui

Cerexagri, Inc.

Abraham J. Tobia

Aventis

Bennard van Ravenswaay

BASF AG

81.1 CHEMISTRY AND FORMULATIONS

Ethylenebisdithiocarbamates (EBDCs) are a group of fungicides that have been used widely throughout the world since the 1940s to protect a wide variety of crops against fungal disease. There are five members of the class, specifically mancozeb, maneb, metiram, zineb, and nabam. All members have an ethylenebisdithiocarbamate backbone, with different metals associated with the individual compounds. The structure of each compound is shown below.

Mancozeb: $[-MnSC(:S)NHCH_2CH_2NHC(:S)S-]_xZn_y$, where $x/y = 11$
Maneb: $[-MnSC(:S)NHCH_2CH_2NHC(:S)S-]_x$
Metiram: $[[-(NH_3)Zn-S-C(:S)NHCH_2CH_2NHC(:S)S-]_3 -S-C(;S)NHCH2CH2NHC(:S)S-]_x$
Zineb: $[-ZnSC(:S)NHCH_2CH_2NHC(:S)S-]_x$
Nabam: $[NaSC(:S)NHCH2CH2NHC(:S)SNa]$

The molecular weights of the individual EBDCs are mancozeb—271, maneb—265, metiram—1088.6, zineb—275, and nabam—256.

At this time mancozeb, maneb, and metiram are the most widely used EBDCs. Zineb is used to a lesser degree and nabam is no longer used in agriculture. Thus, this chapter will focus on mancozeb, maneb, and metiram.

The EBDCs are sold as wettable powder, dry flowable (also called water dispersable granules), and flowable formulations.

EBDCs can also be sold as a premix with various blending partners.

81.2 USES

EBDCs are used to control about 400 fungal pathogens on more than 100 crops. The major EBDC uses around the world include grapes (fresh grapes, grapes grown for juice, and grapes grown for wine), potatoes, citrus, apples, tomatoes, melons, and bananas. EBDCs are also important products for disease control in corn, cereal grains, leafy vegetables, brassica vegetables, cranberries, onions, peanuts, sugar beets, asparagus, and nuts as well as for many other critical crops that are grown on a lower amount of acreage. Diseases of turf and ornamental crops are also controlled by EBDCs. Some of the economically important diseases controlled include early and late blight, downy mildew, and bacterial diseases.

EBDCs are key components of fungicide resistance management programs because they have a multisite mode of action. For example, EBDCs deactivate the sulfhydryl containing enzymes which mediate numerous biosynthesis, mechanical, and transport activities within the fungal cytoplasm. They also inactivate ATP production, the Krebs cycle, the enzymes which convert glucose to pyruvate, and enzymes which convert amino and fatty acids to acetylcoenzyme A.

Thus, resistance will not develop. After over 40 years of use no resistance has developed to any of the EBDCs.

81.3 HAZARD IDENTIFICATION

The toxicology database supporting the assessment of the potential health risks of the EBDCs and their common metabolite ethylenethiourea (ETU) has been upgraded in recent years with a complete set of modern studies of mancozeb, maneb, and metiram conducted in full compliance with OECD and other applicable national and international guidelines and internationally recognized good laboratory practices. These newer studies have superseded the older studies in the published literature and now form the core of the toxicology database relevant for the hazard identification and dose–response assessment of this family of fungicides.

81.3.1 PHARMACOKINETICS AND METABOLISM

Studies of the pharmacokinetics and metabolism of mancozeb, maneb, and metiram in laboratory animals have indicated that the EBDCs are only partially absorbed, then rapidly metabolized and excreted with no evidence of long-term bioaccumulation. Absorption of oral doses is rapid. Most of the administered dose is excreted within 24 hours, with about half eliminated in the urine and half in the feces. Biliary excretion is minimal, indicating that only approximately 50% of oral doses are absorbed. Only low level residues are found in tissues, principally in the thyroid. ETU is the major metabolite. On average 7.5% of an EBDC dose administered to rats is metabolized to ETU on a weight basis. The bioconversion factor in mice is slightly smaller at 5 to 6% (Cameron et al., 1990; DiDonato and Longacre, 1986; Emmerling, 1978b; EPA, 1992; Hawkins et al., 1985; Kocialski, 1989; Longacre, 1986; Nelson, 1986, 1987; Piccirillo et al., 1992; Puhl, 1985).

The spectrum of metabolites produced in laboratory animals points to two common metabolic pathways (Fig. 81.1), which both lead ultimately to the formation of glycine and incorporation into natural products. In the predominant pathway quantitatively, the dithiocarbamate linkages are hydrolyzed to produce ethylenediamine (EDA) directly, and EDA is oxidized to glycine, joining the intermediary metabolic pool at this point. The other pathway is responsible for the toxic effects of the EBDCs and involves oxidation to ethylenebisisothiocyanatesulfide and then to ETU, various derivatives of ETU, and ethyleneurea (EU) before rejoining the main pathway with conversion to EDA, glycine, and other natural products.

ETU metabolism has also been extensively studied in multiple species. As with the EBDCs, oral doses are rapidly absorbed and rapidly excreted, although in this case primarily in the urine and more quickly in mice than in rats. In most species the greater majority (70% or more) of an oral dose is eliminated via the urine within 48 hours. Concentrations in blood and tissues are generally at comparably low levels with the exception of somewhat higher levels in the thyroid; levels in maternal and fetal tissues were similar 3 hours after dosing. Half-lives for elimination from maternal blood were 5.5 and 9.4 hours in

mice and rats, respectively. Unchanged ETU was the principal metabolite in rats and guinea pigs, with small amounts of EU. In mice the principal identified metabolites were ETU and imidazolinylsulfenate, and in cats, S-methyl ETU was the principal metabolite (DiDonato and Longacre, 1987; Emmerling, 1978b; Iverson et al., 1977, 1980; Jordan and Neal, 1979; Kato et al., 1976; Peters et al., 1982; Ruddick et al., 1976a, 1977; Teshima et al., 1981).

Studies of dermal absorption of the EBDCs have been challenging due to the difficulty of small scale preparation of radiolabelled samples representative of their complex polymeric structures. Thus, the reported values of 0.2–6.5% are considered to be overestimates of their actual dermal absorption potential under conditions of use (Craine, 1991; Haines, 1980; Hawkins et al., 1984; Tomlinson and Longacre, 1988). Dermal absorption of ETU increased from 5 to 22% with decreasing applied skin concentrations (DiDonato and Longacre, 1987).

81.3.2 ACUTE TOXICITY

The EBDC's have very low acute toxicity by the oral, dermal, and respiratory routes (Table 81.1). The World Health Organization (WHO) has classified mancozeb, maneb, and metiram as unlikely to present an acute exposure hazard under conditions of normal use (WHO, 1994). Although not irritating to skin on initial contact and only slightly irritating to eyes and mucous membranes, prolonged or repeated skin contact may result in dermatitis due to their weak sensitization potential. ETU is only slightly toxic after oral administration, but it is a moderate to weak sensitizer in the guinea pig maximization test (Matsushita et al., 1976, 1977).

81.3.3 SHORT- AND LONG-TERM TOXICITY AND ONCOGENIC POTENTIAL

The EBDCs share a comparable toxicological profile, primarily based on the toxic effects of their common ETU metabolite. A summary of the critical doses and effects in subchronic and longer term studies is presented for each of the EBDCs in Table 81.2, and a similar summary for ETU is presented in Table 81.3. Results are collected by study type. As is illustrated repeatedly in these tables, the principal target organ upon repeated exposure to all of the EBDCs is the thyroid, which is also the principal target organ of ETU. For example, all three EBDCs (mancozeb, maneb, and metiram) and ETU altered thyroid hormone levels and/or weights at the lowest affected dose after three months of dietary feeding in rats. Most of the other organs affected, such as the liver at generally higher doses or red blood cells usually in dogs, are also common to ETU. Prolonged dietary feeding of ETU produces thyroid and pituitary tumors in rats and mice, and liver tumors in mice.

As normally occurs with toxicological effects due to formation of a metabolite, the effects of ETU are not as strong in the EBDCs. When EBDCs are administered, much higher doses are

Metabolic Pathway of EBDC

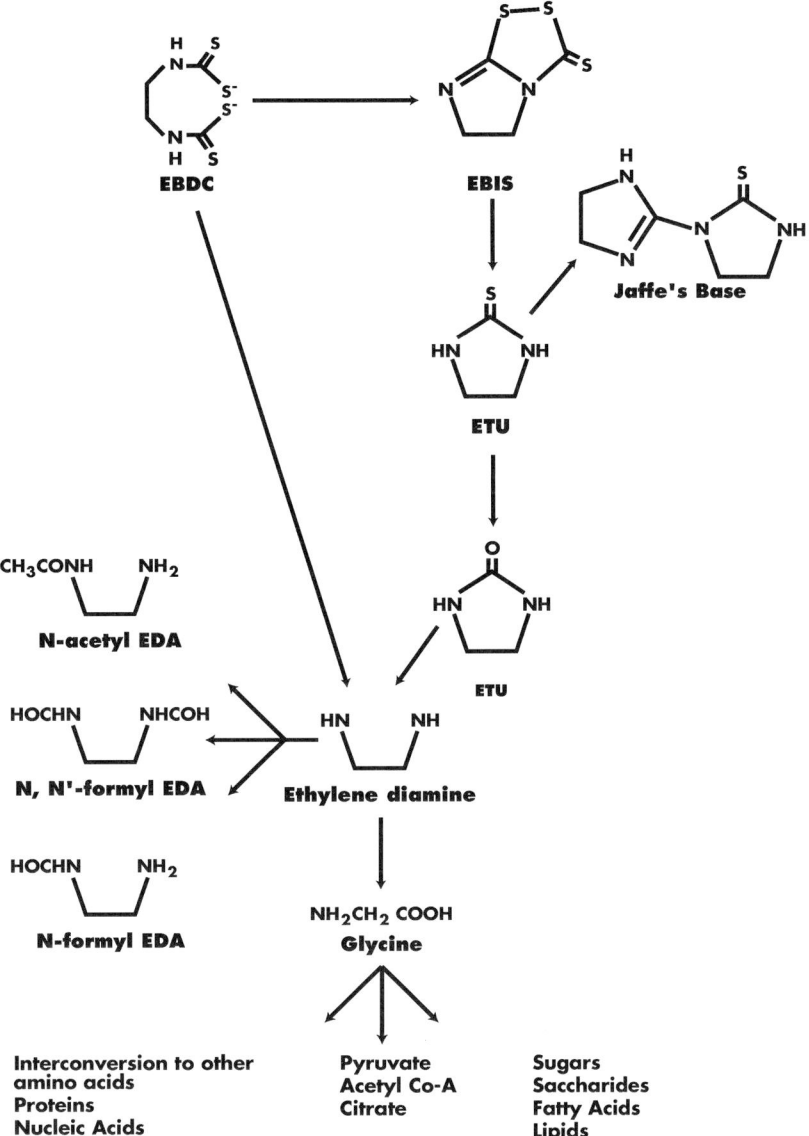

Figure 81.1 Metabolic pathway of EBDC.

required to produce adverse effects, and the effects themselves are generally not as pronounced or may be precluded altogether by high dose limitations.

81.3.3.1 Thyroid Effects

The effects of the EBDCs on the thyroid after either short- or long-term dietary administration are consistent on both a quantitative and a qualitative basis with those of ETU. As described below, it is well accepted that these effects are the result of a secondary mechanism (hormonal imbalance), and that there is a threshold for the resulting tumors Similarly to the structurally related thionamide drugs (propylthiouracil, methimazole, and carbimazole) which are used clinically for treatment of hyperthyroidism in humans, the primary toxicological finding with

ETU in laboratory animals is inhibition of the synthesis of thyroid hormones, thyroxine (T4) and triiodothyronine (T3), leading to elevated serum levels of thyroid stimulating hormone (TSH) via feedback stimulation of the hypothalamus and pituitary (Atterwill and Aylard, 1995; Engler and Burger, 1984; O'Neil and Marshall, 1984) (see Fig. 81.2). Prolonged and continuous elevation of serum TSH levels results in hypertrophy and hyperplasia of the thyroid follicular cells in rats, mice, hamsters, monkeys, and dogs (Briffaux, 1991, 1992; Gak *et al.*, 1976; Chhabra *et al.*, 1992; Freudenthal *et al.*, 1977a; Graham and Hansen, 1972; Graham *et al.*, 1973, 1975; Leber *et al.*, 1978; O'Hara and DiDonato, 1985; Schmid *et al.*, 1992; Ulland *et al.*, 1972), and ultimately in the development of follicular nodular hyperplasia, adenoma, and/or carcinoma in rats and

Table 81.1
Acute Toxicity of Mancozeb, Maneb, Metiram, and ETU

Type of study acute	Active ingredient	Strain–sex	LD(LC)50 mg/kg bw (mg/L)	Reference
Acute oral, rat	mancozeb	F344, M	>5000	Watts and Chan, 1984a, b
	mancozeb	CRCD, M	>5000	DeCrescente and Parsons, 1980
	maneb	Crl:CD BR, M/F	>5000	Naas, 1989a
	metiram	SD, M/F	6500–10,000	Jackh, 1981; Leuschner, 1979a; Hofmann, 1985; Hofmann, 1975
Acute oral, mouse	mancozeb	$B_6C_3F_1$, M	>5000	Watts and Chan, 1984b
Intraperitoneal, rat	mancozeb	Wistar, M/F	380	DeGroot, 1974
	metiram	SD, M/F	318	Hofmann and Munk, 1975
Intraperitoneal, mouse	metiram	NMRI, M/F	80–215	Hofmann, 1974; Leuschner, 1979b
Acute dermal, rat	metiram	SD, M/F	>2000	Grundler, 1979
Acute dermal, rabbit	mancozeb	NZW, M	>5000	DeCrescente and Parsons, 1980
	maneb	NZW, M/F	>2000	Naas, 1989b
Acute inhalation (4 hr)	mancozeb	COBS-CR (SD) BR, M/F	5.14 mg/l	Hagan and Baldwin, 1982
	maneb	Crl:CD BR, M/F	7.38 mg/l	Terrill, 1990
	metiram	SD, M/F	>5.7 mg/l	Klimisch and Zeller, 1980
Acute oral, rat	ETU	M/F	545–ca. 2400	Peters et al., 1980a; Graham and Hansen, 1972; Lewerenz and Plass, 1984; Teramoto et al., 1978
	ETU	F (13 days pregnant)	600	Khera, 1987
Acute oral, mouse	ETU	M/F	ca. 2400–4000	Lewerenz and Plass, 1984; Teramoto et al., 1978; Peters et al., 1980b
	ETU	F (9 days pregnant)	>3000	Khera, 1987
Acute oral, hamster	ETU	F	>3000	Teramoto et al., 1978
	ETU	F (11 days pregnant)	>2400	Khera, 1987

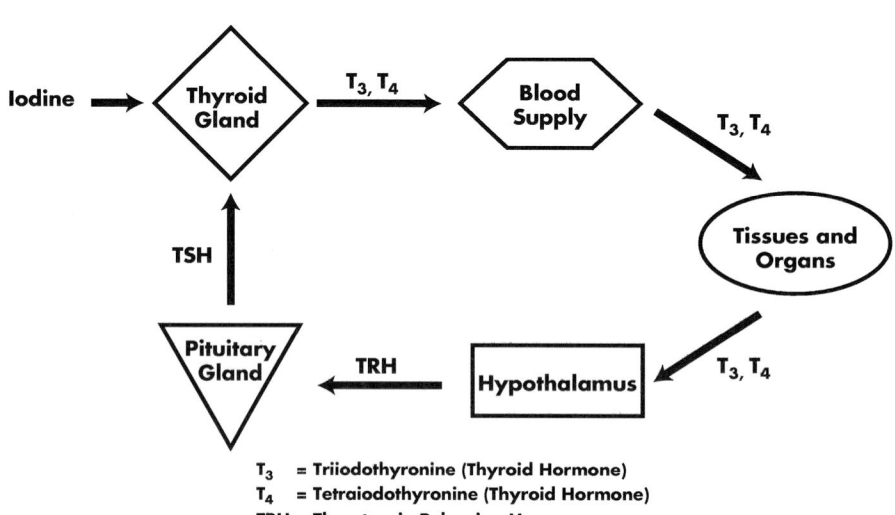

Figure 81.2 Thyroid-pituitary feedback mechanism.

Table 81.2
EBDCs: Critical Findings in the Most Relevant Studies

Study	Active	NOAEL (mg/kg/d)	LOAEL (mg/kg/d)	Effects observed at LOAEL/critical results	Reference
Mouse 3 month oral					
	mancozeb	18	180	Decreased body weight and liver MFO activity; thyroid follicular hypertrophy and hyperplasia	O'Hara and DiDonato, 1985
	metiram	84	302	Decreased T4	Gelbke et al., 1992a
Rat 3 month oral					
	mancozeb	7.4	15	Decreased T4, increased TSH	Goldman et al., 1986
	maneb	5	25	Increased thyroid weight, follicular hyperplasia	Trutter, 1988a
	metiram	6	20	Decreased T4 and iodine uptake, increased thyroid weight; microscopic changes in muscle fibers	Hunter et al., 1977
		5.8	23.2	Slight anemia; decreased T4, increased thyroid weight, general muscle weakness/ataxia and reduced grip strength without histopathological correlate at 70 mg/kg body weight/d	Gelbke et al., 1992b
Rat 1 month dermal					
	mancozeb	1000	none	No systemic toxicity	Trutter, 1988c
Rabbit 1 month dermal					
	maneb	100	300	Increased follicular colloid	Trutter, 1988b
	metiram	250	none	No systemic toxicity	Ullman et al., 1987
Rat 3 month inhalation					
	mancozeb	79 mg/m^3 ×6 hr/d (= 8.3)	326 mg/m^3 ×6 hr (= 34)	Decreased weight gain, T4 levels; thyroid hyperplasia. All effects reversible after 13 weeks recovery	Hagan and Baldwin, 1986; Hagan et al., 1986
	maneb	10 mg/m^3 ×6 hr/d	30 mg/m^3 ×6 hr/d	Decreased weight gain; all effects reversible after 13 weeks recovery	Ulrich, 1986a, 1987
	metiram	2 mg/m^3 ×6 hr/d	20 mg/m^3 ×6 hr/d	Decreased weight gain; alveolar macrophage accumulation due to nonspecific dust reaction	Ulrich, 1986b
Dog 3 month					
	mancozeb	3	30	Decreased weight gain, RBC parameters	Cox, 1986
	maneb	3.7	15	Thyroid follicular hyperplasia	Allen et al., 1989
Rat two generation					
	mancozeb	1.7	10.2	Decreased weight gain; no effect on reproduction below adult toxic levels	Muller, 1992
		7	70	Decreased weight gain, feed consumption; increased thyroid, liver, kidney weights, microscopic changes in thyroid, kidney, and pituitary; no reproductive effect.	Solomon et al., 1988
	maneb	5.6	22.4	Increased liver, kidney weight ratios, thyroid follicular hyperplasia; no reproductive effect below toxic levels	Ryle et al., 1991
	metiram	1.8	14.4	Decreased body weight, feed consumption; no reproductive effect	Cozens et al., 1981

(continues)

Table 81.2

(*continued*)

Study	Active	NOAEL (mg/kg/d)	LOAEL (mg/kg/d)	Effects observed at LOAEL/critical results	Reference
Rat acute neurotoxicity					
	maneb	2000	NA	No adverse effect	Nemec, 1993
Rat 90-day neuropathology					
	mancozeb	8.2	48	Decreased feed consumption; neurohistopathological changes	Stadler, 1991
Rat developmental					
	mancozeb	32	128	Decreased maternal weight gain, feed consumption; teratogenic NOAEL; teratogenicity at 512 mg/kg body weight/d	Gallo *et al.*, 1980
		60	360	Decreased maternal weight gain, feed consumption; maternal "reeling gait" and hindlimb paralysis, embryofetotoxicity	Tesh *et al.*, 1988
	maneb	20	100	Decreased maternal weight gain, feed consumption; embryofetotoxicity	Nemec, 1992
		100	500	Decreased maternal weight gain, feed consumption; hindlimb paresis; embryofetotoxicity and teratogenicity	Kapp *et al.*, 1991
	metiram	80	160	Decreased maternal weight gain, slight decreases in litter size and weight	Palmer and Simons, 1979
Rabbit developmental					
	mancozeb	55	100	Maternal weight loss, decreased feed consumption, increased abortions; no adverse embryofetal effects	Muller, 1991
		30	80	Decreased maternal weight gain, feed consumption, litters; increased abortions, clinical signs, and deaths; no adverse embryofetal effects	Solomon and Holz, 1987; Solomon and Lutz, 1987
	metiram	10	40	Decreased maternal body weight, feed consumption: increased abortions; no adverse embryofetal effects	Gelbke *et al.*, 1988
Dog 12 month					
	mancozeb	7	28	Decreased weight gain, RBC parameters, inc, cholesterol	Shaw, 1990
		2.3	23	Decreased weight gain, feed consumption, T4	Broadmeadow, 1991a, b
	maneb	6.4	32	Thyroid thickening and enlargement, follicular hyperplasia	Corney *et al.*, 1992
	metiram	2.5	31	Decreased T4, increased thyroid size and follicular hyperplasia, focal hepatic lipofuscin deposition, slight anemia, diarrhea, and blood biochemical changes	Corney *et al.*, 1991
Monkey 6 month					
	maneb	7.3	22	Increased thyroid weight	Leuschner *et al.*, 1977
	metiram	5	15	Decreased T3, T4, increased thyroid weight and follicular hyperplasia	Sortwell *et al.*, 1979

(*continues*)

Table 81.2

(*continued*)

Study	Active	NOAEL (mg/kg/d)	LOAEL (mg/kg/d)	Effects observed at LOAEL/critical results	Reference
Mouse oncogenic					
	mancozeb	17	170	Decreased weight gain	Shellenberger, 1991
		13	130	Decreased weight gain, T3, T4	Everett *et al.*, 1992
	maneb	11	44	Decreased body weight, T4; hepatocellular adenomas at 440 mg/kg body weight/day	Tompkins, 1992
	metiram	24	79	Decreased body weight	Hunter *et al.*, 1979
Rat chronic-oncogenic					
	mancozeb	4.8	29	Decreased weight gain, T3, T4; increased TSH, thyroid weight, follicular cell hypertrophy, hyperplasia, nodular hyperplasia, adenoma and carcinoma	Stadler, 1990
		4	16	Decreased weight gain, T4; increased height of thyroid follicular epithelium, prominent microfollicles	Hooks *et al.*, 1992
	maneb	20	67	Decreased body weight, T4; increased ^{131}I half-life, thyroid weight	Leuschner *et al.*, 1979, 1986a, b; Leuschner, 1991
	metiram	3.1	12	Muscular atrophy	Hunter *et al.*, 1981

NOAEL = no observed adverse effect level.
LOAEL = lowest observed adverse effect level.

mice (Chhabra *et al.*, 1992; Graham *et al.*, 1973, 1975; Schmid *et al.*, 1992; Ulland *et al.*, 1972), but not in hamsters (Gak *et al.*, 1976). There is evidence for reversibility of the thyroid effects (Arnold *et al.*, 1983).

The mechanism of the crucial early steps of thyroid tumor formation by ETU is well understood. ETU reversibly inhibits thyroid peroxidase-catalyzed iodination and coupling of tyrosine residues into the thyroid hormone precursor thyroglobulin *in vivo* (Hill *et al.*, 1989). Direct evidence for inhibition of thyroid hormone synthesis by ETU has been obtained in rats *in vivo* (Arnold *et al.*, 1983; O'Neil and Marshall, 1984). ETU also reversibly inhibited thyroid peroxidase-catalyzed iodination reactions *in vitro* (Doerge and Takazawa, 1990). The correlation of the hormonal changes with hyperplasia and neoplasia has been clearly demonstrated in specific studies of ETU (Chhabra *et al.*, 1992; Freudenthal *et al.*, 1977a).

Similarly, the long-term stimulation of the pituitary via hypothalamic thyrotropin-releasing hormone also results in morphologic changes in the pituitary of rats, mice, monkeys, and dogs (Briffaux, 1991; Chhabra *et al.*, 1992; Leber *et al.*, 1978; Schmid *et al.*, 1992), culminating in adenomas of the pars distalis after two years exposure in mice and rats (Chhabra *et al.*, 1992; Schmid *et al.*, 1992).

A regenerative, nonhemolytic anemia that was observed in dogs is considered to be a secondary manifestation of the primary thyroid condition, since anemia is a known manifes-

tation of hypothyroidism in dogs (Duncan *et al.*, 1994; Jain, 1986).

The mechanistic linkage between the prolonged disruption of the hypothalamic–pituitary–thyroid (HPT) axis and thyroid neoplasia has been confirmed in studies of sulfamethazine (Hard, 1998). Indeed, thyroid gland neoplasia can be induced experimentally in laboratory animals simply by a a low iodine diet (Schaller and Stevenson, 1966), i.e., without exogenous agents, indicating that the neoplasia was induced by an internal factor. Supplementing the diet with thyroid hormone abolishes the neoplastic response indicating that the internal factor is TSH (Doniach, 1970).

Thus, the sequence of events relating thyroid hormone inhibition via hormonal imbalance to the onset of pituitary and thyroid follicular neoplasia in rodents is well characterized, resulting in the inference that the threshold for the early steps in the sequence, particularly the key elevation of TSH levels, is necessarily a threshold for the remaining steps in the process including carcinogenesis. For purposes of human oncogenic risk assessment, the principle of the existence of a threshold for thyroid and pituitary neoplasia resulting from thyroid inhibition has been accepted (EPA, 1998; Hard, 1998; Hill *et al.*, 1989, 1998; IPCS, 1990), and the specific relevance of this threshold mechanism to ETU is also accepted (EPA, 1992, 1998; Hurley *et al.*, 1998).

Table 81.3
ETU: Critical Findings in the Most Relevant Studies

Type of study/ species	NOAEL (mg/kg/d)	LOAEL (mg/kg/d)	Effects observed at LOAEL/critical results	Reference
Subchronic dietary				
Mouse 90 day	1.7	17	Thyroid follicular hyperplasia and decreased colloid density in both sexes, and increased liver weights in females	O'Hara and DiDonato, 1985
Rat 90 day	1.7	8.5	Altered thyroid function and follicular hyperplasia	Freudenthal et al., 1977a
Dog 90 day	0.39	6.0	Decreases in rbc parameters and increased cholesterol; thyroid and other effects at 80 mg/kg/d	Briffaux, 1991
Monkey 6 month	0.1–0.5	2.5	Increased iodine uptake, thyroid follicular hyperplasia and pituitary hypertrophy	Leber et al., 1978
Chronic dietary				
1 yr dog	0.18	1.8	Slightly reduced body weight gain, increased thyroid weights and hypertrophy with colloid retention, pigment accumulation in the liver	Briffaux, 1992
2 yr rat	0.25	1.25	Thyroid vacuolarity and hyperplasia	Graham et al., 1973, 1975
2 yr rat	0.37	9.25	Thyroid, pituitary and liver effects, thyroid and pituitary tumors, decreased body weights in males	Schmid et al., 1992
Oncogenicity				
Mouse 2 year	<17	17	Decreased T4, increased TSH and diffuse thyroid follicular cytoplasmic vacuolation at 17 mg/kg/day; tumors of the thyroid, liver and/or pituitary at 56 mg/kg/day and higher	Chhabra et al., 1992; NTP, 1992
Rat 2 year	<1.1	1.1	Decreased T4, increased TSH and thyroid follicular hyperplasia at 1.1 mg/kg/day; thyroid tumors at 3.7 mg/kg/day and higher	Chhabra et al., 1992; NTP, 1992
Reproductive				
Rat 2 generation	0.11–0.43	1.1–4.3	Thyroid follicular hypertrophy and hyperplasia; no reproductive effect at 4.3–21 mg/kg/day, HDT	Dotti, 1992

(continues)

In addition, in comparison to laboratory animals, humans are expected to exhibit a lesser degree of sensitivity to thyroid inhibitors (Costigan, 1998; Hard, 1998; Hill et al., 1998). The reasons for this are threefold: First, humans possess a substantial reserve supply of thyroid hormone, much of which is carried in the serum bound to thyroxine-binding globulin, a serum protein that is missing in laboratory rodents (Odell et al., 1967). Therefore, release of stored thyroid hormones maintains normal serum levels for weeks in euthyroid humans (Martindale, 1972) and for weeks to several months in hyperthyroid individuals (Odell et al., 1967), despite daily doses of antithyroid drugs sufficient to completely block synthesis. This protein is missing in rodents, resulting in comparatively rapid hormone turnover, normally higher levels of TSH, and increased sensitivity to the effects of hormone depletion. Second, the molar concentrations of thiourea compounds required to inhibit thyroid peroxidase activity are far smaller in rats than in monkeys or humans (Takayama et al., 1986), indicating that humans must be exposed at much higher levels to achieve the same degree of enzyme inhibition. Third, under conditions of prolonged thyroid

Table 81.3
(*continued*)

Type of study/ species	NOAEL (mg/kg/d)	LOAEL (mg/kg/d)	Effects observed at LOAEL/critical results	Reference
Developmental toxicity				
Rat	5	10	Anomalies of the brain, neural tube and tail at 10 mg/kg/day; a higher frequency of delayed ossification of the parietal bone at 5 mg/kg/day judged consistent with or close to a NOAEL at this level; maternal NOAEL = 40 mg/kg/day based on maternal lethality at 80 mg/kg/day	Khera, 1973
Rat	10	20	Dilation of the lateral ventricle	Teramoto *et al.*, 1978
Rat	5	10	Decreased fetal weights; hydrocephalus at 20 mg/kg/day. Maternal NOAEL = 40 mg/kg/day based on maternal deaths and reduced weight gain at 80 mg/kg/day	Chernoff *et al.*, 1979
Rat perinatal (exposure from day 7 gestation to day 15 postpartum)	25	30	Hydrocephalus, failure to nurse, increased open field activity in males	Chernoff *et al.*, 1979
Rat	15	25	Dilation of brain ventricles; maternal NOAEL = 35 mg/kg/day, HDT	Saillenfait *et al.*, 1991
Rabbit	40	80	Increased resorptions, decreased brain weights, degeneration of fetal kidney proximal tubules; maternal NOAEL = 80 mg/kg/day, HDT	Khera, 1973
Hamster	90	270	Cleft palate, tail and skeletal anomalies, decreased fetal weight; maternal NOAEL = 810 mg/kg/day, HDT	Teramoto *et al.*, 1978
Hamsters	100	NA	NOAEL	Chernoff *et al.*, 1979
Mice	100	200	Increased supernumerary ribs; maternal NOAEL < 100 mg/kg/day based on increased relative liver weight	Chernoff *et al.*, 1979
Guinea pigs	100	NA	NOAEL	Chernoff *et al.*, 1979
Cat	120	NA	Fetal NOAEL; reported maternal toxicity inconsistent with any other reported studies of ETU	Khera and Iverson, 1978

insufficiency, caused for example by nutritional iodine deficiency, the primary human response is goiter rather than neoplasia (Hill *et al.*, 1989, 1998). Despite extensive epidemiological studies, no convincing evidence has yet emerged to link iodine deficiency with human thyroid cancer (Hard, 1998). Thus, not only is a threshold model appropriate for hazard assessment of the effects of ETU, but also a large uncertainty factor is not needed to insure adequate protection of the human populations.

81.3.3.2 Liver Effects

Although the level of ETU exposure resulting from bioconversion of the EBDCs at maximum tolerated doses is generally insufficient to produce tumors of the liver, ETU given directly does produce tumors of the liver in mice (Chhabra *et al.*, 1992; Innes *et al.*, 1969). Metabolism of the EBDCs to ETU is less extensive in mice (Cameron *et al.*, 1990; Piccirillo *et al.*, 1992), and induction of liver tumors with ETU has been observed only in mice and only at higher dietary levels that were also associated with centrilobular hepatocellular cytomegaly and increased functional demand (i.e., work-related stress to the liver), in addition to thyroid inhibition and sequelae. Hepatocellular tumors have not been seen in rats or hamsters. Although thyroid effects were present, no increase in the incidence of hepatocellular tumors was noted after two years of dietary feeding at 17–18 mg/kg bw/day (Chhabra et al., 1992).

The precise mechanism of liver tumor formation with ETU in mice has not been fully elucidated. One hypothesis is that the liver tumors are related to stress on the HPT axis. The liver is subject to metabolic regulation by thyroid and pituitary hormones, and liver neoplasms have also been produced in mice by two other thionamides, 2-thiouracil and 6-methyluracil, which also produce thyroid neoplasms in rats and mice (IARC, 1974). A second threshold hypothesis notes that ETU exhibits the hallmarks of phenobarbital-type liver promotion, including mixed function oxidase induction, sustained hepatomegaly, eosinophilic foci, and cellular proliferation (McClain, 1995; Whysner et al., 1996). Yet a third notes that redox cycling of ETU, with consumption of glutathione, has been observed with rat liver microsomes in vitro (Decker and Doerge, 1991), and that oxidative damage due to glutathione depletion is a commonly recognized threshold mechanism of tumor formation in animals.

A number of additional factors also lead to the inference that these liver tumors are nonrelevant to human risk. First, there have been no reports associating the use of the structurally related propylthiouracil or other clinically administered thionamide drugs with an excess incidence of primary liver cancer in humans.

Second, there is a wide variability in the incidence of liver tumors among various strains of mice, which is partly dependent on hormonal and/or nutritional factors, in addition to genetic factors. Genetic factors are particularly operative in the case of B6C3F1 and other C3H-derived strains whose high and variable background tumor incidences indicate the presence of a significant population of "initiated" or latent tumor cells whose potential is readily expressed under stressed conditions of various origins. It has been acknowledged by numerous authorities that the induction of these tumors is of questionable or no relevance for assessment of oncogenic potential in human populations, where the background incidence of liver cancer is extremely low (e.g., IPCS, 1990; EU Directive 93/21/EEC; IARC, 1987).

In conclusion, the available information on the pathobiology and mechanism of the ETU-induced liver tumors indicates they are nonrelevant for the assessment of human risk at doses below the threshold for conventional toxic responses in these organs.

81.3.3.3 Genotoxicity

Few materials have been tested for mutagenic potential as exhaustively as the EBDCs and ETU. Among the more than 200 reported studies are more than sufficient numbers of qualified assays to ensure that each of the EBDCs and ETU individually

and collectively have been adequately tested in a wide variety of in vitro and in vivo mutagenicity tests. Care must be taken in the qualification step to exclude flawed or otherwise deficient results. For example, because of the rapid degradation of EBDCs in dimethylsulfoxide (DMSO), and the accompanying rapid liberation of metal ions, EBDC studies in which DMSO has been used as a solvent are invalid. A weight of the evidence evaluation of the scientifically valid studies shows that, when properly tested in higher organism test systems, the EBDCs and ETU are not mutagenic in the two major endpoints used to assess genotoxicity, gene mutations and chromosomal damage, and further, they do not cause adverse effects in ancillary tests of genotoxic damage. Thus, the weight of the evidence indicates that the EBDCs and ETU are not mutagenic in mammalian systems (EBDC/ETU Task Force, 1992; Elia et al., 1995). This conclusion is shared by other organizations, for example, by the NTP (1992) which stated that "ethylenethiourea has been tested extensively for genotoxicity in a variety of in vitro and in vivo test systems, and the results, with few exceptions, are negative," and the WHO (1994) which concluded that ETU was not genotoxic.

81.3.3.4 Bioequivalent Doses of the EBDCs and ETU

The bioconversion factors in rats and mice provide a quantitative basis for comparing the dose–responses of the EBDCs and ETU, and these comparisons provide quantitative support for the concept that the EBDCs' toxic effects are directly related to their conversion to ETU. Example calculations for mancozeb, maneb, and metiram using the 7.5% bioconversion factor in rats and the 6.0% factor in mice are shown in Table 81.4. It is clear that the ETU-equivalent dose levels arising from the feeding of the EBDCs are similar enough to the corresponding LOAELs and NOAELs for ETU to justify the presumption of a cause and effect relationship.

81.3.4 REPRODUCTIVE AND DEVELOPMENTAL TOXICITY

Reproductive outcome is generally unaffected by exposure to EBDCs or ETU. There were no effects on reproductive parameters, the microscopic appearance of the reproductive organs, or neonatal survival or growth resulting from exposure to any of the EBDCs or ETU at levels below those producing frank systemic toxicity in the adults (Tables 81.2 and 81.3). Further, unlike most pesticides, the potential for long-term effects of in utero exposure has been investigated. With the exception of a slight increase in thyroid tumor incidence in rats, in utero and perinatal exposure to ETU did not alter the incidences of tumors produced by postweaning lifetime exposures in either rats or mice (Chhabra et al., 1992).

Developmental toxicity is observed as malformations and embryofetotoxic effects at maternally toxic dose levels with all three EBDCs in the rat (Table 81.2). The effects seen are qualitatively consistent with those produced by ETU, and

Table 81.4
Bioequivalent Doses of the EBDCs and ETU

Critical effect/active	Critical doses (mg/kg/day)		
	EBDC	ETU-equivalent to EBDC[a]	ETU
Rats			
Thyroid tumor LOAEL			
mancozeb	29	2.2	3.7
maneb	90	6.8	
metiram	NA	NA	
Thyroid effect LOAEL			
mancozeb	15	1.1	1.1
maneb	22.4	1.7	
metiram	20	1.5	
NOAEL			
mancozeb	4.8	0.36	0.37
maneb	20	1.5	
metiram	12	0.9	
Mice			
Liver, thyroid tumor LOAEL			
mancozeb	NA	NA	56[c]
maneb	440[b]	26	
metiram	NA	NA	
Thyroid LOAEL			
mancozeb	130	7.8	17
maneb	44	2.6	
metiram	302	18	
NOAEL			
mancozeb	17	1.0	1.7
maneb	11	0.66	
metiram	84	5.0	

[a] EBDC mg/kg bw/day × ETU bioconversion factor of 7.5% in rats, 6% in mice.
[b] Liver adenomas only.
[c] Liver, thyroid, and pituitary tumors.
NA = not applicable.

the dose–response is consistent with their causation by bioconverted systemic ETU doses. Sensitivity varies with the species. Exposure to sufficient doses of ETU at the critical stages of pregnancy produces malformations in rats, predominantly those of the central nervous system and head. Related malformations are produced in hamsters although only at very high doses approaching maternally toxic levels. The mouse and rabbit are far less sensitive. Developmental effects, even at relatively high doses, are limited to findings indicative of embryofetotoxicity. The guinea pig and cat have not shown evidence of teratogenic or other developmental effects (Table 81.3; see also Ruddick and Khera, 1975; Khera, 1987). A relationship of the developmental effects to thyroid inhibition is indicated by several lines of evidence. The malformations produced by ETU exposure *in vivo* are those expected as the result of thyroid insufficiency. They occur

only at doses in excess of those producing significant thyroid inhibition in adults, and they have been prevented, at least in part, by coadministration of thyroxine (Emmerling, 1978a, b).

A key concern with thyroid inhibitors is that impaired thyroid function may alter hormone-mediated events during development, leading to permanent alterations in brain morphology and function (Cooper and Kavlock, 1997). The potential for this type of effect with ETU has been examined in a postnatal behavioral study in rats, resulting in a NOAEL of 25 mg/kg/day, fivefold higher than the 5 mg/kg/day NOAEL for other types of developmental toxicity demonstrated in a companion study (Chernoff *et al.*, 1979).

Consistent with the findings with ETU, no developmental effects were observed with the EBDCs in studies in rabbits. Feed refusal, weight loss, and late-developing abortions observed in these studies are not relevant to human health risk. Being ruminants, rabbits are very sensitive to disruption of their gut microflora by antimicrobials and fungicides (ICH, 1994), and this response is well known to precipitate late term abortions (A. Hoberman, private communication).

81.3.5 NEUROTOXICITY

The one feature of the EBDCs' toxicological profile which is not explainable by the relationship to ETU is hindlimb paralysis and associated effects, including muscular atrophy with mancozeb and metiram and an effect on the retina with mancozeb. Hindlimb paralysis occurs at high doses with all of the EBDCs (LOAELs 60–340 mg/kg bw/day) and is a property of their common primary metabolite, ethylenebisisothiocyanatesulfide (EBIS) (Freudenthal *et al.*, 1977b), presumably related to the ability to release the carbon disulfide moiety (e.g., Johnson *et al.*, 1998). Multiple exposures are generally required to produce the effect. Acute neurotoxicity testing of maneb produced no indication of an adverse effect at doses up to 2000 mg/kg (Nemec, 1993). No evidence of neurotoxicity has been observed with ETU, and a firm chronic NOAEL for neurotoxicity of 8.2 mg/kg/day has been demonstrated in perfusion neuropathology studies of mancozeb (Stadler, 1991).

81.3.6 METABOLITES OTHER THAN ETU

In studies of metabolites other than ETU, EBIS further metabolized in rats and mice to ETU and ETU metabolites (Iverson *et al.*, 1977; Jordan and Neal, 1979), and the thyroid functional changes which would be expected as a result of this metabolism were observed in addition to neurotoxicity (Freudenthal *et al.*, 1977b). No evidence of tumorigenicity was observed with EU (Innes *et al.*, 1969), and neither EU nor any of the other mancozeb and ETU metabolites tested exhibited any teratogenic potential (Ruddick *et al.*, 1976b).

81.3.7 HAZARD CHARACTERIZATION

In summary, based on extensive data, the EBDCs do not pose a hazard of acute intoxication, genetic damage, or reproductive or developmental toxicity below levels that produce other kinds of toxicity in adults, or of *significant* systemic toxicity by the dermal route. There is no evidence of bioaccumulation. Repeated exposures to high doses of the EBDCs affect the thyroid, liver, and nervous systems in laboratory animals. The thyroid and liver effects are due to their metabolism in small amounts to ETU, which interferes with the synthesis of thyroid hormone and induces stress-related liver growth. These effects are reversible when exposures are brief or intermittent, but prolonged exposures can produce secondary changes, including anemia and thyroid, pituitary, and liver tumors in rodents. Available mechanistic information establishes a threshold for the thyroid and pituitary tumors and indicates that none of the tumor types

are relevant for human risk assessment at likely exposure levels. Thus, neither the EBDCs nor ETU pose an oncogenic risk for humans. The EBDCs' neurotoxic effects are shared with their common primary metabolite EBIS, although not with ETU, and a reliable NOAEL well above anticipated human exposure levels has been confirmed in specific neuropathology studies of mancozeb.

81.4 DOSE–RESPONSE

81.4.1 NOAEL AND ACCEPTABLE DAILY INTAKE—ETU

The acceptable daily intake (ADI) or reference dose is defined as the approximate exposure which, if incurred daily over an entire lifetime, appears to be without appreciable risk for the general population, including all subgroups; i.e., it is the exposure level which provides a reasonable certainty of no harm and is therefore safe within the meaning of the U.S. Food Quality Protection Act and the WHO. When clinical studies in humans are inappropriate or unavailable, the ADI is estimated from reliably conducted toxicity studies in laboratory animals by taking the NOAEL associated with the most sensitive endpoint in the most sensitive species, and applying uncertainty factors to account for inter and intraspecies variability, and the need to protect the most sensitive individuals and subgroups, such as infants and children, among the general population.

For ETU, inspection of the critical findings in the comprehensive laboratory animal studies summarized in Table 81.3 readily reveals that thyroid and related parameters are the most sensitive effects. The rat has generally been the most sensitive species to ETU followed closely by the dog and monkey, with the mouse relatively insensitive.

An overall NOAEL of 0.4 mg/kg/day for the effects of ETU on the HPT axis, and therefore for the effects of ETU in laboratory animals, is supported by the 0.39 mg/kg/day NOAEL for hypothyroid changes including anemia in the 90 day and one year study of ETU in dogs (Briffaux, 1991, 1992), the 0.37 mg/kg/day NOAEL for thyroid, pituitary, and liver effects in the two year chronic study in rats (Schmid *et al.*, 1992), and the 0.11–0.43 mg/kg/day NOAEL for thyroid effects among the parents in the rat two-generation reproduction study (Dotti, 1992). Further, it is consistent with the weight of evidence of a comprehensive database, including the 1.1 mg/kg/day NOAEL for induction of thyroid tumors in the two year carcinogen bioassay in rats. The 1.1 mg/kg/day level was a LOAEL for thyroid hormonal changes and follicular hyperplasia (Chhabra *et al.*, 1992).

Taking into account a standard 10-fold safety or uncertainty factor for interspecies variability and a second 10-fold factor for intraspecies variation leads to the ADI of 0.004 mg/kg bw/day for ETU, as recommended by FAO/WHO (1994). Given the known lesser sensitivity of humans to thyroid effects, this is a very conservative assessment, affording extra protection of the public health. A number of factors, among them the unusually complete and reliable database, including chronic effects of *in utero* exposure, the lesser sensitivity of humans to thyroid effects, and the fact that the NOAELs for developmental and reproductive effects are 10-fold or more higher than those for thyroid effects, confirms that no additional uncertainty factor is needed to ensure adequate protection of infants and children.

81.4.2 NOAEL AND ACCEPTABLE DAILY INTAKE—EBDCS

The key requirements to support the identification of an aggregate NOAEL for a group of compounds are a common toxicological profile and a similar dose–response. As noted above, the EBDCs share a comparable toxicological profile, primarily based on the toxic effects of their common metabolite ETU. An issue which deserves some comment in this context is muscular atrophy, which was the critical effect in the two year study of metiram in rats. Muscular atrophy has been seen at high doses with both mancozeb and metiram and is associated in both of these materials with clinically diagnosed hindlimb paralysis at the same or higher doses. Thus, this effect is not an exception to the common toxicological profile in the qualitative

sense, although its appearance at the LOAEL for metiram was not typical of the dose–response seen with the other EBDCs.

With this one possible exception, the three EBDCs exhibit similar dose–effect and dose–response curves, as is illustrated in Fig. 81.3, which presents the NOAELs and LOAELs for the critical studies from Table 81.2 in a graphical format. Inspection of the graph readily reveals that the dose–responses of the three EBDCs are consistent. With only minor exceptions, the NOAELs and LOAELs of the respective materials do not overlap for any particular type of study. Second, no one of the EBDCs is consistently more sensitive than the others. Of the 10 studies conducted with at least two of the three EBDCs, the LOAELs for each study type are evenly divided among the three (4 mancozeb, 3 maneb, 3 metiram), indicating that the apparent differences among the compounds in individual studies are due to dose selection, and not to any intrinsic differences in potency. Similarly, the critical LOAELs for all three compounds are nearly identical, at between 10 and 16 mg/kg bw/day.

Since the toxicological profiles and dose–response are similar for the three EBDCs, it is appropriate to base the determination of the overall NOAEL for the EBDCs on the aggregated dataset for the group. An overall NOAEL of 5.0 mg/kg/day for the EBDCs as an aggregate group is supported by all of the available studies, as presented in Table 81.2 and Fig. 81.2. It

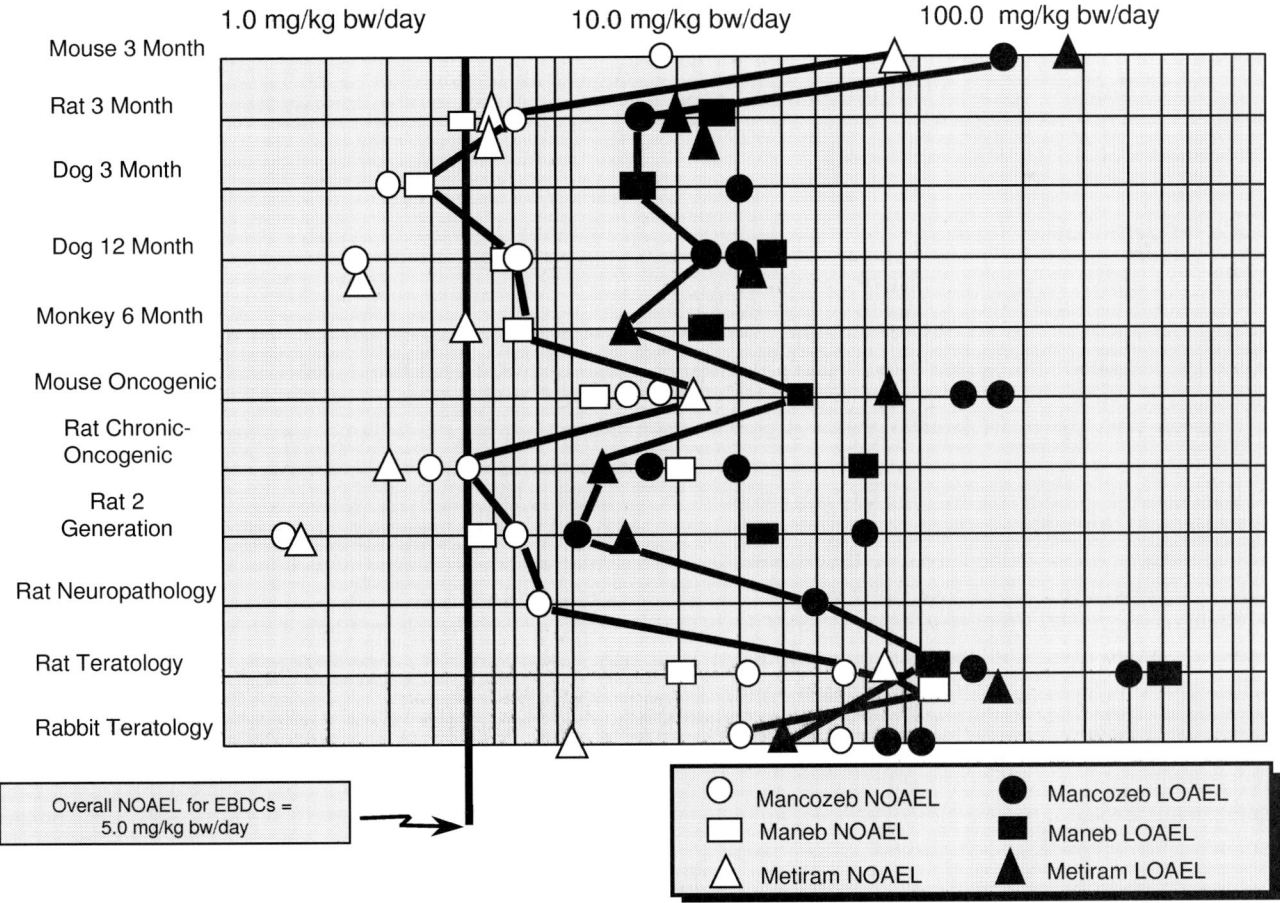

Figure 81.3 Summary of critical doses in toxicology studies of EBDCs.

is further supported by consideration of the dose response and NOAELs for ETU. Taking into account the 7.5% bioconversion factor (EPA, 1992; Kocialski, 1989), a 5.0 mg/kg/day dose of EBDC would result in a systemic dose of 0.4 mg/kg/day of ETU (5.0 mg/kg/day × 0.075 = 0.375 mg/kg/day), precisely equal to the overall NOAEL for ETU determined in independent studies. This comparison lends the support of the full ETU database to the 5.0 mg/kg/day aggregate NOEL for the EBDCs.

In summary, an aggregate evaluation of the individual toxicology databases for the respective EBDCs, mancozeb, maneb, and metiram, and their ETU metabolite indicates an overall NOAEL of 5.0 mg/kg bw/day for the group. Application of a standard 100-fold overall safety factor leads to a recommended acceptable daily intake of 0.05 mg/kg/day. The factors discussed above for ETU, and the unusual reliability of the database, reflecting the combined results of four individually comprehensive databases, confirm that no additional uncertainty factors need be applied.

This aggregate assessment produces a comparable, if slightly higher, estimate of the ADI than the FAO/WHO recommendation. The WHO panel reviewed the data for each of the actives individually and established ADIs of 0.05 mg/kg/day for mancozeb and maneb, and 0.03 mg/kg/day for metiram, resulting in the allocation of a group ADI of 0.03 mg/kg/day for the EBDCs collectively, including mancozeb, maneb, metiram, and zineb. The basis for the establishment of a group ADI was the similarity of the chemical structures of the EBDCs, the comparable toxicological profile of the EBDCs based on the toxic effects of ETU, and the fact that the parent EBDC residues cannot be differentiated using presently available regulatory analytical procedures (FAO/WHO, 1994).

81.4.3 ACUTE REFERENCE DOSE

The acute reference dose (aRfD) is the maximum single day oral exposure which is anticipated to be without appreciable risk for the general population. Toxic effects which might occur as a result of exposures occurring within the period of a single day, or after at most a very few doses, are relevant to the assessment.

For ETU the only relevant acute toxicological endpoint is developmental toxicity. A NOAEL of 5.0 mg/kg/day is supported by the weight of the evidence of multiple studies in the rat, as the most sensitive species (Chernoff *et al.*, 1979; Khera, 1973; Saillenfait *et al.*, 1991; Teramoto *et al.*, 1978). The mechanistic relationship to thyroid inhibition suggests that multiple exposures, producing hormone depletion, would be required for full expression of ETU's developmental toxicity potential in the lower dose range. This and the unusually thorough nature of the database argue that the standard 100-fold uncertainty factor is more than adequate to assure protection of women, infants, and children, indicating an aRfD for ETU of 0.05 mg/kg/day.

For the EBDCs, since expression of their neurotoxic potential requires repeated doses (e.g., Nemec, 1993) and their relevant developmental effects are due to bioconversion to

ETU, the most relevant endpoint for assessment of acute risks is the aRfD for ETU of 0.05 mg/kg bw/day, applied to the combined direct and indirect (7.5% bioconverted EBDC dose) ETU exposure.

81.4.4 ENDPOINTS FOR ASSESSMENT OF DERMAL AND RESPIRATORY EXPOSURE

For assessment of the potential risks of pesticide users and bystanders, and those who encounter exposure after application, the dermal and respiratory routes of exposure are most relevant. Dermatitis due to repeated exposures and irritation of the mucus membranes are prevented by appropriate personal protective equipment. Dermal absorption of the EBDCs is low, 6.5% or less, and consistently with this, the EBDCs are of very low toxicity by the dermal route, with NOAELs in 21-day dermal toxicity studies ranging from 100 mg/kg/day for maneb to 1000 mg/kg/day (limit dose) for mancozeb. Alternatively, the aRfD and ADIs derived from the oral exposure studies may be applied to the estimated systemic exposures from single or multiple doses, respectively, after adjustment for dermal absorption.

Subchronic inhalation studies produced the same kinds of effects as in oral studies of the same length and a generally similar dose–response, with NOAELs of 79, 10, and 2 mg/m^3 for mancozeb, maneb, and metiram, respectively. After correction for respiration rates and respirable fraction, the estimated systemic exposure of 8.3 mg/kg/day at the NOAEL in the mancozeb study was equal to the 7.4–8.2 mg/kg/d NOAELs in the 90-day dietary studies, indicating the relevance of the aRfD and ADIs for systemic exposures. In enclosed spaces, a Workplace Environmental Exposure Limit Guide of 1 mg/m^3 is recommended (AIHA, 1992).

81.4.5 CARCINOGENICITY CLASSIFICATION AND LOW DOSE RISK ASSESSMENT

The criteria for classification of substances as carcinogens differ with the classifying authority. Mancozeb and ETU were evaluated by the EU Commission in 1994, in the context of European classification criteria which assign an important role to the mode of action, and were not classified as carcinogens.

In contrast, the International Agency for Research on Cancer (IARC) classified ETU as category 2B "possibly carcinogenic to humans" based on sufficient evidence in laboratory animals but inadequate evidence in humans (IARC, 1987), and the EPA (1992) cited evidence of carcinogenicity in two species and a weak genotoxic potential in classifying ETU, as a B2 "probable human carcinogen." The Agency's classification of the EBDCs as similar B2 carcinogens was largely due to the metabolic conversion to ETU. Because EPA prefers a probabilistic approach to risk assessment for carcinogens in this class, the linear multistage model was used to calculate an upper

95% confidence limit of 0.06 (mg/kg bw/day)$^{-1}$ on the lifetime risk of cancer from ETU at low exposure levels (q^*) (EPA, 1997).

81.5 TOXICOLOGY IN HUMANS

With the exception of sporadic reports of allergic contact hypersensitivity (Bruze and Fregert, 1983; Crippa *et al.*, 1990; Kleibl and Rackova, 1980; Lee *et al.*, 1981), studies of manufacturing workers and users have not discerned adverse effects of exposure to either ETU or the EBDCs.

In the most comprehensive study of thyroid effects, 153 men currently or previously exposed to EBDC for many years at a manufacturing site were compared for thyroid function to 153 men not exposed to EBDC, its products, or ETU who also worked at the same plant. Workers and controls were carefully matched with respect to age, race, length of employment, and type of employment. Informed consent was obtained from all participants. No significant differences were observed on thyroid palpitation and in thyroid function tests between the EBDC workers and the control men. Urinary excretion of ETU in a subgroup of 42 workers currently exposed to EBDC was 0.002 ppm compared to 0.001 ppm in the control group (41 men), most of whom had undetectable values. The authors concluded that exposure to EBDC manufacture was not associated with an increased prevalence of thyroid abnormalities (Charkes *et al.*, 1985).

Clinical examinations and thyroid function tests were also carried out over a period of 3 years in the United Kingdom on 8 male workers engaged for between 5 and 20 years in the manufacture of ETU and 5 male workers involved for 3 years in the mixing of ETU with rubber, and matched controls. Levels of ETU recorded on personal samplers of manufacturing workers reached 330 $\mu g/m^3$, and levels for mixers ranged from 120 to 160 $\mu g/m^3$. Mixers but not process workers had significantly lower levels of T_4 in their blood compared to controls. With the exception of one mixer with elevated TSH levels, who was evaluated as hypothyroid on further testing, no effects were found on TSH or thyroid binding globulin. The authors concluded that there was no evidence that thyroid function is severely affected by exposure to ETU at the levels experienced by these workers (Smith, 1984). Similarly, no hazard of clinical thyroid depression existed based on medical evidence collected on 51 workers exposed to ETU at a U.S. rubber-processing company (Salisbury and Lybarger, 1977).

No difference was found in the total death rate or deaths due to cancers between 992 male workers involved in the production of EBDCs from 1948 to 1975 and control males from the city of Philadelphia. No thyroid cancer was found in this study (DeFonso, 1976).

Epidemiological studies were conducted on workers in the rubber industry by Parkes (1974) and Smith (1976). Based on examination of national and regional thyroid cancer incidences in the UK, Parkes concluded that, under the conditions in which ETU had been used in the rubber industry, there is no risk of man contracting thyroid cancer as a result of industrial exposure to ethylenethiourea (Parkes, 1974). Similarly, a total of 1929 workers engaged in the production or manufacture of ETU were surveyed retrospectively for thyroid cancer and were compared with the thyroid cancer list of the Birmingham (England) Cancer Registry from 1957 to 1971. No thyroid cancers occurred in these workers. A retrospective study of 699 women who were employed at a rubber manufacturer using ETU assessed the incidence of fetal abnormalities occurring in children to women who had worked with ETU during early pregnancy. No excess incidence was found, and the study did not demonstrate any risk of teratogenesis (Smith, 1976).

81.6 RISK CHARACTERIZATION

81.6.1 DIETARY EXPOSURE AND RISKS

Risk is a function of hazard potential and exposure. The potential risk of consumers of foods derived from chemically protected crops is assessed by comparing the ADI for the particular crop protection chemical, or other indices of its toxicity potential when relevant, to estimated or measured dietary exposure values. Dietary exposure is in turn determined from the level of residues of the crop protection chemical and its toxicologically significant metabolites in foods and food consumption patterns for various population groups.

Dietary intake may be predicted with varying degrees of accuracy. The WHO and the European Union use the International Estimated Dietary Intake (IEDI) for five global diets. The exposure is calculated using average regional food consumption data and the median residue from supervised trials that have been used to assess the maximum residue limit or tolerance consistent with the worldwide labels. Residues of EBDCs and ETU in processed commodities were also calculated. The IEDI was calculated for each of the five global diets using the EBDC and ETU level with the highest dietary contribution. On this basis, the aggregate dietary exposure to the EBDCs ranged from a low of 3% of the ADI in the African diet to 36% of the ADI in the European diet. These levels are well within the criteria of WHO for fully acceptable dietary risk (less than 100% of the ADI) (Ollinger, 1999).

These data overestimate the dietary risks of the EBDCs because the IEDI calculation assumes that 100% of the crop is treated and the residues are measured from crops as they are harvested. More reliable assessments of dietary exposure may be obtained at the national level (National Estimate of Daily Intake, NEDI) . Such a more accurate determination of EBDC and ETU exposure is available from a market basket survey conducted in the United States. In that study, samples of fresh and processed foods were collected every two weeks for one year from grocery stores throughout the United States in a statistically designed survey. Using the most sensitive residue analytical methods achievable, the results from the analysis of almost 6000 samples showed that about 80% of the samples had no measurable residues of EBDC or ETU. The residues that were found were very close to the limit of quantitation in the method. Thus, there is virtually no exposure to the consumer to residues of either EBDCs or ETU.

A reliable NEDI was derived for the United States, a member of the European diet category, from the average consumer level residue values determined in the market basket and related studies, and detailed national data on the consumption of raw and processed food commodities as summarized in the US EPA's Dietary Risk Estimation System. The NEDI for U.S. consumer exposure to EBDCs and ETU was 0.000027 mg/kg bw/day, calculated as ETU, or less than 1% (0.68%) of the 0.004 mg/kg bw/day ADI for ETU. These NEDI values clearly show that actual consumer exposure to residues of the EBDCs is negligible (EBDC/ETU Task Force, 1997b).

Utilization of these market basket data in a Monte Carlo assessment of acute dietary exposure resulted in an acute margin of exposure for women of child-bearing age (13 + years) of 2652 at the 99.9 percentile of exposure, greatly beneath any levels of concern (EBDC/ETU Task Force, 1997b).

EPA calculated the risks to consumers using the market basket data and their standard method of estimating the probability of human cancer risks. They determined that there was only a negligible theoretical dietary risk of 1.2 in one million from the use of EBDCs on 48 crops (EPA, 1992, 1996).

The negligible character of dietary exposure to the EBDCs is further underlined by the nutritional benefits which they confer. The principal use of the EBDCs is the economical protection of fruit and vegetables from disease, making these commodities more widely available in the diet. Overwhelming evidence from epidemiological studies indicates that diets high in fruits and vegetables are associated with a lower risk of numerous cancers, and for this reason, dietary recommendations to increase the intake of citrus fruits, cruciferous vegetables, green and yellow vegetables, and fruits and vegetables high in vitamins A and C have been made by numerous organizations (AICR, 1997; American Cancer Society, 1984, 1996; Block *et al.*, 1992; Giovannucci, 1999; NAS/NRC, 1989; NCI, 1987; Steinmetz and Potter, 1991).

81.6.2 WORKER EXPOSURE AND RISKS

Exposure estimates for mixing, loading, and applying EBDC fungicides during outdoor agricultural applications have been calculated using the predictive operator exposure model of the UK MAFF and also the model of the German BBA as sources of surrogate exposure data. Each of these models represents a synthesis and integration of exposure data obtained in a large number of field trials conducted using various kinds of equipment in a variety of national agricultural settings. The final models were calibrated to insure that the resulting estimates would, if anything, overpredict actual exposures under field conditions. For modeling of EBDC uses, an application rate of 2.4 kg ai/hectare was chosen to represent a typical maximum use rate of EBDC products when used on a standalone basis. Use rates for these products when used as mixtures

are lower. As gloves are recommended as personal protective equipment when handling undiluted product, the use of gloves (during mixing and loading only) is presumed in the models. The exposure estimates obtained using these very conservative models indicate that operator exposures are always below, and in most cases substantially below, acceptable dermal and inhalation exposure limits for workers, even when personal protective equipment is limited to the bare minimum of gloves during mixing and loading. Therefore a significant risk for the operator during the use of EBDC fungicide products appears unlikely.

As in the case of dietary exposure, alternative risk assessment approaches have been used at times by various authorities. At the conclusion of the U.S. Special Review, the EPA concluded there was adequate safety to mixers, loaders, and applicators when proper personal protective equipment is used (EPA, 1992).

Estimates of exposure for other activities, including bystanders, workers reentering treated fields, homeowners, and others reentering treated areas are even lower.

81.6.3 CONCLUSION

Because of their importance to worldwide agriculture, the EBDCs and ETU have been thoroughly tested over many years. Collectively, the data demonstrate that the use of the EBDCs results in essentially negligible exposure to consumers, coupled with a significant contribution to improved nutrition, and low risk to farm workers, production workers, and people who are exposed through recreational activities.

REFERENCES

Allen, T. R., Frei, Th., Biedermann, K., Luetkemeier, H., Terrier, Ch., Vogel, O., and Wilson, J. (1989). "13-Week Oral Toxicity (Feeding) Study with Maneb Technical in the Dog." Rep. 206605 from Research and Consulting Company, Ltd., Itingen, Switzerland. Unpublished report of Elf Atochem North America, Inc.

American Cancer Society (1984). Nutrition and cancer: causation and prevention. An American Cancer Society special report. *CA Cancer J. Clin.* **34**, 5–10.

American Cancer Society (1996). Guidelines on diet, nutrition, and cancer prevention: Reducing the risk of cancer with healthy food choices and physical activity. The American Cancer Society 1996 advisory committee on diet, nutrition and cancer prevention. *CA Cancer J. Clin.* **46**, 325–341.

American Industrial Hygiene Association (AIHA) (1992). "Workplace Environmental Exposure Level Guide: Mancozeb." AIHA, Akron, OH.

American Institute for Cancer Research (AICR) (1997). "Food, Nutrition, and the Prevention of Cancer: A Global Perspective." World Cancer Research Fund and the American Institute for Cancer Research, Washington, DC.

Arnold, D. L., Krewski, D. R., Junkins, D. B., McGuire, P. F., Moodie, C. A., and Munro, I. C. (1983). Reversibility of ethylenethiourea-induced thyroid lesions. *Toxicol. Appl. Pharmacol.* **67**, 264–273.

Atterwill, C. P., and Aylard, S. P. (1995). Endocrine toxicology of the thyroid for industrial compounds. *In* "Toxicology of Industrial Compounds" (H. Thomas, R. Hess, and Waechter, eds.), pp. 257–280. Taylor & Francis, London.

Block, G., Patterson, B., and Subar, A. (1992). Fruit, vegetables, and cancer prevention: a review of the epidemiological evidence. *Nutrition Cancer* **18**, 1–29.

Broadmeadow, A. (1991a). "Mancozeb Technical: Toxicity Study by Oral Administration to Beagle Dogs for 52 Weeks." Rep. 89/PTC004/0015 from Life Science Research Ltd., Suffolk, England. Unpublished report of Elf Atochem North America, Inc.

Broadmeadow, A. (1991b). "Mancozeb Technical: Toxicity Study by Oral Administration to Beagle Dogs for 52 Weeks." Rep. 90/PTC029/0197 from Life Science Research Ltd., Suffolk, England. Unpublished report of Elf Atochem North America, Inc.

Briffaux, J. P. (1991). "ETU: 13-Week Oral (Dietary) Toxicity Study in the Beagle Dog." Project 616/504 from Hazleton Laboratories, Lyon, France. Unpublished report of Rohm and Haas Company.

Briffaux, J. P. (1992). "ETU: 52 Week Oral (Dietary) Toxicity Study in the Beagle Dog." Project 616/505 from Hazleton Laboratories, Lyon, France. Unpublished report of Rohm and Haas Company.

Bruze, M., and Fregert, S. (1983). Allergic contact dermatitis from ethylenethiourea. *Contact Dermatitis* **9**, 208–212.

Cameron, B. D., Clydesdale, K., and Speirs, G. C. (1990). "The Disposition of 14C Mancozeb in the Mouse." Rep. 4909 from Inveresk Research International, Musselburgh, Scotland. Unpublished report of Elf Atochem North America, Inc.

Charkes, N. D., Braverman, L. E., Penko, K. F., Gowers, D. S., Gordon, C. F., Lipworth, L., and Malmud, L. S. (1985). Thyroid function in male workers manufacturing dithane, an agricultural fungicide, and in men not exposed to dithane. *Frontiers Thyroidol.* **2**, 933–936.

Chernoff, N., Kavlock, R. J., Rogers, E. H., Carver, B. D., and Murray, S. (1979). Perinatal toxicity of maneb, ethylenethiourea and ethylenebisisothiocyanate sulphide in rodents. *J. Toxicol. Environmental Health* **5**, 821–834.

Chesterman, H., Heywood, R., Ball, S., Street, A., and Prentice, D. (1978). "Metiram (Active Ingredient) Oral Toxicity Study in Beagle Dogs (Dietary Intake for 4 Weeks)." Rep. BASF 78/0154, BSF 201/76422 from Huntingdon Research Centre, Huntingdon, UK. Unpublished report of BASF Corporation.

Chhabra, R. S., Eustis, S., Haseman, J. K., Kurtz, P. J., and Carlton, B. D. (1992). Comparative carcinogenicity of ethylene thiourea with or without perinatal exposure in rats and mice. *Fundamental Appl. Toxicol.* **18**, 405–417.

Cooper, R. L., and Kavlock, R. J. (1997). Endocrine disruptors and reproductive development: A weight of evidence overview. *J. Endocrinol.* **152**, 159–166.

Corney, S. J., Allen, T. R., Janiak, T., and Springall, C. (1991). "52-Week Oral Toxicity (Feeding) Study with Metiram Premix 95% in the Dog." Rep. 91/10786 from Research and Consulting Company Ltd., Itingen, Switzerland. Unpublished report of BASF Corporation.

Corney, S. J., Allen, T. R., Janiak, T., Frei, Th., Leutkemeier, H., Biedermann, K., Vogel, O., and Springall, C. (1992). "A 52-Week Oral Toxicity Study (Feeding) with Maneb Technical in the Dog." Rep. 206616 from Research and Consulting Company, Ltd., Itingen, Switzerland. Unpublished report of BASF Corporation.

Costigan, M. (1998). "The Relevance of Rat Thyroid Gland Tumors to Humans." United Kingdom Health and Safety Executive, Toxicology Unit, Bootle, UK.

Cox, R. H. (1986). "3-Month Dietary Toxicity Study in Dogs with Mancozeb." Rep. 417-416 from Hazleton Labs, Vienna, VA. Unpublished report of Rohm and Haas Company.

Cozens, D., Simons, R., Clark, R., Offer, J., and Gibson, W. (1981). "Effect of Metiram Technical on Reproductive Function of Multiple Generations in the Rat." Rep. RZ 81/132, BSF 200/80692 from Huntingdon Research Centre, Huntingdon, UK. Unpublished report of BASF Corporation.

Craine, E. M. (1991). "A Dermal Radiotracer Absorption Study in Rats with 14C Maneb." Rep. WIL-134010 from WIL Research Laboratories, Inc., Ashland, OH. Unpublished report of Elf Atochem North America, Inc.

Crippa, M., Misquiih, L., Lunati, A., and Pasollini, G. (1990). Dyshidrotic eczema and sensitization to dithiocarbamates in a florist. *Contact Dermatitis* **23**, 203.

Decker, C. J., and Doerge, D. R. (1991). Rat hepatic microsomal metabolism of ethylenethiourea. Contributions of the flavin-containing monooxygenase and cytochrome P-450 isozymes. *Chem. Res. Toxicol.* **4**, 482–489.

DeCrescente, M. E., and Parsons, R. D. (1980). "Dithane M-45: Acute Oral, and Dermal LD50 and Skin and Eye Irritation." Unpublished Rep. 79R-180 of Rohm and Haas Company.

DeFonso, L. R. (1976). "Mortality Study of Workers Exposed to Dithane from 1948 to 1975." Unpublished report of Rohm and Haas Company.

DeGroot, A. P. (1974). "Determination of Acute IP Toxicity of Dithane M-45 in Rats." Central Institute for Nutrition and Food Research, TNO, the Netherlands. Unpublished report of Rohm and Haas Company.

DiDonato, L. J., and Longacre, S. L. (1986). "Mancozeb Pharmacokinetic Study in Rats." Rep. 31H-86-02. Unpublished Rep. 85R-123 of Rohm and Haas Company. Supplement/appendix to Nelson (1986).

DiDonato, L. J., and Longacre, S. L. (1987). "Ethylene Thiourea: Dermal/Oral Absorption Study in Male Rats." Unpublished Rep. 85R-0206 of Rohm and Haas Company.

Doerge, D., and Takazawa, R. (1990). Mechanism of thyroid peroxidase inhibition by ethylenethiourea. *Chem. Res. Toxicol.* **3**, 98–101.

Doniach, I. (1970). Experimental thyroid tumors. *In* "Tumors of the Thyroid Gland" (D. Smithers, ed.), pp. 73–99. Livingston, Edinburgh.

Dotti, A. (1992). "Ethylene Thiourea (ETU): Two-Generation Reproduction Study in the Rat." Project 252360 from Research and Consulting Company, Ltd., Itingen, Switzerland. Unpublished report of Rohm and Haas Company.

Duncan, J. R., Prasse, K. W., and Mahaffey, E. A. (1994). "Veterinary Laboratory Medicine, Clinical Pathology," 3rd ed., pp. 30 and 196. Iowa State Univ. Press, Ames, IA.

EBDC/ETU Task Force (1992). "EBDCs and ETU Are Not Genotoxic. Comments of the EBDC/ETU Task Force on the EPA Evaluation of the Mutagenic Potential of the EBDCs and ETU."

EBDC/ETU Task Force (1997a). "Reference Doses, Toxicity Endpoints, and Uncertainty Factors, Ethylenethiourea and the Ethylenebisdithiocarbamates, Mancozeb, Maneb and Metiram."

EBDC/ETU Task Force (1997b). "Safety Assessment Regarding Notice of Filing of Pesticide Petitions." Docket PF-751 (62 Federal Register 41379).

Elia, M. C., Arce, G., Hurt, S. S., O'Neill, P. J., and Scribner, H. E. (1995). The genetic toxicology of ethylenethiourea: a case study concerning the evaluation of a chemical's genotoxic potential. *Mutation Res.* **341**, 141–149.

Emmerling, D. C. (1978a). "The Effects of Thyroid Hormones on the Teratogenic Potential of Ethylenethiourea in Rats." Report from Battelle Laboratories, Columbus, OH. Unpublished report of Rohm and Haas Company.

Emmerling, D. C. (1978b). "A Study of the Uptake and Elimination of 14C-Activity after the Oral Ingestion of 14C-Labelled Ethylenethiourea (ETU) and Mancozeb in the Rhesus Monkey." Report from Battelle Laboratories, Columbus, OH. Unpublished report of Rohm and Haas Company.

Engler, D., and Burger, A. G. (1984). The deiodination of the iodothyronines and their derivatives in man. *Endocrine Rev.* **5**, 151–184.

Environmental Protection Agency (EPA) (1992). United States EPA notice announcing final determination, conclusion of the special review of EBDC pesticides. 57 Federal Register 7484, March 2, 1992.

Environmental Protection Agency (EPA) (1996). United States Federal Register of August 14, 1996, pp. 42244–42249.

Environmental Protection Agency (EPA) (1997). United States Office of Pesticide Programs reference dose tracking report of February 19, 1997.

Environmental Protection Agency (EPA) (1998). "Assessment of Thyroid Follicular Tumors." United States Environmental Protection Agency risk assessment forum, EPA/630/R-97/002.

Everett, D. J., Atkinson, C., Perry, C. J., Strutt, A., Millar, P., and Hudson, P. (1992). "Mancozeb 78 Week Dietary Carcinogenicity Study in Mice with 52 Week Interim Kill." Rep. 7561 from Inveresk Research International, Tranent, Scotland. Unpublished report of Elf Atochem North America, Inc.

Food and Agriculture Organization/World Health Organization (1994). "Ethylenethiourea, Ethylenebisdithiocarbamates, Mancozeb, Maneb, Metiram, Zineb." Report of the joint meeting of the FAO panel of experts on pesticide residues in food and the environment and the WHO expert group on pesticide residues, Geneva, 20–29 September 1993. Food and agricultural organization of the United Nations plant production and protection paper 122.

Food and Agriculture Organization (1997). "FAO Manual on the Submission and Evaluation of Pesticide Residues Data for the Estimation of Maximum Residue Levels in Food and Feed." Food and Agriculture Organization of the United Nations, Rome.

Frank, J., and Muller, G. (1988). "ETU: *In Vivo/In Vitro* UDS/s-Phase Assay in Mice." Unpublished Rep. 88R-0047 of Rohm and Haas Company.

Freudenthal, R. I., Kerchner, G., Persing, R., and Baron, R. L. (1977a). Dietary subacute toxicity of ethylene thiourea in the laboratory rat. *J. Environmental Pathol. Toxicol.* **1**, 147–161.

Freudenthal, R. I., Kerchner, G. A., Persing, R. L., Baumel, I., and Baron, R. L. (1977b). Subacute toxicity of ethylenebisisothiocyanate sulfide in the laboratory rat. *J. Toxicol. Environmental Health* **2**, 1067–1078.

Gak, J. C., Graillot, C., and Truhaut, R. (1976). Difference in sensitivity of the hamster and rat to the effects of long term administration of ethylenethiourea. *European J. Toxicol.* **9**, 303–312.

Gallo, M. A., Kam, C., and Stevens, D. R. (1980). "Teratologic Evaluation of Dithane M-45 in the Albino Rat." Unpublished Rep. 81RC-075 of Rohm and Haas Company.

Gelbke, H., Hellwig, J., and Hildebrand, B. (1988). "Report on the Study of the Prenatal Toxicity of Metiram-Premix 95% in Rabbits after Oral Administration (Gavage)." Unpublished Rep. BASF 88/0154 and Supplement BASF 88/0282 of BASF Corporation.

Gelbke, H., Mellert, W., and Hildebrand, B. (1992a). "Study of the Oral Toxicity of Metiram Premix 95% in $B_6C_3F_1$ Mice. Administration in the Diet for 3 Months." Unpublished Rep. 92/11223 of BASF Corporation.

Gelbke, H., Mellert, W., and Hildebrand, B. (1992b). "Study of the Oral Toxicity of Metiram Premix 95% in Wistar Rats. Administration in the Diet for 3 Months Including the Examination of Neurotoxicology (Neurofunctional Observational Battery)." Unpublished Rep. 92/11224 of BASF Corporation.

Giovannucci, E. (1999). Tomatoes, tomato-based products, lycopene, and cancer: Review of the epidemiologic literature. *J. National Cancer Inst.* **91**, 317–331.

Goldman, P., Bernacki, H. J., and Quinn, D. L. (1986). "Mancozeb: Three-Month Dietary Toxicity Study in Rats." Unpublished Rep. 85R-167 of Rohm and Haas Company.

Graham, S. L., and Hansen, W. H. (1972). Effects of short-term administration of ethylenethiourea upon thyroid function of the rat. *Bull. Environmental Contamination Toxicol.* **7**, 19–25.

Graham, S. L., Hansen, W. H., Davis, K. J., and Perry, C. H. (1973). Effects of one-year administration of ethylenethiourea upon the thyroid of the rat. *J. Agr. Food Chem.* **21**, 324–329.

Graham, S. L., Davis, K. J., Hansen, W. H., and Graham, C. H. (1975). Effects of prolonged ethylenethiourea ingestion on the thyroid of the rat. *Food Cosmetol. Toxicol.* **13**, 493–499.

Grundler, O. J. (1979). "Study of the Acute Dermal Toxicity of 'Metiram Technical with 2% ETU' on the Rat." Unpublished Rep. RZ 79/032 of BASF Corporation.

Hagan, J. V., and Baldwin, R. C. (1982). "Dithane M-45: Acute Inhalation Toxicology Study in Rats." Unpublished Rep. 81R-171 of Rohm and Haas Company.

Hagan, J. V., and Baldwin, R. C. (1986). "Mancozeb: Two-Week Range-Finding Inhalation Toxicity Study in Rats." Unpublished Rep. 85R-0190 of Rohm and Haas Company.

Hagan, J. V., Fisher, J. R., and Baldwin, R. C. (1986). "Mancozeb: Subchronic Inhalation Toxicity Study in Rats." Unpublished Rep. 86R-3 of Rohm and Haas Company.

Haines, L. D. (1980). "Dithane M-45 Percutaneous Absorption in Rats." Unpublished Rep. 34F-80-9 of Rohm and Haas Company.

Haines, L. D., and Satterthwaite, S. (1979). "Dithane M-45 Production Worker Exposure Studies." Unpublished Rep. 34F-79-14 of Rohm and Haas Company.

Hard, G. C. (1998). Recent developments in the investigation of thyroid regulation and thyroid carcinogenesis. *Environmental Health Perspectives* **106**, 427–436.

Hawkins, D., Elsom, L., Girkin, R., and Jackson, R. (1984). "Report on the Study of Dermal Absorption of Metiram in Rats." Rep. RZ 85/158, HRC BSF 411/84694 from Huntingdon Research Centre, Huntingdon, UK. Unpublished report of BASF Corporation.

Hawkins, D., Elsom, L., Midgley, I., Biggs, S., and McCay, C. (1985). "The Biokinetics and Metabolism of 14C-Metiram in the Rat." Rep. BASF 85/0470, HRC BSF 410/85720 from Huntingdon Research Centre, Huntingdon, UK. Unpublished report of BASF Corporation.

Hill, R., Erdreich, L., Paynter, O., Roberts, P., Rosenthal, S., and Wilkinson, C. (1989). Review: Thyroid Follicular Cell Carcinogenesis. *Fundamental Appl. Toxicol.* **12**, 629–697.

Hill, R., Crisp, T. M., Hurley, P. M., Rosenthal, S. L., and Singh, D. V. (1998). Risk assessment of thyroid follicular tumors. *Environmental Health Perspectives* **106**, 447–457.

Hofmann, H. (1974). "Acute Intraperitoneal Toxicity of Polyram Combi (Technical Active Ingredient) to the Mouse." Unpublished Rep. RZ 74/011 of BASF Corporation.

Hofmann, H. (1975). "Acute Oral Toxicity of the Technical Active Ingredient Metiram to the Rat." Unpublished Rep. RZ 75/005 of BASF Corporation.

Hofmann, H. (1985). "Report on the Study of the Acute Oral Toxicity of Polyram Combi, Technical Active Ingredient, in the Rat." Unpublished Rep. BASF 85/0485 of BASF Corporation.

Hofmann, H., and Munk, R. (1975). "Acute Intraperitoneal Toxicity of the Technical Active Ingredient Metiram to the Rat." Unpublished Rep. RZ 75/006 of BASF Corporation.

Hooks, W. N., Offer, J. M., Hadley, J. C., Gibson, W. A., Gopinath, C., and Dawe, I. S. (1992). "Mancozeb Technical: Potential Tumorigenic and Toxic Effects in Prolonged Dietary Administration to Rats." Rep. PWT 29/89669 from Huntingdon Research Centre, Huntingdon, UK. Unpublished report of Elf Atochem North America, Inc.

Hunter, B., Barnard, A., Heywood, R., Street, A., and Prentice, D. (1976a). "Preliminary Assessment of Metiram Toxicity in Rats in Dietary Administration for Four Weeks Followed by a Two and a Four Week Withdrawal Period." Rep. RZ 76/024, BSF 172/76245 from Huntingdon Research Centre, Huntingdon, UK. Unpublished report of BASF Corporation.

Hunter, B., Bridges, J., and Prentice, D. (1976b). "Preliminary Assessment of Metiram Toxicity to Mice in Dietary Administration for 4 Weeks." Rep. RZ 76/014, BSF 170/76108 from Huntingdon Research Centre, Huntingdon, UK. Unpublished report of BASF Corporation.

Hunter, B., Barnard, A., Heywood, R., Street, A., Prentice, D., and Offer, J. (1977). "Metiram Toxicity to Rats in Dietary Administration for 13 Weeks Followed by a 6 Week Withdrawal Period." Rep. RZ 77/043, BSF/197/77612 and Addendum BASF 87/0205, BSF 197/8713 from Huntingdon Research Centre, Huntingdon, UK. Unpublished report of BASF Corporation.

Hunter, B., Barnard, A., Prentice, D., and Gregson, R. (1979). "Metiram Tumorigenicity to Mice in Long Term Dietary Administration." Rep. RZ 79/033, BSF 198/78265 from Huntingdon Research Centre, Huntingdon, UK. Unpublished report of BASF Corporation.

Hunter, B., Barnard, A., Street, A., Heywood, R., Prentice, D., Offer, J., and Gibson, W. (1981). "Metiram Toxicity and Tumorigenicity in Prolonged Dietary Administration to the Rat." Rep. RZ 81/280, BSF 199/80391, WNT 77/951, and Addendum BASF 89/0001 from Huntingdon Research Centre, Huntingdon, UK. Unpublished report of BASF Corporation.

Hurley, P. M., Hill, R. N., and Whiting, R. J. (1998). Mode of carcinogenic action of pesticides inducing thyroid follicular tumors in rodents. *Environmental Health Perspectives* **106**, 437–445.

Innes, J. R. M., Ulland, B. M., Valerio, M. G., Petrucelli, L., Fishbein, L., Hart, E. R., Pallotta, A. J., Bates, R. R., Falk, H. L., Gart, J. J., Klein, M., Mitchell, I., and Peters, J. (1969). Bioassay of pesticides and industrial chemicals for tumorigenicity in mice; a preliminary note. *J. National Cancer Inst.* **42**, 1101–1114.

International Agency for Research on Cancer (IARC) (1974). "Ethylenethiourea," Vol. 7, pp. 23–24 and 45—52. Lyon, France.

International Agency for Research on Cancer (IARC) (1987). "Monographs on the Evaluation of Carcinogenic Risks to Humans. Genetic and Related

Effects: An Updating of Selected IARC Monographs from Volumes 1–42," Suppl. 6, pp. 304–307. Lyon, France.

International Conference on Harmonization (ICH) (1994). "Guideline on Detection of Toxicity to Reproduction for Medicinal Products." United States Food and Drug Administration, 59Federal Register 48746, September 22, 1994.

International Programme on Chemical Safety (IPCS) (1990). "Environmental Health Criteria 104. Principles for the Toxicological Assessment of Pesticide Residues in Food," pp. 88–91. World Health Organization, Geneva, Switzerland.

Iverson, F., Newsome, W. H., and Hierlihy, S. L. (1977). Tissue distribution of ethylenethiuram monosulfide (ETM) in the rat. *Bull. Environmental Contam. Toxicol.* **18**, 541–551.

Iverson, F., Khera, K. S., and Hierlihy, S. L. (1980). *In vivo* and *in vitro* metabolism of ethylenethiourea in the rat and the cat. *Toxicol. Appl. Pharmacol.* **52**, 16–21.

Jackh, R. (1981). "Report on the Study of the Acute Oral Toxicity of Metiram Technical Grade in the Rat (Translation)." Unpublished Rep. BASF 92/10669 of BASF Corporation.

Jain, N. C. (1986). In "Schalm's Veterinary Hematology," 4th ed., p. 671. Lea and Febiger, Philadelphia.

Johnson, D. J., Graham, D. G., Amarnath, V., Amarnath, K., and Valentine, W. M. (1998). Release of carbon disulfide is a contributing mechanism in the axonopathy produced by *N,N*-diethyldithiocarbamate. *Toxicol. Appl. Pharmacol.* **148**, 288–296.

Jordan, L. W., and Neal, R. A. (1979). Examination of the *in vivo* metabolism of maneb and zineb to ethylenethiourea (ETU) in mice. *Bull. Environmental Contam. Toxicol.* **22**, 271–277.

Kapp, R. W., Schellhaas, L. J., and Piccirillo, V. J. (1991). "Prenatal Toxicity Study of Maneb in Rats." Unpublished Reps. BASF 88/0522, 88/0523, 88/0524 of BASF Corporation.

Kato, Y., Odanaka, Y., Teramoto, S., and Matano, O. (1976). Metabolic fate of ethylenethiourea in pregnant rats. *Bull. Environmental Contam. Toxicol.* **16**, 546–555.

Khera, K. S. (1973). Ethylenethiourea: Teratogenicity study in rats and rabbits. *Teratology* **7**, 243–252.

Khera, K. (1987). Ethylenethiourea: A review of teratogenicity and distribution studies and as assessment of reproduction risk. *CRC Crit. Rev. Toxicol.* **18**, 129–139.

Khera, K. S., and Iverson, F. (1978). Toxicity of ethylenethiourea in pregnant cats. *Teratology* **18**, 311–314.

Kleibl, K., and Rackova, M. (1980). Cutaneous allergic reactions to dithiocarbamates. *Contact Dermatitis* **6**, 348–349.

Klimisch, H. J., and Zeller, H. (1980). "Report on the Determination of the Acute Inhalation Toxicity LC50 Metiram Technical with 2% ETU as a Dust Aerosol after 4-hr Exposure in Sprague–Dawley Rats." Unpublished Rep. RZ 83/064 of BASF Corporation.

Kocialski, A. (1989). "Establishment of an *In Vitro* Metabolic Conversion Factor of 7.5% for all EBDCs when Converting EBDCs to Ethylenethiourea *In Vivo* and Recalculations of the Previously Considered 20% *In Vivo* Conversion/Exposure Factor for EBDCs to ETU." Memorandum to Caswell file for each EBDC and ETU, Health Effects Division, Office of Pesticide Programs, United States Environmental Protection Agency.

Leber, A. P., Wilkinson, G. E., Persing, R. L., and Holzworth, D. A. (1978). "Effects of Feeding Ethylene Thiourea in the Rhesus Monkey." Contract 68-01-4717 from Battelle Laboratories, Columbus, OH. Unpublished report of Rohm and Haas Company.

Lee, Y. S., Cinn, Y. W., Chang, W. H., and Kim, J. S. (1981). A study on hypersensitivity of Korean farmers to various agrochemicals. 1. Determination of concentration for Patch tests of fruit-tree agrochemicals and hypersensitivity of orange orchard farmers in Che-Ju Do, Korea. *Seoul J. Med.* **22**, 137–142.

Leuschner, F. (1979a). "The Acute Oral Toxicity of the Preparation Metiram, Technical Agent with 2% ETU in Rats." Unpublished Rep. BASF 79/0161, WNT-Nr. 77/951 of BASF Corporation.

Leuschner, F. (1979b). "The Acute Intraperitoneal Toxicity of the Preparation Metiram, Technical Agent with 2% ETU in Mice." Unpublished Rep. BASF 79/0162, WNT-Nr. 77/951 of BASF Corporation.

Leuschner, F. (1991). "Chronic Oral Toxicity of Manganese-ethylene-1,2-bis-dithiocarbamate, 90%—Called for Short 'Maneb'—Sprague–Dawley (SIV) Rats (with Special Attention to Carcinogenic Properties). Amendment 3." Unpublished registration document (BASF) 86/0430 of BASF Corporation.

Leuschner, F., Leuschner, A., Schneider, C., Schwerdtfeger, W., and Dontenwill, W. (1977). "Oral Toxicity of Maneb in the Rhesus Monkey: Six Months Dietary Dosing." Unpublished Rep. WF 1172 of BASF Corporation.

Leuschner, F., Leuschner, A., Klie, R., Dontenwill, W., and Rogulja, P. (1979). "Chronic Oral Toxicity of Manganese-ethylene-1,2-bis-dithiocarbamate, 90%—Called for Short 'Maneb'—Sprague–Dawley (SIV) Rats (with Special Attention to Carcinogenic Properties)." Unpublished registration document (BASF) 86/0430 of BASF Corporation.

Leuschner, F., Dontenwill, W., and Hubschner, F. (1986a). "Chronic Oral Toxicity of Manganese-ethylene-1,2-bis-dithiocarbamate, 90%—Called for Short 'Maneb'—Sprague–Dawley (SIV) Rats (with Special Attention to Carcinogenic Properties). Amendment 1." Unpublished registration document (BASF) 86/0430 of BASF Corporation.

Leuschner, F., Dontenwill, W., and Hubschner, F. (1986b). "Chronic Oral Toxicity of Manganese-ethylene-1,2-bis-dithiocarbamate, 90%—Called for Short 'Maneb'—Sprague–Dawley (SIV) Rats (with Special Attention to Carcinogenic Properties). Amendment 2." Unpublished registration document (BASF) 86/0430 of BASF Corporation.

Lewerenz, H. J., and Plass, R. (1984). Contrasting effects of ethylenethiourea on hepatic monooxygenase in rats and mice. *Arch. Toxicol.* **56**, 92–95.

Longacre, S. (1986). "Summary of ETU and EBDC Analysis in Plasma, Liver, and Thyroid after Mancozeb Administration. Supplement/appendix to Nelson (1986). Rep. 31H-86-02. Unpublished Rep. 86R-1009 of Rohm and Haas Company.

Martindale, W. B. (1972). Carbimazole and other antithyroid agents. *In* "Extra Pharmacopoeia" (N. W. Blacow, ed.), 26th ed., pp. 379–385. Pharmaceutical Press, London.

Matsushita, T., Arimatsu, Y., and Nomura, S. (1976). Experimental study on contact dermatitis caused by dithiocarbamates maneb, mancozeb, zineb, and their related compounds. *Internat. Arch. Occupational Environmental Health* **37**, 169–178.

Matsushita, T., Yoshioka, M., Arimatsu, Y., and Nomura, S. (1977). Experimental study on cross-contact allergy due to dithiocarbamate fungicides. *Industrial Health* **15**, 87–94.

McClain, R. M. (1995). Phenobarbital mouse liver tumors: Implications of hepatic tumor promotion for cancer risk assessment. *In* "Growth Factors and Tumor Promotion: Implications for Risk Assessment," pp. 325–336. Wiley-Liss, New York.

Merkle, J. (1983). "Study to Determine the Prenatal Toxicity of Manganous Ethylenebis (Dithiocarbamate) in Rabbits." Study RZ-No. 83/094 from BASF AG, Ludwigshafen Rhein, Federal Republic of Germany. Unpublished report of Elf Atochem North America, Inc.

Muller, W. (1991). "Mancozeb Oral (Gavage) Teratogenicity Study in the Rabbit." Rep. HLD-853-683-002 from Hazleton Labs, Deutschland Gmbh, Munster, Germany. Unpublished report of Elf Atochem North America, Inc.

Muller, W. (1992). "Mancozeb 2-Generation Oral Reproduction Toxicity Study in the Rat." Rep. HLD-852-683-001 from Hazleton Labs, Deutschland Gmbh, Munster, Germany. Unpublished report of Elf Atochem North America, Inc.

Naas, D. J. (1989a). "Acute Oral Toxicity (LD50) Study in Albino Rats with Maneb Technical." Rep. WIL-134003 from WIL Research Laboratories, Inc., Ashland, OH. Unpublished report of Elf Atochem North America, Inc.

Naas, D. J. (1989b). "Acute Dermal Toxicity (LD50) Study in Albino Rabbits with Maneb Technical." Rep. WIL-134004 from WIL Research Laboratories, Inc., Ashland, OH. Unpublished report of Elf Atochem North America, Inc.

National Academy of Sciences, National Research Council (1989). "Diet and Health: Implications for Reducing Chronic Disease Risk." National Academy Press, Washington, DC.

National Cancer Institute (NCI) (1987). "Diet, Nutrition, and Cancer Prevention: A Guide to Food Choices." United States Government Printing Office, Washington, DC.

National Toxicology Program (NTP) (1992). "Toxicology and Carcinogenesis Studies of Ethylene Thiourea in F344/N Rats and B6C3F1 Mice (Feed Studies)." United States Department of Health and Human Services, Public Health Service, National Institutes of Health Publication 92-2843, United States National Toxicology Program Technical Rep. Ser. 388.

Nelson, S. S. (1986). "Metabolism of 14C Mancozeb in Rats." Unpublished Rep. 31H-86-02 of Rohm and Haas Company.

Nelson, S. S. (1987). "Bioconversion of Mancozeb to ETU in Rat." Unpublished Rep. 31C-87-24 of Rohm and Haas Company.

Nemec, M. D. (1992). "A Developmental Toxicity Study of Maneb Technical in Rats." Rep. WIL-134011 from WIL Research Laboratories, Inc., Ashland, OH. Unpublished report of Elf Atochem North America, Inc.

Nemec, M. D. (1993). "An Acute Neurotoxicity Study of Maneb Technical in Rats." Rep. WIL-134015 from WIL Research Laboratories, Ashland, OH. Unpublished report of Elf Atochem North America, Inc.

Odell, W. D., et al. (1967). Studies of thyrotropin physiology by means of radioassays. In "Proceedings of the 1986 Laurentian Hormone Conference" (G. Pincus, ed.), Vol. 23, pp. 47–85. Academic Press, San Diego.

O'Hara, G. P., and DiDonato, L. J. (1985). "Dithane M-45 and Ethylenethiourea: 3-Month Dietary Toxicity Study in Mice." Unpublished Rep. 80R-124 of Rohm and Haas Company.

Ollinger, J. (1999). "Dithiocarbamates (CCPR Code 105). EBDC/ETU, STMR-P for Apple Juice, EBDC IEDI Calculation." Letter to W. H. van Eck, Codex Committee on Pesticide Residues, EBDC/ETU Task Force.

O'Neil, W., and Marshall, W. (1984). Goitrogenic effects of ethylenethiourea on rat thyroid. Pesticide Biochem. Physiol. 21, 92–101.

Palmer, A., and Simons, R. (1979). "Effect of Metiram Technical on Pregnancy of the Rat." Rep. RZ 79/065, BSF 302/79616 from Huntingdon Research Centre, Huntingdon England. Unpublished report of BASF Corporation.

Parkes, H. G. (1974). Living with carcinogens. J. Inst. Rubber Industry 8, 21–23.

Peters, A. C., Kurtz, P. J., Donorrio, D. J., Thake, D. C., and Cottrill, D. L. (1980a). "Prechronic Studies of Ethylenethiourea: Acute, Repeated Dose and Subchronic in Rats." Unpublished Project G-7186 of Battelle Laboratories, Columbus, OH, for United States National Institute of Environmental Health Sciences.

Peters, A. C., Kurtz, P. J., Donorrio, D. J., Thake, D. C., and Cottrill, D. L. (1980b). "Perchronic Studies of Ethylene Thiourea: Acute, Repeated Dose and Subchronic in Mice." Unpublished Project G-7186 of Battelle Laboratories, Columbus, OH, for United States National Institute of Environmental Health Sciences.

Peters, A. C., Kurtz, P. J., Chin, A. E., Carlton, B. D., Chrisp, C. E., and Dill, G. S. (1982). "Report on the Maximum Neonatal Dose Studies with Ethylenethiourea." Unpublished Contract N01-ES-8-2151 of Battelle Laboratories, Columbus, OH, for United States National Institute of Environmental Health Sciences.

Piccirillo, V. J., Wu, D., and Speirs, G. (1992). "Metabolism of Mancozeb in the Mouse." Rep. T91-3413 from Inveresk Research International, Ltd. Tranent, Scotland. Unpublished report of Elf Atochem North America, Inc.

Puhl, J. R. (1985). "Metabolism of Radiolabelled Maneb in Rats." Rep. 6181-101 from Hazleton Laboratories, America, Inc., Madison, WI. Unpublished report of Elf Atochem North America, Inc.

Rowland, J. (1997). "Toxicity Endpoint Selection Process." Health Effects Division, United States Environmental Protection Agency Office of Pesticide Programs.

Ruddick, J. A., and Khera, K. S. (1975). Pattern of anomalies following single oral doses of ethylenethiourea to pregnant rats. Teratology 12, 277–281.

Ruddick, J. A., Williams, D. T., Hierlihy, L., and Khera, K. S. (1976a). 14C-ethylenethiourea: Distribution, excretion, and metabolism in pregnant rats. Teratology 13, 35–40.

Ruddick, J. A., Newsome, W. H., and Nash, L. (1976b). Correlation of teratogenicity and molecular structure: ethylenethiourea and related compounds. Teratology 13, 263–266.

Ruddick, J. A., Newsome, W. H., and Iverson, F. (1977). A comparison of the distribution, metabolism and excretion of ethylenethiourea in the pregnant mouse and rat. Teratology 16, 159–162.

Ryle, P. R., Bell, P. F., Parker, C., Farmer, H., Offer, J. M., Anderson, A., and Dawe, I. S. (1991). "A Study of the Effect of Maneb (Technical) on Reproductive Function of Two Generations in the Rat." Rep. MNB1/9072 from Huntington Research Centre Ltd., Cambridgeshire, England. Unpublished report of Elf Atochem North America, Inc.

Saillenfait, A. M., Sabate, J. P., Langonne, I., and De Ceaurriz, J. (1991). Difference in the developmental toxicity of ethylenethiourea and three N,N'-substituted thiourea derivatives in rats. Fundamental Appl. Toxicol. 17, 399–408.

Salisbury, S. A., and Lybarger, J. (1977). "Ethylene Thiourea." Health Hazard Evaluation Determination Rep. 77-67-499 from St. Clair Rubber Company, Marysville, MI, United States Department of Health, Education and Welfare.

Schaller, R. T., and Stevenson, J. K. (1966). Development of carcinoma of the thyroid in iodine-deficient mice. Cancer 19, 1063–1080.

Schmid, H., Tennekes, H., Janiak, T., Probst, D., Luetkemeier, H., Pappritz, G., Märki, U., Vogel, O., and Heusner, W. (1992). "Ethylene Thiourea 104 Week Chronic Toxicity (Feeding) Study in Rats." Project 256803 from Research and Consulting Company, Ltd., Itingen, Switzerland. Unpublished report of ETU Task Force.

Shaw, D. (1990). "Mancozeb: 52-Week Oral (Dietary) Study in the Beagle." Project HLA 5913-616/3 from Hazleton Laboratories, UK. Unpublished report of Rohm and Haas Company.

Shellenberger, T. (1991). "Mancozeb: 18-Month Oncogenicity Study in Mice." Project 85051 from Tegeris Labs, Inc., Temple Hills, MD. Unpublished report of Rohm and Haas Company.

Smith, D. (1976). Ethylene thiourea—A study of possible teratogenicity and thyroid carcinogenicity. J. Soc. Occupational Med. 26, 92–94.

Smith, D. (1984). Ethylene thiourea: Thyroid function in two groups of exposed workers. British J. Industrial Med. 41, 362–366.

Solomon, H., and Holz, J. (1987). "Mancozeb: Range-Finding Developmental Study in Rats." Unpublished Rep. 85R-244 from Rohm and Haas Company.

Solomon, H. M., and Lutz, M. F. (1987). "Mancozeb: Oral (Gavage) Developmental Toxicity Study in Rabbits." Unpublished Rep. 86R-021 from Rohm and Haas Company.

Solomon, H. M., Lutz, M. F., and Kulwich, B. A. (1988). "Mancozeb: 2-Generation Reproduction Study in Rats." Unpublished Rep. 87R-020 from Rohm and Haas Company.

Sortwell, R., Heywood, R., Allen, D., Prentice, D., and Cherry, C. (1977). "Metiram Preliminary Oral Toxicity Study in Rhesus Monkeys. Repeated Dosage for 4 Weeks." Rep. BASF 77/0149, BSF 265/77264 from Huntingdon Research Centre, Huntingdon, UK. Unpublished report of BASF Corporation.

Sortwell, R., Allen, D., Heywood, R., and Street, A. (1979). "Metiram (Containing 2.2% Ethylenethiourea) Oral Toxicity Study in Rhesus Monkeys (Repeated Dosage for 26 Weeks with Recovery Period)." Rep. BASF 79/0082, BSF 267/78263 from Huntingdon Research Centre, Huntingdon, UK. Unpublished report of BASF Corporation.

Stadler, J. (1990). "Combined Chronic Toxicity/Oncogenicity 2-Year Feeding Study with Mancozeb in Rats." Unpublished Rep. 259-89 of DuPont Haskell Laboratory.

Stadler, J. (1991). "Neuropathology Study in Rats with Mancozeb." Unpublished Rep. 217-89 of DuPont Haskell Laboratory.

Steinmetz, K. A., and Potter, J. D. (1991). Vegetables, fruit, and cancer. I. Epidemiology. Cancer Causes Control 2, 325–357.

Takayama, S., Aihara, K., Onodera, T., and Akimoto, T. (1986). Antithyroid effects of propylthiouracil and sulfamonomethoxine in rats and monkeys. Toxicol. Appl. Pharmacol. 82, 191–199.

Teramoto, S., Shingu, A., Kaneda, M., and Saito, R. (1978). Teratogenicity studies with ethylenethiourea in rats, mice and hamsters. Congenital Anomalies 18, 11–17.

Terrill, J. B. (1990). "Acute Inhalation Toxicity Study with Maneb in the Rat." Rep. HLA 2567-100 from Hazleton Laboratory, Vienna, VA. Unpublished report of Elf Atochem North America, Inc.

Terrill, J. B. (1991). "A Four-Week Study in the Rat to Determine the Lung Tissue Residue and Effect upon the Thyroid Function with Maneb." Rep. HLA 2567-101 from Hazleton Laboratory, Vienna, VA. Unpublished report of Elf Atochem North America, Inc.

Tesh, J. M., McAnulty, P. A., Willoughby, C. R., Enticott, J., Wilby, O. K., and Tesh, S. A. (1988). "Mancozeb: Teratology Study in the Rat." Rep. 87/PTC 007/365 from Life Science Research Ltd., Suffolk, UK. Unpublished report of Elf Atochem North America, Inc.

Teshima, R., Nagamatsu, K., Kido, Y., and Terao, T. (1981). Absorption, distribution, excretion and metabolism of ethylenethiourea in guinea pigs. *Eisei Kagaku* **27**, 85–90.

Thomas, G. A., and Williams, E. D. (1991). Evidence for and possible mechanisms of non-genotoxic carcinogenesis in the rodent thyroid. *Mutation Res.* **248**, 357–370.

Tomlinson, H. L., and Longacre, S. L. (1988). "Mancozeb Dermal Absorption Study in Male Rats." Unpublished Rep. 88R-218 of Rohm and Haas Company.

Tompkins, C. E. (1992). "An 18-Month Dietary Oncogenicity Study in Mice with Maneb Technical." Rep. WIL-134008 from WIL Research Laboratories, Inc., Ashland, OH. Unpublished report of Elf Atochem North America, Inc.

Trutter, J. A. (1988a). "Subchronic Toxicity Study with Maneb Technical in the Rat." Rep. HLA 153-140 from Hazleton Laboratories, Vienna, VA. Unpublished report of Elf Atochem North America, Inc.

Trutter, J. A. (1988b). "A 21-Day Dermal Toxicity Study in Rabbits with Maneb Technical." Rep. HLA 153-139 from Hazleton Laboratories, Vienna, VA. Unpublished report of Elf Atochem North America, Inc.

Trutter, J. A. (1988c). "Mancozeb: 4-Week Repeat Dermal Toxicity Study in Rats." Rep. HLA 417-432 from Hazleton Laboratories, Vienna, VA. Unpublished report of Rohm and Haas Company.

Ulland, B. M., Weisburger, J. H., Weisburger, E. K., Rice, J. M., and Cypher, R. (1972). Thyroid cancer in rats from ethylenethiourea intake. *J. Nat. Cancer Inst.* **49**, 583–584.

Ullman, L., Sacher, R., Porricello, T., Luetkemeier, H., Vogel, W., Vogel, O., Wilson, J., and Terrier, H. (1987). "Report on the Subacute 21-Day Repeated Dose Dermal Toxicity Study with Polyram DF in Rabbits. Rep. BASF 87/0260, ZNT 86/314 from Research and Consulting Company AG, Ltd., Itingen, Switzerland. Unpublished report of BASF Corporation.

Ulrich, C. E. (1986a). "Thirteen-Week Subchronic Inhalation Toxicity Study on Maneb in Rats (Final Report)." Rep. 550-001 from International Research and Development Corporation, Mattawan, MI. Unpublished report of Elf Atochem North America, Inc.

Ulrich, C. E. (1986b). "Report on the Thirteen Week Subchronic Inhalation Toxicity Study on Metiram in Rats." Rep. RZ 86/407 and Addendum BASF 87/0414 from International Research and Development Corporation, Mattawan, MI. Unpublished report of BASF Company.

Ulrich, C. E. (1987). "Thirteen-Week Subchronic Inhalation Toxicity Study on Maneb in Rats (Addendum to Final Report Covering Recovery Phase)." Rep. 550-001 from International Research and Development Corporation, Mattawan, MI. Unpublished report of Elf Atochem North America, Inc.

Watts, M. H., and Chan, P. K. (1984a). "Dithane M-45: Acute Oral Toxicity Study in Rats." Unpublished Rep. 83R-218 from Rohm and Haas Company.

Watts, M. H., and Chan, P. K. (1984b). "Dithane M-45: Acute Oral Toxicity Study in Rats and Mice." Unpublished Rep. 83R-213A and B from Rohm and Haas Company.

Whysner, J., Ross, P. M., and Williams, G. M. (1996). Phenobarbital mechanistic data and risk assessment: enzyme induction, enhanced cellular proliferation, and tumor promotion. *J. Pharmacol. Therapeutics* **71**, 153–191.

World Health Organization (1994). "The WHO Recommended Classification of Pesticides by Hazard and Guidelines to Classification, 1994–1995." International Program on Chemical Safety, WHO/PCS/94.2.

A Toxicological Assessment
of Sulfur as a Pesticide*

Derek W. Gammon, Thomas B. Moore, and Michael A. O'Malley

Department of Pesticide Regulation, California EPA

82.1 INTRODUCTION

82.1.1 USAGE

Elemental sulfur is the most heavily used crop protection chemical in California (Table 82.1) as well as in the United States. In 1993–1995, for example, annual usage was about 70 million pounds active ingredient (a.i.) in California, which is about one-third of the total weight of pesticides used in agriculture. It is generally applied to crops as a dust to combat fungal disease, at rates of approximately 10 to 30 lbs. per application per acre, as well as being used for postharvest disease control. The range of fungal diseases controlled by sulfur includes brown rot, scab, mildew, powdery mildew, leafspot, and rusts (Farm Chemicals Handbook, 1998). It is also used, to a lesser extent, for the control of mites and insects (fleahoppers) which may be secondary to fungal damage of the plant. Multiple applications are often needed for crops which are particularly susceptible to fungal attack. The main crops on which sulfur is used in California (1995) are grapes (71%), tomatoes (12%), and sugarbeet (8%). It has become an important component of IPM systems since it can be used in "organic" farming.

82.1.2 ENVIRONMENTAL FATE

As a natural substance, environmental fate requirements for sulfur in the United States have been waived by U.S. EPA. In a variety of literature reports, sulfur has been shown to be oxidized, in the presence of water and soil, to the sulfite and then the sulfate, i.e., sulfuric acid. The supplementation of fertilizers with sulfur has been used intentionally to acidify soils which are too alkaline for a particular crop. Conversely, the use of sul-

fur as a fungicide can make the soil too acidic for the continued optimal growth of a particular crop. For example, in Southern Tanzania, sulfur dust was used to control powdery mildew on cashew nut trees. After 4 years, the topsoil pH was reduced by 0.7 units, to below pH 5.5, the ideal pH for cashew nut tree yield (Majule *et al.*, 1997). However, in the case of a 3-year field study on highbush blueberry bushes in mineral soil, sulfur amendment increased both early growth and blueberry yield. It was concluded that the effects of sulfur were probably mediated by a decrease in soil pH with corresponding increases in Mn and Fe levels (Haynes and Swift, 1986). It was also found, in a lysimeter study, that increasing the sulfur content of soil led to a rise in sulfur content of plants, such as corn, wheat, barley, sunflower, and mustard (Gador and Motowicka-Terelak, 1986).

Sulfur is, of course, a natural constituent of plants, as it is of all organisms. In addition to elemental sulfur which may be present from pesticidal exposure, sulfur is commonly found as sulfates and in the amino acids cysteine, methionine, and glutathione. Agricultural practice may introduce elevated sulfur levels into arable land inadvertently by, for example, the use of (animal-derived) manure or other fertilizers as well as from the use of pesticides. By far the greatest contribution in the latter case is likely to be from elemental sulfur used as a fungicide. As described below, there are an increasing number of instances of dermatitis in farm workers and, in many ways more serious, an elevated number of cases of disease in ruminants caused by exposure to high levels of sulfur, and several case reports are given.

Another source of soil acidity caused by sulfur is from industrial pollution. Typically from the burning of coal or oil, sulfur dioxide or hydrogen sulfide can be liberated into the atmosphere. This gaseous sulfur can return to earth following rainfall, producing the so-called "acid rain" phenomenon since sulfuric acid can readily be produced from soil oxidation of sulfur.

---

*The opinions expressed in this chapter represent the views of the authors and do not necessarily reflect the views and policies of the Department of Pesticide Regulation.

Table 82.1
Usage of Elemental Sulfur (a.i.) in California, 1993–1995[a,b]

CROP	1995 in thousands lbs.	acres[d]	1994[c] in thousands lbs.	acres[d]	1993 in thousands lbs.	acres[d]
Alfalfa	294	13.2	227	10.7	139	6.4
Almonds	184	42.4	126	26	48.4	11.0
Bermudagrass	162	5.9	31.2	1.26	62.6	2.2
Cantaloupe	634	31.3	357	17.9	363	20.9
Carrots	177	10.8	347	15.2	454	17.9
Cotton	460	17.3	240	10.9	319	13.3
Date	741	11.3	655	10.9	838	14.1
Grapes, table	26,200	2970	24,900	2660	25,600	2630
Grapes, wine	23,200	2460	23,500	2340	25,700	2450
Lemons	193	4.8	190	5.8	168	5.3
Melons	133	5.8	282	11.8	349	17.0
Nectarines	277	35.3	240	31.0	198	25.5
Peaches	873	83.3	644	69.8	588	66.1
Pears	170	13.6	169	12.9	197	16.2
Peas	204	10.1	305	14.5	281	14.6
Pistachio	500	39.4	592	30.7	846	33.9
Plums	259	25.0	262	23.7	267	26.9
Prunes	224	23.0	135	13.8	157	17.4
Strawberry	238	64.7	262	61.9	256	63.9
Sugarbeet	5300	171	6760	210	6870	218
Tomatoes, fresh	1270	62.8	1620	76.9	1380	70.7
Tomatoes, processing	7250	292	7810	290	7700	219
TOTAL (lbs.)	69.8 million		70.5 million		73.5 million	

[a] DPR, 1995, 1996a, 1996b.
[b] All crops which received more than 100,000 lbs. a.i. in 1995 are included.
[c] 132,000 lbs. of sulfur were applied to 8600 acres of oranges in 1994.
[d] Acres treated include multiple applications to the same land.

82.2 TOXICOLOGY PROFILE OF ELEMENTAL SULFUR

Acute toxicity categories for products containing elemental sulfur were assigned according to FIFRA Pesticide Assessment Guidelines, Subdivision F, Hazard Evaluation: Human and Domestic Animals, Revised Ed., Nov., 1984. The results are summarized in Table 82.2.

82.2.1 ACUTE EXPOSURE ORAL TOXICITY: 81-1

A single-dose limit test was conducted using the rat (five/sex), dosed by gavage at 5000 mg/kg. Lower doses are only required if there is >20% mortality per sex. Seventeen of 20 formulations had a LD_{50} > 5000 mg/kg (Category IV); 3 were between 500 and 5000 mg/kg (Category III).

82.2.2 ACUTE EXPOSURE DERMAL TOXICITY: 81-2

A single-dose limit test was conducted using the rabbit (five/sex), dosed on the skin at 2000 or 5000 mg/kg. Lower doses are only required if there is >20% mortality per sex. There were no compound-related, acute mortalities for any of these formulations at the tested doses of 2000 or 5000 mg/kg. This suggests that it may be more appropriate to consider them all in Category IV rather than III.

82.2.3 ACUTE EXPOSURE INHALATION TOXICITY: 81-3

A single-dose limit test was conducted using the rat (five/sex), dosed by inhalation at 2 mg/l for 4 hours. Lower doses are only required if there is >20% mortality per sex. Fourteen of 17 for-

Table 82.2
Acute Toxicity of Sulfur Formulations used in California

Sulfur product	Oral[a]	Dermal[b]	Inhal.[c]	Eye irrit.[d]	Dermal irrit.[e]	Dermal sensit.[f]
Special Electric Refined Super Adhesive Dusting (98% A.I.)	IV	III	—	III	IV	—
Manufacturing Use (98%)	IV	III	IV	III	IV	—
Spray Sulfur (98%)	IV	III	IV	III	IV	—
Valor Brands products dusting Sulfur (98%)	IV	III	IV	III	IV	0
90% Sulfur WP (90%)	IV	III	IV	III	IV	0
Bensul 85 (85%)	IV	III	IV	III	IV	0
Clean Crop Apple & peach Koloform Fungicide (84%)	IV	III	IV	III	IV	0
LX 112-2 (53%)	IV	III	IV	III	IV	—
Sulfur 6L (51%)	IV	III	IV	III	IV	0
Happy Jack Sarcoptic Mange Medicine (28%)	IV	III	—	III	III	—
Safer Garden Fungicide Concentrate (12%)	IV	III	IV	III	IV	0
Formula 242 (0.4%)	IV	—	—	IV	IV	—
XF-97097 (96.75%), with myclobutanil, 0.5%	IV	IV	IV	III	IV	—
BT 320 Sulfur 50 (50%), with BT, 0.064%	IV	III	IV	III	IV	0
Britz BT50 & Sulfur Dust (50%) BT, 0.064%	IV	III	IV	III	IV	—
Cook/Sevin Plus Multi-purpose Garden Dust (30%) with carbaryl 5%, PBO 0.45%, permethrin 0.03%	III	III	III	IV	IV	—
Britz Botran 6-25 Dust (25%) with dichloran, 6%	IV	III	IV	III	IV	—
Britz Copper Sulfur Dust (25%) 15–25 with Cu, 15%	IV	III	IV	II	IV	—
Copper/Sulfur Flowable (15.5%) with Cu Sulfate, 27.5%	III	III	III	II	IV	—
Kocide 404S (15%) with Cu hydroxide, 26%	III	III	III	I	IV	—

[a]Category IV: $LD_{50} > 5000$ mg/kg; Category III: $LD_{50} = 500$–5000 mg/kg.
[b]Category IV: $LD_{50} > 5000$ mg/kg; Category III: $LD_{50} = 2000$–5000 mg/kg.
[c]Category IV: $LC_{50} > 2$ mg/l; Category III: $LC_{50} > 0.5$–2 mg/l.
[d]Category IV: minimal effects, clearing in <24 hours; Category III: corneal involvement or irritation, clearing in ≤7 days; Category II: corneal involvement or irritation, clearing in 8–21 days; Category I: corrosive (irreversible ocular damage) or corneal involvement or irritation, clearing in >21 days.
[e]Category IV: mild or slight irritation (no irritation or slight erythema); Category III: moderate irritation at 72 hours (moderate erythema).
[f]Buehler test: score of 0 (no erythema) to 3 (severe erythema, with or without edema).

mulations had a $LC_{50} > 2$ mg/l (Category V); 3 were between 0.5 and 2 mg/l (Category III).

82.2.4 PRIMARY EYE IRRITATION: 81-4

A single-dose limit test was conducted using the rabbit (six of either sex), dosed in one eye at 0.1 ml/animal (or 100 mg for a solid). The other eye served as the untreated con-trol and responses were graded (Table 82.2). Two of 20 for-mulations showed minimal effects, clearing within 24 hours (Category IV); 15 showed corneal involvement or irritation, clearing in ≤7 days (Category III); 2 showed corneal involve-ment or irritation, clearing in 8–21 days (Category II); one showed corrosive (irreversible ocular damage) or corneal in-volvement or irritation, clearing in >21 days (Category I), probably as a result of the copper hydroxide in this formula-tion.

82.2.5 PRIMARY DERMAL IRRITATION: 81-5

A single-dose limit test was conducted using the rabbit (six of either sex), dosed at 0.5 ml/inch^2 (or 0.5 g/inch^2) for 4 h. The responses were graded. Nineteen of 20 formulations caused mild or slight irritation (Category IV); 1 showed moderate irritation at 72 h (Category III).

82.2.6 PRIMARY DERMAL SENSITIZATION: 81-6

Using the Buehler test, induction doses were applied to clipped skin at 0.4 mL or 500 mg/guinea pig (*ca.* 1 to 2 g/kg) three times, on a weekly basis, followed two weeks later by a challenge dose, to a naive site. Dermal sensitization was measured, as erythema with or without edema, in response to the challenge dose, at 24 and 48 h, on a scale of 0 to 3. All of the (seven) formulations tested scored zero, i.e., were negative.

82.3 TOXICOLOGY OF SULFUR DIOXIDE

Sulfur dioxide (SO_2) is used as a fumigant because of its antimicrobial properties. It is a colorless gas with a high water solubility. In solution, it hydrates to sulfurous acid (H_2SO_3) which dissociates in turn to form bisulfite (HSO_3^-) and sulfite (SO_3^{2-}) ions. The bisulfite ion is quite reactive by means of ionic and free radical mechanisms (Shapiro, 1977). Sulfur dioxide is used in California for the treatment of grapes held in cold storage to control the fungus *Botrytis cinerea*. The recommended treatment rate is up to a 1% gas concentration for up to 20 treatments with 7 to 10 day intervals between treatments depending on the variety of grape. The main crop uses of SO_2 in California are summarized in Table 82.3.

Sulfur dioxide is used in the United States as a food additive under the authority of the Food and Drug Administration in beer, wine, fruits and vegetables, fruit juices, syrups, meats, and fish. It acts as a preservative in these foods by being both an antimicrobial and an inhibitor of the enzymes which contribute to the discoloration process. Sulfur dioxide has been used in wine

Table 82.3
Usage of Sulfur Dioxide (a.i.) in California, 1993–1995[a]

CROP	1995 (lbs.)	1994 (lbs.)	1993 (lbs.)
Grapes, table	144,000	267,000	194,000
Grapes, wine	24,000	1100	12,000
Commodity fumigation	14,000	11,700	48,100
Other fumigation	4000	5500	6000
Structural pests	13,400	—	15,100
TOTAL (lbs.)	200,000	285,000	276,000

[a]DPR, 1995, 1996a, 1996b.

making to selectively inhibit the growth of acetic acid and lactic acid producing bacteria.

Product registrations for sulfur dioxide in California are for the 100% compressed gas. Precautionary labeling for these products require the signal word "Danger" with the wording "inhalation may be fatal or cause serious illness. Prolonged or repeated exposure may cause impaired lung function.... Liquid or excessive vapor exposure can cause serious skin and eye injury. Harmful if swallowed." When sulfur dioxide is used as a fumigant, respiratory protection is required unless the ambient concentration is less than 2 ppm, which is the threshold limit value for occupational exposure.

Case studies of cats and dogs fed fresh pet food preserved with sulfur dioxide resulted in examples of animals suffering from thiamine deficiency (Studdert and Labuc, 1991). These animals demonstrated a syndrome of depression, pupillary dilation, and ataxia which occasionally progressed to seizures and sudden death caused by acute cardiac failure. In the preserved food samples in which the SO_2 content was greater than 800 mg/kg, the thiamine levels were decidedly reduced. In the presence of sulfiting agents such as sulfur dioxide, thiamine is cleaved into its constituent pyrimidine and thiazole moieties, rendering it inactive. It should be noted that the principal toxic effect of elemental sulfur on the CNS of ruminants is a direct effect of sulfur and not a secondary effect arising from thiamine deficiency.

Other investigators examined pigs fed barley with high moisture content which had been treated with sulfur dioxide (Gibson *et al.*, 1987). Treatment of the barley (1% sulfur dioxide (wt/wt)) demonstrated an enhanced preservation of the barley with a significant time delay before mold growth became evident. However, the thiamine content in the barley was greatly reduced, resulting in a thiamine content in the meat of the treated pigs which was 7.6% that of the control animals. These animals gave evidence of cardiac hypertrophy along with reduced feed intake and body weight gain. Once again, it is possible that direct effects of SO_2 contributed to the toxicity of the barley to the pigs, rather than these being purely secondary consequences of thiamine deficiency. The World Health Organization specifically recommends that foods which are significant sources of thiamine in the human diet should not be treated with sulfur dioxide or other sulfiting agents.

Pollution of the environment has been a major health concern as a consequence of excessive exposures to sulfur dioxide and smoke, for example in the Meuse Valley of Belgium in 1936, in Donora, Pennsylvania in 1948, and in London in 1952. In London where 4000 deaths and numerous incidences of illness were attributed to the exposure, atmospheric sulfur dioxide levels achieved a daily average as high as 1.34 ppm. Pulmonary effects manifested by exposure to sulfur dioxide are attributable to its irritancy. Exposure to sulfur dioxide alone results in direct effects on the nasopharynges and trachea with reduced transport of the mucous layer either due to cessation of ciliary movement in an acute exposure or to an excessive thickening of the mucous as a consequence of chronic exposure. The acute pulmonary response is typical of a irritant effect with bronchial restriction resulting in increased flow resistance. The chronic effect is similar to that of chronic bronchitis without the involvement of a bacterial infection. These effects have been well reviewed by Costa and Amdur (1996).

82.4 VETERINARY EFFECTS OF SULFUR

Probably the major health concern of sulfur for ruminants is the association between excessive sulfur ingestion and polioencephalomalacia (PEM), also known as cerebrocortical necrosis. This was first recognized as a disease in sheep and cattle over 40 years ago (Jensen *et al.*, 1956; Terlecki and Markson, 1961). It involves a softening of the gray matter of the brain and is a major disease worldwide (Olkowski, 1997). Clinical signs can occur from a few hours to several weeks after exposure to excessive sulfur. Signs usually include, initially, mild excitation and restlessness accompanied by loss of appetite. Affected animals avoid light and signs may progress to headpressing, rigidity, blindness, violent convulsions, coma, and death. Young animals are particularly badly affected. Removal of affected animals from the source of sulfur generally reduces the severity of clinical signs.

In the past, the causes of PEM have been ascribed to a variety of agents, including a lack of vitamin B_1 (thiamine) and, more recently, to an excess of dietary sulfur. It has been suggested that the increase in reported cases of PEM over recent years is a result of industrial pollution. However, with the movement away from coal to oil and natural gas, this seems unlikely. For example, according to Beauchamp *et al.* (1984), the ratio of H_2S content of coal, oil, and natural gas, per unit weight of fuel burned, is approximately 35:8:1. Assuming that H_2S liberation is a reasonable marker for possible industrial sulfur exposure, this suggests a reduction, rather than an increase, in environmental exposure to sulfur from industrial sources over the years.

Several reports have described PEM arising from feeding sheep and/or cattle on elevated levels of sulfur in the diet (Hill and Ebbett, 1997; Jeffrey *et al.*, 1994; Low *et al.*, 1996), in drinking water (Hamlen *et al.*, 1993), as well as a case of sheep being allowed to forage on a field of alfalfa which had been treated with elemental sulfur (Bulgin *et al.*, 1996). Reports of field cases have been duplicated in laboratory studies implicating excessive sulfur ingestion as the cause of PEM (e.g., Gould *et al.*, 1991; McAllister *et al.*, 1992; Sager *et al.*, 1990).

PEM was identified in several sheep and cattle farms in England (Jeffrey *et al.*, 1994). It was associated with the use of ammonium sulfate as a feed additive, in place of ammonium bicarbonate, as the usual urinary acidifier. After this was discontinued, there were no further cases of PEM. Necropsy of six calves and two lambs from five of these farms showed lesions in the thalamus and striatum, of great severity, unlike in cases of thiamine deficiency. No lesions were found in PEM-affected animals in the cerebellum, hippocampus, or superior colliculi. Symptoms were similar to those already described and there were deaths on three out of five farms.

On a cattle farm in New Zealand, PEM was diagnosed following gross and histopathological examination of the brain of deceased animals (Hill and Ebbett, 1997). The cattle had been feeding for two months on hay plus a rationed amount of kale (*Brassica oleacea*) when they were transferred to a field of kale. Within two days, neurological signs were observed which were typical of PEM. Twenty-six of 99 heifers (26%) were symptomatic of which 12 died (12%) and 14 recovered (14%) after removal of the cattle from this field. Chemical analysis of the kale revealed that it contained 8500 mg/kg of sulfur (0.85%, DM, dry matter), which is double the maximum range of recommended dietary needs of cattle for sulfur (0.4%, DM).

Examples of sulfur-induced PEM in sheep include an outbreak on a sheep farm in Scotland, after changing from grazing to a ration of pellets containing 0.43% DM sulfur (Low *et al.*, 1996). Clinical signs appeared 15 to 32 days after changing to the artificial diet, and the incidences were 16 of 46 (35%) for Swaledale lambs and 5 of 25 (20%) for Scottish blackface lambs. Clinical signs, which were quite unlike those of vitamin B_1 deficiency, included depression, blindness, head-pressing, nystagmus, and dorsiflexion of the neck or opisthotonus. In some animals, the severity was such that the sheep either died or were killed *in extremis* (4/16 Swaledale; 4/5 Scottish blackface). Histopathological examination of the lambs revealed evidence of PEM in the majority of the animals. The mean intake of pellets during the study period was 880 g/head/day (Swaledale) and 760 g/head/day (Scottish blackface). Because the lambs had an initial average body weight of 20 kg, this intake converts to a food intake of approximately 40 g/kg/day and a sulfur ingestion of approximately 170 mg/kg/day. Administration of vitamin B_1 (by injection) did not reverse the clinical signs, but there were no new cases evident after vitamin B_1 was given combined with removal of the lambs from the high sulfur diet.

An outbreak of PEM was also reported in cattle which had been drinking water containing a high concentration of sodium sulfate, 7200 ppm *vs* a recommended optimal level of 1000 ppm, in Canada (Hamlen *et al.*, 1993). The incidence was 11/110 (10%) and mortality of affected cattle was 4/11 (36%). Clinical signs, which first appeared three days after exposure to the well, and histopathology ($n = 3$), were the same as those reported above, with the additional findings of extensive thrombosis and vascular necrosis in midbrain and thalamus. The blood clinical chemistry for affected animals appeared to be normal from the standpoint of copper and vitamin B_1 levels and transketolase activity (a thiamine-dependent enzyme). The PEM dissipated and no new cases arose after the cattle were moved to a water supply with acceptable levels of sulfur. Unusually, old rather than young animals were affected, but this could have resulted from low exposure to sulfur in calves which were nursing. The level of magnesium in the affected well was also high, 1050 *vs* 200 ppm, recommended.

Another example of sulfur toxicity to livestock is a report (Bulgin *et al.*, 1996) of a flock of sheep grazing on a field of alfalfa stubble which had been sprayed 14 to 16 hours previously with an aqueous suspension of 35% elemental sulfur at

53 lbs./acre, active ingredient.[1] Within two to four hours the sheep became uncoordinated with 91% prostration, despite the sheep being moved to uncontaminated pasture after 2 h, when the problem became apparent. There was 10% (220 out of 2200) mortality after a week, the majority of these sheep (206) dying of acute effects, within 24 hours. Surviving ewes were considered fully recovered at 90 days. Necropsy of sheep which died between 2 and 48 h after the onset of clinical signs revealed a rumen pH of 6.0 to 6.5, a strong smell of rotten eggs (H_2S), but no digestive tract lesions. Necropsy of sheep dying between 5 and 30 days showed PEM, consisting of yellow/tan areas of the cerebral cortex caused by neuronal degeneration and cavitation of cortical grey matter. It should be noted that alfalfa normally is moderately rich in sulfur, having a content of ca. 0.4% DM (Olkowski, 1997), without added extraneous sulfur.

Attempts have been made to study the toxicity of sulfur in laboratory experiments. The appearance of clinical signs of PEM in calves fed on a high sulfate diet coincided with or immediately followed the first odor of H_2S in rumen gas (Sager et al., 1990). PEM was not correlated with copper or thiamine deficiency. These findings were extended by Gould et al. (1991), who fed a high sodium sulfate diet to calves and noted that H_2S accumulation in the stomach was significantly higher in animals with signs of PEM than in asymptomatic calves. Microbes in the rumen readily reduce sulfate to sulfide. The findings were extended to sheep by McAllister et al. (1992). Ten lambs were dosed with sodium hydrogen sulfide (0.94 M) every 20 min, administered directly into the esophagus. Clinical signs of PEM developed within 45 min of first dosing, in all lambs, and PEM was identified in 4/9 brains examined histologically. All (4) animals had visual impairment including blindness, dying at 20 to 96 h. Two lambs had visual impairment without PEM but both died within 90 min of pulmonary congestion and edema (as seen with acute H_2S toxicity in the rat), probably before brain lesions had time to develop.

82.5 HUMAN HEALTH EFFECTS OF SULFUR

There are many cases of dermatitis associated with the agricultural use of elemental sulfur. For example, in California between 1974 and 1985, there were 677 cases reported, more than for any other pesticide (Table 82.4). This would seem to suggest that sulfur is a potent skin irritant in humans. Isolated cases have also been reported in applicators and field workers in Washington State. However, standard (epicutaneous) skin irritation tests in laboratory animals for most agricultural formulations have not shown irritation (Matsushita et al., 1977; Table 82.2). In nonstandard tests though, using subcutaneous injection in the Wistar rat, a 25% aqueous solution of wettable powder or a 22% solution of lime sulfur caused a four

Table 82.4

Summary of Cases of Possible, Probable and Definite Illness Reported to the California Pesticide Illness Registry Involving Exposure to Sulfur as a Primary Pesticide Between 1982 and 1995

Activity	Eye	Eye + other	Skin	Skin + other	Respiratory/ systemic	Total
Clean/fixing pesticide equipment	2		2			3
Handling concentrate	10	1	2	1	2	14
Drift	50	37	11	7	87	148
Emergency response	0	7		4	5	9
Flagger	1		1			2
Handlers	58	10	55	15	34	155
Manufacturing/ formulating	0		1		1	1
Other	19	8	6	6	10	41
Packing/ processing	0		1		1	2
Field residue	81	52	425	51	61	603
Total	221	115	503	85	201	978

(Type of illness spans Eye, Eye + other, Skin, Skin + other, Respiratory/systemic)

or five irritant reaction.[2] Using a similar maximization test with the guinea pig, a 1% or 5% aqueous solution of elemental or lime sulfur was a moderately strong allergen (Matsushita et al., 1977). Limited case reports also implicate elemental sulfur as a human contact allergen. Schneider (1978) reported two cases of contact allergy in patients who used medications containing elemental sulfur to treat superficial fungal dermatoses. Both patients had positive patch test reactions to 5% elemental sulphur in various vehicles. A control series was not reported.

Wilkinson (1975) reported the case of a professional gardener with a previous history of atopic eczema who developed an eczematous eruption involving the elbow flexures and the right hand. He had a positive patch test reaction to 5% sulfur in petrolatum, but a control series was not reported. Gregorczyk and Swieboda (1968) described 15 cases of desquamative dermatitis among 425 Polish sulfur miners in which irritant dermatitis due to elemental sulfur may have played a part. Several instances of apparent allergic reaction to 1% elemental sulfur were also observed in a recent study of California nursery workers (O'Malley and Rodriguez, 1998).

Allergic contact dermatitis was identified in a hospital investigation of patients suffering from eczematous dermatitis (Vena et al., 1994). Patients were subjected to patch tests with (sodium or potassium) metabisulfite ($S_2O_5^{2-}$), bisulfite

---

[1]The restricted entry interval for field workers following sulfur use is 24 hours, i.e., appropriate personal protective equipment must be worn to enter a treated field within 24 h of a sulfur application.

[2]1 = no reaction; 2 = slight hyperemia; 3 = hyperemia; 4 = marked hyperemia and edema; 5 = necrosis.

(HSO_3^-), or sulfite (SO_3^{2-}). Fifty cases of allergic reaction out of 2894 patients of either sex (1.7%) were reported after exposure to metabisulfite, with 100% cross-reactivity between the sodium and potassium salts and with the bisulfite. Only 2 (4%) of these gave a positive reaction to sulfite. Because metabisulfite is readily converted to bisulfite under aqueous conditions, it is not surprising that they showed cross-reactivity. However, because of the low cross-reactivity toward sulfite, it appears unlikely that sulfite is the ultimate allergen, *in vivo*, although it is readily formed from the metabisulfite or bisulfite under acidic conditions. It remains possible that some cases of dermatitis resulting from elemental sulfur are due to the subsequent conversion to one of these derivatives.

A case history of human Sulfur Spring dermatitis from dermal exposure was reported from Taiwan (Sun and Sue, 1995). Over a 10-year period, 44 cases of dermatitis were recorded in visitors to a particular hot springs resort. Two springs were considered, a green sulfur spring (GSS) and a white sulfur one (WSS), and it transpired that all the dermatitis cases had visited the GSS. Of these 44 cases, 32 (70%) had visited the GSS only once, for 10 to 20 min; 25 (57%) had also visited WSS, without signs of dermatitis; and 24 (55%) had a history of skin diseases prior to visiting the GSS. The chemical and physical properties of the GSS and WSS springs were compared with tap water and microbial infection was ruled out as a cause, since no cultures could be grown from water or affected skin. The principal causes of the dermatitis were considered, by the authors, to be soluble sulfur, which was present at 600, 100, and 80 ppm, in the three water sources, respectively; acid irritation, since pH was 1–2, 4, and 7, respectively, was considered a probable contributory factor. It was also noted that there was a large variation in chloride levels, 3000, 20, and 20 ppm. Other factors which could have contributed to the dermatitis in this hot spring were high temperature (100, 50, and 20°C, respectively) and ammonia nitrogen (200, 0.2, and 0.0, respectively). These disparate pieces of information suggest that active irritants (e.g., sulfuric acid or hydrogen sulfide) or allergens (e.g., sulfites or hydrogen sulfide) may be produced by oxidation or reduction of sulfur. Thus, sulfur may be the precursor of dermal irritants and allergens rather than being one *per se*.

82.5.1 OCCUPATIONAL EXPOSURE

For the years between 1982 and 1995, the California illness registry contained 1698 reports of definite, probable, and possible illnesses involving sulfur, including 978 cases (58%) for which sulfur was identified as the primary cause of the reported illness. To evaluate the typical effects of direct exposure to sulfur, the 155 cases involving handlers (mixers, loaders, and applicators cases) are discussed in more detail below. These cases constitute 16% of the cases for which sulfur was identified as the primary cause of the reported illness.

Reactions to elemental sulfur can be broken down by illness type.

82.5.1.1 Eye

Ocular symptoms were present in 68 (44%) of the handler cases, including 58 cases of isolated ocular symptoms, 8 cases of eye and skin symptoms, and 2 cases of respiratory and eye symptoms. The nature of the ocular reaction to sulfur is illustrated by the cases below:

Eye complaints following contact with sulfur

87-310	04/01/1987	Sutter	Peach orchard sprayer had exposure to sulfur in eyes and was diagnosed as having chemical keratitis (superficial corneal injury).
87-508	05/01/1987	Fresno	While dusting with sulfur in a vineyard, the material got into a worker's eye and it became irritated. He was wearing safety glasses but not goggles.
88-944	06/01/1988	Kern	While loading sulfur for helicopter application, this employee experienced eye irritation.

As indicated by the above cases, the relationship between the sulfur exposure and the subsequent ocular irritation is usually simple to evaluate, because the irritation corresponds directly to the site of contact.

82.5.1.2 Skin

Dermatitis was present in 70 (45%) of the handler cases; in 55 it was the only illness reported and in 15 the dermatitis occurred in conjunction with other illness symptoms. As illustrated on next page, some cases appear to have been related to chemical irritation (85-655), while others conceivably could have been related to sulfur allergy (87-174). However, provocation tests to confirm the suspected allergy were not documented in any of the cases reported to the California registry. Figures 82.1 and 82.2 show examples of dermatitis of the arm and torso of an exposed worker. These skin lesions appeared within a few minutes of spending 45 min dosing a rose bed with a mixture of elemental sulfur and malathion; they are typical of sulfur. The worker was wearing a short-sleeved shirt without gloves and was sweating profusely in the 95°F heat. This individual is unlikely to be allergic to sulfur since he has applied elemental sulfur on many occasions since this incident (wearing appropriate protective clothing) without experiencing any ill effects.

82.5.1.3 Respiratory Tract and Systemic Illness

Classification of respiratory symptoms as systemic or purely topical is sometimes difficult. Thirty-four (22%) of the handler cases involved either respiratory or systemic illness. Complaints ranged from principally respiratory (84-726) to nonspecific systemic symptoms such as "vomiting" or "feeling shaky" (82-1436). Some cases had rhinitis (cases 83-595 and 87-1042) or asthma symptoms (84-726, 86-916) that suggested a possible immediate allergy to sulfur (e.g., 85-1134), but no cases had

Dermatitis complaints following exposure to elemental sulfur

85-655	05/14/1985	Sonoma	Employee had applied sulfur with a hand held duster, after which he developed contact dermatitis or a chemical burn.
82-1211	06/29/1982	Madera	Developed skin rash after applying sulfur with wet coveralls.
86-2145	08/29/1986	Riverside	Man was dusting dates with sulfur, wearing a short-sleeve shirt. He experienced contact dermatitis on his upper arms, neck, and back.
87-174	02/28/1987	Tulare	A worker complained of a rash after mixing, loading, and applying Kolospray (81% sulfur powder). He had a 2 year history of sensitivity to the material and reported that the rash occurred despite wearing complete safety gear. The treating physician suspected that the dermatitis was due to an allergic reaction and recommended avoiding sulfur powder in the future.
88-650	04/11/1988	Kern	An employee had been applying flowable sulfur on 04-11-88 and sulfur dust on 04-02-88. He developed a rash on his arms and neck, which he feels was due to the sulfur dust application.

documented provocation tests to demonstrate that the reactions were allergic, rather than irritant, in nature.

82.5.1.4 Trauma or Illness Due to Combustion of Sulfur

The tendency of sulfur to oxidize makes it prone to combustion. Sulfur combustion was involved in several significant illness episodes reported to the California illness registry. These included both spontaneous combustion and combustion following aircraft accidents.

82.6 DISCUSSION

Environmental exposure to sulfur arises from two main anthropogenic sources, industrial automobile emissions and from the use of sulfur in agriculture. This chapter automobile has concentrated on the latter. The extensive use of elemental sulfur as a fungicide in agriculture has, on occasion, led to veterinary problems in animals ingesting toxic levels of sulfur. In addition, sulfur dioxide is used as a fumigant, generally as a preservative for food and drink.

In ruminants, sulfur is converted by microorganisms in the rumen to hydrogen sulfide, which is readily absorbed. Sulfide can then inhibit a variety of enzymes involved in oxidative metabolism. It also inhibits respiration by blocking the carotid body and by combining with hemoglobin to produce sulfhemoglobin, thus reducing the oxygen-carrying capacity of the blood. High concentrations of sulfur may lead to secondary thiamine deficits. Sulfite ion is a strong nucleophile and readily binds to thiamine (to the positively charged nitrogen in the thiazole ring), leading to secondary deficits of vitamin B_1. Veterinary problems associated with the ingestion of excessive sulfur include polioencephalomalacia (PEM), a severe brain disease of ruminants. A combination of anecdotal reports of field incidents and laboratory studies has clearly shown that dietary sulfur in these animals needs to be carefully regulated.

Respiratory and systemic symptoms following sulfur exposure

Upper respiratory symptoms			
83-595	03/29/1983	Merced	Diagnosed as allergic rhinitis; worker did not see doctor until 2 weeks after the reported exposure.
87-1042	06/08/1987	Kern	While dusting grapes with sulfur, he began having an apparent allergic reaction to the sulfur (watery eyes and sneezing).
Systemic and lower respiratory symptoms			
82-1436	07/13/1982	Glenn	A nursery worker was exposed to sulfur drifting from an application to an adjacent field. She began to vomit and "feel shaky."
84-726	04/25/1984	Kern	Experienced breathing difficulties after working with sulfur, triggered asthma attack.
85-1134	06/03/1985	Tulare	Loading plane, experienced breathlessness and burning in eyes. Allergic reaction to sulfur.
86-916	06/05/1986	Stanislaus	Asthmatic response when exposed to sulfur dust. He reported wearing a face mask respirator, gloves, an apron, and hat while applying. M.D. advised him to not spray sulfur anymore.
89-1250	05/25/1989	Napa	Worker was applying sulfur with a power sprayer attached to the rear of a tractor. He was wearing work clothes and Tyvek, boots, (prefitted) respirator with pesticide cartridge. Developed tightness in chest and cough. Diagnosis chemical bronchitis.
90-1214	05/26/1990	Kern	Applicator dusting grapes experienced dizziness, shortness of breath, and fainting spell. Diagnosis exposure to sulfur dust. Off work for injury sustained when fell off tractor due to fainting spell. Wearing coveralls, goggles, and dust mask.

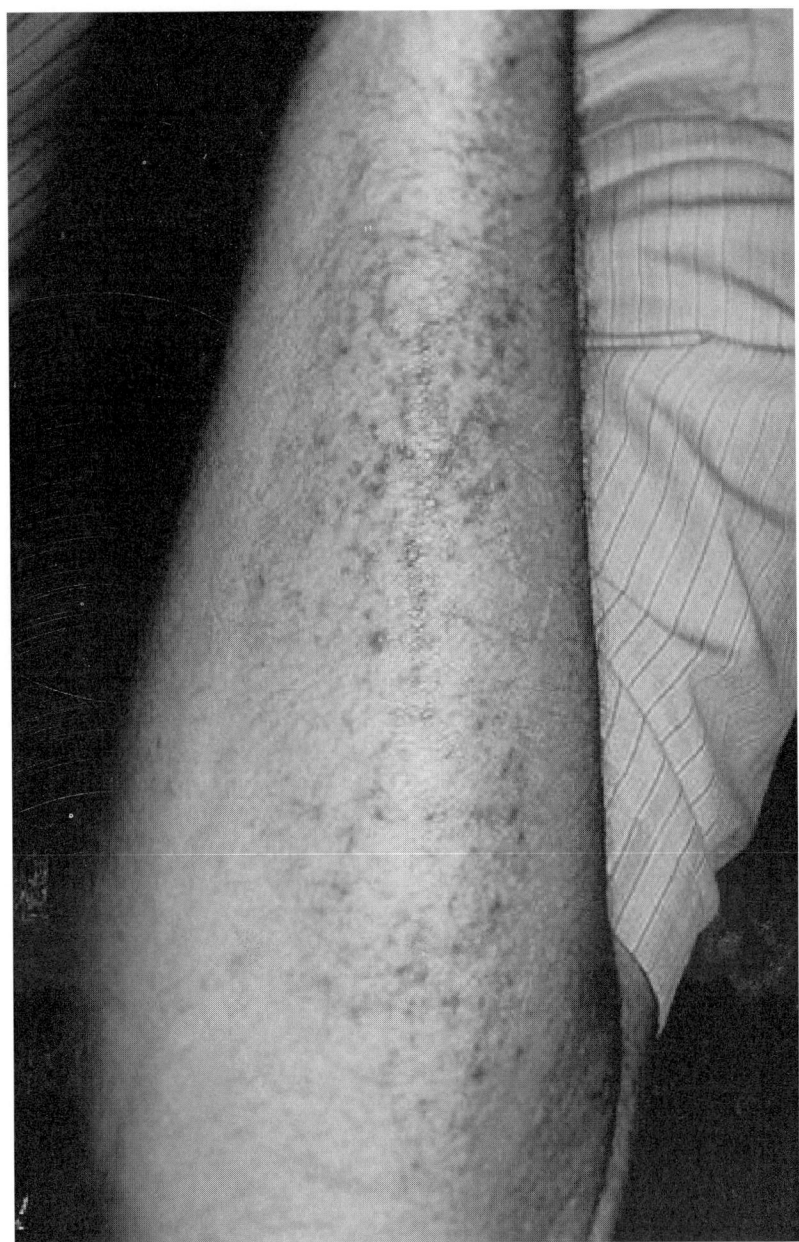

Figure 82.1 Apparent irritant reaction after a sweaty forearm was contaminated with a mixture of sulfur and malathion. Reprinted with permission from M. A. O'Malley (1997), *State of the Art Reviews in Occupational Medicine* **12**, 327–345.

Elemental sulfur appears relatively inert in both the Buehler and Draize skin test models (see above) but is reported to show moderate capacity to cause sensitization in the guinea pig maximization test (Gregorczyk and Swieboda, 1968). This ambiguous response to sulfur in animal tests is contradicted by use experience, where dermatotoxicity in humans appears to be common. A possible explanation may lie in the transformation of sulfur through oxidation and reduction (Matsushita *et al.*, 1977) which may not readily occur in epicutaneous tests in rodents, which thermoregulate by increased respiration rather than by perspiration. The tendency of sulfur to spontaneously transform under field conditions is underscored by the cases of

combustion associated with its use, principally during the summer months in California, where daytime temperatures in the hot, dry inland valleys commonly exceed 100°F (38°C). Current labeling and California regulations prohibit the aerial application of sulfur dust when ambient temperatures exceed 90°F (32°C), in order to reduce combustion incidents due to sulfur.

Data from the California Illness Registry do not clearly indicate how many symptoms of sulfur exposure are due to irritant reactions, how many are possibly due to allergic mechanisms, and how many are due to unknown physiologic mechanisms. No cases were recorded to have provocation testing, the only means of clearly distinguishing between irritant and allergic

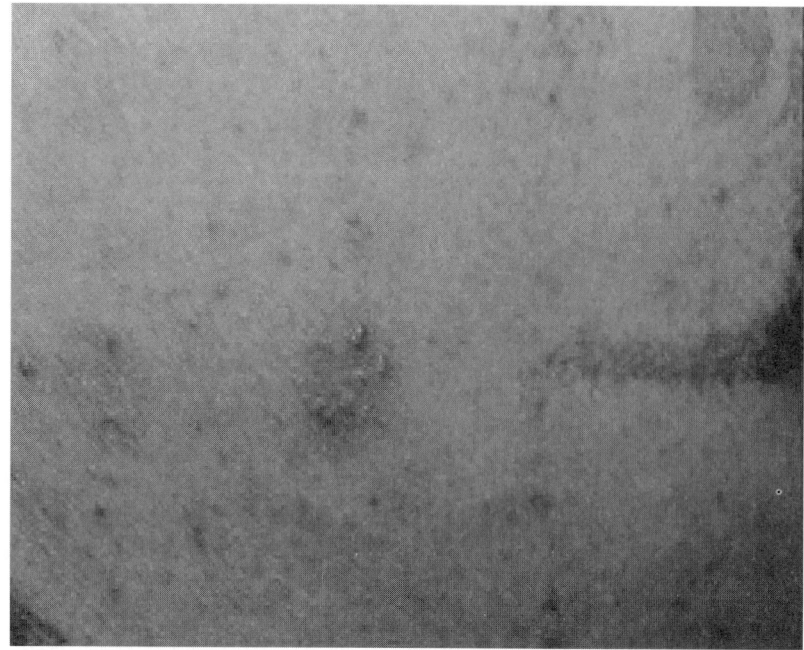

Figure 82.2   A 1+ reaction to sulfur — Subject 43 in a California nursery study. A total of 5 positive reactions to sulfur among 43 subjects. Reprinted with permission from M. A. O'Malley (1997), *State of the Art Reviews in Occupational Medicine* **12**, 327–345.

Post-crash combustion			
90-1220	06/08/1990	Kern	A pilot applying sulfur to sugarbeets crashed when his plane suffered engine failure. The sulfur ignited on impact causing him to inhale the fumes as well as causing burns. He suffered chest tightness, breathing difficulties, and second degree burns over 20% of his body.
88-3029	09/30/1988	Solano	Pilot had just finished applying one load of sulfur to sugar beets when he crashed and died.
85-1461	06/24/1985	San Joaquin	Pilot exposed to burning sulfur when his plane crashed.
Spontaneous combustion			
94-818	06/11/1994	Kern	Pilot was applying sulfur dust to sugar beets when spontaneous combustion of sulfur caused the cockpit to fill with smoke. While trying to land the plane, it flipped over. He crawled out of the cockpit and was taken to a hospital.
94-1278	06/25/1994	Sutter	While standing on the wing of a crop dusting plane, a worker was loading dusting sulfur into the plane's hopper when the sulfur dust ignited. The resulting explosion knocked him off the plane. He suffered respiratory system and skin burns.
93-1220	07/22/1993	Solano	Worker was loading sulfur dust from a hopper into an aircraft. The sulfur dust in the hopper shifted, causing sulfur dust to be dumped onto the airplane fuselage. The sulfur caught fire from the heat of the engine which burned the worker's exposed skin.
91-1252	07/22/1991	Sonoma	An applicator inhaled smoke from a sulfur/grease fire when a bearing on the application equipment burned. He put out the fire with an extinguisher. The fire did not spread to the hopper full of sulfur.
87-772	04/24/1987	Imperial	Aircraft pilot's eyes were burned when the plane caught on fire. Sulfur smoke and fumes were released into the cockpit. The cornea of both eyes were burned.
87-2122	05/14/1987	San Mateo	Worker became ill from burning sulfur fumes while dusting sulfur on ornamentals. He apparently spilled dusting sulfur on the muffler of the motorized hand duster during mixing and loading. Symptoms: nausea, dizziness, vomiting, and wheezing.

reactions. Five instances of apparent allergic reaction to 1% elemental sulfur, ranging from 1+ to 2+/3+,[3] were also observed in a study of California nursery workers. Reactions to sulfur were correlated with a history of working as a pesticide applicator in the nursery business, but none of the participants had a detailed memory of pesticides they had handled or specifically remembered spraying elemental sulfur (O'Malley and Rodriguez, 1998). Two case reports implicate elemental sulfur as a human contact allergen. Schneider (1978) reported two

---

[3]Reactions were scored as 1+ (weak reaction, macular erythema), 2+ (strong reaction, edematous or vesicular), or 3+ (extreme reaction, spreading, bulbous, ulcerative). Equivocal reactions are designated as +/- (Adams, 1990).

cases of contact allergy in patients who used medications containing elemental sulfur to treat superficial fungal dermatoses. Both patients had positive patch test reactions to 5% elemental sulfur in series of vehicles, but a control series was not reported. Wilkinson (1975) reported that a professional gardener with a previous history of atopic eczema developed an eczematous eruption involving the elbow flexures and the right hand. He had a positive patch test reaction to 5% sulfur in petrolatum, but a control series was not reported. Gregorczyk and Swieboda (1968) described 15 cases of desquamative dermatitis among 425 Polish sulfur miners in which irritant dermatitis due to elemental sulfur may have played a part.

REFERENCES

Adams, R. M. (1990). "Occupational Skin Disease." Saunders, Philadelphia.

Beauchamp, R. O., Jr., Bus, J. S., Popp, J. A., Boreiko, C., and Andjelkovich, D. A. (1984). A critical review of the literature on hydrogen sulfide toxicity. *CRC Crit. Rev. Toxicol.* **13**, 25–97.

Bulgin, M. S., Lincoln, S. D., and Mather, G. (1996). Elemental sulfur toxicosis in a flock of sheep. *J. Am. Vet. Med. Assoc.* **7**, 1063–1065.

Costa, D. L., and Amdur, M. O. (1996). *In* Casarett and Doull's "Toxicology, the Basic Science of Poisons" (C. D. Klaassen, ed.), 5th ed. McGraw–Hill, New York.

DPR (1995). "Summary of Pesticide Use Report Data Annual 1993." Department of Pesticide Regulation, California Environmental Protection Agency, Sacramento, CA.

DPR (1996a). "Summary of Pesticide Use Report Data Annual 1994." Department of Pesticide Regulation, California Environmental Protection Agency, Sacramento, CA.

DPR (1996b). "Summary of Pesticide Use Report Data Annual 1995." Department of Pesticide Regulation, California Environmental Protection Agency, Sacramento, CA.

Farm Chemicals Handbook (1998). Volume 84 (R. T. Meister, ed.). Meister Publishing Company, USA.

Gador, J., and Motowicka-Terelak, T. (1986). Effect of contamination with sulfur on soil properties and crop yields in a lysimeter experiment: II Effect of elemental sulphur application to the soil on the yields and chemical compositions of some crops. *Pamietnik Pulawski* **88**, 25–38.

Gibson, D. M., Kennelly, J. J., and Arherra, F. X. (1987). The performance and thiamine status of pigs fed sulfur dioxide treated high-moisture barley. *Can. J. Anim. Sci.* **67**, 841–854.

Gould, D., McAllister, M. M., Savage, J. C., *et al.* (1991). High sulfide concentration in rumen fluid associated with nutritionally induced polioencephalomalacia in calves. *Am. J. Vet. Res.* **52**, 1164–1169.

Gregorczyk, L., and Swieboda, K. (1968). Uber den einfluB von schwefelverbindungen auf die haut und auf die schleimhaute [On the influence of sulfur binding on the skin and mucous membranes]. *Polskie Tygognik Lekarski* **23**, 463–466.

Hamlen, H., Clark, E., and Janzen, E. (1993). Polioencephalomalacia in cattle consuming water with elevated sodium sulfate levels: A herd investigation. *Can. Vet. J.* **34**, 153–158.

Haynes, R. J., and Swift, R. S. (1986). Effects of soil amendments and sawdust mulching on growth, yield and leaf nutrient content of highbush blueberry [*Vaccinium corymbosum* cultivar Bluecrop] plants. *Scientia Hortic.* **29**(3), 229–238.

Hill, F. I., and Ebbett, P. C. (1997). Polioencephalomalacia in cattle in New Zealand fed chou moellier (*Brassica oleracea*). *New Zealand Vet. J.* **45**, 37–39.

Jeffrey, M., Duff, J. P., Higgins, R. J., Simpson, V. R., Jackman, R., Jones, T. O., Mechie, S. C., and Livesey, C. T. (1994). Polioencephalomalacia associated with the ingestion of ammonium sulphate by sheep and cattle. *Vet. Rec.* **134**, 343–348.

Jensen, R., Griner, L. A., and Adams, O. R. (1956). Polioencephalomalacia of cattle and sheep. *J. Am. Vet. Med. Assoc.* **129**, 311–321.

Low, J. C., Scott, P. R., Howie, F., Lewis, M., Fitzsimons, J., and Spence, J. A. (1996). Sulfur-induced polioencephalomalacia in lambs. *Vet. Rec.* **138**, 327–329.

Majule, A. E., Topper, C. P., and Nortcliff, S. (1997). The environmental effects of dusting cashew (*Anacardium occidentale L.*) trees with sulphur in southern Tanzania. *Trop. Agric.* **74**(1), 25–33.

Matsushita, T., Yoshioka, M., Aoyama, K., Arimatsu, Y., and Nomura, S. (1977). Experimental study on contact dermatitis caused by fungicides benomyl and thiophanate-methyl. *Ind. Hlth.* **15**(3-4), 141–148.

McAllister, M. M., Gould, D. H., and Hamar, D. W. (1992). Sulfide-induced polioencephalomalacia in lambs. *J. Comp. Pathol.* **106**, 267–278.

Olkowski, A. A. (1997). Neurotoxicity and secondary metabolic problems associated with low to moderate levels of exposure to excess dietary sulfur in ruminants: A review. *Vet. Human Toxicol.* **39**, 355–360.

O'Malley, M. A., and Rodriguez, H.-P. (1998). "Contact Dermatitis in California Nursery Workers: Part II. Pilot Field Study." California EPA, DPR, Worker Health and Safety Branch HS-1767.

Sager, R. L., Hamar, D. W., and Gould, D. (1990). Clinical and biochemical alterations in calves with nutritionally induced polioencephalomalacia. *Am. J. Vet. Res.* **51**, 1969–1974.

Schneider, H. G. (1978). Schwefelallergie [Sulfur allergy]. *Hautarzt* **29**, 340–342.

Shapiro, R. (1977). Genetic effects of bisulfite (sulfur dioxide). *Mutation Res.* **39**, 149–176.

Studdert, V. P., and Labuc, R. H. (1991). Thiamine deficiency in cats and dogs associated with feeding meat preserved with sulphur dioxide. *Aust. Vet. J.* **68**, 54–57.

Sun, C. C., and Sue, M. S. (1995). Sulfur spring dermatitis. *Contact Dermat.* **32**, 31–34.

Terlecki, S., and Markson, L. M. (1961). Cerebrocortical necrosis in cattle and sheep. *Vet. Rec.* **73**, 2327.

Vena, G. A., Foti, C., and Angelini, G. (1994). Sulfite contact allergy. *Contact Dermat.* **31**, 172–175.

Wilkinson, D. S. (1975). Sulfur sensitivity. *Contact Dermat.* **1**, 58.

Rodenticides

Alain F. Pelfrene
Alain Pelfrene & Associated Consultants

83.1 INTRODUCTION

Rats and mice compete with humans for food. This loss to rodents causes economic loss everywhere. In some developing countries it can cause starvation. Rodents are also hosts for human diseases, including plague, endemic rickettsiosis, leishmaniasis, spirochetosis, tularemia, leptospirosis, tick-borne encephalitis, and listeriosis. Rats occasionally bite people. Finally, rodents do a variety of other damage, mainly by gnawing.

Insofar as possible, rodent populations should be controlled by limiting their access to food and harborage. Individual animals or small groups may be removed conveniently by trapping. However, there will always be a need for poisons in rodent control.

Unfortunately, effective permanent control through poisoning is not simple. The animals must be enticed to ingest a toxicant in sufficient dosage if the effort is to succeed. But rodents rarely or ever constitute an important problem unless they have a supply of food and water. This means that, in spite of containing a foreign substance, the solid or liquid bait used should be at least as attractive to the rodents as their usual supply of food or water. The first problem may be that the intended poison makes the bait unacceptable to animals that have never encountered the poison. This is called primary bait refusal. Because of this common difficulty, many efforts to find better rodenticides have emphasized highly toxic substances of such bland taste and odor that animals always will take a lethal dose the first time. However, this is an impractical objective. At least a few animals will get only a sublethal dose on first encounter and will be conditioned thereby to avoid the poison even though it seems tasteless and odorless at first. This reaction is called secondary bait refusal or bait shyness. There is even some indication that rodents learn from the behavior of their companions in such a way that the manner of death of some of them conditions the behavior of others that have consumed no poison. A third problem with many rodenticides is that they are very nearly as dangerous to humans and useful animals as to rodents. This problem can be minimized by selecting a poison with a wide margin of safety, by coloring the bait, by combining the poison with an emetic, or by restricting the placement of baits. However, all these solutions have their limitations. There is no rat poison that cannot harm humans if sufficiently misused.

Considering all these difficulties, four requirements for an ideal rodenticide may be stated as follows: (*a*) The poison must be surely effective when incorporated into baits in such small quantity that its presence is not detected to an interfering degree. (*b*) Finished baits containing the poison must not excite bait shyness in any way and the necessity of prebaiting must thereby be avoided. (*c*) The manner of death must be such that surviving individuals will not become suspicious of its cause but will remain on the premises and eat freely of the bait until the themselves die. (*d*) The poison, in the concentration used for control, must be specific for the species to be destroyed unless its use can be made safe for humans and domestic animals by some other means.

Part of the safety of the anticoagulant rodenticides is made possible by their cumulative properties and depends on the fact that they are offered to rodents in such a way that a single dose is harmless even to the rodents themselves. Quite aside from the important species differences in susceptibility, which favor human safety, people are protected further by the fact that except in suicide or murder, substantial continuing exposure is far less likely than a single accidental exposure.

Although this chapter is devoted to synthetic organic rodenticides, it is necessary to recall that inorganic and botanical compounds may still be important for rodent control in some areas. Furthermore, some of them, notably arsenic, phosphorus, and strychnine, are very important as sources of human poisoning.

On the contrary, some synthetic rodenticides have other uses. The most important examples are the use of vitamin D and of certain anticoagulants as rodenticides and as drugs in human medicine. In addition, several of the organic fluorine compounds have been used experimentally or in practice as systemic insecticides and/or raticides.

Compared to toxic substances in general, biochemical actions of the synthetic rodenticides that have been studied in humans are unusually well known. This makes it possible to assign them to groups (see the following sections) that are meaningful not only chemically but in terms of biochemical lesions. The same is not true of numerous miscellaneous compounds including crimidine (BSI, ISO) that apparently have not yet produced poisoning in humans and certainly have not been used as drugs or studied experimentally in human subjects.

83.2 FLUOROACETIC ACID AND ITS DERIVATIVES

Sodium fluoroacetate came to prominence in the United States as a result of a search for rodenticides that would not be subject to shortages imposed by World War II (Ward, 1945). This and related compounds had been considered earlier as systemic insecticides. At about the same time, it became known that fluoroacetate is the toxic material in the South African plant "gifblaar" (*Dichapetalum cymosum*). Later it was shown that the same compound is present intermittently in *Acacia georgiana*. The main toxicant in *D. toxicarium* is fluorooleic acid, but fluoropalmitic acid is present also. The ground seeds of *D. toxicarium* have been used by natives as a rat poison. It gave problems with secondary poisoning and human toxicity similar to that later associated with synthetic sodium fluoroacetate.

Under these circumstances, there were practical as well as academic reasons to study the mode of action of organic monofluoro compounds. It appears that the toxicity of all of the compounds depends on the same mechanism. Highly toxic compounds either have two carbon atoms or are metabolized to this form (Chenoweth, 1949; Peters, 1963a; Raasch, 1958; Saunders, 1947).

83.2.1 SODIUM FLUOROACETATE

83.2.1.1 Identity, Properties, and Uses

Chemical Name   Sodium monofluoroacetate is the chemical name.

Structure   See Fig. 83.1.

Synonyms   Sodium monofluoroacetate is also known as Compound-1080 or ten-eighty. The CAS registry number is 62-74-8.

Physical and Chemical Properties   The empirical formula for sodium monofluoroacetate is $C_2H_2FNaO_2$ and the molecular weight is 100.3. Its forms an odorless, white, nonvolatile powder that decomposes at about 200°C. Although the compound is often said to be tasteless, dilute solutions actually tasted like weak vinegar. Sodium fluoroacetate is very water soluble and hygroscopic but is of low solubility in ethanol, acetone, and petroleum oils.

Formulations and Uses   Sodium fluoroacetate is formulated as an aqueous solution containing a warning color. Sodium monofluoroacetate is used to kill rats, mice, other rodents, and predators. It is an intense mammalian poison, and it is used in many countries but only by trained personnel.

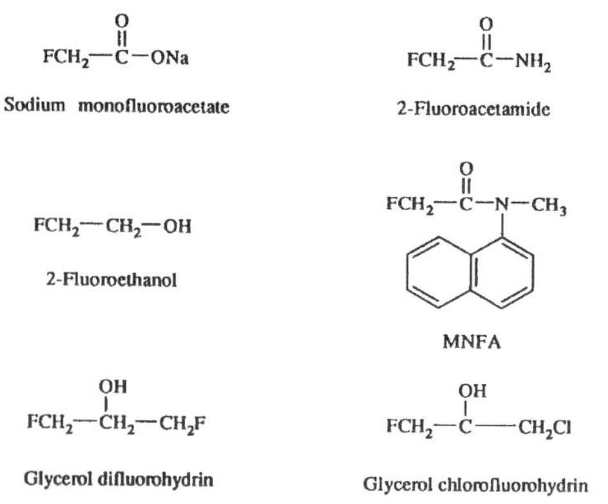

Figure 83.1   Some organic fluorine rodenticides and other organic fluorine pesticides.

83.2.1.2 Toxicity to Laboratory Animals

Basic Findings   The first paper on sodium monofluoroacetate as a rodenticide (Kalmbach, 1945) drew attention to its very high acute toxicity. LD 50 values for ordinary laboratory rats and for wild animals of the same species were reported as 2.5 and 5.0 mg/kg, respectively. The wild black rat (*Rattus rattus*), another commensal species, was much more susceptible (LD 50:0.1 mg/kg). A LD 50 of 0.22 mg/kg has been reported for *Rattus norvegicus* (Dieke and Richter, 1946). The likelihood of danger to people, domestic animals, pets, and nontarget wildlife was pointed out. The acute toxicity of the compound to an extremely wide range of wildlife was reported by Ward and Spencer (1947). See Table 83.1.

Fluoroacetate acts mainly on the central nervous system and the heart. It seems that there are species in which fluoroacetate affects chiefly the heart, such as the rabbit, the goat, and the horse, and others in which only the central nervous system is affected, such as the dog, the guinea pig, and the frog. In the cat, the rhesus monkey, the domestic pig, and birds, both systems are involved. The above results were obtained by Chenoweth and Gilman (1946) using methyl fluoroacetate instead of sodium fluoroacetate. However, since both compounds yield the fluorocitrate ion in the body, where it is converted to fluoroacetate, which is responsible for the induction of pharmacologic and toxic signs (see below), it seems that this experiment is nevertheless interesting in showing a large degree of species variability in the site of action. In all species, there was a delay of 0.5–2 hr or more between administration, either oral or intravenous, and the onset of the symptoms, and the route of administration did not significantly affect the toxicity of fluoroacetate.

Laboratory rats acquire a tolerance to sodium fluoroacetate by ingesting sublethal doses over a period of 5–14 days. However, this tolerance is lost if intake of the compound is interrupted for as little as 7 days (Kalmbach, 1945).

Tolerance of some but not all species was confirmed by several investigators, including Kandel and Chenoweth (1952). These authors found that, whereas small doses of fluoroacetate increased tolerance to challenge doses of fluoroacetate or

Table 83.1
Single-Dose LD 50 for Sodium Fluoroacetate

Species	Route	LD 50 (mg/kg)	Reference
Rat	oral	0.22	Dieke and Richter (1946)
Rat	oral	2.5	Ward and Spencer (1947)
Rat	oral	1–2	Phillips and Worden (1957)
Rat	intraperitoneal	3–5	Ward and Spencer (1947)
Mouse	subcutaneous	19.3	Hutchens *et al.* (1949)
Mouse	subcutaneous	17.0	Tourtellotte and Coon (1951)
Mouse	intraperitoneal	10.0	Ward and Spencer (1947)
Mouse	intraperitoneal	16.5	Tourtellotte and Coon (1951)
Mouse	intraperitoneal	14.7	Raasch (1958)
Guinea pig	oral	0.4	Ward and Spencer (1947)
Guinea pig	intraperitoneal	0.37	Hutchens *et al.* (1949)
Rabbit	subcutaneous	0.28	Hutchens *et al.* (1949)
Dog	oral	0.06	Tourtellotte and Coon (1951)
Cow	oral	0.39	Robinson (1970)
Calf	oral	0.22	Robinson (1970)
Opossum	oral	0.79	Bell (1972)
Mallard duck	oral	4.8	Hudson *et al.* (1972)
South African clawed toad (*Xenopus laevis*)	oral	500	Chenoweth (1949)

4-fluorobutyrate, tolerance to neither could be evoked by small doses of 4-fluorobutyrate. The citrate content of the rat brain appeared to have no relation to tolerance, and the citrate that accumulated after a small dose did not prevent the further accumulation of citrate after a larger dose.

The sensitivity of mice to sodium fluoroacetate depends on temperature. Under otherwise identical conditions, the LD 50 values were 12.1 and 5.16 mg/kg at 23 and 17°C, respectively (Misustova *et al.*, 1969). The survival of individual rats in a particular dosage group may be predicted by following their body temperature. There is a critical level that varies somewhat according to the interval after dosing. Animals that regained their initial temperature within 96 hr usually lived, but those that failed to regain normal temperature within this time usually died (Filip *et al.*, 1970). For groups of animals, the course of the temperature can be described by a computer-generated curve (Hosek and Love, 1952). The temperature change is correlated with citrate metabolism (Kirzon *et al.*, 1970).

Primates and birds are more resistant; rodents and carnivores are most susceptible. In general, cold-blooded vertebrates are less sensitive than warm-blooded ones (Egekeze and Oehme, 1979). Sodium monofluoroacetate in carcasses creates a secondary poisoning hazard to which carnivorous predators are extremely susceptible (Bell, 1972).

Plasma elimination half-life in rabbits was shown to be 1.1 hour and the retention time in tissue greater with larger doses. Tissues residues were substantially lower than in plasma (Gooneratne *et al.*, 1995).

When orally administered to sheep and goats at dose levels of 0.1 mg/kg body weight, the plasma elimination half-life was found to be 10.8 hours in sheep and 5.4 hours in goats. Concentrations of sodium fluoroacetate in muscle, kidney, and liver (0.042, 0.057, and 0.021 µg/g) were clearly lower than those in the plasma (0.098 µg/g) 2.5 hours after administration. After 96 hours, only traces of the compound were detectable in sheep tissues (<0.002 to 0.008 µg/g). The authors concluded that even with accidental exposure to sublethal doses, sodium fluoroacetate would not persist in tissues for more than a few days because of its rapid clearance and because occurrence of residues in meat intended for human consumption would be highly unlikely (Eason *et al.*, 1994).

Absorption, Distribution, Metabolism, and Excretion Using ether as a solvent, it was possible to recover 60–70% of the total dose from the body (including gastrointestinal contents) of rabbits killed by 10 times the LD 50 level. The concentration in the brain was twice that in other organs (Tomiya *et al.*, 1976). Sodium monofluoroacetate is rapidly absorbed by the gastrointestinal tract. It is not well absorbed by the intact skin, but absorption may be greater in the presence of dermatitis or other skin injury.

Biochemical Effects It was in connection with the mode of action of fluoroacetic acid that the term "lethal synthesis" was coined (Peters, 1952). Peters (1963b) later reviewed the research and extended the concept. Very briefly, no mammalian enzyme was found that was inhibited by fluoroacetate *in vitro*. However, *in vivo*, the ion undergoes synthesis to form fluorocitrate and this inhibits mitochondrial aconitase either *in vivo* or *in vitro*. The result is that the Krebs cycle is blocked, which leads to lowered energy production, reduced oxygen consumption, and reduced cellular concentration of ATP; furthermore, since the citrate synthetase continues to work, citrate accumulates in the tissues (Buffa and Peters, 1950). It is thought that toxicity is due not to the accumulation of citrate per se but to the blockage of energy metabolism. However, increased tissue and plasma concentration of citrate is probably responsible for some of the symptoms seen during acute poisoning. Citrate is a potent chelator of calcium ion, and it has been demonstrated that in cats intravenously injected with fluoroacetate at 0.03 mmol/kg the ionized calcium level in blood fell by an average of 27.2%, 40 min after the injection. There was a corresponding prolongation of the QT interval of the electrocardiogram (ECG), and treatment with $CaCl_2$ significantly prolonged the life of the treated animals as compared with unmedicated positive controls (Roy *et al.*, 1980). The characteristic delay at the onset of poisoning by sodium fluoroacetate is accounted for by the time necessary for its metabolism and biochemical mode of action.

The toxicity of fluoroacetate is entirely different from that of inorganic fluorides. It depends on the firmness of the F—C bond such that fluoroacetate is an antimetabolite.

Consistent with the theory that fluorocitrate is the active toxicant, it was found to be at least 100 times more toxic than fluoroacetate when injected directly into the brain under various experimental conditions. An intracerebral dose of 0.115 μg failed to kill rats weighing about 250 gm, and it did not cause convulsions; doses of 0.287 μg (about 0.001 mg/kg) or greater caused convulsions and killed almost all rats (Morselli *et al.*, 1968). On the other hand, a dosage of 40–60 mg/kg is necessary to kill by the intraperitoneal route, and an oral dosage of 40 mg/kg constitutes only an LD 50. The great difference was attributed to failure of fluorocitrate to reach aconitase within critical cells of the brain and heart (Peters and Shorthouse, 1971). Species differ in the degree to which the concentration of citrate increases in different organs and also in the timing of these increases (Kirzon *et al.*, 1973). These biochemical differences presumably underlie the clinical differences between species, especially the relative importance in neurological and cardiac effects.

Accumulation of citrate was evident in mice within 2 hr after intraperitoneal injection of sodium fluoroacetate at a rate of 30 mg/kg, which is about 1.7 times the LD 50 in that species. The concentration of citrate increased from 48 ppm in controls to 74, 101, and 166 ppm within 2, 5, and 24 hr, respectively, after injection. The mice were dead at 24 hr (Matsumura and O'Brien, 1963).

Whereas Williamson *et al.* (1964) agreed that the initial effect of fluoroacetate is to produce fluorocitrate, they considered that the secondary inhibition of phosphofructokinase by the accumulated citrate was actually lethal because it deprived the cell of pyruvate, which would eventually overcome the inhibition of aconitase.

Effects on Organs and Tissues Loracher and Lux (1974) concluded on the basis of studies of neuromembrane depolarization that diminished inhibitory conductance is apparently important as a causative factor in convulsions induced by sodium fluoroacetate. The decreased level of ionized calcium in blood induced by the chelating effect of citrate certainly plays a role in the depolarization of the neuromembrane, as it does on the cardiac cell membranes. The effect of sodium fluoroacetate on the heart rhythm is due, as demonstrated by Noguchi *et al.* (1966), primarily to action on the cells themselves and not on the vagus nerve. Irregularity of rhythm and a condition analogous to fibrillation were produced in cultures of heart cells that had grown until cell-to-cell contact was prevalent and beating was synchronized. The average times necessary to produce irregularity and fibrillation were 9 and 48 hr, respectively, at a concentration of 10 ppm in the medium, but only 2 and 9 hr, respectively, at a concentration of 100 ppm. At a concentration of 1000 ppm, fibrillation was immediate and cytoplasmic vacuoles appeared rapidly.

Effects on Reproduction A dosage of sodium fluoroacetate just below the maternal LD 50 reduced oxygen consumption of the embryos as well as the mother but was not teratogenic (Spielmann *et al.*, 1973).

Treatment of Poisoning in Animals Hutchens *et al.* (1949) demonstrated a significant reduction of mortality in mice, guinea pigs, and rabbits (but not dogs) treated with ethanol at a rate of 800 mg/kg administered subcutaneously as a 10% solution in normal saline. The response occurred when the alcohol was given before signs of poisoning appeared and was best when given within 10 min of poisoning. In mice, sodium acetate and ethanol acted synergistically to antagonize poisoning (Tourtellotte and Coon, 1951). The beneficial effect of ethanol in rodents was confirmed by Chenoweth *et al.* (1951), but these authors found ethanol less effective in the dog and utterly useless in the monkey. In a study of a wide range of chemical substances in mice, rats, rabbits, dogs, and rhesus monkeys, they concluded that commercially available monacetin containing about 60% glycerol monoacetate was superior to any other substance tested as an antidote for poisoning by fluoroacetate. Not only did it reduce mortality, but it was able to normalize heart and brain rhythms as indicated by ECG and electroencephalogram (EEG) tracings.

Light pentobarbital anesthesia for 18–24 hr significantly reduced mortality among dogs poisoned by sodium monofluoroacetate at a rate of 0.10 mg/kg (Hutchens *et al.*, 1949; Tourtellotte and Coon, 1951).

83.2.1.3 Toxicity to Humans

Accidental and Intentional Poisoning Sodium fluoroacetate was introduced in 1946 in the United States for use by pest control operators, including persons hired for the purpose by government agencies. The poison was mixed with a dye. Solutions were supposed to be placed in shallow paper cups made in such a way that they would not tip over. These water baits were supposed to be used only in places that would be unoccupied and locked during exposure of the poison, and all cups and dead rodents were supposed to be collected and incinerated by authorized persons at the end of the exposure period. However, the regulations were not always followed. By the end of the year, at least one child who found an "empty" paper cup had died, and her 3-year-old brother had been severely poisoned. By the end of 1949, there had been at least 12 deaths and 6 cases of nonfatal poisoning. In addition, there had been 4 deaths, all in children, that probably were caused by sodium monofluoroacetate, but other sources of poisoning could not be ruled out. Of the 12 deaths clearly caused by sodium monofluoroacetate, 5 involved small children who had found and often chewed on a poison cup, 3 involved juveniles who had found the poison in a soft drink bottle, and 4 were suicides of adults. Except one, each of the survivors was a child who had found a poison cup. These accidents made such an impression on the few people who had legal access to sodium fluoroacetate that they became far stricter in carrying out the recommended precautions and in selecting situations in which the compound was used at all. As a result, the safety record of the compound in the United States improved greatly.

A typical fatal case involved a 40-year-old man who was found unconscious in his bedroom. He had an 8-year history of severe depression, and his family had been warned of the possibility of suicide. When admitted to hospital, he had slight muscular spasms and nystagmus of both eyes; the heart rate was 92 beats per minute and rhythm was irregular. Following gastric lavage and a soft soap enema, the nystagmus became worse, and the patient had an epileptiform convulsion. The blood pressure fell to 90/40 mm Hg. Treatment consisted of plasma, oxygen, and procaine hydrochloride in the hope of desensitizing the heart. The blood pressure improved to 118/75 mg Hg, but there was no decisive change until the heart and later the respiration stopped about 17 hr after admission (Harrisson *et al.*, 1952a). Another fatal case was remarkable for its combination of prolonged survival following the ingestion of an almost certainly very large dose. Briefly, about 113,000 mg of sodium fluoroacetate was missing from a professional rat exterminator's supplies after his 17-year-old son made a solution and drank it. The boy vomited promptly and then within an hour walked into an hospital emergency room. He gradually became comatose during gastric lavage, and consciousness was never regained. Within less than 3 hr of ingestion, he had a grand mal convulsion associated with fecal incontinence. The clinical course, which lasted slightly over 5 days, was characterized by cardiac irregularity, which responded to a considerable degree to procainamide hydrochloride; dilation and failure of the heart with acute pulmonary edema, which responded surprisingly well to digitalis (lanatoside C); bouts of severe hypotension, which responded only questionably to levarterenol (norepinephrine) but somewhat better to mephentermine; cortical irritability, which responded to barbiturates and later responded more effectively to ethanol; frequent severe carpopedal spasm, controlled somewhat by calcium gluconate; and finally growing evidence of infection including a temperature reaching 42.3°C in spite of efforts to reduce it. The diagnosis based on autopsy was poisoning, bronchopneumonia with septicemia, focal infarction of the right kidney, and mediastinal emphysema (Brockmann *et al.*, 1955).

Serious illness followed by full recovery occurred in a 2-year-old boy who was found licking crystals from the screw cap of a bottle of sodium fluoroacetate solution. The parents did not know whether he drank any of the solution. Almost immediately after he was found, the boy began to vomit. He was brought to hospital about 6 hr later because he began to have generalized convulsive movements and became stuporous. On admission, the boy was comatose and exhibiting carpopedal spasms, tetanic convulsive movements, irregular respiration, and great cardiac irregularity. While a solution of calcium gluconate was being injected, there were a few seconds of cardiac asystole. Thereafter, the irregular cardiac rhythm resumed but at a much slower rate. Tetanic convulsions stopped immediately, and the child became completely flaccid. A few hours after admission, the child became responsive. Very soon the boy suffered a generalized tonic clonic convulsion lasting several minutes and followed by deep coma. Briefly, the boy remained unresponsive for 4 days. Cardiac rhythm continued to change frequently during the first 3 days. Tonic convulsions lasting several minutes occurred many times every hour, sometimes about

every 10 min for many successive hours. During spasm, the pupils dilated and remained inactive to light; between seizures the pupils were miotic but responsive to light. On two occasions respiration stopped and artificial respiration was required briefly.

On the evening of the fourth day, 100 hr after ingestion, the boy began to open his eyes and look about. He tried to talk but was unable to articulate. He could neither sit up nor reach for objects but appeared alert. On the fifth day and sixth days, he rapidly regained all his motor ability, slowly lost his drowsiness, and became articulate. On the evening of the sixth day he was clinically well. He was discharged on the eleventh day. Reexamination 1 year later showed that the boy had had no further neurological trouble, and this mental and physical development has proceeded normally (Gajdusek and Luther, 1950).

In another case in which the initial dosage undoubtedly was smaller, there were no important clinical changes until 20 hr after ingestion, when the 8-month-old girl had a generalized seizure lasting about 1 min. In spite of treatment with phenobarbital, three additional seizures occurred during the next 12 hr. There was no further illness, and the patient was discharged 4 days later. Follow-ups revealed no change in behavior, intellect, or motor performance (Reigart *et al.*, 1975).

Any serious but reversible interference with respiration or general circulation is liable to produce some cases in which the patient survives but with severe brain damage. The cardiac arrhythmias characteristic of poisoning by sodium fluoroacetate are likely to produce such interference. An example involved an 8-year-old boy who was in status epilepticus when he entered hospital. The convulsions were controlled to some degree. There was no striking change until 14 hr after admission, when ventricular asystole occurred. Heart action was renewed but only after sufficient delay that the child suffered brain damage and was clearly mentally defective after a very long and stormy hospital course (McTaggart, 1970).

During the decade 1971–1981, 111 cases of accidental or unintentional poisoning with sodium fluoroacetate were collected by the National Poison Center of Israel. These cases included three cases of death and one case of mass accidental poisoning affecting 30 children, although the great majority of them only consumed a very small number of wheat grain baits impregnated with the compound. These latter cases did not result in clinical symptoms of poisoning (Roy *et al.*, 1982). These authors also described the clinical features of two cases of acute poisoning in which gastrointestinal disorders were rapidly followed by central nervous system manifestations (disorders of consciousness, convulsions, coma) and cardiac disorders, the most frequent cause of death. Ventricular ectopic beats preceded the ventricular arrhythmia, which was then followed by ventricular tachycardia and fibrillation. The electrocardiogram was characterized by a prolonged QT interval. A metabolic acidosis was commonly observed. Chung (1984) reported on five cases collected between 1975 and 1981 in Taiwan. The amount ingested ranged from 8 to 40 ml of a 1% formulation of sodium monofluoroacetate. All five patients survived. All cases had signs of transient cardiac dysfunction, but in addition acute renal failure was seen in three of the five patients, two of them with frank uremia. The acute renal failure was reversible.

In a retrospective study of 38 cases of poisoning collected between 1988 and 1993 in Taiwan by Chi *et al.* (1996), 18% of the patients died. Laboratory symptoms included nonspecific ST-T and T waves on the ECG (72%), hypocalcemia (42%), and hypokalemia (65%). Hypotension, respiratory rate, pulse rate, increased serum creatinine, and decreased pH were considered as the most important predictors of mortality.

Use Experience   In spite of the great toxicity of sodium fluoroacetate, there apparently has been only one case of illness among those who used it without suicidal intent. Even in this case, the kind of illness was so atypical of poisoning and so complicated by the unrelated factor of hypertrophy of the prostate that evaluation of the case is difficult. The patient entered hospital with renal failure and other serious illness. Although he was only 59 years old, he had a 5-year history of symptoms of prostatism but no history of urinary tract infection, renal calculi, or hematuria. He had had gout for 10 years, and he had been digitalized for 12 months. For 6 months he had experienced increasing lassitude, vomiting, and pruritis. Inspection revealed rapid breathing and muscle wasting. More detailed physical examination revealed mild left ventricular failure and evidence of liver disease, hypothyroidism, extrapyramidal disease, and gout, as well as distended bladder, caused by prostatic hypertrophy. These findings were substantiated by laboratory examinations. Following catheter drainage of the bladder, blood urea declined and renal function improved further following prostatectomy 10 days after admission. Recovery was very slow. Neurological and thyroid findings cleared within 6 months. Renal function continued to improve for about 2 years, after which the patient remained well.

Involvement of fluoroacetate was suspected because of the history of exposure, the finding of organic fluorine in the urine, and histological changes found in kidney biopsies. There was no doubt of exposure; the patient had been employed for 10 years as an exterminator of rabbits, and for about 4 weeks each year he had applied sodium fluoroacetate to pieces of carrots that served as bait for the animals. During this work, he had worn rubber gloves and he had never knowingly ingested any of the poison. The report of concentrations of 15.4 and 14.8 ppm of sodium fluoroacetate (analyzed as organic fluoride) in two samples of urine collected 2 weeks after admission and the absence of such organic fluoride in samples collected 5 weeks and 6 months later was accepted as consistent with the history of exposure. A kidney biopsy performed 4 days after admission revealed periglomerular fibrosis, some capsular adhesion and other glomerular changes, plus swelling and vacuolation of tubular cells, increased interstitial fibrous tissue, a few small foci of inflammation, and mild thickening of the arterial walls. A second biopsy 4 weeks later showed little change in the glomerular lesion, but the tubules were no longer vacuolated. However, many tubules had been lost, and many of those remaining were atrophic. Interstitial fibrosis was prominent. The kidney lesions were considered similar to those described in

rats in association with acute poisoning. It was acknowledged that lower urinary tract obstruction may have been a predisposing factor (Parkin *et al.*, 1977). Even if the patient had been exposed to sodium fluoroacetate a short time before he was admitted to hospital, it is difficult to understand why excretion of organic fluoride from this source would continue 2 weeks later. Although no urinary levels of organic fluoride have been reported for other workers, one must note that 15 ppm would indicate a daily output of about 22.5 mg/person/day in a person with average urinary volume. This in turn would indicate a minimal absorption rate of about 0.32 mg/kg/day, an astonishingly high level. The renal changes previously described in rats (Cater and Peters, 1961) followed one or a few very large dosages of fluorocitrate, and the fat droplets were tiny compared to those seen in the human patient.

Dosage Response   In a fatal case, 465 mg (equivalent to a dosage of over 6 mg/kg) was recovered from the stomach contents, urine, brain, liver, and kidneys (Harrisson *et al.*, 1952b). No account was taken of sodium fluoroacetate in other organs and tissues or of that removed by vomiting, lavage, and enema; therefore, the ingested dosage must have been considerably larger.

Several children varying in age from 0.66 to 8.0 years were poisoned seriously or even fatally by chewing on only one paper cup placed earlier for rat control. The cups were made to receive 15 ml of 0.33% solution, that is, 50 mg of sodium fluoroacetate. The average age of the children was 2.37 years, and the weight of such a child is about 13 kg. Thus, the maximal dosage must have been approximately 3.8 mg/kg, but the true dosage must have been considerably smaller because part of the material originally added to the cup may have been lost and not all that dried in the cup would have been ingested. A dosage of 0.5–2.0 mg/kg must be considered highly dangerous. The estimated mean lethal dose in humans ranged from 2 to 10 mg/kg (Gajdusek and Luther, 1950; Harrisson *et al.*, 1952a).

Laboratory Findings   The following concentrations expressed as sodium fluoroacetate were found in samples taken at autopsy from a man who survived about 17 hr after being found unconscious: urine, 368 ppm; liver, 58 ppm; brain, 76 ppm; and kidney, 65 ppm (Harrisson *et al.*, 1952b).

Pathology   In a fatal case, autopsy revealed petechial hemorrhages and congestion of the organs consistent with recent fits. All the findings were nonspecific, but it is interesting that they included diffuse tubular degeneration of the kidneys, which is consistent with the findings in the only case of alleged chronic human poisoning by sodium fluoroacetate.

Treatment of Poisoning   Apparently, most patients who survived poisoning by sodium fluoroacetate as well as those who died of it received no medication that offered any possibility of specific antidotal action. In at least one case (unpublished), a poisoned child was treated with whiskey and survived. Unfortunately, no details are available, and there can be no assurance that the child would not have progressed equally well without treatment.

Although monacetin apparently has not been administered to a human patient, the work of Chenoweth *et al.* (1951) in various animals, especially monkeys, offered good reason to think it would be valuable for treating human poisoning. They recommended that it be injected intramuscularly at least every hour for several hours at the rate of 0.1–0.5 ml/kg per injection. There is no clinical evidence for or against the use of acetate in humans. On the contrary, acetamide has been administered to patients, and it seemed to be the reason for their survival. It is available at Accident and Emergency Departments throughout New Zealand. Acetamide is administered intravenously as a 10% solution in 5% glucose. In severe cases, 500 ml is given in 30 min every 4 hr; in milder cases, 200 ml is given on the same schedule. There can be no doubt that removal of the poison and supportive care are indicated. A number of patients have shown clear-cut poisoning but survived without sequelae following such treatment. Supportive care should include continuous cardiac monitoring. There is strong clinical evidence that the danger of cardiac arrhythmia can be reduced significantly by judicious and continuing use of procainamide hydrochloride. Even so, equipment for defibrillation should be ready. There is reason to hope it would be successful if required because at least one patient was revived with only external massage of the heart. There is also clinical evidence that cortical irritability can be lessened by barbiturates. There is no basis for speculating on the value of diazepam in this connection. Contrary to the evidence in monkeys, clinical evidence in humans has indicated that ethanol is beneficial and perhaps superior to barbiturates. Whereas the effect seemed to involve needed sedation, the possibility of a more fundamental effect in the biochemical lesion was not excluded.

On the basis of laboratory studies, Chenoweth *et al.* (1951) recommended against administration of calcium, potassium, sodium chloride, bicarbonate, or acetate. They considered that any necessary replacement of fluid should be done cautiously with plasma, and they considered digitalization as definitely contraindicated. However, clinical experience argues strongly against two of this prohibitions, and there is no clinical evidence to support some of the others. Calcium gluconate has proved useful in controlling carpopedal spasm, including such spasm in a patient who survived whithout sequelae. Digitalis (lanatoside C) not only improved the function of a poisoned heart that had failed to the point of acute pulmonary edema but also produced no detectable side effects.

Finally, there is clinical evidence that mephentermine is more effective than levarterenol in raising blood pressure if that becomes necessary in the course of poisoning by sodium fluoroacetate.

83.2.2 FLUOROACETAMIDE

83.2.2.1 Identity, Properties, and Uses

Chemical Name 2-Fluoroacetamide is the chemical name.

Structure See Fig. 83.1.

Synonyms Fluoroacetamide is also known as Compound 1081. Trade names for fluoroacetamide include Fuorakil®, Fussol®, Megarox®, and Yancock®. The CAS registry number is 640.19.7.

Physical and Chemical Properties Fluoroacetamide has the empirical formula C_2H_4FNO and a molecular weight of 77.06. It is a crystalline solid that sublimes on heating but melts at 107–109°C. It is very soluble in water, moderately soluble in acetone, and sparingly soluble in aliphatic and aromatic hydrocarbons.

History, Formulations, and Uses At one times fluoroacetamide was used as a systemic insecticide for scale insects, aphids, and mites on fruits; however, it has been considered too toxic to mammals for commercial use as an insecticide. Its use as a rodenticide was suggested by Chapman and Phillips in 1995. It is used as a bait (20 gm active ingredient/kg) in areas to which the public have no access, such as sewers and locked warehouses. It is formulated as dyed cereal-based bait which is mixed with water for use.

83.2.2.2 Toxicity in Laboratory Animals

Basic Findings Fluoroacetamide is a compound of moderate to high acute toxicity depending on the species (see Table 83.2). In the WHO Recommended Classification of Pesticides by Hazards (World Health Organization, 1986), the technical material is listed in class IB, "Highly hazardous."

The compound is absorbed by the skin (Phillips and Worden, 1957). Animals acutely poisoned by this compound show listlessness, irritability, chronic convulsions, abasia, piloerection, and irregular respiration (Araki, 1972). One characteristic usually observed in animals dying from acute poisoning with fluoroacetamide as well as with sodium fluoroacetate is postmortem rigidity (Bentley and Greaves, 1960). Death generally

Table 83.2
Single-Dose LD 50 for Fluoroacetamide

Species	Route	LD 50 (mg/kg)	Reference
Rat	oral	15	Phillips and Worden (1957)
Rat	oral	13	Bentley and Greaves (1960)
Rat	dermal	20[a]	Phillips and Worden (1957)
Mouse	oral	30.62	Araki (1972)
Mouse	subcutaneous	34.20	Araki (1972)
Mouse	intraperitoneal	85	Matsumura and O'Brien (1963)
Rabbit	oral	1.5–2.0	Phillips and Worden (1957)
Rabbit	intravenous	0.25	Buckle *et al.* (1949)
Chicken	oral	4.25	Egyed and Shlosberg (1977)

[a]Lowest lethal dose.

occurs in coma after convulsions have stopped (Phillips and Worden, 1957). There is no obvious difference in susceptibility between the sexes (Bentley and Greaves, 1960). The time that elapses between dosing and the onset of convulsions appears to be related to the dosage level, and fluoroacetamide affects behavior (Bentley and Greaves, 1960). Subacutely poisoned animals show anorexia, emaciation, and alopecia (Araki, 1972).

Perhaps because of strain differences, investigations have reported slightly different thresholds for the largest repeated dosage tolerated by rats without clinical signs. As discussed later, the threshold for testicular injury is much lower. Phillips and Worden (1957) found that 3 mg/kg/day for 20 days was without effect on appetite or general health. Mazzanti *et al.* (1964) found similar results in rats on a dietary level of 50 ppm (about 2.5 mg/kg/day for 90 days). However, Steinberger and Sud (1970) reported that this same dietary level caused a reduction of food intake and of growth.

The poisoning of farm animals by effluent from a factory that manufactured fluoroacetamide caused the Ministry of Agriculture, Fisheries, and Food to recommend that the compound should not be used as an insecticide in agriculture, for home gardens, or food storage in Great Britain, and it was withdrawn from the market (Allcroft and Jones, 1969; Allcroft *et al.*, 1969; Anonymous, 1964a, b).

Absorption, Distribution, Metabolism, and Excretion   Investigators agree that fluoroacetamide is less toxic than fluoroacetate. This has been attributed to the fact that metabolism of the former compared to the latter is slower (Matsumura and O'Brien, 1963). In fact, Phillips and Worden (1957) reported that they recovered, from the urine or rats receiving fluoroacetamide at a rate of 3 mg/kg/day, 62% of the total intake unmetabolized, and they confirmed the identity of the compound by melting point and mixed melting point. This finding raises the possibility that the toxicity of fluoroacetamide (albeit lower than that of fluoroacetate) is in part inherent and does not depend entirely on metabolism to fluoroacetamide on the rat testis, an effect apparently not reported for fluoroacetate.

Biochemical Effects   Evidence that fluoroacetamide has essentially the same mode of action as sodium fluoroacetate is the finding that mammals poisoned by the amide contain greatly elevated levels of citrate (Allcroft *et al.*, 1969; Egyed and Brisk, 1965; Egyed and Miller, 1971; Egyed and Shlosberg, 1977; Matsumura and O'Brien, 1963). Further evidence is offered by the fact that cockroaches convert fluoroacetamide to fluoroacetate as well as to fluorocitrate, and mouse amidase hydrolyzes fluoroacetamide (Matsumura and O'Brien, 1963).

Effects on Reproduction   Selective destruction of the germinal epithelium of the testes of male rats apparently was reported first by Mazzanti *et al.* (1964), who studied only a single dosage level resulting from a dietary level of 50 ppm. On this diet, the body weight of 150–160 gm rats increased by 88% in 90 days but the testes were reduced to slightly less than one-third of the weight in controls. After 64 days, the tubules were almost completely lacking in seminal cells; only some spermatogonia, the Sertoli cells, and the interstitial cells were apparently undamaged. Peculiar giant cells were observed. It was noted that fluoroacetamide acts first on the more mature cells of the germinal epithelium and not on the cells where mitoses are more numerous. Dividing cells in the intestinal mucosa were undamaged.

In a later study, male rats that received a dietary level of 50 ppm (usually calculated as about 2.5 mg/kg/day but said to be about 3.4 mg/kg/day in these rats) showed a marked morphological change in the nucleus of tep-13 spermatids within 24 hours, and the effects became more pronounced and the entire cell became distorted in 5 days. After 10 days of treatment, earlier-step spermatids showed degenerative changes and giant cell formation. Eventually, even spermatocytes were affected. Androgen secretion by the testis apparently was not affected. Dietary levels of 20, 10, and 5 ppm produced characteristic changes in late-stage spermatids but no effect on spermatocytes. The 5 ppm level had no effect on the weight of the testis of rats fed as long as 28 days, but higher levels led to a marked decrease in weight. Subcutaneous administration of fluoroacetamide at a rate of about 1.0 mg/kg/day produced the characteristic change in stage-13 spermatids within 4 days and a 50% reduction in the weight of the testis in 28 days. Spermatogenesis continued, and spermatocytes and young spermatids remained apparently normal, but late spermatids were distinctly abnormal. Subcutaneous doses of about 0.2, 0.04, and 0.02 mg/kg/day produced little or no change in the weight of the testis and produced progressively less histological injury so that change was barely discernible at the lowest dosages. Thus, the effect of fluoroacetamide on spermatogenesis is specific and not secondary to general toxicity, which (in the form of reduced growth) was evident only at the highest oral dosage (Steinberger and Sud, 1970). Testicular degeneration caused by fluoroacetamide has been confirmed in rats and reported in other species (Egyed, 1973).

Fluoroacetamide at an oral dosage of 15 mg/kg also interferes with reproduction in female mice, whether administered 2 days before or 10 days after fertilization; pregnancy was prolonged, prenatal mortality was increased, and the young suffered from cyanonis, respiratory distress, reduced growth, and decreased survival (Tokavera *et al.*, 1971).

Effects on Wildlife and Nontarget Species   In some countries, fluoroacetamide is used to control field rodents, thus exposing nontarget species to either direct toxic effects by feeding on the baits or secondary effects by feeding on carcasses of rodents killed by the compound. Theses effects have been experimentally studied by Braverman (1979) on several nontarget species such as mongoose (*Herpestes ichneumon*), hyena (*Hyaena hyaena*), snakes, birds, cats, and dogs. This experiment showed a degree of susceptibility of the animals similar to that reported for sodium fluoroacetate; it also confirmed that the dog was the most sensitive species. Some species showed a relative tolerance to direct poisoning; this was the case for barn owls, buzzards, and the black kite.

A secondary poisoning study was done by offering the carnivore carcasses of birds (*Meriones tristrami*) which had fed freely on poisoned grains. The results were quite variable; the mongoose was the most susceptible, whereas the risk of secondary poisoning to birds of prey was not high. An outbreak of poisoning by fluoroacetamide in four greylag geese (*Anser anser*) and teal (*Anas crecca*) has been reported in Israel (Shlosberg *et al.*, 1975). Clinical signs in one goose were described as severe convulsions, incoordinated twisting of the neck, total anemia, prostrating depression, and death.

Treatment of Poisoning in Animals Sodium acetate did not protect rats poisoned by fluoroacetamide. However, when administered as a mixture by mouth at a ratio of 4:1 or 9:1, acetamide raised the LD 50 of fluoroacetamide from 15 to 22 mg/kg. When acetamide was administered by mouth at a dosage of 180 mg/kg within 65 min or less after fluoroacetamide at the otherwise fatal oral dosage of 20 mg/kg, all rats survived. The same was true when the ratio (9:1) remained the same, the delay did not exceed 60 min, and the dosage of poison was as high as 35 mg/kg. However, the antidote was ineffective when the delay was 105 min or greater (Phillips and Worden, 1956). The value of acetamide was confirmed by Hashida (1971).

When administered to rats as a mixture by mouth, L-cysteine hydrochloride was antidotal, raising the LD 50 of fluoroacetamide from 15 to 25 and 30 mg/kg, respectively, at dosage ratios of 4:1 and 9:1 (Phillips and Worden, 1957).

Acetamide at an oral dosage of 2500 mg/kg was also effective in treating chickens when given within 20 min after fluoroacetamide at a dosage of 10 mg/kg (slightly more than twice the LD 50 level). The same dosage given 30 min after the poison or 500 mg/kg given with the poison were ineffective (Egyed and Shlosberg, 1977). In limited tests, neither acetamide nor monoacetin was effective in treating poisoned sheep (Egyed, 1971).

The ineffectiveness of sodium acetate and apparently of monoacetin and the effectiveness of acetamide an L-cysteine as antidotes for poisoning by fluoroacetamide raise the possibility that the effective compounds do not prevent biochemical lesions directly but rather competitively retard the conversion of fluoroacetamide to fluoroacetate and thus permit more time for excretion of unmetabolized fluoroacetamide.

83.2.2.3 Toxicity to Humans

Accidental and Intentional Poisoning At about 11:30 hr, an 18-month-old girl removed a 120-ml bottle of 1% fluoroacetamide from a low drawer in the family kitchen and drank some of the contents. On the advice of a pharmacist, the child was given olive oil, the white of an egg, and milk at about noon and was made slightly sick. The child remained lively and played in the garden until her usual bedtime, 18:30. A about 23:30 that evening the child vomited but was put back to bed when she appeared all right. Apparently the child was not checked until 10:30 hr next morning, when she was found

in a semiconscious state. On a physician's order, she was taken to hospital, but convulsions occurred on the way and the patient arrived about 11:30 hr in a shocked state. The child was given about 10 ml acetamide in water once, 3.7 ml of brandy in water each hour, and symptomatic treatment. She continued to have occasional convulsions and remained unconscious until she died almost 96 hr after ingesting the poison. Both the heart and kidney contained 6.3 mg of organic fluoride per gram of dry tissue; the citrate content (108 ppm in heart and 23.9 ppm in kidney) was not considered significantly high. From the evidence available, it was estimated that the baby had consumed about 300 mg of fluoroacetamide or 23 mg/kg (Great Britain Ministry of Agriculture, Fisheries, and Food, 1961; WHO, 1963).

Treatment of Poisoning Treatment of poisoning by fluoroacetamide should be the same as that for fluoroacetate (see Section 83.2.1.3) with due attention to removal of the poison and general care of the patient. Based on animal studies, rapid and energetic treatment with acetamide is recommended. A dosage of 315 mg/kg was effective in rats, but a much higher dosage was required in chickens. It is of special importance that the first dose be given in the earliest possible moment. Repeated administration was not used in the animal experiments but would appear wise. A combination of intravenous monoacetin (glyceryl monoacetate, 0.55 gm/kg), sodium acetate (0.12 gm/kg), and ethanol (0.12 gm/kg) has also been recommended (Dipalma, 1981). Dipalma also suggested as an alternative course the oral administration of 100 ml of monoacetin plus 500 ml of water every hour for about 2 hr.

Hemoperfusion involving fixed-bed uncoated charcoal was used in one case, but it was not helpful and the patient died (de Torrente *et al.*, 1979).

83.2.3 FLUOROETHANOL

83.2.3.1 Identity, Properties, and Uses

Chemical Name 2-Fluoroethanol is the chemical name.

Structure See Fig. 83.1.

Physical and Chemical Properties Fluoroethanol has the empirical formula C_2H_5OF and a molecular weight of 64.07. It is a solid melting at approximately room temperature (26.5°C). It has a density of 1.091, a boiling point of 103°C and a flash point of 31°C.

Use It is used as a rodenticide.

83.2.3.2 Toxicity to Laboratory Animals

Fluoroethanol is a compound of high acute toxicity, as indicated by an intraperitoneal LD 50 of 5 mg/kg in the rat (Bartlett, 1952). According to Bartlett, fluoroethanol is relatively inactive and its toxicity depends on its oxidation to fluoroacetate by tissued alcohol dehydrogenase.

83.2.3.3 Toxicity to Humans

Three cases of poisoning of workers by fluoroethanol occurred in a chemical plant, in at least two instances as the results of accidental rupture of a container and rapid evaporation of the fluid. A typical patient suffered onset in about 90 min and was discharged from hospital in 4 days. All patients had tremor, severe muscular weakness, nausea, headache, and a slight swelling of the liver. (Hemorrhagic gingivitis in one patient and prediabetic hyperglycemia in another were explained by their past histories and were unrelated to poisoning.) Examination of the other 40 workers in the plant failed to reveal any complaints or clinical finding that could be related to the compound (Colamussi *et al.*, 1970).

There is no specific treatment for subacute poisoning except, of course, complete cessation of exposure. If acute poisoning should occur, it should be treated like poisoning by fluoroacetate (see Section 83.2.1.3).

This compound does not seem to be marketed any longer.

83.3 SUBSTITUTED UREAS

One of the compounds that has been promoted as a rodenticide relatively safe for other mammals is pyriminil, as substituted urea (see Fig. 83.2). It is not clear whether this group of compounds has been explored extensively with a view to selecting the one with the best combination of effectiveness for killing rodents and safety for humans and useful animals. However, it has become apparent that pyriminil and some other substituted ureas are specific poisons for the β cells on the pancreas and, therefore, cause diabetes mellitus. This effect may not be related to the mode of action of pyrimidil as a rodenticide, but it has great bearing on the overall safety of the material.

83.3.1 PYRIMINIL

83.3.1.1 Identity, Properties, and Uses

Chemical Name N-(3-pyridylmethyl)-N'-(4-nitrophenyl)-urea is the chemical name.

Structure See Fig. 83.2.

Synonyms Pyriminil is also known as PNU, pyrinuron, and RH-787. It was sold under the trade names Vacor®, Rat Killer®, DLP-787 20% bait, and DLP-787 10% House Mouse Tracking Powder. The CAS registry number is 53558-25-1.

Physical and Chemical Properties Pyriminil has the empiric formula $C_{13}H_{12}N_4O_3$ and a molecular weight of 272.27. It decomposes at 223°C.

History, Formulations, and Uses Pyriminil was introduced in 1975 and developed as an acute rodenticide. It was used to control Norway rats, roof rats, and house mice; it was

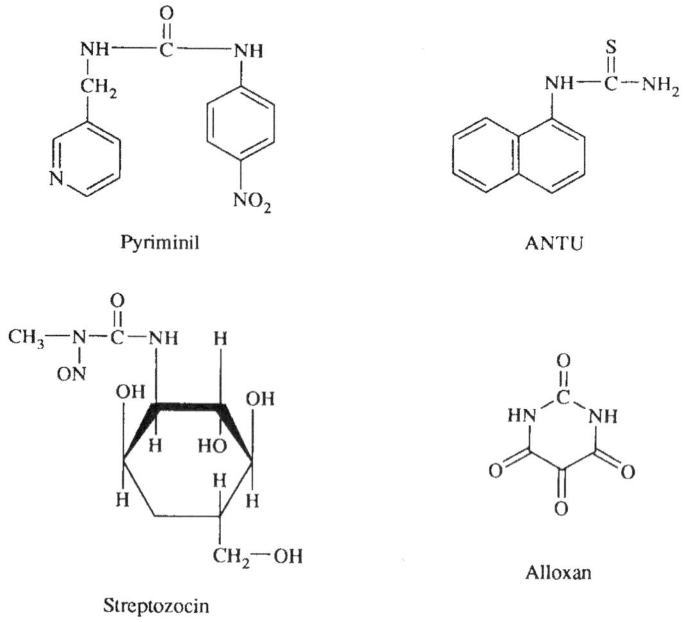

Figure 83.2 ANTU, a thiourea rodenticide, and three substituted ureas known to cause diabetes in one or more species.

especially effective against rodents resistant to anticoagulant poisons. Pyriminil was sold for indoor use only as a prepared bait containing 2% active ingredient and a 10% tracking powder. The product was withdrawn from the market by the U.S. manufacturer in 1979 (Chappelka, 1980), but it is still manufactured on a small scale for local use—in the People's Republic of China, for example.

83.3.1.2 Toxicity in Laboratory Animals

There are greater differences in the susceptibility of different species to pyriminil (technical material) as shown in Table 83.3 (Peardon, 1974).

The marked susceptibility of Norway rats was of course the basis for its use as a rodenticide. Cats also are very susceptible.

Apparently, a good description of the signs of acute poisoning in laboratory animals has not been published. A simple list of signs and symptoms in dogs has been given in the distribution company's technical bulletin. The onset of the symptoms may be delayed 4–48 hr. They include nausea and emesis, depression, initial constriction of pupils followed later by dilated pupils and visual impairment with slow pupillary response to light, ataxia, fine to coarse tremors, hind-limb weakness, decreases reflexes, deep breathing, and dehydration. Similar symptoms have been reported in a horse that had eaten at least 250,000 mg (about 250 mg/kg). The animal showed severe muscular fasciculations, dilated pupils, and profuse sweating within 24 hr after ingestion. Laboratory tests revealed severe hyperglycemia (418 mg/100 ml) and indications of liver injury (elevated liver enzymes). The animal was treated with intravenous nicotinic acid (2.2 mg/kg) followed by four subsequent injections of 1 gm and recovered; it was considered clinically normal 3 months later. Three other poisoned horses showed the

Table 83.3
Single-Dose LD 50 for Pyrimidil in Various Species

Species	Sex	Oral LD 50 (mg/kg)
Albino rat	M	12.30
Norway rat	M	4.75
Roof rat	M	18.00
Cotton rat	M, F	20–60
Albino mouse	M	84
House mouse	M	98
Deer mouse	M	10–20
Guinea pig	M	30–100
Rabbit	M	300
Dog	M	500
Cat	M, F	62
Rhesus monkey	M, F	2000–4000
Pig	M	500
Vole	M, F	205
Chicken	M	710
Pigeon	M, F	1780

same signs as well as intense abdominal pain, hind-limb weakness, ataxia, and persistent inappetence (Russell *et al.*, 1978). Peoples and Maddy (1979) have reported without details poisoning in domestic animals (two horses, three cats, and 17 dogs) in California. The case of a 22-kg dog seen eating a full 30-gm packet of Vacor (780 mg active ingredient) is mentioned. Immediately following ingestion, the dog vomited but became blind 2 days later.

Absorption, Distribution, Metabolism, and Excretion Pyriminil is rapidly absorbed by rats, mice, and dogs after oral administration. Blood levels peaked in 1–6 hr, depending on species and site of the radiolabel ^{14}C. Gastrointestinal transit of ^{14}C is more rapid in dogs than in rats. Urinary and fecal excretions are of similar importance in all three species. Tissue distribution of two ^{14}C labels (nitrophenyl and pyridyl) varied, especially in dogs. The liver contained mor of the dose than any other single organ (Deckert *et al.*, 1978a). Rats tolerated, metabolized, and eliminated single or multiple sublethal dosages (5 mg/kg) but were less efficient than dogs in detoxifying dosages in excess of 20 mg/kg. It was concluded that the tolerance of dogs for the compound depended on their efficient hepatic extraction, metabolism, and excretion of it (Deckert *et al.*, 1978b).

Several metabolites of pyriminil have been identified Deckert *et al.* (1978a, 1979). These include aminopyriminil, *p*-aminophenyl urea, *p*-acetamidophenyl urea, *p*-nitroaniline, *p*-phenylenediamine, *p*-acetamidoaniline, nicotinic acid, nicotinuric acid, and nicotinamide. The concentrations of these metabolites varied from one species to another. The presence of the parent compound in rat and human urine suggests that they may be more sensitive to the compound than the dog because of less efficient metabolism (Deckert *et al.*, 1979).

Biochemical Effects Repeated, sublethal doses of pyriminil increased the urinary and fecal excretion of a later dose of the compound tagged with ^{14}C; however, the same animals showed increased hexobarbital sleeping time and other evidence of inhibition of certain liver microsomal enzymes, especially *p*-nitro-anisole *O*-demethylase. Whatever microsomal enzymes are responsible for metabolism of pyriminil are induced by pretreatment with 3-methylcholanthrene, which increases the biliary excretion of the metabolites and decreases pyriminil toxicity 50-fold Deckert *et al.* (1977, 1978a).

Mild pyriminil-induced hyperglycemia was observed in rats; it was also shown to be reversible by insulin (Deckert *et al.*, 1977). The diabetogenic effects of pyriminil were also confirmed in patients poisoned by the product. This effect is the result of a direct toxic action of the β cells of the pancreas. Wilson and Gaines (1983) have demonstrated that pyriminil at concentrations ranging from 10^{-2} to 10^{-5} M preferentially intoxicates rat pancreatic β cells in culture, whithin 1 hr of contact. It was also shown in the study that nicotinamide can reduce pyriminil-induced β cell injury, thus confirming previous findings by Karam *et al.* (1980) that nicotinamide could partially reverse pyriminil inhibition of glucose-stimulated insulin secretion by freshly isolated islets of Langershans from the rat.

In addition to its diabetogenic effect, pyriminil has a direct effect on glucose metabolism. The erythrocytes of patients poisoned by the compound showed a marked depression of glucose consumption as well as decreased uptake of methylene blue in the presence of glucose. In addition, a 0.1 mM concentration *in vitro* caused decreased utilization of glucose and decreased uptake of methylene blue by erythrocytes from normal people and rabbits (Lee and Lee, 1977).

The mechanism of action has been investigated and it was shown that pyriminil specifically inhibits the NADH:ubiquinone reductase activity of complex I in mammalian mitochondria. The activity of other respiratory enzymes of mitochonrai is unaffected at concentrations that completely inhibit the redox and energetic function of complex I. Inhibition of complex I activity quantitatively correlates with the inhibition of insulin release in insulinoma cells and pancreatic islets and is also consistent with the doses reported in cases of human poisoning. These results indicate that the toxic and diabetogenic action of pyriminil primarily derives from the inhibition of mitochondrial respiration of NAD-linked substrates in the high energy demanding pancreatic islets (Esposi *et al.*, 1996).

Treatment of Poisoning in Animals The mechanism of action of pyriminil remains uncertain, but it is of interest that alloxan, streptozotocin, and dithizone, all which can induce diabetes mellitus in experimental animals, are substituted ureas. However, it would appear that some species such as dogs, cats, and laboratory primates are refractory to both the diabetogenic and neurotoxic effects of pyriminil (Karam *et al.*, 1980).

Whereas 6-aminonicotinamide is not a substitute urea, it is toxic to β cells and it is recognized antagonist of nicotinamide (Herken, 1971). Because nicotinamide can prevent the toxic effect of streptozotocin (Ganda *et al.*, 1976), alloxan (Rossini *et al.*, 1975), and *N*-3-pyridylmethl-*N'*-4nitrophenyl urea (Deckert *et al.*, 1977), it seems possible that all of these compounds act as nicotinamide antagonists.

83.3.1.3 Toxicity to Humans

Accidental and Intentional Poisoning There are many reports on human poisoning in the literature describing the main clinical and laboratory features of those poisonings.

A 25-year-old man with a history of psychiatric disturbances attempted suicide by injecting an unknown amount of pulverized methaqualone tablets and ingesting two packets of rat poison, each containing 737 mg of pyriminil. Seven days later he was admitted to a local hospital for treatment of a staphylococal abscess of the left antecubital fossa. He received antibiotics and had rapid clinical improvement. It was recorded that since attempting suicide the patient had noticed lassitude, anorexia, abdominal bloating, constipation, and the onset of painful paresthesia with numbness of this legs and difficulty in walking. A random plasma glucose level on admission was 309 mg/100 ml, and check samples taken on subsequent days were slightly higher. Ketones and glucose were present in the urine. On the fourth hospital day, insulin therapy was started. The diabetes gradually was controlled, although tolerance for carbohydrate and need for insulin were erratic. An upper gastrointestinal tract series done on the tenth hospital day showed gastric and proximal small bowel hypomobility bordering on atony. The patient was discharged on hospital day 19 on a regimen of insulin and temporary thoridiazine.

The patient remained well for 16 days and then returned because of nausea and vomiting. He was found to have severe autonomic and peripheral polyneuropathy characterized by orthostatic hypotension, greatly diminished response to pinprick and vibratory sensation in the lower extremities, and other changes. Although the diabetes was now better controlled, the serum sodium was low (116 mEq/liter), and the syndrome of inappropriate antidiuretic hormone was demonstrated. The hyponatremia responded to fluid restriction, and the orthostatic hypotension was improved by support stockings.

Ten months after the suicide attempt, the patient experienced two episodes of weakness and lethargy that were relieved by eating. He had lost about 18 kg and appeared cachetic (45 kg, 174 cm) but alert and well oriented. His gait was ataxic and there was substantial muscle wasting. A very thorough examination showed reduced disappearance rate of intravenous glucose and depressed C-peptide response to intravenous glucose when compared with a normal control but no impairment of glucagon release after stimulation by intravenous arginine. Nerve conduction studies demonstrated severe sensory and mild motor neuropathy. Quadricep capillary basement membrane thickness was in the diabetic range. Insulin was discontinued and tolbutamide prescribed. Following discharge, the patient regained 5 kg and experienced subjective improvement of his neuropathy (Prosser and Karam, 1978).

Whereas most clinical studies have place greatest emphasis on the diabetogenic action of pyriminil, its injury to the nervous system was no less remarkable, as emphasized in a paper by LeWitt (1980a). This injury often involved autonomic impairment (postural hypotension often severe enough to cause fainting when the patient sat up, impaired pupillary responses, impotence, decreased sweating, urinary retention, dysphagia, and gastrointestinal hypomobility), peripheral neuropathy (loss of muscle-stretch reflexes, sensory loss, neurogenic myopathy), and encephalopathic and dyskinetic features (loss of cortical function ranging from confusion to coma, cerebellar ataxia, tremor, motor hyperactivity, nystagmus, and diffuse electroencephalographic changes). In addition, some cases involved chest or epigastric pain and some showed ischemic electrocardiographic changes. Cardiac arrhythmias were occasionnally the cause of death. Neurological disorders often appeared within hours after ingestion. Occasionally, onset was delayed or insidious. Symptoms related to different parts of the nervous system began and later improved at different times in the same patient, and the order of progression varied from case to case. Neurological improvement took many months, and full recovery was uncommon, orthostatic hypotension in particular tending to persist. Causes of delayed death included inanition, sepsis, aspiration pneumonia, and insulin-induced hypoglycemia.

Accidental ingestion of pyriminil by a 25-month-old boy resulted in acute vomiting, lethargy, seizures, hypoglycemia (followed by hypreglycemia and glucose intolerance), and autonomic and peripheral neuropathy (Johnson *et al.*, 1980).

A review of reports unpublished in 1978 indicated 7 deaths and 2 nonfatal cases in Korea and 4 fatal and 11 nonfatal cases in the United States. At least in the United States, all the cases were in adults; all but one were attempted suicide; all the survivors developed diabetes mellitus and autonomic nervous system dysfunction, chiefly dysphasia, dystonia, and bowel and bladder dysfunction. Hypothermia and paresthesias were seen. A later review revealed nearly 90 cases in the United States and over 250 in Korea (Frethold *et al.*, 1980).

A case of acute poisoning (approximately 67 mg/kg) in a 42-year-old man with all the signs already described but characterized by a severe orthostatic hypotension with full spontaneous recovery 11 months after hospitalization was reported by Osterman *et al.* (1981). Gallanosa *et al.* (1981) have compared the main features of four cases reported with enough details in the literature with those of one case of their own.

Dosage Response A dose as low as 780 mg was fatal within 150 days. A dose of 2340 mg was fatal within 1 day, but a patient survived 40 days after ingesting 7020 mg. One patient survived 2340 mg, and at least two survived 1560 mg but not without characteristic, persistent illness. The smallest dose known to have produced characteristic illness was 390 mg (about 5.6 mg/kg) (LeWitt, 1980b).

Laboratory Findings The most important findings for guiding treatment and often for diagnosis include nearly transient hypoglycemia followed by persistent hyperglycemia, glycosuria, ketosis, and elevation of serum amylase and lipase activities. *p*-Nitroaniline at a concentration of 5.1 ppm has been reported in the liver of a person who died after accidentally ingesting pyriminil (Osteryoung *et al.*, 1977). In the case of a 7-year-old boy who was found dead a day after another child saw him ingest a packet of pyriminil, unchanged compound at a concentration of 1.5 ppm was found in the urine hydrolysate and two metabolites were found in the liver and some other samples. Aminopyriminil (nitro group metabolized to an amine) was found at concentrations of 5.6, 1.4, 0.3, and 0.6 ppm in liver, kidney, spleen, and urine, respectively. Acetamidopyriminil (amino group conjugated with acetic acid) was found in traces in the blood and liver (Frethold *et al.*, 1980).

Karam *et al.* (1980) reported (in addition to the clinical features) autopsy findings from several cases of acute poisoning, including that of a 7-year-old boy. All three cases showed extensive islet degeneration of the pancreatic tissue with generalized destruction of β cells and sparing of α and Δ cells as well as of the exocrine glandular tissue.

Islet-cell surface antibodies were detected in four of the six reported cases. It may be that these antibodies are the result rather than the cause of β-cell destruction.

Pathology   Loss of β cells of the pancreas has been observed generally in persons killed by pyriminil (Frethold *et al.*, 1980; Karam *et al.*, 1980; LeWitt, 1980a; Prosser and Karam, 1978). Lesions of the nervous system have not been found so regularly. In one case reported by LeWitt (1980a), no lesions of the central or peripheral nervous system were found; in another case, cerebral edema and neuropathic changes restricted to the sensory spinal roots were found. Autopsy of a 39-year-old man who survived 19 days revealed (*a*) severe loss of ganglion cells and rare degenerating neurons in the paravertebral sympathetic ganglia, (*b*) marked loss of neurons in the sensory spinal ganglia with multiple residual nodules of Nageotte, (*c*) marked degeneration of the sensory roots and posterior columns, (*d*) slight perivascular lymphatic infiltrates in both the sympathetic and sensory ganglia, (*e*) swelling of nerve fibers and thinning of the myelin sheaths of the sural nerve, and (*f*) isolated degenerated and regenerating fibers in the skeletal muscles (Papasozomenos, 1980).

Treatment of Poisoning   Patients who develop diabetes mellitus clearly must be treated for that condition in the usual way. There is good reason from animal experiments to believe that diabetes could be prevented if the patient were given large, repeated doses of nicotinamide beginning promptly after ingestion of the poison. However, cases have ended in diabetes and neuropathy when nicotinamide was started 9 and 14 hr, respectively, after ingestion. Nicotinamide was considered possibly beneficial in the case of an infant, even through administration was started something over 12 hr after ingestion of pyriminil (Johnson *et al.*, 1980). However, the fact that the child received the poison "on a piece of gum" offered by another child suggests that the initial dose was small, and complete recovery may have been due to that fact alone (Pont *et al.*, 1979).

The dose and duration of the treatment with nicotinamide are still uncertain (Anonymous, 1979). Nicotinic acid has also been tried as an antidote (Pont *et al.*, 1979), but its use is contraindicated because (*a*) it is toxic in humans, (*b*) it protects animals only against alloxan and not streptozotocin (Ganda *et al.*, 1976), and (*c*) its vasodilatory effects may complicate the control of blood pressure.

Cases that require insulin may progress so that insulin is no longer required but the patient can be maintained on sulfonylureas.

83.4 THIOUREAS

The development of ANTU as a poison for adult Norway rats was described by Richter (1945). The entire development was a result of a chance observation associated with studying the taste of phenylthiourea, which is bitter to most people but tasteless to a few who inherit this specific lack of sensation as a Mendelian recessive trait. When an attempt was made to explore this taste difference in animals, it was found that if a few crystals were placed on the tongues of rats, all of them died overnight. The wide and prolonged use of phenylthiourea for taste and inheritance tests without any untoward effect indicated its safety for humans, whereas the results in rats suggested that it might serve as a rat poison. Further study revealed that rats detect and reject phenylthiourea too effectively for it to be practical as poison. This led to a systematic search of other thiourea derivatives with high toxicity but little or no taste. All monosubstituted thiourea derivatives tested produced pulmonary edema and pleural effusion in the laboratory rat (Dieke *et al.*, 1947). The toxicity of thiourea to wild Norway rats was enhanced by a single aromatic substitution on one of the nitrogen atoms. Two or more substitutions on one or both nitrogen atoms lowered the toxicity, as was also true of substitution on the sulfur atom. ANTU was chosen as the most suitable compound.

Although the dog is susceptible to ANTU, most animals, including monkeys, are resistant. This offered the hope that humans would be resistant also, and extensive field trials in areas of Baltimore led to no toxic symptoms either in workers or in the over 500,000 persons living in the treated areas (Richter, 1945).

A disadvantage of ANTU as a rodenticide is that young Norway rats and roof rats of all ages are too resistant to the compound for it to be practical for their control. Another disadvantage is the prompt appearance of both tolerance and bait refusal in adult Norway rats that have received a nonfatal dose. Tolerance is completely lost within 30 days, but refusal may last longer (Richter (1945, 1946). Gaines and Hayes (1952) found that bait shyness lasted at least 4 months under field conditions.

Several interesting observations were made during the survey of thioureas. All of these compounds produce hyperplasia of the thyroid gland. Whereas nonlethal doses of unsubstituted thiourea have little effect on pigmentation or hair growth, phenylthiourea destroys pigment both in the skin and in the hair but without affecting growth of the hair, and ANTU completely stops pigment production and growth of hair. Withdrawal of the substituted thioureas is followed in less than 10 days by recovery of pigment and hair growth. Finally, different strains of Norway rats on different diets showed thiourea LD 50 values as different as 4 and 1830 mg/kg. The difference was modified but not eliminated by placing the rats on the same diet as that of the most susceptible ones. Age differences in the susceptibility of Norway rats to thiourea are similar to those with ANTU (Dieke and Richter, 1945; Richter, 1945).

83.4.1 ANTU

83.4.1.1 Identity, Properties, and Uses

Chemical name 1-(1-Naphthyl)-2-thiourea is the chemical name.

Structure See Fig. 83.2.

Synonyms ANTU, an acronym for α-naphthylthiourea, is the approved common name (BSI, ISO) for this compound. Trade names include Anturat®, Bantu®, Kill Kantz®, Krysid®, Rattrak®, and Rat-tu®. Code designations for ANTU include Chemical-109 and U-5227. The CAS registry number is 86-88-4.

Physical and Chemical Properties ANTU has the empirical formula $C_{11}H_{10}N_2S$ and a molecular weight of 202.27. Pure

ANTU forms colorless crystals and the technical grade is a gray crystalline powder with a bitter taste. Its melting point is 198°C (pure). Its solubility in water at 25°C is 0.06 gm/100 ml; in acetone, 2.43 gm/100 ml; and in triethylene glycol, 8.6 gm/100 ml (technical).

History, Formulations, and Uses ANTU was discovered as a rodenticide in 1945. The formulations include baits (10–30 gm/kg) and tracking powders (200 gm/kg). It is used specifically against the Norway rat. In some countries it has been withdrawn from use because of the carcinogenicity of β-naphthylamines present as impurities (Worthing and Walker, 1983).

83.4.1.2 Toxicity in Laboratory Animals

Basic Findings Different investigators have been in good agreement about the acute oral toxicity of ANTU to Norway rats. Dieke and Richter (1945) and Lehman (1951, 1952) found oral LD 50 values of 6.9 and 6 mg/kg, respectively. There is a wide variation in susceptibility among different species, especially to intraperitoneal administration (see Table 83.4). The Norway rat is particularly susceptible, the young being slightly more resistant than the adults.

Absorption, Distribution, Metabolism, and Excretion Early studies on the metabolism of phenylthiourea and of

Table 83.4
Single-Dose LD 50 for ANTU[a]

Species	Route	LD 50 (mg/kg)	Reference
Rat	intraperitoneal	10	Boyd and Neal (1976)
Rat	intraperitoneal	7	Lisella *et al.* (1971)
Rat	intraperitoneal	5	DuBois *et al.* (1947)
Norway, domestic I	intraperitoneal	2.5	
Norway, domestic II	intraperitoneal	6.25	
Norway, wild, adult	intraperitoneal	6.20–8.10	
Norway, wild, young	intraperitoneal	16–58	
Alexandrine	intraperitoneal	250	
Norway, wild	oral	6.9	
Mouse	intraperitoneal	56	
Rabbit	intraperitoneal	400	
Guinea pig	intraperitoneal	140	DuBois *et al.* (1947)
Guinea pig	intraperitoneal	350	
Dog	intraperitoneal	16	
Dog	dermal	38	
Cat	oral	500	
Monkey	intraperitoneal	175	
Monkey	oral	4250	
Chicken	intraperitoneal	2500	
Chicken	oral	4250	

[a]From IARC (1983).

diphenylthiourea suggest the basis of the toxicity of monosubstituted thioureas. It was shown by Dieke *et al.* (1947) that the oral LD 50 of the phenyl compound is 8.6 mg/kg, whereas a dosage of 2000 mg/kg of the diphenyl compound did not produce illness. Both rats and rabbits excrete little phenylthiourea as compounds with the —C=S group intact (Carroll and Noble, 1949; Williams, 1959). In rabbits, the proportion of such compounds was only about 12%, but the corresponding proportion was about 70–80% for diphenylthiourea. These observations suggest that toxicity was associated with desulfuration *in vivo* (Williams, 1959). It has been speculated that ANTU acts on the lung by the release of hydrogen sulfide (Petit *et al.*, 1970), but this seems highly unlikely because rats rendered tolerant to ANTU are not tolerant to hydrogen sulfide (or carboxyl sulfide or phosgene) (Carroll and Noble, 1949).

Biochemical Effects By using a mixture of ^{35}S- and ^{14}C-labeled ANTU, it was possible to show that some of the sulfur and a smaller proportion of the carbon were covalently bound to macromolecules of the lung and liver following *in vivo* administration. By contrast, practically no radioactive carbon was bound when an equal amount of the almost nontoxic, ^{14}C-labeled oxygen analog of ANTU (α-[^{14}C]naphthylurea) was administered. In the presence of NADPH, ANTU was metabolized by either lung or liver microsomes *in vitro* in such a way that the rates of binding of ^{35}S or ^{14}C to macromolecules of the microsomes were greater than those associated with boiled microsomes or with normal microsomes without NADPH. Binding in the presence of active enzyme and NADPH was covalent and accompanied by a decrease in the level of cytochrome P-450 detectable as its carbon monoxide complex. Pretreatment of rats at the rate of 2 mg/kg/day for 5 days produced a decrease of their microsomal enzyme activity as measured by metabolism of parathion. All such pretreated rats survived a dosage of ANTU (10 mg/kg) which killed 6 to 10 controls, and binding of ^{35}S by proteins of the liver and especially the lungs of the pretreated animals was less than that of the controls. Pretreatment with 4-ipomeanol protected all rats from an otherwise uniformly fatal dose of [^{35}S]ANTU and cause a slight reduction of covalent binding of ^{35}S to lung (but not liver) proteins. Finally, rats pretreated with dimethylmaleate, which depletes tissue stores of glutathione, were killed by ANTU at 5 mg/kg, a dosage which was harmless to controls. In every instance, rats killed by ANTU showed a hydrothorax of at least 4 ml, whereas those protected by pretreatment with ANTU or ipomeanol developed no hydrothorax. These findings were interpreted as evidence that (*a*) the toxicity of ANTU depends on metabolic activation and on covalent binding of the reactant(s) to lung macromolecules and (*b*) tolerance to ANTU is the result of inhibition of microsomal enzymes and consequent reduction in the metabolic activation of a challenge dose (Boyd and Neal, 1976). An extension of this reasoning would attribute the normal tolerance of young Norway rats to ANTU to their relative lack of microsomal enzyme activity.

Further study showed that about half of the atomic sulfur released from ANTU reacted with cysteine side chains of mi-crosomal protein to form a hydrodisulfide. The other moiety released by microsoma enzymes is α-naphthylurea (Lee *et al.*, 1960).

Effects on Organs and Tissues ANTU induced reverse mutations in *Salmonella typhimurium* strain TA1538 in the presence but not in the absence of Arocolor- or phenobarbital-induced rat liver microsomal preparations. A preparation purified by thin-layer chromatography was as active as a technical grade material, thus excluding the attribution of activity to impurities. ANTU also transformed Syrian hamster embryo cells *in vitro* without the addition of an activating system (Kawalec *et al.*, 1979).

ANTU was tested for carcinogenicity (Fitzburg and Nelson, 1947) in mice (Innes *et al.*, 1969) by administration in the diet. No tumor was reported in either study, but the International Agency for Research of Cancer (IARC) (1983) found that both studies were inadequate to evaluate the carcinogenicity of ANTU to experimental animals.

Pathology As far as the rat lung is concerned, ANTU causes marked edema of the subepithelial spaces of the alveolar walls without erosion or other damage to type I and type II epithelial cells. Thus, edema caused by ANTU differs morphologically and presumably in mechanism from that produced by injection of epinephrine or by an injection of a mixture of fibrinogen and thrombin into the cerebrospinal cistern (Hatakeyama and Shigei, 1971). The edema caused by intraperitoneal ANTU in rats is dosage-related in the range of 3–50 mg/kg. Although interstitial edema was the first observable change, bleeding and scalloping of endothelial cells were observed within 2 hr, and epithelial damage was apparent electron microscopically within 6 hr following 50 mg/kg. The injury was apparently similar to but more rapid than that caused by 99% oxygen at 1 atmosphere pressure (Meyrick *et al.*, 1972). Not only pulmonary edema but also pleural effusion shows a dosage–response relationship (Sobonya and Kleinerman, 1973).

Using a different approach, Böhm (1973) demonstrated changes which he interpreted as indicating increased permeability to colloidal carbon in the pulmonary arteriodes as well as capillaries and venules of rats within 3.25 hr after an intraperitoneal injection of ANTU at a rate of 10 mg/kg.

In anesthetized sheep given 20, 50, 75, or 100 mg/kg ANTU intravenously, the first phase of the response consisted of transient increases in pulmonary artery pressure and plasma and lymph thromboxane B$_2$ concentrations. These changes were not dependent on the dose of ANTU administered. At 2–4 hr after administration, pulmonary artery pressure and thromboxane concentrations were normal or near normal. ANTU produces a two-phase response with the steady state characterized by a dose-dependent increase in lung microvascular permeability (Havill *et al.*, 1982). These authors, on the basis of experimental results in sheep, suggest that the severe pulmonary hypertension that follows ANTU administration may be mediated by vasoconstrictor products of arachidonic acid metabolism and that the complement or coagulation systems may be involved as well, resulting in pulmonary microemboli.

O'Brien *et al.* (1985) have reported that isolated lungs from rats treated 4 hr earlier with ANTU had decreased conversion of angiotension I to angiotension II and that the extent of decrease was related to the dose of ANTU administered and to the perfusate flow rate.

It may be that permeability of membranes of the kidney as well as those of the lung and pleura is increased inasmuch as urinary excretion of albumin occurs (Patil and Radhakrishnamurty, 1977).

Treatment of Poisoning in Animals   Mortality of rats caused by 5 mg/kg of ANTU was reduced when allylthiourea, isopropylthiourea, ethylenethiourea, or ethylidenethiourea was administered simultaneously with or a very short time after the ANTU. The first two compounds reduced the survival time of rats that died, but the last two compounds slightly prolonged it (Meyer and Saunders, 1949). Although the reduction in mortality was statistically significant, the degree of protection was small. Furthermore, these results in the rat may be more closely related to the phenomenon of tolerance than to antidotal action in the usual sense. In any event, Carroll and Noble (1949) found that tolerance to phenylthiourea and ANTU could be produced not only by small dosages of the compounds themselves but also by a number of related and some apparently unrelated compounds. The ability of the effective thiourealike substances to confer protection was unrelated to their acute toxicities ot antithyroid activities. Protected rats failed to develop pulmonary edema or pleural effusion following dosages of toxic thioureas lethal to untreated rats. Thyroidectomized rats could be made tolerant as readily as intact rats. Following a large dose, phenylthiourea was excreted in the urine of a tolerant rat in sufficient quantity to kill a normal animal.

83.4.1.3 Toxicity to Humans

Accidental and Intentional Poisoning   The absence of a report of uncomplicated poisoning is noteworthy in view of the extensive use of ANTU in Baltimore and some other places and the fact that an occasional bait must have been eaten by children.

Several series of cases were reported from France, where chloralose was used either alone for killing crows or rats or in combination with ANTU for killing rats. In one series of 22 cases, all showed some degree of coma and motor agitation, both characteristic of chloralose poisoning; however, more intense pulmonary symptoms were present where ANTU was involved. The low toxicity of ANTU for humans is indicated by the fact that all the patients recovered, although all had ingested the poison with suicidal intent and, therefore, in relatively high dosages (Tempé and Kurtz, 1972). In another series of cases involving chloralose, 14 involved ANTU also, 1 involved chloralose only, and the presence of or absence of ANTU was not established in the remainder. In addition to the respiratory difficulty that may be present with any coma, 11 of

the 14 persons poisoned by a combination of chloralose and ANTU required intubation mainly because of tracheobronchial hypersecretion, and 9 of them required artificial respiration. All survived (Favarel-Garrigues and Boget, 1968). The authors characterized the beginning of tracheobronchial hypersecretion as a secretory storm that started early and sometimes suddenly. The secretion was a white froth that, unlike edema fluid, was not sticky or high in protein. The mildness of X-ray changes contrasted with the clinical gravity of the situation. Oxygenation of the blood was always more nearly complete than in acute pulmonary edema. The hypersecretion disappeared rapidly, often in less than an hour. Apparently, if patients poisoned by a combination of chloralose and ANTU are treated properly, their illness is no more protracted than in poisoning by chloralose alone (see Section 83.1).

Use Experience   Laubstein (1962) reported a case of eczema that he attributed to occupational exposure to ANTU.

On the basis that β-naphthylamine is an impurity in ANTU, Case (1966a) raised the possibility that persons who distribute ANTU may be in danger of bladder cancer. No epidemiological evidence was offered. Later, Case (1966b) mentioned that an investigation of the occupational history of two rodent operators who were suffering from bladder tumors had revealed that different batches of ANTU differed in the degree of contamination with naphthylamine, and some of the contaminant was β-naphthylamine. As a result, the Ministry of Agriculture, Fisheries, and Food recommended in May 1966 that the use of ANTU be restricted to professional operators, and in November 1966 an advisory committee recommended that use of the compound stop until their investigation was complete (Anonymous, 1966).

In 1982, Davis *et al.* reported 14 cases of urothelial tumors observed among 51 rodent operatives exposed to ANTU in the United Kingdom between 1961 and 1980.

In the United States as a whole, the age-adjusted death rate for cancer of the bladder increased from 3.1 to 4.1 per 100,000 from 1931 to 1945, when ANTU was discovered, and it continued to increase more slowly until 1953, when it reached 4.4. Since 1953 the values have varied around slightly over 4.3 as a mean. The *declining* increase in rate from 1945 to 1953 occupied a period less than the average latent period for cancer of the bladder among men with heavy exposure to naphthylamine used in the manufacture of dyes. Thus there is no evidence for any carcinogenic action of ANTU in the general population. Because ANTU had been used so extensively in Baltimore, as described by Richter and his colleagues, the matter was investigated here. Because of the wide fluctuations in rates based on small frequencies, it was not practical to compare death rates for single years; therefore, the data were combined for 3-year periods. For 1949–1965, the rate per 100,000 population varied from the earliest value of 4.4 to 2.9 with no definite trend but certainly with no increase.

Dosage Response   The threshold limit value is 0.3 mg/m³ of air over an 8-hr work shift (OSHA standard).

Treatment of Poisoning   If treatments were required, it would have to be symptomatic.

83.5 ANTI-VITAMIN K COMPOUNDS

As reviewed by Link (1944, 1959), knowledge of the anti-vitamin K compounds began not with vitamin K but with hemorrhagic disease of cattle, which was first recognized in the 1920s on the prairies of North Dakota and neighboring Alberta. It was found that the condition was not caused by a microorganism or a nutritional deficiency but was associated with sweet clover that had gone bad. Hence the condition was known as "sweet clover poisoning." When cattle or sheep had improperly cured hay made from the common varieties of sweet clover (*Melilotus* spp.) as their only food, the clotting power of their blood decreased in about 15 days and they often died of internal hemorrhage in 30–50 days. If the disease had not progressed too far, it could be reversed by substituting good hay or by transfusion of blood freshly drawn from normal cattle. Link first learned of the problem in December 1932. During the following February, a Wisconsin farmer came to his laboratory with a dead heifer, a milk can containing blood with no power to clot, 100 pounds of spoiled sweet clover and the all too common, tragic story of cattle dying on an isolated farm.

In Link's laboratory, a practical bioassay for hemorrhagic effect was developed. It was not until June 1939 that the active poison was isolated and crystallized. Using improved methods of isolation developed after the identity of the compound was known, it was shown that the compound was present in spoiled hay at a concentration of about 60 ppm. The structure was shown to be 3,3'-methylene-bis(4-hydroxycoumarin), later known as dicoumarol or by the trade name Dicumarol®, and it was synthetized in April 1940. The biological synthesis during spoilage of the hay can be rationalized as an oxidation of coumarin (the compound responsible for the characteristic sweet smell and bitter taste of sweet clover) and the subsequent condensation of two molecules of 4-hydroxycoumarin with formaldehyde (see Fig. 83.3).

When synthetic dicoumarol became available in quantity, the essentials of its pharmacological action were established quickly. Between 1940 and 1942, it was rapidly adopted for treatment of thromboembolic disease in humans. About 50 clinical reports were published between 1941 and 1944.

In 1942, Link himself set up field trials to test the suitability of dicoumarol as a rat poison. Tests by O'Connor (1948) using a concentration of 0.44 mg/g were reported as highly successful. However, tests carried out by the U.S. Public Health Service (Hayes and Gaines, 1950) led to the same conclusion as those of Link: that dicoumarol was impractical as a rat poison.

While the medical and possible rodenticidal uses of dicoumarol were being explored, over 100 analogs of the compounds were synthesized in Link's laboratory; they were arranged according to chemical classification and assigned numbers by Overman *et al.* (1944). In the hope of finding a therapeutic agent other than dicoumarol, the anticoagulant activity

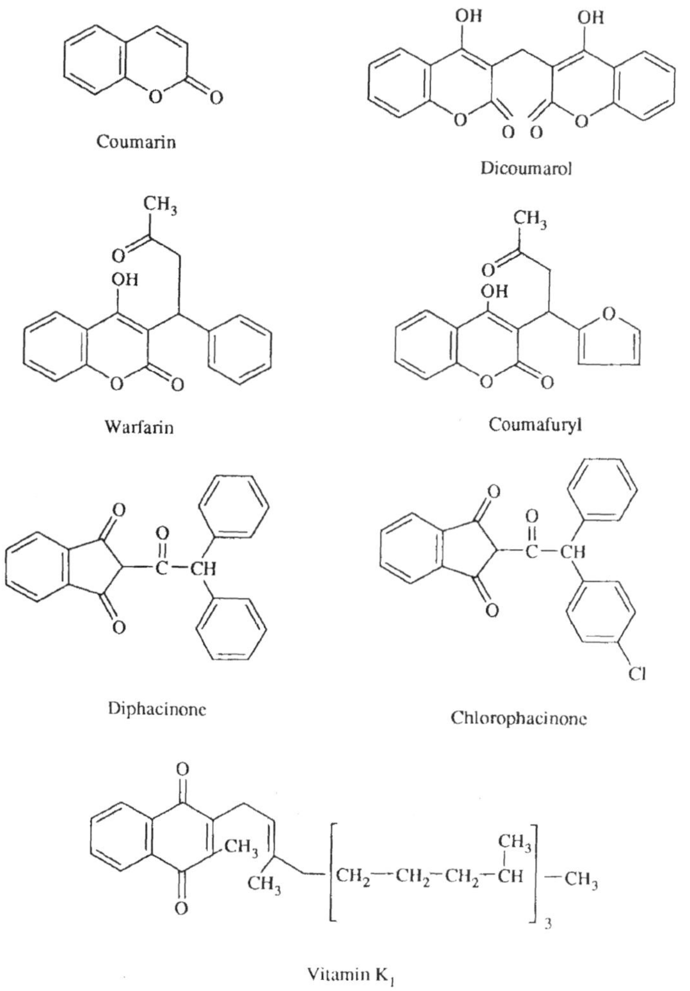

Figure 83.3   Coumarin, dicoumarol, some synthetic rodenticides, and a natural form of vitamin K.

of some of those analogs was reappraised using not only rabbits (the specie used to detect the hemorrhagic agent of sweet clover poisoning) but also rats, mice, and dogs. Work between 1946 and 1948 identified compounds No. 42 and No. 63 as much more potent than dicoumarol in the rat and dog and as capable of producing a more uniform anticoagulant response and of maintaining a more severe hypoprothrombinemia without visible bleeding than was possible with dicoumarol. Partly on the basis of these observations and partly on the basis of lack of taste and odor, ease of manufacturing the pure compound, and convertibility to a stable water-soluble salt, compound No. 42 was selected.

Early in 1948 it was proposed as a rondenticide and promoted by the Wisconsin Alumni Research Foundation. It soon became evident that compound 42 was an important rodenticide.

Link (1959) recalled that, although late in 1950 he proposed warfarin for clinical trial, fear of using a highly successful rat poison as a drug prevented significant progress until April 1951, when knowledge of an unsuccessful suicide effectively treated

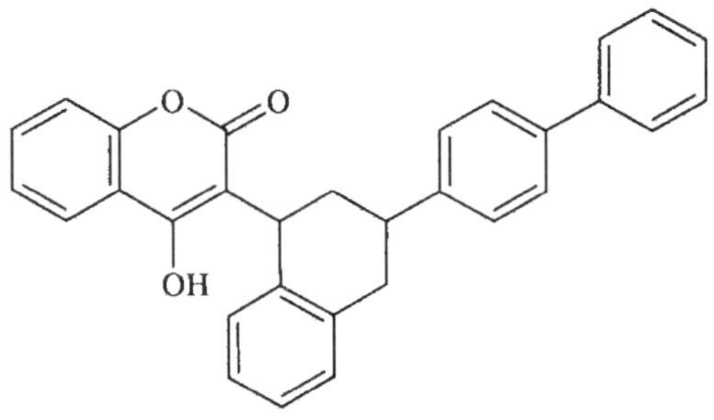

Difenacoum

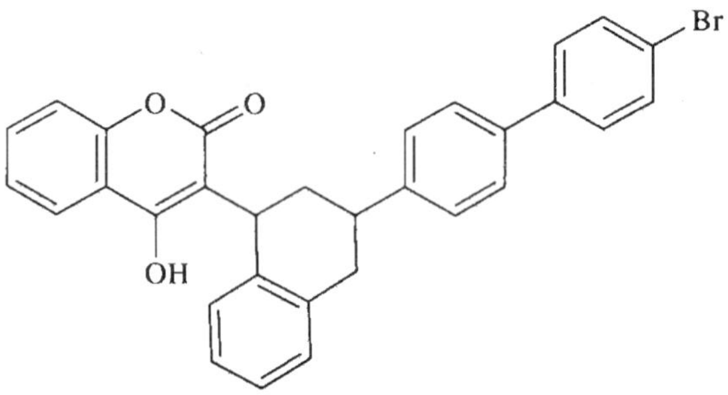

Brodifacoum

Figure 83.4

by vitamin K and transfusion of fresh whole blood (Holmes and Love, 1952) brought reassurance. Progress was so rapid that warfarin was used in 1955 for treating then-President Eisenhower.

The use of Dicumarol as a drug and the use of warfarin as a drug and as a rodenticide did not go unnoticed by those who sought a compound even more effective than warfarin—and free of patent restrictions. The result was a number of alternative compounds available either as drugs or rotenticides, or, in the case of diphacinone, used like warfarin for both purposes.

The appearance of rats resistant to warfarin and to other early anticoagulant rodenticides has stimulated the search for more potent, fast-acting compounds. These are usually called "single-dose-rodenticides" or "second-generation" anticoagulants, among which difenacoum and brodifacoum are coumarin derivatives (Fig. 83.4).

Coumarin compounds are relatively free of untoward effects when used therapeutically and have been given for long periods without signs of toxicity.

83.5.1 WARFARIN

83.5.1.1 Identity, Properties, and Uses

Chemical Name   3(α-acetonylbenzyl)-4-hydroxycoumarin is the chemical name.

Structure   See Fig. 83.3.

Synonyms   The name warfarin (BSI, ICPC, ISO) is in common use except in France, where the compound is called cumafène; in Russia, where it is called zoocoumarin; and in Japan, where it and coumatetralyl both are spoken of as coumarins (JMAF). During development, warfarin was known as Compound-42 or WARF-42. As a drug, the sodium salt is called Coumadin®. Trade names for the rodenticide have included Arthrombine-K®, Dethmore®, and Panwartin®. The CAS registry number is 81-81-2.

Physical and Chemical Properties   Warfarin has the empirical formula $C_{19}H_{16}O_4$ and a molecular weight of 308.32. It forms tasteless, odorless, and colorless crystals with a melting point of 15–161°C. It is practically insoluble in water and benzene, moderately soluble in alcohols, and readily soluble in acetone and dioxane. The sodium salt is fully soluble in water.

History, Formulations, and Uses   The history of warfarin is outlined above. It is formulated as a dust (10 gm of active ingredient per kilogram) for use in holes and runs and as a powder (1 and 5 gm of active ingredient per kilogram) for mixing with bait to a final concentration of 50 ppm for control of the common rat or 250 ppm for control of the ship rat and mice. Warfarin also is available in many forms of prepared bait.

83.5.1.2 Toxicity to Laboratory Animals

Animals intoxicated by warfarin exhibit increasing pallor and weakness reflecting blood loss. Appetite and body weight are not specifically affected. The blood loss may be evident in the form of bloody sputum, bloody or tarry stools, petechiae, or externally visible hematoma. Hematoma formation is more common than free hemorrhage. There is no typical location for hematoma formation, the location of bleeding being apparently a matter of chance in the absence of obvious trauma. Bleeding associated with the central nervous system may be of such location and extent as to cause paralysis of the hindquarters several days before death occurs. Pregnant rats appear slightly more susceptible than nonpregnant ones (Hayes and Gaines, 1950). This may be related to obvious morphological factors, but the decreased metabolism of warfarin in pregnant rats suggests the presence of an inhibitory factor (MacDonald and Kaminsky, 1979).

Warfarin may be the only compound for which a log time-log dosage curve with all three segments has been demonstrated experimentally; the 90-day dose LD 50 in rats is only 0.077 mg/kg/day, and the chronicity index is 20.8. Rats tolerated for 300 days a daily dosage slightly greater than the extrapolated 90-day LD 0.01 dosage, specifically 0.02 mg/kg/day. In spite of its considerable cumulative effect, there is a level of intake that is safe for the rat. The same phenomenon permits the use of warfarin as an anticoagulant drug.

Other investigators have reported completely different results in the same species. Pyorala (1968), who made elaborate studies of the different susceptibility of male and female rats to warfarin, reported LD 50 values of 62–102 mg/kg for males and 21–33 mg/kg for females. Hagan and Radomski (1953) reported values of 323 and 58 mg/kg in males and females, respectively. Why these values differ by one or two orders of magnitude from those reported by others is not clear.

Warfarin is a racemic mixture whether it is used as a rodenticide or as a drug. Almost all published toxicity figures are for the mixture. However, West *et al.* (1961) were able to separate the isomers and to determine their absolute configuration. Based on prothrombin time measured 24 hr after a single oral dose, the $(-)(S)$ isomer was 5.5 times as active as the $(+)(R)$ isomer. Based on mortality within 10 days after starting daily dietary intake, the $(-)(S)$-warfarin was 8.5 times as active as the $(+)(R)$ isomer (Elbe *et al.*, 1966).

Absorption, Distribution, Metabolism, and Excretion Absorption of warfarin from the skin of rats is slow but measurable. Three dermal doses at the rate of 50 mg/kg had about the same pharmacological effect as three oral doses at 0.6 mg/kg (Sanger and Becker, 1975). Because of either species or formulation differences, the results were very different with guinea pigs and rabbits that received a 0.5% solution of the sodium salt in water (with 8% alcohol and 0.1% of a surface-active agent); single applications at rates of 0.7 and 0.25 mg/kg caused a marked change in prothrombin times in guinea pigs and rabbits, respectively. In fact, one dermal dose at the rate of 0.25 mg/kg was about as effective in rabbits as an oral dose of 2.0 mg/kg (Fristedt and Sterner, 1965).

There is great individual variation in the binding of warfarin by the serum proteins of laboratory rats. The rate of excretion showed a strong positive correlation with the concentration of free drug in the plasma (Yacobi and Levy, 1975).

Ninety-six hours after intraperitoneal injection of warfarin, the concentrations of activity in the kidney, liver, and pancreas were 3, 12, and 15 times, respectively, greater than that in the blood (Link *et al.*, 1965). The significance of the pancreatic accumulation remains obscure.

Warfarin is readily hydroxylated *in vitro* and *in vivo* by rat liver microsomal enzymes to form 6-, 8-, and especially 7- hydroxywarfarin. Formation of another metabolite is catalyzed by the soluble fraction of liver in either the presence or absence of oxygen (Ikeda *et al.*, 1968a, b; Ullrich and Staudinger, 1968). Formation of all these metabolites is stimulated by phenobarbital, chlordane, or DDT. The metabolism is a true detoxication. The inducers can increase the LD 50 of warfarin by more than 10-fold (Ikeda *et al.*, 1968a).

A later study of rats that had received [^{14}C]warfarin revealed the following compounds in the urine: unchanged warfarin (6.6%), 4′-hydroxywarfarin (21%), 6-hydroxywarfarin (15.4%), 7-hydroxywarfarin (8.9%), a glucuronide of 7-hydroxywarfarin (3.0%), and an intramolecular condensation product, 2,3-dihydro-2-methyl-4-phenyl-5-oxo-*gamma*-pyranol (3.2c)(1)benzopyran (DHG) (6.6%). These metabolites were found in the feces also but in different relative concentrations (Barker *et al.*, 1970). No radioactive carbon dioxide derived from warfarin has been found in exhaled air (Link *et al.*, 1965). Many of the same metabolites were excreted by guinea pigs,

but the proportions were different. Salicylic acid, not found in the rat, was found in guinea pig urine. Of all metabolites recovered, only 4′-hydroxywarfarin and DHG showed anticoagulant activity. That of 4′-hydroxycoumarin was slight. That of DHG showed two peaks, of which the second was stronger. This suggests metabolism of the compound, perhaps back to warfarin (Deckert, 1973).

Rats injected intraperitoneally with [^{14}C]warfarin excreted approximately 90% of the activity in 14 days, about half in the urine and half in the feces (Link *et al.*, 1965).

Approximately 10% of the activity from [^{14}C]warfarin was excreted in the bile of rats within 5 hr after intraperitoneal injection, but little radioactivity appeared in the feces. Nearly all of the metabolites in the bile were conjugated; they could be released with about equal ease by incubation with β-glucuronidase of with gut flora (Elmer *et al.*, 1977; Powell *et al.*, 1977). The metabolites identified were the same as those found slightly later in the urine.

When guinea pigs were injected with 1 or 2 mg of [^{14}C]warfarin, about 50% of the activity was recovered from urine excreted during the first 12 hr and 87% was found in urine within 7 days. A smaller percentage of large doses was excreted promptly (Deckert, 1973).

The action of warfarin (and of fumarin and coumatetralyl as well) on the smooth muscle of the isolated intestine of the rabbit, of the rat (*Rattus rattus* and *Rattus norvegicus*), and of *Bandicota bengalensis* was studied in vitro. There was a fairly identical reduction in peristaltic activity by all three compounds in all four species. The effect was reversible, thus indicating no permanent damage to the tissue (Renapurkar and Deoras, 1982). Warfarin is bound to albumin but can be displaced from albumin by several compounds, including metals (Brodie, 1964; Chakrabarti, 1978).

Resistance to Warfarin Genetic resistance to warfarin among rodents, lagomorphs, and humans is discussed in Section 83.3.1.3.

Two cases of intriguing warfarin resistance in humans were reported by Kempin (1983). Both patients under anticoagulant therapy could not kept within therapeutic range. The common factor that was found was heavy daily intake of broccoli (250–450 mg/day). Broccoli is an important dietary source of vitamin K (200 μg/100 gm). When the vegetable was removed from the diet, the anticoagulant therapy became effective.

Biochemical Effects Warfarin has two actions: inhibition of synthesis of vitamin K-dependent factors (VII, proconvertin; IX, Christmas factor; and X, Stuart factor) and decrease of the production of prothrombin (factor II) in the liver (Coon and Willis, 1972). In addition, warfarin induces capillary damage. There is unconfirmed evidence that these two actions are produced by the two moieties of the molecule. Thus 4-hydroxycoumarin inhibits the formation of prothrombin and reduces the clotting power of the blood, whereas there is some evidence that at sufficient dosage benzalacetone produces capillary damage and leads to bleeding upon the very slightest trauma. Significantly enough, vitamin K has an antidotal action against both actions of warfarin up to a certain point (Varon and Cole, 1966).

The basis for the change in vitamin K_1 metabolism associated with poisoning and the alteration of this metabolism in resistant animals probably involves a warfarin-binding protein in the microsomal membranes of the liver. Thierry *et al.* (1970) found that ribosomes isolated from the livers of resistant rats bind only one-third to one-fifth as much warfarin as ribosomes from normal rats, regardless of whether warfarin is injected before the rats are killed for study or is added to the *in vitro* preparation. Lorusso and Suttie (1972) found that, when [^{14}C]warfarinat a concentration of 0.786 ppm was incubated with microsomal preparations, the concentrations reached were 42.0 and 17.7 pmol/mg of protein, depending on whether the preparations were prepared from normal or from warfarin-resistant rats, respectively. Furthermore, the warfarin was bound firmly to membranes of normal rats but loosely to those of warfarin-resistant rats. Vitamin K deficiency caused a 24% increase in the amount of warfarin bound, but this was overcome in animals given vitamin K_1 1 hr before being killed for *in vitro* study. Warfarin binding *in vitro* was reduced 90% in animals injected with warfarin 22 hr before being killed. Although the binding protein was a part of microsomal membranes, it seemed unrelated to cytochrome P-450.

A protein which may be the same as the one just discussed has been isolated and shown to have a molecular weight of about 30,000. It may become adherent to ribosomes in the course of their preparation for biochemical study (Searcey and Graves, 1976).

Binding of warfarin to cytochromes P-450 and P-448 occurs also and may help to explain changes in the rate of metabolism of warfarin following induction of microsomal enzymes by phenobarbital and other compounds. The stereochemical aspects of the metabolism of warfarin have been studied in great detail (Kaminsky *et al.*, 1976; Pohl *et al.*, 1976a, b, 1977).

Formation of 7- and 8-hydroxywarfarin is promoted by other cytochromes. The same type of cytochrome is mainly responsible for the formation of each corresponding metabolite, regardless of how the activity of liver microsomal enzymes has been induced (Fasco *et al.*, 1979).

Warfarin has been reported to inhibit (Biezunski, 1970) or to promote (Beracki and Bosmann, 1970) the synthesis of liver microsomal protein and other liver protein. The contradictory results may be explained by differences in procedure, but exactly how is unclear. It is also unclear what bearing the results have on the pharmacological action of warfarin.

Warfarin causes a relative increase in vitamin K_1 oxide in the plasma or liver of people (Shearer *et al.*, 1973) and rats (Matschiner *et al.*, 1970). The oxide is a naturally occurring compound. In vitamin K-deficient but otherwise normal rats, the oxide and vitamin K_1 are equally effective, but the oxide is not therapeutic in warfarin-treated rats. It has been proposed that coumarin and related anticoagulants act by inhibiting the conversion of the oxide back to the active vitamin and that the oxide per se is inhibitory. Involvement of the vitamin K_1–

vitamin K_1 oxide cycle in the action of warfarin seems very likely, since the effect of warfarin on this cycle is greatly reduced in resistant rats. The hypothesis that warfarin inhibits prothrombin synthesis by causing accumulation of the oxide does not appear tenable (Caldwell *et al.*, 1974). However, it seems likely that the brevity of the action of vitamin K in the treatment of poisoning is the result of its irreversible conversion to the epoxide (Shearer and Barkhan, 1979).

The superiority of vitamin K_1 over vitamin K_3 in treating warfarin poisoning has been established experimentally (Penumarthy and Oehme, 1978).

For more detail than can be discussed here regarding vitamin K and vitamin K-dependent proteins a book edited by Suttie is available (1979).

Although L-histidine at a dietary level of 400 ppm was without effect on rats, it potentiated the lethal action of warfarin (50 ppm) in both laboratory and field tests (Rao, 1979). The biochemical basis for this action of histidine should be explored.

Effects on Organs and Tissues   A possible oncogenic effect of prolonged warfarin therapy was speculated by Krauss (1982) based on a report by Gore and associates (1982) of an increased incidence of cancer in patients occurring 3 or more years after a pulmonary embolism. This highly speculative deduction made from a very limited number of cases has been criticized by Zacharski (1982) who cited results from two cohort studies (Annegers and Zacharski, 1980; Michaels, 1974). In those studies, no increased incidence of malignancies was observed in patients who had received long-term anticoagulant treatments and had been followed for several thousand patient-years.

Pathology   Animals killed by warfarin show most extreme pallor of the skin, muscles, and all the viscera. In addition, evidence of hemorrhage may be found in any part of the body but usually only in one location in a single autopsy. Such blood as remains in the heart and vessels is grossly thin and forms a poor clot or no clot. In a report of a boxer dog poisoned with a mixture of warfarin and calciferol, delayed necrosis of the tip of tongue and large areas of necrosed skin were seen. It is difficult, however, to attribute the damaging effect on the walls of the vessels to warfarin alone, since calciferol also can induce such lesions (Edlin, 1982).

Treatment of Poisoning in Animals   A diet containing selenium at a concentration of 2.5 mg/kg of feed was protective against the toxic effects of aflatoxin B_1 (a bifuranocoumarin) and warfarin in pigs given four daily oral doses of 0.2 mg/kg of body weight. Selenium is a component of glutathione peroxidase, an enzyme that prevents the production of free radicals (Davila *et al.*, 1983).

83.5.1.3 Toxicity to Humans

Experimental Exposure   When nine normal men and five normal women were given a single oral dose of warfarin at the rate of 1.5 mg/kg, maximal concentration in plasma was reached in 2–12 hr. Maximal depression of prothrombin activity was between 36 and 72 hr. Their individual increases in prothrombin time were proportional to their half-time for disappearance of warfarin from the plasma. In other words, the pharmacological effect was greates in those with slower excretion. The half-times for disappearance from the plasma varied from 15 to 58 hr with a mean of 42 hr. Absorption of warfarin from the gastrointestinal tract was apparently complete; no warfarin was found in the stool even after massive doses, and plasma levels and prothrombin activity responses were virtually identical following oral and intravenous administration at the same rates (O'Reilly *et al.*, 1963).

Having established the absolute configuration of the four warfarin alcohols, Chan *et al.* (1972) administered them to volunteers. Reduction of the alcohols was stereoselective. The rate of elimination of one of the isomers (*R,S*) was much slower than that of the others, and its effect was more sustained. The resulting metabolites were biologically active but not as active as warfarin itself.

Six normal subjects were given a single dose of warfarin at the rate of 1.5 mg/kg. Three weeks later, the same people were given 200 mg of phenylbutazone three times a day for at least 8 days; on the fourth day, warfarin was repeated at 1.5 mg/kg. Compared to warfarin alone, administration of warfarin with phenylbutazone increased the prothrombin time even though the plasma concentration and biological half-life decreased. The result (in the face of an obvious inactivation of warfarin) was attributed to displacement of warfarin by phenylbutazone from binding to plasma albumin, making more free drug momentarily available to receptor sites in the liver (O'Reilly and Aggeler, 1968). The mutual displacement of phenylbutazone and warfarin from human plasma albumin has been studied *in vitro* (Solomon *et al.*, 1968).

As shown by study in seven volunteers, the action of triclofos (trichloroethyl sodium phosphate) is similar to that of phenylbutazone. A dosage of triclofos at the rate of 22 mg/kg/day prolonged the prothrombin time even though the dosage of warfarin was reduced. Trichloroacetic acid, a metabolie of triclofos, accumulated in the plasma to an average concentration of 80 ppm. The displacement of warfarin from albumin by trichloroacetic acid was sufficient to account for the observed potentiation of warfarin (Sellers *et al.*, 1972). At least in the rat, sodiumsalicylate has a similar effect (Coldwell *et al.*, 1974) but phenobarbital does not significantly influence the binding capacity of the plasma for warfarin (Ikeda *et al.*, 1968a).

In a similar study with 10 male volunteers, both phenobarbital and glutethimide lowered the plasma warfarin concentration and reduced the half-life of warfarin by nearly 50%; chloral betaine had a slight effect also. Phenobarbital and glutethimide significantly reduced the hypoprothrombinemia response of warfarin, but results with chloral betaine were indistinguishable in this regard from results for placebo-treated and untreated controls (MacDonald *et al.*, 1969).

The effects of cimetidine (a drug used to treat peptic ulcer) on the kinetics and dynamics of warfarin were studied in seven volunteers. It was shown clearly that cimetidine acted by inhibition of drug metabolism without significant effect on the binding of warfarin to plasma protein (Breckenridge *et al.*, 1979).

Therapeutic Use Use of warfarin as a drug offers greater dosage and, therefore, greater opportunity for side effects than pest control operators encounter. Of course, bleeding is the most common complication of treatment. Most of it is clinically insignificant. Probably many cases remain unpublished. According to one study, the incidence among hospitalized patients was 10%, and it was 40% among ambulatory patients. The incidence of serious hemorrhage was estimated at 2–10% in hospitalized and ambulatory patients, respectively. A series of case reports illustrated some of the circumstances leading to serious hemorrhage. It was concluded that the complication can be kept at a minimum by careful selection of patients, informed and adequate supervision by the physician, and reliable laboratory control (Pastor *et al.*, 1962).

Although the diagnosis in most cases of hemorrhage is obvious, there are exceptions. For example, two cases of intestinal hemorrhage leading to an initial diagnosis of acute abdomen have been reported (Cocks, 1960).

Macular, papular, pruritic, or vesicular rashes due to warfarin are unusual, but those that do occur often are in patients who had taken the drug without untoward effect for 3 or more months. The skin returned to normal slowly after medication was stopped, but the dermatitis recurred within 2 or 3 days when medication was renewed (Schiff and Kern, 1968).

Necrosis of the skin and subcutaneous tissues of localized areas has been attributed to warfarin only rarely and not always convincingly. For example, in a case reported by Vaughan *et al.* (1969), a totally unexplained illness suggestive of but not proved to be thrombophlebitis and pulmonary embolism preceded warfarin therapy by 6 weeks and may have been the underlying cause of the complication attributed circumstantially to warfarin. In two other cases, a more persuasive interpretation was made, namely that anticoagulants (heparin and warfarin) acted as neither the preparatory nor the provoking substance for the localized necrosis attributed to their use, but that underlying disease processes, including intravascular coagulation, sepsis, or localized inflammation, triggered a localized purpuric reaction that was then intensified by the warfarin therapy (Martin *et al.*, 1970).

An entirely different kind of complication has involved potentiation of warfarin by disulfiram (Rothstein, 1968) or interference with its action by other drugs including griseofulvin (Cullen and Catalano, 1967) and phenobarbital (Robinson and MacDonald, 1966) or by insecticides. In one case, medical use of warfarin was nullified by use of 5% toxaphene and 1% lindane to dust sheep. Response to warfarin returned to normal within about 3 months after exposure to the insecticides (Jeffery *et al.*, 1976). Of course, discontinuing a drug that promotes the metabolism of warfarin has the same effect as introducing a drug such as disulfiram that interferes with metabolism of the anticoagulant.

The success of cardiac value prostheses requires anticoagulation to prevent immobilization of the valve by thrombi and to minimize the chance of emboli. Installation of such prostheses in young women to correct rheumatic mitral or aortic stenosis increases their chance of surviving and reproducing, but it necessarily complicates any pregnancies they may have.

Anticoagulants also may be used in women of childbearing age to treat thrombophlebitis, embolic disease, and a few other conditions. It has long been recognized that administration of any anticoagulant during pregnancy increases the danger of hemorrhage either during the course of gestation or during delivery. It gradually has become evident that warfarin also is teratogenic in humans (Beckert *et al.*, 1975; DiSaia, 1966; Keber *et al.*, 1968; Pettifor and Benson, 1975; Shaul *et al.*, 1975; Sherrod and Harrod, 1978; Tejani, 1973). At least 29 cases of congenital anomaly have been attributed to warfarin (Hall *et al.*, 1980). Most if not all of the recognized cases have involved nasal hypoplasia ranging from barely recognizable to very severe. Many of the babies had chondrodysplasia punctata, and this defect of cartilage development may be the basis not only of the nasal deformity but also of defects of the bones such as meningocele, deformities of the limbs, and a high arched palate seen much more rarely in babies of women treated with warfarin during the first trimester. Other teratogenic effects reported in one or more cases include microphthalmia, blindness, hydrocephalus, persistent truncus arteriosus, and mental retardation. Of 423 reported pregnancies in which coumarin derivatives were used, not over two-thirds resulted in apparently normal infants, one-sixth resulted in abortion or stillbirth, and one-sixth resulted in abnormal liveborn infants of which 29 showed fetal embryopathy. The critical period of exposure seemed to be between 6 and 9 weeks of gestation. Five cases of typical embryopathy and eight other cases showed central nervous system abnormalities following exposure to coumarin derivatives during gestation, but no critical period of exposure was evident (Hall *et al.*, 1980; Stevenson *et al.*, 1980).

Twenty-nine of 423 pregnancies is a high incidence of teratogenic effect even if one takes into account that only medically reported cases were available for consideration. A different kind of evidence for the teratogenic action of warfarin involved a family with no history of consanguinity, birth defects, or mental retardation that produced one normal child in a pregnancy without warfarin and two deformed children in separate pregnancies in which warfarin was used (Sherrod and Harrod, 1978). On the other hand, inasmuch as defects occur in only about one-third of instances, none may be found in some small series of cases (Chong *et al.*, 1984).

The use of heparin during gestation does not result in a significantly better outcome of pregnancy than that obtained with warfarin. In 135 published cases, about two-thirds were apparently normal, one-eighth were stillborn, and one-fifth (of whom one-third died) were premature (Hall *et al.*, 1980).

Kaplan (1985) and Zakzouk (1986) reviewed the subject of warfarin-associated malformations and established that, based on the timing of warfarin exposure, second- and third-trimester exposure predisposes to central nervous system abnormalities

whereas first-trimester exposure is associated with the warfarin embryopathy: midface and nasal hypoplasia, optic atrophy, hypoplasia of the digits, and mental impairment. In addition, Kaplan reports a case of Dandy–Walker malformation associated with warfarin exposure confined to weeks 8–12 of gestation. Four previous cases of such association were known but the gestational exposure period was much longer.

Not only has hereditary resistance of people to warfarin been observerd (O'Reilly, 1970) but also exceptional susceptibility, also presumably on a hereditary basis, has been reported (Solomon, 1968).

Accidental and Intentional Poisoning   A 32-year-old man was murdered by feeding him warfarin for 13 days. On the fourth day after intake started, the victim began having severe nosebleeds. Later, he bled from the mouth. Two days before death, he complained of pain in his limbs. His symptoms became worse and he died of circulatory failure on day 15 (Pribilla, 1996).

The initial symptoms in an attempted suicide using warfarin were back pain and abdominal pain. The onset occurred 1 day after the sixth daily dose. A day after onset, vomiting and attacks of nose bleeding occurred. On the second day of illness, when admitted to hospital, the patient was observed to have a generalized petechial rash (Holmes and Love, 1952).

In Korea, a family of 14 persons lived for a period of 15 days on a diet consisting almost entirely of corn (maize) meal containing warfarin. The first symptoms appeared 7–10 days after the eating of warfarin was begun. Massive bruises or hematomata developed at the knee and elbow joints and on the buttocks in all cases. Extensive gum and nasal hemorrhage usually appeared about a day later, and by days 15 blood loss was extensive (Lange and Terveer, 1954).

A suicidal gesture that was reported and treated after only a single ingestion of a heaping tablespoonful of 0.5% wafarin produced no illness and not even an increase in prothrombin time (Kellum, 1952).

There have been at least two attempted murders with warfarin (Ikkala *et al.*, 1964; Nilsson, 1957). In each instance there were recurrent bouts of hemorrhagic difficulty, including hematuria, epistaxis, severe bruises without any history of trauma, and intestinal hemorrage. Abdominal or back pain was present. Each patient recovered promptly in hospital, but one had relapses for nearly a year and the other had bouts of poisoning of 2.5 years following repeated doses. An anticoagulant drug was suspected from the first in both cases, but finding the source proved difficult. Solution of each case was essentially epidemiological, but measurement of warfarin in the plasma was decisive in one case. Faced with the evidence, the daughter-in-law of a 72-year-old woman and the wife of a 69-year-old man both confessed to the police.

Although numerous accidental ingestions by children and adults have been reported to the New York Poison Control Center, no known injury from these ingestions has been observed (Jacobziner and Raybin, 1960).

An outbreak of hemorrhagic disease due to the use of warfarin-contaminated talcum was described in Vietnam (Martin-Bouyer *et al.*, 1983). Of the 741 cases located in Ho-Chi-Minh City, all in infants (55% under 2 months of age), 177 died. Eleven samples of baby powder were analyzed and concentrations of warfarin ranged from 1.7 to 6.5%. The percutaneous penetration of warfarin contained in the contaminated talc was studied in a young healthy female baboon, treated twice daily with a topical application of 3 gm of talc containing 3% warfarin (188 mg/kg/day of warfarin). One control animal was treated with uncontaminated talc. On the fifth day, the treated animal began to show signs of intoxication with profuse bleeding and died. At necropsy there were two large subcutaneous hematomata on the skull and the peritoneal cavity with filled with unclotted blood. On day 3 of treatment, a blood sample showed severe disturbances of the hepatic coagulation factors. Electron microscopy showed an increased number of swollen and misshapen mitochondria in the hepatocytes (Dreyfus *et al.*, 1983).

Warfarin was administered to an 11-month-old baby girl by her psychologically disturbed mother. Upon hospitalization the parameters of coagulation were elevated (prothrombin time 53 sec, control 12 sec); the child had multiple hematomata and had a bloody discharge from her left ear. Treatment with vitamin K_1 and infusion of fresh frozen plasma stopped the bleeding (White, 1985).

Use Experience The safety record of warfarin used as a rodenticide has been excellent. One case of poisoning has been attributed to extensive, prolonged skin contact in the process of preparing and distributing baits. Unlike most solid bait, which is prepared by mixing ground grain with starch containing warfarin powder, this bait was prepared by pouring a 0.5% solution of the sodium salt over dried bread. The hands of the 23-year-old farmer who used this method were wet with the solution each of the 10 times he made bait during a 24-day period, and he did not wash his hands until several hours after each application.

Two days after the last contact with rodenticide, gross hematuria appeared. Next day hematomata were noticed on the arms and legs; there was dull pain in both groins. The hematuria subsided after 3 days of rest but recurred along with nose bleeding when the man returned to work. When he was admitted to hospital, prothrombin, clotting, and bleeding times were abnormally long and anemia was severe (hemoglobin, 8.2%; red cell count, 2.9 million/mm^3). The patient responded promptly to treatment with vitamin K_1 (Fristedt and Sterner, 1965).

Atypical Cases of Various Origins Mogilner *et al.* (1974) described three fatal cases of what they considered to represent Reye's syndrome. One of the young children was said to have ingested warfarin that she found by the road on her way to kindergarten 4 days before hospital admission; warfarin was found in the urine and traces were present in the blood. In another case, "significant amounts of warfarin were found in the urine and also in autopsy samples of liver and kidney tissue;"

no source of the rotendicide was reported, and no information was given that would permit evaluation of the validity of the chemical analysis. There was no indication of warfarin in the third case. The authors considered that it was justified "to add warfarin to the long and varied list of etiological or precipitating factors in Reye's syndrome."

The death of a 2-year-old boy was attributed to warfarin poisoning on his death certificate but probably was the result of beating, with pneumonia as a terminal event (Hayes and Vaughn, 1977).

Dosage Response A total dose of 1000 mg of warfarin consumed in 13 days (about 1.1 mg/kg/day) was fatal (Pribilla, 1996).

Serious illness followed the ingestion of 1.7 mg warfarin/kg/day for 6 consecutive days with suicidal intent. This would correspond to eating almost 1 pound of bait (0.025% warfarin) each day for 6 days. All signs and symptoms were caused by hemorrhage and, following multiple small transfusions and massive doses of vitamin K, recovery was complete (Holmes and Love, 1952).

In the Korean cases, the dosage of the different individuals was determined to vary from about 1 to 2 mg warfarin/kg/day. As a result of this exposure and without benefit of treatment, 2 of the 14 persons died. A 19-year-old girl, who was in a state of shock and severe hemorrhage 2 days after the warfarin diet was discontinued, recovered following a blood transfusion and small daily doses of vitamin K. The remaining 11 members of the family recovered within a week after exposure, although only small daily doses of vitamin K were given and they all had shown marked signs of poisoning when they first accepted treatment. There was reason to think that those who died had received slightly higher dosages than those who survived (see Table 2.9 in Hayes, 1975). Recovery of the 12 survivors was complete. The entire episode was made possible only by a series of unusual events and by the extraordinary apathy of the family, resulting in their totally ignoring unmistakable signs of illness (Lange and Terveer, 1954).

A single intravenous therapeutic dose of the sodium derivative (40–60 mg or about 0.7 mg/kg) in humans may produce some increase in prothrombin time within 2 hr and usually produces a substantial increase within 14 hr. The average maximal response is on the fourth day. Spontaneous recovery to normal occurs about 8 days after a single therapeutic dose. Thus significant depression of prothrombin level is maintained for 3–6 days. In the treatment of thromboembolic disease, a maintenance dose of about 2–10 mg/day is required to keep the prothrombin level between 10 and 30% of normal. Patients have been thus maintained for years. If human susceptibility to warfarin were different (as it is in a few genetically determined cases), the therapeutic dosage could be adjusted accordingly. It is interesting, however, that the upper limit of the usual maintenance dosage for humans (about 0.14 mg/kg/day) is an LD 95 for the rat. The inherently lesser susceptibility of humans to the compound undoubtedly contributes to its safety as a rodenticide. The threshold limit value of 0.1 mg/m^3 indicates that occupational intake of warfarin at the rate of 0.014 mg/kg/day is considered safe.

Laboratory Findings Metabolites of warfarin including 5-, 6-, 7-, and 8-hydroxywarfarin and two aliphatic side-chain alcohols have been identified in the urine of normal volunteers who had received a single oral dose at the rate of 1.5 mg/kg (Chan *et al.*, 1972; Lewis and Traeger, 1970). This is, however, not a common way to confirm poisoning.

Adequacy of treatment with warfarin usually is followed by measuring prothrombin time. In case of poisoning, the prothrombin time is greatly prolonged. The coagulation time is definitely increased by the Lee–White method and slightly increased by the capillary tube method. Bleeding time often is normal. Urine may be normal in appearance but may contain many red cells on microscopic examination, or it may be grossly hemorrhagic. The red cell count and hemoglobin gradually fall if bleeding continues. In terminal cases a state of shock develops.

Sixty-nine euthyroid patients being treated with warfarin for thromboembolic disease showed no evidence of hyperthyroid condition, and 14 of them showed a hypothyroid tendency associated with an elevation of the thyroxine-binding capacity of plasma globulin. However, no clinical evidence of thyroid dysfunction was reported, and it was uncertain whether the small changes in laboratory tests of thyroid function were caused by warfarin (Braverman and Foster, 1969).

Plasma levels of warfarin were 6.8 and 11.2 ppm 4 and 7 hr, respectively, after the ingestion of 50 mg of warfarin sodium in a suicide attempt. Plasma levels declined thereafter, and the half-time disappearance was calculated as 46 hr. Part of the dose was removed by gastric lavage soon after ingestion. This and other appropriate treatment prevented any increase in bleeding tendency (Cole and Bachmann, 1976).

Pathology Apparently there is only one complete description of human pathology associated with uncomplicated warfarin poisoning, that of Pribilla (1996). The findings in that case were strikingly different from typical findings in the rat: exsanguination was less complete, as indicated by the fact that the liver was not tan in color and bleeding was far more generalized and not restricted to one or a few large hematomata. The two factors may be related in that bleeding into the organs may have interfered with their function and hastened death. In addition to generalized bleeding (due mainly to deficiency of coagulation), evidence of capillary damage and of parenchymal injury of the liver was found in the human case. In spite of the obvious differences between the findings in human and rat, the similarity was also striking because subserosal and intraseptal bleeding was prominent in the human case.

Treatment of Poisoning After blood has been taken for prothrombin and other differential diagnostic tests, vitamin K_1 in a dose of 5–10 mg should be given three times on the first days of treatment irrespective of symptoms. The vitamin should be given intravenously slowly, usually by infusion. Smaller doses

should be continued until the prothrombin time has reached normal. In a seriously ill patient, a small transfusion of carefully matched whole blood should be given initially and repeated daily until the patient has returned to normal. Such a patient should be given vitamin K_1 also. If it were ever necessary to treat a patient in shock from blood loss resulting from warfarin poisoning, frequent small transfusions and a complete consideration of the blood chemistry would be in order. Any large hematomata should be the subject of a surgical consultation, but any surgical action should be taken only after the clotting power of the blood is restored to normal.

The progress of the patient should be followed by the prothrombin test. Tests should be made at least twice daily until a return to normal is clearly established and stable.

83.5.2 COUMAFURYL

83.5.2.1 Identity, Properties, and Usses

Chemical Name 3-[-1(2-furanyl)-3-oxobutyl]-4-hydroxy-2H-1-benzopyran-2-one in the chemical name.

Structure See Fig. 83.3.

Synonyms Coumafuryl is the common name approved by ISO. Other names for the compound include fumarin (BSI) and tomarin (Turkey). Trade names include Fumarin®, Fumasol®, Krumkil®, Lurat®, Ratafin®, Rat-a-way®, and Tomarin®. The CAS registry number is 117-52-2.

Physical and Chemical Properties The empirical formula for coumafuryl is $C_{17}H_{14}O_5$, and the molecular weight is 298.28. It is a crystalline solid melting at 214°C.

Use Coumafuryl is an anticoagulant rat poison.

83.5.2.2 Toxicity in Laboratory Animals

Coumafuryl is very similar to warfarin (see Fig. 83.3). The oral LD 50 for rats is quoted as 0.4 mg/kg (Wiswesser, 1976).

Coumafuryl poisoning was observed in young chicks (less than 1 week old) with a mortality rate of 100%. Hemorrhage and unclotted blood was noted in the abdominal and thoracic cavities. At necropsy, crops and gizzards contained feed. Analysis of the content detected approximately 340 mg/kg of coumafuryl. Investigations found coumafuryl was present in the wood-straw mats in the chicken boxes (Munger *et al.*, 1993).

83.5.2.3 Toxity to Humans

It is inevitable that a number of children and perhaps others have ingested coumafuryl. In fact, McLeod (1970) reported that coumafuryl and warfarin were among the pesticides most often ingested by persons (mainly children) admitted to a large hospital in New Orleans. However, these two compounds were the least hazardous pesticides in terms of morbidity.

Treatment of Poisoning Treatment is the same as that for warfarin (see Section 83.5.1.3).

83.5.3 DIPHACINONE

83.5.3.1 Identity, Properties, and Usses

Chemical Name 2(Diphenylacetyl)indan-1,3-dione is the chemical name.

Structure See Fig. 83.3.

Synonyms Diphacinone (ANSI, BSI, ISO) is the common name in use except in Turkey and Italy, where diphacin is used, and in Russia where ratindan is used. Other nonproprietary names include dipazin and diphenacin. As a drug, the compound is known as diphenadione. Trade names for formulated baits containing diphacinone include Diphacine®, Ramik®, Promar®, and Gold Crest®. The CAS registry number is 82-66-6.

Physical and Chemical Properties Diphacinone has the empirical formula $C_{23}H_{16}O_3$ and a molecular weight of 340.40. Its technical grade is a yellow crystalline powder melting at 145°C; it is slightly soluble in water (0.3 mg/liter) and soluble in acetone (29 gm/liter) and toluene (73 gm/liter). Diphacinone is rapidly decomposed in water by sunlight.

History, Formulation, and Uses The rodenticidal activity of diphacinone was described in 1952. It is formulated as prepared weather-resistant baits (pellets or meal) in concentrations of 50 mg/kg. A dry concentrate (1 gm/kg) for mixing with cereal bait is also available. All formulations are for professional application only. Diphacinone is used to control mice, rats, pairie dogs (*Cynomys* spp.), ground squirrels, voles, and other rodents.

83.5.3.2 Toxicity in Laboratory Animals

In a study of bishydroxycoumarin, ethyl biscoumacetate, and 17 analogs of indandione in rabbits, diphacinone was found to be the most hypoprothrombinemic. A marked response lasting about 7 days was produced by a dosage of only 0.05 mg/kg. The acute oral LD 50 ranges from 0.3 to 2.3 mg/kg in the rat and from 3.0 to 7.5 mg/kg in the dog. It was found to be 14.7 mg/kg for cats and 150 mg/kg for pigs. In mice and rabbits, the oral LD 50 is 340 and 35 mg/kg, respectively. For the mallard duck, it is 3158 mg/kg. The LD 50 associated with 14 daily oral doses in rats was 0.1 mg/kg (Correll *et al.*, 1952). Acute percutaneous LD 50 for rats is less than 200 mg/kg. In a 21-day subchronic percutaneous study in rabbits, the no-effect level was 0.1 mg/kg daily. Diphacinone is neither a skin and eye irritant nor a skin sensitizer. An acute inhalation of diphacinone dust in the rat as shown an LC 50 of less than 2000 mg/m3 of air. Diphacinone is not mutagenic in the Ames test.

Sprague–Dawley rats were fed for 21 days on a diet containing 1, 2, or 4 ppm diphacinone. All animals in the 2 and 4 ppm groups died and postmortem examination revealed massive internal hemorrhages. On day 21, the prothrombin clotting time of the animals in the 1 ppm group was not affected. A second study was performed in which the rats were fed for 90 days on a diet containing 0.0313, 0.625, 0.125, 0.25, or 0.5 ppm of diphacinone, or approximately 0.002, 0.003, 0.006, 0.013, and 0.025 mg/kg/day. One male in the 0.25 ppm group died on day 17 of treatment and another male in the 0.0625 ppm group on day 20 from a subdural hemorrhage. However, the mean prothrombin clotting times of the animals surviving the treatment period were not affected. The only parameter that showed some variation was the fibrinogen level, which was lower in the 0.5 ppm group (Elias and Johns, 1981).

The most interesting aspect of the toxicity of diphacinone involves species difference. The oral LD 50 of the compound for vampire bats (*Desmodus rotundus*) was 0.91 mg/kg, whereas a dosage of 5 mg/kg produced no sign of illness in cattle (Elias *et al.*, 1978). The blood of beef cattle given a single intraruminal injection of the compound at a rate of 1 mg/kg became toxic to these bats and remained toxic for 3 days without harming the cattle. As indicated by examination before and 2 weeks after treatment, cattle dosed in this way on three ranches in Mexico experienced a 93% reduction in vampire bat bites. Bioassays of milk and liver indicated that there was no residue problem (Thompson *et al.*, 1972). Residue studies indicated that people may safely eat meat, including liver and kidney, from treated cattle (Bullard *et al.*, 1976).

Absorption, Distribution, Metabolism, and Excretion When ^{14}C-labeled diphacinone was administered orally to mice, radioactivity reached its highest levels in the liver and lungs. The concentration in the liver reached its maximum in 7.5 and 3.0 hr in males and females, respectively (Cahill and Crowder, 1979). In another study, rats and mice were orally administered ^{14}C-labeled diphacinone at dosages of 0.2 and 1.5 mg/kg. In rats, about 70% of the dose was excreted in the feces and 10% in urine in 8 days. The same elimination pattern was observed in mice. Eight days after the administration of the compound in rats and 4 days in mice, the liver had the highest level of residues, but kidneys and lung also contained significant levels of residues; brain, fat, and muscles had the lowest levels. Diphacinone is not extensively metabolized in rats, less than 1 % of the dose being expired as CO_2 hr. The metabolism pattern in rats involved mainly hydroxylation and conjugation reactions (Yu *et al.*, 1982).

Mode of Action Diphacinone inhibits the K-enzyme complex (liver-synthesized coagulation proteins: factors II, VII, and X), and this inhibition phase lasts approximately 30 days in dogs, as opposed to the relatively short effect of warfarin (Mount and Feldman, 1983). The prolonged action of diphacinone may be due to protein binding in the liver or low excretion rate or a combination of both factors.

Treatment of Poisoning in Animals In dogs, the results of the usual vitamin K oral therapy after diphacinone poisoning ware poor. Dogs treated with a sufficient quantity of vitamin K relapsed fatally several days after the corrective treatment stopped. The response to treatment seems to vary according to the amount of exposure to the rodenticide. The recommended therapeutic dose of vitamin K_1 is 5 mg/kg of body weight in subcutaneous injections for at least 5 consecutive days (Mount and Feldman, 1983).

83.5.3.3 Toxicity to Humans

Therapeutic Use   Diphacinone has been used as a therapeutic agent because it has a relatively long duration of action. Its half-life in humans is 15–20 days. A single oral dose of diphacinone of 4 mg/person produced a clearly detectable reduction of prothrombin about 14 hr after ingestion and slightly more reduction a day later, with recovery to normal by the third day. A smaller, uncertain reduction was produced by 2 mg/person. A single 20-mg dose caused hypoprothrombinemia that was definite in 14 hr, marked in 48 hr, and persisted from 6 to 10 days. The recommended initial dose for therapy was 20 mg followed by daily doses of 2–4 mg (Field *et al.*, 1952). The drug was in use until a few years ago. Although there were no adverse effects except occasional nausea and not unexpected hemorrhagic complications at high dosage levels, caution was advised because of its close relation to phenidione, which has caused agronulocytosis, hepatitis with jaundice, nephropathy with actue renal tubular necrosis, severe exfoliative dermatitis, and massive generalized edema (American Medical Association (AMA), 1977). The drug ceased to be listed in the AMA Drug Evaluations of 1980.

Treatment of Poisoning   Treatment is the same as that for warfarin, but based on experimental data from animals it would seem advisable to increase the dose of vitamin K as well as the duration of the corrective treatment.

83.5.4 BRODIFACOUM

83.5.4.1 Identity, Properties, and Usses

Chemical name   3-[3-(4′-bromo-[1,1′-biphenyl]-4-yl)-1,2,3, 4-tetrahydro-1-naphthylenyl]-4-hydroxy-2H-1-ben-zopyran-2-one is the chemical name.

Structure   See Fig. 83.4.

Synonyms   Brodifacoum is the approved common name (ISO-BIS). Trade names for the formulated material include Ratak®, Volak®, and Talon®. The code names are WBA 8119 and PP 581. The CAS registry number is 56073-10-0.

Physical and Chemical Properties   The empirical formula for brodifacoum is $C_{31}H_{23}BrO_3$ and the molecular weight is 523.4. It is an off-white to fawn-colored odorless powder with a melting point of 228–232°C. It is of very low solubility in water (less than 10 mg/liter at 20°C and pH 7). Brodifacoum is

slightly soluble in alcohols and benzene and soluble in acetone. It is stable at room temperature. It has a very low vapor pressure of less than 1.33×10^{-7} kPa (1×10^{-6} mm Hg) at 25°C.

History, Formulation, and Uses   The rodenticidal properties of brodifacoum were described in 1976. It is an indirect anticoagulant active against rats and mice including strains resistant to warfarin and other anticoagulants (Rennison and Hadler, 1975). It is also used to control other wild rodents. Brodifacoum is formulated as ready-to-used baits of low concentration (20 and 50 mg/kg of bait). A single ingestion is usually sufficient to kill.

83.5.4.2 Toxicity to Laboratory Animals

Brodifacoum is extremely toxic to a number of mammalian species. The oral and dermal LD 50 values of the technical material are given in Table 83.5.

In chicken, the oral LD 50 is reported to be 4.5 mg/kg and in the mallard duck it is 2.0 mg/kg.

In a 42-day feeding study in rats, a concentration of 0.1 ppm did not induce any adverse effect (Worthing and Walker, 1983).

Several cases of poisoning in domestic animals have been reported. One day after being seen to ingest brodifacoum-containing bait, a 17-kg cocker spaniel developed depression and icterus accompanied by accelerated pulse and rapid and labored respiration. Despite supportive therapy, the dog died the same day. The autopsy confirmed the icter and showed approximately 1 liter of unclotted blood in the thoracic cavity and 100 ml in the pericardiac sac. Numerous hemorrhagic areas were seen in the serous membranes (Stowe *et al.*, 1983). A 4-year-old cross-bred bitch was noticed to be depressed and weak the day following the laying of Talon® bait (0.005% brodifacoum); she was found dead in her kennel the next morning. The actual dose of brodifacoum ingested was unknown but it was estimated that the maximum quantity of bait eaten could have been 900 gm, resulting in an intake of 45 mg of active ingredient. At autopsy, the thoracic cavity contained approximately 1.8 liter of unclotted blood and a single clot was adherent to the base of the heart and to the aorta. Subcutaneous bruising was present on the rib cage. Brodifacoum was found in the liver at a concentration of 0.8 mg/kg (McSporran and Phillips, 1983).

Table 83.5
Single-Dose LD 50 for Brodifacoum

Species	Route	LD 50 (mg/kg)	Reference
Rat, M	oral	0.27	
Rat	dermal	50.00	
Mouse, M	oral	0.40	
Guinea pig, F	oral	0.28	
Rabbit, M	oral	0.30	
Dog	oral	0.25–1.0	
Cat	oral	≈0.25	

The acute oral toxicity of brodifacoum was examined in sheep. An LD 50 of 11 mg/kg was considered a good estimate (Godfrey *et al.*, 1985).

A white-winged duck (*Cairina sculata*) of a zoological setting was found with bilateral epistaxis and anemia. Brodifacoum was detected in the blood at a level of 0.002 ppm. The bird was treated with injectable and oral vitamin K_1 and transfused with 40 ml of whole blood and fully recovered (James *et al.*, 1995).

Absorption, Distribution, Metabolism, and Excretion Brodifacoum is absorbed through the gastrointestinal tract. When orally administered to male Sprague–Dawley rats at doses ranging from 0.1 to 0.33 mg/kg, brodifacoum exhibited a remarkably steep dose–response curve; 0.1 mg/kg failed to show an effect on the plasma prothrombin level within 24 hr, whereas 0.2 mg/kg reduced the prothrombin complex activity to 7% of normal values and 0.33 mg/kg reduced it to 4% of normal. Concentrations in the liver were rapidly established and remained relatively constant for at least 96 hr. The mean liver/serum concentration ratio is approximately 20. Disappearance from serum is slow with a half-life of 156 hr or even more. The slow disappearance from the plasma and liver and the large liver/serum ratio probably contribute to the higher toxicity of brodifacoum than of warfarin. These particular features may also explain the efficacy of brodifacoum against warfarin-resistant rats (Bachmann and Sullivan, 1983).

Six weeks after intravenous administration of a single 1 mg/kg dose of brodifacoum to male New Zealand White rabbits, the prothrombin complex activity was still lower than 30% of normal (in the early part of the study, subcutaneous injections of vitamin K were given to prevent lethal hemorrhage). In the same study (Park and Leck, 1982), it was shown that in the rabbit, the maximal antagonism of vitamin K_1 by warfarin was produced by a dose of 63 mg/kg, whereas a similar result was obtained with only 1 mg/kg brodifacoum. It was shown that, in warfarin-resistant and warfarin-sensitive rats, brodifacoum produced the same rate of degradation of prothrombin complex activity as warfarin and significantly reduced the activity of clotting factors II, VII, and X without affecting factor V. It was also demonstrated that brodifcacoum has the same mechanism of action as warfarin: reduction of vitamin K-dependent clotting factor synthesis by interruption of the vitamin K–epoxide cycle (Leck and Park, 1981). In mongrel dogs, the elimination of brodifacoum follows a classical experimental decay with a distributive half-life of 1.4 days and an elimination half-life phase of 8.7 days (Murphy *et al.*, 1985).

Brodifacoum was fed to four dogs for 3 consecutive days, producing a cumulative dose of 1.1 mg/kg body weight. Serum brodifacoum concentrations were monitored. Inappetence and hemorrhagic tendencies were exhibited by day 5 postrodenticide exposure. One-stage prothrombin time, APTT, and ACT were 25% greater than time zero values at 24, 24, and 72 hours postdosing, respectively. All laboratory parameters returned to normal within 48 hours of initiating vitamin K_1 therapy (0.83 mg/kg orally for 5 days). Serum brodifacoum concentrations were highest (1065–1215 ng/mL) during the 3 days after dosing and were detectable (3.0–7.5 ng/mL) until day 24 brodifacoum postexposure. A mean brodifacoum elimination half-life of 6 ± 4 days was observed (Woody *et al.*, 1992).

Factors Influencing Toxicty Pretreatment of rats daily by intraperitoneal injection of phenobarbital at 80 mg/kg for 2 consecutive days followed by a single administration of brodifacoum at 0.2 mg/kg by stomach tube reduced the anticoagulant effects, although the reduction was less marked than in the case of warfarin (Bachmann and Sullivan, 1983). It is also known that a very large number of drugs of different chemical structures can interact with coumarin anticoagulant therapy in humans (Koch-Weser and Sellers, 1971).

Pathology Necropsies of poisoned dogs have shown that, in addition to large collections of unclotted blood, a number of lesions were also present, including bile statis with large amounts of brown pigment accumulated in the portal triads and in the macrophages of the periportal regions and congestion of the spleen with accumulation of golden brown pigment, believed to be hemosiderin, in the red pulp (Stowe *et al.*, 1983).

Treatment of Poisoning in Animals Treatment should be as for other anticoagulant rodenticides: vitamin K^1 at dosage of 2.5–5.0 mg/kg and transfusion of fresh whole blood. Because of the long-lasting effect of brodifacoum, vitamin K therapy must be continued for at least 2–3 weeks.

83.5.4.3 Toxicity to Humans

Brodifacoum has not been used therapeutically in humans. Cases of attempted suicide have been reported. A 31-year-old mentally disturbed woman ingested over a 2-day period approximately thirty 50-gm packages of Talon® (approximately 75 mg of brodifacoum). Two days later she was brought to the hospital's psychiatric unit, without any physical signs or symptoms. The routine laboratory tests showed a prothrombin time of 72 sec (control, 12 sec) and an activated partial thromboplastin time greater than 100 sec (normal, 25–35 sec). In spite of prolonged administration of large amounts of vitamin K_1 and repeated infusion of fresh frozen plasma, the depression of the prothrombin complex activity persisted for more than 45 days after the ingestion (Lipton and Klass, 1984). Jones *et al.* (1984) have reported a similar case in a 17-year-old boy who attempted suicide by ingesting approximately 7.5 mg (0.12 mg/kg) brodifacoum. He was first seen for a gross hematuria, rapidly followed by epistaxis and gum bleeding. The prothrombin time and the activated partial thromboplastin time were considerably prolonged. The levels of plasma clotting factors II, VII, IX, and X were decreased. Factor V was normal. Vitamin K_1 and plasma therapy were instituted and had to be continued for 55 days until the patient's coagulation remained normal and stable.

Dosage Response From the two cases of poisoning reported above, it can be seen that the total doses ingested were in one case 75 mg and in the second one 7.5 mg and that the effects on the clotting factors were maximum in both cases, the clinical signs being almost absent in the woman who absorbed 75 mg of brodifacoum (although it was ingested over a 48-hr period). Therefore it would seem that, above a certain threshold, the response is maximum. This was also shown in rabbits given 1 and 10 mg/kg brodifacoum (Park and Leck, 1982). Murphy *et al.* (1985) have shown that in dogs serum concentrations below 12 mg/ml caused no measurable coagulopathic effects after cessation of vitamin K therapy.

Plasma brodifacoum concentration was compared to prothrombin levels over time in a case of brodifacoum poisoning. Brodifacoum was eliminated according to a two-compartment model, with an initial half-life of 0.75 days and a terminal half-life of 24.2 days. On admission, the brodifacoum level was 731 micrograms/L and the patient suffered severe urinary tract hemorrhage, requiring transfusion of blood products. Persistently increased prothrombin times necessitated treatment with phytonadione up to 80 mg/day for 4 months, until the brodifacoum level reached 10 micrograms/L (Hollinger *et al.*, 1993).

The plasma concentration, plasma half-life, and mean retention time of brodifacoum (among other anticoagulant rodenticides) were determined in dogs in which preliminary diagnosis of anticoagulant poisoning had been made. Analysis was performed with high performance liquid chromatography (HPLC) on the plasma. In 7 dogs, the estimated half-time of brodifacoum ranged from 0.9 to 4.7 (median 2.4) days with a mean retention time of 1.9 to 3.7 (median 2.8 days) (Robben *et al.*, 1998).

The case of a voluntary ingestion of brodifacoum by a 39-year-old man was reported by Sheen *et al.* (1994). His prothrombin and partial thromboplastin times were respectively 150 and 113 seconds. Treatment with a daily dose of 200 mg of phytonadione for 5 months corrected the coagulopathy with no side effects occurring.

Prolonged follow-up and vitamin K treatment were necessary in a child with spontaneous hemorrhage from her nose, mouth, and urinary tract following accidental ingestion of brodifacoum (Travis *et al.*, 1993).

83.5.5 CHLOROPHACINONE

83.5.5.1 Identity, Properties, and Usses

Chemical Name 2-[4-(chlorophenyl)phenylacetyl]-1*H*-indene-1,3(2*H*)-dione is the chemical name.

Structure See Fig. 83.3.

Synonyms Chlorophacinone is the approved common name (BSI-ISO). Trade names for the formulated products include Caid®, Liphadione®, Raviac® , Drat®, Quick®, Lepit®, Rozol®, and Saviac®. The CAS registry number is 3691-35-8.

Physical and Chemical Properties Chlorophacinone has the empirical formula $C_{23}H_{15}ClO_3$ and the molecular weight of 364.8. It forms a yellow crystalline solid with a melting point of 140°C. It is slightly soluble in water (100 mg/liter at 20°C) and soluble in acetone, ethanol, and methanol. It is stable under normal storage conditions and noncorrosive.

History, Formulation, and Uses Chlorophacinone is an anticoagulant rodenticide used to control rats, mice, voles, and other wild rodents. It is formulated as ready-to-use baits based on whole, cracked, or milled grain at concentrations of active ingredient ranging from 0.005 to 0.25%. It can also be used as a tracking powder. An oil concentrate is also available.

83.5.5.2 Toxicity to Laboratory Animals

The acute oral LD 50 is reported to be 2 mg/kg in the rat, 1 mg/kg in the mouse, and 50 mg/kg in the rabbit. In the duck, the oral LD 50 is 100 mg/kg. Chlorophacinone is of low acute toxicity to wild birds (LD 50 of 430 mg/kg). The acute dermal LD 50 in the rabbit is 200 mg/kg (Sax, 1984). It is absorbed through the skin of the rabbit; a solution of 5 mg in 2 ml of liquid paraffin applied to 100 cm^2 of shaved skin of a rabbit caused a slight reduction of prothrombin (Worthing and Walker, 1983). Administration of 15 daily doses of 2.25 mg to gray partridges produced no detectable ill effects. Chlorophacinone is not an eye or skin irritant.

Absorption, Distribution, Metabolism, and Excretion Chlorophacinone is absorbed through the gastrointestinal tract. After oral administration, 90% is eliminated in the feces within 48 hr in the form of metabolites (Hartley and Kidd, 1983).

Mode of Action Chlorophacinone is an anticoagulant agent depressing hepatic synthesis of prothrombin and clotting factors VII, IX, and X. Direct damage to capillary permeability occurs concurrently. The ultimate effect of these actions is to induce widespread internal hemorrhage. In addition, chlorophacinone is an uncoupler of oxidative phosphorylation. Unlike the coumarin derivatives, chlorophacinone may causes symptoms and signs of neurologic and cardiopulmonary injury in laboratory rats, which often lead to death before hemorrhage occurs. Chlorophacinone is characterized by its long-lasting depressive action on coagulation.

83.5.5.3 Toxicty to Humans

Chlorophacinone has not been used therapeutically. Only two reports of human intoxication are known. They both involve suicidal attempts. One of them concerns a 37-year-old woman who ingested about 250 ml of a 0.25% concentrate formulation (about 625 mg of chlorophacinone). Despite intensive therapy with vitamin K_1 (phytomenadione, natural form of vitamin K), the anticoagulant effect of chlorophacinone persisted for at least 45 days. An interesting fact is that it was discovered during this episode that the synthetic analog of vitamin K was ineffective (Murdoch, 1983). The second report concerns a 28-year-old man who ingested an unknown amount of chlorophacinone-based rodenticide. Again, the most striking feature in this case was the unusually prolonged and severe anticoagulant effect, even under adequate therapy; it required 4 weeks for prothrombin level to come back to normal (Dusein *et al.*, 1984).

Treatment of Poisoning   Intoxication by chlorophacinone is treated by massive and prolonged administration of natural vitamin K.

83.5.6 DIFENACOUM

83.5.6.1 Identity, Properties, and Usses

Chemical Name   3-[3-(1,1'-biphenyl)4-yl-1,2,3,4-tetrahydro-1-naphthalenyl]-4-hydroxy-2H-1-benzopyran-2-one   is   the chemical name.

Structure   See Fig. 83.4.

Synonyms   Difenacoum is the approved common name. Trade names include Neoxorexa® and Ratak®. The CAS registry number is 56073-07-5.

Physical and Chemical Properties   Difenacoum has the empirical formula $C_{31}H_{24}O_3$ and a molecular weight of 444.5. It is an off-white powder with a melting point of 215–219°C. It is slightly soluble in water (less than 10 mg/liter at pH 7) and soluble in organic solvents (50 g/liter in acetone and chloroform and 600 mg/liter in benzene).

History, Formulations, and Uses   The rodenticidal properties of difenacoum were first described in 1975. It is formulated as a 1 gm/kg concentrate and as a ready-to-use bait containing 50 mg of active ingredient per kilogram of bait. It is an indirect anticoagulant, more potent than the early compounds. It is used to control rats and mice resistant to other anticoagulants with varying degrees of activity.

83.5.6.2 Toxicity to Laboratory Animals

The oral LD 50 is 1.8 mg/kg in male rats, 0.8 mg/kg in male mice, and 50 mg/kg in female guinea pigs. The LD 50 value for oral administration in pigs is reported to be above 80 mg/kg and it is 100 mg/kg in cats. The acute dermal LD 50 is 50 mg/kg in rats and 1000 mg/kg in rabbits. The cumulative oral LD 50 in male rats over a 5-day period is 0.16 mg/kg/day.

Difenacoum and brodifacoum have been suspected of being responsible for secondary toxicity in barn owls feeding on rodents poisoned by these "second-generation" anticoagulants, a phenomenon which was not seen with warfarin baits (Wenz, 1984).

Biochemical Effects   Like brodifacoum and warfarin, difenacoum was shown to inhibit K-dependent steps in the synthesis of clotting factors II, VII, IX, and X, and it is suspected that

coumarin anticoagulants block the vitamin K_1 epoxide cycle by inhibiting the vitamin K_1 epoxide reductase. The latter is confirmed by the observation that difenacoum and brodifacoum produce an accumulation of tritiated vitamin K_1 epoxide in rats and rabbits administered tritiated vitamin K_1 (Park and Leck, 1982). Like brodifacoum, difenacoum has a much longer duration of action than warfarin.

Treatment of Poisoning in Animals   Prolonged administration of vitamin K_1 over several weeks is the treatment of choice. Since the effect of vitamin K_1 is usually delayed as it only permits the formation of new prothrombin, initial treatment with transfusion of fresh-frozen plasma or a small quantity of matched fresh blood is recommended in order to provide enough protrhombin to prevent further hemorrhage (Barlow *et al.*, 1982; Park and Leck, 1982).

83.5.6.3 Toxicity to Humans

A case of an attempted suicide in a 17-year-old girl is reported in the literature. She was admitted to hospital having ingested 500 gm of the rat bait Neosorexa or about 25 mg of difenacoum. Upon admission she had a prolonged prothrombin time. She was treated with vitamin K1 for 45 days. The clotting activity returned to normal 30 days after the beginning of treatment (Barlow *et al.*, 1982).

The coumarin anticoagulant difenacoum was detected by HPLC with multiwavelengh ultraviolet detection in plasma from a 41-years-old man who presented with a severe deficiency of vitamin K-dependent clotting factors of unknown aetiology. Plasma concentrations of difenacoum declined from 0.97 to 0.11 mg l^{-1} in 47 days with a terminal half-life of 11.7 days. Subsequently, plasma concentrations of difenacoum and descarboxyprothrombin unexpectedly increased. Seven months after exposure, clotting times were still prolonged. The patient continued to have episodes of epistasix, haematoma, purpurae, and bruising and he required frequent treatment with fresh-frozen plasma in additional to oral phylloquinone (200 mg/days^{-1}). Intermittent and unexpected increases in plasma concentrations of difenacoum and descarboxyprothrombin suggested that covert, repeated ingestion of the anticoagulant was the most likely cause of the poisoning. The measurement of low concentrations of plasma phylloquinone except following supervised ingestion of the vitamin indicated that as an outpatient, the subject was not compliant with treatment despite his protestations on the contrary. He continued to deny this even when confronted by laboratory findings and at no time did he ever admit to self-poisoning (McCarthy *et al.*, 1997).

Treatment of Poisoning   In case of threatening hemorrhage transfusion of fresh blood of fresh-frozen plasma is the initial step. Intravenous and oral administration of vitamin K_1 for a prolonged period of time (several weeks) with regular monitoring of coagulation is necessary.

83.5.7 BROMADIOLONE

83.5.7.1 Identity, Properties, and Uses

Chemical   Name   3-[3-bromo[1,1'-biphenyl-4-yl)-3-hyd-roxy-1-phenylpropyl]-4-hydroxy-2H-1-benzopyran-2-one   is the chemical name. The CAS registry number is 28772-56-7.

Structure   See Fig. 83.3.

Synonyms   Bromadiolone is the approved common name (BSI, E-ISO, F-ISO). Trade names include Deadline®, Lanirat®, Maki® and SuperCaid®.

Physical and Chemical Properties   Bromadiolone has the empirical formula $C_{30}H_{23}BrO_4$ and a molecular weight of 527.4. The technical material is a yellowish powdered mixture of two diastereoisomers of a minimum purity of 97% and a melting point of 200–210°C. Its water solubility is in the or-der of 20 mg/l at 20°C. Solubility in organic solvents is (20°C) 730 g/l for dimethyl formamide, 25 mg/l for ethyl acetate, 8 mg/l for ethanol. It is stable under normal storage conditions.

History, Formulations, and Uses   Bromadiolone is a second-generation anticoagulant of the hydroxy-4-coumarin that was patented in 1967 for the control of commensal rats and mice, including those resistant to warfarin and first-generation antico-agulants, voles, and water voles. It is formulated as ready-to-use cereal and paraffine based baits containing 0.005% bromadi-olone.

83.5.7.2 Toxicity to Laboratory Animals

Single dose acute toxicity of bromadiolone is in the same order of magnitude as other second-generation anticoagulants: in the wild rat (*Rattus norvegicus*) 1.1–1.8 mg/kg and in the mouse (*Mus musculus*) 1.75 mg/kg (Buckle *et al.*, 1972). The toxicity to nonrodent species has been reported to be 0.3 mg/kg in the rabbit, 25 mg/kg in the cat, 0.15 to 1.0 in the dog, and 0.5 to 2.0 in the pig (Meehan, 1984). Birds appear to be somewhat less susceptible with acute oral LD 50s of 1600 mg/kg for quails (Tomlin, 1994).

The acute percutaneous LD 50 is reported to be 2.1 mg/kg in the rabbit (Tomlin, 1994).

Toxicity to Wildlife   A recent survey of the effects of anti-coagulant rodenticides on nontarget wild species in France has shown that this category of compounds is responsible for a very limited number of identified causes of death in most species: 1 to 3% (Berny *et al.*, 1997).

Mode of Action   Bromadiolone is an anticoagulant with the same mechanism of action as the other second-generation ro-denticides.

83.5.7.3 Toxicity to Humans

It seems that so far no cases of human poisoning by bromadi-olone have been reported in the literature.

Treatment of Poisoning   Intoxication by bromadiolone, like with other second-generation anticoagulant rodenticides, re-quires massive and prolonged administration of vitamin K.

83.5.8 DIFETHIALONE

83.5.8.1 Identity, Properties, and Uses

Chemical   Name   3-[3-(4'-bromo[1,1'-biphenyl]-4-yl)-1,2,3, 4-tetrahydro-1-naphthalenyl]-4-hydroxy-2H-1-[benzothiopy-ran-2-one] is the chemical name. The CAS registry number is 104653-34-1.

Structure   See Fig. 83.3.

Synonyms   Difethialone is the approved common name (BSI). Trade names include Frap®, Baraki®, and Operats Plus®.

Physical and Chemical Properties   Difethialone has the em-pirical formula $C_{31}H_{23}BrO_2S$ and a molecular weight of 539.5. It forms a whitish powder with a vapor pressure of 0.074 mPa at 25°C. It is practically unsoluble in water: 0.39 mg/l at 25°C. Its solubility in ethanol, methanol, hexane, chloroform, and ace-tone in mg/l at 25°C is respectively 0.7, 0.47, 0.2, 40.8, and 4.3. The octanol/water partition coefficient is 1.41×10^5. It is stable at temperatures up to 230°C. It is highly sensitive to phytolysis in aqueous solutions. It is strongly adsorbed in soils.

History, Formulations, and Uses   Difethialone was intro-duced as a second-generation anticoagulant rodenticide in 1986 for the control of commensal rats and mice including those resistant to firs-generation anticoagulants. It is formulated as ready-to-use whole grain cereals and husked oat grain baits con-taining 0.0025% active substance.

83.5.8.2 Toxicity to Laboratory Animals

The acute single dose oral LD 50 of technical grade difethialone (97.6% purity) has been reported as 0.56 mg/kg for rats, 1.29 mg/kg for mice, 4 mg/kg for dogs, and 2 to 3 mg/kg for pigs. The percutaneous acute LD 50 was determined in rabbits at 5.3 mg/kg, 6.5 mg/kg in male rats, and 5.3 mg/kg for females. By inhalation in rats exposed for 4 hours, the LC 50 is between 5 and 19.3 mg/m³. It is not irritant to the rabbit skin and only slightly irritant to the eyes. It is not a skin sensitizer. It has no mutagenic or teratogenic potential. The only effects seen in a 90-day feeding study in the rate were those expected on blood coagulation.

Absorption, Distribution, Metabolism, and Excretion   In rats treated by oral administration difethialone has a short half-life in blood and a longer half-life in the liver. It is essentially eliminated in the feces as the unchanged parent compound, indicating a very limited metabolization (Tomlin, 1994).

Mode of Action Difethialone is an anticoagulant with the same mode of action as the other second-generation compounds.

83.5.8.3 Toxicity to Humans

It seems that so far no cases of human poisoning by difethialone have been reported in the literature.

Treatment of Poisoning Intoxication by difethialone, like with other second-generation anticoagulant rodenticides, requires massive and prolonged administration of vitamin K.

83.6 VITAMIN D-RELATED COMPOUNDS

83.6.1 ERGOCALCIFEROL

83.6.1.1 Identity, Properties, and Uses

Chemical Name 9,10-Secoergosta-5,7,10(19),22-tetraen-3-01 is the chemical name.

Structure See Fig. 83.5.

Synonyms The common name calciferol is approved by BPC (British Pharmacopeia Commission); ergocalciferol is approved by USP (U.S. Pharmacopeia). It is also known as vitamin D_2, but for safety reasons it is prohibited in some countries to mention the identity of these compounds as vitamin D on rodenticides labels [Food and Agriculture Organization (FAO), 1979]. Other names include activated ergosterol, Derat Concentrate®, Deratol®, and Hi-Deratol®. The trade name is Sorexa C.R.® for a combination of calciferol and warfarin.

Physical and Chemical Properties The empirical formula is $C_{28}H_{44}O$ and the molecular weight is 396.63. It forms colorless prismatic crystals. The melting point is 115–118°C. It is insoluble in water and soluble in most organic solvents; solubility at 7°C is 69.5 g/l in acetone. It is slightly soluble in vegetable oils. Deterioration of pure, crystalline vitamin D_2 is negligible after storage for 9 months in evacuated amber ampules at refrigerator temperature. However, calciferol tends to decompose in the presence of air and moisture. The stability of corn oil solutions is, however, satisfactory (Greaves *et al.*, 1974).

History, Formulations, and Uses The rodenticidal properties of calciferol were described by Greaves *et al.* (1974). The commercial rodenticide was introduced in the United Kingdom in 1974 as a combination of calciferol and warfarin formulated as a ready-to-use bait on canary seed (1 gm of calciferol and 250 mg of warfarin per kilogram). It is also available as an oil concentrate (20 gm/liter). Calciferol is used as a rodenticide for control of commensal rats and mice. Toxicity tests with calciferol combined with warfarin suggest that an additive effect between the compounds could exist. One interesting advantage of calciferol is that it is toxic to warfarin-resistant rodents. A second advantage is that it kills more rapidly—within 1 week instead of 1–3 weeks that are often required with anticoagulants (Greaves *et al.*, 1974).

83.6.1.2 Toxicity to Laboratory Animals

Basic Findings The acute oral LD 50 of calciferol is 56 mg/kg for rats and 23.7 mg/kg for mice. When administered daily for 5 consecutive days to laboratory rats, the LD 50 falls to 7 mg/kg/day. Lethal doses have also been reported by Gill and Redfern (1979) for the multimammate rats *Mastomys natalensis*; they range from 78 to 107 mg/kg (mean 96 mg/kg) in males and from 108 to 137 mg/kg (mean 119) in females when administered for 1 days at a concentration of 0.1% in bait. Similar values were reported by Greaves *et al.* (1974) for wild rodents. When calciferol was given at doses of 100 mg/kg by stomach tube on one or more days, laboratory rats and mice became visibly ill within 3 days. The clinical signs are characterized by loss of appetite, listlessness, piloerection, hunched position, absence of reaction to external stimuli, weight loss, priapism, and frequent micturition (Gillman *et al.*, 1960).

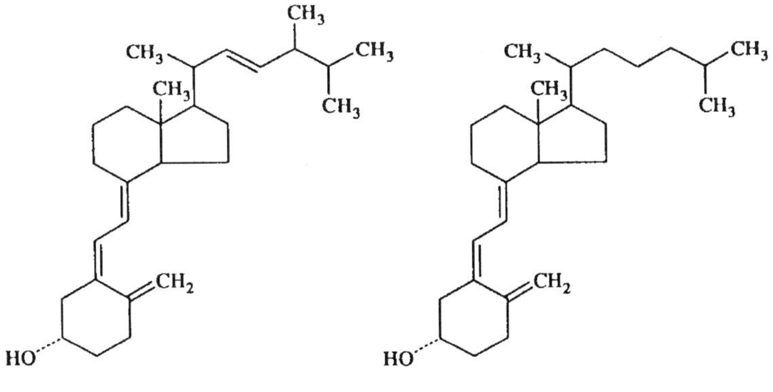

Figure 83.5 Two forms of vitamin D used as rodenticides.

Absorption, Distribution, Metabolism, and Excretion The action of calciferol is to raise blood calcium levels by stimulating the absorption of calcium from the intestine and mobilizing skeletal reserves. This mechanism is slow and takes many hours to build up an effective level; the period of latency between the ingestion of calciferol and the development of hypercalcemia and occurrence of lethal lesions is of the order of several days, usually 4 or 5 (Greaves *et al.*, 1974).

Calciferol has a long biological half-life in mammals and hypercalcemia induced by overdosage may continue for 6–9 months (Buckle *et al.*, 1972). The various tissues of the body store vitamin D for varying periods. The depletion of stores in the body is caused partly by its fecal excretion and partly by its destruction in the body.

Biochemical Effects Calciferol is the most important factor for the optimal absorption of calcium. It is responsible for the synthesis of a protein that binds calcium in the intestinal mucosa, especially in the duodenum. In the absence of calciferol, calcium cannot be absorbed.

Effects on Organs and Tissues All forms of vitamin D are toxic when given in sufficiently large amounts. Excessive doses of calciferol mobilize the phosphorus and calcium from the tissues, thus broadly having an opposite effect to normal doses. The soft tissues tend to become calcified while the bone tends to be rarefied.

The soft tissues most affected are the renal tubules and the media of the small renal arteries and of the large vessels, especially the aorta. The bronchi, lungs, heart and coronaries, and the stomach also are affected. In dogs, there is atrophy of the testes and the prostate while the parathyroids are smaller than normal. The histochemical effects of vascular injuries induced by calciferol orally administered to male and female Wistar rats for 5 consecutive days at doses ranging from 25,000 to 150,000 IU (1 mg of calciferol is equivalent to 40,000 IU) were studied by Gillman *et al.* (1960). By day 15 of the experiment—that is, day 10 after the last day of calciferol administration—necrosis of the spleen was observed in many rats that died or were sacrificed. Among the survivors, there were indications that the damaged spleen had been regenerated completely by day 25. The heart was severely injured very early in the experiments. Similarly, the coronary arteries were observed showing early dilation, injury to the internal elastic membranes, and associated early calcification. These changes were associated with sclerotic repair. In the aorta, there was an apparent relationship between the intensity of the reaction and the doses of calciferol received by the rats. By day 20, a very large concentration of calcium accumulated in the aorta (13–14% calcium compared to 22% in the femur). Similar observations were made by Grant *et al.* (1963) who also showed that this phenomenon was a three-step process involving early widespread alterations in many organs and tissues, followed by spontaneous recurrent resolution and reappearance of calcification for many months, even after a single episode of acute intoxication. These authors also showed distinct differences in the time of onset and rate and extent of calcification of various tissues.

Nikodemusz *et al.* (1981) have shown that in six male and six female common vole (*Microtus arvalis*), single acute oral dosing with calciferol (80–620 mg/kg) induced morphological changes representing varying degrees of parenchymal degeneration and calcification in the kidneys, lungs, and heart. Calcium deposits were observed in the esophageal and gastric mucosae, as well as in the aortic media. These lesions were not observed in the group receiving 80 mg/kg of calciferol. The approximate lethal dose by the oral route was estimated as 120 mg/kg in males and 280 mg/kg in females. The survival time ranged from 53 to 94 hr. Tarrant and Westlake (1984) have also shown that feeding laboratory-reared male rats (*Rattus norvegicus*) and male and female quail (*Coturnix coturnix japonica*) a diet containing 0.1% calciferol (the recommended field concentration) for 2 days induced in both species a similar pattern of calcium deposits in the kidneys, beginning on the second day after the animals were returned to a standard, calciferol-free diet.

Effects on Reproduction Adult female New Zealand White rabbits had been intramuscularly treated with ergosterol in cottonseed oil in divided doses every other day for a total of 1.5 million IU. Three other groups of five rabbits each received intramuscular injections of ergosterol daily for the duration of the gestational period for a total of 2.5–3.5 million and 4.5 million IU. At autopsy all the females given 2.5 million IU and above died spontaneously within 65 days after their first injection of calciferol and all that were pregnant aborted during the first 12 days of pregnancy or delivered macerated fetuses. All aortas had various degrees of pathological changes, including those from females treated with 1.5 million IU. A total of 14 abnormalities of the aorta were observed in the 34 offspring whose mothers had been treated with excessive levels of ergocalciferol. Aortic lesions that appeared similar to the supravalvular aortic stenosis seen in humans were noted in six rabbits. The blood levels of ergocalciferol in the mothers and their offspring were seven and nine times greater than those in the control classes and their offspring, respectively, indicating that transplacental passage occurred (Friedman and Roberts, 1966). A similar experiment was carried out by Friedman and Mills (1969) on 15 pregnant New Zealand White rabbits given divided doses of intramuscular ergocalciferol every other day, starting on the second day of insemination and throughout the pregnancy for a total of 750,000 IU. Characteristic malformations were observed in the offspring. These were represented by premature closure of cranial structures, small skulls compared with the controls, and narrowing of the body of the mandible. The maxillary and mandibular central incisors showed severe enamel hypoplasia. Some cases of anodontia and abnormal palatal shape were noted. Similar craniofacial malformations are frequently associated with supravalvular aortic stenosis in children.

Several additional studies of the effects of vitamin D on reproduction and fetal development in rats and rabbits have been reported. Latore (1961) found that excess ergocalciferol reduces fertility in rats when administered on days 0–7 of gestation but not when administered on days 8–21. Nebel and Ornstein (1966) have demonstrated that ergocalciferol administered to rats (*Rattus rattus*) in daily doses of 20,000 IU for 1–3 weeks significantly affected the genital cycle, fertility, and early pregnancy from both the morphological and functional points of view in direct relation to the beginning and duration of ergocalciferol administration. Ornoy *et al.* (1968) showed that vitamin D_2 (ergocalciferol) given to pregnant albino rats at daily doses of 4000, 20,000, or 40,000 IU from day 9 to days 21 of pregnancy crosses the placental barrier and induces alterations of the mineral composition in the fetal bones at the 40,000 IU level only. In the same treated group, placentas, fetuses, and fetal bones were found to be smaller than those in the untreated groups. However, it seems from the experimental data that pregnant rats are more tolerant to rather high levels of ergocalciferol than nonpregnant females (Ornoy *et al.*, 1968; Potvliege, 1962).

Factors Influencing Toxicity   In commercially available preparations, calciferol is often associated with warfarin in a 4:1 ratio because it has been shown that this mixture produced a marked increase in mortality in Norway rats (Greaves *et al.*, 1974), thus suggesting an additive effect of the two compounds. At the LD 50 level, toxicity of the mixture is intermediate between the toxicities of calciferol and warfarin.

Treatment of Poisoning in Animals   It seems that the only case of poisoning of a domestic animal reported is that of a 4-year-old boxer dog seen several days following ingestion of a warfarin-calciferol mixture. Despite treatment with vitamin K, antibiotics and vitamins, the end of the tongue became necrotic and had to be removed and large areas of the skin were also necrosed, indicating generalized vascular damage. The dog made a slow recovery (Edlin, 1982). It is likely that treatment with vitamin K had prevented the hemorrhagic manifestations of warfarin toxicity from showing but that the vascular injuries due to calciferol were responsible for the necrotic effects.

83.6.1.3 Toxicity to Humans

Therapeutic Use   As a vitamin, calciferol is used to prevent and to cure rickets, tetany, spasmophilia and osteoporomalacia. Several decades ago, vitamin D was recommended for the treatment of lupus vulgaris (skin tuberculosis limited to the face); massive doses were used, sufficient to provoke a mild degree of hypervitaminosis. The purpose was to induce calcification of the subcutaneous lesions in order to stop their progression. In the case of rickets, the recommended preventive dose was 500–1500 IU/day, and the curative dose was 1000–3000 IU/day; it was estimated that 10,000 IU represents a toxic dose. The minimal toxic overdose does not appear to be many times greater than the optimum curative dose (Harris, 1955).

Many cases of vitamin D_2 as well as D_3 poisoning in humans have been reported. The oldest ones were analyzed by Bicknell and Prescott (1953). More recent cases have been reported, all related to accidental or inadvertent overdosing. A 69-year-old women with hypoparathyroidism was treated with a twice-weekly dose of 50,000 IU of calciferol. However, for 4 weeks before admission to hospital she had mistakenly taken 300,000 IU (7.5 mg) a day. On examination she was lethargic and mentally confused, with muscular hypotonia. In this report, two other similar cases concerning elderly women are reported; one had received 100,000 IU (2.5 mg) calciferol orally on alternate days for 3 months and the other had received 400,000 IU (10 mg) a day by mouth and 600,000 IU of calciferol once a week by injection during the 2 months before admission to hospital. All three patients had elevated serum calcium. All three of them were treated with intravenous injections of porcine calcitonin, which caused serum calcium to fall back to a normal level within 2–3 days (Buckle *et al.*, 1972). Davies and Adams (1978) have also reported eight cases of severe vitamin D poisoning. In six patients the therapy was unnecessary, and in two others inadequate supervision of treatment resulted in overdosage. Paterson (1980) reported 21 cases of hypercalcemia due to vitamin D poisoning; among them two patients died while intoxicated. Overall, the clinical symptoms induced by chronic poisoning include, in various associations and intensity, loss of appetite, loss of weight greater than would be expected from the loss of appetite, nausea, vomiting, and constipation or diarrhea. Abdominal pain may be so severe as to lead to unnecessary laparotomies. Headaches are usual and one special form has been noticed. This is a tightness across the back of the head which goes on to acute sensitiveness of the scalp. Mental confusion and loss of memory may also be seen. Epileptiform fits are a rare complication. Metastatic calcification has been described along with vascular and renal calcification. An unusual, albeit typical case has been reported by Cohen *et al.* (1979): a case of a deafness due to a long-term overdosage for the treatment of pseudohypoparathyroidy (2.5 mg of calciferol daily for 4 years). The patient had a 3-month history of deafness, weight loss, anorexia, and weakness. She had extensive calcification of the tympanic membranes, corneas, kidneys, and blood vessels. She had also, of course, high serum calcium, which was successfully treated with calcitonin and prednisolone and a low-calcium diet. She was discharged from hospital symptom-free except for the deafness. Hypercalcemia is the earliest sign of vitamin D overdosage. It was suggested at one point that increased intake of vitamin D through consumption of fish liver in Norway might be correlated with an increased probability of myocardial infarction (Linden, 1974). However, this hypothesis, based on a retrospective study of a number of patients with myocardial infarction, angina pectoris, and degenerative joint diseases, was later criticized because of serious bias and shortcomings in the methodology (Lindahl and Lindwall, 1975). A prospective study, performed in the same area of northern Norway, has not confirmed the existence of a higher risk of myocardial infraction related to vitamin D intake or status of the population (Vik *et al.*, 1979).

Use Experience and Dosage Response   There is no known report of accidents occurring with calciferol used as a rodenticide. It is difficult to estimate the minimum toxic dose in humans; however, from the reported cases of overdosage, it would seem that 0.15 mg/kg/day for 3 weeks may lead to clinical signs of poisoning.

Treatment of Poisoning Treatment of acute and chronic overdosages with calciferol requires that hypercalcemia be brought down to a normal level quickly; intravenous injection of calcitonin is the specific treatment to be applied under close monitoring of the serum calcium level. Steroid therapy is also often effective but slower, normocalcemia being achieved after 5–7 days. Other methods are available but they are not devoid of problems: Chelation with sodium ededate is only temporary in its effect and is nephrotoxic. Sodium phosphate is also effective but may be responsible for metastatic calcifications (Buckle *et al.*, 1972). One case of vitamin D_2 poisoning in an elderly woman was successfully treated by inducing the hepatic microsomal enzymes with 500 mg/day of glutethimide. The mechanism of action is still unknown (Iqbal and Taylor, 1982), but this approach is rather slow since the serum calcium level did not fall back to normal values until day 12 of treatment.

83.6.2 CHOLECALCIFEROL

83.6.2.1 Identity, Properties, and Uses

Chemical name 9,10-secocholesta-5,7,10(19)-trien-3-betaol is the chemical name.

Structure See Fig. 83.5.

Synonyms Some synonyms are activated 7-dehydrocholesterol, oleovitamin D_3, cholecalcifero natural vitamin D_3. The trade name for the rodenticide is Quintox®.

Physical and Chemical Properties The empirical formula is $C_{27}H_{44}O$ and the molecular weight is 384.62. It forms tine needles. The melting point is 84–86°C. It is practically insoluble in water, soluble in the usual organic solvents, and only slightly soluble in vegetable oils. It is oxidized and inactivated by moist air within a few days. However, the formulated product is stable over 1 year at ambient temperatures in sealed packages.

History, Formulations, and Uses Cholecalciferol is formulated for use ad a rodenticide as a grain bait containing 750 ppm (0.075%) of active ingredient and commercialized under the trade name Quintox®. It is a single-feeding and multifeeding rodenticide used for controlling anticoagulant-resistant rats and mice. There is a period of time between feeding and death similar to but perhaps shorter than the observed with anticoagulant rodenticides. The rodenticidal activity of cholecalciferol is comparable to that of ergocalciferol.

83.6.2.2 Toxicity to Laboratory Animals

The two forms of calciferol are equally toxic to most mammals. The acute oral LD 50 of cholecalciferol is 43.6 mg/kg for *Rattus*

norvegicus and 42.5 mg/kg for mice (*Mus musculus*). In the dog, the oral LD 50 is 88 mg/kg. However, deaths have been observed with doses of 10 to 20 mg/kg (El Bahri, 1990).

Absorption, Distribution, and Excretion Cholecalciferol after absorption from the intestine is transported to the liver, where it is metabolized to 25-hydroxycholecalciferol by an NADPH-dependent reaction. This metabolite is then transferred to the kidney and converted to 24-, 25-, or 1,25-dihydrocholecalciferol by mitochondrial mixed-function oxidases (McClain *et al.*, 1980). After their intestinal absorption, ergocalciferol (vitamin D_2) and cholecalciferol (vitamin D_3) undergo an identical metabolic C pathway (Fournier *et al.*, 1985). The metabolism and pharmacokinetics of one metabolite of cholecalciferol, 24,25-dihydrocholecalciferol, have been reviewed by Jarnargin *et al.* (1985); the excretion curve shows an initial fast phase with a plasma half-life of 0.55 hr and a second slow phase with a plasma half-life of 73.8 hr in the rat. The clearance from plasma, liver, and kidney but not intestine follows a two-compartment model. The most potent form of vitamin D_3, 1,25-dihydrochlolecalciferol, has been shown to be responsible for the stimulation of intestinal absorption of calcium and the metabolism of calcium in bone. However, Frolick and Deluca (1973) have shown that when given orally to rats, 1,25-dihydrocholecalciferol is rapidly modified during its passage through the intestine, thus reducing its physiological activity to a large extent.

Effects on Organs and Tissues Moderately excessive doses of cholecalciferol, 100, 300, 2000, and 4000 IU/kg of feed, given for 4 months to experimental Yorkshire pigs rapidly produced gross arterial lesions (fibromuscular interstitial thickening of the coronaries, especially at the branching sites). Macrophages, plasma cells, and mast cells were observed to accumulate in the subendothelial space. The extent of these lesions, resembling those commonly seen in atmosceloris in humans, was more or less dose-related (Toda *et al.*, 1985). Since both forms of vitamin D (ergocalciferol and cholecalciferol) follow the same metabolic pathway, it is expected that they are responsible for inducing the same lesions.

Effects on Reproduction Calcitriol (1,25-dihydrocholecalciferol), which is the most biologically active metabolite of cholecalciferol, has been administered to pregnant rats and rabbits at daily doses of 0.02–0.08 and 0.30 μg/kg from days 7–15 of gestation in the rat and from days 7–18 in the rabbit. In rats no adverse effect on fertility, litter parameters and offspring was observed. Hypercalcemia and hypophosphatemia were observed in pregnant rats of the middle an high-dose groups, as well as hypercalcemia in pups. Calcitriol induced maternal mortality and fetotoxicity in rabbits treated with 0.3 μg/kg/day. Two litters at the highest dose and one litter at the middle dose levels contained fetuses with multiple abnormalities (McClain *et al.*, 1980).

83.6.2.3 Toxicity to Humans

Experimental Oral Exposure The active metabolite 1,25-dihydrocholecalciferol was administered either orally or intravenously to four healthy volunteers and three patients with hypoparathyroidism. After an oral dose, the highest serum concentration of radioactivity was reached after 4 hr. The route of administration had little apparent effect on the serum concentration or on the rapid phase of elimination, but the slow phase of excretion was longer after oral administration. The highest urinary excretion rate was observed during the first 24 hr and was little affected by the route of administration. The half-life of 1,25-dihydrochole-calciferol was 3–5 days. On average, 40% of the dose of 1,25-dihyrocholecalciferol was excreted within 10 days (Mawer *et al.*, 1976).

Therapeutic Use Cholecalciferol being the natural form of vitamin D, the therapeutic uses are those outlined for ergocalciferol.

Accidents and Use Experience These are the same as those mentioned for ergocalciferol. There is no known report on an accident specifically attributable to cholecalciferol used as a rodenticide. However, intoxication from overdosage during therapeutic use of vitamin D_3 is well known and signs and symptoms have been well studied (Navarro *et al.*, 1985).

83.7 MISCELLANEOUS SYNTHETIC ORGANIC RODENTICIDES

As far as is known, the miscellaneous synthetic organic rodenticides (see Fig. 83.6) are unrelated to one another or to other groups of pesticides either pharmacologically or chemically. The two that have been studied in humans are remarkable. Chloralose is an anesthetic, albeit one with the property of inducing myoclinic seizures. With the possible exception of this compound, anesthetics have nothing to offer for killing vertebrate pests. Far too many animals become anesthetized before consuming a fatal dose, and they later recover. In fact, the possibility of recovery seems to be taken into account in the British practice of recovering birds affected by the compound.

Norbomide is of interest as one of the most selective poisons known. Its limitation is not any lack of toxicity to species of the genus *Rattus* but the problem of secondary bait refusal (Greaves, 1966).

83.7.1 CHLORALOSE

83.7.1.1 Identity, Properties, and Uses

Chemical Name 1,2-*O*-(2,2,2-trichloroethylidene)-α-D-glucofuranose is the chemical name.

Structure See Fig. 83.6.

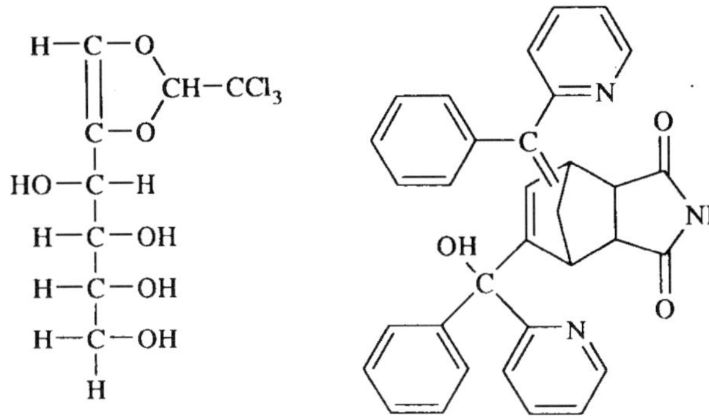

α-Chloralose   Norbormide

Figure 83.6 Miscellaneous synthetic organic rodenticides.

Synonyms Chloralose (BSI) is the common name in use. Other nonproprietary names include α-chloralose, α-D-glucochloralose, anhydroglucochloral, chloro-alosane, and glucochloral. Trade names include Alphakil® and Somio®. The CAS registry number is 15879-93-3.

Physical and Chemical Properties Chloralose has the empirical formula $C_8H_{11}Cl_3O_6$ and a molecular weight of 309.54. It forms a crystalline powder that melts at 187°C. It is soluble in ether and glacial acetic acid, slightly soluble in chloroform, and almost insoluble in petroleum ether. Its solubility in water at 15°C is 0.44%. Chloralose reduces Fehling's solution only after prolonged heating. It is hydrolyzed into its two components by acids.

History, Formulations, and Uses Chloralose has been in use in Europe for many years. Its narcotic properties are employed to immobilize depredating birds and render them easier to kill by other means. Baits contain about 1.5% of the compound.

It has been reported that chloralose is also used on seed grain as a bird repellent. It is used against mice in baits of up to 40 gm/kg. All baits should contain a warning dye.

Chloralose is used in medicine as a soporific and formerly was used as an anesthetic.

83.7.1.2 Toxicity to Laboratory Animals

The oral LD 50 values of chloralose in rats and mice are in the range of 300–400 mg/kg. Cats are more susceptible (100 mg/kg) and dogs more resistant (600–1000 mg/kg) (Cornwell, 1969). The compound is more toxic to many birds than to mammals. Oral LD 50 values have been determined for the starling (75 mg/kg), redwing blackbird (32 mg/kg), yellow-headed blackbird (133 mg/kg), crow (42 mg/kg), pigeon (178 mg/kg), house finch (56 mg/kg), house sparrow (42 mg/kg), mallard duck (42 mg/kg), mourning dove (42 mg/kg), and white-crowned sparrow (56 mg/kg) (Schafer, 1972).

Hanriot and Richet, who advocated chloralose as a soporific, found that dogs survived oral dosages as high as 610 mg/kg but were killed by dosages of 660 mg/kg and greater. Cats survived oral dosages of 65 mg/kg or lower but one was killed by a dosage of 71 mg/kg and all were killed by 140 mg/kg or more. Dogs survived intravenous injection of 120 mg/kg or less but were killed by 150 mg/kg. A dosage of 12.5 mg/kg produced severe symptoms in a cat (Hanriot and Richet, 1897).

After some delay, animals poisoned by chloralose show incoordination, vertigo, tremor, and failure to recognize objects. The sense of pain is lost but there is increased reactivity to touch, sound, or electric shock. If stimulated, the animals respond reflexively and with full force. If artificial respiration is withheld, animals that have received a sufficient dosage die of respiratory failure (Hanriot and Richet, 1897). Thus it was recognized very early that although response to chloralose is somewhat similar to that to chloral, it is also similar to the response to strychnine in the sensitization to external stimuli.

Chloralose is metabolized to chloral, $CH(OH)_2-CCl_3$ (Cornwell, 1969), oxidized to trichloroacetic acid, and reduced to trichloroethanol (Marshall and Owens, 1954; Owens and Marshall, 1955). The latter metabolite is responsible for much of the hypnotic effect of chloral hydrate; all tissues studied so far are capable of forming it from chloral hydrate (Butler, 1949). Trichloroethanol combines with glucuronic acid in the liver to form the pharmacologically inactive urochloralic acid, which is readily excreted in the urine (Lees, 1972).

Chloralose was not tumorigenic in two strains of mice that received it at the highest tolerated level for 18 months (Innes *et al.*, 1969).

Treatment of Poisoning in Animals   Administration of analeptic drugs or stimulants of the central nervous system such as methylamphetamine (0.5–4 mg/kg of body weight, orally or intramuscularly) or ephedrine (2.5 mg/kg of body weight subcutaneously) has been recommended and successfully applied in poisoned dogs (Bennett, 1972; Smith and Boyd, 1972), although his had already been criticized (Shepherd, 1971) on pharmacological and biochemical grounds. In addition, supportative therapy to correct any hypothermia and respiratory problems may be indicated in severely poisoned animals.

83.7.1.3 Toxicity to Humans

Therapeutic Use   Chloralose was introduced in 1888 and 1893 as an anesthetic and soporific. Its anesthetic use was soon dropped, presumably because an effective dosage tended to cause excessive muscular activity. However, this same feature was regarded as an advantage in connection with a soporific. Thus Sollman (1901) considered chloralose preferable to chloral except for insomnia due to exaggerated reflex irritability. He pointed out that chloralose is a stronger hypnotic, heightens the reflexes, has less action on the heart, and produces practically no local irritation.

Chloralose has gone out of fashion in the United States because its action is somewhat delayed compared to that of chloral (Sollman, 1942) and perhaps because activation of reflexes was not considered an appropriate property of a soporific.

Accidental and Intentional Poisoning   Most reported cases of poisoning by chloralose have occurred in France, where the compound is used medically as a soporific and sedative and also is used as a poison to kill crows and rats. Tempé and Kurtz (1972) listed 60 brands of poison based on chloralose, of which 31 also contained ANTU (see Section 83.4.1.3). In their series of 22 acute intoxications by chloralose, only one was caused by the compound intended for use as a drug; the others were caused by rat poisons.

Most cases of poisoning have involved attempted—generally unsuccessful—suicide. A few cases of mild accidental poisoning of children have been recorded (Gaultier *et al.*, 1962).

The characteristic effect of chloralose is coma, which may be preceded by vomiting, vertigo, trembling, and a sensation of inebriation. In massive intoxication, the coma may appear in some minutes but usually appears in one to several hours after ingestion of chloralose (Favarel-Garrigues and Boget, 1968; Tempé and Kurtz, 1972). The patient may be calm and limp or may be agitated. Cornette and Franck (1970) saw only cases in agitated coma with varying degrees of myoclonia. The myoclonia was always reinforced by stimulation and it occurred predominantly in the arm or leg that was stimulated. There was a bilateral, symmetrical seizure, occasionally with hypersalivation and incontinence of urine. However, tonic spasm or tonic clonic convulsions were not seen. These authors never encountered a case of hypotonic or "calm" coma seen by some others. The attributed the difference to better treatment, but it would seem difficult to exclude differences in dosage as a cause. Favarel-Garrigues and Boget (1968) specifically noted that this form of coma usually but not always occurred in massive intoxications, and one almost always saw hyperreactivity, clonic jerks, and a state of agitation in such cases during recovery. Tempé and Kurtz (1972) reported similar experience. The reflexes are active in agitated coma. In 9 of the 22 cases reported by Tempé and Kurtz (1972), 6 showed a positive Babinski test bilaterally. Reflexes are diminished or absent in massive intoxication.

Authors have not agreed on whether the most severe seizures caused by chloralose are truly epileptic (Moene *et al.*, 1969) or are bilateral, synchronous myoclonic disturbances (Cornette and Franck, 1970). That the latter view is correct seems to depend not on any difference in clinical severity but on a lack of correlation of the EEG with the physical disturbance.

Hypersecretion of the respiratory tract apparently is the most life-threatening aspect of intoxication. It may occur in the absence of ANTU but is more common and more severe when ANTU is involved. This hypersecretion may appear early, suddenly, and severely, but it also disappears in less than an hour. Unlike pulmonary edema, the secretion is not sanguineous and it is poor of albumin. The mild appearance on X-ray contrasts with the clinical severity (Favarel-Garrigues and Boget, 1968).

Even in the apparent absence of injection, the temperature may be elevated as high as 41°C (Moene *et al.*, 1969).

Reawaking requires several hours in mild poisoning, 12–14 hr in severe poisoning, and as much as 96 hr in massive poisoning. The return of consciousness may be gradual but usually is sudden and may be accompanied by headache, stiffness, and weakness. Recovery without sequelae is the rule (Favarel-

Garrigues and Boget, 1968; Tempé and Kurtz, 1972). Moene *et al.* (1969) reported a death caused by uncomplicated poisoning, but it is indicative of the toxicity of chloralose that the victim succeeded in his suicide with this compound only on his third attempt within a period of about 4 months. Death due to circulatory collapse occurred on the evening of the fifth hospital day.

Dosage Response   Eleven patients, who were thought to have taken doses ranging from 640 to 2880 mg, all survived with appropriate treatments (Cornette and Franck, 1970). In another case involving chloralose intended as a rat poison, a dose thought to be 3000–4000 mg was survived (Boudouresque *et al.*, 1966). Other reports of nonfatal dosages have fallen within the range of 2000–9000 mg, but one kind of rat poison came in 20-gm packets and at least one person may have survived that dose. The dose in a fatal case was unknown (Moene *et al.*, 1969; Gras *et al.*, 1975). Tempé and Kurtz (1972) considered that toxic signs could result from 400 mg but that most cases resulted from ingestion of about 1000 mg.

Laboratory Findings   In two cases in which the dosage was known with considerable certainty, about 45% of the amount ingested was recovered from urine passed within the first 24 hr, about 90% in the form of the glucose conjugate (Gras *et al.*, 1975).

The EEG picture in acute poisoning by chloralose is characteristic, involving slow waves and numerous spikes that usually are bilaterally symmetrical and synchrounous. The pattern is changed dramatically by diazepam, which converts it to delta activity without the rapid rhythms commonly seen with that medication. The tracing always become normal, often within 24 hr. The acute EEG record does not correspond to the myoclonic movements that, as observed visually or by EMG, are usually isolated, brief asymmetrical, and asynchronous (Boudouresque *et al.*, 1966; Cornette and Franck, 1970; Tempé and Kurtz, 1972).

Treatment of Poisoning   The myoclonic seizures respond to intravenous injection of 10 mg of diazepam, but this may have to be repeated once or twice. Recovery without sequelae is the rule (Boudouresque *et al.*, 1966; Cornette and Franck, 1970; Tempé and Kurtz, 1972).

83.7.2 NORBORMIDE

83.7.2.1 Identity, Properties, and Uses

Chemical Name   6-(α-hydroxy-α-2-pyridylbenzyl)-7-(α-2-pyridylbenzylidene)-norbor-5-ene-2,3-dicarboximide is the chemical name.

Structure   See Fig. 83.6.

Synonyms   Norbormide (ANSI, BSI, ISO) is the common name for this compound. Trade names include Shoxin® and Raticate®. Code designations include McN-1,025 and S-6,999. The CAS registry number is 991-42-4.

Physical and Chemical Properties   Norbormide has the empirical formula $C_{33}H_{25}N_3O_3$ and a molecular weight of 511.55. It is a white crystalline powder melting at 190–198°C. Its solubility at 30°C in ethanol is 14 mg/liter; in chloroform, more than 150 mg/liter; in diethyl ether, 1 mg/liter; and in 0.1 N CHl, 20 mg/liter. Norbormide is stable at room temperature and to boiling. It is hydrolyzed by alkali and is noncorrosive.

History, Formulations, and Uses   Norbormide was introduced in 1964 by the McNeil Laboratories, Inc. It is a selective rodenticide, lethal to rats but not to other rodent species. It usually is concentrated in prepared baits of cereal at 5–10 gm/kg. Baits containing the compound should contain a warning dye.

Basic Findings   Norbormide shows a remarkable selectivity both in toxicity and in pharmacological effect. Oral LD 50 values for both wild and domestic Norway rats ranged from 5.3 to 15.0 mg/kg (Greaves, 1966; Niu, 1970; Roszkowski, 1965; Roszkowski *et al.*, 1964). Corresponding values for roof rats and Hawaiian rats were 52 and about 10 mg/kg, respectively. Oral LD 50 values were much higher in other rodents and lagomorphs—for example, hamster, 140 mg/kg; guinea pig, 620 mg/kg; mouse, 2250 mg/kg; and rabbit, about 1000 mg/kg. The oral toxicity was low in all other species tested; in the dog, cat, monkey, sheep, pig, and chicken, no effect was detectable at 1000 mg/kg (Niu, 1970; Roszkowski, 1965; Roszkowski *et al.*, 1964).

Rats given an overdose of norbormide died within 15 min to 4 hr. At first, the animals assumed a hunched position. Later there was locomotor impairment due to weakness but not paralysis of the hind legs. Struggling, labored breathing and, in some instances, a mild convulsion preceded death (Roszkowski *et al.*, 1964).

Many analogs have been studied and none was found as toxic to rats as norbormide (Poos *et al.*, 1996).

Dogs survived daily doses of norbormide corresponding to a dietary level of 10,000 ppm for 15–60 days, but they lost appetite and looked ill. Dogs tolerated a dosage corresponding to a dietary level of 1000 ppm for 60 days without ill effect (Roszkowski *et al.*, 1964).

Even in laboratory rats, susceptibility to the compounds was greatly reduced when it was mixed in the diet rather than being given by stomach tube. This may be explained in part by tolerance. The oral LD 50 determined after a 1-day rest period was less than doubled in rats pretreated for 1–7 days at the rate of 2 mg/kg/day. The degree of tolerance was small, but it was statistically significant. When the rest period was 5 days, no tolerance remained (Roszkowski, 1965). In any event, primary bait refusal can be a very serious problem in the use of norbormide (Maddock and Schoff, 1967).

Mode of Action and Cause of Death   Some sex and species differences in susceptibility could be explained by differences in metabolism or absorption. For example, the oral LD 50 values for male and female laboratory rats were 5.3 and 15.0 mg/kg, respectively, although the intravenous values (0.65 and 0.63 mg/kg, respectively) did not differ significantly. The very low susceptibility of mice to oral doses (LD 50, 2250 mg/kg) was due in part to poor absorption, as indicated by the intraperitoneal LD 50 of only 390 mg/kg. However, differences in absorption could not account for many observed species differences. For example, anesthetized dogs showed no detectable response to intravenous injection at the rate of 40 mg/kg.

Species differences in response of the peripheral blood vessels to norbormide seemed to account for most of the observed species differences in its toxicity. The compound caused an extreme, irreversible vasoconstriction in laboratory rats, and this was considered the cause of death. The effect was demonstrated by direct observation of flow experiments, or both, in the ear, eye, skin, mesentary, and heart and undoubtedly occurred in other organs. It resulted from either systemic or appropriate local administration. Only vessels of relatively small caliber were visibly constricted. Spiral rat aortic segments and duodenal strips did not respond to norbormide.

The mechanism of action was best demonstrated in the heart. Isolated myocardial strips showed no loss of contraction or responsiveness when norbormide was added to the bath. However, when norbormide was injected into the aorta of isolated rat hearts, the coronary flow rate decreased greatly and the heart slowed and developed arrhythmia. The effects were not inhibited or reversed by sodium nitrite or other vasodilators.

Following vasoconstriction and presumably as a result of vascular injury, an erythematous but not typically inflammatory lesion began to develop in the rat skin 6 hr after intradermal injection of 0.1 ml of 0.1% solution. The lesion became maximal in 24–48 hr. Sometimes an area of central necrosis was observed. A concentration of 0.01% produced the effect only inconsistently.

Except in rats, vasoconstriction was not seen even at high dosage levels. Why rats respond differently remains obscure (Roszkowski, 1965). A number of the observations just discussed were confirmed by Niu (1970), who reached the same general conclusion regarding the importance of vasoconstriction in the rat.

An oral or intraperitoneal dosage of 1020 mg/kg caused a doubling of blood glucose levels and a decrease of liver and muscle glycogen when coma began 0.5–2 hr after treatment. The same dosage had no effect on the glucose levels of two strains of mice, nor did it produce illness. Insulin counteracted the hyperglycemic effect or norbormide in rats but did not protect against toxic manifestations and death, suggesting that the hyperglycemia is secondary (Patil and Radhakrishnamurty, 1973).

83.7.2.2 Toxicity to Humans

Because the toxicity of norbormide to different species corresponds to its ability to cause peripheral vasoconstriction in

them, it was a meaningful test to inject three volunteers intradermally with 0.1 ml of 0.1% solution. Skin treated in this was showed no response not seen in controls (Roszkowski, 1965).

In a study that has been cited for many years but apparently was first published by Hayes (1975), Dr Kazwya Kamoya of the Showa Medical School in Tokyo administered norbormide to volunteers orally at doses ranging from 20 to 300 mg. No sign or symptom was produced. It was concluded that body temperature and blood pressure decreased slightly and temporarily following the larger dose. Actually, the largest fall in temperature observed at any dose was 0.7°C, and this occurred after doses of 20 to 80 mg, whereas the largest fall after a dose of 120 mg or more was only 0.3°C. Systotic (but not diastolic) blood pressure possibly fell after 120 mg of norbormide and certainly fell after larger doses. The largest decreases recorded were from 1332/76 to 100/74 after 200 mg and from 120/80 to 96/80 after 300 mg. The lowest values were measured 1 hr after ingestion, and the values were essentially normal at 2 hr in each instance.

It seems unlikely that poisoning by norbormide will occur. If it does, treatment must be symptomatic.

REFERENCES

Allcroft, R., and Jones, J. S. L. (1969). Fluoroacetamide poisoning. I. Toxicity in dairy cattle: Clinical history and preliminary investigations. *Vet. Rec.* **84**, 399–402.

Allcroft, R., Salt, F. J., Peters, R. A., and Shorthouse, M. (1969). Fluoroacetamide poisoning. II. Toxicity in dairy cattle: Confirmation of diagnosis. *Vet. Rec.* **84**, 403–409.

American Medical Association (AMA) (1977). "AMA Drug Evaluations," 3rd ed. Publishing Sciences Group, Littleton, MA.

American Medical Association (AMA) (1980). "AMA Drug Evaluations," 4th ed. Am. Med. Assoc., Chicago.

Annegers, J. F., and Zacharski, L. R. (1980). Cancer morbidity and mortality in previously andicoagulated patients. *Thromb. Res.* **18**, 399–403.

Anonymous (1964a). Fluoroacetamide. *Lancet* **1**, 442–443.

Anonymous (1964b). Fluoroacteamide. *Lancet* **1**, 759.

Anonymous (1966). A dangerous rodenticide. *Lancet* **2**, 1183.

Anonymous (1979). Pesticidal diabetes (editorial). *Br. Med. J.* **2**, 292–293.

Araki, S. (1972). Studies on organofluorine pesticides from the medico-legal viewpoint. *Jpn. J. Leg. Med.* **26**, 203–219 [in Japanese].

Bachmann, K. A., and Sullivan, T. J. (1983). Dispositional and pharmacodynamic characteristics of brodifacoum in warfarin-sensitive rats. *Pharmacology* **27**, 281–288.

Barker, W. M., Hermodson, M. A., and Link, K. P. (1970). The metabolism of 4-C[14] warfarin sodium by the rat. *J. Pharmacol. Exp. Ther.* **171**, 307–313.

Barlow, A. M., Gay, A. L., and Park, B. K. (1982). Difenacoum (Neosorexa) poisoning. *Br. Med. J.* **285**, 541.

Bartlett, G. R. (1952). The mechanism of action of monofluoroethanol. *J. Pharmacol. Exp. Ther.* **106**, 464–467.

Beckert, M. H., Genieser, N. B., Finegold, M., Miranda, D., and Spacman, T. (1975). Chondrodysplasia punctata. Is maternal warfarin a factor? *Am. J. Dis. Child.* **129**, 356–359.

Bell, J. (1972). The acute toxicity of four common poisons to the opossum, *Trichosurus vulpecula*. *N. Z. Vet. J.* **20**, 212–214.

Bennett, D. (1972). Accidental poisoning in a retriever puppy by a new rodenticide. *Vet. Rec.* **91**, 609–610.

Benowitz, N. L., Byrd, R., Schambelan, M., Rosenberg, J., and Roizen, M. (1979). Rodenticide induced orthostatic hypotension and its successful management with dihydroergotamine. *Clin. Res.* **27**, 73a.

Bentley, E. W., and Greaves, J. H. (1960). Some properties of fluoroacetamide as a rodenticide. *J. Hyg.* **58**, 125–132.

Beracki, R. J., and Bosmann, H. B. (1970). Warfarin and vitamin K accelerate protein and glycoprotein synthesis in isolated rat liver mitochondria *in vitro*. *Biochem. Biophys. Res. Commun.* **41**, 498–505.

Berny, P. J., Buronfosse, T., Lamarque, F., and Lorgue, G. (1997). Field evidence or secondary poisoning of foxes (*Vulpes vulpes*) and buzzards (*Buteao buteo*) by bromadiolone, a 4-year survey. *Chemosphere* **35(8)**, 1817–1829.

Bicknell, F., and Prescott, F. (1953). "The Vitamins in Medicine," 3rd ed. Heinemann, London.

Biezunski, N. (1970). Action of warfarin injected into rats on protein synthesis *in vitro* by liver microsomes as related to its anticoagulating action. *Biochem. Pharmacol.* **19**, 2645–2652.

Blus, L. J., Henny, C. J., and Groove, R. A. (1985). Effects of pelletized anticoagulant rodenticides in California quail. *J. Wildl. Dis.* **21**, 391–395.

Böhm, G. M. (1973). Changes in lung arteriodes in pulmonary oedema induced in rats by alpha-naphthyl-thiourea. *J. Pathol.* **110**, 343–345.

Boudouresque, J., Roger, J., Naquet, R., Billé, J., Guin, P., Vigouroux, R., and Gosset, A. (1966). Acute chloralose poisoning. Myoclonic seizures. EEG follow-up. *Rev. Neurol.* **114**, 312–317 [in French].

Boyd, M. R., and Neal, R. A. (1976). Studies on the mechanism of toxicity and of development of tolerance to he pulmonary toxin, α-naphthylthiourea (ANTU). *Drug. Metab. Dispos.* **4**, 314–322.

Boyle, C. M. (1960). Case of apparent resistance of *Rattus norvegicus* Berkenhout to anticoagulant poisons. *Nature (London)* **188**, 517.

Braithwaite, G. B. (1982). Vitamin K and brodifacoum. *J. Am. Vet. Med. Assoc.* **181**, 531–534.

Braverman, L. E., and Foster, A. E. (1969). Effect of chronic coumadin administration on thyroid hormon in serum. *J. Nucl. Med.* **10**, 511–513.

Braverman, Y. (1979). Experiments on direct and secondary poisoning by fluoroacetamide (1081) in wildlife and domestic carnivores. *J. Wildl. Dis.* **15**, 319–325.

Breckenridge, A. M., Challiner, M., Mossman, S., Park, B. K., Serlin, M. J., Siberon, R. G., Williams, J. R. B., and Willoughby, J. M. T. (1979). Cimetidine increases the action of warfarin in man. *Br. J. Clin. Phamarcol.* **8**, 329P–393P.

Brockmann, J. L., McDowell, A. V., and Leeds, W. G. (1955). Fatal poisoning with sodium fluoroacetate. Report of a case. *J. Am. Med. Assoc.* **159**, 1529–1532.

Brodie, B. B. (1964). Displacement of one drug by another from carrier or receptor sites. *Proc. Roy Soc. Med.* **58**, 946–955.

Buckle, F. J., Heap, R., and Saunders, B. C. (1949). Toxic fluorine compounds containing the C–F link. Part III. Fluoroacetamide and related compounds. *J. Chem. Soc. London* 912–916.

Buckle, R. M., Gamber, T. R., and Pullen, I. M. (1972). Vitamin D intoxication treated with porcine calcitonin. *Br. Med. J.* **3**, 205–207.

Buffa, P., and Peters, R. A. (1950). The *in vivo* formation of citrate induced by fluoroacete poisoning and its significance. *J. Physiol. (London)* **110**, 488–500.

Bullard, R. W., Thompson, R. D., and Holguin, G. (1976). Diphenadione residues in tissues of cattle. *J. Agric. Food Chem.* **24**, 261–263.

Butler, T. C. (1949). Reduction and oxidation of chloral hydrate by isolated tissues *in vitro*. *J. Pharmacol. Exp. Ther.* **95**, 360–362.

Cahill, W. P., and Crowder, L. A. (1979). Tissue distribution and excretion of diphacinone in the mouse. *Pestic. Biochem. Physiol.* **10**, 259–267.

Caldwell, P. T., Ren, P., and Bell, R. G. (1974). Warfarin and metabolism of vitamin K. *Biochem. Pharmacol.* **23**, 3353–3362.

Carroll, K., and Noble, R. L. (1949). Resistance to toxic thioureas in rats treated with anti-thyroid compounds. *J. Pharmacol. Exp. Ther.* **97**, 478–483.

Case, R. A. M. (1966a). Tumours of the urinary tract as an occupational disease in several industries. *Ann. R. Coll. Surg. Engl.* **39**, 213–235.

Case, R. A. M. (1966b). Occupational bladder cancers (Discussion). *Proc. Roy. Soc. Med.* **59**, 1252.

Cater, D. B., and Peters, R. A. (1961). The occurrence of renal changes resembling nephrosis in rats poisoned by fluocitrate. *Br. J. Exp. Pathol.* **42**, 278–279.

Chakrabarti, S. K. (1978). Influence of heavy metals on the *in vitro* interaction between human serum albumin and warfarin. *Biochem. Pharmacol.* **27**, 2957–2959.

Chan, K. K., Lewis, R. J., and Trager, W. F. (1972). Absolute configuration of the four warfarin alcohols. *J. Med. Chem.* **15**, 1265–1270.

Chapman, C., and Phillips, M. A. (1955). Fluoroacetamide as a rodenticide. *J. Sci. Food Agri.* **6**, 231–232.

Chappelka, R. (1980). The rat poison Vacor. Letter to the editor. *N. Engl. J. Med.* **302**, 1147.

Chenoweth, M. B. (1949). Monofluoroacetic acid and related compounds. *Pharmacol. Rev.* **1**, 383–384.

Chenoweth, M. B., and Gilman, A. (1946). Studies on the pharmacology of fluoroacetate. *J. Pharmacol. Exp. Ther.* **87**, 90–103.

Chenoweth, M. B., Kandel, A., Johnson, L. B., and Bennett, D. R. (1951). Factors influencing fluoroacetate poisoning. Practical treatment with glycerol monoacetate. *J. Pharmacol. Exp. Ther.* **102**, 31–49.

Chi, C. H., Chen, K. W., Chan, S. H., Wu, M. H., and Huang, J. J. (1996). Clinical presentation and prognostic factors in sodium monofluoroacetate intoxication. *J. Toxicol. Clin. Toxicol.* **34(6)**, 707–712.

Chong, M. K. B., Harvey, D., and DeSwiet, M. (1984). Follow-up study of children whose mothers were treated with warfarin during pregnancy. *Br. J. Obstet. Gynaecol.* **91**, 1070–1073.

Chung, H. M. (1984). Acute renal failure caused by acute monofluoroacetate poisoning. *Vet. Hum. Toxicol.* **26**, 29–32.

Cocks, J. R. (1960). Anticoagulants and the acute abdomen. *Med. J. Aust.* **1**, 1138–1141.

Cohen, H. N., Fogelman, I., Boyle, I. T., and Doig, J. A. (1979). Deafness due to hypervitaminosis D. *Lancet* **1**, 985.

Colamussi, V., Bonari, R., and Benini, F. (1970). Minor poisoning from fluoroethanol (description of three cases). *Arcisp. S. Anna Ferrara* **23**, 447–458.

Coldwell, B. B., Buttar, H. S., Paul, C. J., and Thomas, B. H. (1974). Effect of sodium salicylate on the fate of warfarin in the rat. *Toxicol. Appl. Pharmacol.* **28**, 374–384.

Cole, E. R., and Bachmann, F. (1976). Spectrophotometric assays for warfarin sodium and dicumarol. *Arch. Intern. Med.* **136**, 474–479.

Coon, W. W., and Willis, P. W. (1972). Some aspect of the pharmacology of oral anticoagulants. *Clin. Pharmacol. Ther.* **11**, 312–336.

Cornette, M., and Franck, G. (1970). Clinical and electroencephalographical aspects of acute chloralose poisoning. Review of 11 recent cases. *Rev. Neurol.* **123**, 268–272 [in French].

Cornwell, P. B. (1969). Alphakil—A new rodenticide for mouse control. *Pharm. J.* **202**, 74–75.

Correll, J. T., Coleman, L. L., Long, S., and Willy, R. F. (1952). Diphenylacetyl-1,3-indandione as a potent hypoprothrombinemic agent. *Proc. Soc. Exp. Biol. Med.* **80**, 139–143.

Cullen, S. I., and Catalano, P. M. (1967). Griseofulvin-warfarin antagonism. *J. Am. Med. Assoc.* **199**, 582–583.

Davies, J. M., Thomas, H. F., and Manson, D. (1982). Bladder tumours among rodent operatives handling ANTU. *Br. Med. J.* **285**, 927–931.

Davies, M., and Adams, P. H. (1978). The continuing risk of vitamin D intoxication. *Lancet* **2**, 621–623.

Davila, J. C., Edds, G. T., Osona, O., and Simpson, C. F. (1983). Modification of the effects of aflatoxin B1 and warfarin in young pigs given selenium. *Am. J. Vet. Res.* **44**, 1877–1883.

Deckert, F. W. (1973). Warfarin metabolism in the guinea pig. I. Pharmacological studies. *Drug. Metab. Dispos.* **1**, 704–710.

Deckert, F. W., Moss, J. N., Sambuca, A. S., Seigel, M. C., and Steigerwalt, R. B. (1977). Nutritional and drug interactions with Vacor rodenticide in rats. *Fed. Proc., Fed. Am. Soc. Exp. Biol.* **36**, 990.

Deckert, F. W., Godfrey, W. J., Lisk, D. C., Steigerwalt, R. B., and Udinsky, J. R. (1978a). Metabolic interactions with RH-787 (Vacor rodenticide). *Fed. Proc., Fed. Soc. Exp. Biol.* **37**, 424.

Deckert, F. W., Hagerman, L. M., Lisk, D. C., Steigerwalt, R. D., and Udinsky, J. R. (1978b). The disposition of (^{14}C)-RH-787 (Vacor rodenticide) in rodents and dogs. *Toxicol. Appl. Pharmacol.* **45**, 313.

Deckert, F. W., Geyer, W., Godfrey, W. J., Lisk, D. C., Steigerwalt, R. B., and Udinski, J. R. (1979). Partial metabolic fate of ^{14}C-RH-787 (Vacor rodenticide) in dogs, rats and humans. *Toxicol. Appl. Pharmacol.* **48**, A163.

de Torrente, A., Rumack, B. H., Blair, D. T., and Anderson, R. J. (1979). Fixed-bed uncoated charcoal hemoperfusion in the treatment of intoxications. Animal and patient studies. *Nephron* **24**, 71–77.

Dieke, S. H., and Richter, C. P. (1945). Acute toxicity of thioureas to rats in relation to age, diet, strain, and species variation. *J. Pharmacol. Exp. Ther.* **83**, 195–202.

Dieke, S. I•., and Richter, C. P. (1946). Comparative assays of rodenticides on wild Norway rats. *Public Health Rep.* **61**, 672–679.

Dieke, S. ʼ•l., Allen, G. S., and Richter, C. P. (1947). The acute toxicity of thioureas and related compounds to wild and domestic Norway rats. *J. Pharmacol. Exp. Ther.* **90**, 260–270.

Dipalma, J. R. (1981). Human toxicity from rat poisons. *Am. Fam. Physician* **24**, 186–189.

DiSaia, P. J. (1966). Pregnancy and delivery of a patient with a Starr-Edwards mitral valve prothesis. *Obstet. Gynecol. (N.Y.)* **28**, 469–471.

Dreyfus, M., Dubouch, P., Pierson, K., Neveu, Y., Martin, E., and Techernia, G. (1983). Warfarin-contaminated talc. *Lancet* **1**, 1110.

DuBois *et al.* (1947).

Dusein, P., Manigaud, G., and Taillandier, J. (1984). Severe and prolonged hypoprothrombinemia following chlorophacinone poisoning. *Presse Med.* **13**, 1845 [in French].

Eason, C. T., Goonerathne, R., Fitzgerald, H., Wright, G., and Frampton, C. (1994). Persistence of sodium monofluoroactetate in livestock animals and risk to humans. *Human Experimental Toxicol.* **13**(2), 119–122.

Edlin, J. (1982). Rat bait poisoning in a boxer. *Vet. Rec.* **110**, 136.

Egekeze, J. O., and Oehme, F. W. (1979). Sodium monofluoroacetate (SMFA, compound 1080): A literature review. *Vet. Hum. Toxicol.* **21**, 411–416.

Egyed, M. N. (1971). Experimental acute fluoroacetamide poisoning in sheep. III. Therapy. *Refuah Vet.* **28**, 70–73.

Egyed, M. N. (1973). Clinical, pathological, diagnosis and therapeutic aspects of fluoroacetate research in animals. *Fluoride* **6**, 215–224.

Egyed, M. N., and Brisk, Y. (1965). Experimental fluoroacetamide poisoning in mice, rats and sheep. *Refuah Vet.* **22**, 273–274.

Egyed, M. N., and Miller, G. W. (1971). Experimental acute fluoroacetamide poisoning in guinea pig and sheep. *Fluoride* **4**, 137–142.

Egyed, M. N., and Shlosberg, A. (1977). The efficiency of acetamide in the prevention and treatment of fluoroacetamide poisoning in chickens. *Fluoride* **10**, 34–37.

El Bahri, L. (1990). Poisoning in dogs by vitamin D3-containing rodenticides. *Compendium Small Animals* **12**(10), 1414–1417.

Elbe, J. N., West, B. D., and Link, K. P. (1966). A comparison of the isomers of warfarin. *Biochem. Pharmacol.* **15**, 1003–1006.

Elias, D. J., and Johns, B. E. (1981). Response of rats to chronic ingestion of diphacinone. *Bull. Environ. Contam. Toxicol.* **27**, 559–567.

Elias, D. J., Thompson, R. D., and Savarie, P. J. (1978). Effects of the anticoagulant diphacinone on suckling calves. *Bull. Environ. Contam. Toxicol.* **20**, 71–78.

Elmer, G. W., Powell, M. L., and Trafer, W. F. (1977). Warfarin metabolism by rat intestinal microflora. *Lloydia* **40**, 610–611.

Esposi, M. D., Ngo, A., and Myers, M. A. (1996). Inhibition of mitochondrial complex I may account for IDDM induced by intoxication with the rodenticide Vacor. *Diabetes* **45**(11), 1531–1534.

Fasco, M. J., Piper, L. J., and Kaminsky, L. S. (1979). Cumene hydroperoxide-supported microsomal hydroxylations of warfarin. A probe of cytochrome P-450 multiplicity and specificity. *Biochem. Pharmacol.* **28**, 97–103.

Favarel-Garrigues, J. C., and Boget, J. C. (1968). Acute poisonings by chloralose and ANTU-based rodenticides. *Concours Med.* **90**, 2289–2298 [in French].

Field, J. B., Goldfarb, M. S., Ware, A. G., and Griffith, G. C. (1952). Effect n man of an new indandione anticoagulant. *Proc. Soc. Exp. Biol. Med.* **81**, 678–381.

Filip, J., Novak, L., Sikulova, J., and Kolacny, I. (1970). Body temperature during fluoroactetate poisoning in rats. *Physiol. Bohemoslov.* **19**, 123–127.

Fitzburg, O. G., and Nelson, A. A. (1947). Chronic oral toxicity of alphanaphthylurea. *Proc. Soc. Exp. Biol. Med.* **64**, 305–310.

Food and Agriculture Organization (FAO) (1979). "Rodenticides: Analyses, Specifications, Formulations." FAO Plant Prod. Prot. Pap. No. 16, Food Agric. Organ. U. N., Rome.

Fournier, A., Garabedian, M., Grégoire, I., Sebert, J. L., and Pruna, A. (1985). Vitamin D: Its metabolism and its biological properties. *Ann. Med. Interne* **136**, 154–163 [in French].

Frethold, D., Undinsky, J. R., Deckert, F. W., and Sunshine, I. (1980). Postmortem findings for a Vacor poisoning case. *Clin. Toxicol.* **16**, 175–180.

Friedman, W. F., and Mills, L. F. (1969). The relationship between vitamin D and the craniofacial and dental anomalies of the supravalvular aortic stenosis syndrome. *Pediatrics* **43**, 12–18.

Friedman, W. F., and Roberts, W. C. (1966). Vitamin D and the supravalvular aortic stenonis syndrome. The transplacental effects of vitamin D on the aorta of the rabbit. *Circulation* **34**, 77–85.

Fristedt, B., and Sterner, N. (1965). Warfarin intoxication from percutaneous absorption. *Arch. Environ. Health* **11**, 205–208.

Frolick, C. A., and Deluca, H. F. (1973). The stimulation of 1,25 dihydrocholecalciferol metabolism in vitamin D-deficient rat by 1,25 dihydrocholecalciferol treatment. *J. Clin. Invest.* **52**, 543–548.

Gaines, T. B., (1969). Acute toxicity of pesticides. *Toxicol. Appl. Pharmacol.* **4**, 515–534.

Gaines T. B., and Hayes, W. J., Jr. (1952). Bait shyness to ANTU in wild Norway rats. *Public Health Rep.* **67**, 306–311.

Gajdusek, D. C., and Luther, G. (1950). Fluoroacetate poisoning. A review and report of a case. *Am. J. Dis. Child.* **79**, 310–320.

Gallanosa, A. G., Spyker, D. A., and Curnow, R. T. (1981). Diabetes mellitus associated with autonomic and peripheral neuropathy after Vacor rodenticide poisoning. A review. *Clin. Toxicol.* **18**, 441–449.

Ganda, O. P., Rossini, A. A., and Like, A. A. (1976). Studies on streptozotocin. *Diabetes* **25**, 596–603.

Gaultier, M., Fournier, E., and Gervais, P. (1962). Pesticides poisonings: Activities of an antipoison center over an eighteen-month period. *Concours Med.* **84**, 6505–6512 [in French].

Gill, J. E., and Redfern, R. (1979). Laboratory test of seven rodenticides for the control of *Mastomys natalensis*. *H. Hyg.* **8**, 345–352.

Gillman, T., Grant, R. A., and Hathorn, M. (1960). Histochemical and chemical studies of calciferol induced vascular injuries. *Br. J. Exp. Pathol.* **41**, 1–18.

Godfrey, M. E. R., Laas, F. J., and Rammel, C. G. (1985). Acute toxicity of brodifacoum to sheep. *N. Z. J. Exp. Agric.* **13**, 23–25.

Gooneratne, S. R., Eason, C. T., Fitzgerald, H., and Wright, G. (1995). Persistence of sodium fluoroacetate in rabbits and risk to non-target species. *Human Experimental Toxicology* **14**(2), 212–216.

Gore, J. M., Appelbaum, J. S., Greene, H. L., Dexter, L., and Dalen, J. E. (1982). Occult cancer in patients with acute pulmonary embolism. *Ann. Intern. Med.* **96**, 556–560.

Grant, R. A., Gillman, T., and Hathorn, M. (1963). Prolonged chemical and histochemical changes associated with widespread calcifications of soft tissues following brief acute calciferol intoxication. *Br. J. Exp. Pathol.* **44**, 220–232.

Gras, G., Pellissier, C., and Fauran, F. (1975). Analytical toxicology of chloralose. Application to 3 cases of acute poisoning. *Eur. J. Toxicol.* **8**, 371–377 [in French].

Great Britain Ministry of Agriculture, Fisheries and Food (1961). "Memorandum on the Working of the Agriculture (Poisonous Substances) Regulations During 1960." Reissued in *WHO Inf. Circ. Toxic. Pestic. Man* **9**, 51–55.

Greaves, J. H. (1966). Some laboratory observations on the toxicity and acceptability of norbormide to wild *Rattus norvegicus* and on feeding behavior associated with sublethal dosing. *J. Hyg.* **64**, 275–285.

Greaves, J. H., Redfern, R., and King, R. E. (1974). Some properties of calciferol as a rodenticide. *J. Hyg.* **73**, 341–351.

Hagan, E. C., and Radomski, J. L. (1953). The toxicity of 3-(acetonyl-benzyl)-4-hydroxycoumarin (warfarin) to laboratory animals. *J. Am. Pharm. Assoc.* **42**, 379–382.

Hall, J. G., Pauli, R. M., and Wilson, K. M. (1980). Maternal and fetal sequelae of anticoagulation during pregnancy. *Am. J. Med.* **68**, 122–140.

Hanriot and Richet, C. (1897). Chloralose. *Arch. Int. Pharmacodyn.* **3**, 191–211 [in French].

Harris, L. J. (1955). "Vitamins in Theory and Practice," 4th ed. Cambridge Univ. Press, London/New York.

Harrisson, J. W. E., Ambrus, J. L., Ambrus, C. M., Rees, E. W., Peters, R. H., Reese L. C., and Baker, T. (1952a). Acute poisoning with sodium fluoroacetate (compound 1080). *J. Am. Med. Assoc.* **149**, 1520–1522.

Harrisson, J. W. E., Ambrus, J. L., and Ambrus, C. M. (1952b). Fluoroacetate (1090) poisoning. *Ind. Med. Surg.* **21**, 440.

Hartley, D., and Kidd, H. (1983). "The Agrochemicals Handbook." The Royal Society of Chemistry, Nottingham, UK.

Hashida (1971).

Hatakeyama, H., and Shigei, T. (1971). Fine-structured changes of alveolar walls in fibrin-induced, so-called neurogenic pulmonary edema of the rat: Comparative representation with adrenaline and ANTU-induced edema. *Jpn. J. Pharmacol.* **21**, 673–675.

Havill, A. M., Gee, M. H., Washburne, J. D., Premkumar, A., Ottavianon, R., Flynn, J. J., and Spath, J. A. (1982). Alpha-naphthylthiourea produces dose-dependent lung vascular injury in sheep. *Am. J. Physiol.* **243**, 505–511.

Hayes, W. J., Jr. (1975). "Toxicology of Pesticides." Williams & Wilkins, Baltimore.

Hayes, W. J., Jr., and Gaines, T. B. (1950). Control of Norway rats with residual rodenticide warfarin. *Public Health Rep.* **65**, 1537–1555.

Hayes, W. J., Jr., and Vaughn, W. K. (1977). Mortality from pesticides in the United States in 1973 and 1974. *Toxicol. Appl. Pharmacol.* **42**, 235–252.

Herken, H. (1971). Antimetabolic action of 6-aminonicotinamide on the pentose phosphate pathway in the brain. *In* "Mechanisms of Toxicity" (W. N. Aldridge, ed.). Macmillan, London.

Hollinger *et al.* (1993).

Holmes, R. W., and Love, J. (1952). Suicide attempt with warfarin, a bishydroxycoumarin-like rodenticide. *J. Am. Med. Assoc.* **148**, 935–937.

Hosek, R. W., and Love, J. (1952). Mathematical evaluation of the course of body temperature in mice after the administration of sodium fluoroacetate. *Physiol. Bohemoslov.* **19**, 129–133.

Hudson, R. H., Turcker, R. K., and Haegele, M. A. (1972). Effect of age on sensitivity: Acute oral toxicity of 14 pesticides to mallard ducks of several ages. *Toxicol. Appl. Pharmacol.* **22**, 556–561.

Hutchens, J. O., Wagner, H., Podolsky, B., and McMahon, T. M. (1949). The effect of ethanol and various metabolites in fluoroacetate poisoning. *J. Pharmacol. Exp. Ther.* **95**, 62–70.

Ikeda, M., Conney, A. H., and Burns, J. J. (1968a). Stimulatory effect of phenobarbital and insecticides on warfarin metabolim in the rat. *J. Pharmacol. Exp. Ther.* **162**, 338–343.

Ikeda, M., Ullrich, V., and Staudinger, H., (1968b). Metabolism *in vitro* of warfarin by enzymic and nonenzymic systems. *Biochem. Pharmacol.* **17**, 1663–1669.

Ikkala, E., Myllyla, G., Nevanlinna, H. R., Pelkonen, K., and Pyorala, K. (1964). Hemorrhagic diathesis due to criminal poisoning with warfarin. *Acta Med. Scand.* **176**, 201–203.

Innes, J. R. M., Ulland, B. M., Valerio, M. G., Petrucelli, L., Fishbein, L., Hart, E. R., Pallotta, A. J., Bates, R. R., Falk, H. L., Gart, J. J., Klein, M., Mitchell, I., and Peters, J. (1969). Bioassay of pesticides and industrial chemicals for tumorigenicity in mice: A preliminary note. *J. Natl. Cancer Inst. (U.S.)* **4**, 1101–1114.

International Agency for Research in Cancer (IARC) (1983). "Monograph on the Evaluation of the Carcinogenic Risk of Chemicals to Humans. Miscellaneous Pesticides," Vol. 30. Int. Agency Res. Cancer, Lyon, France.

Iqbal, S. J., and Taylor, W. H. (1982). Treatment of vitamin D2 poisoning by induction of hepatic enzymes. *Br. Med. J.* **285**, 541–542.

Jacobziner, H., and Raybin, H. W. (1960). Oil of wintergreen, warfarin sodium and potassium permanganate intoxications. *N. Y. State J. Med.* **60**, 3873–3875.

James, S. R., Eason, C. T., Fitzgerald, H., and Wright, G. (1995). Persistence of sodium fluoroacetate in rabbits and risk to non-target species. *Human Experimental Toxicol.* **14**(2), 212–216.

Jarnargin, K., Zeng, S. Y., Phelps, M., and Deluca, H. F. (1985). Metabolism and pharmacokinetics of 24,25-dihydroxyvitamin D3 in the vitamin D3-replete rat. *J. Biol. Chem.* **260**, 13625–13630.

Jeffery, W. H., Ahlin, T. A., Goran, C., and Hardy, W. R. (1976). Loss of warfarin effect after occupational insecticide exposure. *J. Am. Med. Assoc.* **236**, 2881–2882.

Johannsen, . F. R., and Knowles, C. O. (1972). Citrate accumulation in twospotted spider-mites, house flies, and mice following treatment with the acaricide 2-fluoro-*N*-methyl-*N*-(1-naphthyl-acetamide. *J. Econ. Entomol.* **65**, 1754–1756.

Johnson, D., Kubic, P., and Levitt, C. (1980). Accidental ingestion of Vacor rodenticide. The symptoms and sequelae in a 25-month-old child. *Am. J. Dis. Child.* **134**, 161–164.

Jones, E. C., Growe, G. H., and Naiman, S. C. (1984). Prolonged anticoagulation in rat poisoning. *J. Am. Med. Assoc.* **252**, 3005–3007.

Kalmbach, E. R. (1945). "Ten-eighty," a war-produced rodenticide. *Science* **102**, 232–233.

Kaminsky, S. S. S., Piper, L. J., and Fasco, M. J. (1976). The binding of R and S warfarin to hepatic cytochromes P-450. *Fed. Proc., Fed. Am. Soc. Exp. Biol.* **35**, 1709.

Kandel, A., and Chenoweth, M. B. (1952). Tolerance to fluoroacetate and fluorobutyrate in rats. *J. Pharmacol. Exp. Ther.* **104**, 248–252.

Kaplan, L. C. (1985). Congenital Dandy-Walker malformation associated with first trimester warfarin: A case report and literature review. *Teratology* **32**, 333–337.

Karam, J. H., Prosser, P. R., and LeWitt, P. A. (1978). Islet cell surface antibodies in a patient with diabetes mellitus after rodenticide ingestion. *N. Engl. J. Med.* **299**, 1191.

Karam, J. H., LeWitt, P. A., Young, C. W., Nowlain, R. E., Frankel, B. J., Fujiya, N., Freedman, Z. R., and Grodsky, G. M. (1980). Insulinopenic diabetes after rodenticide (Vacor) ingestion. A unique model of acquired diabetes in man. *Diabetes* **29**, 971–978.

Kawalec, J. C., Andrews, A. W., and Pienta, R. J. (1979). 1-Naphthylthiourea: A mutagenic rodenticide that transforms hamster embryo cells. *Mol. Pharmacol.* **15**, 678–684.

Keber, I. J., Warr, O. S., III, and Richardson, C. (1968). Pregnancy in a patient with a prosthetic mitral valve associated with a fetal anomaly attributed to warfarin sodium. *J. Am. Med. Assoc.* **203**, 223–225.

Kellum, J. M. (1952). Warfarin for suicide. *J. Am. Med. Assoc.* **148**, 1443.

Kempin, S. J. (1983). Warfarin resistance caused by broccoli. *N. Engl. J. Med.* **308**, 1229–1230.

Kirzon, M. V., Timeiko, V. N., and Artiushkova, V. A. (1970). The content of citric acid in various organs of rats in fluoroacetate poisoning. *Vopr. Med. Khim.* **16**, 543–549 [in Russian].

Kirzon, M. V., Timeiko, V. N., and Artiushkova, V. A. (1973). Accumulation of citric acid in different organs of rabbits and cats in sodium fluoroacetate poisoning. *Vopr. Med. Khim.* **19**, 471–474 [in Russian].

Koch-Weser, J., and Sellers, E. M. (1971). Drug interactions with coumarin anticoagulants. Parts I and II. *N. Engl. J. Med.* **285**, 487–498, 547–558.

Krauss, J. S. (1982). Warfarin, pulmonary embolism and cancer. *Ann. Intern. Med.* **97**, 282.

Lange, P. F., and Terveer, J. (1954). Warfarin poisoning. *U. S. Armed Forces Med. J.* **5**, 872–877.

Latore, G. (1961). Effect of overdose of vitamin D2 on pregnancy in the rat. *Fertil. Steril.* **12**, 343–345.

Laubstein, H. (1962). Contact dermatitis from a rodenticide. *Berufs-Dermatosen* **10**, 154–160 [in German].

Leck, J. B., and Park, B. K. (1981). A comparative study of the effects of warfarin and brodifacoum on the relationship between vitamin K1 metabolism and clotting factor activity in warfarin-resistant rats. *Biochem. Pharmacol.* **30**, 123–128.

Lee, P. W., Arnau, T., and Neal, R. A. (1960). Metabolism of α-naphthylthiourea by rat liver and rat lung microsomes. *Toxicol. Appl. Pharmacol.* **53**, 164–178.

Lee, T. H., and Lee, M. W. (1977). Inhibitory effect of a rodenticide RH-787 on the glucose metabolism of erythrocytes. *Korean J. Intern. Med.* **20**, 597–601 [in Japanese].

Lees, P. (1972). Pharmacology and toxicology of alphachloralose: A review. *Vet. Rec.* **91**, 330–333.

Lehman, A. J. (1951). Chemicals in foods. A report to the Association of Food and Drug Officials on current developments. Part II. Pesticides. Section I. Introduction. *Q. Bull. Assoc. Food Drug Off.* **15**(1), 122–123.

Lehman, A. J. (1952). Chemicals in foods. A report to the Association of Food and Drug Officials on current developments. Part II. Pesticides. Section II. Dermal toxicity. Section III. Subacute and chronic toxicity. Section IV. Biochemistry, Section V. Pathology. *Q. Bull. Assoc. Food Drug Off.* **16**(II), 3–9; (III), 47–53; (IV), 85–91; (V), 126–132.

Lewis, R. J., and Traeger, W. F. (1970). Warfarin metabolism in man: Identification of metabolites in urine. *J. Clin. Invest.* **49**, 907–913.

LeWitt, P. A. (1980a). The neurotoxicity of the rat poison Vacor: A clinical study of 12 cases. *N. Engl. J. Med.* **302**, 73–77.

LeWitt, P. A. (1980b). The rat poison Vacor. *N. Engl. J. Med.* **302**, 1147.

Lindahl, O., and Lindwall, L. (1975). Vitamin D and myocardial infarction. *Br. Med. J.* **2**, 560.

Linden, V. (1974). Vitamin D and myocardial infarction. *Br. Med. J.* **3**, 647–650.

Link, K. P. (1944). The anticoagulant from spoiled sweet clover hay. *Harvey Lect.* **39**, 162–216.

Link, K. P. (1959). The discovery of dicumarol and its sequels. *Circulation* **19**, 97–107.

Link, K. P., Berg, D., and Barker, W. M. (1965). Partial fate of warfarin in the rat. *Science* **50**, 378.

Lipton, R. A., and Klass, E. M. (1984). Human ingestion of a "superwarfarin" rodenticide resulting in a prolonged anticoagulant effect. *J. Am. Med. Assoc.* **252**, 3004–3005.

Lisella *et al.* (1971).

Loracher, C., and Lux, H. D. (1974). Impaired hyperpolarising inhibition during insulin hypoglycemia and fluoroacetate poisoning. *Brain Res.* **69**, 164–169.

Lorusso, D. J., and Suttie, J. W. (1972). Warfarin binding to microsomes isolated from normal and warfarin-resistant rat liver. *Mol. Pharmacol.* **8**, 197–203.

Lund, M. (1964). Resistance to warfarin in the common rat. *Nature (London)* **203**, 778.

Lund, M. (1967). Resistance of rodents to rodenticides. *World Rev. Pest Control* **6**, 131–138.

MacDonald, M. G., and Kaminsky, L. S. (1979). Development of the hepatic monoxygenase system and metabolism of warfarin in the perinatal rat. *Pediatr. Res.* **13**, 370.

MacDonald, M. G., Robinson, D. S., Sylvester, D., and Jaffe, J. J. (1969). The effects of phenobarbital, chloral betaine and glutethimide administration on warfarin plasma level and hypoprothrombinemic responses in man. *Clin. Pharmacol. Ther.* **10**, 80–84.

Maddock, D. R., and Schoff, H. F. (1967). Laboratory and field evaluation of norbormide against wild rats. *Pest Control* **35**(8), 22, 24, 26, 28.

Marshall, E. K., and Owens, A. H. (1954). Absorption, excretion and metabolic fate of chloral hydrate. *Bull. Johns Hopkins Hosp.* **95**, 1–18.

Martin, C. M., Engström, P. F., and Chandro, S. B. (1970). Skin necrosis associated with warfarin sodium. *Calif. Med.* **113**, 78–80.

Martin-Bouyer, G., Linh, P. D., Tuan, L. C., Barin, C., Khahn, N. B., Hoa, D. Q., Tourneau, J., and Guerbois, H. (1983). Epidemic of haemorrhagic disease in Vietnamese infants caused by warfarin-contaminated talc. *Lancet* **1**, 230–232.

Matschiner, J. T., Bell, R. G., Amoletti, J. M., and Knauer, T. E. (1970). Isolation and characterization of a new metabolite of phylloquinone in the rat. *Biochem. Biophys. Acta* **210**, 309–315.

Matsumura, F., and O'Brien, R. D. (1963). A comparative study of the modes of action of fluoroacetamide and fluoroacetate in the mouse and American cockroach. *Biochem. Biophys.* **12**, 1201–1205.

Mawer, E. B., Backhouse, J., Davie, M., Hill, L. F., and Taylor, C. M. (1976). Metabolic fate of administered 1,25-dihydrocholecalciferol in controls and in patients with hypoparathyroidism. *Lancet* **1**, 1203–1205.

Mazzanti, L., Lopez, M., and Berti, M. G. (1964). Selective destruction in testes induced by fluoroacetamide. *Experientia* **20**, 492–493.

McCarthy, P. T., Cox, A. D., Harrington, D. J., Evely, R. S., Hampton, E., Al-Sabah, A. I., Masey, E., Jackson, H., and Ferguson, T. (1997). Covert poisoning with difenacoum: Clinical and toxicological observations. *Human Experimental Toxicol.* **16**(3), 166–170.

McClain, R. M., Langhoff, L., and Hoar, R. M. (1980). Reproduction studies with 1α, 25-dihydroxyvitamin D3 (calcitriol) in rats and rabbits. *Toxicol. Appl. Pharmacol.* **52**, 89–98.

McLeod, A. R. (1970). An epidemiological study of pesticide poisonings admitted to Charity Hospital, New Orleans. *J. La. State Med. Soc.* **122**, 337–343.

McSporran, K. D., and Phillips, C. A. (1983). Brodifacoum poisoning in a dog. *N. Z. Vet. J.* **31**, 185–186.

McTaggart, D. R. (1970). Poisoning due to sodium fluoroacetate ("1080"). *Med. J. Aust.* **2**, 641–642.

Medved, L. I., ed. (1974). "Handbook of Pesticides (Hygiene of Use and Toxicology)." Urogai Publishing House, Kiev, U. S. S. R.

Meehan (19984).

Meyer, B. J., and Saunders, J. P. (1949). The effects of thioureas and related compounds on alphanaphthylthiourea (ANTU) toxicity to rats. *J. Pharmacol. Exp. Ther.* **97**, 432–440.

Meyrick, B., Miller, J., and Reid, L. (1972). Pulmonary oedema induced by ANTU, or by high or low oxygen concentrations in rat—An electron microscopic study. *Br. J. Exp. Pathol.* **45**, 347–358.

Michaels, L. (1974). The incidence and course of cancer in patients receiving anticoagulant therapy: Retrospective and prospective study. *J. Med.* **5**, 98–106.

Misustova, J., Novak, L., and Hosek, B. (1969). Influence of lowered environmental temperature on metabolic and lethal effects of sodium fluoroacetate in mice. *Physiol. Bohemoslov.* **18**, 319–324.

Moene, Y., Cuche, M., Trillet, M., Motin, J., and Michel, D. (1969). Diagnostic problems for acute poisoning by chloralose (review of 6 cases). *J. Med. Lyon* **50**, 1483–1484; 1487–1488; 1491–1493.

Mogilner, B. M., Freeman, J. S., Blashar, Y., and Pincus, F. E. (1974). Reye's syndrome in three Israeli children. Possible relationship to warfarin toxicity. *Isr. J. Med. Sci.* **10**, 1117–1125.

Morselli, P. L., Garattini, S., Marucci, F., Mussini, E., Rewersky, W., Valzelli, L., and Peters, R. A. (1968). The effect of injections of fluorocitrate into the brains of rats. *Biochem. Pharmacol.* **17**, 195–202.

Mount, M. E., and Feldman, B. F. (1983). Mechanism of diphacinone rodenticide toxicosis in the dog and its therapeutic implications. *Am. J. Vet. Res.* **44**, 2009–2017.

Munger, L. L., Su, J. J., and Barnes H. J. (1993). Coumafuryl (Fumarin) toxicity in chicks. *Avian Diseases* **37**(2), 622–624.

Murdoch, D. A. (1983). Prolonged anticoagulation in chlorophacinone poisoning. *Lancet* **1**, 355–356.

Murphy, M. J., Ray, A. C., Woody, B., and Reagor, J. C. (1985). Serum brodifacoum concentrations and coagulopathic effects in anticoagulant poisoned dogs treated with vitamin K1. *Toxicologist* **5**, 88.

Navarro, M., Acevedo, C., Espinosa, L., Pena, A., Picazo, M. L., and Larraudi, M. (1985). Vitamin D3 intoxication with irreversible sequelae. *An. Esp. Pediatr.* **22**(2), 99–106.

Nebel, L., and Ornstein, A. (1966). Effect of hypervitaminosis D2 on fertility and pregnancy in rats. *Isr. J. Med. Sci.* **2**, 14–21.

Nikodemusz, E., Nechay, G., and Imre, R. (1981). Histophatological changes resulting from intoxication by some pesticides in the common vole (*Microtus arvalis* Pallas). *Acta Vet. Acad. Sci. Hung.* **29**, 317–326.

Nilsson, I. M. (1957). Recurrent hypoprothrombinaemia due to poisoning with a dicumarol-containing rat killer. *Acta Haematol.* **17**, 176–182.

Niu, M. (1970). Pharmacological action of norbormide. *Jpn. J. Pharmacol.* **66**, 224–236 [in Japanese].

Noguchi, T., Ohnyki, Y., and Okigaki, T. (1966). Effect of sodium fluoroacetate on myocardial cells *in vitro*. *Nature (London)* **209**, 1197–1198.

O'Brien, R. F., Makarski, J. S., and Rounds, S. (1985). Studies of the mechanism of decreased angiotensin I conversion in rat lungs injured with alphanaphthylthiourea. *Exp. Lund Res.* **8**, 243–259.

O'Connor, J. A. 51948). The use of blood anti-coagulants for rodent control. *Research (London)* **1**, 334–336.

O'Reilly, R. A. (1970). The second reported kindred with hereditary resistance to oral anticoagulant drugs. *N. Engl. J. Med.* **282**, 1448–1451.

O'Reilly, R. A., and Aggeler, P. M. (1968). Phenylbutazone potentiation of anticoagulant effect: Fluorometric assay of warfarin. *Proc. Soc. Exp. Biol. Med.* **128**, 1080–1081.

O'Reilly, R. A., Aggeler, P. M., and Leong, LS. (1963). Studies on the coumarin anticoagulant drugs: The pharmacodynamics of warfarin in man. *J. Clin. Invest.* **42**, 1542–1551.

Ornoy (Ornstein), A., Menczel, J., and Nebel, L. (1968). Alterations in the mineral composition and metabolism of rat fetuses and their placentas induced by maternal hypervitaminosis D2. *Isr. J. Med. Sci.* **4**, 827–832.

Osterman, J. Zmyslinski, R. W., Hopkins, C. B., Cartee, W., Lin, T., and Nankin, H. R. (1981). Full recovery from severe orthostatic hypotension after Vacor rodenticide ingestion. *Arch. Intern. Med.* **141**, 1505–1507.

Osteryoung, J. G., Whittaker, J. W., Tessari, J., and Boyes, V. (1977). The identification of *p*-nitroaniline as a metabolite of the rodenticide Vacor in human liver. *In* "Fate of Pesticides in Larger Animals" (G. W. Ivie and H. G. Dorough, eds.), pp. 253–256. Academic Press, New York.

Overman, R. S., Stahmann, M. A., Huebner, C. F., Sullinvan W. R., Spero, L. Doherty, D. G., Miyoshi, I., Grae, L., Roseman, S., and Link, K. P. (1944). Studies on the hemorrhagic sweet clover disease. XIII. Anticoagulant activity and structure in the hydroxycoumarin group. *J. Biol. Chem.* **153**, 5–24.

Owens, A. H., and Marshall, E. K. (1955). Further studies on the metabolic fate of chloral hydrate and trichlorethanol. *Bull. Johns Hopkins Hosp.* **97**, 320–326.

Papasozomenos, S. (1980). The rat poison Vacor. *N. Engl. J. Med.* **302**, 1146–1147.

Park, B. K., and Leck, J. B. (1982). A comparison of vitamin K antagonism by warfarin, difenacoum and brodifacoum in the rabbit. *Biochem. Pharmacol.* **31**, 3635–3639.

Parkin, P. J., McGiven, A. R., and Bailey, R. R. (1977). Chronic sodium monofluoroacetate (compound 1080) intoxication in a rabbit. *N. Z. Med. J.* **85**, 93–96.

Pastor, B. H., Resnick, M. E., and Rodman, T. (1962). Serious hemorrhagic complications of anticoagulant therapy. *J. Am. Med. Assoc.* **180**, 747–751.

Paterson, C. R. (1980). Vitamin D poisoning: Survey of causes in 21 patients with hypercalcemia. *Lancet* **1**, 1164–1165.

Patil, T. N., and Radhakrishnamurty, R. (1973). Effect of norbormide on blood glucose levels in albino rats. *Indian J. Biochem. Biophys.* **10**, 206–208.

Patil, T. N., and Radhakrishnamurty, R. (1977). Biochemical changes induces by α-naphthylthiourea in albino rats. *Indian J. Biochm. Biophys.* **14**, 24.

Peardon, D. L. (1974) RH-787, a new selective rodenticide. *Pest Control* **42**(9), 14, 16, 18, 27.

Penumarthy, L., and Oehme, F. W. (1978). Treatment of prothrombin responses during warfarin toxicosis in rats and mice. *Toxicology* **10**, 377–401.

Peoples, S. A., and Maddy, K. T. (1979). Poisoning of man and animals due to ingestion of the rodent poison Vacor. *Vet. Hum. Toxicol.* **21**(4), 266–268.

Peters, R. A. (1952). Significance of biochemical lesions in the pyruvate oxidase system. *Br. Med. Bull.* **9**, 116–122.

Peters, R. A. (1963a). Organo-fluorine compounds present in certain plants and their effect on animals. *Biochem. J.* **88**, 55P.

Peters, R. A. (1963b). "Biochemical Lesions and Lethal Synthesis." Macmillan, New York.

Peters, R. A., and Shorthouse, M. (1971). Oral toxicity of fluoroacetate and fluorocitrate in rats. *J. Physiol. (London)* **216**, 40P–41P.

Petit, L., Leperchey, F., and Fournier, E. (1970). Experimental toxicology of isothioureas. *Poumon Cœur* **26**, 893–894 [in French].

Pettifor, J. M., and Benson, R. (1975). Congenital malformation associated with the administration of oral anticoagulants during pregnancy. *J. Pediatr.* **86**, 459–462.

Phillips, M. A., and Worden, A. N. (1956). Toxicity of fluoroacetamide. *Lancet* **2**, 731.

Phillips, M. A., and Worden, A. N. (1957). The mammalian oral toxicity of fluoroacetamide. *J. Soc. Food Agric.* **8**, 653–657.

Pohl, L. R., Nelson, S. D., Porter, W. R., Trager, W. F., Fasco, M. J., Baker, F. D., and Fenton, J. W., II (1976a). Warfarin-stereochemical aspects of its metabolism by rat liver microsomes. *Biochem. Pharmacol.* **25**, 2153–2162.

Pohl, L. R., Bales, R., and Trager, W. F. (1976b). Warfarin: Stereochemical aspects of its metabolism *in vivo* in the rat. *Res. Commun. Chem. Pathol. Pharmacol.* **15**, 233–236.

Pohl, L. R., Porter, W. R., Trager, W. F., Fasco, M. J., and Fenton, J. W., III (1977). Stereochemial biotransformation of warfarin as a probe of the homogeneity and mechanism of microsomal hydroxylases. *Biochem. Pharmacol.* **26**, 109–114.

Pont, A., Rubino, J. M., Bishop, D., and Peal, K. (1979). Diabetes mellitus and neuropathy following Vacor ingestion in man. *Arch. Intern. Med.* **139**, 185–187

Poos, G. I., Mohrbacher, R. J., Carson, E. L., Paragamian, V., Puma, B. M., Rasmussen, C. R., and Roszkowski, A. P. (1996). Structure-activity studies with the selective rat toxicant norbormide. *J. Med. Chem.* **9**, 537–540.

Potvliege, P. R. (1962). Hyperviaminosis D2 in gravid rats. *Arch. Pathol.* **73**, 371–382.

Powell, M. L., Pope, B., Elmer, G. W., and Trager, W. F. (1977). Biliary excretion of warfarin metabolites and their metabolism by rat gut flora. *Life Sci.* **20**, 171–178.

Pribilla, O. (1996). Murder caused by warfarin. *Arch. Toxicol.* **21**, 235–249.

Prosser, P. R., and Karam, J. H. (1978). Diabetes mellitus following rodenticide ingestion in man. *J. Am. Med. Assoc.* **239**, 1148–1150.

Pyorala, K. (1968). Sex differences in the clotting factor response to warfarin and in the rate of warfarin metabolism in the rat. *Ann. Med. Exp. Biol. Fenn.* **46**, 23–34.

Pyorala K., and Nevanlinna, H. R. (1968). The effect of selective and nonselective inbreeding on the rate of warfarin metabolism in the rat. *Ann. Med. Exp. Biol. Fenn.* **46**, 35–44.

Raasch, M. S. (1958). 5-Fluoronorvaline and 6-fluoronorleucine. *J. Org. Chem.* **23**, 1567–1568.

Rao, M. B. K. (1979). Potentiation of warfarin toxicity of roof rats (*Rattus rattus*) by L-histidine and by vitamin K adsorbers. *Pestic. Sci.* **10**, 221–226.

Reigart, J. R., Brueggeman, J. L., and Keil, J. E. (1975). Sodium fluoroacetate poisoning. *Am. J. Dis. Child* **129**, 1224–1226.

Renapurkar, D. M., and Deoras, P. J. (1982). Effects of anticoagulant rodenticides on rat intestine *in vitro*. *Pestology* **6**, 11–13.

Rennison, B. D., and Hadler, M. R. (1975). Field trials of difenacoum against warfarin-resistant infestations of *Rattus norvegicus*. *J. Hyg.* **74**, 449–455.

Richter, C. P. (1945). The development and use of alpha-naphthyl thiourea (ANTU) as a rat poison. *J. Am. Med. Assoc.* **129**, 927–931.

Richter, C. P. (1946). Biological factors involved in poisoning rats with alphanaphthyl thiourea (ANTU). *Proc. Soc. Exp. Biol. Med.* **63**, 364–372.

Robben, J. H., Kuijpers, E. A., and Mout, H. C. (1998). Plasma superwarfarin levels and vitamin K1 treatment in dogs with anticoagulant rodenticide poisoning. *Vet. Quart.* **20**(1), 24–27.

Robinson, D. S., and MacDonald, M. G. (1966). The effect of phenobarbital administration on the control of coagulation achieved during warfarin therapy in man. *J. Pharmacol. Exp. Ther.* **153**, 250–253.

Robinson, W. H. (1970). Acute toxicity of sodium monofluoroacetate to cattle. *J. Wildl. Manage.* **34**, 647–348.

Rossini, A. A., Arcangeli, M. A., and Cahill, G. F. (1975). Studies on alloxan toxicity on the beta cell. *Diabetes* **24**, 516–522.

Roszkowski, A. P. (1965). The pharmacological properties of norbormide, a selective rat toxicant. *J. Pharmacol. Exp. Ther.* **149**, 288–299.

Roszkowski, A. P., Poos, G. I., and Mohrbacher, R. J. (1964). Selective rat toxicant. *Science* **144**, 412–413.

Rothstein, E. (1968). Warfarin effect enhanced by disulfiram. *J. Am. Med. Assoc.* **206**, 1574–1575.

Roy, A., Teitelman, U., and Bursztein, S. (1980). Evaluation of the role of ionized calcium in sodium fluoroacetate ("1080") poisoning. *Toxicol. Appl. Pharmacol.* **56**, 216–220.

Roy, A., Raikhlin-Eisenkraft, B., Teitelman, U., and Hazani, A. (1982). Poisoning by fluoroacetate and fluoroacetamide. A description of two cases. *Harefuah* **48**, 523–524.

Russell, S. H., Monin, T., and Edward, W. C. (1978). Rodenticide toxicosis in a horse. *J. Am. Vet. Med. Assoc.* **172**, 270–271.

Sanger, G., and Becker, K. (1975). Dermal absorption of warfarin in man and rat. *Umwelthygiene* **1**, 156–158 [in German].

Saunders (1947).

Sax, I. N. (1984). "Dangerous Properties of Industrial Material," 6th ed. Van Nostrand–Reinhold, New York.

Schafer, E. W. (1972). The acute oral toxicity of 369 pesticidal, pharmaceutical and other chemicals to wild birds. *Toxicol. Appl. Pharmacol.* **21**, 315–330.

Schiff, B. L., and Kern, A. B. (1968). Cutaneous reactions to anticoagulants. *Arch. Dermatol.* **98**, 136–137.

Searcey, M. T., and Graves, C. B. (1976). Subcellular distribution and warfarin-binding protein from Sprague-Dawley and Warfarin-resistant rats. *Fed. Proc., Fed. Am. Soc. Exp. Biol.* **35**, 1763.

Sellers, E. M., Lang, M., Koch-Weser, J., and Coleman, R. W. (1972). Enhancement of warfarin-induced hypoprothrombinemia by trichlofos. *Clin. Pharmacol. Ther.* **13**, 911–915.

Shaul, W. L., Emery, H., and Hall, J. G. (1975). Chondrodysplasia punctata and maternal warfarin use during pregnancy. *Am. J. Dis. Child.* **129**, 360–362.

Shearer, M. J., and Barkhan, P. (1979). Vitamin K, and therapy of massive warfarin overdose. *Lancet* **1**, 266–267.

Shearer, M. J., McBurney, A., and Barkhan, P. (1973). Effect of warfarin anticoagulation on vitamin-K metabolism in man. *Br. J. Haematol.* **24**, 471–479.

Sheen, S. R., Spiller, H. A., and Grosman, D. (1994). Symptomatic brodifacoum ingestion requiring high dose phytonadione therapy. *Vet. Human Toxicol.* **36**(3), 216–217.

Shepherd, D. (1971). Bemegride sodium and alphachloralose poisoning. *Vet. Rec.* **88**, 375.

Sherrod, P. S., and Harrod, M. J. E. (1978). Warfarin embryopathy in siblings. *Am. J. Hum. Genet.* **30**, 104A.

Shlosberg, A., Egyed, M. N., Mendelsohn, H., and Langer, B. (1975). Fluoroacetamide (1081) poisoning in wild birds. *J. Wildl. Dis.* **11**, 534–536.

Smith, I. A., and Boyd, J. H. (1972). Another case of poisoning by alphachloralose. *Vet. Rec.* **91**, 662.

Sobonya, R. E., and Kleinerman, J. (1973). Recurrent pulmonary edema induced by α-naphthyl thiourea. *Am. Rev. Respir. Dis.* **108**, 926–932.

Sollman, T. (1901). "A Text-Book of Pharmacology and Some Allied Sciences." Saunders, Philadelphia.

Sollman, T. (1942). "A Manual of Pharmacology and Its Applications to Therapeutics and Toxicology." Saunders, Philadelphia.

Solomon, H. M. (1968). Variations in metabolism of coumarin anticoagulant drugs. *Ann. N.Y. Acad. Sci.* **15**, 932–935.

Solomon, H. M., Schrogie, J. J., and Williams, D. (1968). The displacement of phenylbutazone-^{14}C and warfarin-^{14}C from human albumin by various drugs and fatty acids. *Biochem. Pharmacol.* **17**, 143–151.

Spielmann, H., Meyer-Wendecker, R., and Spielmann, F. (1973). Influence of 2-deoxy-D-glucose and sodium fluoroacetate on respiratory metabolism of rat embryos during organogenesis. *Teratology* **7**, 127–134.

Steinberger, E., and Sud, B. N. (1970). Specific effects of fluoroacetamide on spermiogenesis. *Biol. Reprod.* **2**, 369–375.

Sterner, R. T. (1979). Effects of sodium cyanide and diphacinone in coyotes (*Canis latrans*): Applications as predaticides in livestock toxic collars. *Bull. Environ. Contam. Toxicol.* **23**, 211–217.

Stevenson, R. E., Burton, M., Ferlanton, G. J., and Taylor, H. A. (1980). Hazards of oral anticoagulants during pregnancy. *J. Am. Med. Assoc.* **243**, 1549–1551.

Stowe, C. M., Metz, A. L., Arendt, T. D., and Schultman, J. (1983). Apparent brodifacoum poisoning in a dog. *J. Am. Med. Assoc.* **182**, 817–818.

Suttie, J. W., ed. (1979). "Vitamin K Metabolism and Vitamin K-Dependent Proteins." University Park Press, Baltimore.

Tarrant, K. A., and Westlake, G. E. (1984). Histological technique for the identification of poisoning in wildlife by the rodenticide calciferol. *Bull. Environ. Contam. Toxicol.* **32**, 175–178.

Tejani, N. (1973). Anticoagulant therapy with cardiac valve prothesis during pregnancy. *Obstet. Gynecol.* **42**, 785–793.

Tempé, J. D., and Kurtz, D. (1972). Acute chloralose poisoning. *Concours Med.* **94**, 801–813 [in French].

Thierry, M. J., Hermodson, M. A., and Suttie, J. W. (1970). Vitamin K and warfarin distribution and metabolism in the warfarin-resistant rat. *Am. J. Physiol.* **219**, 854–859.

Thompson, R. D., Mitchell, G. C., and Burns, R. J. (1972). Vampire bat control by systemic treatment of livestock with an anticoagulant. *Science* **177**, 806–807.

Toda, T., Ito, M., Toda, Y., Smith, T., and Kummerov, F. (1985). Angiotoxicity in swine of a moderate excess of dietary vitamin D3. *Food Chem. Toxicol.* **23**, 585–592.

Tokavera, T. G., Turov, I. S., and Alekseyev, A. N. (1971). The action of fluoroacetamide on albino mouse fecundity (preliminary report). *Zh. Mikrobiol. Epidemiol. Immunobiol.* **48**, 24–26 [in Russian].

Tomiya, K., Shimoda, R. Kakihara, Y., and Kanda, M. (1976). Studies on extraction of toxic materials from organs of victims of fatal intoxication by organofluorine pesticides. *Jpn. J. Leg. Med.* **29**, 237–238 [in Japanese].

Tomlin (1994).

Tourtellotte, W. W., and Coon, J. M. (1951). Treatment of fluoroacetate poisoning in mice and dogs. *J. Pharmacol. Exp. Ther.* **101**, 82–91.

Travis, S. F., Warfield, W., Greenbaum, B. J., Moloskier, M., and Siegel, J. E. (1993). Spontaneous hemorrhage associated with accidental brodifacoum poisoning in a child. *J. Pediatrics* **122**(6), 982–984.

Ullrich, V., and Staudinger, H. (1968). Metabolism *in vitro* of warfarin by enzymic and nonenzymic systems. *Biochem. Pharmacol.* **17**, 1663–1669.

Varon, M. L., and Cole, L. J. (1966). Heopoietic colony-forming units in regenerating mouse liver suppression by anticoagulants. *Science* **153**, 643–644.

Vaughan, E. D., Jr., Moore, R. A., Warren, H., Moler, D. N., and Gillenwater, J. Y. (1969). Skin necrosis of genitalia and warfarin therapy. *J. Am. Med. Assoc.* **210**, 2282–2283.

Vik, T., Try, K., Thelle, D. S., and Forde, O. H. (1979). Tromso heart study: Vitamin D metabolism and myocardial infarction. *Br. Med. J.* **2**, 176.

Ward, J. C. (1945). Rodenticides—Present and future. *Soap Sanit. Chem.* **21**(9), 117, 119, 127.

Ward, J. C., and Spencer, D. A. (1947). Notes on the pharmacology of sodium fluoroacetate-compound 1080. *J. Am. Pharm. Assoc. Sci. Ed.* **36**, 59–62.

Wenz, C. (1984). New chemicals under fire. *Nature (London)* **1**, 741.

West, B. D., Preist, S., Schroeder, C. H., and Link, K. P. (1961). Studies on the 4-hydroxycoumarin. XVII. The resolution and absolute configuration of warfarin. *J. Am. Chem. Soc.* **83**, 2676–2679.

White, S. T. (1985). Surreptitious warfarin ingestion. *Child Abuse Neglect* **9**, 349–352.

Williams, R. T. (1959). "Detoxication Mechanisms," 2nd ed. Wiley, New York.

Williamson, J. R., Jones, E. A., and Azzone, G. F. (1964). Metabolite control in perfused rat heart during fluoroacetate poisoning. *Biochem. Biophys. Res. Commun.* **17**, 696–702.

Wilson, G. L., and Gaines, K. L. (1983). Effects of the rodenticide Vacor on cultured rat pancreatic beta cells. *Toxicol. Appl. Pharmacol.* **68**, 375–379.

Wiswesser, W. J. (1976). "Pesticide Index," 5th ed. Entomol. Soc. Am., College Park, MD.

Woody, B. J., Murphy, M. J., Ray, A. C., and Green, R. A. (1992). Coagulopathic effects and therapy of brodifacoum toxicosis in dogs. *J. Vet. Intern. Med.* **6**(1), 23–28.

World Health Organization (WHO) (1986). "The WHO Recommended Classification of Pesticides by Hazards." VBC/86.1, World Health Organ., Geneva.

World Health Organization (WHO) (1963). Fluoroacetamide poisoning case. *WHO Inf. Circu. Toxic. Pestic. Man* **11**, 9.

Worthing, C. R., and Walker, S. B. (1983). "The Pesticide Manual," 7th ed. Br. Crop Prot. Counc., Lavenham, UK.

Yacobi, A., and Levy, G. (1975). Comparative pharmacokinetics of coumarin anticoagulants. XIV. Relationship between binding, distribution and elimination kinetics of warfarin in rats. *J. Pharm. Sci.* **64**, 1660–1664.

Yu, C. C., Atallah, Y. H., and Whitacre, D. M. (1982). Metabolism and disposition of diphacinone in rats and mice. *Drug Metab. Dispos.* **10**, 645–648.

Zacharski, L. R. (1982). Warfarin and cancer. *Ann. Inter. Med.* **97**, 784.

Zakzouk, M. S. (1986). The congenital warfarin syndrome. *J. Laryngol. Otol.* **100**, 215–219.

Zimmerman, A., and Matschiner, J. T. (1972). The biochemical basis of hereditary resistance to warfarin in the rat. *Fed. Proc. Fed. Am. Soc. Exp. Biol.* **21**, 714.

Methyl Bromide

Vincent J. Piccirillo
NPC Incorporated

84.1 INTRODUCTION

Methyl bromide is a broad spectrum pesticide primarily used for soil fumigation, commodity/quarantine treatment, and structural fumigation. Since human exposure is more likely to occur by the inhalation route, the majority of the toxicologic evaluations for methyl bromide are inhalation studies. Ingestion of fumigated commodities is a secondary route of human exposure. Chronic dietary studies in rats and dogs show no concern for long term oral ingestion of methyl bromide. This chapter briefly describes many of the published studies and elaborates the results from a number of contemporaneous methyl bromide toxicity studies by the oral and inhalation routes which were conducted to support the pesticide registration and other regulatory needs of the U.S. Environmental Protection Agency as well as State and international regulatory bodies. A primary focus in this chapter is methyl bromide induced neurotoxicity. From a risk characterization standpoint, clinical observations of neurotoxicity are considered as the primary endpoint of concern from inhalation exposure. Review of the overall toxicity of methyl bromide shows that methyl bromide induced toxicity is a function of both the concentration and the duration of exposure. This is an important consideration for human exposure assessments.

84.2 CHEMICAL PROPERTIES AND PESTICIDAL USES OF METHYL BROMIDE

Methyl bromide (CH_3Br, bromomethane, CAS no. 74-83-9) is a colorless, odorless gas at normal temperature and pressure. Methyl bromide is produced by the interaction of methanol (CH_3OH) and hydrogen bromide (HBr). It is made commercially but also is produced natually by marine algae and other plants and as a by-product of the combustion of plant materials (i.e., forest fires). Under increased pressure or below 3°C, methyl bromide is a clear to straw colored liquid and it is usually shipped as a liquified, compressed gas. Methyl bromide has a boiling point of 38.5° Fahrenheit and is nonflammable in air. Methyl bromide formulations contain chloropicrin, an irritant and lacrimator, as a warning agent.

Methyl bromide is a broad spectrum pesticide primarily used for soil fumigation, commodity/quarantine treatment and structural fumigation. It is also used as an intermediate in the manufacture of other chemicals. Methyl bromide has been used as a fumigant for more than 50 years and is strictly controlled by the U.S. Environmental Protection Agency (EPA) under the Federal Insecticide, Fungicide, and Rodenticide Act. Its application and use are also controlled by various state regulatory authorities.

For soil fumigation, methyl bromide is injected directly into the soil, which is then covered with plastic sheeting. The sheeting is sealed, kept in place for several days, and then removed. Soil fumigation with methyl bromide enhances the quality of the crops and increases yield by eliminating fungal diseases, nematodes, weed seeds, and other soil borne pests. The primary crops grown in methyl bromide treated soil are peppers, strawberries, tomatoes, and grapes.

Methyl bromide is widely used for fumigating postharvest commodities, such as wheat and cereals, spices, nuts, and dried and fresh fruits to eradicate pest infestations. Fumigation typically occurs where the commodities are stored, such as in ship holds, grain elevators, warehouses, special fumigation chambers, and on shipping piers/docks. Commodity fumigation typically involves the use of specially designed and permanently installed chambers into which the methyl bromide is released. After treatment, mechanical ventilation is used to continuously aerate the commodity until the concentration of methyl bromide in the vented air is at established safety levels. Another type of commodity fumigation involves the sealing of the commodity under a tarpaulin followed by injection of the methyl bromide. Aeration and ventilation occurs after the tarpualin is removed. In structural fumigation, all openings in the structure are sealed.

All types of commercial and residential structures may be fumigated with methyl bromide to control or eradicate pests, such as termites. The structure is covered by a "tent" or tarpaulin and the methyl bromide gas is released inside the structure. After a specified period, the tarpaulin is removed and the structure is aerated until the concentration of methyl bromide inside the structure reaches safe levels.

Methyl bromide may only be applied and used by professional, certified applicators. All persons working with methyl bromide are required to be knowledgeable about its hazards and trained in the use of required respiratory protection equipment, detector devices, and emergency procedures. Applicators and other persons in the fumigation area must wear appropriate personal protective equipment (PPE) as required by the label and U.S. EPA regulations. Such PPE typically includes full eye/face shields, safety shoes, and respirators. If the concentration of methyl bromide in the work area exceeds establishes safety levels, all persons in the fumigated area must wear approved, self-contained breathing apparatus or evacuate the area. The placarding and posting of warning notices at all entrances to an area undergoing fumigation is required. No one is permitted in a structure or area undergoing fumigation, unless they are involved in the fumigation and are wearing appropriate PPE. Re-entry into fumigated areas or structures is prohibited until the air concentration of methyl bromide is shown to be at safe levels. Individuals living in close proximity to fumigated fields, greenhouses, or structures are unlikely to be exposed to unsafe levels of methyl bromide because the application restrictions and the rapid dissipation of methyl bromide in the atmosphere. Additional regulatory controls further limit this possibility. For example, in California, maximum air concentration levels have been established for state-mandated buffer zones surrounding fumigated areas.

84.3 TOXICOLOGY OF METHYL BROMIDE

The toxicology of methyl bromide has been extensively reviewed (ATSDR, 1991; WHO, 1995). This chapter briefly describes many of the published studies and elaborates the results from a number of contemporaneous toxicity studies with methyl bromide which were conducted to support the EPA reregistration and to provide specific data to meet various state registration/regulatory requirements. A primary focus in this chapter is methyl bromide induced neurotoxicity. From a risk characterization standpoint, clinical observations of neurotoxicity are considered as the primary endpoint of concern from inhalation exposure. Reviewing of the overall toxicity of methyl bromide shows that methyl bromide induced toxicity is a function of both the concentration and the duration of exposure. This is an important consideration in evaluating potential human risks.

84.3.1 ACUTE TOXICITY

84.3.1.1 Oral

The acute LD50 for methyl bromide in rats was reported as 214 mg/kg (Danse *et al.*, 1984). Prior to conducting longer term toxicity studies, an acute oral toxicity study was conducted which compared liquid methyl bromide to a microencapsulated form. Similar oral toxicity was noted for both forms of methyl bromide; the oral LD50 values were 104 mg/kg for liquid methyl bromide and 133 mk/kg for microencapsulated methyl bromide (Kiplinger, 1994).

In beagle dogs, 500 mg/kg produced severe signs of toxicity and vomiting followed by death within 24 hours of dosing. A 50 mg/kg dose elicited signs of toxicity and vomiting of reddish material but no deaths. At low doses of 5 and 3 mg/kg, dogs vomited shortly after dosing. An oral LD50 study could not be conducted since dogs vomited the dose (Naas, 1990).

84.3.1.2 Inhalation

Overt toxicity (i.e., death) from acute inhalation exposures to methyl bromide has been extensively evaluated in rodents (Alexeeff and Kilgore, 1985; Irish *et al.*, 1940; Japanese Ministry of Labour, 1992; Zwart, 1988). The majority of the acute inhalation studie in mice and rats demonstrate that methyl bromide exposure related effects and mortality are a function of both the concentration and the duration of exposure. Inhalation LC50 values for methyl bromide in mice have been reported as 1700 ppm for a 30 minute exposure (Bakhishev, 1973), 1200 ppm for a 60 minute exposure (Alexeeff and Kilgore, 1985), 397 ppm for a 120 minute exposure (Balander and Polyak, 1962), and 405 ppm for a 240 minute exposure (Yamano, 1991). Similarly, inhalation LC50 values for rats were 2833 ppm for 30 minute exposure (Bakhishev, 1973), 1880 ppm for a 60 minute exposure (Zwart, 1988; Zwart *et al.*, 1992), 781 ppm for a 240 minute exposure (Kato *et al.*, 1986), and 302 ppm for an eight hour exposure (Honma *et al.*, 1985).

A number of acute inhalation study provide results which clearly demonstrate the concentration and the duration of exposure relationship for methyl bromide.

In an acute inhalation study, groups of F344 rats were exposed to methyl bromide at concentrations of 150, 225, 338, 506, 760, or 1140 ppm for four hours (Japanese Ministry of Labour, 1992). This single exposure resulted in decreased locomotor activity, ataxia, nasal discharge, lacrimation, diarrhea, irregular breathing, and bradypnea in rats exposed to 338 ppm and greater. No clinical signs of toxicity were evident in animals exposed to 225 ppm methyl bromide or less. Histologic evaluations revealed metaplasia of the olfactory epithelium for rats exposed to 225, 338, and 506 ppm methyl bromide.

Honma *et al.* (1985) conducted a series of acute inhalation toxicity studies to evaluate methyl bromide-induced effects on locomotor activity, body temperature, body weight gain, and enhancement of thiopental-induced sleep. Rats were exposed to methyl bromide concentrations of 63, 125, 188, or 250 ppm for eight hours. At 63 ppm and greater, enhanced thiopental sleep potentiation, measured by time to loss of righting reflex upon thiopental injection, was noted. Body weight gain and body temperature were decreased in rats exposed to methyl bromide concentrations of 125 ppm and greater. Neurotoxicity, indicated by reduced locomotor activity, was seen at concentrations of 188 and 250 ppm methyl bromide. These effects were reversible within 24 hours of exposure.

In a study that evaluated histologic changes from acute inhalation of methyl bromide (Hurtt *et al.*, 1987), Fischer 344 rats were exposed to methyl bromide concentrations of 0, 90, 175, 250, or 325 ppm on a six hours/day, five consecutive day regimen. Diarrhea was noted by the end of the second day of exposure for 250 and 325 ppm animals. By the end of the third exposure, animals from these groups showed ataxia. Two of the 325 ppm rats exhibited tremors and/or convulsions during the fourth exposure. Subsequently, three animals from this group succumbed after the fourth exposure. Clinical signs of neurotoxicity were not observed in the 250 and 325 ppm animals after a single (or second) exposure to methyl bromide.

Irish *et al.* (1940) exposed rats and rabbits to methyl bromide concentration ranging from 108 to 12,850 ppm. The study results showed clear concentration and exposure duration dependence. Rabbits tolerated exposure to 220 ppm methyl bromide for 20 hours but exposure at this concentration for 32 hours resulted in 100% mortality. At 2570 ppm, rabbits survived a 1 hour exposure to while 100% mortality was observed after 2.2 hours exposure.

Groups of mice were exposed for four hours via whole body exposure to methyl bromide atmospheric concentrations of 100, 150, 225, 338, 506, or 760 ppm (Japanese Ministry of Labour, 1992). Concentration dependent clinical signs of toxicity consisting of decreased locomotor activity, tremors, convulsions, diarrhea, dyspnea, and bradypnea were seen at concentrations of 506 and 760 ppm methyl bromide. The acute inhalation NOAEL for clinical signs of neurotoxicity in mice exposed to methyl bromide was 338 ppm.

Alexeeff and Kilgore (1985) conducted a series of one-hour inhalation exposure studies in which mice were exposed to methyl bromide concentrations ranging from 225 to 1530 ppm. Based on all signs of neurotoxicity, the NOEL was 560 ppm.

In a series of inhalation studies (Newton, 1994a), beagle dogs received one to four days exposure to methyl bromide. The purpose of this study was to determine tolerable inhalation exposure levels to be used in a four-week inhalation study. In the initial phase of the study, three males and three females were exposed for six to seven hours to methyl bromide concentrations of 233 (one male), 314 (one male, one female), 345/350 (one male, one female), or 394 ppm (one female). Signs of toxicity were observed at all concentrations, therefore, the one-day NOAEL was <233 ppm. In the second phase of the study, dogs were exposed to either 55 ppm (one male, one female), 156 (one male, one female), 268 (one male, two females),or 283 ppm (two males, one female) for seven hours/day for up to four days. The 268 ppm and 283 ppm dogs were exposed to methyl bromide for two days and developed clinical signs of toxicity. Therefore, the two-day NOAEL for beagle dogs exposed to methyl bromide was <268 ppm. The 55 ppm and 156 ppm dogs were exposed to methyl bromide seven hours/day for four consecutive days. No effects were seen in either the 55 or 156 ppm dogs during days 1 and 2 of exposure. However, the 156 ppm animals showed decreased activity during exposure on days 3 and 4 and irregular gait during the postexposure period on day 4.

84.3.2 SUBCHRONIC TOXICITY

84.3.2.1 Oral

In a subchronic toxicity study (Danse *et al.*, 1984), Wistar rats were dosed with methyl bromide via gavage at doses of 0, 0.4, 2, 10, or 50 mg/kg/day for 90 days. At 50 mg/kg/day, marked, diffuse hyperplasia of the epithelium of the forestomach was seen in all animals. Squamous cell carcinoma of the forestomach was diagnosed in 13 of 20 animals receiving methyl bromide at 50 mg/kg/day. Upon subsequent evaluation of the histology slides, it was concluded that the forestomach lesions represented inflammation and hyperplasia rather than malignant lesions. Inflammatory lesions of the forestomach were also seen in animals treated with 2 and 10 mg/kg/day.

84.3.2.2 Inhalation

Table 84.1 summarizes the results from a number of subchronic inhalation studies in rats and mice. For comparison purposes, the study results have been presented to show the overall study NOEL, the NOEL for neurotoxicity, and the LOEL for neurotoxicity.

Beagle dogs were exposed to either 55 ppm (one male, one female), 156 (one male, one female), 268 ppm (one male, two females), or 283 ppm (two males, one female) for seven hours/day for up to four days (Newton, 1994a). Clinical signs of toxicity were seen in the 268 and 283 ppm dogs after two exposures. The 156 ppm animals showed decreased activity during exposure on days 3 and 4 and irregular gait during the post exposure period on day 4. The 55 ppm concentration was the four-day NOEL.

In a four-week inhalation study (Newton, 1994b), beagle dogs (four/sex/group) were exposed for five days/week, seven hours/day to methyl bromide at concentrations of 0, 5, 10, 25, 50, or 100 ppm. No clinical evidence of neurotoxicity was seen in any group throughout the four weeks of exposure. After four weeks, four of the controls (two females and two males) and all dogs in the 5 ppm group continued the test for an additional two weeks and the exposure concentration for the 10 ppm group was increased to 150 ppm. Dogs exposed to 150 ppm methyl bromide showed severe body weight loss over the first few days of exposure. After five or six exposures, evaluation of the 150 ppm animals by a veterinary neurologist revealed ataxia, a base-wide stance, intention tremor, nystagmus, marked depression, and inability (unwillingness) to stand and perform postural responses. Due to the severity of these effects, the dogs were sacrificed. Neurologic evaluation revealed no treatment related neurologic effects for dogs exposed at the lower methyl bromide concentrations. Microscopic findings were limited to the 150 ppm group in which significant neurologic effects were seen and consisted of vacuoles in the granular layer of the cerebellum.

84.3.3 GENETIC TOXICITY

Methyl bromide has been tested in numerous *in vitro* and *in vivo* genetic toxicity studies with variable results.

Table 84.1
Summary of Subchronic Inhalation Toxicity Studies with Methyl Bromide

Study	Species (Strain)	Exposure (hours/days/weeks)	Overall NOEL	Neurotoxicity NOEL (effect)	Neurotoxicity LOEL
Subchronic neurotoxicity (Norris et al., 1993)	Rat (SD)	6/5/13	30 ppm	30 ppm	70 ppm
Subchronic toxicity (NTP, 1992)	Rat (SPF Wistar)	6/5/3; 6/7/1	18 ppm	18 ppm	51 ppm
Subchronic toxicity (Kato et al., 1986)	Rat (SD)	4/5/6	<150 ppm	200 ppm (dec. body weight)	300 ppm
Subchronic toxicity (Haber et al., 1985) (NTP, 1992)	Rat (F344/N)	6/5/13	30 ppm	60 ppm (dec. body weight)	120 ppm
Subchronic toxicity (Japanese Ministry, 1992)	Rat (F344/DuCrj)	6/5/13	7.5 ppm	117 ppm (clinical pathology)	293 ppm
Subchronic toxicity (Wilmer et al., 1983)	Rat (Wistar)	6/5/13	6.4 ppm	42 ppm (liver pathology)	no neurotoxicity
Subchronic toxicity (NTP, 1992)	Mouse (B6C3F1)	6/5/13	20 ppm	80 ppm (hematology)	120 ppm
Subchronic toxicity (Japanese Ministry, 1992)	Mouse (Crj:BDF1)	6/5/13	30 ppm	60 ppm (body weight, hematology, urinalysis)	no neurotoxicity

Methyl bromide has been reported to induce mutagenic effects in bacterial tests with *Salmonella typhimurium* (TA100 and TA1535), *E. coli*, and *Klebsiella pneumoniae* (Djalali-Behzad et al., 1981; Kramers et al., 1985a; Moriya et al., 1983; Simmon et al., 1977). No evidence of mutagenicity was seen when methyl bromide was tested in a modified Ames test using an *in situ* impingement test system but a significant response was seen with the SOS repair test (Ong et al., 1987).

A sex-related recessive lethal assay was conducted with male strain Oregon K Drosophila melanogaster (McGregor, 1981). The Drosophila were exposed to methyl bromide concentrations of 20 or 70 ppm for 5 hours and then allowed to mate on days 1, 3, or 8 following exposure. The F1 progeny were mated brother to sister, 1 to 4 days after emergence. The resulting F2 generation was then examined for the absence of wild-type males. No compound-related increases in the frequency of lethal mutations in the F2 generation were noted.

In a second sex-related recessive lethal assay, Drosophilia melanogaster of the Berlin K strain were exposed to methyl bromide concentrations ranging from 18 to 192 ppm for varying exposure intervals (Kramers et al., 1985a, b). As was noted for the acute inhalation studies in mammalian species, mutagenic responses were related to both exposure concentration and duration. No increase in mutation frequency was seen in Drosophila exposed to 192 ppm for six hours at 192 ppm. Exposure at 155 ppm resulted in all flies dying during the fourth day of exposure. At lower concentrations, prolonged exposure resulted in mutagenic responses. Exposure at 125 ppm for five days (six hours per day) and at 50 ppm for 15 days (six hours per day) were considered mutagenic.

Exposure of L5178Y mouse lymphoma cells to methyl bromide concentrations ranging from 7.7 to 7710 ppm resulted in dose-related increases in 6-thioguanine- and bromodeoxyuridine-resistant mutants (Kramers et al., 1985a).

Sister chromatid exchanges (SCEs) and chromosomal aberrations in human lymphocytes exposed to methyl bromide were evaluated. Exposure of human lymphocyte cultures to an atmosphere of 4.3% methyl bromide for 100 seconds increased the frequency of SCEs from 10.0 to 16.8 per cell (Tucker et al., 1986). When human lymphocytes were treated with methyl bromide (0–24 μg/ml) for 30 minutes, dose-related increases in SCEs and chromosomal aberration were found. Metabolic activation (S9) significantly induced chromosomal aberrations (Garry et al., 1990).

Drosophila melanogaster (third instar larvae trans-dihybrid for two recessive wing hair mutations) were exposed to methyl bromide vapor concentrations ranging up to 5140 ppm for one hour in a mitotic recombination assay in somatic cells (somatic wing spot assay). Wings of surviving adults were evaluated for the presence of cellular clones with malformed wing hairs. Methyl bromide induced mitotic recombination as exhibited by the observation of small and large single as well as twin spots (Katz, 1985, 1987).

A rodent micronucleus (MN) study was conducted in BDF1 mice and F344 rats (10/sex/group) exposed via vapor inhalation to methyl bromide concentrations of 0, 154, 200, 260, 338, or 440 ppm for six hours/day, five days/week for two weeks (Araki et.al, 1995). Bone marrow of rats and peripheral blood of mice were evaluated for MN induction. In mice, significantly increased incidences of micronuclei in bone marrow polychromatic erythrocytes (PCE) were observed in males at 154 and

200 ppm and in females at 154 ppm; smaller increases in MN frequency were observed in normochromatic erythrocytes. Peripheral blood showed significant increases in MN at 200 ppm in males and 154 ppm in females. Due to excessive mortality, mice exposed to methyl bromide concentrations of 260 ppm and greater were not assayed. In rats, a statistically significant increase of MN in PCE was seen for males exposed at 338 ppm. A nonstatistically significant increase of MN in PCEs was seen in female rats exposed at 260 and 338 ppm. Rats exposed at 400 ppm were not assayed due to excessive mortality.

Methyl bromide was selected by the National Institutes of Occupational Safety and Health for evaluation in a Tier II Mutagenic Screening (McGregor, 1981). The testing program included: (1) unscheduled DNA synthesis (UDS) assay in human diploid fibroblasts, (2) sex-linked recessive lethal test in Drosophila melanogaster, (3) cytogenetic test in bone marrow cells of male and female rats, (4) sperm abnormality test in male mice, and (5) dominant lethal test in male rats. Summary results from this screening battery show that:

- Human diploid fibroblasts exposed for three hours to methyl bromide concentrations of up to 70% in air over a minimal volume of culture medium in a UDS resulted in no increase in UDS.
- Drosophila melanogaster exposed to methyl bromide concentrations of 20 or 70 ppm for five hours did not have an increased frequency of sex linked recessive mutations.
- Cytogenetic analysis of bone marrow cells derived from male and female Sprague Dawley rats that were exposed for one or five days (seven hours/day) to methyl bromide concentrations of 20 or 70 ppm showed no treatment related increases in the frequency of chromosomal aberrations in any of the methyl bromide exposed groups.
- Evaluation and characterization of sperm from male B6C3F1 mice exposed to 20 or 70 ppm methyl bromide for seven hours/day on five consecutive days then sacrificed five weeks later showed no significant increase in the frequency of abnormal sperm.
- In the dominant lethal study, male Sprague Dawley rats were exposed to methyl bromide concentrations of 0 (air), 20, or 70 ppm for seven hours per day for five consecutive days then allowed to breed with two virgin females weekly for 10 weeks. The females were sacrificed on Day 14 after presumed mating. Examination of the ovaries and the uterine contents showed no evidence of genotoxicity.

In a separate study, methyl bromide was evaluated for its ability to induce single strand breaks in rat testicular DNA using alkaline elution techniques (Bentley, 1994). In this study, groups of 10 male Fischer 344 rats were exposed to methyl bromide vapor concentrations of 0, 75, 150, or 250 ppm for six hours per day over five consecutive days. The negative control group was exposed to room air only. A positive control group received a single intraperitoneal injection of 50 mg/kg methyl methanesulfonate in phosphate buffered saline. Five animals

from each group were sacrificed at 1 and 24 hours postexposure. Significant toxicity was seen in the 250 ppm rats. Two males from this group died and a third male was sacrificed in extremis with the 1-hour post treatment animals. Surviving rats showed decreased body weight and clinical signs of toxicity characterized by ataxia, spasms, diarrhea, lethargy, and prostration. At 150 ppm, the male rats showed slight body weight loss, nasal and/or ocular discharge and wet and/or stained perineum during the five-day exposure. A statistically significant increase in the mean elution rate of testicular cell DNA was observed at both sacrifice times only in rats exposed to the highly toxic 250 ppm concentration.

84.3.4 DEVELOPMENTAL AND REPRODUCTIVE TOXICITY

In a developmental toxicity study (Sikov et al., 1981), pregnant female Wistar rats were exposed to methyl bromide concentrations of 0, 20, or 70 ppm for seven hours/day on gestation days 1 to 19. In addition, some groups were exposed pregestationally to 20 or 70 ppm on a for three weeks (five days per week) immediately prior to mating. The distribution of dose groups (pregestational exposure concentration/gestational exposure concentration) was 0/0, 0/20, 0/70, 20/0, 20/20, 70/0, and 70/70 ppm. Cesarean sacrifice was performed on gestation day 19. No clinical evidence of maternal toxicity, fetotoxicity or developmental toxicity was observed in any exposure scenario.

Artificially inseminated New Zealand White rabbits (24 per group) were exposed daily on gestation days 1 through 24 to methyl bromide concentrations of 0 and 20 ppm; a group of inseminated rabbits exposed to 70 ppm methyl bromide were terminated due to excessive mortality and neurotoxicity characterized by convulsions and paresis in the hindlimbs seen after one week of treatment (Sikov et al., 1981). Control and 20 ppm exposed rabbits were sacrificed on gestation day 30. No fetoxicity nor developmental toxicity was noted for the 20 ppm group.

In probe studies (Breslin et al., 1990a), pregnant rabbits were exposed to methyl bromide concentrations of 0, 10, 30, or 50 ppm in one study and concentrations of 0, 50, 70, or 140 ppm in a second study. Exposure was for six hours/day on gestation days 7 to 19. Evidence of toxicity was observed only in the 140 ppm group does. All does exposed to methyl bromide at this concentration showed lethargy and decreased food consumption after eight exposures. With continued exposure signs of neurotoxicity were apparent and resulted in sacrifice of the does on gestation day 17. No apparent embryotoxicity was observed at any exposure level. The subsequent developmental toxicity study in rabbits was conducted in two phases (Breslin et al., 1990a, 1990b). In the initial phase, pregnant New Zealand White rabbits were exposed for six hours/day to methyl bromide concentrations of 0, 20, 40, and 80 ppm on days 7 through 19 of gestation. In the second phase, pregnant does were exposed to 0 or 80 ppm only. Cesarean delivery was performed on day 28 of gestation. In the first phase, maternal toxicity, evidenced by decreased bodyweight gain and clinical signs of neurotoxicity, was observed in three of the does from the 80 ppm group. The clinical signs consisted of right-sided head tilt, ataxia, slight lateral recumbency, and lethargy. In the second study, a significant decrease in bodyweight during gestation was the only evidence of maternal toxicity in the 80 ppm group. Developmental effects were limited to the maternally toxic 80 ppm group only. In phase 1, fetal findings consisted of low incidences of omphalocele, hemorrhaging with or without hydrops (edema), retroesophogeal right subclavian artery, gall bladder agenesis, and fused sternebra. Fetal effects in phase 2 were limited to decreased fetal weight, hemorrhaging with or without hydrops and gall bladder agenesis.

Male and female Sprague Dawley rats were exposed to methyl bromide by whole body inhalation exposure, six hours/day, five days/week at concentrations of 0, 3, 30, or 90 ppm in a two-generation reproduction study (American Biogenics Corporation, 1986). Two litters were produced for each generation. No deaths nor noteworthy antemortem clinical finding were observed over the course of the study. The 90 ppm F0 males had significantly decreased body weights at five of the 10 premating intervals and at final sacrifice. No other decreases in body weights were observed among the F0 generation or during the F1 generation prior to the gestational period for the F2a litter. A slight depression of body weight was noted during the gestation and lactation periods for the 90 ppm F1 dams. Reproductive performance was not altered by methyl bromide exposure and there were no significant differences in pup survival. No methyl bromide related anomalies were noted for the progeny. Gross pathologic examination revealed no treatment related lesions in either the parental animals or their progeny. Mean brain weight for the 90 ppm males (P0 and F1) and females (F1) were decreased Increased liver to body weight ratio for the 90 ppm P0 males and females and increased heart to brain weight ratios for the 90 ppm F1 females were noted. No other significant differences were seen in the parent organ weight data. No significant differences in the F1b progeny body and organ weights were noted but statistically significant decreases in final body weights were observed for the 90 ppm F2b males and females and the 30 ppm F2b females. F2b progeny organ weights were significantly reduced for the 90 ppm female brain, heart, kidney, and liver weights, the 30 ppm female liver weight, and the 30 and 90 ppm female liver to brain weight ratio. The 30 and 90 ppm F2b female brain to body weight ratio was increased. There were no other significant differences noted for progeny. Microscopic examination of the reproductive organs and abnormal tissues revealed no treatment related lesions.

84.3.5 CHRONIC TOXICITY AND ONCOGENICITY—INHALATION

Wistar rats were exposed (whole body) to methyl bromide at atmospheric concentrations of 0, 3, 30, or 90 ppm on a six hour/day, five days/week basis for 29 months (Reuzel *et al.*, 1987, 1991). At the 90 ppm concentration, decreased survival was noted for both the males and females from the end of the second year through termination at 29 months. Also, at this concentration, body weights, especially for females, were lower than the control group from week 4 and throughout the remainder of the study, and decreased absolute brain weight was noted for females. No differences in hematology, clinical pathology, or urinalysis were seen at either the 3 month or one year intervals. No treatment related evidence of neoplasia was observed in the study. Treatment related nonneoplastic pathology consisted of an increased incidence of thrombi in the heart, and myocardial degeneration for both sexes from the 90 ppm group. Irritation of the nasal cavity characterized by hyperplasia of the olfactory epithelium was seen in a time-related fashion for all methyl bromide treated groups. Dose-dependent increases in the incidences of degenerative and hyperplastic changes of the nasal olfactory epithelium were observed. The lesions were characterized as very slight, slight, or moderate. A statistically significant increase was found between controls and the low-dose group (3 ppm) at the end of the exposure period (29 months). However, the frequency of this lesion also increased in the controls (age dependence) from 12 through 24 months to 29 months of age. In addition, all but one of the lesions in the 3 ppm exposure level group were described as slight or very slight. Moreover, one moderate lesion of the nasal mucosa was also observed in a control animal at the 24-month sacrifice interval. The NOEL for this lesion was >90 ppm after 12 months of exposure, 3 ppm after 24 months of exposure, and <3 ppm after 29 months of exposure.

The Gotoh *et al.* (1994) study directly correlate with the Reuzel *et al.* (1987, 1991) study at the 24-month interval. Gotoh *et al.* exposed F344 rats to methyl bromide concentrations of 0, 4, 20, and 100 ppm on a six hour/day, five day/week basis for 104 weeks. After 24 months of exposure, increased incidences of necrosis and respiratory metaplasia of the olfactory epithelium were seen for male rats exposed to 100 ppm methyl bromide; these findings were marginally increased for the female rats at 100 ppm. Metaplasia was noted for 22% of the control males and 6% of the control females at the 24-month terminal interval. These results show that metaplasia produced in the rat olfactory epithelium was a threshold response upon chronic inhalation exposure to methyl bromide and that a high control incidence of metaplasia is noted in aged rats.

B6C3F1 mice were exposed via inhalation (whole body) to concentrations of 0, 10, 33, or 100 ppm methyl bromide on a six hours/day, five days/week basis for two years (NTP, 1992). The 100 ppm exposure concentration clearly exceeded an acceptable maximum tolerated dose for carcinogenicity testing. This exposure concentration was terminated after 20 weeks due to debilitating neurotoxicity and mortalities; these animals were exposed to untreated air for the remainder of the two-year study period. Interim sacrifice of 10 mice per sex/treatment level was performed after 6 and 15 months of exposure. Neurobehavioral testing was performed on selected animals every 3 months. Clinical signs of neurotoxicity, consisting of tremors, paralysis, gait disturbances, and abnormal posture, were noted for 100 ppm males (78%) and females (43%). Similar findings were seen for a few (2 to 3%) of the 33 ppm exposed animals. After 3 months of exposure, neurobehavioral changes were noted for the 100 ppm males and females. Neurobehavioral testing also revealed changes in the 10 and 33 ppm groups after 6 months of exposure. Decreased body weights were observed in females dosed at 33 ppm and in both sexes dosed at 100 ppm. Exposure related histologic changes were generally limited to the 100 ppm animals and consisted of findings in the brain (degeneration of the cerebrum and cerebellum), heart (degeneration and cardiomyopathy), sternal dysplasia, and either necrosis or metaplasia of the olfactory epithelium.

84.3.6 CHRONIC TOXICITY AND ONCOGENICITY—DIETARY

Methyl bromide was evaluated for chronic toxicity and oncogenicity in a 24-month dietary toxicity study (Mertens, 1997) in Sprague Dawley rats. Because of the volatile nature of methyl bromide and the feeding characteristics of rats, it was not possible to conduct the study using feed fumigated with methyl bromide. For purposes of this study, methyl bromide was microencapsulated and mixed into the rodent diet. Methyl bromide dietary concentrations were 0.5, 2.5, 50, and 250 ppm (0.02, 0.11, 2.20, and 11.10 mg/kg/day for males and 0.3, 0.15, 2.92, and 15.12 mg/kg/day for females, respectively). Basal diet and placebo (microcapsules without methyl bromide) control groups were treated on a comparable regimen. No methyl bromide related effects were seen on survival, clinical condition, hematology, serum chemistry, urinalysis, organ weights, ophthalmologic assessments, or macroscopic and microscopic pathology evaluations. Food consumption, mean body weights, and mean body weight gains were reduced in the 250 ppm males and females during the rapid growth phase for the animals during the first 12 to 18 months of the study. During the first 18 months of the study, mean body weight gain for males were 9% to 21% lower than the male control groups while mean body weight gain for females was 7% to 22% lower than the female control groups. Typical of chronic toxicity studies, food consumption and body weight gains during the second year of the study were comparable to controls as the mature animals reached adult body weight plateau. No evidence of oncogenicity was seen in this study.

In a 12-month dietary safety study (Newton, 1995), beagle dogs were exposed to methyl bromide fumigated feed at dietary concentrations of 0, 0.5, 1.5, or 5 ppm (0, 0.06, 0.13, and 0.27 mg/kg/day for males and 0, 0.07, 0.12, and 0.26 mg/kg/day for females, respectively). Prestudy trials were conducted to determine the methyl bromide fumigation concentrations and postfumigation intervals required to achieve the desired concentrations over a 1-hour feeding period. No toxicologically significant methyl bromide effects were seen in clinical observations, body weight, body weight gain, food consumption, clinical pathology, urinalysis, ophthalmology, absolute or relative organ weights, and macroscopic or microscopic pathology. Based on the results of this study, the NOEL for methyl bromide when administered via fumigated feed to beagle dogs

was greater than 5 ppm (>0.27 mg/kg/day for males and >0.26 mg/kg/day for females).

84.3.7 NEUROTOXICITY

In an acute neurotoxicity study (Driscoll and Hurley, 1993), male and female CD (Sprague Dawley) rats were exposed via inhalation for six hours to methyl bromide at concentrations of 0, 30, 100, or 350 ppm. Animals were assessed for clinical signs and changes in body weights. Neurobehavioral evaluations were performed within three hours of exposure and at 7 and 14 days postexposure. These evaluations included the functional observation battery and motor activity assessments. After 15 days, animals were euthanized, necropsied, and examined for gross pathologic changes, and brains were weighed. In addition, microscopic evaluations were performed on central and peripheral nervous tissue. All animals survived to study termination. No methyl bromide induced effects were noted for body or brain weights. Neurobehavioral effects were observed only in the 350 ppm exposed group and were limited to the three-hour postexposure assessment. Effects noted in male and female rats consisted of decreased arousal, increased incidences of drooping or half-shut eyelids, piloerection, decreased rearing, depressed body temperature, and markedly decreased motor activity. The 350 ppm males had a decreased tail pinch response while females from this group showed increased urination and abnormal air righting response. No treatment related histological findings were seen in nervous system or nasal tissues.

In a subchronic inhalation neurotoxicity study (Norris et al., 1993) CD (Sprague Dawley) rats were exposed to methyl bromide concentrations of 0, 30, 70, or 140 ppm. Exposure was six hours/day, five days/week for 13 weeks. At the 140 ppm concentration, two male rats died during the first month. Clinical signs observed for these rats included convulsions, tremors, hyperactivity, rapid respiration, and salivation. Mean body weights were significantly lower than the controls. Neurologic evaluations for males revealed increased hind limb splay (weeks 4, 8, 13), abnormal air righting reflex (week 13), and decreased forelimb grip strength (week 13). Female rats demonstrated lower arousal scores (weeks 8, 13), decreased rearing (weeks 4, 8, 13) and significantly decreased motor activity (week 13). Mean absolute brain weights were significantly lower for both sexes; no differences were noted for the relative brain weights, indicating that lower absolute brain weight was a reflection of the generally lower body weights for the treated animals. Gross lesions were limited to moderate to severe brain hemorrhage in the two 140 ppm male animals which died. Microscopic lesions in the brain were found in these two males and in one 140 ppm male that survived the 13-week exposure. Microscopic lesions in the brain were seen in these three males and consisted of neuronal necrosis in the hippocampus, necrosis and malacia in the cerebral cortex and basal ganglia, and malacia and/or necrosis in the thalamus and midbrain. The lesions were more severe for one of the males which was found dead and the male that survived the 13-week exposure; both of these animals were noted with convulsions during the study, suggesting that some of the microscopic brain findings may have been secondary effects of brain swelling related to the convulsions. One additional 140 ppm male had slight neuronal edema in the hippocampus. Other lesions in the 140 ppm group consisted of minimal regenerative dysplasia of the olfactory epithelium of the nasal cavity in three males and three females and minimal peripheral nerve degeneration in two males and two females. In the 70 ppm group, lower mean body weights and weight gain were seen for females from week 9 onward of the study. Neurologic findings were limited to slightly decreased forelimb grip strength (week 13) in males and decreased motor activity (week 13) in females. Although the mean absolute brain weight for females was statistically significantly decreased (5% lower than the control group), no difference was seen for the relative brain weight and no microscopic pathology was seen. At 30 ppm, the mean absolute brain weight for females was statistically significantly lower than control (5% lower than the control group); however, no difference was seen in relative brain weight and no microscopic pathology in the brain was seen. Peripheral nerve degeneration was observed in one female rat. This finding was considered incidental since nerve degeneration was not seen in animals from the 70 ppm group.

84.3.8 SPECIFIC TARGET ORGAN EFFECTS

Methyl bromide is an unusual respiratory toxicant in the rat in that it is specifically toxic to the olfactory epithelium while other nasal epithelia are unaffected (Hurtt et al., 1988). Within the olfactory epithelium, methyl bromide only affects specific cell types. The major components of the rat olfactory epithelium are the basal cells, the long ducts of Bowman's glands, sensory cells, and the sustenacular or support cells. Studies using histochemical techniques clearly showed that methyl bromide specifically induced degeneration of the sensory and sustenacular cells while sparing the basal cells from which the sensory and sustenacular cells are regenerated.

Hurtt et al. (1988) evaluated the time course for the regeneration of the olfactory epithelium following short term exposures to methyl bromide. Male rats were exposed to 200 ppm methyl bromide for six hours/day for one to five days. Air-exposed animals served as controls. In a companion study, animals were exposed to 0, 90, or 200 ppm for six hours and olfactory function assessed by the ability of food deprived animals to locate buried food pellets. Destruction of the olfactory epithelium was evident after a single six-hour exposure to 90 or 200 ppm. As discussed previously, severe effects were seen in the sustenacular and mature sensory cells while basal cells remained intact. Regeneration of the olfactory epithelium was seen as early as day 3 of exposure despite continued exposure at these high methyl bromide concentrations. The recovery of the olfactory epithelium was essentially complete by 10 weeks after exposure. The rapid recovery would be expected since the non-affected basal cells regenerate sensory and sustenacular cells.

Olfactory function, as measured by food finding activity, was impaired in animals exposed to 200 ppm only. Recovery of this function was evident by four to six days postexposure, much earlier than the time course for histological recovery.

In another study (Hastings et al., 1994), morphologic and biochemical (carnosine content of the olfactory bulb, a biomarker for integrity of the olfactory epithelium) evaluations were conducted to further explore methyl bromide exposure effects and recovery. Prior to treatment, rats were food-deprived and trained to find buried food pellets as a measure of olfactory function. The rats were exposed to a methyl bromide concentration of 200 ppm on a four hour/day, four days/week, two-week regimen. After a single exposure, extensive damage to the olfactory epithelium, reduced carnosine content, and impaired olfactory function were observed. Even though exposure continued, olfactory function began to improve after the first exposure. This recovery proceeded even though persistent thinning and disorganization of the olfactory epithelium and decreased carnosine levels in the olfactory bulb were present. Regeneration of the olfactory epithelium was complete approximately 30–40 days after the last exposure.

84.4 METABOLISM

Inhalation was the primary route of exposure for the majority of the methyl bromide toxicology studies and is the most probable route of exposure for humans. As a result, the metabolism of methyl bromide has been almost exclusively evaluated by inhalation.

84.4.1 ABSORPTION

Medinsky et al. (1984, 1985) evaluated the uptake of methyl bromide upon six-hour exposure of rats to concentrations of 1.6, 9.0, 170, or 310 ppm. Methyl bromide uptake was found to be linear over all exposure concentrations with the exception of the 310 ppm concentration. It was noted that suspected nasal irritation at 310 ppm may have reduced the total amount of methyl bromide inhaled due to decreased tidal and minute volumes (Medinsky et al., 1985). Total methyl bromide absorbed was 9 or 40 μmol/kg body weight after exposure to 1.6 ppm (50 nmol/liter) or 9.0 ppm (300 nmol/liter), respectively. Uptake at the lower levels was approximately 48%. Uptake at 5700 (170 ppm) and 10,400 (310 ppm) nmol/liter was 37% and 27%, respectively (Medinsky et al., 1985).

Andersen et al. (1980) found methyl bromide to exhibit rapid, first-order uptake kinetics. Saturation was not reached until concentrations causing animal death were achieved. Gargas and Andersen (1982) also demonstrated that methyl bromide uptake and metabolism followed first order over a broad range of exposure concentration (100–3000 ppm). Honma et al. (1985) also found methyl bromide to be rapidly absorbed and distributed. Methyl bromide concentrations in blood, liver, adipose, and brain reached maximum levels within one hour after the start of exposure and maintained almost the same levels during the eight hour exposure. Equilibrium between methyl bromide air and tissue concentrations occurred rapidly.

84.4.2 DISTRIBUTION

Methyl bromide is rapidly and widely distributed in tissues immediately after exposure.

Bond et al. (1985) investigated the tissue distribution of 14C methyl bromide. Radioactivity was widely distributed in tissues immediately following exposure with highest levels of 14C found in lung, adrenal, kidney, liver, and nasal turbinates. Low concentrations of 14C were also detected in other tissues. The liver was the only tissue examined immediately after exposure that contained a large percentage (about 17%) of the absorbed methyl bromide. Approximately 80% of the initial amount of tissue radiolabel was eliminated by 65 hours. Elimination half-lives varied from 1.5 to 8 hours with the exception of the liver with an elimination half-life of 33 hours.

Using non-radiolabelled methyl bromide, Honma et al. (1985) investigated the distribution of methyl bromide into liver, fat, brain, muscle, kidney, and blood upon inhalation exposure of rats to 250 ppm for 8 hours. Methyl bromide concentrations in all tissues listed reached maximum levels within 1 hour after the start of the exposure and was found at approximately the same tissue concentration through the remainder of exposure period. The highest tissue concentration was found in fat. Methyl bromide was rapidly eliminated from rat tissues following the cessation of exposure, with a half-life of about 30 minutes in the early postexposure period. At 48 hours postexposure, methyl bromide was not detected in any tissue examined.

Medinsky et al. (1985) evaluated tissue distribution of methyl bromide 66 hours after exposure to range of vapor concentrations. Significant levels of 14C (approximately 20% of the absorbed methyl bromide dose) remained in tissues 66 hours after exposure. The highest level (approximately 20% of the 14C) was associated with the liver. Other tissues having appreciable concentrations of 14C included the lungs, nasal turbinates, and kidneys. Very low concentrations of 14C (less than 1 µmol of methyl bromide equivalents/g of tissue) were found in nervous tissues (spinal cord and brain).

Tissue disposition after oral or intraperitoneal (IP) injection of 250 µmol/kg 14C-methyl bromide was also evaluated (Medinsky et al., 1984). Approximately 14–17% of the radioactivity administered was found in the tissues and carcass 72 hours after oral and IP dosing, respectively. Analysis of individual tissues indicated liver was the major organ for retention of radioactivity after administration of methyl bromide. Other tissues containing significant amounts of radioactivity (>10 nmol or 1% of the total dose) included kidney, testes, lung, heart, stomach, and spleen. As expected, the only tissue showing significantly higher radioactivity level after oral administration, as compared to IP injection, was the stomach.

84.4.3 IDENTIFICATION AND QUANTITATION OF METABOLITES

In all methyl bromide metabolism studies, carbon dioxide was the major metabolite. Approximately 47% of the total methyl bromide dose was excreted as 14CO2 in expired air (Bond et al., 1985). About 1% of the total 14C-methyl bromide absorbed was exhaled as 14C-methyl bromide. Smaller quantities of the radiolabelled material were excreted in the urine and feces, with about 22% and 2% of the total absorbed 14C-methyl bromide excreted by these routes, respectively. All radioactivity in excreta was identified as methyl bromide degradates/metabolites. No evidence of parent chemical was found in any of the excreta samples (Bond et al., 1985).

Gargas and Andersen (1982) showed that bromine ion is released in the initial metabolism of a variety of brominated hydrocarbons. The study results showed that bromine ion is retained in extracellular fluid, is stable to further biotransformation, and is very slowly excreted. The first-order rate constant for the release of bromine from methyl bromide is 0.32/kg/hour. The elimination of bromine from rat tissue is slower than that of methyl bromide (Honma et al., 1985). Peak concentrations of bromine in blood, kidneys, and liver occurred four to eight hours after methyl bromide exposure, and the half-life of bromine in these tissues was about five days. There was no correlation between the duration of bromine retention and observed signs of neurotoxicity (Gargas and Andersen, 1982).

In a methyl bromide inhalation study in mice, Alexeeff and Kilgore (1985) followed mouse tissue bromine concentrations through 7 days postexposure. No bromide ion was detected in any tissue one week after exposure to concentrations up to 2.72 mg/l air. Over 95% of the bromide ion in exposed mice was eliminated within 2.5 days. The bromide ion levels were highest in liver and kidney and lowest in whole blood. Lung and brain bromide ion levels were intermediate.

Honma et al. (1985) also investigated bromine and methanol concentrations in response to treatment with methyl bromide. Peak concentrations of bromine in blood, kidneys, and liver occurred four to eight hours after methyl bromide exposure, and the half-life of bromine in these tissues was about five days. Methanol production was not significant.

84.4.4 EXCRETION

Excretion of methyl bromide is primarily as exhaled CO2. Very low levels of parent methyl bromide are found in expired air. Greater than 85% of the total amount of 14C that was exhaled as CO2 and excreted in urine and feces was eliminated within 24 hours (Bond et al., 1985). CO2 excretion exhibited a biphasic elimination pattern with 85% of the 14CO2 excreted with a half-life of about 4 hours and 15% excreted with a half-life of about 11 hours. The elimination half-life of 14C in urine was approximately 10 hours and in feces was approximatley 16 hours. Analysis of excreta samples in which there was sufficient radioactivity showed no evidence parent methyl bromide.

84.5 HUMAN EXPOSURE

The potential routes of human exposure to methyl bromide are oral (through consumption of fumigated food products), dermal (skin contact), or inhalation (exposure to methyl bromide gas). Extensive studies have shown that residues of methyl bromide found in crops grown on fumigated soils are virtually nondetectable. In addition, methyl bromide concentrations in commodities treated postharvest, decrease rapidly after required aeration, and are nondetectable after relatively short periods of time. Tolerance levels for the metabolite of methyl bromide (inorganic bromide) in treated foods have been established by the EPA. These tolerances further ensure that humans are not exposed to unsafe levels of methyl bromide's metabolite in foods. In summation, there is no significant likelihood of oral exposure to methyl bromide through consumption of treated food.

Human exposure is more likely to occur by inhalation. People living in close proximity to fumigated fields, greenhouses, or structures are protected from the risk of significant inhalation exposure through special notice requirements, safety precautions, and the use of buffer zones. The potential for dermal or inhalation exposure to methyl bromide is highest for applicators and other personnel who are involved in manufacturing, filling, handling, or application of methyl bromide. Strictly applied safety measures in manufacturing and filling installations limit the potential risk of exposure to plant personnel. In addition, fumigators/applicators are protected from dermal and inhalation exposures through adherence to strict safety procedures and the use of protective equipment.

REFERENCES

Alexeeff, G. V., and Kilgore, W. W. (1983). Methyl bromide. *Residue Rev.* **88**, 101–153.

Alexeeff, G. V., and Kilgore, W. W. (1985). Determination of acute toxic effects in mice following exposure to methyl bromide. *J. Toxicol. Environ. Health* **15**, 109–123.

American Biogenics Corporation (1986). "Two-Generation Reproduction Study via Inhalation in Albino Rats Using Methyl Bromide." Unpublished report from Study 450–1525.

Andersen, M., Gargas, M., Jones, R., and Jenkins, L. (1980). Determination of the kinetic constants for metabolism of inhaled toxicants in vivo using gas uptake measurements. *Toxicol. Appl. Pharmacol.* **54**, 100–116.

Anger, W. K., Setzer, J. V. Russo, J. M., Brightwell, W. S., Wait, R. G., and Johnson, B. L. (1981). Neurobehavioral evaluation of soil and structural fumigators using methyl bromide and sulfuryl fluoride. *NeuroToxicology* **7**, 137–156.

Araki, A., Kato, F. Matsushima, T., Ikawa, N., and Nozaki, K. (1995). Methyl bromide—micronuclei induction of methyl bromide in rats and mice by subchronic inhalation test. *Environ. Mut. Commun.* **17**, 47–56.

ATSDR (1991). "Toxicological Profile for Bromomethane." U.S. Department of Health and Human Services, Public Health Services Agency for Toxic Substances and Disease Registry, Publication 91-06.

Bakhishev, G. N. (1973). Relative toxicity of aliphatic halohydrocarbons to rats. *Farmakol Toksikol.* **8**, 140–142. [In Russian]

Balander, P. A., and Polyak, M. G. (1962). Toxicological characteristics of methyl bromide. *J. Gig. I Toksikol.* **60**, 412–419.

Bentley, K. S. (1994). "Detection of Single Strand Breaks in Rat Testicular DNA by Alkaline Elution Following *In Vivo* Inhalation Exposure to Methyl Bromide." Unpublished report from E. I. DuPont Haskell Laboratories, Project 9714-001: MBIP/21/ALK/HASK: 999.

Bond, J. A., Dutcher, J. S., Medinsky, M. A., Henderson, R. F., and Birnbaum, L. S. (1985). Disposition of [14C]methyl bromide in rats after inhalation. *Toxicol. Appl. Pharmacol.* **78**, 259–267.

Breslin, W. J., Zablotny, C. L., Bradley, G. J., Nitschke, K. D., and Lomax, L. G. (1990a). "Methyl Bromide Inhalation Teratology Probe Study in New Zealand White Rabbits." Unpublished study from Dow Chemical Company Toxicology Laboratory.

Breslin, W. J., Zablotny, C. L., Bradley, G. J., and Lomax, L. G. (1990b). "Methyl Bromide Inhalation Teratology Study in New Zealand White Rabbits." Unpublished study from Dow Chemical Company Toxicology Laboratory.

Danse, L. H. J. C., van Velsen, F. L., and vander Heijden C. A. (1984). Methyl bromide: Carcinogenic effect in the rat forestomach. *Toxicol. Appl. Pharmacol.* **72**, 262–271.

Djalali-Behzad, G., Hussain, S., Ostermann-Golker, S., and Segerbaeck, D. (1981). Estimation of genetic risks of alkylating agents. VI. Exposure of mice and bacteria to methyl bromide. *Mutat. Res.* **84**, 1–9.

Driscoll, C. D., and Hurley, J. M. (1993). "Methyl Bromide: Single Exposure Vapor Inhalation Neurotoxicity Study in Rats." Unpublished report from Bushy Run Research Center, Project 92N1197.

Eustis, S. L., Haber, S. B., Drew, R. T., and Yang, R. S. H. (1988). Toxicology and pathology of methyl bromide in F344 rats and B6C3F1 mice following repeated inhalation exposure. *Fundam. Appl. Toxicol.* **11**, 594–610.

Gargas, M., and Andersen, M. (1982). Metabolism of inhaled brominated hydrocarbons: validation of gas uptake results by determination of stable metabolite. *Toxicol. Appl. Pharmacol.* **66**, 55–68.

Garry, V. F., Nelson, R. L., Griffith, J., and Harkins, M. (1990). Preparation of human study of pesticide applicators: sister chromatid exchanges and chromosomal aberrations in cultured human lymphocytes exposed to selected fumigants. *Teratolog. Carcinog. Mutagen.* **10**, 21–29.

Gotoh, K, Nishizawa, T., Yamaguchi, T, Kanou, H., Kasai, T., Ohsawa, M., Ohbayyashi, H., Aiso, S., Ikawa, N., Yamamoto, S., Noguchi, T., Nagano, K., Enomoto, M., Nozaki, K., and Sakabe, H. (1994). Two year toxicological and carcinogenesis studies of methyl bromide in F344 rats and BDF1 mice—Inhalation studies. In "Proceedings: Second Asia–Pacific Symposium on Environmental and Occupational Health."

Haber *et al.* (1985).

Hastings, L., Andringa, A., and Miller, M. A. (1994). Exposure of the olfactory system to toxic compounds: structural and functional consequences. *Inh. Toxicol.* **6**, 437–440.

Hine, C. H. (1969). Methyl bromide poisoning: A review of ten cases. *J. Occup. Med.* **11**, 1–10.

Honma, T., Miyagawa, M., Sato, M., and Hasegawa, H. (1985). Neurotoxicity and metabolism of methyl bromide in rats. *Toxicol. Appl. Pharmacol.* **81**, 183–191.

Hurtt, M. E., Morgan, K. T., and Working, P. K. (1987). Histopathology of acute toxic responses to selected tissues from rats exposed by inhalation to methyl bromide. *Fundam. Appl. Toxicol.* **9**, 352–365.

Hurtt, M. E., Thomas, D. A., Working, P. K., Monticello, T. M., and Morgan, K. T. (1988). Degeneration and regeneration of the olfactory epithelium following inhalation exposure to methyl bromide: Pathology, cell kinetics and olfactory function. *Toxicol. Appl. Pharmacol.* **94**, 311–328.

Irish, D. D., Adams, E. M., Spencer, H. C., and Rowe, V. K. (1940). The response attending exposure of laboratory animals to vapors of methyl bromide. *J. Ind. Hyg. Toxicol.* **22**, 218–230.

Japanese Ministry of Labour (1992). "Toxicology and Carcinogenesis Studies of Methyl Bromide in F344 Rats and BDF Mice (Inhalation Studies)." Unpublished report from the Industrial Safety and Health Association, Japanese Bioassay Laboratory, Tokyo.

Kato, N., Morinobu, S., and Ishizu, S. (1986). Subacute inhalation experiment for methyl bromide in rats. *Ind. Health* **24**, 87–103.

Katz, A. J. (1985). Genotoxicity of methyl bromide in somatic cells of Drosophila larvae. *Environ. Mutagen.* **7**, 13.

Katz, A. J. (1987). Inhalation of methyl bromide gas induces mitotic recombination in somatic cells of Drosophila melanogaster. *Mutat. Res.* **192**, 131–135.

Kiplinger, G. A. (1994). "Methyl Bromide: Acute Oral Toxicity Comparison Study of Microencapsulated Methyl Bromide and Liquid Methyl Bromide in Albino Rats." Unpublished report from WIL Research Laboratories, Project WIL-49011.

Kramers, P. G. N., Voogd, C. E., Knaap, A. G. A. C., and Van der Heijden, C. A. (1985a). Mutagenicity of methyl bromide in a series of short term assays. *Mutat. Res.* **155**, 41–47.

Kramers, P. G. N., Bissumbhar, B., and Mout, H. C. A. (1985b). Studies with gaseous mutagens in Drosophila melanogaster. *In* "Short Term Bioassays in the Analysis of Complex Environmental Mixtures IV" (M. D. Waters, S. S. Sandhu, J. Lewtas, L. Claxton, G. Straus, and S. Nesnow, eds.), pp. 65–73. Plenum, New York/London.

McGregor, D. B. (1981). "Tier II Mutagenic Screening of 13 NIOSH Priority Compounds. Report 32. Individual Compound Report: Methyl Bromide." National Institute of Occupational Safety and Health, Cincinnati, OH, PB83-130211.

Medinsky, M., Bond, J., Dutcher, J., and Birnbaum, L. (1984). Disposition of [14C]-methyl bromide in rats after inhalation. *Toxicology* **32**, 187–196.

Medinsky, M., Dutcher, J., Bond, J., Henderson, R., Mauderly, J., Snipes, M., Mewhinney, J., Cheng, Y., and Birnbaum, L. (1985). Uptake and excretion of [14C]-methyl bromide as influenced by exposure concentration. *Toxicol. Appl. Pharmacol.* **78**, 215–225.

Mertens, J. J. W. M. (1997). "A 24-Month Chronic Dietary Study of Methyl Bromide in Rats." Unpublished report from WIL Research Laboratories, Project WIL-49014.

Moriya, M., Ohta, T., Watanabe, K., Miyazawa, T., Kato, K., and Shirasu, Y. (1983). Further mutagenicity studies on pesticides in bacterial reversion assay systems. *Mutat. Res.* **116**, 185–216.

Naas, D. J. (1990). "Acute Oral Toxicity Study in Beagle Dogs with Methyl Bromide." Unpublished report from WIL Research Laboratories, Inc., Project WIL-49006.

Newton, P. E. (1994a). "An Up-and-Down Acute Inhalation Toxicity Study of Methyl Bromide in the Dog." Unpublished report from Pharmaco-LSR, Project 93-6067.

Newton, P. E. (1994b). "A Four Week Inhalation Toxicity Study of Methyl Bromide in the Dog." Unpublished report from Pharmaco LSR, Project 93-6068.

Newton, P. E. (1995). "A Chronic (12-Month) Toxicity Study of Methyl Bromide Fumigated Feed in the Dog." Unpublished report from Pharmaco-LSR, Project 94-3186.

Norris, J. C., Driscoll, C. D., and Hurley, J. M. (1993). "Methyl Bromide: Ninety-Day Vapor Inhalation Neurotoxicity Study in CD Rats." Unpublished report from Bushy Run Research Center, Project 92N1172.

NTP (1992). "Toxicology and Carcinogenesis Studies of Methyl Bromide (CAS No. 74-83-9) in B6C3F1 Mice (Inhalation Studies)." National Toxicology Program Technical Report Series 385.

Ong, J. M., Stewart, J., Wen, Y., and Whong, W. (1987). Application of SOS umu-test for the detection of genotoxic volatile chemicals and air pollutants. *Environ. Mutagen.* **9**, 171–176.

Reuzel, P. G. J., Kuper, C. F., Dreef-van der Meulen, H. C., and Hollanders, V. M. H. (1987). "Chronic (29-Month) Inhalation Toxicity and Carcinogenicity Study of Methyl Bromide in Rats." Unpublished Report From CIVO Institutes TNO.

Reuzel, P. G. J., Dreef-van der Meulen, H. C., Hollanders, V. M. H., Kuper, C. F., Feron, V. J., and van der Heijden, C. A. (1991). Chronic inhalation toxicity and carcinogenicity study of methyl bromide in Wistar rats. *Food Chem. Toxicol.* **29**, 31–39.

Sikov, M. R., Cannon, W. C., Carr D. B., Miller, R. A., Montgomery, L. F., and Phelps, D. W. (1981). "Teratologic Assessment of Butylene Oxide, Styrene Oxide and Methyl Bromide." Battelle Pacific Northwest Laboratories, Contract 210-78-0025, Division of Biomedical and Behavioral Science, National Institute for Occupational Safety and Health, U. S. Department of Health and Human Services.

Simmon, V. F., Kauhanen, K., and Tardiff, R. G. (1977). Mutagenic activity of chemicals identified in drinking water. *In* "Progress in Genetic Toxicology" (D. Scott, B. A. Bridges, and F. M. Sobels, eds.), pp. 249–258. Elsevier/North-Holland Biomedical Press, Amsterdam.

Tucker, J. D., Xu, J., Stewart, J., Baciu, P. C., and Ong, T. (1986). Detection of sister chromatid exchanges induced by volatile genotoxicants. *Teratog. Carcinog. Mutagen.* **6**, 14–21.

WHO (1995). "Environmental Health Criteria 166, Methyl Bromide." Published under the joint sponsorship of the United Nations Environment Programme, the International Labour Organisation, and the World Health Organization, Geneva.

Wilmer *et al.* (1983).

Yamano, Y. (1991). Experimental study on methyl bromide poisoning in mice. Acute inhalation study and the effects of glutathione as an antidote. *Jpn. J. Ind. Health* **33**: 23–30. [in Japanese]

Zwart, A. (1988). "Acute Inhalation Study of Methyl Bromide in Rats." CIVO Rep. V88. 127/27. CIVO Institutes, TNO, Zeist, The Netherlands.

Zwart, A., Arts, J. H. E., Ten Berge, W. F., and Appelman, L. M. (1992). Alternative acute inhalation toxicity testing by determination of the concentration-time-mortality relationship: Experimental comparison with standard LC50 testing. *Regul. Toxicol. Pharmacol.* **15**, 278–290.

1,3-Dichloropropene

W. T. Stott and B. B. Gollapudi
Dow Chemical Company

85.1 CHEMISTRY AND FORMULATIONS

85.1.1 CHEMICAL NAME

1,3-Dichloro-1-propene is the chemical name. The pesticide is typically marketed either as a relatively pure *cis*-isomer or as a mixture of *cis*- (E) and *trans*- (Z) isomers.

85.1.2 STRUCTURE

85.1.3 SYNONYMS

1,3-Dichloropropene also is known as α-chloroallyl chloride and 1,3-dichloropropylene. The CAS registry number for 1,3-dichloropropene is 542-75-6. The number for the *trans*-isomer is 10061-02-6; that of the *cis*-isomer is 10061-01-5.

85.1.4 PHYSICAL AND CHEMICAL PROPERTIES

1,3-Dichloropropene has the empirical formula $C_3H_4Cl_2$ and a molecular weight of 110.98. It is a white to amber-colored liquid with a sweet-penetrating odor. The density at 25°C is 1.217. The boiling points of the *cis*- and *trans*-isomers are 104 and 112°C, respectively. The flash point is 28°C. The solubility in water at 25°C is approximately 2 g/kg. The compound is miscible with acetone, benzene, carbon tetrachloride, heptane, and methanol.

85.1.5 FORMULATIONS

Commercial formulations, containing varying amounts of a mixture of *cis*- and *trans*-isomers, have historically been mar-

keted under the trademarks Dorlone® (admixture with 1,2-dibromoethane), D-D® Soil Fumigant, Nemex®, Telone®, and Vidden D®. More recent trademarks include Vorlex® (admixture with methylisothiocyanate), Di-Trapex®, D-D® Super, Telone® II Soil Fumigant, and Telone® C-17 Soil Fungicide and Nematicide (admixture with chloropicrin). Purified *cis*-isomer 1,3-dichloropropene has also been marketed under the trademarks Telone-*cis*® and Nematrap®. Formulations have typically contained 1–2% of an acid scavenger. Older formulations were often stabilized using epichlorohydrin while epoxidized soybean oil has been utilized in more recent formulations.

85.2 USES

Introduced in 1945, 1,3-dichloropropene is a soil fumigant nematocide, for preplanting control of parasitic plant nematodes in numerous food and nonfood crops including deciduous fruit and nuts, vines, strawberries, field crops, vegetables, tobacco, tree nurseries, and numerous other specialty crops. Formulated 1,3-dichloropropene is injected into the soil using chisels prior to crop planting at a minimum depth of 10–12 inches below the soil surface. The injected zone is subsequently capped off with soil which is often then covered with plastic to help maintain concentrations in the soil. Injected 1,3-dichloropropene is believed to volatilize, move through the soil air space, and redissolve into the film of water that surrounds soil particles, where it may exert its toxic effect on soil nematodes. 1,3-Dichloropropene in the soil is lost via chemical hydrolysis in water, metabolism by soil biotica, and evaporation. Efficacy is thus dictated not only by target organism sensitivity, but also by the vapor pressure, diffusion coefficient, distribution in air, water, and soil phases of the soil matrix, and the temperature and moisture content of the treated soil.

85.3 HAZARD IDENTIFICATION

85.3.1 ACUTE TOXICITY

1,3-dichloropropene is irritating to eyes and skin of animals. As reviewed by Torkelson (1994), application of mixed isomers of

1,3-dichloropropene to the skin of rabbits up to 4 hours (occluded application site) caused a moderate erythema and moderate to severe edema. Mixed isomers of 1,3-dichloropropene also caused a marked redness and slight to moderate chemosis of the conjunctivae immediately following instillation of 0.1 mL into the eyes of rabbits. These effects were gradually reversible and, in most instances, washing with water was effective in averting injury. Similar dermal and ocular effects have been reported for cis-1,3-dichloropropene (Gardner, 1989) and a formulation of 1,3-dichloropropene containing approximately 30% 1,2-dichloropropane (D-D®) (Hine et al., 1953). Both mixed isomer 1,3-dichloropropene and cis-1,3-dichloropropene have tested positive in Guinea pig skin sensitization assays (Gardner, 1989; Jones, 1988a; Torkelson, 1994).

The acute oral, dermal, and inhalation lethality of both mixed isomers of 1,3-dichloropropene and cis-1,3-dichloropropene in laboratory animals have also been established (Gardner, 1989; Hine et al., 1953; Jones, 1988b, c; Jones and Collier, 1986a, b; Nitschke et al., 1990a; Torkelson, 1994). The oral LD_{50} of mixed isomers of 1,3-dichloropropene in rats ranges from 130 to 713 mg/kg in males and 110–250 to 510 mg/kg in females dependent upon vehicle and strain used. The oral LD_{50} for cis-1,3-dichloropropene in rats has been calculated to be 85 to 126 and 117 in males and females, respectively. The dermal LD_{50} has been reported as greater than 1211 mg/kg mixed isomers in both sexes of rats (unoccluded application site); 1000 and 1300-2000 mg/kg mixed isomers in male and female rats, respectively (occluded application site); 333–540 mg/kg mixed isomers for both sexes of rabbits (occluded application site); and 758–1090 mg/kg cis-1,3-dichloropropene for both sexes of rats (occluded application site). The acute 4-hour LC_{50} value for mixed isomers of 1,3-dichloropropene vapor in rats was 855–1035 ppm for males and 904 ppm for females. Exposed animals had a distinct "garlic" odor and suffered eye and nasal irritation. The acute 4-hour LC_{50} value for cis-1,3-dichloropropene vapor in rats was 670 and 744 ppm for males and females, respectively. Grossly observable eye and respiratory tract irritation was absent following a 2-week observation period. Brief exposure to concentrations in excess of 2700 ppm mixed isomer vapor also caused severe lung, liver, and kidney injury.

85.3.2 REPEATED DOSE TOXICITY

The subacute and subchronic toxicity of 1,3-dichloropropene has been examined both orally, via gavage or mixed in feed, and via inhalation. Subacute and subchronic oral toxicity studies on relatively modern formulations have been carried out in rats, mice, and dogs by stabilizing the 1,3-dichloropropene by microencapsulation in a starch–sucrose matrix and then mixing the encapsulated material into the feed of test animals. Studies reported by Stott et al. (1988) have demonstrated the ready bioavailability of this material once ingested by test animals.

Relatively short-term oral dietary toxicity studies employing microencapsulated 1,3-dichloropropene were conducted as a prelude to the subchronic studies summarized below (Haut et al., 1992a, b). Male and female Fischer 344 rats and B6C3F1 mice were administered dosages of 10, 25, 50, or 100 (rats) or 175 (mice) mg/kg/day of microencapsulated 1,3-dichloropropene (mixed isomers) via their diet for 2 weeks. The body weights of both sexes of rats ingesting ≥50 mg/kg/day and male mice and female mice ingesting ≥100 and 175 mg/kg/day, respectively, were decreased. Histopathological changes were restricted to rats and consisted of hyperplasia and hyperkeratosis of the nonglandular mucosa of the stomachs of both sexes of rats ingesting ≥ 50 mg/kg/day and a single male ingesting 25 mg/kg/day.

In a subsequent subchronic rat study, male and female Fischer 344 rats were administered dosages of 5, 15, 50, or 100 mg/kg/day of microencapsulated 1,3-dichloropropene (mixed isomers) via their diet for 13 weeks (Haut et al., 1996).

The body weights of males and females ingesting ≥5 and ≥15 mg/kg/day, respectively, were decreased. A number of changes in serum biochemical parameters and decreases in organ weights accompanied the depressed body weights of these animals. Histopathological changes were restricted to basal cell hyperplasia and/or hyperkeratosis of the nonglandular mucosa of the stomach of both sexes ingesting ≥50 mg/kg/day and a single male ingesting 15 mg/kg/day. These changes were at least partially reversible upon ingestion of control feed for 4 weeks.

In a subsequent subchronic mouse study, male and female B6C3F1 mice were administered dosages of 15, 50, 100, or 175 mg/kg/day of microencapsulated 1,3-dichloropropene (mixed isomers) via their diet for 13 weeks (Haut et al., 1996). A dose-related decrease in the body weights of males and females ingesting ≥50 mg/kg/day was observed. Histologic changes consistent with decreased cytoplasmic glycogen and with decreased lipid content were observed in the liver of all treated mice and the kidneys of high dose group mice. No treatment-related histopathologic effects were reported.

Male and female Beagle dogs were administered microencapsulated 1,3-dichloropropene via their diets for 13 weeks at concentrations which resulted in mean dosages of 5, 15–16, or 41 mg/kg/day (Stebbins et al., 1999). The body weights of both sexes of dogs were decreased in a dose-related manner relative to controls. The primary effect of 1,3-dichloropropene ingestion was upon erythroid parameters measured in peripheral blood. Calculated erythroid indices and morphologic changes in stained peripheral blood of male and females ingesting ≥15–16 mg/kg/day indicated the presence of a hypochromic, microcytic anemia.

In an early oral toxicity study, male and female Wistar rats were administered dosages of 1, 3, 10, or 30 mg/kg/day of a roughly 78% pure mixed isomer 1,3-dichloropropene formulation 6 days/week for 13 weeks via oral gavage (see Stott et al., 1988; Til et al., 1973). The kidney weights of both sexes of high dose group animals and males administered 10 mg/kg/day mixed isomer 1,3-dichloropropene were elevated relative to controls. However, no gross or histopathologic changes or alterations in hematologic indicies, urinalysis, or serum enzymes accompanied these changes. It was not clear whether toxicity was dictated by 1,3-dichloropropene or of some impurity, possibly 1,2-dichloropropane, which was present at a concentration of nearly 20%. The latter chemical reportedly causes increased liver and kidney weights and hepatic histopathologic changes in rats (Bruckner *et al.*, 1989; IPCS, 1993).

The toxicity of inhaled 1,3-dichloropropene in several formulations has also been evaluated over the years. Formulations of >90% purity have been studied in which both sexes of Fischer 344 rats and CD-1 mice were exposed 6 hours/day, 5 days/week to mixed-isomer vapor concentrations of 5, 10, or 30 ppm for 4 weeks; 10, 30, or 90 ppm for 13 weeks; and 10, 30, 90, or 150 ppm for 13 weeks (Coate, 1979a, b; Stott *et al.*, 1988). No treatment-related effects were observed in rats or mice following a 4-week exposure to up to 30 ppm vapor. However, decreases in body weights were noted and the nasal mucosa and urinary bladder (female mice) were identified as potential target tissues of inhaled 1,3-dichloropropene for 13 weeks. Nasal effects consisted of degeneration of olfactory epithelium and/or hyperplasia of respiratory epithelium in both sexes of rats (≥30 ppm) and mice (≥90 ppm) and respiratory metaplasia in olfactory regions of mice (150 ppm). Bladder effects consisted of hyperplasia of the transitional epithelium in female mice only (≥90 ppm). Subsequent studies were undertaken in which Fischer 344 rats were similarly exposed to *cis*-1,3-dichloropropene vapor concentrations of 10, 60, or 150 ppm for 2 weeks or 10, 30, or 90 ppm for 13 weeks (Nitschke *et al.*, 1990b; Nitschke and Lomax, 1990). These latter studies also identified body weight changes and/or histopathological changes in the nasal respiratory and olfactory epithelium in both sexes of rats (≥60–90 ppm).

In contrast, in an early inhalation study conducted in 1958, male and female rats, guinea pigs, rabbits, and dogs (females only) were exposed to 1 or 3 ppm mixed isomer 1,3-dichloropropene vapor 7 hr/day, 5 days/week, for 6 months (Torkelson and Oyen, 1977). The only effect of exposure which was reported was a "foamy vacuolation or proximal tubule epithelium" in high exposure group male rats. The significance of this change has been questioned in view of findings from more recent studies and the diagnosis was characteristic of nephropathy endemic in the site-bred rats used during this early period (Stott *et al.*, 1988). No effects were reported in female rats or other animals exposed to 1 ppm vapor.

Exposure of rats and mice to 5, 15, or 50 ppm D-D®, an admixture of 1,3-dichloropropene and 1,2-dichloropropene, for 12 weeks revealed liver and kidney weight changes in high exposure male and female rats, respectively, and diffuse hepatocellular swelling in high exposure male mice (urinary bladders were not examined) (Parker *et al.*, 1982). As noted, increased liver and kidney weights and hepatic histopathologic changes have been a consistent finding in 1,2-dichloropropene toxicity studies (Bruckner *et al.*, 1989; IPCS, 1993).

85.3.3 EFFECTS ON REPRODUCTION

Mixed isomer vapors of 1,3-dichloropropene were not embrytotoxic or teratogenic in bred rats or inseminated rabbits exposed to 20, 60, or 120 ppm vapors, 6 hours/day, during gestation days 6–15 (rats) or 6–18 (rabbits) (Hanley *et al.*, 1987). Maternal toxicity was evidenced at all exposure levels. Exposure of male and female rats to 10, 30, or 90 ppm 1,3-dichloropropene vapors for two generations did not adversely affect reproduction or neonatal growth or survival even though 90 ppm proved to be a toxic exposure level (Breslin *et al.*, 1989). Consistent with these results, no treatment-related changes in testes weight, sperm count, or sperm morphology occurred in mice 30 days after being injected i.p. with 10, 19, 38, 75, 150, 300, or 600 mg/kg/day 1,3-dichloropropene daily, for 5 days (Osterloh and Feldman, 1993). Finally, exposure of male and female rats to 14, 32, or 96 ppm D-D®, a low purity 1,3-dichloropropene formulation containing approximately 30% 1,2-dichloropropane, 6 hours/day, for 10 weeks did not affect animal mating behavior or fertility (Linnett *et al.*, 1988).

85.3.4 ABSORPTION, DISTRIBUTION, METABOLISM, AND EXCRETION

Toxicity and pharmacokinetic data indicate that 1,3-dichloropropene is absorbed from the skin, respiratory tract, and gastrointestinal tract. Both inhaled and ingested *cis*- and *trans*-isomers were rapidly eliminated from the bloodstream of rats in a biphasic manner consisting of a prominent initial phase with a half-life of approximately 4–7 minutes followed by a slower phase with a half-life of 22–43 minutes (Stott and Kastl, 1986; Stott *et al.*, 1988). The predominant routes of excretion of radioactivity in male and female rats following a single or repeated oral dose(s) of *cis*, *trans*, or mixed 1,3-dichloropropene were via the urine (*cis*, 82–84%; *trans*, 56–61%; mixed, 51–61%), feces (*cis* or *trans*, 2–3%; mixed, 17–21%), and expiration of CO_2 (*cis*, 2–5%; *trans*, 23–24%; mixed, 15%) (Bartels *et al.*, 1999; Dietz *et al.*, 1984a; Hutson *et al.*, 1971; IPCS, 1993). Excretion and distribution of 1,3-dichloropropene was independent of dose in rats and mice administered up to 50 and 100 mg/kg, respectively (Dietz *et al.*, 1984a). In both species, greater than 80% of the administered dosages were excreted within 24 hours of dosing. There were no remarkable sex-related differences in excretion routes, kinetics of excretion, or tissue distribution of administered radioactivity in rats (Bartels *et al.*, 1999; Hutson *et al.*, 1971).

Humans also rapidly metabolize and excrete inhaled 1,3-D vapor (Waechter *et al.*, 1992). Human volunteers exposed to 1.0 ppm mixed isomer vapor for 6 hours asorbed roughly 80% of inhaled 1,3-D. Blood concentrations of 1,3-D rapidly fell following postexposure, resulting in no quantifiable concentrations by the first sampling time point post exposure, 10 minutes, establishing a blood half-life of less than this value. Approximately 90% of the estimated dose of inhaled Telone II was excreted within 36 hours of exposure. Dermal absorption of

1,3-D vapor does not appear to be a factor in exposed humans as whole-body uptake has been estimated to be roughly only 2–5% of that absorbed via inhalation (Kezic *et al.*, 1996).

The mercapturic acid conjugate of 1,3-dichloropropene and its further oxidation product, a sulfoxide, were the primary excretion products identified in the urine of treated animals (Bartels *et al.*, 1999; Climie *et al.*, 1979; Dietz *et al.*, 1984a; Fisher and Kilgore, 1988a). Approximately 32–36% of acute 5 or 50 mg/kg oral doses of mixed isomers were excreted in male rats in an isomeric ratio of *cis*- to *trans*-mercapturate of approximately 4 : 1 (Bartels *et al.*, 1999; Dietz *et al.*, 1984a). Repeated dosing of rats at 5 mg/kg/day for several weeks appeared to increase the percentage excretion of these metabolites to roughly 43% of the dose (Bartels *et al.*, 1999). In contrast, Onkenhout *et al.* (1986) reported that approximately 45–55% of a range of dosages from 0.05 to 4.5 mg/kg mixed isomers administered via interperitoneal injection to rats were excreted as the mercapturate conjugate at an isomeric ratio of only 1.2 : 1. Several additional glutathione conjugate degradates have been observed in the urine of rats and, to a greater extent, mice (Bartels *et al.*, 1999; Dietz *et al.*, 1984a). These have included the mercaptoacetate, mercaptopyruvate, and cysteine conjugates of 1,3-dichloropropene.

The mercapturic acid conjugate of 1,3-D has also been identified in the urine of human subjects exposed to mixed isomer vapors of 1,3-D under field application or laboratory conditions and has been utilized as a biomonitor of 1,3-D exposure (Kezic *et al.*, 1996; Osterloh *et al.*, 1984; Osterloh and Feldman, 1993; van Welie *et al.*, 1991; Waechter *et al.*, 1992). Consistent with the earlier rat data, Waechter *et al.* (1992) found that humans excrete approximately 45% and 14% of absorbed *cis*- and *trans*-isomers of 1,3-dichloropropene, respectively, as the *cis*- and *trans*-mercapturates, a 3.2 : 1 ratio.

Based upon these data, it has been proposed that 1,3-dichloropropene is primarily metabolized in rats and mice, and likely humans, by conjugation with glutathione and by hydrolysis of the 3-position chlorine (Dietz *et al.*, 1984b; Hutson *et al.*, 1971; IPCS, 1993; Onkenhout *et al.*, 1986). The end product of the latter pathway is CO_2. Several other minor metabolites suggestive of oxidative metabolism (epoxidation) have also been reported in the liver of rats administered a very high, lethal, dosage of 1,3-dichloropropene (700 mg/kg) via i.p. injection (Schneider *et al.*, 1998). However, a disproportionately lower yield of epoxide was reported at a lower, nonleathal, i.p. dosage and none was detected upon oral dosing (Bartels *et al.*, 1999). The toxicity of 1,3-dichloropropene thus appears to reflect the balance between inherent chemical reactivity and competing enzymatic activation, and spontaneous and enzymatic detoxification pathways, some or all of which are saturable.

A relatively small amount of mixed isomers have been found to bind to macromolecules in the forestomach and, to a lesser extent, in the glandular stomach of rats and mice following acute oral dosing with 1,3-dichloropropene (Dietz *et al.*, 1984b). Macromolecular binding correlated with a dose and time-related depression in the nonprotein sulfhydryl content, presumably of glutathione, as a result of direct or enzymatic,

of stomach and liver tissues of these latter animals. Similar exposure-related decreases in the sulfhydryl content of a number of tissues of rats inhaling 1,3-dichloropropene vapor for one hour have also been reported (Fisher and Kilgore, 1988b). Initial losses in sulfhydryl levels, however, may be offset somewhat by a significant rebound effect which was observed in livers of rats and lungs of mice repeatedly administered 1,3-dichloropropene via oral gavage and inhalation, respectively (W. Stott, unpublished data). Indeed, no DNA adducts were reported by Gollapudi *et al.* (1999) in a relatively sensitive ^{32}P-postlabeling assay of these same hepatic and pulmonary tissues and Schneider *et al.* (1998) reported a seven-fold decrease in formation of epoxide *in vitro* in the presence of glutathione. Significantly, the net activities of glutathione-S-*trans*ferase isozymes to metabolize 1,3-dichloropropene also appear to determine responses in *in vitro* assays of genotoxicity. In general, target organisms utilized in *in vitro* assays, especially bacteria, conjugate 1,3-dichloropropene very poorly relative to mammalian tissue extracts, especially when the latter are fortified with physiological levels of glutathione (Creedy *et al.*, 1984; Stott, *et al.*, 1992).

85.3.5 SHORT TERM ASSAYS

1,3-Dichloropropene has been tested in a wide variety of genotoxicity assays with variable results. A number of early *in vitro* assays reporting positive responses for 1,3-dichloropropene in bacteria (De Lorenzo *et al.*, 1977; Eder *et al.*, 1982; Neudecker *et al.*, 1977; Stolzenberg and Hine, 1980) were confounded by the presence of mutagenic impurities and/or stabilizing agent (e.g., epichlorohydrin) or by the generation of mutagenic oxidation products during gas chromatographic purification procedures (Talcott and King, 1984; Watson *et al.*, 1987). Subsequent studies, using 1,3-dichloropropene purified by passage through a silicic acid column, were weakly positive only in the presence of liver microsomes (100,000 × g pellet) from rats induced with polychlorinated biphenyls. Addition of cytosolic fractions, which contain glutathione-S-*trans*ferase, and physiological levels of glutathione, eliminated activity. Metabolically active fractions (S9) obtained from the lungs or kidneys of naïve mice or from the lungs of mice repeatedly exposed to 1,3-dichloropropene vapor also did not metabolize purified 1,3-dichloropropene to a mutagen in *Salmonella* mutagenicity assays (Gollapudi *et al.*, 1999; Stott, *et al.*, 1992).

Assays employing mammalian cell lines have also resulted in mixed evidence of genotoxicity. Negative results have been obtained using an epoxidized soybean oil-stabilized mixed isomer formulation of 1,3-dichloropropene in the Chinese hamster ovary (CHO) HGPRT forward mutation and rat hepatocyte unscheduled DNA synthesis assays (Gollapudi *et al.*, 1999). 1,3-Dichloropropene samples of unknown purity or stabilizing agent were negative in chromosomal aberration assays in CHO cells, and rat liver cell lines (Dean *et al.*, 1985; Loveday *et al.*, 1989) and negative sister chromatid exchange assays in V79 lung fibroblasts with S9 have also been reported (Loveday *et al.*, 1989). However, similar samples of single or mixed isomeric 1,3-dichloropropene induced unscheduled DNA synthesis in HeLa cells (Schiffman *et al.*, 1983), sister chromatid exchanges in V79 lung fibroblasts (von der Hude *et al.*, 1987), DNA fragmentation and repair in V79 cells and rat and human hepatocytes (Dean *et al.*, 1985; Martelli *et al.*, 1993), chromosomal aberrations in CHL and CHO cells (Loveday *et al.*, 1989), and mutations at the tk locus in L5178Y mouse lymphoma cells (Myhr and Caspary, 1991).

In contrast to the results of in vitro genotoxicity assays, in vivo assays of 1,3-dichloropropene have been generally negative. Negative results were obtained in mouse bone marrow micronucleus assays using relatively high oral or i.p. dosages of 1,3-dichloropropene (Gollapudi *et al.*, 1999; Shelby *et al.*, 1993). However, Kevekordes *et al.* (1996) reported that 1,3-dichloropropene induced micronuclei in bone marrow erythrocytes of female, but not male, mice. Inhaled 1,3-dichloropropene vapors did not cause dominant lethal effects in rat germ cells in two separate assays (Gollapudi *et al.*, 1998; Linnett *et al.*, 1988) nor did they cause point mutations in somatic tissues (lung and liver) of Big Blue™ transgenic mice (Gollapudi *et al.*, 1999). In addition, negative results have been obtained for a 1,3-dichloropropene formulation (stabilizer unknown) in several host-mediated bacterial mutagenicity assays in mice (Shirasu *et al.*, 1981; Sudo *et al.*, 1979). A ^{32}P-postlabelling assay of liver tissue from rats dosed orally and of lung tissue of mice exposed via inhalation (target tissues for tumor formation) for the potential formation of DNA adducts was also negative (Gollapudi *et al.*, 1999). Positive results, however, have been reported to cause single strand breaks in the DNA of several tissues and DNA repair in hepatocytes of rats following oral or intraperitoneal dosing (Ghia *et al.*, 1993; Kitchin and Brown, 1994). Finally, when fed to *Drosophila* at a high concentration, an epoxide-stabilized 1,3-dichloropropene formulation caused an increased incidence of sex-linked recessive lethal mutations but not reciprocal translocations (Valencia *et al.*, 1985).

85.3.6 CHRONIC TOXICITY AND ONCOGENICITY ASSAYS

Chronic toxicity and oncogenicity studies of 1,3-dichloropropene via several routes have been conducted. In a recent study using an epoxidized soybean oil stabilized and weakly *in vitro* mutagenic formulation of 1,3-dichloropropene, Fischer 344 rats, and B6C3F1 mice were administered dosages of 2.5, 12.5, or 25 mg/kg/day and 2.5, 25, or 50 mg/kg/day, respectively, as a microencapsulated preparation via their diet, 7 days/wk, for 2 years (Stott *et al.*, 1996). In both sexes of rats and mice, body weights were decreased and hyperplasia of the nonglandular stomach mucosa was reported to occur in a dose-related manner. An increased incidence of foci of altered cells was also noted in the livers of treated rats following 24 months dosing. The only tumorigenic response observed in rats was an increase in the incidence of benign liver tumors in high dose males and females and intermediate dose males. No tumorigenic response was reported in either sex of mice.

In contrast, an early study involving the administration of an older, highly *in vitro* mutagenic, mixed-isomer epichlorohydrin-stabilized formulation of 1,3-dichloropropene to rats (25 or 50 mg/kg/day) and mice (50 or 100 mg/kg/day) via gavage, 3 days/week, for up to 2 years resulted in increases in several benign and malignant tumor types in both species (NTP, 1985; Yang *et al.*, 1986). These included forestomach and liver tumors in male rats (25 or 50 mg/kg/day or both), forestomach tumors in female rats (50 mg/kg/day), and forestomach, lung, and urinary bladder tumors in female mice (50 or 100 mg/kg/day or both). The gavage bioassay in male mice was judged to be an "inadequate study of carcinogenicity" due to excessive early mortality of controls. Nontumorigenic responses were limited to hyperplasia of the nonglandular portion of the stomachs of mice and rats and hyperplasia of the urinary bladder epithelium of mice.

The chronic toxicity of orally administered epoxidized soybean oil stabilized formulation of 1,3-dichloropropene has also been evaluated in male and female Beagle dogs administered 0.5, 2.5, or 15 mg/kg/day of microencapsulated 1,3-dichloropropene via their diets for one year (Stebbins *et al.*, 1999). The primary effect in both sexes of dogs ingesting 15 mg/kg/day 1,3-dichloropropene was a regenerative, hypochromic, microcytic anemia. Histologic changes in bone marrow and spleen consistent with increased hematopoiesis and extramedullary hematopoisis were consistent with this diagnosis. The latter changes along with increases in reticulocytes in these animals confirmed the regenerative nature of this effect. Anemia was observed following 3 months of dosing and remained relatively constant or improved somewhat over the remainder of the dosing period. The only other treatment-related effect observed in the study was a slight inflammation of the tongue of several high dose males suggestive of irritation by ingestion of 1,3-dichloropropene.

Inhalation exposure of rats and mice to 5, 20 or 60 ppm of an epoxidized soybean oil stabilized formulation of 1,3-dichloropropene 6 hours/day, 5 days/week, for 2 years resulted in nontumorigenic lesions of the nasal mucosa in both sexes of rats and mice exposed to 60 ppm and female mice exposed to 20 ppm, the urinary bladder epithelium of both sexes of mice exposed to 60 ppm and the forestomach of male mice exposed to 60 ppm (Lomax *et al.*, 1988). Slight changes in the morphology of renal and hepatic tissues of male and female mice exposed to 60 ppm, respectively, indicative of decreased lipid and glycogen content, respectively, were also observed. An increased incidence of benign lung tumors in high exposure group male mice was the only tumorigenic response observed (44% vs 18% in controls; historical incidence of adenomas = 7–32%).

Cis-1,3-dichloropropene was negative in a mouse skin initiation–promotion bioassay when tested with phorbol myristate as a promoter and was not carcinogenic following repeated dermal application of 122 mg to the backs of Ha:ICR Swiss mice 3 times/week for up to 85 weeks (Van Duuren *et al.*, 1979). An increase in local fibrosarcomas (6 of 30 mice vs 0 of 30 controls) was reported in mice following repeated subcutaneous injections of 3 mg/animal/week (1/week) for up to 83 weeks.

85.4 DOSE–RESPONSE

The toxicity of 1,3-dichloropropene in a number of laboratory animals displays both a clear dose–response and clearly defined no-observed-effect levels (NOELs). This is true for both acute and repeated dose (subacute, subchronic, and chronic) non-neoplastic treatment-related effects as well as neoplastic effects in rodents upon chronic exposure (see above discussion of individual studies). A number of toxicity studies with their lowest effect levels (LEL), NOELs, and target tissues/effect at the LELs are summarized in Table 90.1. It can be seen that the most sensitive target tissues/effects (i.e., those observed at LELs) are consistent between studies of differing durations for a given species of test animal. Increasing the duration of the dosing period from 2 to 13 weeks to 2 years did not appear to significantly change the potential toxicity of 1,3-dichloropropene relative to nonneoplastic pathological effects. Changes in NOELs or no-observed-adverse-effect levels (NOAELS) obtained in studies in which 1,3-dichloropropene was ingested or inhaled were generally within less than half a log unit of each other. An exception to this was the series of oral dietary toxicity studies in mice in which body weight depression was the major treatment-related change noted. In this case, more significant duration of treatment dependent decreases in NOELs occurred.

The most sensitive treatment-related effects observed in animals ingesting or inhaling 1,3-dichloropropene were quite similar between studies for a given species and method of administration. Affected tissues often represented portal-of-entry tissues, for example gastric mucosa for ingested and nasal mucosa for inhaled 1,3-dichloropropene, consistent with the irritant nature of this chemical. Exceptions to this were the occurrence of hyperplasia of the transitional epithelium of the urinary bladders of both sexes of mice inhaling vapors or dosed orally via gavage, and anemia in dogs ingesting 1,3-dichloropropene. In most bioassays, tumorigenic responses, when present, have involved portal-of-entry tissues. Ingestion or inhalation of relatively recent formulations of 1,3-dichloropropene resulted in tumors in the livers, often regarded as a portal-of-entry tissue of the enteric tract, of rats and the lungs of male mice, respectively. However, chronic gavage of an older and highly mutagenic, epoxide stabilized formulation of 1,3-dichloropropene, while causing forestomach and liver tumors in rats and mice, also caused urinary bladder and lung tumors in mice.

The effect of 1,3-dichloropropene upon portal-of-entry tissues is consistent with a direct toxicity of the molecule and its removal by saturable metabolic pathways. As noted, a major pathway for 1,3-dichloropropene metabolism is via glutathione-S-*trans*ferase dependent conjugation with glutathione. As reviewed by Watson *et al.* (1987) and in the IPCS (1993) review, this metabolism provides for practical thresholds in the dose–response of toxicity, and even mutagenicity, of 1,3-dichloropropene in test organisms. The saturation of this pathway may result in a nonlinear elevation in concentrations of 1,3-dichloropropene in cells of an *in vitro* mutagenicity or clastogenicity assay or tissues of an exposed animal, especially in portal-of-entry tissues, and subsequent toxicological consequences.

85.5 TOXICOLOGY IN HUMANS

85.5.1 EXPERIMENTAL EXPOSURE

Seven out of 10 volunteers detected 1,3-dichloropropene at an air concentration of 3 ppm; some reported fatigue of the sense of smell after a few minutes. The same proportion of volunteers detected 1 ppm, but the odor was noticeably fainter (Torkelson and Oyen, 1977). In a population of 22 persons, the concentration at which odor was detected was 4.4 ± 3.1 ppm (mean $\pm$ S.D.) (Rick and McCarty, 1987).

85.5.2 ACCIDENTAL POISONING

Forty-six people were treated for exposure to 1,3-dichloropropene fumes following a traffic accident in 1975 involving spillage of 4500 liters of a formulated product (Flessel *et al.*, 1978). Twenty-four of these, 3 of whom had lost consciousness, were hospitalized overnight with symptoms including headache, irritation of mucous membranes, and chest discomfort. All patients took showers and were given intravenous fluids and three received oxygen and corticosteroids because of chest pain and cough. Eleven of 41 persons tested had slightly higher than average serum SGOT and/or SGPT values which reverted to normal within 48–72 hours, except for 5 which still had slightly higher than average SGOT values. Follow-up interviews with patients 1–2 weeks later revealed symptoms including headache, abdominal, and chest discomfort and malaise. One was diagnosed as having had pneumonia. Symptoms were reported more frequently in those most heavily exposed to the fumes. Patient interviews conducted approximately two years after the accident revealed complaints of headache, chest pain or discomfort, and "personality changes" (fatigue, irritability, difficulty in concentrating, or decreased libido). Two had undergone cardiac catheterizations but their arteriograms were normal. There was no correlation of these long-persisting symptoms with intensity of exposure.

Two fatalities involving 1,3-dichloropropene have been confirmed. Accidental ingestion of D-D® (admixture with 1,2-dichloropropane) resulted in abdominal pain and vomiting, muscular twitching, pulmonary edema, and death (Gosselin *et al.*, 1976). Accidental ingestion of TELONE II® by a farm worker in Spain resulted in abdominal pain and vomiting, adult respiratory distress syndrome, hematologic changes, hepatorenal impairment, muscular twitching followed by coma, and death (Hernandez *et al.*, 1994). A possible association between overexposure to 1,3-dichloropropene and the development of hematologic malignancy has also been suggested by Markovitz and Crosby (1984). The latter was based upon the development of histiocytic lymphoma in a farm worker and two firemen accidentally exposed (acute) to high levels TELONE II® and D-D®,

Table 85.1
Summary of Lowest Effective Levels, No-Observed-Effect Levels, and Most Sensitive Treatment-Related Effects for Toxicity Studies of Mixed and *cis*-Isomer 1,3-Dichloropropene Formulations

Route species	Sex	Study duration	LEL[a]	NOEL[b]	Target tissue at LEL	Reference
Oral (diet)						
Rats	Males	2 Weeks	25 mkd[c]	10 mkd	Body wt., gastric mucosa	Haut *et al.* (1992a)
	Females		50 mkd	25 mkd	Body wt., gastric mucosa	
	Males	13 Weeks	15 mkd	5* mkd	Body wt., gastric mucosa	Haut *et al.* (1996)
	Females		15 mkd	5 mkd	Body wt., gastric mucosa	
	Males	2 Years	12.5 mkd	2.5 mkd	Body wt., gastric mucosa, liver AD[d]	Stott *et al.* (1996)
	Females		12.5 mkd	2.5 mkd	Body wt., gastric mucosa	Stott *et al.* (1996)
Mice	Males	2 Weeks	100 mkd	50 mkd	Body wt.	Haut *et al.* (1992b)
	Females		175 mkd	100 mkd	Body wt.	
	Males and females	13 Weeks	50 mkd	15* mkd	Body wt.	Haut *et al.* (1996)
	Males and females	2 Years	25 mkd	2.5 mkd	Body wt.	Haut *et al.* (1996)
Dogs	Males	13 Weeks	15 mkd	5* mkd	Anemia	Stebbins *et al.* (1999)
	Females		16 mkd	5* mkd	BW, anemia	
	Males and females	1 Year	15 mkd	2.5 mkd	Anemia	Stebbins *et al.* (1999)
Oral (gavage)						
Rats	Males	2 Years	25 mkd	ND[e]	Gastric mucosa, liver AD	NTP (1985)
	Females		25 mkd	ND	Gastric mucosa, stomach AD	
Mice	Females	2 Years	50 mkd	ND	Gastric and u. bladder (CA[f]) mucosa, lung AD and CA	NTP (1985)

(*continues*)

Table 85.1

(*continued*)

Route species	Sex	Study duration	LEL	NOEL	Target tissue at LEL	Reference
Inhalation						
Rats	Males and females	4 Weeks	ND	30 ppm	ND	Coate (1979a)
	Males	13 Weeks	90 ppm	30 ppm	Body wt., nasal mucosa	Coate (1979b); Stott *et al.* (1988)
	Females		30 ppm	10 ppm	Nasal mucosa	
	Males and females	13 Weeks	30 ppm (90 ppm)*g*	10 ppm	Body wt., (nasal mucosa)	Stott *et al.* (1988)
	Males and females	2 Years	60 ppm	20 ppm	Body wt., nasal	Lomax *et al.* (1988)
Mice	Males and females	4 Weeks	ND	30 ppm	ND	Coate (1979a)
	Males and females	13 Weeks	90 ppm	30 ppm	Body wt., nasal mucosa (females)	Coate (1979b); Stott *et al.* (1988)
	Males and females	13 Weeks	30 ppm	10 ppm	Body wt., nasal & u. bladder mucosa	Stott *et al.* (1988)
	Males and females	2 Years	20 ppm	5 ppm	Nasal mucosa	Lomax *et al.* (1988)

*Signifies no-observed-adverse-effect level.

a Lowest effect level.

b No-observed-effect level.

c mkd = mg/kg/day.

d AD = adenoma (bening tumors).

e ND = not determined.

f CA = carcinomas (malignant tumors).

g Exposure level in parenthesis reflects exposure level at which effects on nasal mucosa were observed.

respectively; however, it was subsequently established that the farm worker had leukemia prior to the incident (public records, State of California, Court of Appeal, Case No. 28344).

85.5.3 USE EXPERIENCE

1,3-Dichloropropene causes edema, redness, and necrosis of the skin (Torkelson and Oyen, 1977) and in one documented case was believed to have caused a contact hypersensitivity in a repeatedly exposed farmer (Nater and Gooskens, 1976). A fertility study of 64 employees engaged in the production of chlorinated 3-carbon compounds, including 1,3-dichloropropene, revealed no effects upon hormone levels (LH, FSH, testosterone), sperm count, sperm motility, and % normal and ab-

normal sperm regardless of duration or magnitude of exposure (Venable *et al.*, 1980).

Several studies have also been undertaken to evaluate potential biological effects of 1,3-dichloropropene vapors in fumigation workers. In a California study, urinary parameters were measured over time in the same workers following single or repeated occupational exposure(s) to a range of 0.3–9.4 mg/m^3 mixed isomers of 1,3-dichloropropene during soil fumigation operations (Osterloh and Feldman, 1993). Exposure was reportedly associated with elevated urinary excretion of *N*-acetylglucosamidase (NAG) and retinol binding protein (RBP). No changes were observed in albumin (ALB) excretion. These findings were interpreted to suggest a "subclinical" renal toxicity. In a Dutch study, several urinary and serum parameters were measured in the same workers occupationally exposed to 1.9–18.9 mg/m^3 *cis*-1,3-dichloropropene products once before and once after the tulip bulb field fumigation season (about three months duration) (Brouwer *et al.*, 1991). A number of slight changes in several parameters were reported after relative to before the "season:" excretion of urinary NAG and ALB, decreased serum creatinine (CREAT-S), and decreased total bilirubin (TBILI) levels in combination with increased serum γ-glutamyltranspeptidase (GGT). No differences were reported in serum (β_2-microglobulin (β_2M), alanine aminopeptidase (AAP), β-galactosidase, alkaline phosphatase (ALP), aspartate aminotransferase (AST), alanine aminotransferase (ALT), or lactate dehydrogenase. These data were interpreted by Brouwer *et al.* (1991) to reflect a slight degree of liver and kidney toxicity. Both of these studies have been strongly criticized for perceived study design and data interpretation flaws (Stott *et al.*, 1990; van Sittert *et al.*, 1991).

A subsequent comprehensive study in Dutch potato field fumigation workers conducted over the whole of the fumigation season failed to observe treatment-related toxicity (Verplanke *et al.*, 1995). Workers were exposed to a range of 0.1–9.5 mg/m^3 *cis*-1,3-dichlororporpene and a number of parameters were measured before, during, and following the fumigation season. Unlike previous studies, this study employed a matched control group of individuals. Parameters measured included urinary AAP, NAG, RBP, and ALB, and serum β_2M, CREAT-S, ALT, AST, GGT, ALP, and TBILI. The only change observed was a slightly lower urinary ratio of 6-β-hydroxycortisol to free cortisol ratio which was not considered to be related to 1,3-dichloropropene exposure. It was concluded that no adverse effects on liver or kidney function were suggested by the data.

Additional reviews of the human toxicity data for 1,3-dichloropropene have been published by Yang (1986) and IPCS (1993).

85.6 SUMMARY RISK CHARACTERIZATION

1,3-Dichloropropene has found use for over 45 years and remains one of the few remaining compounds available to agriculture for fumigating soils to eliminate parasitic nematodes. This compound has been extensively evaluated in a number of test organisms for acute, subchronic, and chronic toxicity, reproductive and developmental toxicity, carcinogenicity, and genotoxicity. Its metabolism in animals, including humans, has also been extensively studied and is relatively well understood. 1,3-Dichloropropene is moderately to highly acutely toxic to animals. It is irritating to skin and if occluded can cause a chemical burn and death in rabbits; however, its relatively high vapor pressure results in much lower toxicity if left on skin unoccluded. Orally administered 1,3-dichloropropene, either neat or in an aqueous vehicle, may be lethal to rodents at roughly 100 mg/kg or greater. Two human fatalities from accidental imbibition of 1,3-dichloropropene formulations, a relatively purified 1,3-dichloropropene and an admixture with

1,2-dichloropropane, have been reported. Toxic effects observed in humans exposed to high levels of vapors or having extended dermal contact with the liquid appear to reflect the irritant nature of 1,3-dichloropropene. In animal models, the results of subchronic and chronic toxicity studies of this chemical reflect both its irritant properties, as evidenced by effects on portal-of-entry tissues, and potential toxicity of a metabolite(s), as evidenced by effects upon distal tissues (e.g., urinary bladder mucosa). Despite this, studies have demonstrated a lack of reproductive or developmental effects, even at toxic dosages.

1,3-Dichloropropene is rapidly and extensively metabolized upon absorption by animals, including humans. Elimination from the blood of rats occurs in a biphasic manner, with half-lives for both isomers in the prominent α-phase of approximately 4–7 minutes and the β-phase of approximately 25–45 minutes. No appreciable excretion of parent chemical occurs and metabolites are primarily eliminated via the urine as products of a glutathione conjugation metabolic pathway or via exhalation of CO_2, product of a hydrolytic pathway. Evidence of the former pathway has been dose-related decreases in tissue glutathione levels of rats and mice administered 1,3-dichloropropene via oral or inhalation routes. The major urinary metabolite, the mercapturate conjugate of 1,3-dichloropropene, has represented a useful biomarker by which to estimate the exposure of workers to this molecule during soil fumigation operations.

Genotoxicity tests of 1,3-dichloropropene have often provided contradictory results. Many short-term assays of genotoxicity have been confounded by the presence of a known mutagen, epichlorohydrin, in the formulated material tested which was historically added as a stabilizing agent. The potential of 1,3-dichloropropene to undergo autooxidation to generate a mutagenic epoxide has further complicated interpretation of the *in vitro* genotoxicity data. Epoxide may be formed upon prolonged exposure to oxygen or during gas-chromatographic "purification" proceedures carried out prior to testing. *In vivo* assays of mutagenic or clastogenic activity, with their intact compliment of metabolizing enzymes, have almost uniformly been negative, especially at nontoxic dosages or at dosages which do not deplete tissue glutathione levels. It has been proposed that the genotoxic potential of 1,3-dichloropropene is directly related to the extensive depletion of glutathione in target organisms and tissues (IPCS, 1993). Based upon a weight-of-the-evidence analysis inclusive of in vivo assay data, 1,3-dichloropropene lacks significant genotoxic activity.

Bioassay data have provided an equally complicated assessment of the potential of 1,3-dichloropropene to cause tumors in animals. Inhalation of vapor, the primary route of occupational exposure to this chemical, has been shown to cause an increase in the incidence of benign lung tumors in male mice. Ingestion of this chemical via the diet as a stabilized microencapsulated product has been shown to cause a low incidence of benign liver tumors in rats. These results contrast with those of a previous oral oncogenicity study conducted by repeated bolus dosing (gavage) of an older, epichlorohydrin stabilized, and highly mutagenic formulation of 1,3-dichloropropene which resulted in numerous benign and maligant tumors in both rats and mice.

REFERENCES

Bartels, M. J., Waechter, J. M., Katl, P. E., Dietz, F. K., and Hansen, S. C. (1999). Pharmacokinetics and metabolism of 1,3-dichloropropene in the rat and mouse. Unpublished.

Breslin, W. J., Kirk, H. D., Streeter, C. M., Quast, J. F., and Szabo, J. R. (1989). 1,3-Dichloropropene: Two-generation inhalation reproduction study in Fischer 344 rats. *Fund. Appl. Pharmacol.* **12**, 129–143.

Brouwer, E. J., Evelo, C. T. A., Verplanke, A. J. W., van Welie, R. T. H., and de Wolff, F. A. (1991). Biological effect monitoring of occupational exposure to 1,3-dichloropropene: Effects on liver and renal function and on glutathione conjugation. *Brit. J. Ind. Med.* **48**, 167–172.

Bruckner, J. V., MacKenzie, W. F., Ramanathan, R., Muralidhara, S., Kim, H. J., and Dallas, C. E. (1989). Oral toxicity of 1,2-dichloropropane: Acute, short-term and long-term studies in rats. *Fund. Appl. Toxicol.* **12**, 713–730.

Climie, I., Hutson, D., Morrison, B., and Stoydin, G. (1979). Glutathione conjugation in the detoxication of (Z)-1,3-dichloropene (a component of the nematocide D-D) in the rat. *Xenobiotica* **9**, 149–156.

Coate, W. B. (1979a). "Subacute Inhalation Study in Rats and Mice: TELONE II." Report of The Dow Chemical Company.

Coate, W. B. (1979b). "90-Day Inhalation Study in Rats and Mice: TELONE II." Report of The Dow Chemical Company.

Creedy, C., Brooks, T., Dean, B., Hutson, D., and Wright, A. (1984). The protective action of glutathione on the microbial mutagenicity of the Z- and E-isomers of 1,3-dichloropropene. *Chem.–Biol. Interact.* **50**, 39–48.

Dean, B. J., Brooks, T. M., Hodson-Walker, G., and Hutson, D. H. (1985). Genetic toxicology testing of 41 industrial chemicals. *Mut. Res.* **153**, 57–77.

De Lorenzo, F., Degl'Innocenti, S., Ruocco, A., Silengo, L., and Cotese, R. (1977). Mutagenicity of pesticides containing 1,3-dichloropropene. *Cancer Res.* **37**, 1915–1917.

Dietz, F., Hermann, E., and Ramsey, J. (1984a). The pharmacokinetics of ^{14}C-1,3-dichloropropene in rats and mice following oral administration. *Toxicologist* **4**, Abst. No. 585.

Dietz, F., Dittenber, D., Kirk, H., and Ramsey, J. (1984b). Non-protein sulfhydryl content and macromolecular binding in rats and mice following administration of 1,3-dichloropropene. *Toxicologist* **4**, Abst. No. 586.

Eder, E., Neudecker, T., Lutz, D., and Henschler, D. (1982). Correlation of alkylating and mutagenic activities of allyl and allylic compounds: standard alkylation test vs. kinetic investigation. *Chem.–Biol. Interact.* **38**, 303–315.

Fisher, G. D., and Kilgore, W. W. (1988a). Mercapturic acid excretion by rats following inhalation exposure to 1,3-dichloropropene. *Fund. Appl. Toxicol.* **11**, 300–307.

Fisher, G. D., and Kilgore, W. W. (1988b). Tissue levels of glutathione following acute inhalation of 1,3-dichloropropene. *J. Toxicol. Environ. Hlth.* **23**, 171–182.

Flessel, P., Goldsmith, J., Kahn, E., Wesolwski, J., Maddy, K., and Peoples, S. (1978). Acute and possible long-term effects of 1,3-dichloropropene—California. *Morbidity Motality Weekly Rep.* **27**, 50–55.

Gardner, J. R. (1989). "Cis-1,3-Dichloropropene: Acute Oral and Dermal Toxicity, Skin and Eye Irritancy and Skin Sensitisation Potential." Report of Sittingbourne Research Center.

Ghia, M., Robbiano, L., Allavena, A., Martelli, A., and Brambilla, G. (1993). Genotoxic activity of 1,3-dichloropropene in a battery of *in vivo* short-term tests. *Toxicol. Appl. Pharmacol.* **120**, 120–125.

Gollapudi, B. B., Cieszlak, F. S., Day, S. J., and Carney, E. W. (1998). Dominant lethal test with rats exposed to 1,3-dichloropropene. *Environ. Mol. Mut.* **32**, 351–359.

Gollapudi, B. B., Mendrala, A. M., Linscombe, A., and Stott, W. T. (1999). Lack of genotoxicity of 1,3-dichloropropene in *in vitro* and *in vivo* genotoxicity tests. Unpublished.

Gosselin, R., Hodge, H., Smith, R., and Gleason, M. (1976). "Clinical Toxicology of Commercial Products," 4th ed., pp. 119–121. Wilkins-Williams, Baltimore.

Hanley, T. R., John-Greene, Young, J. T., Calhoun, L. L., and Rao, K. S. (1987). Evaluation of the effects of inhalation exposure to 1,3-dichloropropene on fetal development in rats and rabbits. *Fund. Appl. Toxicol.* **8**, 562–570.

Haut, K. T., Stebbins, K. E., Kropscott, B. E., and Stott, W. T. (1992a). "TELONE®II Soil Fumigant: Palatability and Two-Week Dietary Probe Studies in Fischer 344 Rats." Report of The Dow Chemical Company, Midland, MI.

Haut, K. T., Stebbins, K. E., Kropscott, B. E., and Stott, W. T. (1992b). "TELONE®II Soil Fumigant: Palatability and Two-Week Dietary Probe Studies in B6C3F1 Mice." Report of The Dow Chemical Company, Midland, MI.

Haut, K. T., Johnson, K. A., Shabrang, S. N., and Stott, W. T. (1996). Subchronic toxicity of ingested 1,3-dichloropropene in rats and mice. *Fund. Appl. Toxicol.* **32**, 224–232.

Hernandez, A. F., Martin-Rubi, J. C., Ballesteros, J. L., Oliver, M., Pla, A., and Villanueva, E. (1994). Clinical and pathological findings in fatal 1,3-dichloropropene intoxication. *Hum. Exptl. Toxicol.* **13**, 303–306.

Hine, C. H., Anderson, H. H., Moon, H. D., Kodama, J. K., Morse, M., and Jacobson, N. W. (1953). Toxicology and safe handling of CBP-SS (technical 1-chloro-3-bromopeopene-1). *Arch. Ind. Hyg. Occ. Med.* **7**, 118–136.

Hutson, D. H., Moss, J. A., and Pickering, B. A. (1971). Components of the soil fumigant D-D* and their metabolites in the rat. *Fd. Cosmet. Toxicol.* **9**, 677–680.

IPCS (International Programme on Chemical Safety) (1993). "1,3-Dichloropropene, 1,2-Dichloropropane and Mixtures." Environmental Health Criteria No. 146, World Health Organization, Geneva.

Jones, J. R. (1988a). "1,3-Dichloropropene *cis*-Isomer: Modified Nine-Induction Buehler Contact Sensitisation Study in the Guinea Pig." Report of Safepharm Laboratories Limited, Derby, UK.

Jones, J. R. (1988b). "1,3-Dichloropropene *cis*-Isomer: Acute Oral Toxicity Test in the Rat." Report of Safepharm Laboratories Limited, Derby, UK.

Jones, J. R. (1988c). "1,3-Dichloropropene *cis*-Isomer: Acute Dermal Toxicity Test in the Rat." Report of Safepharm Laboratories Limited, Derby, UK.

Jones, J. R., and Collier, T. A. (1986a). "TELONE II: Acute Oral Toxicity in the Rat." Report of The Dow Chemical Company.

Jones, J. R., and Collier, T. A. (1986b). "TELONE II: Acute Dermal Toxicity Test in the Rat." Report of The Dow Chemical Company.

Kevekordes, S., Gebel, T., Pav, K., Edenharder, R., and Dunkelberg, H. (1996). Genotoxicity of selected pesticides in the mouse bone marrow micronucleus test and in the sister-chromatid exchange test with human lymphocytes *in vitro*. *Toxicol. Lett.* **89**, 35–42.

Kezic, S., Monster, A. C., Verplanke, J. W., and de Wolff, F. A. (1996). Dermal absorption of *cis*-1,3-dichloropropene vapour: human experimental exposure. *Hum. Exp. Toxicol.* **15**, 396–399.

Kitchin, K. T., and Brown, J. L. (1994). Dose–response relationship for rat liver DNA damage caused by 49 rodent carcinogens. *Toxicology* **88**, 31–49.

Linnett, S. L., Clark, D. G., Blair, D., and Cassidy, S. L. (1988). Effects of subchronic inhalation of D-D (1,3-dichloropropene/1,2-dichloropropane) on reproduction in male and female rats. *Fund. Appl. Toxicol.* **10**, 214–223.

Lomax, L. G., Stott, W. T., Johnson, K. A., Calhoun, L. L., Yano, B. L., and Quast, J. F. (1988). The chronic toxicity and oncogenicity of inhaled technical grade 1,3-dichloropropene in rats and mice. *Fund. Appl. Toxicol.* **12**, 418–431.

Loveday, K. S., Lugo, M. H., Resnick, M. A., Anderson, B. E., and Zeiger, E. (1989). Chromosome aberration and sister chromatid exchange tests in Chinese hamster ovary cells *in vitro*: II. Results with 20 chemicals. *Environ. Mol. Mutag.* **13**, 60–94.

Martelli, A., Allavena, A., Ghia, M., Robbiano, L., and Brambilla, G. (1993). Cytotoxic and genotoxic activity of 1,3-dichlororporpene in cultured mammalian cells. *Toxicol. Appl. Pharmacol.* **120**, 114–119.

Markovitz, A., and Crosby, W. H. (1984). Chemical carcinogenesis. A soil fumigant, 1,3-dichloropropene, as possible cause of hematologic malignancies. *Arch. Intern. Med.* **144**, 1409–1411.

Myhr, B. C., and Caspary, W. J. (1991). Chemical mutagenesis at the thymidine kinase locus in L5178Y mouse lymphoma cells: Results for 31 coded compounds in the National Toxicology Program. *Environ. Mol. Mutag.* **18**, 51–83.

Nater, J. P., and Gooskens, V. H. J. (1976). Occupational dermatosis due to a soil fumigant. *Contact Dermat.* **2**, 227–229.

National Toxicology Program (NTP) (1985). "Toxicology and Carcinogenesis Studies of TELONE II® in F344/N Rats and B6C3F1 Mice (Gavage Studies)." NTP Tech. Rep. 269, Government Printing Office, Washington, DC.

Neudecker, T., Stefani, A., and Henschler, D. (1977). *In vitro* mutagenicity of soil nematocide 1,3-dichloropropene. *Experientia* **33**, 1084–1085.

Nitschke, K. D., and Lomax, L. G. (1990). "*Cis*-1,3-Dichloropropene: 2-Week Vapor Inhalation Toxicity Study in Fischer 344 Rats." Report of The Dow Chemical Company, Midland, MI.

Nitschke, K. D., Crissman, J. W., and Schuetz, D. J. (1990a). "*Cis*-1,3-Dichloropropene: Acute Inhalation Toxicity Study with Fischer 344 Rats." Report of The Dow Chemical Company, Midland, MI.

Nitschke, K. D., Lomax, L. G., and Sanderson, T. G. (1990b). "*Cis*-1,3-Dichloropropene: 13-Week Vapor Inhalation Toxicity Study in Fischer 344 Rats." Report of The Dow Chemical Company, Midland, MI.

Onkenhout, W., Mulder, P. P. J., Boogaard, P. J., Buijs, W., and Vermeulen, N. P. E. (1986). Identification and quantitative determination of mercapturic acids formed from Z- and E-1,3-dichloropropene by the rat, using gas chromatography with three different detection techniques. *Arch. Toxicol.* **59**, 235–241.

Osterloh, J. D., and Feldman, B. J. (1993). Urinary protein markers in pesticide applicators during a chlorinated hydrocarbon exposure. *Environ. Res.* **63**, 171–181.

Osterloh, J., Letz, G., Pond, S., and Becker, C. (1983). An assessment of the potential testicular toxicity of 10 pesticides using the mouse-sperm morphology assay. *Mut. Res.* **116**, 407–415.

Osterloh, J. D., Cohen, B. S., Popendorf, W., and Pond, S. M. (1984). Urinary excretion of the *N*-acetyl cysteine conjugate of *cis*-1,3-dichloropropene by exposed individuals. *Arch. Environ. Hlth.* **39**, 271–275.

Parker, C., Coate, W., and Voelker, R. (1982). Subchronic inhalation toxicity of 1,3-dichloropropene/1,2-dichloropropane (D-D®) in mice and rats. *J. Toxicol. Environ. Hlth.* **9**, 899–910.

Rick, D. L., and McCarty, L. P. (1987). "The Determination of the Odor Threshold of Vapors and Gases." Report of The Dow Chemical Company.

Schiffman, D., Eder, E., Neudecker, T., and Henschler, D. (1983). Induction of unscheduled DNA synthesis in HeLa cells by allylic compounds. *Can. Let.* **20**, 263–269.

Schneider, M., Quistad, G. B., and Casida, J. E. (1998). 1,3-Dichloropropene epoxides: Intermediates in bioactivation of the promutagen 1,3-dichloropropene. *Chem. Res. Toxicol.* **11**, 1137–1144.

Shelby, M. D., Erexson, G. L., Hook, G. J., and Tice, R. R. (1993). Evaluation of a three-exposure mouse bone marrow micronucleus protocol: Results with 49 chemicals. *Environ. Mol. Mut.* **21**, 160–179.

Shirasu, Y., Moriya, M., Tequka, H., Teramoto, S., Ohata, T., and Inoue, T. (1981). Mutagenicity screening studies on pesticides. *In* "Environmental Mutagens and Carcinogens: Proceedings of the Third International Conference on Environmental Mutagens," Tokyo, Mishima, and Kyoto, September 21–27, pp. 331–335.

Stebbins, K. E., Stott, W. T., Haut, K. T., Quast, J. F., and Shabrang, S. N. (1999). Subchronic and chronic toxicity of ingested 1,3-dichloropropene in beagle dogs. Unpublished.

Stolzenberg, S., and Hine, C. (1980). Mutagenicity of 2- and 3-carbon halogenated compounds in the Salmonella/mammalian-microsome test. *Environ. Mut.* **2**, 59–66.

Stott, W. T., and Kastl, P. L. (1986). Inhalation pharmacokinetics of technical grade 1,3-dichloropropene in rats. *Toxicol. Appl. Pharmacol.* **85**, 332–341.

Stott, W., Young, J., Calhoun, L., and Battjes, J. (1988). Subchronic toxicity of inhaled technical grade 1,3-dichloropropene in rats and mice. *Fundam. Appl. Toxicol.* **11**, 207–220.

Stott, W. T., Waechter, J. M., and Quast, J. T. (1990). Letter to the editor. *Arch. Environ. Hlth.* **45**, 250–253.

Stott, W. T., Mendrala, A. M., Redmond, J. M., Nwosu, A. F., and Lomax, L. G. (1992). Mechanism of 1,3-dichloropropene (1,3-D) induced toxicity in urinary bladder epithelium of mice. *Toxicologist* **12**, Abstr. No. 415.

Stott, W. T., Johnson, K. A., Stebbins, K. F., Redmond, J. M., and Jeffries, T. K. (1996). Dietary chronic toxicity/oncogenicity study of microencapsulated 1,3-dichloropropene (1,3-D) in rats and mice. *Toxicologist* **30**, Abstr. No. 276.

Stott, W. T., Gilbert, J. R., McGuirk, R. J., Brzak, K. A., Alexander, L. M., Dryzga, M. D., Mendrala, A. L., and Bartels, M. J. (1998). Bioavailability and pharmacokinetics of microencapsulated 1,3-dichloropropene in rats. *Toxicol. Sci.* **41**, 21–28.

Sudo, S., Kimura, Y., Yamamoto, K., and Ichihara, S. (1979). "The Mutagenicity Test on 1,3-Dichloropropene in Bacteria Test System." Report of The Dow Chemical Company, Midland, MI.

Talcott, R., and King, J. (1984). Mutagenic impurities in 1,3-dichloropropene preparations. *J. Natl. Cancer Inst.* **72**, 1113–1116.

Til, H. P., Spanjers, M. T., Feron, V. J., and Reuzel, P. J. C. (1973). "Sub-chronic (90-Day) Toxicity Study with TELONE* in Albino Rats." Report of The Dow Chemical Company, Horgen, Switzerland.

Torkelson, T. R. (1994). Halogenated aliphatic hydrocarbons containing chlorine, bromine, and iodine. *In* "Patty's Industrial Hygiene and Toxicology" (G. D. Clayton and F. E. Clayton, eds.), 4th ed., pp. 4007–4251. Wiley, New York.

Torkelson, R., and Oyen, F. (1977). The toxicity of 1,3-dichloropropene as determined by repeated exposure of laboratory animals. *Am. Ind. Hyg. Assoc. J.* **38**, 217–223.

Valencia, R., Mason, J. M., Woodruff, R. C., and Zimmering, S. (1985). Chemical mutagenesis testing in *Drosophila*. III. Results of 48 coded compounds tested for the national toxicology program. *Environ. Mut.* **7**, 325–348.

Van Duuren, B. L., Goldschmidt, B. M., Loewengart, G., Smith, A. C., Melchionne, S., Seidman, I., and Roth, D. (1979). Carcinogenicity of halogenated olefinic and aliphatic hydrocarbons in mice. *J. Natl. Cancer Inst.* **63**, 1433–1439.

van Sittert, N. J., Veenstra, G. E., Dumas, E. P., and Tordoir, E. F. (1991). Letter to the editor. *Br. J. Med.* **48**, 646–648.

van Welie, R. T. H., van Duyn, P., Brouwer, D. H., van Hemmen, J. J., Brouwer, E. J., and Vermeulen, N. P. E. (1991). Inhalation exposure to 1,3-dichloropropene in the Dutch flower-bulb culture. Part II. Biological monitoring by measurement of urinary excretion of two mercapturic acid metabolites. *Arch. Environ. Contam. Toxicol.* **20**, 6–12.

Venable, J. R., McClimans, C. D., Flake, R. E., and Dimick, D. B. (1980). A fertility study of male employees engaged in the manufacture of glycerine. *J. Occ. Med.* **22**, 87–91.

Verplanke, A. J. W., Bloemen, L. J., Brouwer, E. J., Van Sittert, N. J., Boogaard, P. J., Herber, R. F. M., and De Wolff, F. A. (1998). Monitoring of occupational exposure to *cis*-1,3-dichloropropene and effects on liver and kidney. Part 2. Effects on liver and kidney. Unpublished.

von der Hude, W., Scheutwinkel, M., Gramlich, U., Fibler, B., and Basler, A. (1987). Genotoxicity of three-carbon compounds evaluated in the SCE test *in vitro*. *Environ. Mutag.* **9**, 401–410.

Watson, W. P., Brooks, T. M., Huckle, K. R., Hutson, D. H., Land, K. L., Smith, R. J., and Wright, A. S. (1987). Microbial mutagenicity studies with (Z)-1,3-dichloropropene. *Chem.–Biol. Interact.* **61**, 17–30.

Waechter, J. M., Brzak, K. A., McCarty, L. P., LaPack, M. A., and Brownson, P. J. (1992). *Cis/trans* 1,3-dichloropropene (1,3-dichloropropene): Inhalation pharmacokinetics and metabolism in human volunteers. *Toxicologist* **13**, Abstr. No. 1090.

Yang, R. S. H. (1986). 1,3-dichloropropene. *Residue Rev.* **97**, 19–35.

Yang, R. S. H., Huff, J. E., Boorman, G. A., Haseman, J. K., Kornreich, M., and Stookey, J. L. (1986). Chronic toxicology and carcinogenesis studies of TELONE II by gavage in Fischer 344 rats and B6C3F1 mice. *J. Toxicol. Environ. Hlth.* **18**, 377–392.

Phosphine

V. F. Garry and A. V. Lyubimov
University of Minnesota

86.1 IDENTITY, PROPERTIES, AND USES

Chemical Name: Hydrogen Phosphide

Structure: PH_3.

Synonyms: Phosphoretted hydrogen, phosphorus hydride, Phosphorus trihydride.

The CAS Registry No.: 7803-51-2.

Conversion factor: 1 ppm = 1.39 mg/m^3. The most common commercial fumigants generating phosphine are aluminum phosphide and magnesium phosphide. Aluminum Phosphide (AIP) is sold under the following trade names: Phostoxin, Fumitoxin, Agtoxin, Weevilcide, Detia, Gastoxin, Max-Kill, Phosfume, Fastphos. Common trade names for Magnesium Phosphide (Mg_3P_2) are Fumi-Cel, Fumi Strip, Magtoxin, Magnaphos, Magphos.

86.1.1 PHYSICAL PROPERTIES

Pure phosphine is an odorless and colorless gas with a molecular weight of 34.00 and density of 1.17 at 25°C. Commercial grade phosphine derived from aluminum or magnesium phosphide can contain to a variable degree higher molecular weight phosphines including diphosphines. These higher phosphines give commercial grade fumigants containing aluminum or magnesium phosphide odor characteristics described as decaying fish or "garlic–like." Commercial grade phosphine containing diphosphines can ignite and form explosive mixtures at concentrations exceeding 1.8% phosphine in air. The rate of conversion of the phosphide to phosphine is temperature and humidity dependent. Similarly, metal phosphides readily hydrolyze in water to yield phosphine, which is poorly soluble in water. Major products resulting from the oxidation of phosphine in water are hypophosphorous and phosphoric acids (Van Wazer, 1958; WHO, 1988).

86.1.2 CHEMISTRY

Phosphine is a nucleophile and acts as a strong reducing agent (Lam *et al.*, 1991). Under standard conditions of temperature, pressure, and humidity PH_3 is stable and does not undergo autoxidation. Very early work suggests that under conditions of increased atmospheric pressure and oxygen content autoxidation can occur (Van Wazer, 1958). Further, in the presence of trace levels of diphosphine and perhaps other higher phosphines in air, PH_3 will undergo a branched chain oxidation reaction (Green *et al.*, 1984; Osadchenko and Tomilov, 1969), a form of autoxidation. Similarly, under experimental conditions the reaction can be induced photolytically by ultraviolet (UV) light or ammonia (Buchanan and Hanrahan, 1970; Woller, 1965). The branched chain reaction when it occurs is a generator and a good source of free radicals (see below) (Green *et al.*, 1984):

Propagation

$O_2 + PH_2\cdot$	$\Rightarrow$	$HPO + OH\cdot$
$OH\cdot + PH_3$	$\Rightarrow$	$PH_2\cdot + H_2O$
$O_2 + PH_2\cdot$	$\Rightarrow$	$PH + HO_2\cdot$
$O_2 + PH$	$\Rightarrow$	$HPO + O$

Branching

$O + PH_3$	$\Rightarrow$	$PH_2\cdot + OH\cdot$

Termination

$O + O_2 + M$	$\Rightarrow$	$O_3 + M$
Radical + Wall	$\Rightarrow$	Compound

Secondary Reactions

$HPO + O_2$	$\Rightarrow$	HPO_3
$HPO_3 + H_2O$	$\Rightarrow$	H_3PO_4

86.2 SOURCES, USES, AND FORMULATIONS

86.2.1 NATURAL SOURCES

Phosphine can be generated in decaying organic matter in open air sewage treatment plants (Dévai *et al.*, 1998) and other sources of decaying organic material (Glindemann *et al.*, 1996) including landfills, compost processing, and river sediments. Maximum concentrations detected were approximately 20 ppb.

86.2.2 COMMERCIAL SOURCES

Metal phosphides, notably aluminum, magnesium, and zinc phosphide, are the most common commercial sources of phosphine. Aluminum and magnesium phosphides are commonly used fumigants supplied as pellets, tablets, sachets, ropes, or strips (Meister, 1999) for insect control in stored grains and other products. Zinc phosphide baits are commonly used for rodent control. Ammonia from ammonium carbamate is sometimes used as a warning odorant in some fumigant formulations. Phosphine gas is also used in the synthesis of flame retardants, as a dopant in the semiconductor industry, and as a polymerization initiator and catalyst (U.S. DHHS, 1993).

86.3 TOXICOLOGY

86.3.1 OVERVIEW

The modern history of our understanding of the biologic effects of the toxicant phosphine begins with the works of O. R. Klimmer (1969, 1970). In these works the investigator established the dose related lethal effects of phosphine in multiple species, determined the dose threshold for lethality, and explored possible mechanisms for lethality including effects on hemoglobin. From these works, there is ample evidence that the acute lethal effects of phosphine can occur at levels less than 8 mg/m³. Since that time, work by others has gone forward to explore the avenues for the lethal effects of this toxicant gas in insects, mammals, and humans *in vivo* and *in vitro*. Genotoxicity and reproductive effects have also been considered. Because phosphine is an explosive hazard, many of the laboratory-based studies have been conducted under exposure conditions to eliminate or reduce the possibility of the branched chain oxidation reaction in air. Thus, these studies reflect the effects of phosphine in the unoxidized state. Human case and field population studies and some *in vitro* studies may reflect to a greater or lesser degree the toxicant effects of phosphine and its auto-oxidation products induced by the contaminant diphosphine in the commercial product, and uncontrolled environmental conditions including UV light, humidity, temperature, and/or ammonia as well. The studies reviewed below emerge as a complex picture of the toxicant effects of phosphine.

86.4 TOXICITY AND MODE OF ACTION

86.4.1 ACUTE TOXICITY

86.4.1.1 Symptoms

Early on, Klimmer found that animals exposed to high concentrations of phosphine quickly develop lassitude, ataxia, apnea, and cardiovascular collapse resulting in death within one half-hour (Klimmer, 1969). At lower concentrations (range studied 7.5 to 564 mg/m³) time to death varied with dose (Fig. 86.1). Concentrations as low as 7 mg/m³ are lethal over a period of 820 hours.

In humans, case studies involving suicide and suicide attempts by ingestion of pellets of aluminum phosphide are instructive. Rapid onset of epigastric distress, hypotension, cardiovascular collapse, and death are a recurrent pattern. In those who reach a hospital, altered sensoria, vomiting, severe acidosis, hypotension, cardiac arrhythmia, jaundice, and pulmonary crepitation were common occurrences (Banjaj and Wasir, 1988; Misra *et al.*, 1988a, b; Singh *et al.*, 1996). In a review of 195 intentional intoxication cases, Singh *et al.* (1985) concluded that ingestion of 1.5 g aluminum phosphide can be lethal in adults. Autopsy findings from published accidental death investigations (Garry *et al.*, 1993; Heyndrickx *et al.*, 1976; Wilson *et al.*, 1980) show microscopic pulmonary congestion with edema and alveolar cell necrosis, individual myocardial cell and liver cell necrosis, and anoxic changes in the brain. Klimmer (1970) noted earlier in autopsied animals a peculiar crimson color to the blood. These findings were variably recorded in the human autopsy and in clinical case studies. These human case studies and early animal acute toxicity studies provide some insights for formal mechanistic studies.

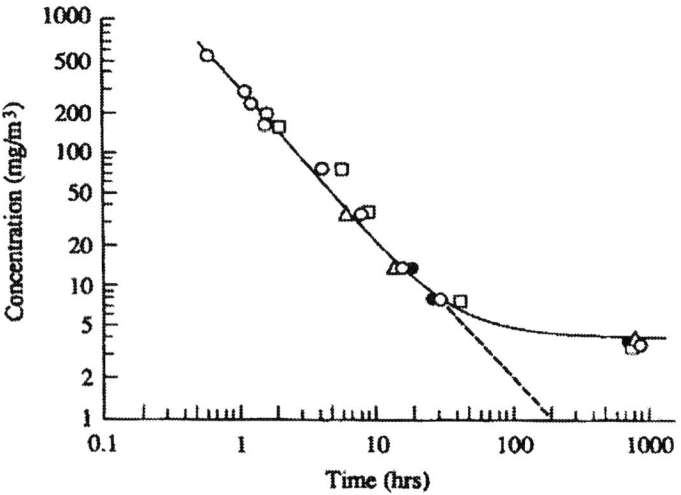

Figure 86.1 Comparison of dose and time to death in different species. Response of rats (○), rabbit (△), guinea pigs (●) and cats (□) to phosphine. Each point indicates the concentration of phosphine to which a group of animals was exposed and the average time to death. From data of Klimmer (1969) and Hayes and Laws (1991). Reproduced with permission.

86.5 ANIMAL DOSE/RESPONSE

86.5.1 THRESHOLD FOR LETHALITY

The early studies of Klimmer (1969) as illustrated previously show that for rats, rabbits, cats, and guinea pigs, a threshold for acute lethality by the inhalation route occurs at about 7 mg/m^3. Similarly, Newton *et al.* (1993), demonstrated in pregnant Fischer 344 female rats, exposed six hours daily, four days was the median lethal time at a concentration of 9.7 mg/m^3. Concentrations below 7 ppm showed no lethality. In mice (both sexes) the Median Lethal Dose after two weeks exposure is 9 mg/m^3 (Barbosa *et al.*, 1994). Concentrations below this level were not lethal. As indicated before, there are only minor differences in the mortality data from earlier to more recent studies regarding duration time-dose threshold for acute lethality.

86.5.2 ACUTE AND SUBACUTE DOSE/RESPONSE

Given the time-duration effects noted above and other factors, the LC$_{50}$ for inhaled phosphine is somewhat variable. Early studies by Waritz and Brown (1975) showed a four hour LC$_{50}$ of 11 ppm in male rats. Using highly purified phosphine, Omae *et al.* (1996) reported a four hour LC$_{50}$ between 26.5 and 33.4 ppm in male mice. Newton *et al.* (1993) reported no lethality in male and female rats acutely exposed to 10 ppm phosphine for six hours. In subacute studies in Fischer 344 female rats these authors indicate that three day exposure to 10 ppm phosphine was lethal. They further demonstrated that female rats were more sensitive to the lethal effects of the inhaled gas.

86.6 ABSORPTION, DISTRIBUTION, METABOLISM, AND EXCRETION

Aside from empirical observations regarding ingestion and respiratory exposure, there is little toxicokinetic data regarding absorption, distribution, and excretion of phosphine and its reaction products. In one study, ^{32}P labeled phosphine as reaction product residues (hypophosphite and phosphite) in flour were fed to mice. Labeled material in excreta was found to persist for periods up to three weeks (Robinson and Bond, 1970).

86.7 CELLULAR AND MOLECULAR STUDIES

86.7.1 GENERAL

Much of the work regarding phosphine as a metabolic poison centers on the concept that reactivity of phosphine as a nucleophile, and/or the electrophilic character of the intermediates arising from oxidation, could lead to derivatization of critical biomolecules (Lam *et al.*, 1991). Certain critical biologic

endpoints including the cytochromes and cytochrome oxidase system, hemoglobin, peroxidases and lipid peroxidation, catalase, cholinesterase, and DNA have been studied in some detail. The reported phosphine effects in each of these systems will be discussed below. As part of the discussion, the importance of oxygen as a modifier enhancing toxicity and the reduction of toxicity in reduced oxygen atmospheres will be considered.

86.7.2 CYTOCHROMES AND CYTOCHROME OXIDASE

Early on, the requirement for oxygen to mediate the toxicity of phosphine was identified in insects (Bond *et al.*, 1969) indicating that the gas may be an aerobic mitochondrial respiratory poison. Since that time, *in vitro* studies, both animal and insect, have shown that the respiratory enzyme, cytochrome c oxidase, may be the specific site of action (Bolter and Chefurka, 1990; Chaudhry, 1997; Kashi and Chefurka, 1976; Price, 1980). On the other hand, *in vivo* treatment of insects with lethal dose levels of phosphine (Nakakita, 1987) showed no more than 50% inhibition of the enzyme. Further work showed that this level of respiratory enzyme inhibition was sufficient to generate superoxide anions (Bolter and Chefurka, 1990) and these authors suggested that the toxicity of phosphine was due to free radical damage.

86.7.3 HEMOGLOBIN

In seminal efforts Trimborn and Klimmer (1962) described phosphine-induced hemoglobin denaturation, oxidation to methemoglobin, and formation of a peculiar pigmented form of hemoglobin "Verdichromogen." Studies of purified hemoglobin by Potter *et al.* (1991) and Chin *et al.* (1992) showed that with increasing duration of exposure, phosphine in concentrations as low as 0.11 μM gradually resulted in the formation of hemichrome pigment. In intact red blood cells, Potter *et al.* (1991) noted formation of Heinz bodies (hemoglobin protein aggregates) at PH$_3$ concentrations as low as 2 μg/ml. The toxicant effects both in intact cells and in purified hemoglobin were abolished by incubation in a reduced oxygen atmosphere, indicating an oxygen requirement for phosphine hemoglobin toxicity.

86.8 PEROXIDASES, LIPID PEROXIDATION, CATALASE, AND CHOLINESTERASE

Because phosphine is a strong reducing agent, peroxidation and formation of peroxides and their reduction are concerns mechanistically and therapeutically. Studies by Pazynich *et al.* (1984) in animals showed that the gas inhibited myeloperoxidase enzyme at concentrations of 8 mg/m^3. More recently in the occupational setting, Garry *et al.* (1990) noted histochemically a 50% reduction in myeloperoxidase activity in neutrophils from exposed workers compared to control subjects. Ambient air monitoring data obtained at the time varied from 0.4 to 5.8 mg/m^3. The permissible exposure limit (PEL) for phosphine at the time in the US was 0.4 mg/m^3. In other human studies by Chugh *et al.* (1996) in 45 patients recovering from phosphine poisoning, serial studies of serum levels of superoxide dismutase (SOD), malondialdehyde (MDA), and catalase were performed. Increased levels of SOD and MDA were found in nonsurvivors while catalase was inhibited. Remarkably similar findings (i.e., decreased peroxidase and catalase and increased superoxide dismutase) were reported by Bolter and Chefurka (1990) and Chaudhry and Price (1990) in insects. Taken together, the works cited above indicate that phosphine intoxication can lead to accumulation of cellular peroxides. Further, the oxidation of phosphine (Lam *et al.*, 1991) can lead to formation of reactive phosphorylating species. As such effects on cholinesterase are also possible. Significant inhibition of cholinesterase was detected in animals (Pazynich *et al.*, 1984). Occupational studies of grain fumigant applicators (Potter *et al.*, 1993) and *in vitro* studies in human red blood cells (Potter *et al.*, 1991) demonstrate that significant phosphine-induced inhibition of red cell cholinesterase occurs at concentrations exceeding 10 µg/ml.

86.9 GENOTOXICITY, CANCER AND REPRODUCTIVE EFFECTS

Studies in the occupational setting (Garry *et al.*, 1989, 1990, 1992) suggest that in enclosed space applications where PH$_3$ ambient air concentrations exceed the permissible exposure limit of 0.4 mg/m^3 (range 0.4–5.8 mg/m^3) for a duration of more than 20 minutes, increased chromosome aberrations are detectable in human lymphocytes from exposed workers. Studies by Barbosa and Bonin (1994) using micronucleus assay found no increase in micronucleus frequency in exposed workers where ambient exposures were less than the PEL. Later follow up studies by Garry *et al.* (1996) of the same worker population did not show increased chromosome aberrations. During the interim, changes in application practice from manual probe application to more automated methods and nonuse of phosphine in pesticide applications were noted (unpublished). In subacute tightly controlled animal studies (Kligerman *et al.*, 1994b) using purified PH$_3$ mixed with nitrogen, no increased numbers of micronuclei or chromosome aberrations were found in spleen cells cultured from animals exposed to phosphine for six hours per day for 9 days at concentrations as high as 7 mg/m^3 in ambient air. A single 6 hours 20 mg/m^3 study by this investigator showed similar negative results (Kligerman *et al.*, 1994a). In similarly constructed subchronic studies, Barbosa *et al.* (1994) found significantly increased numbers of micronuclei at the highest concentration tested (6.3 µg/m^3). Cast in the light of these *in vivo* studies (both animal and human) one can conclude that in regard to genotoxicity, phosphine may be a genotoxin. From a mechanistic view, *in vitro* studies of genotoxicity offer some additional insights. In these studies (Garry

et al., 1989; Hsu *et al.*, 1998) aluminum or magnesium phosphide was used as a phosphine generating system. Exposure of human lymphocytes (Garry *et al.*, 1989) to concentrations of phosphine (1.4–4.5 µg/l) derived from AlP for 20 minutes yielded increased chromosome aberrations after 96 hours of lymphocyte culture, indicating that the expression of genotoxicity of phosphine is delayed. In a much more detailed mechanistic examination of the genotoxicity of phosphine derived from AlP or Mg$_3$P$_2$ in Hepa cells at a nominal concentration of 1 mM PH$_3$, Hsu *et al.* (1998) found that reactive oxygen species were maximally generated between 0.5 to 1.5 hr, while damage to DNA expressed as 8-hydroyguanine adducts occurred between 4 and 6 hours. Both of these *in vitro* studies demonstrate that phosphine or its reaction products derived from AlP can generate DNA damage and that expression of these effects is delayed, probably indirectly and dependent on generation of hydrogen peroxides (Hsu *et al.*, 1998).

No completed long term animal studies were noted in this review regarding carcinogenicity. One preliminary report (U.S. EPA, 1998) noted no carcinogenic effects in rats chronically exposed to an inhaled dose of 3 ppm phosphine after one year. One human epidemiologic study of grain worker mortality (Alavanja *et al.*, 1987a, b) shows an excess of cancers of the lymphatic and hematopoietic system in this occupational setting where exposure to phosphine and other chemicals and biologic agents occurs. One study of animal teratogenicity (Newton *et al.*, 1993) with exposure concentrations as high as 4.9 ppm during days 6–15 of gestation in rats showed neither maternal toxicity nor developmental toxicity. No other reproductive endpoint studies were available for review.

86.10 TREATMENT OF POISONING

There is no current medical standard of treatment for acute phosphine intoxication. In general, support of vital functions, prevention and/or treatment of shock, and early gastric lavage for ingested poison are suggested (Singh *et al.*, 1985). Few clinical research efforts have been devoted to evaluation of antiperoxidants use (Chugh *et al.*, 1996; Gupta and Ahlawat, 1995) such as magnesium sulfate for treatment of acute intoxication. Finally, there is clear need to fully evaluate use of antioxidants as potential therapeutic agents in light of the current toxicologic findings.

86.11 REGULATORY NOTES (EXPOSURE GUIDELINES)

NIOSH REL: TWA 0.3 ppm (0.4 mg/m^3), STEL 1 ppm (1.4 mg/m^3)

OHSHA PEL: TWA 0.3 ppm (0.4 mg/m^3)

1993–1994 AGGIH TLV: 0.3 ppm (0.42 mg/m^3) TWA, 1 ppm (1.4 mg/m^3) STEL

Revised IDHL (immediately dangerous to health or life): 50 ppm (NIOSH, 1996)

Acute reference dose (RfD) was established as 0.018 mg/kg/day (U.S. EPA, 1998). Chronic reference dose was found to be 0.0113 mg/kg/day. Earlier EPA established RfD for phosphine was 0.0003 mg/kg/d based on body weight and clinical parameters (U.S. EPA, 1995).

86.12 SUMMARY AND COMMENTS

Phosphine is a toxicant gas with strong reducing properties capable of chemical and biologic oxidant effects. The signature threshold for lethality over a narrow dose range and slow evolution of mortality at lower doses indicates that the chemical induces a cumulative biologic oxidant cascade involving progressive alteration of a number of critical biologic endpoints. The critical threshold for these effects may be moderated by environmental–chemical interactions affecting conditions of exposure. As O. R. Klimmer (1969) said "It is a most peculiar poison."

REFERENCES

Alavanja, M. C., Malker, H., and Hayes, R. B. (1987a). Occupational cancer risk associated with the storage and bulk handling of agricultural foodstuff. *J. Toxicol. Environ. Health* **22**, 247–254.

Alavanja, M. C., Rush, G. A., Stewart, P., and Blair, A. (1987b). Proportionate mortality study of workers in the grain industry. *J. Natl. Cancer I.* **78**, 247–252.

Banjaj, R., and Wasir, H.S. (1988). Epidemic caluminium phosphide poisoning in northern India. *Lancet* **1**, 820–821.

Barbosa, A., and Bonin, A. M. (1994). Evaluation of phosphine genotoxicity at occupational levels of exposure in New South Wales, Australia. *Occup. Environ. Med.* **51**, 700–705.

Barbosa, A., Rosinova, E., Dempsey, J., and Bonin, A. M. (1994). Determination of genotoxic and other effects in mice following short term repeated-dose and subchronic inhalation exposure to phosphine. *Environ. Mol. Mutagen.* **24**, 81–88.

Bolter, C. J., and Chefurka, W. (1990). Extramitochondrial release of hydrogen peroxide from insect and mouse liver mitochondria using the respiratory inhibitors phosphine, myxothiazol, and antimycin and spectral analysis of inhibited cytochromes. *Arch. Biochem. Biophys.* **278**, 65–72.

Bond, E. J., Robinson, J. R., and Buckland, C. T. (1969). The toxic action of phosphine: Absorption and symptoms of poisoning in insects. *J. Stored Prod. Res.* **5**, 289–298.

Buchanan, J. W., and Hanrahan, R. J. (1970). The radiation chemistry of phosphine–ammonia mixtures in the gas phase. *Mutat. Res.* **44**, 206–304.

Chaudhry, M. Q. (1997). A review of the mechanisms involved in the action of phosphine as an insecticide and phosphine resistance in stored-product insects. *Pestic. Sci.* **49**, 213–228.

Chaudhry, M. Q., and Price, N. R. (1990). A spectral study of the biochemical reactions of phosphine with various haemproteins. *Pestic. Biochem. Physiol.* **36**, 14–21.

Chin, K. L., Meaklim, M. J., Scollary, G. R., and Leaver, D. D. (1992). The interaction of phosphine with haemoglobin and erythrocytes. *Xenobiotica* **22**, 599–607.

Chugh, S. N., Arora, V., Sharma, A., and Chugh, K. (1996). Free radical scavengers and lipid peroxidation in acute aluminum phosphide poisoning. *Indian J. Med. Res.* **104**, 190-193.

Dévai, I., Felföldy, L., Wittner I., and Plösz, S. (1998). Detection of phospine: New aspects of the phosphorous cycle in the hydrosphere. *Nature* **333**, 343–345.

Garry, V. F., Danzl, T. J., Nelson, R. L., Cervenka, J., Krueger, L. A., Griffith, J., and Whorton, E. (1989). Human genotoxicity: Pesticide applicators and phospine. *Science* **246**, 251–255.

Garry, V. F., Nelson, R. L., Danzl, T. J., Cervenka, J., Krueger, L. A., Griffith, J., and Whorton, E. (1990). Human genotoxicity in phosphine-exposed fumigant applicators. *Prog. Clin. Biol. Res.* **340C**, 367–376.

Garry, V. F., Danzl, T. J., Tarone, R., and Griffith, J. (1992). Chromosome rearrangements in fumigant appliers: possible relationship to non-Hodgkin's lymphoma risk. *Canc. Epi. Biomark. Prev.* **1**, 287–291.

Garry, V. F., Good, P. F., Manivel, C., and Perl, D. (1993). Investigation of a fatality from nonoccupational aluminum phosphide exposure: Measurement of aluminum in tissue and body fluids as a marker of exposure. *J. Lab. Clin. Med.* **122**, 739–747.

Garry, V. F., Tarone R. E., Long, L., Griffith, J., Kelly, J. T., and Burroughs, B. (1996). Pesticide appliers with mixed pesticide exposure: G-banded analysis and possible relatonship to non-Hodgkin's lymphoma. *Canc. Epi. Biomark. Prev.* **5**, 11–16.

Glindemann, D., Stottmeister, U., and Bergmann, A. (1996). Free phosphine from the anaerobic biosphere. *Environ. Sci. Pollut Res. Intern.* **3**, 17–19.

Green, A. R., Sheldon, S., and Banks, H. J. (1984). The flammability limit of pure phosphine-air mixtures at atmospheric pressure. *In* "Controlled Atmosphere and Fumigation in Grain Storage" (B. E. Ripp, ed.), Vol. 5, pp. 433–451. Elsevier, Amsterdam.

Gupta, S., and Ahlawat, S. K. (1995). Aluminum phosphide poisoning: A review. *J. Toxicol. Clin. Toxicol.* **33**, 19–24.

Hayes, W. J., and Laws, E. R., ed. (1991). "Handbook of Pesticide Toxicology," Vol. 2, p. 657.

Heyndrickx, A., Van Peteghem, C., Van Den Heede, M., and Lauwaert, R. (1976). A double fatality with children due to fumigated wheat. *Eur. J. Toxicol.* **9**, 113–118.

Hsu, C.-H., Quistad, G. B., and Casida, J. E. (1998). Phosphine induced oxidative stress in Hepa 1c1c7 cells. *Toxicol. Sci.* **46**, 204–210.

Kashi, K. P., and Chefurka, W. (1976). The effect of phosphine on the absorption and circular dichroic spectra of cytochrome c and cytochrome oxidase. *Pestic. Biochem. Physiol.* **6**, 350–362.

Kligerman, A. D., Bryant, M. F., Doerr, C. L., Erexson, G. L., Kwanyuen, P., and McGee, J. K. (1994a). Cytogenic effects of phosphine inhalation by rodents: I. Acute 6 hour exposure of mice. *Environ. Mol. Mutagen.* **23**, 186–189.

Kligerman, A. D., Bishop, J. B., Erexson, G. L., Price, H. C., O'Connor, R. W., Morgan, D. L., and Zeiger, E. (1994b). Cytogenic and germ cell effects of phosphine inhalation by rodents. II. Subacute exposures to rats and mice. *Environ. Mol. Mutagen.* **24**, 301–306.

Klimmer, O. R. (1969). Beitrag zur Wirkung des Phosphorwasserstoffes (PH₃). Zur Frage der sog chronischen Phosphorwasserstoffvergiftung. *Arch. Toxikol.* **24**, 164–187 [in German].

Klimmer, O. R. (1970). Akute Vergiftungen durch Insektizide und Herbizide. *Z. Allgemeinmedizin* **46**, 1731–1734 [in German].

Lam, W. W., Toia, R. F., and Casida, J. E. (1991). Oxidatively initiated phosphorylation reactions of phosphine. *J. Agric. Food Chem.* **39**, 2274–2278.

Meister, R. T. (1999). "Farm Chemicals Handbook." Meister, Wikkoughby.

Misra, U. K., Bhargave, S. K., Nag, D., Kidwai, M. M., and Lal, M. M. (1988a). Occupational phosphine exposure in Indian workers. *Toxicol. Lett.* **42**, 257–263.

Misra, U. K., Tripathi, A. K., Pandey, R., and Bhargwa, B. (1988b). Acute phosphine poisoning following ingestion of aluminum phosphide. *Human Toxicol.* **7**, 343–345.

Nakakita, H. (1987). The mode of action of phosphine. *J. Pestic. Sci.* **12**, 299–309.

Newton, P. E., Schroeder, R. E., Sullivan, J. B., Busey, W. M., and Banas, D. A. (1993). Inhalation toxicity of phosphine in the rat: Acute, subchronic, and developmental. *Inhal. Toxicol.* **5**, 223–239.

NIOSH Pocket Guide to Chemical Hazards (1996). "Documentations for Immediately Dangerous to Life or Health Concentrations (IDLH): Phosphine."

Omae, K., Ishizuka, C., Nakashima, H., Sakurai, H., Yamazaki, K., Mori, K., Shibata, T., Kanoh, H., Kudo, M., and Tati, M. (1996). Acute and subacute inhalation toxicity of highly purified phosphine (PH_3) in male ICR mice. *J. Occup. Health* **38**, 36–42.

Osadchenko, I. M., and Tomilov, A. P. (1969). Phosphorous hydrides. *Russian Chem. Rev.* **33**, 495–504.

Pazynich, V. M., Mazur, I. A., Podlozny, A. V., Chinchevich, V. I., and Mandrichenko, B. E. (1984). Experimental substantiation and prediction of time related maximum permissible concentration of phosphine in the air. *Gig. Sanit.* **1**, 13–15 [in Russian].

Potter, W. T., Rong, S., Griffith, J., White, J., and Garry, V. F. (1991). Phosphine mediated Heinz Body formation and hemoglobin oxidation in human erythrocytes. *Toxicol. Lett.* **57**, 37–45.

Potter, W. T., Garry, V. F., Kelly, J. T., Taronef, R., Griffith, J., and Nelson, R. L. (1993). Radiometric assay of red cell and plasma cholinesterase in pesticide appliers from Minnesota. *Toxicol. Appl. Pharmacol.* **119**, 150–155.

Price, N. R. (1980). Some aspects of the inhibition of cytochrome *c* oxidase by phosphine in susceptible and resistant strains of Rhyzopertha Dominicia. *Insect Biochem.* **10**, 147–150.

Robinson, J. R., and Bond, E. J. (1970). The toxic action of phosphine: Studies with [32]PH_3; terminal residues in biological materials. *J. Stored Prod. Res.* **6**, 133–146.

Singh, S., Dilawari, J. B., Vashist, R., Malhotra, H. S., and Sharma, B. K. (1985). Aluminum phosphide ingestion. *Br. Med. J. (Clin. Res.)* **290**, 1110–1111.

Singh, S., Singh, D., Wig, N., Jit, I., and Sharma, B. K. (1996). Aluminum phosphide ingestion—A clinico-pathologic study. *J. Toxicol. Clin. Toxicol.* **34**, 703–706.

Trimborn, H., and Klimmer, O. R. (1962). Experimentelle untersuchungen über chemische veränderungen des blutfarbstoffs in vitro durch phosphorwasserstoff. *Arch. Int. Pharmacodyn.* **CSSSVII**, 331–347.

U.S. Department of Health and Human Services (1993). "Hazardous Substances Data Bank" (HSDB, online database). National Toxicilogy Information Program, National Library of medicine, Bethesda.

U.S. EPA (1995). "Integrated Risk Information System (IRIS) on Phosphine." Environmental Criteria and Assessment Office, Office of Health and Environmental Assessment, Office of Research and Development, Cincinnati, OH.

U.S. EPA (1998). "Prevention, Pesticides And Toxic Substances (7508C). Reregistration Eligibility Decision (RED) Aluminum and Magnesium Phosphide." EPA 738-R-98-017.

Van Wazer, J. R. (1958). "Phosphorus and Its Compounds," Vol. I. Chemistry. Interscience Publishers, New York.

Waritz, R. S, and Brown, R. M. (1975). Acute and subacute inhalation toxicities of phosphine, phenylphosphine and triphenylphosphine. *Am. Ind. Hyg. Assoc. J.* **36**, 452–458.

Wilson, R., Lovejoy, F. R., Jaeger, R. J., and Landrigan, P. L. (1980). Acute phosphine poisoning aboard a grain freighter. *JAMA, J. Am. Med. Assoc.* **244**, 148–150.

Woller, C. R. (1965). Aliphatic Compounds of Some Elements. *In* "Chemistry of Organic Compounds" (W. B. Saunders, ed.), pp. 317–323.

World Health Organization (1988). Phosphine and selected metal phosphides. *Environmental Health Criteria* **73**, 17–19.

Metam-Sodium

Linda L. Carlock
Toxicology and Regulatory Consulting
Timothy A. Dotson
UCB Chemicals Corporation

87.1 INTRODUCTION

Metam-sodium ($C_2H_4NNaS_2$, CAS no. 137-42-8), also known as metham sodium, sodium metam, sodium-N-methyldithio-carbamate, methylcarbamodithioic acid sodium salt, methyl-dithiocarbamic acid sodium salt, carbam, and SMDC, is a white crystalline powder in the pure form but is normally found as a clear yellow liquid with a strong sulfurlike odor (Merck, 1989). Metam-sodium is prepared from methylamine, carbon disulfide, and sodium hydroxide in an aqueous solution. Metam-sodium has a molecular weight of 129.18. Metam-sodium is stable in its dry, crystalline state, and in concentrated aqueous solution. In solution, metam-sodium has a vapor pressure of 21 mg Hg at 25°C (U.S. EPA, 1994a). Metam-sodium is very stable at a pH greater than 8.8, but at pH 7 and below it readily hydrolyzes. In soil or when diluted with water, metam-sodium is converted to methyl isothiocyanate (MITC). Other degradates of metam-sodium include carbon disulfide (CS_2) and hydrogen sulfide (H_2S).

Metam-sodium is an agricultural general use pesticide used primarily as a broad spectrum preplant soil fumigant to control weeds, weed seeds, fungi, nematodes, and soil insects. End use products are formulated as 18–42% aqueous solutions sold under the trade names of Metam CLR, Vapam, and Sectagon. Metam-sodium has been registered since 1954. Registered uses of metam-sodium include agricultural soil fumigation, wood preservative, slimicide, tree-root killer, and aquatic weed control. Approximately 10 million pounds of metam-sodium were used in 1990, with 40–45% used for agricultural purposes (U.S. EPA, 1994a).

As a soil fumigant, metam-sodium is applied after harvest and/or 14 to 21 days prior to planting by shank injection, disc, rotary tiller, drip irrigation, solid set sprinkler, or center pivot chemigation. In some parts of North America, fall applications are preferred because metam-sodium volatilizes over the winter and clears the soil, allowing planting to begin as soon as favorable springtime conditions arrive. By treating the soil with metam-sodium, fruit and vegetable growers can control weeds, reduce nematode populations, and control soil-borne pests. Metam-sodium may be used on all crops but is particularly important in the production of melons, peppers, tomatoes, potatoes, strawberries, citrus, grapes, almonds, artichokes, asparagus, carrots, lettuce, spinach, squash, forest tree seedlings, ornamentals, and cut flowers. By reducing competition from soil pests, metam-sodium promotes healthier plants and increased yields.

The U.S. EPA (1997) considers metam-sodium to be a commercially viable alternative to methyl bromide fumigation for fruit and vegetable production due to its low cost, wide range of control, and long record of safe use. It can be used to control weeds (e.g., bluegrass, Bermuda grass, chickweed, dandelion, ragweed, henbit, nutsedge, and wild morning glory), nematodes, and soil diseases caused by species of *Rhizoctonia, Fusarium, Pythium, Phytophthora, Verticillium,* and *Sclerotinia* (U.S. EPA, 1997). Metam-sodium has also been shown to be useful in integrated pest management systems as it can be used in conjunction with other treatment methods such as biological controls and soil pasteurization.

Metam-sodium is a slightly to moderately toxic compound that when used according to label directions has been shown to be a safe and versatile product for over 45 years. For agricultural use, metam-sodium must be applied in a manner where there is no contact with workers or other persons, either directly or through drift. Only handlers equipped with the proper personal protection equipment may be in the area during application. In California, application must also be in compliance with the Technical Information Bulletin "Guidelines for All Application Methods for Metam-sodium in California."

The potential routes of human chemical exposures are oral (ingestion), dermal (direct skin contact), and inhalation, however, the chance for nonoccupational exposure to metam-sodium is minimal. Approved agricultural uses of metam-sodium do not leave residues on crops, thus eliminating diet as a source of exposure. The primary means of exposure to metam-sodium is through dermal occupational exposure. Most of the potential for exposure to metam-sodium itself comes from transloading and handling the liquid when preparing for application. The use of required protective gloves, boots, and clothing minimizes or eliminates dermal exposure to metam-sodium. The U.S. EPA's Occupational and Residential Exposure Branch assumes that dermal exposure is minimal for handlers and nonexistent for nearby residents and bystanders (U.S. EPA, 1994a). There is little potential for inhalation exposure to metam-sodium, which has been proven through extensive monitoring and in a number of worker exposure studies. Proper protective equipment such as in-cab filtering systems and NIOSH-approved respirators that are used by workers provide protection in the unlikely situation that the liquid compound becomes aerosolized.

The toxicology of "technical grade" or formulated metam-sodium (approximately 42% a.i.) is well established. Metam-sodium is synthesized in aqueous solution and then diluted with water, as necessary, to achieve the desired concentration and meet the label guarantee for the formulated product. Thus, "technical grade" is synonymous with the formulated material. Little toxicity information is available regarding pure or analytical-grade metam-sodium.

The following discussion of technical grade/formulated metam-sodium toxicity briefly covers a number of published studies and the results of toxicity studies submitted to governmental agencies in support of metam-sodium registration.

87.2 ACUTE TOXICITY

Metam-sodium is slightly to moderately acutely toxic depending on the route of exposure. The following toxicity values pertain to technical grade metam-sodium (U.S. EPA, 1994a). All of the following values were obtained with standard acute toxicity studies designed to determine the dose or concentration that causes death to 50% of the test animals (LD50 or LC50):

- The acute LD50 for technical grade metam-sodium (43.7% a.i.) is reported as 870 mg/kg for male rats and 924 mg/kg for female rats. The combined (male and female) LD50 is 896 mg/kg (placing the compound into Toxicity Category III (U.S. EPA, 1994a) or similarly classified as slightly toxic (LD50 = 5–15 g/kg; Klaassen, 1986).
- The acute dermal LD50 of technical grade metam-sodium (43.7%) applied to male and female rabbits is 368 mg/kg (Toxicity Category III).
- The acute inhalation LC50 of aerosolized technical grade metam-sodium (42%) in rats is 2.275 mg/l (Toxicity Category III).
- Technical grade metam-sodium (42%) was found to be slightly irritating to the eyes of New Zealand White rabbits (Toxicity Category III).
- Technical grade metam-sodium (42%) is irritating to the shaved skin of male and female rabbits (Liggett and McRae, 1991) and is classified as a moderate to severe dermal irritant (Toxicity Category II).

- Metam-sodium (42%) was also found to be a skin sensitizer to guinea pigs using the delayed contact hypersensitivity test (Parcell and Denton, 1991).

Acute studies conducted with 32.7% metam-sodium showed similar but milder results than the above cited data for the 42% formulated compound. Jowa (1998) reported the following values for multiple studies conducted with metam-sodium:

- The acute oral LD50 for 32.7% metam-sodium varied from 1294 to 1415 mg/kg for male rats and 1350 to 1428 mg/kg for female rats.
- The acute dermal LD50 for 32.7% metam-sodium varied from 1012 to 3500 mg/kg in rabbits.
- The acute inhalation LC50 varied from >4.7 to >5.4 mg/l for male rats exposed to 32.7% metam-sodium for four hours.
- In one eye irritation study with rabbits, 32.7% metam-sodium was found to be a mild irritant, but in another study it was found to be nonirritating.
- Dermal irritation studies with rabbits exposed to 32.7% metam-sodium showed that the compound was a severe irritant in one study and was corrosive in another study.
- Testing guinea pigs with 32.5% metam-sodium in the Buehler test resulted in sensitization.

Standardized acute toxicity studies provide limited information regarding subtle toxic effects and are not designed to establish a no observed effect level (NOEL). To further understand the sublethal effects of a compound, lower dose levels or concentrations are required.

87.3 SUBCHRONIC TOXICITY

Effects of metam-sodium exposure over longer periods vary with the species tested and route of administration. A variety of toxicity studies have shown that there is a definite dose–response effect to metam-sodium (U.S. EPA, 1992, 1993). At very low doses levels there is no evidence of toxicity, but as the dose level increases the prevalence and severity of toxic effects increases.

In a 90-day study (Whiles, 1991), male and female mice were administered metam-sodium in drinking water at dose levels of 0, 0.018, 0.088, 0.35, or 0.62 mg/ml (2.7, 11.7, 52.4, or 78.7 mg/kg/day for males; 3.6, 15.2, 55.4, or 83.8 mg/kg/day for females). No treatment-related mortality, morbundity, or clinical signs of toxicity were observed during the 90-day study period. Treatment-related statistically significant decreases in mean body weight were observed in both males and females at dose levels of 0.35 and 0.62 mg/ml. Treatment-related changes in hematology parameters were noted at doses as low as 0.088 mg/ml for females and 0.62 mg/ml for males. The lowest effect level was determined to be 0.088 mg/ml (11.7 mg/kg/day for males, 15.2 mg/kg/day for females) based on urinary bladder lesions observed in both males and females and in statistically significant decreases in hemoglobin, red blood cell, and hematocrit in females. The NOEL for systemic toxicity was 0.018 mg/ml (2.7 and 3.6 mg/kg/day for males and females, respectively).

In another 90-day metam-sodium study (Allen, 1991), male and female rats received metam-sodium in the drinking water at nominal dose levels of 0, 0.018, 0.089, and 0.443 mg/ml (1.7, 8.1 and 26.9 mg/kg/day for males; 2.5, 9.3, and 30.6 mg/kg/day for females). Systemic toxicity was evident by significant decreases in food and water consumption, decreased body weight gain, and histological changes in the nasal cavity olfactory epithelium in both males and females receiving metam-sodium at 0.443 mg/ml. Renal tubular dilation and basophilia along with increases in blood and protein in the urine were also observed in 0.443 mg/ml rats. In both males and females receiving 0.089 mg/ml there were significant decreases in red blood cell count and hematocrit. Females at the 0.089 mg/ml dose level also had a significant decrease in group mean body weight and decreased body weight gain (11%) when compared to controls. Based on the results of this study the NOEL was 0.018 mg/ml (1.7 mg/kg/day for males; 2.5 mg/kg/day for females).

In a subchronic dog study (Brammer, 1992), metam-sodium (43.15% purity) was administered by gelatin capsule to male and female beagles at nominal dose levels of 0, 1, 5, or 10 mg/kg/day once daily for 13 weeks. Toxic effects were observed at all dose levels tested but were primarily evident at the 5 and 10 mg/kg/day dose levels. Decreased body weight and body weight gain were observed in males and females receiving metam-sodium at 10 mg/kg/day. There were no significant clinical effects at 1 or 5 mg/kg/day and no ophthalmoscopic abnormalities in any animals. Regurgitation within 30–60 minutes of dosing occurred throughout the study in the 10 mg/kg/day group and on isolated occasions in the 5 mg/kg/day dogs. There was no regurgitation in the 1 mg/kg/day dosing group. In dogs receiving 5 and 10 mg/kg/day there were changes in hematologic parameters (increases in cell volume, cell hemoglobin, neutrophils, and monocytes; decreases in mean corpuscular hemoglobin concentration); significant increases in plasma alanine aminotransferase (ALT), aspartate aminotransferase (AST), alkaline phosphatase (ALP), and gamma-glutamyltransferase; increased blood, urobilinogen, bilirubin, and protein in the urine; and microscopic evidence of hepatitis). One female receiving 1 mg/kg/day showed increased plasma ALT. Biliary duct proliferation with inflammatory cell infiltration (less severe than hepatitis) was observed in one male and one female at the 5 mg/kg/day dose level and in one female at the 1 mg/kg/day dose level. No evidence of tumors were found in this study. Toxic effects appeared to be dose- and time-related. For female dogs, no systemic NOEL was established (NOEL < 1 mg/kg/day) due to increases in plasma ALT and biliary duct proliferation with inflammatory cell infiltration observed in a single female from the 1 mg/kg/day dose group. For male dogs, the systemic NOEL is 1 mg/kg/day. The lowest observed effect level (LOEL) of 5 mg/kg/day is based on statistically significant increases in plasma ALT, AST, and alkaline

phosphatase, and the increased incidence of hepatitis and bile duct proliferation.

In order to further study the effects of metam-sodium on the liver of dogs, a study was conducted at the dose level that caused moderate to marked hepatitis in all dogs during the 90-day study described above (Brammer, 1993). One male and one female beagle dog received metam-sodium (43.14% purity) in a gelatin capsule daily at a dose level of 10 mg/kg. Dosing of each dog continued until there were elevations in plasma enzyme activities (or other clinical signs) indicative of liver toxicity. Following cessation of dosing, each dog was monitored until the enzyme activities returned to normal or prestudy levels. Dosing ceased after 12 weeks of dosing for the female and after 13 weeks for the male. Recovery was monitored for 8 weeks. After Week 6 the plasma ALT levels in the female began to increase and by Week 10 they were over 200 IU/L. In the male, elevated plasma ALT was noted at Week 9 and exceeded 200 UI/L by Week 11. In both dogs, plasma ALP levels gradually increased until dosing ceased. Following cessation of dosing, ALT levels increased during the first recovery week then gradually declined to normal levels after 8 weeks. Plasma ALP decreased in the female dog immediately after cessation of dosing and by Recovery Week 4 was less than prestudy values. In the male, ALP continued to rise during the first recovery week then gradually decreased so that by Recovery Week 5, ALP values were less than prestudy values. In both dogs, ALP levels continued to fall until study termination. At study termination, there were no macroscopic abnormalities in either dog and liver weights were normal. Microscopic evaluations revealed that there was a minimal or slight increase in the number of pigmented macropahges/Kupffer cells in the liver, but this is a common finding in beagle dogs of this strain (Alderley Park).

The significant elevations in plasma ALT and ALP levels found in this study are consistent with the findings of the previous 90-day dog study at the same dose level (10 mg/kg/day) and are indicative of liver injury. However, after cessation of exposure, enzyme levels returned to normal, with full recovery eight weeks after the last exposure to metam-sodium. There was no evidence of liver injury at the end of the study. These findings confirm the reversible nature of induced liver effects from subchronic exposure to relatively high levels of metam-sodium.

87.4 GENETIC TOXICITY

Metam-sodium is not mutagenic but has been shown to be directly cytotoxic to bacteria, fungi, and mammalian cells. Metam-sodium has been tested and found to be negative in both *in vitro* and *in vivo* genetic toxicology assays covering a range of genetic toxicology endpoints including mutations, cytogenetics, and DNA repair. There is evidence that at high enough dose levels, exposure to metam-sodium can be immunotoxic, with response evident in a dose-dependent manner.

A review of metam-sodium genetic toxicity studies (Mackay, 1996) concluded that "[M]etam sodium shows no *in vitro* or *in vivo* genotoxic activity in a series of assays conducted up to concentrations/dose levels inducing significant toxicity in the target cells/animals."

- In a bacterial gene mutation assay using *Salmonella typhimurium* strains TA92, TA98, TA100, TA1535, TA1537, and TA1538 in the presence and absence of metabolic activation (AROCHLOR 1254-induced rat liver S9 mix) there were no significant increases in the number of revertant colonies in any of the strains or S9 combinations tested.
- In a Chinese hamster ovary mammalian cell gene mutation (HGRPT locus) assay metam-sodium was tested in the presence and absence of metabolic activation. There was no evidence of any reproducible dose-related effects of metam-sodium on mutation frequency or evidence of *in vitro* mutagenic activity.
- In two *in vitro* cytogenetic assays using human lymphocytes there was no evidence of clastogenic activity from metam-sodium treatment when tested at concentrations up to those limited by toxicity and/or cytotoxic effects on chromosomal morphology.

  - The first study found an increase in aberrant cells at concentration levels that caused severe cytotoxicity (20 µg/ml without S9 mix; 40 and 20 µg/ml with S9 mix) and therefore were unsuitable to be included in the evaluation of clastogenic potential. At concentration levels of 1, 5, and 10 µg/ml with and without S9 mix, there were no increases in the percentage of aberrant cells.
  - In the second *in vitro* human lymphocyte clastogenic study, metam-sodium at concentrations of 2.5, 20, and 30 µg/ml in the absence of S9 mix and 5, 20, and 40 µg/ml with S9 were tested. No statistically or biologically significant increases in the percentage of aberrant cells were observed at any of the metam-sodium concentrations tested in the absence of the S 9 mix. There was a small statistical increase in the number of aberrations observed in the 40 µg/ml test concentration with the S9 mix, but the values observed were well within the historical solvent control range and do not indicate clastogenic activity.

- In an *in vitro* unscheduled DNA synthesis assay using primary rat hepatocytes treated with metam-sodium there was no evidence of induction of DNA repair, even in cultures treated with toxic concentrations of metam-sodium.
- In an *in vivo* Chinese hamster bone marrow chromosomal aberration assay there was no evidence of any polyploidy inducing effect of metam-sodium nor was there evidence of any clastogenic activity.
- When metam-sodium was administered to CD-1 mice in an *in vivo* mouse bone marrow micronucleus test, there was no evidence of clastogenic activity in the mouse bone marrow when tested up to the maximum tolerated dose level for both male and female mice. There were no statistically or biologically significant increases in the incidence of micronucleated polychromatic erythrocytes.

U.S. EPA Tox Oneliners report on the results of genetic studies submitted to and reviewed by the U.S. EPA. Jowa (1998) reported on the same genetic studies submitted to and reviewed by the California Environmental Protection Agency (Cal EPA). In some cases, the results presented by Jowa did not agree with conclusions of the U.S. EPA.

- In two separate Ames studies using multiple strains of *Salmonella typhimurium* (TA 1535, 1537, 1538, 92, 98, and 100) up to 2500 µg/plate with and without activation (S9 mix), metam-sodium did not induce mutations and the results were negative.
- In a study with yeast (*Sacchromyces cerevisiae* strain D4) with and without S9 mix, metam-sodium did not induce mutations and the results were negative.
- In an *in* vitro study with *Bacillus subtilis*, metam-sodium did not cause DNA damage.

  - According to the Cal EPA review, equivocal results were obtained for a *REC* assay in *Bacillus subtilis* H17 and M45 (+/− S9).
  - According to the U.S. EPA review, metam-sodium (42.2%) is not a recombinogenic agent (i.e., causes DNA damage) to *Bacillus subtilis* strains H17 and M45 at concentrations up to 150 µl/well.

- In an *in vitro* study using cultured lymphocytes procured from a single male human donor, there was evidence of possible aberrant chromosomes. However, according to the Metam-sodium Task Force, the scientific validity of this study is under question since the aberrant chromosomes were observed only at concentration levels that were clearly cytotoxic to the cells. When the cells from noncytotoxic concentration levels were evaluated, there was no indication of any clastogenic activity.
- In a mammalian cytogenetic study with Chinese hamsters, metam-sodium did not induce cytogenic effects.

  - According to the Cal EPA review, there was evidence of polyploidy in Chinese hamster ovary cells at dose levels of 150 and 300 mg/kg.
  - According to the US EPA review, metam-sodium (42.2%) had a negative response (no effect) in the Chinese hamster bone marrow cytogenetic assay at concentrations of 150, 300, and 600 mg/kg.

- Metam-sodium was found to be negative in an unscheduled DNA synthesis study with primary rat hepatocyte culture.

A study was conducted to assess the immunotoxicological and selected general toxicological effects of metam-sodium

(Pruett *et al.*, 1992). Metam-sodium was administered to female B6C3F1 mice at 200 mg/kg/day for 3, 5, 10, or 14 days. Selected organ weights were measured, hematological and bone parameters were examined, changes in thymus and spleen lymphocyte subpopulations were evaluated, and production of antibody-forming cells *in vitro* was measured. Major effects of metam-sodium administration included decreased thymus weight at all time points; increased spleen weight and bone marrow cellularity after 10 or 14 days of exposure; significant decreases in mature lymphocytes in the thymus and spleen; decrease in thymocytes; and decreased body weight. According to Pruett and co-workers (1992), overall patterns of change indicate that metam-sodium rapidly depletes most CD4 + CD8 + thymocytes, more slowly depletes a smaller number of mature lymphocytes in the thymus and spleen, and induces compensatory and/or detoxication mechanisms after 10–14 days of exposure.

Pruett and co-workers (1992) conducted subsequent experiments to assess selected immune function parameters after exposure to metam-sodium. Metam-sodium was administered for seven days (either orally or dermally) and immunological assays were conducted on Day 8. Mice receiving metam-sodium orally at dose levels of 50 to 300 mg/kg showed substantial, dose-dependent suppression of NK cell activity. Evaluation of humoral responses indicated that the cellular and molecular components required for humoral immune responses are not major targets for the acute effects of metam-sodium. There was no suppression of antibody production *in vivo* or splenocyte responses to mitogens or allogeneic lymphocytes *in vitro*, which indicates that the lymphocytes which survive metam-sodium exposure are still able to proliferate and differentiate and are not significantly impaired with regard to function. The authors also noted that the pattern of thymic subpopulation changes is consistent with direct or indirect induction of apoptosis. These studies showed that immunological parameters could be significantly suppressed in the absence of a significant decrease in body weight, suggesting that most of the effects of metam-sodium on the immune system are not secondary to generalized toxicity.

In response to reports that metam-sodium is immunotoxic, a series of *in vivo* and *in vitro* studies was conducted with metam-sodium and other dithiocarbamates (Padgett *et al.*, 1992). Metam-sodium in distilled water was administered orally via daily gavage to female mice for seven days at dose levels of 0, 150, 225, or 300 mg/kg. Body weight was not significantly decreased at any dose level, but thymus weight was significantly decreased in mice receiving metam-sodium at dose levels of 225 and 300 mg/kg. In tests of splenic NK cell activity, metam-sodium at dose levels of 225 and 300 mg/kg was found to significantly inhibit NK activity. This study also demonstrated that metam-sodium was directly cytotoxic to lymphoid cells *in vitro*, but that cytotoxic potency *in vitro* does not correlate well with immunological changes *in vivo*.

87.5 DEVELOPMENTAL AND REPRODUCTIVE TOXICITY

Developmental studies in two different species found evidence of increased fetal loss, increased skeletal variations, and developmental delays from oral administration of metam-sodium to pregnant animals at dose levels that also caused overt maternal toxicity. Visceral or skeletal abnormalities were not present at low dose levels but increased in incidence and severity with increasing dose (U.S. EPA, 1991). In a multigeneration reproductive study, metam-sodium did not affect reproductive performance, even at toxic dose levels (U.S. EPA, 1994a).

A developmental study with rats receiving metam-sodium (Hellwig and Hildebrand, 1987) indicated that there were significant maternal and fetal effects at higher dose levels and that these effects were dose-related. An aqueous solution of metam-sodium (42.2%) was administered at 0, 10, 40, or 120 mg/kg by gavage to pregnant Wistar rats on Days 6–15 of gestation. Body weight gains were significantly decreased in dams receiving metam-sodium at dose levels of 40 and 120 mg/kg during the dosing period. Cesarean section observations revealed that there was a statistically significant increase in the percentage of postimplantation loss and a significant decrease in the percentage of live fetuses per dam at the 10 and 120 mg/kg dose levels, but not at the 40 mg/kg dose level. It is possible that the effects observed at the 10 mg/kg dose level were statistical anomalies, but this remains unconfirmed in the absence of a review of the individual data, which were not available. All other parameters in the 10 mg/kg group were comparable to controls, including the total number of live fetuses and live fetuses per dam. Since there were no statistically significant changes in Cesarean section observations in the 40 mg/kg group, it is likely that the statistically significant changes in percentage of live fetuses per dam and the percentage of postimplantation loss in the 10 mg/kg group are not treatment-related. The only abnormal finding observed during the macroscopic examination of the fetuses was meningocele (hernial protrusion of the meniges through a bony defect) in two fetuses from one litter in the 120 mg/kg dose group. Since this is a rare finding that was not present in historical controls, this anomaly was considered to be treatment-related. Skeletal evaluations of the fetuses revealed an increased incidence of variations and a delay in the development of fetuses in the 40 and 120 mg/kg dose groups. Fetal weights were significantly reduced in the 120 mg/kg group. The NOEL for fetal and maternal effects was 10 mg/kg.

In another rat developmental toxicity study (Tinston, 1993) groups of pregnant rats were administered metam-sodium at dose levels of 0, 5, 20, or 60 mg/kg/day on Days 7–16 (inclusive) of gestation. Maternal toxicity evidenced by reduced body weight gain, reduced food consumption, and the presence of clinical signs (piloerection, salivation, and urinary incontinence) occurred at the 20 and 60 mg/kg/day dose levels. Body weight gain and food consumption were marginally reduced at the 5 mg/kg/day dose level but there were no treatment-related clinical signs. In both the 20 and 60 mg/kg/day dose groups

Table 87.1
Summary of Metam-Sodium No Observed Effect Levels (NOELs) and Lowest Observed Effect Levels (LOELs)

Study	Species	Dosing duration	Dose levels	NOEL	LOEL effects
90-day drinking water	Mouse	90 days	0, 0.018, 0.088, 0.35, and 0.62 mg/ml	0.018 mg/ml	0.088 mg/ml • urinary bladder lesions
			0, 2.7, 11.7, 52.4, and 78.7 mg/kg/day (♂)	2.7 mg/kg/day	• decreases in hemoglobin, RBC, and hematocrit
			0, 3.6, 15.2, 55.4, and 83.8 mg/kg/day (♀)	3.6 mg/kg/day	
90-day drinking water	Rat	90 days	0, 0.018, 0.089, and 0.443 mg/ml	0.018 mg/ml	0.089 mg/ml • decreased body weight and body weight gain
			0, 1.7, 8.1, and 26.9 mg/kg/day (♂)	1.7 mg/kg/day	• decreases in RBC and hematocrit
			0, 2.5, 9.3, and 30.6 mg/kg/day (♀)	2.5 mg/kg/day	
90-day oral	Dog	90 days	0, 1, 5, and 10 mg/kg/day	1 mg/kg/day ♂	♂ 5 mg/kg/day • increased plasma ALT, AST, and ALP • hepatitis and bile duct proliferation
				<1 mg/kg/day ♀	♀ 1 mg/kg/day • increased plasma ALT • bile duct proliferation
Developmental toxicity	Rat	10 days	0, 10, 40, and 120 mg/kg/day	10 mg/kg/day	40 mg/kg/day • decreased maternal weight gain • increased fetal skeletal variations • delay in development
Developmental toxicity	Rat	10 days	0, 5, 20, and 60 mg/kg/day	5 mg/kg/day	20 mg/kg/day • decreased maternal weight gain • reduced food consumption • maternal clinical signs • increased fetal skeletal variations • reduced ossification of manus and pes • reduced fetal weights
Developmental toxicity	Rabbit	13 days	0, 10, 30, and 100 mg/kg/day	10 mg/kg/day—fetal	30 mg/kg/day—fetal • decreases in live fetuses • increased resorptions
				30 mg/kg/day—maternal	100 mg/kg/day—maternal • decreased body weight gain
Developmental toxicity	Rabbit	13 days	0, 5, 20, and 60 mg/kg/day	5 mg/kg/day	20 mg/kg/day • reduced maternal body weights • change in fetal ossification pattern

(continues)

Table 87.1

continued

Study	Species	Dosing duration	Dose levels	NOEL	LOEL effects
Multigeneration	Rat	Chronic	0, 0.01, 0.03, and 0.1 mg/ml 0, 1.2, 3.2, and 11.5 mg/kg/day (♂) 0, 1.8, 3.9, and 13.5 mg/kg/day (♀)	0.03 mg/ml—systemic 0.1 mg/ml—reproductive	0.1 mg/ml—systemic toxicity • changes in Bowman's gland and olfactory epithelium (adults) • decreased mean pup weight >0.1 mg/ml
Carcinogenicity: two-year drinking	Rat	Chronic	0, 0.019, 0.056, and 0.19 mg/ml 0, 1.3, 3.9, and 12.0 mg/kg/day (♂) 0, 2.3, 6.2, and 16.2 mg/kg/day (♀)	0.056 mg/ml	0.19 mg/ml • decreased body weight gain • decreased food consumption, food efficiency and water consumption • changes in hematology and clinical chemistry • abnormalities in nasal cavity, voluntary muscle and sciatic nerve
Carcinogenicity: two-year drinking	Mouse	Chronic	0, 0.019, 0.074, and 0.23 mg/ml 0, 1.6, 6.5, and 27.7 mg/kg/day (♂) 0, 2.3, 8.7, and 29.9 mg/kg/day (♀)	0.019 mg/ml	0.074 mg/ml • increased liver weight • changes in kidney and epididymis weights
1-year oral	Dog	Chronic	0, 0.05, 0.1, and 1.0 mg/kg/day	0.1 mg/kg/day	1.0 mg/kg/day • increase in hepatocyte and liver macrophage/ Kupffer cells • increased plasma ALT
Acute neurotoxicity	Rat	Single dose	0, 22, 324, and 647 mg/kg	<22 mg/kg	22 mg/kg • reduced ambulatory and total motor activity
Subchronic neurotoxicty	Rat	13 weeks	0, 0.02, 0.06, and 0.2 mg/ml 0, 1.4, 5.0, and 12.8 mg/kg/day (♂) 0, 2.3, 7.0, and 15.5 mg/kg/day (♀)	0.06 mg/ml (♂) 0.02 mg/ml (♀)	0.2 mg/ml (♂) 0.06 mg/ml (♀) • decreased body weight gain

there was an increase in fetal effects (reduced fetal weights, reduced ossification of *manus* and *pes*, and increased incidences of minor skeletal defects and/or variants). The no observed adverse effect level (NOAEL) for maternal toxicity or fetal effects in this study was 5 mg/kg/day.

In a teratology/developmental study (Hellwig, 1987), pregnant Himalayan rabbits were administered a 42.2% aqueous solution of metam-sodium at dose levels of 0, 10, 30, or 100 mg/kg by gavage from gestation Days 6 through 18. Evaluation of body weight data revealed a treatment-related decrease in body weight gain in the 100 mg/kg dams. There were no statistically significant treatment-related effects noted in food consumption or food efficiency. Cesarean section observations revealed statistically significant decreases in the total number of live fetuses and statistically significant increases in total resorptions in the 30 and 100 mg/kg/day groups. Macroscopic fetal examinations revealed meningocele and spina bifida in one rabbit in one litter in the 100 mg/kg/day group (it is not clear from the data if the findings were in the same rabbit or in two separate rabbits). Due to the rarity of this event and that it was also present in the rat developmental study, this abnormality is considered to be treatment-related. There were no treatment-related effects noted from the visceral examinations. Skeletal examinations revealed no treatment-related effects. However, these examinations were done using acceptable European methods that have not been validated by EPA and are not considered to be comparable with U.S. EPA-accepted methods.

In another rabbit developmental toxicity study (Hodge, 1993) groups of pregnant rabbits were administered metam-sodium at dose levels of 0, 5, 20, or 60 mg/kg/day on Days 8–20 (inclusive) of gestation. At the 60 mg/kg/day dose level, dams showed marked weight loss and reduced food consumption. At 20 mg/kg/day, body weight of dams was slightly reduced. There were no observable effects noted on dams at the 5 mg/kg/day dose level. Fetal examinations revealed a marked increase in embryonic lethality at the 60 mg/kg/day maternal dose level and changes in ossification pattern at the 20 and 60 mg/kg/day maternal dose levels. The NOAEL for maternal and developmental toxicity was 5 mg/kg/day.

In a multigeneration reproduction study (Milburn, 1993), Alpk:ApfSD rats received metam-sodium in drinking water at the following concentrations: 0, 0.01, 0.03, or 0.1 mg/ml. These concentrations corresponded to dose levels of 0, 1.2, 3.2, or 11.5 mg/kg/day for males and 0, 1.8, 3.9, or 13.5 mg/kg/day for females. After the first 10 weeks of treatment, animals were mated on a one-to-one ratio. Males were then removed from their cages and females were allowed to give birth and raise pups. At 21 days of age, pups from the parental (F0) generation were selected as parents for the F1 generation.

In parents, body weights were marginally reduced in rats receiving 0.10 mg/ml (the highest concentration tested) during the premating period and markedly reduced during pregnancy and lactation. Water consumption was reduced in the 0.10 mg/ml rats throughout the study and to a lesser extent in the 0.03 mg/ml group. In offspring, there was a marginal reduction in food consumption during the premating period in the F0 and F1 rats in the 0.10 mg/ml group, but there were no effects on food consumption in the 0.01 and 0.03 mg/ml treatment groups. Offspring body weights and total litter weights were reduced in the 0.10 mg/ml group in both generations. There were no effects on any of the reproductive parameters at any treatment level for parents or offspring. Histopathological evaluations indicated increased changes in the epithelium of the nasal passages of the F0 and F1 adult females in the 0.10 mg/ml groups. This effect was not observed in 0.10 mg/ml adult males or in male or female offspring of either generation. No treatment-related histopathological changes were observed in rats receiving metam-sodium at concentrations of 0.01 or 0.03 mg/ml.

Metam-sodium did not affect reproductive performance at any dose level tested. Evidence of toxicity was observed only at the highest concentration level tested, i.e., 0.1 mg/ml. In adult female rats receiving metam-sodium at the 0.1 mg/ml concentration level (13.5 mg/kg/day), evidence of systemic toxicity consisted of (1) duct hypertrophy of Bowman's gland with loss of alveolar cells, (2) degeneration, disorganization, and/or atrophy of the olfactory epithelium, and (3) dilation of the Bowman's gland ducts. Changes in Bowman's glands were accompanied in all affected animals by degeneration, disorganization, and/or atrophy of the olfactory epithelium. In pups in the 0.1 mg/ml group, evidence of toxicity consisted of a 14% decrease in mean pup weight on Day 22 for the F1 generation,

a 16% decrease in mean body weight gain for F2 litters, and decreases of 8–9% in testes and epididymis weight in male pups in the F1a and F2a litters. The NOEL for systemic toxicity (adults and pups) was 0.03 mg/ml. The NOEL for reproductive effects was 0.1 mg/ml (11.5 mg/kg/day for males, 13.5 mg/kg/day for females).

87.6 CHRONIC/ONCOGENICITY TOXICITY

A two-year combined chronic toxicity/carcinogenicity study demonstrated that metam-sodium shows no carcinogenic potential in rats (Thomassen, 1998; U.S. EPA, 1994b). However, a two-year carcinogenicity study in mice revealed an increased incidence of angiosarcoma in mice at higher dose levels (U.S. EPA, 1994c). A one-year study with dogs showed no evidence of carcinogenicity but evidence of liver damage similar to but less severe than the effects (that were shown to be reversible) observed in previous subchronic metam-sodium dog studies.

In a two-year combined chronic toxicity/carcinogenicity study with Wistar rats (Rattray, 1994), metam-sodium (43.14% a.i.) was administered in drinking water at concentration levels of 0, 0.019, 0.056, or 0.19 mg/ml (achieved dosages of 0, 1.3, 3.9, or 12.0 mg/kg/day for males and 0, 2.3, 6.2, or 16.2 mg/kg/day for females). There was no evidence of an adverse effect of metam-sodium on the survival or rats. There were no ophthalmological changes associated with metam-sodium treatment.

Evidence of toxicity was present in both males and females at the highest concentration level tested, i.e., 0.19 mg/ml. At 0.19 mg/ml, male and female rats had decreased mean body weight gain for Weeks 1–13 (12% for males, 16% for females) and for Weeks 1–105 (18% for males, 20% for females). Food consumption, food efficiency, and water consumption were significantly decreased for both males and females receiving 0.19 mg/ml metam-sodium. Effects were also observed in 0.19 mg/ml male and female hematology (decreased red blood cells, hemoglobin, and hematocrit) and clinical chemistry (decreased cholesterol and triglycerides). Nasal passages were identified as the target organ. Microscopic abnormalities of the nasal cavity were mainly confined to 0.19 mg/ml animals. These changes included (1) an increased incidence of rhinitis, (2) hypertrophy of Bowman's ducts/glands, (3) atrophy and adenitis of Steno's gland, and (4) hyperplasia and degeneration of olfactory epithelium. The incidence of degenerative myopathy of voluntary muscle was similar in all groups, including controls. However, there was an increase in the severity of myopathy in animals in the 0.019 mg/ml group. There was no indication of an increased incidence of neoplasia or early onset of tumors from treatment with metam-sodium. Evaluation of the tumor incidence demonstrated that metam-sodium shows no carcinogenic potential in rats (Rattray, 1994; U.S. EPA, 1994b). The NOEL for both male and female Wistar rats was 0.056 mg/ml.

The Cal EPA, Department of Pesticide Regulation evaluated the tumor data from the two-year metam-sodium drinking-water study in rats and concluded that there was a possible tumorigenic effect at the 0.056 mg/ml concentration level (U.S. EPA, 1995). According to the Cal EPA review, the incidence of hemangiosarcoma (8/64) was increased at this dose, in relation to the control incidence (0/64) and the high dose (0.19 mg/ml) incidence (3/64). The hypothesis that this could be a positive response was based on the positive findings in the two-year mouse study and that this increased incidence could be based on decreased body weight observed at the high dose in relation to other doses.

When the U.S. EPA (1995) re-evaluated the tumor data for their Carcinogenicity Classification, they did not find the effect that the Cal EPA found (presumably because the Cal EPA analysis did not exclude animals that died before observation of the first tumor). However, there was a significant pairwise comparison in the incidence of hemangiosarcoma in male rats at the 0.019 and 0.056 mg/ml (1.3 and 3.9 mg/kg/day) levels when compared to controls. The U.S. EPA also considered debatable the hypothesis of increased incidence of hemangiosarcoma at the mid-dose level based on decreased body weight in male rats at the high dose level. Rats in this study were not fed a calorie-restricted diet, nor was their access to food controlled. In addition, the decreases in body weight gain were observed for both male *and* female rats, although the preponderance of hemangiomas/hemangiosarcomas was observed only in male rats. In addition, the time to tumor formation was observed at approximately the same time in all dose levels. In calorie-restricted studies, the numbers of tumors are often reduced in conjunction with a delay in the time to tumor formation.

In response to the position taken by Cal EPA, the two-year drinking water study with Wistar rats was reviewed and compared to an expanded historical control data base for Wistar rats that at the time of their original review was not available (Thomassen, 1998). Hemangiomatous tumors (hemangioma and/or hemangiosarcoma) were observed only in rats sacrificed at termination of the study (Study Week 105) or in rats that were found dead or were euthanized due to their clinical condition (moribund or to prevent suffering). No hemangiomatous tumors were observed in rats euthanized during the interim sacrifice at Study Week 53. Therefore, tumor analysis (as was done by the U.S. EPA) should exclude animals that were sacrificed or died prior to the first observance of a hemangioma or hemangiosarcoma. Statistically significant increased incidence of hemangiosarcomas occurred only in the 0.019 and 0.056 mg/ml males and not in the 0.19 mg/ml males, although the actual numbers were very similar (3/49 at 0.019 mg/ml and 3/51 at 0.19 mg/ml). Three possible explanations for reduced tumor incidence with an increase in treatment are: (1) the high dose of metam-sodium exceeded the maximum tolerated dose and had a negative impact on the tumor response in the high dose males; (2) reduced body weight associated with reduced tumor incidence accounted for the difference (as suggested by the Cal EPA reviewer); or (3) biological variability was responsible. Neither the U.S. EPA nor the Cal EPA thought the maximum tolerated dose had been exceeded. The U.S. EPA carcinogenicity peer review panel did not believe that reduced body weight accounted for the reduced tumor incidence (U.S.

EPA, 1995). However, the possibility that biological variability could account for the effect was hampered by the lack of historical control data for Wistar rats.

Hemangiomatous tumors (variously diagnosed as angiomas and angiosarcomas, hemangiomas and hemangiosarcomas, and lymphangiomas and lymphangiosarcomas) are common in some but not all strains of Wistar rats (Bomhard, 1992; Bomhard *et al.*, 1986; Crain, 1958; Deerberg *et al.*, 1980; Kroes *et al.*, 1981; Rehm *et al.*, 1984). The reported incidences of these tumors in Wistar-derived rats used in European laboratories vary considerably, but there are reports of up to a 74% incidence for males and 44% for females (Rehm *et al.*, 1984). These reports also indicate that there is a definite propensity for development of tumors in the lymph nodes, particularly the mesenteric lymph nodes of male Wistar rats. Although Zeneca Central Toxicology Laboratory did not have an historical control data base for Wistar rats used in this study, there was a large historical control tumor data base compiled by several European laboratories utilizing Wistar-derived rats (49 studies ranging in duration from 24 to 31 months). This data base was published as the RITA Wistar Rat Control Tumor Data Base (Thomassen, 1998). Information presented in the RITA control data base is consistent with the types and numbers of tumors observed in the metam-sodium two-year rat study. Based on a thorough review of the original study and comparisons with the RITA control data base for Wistar rats, it was concluded that:

- Metam-sodium is not a carcinogen in the rat.
- The reduced number of hemangiosarcomas in the high dose male rats in the metam-sodium study is not due to reduced caloric intake.
- The natural distribution and incidence of spontaneously occurring hemangiosarcomas in untreated male Wistar rats can account for the distribution and incidence of hemangiosarcomas observed in male rats treated with metam-sodium.

In a two-year carcinogenicity study in mice (Horner, 1994), metam-sodium (43.15%) was administered in the drinking water to C57BL/10JfCD-1/Alpk mice for 104 weeks at nominal concentration levels of 0, 0.019, 0.074, or 0.23 mg/ml (actual achieved doses of 0, 1.6, 6.5, or 27.7 mg/kg/day for males and 0, 2.3, 8.7, or 29.9 mg/kg/day for females). Metam-sodium did not adversely affect survival of mice at any dose level. Clinical signs of toxicity were considered to be unremarkable. Male and female mice receiving metam-sodium at 0.074 and 0.23 mg/ml had dose-related and statistically significant increases in absolute liver weight when compared to controls (111% and 119% for 0.074 mg/ml males and females, respectively; 135% and 122% for 0.23 mg/ml mice). At 0.23 mg/ml, male mice had decreased body weight gain of 14% for Weeks 1–13 and 20% for Weeks 1–104. Food consumption was unaffected during the early part of the study, but during Weeks 24 to 52 there were statistically significant decreases in food consumption for the 0.074 and 0.23 mg/ml male mice. Decreases in food consumption were not observed for female mice. Water consumption was significantly decreased for both males and females in the 0.23 mg/ml group during the study's first week, but by Week 9, males in the 0.23 mg/ml group had significantly increased water consumption. By Week 11, water consumption was significantly increased for both 0.074 and 0.23 mg/ml males. By Week 48, water consumption for all groups (male and female) were approximately equal to controls. Hematological investigations showed no significant treatment-related effects at any dose level. Macroscopic observations revealed several changes in 0.23 mg/ml mice including liver appearance (accentuated lobular pattern, pale), subcutaneous tissue masses, urinary bladder wall thickening, and reduced incidence of enlarged seminal vesicles. Several changes were noted in liver, kidney, and epididymis weights at 0.074 and 0.23 mg/ml treatment levels. Microscopic evaluations revealed several non-neoplastic effects in 0.23 mg/ml mice but also revealed evidence of neoplastic changes at this same dose level.

There was evidence of dose-dependent metam-sodium induced carcinogenicity in mice. In both males and females at the 0.23 mg/ml treatment level, there was an increased incidence of hepatic adenoma and angiosarcoma, splenic angiosarcoma, subcutaneous tissue angiosarcoma, and a single incidence of a urinary bladder transitional cell papilloma in one high dose male and a single incidence of urinary bladder transitional cell carcinoma in one high dose female. The overall incidence of angiosarcoma, regardless of site, increased for both males and females in the 0.23 mg/ml treatment group when compared to concurrent as well as historical controls. The no observed effect level for neoplastic changes is 0.074 mg/ml.

According to the U.S. EPA (1994c), there was equivocal evidence of a possible increase in splenic angiosarcoma at 0.074 mg/ml [something that the study author and registrants believe is related to the difficulty in determining the primary site(s) of angiosarcoma]. There was no evidence of increased tumors at the lowest dose level. In the U.S. EPA's (1994c) evaluation of the two-year mouse study, the reviewers suggested that the dosing levels in this study were adequate due to the degree of toxicity (increased liver weights, non-neoplastic changes in bladder, and tumors) observed in both males and females at the 0.23 mg/ml treatment level. According to the U.S. EPA (1994c) based on the significant increase observed in liver weight in male and female mice, the LOEL is considered to be 0.074 mg/ml, which is the NOAEL for neoplastic changes.

In a one-year toxicity study (Brammer, 1994), metam-sodium was administered orally to beagle dogs at dose levels of 0, 0.05, 0.1, or 1.0 mg/kg/day. Animals were observed daily for food consumption, evidence of gastro-intestinal upset, and changes in clinical condition. Animals also received detailed clinical evaluations weekly and complete veterinary examinations (including ophthalmoscopy) every three months. Blood chemistry, hematology, urine chemistry, and cytology evaluations were conducted at regular intervals throughout the study. At study termination, each animal received a full necropsy and histopathological evaluation of selected tissues. Throughout the study, there were no overt signs of toxicity at any dose level and all dogs remained in good health. There were no toxico-

logically significant effects on body weight, food consumption, clinical condition, or on the incidence of gastro-intestinal effects (i.e., vomiting, loose stools, etc.). There were no ophthalmoscopic abnormalities nor were there significant changes in hematology or urinalysis or in organ weights. There were no macroscopic findings that could be attributed to treatment with metam-sodium. Microscopic evaluations revealed a slight increase in hepatocyte and macrophage/Kupffer cells in the liver of one female dog dosed at 1.0 mg/kg/day. This same female also had significant elevations in plasma alanine transaminase activity. These changes were similar to but less severe than those observed in previous subchronic dog studies with metam-sodium and are considered to be treatment-related. Therefore, the NOEL for this study was 0.1 mg/kg/day.

87.7 NUROTOXICITY

Metam-sodium is not neurotoxic based on evidence from neurotoxicity studies.

In an acute neurotoxicity study (Lamb, 1993), male and female Sprague–Dawley Crl : CD®BR rats received metam-sodium (43.15%) orally at doses of 0, 50, 750, or 1500 mg formulated metam-sodium/kg body weight or 0, 22, 324, or 647 mg a.i./kg. Mortality was observed at the 1500 mg/kg dose level (males 31%, females 19%). Signs of systemic toxicity were observed at the 750 and 1500 mg/kg dose levels and included changes in posture, palpebral closure, respiratory rate, arousal, rearing activity, time to first step, olfactory and pupil responses, tail pinch response, hindlimb strength, body temperature, and body weight. Lacrimation and salivation were also noted among some animals at both the 750 and 1500 mg/kg dose levels. Reductions in ambulatory and motor activity were observed at the 50 mg/kg dose level and above on Day 0 (day of dosing) yet there were no treatment-related effects on the functional observational battery in the 50 mg/kg dose group. No signs indicative of neurotoxicity were observed at any dose level. There was no significant change in brain cholinesterase (ChE) activity at any dose level and there were no signs of cholinergic effects at any dose level. There were no treatment related differences in brain weight or dimensions in any treatment group. Histopathological evaluations of brain and nervous system tissues showed no evidence of neurotoxicity.

According to the U.S. EPA (1994d), plasma and RBC ChE activity levels were reduced in 1500 mg/kg male and female rats 24 hours postdose (6% and 12% for male plasma and RBC ChE, respectively; 24% and 14% for females). [Although statistically significant, none of these decreases in ChE activity are considered to be biologically relevant as all decreases are well within the range of normal variation and are below the thresholds set by the World Health Organization (JMPR, 1995; WHO, 1990) and other regulatory agencies (Carlock et al., 1999).]

Based on the results of this study, the 1500 mg/kg dose level was considered the NOAEL in males and females for acute neurotoxicity while the 50 mg/kg/day dose level was considered the LOEL for acute systemic toxicity (based on reduced motor activity).

In a subchronic neurotoxicity study (Allen, 1991), male and female Sprague–Dawley rats were given metam-sodium (43.15%) in drinking water at concentration levels of 0, 0.02, 0.06, or 0.2 mg/ml for 13 weeks (achieved dosages of 0, 1.4, 5.0, or 12.8 mg/kg/day for males and 0, 2.3, 7.0, and 15.5 mg/kg/day for females). Male and female rats administered 0.2 mg metam-sodium/ml drinking water showed reductions in body weight, food consumption, and water consumption. Similar effects were observed in females at the 0.06 mg/ml concentration level. Body weight gain was reduced 14% for the 0.2 mg/ml males and the 0.06 mg/ml females, and 18–21% for the 0.2 mg/ml females. Food utilization was slightly reduced in males at the 0.2 mg/ml level. Reduced water consumption was also observed in males at the 0.06 mg/ml level and in females at the 0.02 mg/ml level. All of these effects were considered to be a consequence of poor potability of the drinking water rather than toxicity of metam-sodium.

A functional observational battery and comprehensive neuropathological examination of the peripheral and central nervous systems revealed no evidence of any effects attributable to treatment with metam-sodium. Since there was no evidence of a neurotoxic effect from metam-sodium, the NOAEL for neurotoxicity is 0.2 mg/ml.

87.8 OTHER STUDIES (MAMMALIAN)

In vitro percutaneous absorption of metam-sodium through rat and human skin was evaluated (Clowes, 1993). Metam-sodium was applied at dose levels of 940 and 94.0 $\mu g/cm^2$. Ten hours after dermal application, the skins were washed to determine how much of the dose could be removed from the skin surface, receptor fluid was analyzed, and the proportion of the dose remaining associated with the skin after washing and the amount absorbed were quantified. The absorption of metam-sodium was found to be dose and time dependent through both rat and human skin. The highest amount of metam-sodium absorbed was through rat skin from the 940 $\mu g/cm^2$ application (mean 200 $\mu g/cm^2$; 21.3% of the applied dose at 10 hours). A correspondingly smaller amount was absorbed from the 94.0 $\mu g/cm^2$ application through rat skin (mean 18.2 $\mu g/cm^2$; 19.4% at 10 hours). Absorption through cadaver human skin was 2.19% for the 940 $\mu g/cm^2$ dose (mean 20.6 $\mu g/cm^2$) and 12.2% (mean 11.5 $\mu g/cm^2$) of the applied dose. Absorption of metam-sodium through both rat and human skin increased with time but at a decreasing rate over the 10 hour period. The percentage of the dose remaining in the skin increased with decreasing dose. There was less metam-sodium absorbed through human skin than rat skin, and at the highest dose level there was approximately a 10-fold decrease in absorption of metam-sodium by human skin when compared to rat skin.

An *in vivo* percutaneous (dermal) absorption study in the rat (Stewart, 1992) showed that metam-sodium and/or its radiolabeled degradation products are only poorly absorbed following a single dermal application to the rat. Radiolabeled ^{14}C metam-sodium was applied to male rats in aqueous solution at nominal dose levels of 0.1, 1, and 10 mg/animals. A glass saddle containing an activated charcoal filter to adsorb any volatile radioactivity evaporating from the skin surface protected the application site. Four animals from each group were evaluated at 1, 2, 10, and 24 hours after treatment for radioactivity in the excrement, in and on the skin, and in the body. Another four animals per group had the treatment area washed 10 hours after administration. Radioactivity in the excrement was monitored over a total of 72 hours prior to evaluations of the skin and body. Overall mean recoveries of radioactivity were in the range of 83.5 to 95.7% of the applied dose. The extent of absorption was similar at each dose level with an overall mean of approximately 3%. In general, absorption increased with time. Levels of absorbed material 24 hours postapplication for the 0.1, 1, and 10 mg/animal dose levels were approximately 7.5, 50, and 231 μg equivalents of ^{14}C metam-sodium, respectively. Substantial quantities of the nonabsorbed dose were recovered from the charcoal, suggesting that metam-sodium or its degradation products are highly volatile. At the 0.1, 1, and 10 mg/animal dose levels, the amounts of metam-sodium absorbed over a 10 hour exposure period were 2.4, 3.7, and 1.5% of the applied dose, respectively. Absorbed radioactivity was either eliminated in urine or exhaled and subsequently trapped in expired air traps. Less than 0.7% of the applied dose was recovered in feces and the recovery of radioactivity from the carcass ranged from below the limit of detection to 1.2%. Following applications of metam-sodium at 1 and 10 mg/animal, concentrations of radioactivity in blood and plasma peaked at one hour postdose. Levels of radioactivity in blood and plasma in the 0.1 mg/animal group were below the limit of detection. This study showed that (1) metam-sodium is poorly absorbed following a single dermal application; (2) absorbed radioactivity is rapidly excreted, primarily via the urine and expired air; and (3) washing the application site with soap and water effectively removes the majority of the applied dose.

A further dermal absorption study with metam-sodium showed that absorption for rats was only 2.5% of the applied dose (U.S. EPA, 1994a). Radiolabeled ^{14}C metam-sodium was applied to shaved dorso-lumbar skin sites of rats at concentrations of 8.6, 86.2, or 862 $\mu g/cm^2$. Animals were exposed to metam-sodium for 1, 2, 10, 24, or 72 hours. At the end of the study, total dermal absorption after 72 hours was determined to be 2.5% of total applied dose.

Since metam-sodium is poorly absorbed dermally, human skin surfaces are acidic, and sweat is approximately pH5, metam-sodium that may come in contact with skin is expected to rapidly degrade prior to absorption.

87.9 METABOLISM

After oral ingestion, metam-sodium is rapidly absorbed, metabolized, and excreted from the body. Exhalation and excretion in the urine are the major elimination pathways after oral exposure. Metam-sodium is poorly absorbed following dermal application but the metam-sodium that is absorbed is rapidly excreted, primarily through the urine and expired air.

In study of biokinetics and metabolism, radiolabeled metam-sodium [^{14}C] (purity > 99%) was administered to Sprague–Dawley rats at dose levels of 10 or 100 mg/kg (Hawkins *et al.*, 1987). Blood, urine, and feces were tested for radioactivity for up to seven days postdosing while expired air was collected up to 72 hours postdose. The results of this study showed that metam-sodium was rapidly and completely absorbed after oral ingestion. Radioactivity in plasma reached a maximum level in 1 hour and decreased to near background levels by 24 hours. Animals receiving [^{14}C] metam-sodium at 10 mg/kg eliminated approximately 25% of the total radioactivity through the urine during the first 8 hours. By 168 hours, 55% of the total activity had been eliminated through the urine and 3–4% through feces. At the 100 mg/kg dose, 18% of the total activity had been eliminated in the urine by 8 hours and 40% by 168 hours. Within 24 hours, expired air from 10 mg/kg rats contained approximately 32% of the radioactivity with 1% MITC, 15% carbon disulfide (CS_2)/carbonyl sulfide (COS), and 17% carbon dioxide. At 24 hours for the 100 mg/kg dose level, expired air contained approximately 48% of the total radioactivity with 24% MITC, 18% CS_2/COS, and 6% CO_2. Negligible amounts of radiolabeled material were expired from 24 to 72 hours at either dose level. Approximately 98% of the radioactivity had been eliminated by the seventh day, with only 2% of the activity remaining in the tissues. The highest concentration of radioactivity was found in the thyroid, but significant concentrations were also found in the liver, kidneys, and lungs.

Analysis of the urinary metabolites found that glutathione conjugation with MITC is the source of the major urinary metabolite, *N*-acetyl-*S*-(*N*-methylthiocarbamoyl)-l-cysteine, which accounted for 21% of the excreted dose. No evidence for glucuronide or sulfate conjugates of the metabolites of metam-sodium was found. Based on the results of this study, it appears that metam-sodium degrades to either CS_2 or MITC in the stomach (accelerated by the stomach pH). MITC is eliminated either through exhalation or in the urine after glutathione conjugation in the liver. CS_2 is eliminated by exhalation or further metabolized in the liver to CO_2 prior to elimination. Therefore, two different metabolic pathways, CS_2 metabolism and MITC conjugation, are involved in urinary elimination. At higher dose levels, saturation of the metabolic processes results in greater exhalation of unmetabolized products.

The *in vivo* dermal absorption study conducted by Stewart (1992), which was described previously, further demonstrated that (1) metam-sodium is poorly absorbed following a single dermal application; (2) absorbed radioactivity is rapidly excreted, primarily via the urine and expired air; and (3) washing the application site with soap and water effectively removes the majority of the applied dose. In both this study and the Hawkins *et al.* (1987) metabolism study, peak blood and plasma radioactivity levels occurred one hour after dosing.

REFERENCES

Allen (1991).

Bomhard, E. (1992). Frequency of spontaneous tumors in Wistar rats in 3-month studies. *Exp. Toxic. Pathol.* **44**, 381–392.

Bomhard, E., Karbe, E., and Loesser, E. (1986). Spontaneous tumors of 2000 Wistar TNO/W.70 rats in two-year carcinogenicity studies. *J. Environ. Path. Toxicol. Oncol.* **7**, 35–52.

Brammer, A. (1992). "Metam-Sodium: 90-Day Oral Dosing Study in Dogs." Unpublished study (Rep. CTL/P/3679) conducted by Zeneca Central Toxicology Laboratory, Alderley Park, Macclesfield, Cheshire, UK. Submitted by Metam-sodium Task Force.

Brammer, A. (1993). "Metam-Sodium: Assessment of Recovery in Dogs." Unpublished study (Rep. CTL/L/5204) conducted by Zeneca Central Toxicology Laboratory, Alderley Park, Macclesfield, Cheshire, UK. Submitted by Metam-sodium Task Force.

Brammer, A. (1994). "Metam-Sodium: 1-Year Oral Toxicity Study in Dogs." Unpublished study (Rep. CTL/P/4196) conducted by Zeneca Central Toxicology Laboratory, Alderley Park, Macclesfield, Cheshire, UK. Submitted by Metam-sodium Task Force.

Carlock, L. L., Chen, W. L., Gordon, E. B., Killeen, J. C., Manley, A., Meyer, L. S., Mullin, L. S., Pendino, K. J., Percy, A., Sargent, D. E., Seaman, L. R., Svanborg, N. K., Stanton, R. H., Tellone, C. I., and Van Goethem, D. L. (1999). Regulating and assessing risks of cholinesterase-inhibiting pesticides: Divergent approaches and interpretations. *J. Toxicol. Environ. Health. B* **2**, 105–160.

Clowes, H. M. (1993). "Metam Sodium: *In Vitro* Absorption through Rat and Human Skin." Unpublished study (Rep. CTL/P/4118) conducted by Zeneca Central Toxicology Laboratory, Alderley Park, Macclesfield, Cheshire, UK. Submitted by Metam-sodium Task Force.

Crain, R. C. (1958). Spontaneous tumors in the Rochester strain of the Wistar rat. *Amer. J. Pathol.* **34**, 311–335.

Deerberg, F., Rapp, K., Rehm, S., and Pitterman, W. (1980). Genetic and environmental influences on lifespan and diseases in Han : Wistar rats. *Mech. Ageing Devel.* **14**, 333–343.

Hawkins, D. B., Elsom, L. F., and Girkin, G. (1987). "The Biokinetics and Metabolism of ^{14}C-Metam in the Rat." Unpublished study conducted by Huntingdon Research Centre, UK. Submitted by BASF Corporation, Research Triangle Park, NC.

Hellwig, J. (1987). "Report on the Study of the Prenatal Toxicity of Metam-Sodium (Aqueous Solution) in Rabbits after Oral Administration (Gavage)." Unpublished study (Project 38R0232/8579) conducted by BASF Aktiengesellschaft, Federal Republic of Germany. Submitted by BASF Corporation Chemicals Division, Parsippany, NJ.

Hellwig, J., and Hildebrand, B. (1987). "Report on the Study of the Prenatal Toxicity of Metam-Sodium in Rats after Oral Administration (Gavage)." Unpublished study (Rep. 87/0128) conducted by BASF Aktiengesellschaft, West Germany. Submitted by BASF Corporation, Research Triangle Park, NC.

Hodge, M. C. E. (1993). "Metam Sodium: Developmental Toxicity Study in the Rabbit." Unpublished study (Rep. CTL/P/4035) conducted by Zeneca Central Toxicology Laboratory, Alderley Park, Macclesfield, Cheshire, UK. Submitted by Metam-sodium Task Force.

Horner, S. A. (1994). "Metam-Sodium: Two Year Drinking Study in Mice." Unpublished study (Rep. CTL/P/4095) conducted by Zeneca Central Toxicology Laboratory, Cheshire, UK. Submitted by Metam-sodium Task Force.

JMPR (Joint Meeting on Pesticide Registrations, World Health Organization) (1995). "Pesticide Residues in Food—1995." FAO Plant Production and Protection Paper 133, p. 4.

Jowa, L. (1998). Metam: Animal toxicology and human risk assessment. *In* "Toxicology and Risk Assessment: Principles, Methods, and Applications" (A. M. Fan and L. W. Chang, eds.), p. 619. Dekker, New York.

Klaassen, C. D. (1986). Chapter 2: Principles of toxicology. *In* "Cassarett and Doull's Toxicology: The Basic Science of Poisons" (C. D. Klaassen, M. O. Amdur, and J. Doull, eds.), pp. 11–32. McGraw–Hill, New York.

Kroes, R., Garbis-Berkvens, J. M., de Vries, T., and van Nesselrooy, H. J. (1981). Histopathological profile of a Wistar rat stock including a survey of the literature. *J. Gerontol.* **36**, 259–279.

Lamb, I. C. (1993). "An Acute Neurotoxicity Study of Metam-Sodium in Rats (Definitive)." Unpublished study (Study WIL-188009) conducted by WIL Research Laboratories, Inc., Ashland, OH. Submitted by Metam-sodium Task Force, Los Angeles, CA.

Liggett, M. P., and McRae, L. A. (1991). "Skin Irritation to Rabbits with Metam-Sodium." Unpublished study (Study 90997D/UCB 368/SE) conducted by Huntingdon Research Centre, Ltd., UK. Submitted by UCB Chemicals Corporation, Norfolk, VA.

Mackay (1996).

Merck (1989). Metham sodium. *In* "The Merck Index" (S. Budavari, M. L. O'Neil, A. Smith, and P. E. Heckelman, eds.), 11th ed., p. 937. Merck, Rahway, NJ.

Milburn, G. M. (1993). "Metam Sodium: Multigeneration Study in the Rat." Unpublished study (Rep. CTL/P/3788) conducted by Zeneca Central Toxicology Laboratory, Alderley Park, Macclesfield, Cheshire, UK.

Padgett, E. L., Barnes, D. B., and Pruett, S. B. (1992). Disparate effects of representative dithiocarbamates on selected immunological parameters *in vivo* and cell survival *in vitro* in female B6C3F1 mice. *J. Toxicol. Environ. Health* **37**, 559–571.

Parcell, B. I., and Denton, S. M. (1991). "Delayed Contact Hypersensitivity in the Albino Guinea Pig." Unpublished report (Rep. 901002D/UCB370/SS) conducted by Huntingdon Research Centre, Ltd., UK. Submitted by UCB Chemicals Corporation, Norfolk, VA.

Pruett, S. B., Barnes, D. B., Han, Y. C., and Munson, A. E. (1992). Immunotoxicological characteristics of sodium methyldithiocarbamate. *Fund. Appl. Toxicol.* **18**, 40–47.

Rattray, N. J. (1994). "Metam-Sodium: Two Year Drinking Study in Rats." Unpublished study (Project PR0838) conducted by Zeneca Central Toxicology Laboratory, Cheshire, UK. Submitted by Metam-sodium Task Force.

Rehm, S., Deerberg, F., and Rapp, K. G. (1984). A comparison of life-span and spontaneous tumor incidence of male and female Han : WIST virgin and retired breeder rats. *Lab. Anim. Sci.* **34**, 458–464.

Stewart, F. P. (1992). "Metam-Sodium: *In Vivo* Percutaneous Absorption Study in the Rat." Unpublished study (Report 7268-38/142) conducted by Hazleton UK, Harrogate, North Yorkshire, UK.

Thomassen, R. W. (1998). "Review of the 2-Year Drinking Water Study with Metam-Sodium in the Wistar Rat." Unpublished report submitted to the California Office of Environmental Health Hazard Assessment. Reviewed with California Office of Environmental Health Hazard Assessment at a conference on July 29, 1998.

Tinston, D. J. (1993). "Metam Sodium: Developmental Toxicity Study in the Rat." Unpublished study (Report CTL/P/4052) conducted by Zeneca Central Toxicology Laboratory, Alderley Park, Macclesfield, Cheshire, UK.

United States Environmental Protection Agency (U.S. EPA) (1991). "Metam-Sodium—Review of Two Developmental Toxicity Studies in Rats and Rabbits Submitted by the Registrant." Memorandum from Y. M. Ioannou to S. Lewis.

United States Environmental Protection Agency (U.S. EPA) (1992). "Metam-Sodium—Review of a 90-Day Study in Mice." Memorandum from Y. M. Ioannou to S. Lewis.

United States Environmental Protection Agency (U.S. EPA) (1993). "Sodium *N*-Methyldithiocarbamate (Metam-Sodium)." Memorandum from T. F. McMahon to A. Mehta.

United States Environmental Protection Agency (U.S. EPA) (1994a). "Worker and Residential/Bystander Risk Assessment of Metam-sodium During Soil Applications." Memorandum from A. Mehta to J. Ellenberger and J. Housenger.

United States Environmental Protection Agency (U.S. EPA) (1994b). "Metam-Sodium: Review of a Chronic Toxicity/Carcinogenicity Study in Rats and Chronic Toxicity Study in Dogs Submitted by the Registrant." Memorandum from T. F. McMahon to T. Myers.

United States Environmental Protection Agency (U.S. EPA) (1994c). "Metam-Sodium: Review of a Mouse Carcinogenicity Study Submitted under FIFRA Section 6(a)(2) by the Registrant." Memorandum from T. F. McMahon to T. Myers.

United States Environmental Protection Agency (U.S. EPA) (1994d). "Metam-Sodium: Review of an Acute Neurotoxicity Study Submitted by the Registrant." Memorandum from T. F. McMahon to T. Myers.

United States Environmental Protection Agency (U.S. EPA) (1994e). "Metam-Sodium: Review of a Subchronic Neurotoxicity Study in Rats." Memorandum from T. F. McMahon to T. Myers.

United States Environmental Protection Agency (U.S. EPA) (1995). "Carcinogenicity Peer Review of Metam-Sodium." Memorandum from T. F. McMahon and E. Rinde to L. Cole and T. Myers.

United States Environmental Protection Agency (U.S. EPA) (1997). "Case Study—Methyl Bromide Alternative: Metam-Sodium as an Alternative to Methyl Bromide for Fruit and Vegetable Production." US EPA document posted at http://earth1.epa.gov/ozone/mbr/metams.htm.

Whiles, A. J. (1991). "Metam-Sodium: 90-Day Drinking Water Study in Mice with a 28-Day Interim Kill." Unpublished Report (Rep. CTL/P/3185) conducted at ICI Central Toxicology Laboratory, Alderley Park, Macclesfield, Cheshire, UK.

World Health Organization (WHO) (1990). "Environmental Health Criteria 104. Principles for the Toxicological Assessment of Pesticide Residues in Food." International Program on Chemical Safety, World Health Organization, Geneva.

Sulfuryl Fluoride

Kenneth D. Nitschke

The Dow Chemical Company

David L. Eisenbrandt

Dow AgroSciences LLC

88.1 CHEMISTRY AND FORMULATIONS

Sulfuryl fluoride, SO_2F_2, is manufactured and sold under the trade name Vikane* Gas Fumigant. The CAS registry no. is 2699-79-8. The molecular weight of sulfuryl fluoride is 102.07 and it is a colorless, odorless gas with a melting point of $-135.82°C$ and a boiling point of $-55.38°C$. The vapor pressure is 13×10^3 Torr at 25°C. The solubility in water is 0.75 g/kg at 25°C. Sulfuryl fluoride is of low solubility in most organic solvents but is miscible with methyl bromide. It is stable and noncorrosive by DOT definitions. Sulfuryl fluoride is not hydrolyzed by water but is hydrolyzed by NaOH solution.

88.2 USES

Since first marketed in 1961 as Vikane gas fumigant, sulfuryl fluoride has been used to fumigate over one million buildings, including houses, museums, historical landmarks, rare book libraries, government archives, and scientific and medical research laboratories (Dow AgroSciences, 1997). Initial concentrations in fumigated structures are typically 2000–4000 ppm although other concentrations may be used depending upon the target pest to be controlled, temperature, and the length of the exposure period. Sulfuryl fluoride can be used to control a wide variety of household pests, including cockroaches, rodents, clothes moths, bedbugs, and carpet beetles.

The activity of sulfuryl fluoride is dependent on the concentration reaching the target pest and the duration of exposure. Insect eggs require a higher dosage of sulfuryl fluoride compared to postembryonic life stages. Since the immature stages of some insects, such as termites and ants, cannot survive without adult care, dosages substantially less than required for egg control are effective.

Prior to fumigation with sulfuryl fluoride, a small amount of chloropicrin is introduced into the structure to warn people and animals that the structure is being fumigated (Dow AgroSciences, 1997). Chloropicrin has a noticeable disagreeable pungent odor at less than 1 ppm and causes irritation of the eyes, tears, and noticeable discomfort. Since chloropicrin diffuses from structures more slowly than sulfuryl fluoride, building occupants may experience eye irritation immediately after entering previously fumigated buildings.

The ACGIH threshold limit value and OSHA permissible exposure level for sulfuryl fluoride are 5 ppm TWA, 10 ppm STEL (ACGIH, 1998).

88.3 HAZARD IDENTIFICATION—TOXICITY TO LABORATORY ANIMALS (PRE-1980)

88.3.1 ACUTE TOXICITY

Liquid sulfuryl fluoride directly contacting skin can result in frostbite (Torkelson *et al.*, 1966). Animals exposed to lethal doses of sulfuryl fluoride had tremors and convulsions. The convulsions were characterized by stiffening of the animal to a very rigid position and then toppling over backward. Excessive salivation, loss of bladder control, and chromodacryorrhea were observed also. A 1 hour LC_{50} in male and female rats was 3020 and 3730 ppm, respectively (Vernot *et al.*, 1977).

88.3.2 SUBCHRONIC TOXICITY

Lung, kidney, and liver microscopic changes were observed within 3 weeks in rats, guinea pigs, and rabbits exposed to 400 ppm sulfuryl fluoride for 7 hours/day, 5 days/week (Torkelson, 1959). In studies at 20, 50, 100, 150, and 200 ppm for up to 6 months, lung pathology was the most significant effect observed. In addition, slight central lobular degeneration and vacuolation of the liver and slight cloudy swelling of the tubular epithelium of the kidney were observed. Increased levels of fluoride in the blood, lungs, bone, and teeth as well as fluorosis of the teeth were observed.

Groups of male and female rats (10/sex/dose) were maintained for 66 days on diets fumigated with 0 (control), 2, 10, 100, or 200 pounds/1000 cu. ft. of sulfuryl fluoride (Lockwood,

1958). The animals were weighed twice weekly for the first 28 days and then once a week thereafter and food consumption was recorded for the first month. They were observed frequently for gross changes in appearance or behavior and the teeth were examined for visual evidence of fluorosis. Samples of urine were obtained from all male rats for fluoride analysis. Terminal hematological values were obtained from five female rats in the 0, 2, and 10 pounds/1000 cu. ft. levels and from two male rats at each dietary level. Animals were autopsied at study termination and the lungs, heart, liver, kidneys, spleen, and testes were weighed. Portions of these organs as well as pancreas and adrenals were preserved and prepared for histological examination. Two additional rats of each sex were included in each dose group for collection of samples at 30 days of blood, urine (male), kidney, lung, liver, and bones and subsequent analysis for fluorides.

Control diets averaged 36 ppm of fluoride while diets fumigated with 2, 10, 100, or 200 pounds/1000 cu. ft. sulfuryl fluoride contained 55, 89, 386, or 740 ppm fluoride, respectively. Male and female rats tolerated a diet fumigated with sulfuryl fluoride at the rate of 2 pounds/1000 cu. ft. with no evidence of adverse effects, although fluoride content of bone was increased somewhat. Diets fumigated with higher levels of sulfuryl fluoride resulted in retardation of growth and evidence of fluorosis in the teeth. The severity of the effects was directly proportional to the fluoride content of the diet. Fluoride analysis of urine and bones showed increased amounts of fluorides in proportion to the amount of sulfuryl fluoride exposure to the diet (in males, concentration of fluoride in bone was 260, 408, 413, 1615, and 1920 ppm and in urine was 9.9, 11.9, 13.3, 85.6, and 174.4 ppm for diets containing 36, 55, 89, 386, or 740 ppm fluoride, respectively); analysis of blood, kidney, lung, and liver for fluorides was inconsistent with dosage levels.

88.4 TOXICITY TO LABORATORY ANIMALS (POST-1980)

88.4.1 ACUTE TOXICITY

The 4 hour LC_{50} in male and female Fischer 344 rats was 1122 and 991 ppm, respectively (Miller *et al.*, 1980). Gross pathologic changes were observed primarily in the upper and lower respiratory tract. Histopathologic examination of animals exposed to 1200–1250 ppm revealed liver and kidney and possibly lung, heart, and spleen effects. Animals that survived for two weeks following exposure to 1200–1250 ppm exhibited regenerative responses in the kidney. The highest concentration at which all animals survived was 450 ppm for males and 790 ppm for females.

B6C3F1 mice were exposed to 400, 600, or 1000 ppm for 4 hours (Nitschke and Lomax, 1989). All animals died within 90 minutes after termination of the exposure to 1000 ppm and within 6 days following exposure to 600 ppm. Body tremors were observed in several female mice shortly after exposure to 600 ppm and animals surviving after the exposure period were

lethargic prior to death. There were no clinically visible effects noted in mice exposed to 400 ppm. In the B6C3F1 mouse, the 4-hour LC_{50} was between 400 and 600 ppm for both males and females.

CD-1 mice were exposed to 600, 700, or 800 ppm for 4 hours to determine the LC_{50} (Nitschke and Quast, 1990). Effects noted in the CD-1 mouse were similar to those observed in the B6C3F1 mouse, but they occurred at slightly higher concentrations. The 4-hour LC_{50} was 660 and 642 ppm for males and females, respectively.

Acute dermal exposure to sulfuryl fluoride was evaluated in rats exposed to 1000 or 9600 ppm for 4 hours (Bradley *et al.*, 1990). These concentrations are 1 and 10 times greater than the 4-hour LC_{50} in rats identified by Miller *et al.* (1980). The exposures occurred in a Rochester-type chamber equipped with a door modified to allow the head of rats to protrude outside of the chamber. In the door, an elastic dental dam surrounded the neck of the rats and served as a barrier between the chamber air containing sulfuryl fluoride and the breathing air outside of the chamber. In addition, the backs of the rats were shaved prior to exposure to maximize dermal exposure. The only clinical effects during the exposure were chromodacryorrhea and fecal soiling. The incidence of chromodacryorrhea and fecal soiling was comparable between the two exposure groups and the effects were considered to be stress related, due to the method of restraint used during the exposure. There was no evidence of body tremors in these rats. Histopathologic examination of the skin and brain revealed no treatment-related lesions. Thus the dermal route does not appear to play a significant role in the toxicity of sulfuryl fluoride.

88.4.2 NEUROTOXICITY

Rats were exposed to 0, 100, or 300 ppm sulfuryl fluoride for 6 hours/day for 2 consecutive days (Albee *et al.*, 1993). A functional observational battery, grip performance, landing foot splay, motor activity, and a battery of electrodiagnostic tests, including flash evoked potentials, somatosensory evoked potentials, and auditory brainstem responses, were conducted pre- and postexposure. Except for motor activity data, postexposure data were collected within 5 hours after the second exposure. Motor activity data were collected 18 hours after exposure. There were no exposure-related effects in any of the parameters.

88.4.3 TIME TO INCAPACITATION

In an effort to understand the mode of action of sulfuryl fluoride, rats were exposed to 4000, 10,000, 20,000, or 40,000 ppm to determine the time to incapacitation (Nitschke *et al.*, 1986). Rats were exposed to sulfuryl fluoride in a 14 liter cylindrical chamber equipped with a motor-driven activity wheel. Animals were forced to walk on the activity wheel for designated intervals during the exposure. Exposures were terminated when incapacitation or convulsions occurred. All rats either died or were moribund within 3 hours following the end of the exposure. At the two highest concentrations, 20,000 and 40,000 ppm, rats were incapacitated within 12 minutes and died within 10 minutes after terminating exposure. At 10,000 ppm, rats were incapacitated after 16 minutes and, at 4000 ppm, rats were incapacitated after 40 minutes. At the lowest concentration, the mean survival time was 2.5 hours after incapacitation occurred. Animals exposed to 10,000 ppm and higher appeared to be slightly cyanotic shortly after exposure occurred. The bluish skin discoloration disappeared within 10 minutes after purging the chamber with room air following exposure to 10,000 ppm. The skin discoloration did not appear to be reversible at higher concentrations. The cause of death at all concentrations appeared to be cardiovascular failure and acute death. Pulmonary congestion increased in severity as the concentration of the test chemical was increased in the atmosphere and at the two highest exposure concentrations, the pulmonary lesions appeared to contribute significantly to the death of the animals. At the two lowest concentrations, the pulmonary effects were not severe enough to be the major factor in the death of these animals (Nitschke *et al.*, 1986).

The lungs of rats exposed to 4000 or 20,000 ppm sulfuryl fluoride until incapacitation occurred were examined by light and electron microscopy (Eisenbrandt *et al.*, 1987). Histopathologic examination of the lungs from rats exposed to 4000 ppm revealed minimal congestion, edema, and hemorrhage. Rats exposed to 20,000 ppm had more severe changes. Swelling and focal disruptions in alveolar epithelial cells were observed by electron microscopic examination of the lung. In addition, multifocal destruction of the alveolar wall with associated thrombosis was present in the lungs of rats exposed to 20,000 ppm. Both concentrations increased permeability of the alveolar wall as evidenced by the presence of edema, red blood cells, and fibrin in alveoli and interstitial spaces.

In another study to understand the mode of action of sulfuryl fluoride, rats were exposed to 4000 or 10,000 ppm sulfuryl fluoride to determine the effect on respiration (Landry and Streeter, 1983). Respiratory frequency as well as tidal and minute volume were measured at 1 minute intervals for 10 minutes prior to exposure and during a 20 minute exposure. At 4000 ppm, there was a rapid initial increase in mean respiratory frequency and a decrease in mean tidal volume and mean minute volume relative to pre-exposure values. These respiratory parameters peaked after 2 minutes of exposure; there was a 39% increase in frequency, a 40% decrease in tidal volume, and a 23% decrease in minute volume. After approximately 10 minutes of exposure, frequency and tidal volume were near pre-exposure levels. These effects were considered to be insufficient to have resulted in mortality.

Body temperature, heart rate, blood pressure, and electroencephalogram were monitored in rats exposed to 4000 or 20,000 ppm sulfuryl fluoride until rats expired (Gorzinski and Streeter, 1985). At 4000 and 20,000 ppm animals survived for 79 and 14 minutes, respectively. A decrease in heart rate, a gradual increase in blood pressure, decreased respiration, occasional spiking and high frequency loss in the EEG, and power loss in the EEG were observed at both levels. All physiological parameters ceased to function at about the same time when the animals died regardless of the concentration of sulfuryl fluoride and did not help explain the cause of death in these animals.

88.4.4 THERAPEUTIC/AMELIORATION OF TOXICITY

Therapeutic treatment with calcium gluconate was evaluated because sulfuryl fluoride is extensively dehalogenated in termites (Meikle *et al.*, 1963) and the similarity of effects in the mammalian incapacitation studies suggested fluoride toxicity (Nitschke *et al.*, 1986). Rats were exposed to 4000 or 10,000 ppm sulfuryl fluoride for 45 or 16 minutes (sufficient to result in 100% lethality within 3 hours), respectively, or were treated i.p. with calcium gluconate prior to and after exposure to sulfuryl fluoride. Animals which were still alive 3 days after exposure to sulfuryl fluoride were considered to have survived. In separate groups of rats, serum fluoride levels were determined in rats exposed to sulfuryl fluoride alone or pretreated with calcium gluconate. Four of five rats pretreated with calcium gluconate prior to exposure to 4000 ppm sulfuryl fluoride survived 3 days after dosing. The other rat died 90 minutes after exposure. Treatment with calcium gluconate after exposure to sulfuryl fluoride was not effective. While survival was increased in rats pretreated with calcium gluconate, the surviving animals were extremely debilitated with no apparent protection from convulsions. Animals pretreated with calcium gluconate did not survive exposure to 10,000 ppm sulfuryl fluoride.

Administration of calcium gluconate resulted in approximately 10% increase in serum calcium levels and did not appear to affect serum fluoride or magnesium levels (Nitschke *et al.*, 1986).

Since the cause of death in rats pre- or postexposure treated with calcium gluconate appeared to be due to convulsions, rats were pretreated with one of three anticonvulsants (phenobarbital, diazepam, or diphenylhydantoin) prior to exposure to 4000 ppm sulfuryl fluoride or were treated postexposure with phenobarbital and diazepam (Nitschke *et al.*, 1986). These three anticonvulsants were selected due to their ready availability and different mechanisms of action. Phenobarbital was the most effective anticonvulsant followed by diazepam with five of five and four of five pretreated with phenobarbital and diazepam surviving exposure to 4000 ppm for 50 minutes. Diphenylhydantoin accentuated the adverse effects of sulfuryl fluoride. At higher concentrations of sulfuryl fluoride, 10,000 ppm phenobarbital was also ineffective.

88.4.5 REPEATED EXPOSURES

The study design of several repeated exposure studies followed the appropriate EPA Test Guidelines (FIFRA Guideline Nos. 82-1, 82-4, 83-1, 83-2, and 83-5). For example, the study designs for several of these studies are detailed by Eisenbrandt and Nitschke (1989) and Hanley *et al.* (1989). Briefly, animals were exposed to 99.8% pure sulfuryl fluoride for 6 hours/day, 5 days/week for various time intervals. The analytical concentrations of sulfuryl fluoride in the air were measured by infrared spectrophotometry and analytical and nominal concentrations were in very close agreement. In general, animals were observed after exposure for changes in appearance or behavior. Animals were weighed periodically. Blood samples were obtained for hematological and clinical chemistry determinations. Urine was collected from rats and various parameters were measured. Animals were sacrificed the day following the last exposure to sulfuryl fluoride. Terminal body weights and selected organ weights were recorded. All animals were examined for gross pathological alterations by a veterinary pathologist. Animals that died or were moribund prior to the scheduled sacrifice were necropsied as soon as possible. An extensive set of tissues was collected and processed for light microscopy by conventional techniques and was stained with hematoxylin and eosin. In some cases special stains were used for selected tissues.

88.4.6 SUBCHRONIC TOXICITY—MICE

Groups of 5 mice/sex were exposed to 0, 30, 100, or 300 ppm sulfuryl fluoride for 6 hours/day, 5 days/week for two weeks (Nitschke and Quast, 1995). All male mice and 4 of 5 female mice exposed to 300 ppm sulfuryl fluoride died during the second week of the study. These animals lost weight and many had tremors. Vacuoles were observed in the cerebrum and/or

Table 88.1

Serum Fluoride Levels in Mice Following 13-Week Exposure to Sulfuryl Fluoride

Concentration SO$_2$F$_2$ (ppm)	Fluoride (ppm)	
	Males	Female
0	0.107 ± 0.017	0.090 ± 0.015
10	0.112 ± 0.027	0.088 ± 0.019
30	0.156 ± 0.019	$0.132 \pm 0.020^*$
100	$0.259 \pm 0.073^*$	$0.233 \pm 0.022^*$

*Statistically different from control mean by Dunnett's test, alpha = 0.05. $N = 4$.

medulla of 8 of 10 mice exposed to 300 ppm and varied from very slight to moderate in severity. Four male and 2 female mice exposed to 100 ppm had very slight vacuoles in the cerebrum. The no-observed-effect-level (NOEL) was 30 ppm.

Groups of 14 mice/sex were exposed to 10, 30, or 100 ppm for 6 hours/day, 5 days/week for 13 weeks (Nitschke and Quast, 1993). Four animals/sex/exposure level were used to measure serum fluoride levels. In addition, tissues of these 4 animals/sex/exposure level were perfused with glutaraldehyde/formaldehyde fixative and neural tissues were examined histopathologically. Standard parameters were evaluated in the main group of 10 mice/sex/concentration. At the highest concentration, 100 ppm, there was approximately a 10% body weight decrease in male and female mice from control values. Except for elevated serum fluoride levels (Table 88.1) which

Table 88.2

Histopathologic Observations in Brains of Males Exposed to Various Concentrations of Sulfuryl Fluoride for 13 Weeks

Species	Concentration			
	Control	Low	Middle	High
Mice				
Brain—cerebrum—number of tissues examined	10	10	10	10
vacuolation caudate putamen very slight	0	0	0	7
vacuolation caudate putamen slight	0	0	0	2
vacuolation external capsule very slight	0	0	0	7
vacuolation external capsule slight	0	0	0	2
Rats				
Brain—cerebrum—number of tissues examined	10	10	10	10
vacuolation cerebrum slight	0	0	0	10
Rabbits				
Brain—cerebrum—number of tissues examined	7	7	7	7
malacia severe	0	0	0	3
vacuolation very slight	0	0	0	3
Dogs				
Brain—midbrain—number of tissues examined	4	4	4	4
vacuolation very slight	0	0	0	1

Animals were exposed to sulfuryl fluoride for 6 hrs/day, 5 days/week for 13 weeks. The low, middle, and high concentrations corresponded to targeted concentrations of 10, 30, and 100 ppm in mice, 30, 100, and 300 ppm in rats, 30, 100, and 300 ppm in rabbits, and 30, 100, and 200 ppm in dogs, respectively.

followed a dose–response relationship, there were no exposure-related effects on clinical chemistry, hematology, urinalysis, organ weight, or gross pathology.

Histopathologic examination of mice exposed to 100 ppm sulfuryl fluoride for 13 weeks revealed effects in the brain and thyroid gland (Tables 88.2 and 88.3). In the cerebrum, microvacuolation in male and female mice was observed in the external capsule and the caudate putamen. The effect was very slight to slight in severity and was bilaterally symmetrical. Microvacuoles were also observed in the region of the thalamus/hypothalamus of these animals. In this region, the microvacuoles usually extended from the external capsule and involved the adjacent amygdaloid region. There were no recognizable inflammatory or degenerative changes associated with the microvacuoles. The single male mouse from the 100 ppm group without microvacuoles in the brain died during the course of the study due to accidental trauma. Microscopic changes in the thyroid gland were characterized by very slight hypertrophy of the follicular epithelial cells associated with a decrease in the amount of colloid present. The NOEL was 30 ppm in mice exposed to sulfuryl fluoride for 6 hours/day, 5 days/week for 13 weeks.

88.4.7 SUBCHRONIC TOXICITY—RATS

Groups of five animals of each sex were exposed to 100, 300, or 600 ppm sulfuryl fluoride for 6 hr/day, 5 days/week for nine exposures in two weeks (Eisenbrandt and Nitschke, 1989). Nine of 10 rats in the 600 ppm exposure group were moribund and/or died between the second and sixth exposures. One female rat exposed to 600 ppm survived the nine exposures in the two week period. These animals had severe weight loss with body weights less than 70% of control values by the fifth exposure. Severe kidney lesions were observed in all rats exposed to 600 ppm. The papillary epithelium was necrotic over the tip of the papillae and the remainder of the epithelium was moderately hyperplastic. Subacute inflammation was associated with the necrosis and collecting ducts throughout the kidneys were dilated as a result of obstruction of the papillae. There was degeneration and necrosis of epithelial cells of the collecting ducts with regeneration of surviving epithelial cells. Several rats had mineralization at the junction of the inner and outer medulla which was accompanied by chronic interstitial inflammation in some animals. Degenerative and regenerative changes in the proximal tubules were also observed. Minimal kidney changes were observed in rats exposed to 300 ppm; there were no exposure-related kidney lesions observed in rats exposed to 100 ppm.

Severe effects were observed in the upper respiratory tract and, to a lesser extent, larynx, trachea, and lungs in the sole surviving female rat exposed to 600 ppm. Also, severe, diffuse inflammation was noted in the nasal mucosa and was accompanied by multifocal ulceration of the mucosa and slight bronchioalveolar inflammation was present in the lungs. The

Table 88.3
Histopathologic Observations in Brains of Females Exposed to Various Concentrations of Sulfuryl Fluoride for 13 Weeks

Species	Concentration			
	Control	Low	Middle	High
Mice				
Brain—cerebrum—number of tissues examined	10	10	10	10
vacuolation caudate putamen very slight	0	0	0	3
vacuolation caudate putamen slight	0	0	0	5
vacuolation external capsule very slight	0	0	0	6
vacuolation external capsule slight	0	0	0	4
Rats				
Brain—cerebrum—number of tissues examined	10	10	10	10
vacuolation cerebrum slight	0	0	0	10
Rabbits				
Brain—cerebrum—number of tissues examined	7	7	7	7
malacia severe	0	0	0	1
vacuolation very slight	0	0	0	3
vacuolation slight	0	0	0	2
vacuolation moderate	0	0	1	0
Dogs				
Brain—midbrain—number of tissues examined	4	4	4	4
vacuolation very slight	0	0	0	1

Females were exposed to same concentrations as males in Table 88.2.

NOEL was 100 ppm in rats exposed to sulfuryl fluoride for two weeks.

Groups of 10 rats/sex were exposed to 0, 30, 100, or 300 ppm for 6 hr/day, 5 days/week for 13 weeks (Eisenbrandt and Nitschke, 1989). Effects attributed to sulfuryl fluoride toxicity included mottled teeth in rats exposed to 100 or 300 ppm, decreased specific gravity of the urine, and histopathological changes in the respiratory tract, brain, and kidneys of rats exposed to 300 ppm. The respiratory tract effects consisted of very slight to severe inflammation in the nasal tissue with mucopurulent exudate in the nasal passages in the more severe cases. The more extensive inflammation was accompanied by degeneration and reactive changes in the mucosa. Slight subpleural histiocytosis also was observed in the lungs of rats exposed to 300 ppm sulfuryl fluoride.

In the brain, minimal vacuolation in the area of the caudate-putamen nuclei was observed in rats exposed to 300 ppm and was more prominent in the white fiber tracts of the internal capsule than in the adjacent neuropil (Tables 88.2 and 88.3). Special stains of the brain with LFB-PAS or Sevier Munger stain did not reveal any additional effects.

Very slight hyperplasia of the renal collecting ducts was most apparent in the outer portion of the inner zone of the medulla of most female rats exposed to 300 ppm.

As a separate part of the above mentioned 13 week study, groups of 7 rats/sex were exposed to 0, 30, 100, or 300 ppm for the same time period for the specific purpose of evaluating neurological function (Mattsson *et al.*, 1988). After 13 weeks of exposure to sulfuryl fluoride, hindlimb grip strength, observation battery, visual evoked response, cortical flicker fusion, auditory brainstem response to tone pips, auditory brainstem response to clicks, cerebellar evoked response, somatosensory evoked response, and caudal nerve action potential were measured approximately 12 hours after the last exposure to sulfuryl fluoride. All but two males and two females from the 0 and 300 ppm exposure groups were subjected to a gross pathologic examination at the end of the 13 week study. The 2 animals/sex from the 0 and 300 ppm exposure group were evaluated with an auditory brainstem response approximately 8 weeks after the last exposure to sulfuryl fluoride and then sacrificed.

Hindlimb grip strength was normal for all rats, but evoked responses were clearly altered at 300 ppm and slightly altered at 100 ppm. The principal effect was decrease in flicker fusion and a slowing of all waveforms at 300 ppm, and a slowing of the visual evoked response and the somatosensory evoked response of female rats at 100 ppm. Histopathologic changes in the brain consisted of vacuoles in the white fiber tracts of the caudate-putamen. No necrosis or neuronal destruction were noted. The two rats exposed to 300 ppm in the recovery group had normal auditory brainstem responses and normal brain histopathology. The fact that all of the evoked responses in rats exposed to 300 ppm for 13 weeks were affected suggested a widespread functional CNS effect. The electrophysiologic slowing of the evoked responses was felt to be due to some mechanism other than the minor vacuolization observed in the caudate-putamen. The NOEL was 30 ppm in rats exposed to sulfuryl fluoride for 13 weeks in the standard subchronic and neurological studies.

88.4.8 SUBCHRONIC TOXICITY—RABBITS

Groups of three rabbits of each sex were exposed to 100, 300, or 600 ppm sulfuryl fluoride for 6 hr/day, 5 days/week for nine exposures in two weeks (Eisenbrandt and Nitschke, 1989). All rabbits exposed to 600 ppm were hyperactive and one animal had a convulsion which resulted in a fractured tibia. A second rabbit had a fractured vertebra which may have been the result of a convulsion.

Treatment-related malacia (necrosis) was present in the cerebrum of all rabbits exposed to 600 ppm and one male and one female rabbit exposed to 300 ppm. Reactive gliosis and demyelination accompanied the malacia. Rabbits exposed to 300 or 600 ppm also had vacuoles in the globus pallidus and putamen as well as the external and internal capsules of the brain.

Moderate, subacute, to chronic inflammation of nasal tissues with mucopurulent exudate in the nasal cavities was observed in most rabbits exposed to 300 or 600 ppm sulfuryl fluoride. The inflammation was probably from irritation of the nasal mucosa due to the test material. At the higher concentration, acute inflammation was observed in the trachea, bronchi, and bronchioles of some rabbits and may have been treatment-related. The NOEL was 100 ppm in rabbits exposed to sulfuryl fluoride for two weeks.

In a 13 week study, groups of 7 rabbits/sex were exposed initially to 30, 100, or 600 ppm for 6 hours/day, 5 days/week (Eisenbrandt and Nitschke, 1989). After 2 weeks exposure to 600 ppm, the target concentration was reduced to 300 ppm, which resulted in an average concentration over the 13 week period of 337 ppm. The exposure concentration was reduced from 600 to 300 ppm due to convulsions observed in one male and one female. A second female rabbit exposed to 600 ppm was euthanized after eight exposures due to a fractured vertebra. No clinically visible effects were noted in rabbits exposed to 300 ppm or lower concentrations. Except for elevated serum fluoride levels which followed a dose–response relationship, there were no clinical chemistry, hematology, urinalysis, organ weight, or gross pathologic changes observed.

Histopathologic changes were noted in the nasal tissues and brain of rabbits exposed to 300 and in the nasal tissue of one male and in the brain of one female exposed to 100 ppm (Tables 88.2 and 88.3). In the nasal tissues, varying degrees of purulent nasal exudate, olfactory epithelial degeneration, and hyperplasia and hypertrophy of the respiratory epithelium in the nasal turbinates were observed. The brain changes consisted of vacuolation of the white matter at 100 ppm. In rabbits exposed to 300 ppm, malacia of the internal and external capsules, putamen, and globus pallidus were observed. Some animals exposed to 300 ppm had gliosis and/or hypertrophy of vascular endothelial cell in the same area. Special stains of the brain with LFB-PAS or Sevier Munger stain were not remarkable. The NOEL was 30 ppm in rabbits exposed to sulfuryl fluoride for 13 weeks.

88.4.9 SUBCHRONIC TOXICITY—DOGS

Groups of one male and one female dog were exposed to target concentrations of 0, 30, 100, or 300 ppm for 6 hr/day 5 day/week for nine exposures (Nitschke and Quast, 1991). At 300 ppm, infrequent intermittent episodes of tremors and tetany were observed in both dogs beginning with the fifth exposure. On test day 9, during the seventh exposure, the tremors and tetany were severe enough that the exposure was terminated after approximately 5.5 hours. Within 30 minutes after terminating the exposure, both dogs appeared to be normal. Similar clinical effects were noted during subsequent exposure periods and were rapidly reversible even during the exposure period. There were no exposure-related clinical effects in dogs exposed to 30 or 100 ppm. The female dog exposed to 300 ppm sulfuryl fluoride lost approximately 500 grams body weight over the nine exposures. Serum fluoride levels of dogs exposed to 100 or 300 ppm were approximately 2–4 fold higher than control values. Serum calcium levels measured shortly after exposure on test days 5 and 9 when the animals appeared to be clinically normal were comparable to control levels. There were no exposure-related hematological, organ weight, or gross pathological effects noted in dogs exposed to concentrations as high as 300 ppm. Minimal microscopic inflammatory changes were observed in the nasal turbinates of the male and female dog and trachea of the female dog exposed to 300 ppm. Although numerous microscopic sections were examined from the cerebral cortex, brainstem, cerebellum, and medulla oblongata, there were no histopathologic changes detected in dogs exposed to 300 ppm. The NOEL was 100 ppm in dogs exposed to sulfuryl fluoride for two weeks.

In a 13-week study, groups of four male and four female beagle dogs were exposed to 0, 30, 100, or 200 ppm sulfuryl fluoride for 6 hours/day, 5 days/week for 13 weeks (Nitschke et al., 1992). One male dog exposed to 200 ppm was laterally recumbent with tetany, tremors, salivation, and incoordination 75 minutes after exposure on test day 19. An hour later the activity of this animal was decreased relative to controls but was otherwise normal. Similar effects were not observed during the remainder of the study. After 13 weeks of exposure to sulfuryl fluoride, the mean body weight values of male and female dogs exposed to 200 ppm were 88 and 96%, respectively, of control values. Mean body weight values of male and female dogs exposed to lower concentrations of sulfuryl fluoride were comparable to control values. There were no exposure-related hematological, clinical chemistry, urinalysis, organ weight, and gross pathological effects observed. Histopathologically, a single small bilaterally symmetrical focal change was noted in the putamen of the midbrain of one male and one female dog exposed to 200 ppm (Tables 88.2 and 88.3). The minimal focal change was characterized by vacuolation, gliosis, perivascular

cuffing, and hypertrophy of endothelial cells, and individual cells showed nuclear pyknosis and karyorrhexis. The focal reaction was slightly more prominent in the male compared to the female. All other microscopic observations were considered to be incidental findings unrelated to exposure to sulfuryl fluoride. The NOEL was 100 ppm in dogs exposed to sulfuryl fluoride for 6 hours/day, 5 days/week for 13 weeks.

88.4.10 CHRONIC TOXICITY—MICE

Groups of 50 mice/sex were exposed to measured vapor concentrations of 0, 5, 20, or 80 ppm sulfuryl fluoride for 6 hours/day, 5 days/week for 18 months (Quast et al., 1993a). Ten additional mice/sex/exposure level were randomly designated as a satellite group for necropsy after 12 months of exposure to evaluate chronic toxicity. During the first year of exposure a slightly earlier onset of mortality was observed in the 80 ppm males; however, mortality at the end of the 18 months of exposure was not statistically identified as increased in any of the sulfuryl fluoride exposed groups of male mice (Fig. 88.1a). The female mortality rate during the first year of exposure was comparable in all groups (Fig. 88.1b). In both males and females exposed to 80 ppm the incidence of exudative rhinitis and aspiration pneumonia accompanied by an impacted esophagus was increased from control values.

Body weight of 80 ppm male mice was 10% lower than control values after 6 months and body weights of female mice exposed to 80 ppm were significantly decreased from control values after 1 month exposure (Fig. 88.2a and b, resp.). In general, the effect in the female mice was not as severe as in the male mice during the first 12 months. During the last several months of exposure, the body weight difference between control and high dose female mice ranged from 10–15%. The body weights of male and female mice exposed to 5 or 20 ppm were comparable to control values throughout the study.

Clinical chemistry and hematology values of male and female mice exposed to the various concentrations of sulfuryl fluoride were comparable to control values at the 12 month and terminal sacrifice. Although terminal body weight effects were observed in male and female mice exposed to 80 ppm sulfuryl fluoride for 12 or 18 months, the organ weight effects observed were considered to be due to the marked body weight differences and not indicative of target organ toxicity. There were no treatment-related gross pathological effects noted in mice at 12 months. There was a decreased incidence of normally occurring spontaneous gross lesions observed in animals exposed to 80 ppm and included a marked decrease in the incidence of cystic ovaries and cystic endometrial hyperplasia of the uterus in females and a decreased incidence of dilated kidney pelvis. Based upon the necropsy findings, there were no target organs identified in the mice after 12 or 18 months.

At the 12 month interim sacrifice, histopathologic examination of male and female mice exposed to various concentrations of sulfuryl fluoride revealed changes in the brain and thyroid gland of animals exposed to 80 ppm only. Essentially all

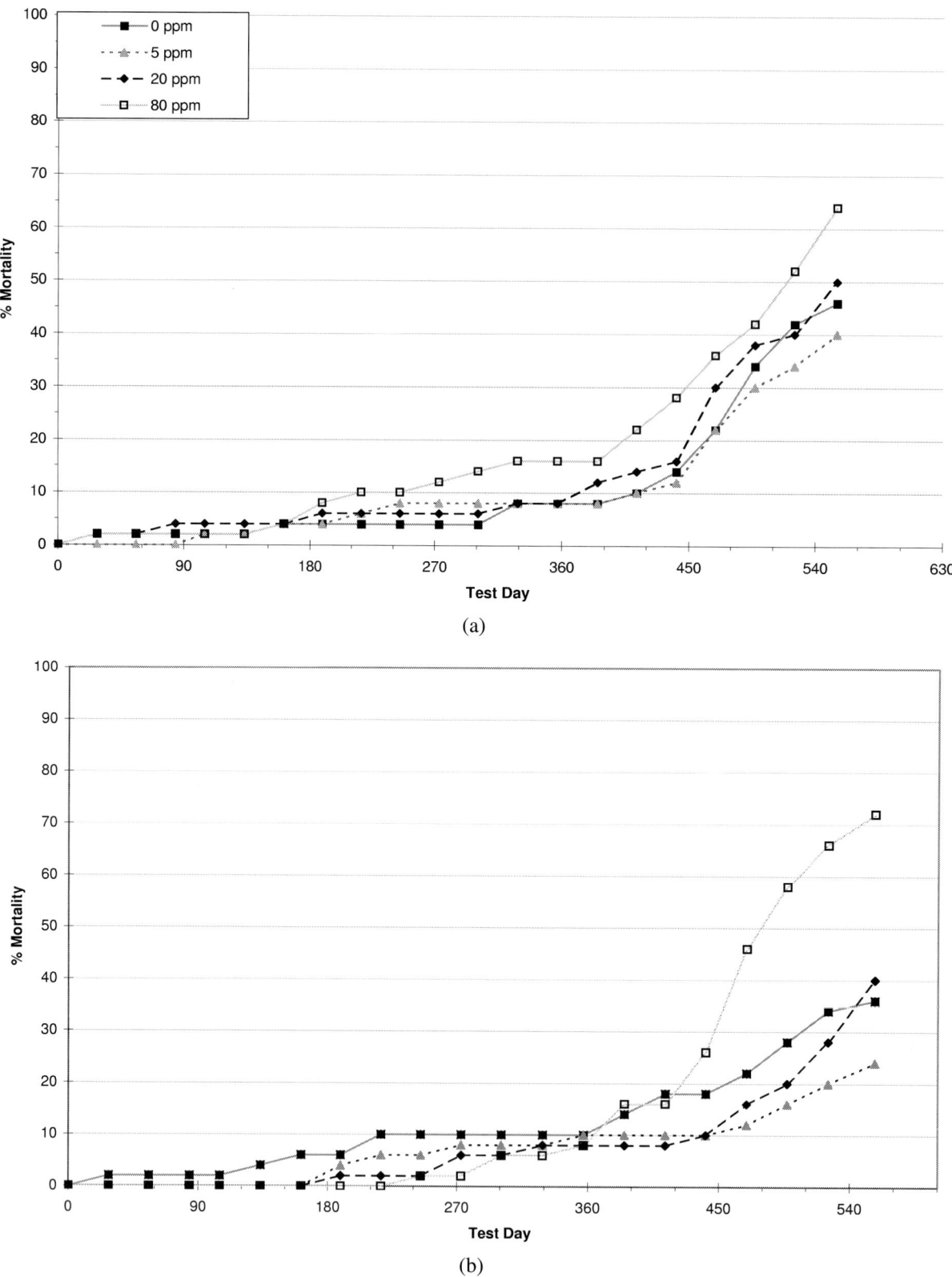

Figure 88.1 Mortality in (a) male and (b) female mice.

80 ppm exposed mice had very slight or slight microscopic vacuolation of the cerebrum in the region of the external capsule. The caudate-putamen was only affected in one male mouse in the 80 ppm group. The amygdaloid adjacent to the external capsule was not affected. The vacuolation in the cerebrum was suggestive of edematous change and was not associated with an

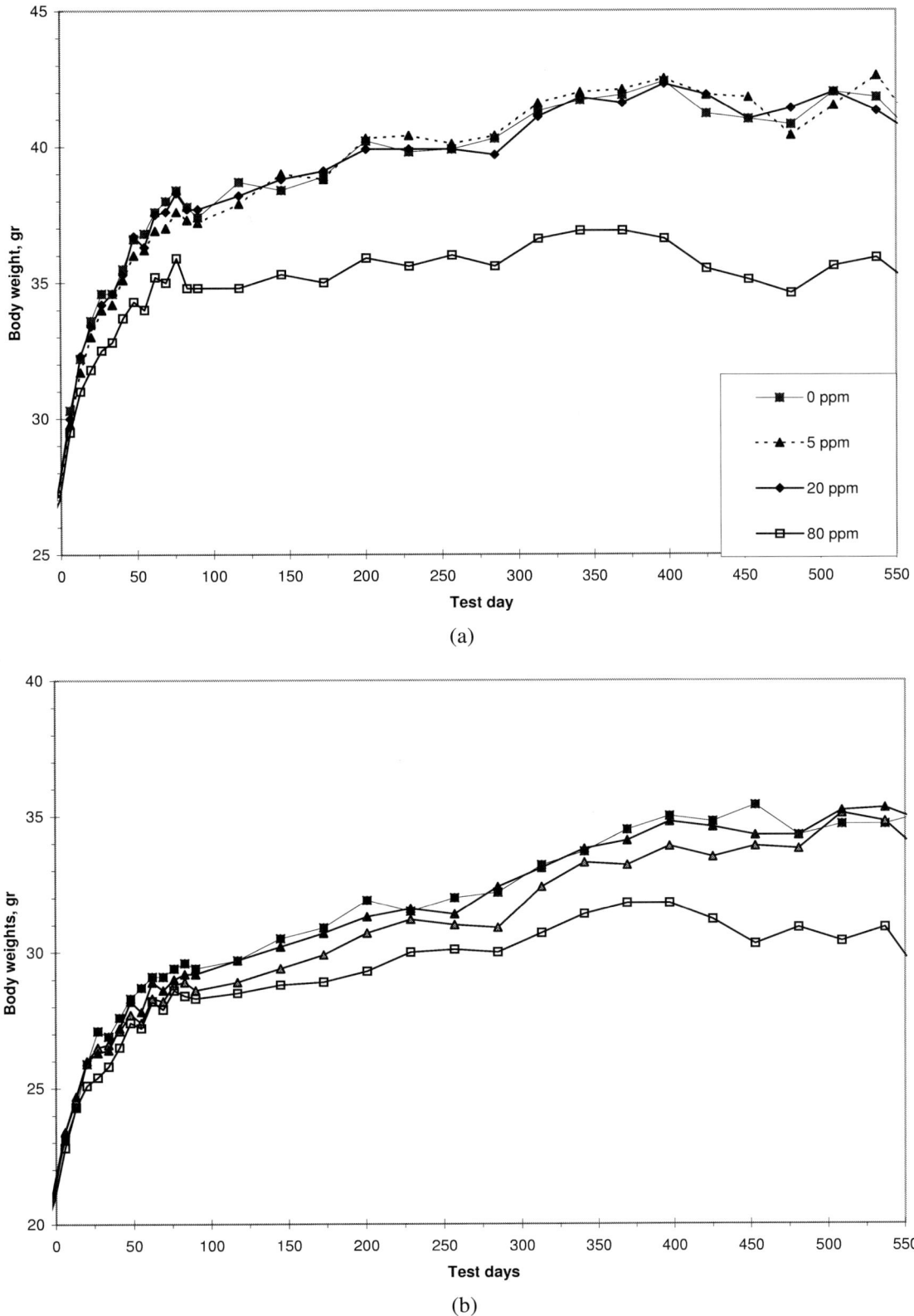

Figure 88.2   Body weights of (a) male and (b) female mice.

inflammatory cell reaction. Very slight hypertrophy of the thyroid follicular epithelial cells was observed. More male mice were affected than female mice. Interestingly, mice exposed to 80 ppm for 12 or 18 months exhibited a lower incidence and severity of brain effects than mice exposed to 100 ppm for 13 weeks (Nitschke and Quast, 1993).

In the oncogenicity group, target organs were limited to those previously defined after 12 months and consisted of the brain and thyroid gland of mice exposed to 80 ppm only. Only a quarter of the mice exposed to 80 ppm sulfuryl fluoride had histopathologic changes in the external capsule of the brain. There were no recognizable changes in the caudate-putamen or amygdaloid regions of the brain. Thyroid changes in mice exposed to 80 ppm were characterized by hypertrophy of follicular epithelial cells. These thyroid changes occurred at a much lower incidence in mice at 18 months when compared to 12 months with males having a higher incidence than females. All other microscopic changes were considered to be unrelated to sulfuryl fluoride exposure. There was no increase in the incidence of any tumor in male or female mice exposed to concentrations as high as 80 ppm sulfuryl fluoride.

88.4.11 CHRONIC TOXICITY—RATS

Groups of 50 male and 50 female rats were exposed to 0, 5, 20, or 80 ppm sulfuryl fluoride for 6 hr/day, 5 days/week for two years (Quast et al., 1993c). Fifteen additional rats/sex/exposure level were randomly designated at the beginning of the study as a satellite group for assessment of general toxicity and neurotoxicity (functional observational battery, motor activity, and perfusion-fixed histopathology of nervous system tissues) following one year of exposure. Mortality of rats exposed to sulfuryl fluoride through the first 16 months of the study was similar to the control group in both male and female rats (Fig. 88.3a and b). After 16 months of exposure to 80 ppm, mortality of both males and female rats was increased from control values. The mortality rate of female rats exposed to 5 or 20 ppm was lower than control values from 20 months until the end of the study. Slight body weight effects were observed in female rats exposed to 80 ppm throughout the first year; body weights of male and female rats exposed to 80 ppm became progressively more severe after one year (Fig. 88.4a and b). There were no consistent effects observed during the first year in urinary specific gravity values of males or females exposed to sulfuryl fluoride. However, urinary specific gravity values of male and female rats exposed to 80 ppm for 19 or 21 months were significantly decreased from control values. Several clinical chemistry parameters commonly associated with kidney toxicity were affected in rats exposed to 80 ppm for 19 and 21 months. These included increased urea nitrogen, cholesterol, triglycerides, creatinine, and phosphorus and decreased total protein, albumin, and chloride. In addition, albumin levels of male rats exposed to 80 ppm for 12 months were also affected. At the 12 month sacrifice, increases in the relative kidney and liver weights of male rats exposed to 80 ppm were the only organ weight differences noted in rats exposed to sulfuryl fluoride.

Histopathologic changes were noted in the kidneys, lungs, and teeth of rats exposed to 80 ppm sulfuryl fluoride for 12 months. A very slight to slight degree of chronic progressive glomerulonephropathy was noted in males and females with the effects observed in females generally less severely affected (Table 88.2). In the lungs, very slight to slight aggregates of alveolar macrophages were noted in rats. These effects were very minimal and were not considered to significantly impair pulmonary function. Very slight to slight dental fluorosis involving the upper incisor teeth was observed also. The molars of these animals were unaffected. There were no exposure related histopathologic changes noted in rats exposed to 5 or 20 ppm.

As in rats exposed to sulfuryl fluoride for 12 months, gross and histopathologic changes were noted in the kidneys, lungs, and teeth of rats exposed to 80 ppm sulfuryl fluoride for a lifetime. While there was no apparent difference in the gross and histopathologic changes noted in the lungs and teeth of rats exposed for 12 or 24 months, the kidney changes had progressed from very slight or slight to severe or very severe chronic progressive glomerulonephropathy (Table 88.2). These kidney changes have been commonly observed in control animals from lifetime studies, however, the incidence rate was much higher in the high exposure animals. Along with the kidney changes, secondary changes, such as hyperparathyroidism and mineralization of many tissues were observed. These changes have been described previously by Boorman et al. (1990) and Mohr et al. (1992). Except for a very slight fluorosis of the teeth of male rats exposed to 20 ppm, there were no effects observed in male or female rats exposed to 5 or 20 ppm.

There was no increase in the incidence of any tumor in male or female rats exposed to concentrations as high as 80 ppm sulfuryl fluoride. There was no evidence of a nervous system effect based on functional observational battery, motor activity or histopathological examination of perfusion-fixed nervous system tissues (Spencer et al., 1994). The no-observed-adverse-effect level (NOAEL) for chronic toxicity was 20 ppm. The NOEL was 5 ppm in males and 20 ppm in females due to several rats with very slight fluorosis.

88.4.12 CHRONIC TOXICITY—DOGS

Groups of 4 dogs/sex were exposed to 0, 20, 80, or 200 ppm for 6 hours/day, 5 days/week for one year (Quast et al., 1993b). Body weight gains in the highest exposure group of males and females were less than controls within the first two weeks of exposure to sulfuryl fluoride and the differences became greater throughout the study until the dogs were removed due to morbidity or death. Although no clinical effects were noted in dogs exposed to 200 ppm for the first eight months, clinical effects were observed in these animals at approximately nine months into the study. Observations in these animals included labored breathing, shallow, rapid respiration, and pale or blue mucous membranes. The onset of these observations was relatively swift; in the first dog, effects were noted on test day 263 and the animal died on test day 267. Due to the relatively swift onset, the last dog was sacrificed on test day 282 when the exposure was stopped due to excessive toxicity.

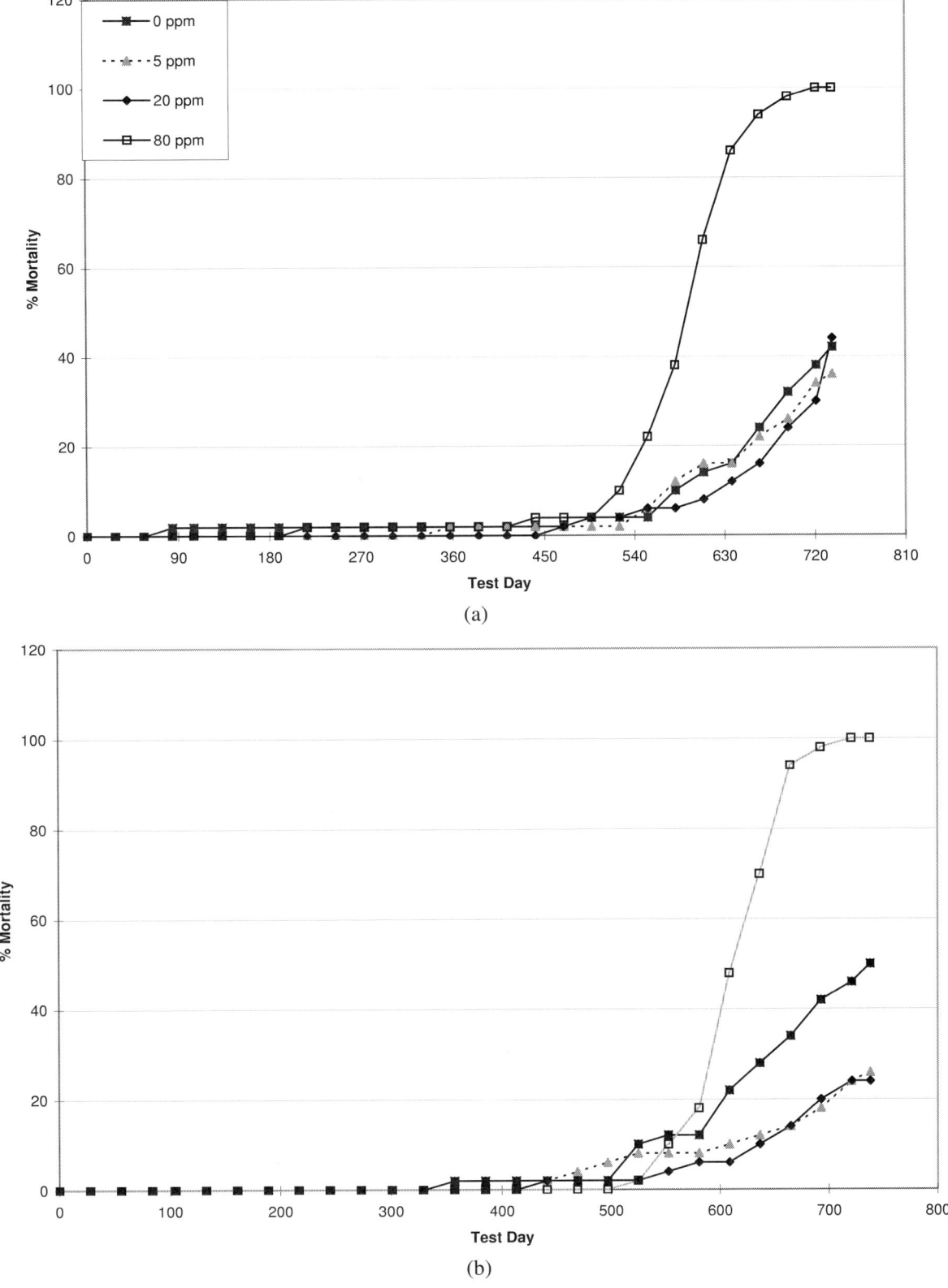

Figure 88.3   Mortality in (a) male and (b) female rats.

There were no exposure-related effects noted in dogs exposed to 20 or 80 ppm sulfuryl fluoride for one year or dogs exposed to 200 ppm through six months. Effects were noted in hematological or clinical chemistry values of dogs exposed to 200 ppm for approximately nine months. However, by this point, these dogs were starting to show signs of

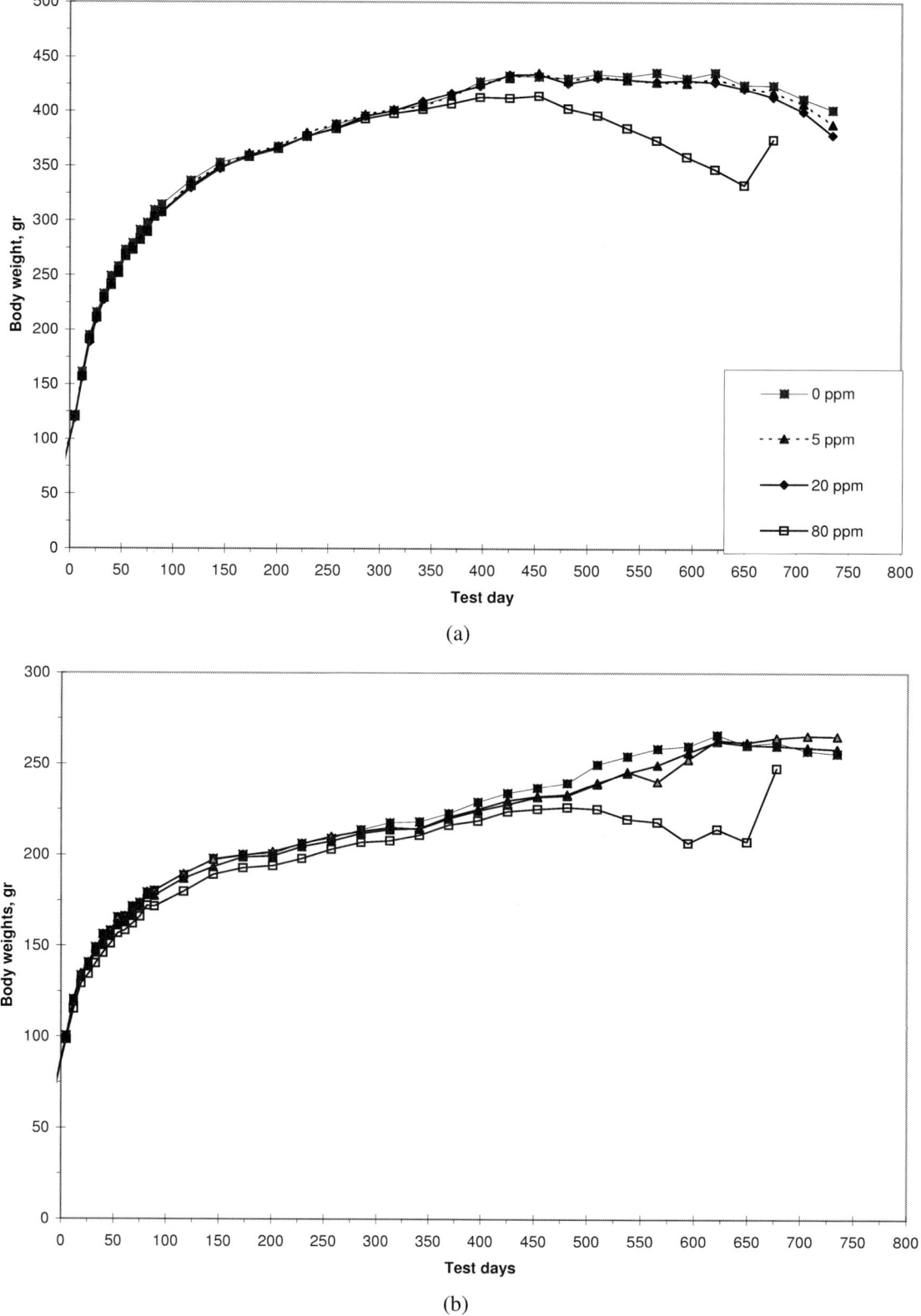

Figure 88.4 Body weights of (a) male and (b) female rats.

respiratory distress and the observed effects were considered to be minor secondary hematological and clinical chemistry changes.

Gross examination of dogs exposed to 200 ppm revealed dark colored lungs which appeared to be consolidated. There were no other tissues affected in dogs exposed to 200 ppm for approximately nine months or dogs exposed to concentrations of 20 or 80 ppm for one year.

Histopathologic changes were noted in the lungs, brain, thyroid gland, and canine teeth of dogs exposed to 200 ppm and in the lungs and canine teeth of dogs exposed to 80 ppm. The pulmonary changes appeared to be a chronic active inflammation which primarily involved the peripheral regions of the lung of animals exposed to 200 ppm without recognizable alterations in the major airways. An increased number of alveolar macrophages was observed in scattered alveoli. In the more advanced stages of the chronic active inflammation process these foci apparently increased in size and hypertrophied type II pneumocytes were observed. In addition, epithelial cells were hypertrophied and hyperplastic. In the more severe cases, a focal thickening of the pleura and interalveolar septae was observed also. Dogs exposed to 80 ppm had a very slight increase in the aggregates of alveolar macrophages with several dogs exhibiting a very slight degree of the chronic active inflammatory process. In the brain, a focus of malacia was observed in five of eight dogs inhaling 200 ppm. Although inflammatory cells were noted, they appeared to be an insignificant factor. Very slight hypertrophy of the follicular epithelium was observed in the thyroid gland of all male and three female dogs. Since the dogs were approximately five months of age when initially exposed to sulfuryl fluoride, the teeth of these animals were still growing. Consequently during the beginning of the study, concentric rings were observed for each exposure period. Thus five concentric rings were observed for each week of exposure. However, as these animals matured it was more difficult to recognize the concentric rings. There were no exposure-related effects noted in dogs exposed to 20 ppm sulfuryl fluoride.

88.4.13 TERATOLOGY STUDIES—RATS

Groups of 35-36 bred Fischer 344 rats were exposed to 0, 25, 75, or 225 ppm sulfuryl fluoride for 6 hr/day on days 6–15 of gestation (Hanley *et al.*, 1989). There was no evidence of embryotoxicity, fetotoxicity, or teratogenicity noted in rats exposed to concentrations as high as 225 ppm sulfuryl fluoride.

88.4.14 TERATOLOGY STUDIES—RABBITS

Groups of 28-29 inseminated New Zealand White rabbits were exposed to 0, 25, 75, or 225 ppm sulfuryl fluoride for 6 hr/day on days 6–18 of gestation (Hanley *et al.*, 1989). Pregnant rabbis exposed to 225 ppm lost weight during the exposure period and did not gain weight in the postexposure period (days 19–29 of gestation). Body weights of rabbits exposed to 25 or 75 ppm were unaffected. Body weights of the fetuses from dams exposed to 225 ppm were significantly lower (14% decrease) than in the control group. Fetal crown-rump length was also slightly decreased in this group. There was no evidence of embryotoxicity, fetotoxicity, or teratogenicity noted in rabbits exposed to concentrations as high as 225 ppm sulfuryl fluoride.

88.4.15 REPRODUCTION TOXICITY—RATS

Groups of 30 male and 30 female Sprague–Dawley rats were exposed to 0, 5, 20, or 150 ppm sulfuryl fluoride for 6 hours/day, 5 days/week for 10 weeks for the F0 and 12 weeks for the F1 generation prior to mating and 6 hours/day, 7 days/week during mating, gestation, and lactation through two generations (Breslin *et al.*, 1993). Body weights of F0 male and female rats exposed to 150 ppm were significantly decreased from control values during most of the premating period. The body weight gain of these female rats during gestation was also decreased. However, during the lactation period, the body weight gain was increased possibly as a compensatory mechanism. There was no exposure-related effect on the F0 male or female conception index, fertility indices, length of gestation, time to mating, pup survival indices, or pup sex ratio. Similarly, there was no exposure-related effect on the number of F1 pups born dead or alive, or on the litter size at any exposure level. However, the litter size of live pups at birth and on days 1 and 4 before culling were increased 2.0 pups/litter in the 5 ppm exposure group and 1.5 pups/litter in the 20 ppm exposure group when compared to the control group. While these increases in litter size were not considered exposure-related, as a dose–response was not observed and no effects on litter size were observed in animals exposed to 150 ppm, the increase in litter size above control values has biological significance in that average pup weights are known to decrease with increasing litter size (Tyle, 1988). Indeed, F1 female pup body weights were occasionally decreased in the 5 ppm exposure group. On the other hand, the body weights of F1 male and female pups from dams exposed to 150 ppm were statistically decreased throughout most of the lactation period. While the decreases in body weight of F1 pups from the 150 ppm exposure group were attributed to treatment, these body weight effects were considered secondary to the decreased maternal growth observed throughout the premating and gestation periods.

Body weight effects in the F1 adults were similar to those observed in the F0 generation. Exposure-related effects were noted in body weights of male and female F1 rats exposed to 150 ppm during premating and female F1 rats exposed to 150 ppm during gestation and lactation but not at lower exposure levels. No exposure-related effects were observed on the F1 male or female fertility indices, length of gestation, time to mating, pup survival indices, or pup sex ratio in any exposure group. Similarly, no exposure-related effects on the number of F2 pups born alive or dead, or on the litter size were observed at any exposure level. No exposure-related effects on the body weights of male or female F2 pups from dams exposed to 5 or 20 ppm were observed at any time during the lactation period. However, body weights of male and female pups from dams exposed to 150 ppm were significantly decreased on lactation Days 14 and 21. This was considered to be secondary to the decreased maternal growth observed during the premating and gestation periods. The decreased growth of F2 pups from dams exposed to 150 ppm sulfuryl fluoride was less severe than the decreased weights observed in the F1 pups at the same exposure level.

The pathologic changes in the teeth, lungs, and brain in the adult F0 and F1 Sprague–Dawley rats in this study were essentially identical to those observed in a subchronic study in Fischer 344 rats previously mentioned (Eisenbrandt and Nitschke, 1989). Minor changes in the lung and brain were present at lower exposure concentrations in this study (20 ppm in the lung and 150 ppm in the brain) than previously noted in Fischer 344 rats. Interestingly, the effects observed in the brain of the F1 adults occurred in fewer animals than in the F0 adults even though the length of exposure to sulfuryl fluoride was increased. Female rats had a higher incidence of brain and lung lesions than did males at a given exposure level. The parental NOEL was 5 ppm, the NOEL for neonatal growth was 20 ppm, and the NOEL for reproductive toxicity and fertility was 150 ppm.

88.5 GENETIC TOXICITY

88.5.1 AMES TEST

Sulfuryl fluoride was tested in strains TA98, TA100, TA1535, and TA1537 with and without metabolic activation (Gollapudi et al., 1990a). Petri plates were exposed for 4 hours at 37°C to nominal concentrations of 300, 1000, 3000, 10,000, and 30,000 ppm sulfuryl fluoride. The plates were incubated for an additional two days prior to determining the frequencies of mutants/plate. Sulfuryl fluoride was not mutagenic in any of the tester strains.

88.5.2 UNSCHEDULED DNA SYNTHESIS

The genotoxicity of sulfuryl fluoride was evaluated in the rat hepatocyte unscheduled DNA synthesis (UDS) assay (Gollapudi et al., 1991). In two separate assays, sulfuryl fluoride did not elicit a positive UDS response at nominal concentrations ranging from 204 to 1020 ppm.

88.5.3 MICRONUCLEUS TEST

Sulfuryl fluoride was evaluated in the mouse bone marrow micronucleus test (Gollapudi et al., 1990b). Groups of mice were exposed to 0, 50, 175, or 520 ppm sulfuryl fluoride. Mice were sacrificed at 24, 48, or 72 hours after exposure to sulfuryl fluoride. There were no significant increases in the frequencies of micronucleated polychromatic erythrocytes in the bone marrow of mice.

88.5.4 METABOLISM

The metabolism, disposition, and the relationships, if any, of the metabolites to the mechanism of action of SO2F2 have not

as yet been determined in mammals. However, sulfuryl fluoride has been shown to be fairly stable in saline (Waechter, 1991). At concentrations of 1000 and 5000 ppm in saline, 93% sulfuryl fluoride remained after 240 minutes at 37°C. Sulfuryl fluoride was less stable in rat blood. At concentrations of 1000 and 5000 ppm, 50 and 84% sulfuryl fluoride, respectively, remained after 220 and 255 minutes at 37°C.

Studies in termites have demonstrated extensive dehalogenation of ^{35}S-labeled sulfuryl fluoride (Meikle et al., 1963). The fluoride ion may play a role in the mechanism of action of sulfuryl fluoride in insects and possibly also in mammals. Serum fluoride levels have been elevated from control values in several species, including mice, rats, rabbits, and dogs, following acute or subchronic exposure to sulfuryl fluoride. Many of the observations in rodents overexposed to sulfuryl fluoride seem to be typical of acute fluoride poisoning (Drill, 1954; Goodman et al., 1980; Greenwood, 1940).

88.5.5 TOXICOLOGY IN HUMANS

There have been a few case reports of individuals exposed to sulfuryl fluoride. A 30-year-old male was exposed to unknown concentrations of sulfuryl fluoride in air containing 1% chloropicrin for 4 hours (Taxay, 1966). Nausea, vomiting, cramps, abdominal pain, and itching were observed while exposed to sulfuryl fluoride. Vital signs were normal upon admittance to the hospital, however, reddening of the conjunctival, pharyngeal, and nasal mucosae; diffuse rhonchi; and paresthesia of the lateral surface of the right leg were observed. Serum fluoride levels were elevated above normal values. The signs and symptoms resolved quickly and the patient was discharged from the hospital after four days. In a second case report, an elderly couple returned to their home approximately 5–8 hours after their house was ventilated to remove any remaining sulfuryl fluoride following approximately 24 hour fumigation of their home (Nuckolls et al., 1987). Within 24 hours of their return, the wife experienced weakness, nausea, and repeated vomiting and her husband complained of dyspnea and restlessness. Within 48 hours the husband had a generalized seizure followed by cardiopulmonary arrest. The wife died within seven days due to ventricular fibrillation. Serum fluoride level of the wife six days after the house was fumigated was 0.5 mg/liter (background levels are highly dependent upon fluoride levels in drinking water and range from 0.010 to 0.2 mg/liter) (Burtis and Ashwood, 1999). A couple of individuals have entered structures under fumigation with sulfuryl fluoride (Scheuerman, 1986). These individuals were found dead or died shortly after exposure. The cause of death appeared to be severe pulmonary edema with congestion. Serum fluoride levels in two individuals were elevated above normal values.

Structural fumigators using sulfuryl fluoride were evaluated in a neurobehavioral battery (Anger et al., 1986). While there were no significant differences from a reference group, a greater number of symptoms and slightly reduced performance on cognitive tests was observed in the fumigator group. However, educational levels, race, and use of illegal drugs were different between the sulfuryl fluoride workers and the referent group. Thus, the slight difference in cognitive test results was very likely due to differences other than exposure to sulfuryl fluoride.

88.5.6 SUMMARY RISK CHARACTERIZATION

In the toxicity studies reported here, the NOEL ranged from 600 to 20 ppm (Table 88.4). The highest value is the two-week rat neurotox NOEL. In general, neurotox NOELs were higher than general tox NOELs. Remarkably little difference was observed in all four species exposed in two-week to chronic studies.

The label instructions approved by the EPA specify instructions for sealing structures to confine the gas during the fumigation with tarps and/or sealing (Dow AgroSciences, 1996). After the appropriate fumigation period, the building is aerated using one of two specified aeration procedures and is dependent upon the concentration used. Depending upon which aeration procedure is used, the building must be secured for either 6 or 8 hours. After this waiting period, the concentration of Vikane in the breathing zones must be determined. If the concentration of Vikane is greater than 5 ppm, the structure must be ventilated until the concentration is less than 5 ppm, at which point the structure may be reoccupied. The fumigation site cannot be reoccupied until aeration is complete. Only an approved detection device of sufficient sensitivity, such as the INTERSCAN or MIRAN gas analyzer, can be used to confirm a concentration of sulfuryl fluoride is 5 ppm or less. Warning signs must remain posted until aeration is determined to be complete.

Table 88.4
Summary of NOAELs for Various Species Exposed to Sulfuryl Fluoride

Repeated exposure studies	General Tox NOEL (ppm)	Neuro Tox NOEL (ppm)
2-week rat	100	600
2-week rabbit	100	100
2-week mouse	30	30
2-week dog	100	100
13-week rat	30	30
13-week rat (electrophysiology)	30	30
13-week rabbit	30	100 (M), 30 (F)
13-week mouse	30	30
13-week dog	100	100
12-month rat	5 (M)*, 20 (F)	80
12-month rat (Neurotox guideline)	80	80
12-month mouse	20	20
12-month dog	20	20
24-month rat	5 (M)*, 20 (F)	80
18-month mouse	20	20
Two-generation rat reproduction	5	20

*Microscopic dental fluorosis was observed in several 20 ppm male rats.

REFERENCES

ACGIH (1998). "TLVs and other Occupational Exposure Values—1998."

Albee, R. R., *et al.* (1983). "Sulfuryl Fluoride (Vikane*): Induced Incapacitation in Rats." Unpublished report of The Dow Chemical Company.

Albee, R. R., *et al.* (1993). "Sulfuryl Fluoride: Electrodiagnostic, FOB, and Motor Activity Evaluation of Nervous System Effects from Short-Term Exposure." Unpublished report of The Dow Chemical Company.

Anger, W. K., *et al.* (1986). Neurobehavioral evaluation of soil and structural fumigants using methyl bromide and sulfuryl fluoride. *Neurotoxicology* **7**, 137–156.

Boorman, G. A., Eustis, S. L., Elwell, M. R., Montgomery, Jr., C. A., and MacKenzie, W. F. (1990). "Pathology of the Fischer Rat. Reference and Atlas." Academic Press, San Diego.

Bradley, G. J., *et al.* (1990). "Sulfuryl Fluoride: Four-Hour Dermal Vapor Exposure in Fischer 344 Rats." Unpublished report of The Dow Chemical Company.

Breslin, W. J., Liberacki, A. B., Kirk, H. D., Bradley, G. J., and Crissman, J. W. (1993). Sulfuryl fluoride: Two-generation inhalation reproduction study in Sprague–Dawley rats. *Toxicologist* **13**, 368.

Burtis, C. A., and Ashwood, E. R. (1999). "Tietz Textbook of Clinical Chemistry," 3rd ed. Saunders, Philadelphia.

Dow AgroSciences (1996). Vikane Specialty Gas Fumigant Label.

Dow AgroSciences (1997). "General Information on Vikane Gas Fumigant Product." Brochure 311-56-077.

Drill, V. A. (1954). "Pharmacology in Medicine." McGraw–Hill, New York.

Eisenbrandt, D. L., and Nitschke, K. D. (1989). Inhalation toxicity of sulfuryl fluoride in rats and rabbits. *Fundam. Appl. Toxicol.* **12**, 540–557.

Eisenbrandt, D. L., Williams, D. M., Albee, R. R., and Streeter, C. M. (1987). "Sulfuryl Fluoride (Vikane* Gas Fumigant): An Ultrastructural Assessment of the Lungs of Rats Exposed to High Concentrations of Sulfuryl Fluoride." Unpublished report of The Dow Chemical Company.

Gollapudi, B. B., Samson, Y. E., and Zempel, J. A. (1990a). "Evaluation of Sulfuryl Fluoride in the Ames Salmonella/Mammalian Microsome Bacterial Mutagenicity Assay." Unpublished report of The Dow Chemical Company.

Gollapudi, B. B., McClintock, M. L., and Nitschke, K. D. (1990b). "Evaluation of Sulfuryl Fluoride in the Mouse Bone Marrow Micronucleus Test." Unpublished report of The Dow Chemical Company.

Gollapudi, B. B., McClintock, M. L., and Zempel, J. A. (1991). "Evaluation of Sulfuryl Fluoride in the Rat Hepatocyte Unscheduled DNA Synthesis (UDS) Assay." Unpublished report of The Dow Chemical Company.

Goodman, A. G., Goodman, L. S., and Gilman, A. (1980). "The Pharmacological Basis of Therapeutics," 6th ed. Macmillan, New York.

Gorzinski, S. J., and Streeter, C. M. (1985). "Effect of Acute Vikane Exposure on Selected Physiological Parameters in Rats." Unpublished report of The Dow Chemical Company.

Greenwood, D. A. (1940). Fluoride intoxication. *Physiol. Rev.* **20**, 582–616.

Hanley, Jr., T. R., Calhoun, L. L., Kociba, R. J., and Greene, J. A. (1989). The effects of inhalation exposure to sulfuryl fluoride on fetal development in rats and rabbits. *Fundam. Appl. Toxicol.* **13**, 79–86.

Landry, T. D., and Streeter, C. M. (1983). "Sulfuryl Fluoride: Effects of Acute Exposure on Respiration in Rats." Unpublished report of The Dow Chemical Company.

Lockwood, D. L. (1958). "Results of Dietary Feeding of Rats with Feed Fumigated with Sulfuryl Fluoride (Vikane)." Unpublished report of The Dow Chemical Company.

Mattsson, J. L., Albee, R. R., Eisenbrandt, D. L., and Chang, L. W. (1988). Subchronic neurotoxicity in rats of the structural fumigant, Sulfuryl Fluoride. *Neurotoxicol. Teratol.* **10**, 127–133.

Meikle, R. W., Steward, D., and Globus, O. A. (1963). Fumigant mode of action, drywood termite metabolism of Vikane fumigant shown by labelled pool technique. *J. Agr. Food Chem.* **11**, 226–230.

Miller, R. R., *et al.* (1980). "Sulfuryl Fluoride (Vikane Fumigant): An LC$_{50}$ Determination." Unpublished report of The Dow Chemical Company.

Mohr, U., Dungworth, D. L., and Capen, C. C. (1992). "Pathobiology of the Aging Rat," Vol. 1. International Life Sciences Institute, Washington, DC.

Nitschke, K. D., and Lomax, L. G. (1989). "Sulfuryl Fluoride: Acute LC$_{50}$ Study with B6C3F1 Mice." Unpublished report of The Dow Chemical Company.

Nitschke, K. D., and Quast, J. F. (1990). "Sulfuryl Fluoride: Acute LC50 Study with CD-1 Mice." Unpublished report of The Dow Chemical Company.

Nitschke, K. D., and Quast, J. F. (1991). "Sulfuryl Fluoride: Two-Week Inhalation Toxicity Study in Beagle Dogs." Unpublished report of The Dow Chemical Company.

Nitschke, K. D., and Quast, J. F. (1993). "Sulfuryl Fluoride: Thirteen-Week Inhalation Toxicity Study in CD-1 Mice." Unpublished report of The Dow Chemical Company.

Nitschke, K. D., and Quast, J. F. (1995). "Sulfuryl Fluoride: Two-Week Inhalation Toxicity Study in CD-1 Mice." Unpublished report of The Dow Chemical Company.

Nitschke, K. D., Albee, R. R., Mattsson, J. L., and Miller, R. R. (1986). Incapacitation and treatment of rats exposed to a lethal dose of sulfuryl fluoride. *Fundam. Appl. Toxicol.* **7**, 664–670.

Nitschke, K. D., Beekman, M. J., and Quast, J. F. (1992). "Sulfuryl Fluoride: 13-Week Inhalation Toxicity Study in Beagle Dogs." Unpublished report of The Dow Chemical Company.

Nuckolls, J. G., Smith, D. C., Walls, W. E., Oxley, D. W., Hackler, R. L., Tripathi, R. K., Armstron, C. W., and Miller, G. B. (1987). Fatalities resulting from sulfuryl fluoride exposure after home fumigation—Virginia. *JAMA* **258**, 2041–2044.

Quast, J. F., Bradley, G. J., and Nitschke, K. D. (1993a). "Sulfuryl Fluoride: 18-Month Inhalation Oncogenicity Study in CD-1 Mice." Unpublished report of The Dow Chemical Company.

Quast, J. F., Beekman, M. J., and Nitschke, K. D. (1993b). "Sulfuryl Fluoride: One-Year Inhalation Toxicity Study in Beagle Dogs." Unpublished report of The Dow Chemical Company.

Quast, J. F., Bradley, G. J., and Nitschke, K. D. (1993c). "Sulfuryl Fluoride: 2-Year Inhalation Chronic Toxicity/Oncogenicity Study in Fischer 344 Rats." Unpublished report of The Dow Chemical Company.

Scheuerman, E. H. (1986). Suicide by exposure to sulfuryl fluoride. *J. Forensic Sci.* **31**, 1154–1158.

Spencer, P. J., Bradley, G. J., and Quast, J. F. (1994). "Sulfuryl Fluoride: Chronic Neurotoxicity Study in Fischer 344 Rats—Final Report." Unpublished report of The Dow Chemical Company.

Taxay, E. P. (1966). Vikane inhalation. *J. Occup. Med.* 425–426.

Torkelson, T. R. (1959). "Summary Report of Toxicological Studies with Vikane (Sulfuryl Fluoride, SO2F2)." Unpublished report of The Dow Chemical Company.

Torkelson, T. R., Hoyle, H. R., and Rowe, V. K. (1966). Toxicological hazards and properties of commonly used space, structural and certain other fumigants. *Pest Control* 1–8.

Tyle, R. W. (1988). "Perspectives in Modern Toxicology," Chap. 8. Wright, London.

U. S. Environmental Protection Agency (1982). "Pesticide Assessment Guidelines, Subdivision F, Hazard Evaluation: Human and Domestic Animals," pp. 98–100. U.S. Environmental Protection Agency, Washington, DC.

Vaccaro, (1988). Unpublished data of The Dow Chemical Company.

Vernot, E. H., *et al.* (1977). Acute toxicity and skin corrosion data for some organic and inorganic compounds and aqueous solutions. *Toxicol. Appl. Pharmacol.* **42**, 417–423.

Waechter, J (1991). Personal communication. Unpublished data of The Dow Chemical Company.

Index

ISBN 0-12-426262-7

90038

9 780124 262621